SECOND EDITION

Kinn's

MEDICAL ASSISTING
FUNDAMENTALS

Administrative and Clinical Competencies with Anatomy & Physiology

BRIGITTE NIEDZWIECKI, MSN, RN, RMA
Medical Assistant Program Director & Instructor
Chippewa Valley Technical College
Eau Claire, Wisconsin

ELSEVIER

ELSEVIER
3251 Riverport Lane
St. Louis, Missouri 63043

KINN'S MEDICAL ASSISTING FUNDAMENTALS, SECOND EDITION   ISBN: 978-0-323-82450-7

Notice

Previous edition copyrighted 2019

Library of Congress Control Number: 2021944944

Publishing Director, Education Content: Kristin Wilhelm
Director, Content Development: Laurie Gower
Senior Content Development Specialist: Rebecca Leenhouts
Publishing Services Manager: Julie Eddy
Senior Project Manager: Cindy Thoms
Book Designer: Renee Duenow

Printed in the United States of America

Last digit is the print number: 9   8   7   6   5   4   3   2   1

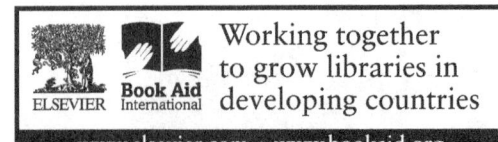

Angela Belnap, DHPE, CMA (AAMA)
Medical Assistant Program Coordinator & Associate Professor
Salt Lake Community College
West Jordan, Utah
Infection Control
Vital Signs
Patient Interview
Physical Examination
Assisting in Obstetrics and Gynecology
Assisting in Pediatrics
Assisting in Geriatrics
Surgical Equipment and Supplies
Surgical and Special Procedures
Assisting with Radiology
Radiological Positioning

Letitia Patterson, MPA, RHIA, CCS-P, CPC, CPB, CPMA, CRC, CPC-I
President
A Coder's Resource
Chicago, Illinois
Health Insurance Basics
Diagnostic Coding Basics
Procedural Coding Basics
Billing and Reimbursement

Pamela B. Primrose, PhD, MLS, ASCP
Professor Life Sciences
Ivy Tech Community College
South Bend, Indiana
Assisting in the Clinical Laboratory
Assisting in the Analysis of Urine
Assisting in Blood Collection
Assisting in the Analysis of Blood
Assisting in Microbiology and Immunology

REVIEWERS

Kyle James Brownfield
University of Illinois at Chicago – Bachelor of Science in Kinesiology
EMT-B Licensure
BLS-CPR/AED Certified
Chicago, Illinois

Candace S. Crump, CMA (AAMA)
Department Chair: Medical Assisting
Asheville-Buncombe Technical Community College
Asheville, North Carolina

Deborah S. Gilbert, RHIA, MBA
Retired Health Information Program Director
Dalton State College
Dalton, Georgia

Jolene Guenthner, BS, CMA (AAMA)
Medical Assistant Program Director
Nicolet College
Rhinelander, Wisconsin

Kathy A. Harris, LPN, MBA, RMA (AMT)
Program Director Medical Assisting
Clark State Community College
Springfield, Ohio

Starra Herring, MBA, MHA, BSAH, BSHA, CMA (AAMA)-MA, AHI
Program Director Medical Assisting Program
Program Director Medical Billing & Coding Program
Program Director MOA Program
Program Director AAS in Applied Science Medical Assisting
Stanly Community College
Chaffey College
Locust, North Carolina
Rancho Cucamonga, California

Mandy Hunter, CCMA
Medical Assistant Instructor
Putnam Career and Technical Center
Eleanor, West Virginia

LaToya Nicole Mason, CMA (AAMA), MBA, MHA
Director, Health Sciences
Lake Michigan College
Benton Harbor, Michigan

Melody Miller, LPN
Medical Assistant Instructor
Lancaster Career and Technology Center
Willow Street, Pennsylvania

Linda Mollino, MSN, RN
Director of Career and Technical Programs
Oregon Coast Community College
Newport, Oregon

Genesee Marie Osuna
Certified Clinical Medical Assistant
Chaffey College
Rancho Cucamonga, California

Kristen Schoville, RN/BSN
Medical Assistant Instructor
Southwest Wisconsin Technical College
Fennimore, Wisconsin

Candice Spaulding, CMA, MS
Medical Assistant Program Director
Manchester Community College
Manchester, New Hampshire

Angela Belnap, MS, CMA (AAMA)
Master of Science in Integrated Healthcare Management
Bachelor of Science in Applied Management
Associate of Applied Science in Medical Assistant
Doctoral student in Health Professional Education
Certified Medical Assistant through the AAMA since 2005
Assistant Professor of Health Science
Medical Assisting Department
Salt Lake Community College
School of Health Sciences
Division of Allied Health
Department of Medical Assisting
Salt Lake Community College
Salt Lake City, Utah

Amber Dunn, LPN, RMA, AHI
BS Health Science, Community Development
Director of the Medical Assistant Program
Allied Health
East Central College
Union, Missouri

Bryan Quincy Edmonds, Sr, MBA-H, RMA (AMT), EMT
Medical Assisting Program Coordinator/Instructor
Medical Assisting
Milwaukee Area Technical College
Milwaukee, Wisconsin

Lyndsay Evans, CMAA, CBCS, CEHRS
CTT Instructor
Medical Administrative Assisting
Sierra Nevada Job Corps Center
Reno, Nevada

Deborah S. Gilbert, RHIA, MBA, CMA
Program Director Health Information Management
Health Professions
Dalton State College
Dalton, Georgia

Pamela Harvey, RN, ASN, BSN, MSN, BLS
Instructor in the Medical Assistant Program
Bradford Union Career Technical Center
Starke, Florida

Kimberly Head, BA, BS, DC
Director of Healthcare Programs
Continuing Education
Collin College
Plano, Texas

Starra R. Herring, BSAH, BSHA, CMA (AAMA)-MA, AHI
Medical Assisting Program Director & Practicum Coordinator of
    the Medical Assisting Program & Billing and Coding Program
    Director
Medical Assisting/Allied Health and Public Service
Stanly Community College
Locust, North Carolina

Judith Kimelman Kline, NCRMA
Medical Assistant Instructor
Health Science
Miami Lakes Educational Center and Technical College–Miami Dade
    Public School
Miami Lakes, Florida

LaToya Nicole Mason, CMA (AAMA), MBA, MHA
Director, Healthcare Education Institute
Health Sciences
Lake Michigan College
Benton Harbor, Michigan

Jillian J. McDonald, BS, RMA (NHA), EMT, CPT (NPA)
Medical Assisting Program Director
Health and Natural Sciences (Medical Assisting)
Goodwin College
East Hartford, Connecticut

Melody A. Miller, LPN
Medical Assistant Instructor
Lancaster County Career and Technology Center
Willow Street, Pennsylvania

Kristen Schoville, RN/BSN
Medical Assistant Instructor
Southwest Wisconsin Technical College
Fennimore, Wisconsin

Kathy Elisa Smith-Stillson, PhD, MSN, RN
Doctor of Philosophy in Human Resource Development and Educational Leadership
Nursing
Colorado Christian University
Northglenn, Colorado

Bobbi Jane Steelman, BSEd, MAEd, CPhT
Director of Education, Pharmacy Technician Program Director
Academics
Daymar College
Bowling Green, Kentucky

Audrey Jean Theisen, BS, RHIA, MSCIS, PhD
Adjunct Professor
Medical Assistant Program
Community College of Denver
Denver, Colorado

Debra Van Den Bussche
Instructor
Medical Office Assisting/Unit Clerk
Bredin College of Business and Health Care
Spruce Grove, Alberta, Canada

Shaili N. Vora, MD
Manager of Training & Development
Staff Training
Baylor Scott & White Health
Temple, Texas

Jessica Weinoldt, RT(R)(M) (CMA)
Radiographer, Medical Assistant Instructor
Medical Assistant Class
Lancaster County Career and Technology Center
Willow Street, Pennsylvania

Petra M. York, BS, CMA (AAMA), CET, CPT, AHI, CMAA, CPhT
Program Director
Medical Assistant
Western Technical College
El Paso, Texas

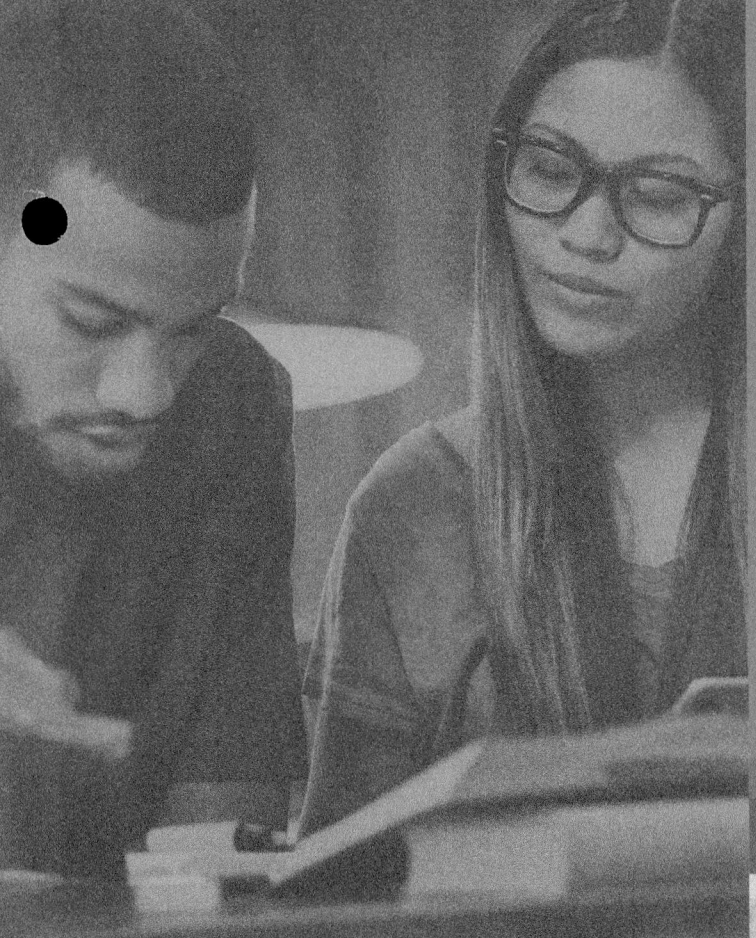

A tailored education experience —

Sherpath book-organized collections

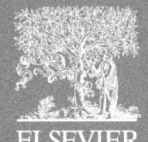
ELSEVIER

Sherpath book-organized collections offer:

Objective-based, digital lessons, mapped chapter-by-chapter to the textbook, that make it easy to find applicable digital assignment content.

Adaptive quizzing with personalized questions that correlate directly to textbook content.

Teaching materials that align to the text and are organized by chapter for quick and easy access to invaluable class activities and resources.

Elsevier ebooks that provide convenient access to textbook content, even offline.

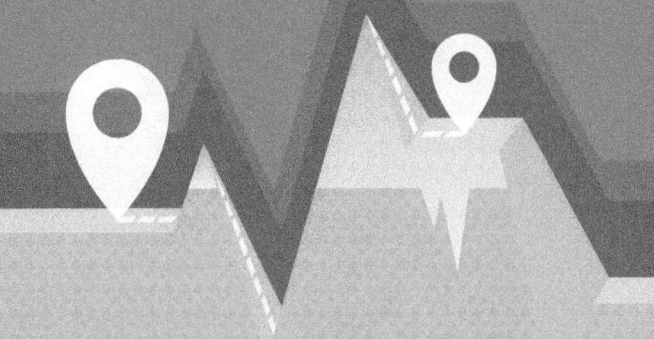

Sherpath is the digital teaching and learning technology designed specifically for healthcare education.

Medical assisting as a profession has dramatically changed over the past 60 years. You are entering the profession at an exciting time. With the advances in technology, the medical assistant role has expanded. With those changes, medical assistants need a strong foundation in anatomy, disease, medical terminology, math, and soft skills as they apply to administrative and clinical responsibilities.

FEATURES OF THIS TEXTBOOK FOR STUDENTS

Following in the tradition of *Kinn's* product suite, *Kinn's Medical Assisting Fundamentals: Administrative and Clinical Competencies with Anatomy & Physiology* offers a comprehensive, up-to-date, and innovative approach to learning the medical assistant role. The easy-to-understand writing style and the tables with concise information will help you build a strong foundation of knowledge. The extensive figures provide examples, illustrate skills, and showcase ambulatory equipment and supplies. Features we have incorporated into the textbook include:

- *Emphasis on anatomy, physiology, and pathology*, including signs/symptoms, diagnostic procedures, and treatments.
- *Strong focus on medical terminology,* including a chapter focused on the basics of medical terminology and feature boxes highlighting chapter-related medical terminology throughout the textbook.
- *Embedded math exercises* to help you build your math skills.
- *Patient-Centered Care boxes* incorporate the importance of providing patient-focused care in a team environment.
- *Being Professional boxes* provide information on professional behavior with a related role-play example to allow students to apply the professionalism concepts.
- *Applied learning approach* introduces a case scenario at the beginning of each chapter and then revisits it throughout the chapter to help you understand new concepts as they are presented.
- *Chapter learning tools* include vocabulary with definitions, critical thinking applications, and content that ties directly to the order of learning objectives.
- *Pharmacology glossary* of the top 150 most common over-the-counter and prescription medications gives you quick access to pronunciation guides, generic and trade names, and drug classification.
- *Trusted Kinn's content* supports the following exam plans: CMA from the American Association of Medical Assistants; RMA and CMAS from American Medical Technologist; CCMA and CMAA from the National Healthcareer Association; NCMA from the National Center for Competency Testing; and CMAC from the American Medical Certification Association.

ORGANIZATION OF THIS TEXTBOOK

To provide you with a solid understanding of the basics, Unit 1 addresses medical terminology, anatomy, physiology, and pathology. Unit 2 focuses on the professional medical assistant. This content is critical to you as you begin your career. Being professional starts in the classroom and extends into the practicum and beyond. Besides professional attributes, communication skills and legal and ethical concepts will be discussed.

Unit 3 covers administrative medical assistant topics. Reception duties, including working with the health record, answering telephones, and scheduling appointments, are addressed. Insurance, coding, billing, collections, and banking principles are also discussed. Often in larger ambulatory care facilities, these activities are done in the business department.

Units 4 through 7 address the clinical medical assistant duties. Unit 4 covers skills related to infection control procedures, obtaining vital signs, assisting with physical exams, and assisting with minor surgery. Unit 5 includes advanced clinical procedures. The medical assistant's role with advanced clinical procedures depends on the state's law and the agency where the medical assistant is employed. Advanced clinical procedures include coaching patients, administering medications, performing cardiopulmonary procedures, and assisting with medical emergencies. Unit 6 addresses limited scope radiology, and Unit 7 focuses on procedures performed in the medical laboratory setting. These skills include collecting specimens, performing Clinical Laboratory Improvement Amendments (CLIA)-waived laboratory tests on urine, blood, and other body fluids.

Unit 8 focuses on employment. As you complete your program, learning how to market yourself to potential employers is important. This unit addresses the skills to secure employment.

STUDY GUIDE FEATURES FOR STUDENTS AND INSTRUCTORS

The Study Guide provides students with the opportunity to review and build on information they have learned in the text through medical terminology and vocabulary reviews, review of concepts, chapter review multiple-choice questions, case scenarios, and online activities. Students also have the opportunity to review and practice procedures for psychomotor and affective competencies, with clear steps and behaviors indicated.

For instructors, the Study Guide offers unique, time-saving tools, including specific mapping of assessments to competencies of both the Commission on Accreditation of Allied Health Education Programs (CAAHEP) and the Accrediting Bureau of Health Education Schools (ABHES).

- Specific assessment questions and procedure steps are mapped to competencies, helping to eliminate hours of program management for national accreditation.
- Procedures are designed to be conveniently performed in the classroom.
- Procedure Checklists for psychomotor competencies are easy to use and address multiple competencies in many cases.

- Uniquely designed Procedure Checklists for affective competencies allow instructors to quickly identify a student's professional and nonprofessional behaviors while assessing the range of performance with ease.
- Clearly written Procedure Checklists for psychomotor and affective competencies help students identify what steps and behaviors are required for success.

EVOLVE

The Evolve site features a variety of student resources, including Chapter Review Quizzes, Procedure Videos, practice CMA and RMA exams, and much more! The Instructor Resources consists of TEACH Instructor Resources, including Lesson Plans, PowerPoint Presentations, Answer Keys for Chapter Review Quizzes, and a Test Bank.

FEATURES

LEARNING OBJECTIVES

1. Describe the composition of blood.
2. List the major organs and structures for the lymphatic and immune systems. Also identify the anatomic location of these major organs and structures.
3. Describe coagulation and hemostasis.
4. Differentiate between innate and acquired immunity and the types of acquired immunity.
5. Identify the etiology, signs and symptoms, diagnostic procedures, treatment, prognosis, and prevention of blood, lymphatic, and immune system diseases and disorders.
6. Compare the structure and function of the lymphatic and immune systems across the life span.

Learning Objectives emphasize the cognitive and performance objectives presented in the chapter.

Chapter Outlines present a guide for the chapter content and a quick reference for the topics covered.

OUTLINE

▶ OPENING SCENARIO

Marie Rodríguez, CMA (AAMA), has been working at Walden-Martin Family Medical (WMFM) Clinic. She was hired at WMFM Clinic shortly after passing her CMA exam 4 years ago. She has recently accepted a position helping the obstetrics/gynecology (OB/GYN) outreach providers. Marie will still work with the family medicine providers when the outreach providers are not at the clinic.

As a medical assistant over the last 4 years, Marie has worked with patients who have had reproductive disorders. Both male and female patients with reproductive system concerns are commonly seen in family medicine. Marie anticipates that her new position will allow her to learn more about pregnancy, pregnancy disorders, and infertility. She is excited to expand her knowledge in these areas. As she learns her new position, she has an opportunity to shadow with the medical assistants who assist the OB/GYN providers.

Opening Scenarios present a real-world situation for students to envision while reading the chapter content.

Vocabulary boxes highlight terms and definitions found in the chapter.

VOCABULARY

intrinsic factor Secreted by the parietal cells of the stomach; necessary for the absorption of vitamin B_{12} to prevent pernicious anemia.

rugae Folds in the wall of an organ; when an organ (e.g., stomach, bladder, uterus) fills or needs to expand, the rugae unfold.

MEDICAL TERMINOLOGY

cheil/o, labi/o	lips
bol/o	bolus
bucc/o	cheek
corpor/o	body, corporis
dent/i, odont/o	teeth
esophag/o	esophagus
fund/o	fundus
gastr/o	stomach
gingiv/o	gums
gloss/o, lingu/o	tongue
laryng/o	voice box, larynx
mucos/o, myx/o	mucus, mucosa
nas/o	nose
or/o, stomat/o, stom/o	mouth, oral cavity
palat/o	palate
pharyng/o	throat, pharynx
pylor/o	pylorus
sial/o	saliva
sialaden/o	salivary glands
peri-	surrounding
-al	pertaining to
-stalsis	contraction

Medical Terminology boxes provide review of word parts to help students learn how medical terms are built.

CRITICAL THINKING 42.1

Kayla wants to help Tim review carbohydrates. She asks him to list two foods from each category: simple sugars, starches, and fiber. What foods would you list?

Critical Thinking boxes prompt students to apply what they have learned as they read and study the chapter.

Study Tip boxes provide pointers and tips on remembering and distinguishing topics that are easily confused in practice.

✳ STUDY TIP

Think of the three states as:
- Polarized state – resting state
- Depolarized state – discharge (impulse) state
- Repolarized state – recovery state

Remember when discussing these three states that the cardiac chamber comes before the word (e.g., atrial polarization).

PROCEDURE 32.3   Remove Contaminated Gloves and Discard Biohazardous Material

Task
Minimize exposure to pathogens by medical aseptically removing and discarding contaminated gloves.

Equipment and Supplies
- Disposable gloves
- Biohazardous waste container with labeled red biohazard bag

Procedural Steps
1. With the dominant hand, grasp the glove of the opposite hand near the palm and begin removing the first glove (Fig. 1). The arms should be held away from the body with the hands pointed down.
   Purpose: Holding the hands down and away from the body helps prevent possible contamination.

2. Pull the glove inside out (Fig. 2). After removal, ball it into the palm of the remaining gloved hand.
   Purpose: Taking off the glove inside out prevents transmission of pathogens to another surface.

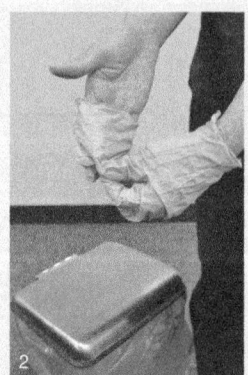

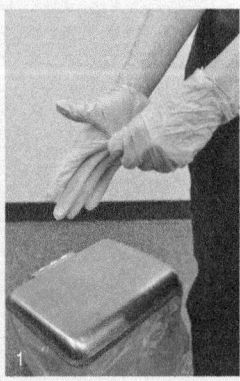

Step-by-step Procedure boxes demonstrate how to perform and document procedures encountered in the healthcare setting.

The Scenario Wrap-Up brings together the content of the chapter and the opening scenario in a real-world context.

The Chapter Review at the end of each chapter reviews and reinforces the important points of the chapter's focus to help students with content mastery.

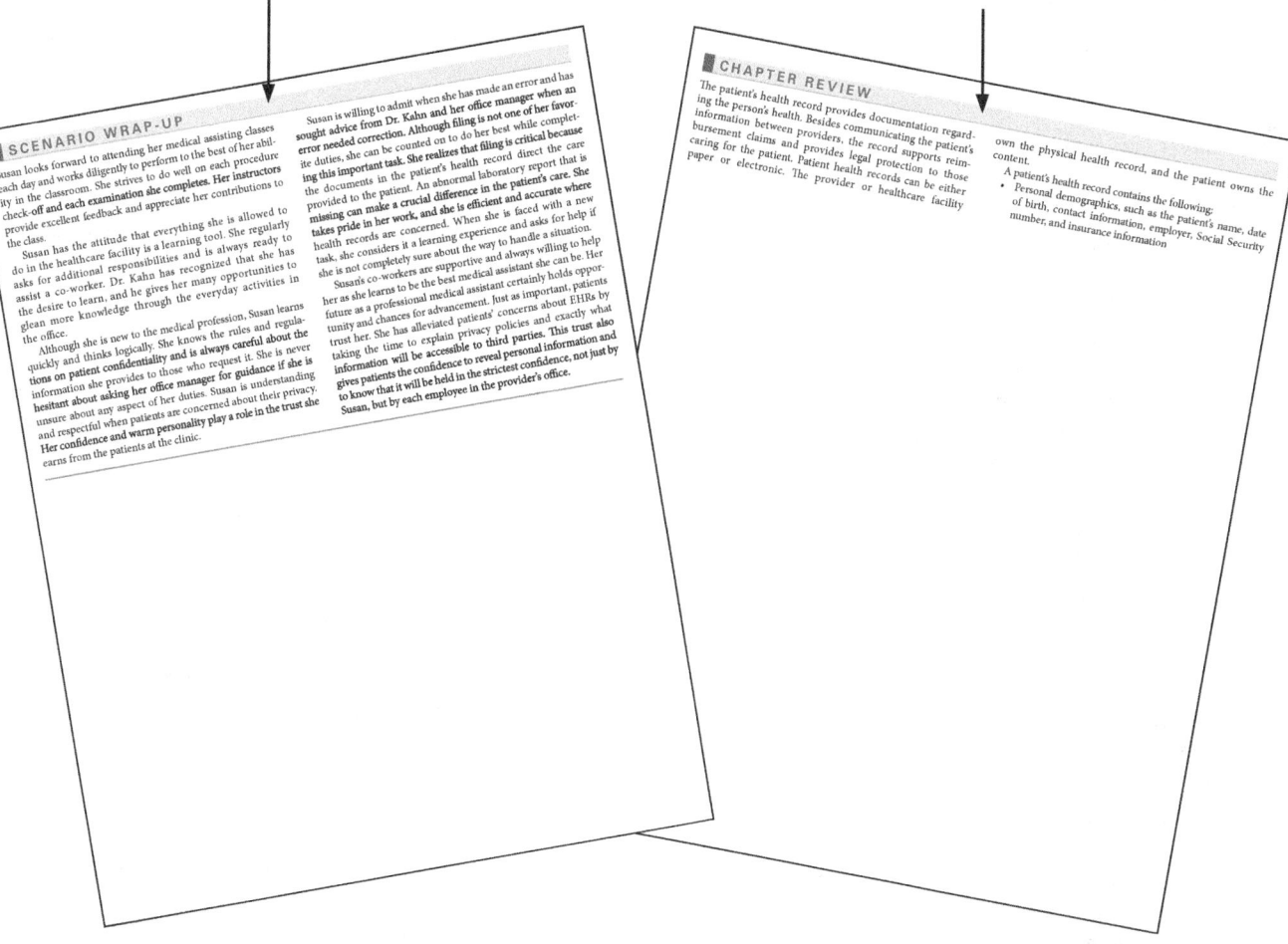

SCENARIO WRAP-UP

Susan looks forward to attending her medical assisting classes each day and works diligently to perform to the best of her ability in the classroom. She strives to do well on each procedure check-off and each examination she completes. Her instructors provide excellent feedback and appreciate her contributions to the class.

Susan has the attitude that everything she is allowed to do in the healthcare facility is a learning tool. She regularly asks for additional responsibilities and is always ready to assist a co-worker. Dr. Kahn has recognized that she has the desire to learn, and he gives her many opportunities to glean more knowledge through the everyday activities in the office.

Although she is new to the medical profession, Susan learns quickly and thinks logically. She knows the rules and regulations on patient confidentiality and is always careful about the information she provides to those who request it. She is never hesitant about asking her office manager for guidance if she is unsure about any aspect of her duties. Susan is understanding and respectful when patients are concerned about their privacy. Her confidence and warm personality play a role in the trust she earns from the patients at the clinic.

Susan is willing to admit when she has made an error and has sought advice from Dr. Kahn and her office manager when an error needed correction. Although filing is not one of her favorite duties, she can be counted on to do her best while completing this important task. She realizes that filing is critical because the documents in the patient's health record direct the care provided to the patient. An abnormal laboratory report that is missing can make a crucial difference in the patient's care. She takes pride in her work, and she is efficient and accurate where health records are concerned. When she is faced with a new task, she considers it a learning experience and asks for help if she is not completely sure about the way to handle a situation.

Susan's co-workers are supportive and always willing to help her as she learns to be the best medical assistant she can be. Her future as a professional medical assistant certainly holds opportunity and chances for advancement. Just as important, patients trust her. She has alleviated patients' concerns about EHRs by taking the time to explain privacy policies and exactly what information will be accessible to third parties. This trust also gives patients the confidence to reveal personal information and to know that it will be held in the strictest confidence, not just by Susan, but by each employee in the provider's office.

CHAPTER REVIEW

The patient's health record provides documentation regarding the person's health. Besides communicating the patient's information between providers, the record supports reimbursement claims and provides legal protection to those caring for the patient. Patient health records can be either paper or electronic. The provider or healthcare facility own the physical health record, and the patient owns the content.

A patient's health record contains the following:
- Personal demographics, such as the patient's name, date of birth, contact information, employer, Social Security number, and insurance information

---

PATIENT-CENTERED CARE

Most patients know little about medical coding, so they may not understand how the codes on their encounter forms relate to their diagnosis. If the patient has questions, explain that the codes represent their diagnosis to the most specific and accurate level. Because the coding system is much like a foreign language to patients, be patient when explaining this process and answering questions. This will help the patient to understand the insurance billing process.

The Patient-Centered Care feature incorporates the importance of providing patient-focused care in a team environment.

The Being Professional feature provides information on professional behavior with a related role-play example to allow students to apply the professionalism concepts.

BEING PROFESSIONAL

Although providers may be overly concerned about the need to maximize insurance reimbursements, coders should never feel coerced into fraudulent coding practices. Successful coders rely solely on medical documentation as the source of diagnostic statements. Coders should never assume that additional complications or conditions exist if they are not documented. In these cases, strong communication between the coder and the provider is necessary to clarify the appropriate diagnoses.

Role-play the following scenario with a peer: You are a medical assistant who is doing a provider's coding, and the peer is the provider. The provider is encouraging you to code to the maximum reimbursement, yet you do not see the documentation supporting the reimbursement they are pushing for. Respond to the provider in a respectful and professional manner.

CONTENTS

UNIT 8 Employment Seeking

Medical Terminology Basics

LEARNING OBJECTIVES

1. Describe eponyms, abbreviations, acronyms, and symbols.
2. Identify common medical prefixes and suffixes.
3. List the functions and major organs of each body system.
4. Define common combining forms for each body system.
5. Use the given rules to build, spell, and pronounce medical terms.
6. Explain how to define medical terms.

OUTLINE

⟫ OPENING SCENARIO

Daniela Garcia was recently hired as a part-time float receptionist at Walden-Martin Family Medical (WMFM) Clinic. Daniela has also recently started the medical assistant program at the local community college. She is currently taking a medical terminology course along with a human body and disease course.

As a float receptionist, she works in many different departments. Her job duties are consistent between the departments. She greets and checks in patients and also updates their information in the computer. The most challenging part of her new job is the medical terminology. The different diagnoses and procedures can get confusing. So she makes a list of new words that she hears. During her breaks, she looks up the words using an online medical dictionary. Audio pronunciation tools help her learn how to say the words.

YOU WILL LEARN

1. To describe the difference between eponyms, abbreviations, acronyms, and symbols.
2. To identify the prefix, suffix, root, and combining vowels of medical terms.
3. To describe each body system, including the functions and major organs.
4. To identify the meaning of combining terms for the body systems.
5. To build singular and plural medical terms.
6. To identify the meanings of medical terms.

INTRODUCTION

One of the first things students encounter in a medical assistant program is the language of healthcare. Medical terminology relates to anatomy, diseases, diagnostic tests, procedures, and so on. Having a strong understanding of medical terminology is not only helpful in your program, but critical as a healthcare professional.

This chapter discusses the parts of medical terms. It introduces students to common word parts related to the different body systems. You will learn how to label, identify, and define medical terms. These skills will help you as you progress through your program and start your new career in medical assisting.

FOUNDATIONS OF MEDICAL TERMINOLOGY

To many healthcare students, the vocabulary used in the medical environment may seem like words in a foreign language. The vocabulary used is a combination of eponyms, abbreviations, acronyms, symbols, and medical terminology.

> **VOCABULARY**
> **acronym** An abbreviation formed from the first letter of each word of a phrase and pronounced as a word.
> **eponym** A word that comes from the name of a person, place, or thing associated with the word.

Eponyms

Diseases and medical instruments are just a few of the areas where eponyms are used. Eponyms in medicine have been developed to honor scientists and providers who have created an innovative device or researched a new disease. Eponyms must be memorized. Examples of eponyms include:

- Parkinson disease was named after James Parkinson.
- Graves disease was named after Dr. Robert James Graves.
- Hashimoto disease was named after Dr. Hakaru Hashimoto.
- Cushing disease was named after Dr. Harvey Cushing.
- The Jackson-Pratt drain, used in some surgical procedures, was named after its inventors, Dr. Fredrick Jackson and Dr. Richard Pratt.
- The Snellen eye chart was named after its inventor, Dr. Herman Snellen.

Abbreviations, Acronyms, and Symbols

An *abbreviation* is a shortened version of a word or phrase. The abbreviation can be derived from the letters in the word or from combining the first letter of each word. Examples of medical abbreviations include:

- BP: Blood pressure
- CBC: Complete blood count
- CC: Chief complaint
- HTN: Hypertension
- Ca: Cancer
- HA: Headache
- PT: Physical therapy

Acronyms are also abbreviations that become pronounceable words. Examples of acronyms include:

- ACE: angiotensin-converting enzyme
- AIDS: acquired immunodeficiency syndrome
- ARDS: acute respiratory distress syndrome
- HIPAA: Health Insurance Portability and Accountability Act
- LASER: light amplification by stimulated emission of radiation

> **BOX 1.1   Symbols**
>
> $\bar{s}$ = without
> $\bar{p}$ = after
> $\bar{a}$ = before
> ↑ = increase
> ↓ = decrease
> △ = change

- RICE: rest, ice, compression, elevation
- SIDS: sudden infant death syndrome

A *symbol* is a picture that represents a word or phrase (Box 1.1). Symbols were used more often with paper health records. Using symbols increases the speed of documentation and reduces the amount of paper required. The use of symbols has decreased with the use of electronic health records.

Throughout the textbook, abbreviations and acronyms are listed. It is important to learn these. Making and using flashcards to study these can be useful.

Most healthcare facilities have lists of approved abbreviations and symbols that the healthcare professionals can use. Make sure to use only the approved abbreviations and symbols. Using unapproved abbreviations and symbols in messages and documentation may lead to confusion and patient care errors.

> **CRITICAL THINKING 1.1**
>
> Everyday Daniela hears abbreviations and acronyms at her job. List a medical abbreviation and an acronym and provide the meanings for both.

Medical Terminology

Medical terms used in healthcare can be divided into two groups, depending on whether they are made of word parts or not. Medical terms not made up of word parts need to be memorized. Medical terms made up of word parts can be literally defined.

Medical term word parts have either a Greek or Latin origin. By knowing the meaning of the word parts, a person can easily create or define medical terms. Four common word parts include:

- *Prefix*: A word part found at the beginning of the word. Prefixes modify the meaning of the word. In this textbook, prefixes are listed with a hyphen, such as "bi-" and "mal-."
- *Suffix*: A word part found at the end of the word. Suffixes follow a hyphen, such as "-is" and "-tic."
- *Root*: A word part that is the foundation of the term.
- *Combining vowel*: A vowel that links the root to the suffix or a root to a root. Typically, the combining vowel is an "o."

When the root is added to the combining vowel, the result is called a *combining form*. Combining forms can be given by stating the root word part followed by a slash and the vowel (e.g., oste/o and arthr/o).

PREFIXES AND SUFFIXES

The prefix is added to the beginning of the word. Not all medical terms have prefixes. Table 1.1 lists prefixes and their meanings.

TABLE 1.1 Prefixes

Prefix	Meaning	Prefix	Meaning
a-, an-	without, no, not	intra-	within
ab-	away from	ipsi-	same
ad -	near, toward	macro-	very large
af-	toward	mal-	bad
ana-	up, apart	megalo-	large
ante-	before, forward, in front of	meta-	change, beyond
anti-	against	micro-	small
bi-	two, both	neo-	new
brady-	slow	par-	near, beside
con-	together, with	para-	near, abnormal, beside
contra-	opposite	per-	through
dia-	complete, through	peri-	surrounding, around
dys-	difficult, painful, abnormal, bad	poly-	many, much, excessive, frequent
ec-	outside, out	post-	after, behind
echo-	using ultrasonic waves	pre-	before, in front of
ef-	away from	pro-, pros-	forward, before
electro-	using electricity	quadri-	four
end-, endo-	in, inner, within	re-, retro-	behind, back
epi-	above, upon	sub-	under, less than
ex-	out	supra-	upward, above
extra-	outside of	syn-	together, with
hemi-	half	tachy-	fast
hyper-	excessive, too much, above	trans-	through, across
hypo-	deficit, too little, below	tri-	three
in-	into, in	ultra-	beyond
inter-	between	uni-	one

Some prefixes have more than one meaning. The prefix modifies the root by describing the:
- Location or position: peri- (surrounding, around) and endo- (within, in, inner)
- Number: bi- (two, both) and tri- (three)
- State or problem: mal- (bad) and an- (without, no, not)
- Size: macro- (very large) and micro- (small)
- Speed or level: hyper- (above normal) and hypo- (below normal)

The suffix is added to the end of the word. Table 1.2 lists suffixes and their meanings.

CRITICAL THINKING 1.2

Look at Table 1.1, Prefixes, and Table 1.2, Suffixes. List four words you can think of that contain either a prefix or suffix from the tables.

COMBINING FORMS

A combining form contains both the root word part and the combining vowel. A combining form is linked to a root or a suffix.

Learning combining forms by body system can be helpful. The following sections describe the body systems and list the related combining forms. Table 1.3 provides the directional combining forms.

Cardiovascular System

The function of the cardiovascular (kar dee oh VASS kyoo lur) system is to transport materials throughout the body using the blood. The blood transports oxygen and nutrients and collects wastes through the body. Components in the blood also fight infections and form clots. The cardiovascular system includes the heart, arteries, arterioles, veins, venules, and the blood. Combining terms related to the cardiovascular system include:
- angi/o (vessel, blood vessel)
- aort/o (aorta)
- apic/o (apex)
- arteri/o (artery)
- cardi/o, coron/o (heart)
- hemat/o (blood)
- phleb/o, ven/o (vein)
- plasm/o (plasma)
- valv/o (valve)
- ventricul/o (ventricle)

Digestive System

The digestive system, also called the gastrointestinal (gass troh in TESS tih nul) system, breaks down, digests, and absorbs nutrients. The digestive system includes the mouth, tongue, teeth, pharynx, esophagus, stomach, small intestine, large intestine,

TABLE 1.2 Suffixes

Type	Suffix	Meaning	Type	Suffix	Meaning
Adjective	-ac	pertaining to		-pnea	breathing
	-al			-rrhagia	rapid flow of blood
	-ar			-rrhea	flow, discharge
	-ary			-sclerosis	abnormal condition of hardening
	-eal			-stenosis	abnormal condition of narrowing
	-ent			-thesis	to put, place (state of putting or placing)
	-ic				
	-ine			-uria	urine condition
	-ous			-y	process of, condition
	-tic		Instruments/recording	-graph	instrument to record
Body structure and function	-crine	secretion		-gram	record or recording
	-dipsia	thirst		-meter	instrument to measure
	-gen	to produce		-scope	instrument to view
	-is	structure	Noun ending	-icle	small or tiny structure
	-lapse	to fall, slide		-ole	
	-partum	birth		-ule	
	-phagia	to eat, swallow	Procedures	-cision	process of cutting
	-phasia	to speak		-centesis	surgical puncture and aspiration of fluid
	-plasm	formation		-ectomy	surgical removal, excision, resection
	-stasis	to stand, place, stop, control			
	-tension	pressure		-graphy	process of recording
	-trophy	nourishment; development		-metry	process of measuring
	-um	structure, membrane		-opsy	process of viewing
Conditions and diseases	-algia	pain		-pexy	surgical fixation
	-ation	process, condition		-plasty	surgical repair
	-cele	herniation		-rrhaphy	suture repair
	-emia	blood condition		-scopic	pertaining to visual examination
	-ia	diseased or abnormal condition		-scopy	process of visual examination
	-ism	condition, process		-section	to cut
	-itis	inflammation		-stomy	surgical creation of artificial opening
	-lysis	loosening, breakdown, separation, destruction			
				-tomy	incision, cut into
	-malacia	softening		-tripsy	crushing
	-megaly	enlargement	Specialty	-ist	one who specializes
	-oma	tumor, mass		-logist	one who specializes in the study of
	-osis	abnormal condition		-logy	study of
	-pathy	disease condition	Miscellaneous	-ad	toward
	-plegia	paralysis			

TABLE 1.3 Directional Combining Forms

Combining Form	Meaning	Combining Form	Meaning
anter/o	front	infer/o	downward
caud/o	tail	later/o	side
cephal/o	head	medi/o	middle
cubit/o	elbow	poplit/o	back of knee
dextr/o	right	poster/o	back
dist/o	far	proxim/o	near
dors/o	back	sinistr/o	left
fer/o	to carry	super/o	upward
front/o	front	ventr/o	belly
glute/o	buttocks		

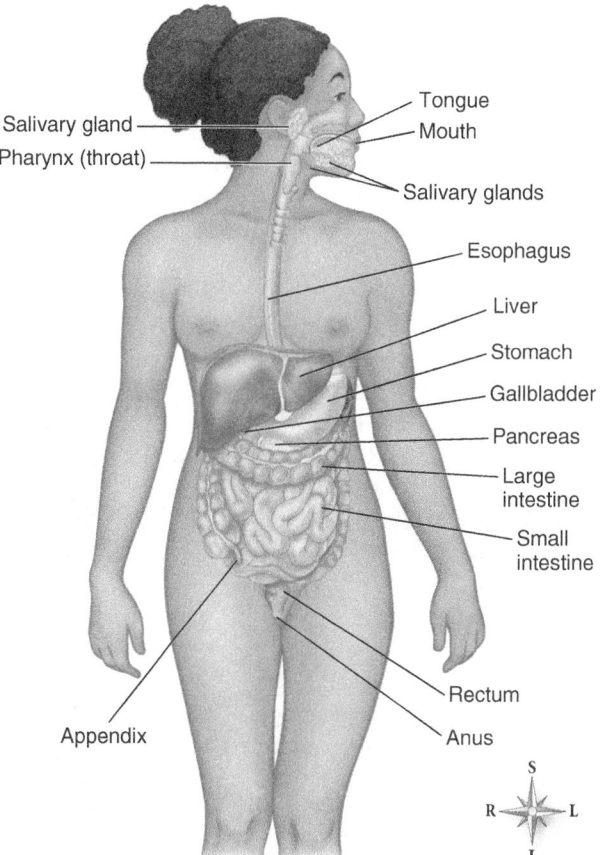

Fig. 1.1 Digestive System. (From Patton KT, Thibodeau GA: *The human body in health and disease*, ed 7, St. Louis, 2018, Elsevier.)

liver, gallbladder, pancreas, and appendix (Fig. 1.1). Combining terms related to the digestive system include:
- abdomin/o (abdomen)
- an/o (anus)
- append/o, appendic/o (appendix)
- chol/e (gall, bile)
- col/o, colon/o (colon)
- corpor/o, som/o, somat/o (corporis, body)
- enter/o (small intestine)
- esophag/o (esophagus)
- gastr/o (stomach)
- gingiv/o (gum)
- hepat/o (liver)
- lumin/o (lumen)
- or/o, stomat/o (mouth)
- pancreat/o (pancreas)
- pharyng/o (pharynx)
- rect/o (rectum)

Endocrine System

The endocrine (EN doh krin) system produces hormones that circulate in the blood. These hormones go to target tissues, which stimulate a particular action. The endocrine system includes the pituitary gland, pineal gland, hypothalamus, thyroid gland, pancreas, adrenal cortex and medulla, parathyroid gland, thymus gland, ovaries, and testes. Combining terms related to the endocrine system include:

- adren/o (adrenal gland)
- hypophys/o (pituitary gland)
- oophor/o, ovari/o (ovary)
- orch/o, orchi/o (testis)
- pancreat/o (pancreas)
- parathyroid/o (parathyroid gland)
- pituitary/o (pituitary gland)
- thyroid/o (thyroid gland)

CRITICAL THINKING 1.3

Using the combining forms for the cardiovascular, endocrine, and gastrointestinal systems, list four words that contain a combining form listed.

Integumentary System

The integumentary (in teg yoo MEN tuh ree) system is a barrier that protects the body and acts as a sense organ. It helps to retain body fluids, protect against infection, and helps regulate the body temperature. The integumentary system includes the skin, subcutaneous tissue, sweat and sebaceous glands, hair, nails, and sense receptors. Combining terms related to the integumentary system include:
- cutane/o, derm/o, dermato/o (skin)
- hidr/o (sweat)
- myc/o (fungus)
- necr/o (death - cells, body)
- onych/o, ungu/o (nail)
- pachy/o (thick)
- pil/o, trich/o (hair)
- seb/o (sebum, oil)
- xer/o (dry)

Lymphatic and Immune Systems

The lymphatic (lim FAT tick) system maintains fluid balance. The immune system provides immunity to some diseases. Both systems protect the internal environment of the body. The lymphatic and immune systems include the lymph, lymph vessels, lymph nodes, thymus, tonsils, spleen lymphocytes, and antibodies (Fig. 1.2). Combining terms related to the lymphatic and immune systems include:
- lymph/o (lymph)
- lymphaden/o (lymph node)
- lymphangi/o (lymph vessel)
- myel/o (bone marrow, spinal cord)
- splen/o (spleen)
- thym/o (thymus)

Musculoskeletal System

The musculoskeletal (muss kyoo loh SKELL uh tul) system is involved with movement, heat production, support, and protection of the body. The musculoskeletal system includes the bones, joints, muscles, tendons, ligaments, and cartilage. Combining terms related to the musculoskeletal system include:
- acromi/o (acromion)
- ankyl/o (stiff, bent)
- arthr/o (joint)
- carp/o (carpals)
- chondr/o (cartilage)
- cost/o (rib)

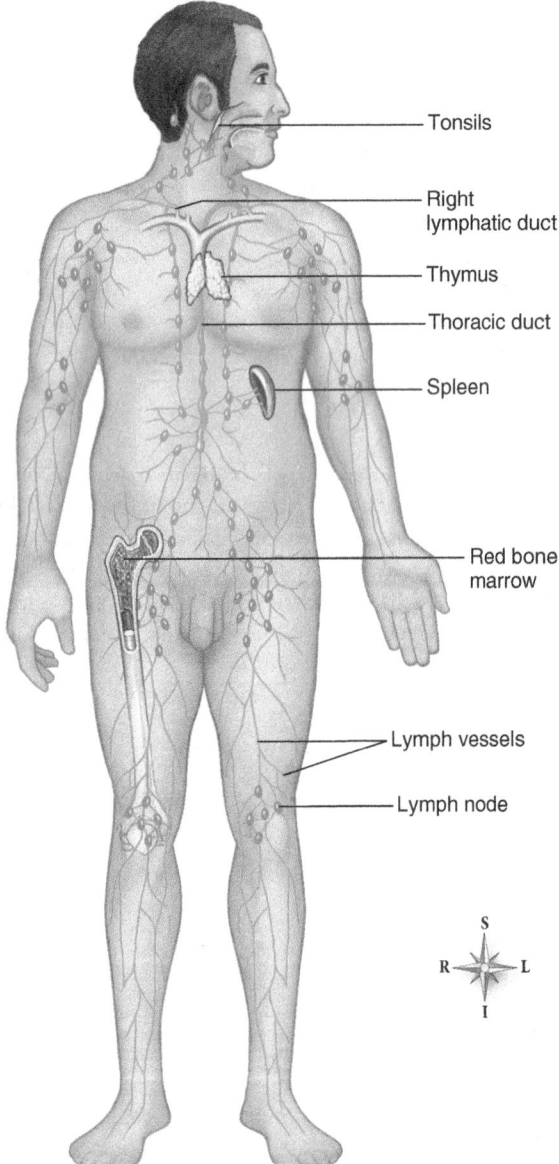

Fig. 1.2 Lymphatic and Immune Systems. (From Patton KT, Thibodeau GA: *The human body in health and disease*, ed 7, St. Louis, 2018, Elsevier.)

- cox/o (hip)
- crani/o (skull)
- digit/o (finger/toe)
- femor/o (thigh)
- ligament/o (ligament)
- lumb/o (lumbar)
- muscul/o, my/o, myos/o (muscle)
- oste/o (bone)
- patell/o, patell/a (kneecap)
- pelv/i, pelv/o (pelvis)
- pub/o (pubis)
- sacr/o (sacral)
- scapul/o (scapula)
- scoli/o (crooked, curved spine)
- stern/o (sternum)
- ten/o, tendin/o (tendon)

- thorac/o (chest)
- vertebr/o (vertebra)

> ## CRITICAL THINKING 1.4
>
> Using the combining forms for the integumentary, lymphatic, immune, and musculoskeletal systems, list four words that contain a combining form listed.

Nervous System

The nervous (NER vus) system controls body structures to maintain homeostasis. It receives and processes information from other body structures. The nervous system includes the brain, spinal cord, neurons, neuroglial cells, peripheral nerves, and autonomic nerves. Combining terms related to the nervous system include:

- cerebell/o (cerebellum)
- cerebr/o (cerebrum)
- dur/o (dura mater)
- encephal/o (brain)
- gangli/o, ganglion/o (ganglion)
- gli/o (glia)
- mening/o, meningi/o (meninges)
- myel/o (spinal cord, bone marrow)
- neur/o (nerve)

> **VOCABULARY**
>
> **homeostasis** The internal environment of the body that is compatible with life. A steady state that is created by all the body systems working together to provide a consistent and an unvarying internal environment.

Reproductive System

The reproductive system produces hormones and is involved with reproduction. The female reproductive system includes the ovaries, fallopian tubes, uterus, vagina, vulva, mammary glands, ovum, estrogen, and progesterone. The male reproductive system includes the epididymis vas deferens, prostate gland, testes, scrotum, penis, urethra, sperm, and testosterone. Combining terms related to the reproductive system include:

- cervic/o (cervix)
- colp/o, vagin/o (vagina)
- fund/o (fundus)
- mamm/o, mast/o (breast)
- men/o (menstruation)
- oophor/o, ovari/o (ovary)
- orch/o, orchi/o, orchid/o, test/o, testicul/o (testis)
- prostat/o (prostate gland)
- salping/o (fallopian tube)
- scrot/o (scrotum)
- umbilic/o (umbilical)
- uter/o, hyster/o, metri/o, metr/o (uterus)

Respiratory System

The respiratory (RESS pur ah tore ee) system delivers oxygen to the cells and removes carbon dioxide from the body. The respiratory system includes the nose, sinuses, pharynx, larynx, trachea,

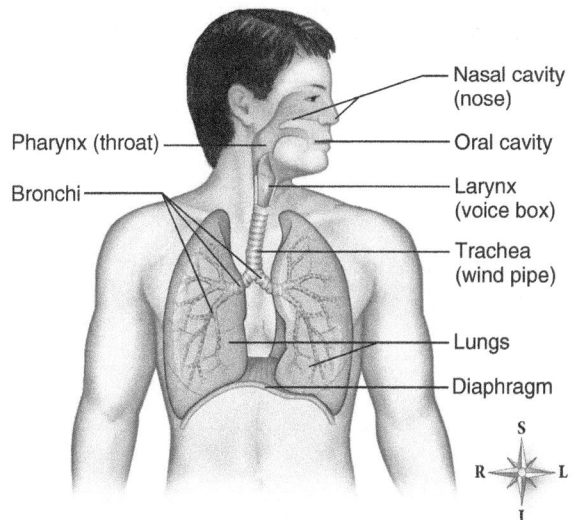

Fig. 1.3 Respiratory System. (From Patton KT, Thibodeau GA: *The human body in health and disease*, ed 7, St. Louis, 2018, Elsevier.)

bronchi, lungs, bronchioles, and alveoli (Fig. 1.3). Combining terms related to the respiratory system include:
- alveol/o (alveolus, air sac)
- bronch/o, bronchi/o (bronchial tube)
- cyan/o (blue)
- epiglott/o (epiglottis)
- laryng/o (larynx)
- nas/o, rhin/o (nose)
- pector/o, steth/o, thorac/o (chest)
- pharyng/o (pharynx)
- phren/o (diaphragm)
- pneumon/o, pulmon/o, pneum/o (lung)
- sin/o, sinus/o (sinus)
- trache/o (trachea)

CRITICAL THINKING 1.5

Using the combining forms for the nervous, reproductive, and respiratory systems, list four words that contain a combining form listed.

Sensory System

The sensory system gathers information through the senses of vision, hearing, balance, taste, and smell. The sensory system consists of the eyes, ears, taste buds, olfactory receptors, and sensory receptors. Combining terms related to the sensory system include:
- audi/o (hearing)
- aur/i, aur/o (ear)
- blephar/o (eyelid)
- cochle/o (cochlea)
- conjunctiv/o (conjunctiva)
- corne/o (cornea)
- dipl/o (two, double)
- ir/o, irid/o (iris)
- myring/o (tympanic membrane, eardrum)

- ocul/o, ophthalm/o (eye)
- opt/o (vision)
- ot/o (ear)
- retin/o (retina)
- scler/o (sclera)
- vestibul/o (vestibule)

Urinary System

The urinary (YOOR ih nair ee) system eliminates nitrogenous waste and maintains the electrolyte, water, and acid-base balances. The urinary system includes the nephron unit, kidneys, ureters, bladder, and urethra. Combining forms related to the urinary system include:
- cyst/o, vesic/o (urinary bladder)
- glyc/o, glycos/o (sugar)
- hil/o (hilum)
- hydr/o (water)
- lith/o (stone)
- noct/i (night)
- nephr/o (kidney)
- olig/o (scanty)
- pyel/o (renal pelvis)
- ren/o (kidney)
- ureter/o (ureter)
- urethr/o (urethra)
- urin/o, ur/o (urinary)

CRITICAL THINKING 1.6

Using the combining forms for the sensory and urinary systems, list four words that contain a combining form listed.

BUILDING MEDICAL TERMS

Using Combining Vowels

When building a medical term, it is important to know when to use a combining vowel. When combining a root with a suffix, remember these guidelines:
- If the suffix begins with a consonant, use a combining vowel between the root and the suffix.
- If the suffix begins with a vowel, do not use a combining vowel. Furthermore, if the root ends in a vowel and the suffix starts with the same vowel, one of the vowels is dropped.

See Table 1.4 for examples of building medical terms following these root-suffix guidelines.

Additional guidelines include:
- When adding a root to a root, use a combining vowel. Fig. 1.4 shows how cholangiopancreatography and pyloromyotomy are built. A combining vowel is used even if the second root begins with a vowel.
- Do not use a combining vowel between a prefix and a root (Fig. 1.5).

Ordering of Combining Forms

Some medical terms have two or more combining forms. With some terms, the order of the combining forms follows the

TABLE 1.4   Use of a Combining Vowel

Combining Vowel	Combining Form (Meaning)	Suffix (Meaning)	Medical Term
When the suffix begins with a consonant, the combining vowel is used.	arteri/o (artery)	-sclerosis (abnormal condition of hardening)	arteriosclerosis (ar teer ee oh sklah ROH sis)
	neutr/o (neutral)	-phil (attraction)	neutrophil (NOO tro fil)
	hem/o (blood)	-stasis (to stand, place, stop, control)	hemostasis (hee muh STEY sis)
	thromb/o (clot, clotting)	-cyte (cell)	thrombocyte (THROM bow site)
When the suffix begins with a vowel, the combining vowel is not added.	sept/o (septum)	-al (pertaining to)	septal (SEP tal)
	esophag/o (esophagus)	-eal (pertaining to)	esophageal (eh sah fah JEE ul)
	ventricul/o (ventricle)	-ar (pertaining to)	ventricular (ven TRIK yah lar)
	coron/o (heart)	-ary (pertaining to)	coronary (KORE ih nair ee)
When the suffix begins with a vowel and the root ends in the same vowel, one of the vowels is dropped.	arteri/o (artery)	-itis (inflammation)	arteritis (ahr ter EYE tis)
	cardi/o (heart)	-itis (inflammation)	carditis (kar DYE tis)
	ovari/o (ovary)	-itis (inflammation)	ovaritis (OH vah rie tis)

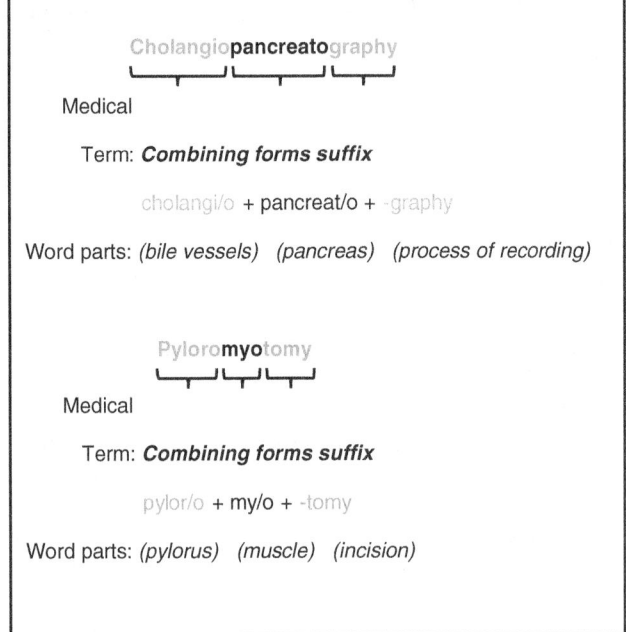

Fig. 1.4 Combining Roots.

sequence of the procedure. For instance, when a proctosigmoidoscopy is performed, an endoscope is used. (Remember, -scopy means process of visual examination.) An endoscope is a thin flexible tube with a light. At the start of the procedure, the provider inserts the endoscope into the anus. The endoscope enters the rectum (proct/o) and then is advanced into the sigmoid colon (sigmoid/o).

Singular and Plural Terms

When singular Latin and Greek terms are changed to the plural forms, special rules apply. Table 1.5 shows how to change these terms to plural forms. When Latin terms that consist of a noun and an adjective are pluralized, both terms need to be pluralized. For example, placenta previa would become placentae previae.

It is also helpful to remember these English rules for pluralizing nouns:

- Most words can be made into the plural form by adding -s. For example, the plural form of heart is hearts.
- If the term ends in -s, -x, -ch, or -sh, add -es. For example, the plural form of stitch is stitches.
- If the term ends in -y after a consonant, drop the -y and add -ies. For example, the plural form of artery is arteries.
- If the term ends in -o after a consonant, add -nes. For example, the plural form of comedo is comedones.

There are some exceptions to these rules, and the spelling of those terms must be memorized.

CRITICAL THINKING 1.7

Using English rules for pluralizing nouns, list four (nonmedical) words that follow one of these rules.

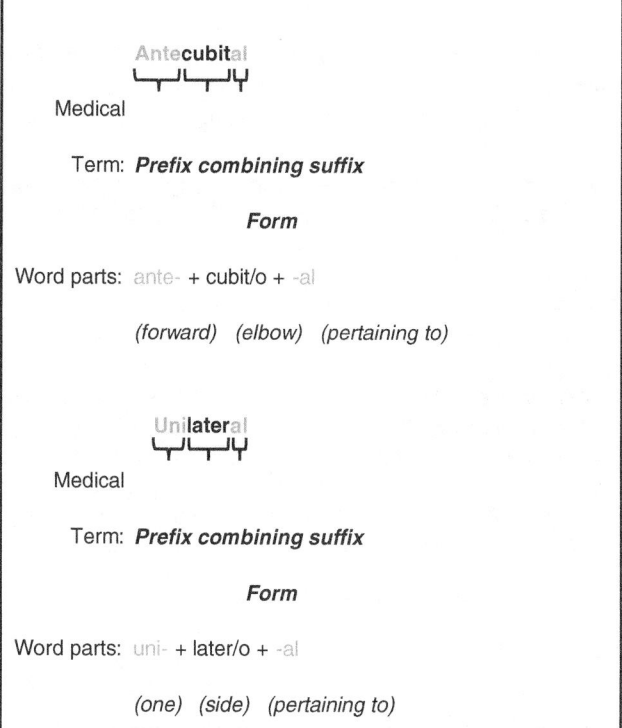

Fig. 1.5 Prefixes.

1. Divide the term into word parts. For example, divide vasculitis into word parts.
   vascul/itis
2. Label each word part and combining form.
   vascul/o -itis
   combining form, suffix
3. Define each word part.
   vascul/o -itis
   combining form – vessel; suffix – inflammation
4. Define the term. Start with the suffix definition. Then add the definition(s) for the rest of the word, starting at the beginning of the term.
   inflammation of the (blood) *vessel*

PRONOUNCING UNUSUAL LETTER COMBINATIONS

As a medical assistant, it is important to accurately pronounce medical terms. Some medical terms are easy to pronounce, whereas others are more difficult. Use the following tips when learning medical term pronunciations:

- Listen to the pronunciation. Many online medical dictionaries have pronunciation tools available.
- Break apart unfamiliar terms. Pronounce each section separately.
- Think about similar looking terms and how they are pronounced.
- Focus on letter combinations that have different sounds (Table 1.6).
- Practice saying the terms out loud.

TABLE 1.5 Changing Latin and Greek Terms to Plural Terms

Singular Term Ends in	Change to a Plural Term	EXAMPLES Singular Form	Plural Form
-a	add e	bursa	bursae
-ax	change the x to a c and add es	thorax	thoraces
-ex -ix	drop -ex or -ix and add -ices	appendix	appendices
-is	drop -is and add -es	diagnosis	diagnoses
-ma	add -ta	fibroma	fibromata
-nx	change the x to a g and add es	larynx	larynges
-on	drop the -on and add -a	spermatozoon	spermatozoa
-um	drop -um and add -a	atrium	atria
-us	drop -us and add -i	bronchus	bronchi
-yx	change the x to a c and add es	calyx	calyces

TABLE 1.6 Pronouncing Letter Combinations

Letter Combination	Sound	Example
C before the vowel e or i	S	cilia
G before the vowel e or i	J	gene
C before the vowels a, o, or u	K	cochlear
G before the vowels a, o, or u	G	gallbladder
eu	you	eustachian tube
ch	K	cholangiogram
ph	F	physiology
pn	N	pneumothorax
ps	S	psychosis
pt	T	ptosis
rh, rrh	R	rhinorrhagia
x-	Z	xenograft
cy	ss	cyanosis
qu	kw	quadrant

DEFINING MEDICAL TERMS

When you encounter an unknown medical term, take the following steps to identify the meaning.

CLOSING COMMENTS

Having a strong understanding of medical terminology will help you as you complete your medical assistant program and practicum. As you move through your career, you will continue to learn new medical terms. Always remember to break down the terms into word parts and then define the word parts. This strategy will help you successfully define new medical terms.

PATIENT-CENTERED CARE

Patient-centered care means patients are partners in their healthcare. Patients often get overwhelmed by the continual use of medical terms. The use of unfamiliar medical terms can reduce what the patients and families understand about the diseases and treatments. This limits their ability to be true partners in their healthcare. It is important for medical assistants to remember to limit the use of medical terms when talking with patients. If medical terms need to be used, the medical assistant should explain what they mean.

BEING PROFESSIONAL

It is important for the medical assistant to help patients understand the medical terms they encounter during their care. The medical assistant should use easy to understand terms to define the words to patients. If pictures or images are available, those can also help patients understand complicated terminology.

Anna Richardson comes to the reception desk after her visit. She hands you the visit summary notes. You see she needs to be scheduled for an esophagogastroduodenoscopy. She also needs a referral visit scheduled with the gastroenterologist. Anna comments that she is not familiar with the test and gastroenterologists. "I wish they would use words I can understand," she says. What should you do and say to help Anna have a better patient experience? Role-play this scenario with a peer.

CHAPTER REVIEW

The vocabulary used in healthcare is a combination of eponyms, abbreviations, acronyms, symbols, and medical terminology. Four common word parts make up medical terms. A prefix, which is found at the beginning of the word, modifies the meaning of the word. A suffix is found at the end of the word. A root is the foundation of the term. A combining vowel links the root to another root or a suffix. The root and a combining vowel make up a combining form.

Many of the combining terms can be organized by body systems. Some of the related combining terms for each body system include:
- Cardiovascular system: angi/o, cardi/o, hemat/o, and phleb/o
- Digestive system: abdomin/o, chol/e, col/o, and hepat/o
- Endocrine system: adren/o, ovari/o, pancreat/o, and thyroid/o
- Integumentary system: cutane/o, derm/o, pil/o, and seb/o
- Lymphatic and immune systems: lymph/o, myel/o, splen/o, and thym/o
- Musculoskeletal system: arthr/o, cost/o, my/o, and ten/o
- Nervous system: cerebell/o, cerebr/o, mening/o, and neur/o
- Reproductive system: cervic/o, mamm/o, orch/o, and uter/o
- Respiratory system: bronch/o, laryng/o, nas/o, and pneumon/o
- Sensory system: audi/o, aur/o, ocul/o, and ot/o
- Urinary system: cyst/o, ren/o, ureter/o, and urethr/o

When identifying the meaning of a medical term, first divide the term into word parts. Label and define each word part, and then define the term as a whole. When defining the term, start with the suffix definition and follow with the rest of the term, beginning with the start of the term.

SCENARIO WRAP-UP

By looking up the medical terms she is unfamiliar with, Daniela is starting to learn more of the common diagnoses and procedures. While floating to the different departments, she is learning medical terms related to the different body systems.

Daniela is looking forward to learning more in her medical terminology class, so she can use the information in her job. She hopes after graduation to obtain a medical assistant job at WMFM Clinic.

Anatomy and Pathology Basics

LEARNING OBJECTIVES

1. Describe the structural organization of the human body.
2. Use surface anatomy, positional, and directional terminology.
3. Describe body cavities, abdominopelvic quadrants, and body planes.
4. Discuss the acid-base balance in the human body.
5. Discuss pathology basics, including pathology terminology, protection mechanisms, predisposing factors, the causes of disease, and diagnostic procedures.

OUTLINE

⫸ OPENING SCENARIO

Daniela Garcia is a part-time float receptionist at Walden-Martin Family Medical (WMFM) Clinic. As a float receptionist, she moves between the family medicine and outreach services. At WMFM Clinic, the providers see family practice patients. When patients need to see specialists, the WMFM providers refer them to outreach specialty providers. The outreach specialty providers come to WMFM Clinic on a rotating schedule to provide services beyond those of the WMFM providers.

Besides working, Daniela is pursuing a medical assistant diploma. She is currently taking courses in medical terminology and the human body. Daniela really enjoys working with the outreach providers, because she continues to learn new information that is helping her in the human body course.

YOU WILL LEARN

1. To recognize and use terms related to the basic anatomy and pathology concepts.
2. To describe the organization of the body.
3. To describe body systems.
4. To recognize and use surface anatomy, directional, and positional terms.
5. To describe body cavities and abdominopelvic quadrants.
6. To describe predisposing factors and causes of disease.

INTRODUCTION

It is important for medical assistants to understand the anatomy and physiology of the body. *Anatomy* (ah NAT uh mee) is the study of how the body is shaped and structured. It includes the structures, levels of organization, and the relationships between different body parts. *Physiology* (fi zee ALL uh jee) is the study of body functions. Anatomy and physiology information is used in many ways in clinical and administrative settings. From coding and billing to entering diagnostic orders, having a strong understanding of this information will help medical assistants perform their roles more efficiently.

This chapter discusses the organization of the body, along with body cavities and directional terms. In the coming body system chapters, you will learn the anatomy and physiology of each body system. You will also be introduced to diseases that affect each system. To help you understand this content, this chapter also provides the basics for understanding pathology (pah THOL uh jee), diagnostic procedures, and treatments.

> **MEDICAL TERMINOLOGY**
>
> | path/o | disease |
> | physi/o | growth |
> | ana- | apart, away, up |
> | -logy | study of |
> | -tomy | cutting, incision |

> **VOCABULARY**
>
> **diagnostic procedures** Tests and procedures used to help diagnose or monitor a condition.
> **pathology** Study of disease.

ANATOMY BASICS

Structural Organization of the Body

If we were to break apart the body, we would have many body systems. Examples include the digestive, cardiovascular, musculoskeletal, and respiratory systems. Each system is composed of different organs. For instance, the stomach and intestines are digestive system organs. Each organ is made up of combinations of tissues, and these tissues are composed of cells. So, when studying the organization of the body, it is easier to start at the level of cells and work up to the organism (human body) level.

Cells. The basic unit of life is the cell. Cells determine the functional and structural characteristics of the entire body. Cells are microscopic in size. They have a variety of shapes and perform a vast array of functions. A cell is covered by a plasma membrane. The cell contains cytoplasm and *organelles* (ORE ga nels), or structures inside of the cell. See Table 2.1 and Fig. 2.1 for the parts of the cells.

Most human cells reproduce by *mitosis* (my TOE sis). Mitosis is a process in which one cell splits into two identical daughter cells. The two cells are genetically identical to the parent cell. Prior to the mitosis process, the cell enters the interphase stage. During this stage, the genetic information, chromosomes (KROE mah somes), replicate. Each sister pair of chromosomes (called *chromatids*) are joined together until they are pulled apart later in the mitosis process. The point where the two chromatids are joined is called the *centromere*. The centromere is also the

TABLE 2.1   Cell Parts

Cell Part	Description
Plasma membrane (PLAZ ma mem BRAIN)	Outer covering surrounding the cell that allows certain substances to enter the cell and blocks other substances. Can also be called the *cell membrane*.
Cytoplasm (SYE toh plaz um)	Jelly-like substance the surrounds the nucleus and fills the cells. *Organelles* (structures in the cell) are suspended in the cytoplasm.
Ribosome (RYE boh sohm)	Free-floating organelle that makes enzymes and proteins. Contains ribonucleic acid (RNA). Considered the cell's "protein factories."
Rough endoplasmic reticulum (ER) (en doe PLAZ mik ri TIK ue lum)	Organelle that is a network of membranes; connects to the nucleus. Ribosomes are attached to the ER, causing the rough appearance. Involved with making protein.
Smooth endoplasmic reticulum (ER) (en doe PLAZ mik ri TIK ue lum)	Tubelike organelle; role differs based on the type of cell. Roles may include storage of calcium and making steroids and lipids.
Golgi apparatus (GOLE jee)	Organelle that processes and packages the proteins and lipids made by the cell. Considered to be the cell's "processing plant."
Lysosomes (LYE soh sohm)	Organelles that contain enzymes and are involved with digesting nutrients and other substances in the cell. Considered to be the cell's "waste collectors."
Mitochondrion (pl. mitochondria) (mye toh KAHN dree un)	Organelle that produces the energy for the cell. Called the cell's "power plant."
Nucleus (pl. nuclei) (NOO klee us)	Control center of the cell; contains chromosomes that are made up of deoxyribonucleic acid (DNA), which carries genetic information. Called the "control center."
Nucleolus (NOO klee o lus)	Inside of the nucleus; produces ribosomes.
Centrioles (SEN tree ol)	Tubelike structures that help with cell division and with the formation of the spindle fibers (a type of microtubule).
Cilia (SIL ee ah)	Fine, hairlike extensions on the surface of the cell. Used to detect surroundings or chemicals.
Microvilli	Small projections on the surface of the cell. This increases the surface area, which allows for additional absorption.
Flagellum (fla JEL uhm)	Single long hairlike extension on the surface of the cell. Used to propel or move cell.

attachment point for spindle fibers, which will be involved in the mitosis process. The mitosis process consists of four phases:

- *Prophase*: The membrane around the nucleus starts to break down. Centrioles produce spindle fibers and start to move toward opposite sides of the cell.
- *Metaphase*: Each pair of chromatids lines up, and each chromatid is attached to a spindle fiber.
- *Anaphase*: Spindle fibers pull the sister chromatids apart.
- *Telophase*: The nucleus reforms around each set of chromosomes. The cell continues to separate into two daughter cells.

STUDY TIP

Remember the phases of mitosis as PMAT:
- Prophase – PREPARES
- Metaphase – chromosomes MEET in the MIDDLE
- Anaphase – chromosome pulls APART
- Telophase – the cell TEARS in TWO

CRITICAL THINKING 2.1

Daniela is learning about the cell structures in school. While on break one night, she talked to Bella. Bella is a new CMA (AAMA) who just graduated. Daniela mentioned she was learning about cell parts. Bella encouraged Daniela to associate the cell parts to the things she might see in an old city. For instance, she stated, "The plasma membrane could be the walls around the city." What other associations could be made between the cell structures and a city?

VOCABULARY

chromosomes Rod-shaped structures found in the cell's nucleus; they contain genetic information.

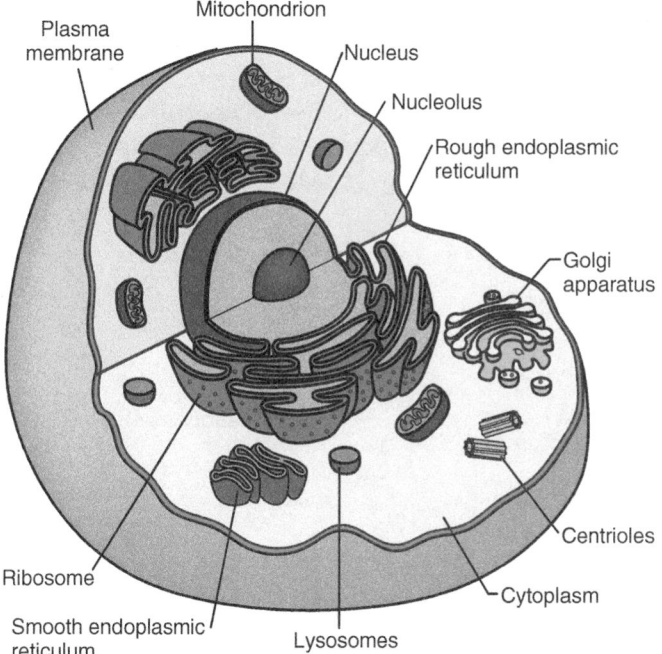

Plasma membrane
Mitochondrion
Nucleus
Nucleolus
Rough endoplasmic reticulum
Golgi apparatus
Centrioles
Cytoplasm
Ribosome
Smooth endoplasmic reticulum
Lysosomes

Fig. 2.1 Cell Structure.

Tissues. A *tissue* is a group of similar cells from the same source that together carry out a specific function. The microscopic study of body tissues is known as *histology* (hi STOL uh jee). All of the body tissues are grouped into four types. The four types of tissue include:

1. *Epithelial* (eh puh THEE lee ul) *tissue:* Acts as an internal or external covering for organs. Examples of epithelial tissue include the outer layer of the skin, glands, and linings of body cavities and organs. In epithelial tissue, the cells are packed so closely together that there is little to no intercellular material. Two types of epithelial tissue include simple and stratified. *Simple epithelium* is a single layer of the same shaped cells. *Stratified epithelium* contains multiple layers of cells. Epithelial tissue is classified according to shape:
   - *Squamous*: Flat in appearance
   - *Cuboidal*: Square in appearance
   - *Columnar*: Long and narrow in appearance
   - *Transitional*: Varying shapes that can stretch
2. *Connective tissue*: Supports and binds other body tissues. Examples of connective tissue include bone, blood, fat, fibrous tissue, areolar tissue, and cartilage. Connective tissue is the most frequently occurring tissue in the body.
3. *Muscle tissue*: Produces movement. Classifications of muscle tissue include:
   - *Skeletal*: Voluntary muscles that appear *striated* or striped. Attached to bones and produce voluntary body movements when contracted.
   - *Cardiac*: Involuntary muscles that appear striated and form the heart muscle wall.
   - *Smooth*: Involuntary nonstriated muscles. Line the blood vessel walls and hollow organs and cause peristalsis (per uh STAHL suhs) and vasoconstriction (va zo kuhn STRIK shun).
4. *Nervous tissue*: Includes cells that provide transmission of information to control a variety of functions. Nervous tissue controls the body's functions to maintain homeostasis (hoh mee oh STAY sis). Nervous tissue is made up of **neurons (nerve cells)** and supportive structures called *neuroglial cells.*

MEDICAL TERMINOLOGY

cyt/o	cell
hist/o	tissue
home/o	same
my/o	muscle
neur/o	nervous
nucle/o	nucleus
endo-	within, inner
-plasm	formation
-stasis	controlling

VOCABULARY

homeostasis The internal environment of the body that is compatible with life. A steady state that is created by all the body systems working together to provide a consistent and unvarying internal environment.

intercellular Located between cells.

peristalsis Rhythmic contraction of involuntary muscles lining the gastrointestinal tract.

vasoconstriction Contraction of the muscles causing narrowing of the inside tube of the vessel.

Organs. An organ is a structure composed of two or more types of tissue. An organ may have one or more functions. For instance, the pancreas has two functions: it produces insulin, and it produces digestive enzymes (EN zimes). Organs are grouped within body systems. An organ may be part of one or more systems. For instance, the pancreas is part of the endocrine system and also part of the digestive system.

Body Systems. A body system is composed of several organs and their related structures. These structures work together to perform a specific function in the body. Body systems were described in the prior chapter. Body systems include the cardiovascular, respiratory, nervous, endocrine, gastrointestinal, integumentary, lymphatic, immune, muscular, skeletal, reproductive, sensory, and urinary systems.

Organism. The organism of the body is made up of many body systems. These work together to maintain a steady environment in the body called *homeostasis*. If the balance is off or if the environment moves out of the normal range, diseases can occur.

To summarize the structural organization of the body from simple to complex:
- Cells are the most basic unit.
- Tissues are groups of similar cells from the same source that carry out a specific function.
- Organs are structures made up of two or more types of tissues.
- Body systems are made up of several organs and their related structures.

- An organism is made up of many body systems that work together for homeostasis in the body.

CRITICAL THINKING 2.2

Bella's tip really helped Daniela with the cell structures. Now Daniela needs to remember the organization of the body in order from the simplest to the most complex. Bella encourages Daniela to create a phrase or word that would help her remember cells, tissues, organs, body system, and organism. What might be a way to remember these five items in order?

Anatomic Position and Body Planes

The *anatomic position* is a standard frame of reference. This means the body stands erect with the face forward, arms at the sides, palms forward, and toes pointed forward. Fig. 2.2 shows the body in this position.

Using the anatomic position, the body can be divided into planes as another frame of reference. *Planes* are imaginary cuts or sections through the body. The use of plane terminology is common when discussing diagnostic imaging (e.g., computed tomography [CT] scan) of the body. Diagnostic imaging will be discussed in more detail later in the chapter. Planes include the coronal, midsagittal, and transverse planes (Fig. 2.3).

The *coronal* (koh ROH nul) *plane* or *frontal plane* divides the body into front and back portions. The front of the body is referred to as the *anterior* or *ventral*. The back of the body is referred to as the *posterior* or *dorsal*.

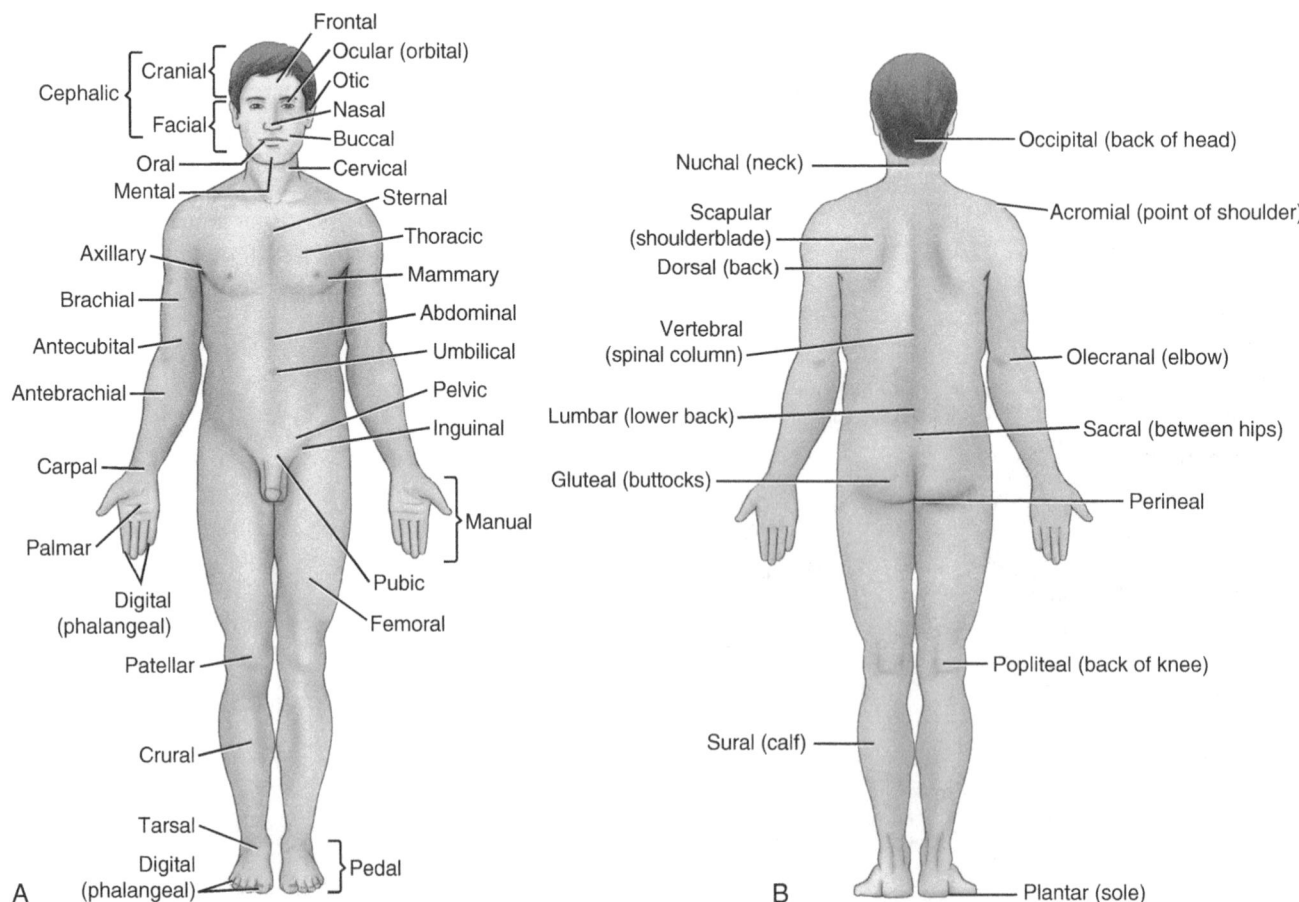

Fig. 2.2 A, Ventral surface anatomy. B, Dorsal surface anatomy. (From Shiland B: *Mastering healthcare terminology*, ed 5, St. Louis, 2016, Elsevier.)

The *midsagittal* (mid SAJ ih tul) *plane* or *median plane* separates the body into equal right and left halves. The medial line starts at the top of the head (cranium) and continues down the body to between the legs to the ground. This is also referred to as the *midline* of the body. Closer to the midline is referred to as *medial*, and farther away from the midline is called *lateral*.

The *transverse plane* or *horizontal plane* divides the body horizontally into upper and lower sections. The area above the plane is called *superior* (pertaining to upward) or *cephalad* (toward the head). The area below the plane is called *inferior* (pertaining to downward) or *caudad* (toward the tail).

Directional and Positional Terms. Besides the directional terms discussed in the prior section (e.g., anterior, posterior, superior), additional terms can be used to indicate a position on the patient. Additional positional and directional terms include:
- *Unilateral* pertains to one side; *bilateral* pertains to two sides.
- *Dextrad* (DEKS trad) means toward the right side and *sinistrad* (SIN is trad) means toward the left side. Dextrad and sinistrad are opposites.
- *Afferent* (AF fur ent) pertains to carrying toward a structure. *Efferent* (EF fur ent) pertains to carrying away from a structure. Examples: The afferent arteriole brings blood to the glomerulus. The efferent arteriole carries blood away from the glomerulus.
- *Ipsilateral* (ip see LAT er uhl) pertains to the same side. *Contralateral* (kon trah LAT er uhl) pertains to the opposite side. Example: The right leg is ipsilateral to the right arm, but contralateral to the left arm.

- *Superficial* (soo per FISH uhl) is toward the surface of the body. *Deep* is away from the surface of the body. Example: The skin is superficial, whereas bones are deep in the body.
- *Proximal* (PROCK sih muhl) pertains to near the origin or toward the trunk of the body. *Distal* (DISS tuhl) pertains to far from the origin or farthest from the trunk of the body. Examples: The toes are distal to the knee. The hip is proximal to the knee.
- Body positions refer to the physical orientation of the body. *Supine* (SOO pine) means a person is lying face up, and *prone* (PROHN) is lying face down. Lying on one's side is called the *lateral* (LAT er uhl) position.

MEDICAL TERMINOLOGY	
anter/o	front
caud/o	tail
cephal/o	head
dextr/o	right
dist/o	far
dors/o	back
fer/o	to carry
front/o	front
infer/o	downward
later/o	side
medi/o	middle
poster/o	back
proxim/o	near
sinistr/o	left
super/o	upward
ventr/o	belly

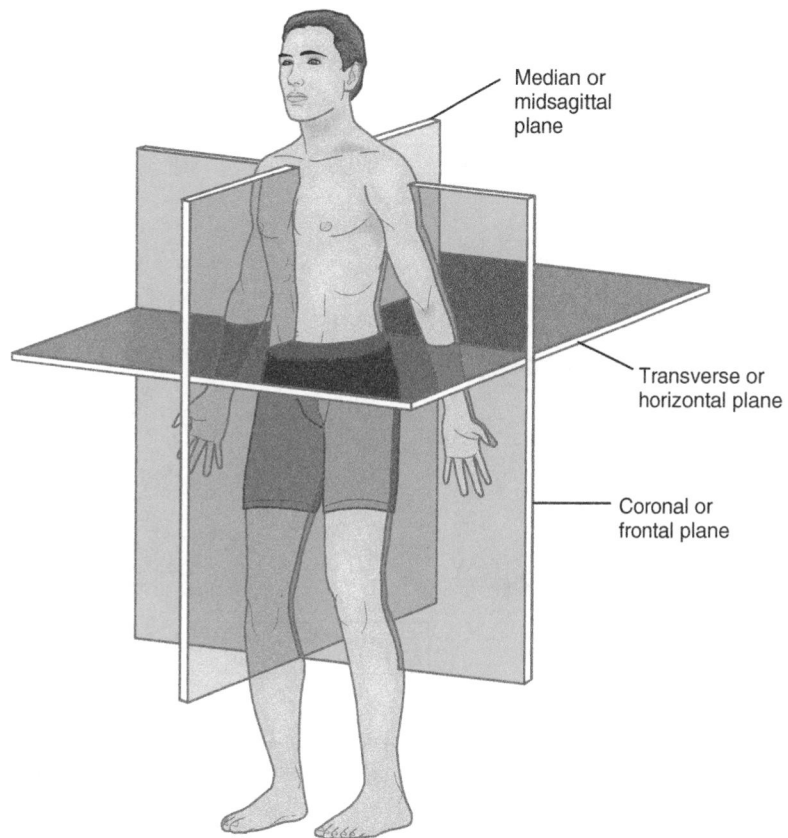

Fig. 2.3 Body Planes. (From Proctor D, et al: *Kinn's the medical assistant*, ed 13, St. Louis, 2017, Elsevier.)

Median or midsagittal plane

Transverse or horizontal plane

Coronal or frontal plane

CRITICAL THINKING 2.3

Bella continues to help Daniela on breaks during work. Today, Daniela is learning directional terms. Bella encourages Daniela to repeat the term and definition as she points to that part of her body. How else might Daniela learn the directional terms and the opposite pairs?

VOCABULARY

diaphragm A broad dome-shaped muscle used for breathing that separates the thoracic and abdominopelvic cavities.

Body Cavities. The body contains cavities or hollowed areas that are filled with organs. The body is separated into the *dorsal* (posterior) and *ventral* (anterior) body cavities. The dorsal body cavity protects nervous system organs. It contains the cranial cavity and the spinal cavity. The ventral body cavity is divided into the thoracic and abdominopelvic cavities. The diaphragm (DYE uh fram) creates a physical separation between the thoracic and the abdominopelvic cavities (Fig. 2.4). Table 2.2 summarizes the structures found in each body cavity.

Abdominopelvic Quadrants and Regions. The abdominopelvic cavity is extensive. To help describe a location in the abdominopelvic area, either the four quadrants or the nine

TABLE 2.2   Body Cavities

Main Body Cavities	Subcategories	Description
Dorsal body cavity	Cranial cavity	Contains the brain; surrounded and protected by the cranium (skull)
	Spinal cavity	Contains the spinal cord; surrounded and protected by the vertebrae (bones of the spine)
Ventral body cavity	Thoracic cavity	Contains the heart, lungs, esophagus, and trachea (windpipe). Protected by the ribs, the sternum (breastbone), and the vertebrae (backbones)
	Abdominopelvic cavity	Can be divided as follows: • Abdominal cavity: Contains the abdominal organs (e.g., stomach, liver, gallbladder, intestines) • Pelvic cavity: Contains the urinary bladder and the reproductive organs. Nothing separates the abdominal and pelvic cavities.

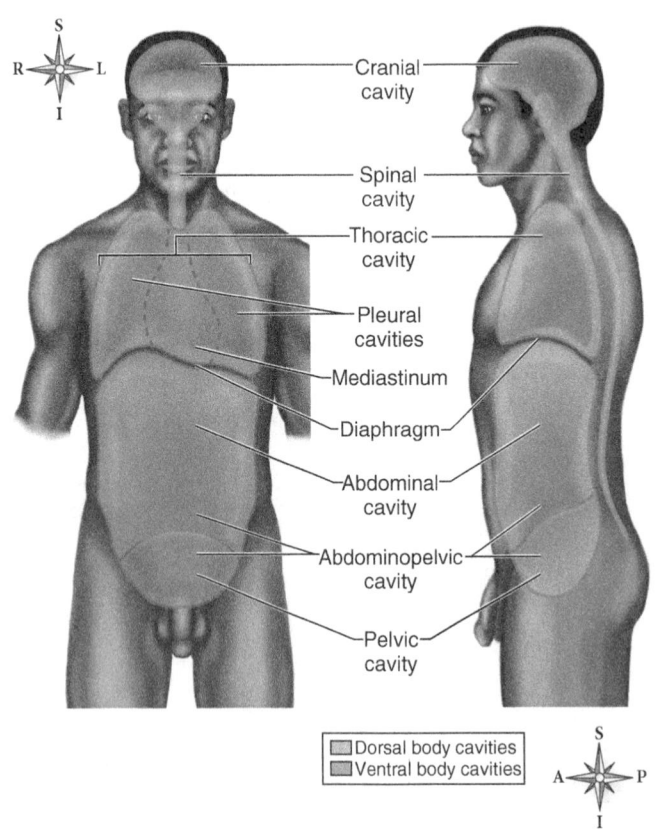

S
R — L
I

Cranial cavity
Spinal cavity
Thoracic cavity
Pleural cavities
Mediastinum
Diaphragm
Abdominal cavity
Abdominopelvic cavity
Pelvic cavity

☐ Dorsal body cavities
☐ Ventral body cavities

S
A — P
I

Fig. 2.4 Body Cavities. Location and subdivisions of the dorsal and ventral body cavities as viewed from the front (anterior) and from the side (lateral). (From Patton KT, Thibodeau GA: *The human body in health and disease*, ed 7, St. Louis, 2018, Elsevier.)

regions can be used. Descriptions that focus on the quadrants are simpler to understand and may be used with patients. The regions are more specific and are typically used by healthcare providers.

With the abdominopelvic quadrants, an imaginary line is drawn down the midline of the body. A horizontal line is drawn across the abdominopelvic cavity, intersecting at the naval (Fig. 2.5). These quadrants are referred to as either right or left and upper or lower. Typically, abbreviations are used when documenting information about the patient. The four quadrants are:

- *Right upper quadrant* (RUQ): Includes the right lobe of the liver and the gallbladder, right kidney, small intestine (duodenum), large intestine (ascending and transverse colon), and head of the pancreas
- *Left upper quadrant* (LUQ): Includes the stomach, spleen, left lobe of the liver, pancreas, left kidney, and large intestine (transverse and descending colon)
- *Right lower quadrant* (RLQ): Includes the appendix, cecum, right ovary, right ureter, right spermatic cord, large intestine (ascending colon), and right kidney
- *Left lower quadrant* (LLQ): Includes the small intestine, large intestine (descending and sigmoid colon), left ovary, left ureter, left spermatic cord, and left kidney

The nine abdominopelvic regions lie over the abdominopelvic cavity. They provide a more specific location than the quadrants. Refer to Fig. 2.6 and Table 2.3 for the nine regions and the related organs.

MEDICAL TERMINOLOGY

abdomin/o	abdomen
chondr/o	cartilage
gastr/o	stomach
pelv/o	pelvis
epi-	above, upon
hypo-	under
-ic, -iac	pertaining to

ACID-BASE BALANCE

The *pH* refers to the acid-base level of a solution on a scale of 1 to 14. A neutral pH is 7. An acidic solution has a pH under 7 and contains more hydrogen ions. A base or an alkaline solution has a pH over 7 and contains fewer hydrogen ions. To maintain homeostasis, the body attempts to keep the pH between 7.35 and

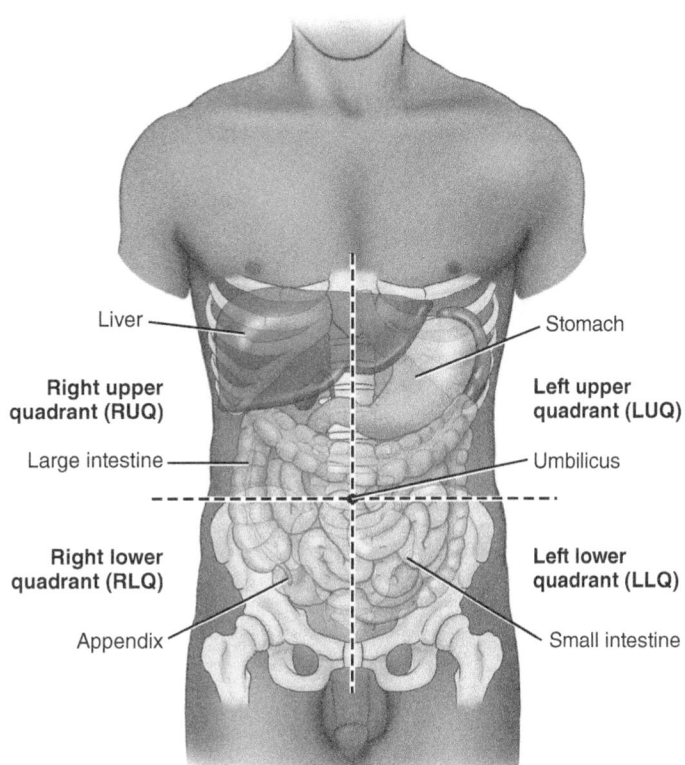

Fig. 2.5 Abdominopelvic Quadrants. (From LaFleur Brooks M, LaFleur Brooks D: *Exploring medical language*, ed 10, St. Louis, 2018, Elsevier.)

7.45. To maintain the acid-base range in the body, the concentration of hydrogen ions must remain constant. If the pH moves outside of this range, serious illness or even death can occur.

The pH of our bodies can change based on the food we eat, the air we breathe, and the urine we excrete. To help maintain the pH range, the urinary system, the respiratory system, and chemical buffers must all work together. *Buffers* (e.g., bicarbonate) work to prevent changes in the pH. If there are more hydrogen ions, which lowers the pH, buffers will absorb some of the hydrogen ions. This will raise the pH. If the pH is too high, the buffers will "donate" hydrogen ions, bringing the pH down to the normal range.

The respiratory system regulates the carbon dioxide (CO_2) in our blood. CO_2 in the blood can combine with water to form the buffer bicarbonate. If a person *hyperventilates* (breathes rapidly), the CO_2 levels in the blood decrease, which also causes a decrease in the bicarbonate levels in the blood. This causes the pH of the body to rise.

The urinary system also has a role in the acid-base levels. The kidneys can absorb more base or more acid, depending on what the body needs for homeostasis. The kidneys can also produce bicarbonate if needed.

PATHOLOGY BASICS

Pathology is the study of diseases. In the ambulatory care setting, many patients' visits relate to the diagnosis or treatment of one or more disease processes. As a person ages, it is common to have more than one chronic illness. Understanding common diseases is important for medical assistants. The body system chapters that follow will cover the most common diseases affecting the system discussed. This chapter provides you with the basics to help you understand the concepts discussed in the future chapters. Common pathology terminology, protective mechanisms in the body, predisposing factors for disease, and causes of disease will be discussed.

Pathology Terminology

As you learn more about diseases, you will notice different terms used. Here is a list of terms commonly used when discussing pathology:

- *Disease*: A specific illness with a recognizable group of signs and symptoms and a clear cause (e.g., infection, environment)
- *Syndrome*: A group of signs and symptoms that occur together and are associated with a condition
- *Disorder*: A disruption of the function or structure of the body. Many times, the words *disorder* and *disease* are used interchangeably in healthcare
- *Prevalence*: How often the disease occurs
- *Incidence*: Reflects the number of people newly diagnosed with the disease
- *Morbidity:* Illness
- *Mortality:* Death
- *Acute*: A severe, sudden onset of a disease
- *Chronic*: A disease, disorder, or syndrome that lasts longer than 6 months
- *Prognosis*: Medical prediction of the outcome of the disease or disorder process
- *Prevention*: Methods to avoid getting the disease

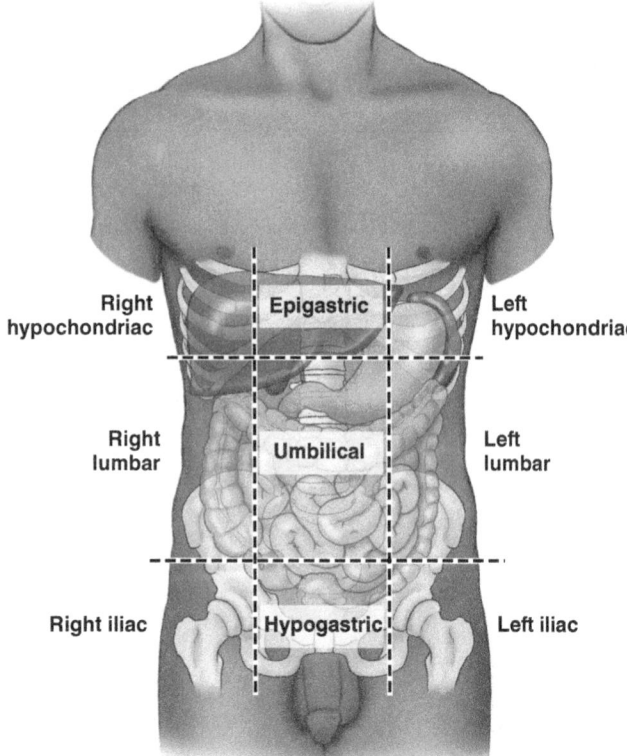

Fig. 2.6 Abdominopelvic Regions. (From LaFleur Brooks M, LaFleur Brooks D: *Exploring medical language*, ed 10, St. Louis, 2018, Elsevier.)

TABLE 2.3	Abdominopelvic Regions With the Underlying Organs	
Right Hypochondriac Region	**Epigastric Region**	**Left Hypochondriac Region**
(hye poh KON dree ack) Liver, gallbladder, right kidney	(eh pee GASS trick) Kidneys, pancreas, liver, stomach	(hye poh KON dree ack) Stomach, liver, left kidney, spleen
Right Lumbar Region	**Umbilical Region**	**Left Lumbar Region**
(LUM bar) Small intestine, large intestine (ascending colon), liver, right kidney	(um BILL ih kul) Small intestine, large intestine (transverse colon), pancreas, stomach	(LUM bar) Small intestine, large intestine (descending colon), left kidney
Right Iliac Region	**Hypogastric Region**	**Left Iliac Region**
(ILL ee ack) Appendix, small intestine, large intestine (cecum and ascending colon)	(hye poh GASS trick) Small intestine, large intestine (sigmoid colon), bladder	(ILL ee ack) Small intestine, large intestine (descending and sigmoid colon)

The coming chapters regarding the body systems will discuss common diseases. For most of the diseases, the following sections will be discussed. It is important for the medical assistant to be familiar with the terminology used:

- *Etiology*: The cause of the disorder or disease.
- *Sign*: Something that is measured or observed by others; also called *objective data*. Examples of signs include redness, swelling or edema, blood pressure, and pulse.
- *Symptom*: Something that is only perceived by the patient; also called *subjective data*. Examples include pain, headache, dizziness, and nausea. Many times, *signs* and *symptoms* are used interchangeably, but there is a difference in their definitions.
- *Diagnostic procedures*: Tests and procedures that are used to help diagnose or monitor a condition. See Table 2.4 for common diagnostic procedures.
- *Treatments*: Management of a disease or disorder; can include follow-up care and home treatments (e.g., medications, special diets, testing).

CRITICAL THINKING 2.5

Daniela is struggling to remember the difference between signs and symptoms. What might be ways to remember these two terms? What are some examples of signs and symptoms?

MEDICAL TERMINOLOGY

tom/o	section
-gram	record, recording
-graphy	process of recording
-scope	instrument to view
-scopy	process of viewing

Protection Mechanisms

The body has built-in mechanisms that protect against infection. The body's first line of defense includes chemical and physical barriers; for example:

- Skin forms a waterproof barrier.
- Tears and saliva contain an enzyme that breaks the cell wall of the pathogen (PATH oe jen).
- Mucus is a slick secretion produced in the respiratory, reproductive, and digestive systems. It protects the tissues and traps substances (e.g., bacteria, dust).
- Cilia are fine hairs that work closely with the mucus in the respiratory tract, trapping substances.
- Stomach acid is a very strong acid that kills bacteria, parasites, and other invaders that are swallowed.
- "Good" bacteria found on the skin and in the digestive system prevent "bad" bacteria from taking over.
- Urine flushes pathogens from the bladder and urethra.

If the structures are altered (e.g., a cut in the skin), pathogens can get into the body. When this happens, the second line of defense, the immune system, kicks in. White blood cells and the lymphatic system work together to protect the body. The immune system will be covered in Chapter 9.

VOCABULARY

endoscope A scope with a camera attached to a long, thin tube that can be inserted into the body.

endoscopy A nonsurgical procedure that uses an endoscope to view the inside of the body.

pathogen A disease-causing organism.

Predisposing Factors

Predisposing factors are risk factors for disease. These factors make it more likely or increase the risk that the person may develop the disease or condition. Some predisposing factors can be changed to reduce the risk of developing a disease, whereas others cannot be changed. Predisposing factors include:

- *Hereditary or genetic factors*: Certain diseases can be inherited, or members of a family can have a higher than normal risk for getting a specific disease.
- *Age*: Certain diseases occur in childhood, whereas others occur more often in older adults. Some diseases occur as a result of changes in the body structures with age. For instance, the ear structures in an infant are different from those of an older person. Degenerative diseases occur in the older generations due to the wear and tear on the structures.
- *Gender*: Certain diseases occur more in one gender than the other. For instance, testicular cancer affects males, whereas uterine cancer affects females. Sometimes both genders may get a disease, but one gender has a higher risk factor. Women are at higher risk for breast cancer than men.
- *Environmental factors*: Certain diseases are more common when a person has been exposed to pollutants in the air, land, or water. Though pesticides can reduce the risk of disease (e.g., West Nile virus disease and rabies), exposure to certain pesticides has been found to increase the risk of cancer.
- *Lifestyle*: Stress, poor diet, infrequent exercise, or abuse of nicotine, alcohol, or drugs can increase the risk for disease.

CRITICAL THINKING 2.6

While on break at work Daniela works on an assignment. She needs to determine which predisposing factors to disease can be changed and how they can be changed. What might be her answers?

Causes of Disease

Disease can result from a change in homeostasis or can be the result of the body's response to a perceived threat. There are several common causes of diseases, including genetics, infectious pathogens, inflammatory processes, immunity, nutritional imbalance, trauma and environmental agents, and neoplasms. The following sections describe these causes.

Genetics. Each person is made up of 46 chromosomes, which carry genetic information (genes). We get 23 chromosomes from each of our parents. Genes are the basic units of heredity, or the instructions on how our bodies should develop and function. Genes provide the differences among us and the similarities in

TABLE 2.4   Common Diagnostic Procedures in Ambulatory Care

Done by/Type of Test	Procedure	Description
Medical laboratory blood tests	Blood glucose	Used to detect high or low blood sugar (glucose)
	C-reactive protein (CRP)	Detects inflammation
	Complete blood count (CBC)	Measures red blood cells (RBCs) and white blood cells (WBCs), hemoglobin (Hgb), hematocrit (HCT), and platelets; CBC with differential test provides a breakdown of the number of each type of white blood cell
	Comprehensive metabolic panel (CMP)	Includes different tests that evaluate, for instance, liver function, kidney function, glucose, and electrolytes
	Electrolyte panel (Lytes)	Used to check for electrolyte (e.g., sodium, potassium, chloride) imbalances
	Erythrocyte sedimentation rate (ESR)	Used to measure the degree of inflammation in the body
	Follicle-stimulating hormone (FSH)	Measures the follicle-stimulating hormone, a reproductive hormone
	Glycated hemoglobin test or hemoglobin glycosylated test (HbA$_{1C}$ or A$_{1C}$)	Measures the average blood glucose (sugar) over the last 2 to 3 months
	Lipid profile	Used to check cholesterol and triglycerides
	Liver function panel	Measures specific proteins and enzymes to provide information on the liver's functioning; also called the hepatic function test
	Partial thromboplastin time (PTT), prothrombin time (PT), and international normalized ratio (INR)	Measures blood clotting time
	Thyroid-stimulating hormone (TSH) test	Measures the amount of thyroid-stimulating hormone in the blood; also, part of the thyroid panel, which includes additional tests
Medical laboratory tests	Culture and sensitivity (C & S)	Culture detects organism in body fluid (e.g., blood, sputum, urine) or on tissue; sensitivity testing determines antibiotics that would inhibit (kill) the bacteria
	Fecal immunochemical test (FIT) (also called immunochemical fecal occult blood test [iFOBT])	Uses antibodies to detect human hemoglobin proteins.
	Guaiac fecal occult blood test (gFOBT)	Used to detect blood in stool
	Multi-targeted stool DNA test (Cologuard)	Computer analysis looks at the DNA in the stool, checking for cancer and precancerous cells
	Stool parasitic examination (O & P)	Used to detect ova and parasites in the stool
	Urinalysis (UA)	Detects abnormalities in the urine that can be used to diagnose many conditions
Endoscopy	Arthroscopy	An arthroscope is inserted in a small incision to view a joint
	Bronchoscopy	A bronchoscope is inserted through the mouth to visualize the trachea and bronchi
	Capsule endoscopy	A camera in a capsule is swallowed and provides pictures of the gastrointestinal tract
	Colonoscopy and sigmoidoscopy	An endoscope is inserted through the anus and used to visualize the large intestine and colon
	Colposcopy	A colposcope is inserted into the vagina to visualize the cervix and vagina
	Cystoscopy and ureteroscopy	An endoscope is inserted into the urethra and used to look at the urinary system
	Endoscopic retrograde cholangiopancreatography (ERCP)	An endoscope is inserted into the mouth and passed to the duodenum; a thin tube, called a catheter, is passed through the endoscope and is used to inject dye into the ducts that lead to the pancreas and gallbladder, then x-rays are used to detect narrowing of structures
	Esophagogastroduodenoscopy (EGD)	An endoscope is inserted through the mouth to visualize the lining of the esophagus, stomach, and duodenum (small intestine)

TABLE 2.4   Common Diagnostic Procedures in Ambulatory Care—cont'd

Done by/Type of Test	Procedure	Description
Imaging procedures	*Computed tomography* (CT, CAT) *scan*	A computerized x-ray imaging modality that provides axial and three-dimensional scans; the patient lies on a table that slides into the circular device that takes the x-rays
	CT colonography or *virtual colonoscopy*	A small tube is inserted into the rectum. The lower colon is inflated with gas. CT images are taken of the colon and rectum
	Fluoroscopy	Direct observation of an x-ray image in motion
	Magnetic resonance imaging (MRI)	An imaging modality that uses a magnetic field and radiofrequency pulses to create computer images of both bones and soft tissues in multiple planes
	Nuclear scans	A radioactive substance is injected or ingested and then is detected by a special camera as it to moves through a body structure
	Positron emission tomography (PET) *scan*	Imaging test that uses a radioactive drug (tracer) to show the activity of tissues and organs
	Ultrasound (US) (also called *sonography*)	A transducer is moved over the body and sends out high-frequency sound waves; waves bounce off of tissues and the transducer captures the waves • 2D US: creates a flat two-dimensional picture (Fig. 2.7) • 3D US: creates a three-dimensional (3D) picture (Fig. 2.8) • 4D US: creates a 3D picture with sound and motion • Doppler US: assesses blood flow through blood vessels

	X-ray (also called *radiograph*)	Uses electromagnetic waves to take pictures of the inside structures of the body; creates black-and-white images based on the amount of radiation that is absorbed
		• White areas: absorb more radiation (e.g., bones)
		• Gray areas: absorb less (e.g., soft tissue and fat)
		• Black areas: absorb none (e.g., air)
		  • Different views can be ordered
		    • PA (posteroanterior) films: x-ray passes from the back to the front of the person
		    • AP (anteroposterior) films: x-ray passes from the front to the back of the person

	Contrast media	Can be used with x-rays, CT, MRI, and US to improve the clarity of the soft tissue picture; ingested, administered by enema, or by injection (via blood vessels) and eliminated via the urine or stool; common contrast media include: • X-rays and CT scans: barium and iodine • MRIs: gadolinium • US: saline (salt water) and air

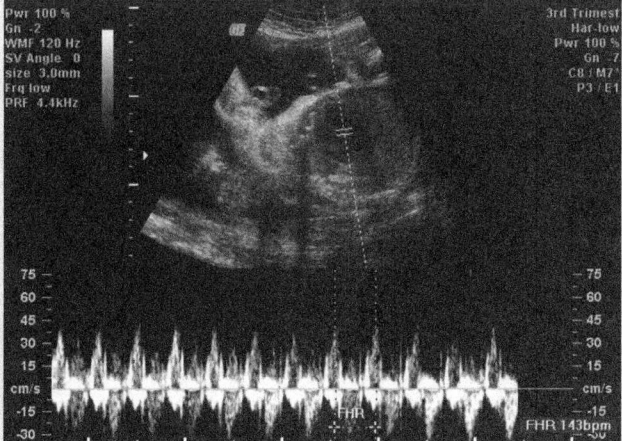

Fig. 2.7 2D Ultrasound.

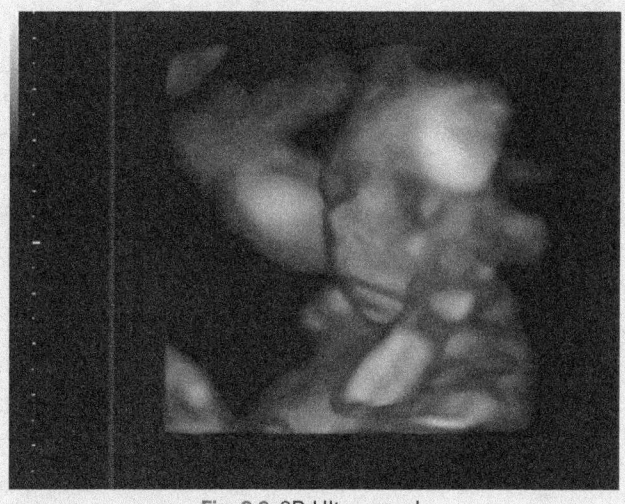

Fig. 2.8 3D Ultrasound.

families. From genes we get our physical appearance and our susceptibility to disease.

Recall that chromosomes are found in the cell's nucleus. During the process of conception and the cell division that follows, an extra chromosome or a change in the chromosome structure may occur. A genetic disease may result from a chromosomal error or from the patient inheriting a defective gene from either parent. Types of genetic disease include the monogenic disorders and chromosomal disorders.

A *monogenic disorder* is caused by a single defective gene that is inherited from one or both parents. There are three main categories of monogenic disorders:

- *Dominant.* The child only needs to inherit one defective dominant gene to get the disease. Examples of autosomal dominant disorders include Huntington disease, Marfan syndrome, and neurofibromatosis type 1 (NFI).
- *Recessive.* The child would need to inherit a defective recessive gene from both parents to get the disease. Examples of autosomal recessive disorders include cystic fibrosis, Tay-Sachs disease, sickle cell anemia, albinism (Fig. 2.9), and phenylketonuria (PKU).
- *X-linked.* Sex determination is based on the father (Box 2.1).
  - Dominant X-linked traits appear in a person who inherits one defective X chromosome. Fragile X syndrome (FXS) is an example of a dominant X-linked disorder. Both males and females are affected, but females usually have milder symptoms.
  - For recessive X-linked traits, the female would need two recessive X-linked genes to get the disorder. Because the male only has one X chromosome, inheriting one recessive X-linked gene will produce the recessive trait. Red-green color blindness and hemophilia A are examples of X-linked recessive conditions (Fig. 2.10).

> ## BOX 2.1   X and Y Chromosomes
>
> The X and Y chromosomes are sex chromosomes. A biological female will have two X chromosomes, one from each parent. A biological male will have an X chromosome and a Y chromosome. The X chromosome comes from the mother and the Y chromosome from the father.
>
> The X chromosome is about three times the size of the Y chromosome. The X chromosome contains more than 900 genes, also called *X-linked genes*. The Y chromosome only has about 55 genes, which are called *Y-linked genes*. These traits are only expressed in males.

With a *chromosomal disorder*, an abnormal number of chromosomes or a change in the chromosomal structure causes the disease. Examples of chromosomal disorders include:

- Down syndrome – the person has an extra chromosome.
- Trisomy X syndrome – the female has three X chromosomes.
- Turner syndrome – the female inherits only one copy of the X chromosome.

Infectious Pathogens. Many microorganisms are nonpathogenic, which means they do not cause disease. They can be found in our body, maintaining homeostasis. Other microorganisms are pathogenic, which means disease causing (Table 2.5). These pathogens enter our bodies through direct contact, indirect contact, or by vectors (Table 2.6).

When a pathogen enters our body and starts to multiply, an infection occurs. Changes occur in our body, yet we do not feel any different. This is the *incubation period*. It starts at the time of exposure and ends when the signs and symptoms appear. The incubation period is different for each disease. For instance, strep throat has an incubation period of 2 to 5 days, whereas varicella (chickenpox) has an incubation period of 14 to 16 days. As our body tissues become damaged from the infection,

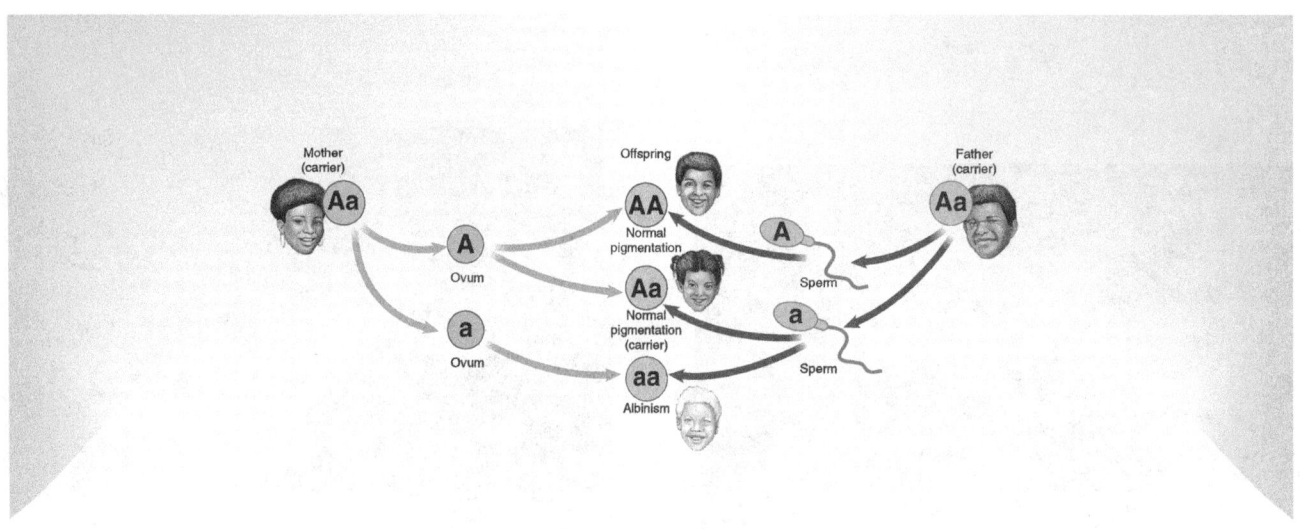

Fig. 2.9 Inheritance of Albinism. Albinism is a recessive trait, producing abnormalities only in those with two recessive genes *(a)*. Presence of the dominant gene *(A)* prevents albinism. (From Patton KT, Thibodeau GA: *The human body in health and disease*, ed 7, St. Louis, 2018, Elsevier.)

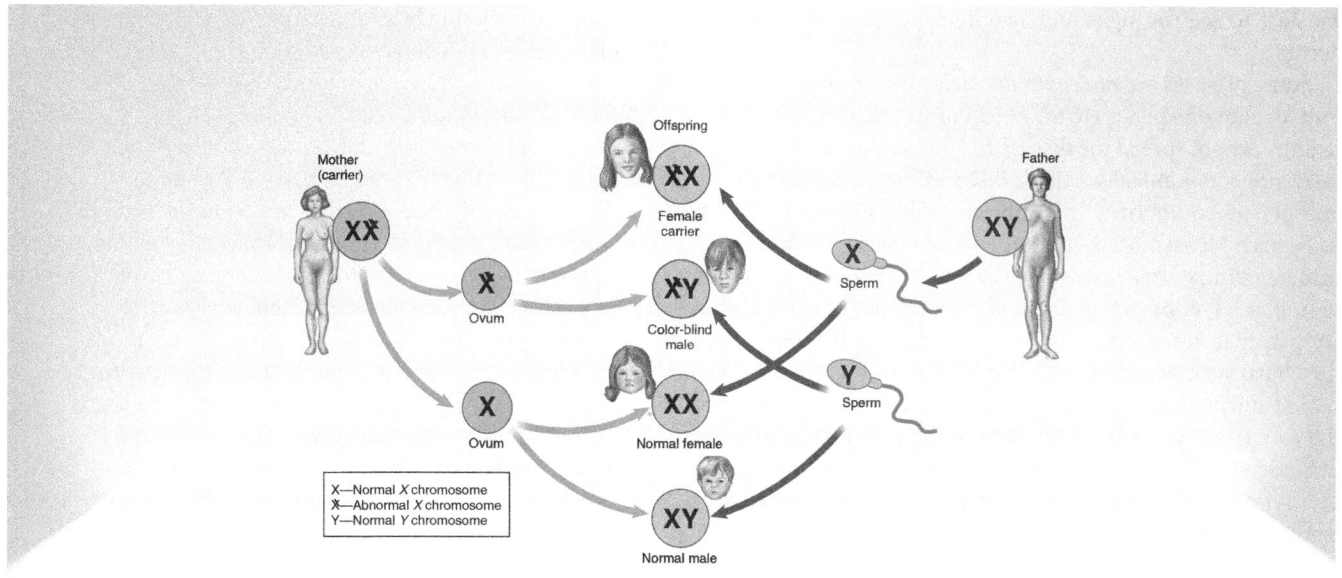

Fig. 2.10 Sex-Linked Inheritance. Some forms of color blindness involve recessive X-linked genes. In this case, a female carrier of the abnormal gene can produce male children who are color blind. (From Patton KT, Thibodeau GA: *The human body in health and disease,* ed 7, St. Louis, 2018, Elsevier.)

TABLE 2.5 Common Pathogens

Pathogen	Description	Related Diseases
Fungi	Yeast and molds; only a few cause fungal disease or mycoses	Tinea corporis (ringworm), tinea pedis (athlete's foot), thrush
Protozoa	One-celled organism	Trichomoniasis, malaria, amebic dysentery
Viruses	Smallest microorganism that requires a host cell to multiply	Common cold, measles, mumps, varicella, influenza
Bacteria	Single-celled organisms; classified by shape: bacilli (rod shaped), spirilla (spiral shaped), cocci (dot shaped) Many disease-causing bacteria produce **toxins** (TOK sins) that create the illness	Bacilli: tuberculosis, whooping cough, *Escherichia coli*, salmonella Spirilla: cholera, syphilis, Lyme disease Cocci: gonorrhea, meningitis, strep throat
Helminths	Large, multicellular parasites that can live in the body.	Flatworms (including flukes and tapeworms), thorny-headed worms, and roundworms
Ectoparasite	A parasite that lives on the body	Lice, scabies

TABLE 2.6 Modes of Transmission for Pathogens

Modes of Transmission	Definition	Examples of Diseases
Direct contact	Susceptible person comes in contact with an infected person; spread via contact with blood, body fluids, and excretions (e.g., stool, urine, and saliva) Methods of direct contact include: • Person to person (sneezing, touching, coughs) • Animal to person (being bitten or scratched or handling animal waste) • Mother to unborn child	Influenza Pertussis Varicella Rabies Gonorrhea Tuberculosis
Indirect contact	Through contact with a contaminated object (e.g., water, food, drinking glass, airborne transmission)	*Escherichia coli* Botulism
Vectors (insects)	Most blood-sucking insects consume the disease-causing microorganism from one host and transmit it during a "meal" to another host	*Mosquitoes:* yellow fever, malaria, West Nile fever, Zika virus *Ticks:* Lyme disease, tick-borne encephalitis, rickettsial diseases *Fleas:* plague

we start to see the signs and symptoms. This is when disease occurs.

Some diseases are *noncommunicable*. They cannot be transmitted from one person to another. For instance, a person with tetanus cannot spread the disease to another person. Other diseases are *communicable*. These diseases are transmitted from one person to another. If a communicable disease is known to be easily transmitted, it is called a *contagious disease*. Strep throat, coronavirus disease (COVID-19), and influenza are examples of contagious diseases. For instance, people with strep throat are contagious from the start of the fever until they have been on the appropriate antibiotics for 24 hours. The period during which a disease can spread to another is called the *contagious period*. It is important for people in healthcare to understand the ways diseases are spread. Taking required precautions will minimize your risk of "catching something" from your patients.

VOCABULARY

toxins Substances created by microorganisms, plants, or animals that are poisonous to humans.

CRITICAL THINKING 2.7

At school Daniela is learning about the transmission of pathogens. As a receptionist she sees a lot of sick people stopping at her desk. She encourages those who cough to wear a mask. Hand sanitizer and tissues are also available. In light of disease transmission, why are these three items important in the prevention of disease?

Inflammatory Processes. The inflammatory response is the body's efficient way of protecting itself. Inflammation occurs when the tissues are injured. The injury could be the result of bacteria, trauma, heat, toxins, or other causes. The cells damaged release the chemicals histamine, prostaglandins, and bradykinin. These chemicals cause the following responses:
- Blood vessels at the site dilate. This causes more local blood flow. With the increase in blood flow, *erythema* (ER i thee mah) (redness) and warmth occur in that area.
- Blood vessel walls allow more white blood cells and plasma to move out of the vessel into the surrounding tissues. The white blood cells work to protect the cells and clean up the dead tissue. The extra fluid from the blood causes *edema* (eh DEE mah) (swelling), pain, and loss of movement. For instance, if the injury occurred in the finger joint area, the edema may be so great that it prevents you from moving your finger.

Five key signs of inflammation are erythema, edema, pain, warmth, and loss of function.

Even though the inflammatory process can be efficient, it can also be the cause of disease. *Autoinflammatory diseases* (e.g., familial Mediterranean fever) differ from autoimmune diseases, which will be described later in the chapter. Autoinflammatory diseases result from a genetic mutation that causes the inflammatory process to activate without a reason. The person may

experience recurring brief attacks of pain and fevers, and blood work indicates systemic inflammation.

Immunity. Our immune system protects our bodies against potentially harmful substances. Our immune system "remembers" the antigens (an TIE jens) from diseases and responds with specific antibodies (AN tih bod ees). The antibodies destroy or attempt to destroy the harmful substances. As with the autoinflammatory conditions, at times the immune response can work against us. These malfunctions are classified as follows:
- *Allergies* (AL ur jee): Reactions occur if a person is exposed to a food (e.g., milk, tree nuts, peanuts, eggs, soy, and wheat), pollen, dust mites, latex, mold, pet dander, inhalants, or other substances.
- *Autoimmunity*: The immune system does not recognize the body's own antigens and starts attacking itself. Rheumatoid arthritis, lupus, and psoriasis are examples of autoimmune disorders.
- *Immunodeficiency* (ih myoo noh deh FIH shun see): This is caused by a deficiency in one or more of the immune system key players (e.g., white blood cells, such as the B cells and T cells). A person with immunodeficiency has impaired resistance to infections.

VOCABULARY

antibodies Protein substances produced in the blood or tissues, in response to a specific antigen, that destroy or weaken the antigen. Part of the immune system.

antigens Substances that stimulate the production of an antibody when introduced into the body. Antigens include toxins, bacteria, viruses, and other foreign substances.

MEDICAL TERMINOLOGY

erg/o	work
immun/o	safety, protection
allo-	different, other
anti-	against
auto-	self
-gen	producing
-y	condition

Nutritional Imbalance. Nutritional imbalances include too little or too much of a nutrient. Nutritional imbalances can affect growth, disease, and death. Causes of nutritional imbalances include:
- *Vitamin and mineral deficiencies*: Some of these deficiencies can be caused by alcoholism, disease, dietary deficiencies (and poverty), weight loss surgery, and metabolic disorders.
- *Vitamin and mineral excesses*: Vitamin excesses can occur when a person takes too much of a vitamin. The water-soluble vitamins (vitamins B and C) pass through the body fairly quickly. The fat-soluble vitamins (vitamins A, D, E, and K) can accumulate in the body. This can lead to toxic conditions. Mineral excess can be caused by diet, medication, or a metabolic error.

- *Obesity*: This is caused by eating too many calories, getting too little exercise, or having an endocrine or metabolic condition. Obesity can increase a person's risk for other diseases, including heart disease, diabetes, hypertension (high blood pressure), and stroke.
- *Starvation*: Eating too little food can result from disease or poverty.

Trauma and Environmental Agents. Trauma from auto accidents, violence, falls, and other events can cause disease. Common traumatic injuries include fractures, lacerated and ruptured organs, bleeding, neck and spinal injuries, and head injuries. Psychological trauma can also cause disorders.

Environmental changes, such as severe hot or cold temperatures and extremes of atmospheric pressures, can affect health. Poisonings, insect and animal bites, burns, electric shock, and near drownings can also cause diseases.

Neoplasms. When cells grow quicker than normal or do not die as fast as they should, an abnormal mass is created. This mass is called a *neoplasm* (NEE oh plaz uhm) or *tumor* (too mohr). Tumors can be *benign* (bi NINE) (noncancerous) or *malignant* (mah LIG nahnt) (cancerous). Table 2.7 shows the difference between benign and malignant tumors.

There are more than 100 different types of cancer. Cancers are classified based on the type of tissue from which they originate. The six major classifications are:

- *Carcinoma* (kar sih NOH mah): A cancer of epithelial origin or cancer of the internal or external lining of the body. Carcinoma can originate from many areas of the body, including the skin, lungs, breast, colon, and prostate. Carcinomas makes up about 80% to 90% of all cancer cases. Two major subtypes of carcinomas are:
  - *Squamous* (SKWAY muss) *cell carcinoma*: A cancer that originated from squamous epithelium. Example: squamous cell carcinoma of the lung
  - *Adenocarcinoma* (ad en noh kar seh NOH mah): A cancer that started in an organ or a gland. Example: gastric adenocarcinoma
- *Sarcoma* (sar KOH mah): A cancer that started in supportive and connective tissues (e.g., bones, tendons, cartilage, fat, and muscle). Examples: osteosarcoma, chondrosarcoma, hemangiosarcoma, mesothelioma, and glioma
- *Myeloma* (mye eh LOH mah): A cancer that originated in the plasma cells (a type of white blood cells) in the bone marrow. Example: multiple myeloma

- *Leukemia* (loo KEE me ah): A cancer of the bone marrow. Example: acute myelocytic leukemia
- *Lymphoma* (limf OH mah): A cancer that originated in the lymphatic system. There are two types of lymphomas:
  - *Hodgkin lymphoma*: Diagnosed by the detection of Reed-Sternberg cells, a cell specific only to this disease
  - *Non-Hodgkin lymphoma*: All lymphomas other than Hodgkin lymphoma
- *Mixed types*: Cancer that has a combination of cells from within one classification or between two cancer classifications. Examples: teratocarcinoma and carcinosarcoma

As the malignant cells grow, they can break through the *basement membrane*. This delicate membrane separates the epithelial cells from connective tissues. Once this occurs, the cancerous cells can invade blood and lymph vessels. The circulating fluid (blood, lymph fluid) can then carry the cancerous cells to another location in the body. Thus cancerous cells from the *primary tumor* (original site) can metastasize to another location in the body, creating a *secondary tumor*.

If a provider suspects a patient may have cancer, a number of blood tests and imaging tests will be ordered. A biopsy (bye OP see) may be performed. The surgeon may also take a biopsy of nearby lymph nodes so the tissue can be checked for malignant cells. Based on the diagnostic results, the oncologist (on KOL uh jest) or pathologist (pa THOL uh jest) will grade and stage the cancer.

MEDICAL TERMINOLOGY

aden/o	gland
carcin/o	cancer
lymph/o	lymph
sarc/o	connective tissue
-oma	tumor, mass

VOCABULARY

anaplastic Describes a rapidly dividing cancer cell that has little to no similarity to normal cells.

biopsy Process of viewing living tissue that has been removed for the purpose of diagnosis or treatment.

differentiated Describes how malignant tissue or cells looks like the normal tissue or cells it came from; poorly differentiated means it does not look like the normal tissue or cells, and well differentiated means it looks like the normal tissue or cells.

metastasize To spread from one part of the body (the primary tumor) to another part of the body, forming a secondary tumor.

oncologist A specially trained physician who diagnoses and treats cancer.

pathologist A physician specially trained in the nature and cause of disease.

TABLE 2.7 Differences Between Benign and Malignant Tumors

Characteristic	Benign Tumor	Malignant Tumor
Cellular structure	Same as surrounding tissue	Anaplastic (a NAH plas tik) changes and poorly differentiated (dif EH ren shee ated)
Type of growth	Grows within a "shell" (encapsulated)	Infiltrates and metastasizes (MEH tas tuh sizes); spreads to distant site(s) in the body via the bloodstream or lymph system
Rate of growth	Usually slow; rarely fatal	May be slow, rapid, or very rapid; almost always fatal if left untreated
Destruction of localized tissue	None	Common; invades and takes over the surrounding tissue

Grade. *Grade* refers to how abnormal the malignant cells look. If the malignant cells and tissues closely resemble normal cells and tissue, the tumor is called *well differentiated*. These are more slow-growing tumors. If the malignant cells and tissues do not look like normal cells and tissue, they are called *undifferentiated* or *poorly differentiated*. The microscopic look of the cell is graded using 1, 2, 3, or 4 to indicate the appearance. Grade 1 means well differentiated, or the cells and organization of the malignant tissue look close to that of normal tissue. Grade 2 means moderately differentiated, or the tissue does not look like normal tissue. The cells are also growing at a faster rate than normal. Grades 3 and 4 do not look like normal tissue and tend to spread quicker.

Stage. *Stage* refers to the extent of the cancer, including its size and whether it has spread. A cancer is referred to by this stage. Several staging systems are used, and various factors must be taken into consideration with staging systems:

- Location of the tumor
- Type of cell
- Size of the tumor
- Whether it has spread to nearby lymph nodes
- Whether it has spread to other locations in the body
- Tumor grade, or how abnormal the cells look compared with normal sizes and how quickly it grows and spreads

The TNM staging system is widely used (Box 2.2). Table 2.8 describes another type of staging system.

BOX 2.2   Staging Systems

TNM Staging System

The letters T, N, and M are followed by a number or letter. X after T, N, or M indicates that it cannot be measured.

T: refers to the size and extent of the primary tumor
- T0: primary tumor cannot be found
- T1, T2, T3, and T4: refer to the size and extent of the primary tumor; the higher the number the larger or more extensive the tumor

N: refers to the number of nearby lymph nodes affected by the malignant cells
- N0: no cancer in the nearby lymph nodes
- N1, N2, N3, and N4: refers to the location and number of nearby lymph nodes that have cancer; the higher the number, the more nodes are affected

M: refers to whether the tumor has metastasized
- M0: no metastasis has occurred
- M1: metastasis has occurred

Stage Grouping

Once TNM staging has been done, the three elements are combined for an overall stage.
- Stage 0: Abnormal cells are present; no spreading has occurred.
- Stages I, II and III: Malignancy is present. The number is greater for larger tumors and tumors that have spread to nearby tissues.
- Stage IV: Cancer has metastasized.

TABLE 2.8   Stages of Cancer

Stage	Definition
In situ	Abnormal cells are present; no spreading has occurred.
Localized	Cancer cells are present; no spreading has occurred.
Regional	Cancer has spread to nearby lymph nodes, organs, or tissues.
Distant	Cancer has metastasized.
Unknown	Not enough information is available.

CLOSING COMMENTS

Understanding the structural organization of the body will help as you learn about each system. Knowing the medical terminology that relates to body organization, cavities, quadrants, regions, and planes is important. As a medical assistant, you will be communicating with providers and peers. Using correct medical terminology and having a strong understanding of the body systems will help you communicate clearly and accurately in the ambulatory care setting.

PATIENT-CENTERED CARE

"The patient has pain in the epigastric region." "The provider ordered an anteroposterior (AP) chest x-ray." The use of directional terms is common in healthcare as procedures are ordered and patients' signs and symptoms are described. Using directional terms while documenting is appropriate, but medical assistants must limit the use of such terms when talking with patients. If these terms are used, make sure to describe what the terms mean to the patient. This will help the patient understand what is occurring, thus increasing the patient's satisfaction with the healthcare experience.

BEING PROFESSIONAL

As discussed in Chapter 1, it is important for the medical assistant to help patients understand medical terms that they encounter during their care.

Dr. Martin just finished seeing Mr. Green. You are in the room with them. Dr. Martin turns to you and orders an abdominal ultrasound for right iliac region pain. He leaves the room. Mr. Green, appearing to be confused, asks you what Dr. Martin just said. "What is an ultrasound? What did he mean by right iliac region pain?" What should you say to Mr. Green? Role-play this scenario with a peer.

CHAPTER REVIEW

Cells are the basic units of life. Groups of similar cells from the same source that carry out a specific function are called *tissues*. A structure composed of two or more types of tissues is an organ. Several organs and their related structures make up a body system. The most complex level, the organism (body), is made up of many body systems that work together to maintain homeostasis in the body.

The anatomic position provides a reference when using directional and positional terms. In the anatomic position, the body stands erect with the face forward, arms at the sides, palms forward, and toes pointed forward.

Body cavities are hollowed areas filled with organs. The body has dorsal and ventral body cavities. The dorsal body cavity protects nervous system organs and contains the cranial cavity and spinal cavity. The ventral body cavity is divided into the thoracic cavity and the abdominopelvic cavity.

With the abdominopelvic quadrants, an imaginary line is drawn down the midline of the body. A horizontal line is drawn across the abdominopelvic cavity, intersecting at the naval. These quadrants are referred to as either right or left and upper or lower. The abdominopelvic regions are nine regions that lie over the abdominopelvic cavity. They provide a more specific location than the quadrants.

The body's first line of defense includes chemical and physical barriers. These include skin, tears, saliva, mucus, cilia, stomach acid, good bacteria, and urine. If the structures are altered, pathogens can get into the body. When this happens, the second line of defense, the immune system, kicks in. White blood cells and the lymphatic system work together to protect the body.

Predisposing factors to disease include genetic factors, age, gender, environmental factors, and lifestyle. Diseases can be caused by genetics, pathogens, nutritional imbalances, trauma, environmental agents, and neoplasms. Normal body processes, including the inflammatory processes and immunity, can also function improperly and cause disease.

SCENARIO WRAP-UP

Daniela continues in her position as a float receptionist. She is gaining a lot of experience in the WMFM Clinic. Bella continues to help Daniela with her medical terminology and human body courses. Daniela really appreciates the study tips and reviewing assistance that Bella gives her. Some of her favorite ways to study these courses include:

- Daniela made flashcards with the term or word part on one side and its definition on the other. Bella warned her to keep the definition short and simple. For nonmedical terminology, Daniela figured out that she learned more when she wrote her own definition. She realized the tests did not always use the exact words used in the textbook.

- Daniela realized that she learned better when she listened to the content. So, she recorded herself going through her flashcards and review sheets. She found that if she stated the term or question and then paused, when she listened, she could fill in the blank before hearing the answer.
- Daniela learned that she sometimes felt she knew the content but was not always certain about it until it came to the test. So, she decided to test herself on the content during her study times to see what she really knew.

Daniela is very excited to complete her human body and disease course and medical terminology course. She is also excited to apply the study practices she is learning to her future medical assistant courses.

3

Skeletal System

LEARNING OBJECTIVES

1. Describe the anatomy of the skeletal system.
2. Explain how joints are classified, including the classifications of synovial joints.
3. Discuss the three roles of the skeletal system, including development of new bone, regulation of the blood calcium level, and hematopoiesis.
4. Explain the common diagnostic procedures and treatments for skeletal system disorders.
5. Describe common skeletal system disorders, including common signs and symptoms, etiology, diagnostic procedures, and treatments.
6. Compare the structure and function of the skeletal system across the life span.

OUTLINE

▶ OPENING SCENARIO

Suzanne Peterson, CMA (AAMA), works with Dr. Kahn at the Walden-Martin Family Medical (WMFM) Clinic. Dr. Kahn hired Suzanne right out of school as a new graduate. She has seen a lot in her 20 years as a medical assistant (MA). Many aspects of her day have changed from when she first started as an MA, but one thing that has not changed is her love for helping patients.

Another busy day is scheduled, and Suzanne's first patient is Walter Biller. Walter is in his late 40s, is in good general health, is near his ideal weight, and has no chronic conditions. He saw Dr. Kahn a few weeks ago when he experienced worsening pain in his hands and knees. He had been planting in his garden and noticed the next day that he had more pain and stiffness in his hands than usual. Bending down on his hands and knees in the garden was not as easy as it used to be. Dr. Kahn performed a physical exam and ordered lab tests. He asked Walter to make a follow-up appointment to go over the results. Today Walter is back at the clinic, and Suzanne is ready to room him for his appointment.

YOU WILL LEARN

1. To identify the structures that make up the axial and appendicular skeleton.
2. To explain the difference between synarthrotic, amphiarthrotic, and diarthrotic joints (synarthroses, amphiarthroses, and diarthroses), along with describing the six classifications of diarthrotic joints.
3. To describe the skeletal system's role with new bone development, blood calcium regulation, and hematopoiesis.
4. To describe common skeletal system disorders, including etiology, signs and symptoms, diagnostic procedures, and treatments.
5. To discuss life span changes in the skeletal system.

INTRODUCTION

Skeletal system disorders are common in the ambulatory care facility. Patients with skeletal concerns are typically seen in primary care and urgent care settings, before being referred to the orthopedic department.

Orthopedics (ORE thoe PEE diks) is the healthcare specialty that deals with most skeletal disorders and associated muscle, joint, and ligament conditions. An *orthopedist* is a physician who is specially trained to diagnose and treat skeletal system disorders. Some orthopedists specialize in certain areas of the body, such as hand, ankle, and foot injuries. An *orthopedic surgeon* is a specially trained physician who medically, surgically, and physically treats musculoskeletal disorders. A *physiatrist* (FIZ ee at rist) is a physician who specializes in physical medicine and rehabilitation, which includes treating patients with musculoskeletal disorders. *Podiatry* (pah DIE ah tree) is the branch of medicine that deals with the diagnosis, treatment, and prevention of foot disorders. A *podiatrist* is a physician who specializes in treating the foot and ankle.

Rheumatology (roo muh TOL oh gee) is a specialty that deals with disorders of connective tissue, including bone and cartilage. Rheumatology also deals with many diseases that are classified as autoimmune disorders. A *rheumatologist* (roo muh TOL uh jist) is a physician who specializes in internal medicine and rheumatology. A rheumatologist treats patients with diseases of joints, muscles, bones, and tendons.

> **VOCABULARY**
> **autoimmune** An immune response against a person's own tissues, cells, or cell parts, as in autoimmune disease, leading to the deterioration of tissue.

ANATOMY OF THE SKELETAL SYSTEM

The skeletal system consists of bones, joints, and supportive connective tissues. The supportive connective tissues include:
- *Cartilage* (KAR tih lij), which is flexible connective tissue that covers the ends of many bones at the joint.

- *Tendons* (TEN duns), which attach muscles to bones.
- *Ligaments* (LIH gah ments), which connect bones at a joint.

Bones

Human bones appear in a variety of shapes and sizes that suit their function in the body. Bones generally are categorized by shape.
- *Flat bones* protect internal organs. Examples include the cranium, ribs, and sternum.
- *Short bones* provide stability with their cube shape. Examples include carpals and tarsals.
- *Long bones* support weight and help with movement. Examples include the humerus, radius, femur, and tibia.
- *Irregular bones* have an irregular shape and help protect internal organs. The vertebrae are an example of irregular bones.
- *Sesamoid bones* are embedded in the tendons and help protect the tendons. The patella is the largest sesamoid bone in the body.

The human skeleton is composed of more than 200 bones. Bones are divided into two categories, the axial skeleton and the appendicular skeleton (Fig. 3.1).

Axial Skeleton. The axial skeleton is composed of 80 bones and includes the skull, hyoid bone, vertebral column, and the rib cage.
- The skull is made up of the following structures:
  - *Cranium* (KRAY nee um), which encloses and protects the brain. The eight bones that make up the cranium include the frontal, parietal (2), temporal (2), occipital, sphenoid, and ethmoid bones (Box 3.1 and Fig. 3.2).
  - *Facial bones*, which include the mandible and vomer bone, and two each of the following bones: nasal, zygomatic, lacrimal, palatine, inferior nasal conchae, and maxillary (also called the maxilla or upper jawbone) (Fig. 3.3).
  - *Ossicles* (OS i kahls), or the three small bones of the middle ear that transmit sound vibrations from the eardrum to the inner ear. The small bones include the malleus (hammer), incus (anvil), and stapes (stirrup).
- The *hyoid bone*, in the neck above the larynx, is the attachment point for the extrinsic tongue muscle and other mouth muscles.
- The *spinal* or *vertebral column* is divided into five regions: cervical, thoracic, lumbar, sacral, and coccygeal. The spinal column is composed of 26 vertebrae (VUR teh bray) (Fig. 3.4). Soft disks filled with a jellylike substance are between the vertebrae to cushion and keep them in place.
- The rib cage is made up of these structures:
  - *Sternum* (breastbone), which is made up of the manubrium, body, and xiphoid process (Fig. 3.5).
  - Seven pairs of *true ribs*, which attach to the sternum by costal cartilage.
  - Five pairs of *false ribs*. The first three pairs of false ribs attach to the seventh rib and indirectly to the sternum by costal cartilage. The last two pairs of false ribs are called *floating ribs*, because they are not attached in the front of the body.

The ribs, thoracic vertebral column, and sternum form the thorax.

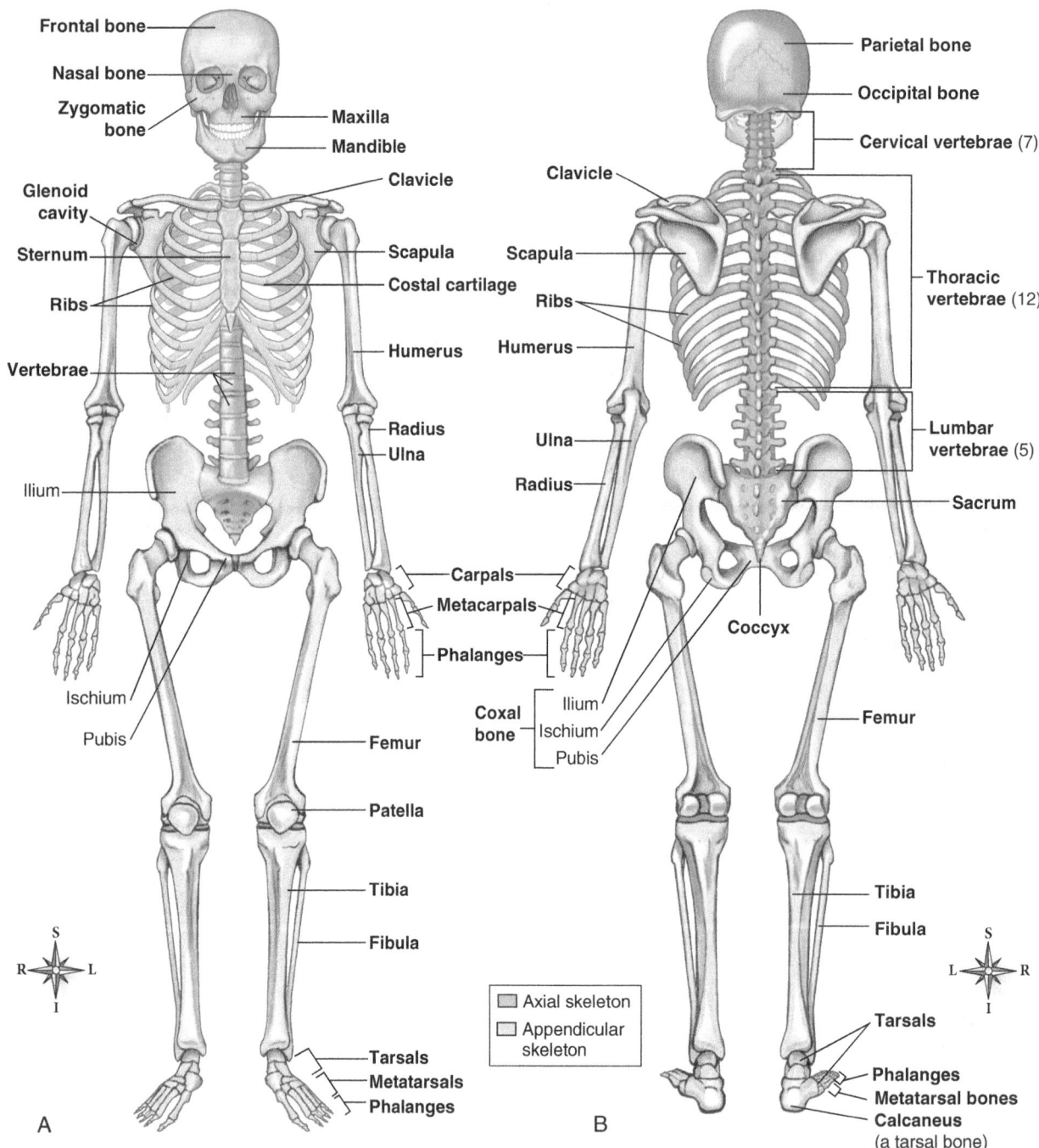

Fig. 3.1 Human Skeleton. The axial skeleton is distinguished by a blue tint. A, Anterior view. B, Posterior view. (From Patton KT, Thibodeau GA: The human body in health and disease, ed 7, St. Louis, 2018, Elsevier.)

BOX 3.1 Paranasal Sinuses

The *paranasal sinuses* are mucous membraned–lined, air-filled spaces or cavities in the skull that connect to the nasal cavity. The paranasal sinuses include the frontal sinuses, the sphenoid sinus, and the maxillary sinuses.

VOCABULARY

process A prominence or projection on a bone.

vertebrae A series of small, irregularly shaped bones that form the spine. Each vertebra has several projections, joint surfaces, areas for muscle attachment, and a hole where the spinal cord passes.

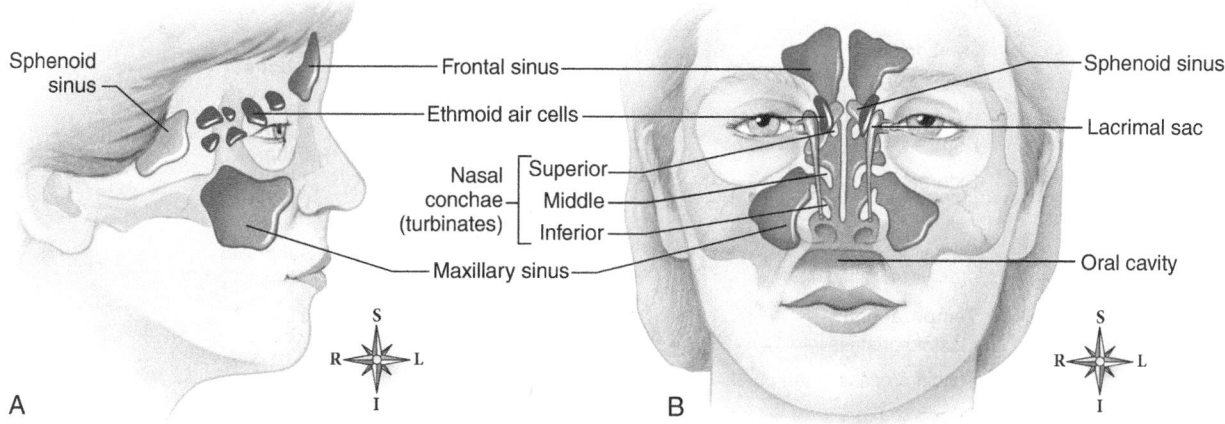

Fig. 3.2 Paranasal Sinuses. A, Lateral view of the face shows the position of the paranasal sinuses. B, Anterior view shows the relationship of the sinuses to each other and the nasal cavity. (From Patton KT, Thibodeau GA: *The human body in health and disease,* ed 7, St. Louis, 2018, Elsevier.)

MEDICAL TERMINOLOGY	
cervic/o	neck
chondr/o, cartilag/o	cartilage
coccyg/o	coccyx
cost/o	rib
crani/o	cranium, skull
ethmoid/o	ethmoid
front/o	frontal
lacrim/o	tears, lacrimal
mandibul/o	mandible
maxill/o	maxilla
occipit/o	occipital
oste/o, osse/o, oss/i	bone
palat/o	palatine
pariet/o	parietal
sacr/o	sacrum
scapul/o	scapula, shoulder blade
skelet/o	skeleton
sphenoid/o	sphenoid
spin/o, vertebr/o	spine, spinal column
stern/o	sternum
tempor/o	temporal
tendin/o, tend/o, ten/o	tendon
thorac/o	thorax
vertebr/o, spondyl/o	vertebra
vomer/o	vomer
zygom/o, zygomat/o	zygoma, cheekbone, zygomatic bone

Appendicular Skeleton. The appendicular skeleton is composed of 126 bones. It can be divided into the upper and lower extremities. The upper extremities are made up of these structures:

- *Clavicle* (collarbone).
- *Scapula* (shoulder blade). The *acromion process* is the lateral tip of the scapula. The acromion process is used as a landmark when injections are given in the deltoid muscle.
- *Humerus* (upper arm bone) (see Fig. 3.1).
- *Radius* and *ulna* (lower arm bones). The radius is the bone on the thumb side, and the ulna is the little finger side of the forearm.
- *Carpals* (wrist bones), *metacarpals* (in the palm of the hand), and the *phalanges* (finger bones) (see Fig. 3.1).

The lower extremities are made up of these structures:

- Pelvic girdle (coxal bone), which includes the *ilium*, *ischium*, and *pubis* (see Fig. 3.1). The male pelvis is deep and narrow. The female pelvis is broad and shallow. The pelvic inlet is wider to accommodate the birth of the baby (Fig. 3.6).
- *Femur* (thigh bone), which is the longest and heaviest bone in the body. The *greater trochanter* is a protrusion near the neck of the femur. The greater trochanter is used as a landmark when ventrogluteal injections are given.
- *Patella* (kneecap), which is the largest sesamoid bone.
- *Tibia* (shin bone) and *fibula* (lower leg bones). The tibia is larger and stronger than the fibula, which is on the outer side of the leg. The protrusions on the ankle include:
  - *Medial malleolus*, part of the tibia and located on the inner side of the ankle.
  - *Posterior malleolus*, part of the tibia and located on the back of the ankle.
  - *Lateral malleolus*, part of the fibula and located on the outer side of the ankle.
- *Tarsals*, which form the heel and the posterior side of the foot. The tarsals include the calcaneus (heel bone), talus, navicular, cuboid, medial cuneiform, intermediate cuneiform, and the lateral cuneiform.
- *Metatarsals* (feet bones) and the *phalanges* (toe bones).

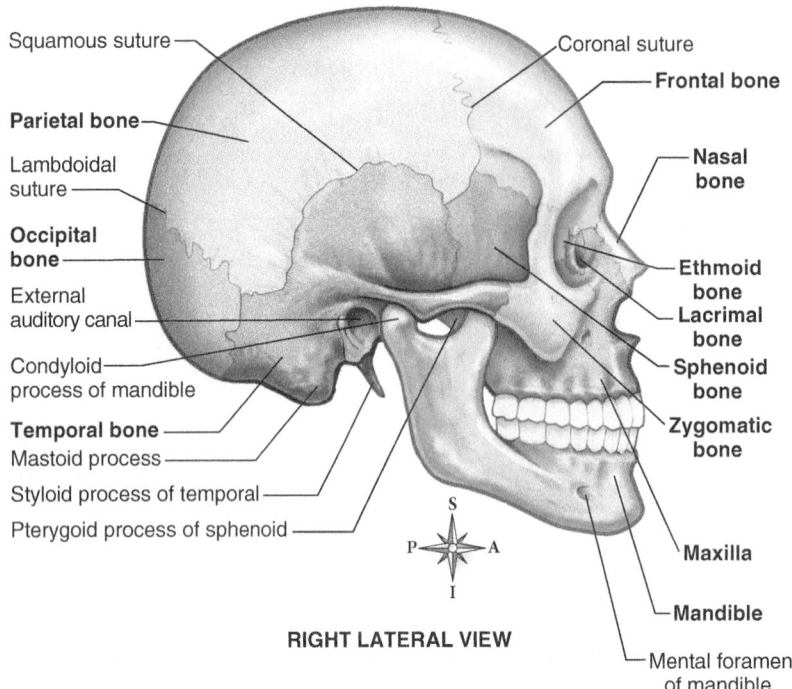

Fig. 3.3 Skull. Right side. (From Patton KT, Thibodeau GA: *The human body in health and disease,* ed 7, St. Louis, 2018, Elsevier.)

RIGHT LATERAL VIEW

Squamous suture
Coronal suture
Parietal bone
Frontal bone
Lambdoidal suture
Nasal bone
Occipital bone
Ethmoid bone
External auditory canal
Lacrimal bone
Condyloid process of mandible
Sphenoid bone
Temporal bone
Zygomatic bone
Mastoid process
Styloid process of temporal
Pterygoid process of sphenoid
Maxilla
Mandible
Mental foramen of mandible

Right lateral view

Cervical curvature
Thoracic curvature
Lumbar curvature
Intervertebral foramina
Sacral curvature

A

Anterior view

Atlas
Axis
Cervical vertebrae (7)
Thoracic vertebrae (12)
Lumbar vertebrae (5)
Sacrum
Coccyx

B

Posterior view

C

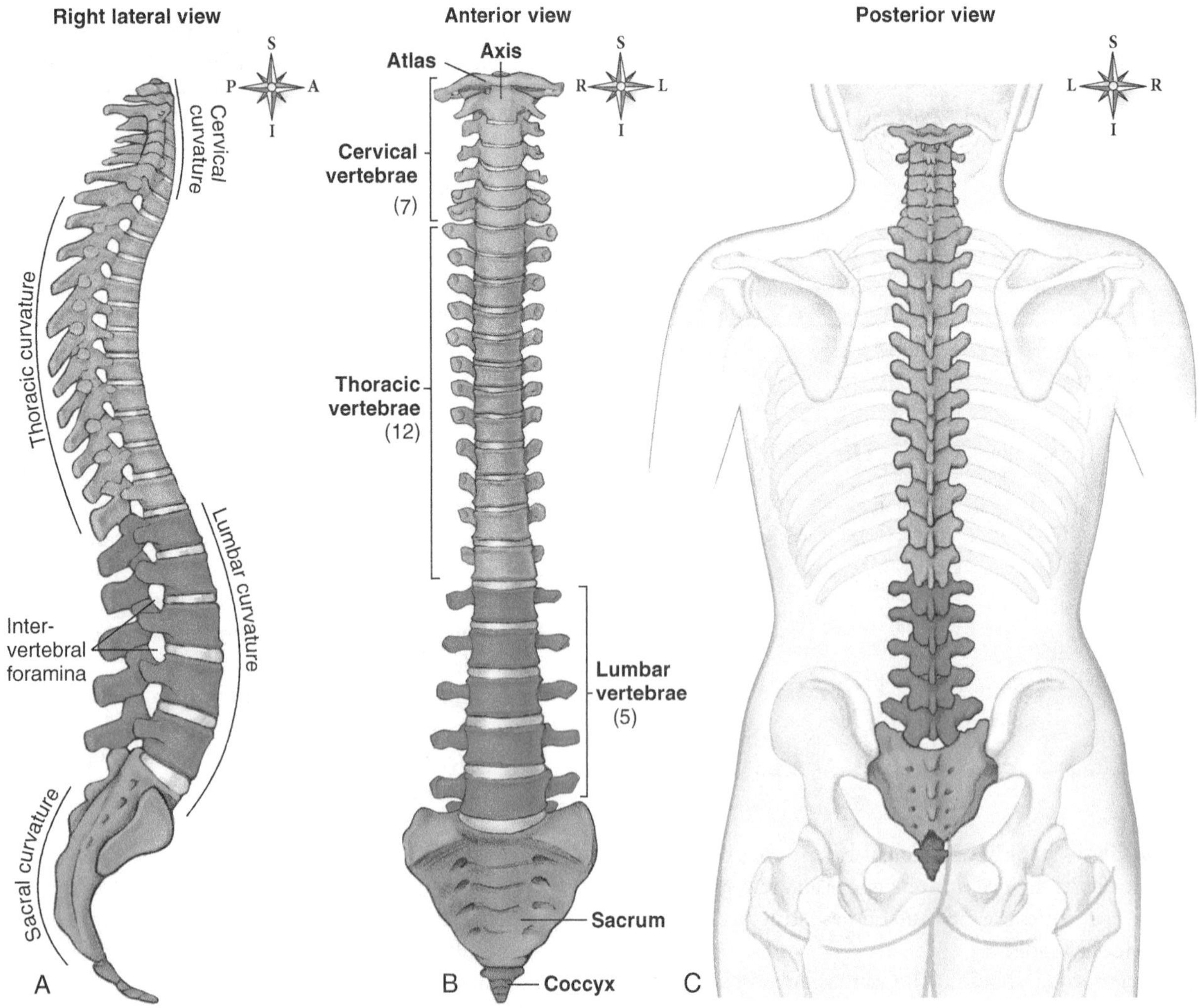

Fig. 3.4 The Vertebral Column. (From Patton KT, Thibodeau GA: *The human body in health and disease,* ed 7, St. Louis, 2018, Elsevier.)

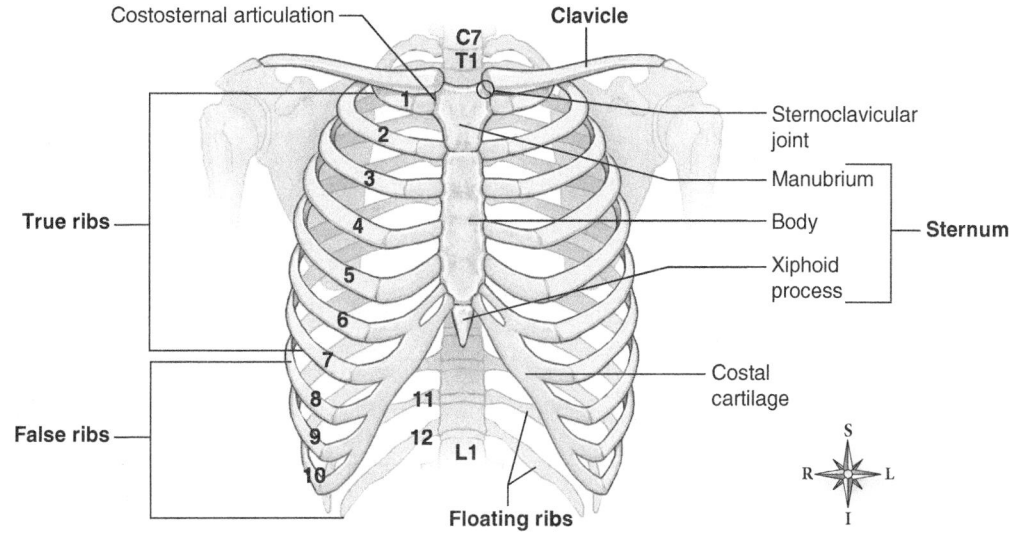

Fig. 3.5 Thorax. (From Patton KT, Thibodeau GA: *The human body in health and disease,* ed 7, St. Louis, 2018, Elsevier.)

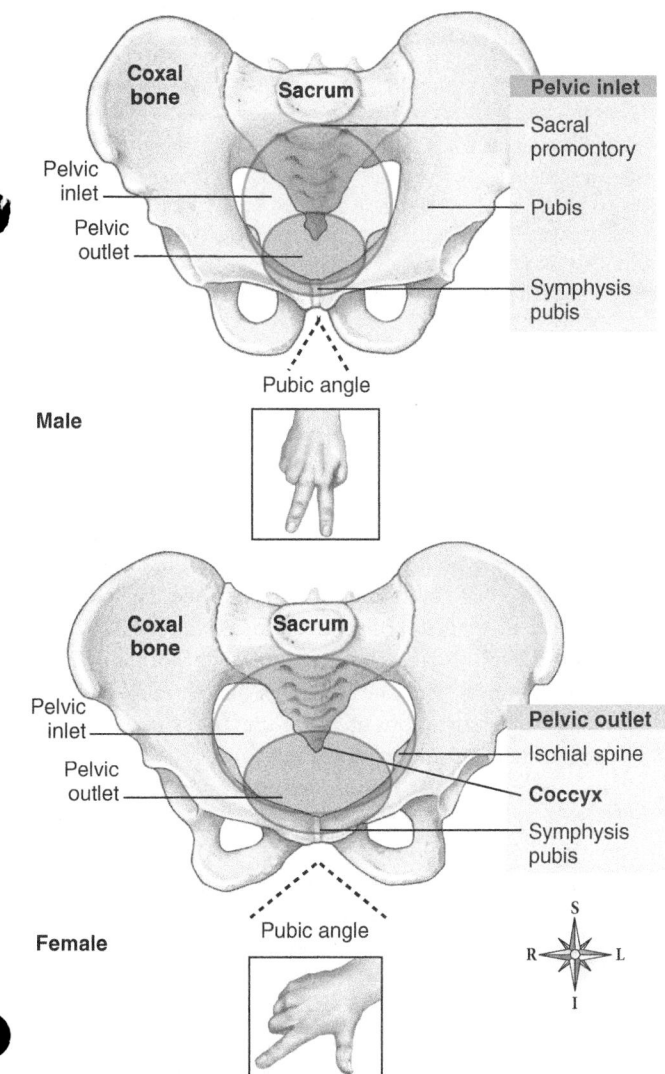

Fig. 3.6 Comparison of the Male and Female Pelvises. (From Patton K: *Structure and function of the body,* ed 15, St. Louis, 2016, Elsevier.)

CRITICAL THINKING 3.1

Suzanne is thinking about Walter as she prepares the exam room for his appointment. Walter's hands and knees are bothering him. The hands and knees are both part of the appendicular skeleton. She thought for a moment and quickly named the major structures in the appendicular and axial skeleton. Can you name them, too?

MEDICAL TERMINOLOGY	
burs/o	bursa
calcane/o	calcaneus
carp/o	carpal bone
clavicul/o, cleid/o	clavicle
fibul/o, perone/o	fibula
humer/o	humerus
ischi/o	ischium
metacarp/o	metacarpus
metatars/o	metatarsus
patell/o, patell/a	patella
pelv/i, pelv/o	pelvis
phalang/o	phalanx
pub/o	pubis
radi/o	radius
tars/o	tarsal
tibi/o	tibia
uln/o	ulna

Long Bones

The outer covering of a long bone is called the *periosteum,* and the inner lining is called the *endosteum.* The long bone is composed the following parts:

- *Diaphysis:* The long shaft, which is made of hard compact bone (Fig. 3.7).
- *Medullary cavity:* The hollow space inside the diaphysis. *Yellow bone marrow* is found in the medullary cavity. Yellow

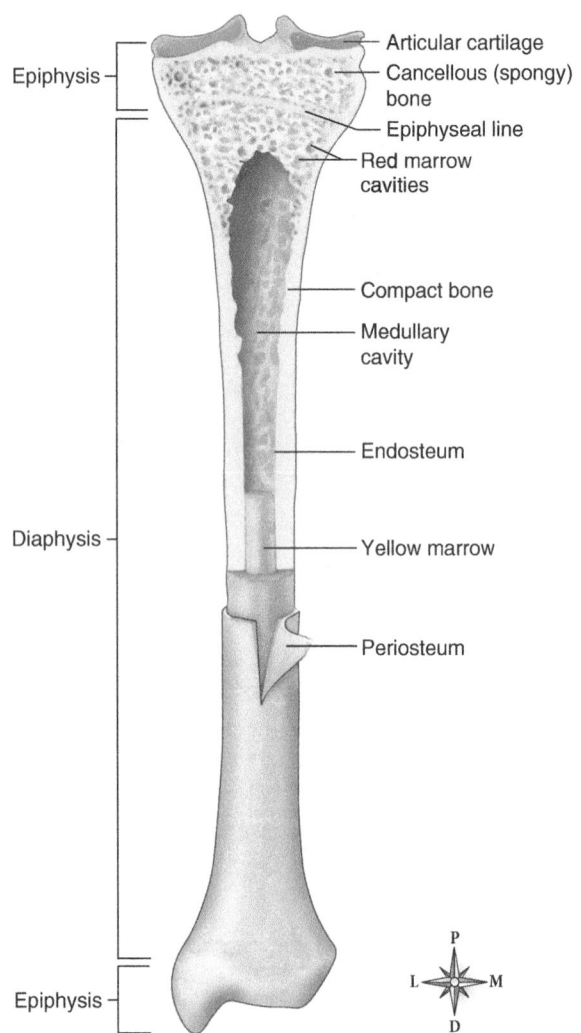

Epiphysis —

— Articular cartilage
— Cancellous (spongy) bone
— Epiphyseal line
— Red marrow cavities

— Compact bone

— Medullary cavity

— Endosteum

Diaphysis —

— Yellow marrow

— Periosteum

Epiphysis —

P
L ⬥ M
D

Fig. 3.7 Long Bone. Frontal section (partial) of a tibia. (From Patton KT, Thibodeau GA: *The human body in health and disease,* ed 7, St. Louis, 2018, Elsevier.)

bone marrow is a soft, gelatinous tissue that consists mostly of fat cells and a small amount of primitive blood cells.

- *Epiphysis:* The end of the long bone, which is made of spongy bone. The epiphysis is covered with articular cartilage and is attached by ligaments to the epiphysis of another bone, forming a joint. Articular cartilage reduces the stress of weight bearing and the friction of movement. The thickness of the cartilage depends largely on the amount of stress placed on a particular joint.
- *Metaphysis:* The narrow strip between the diaphysis and epiphysis. The metaphysis contains the *epiphyseal plates* (also called *growth plates*). This is where bone growth normally occurs.

Compact bone is made up of structural units called *osteons.* Osteons are composed of *osteocytes* (bone cells) and calcified matrix. The matrix stores phosphorus and calcium for the body to use. The *nutrient foramina* are small passageways that contain blood vessels that supply osteocytes with nutrients.

Joints

Bones are connected to each other at junctions known as *joints (articulations).* The range through which a joint can extend and flex is called its *range of motion* (ROM). Joints can be classified by their ROM:

- *Synarthroses:* Immovable (no ROM) joints held together by fibrous cartilaginous tissue. An example of this joint is the suture lines of the skull.
- *Amphiarthroses:* Limited ROM joints, which are joined together by cartilage that is slightly movable. Examples of these joints include the vertebrae and the pubic bones of the pelvic girdle.
- *Diarthroses* (or *synovial joints*): Full ROM joints. Examples include the hinge joints in the knee and the ball-and-socket joint in the hip. The following section will provide more details on diarthrotic joints.

CRITICAL THINKING 3.2

As Dr. Kahn examines Walter's hands, he has Walter open and close his hands, wiggle his fingers, grip tightly around two of Dr. Kahn's fingers, and move his wrist. Throughout the whole exam, Dr. Kahn is watching Walter's hands and wrists. Dr. Kahn is looking at the range of motion (ROM) in Walter's hands. Describe in your own words what the acronym ROM means. List the three joint types (based on ROM) and give one example of each.

Diarthrotic Joints. Many of the diarthroses, or synovial joints, have *bursae.* Bursae are sacs of *synovial fluid* located between the bones of the joint and the tendons that hold the muscles in place. Bursae help cushion and support the joints when they move. Synovial joints also have joint capsules that enclose the ends of the bones (Fig. 3.8). A synovial membrane lines the joint capsules. This membrane secretes synovial fluid that lubricates the joint. Joints also have cartilage that covers and protects the bone. The *meniscus* consists of crescent-shaped cartilage in the knee joint that also cushions the joint. Ligaments are strong bands of white, fibrous connective tissue that connect one bone to another bone at the joints.

There are six classifications of *diarthroses* (or synovial joints). Each type has its own unique movement.

- *Hinge joint:* Permits flexion and extension (Fig. 3.9 and Table 3.1). Examples include the elbow, knee, and finger joints.
- *Pivot joint:* Permits rotation. Pivot joints are found between the atlas and the axis (first and second cervical vertebrae).
- *Saddle joint:* Allows for flexion, extension, and other movement. An example is the thumb crossing over the palm of the hand.
- *Condyloid joint:* Permits flexion, extension, and circular motion. An example would be the movement of the atlas.
- *Ball-and-socket joint:* Allows free movement (rotation). Examples include the shoulder and hip joints.

When a fracture occurs, a protective blood clot and callus (KAL us) form at the break (Fig. 3.10). During the healing process, new bone cells start to grow on both sides of the break. Eventually, the new bone from both sides meets, closing the fracture, and the callus is absorbed.

> **VOCABULARY**
>
> **callus** Hard bony tissue that forms at the ends of fractured bones during the healing process.

Regulation of the Blood Calcium Level

About 98% of the body's calcium is stored in the bones. Calcium is moved between the blood and bones through the work of the osteoblasts and osteoclasts. It is removed from the blood as the osteoblasts form new bone. This lowers the blood calcium level. When the osteoclasts break down bone, calcium is released into the blood, thus increasing the blood calcium level.

Two hormones work to maintain the blood calcium level. The *parathyroid hormone* from the parathyroid gland increases the activity of the osteoclasts when the blood calcium level is decreased. *Calcitonin*, which is produced in the thyroid, helps to lower the blood calcium level. Calcitonin promotes bone formation by the osteoblasts and inhibits the bone breakdown by the osteoclasts.

Hematopoiesis

Spongy bone is found at the center of most bones. It is less dense than compact bone and has a network of open spaces that contain *red bone marrow*. The red bone marrow is a soft, gelatinous tissue that consists of blood stem cells. These stem cells can become white or red blood cells or platelets.

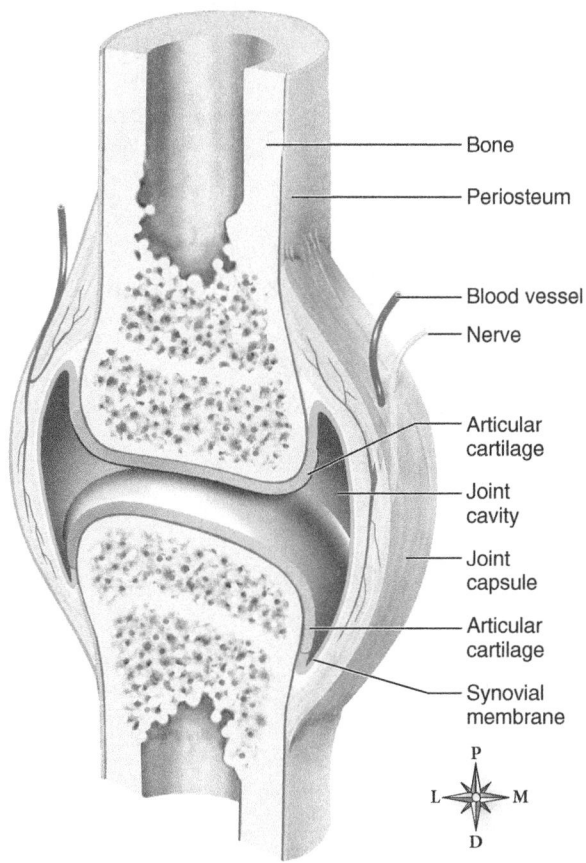

Fig. 3.8 Diarthrotic Joint Structure. Each diarthrosis has a joint capsule, a joint cavity, and a layer of cartilage over the ends of the joined bones. (From Patton KT, Thibodeau GA: *The human body in health and disease*, ed 7, St. Louis, 2018, Elsevier.)

- *Gliding joint*: Allows a bone to slide over another bone. This occurs in the wrist and between the vertebrae.

PHYSIOLOGY OF THE SKELETAL SYSTEM

The skeletal system has several important roles in the body:
- Protecting, supporting, and providing a framework for organ systems of the body
- Helping with movement
- Developing new bone
- Regulating the blood calcium level
- *Hematopoiesis* (hee mah toh poh EE sis), the formation of blood cells and platelets

The last three roles will be addressed in more depth in the following sections.

Development of New Bone

Between the periosteum and the endosteum, the osteoclasts (OS tee oh clasts) and osteoblasts (OS tee oh blasts) continuously remodel bones. The *osteoclasts* are bone cells that break down bone. The *osteoblasts*, bone-forming cells, make the bones strong, durable, and able to heal. Because bones have a good blood supply, they easily heal after trauma or a break *(fracture)* (Box 3.2).

> **BOX 3.2 Healthy, Strong Bones**
>
> Peak bone mass is usually achieved around age 30. After that time, a little more bone is lost through remodeling than what is gained. This leads to a decrease in bone mass or density. For good bone health, it is important to do the following:
> - Eat a diet rich in calcium. Good sources of calcium include dairy products, canned salmon with bones, soy products (e.g., tofu), broccoli and kale, and almonds.
> - Take in adequate amounts of vitamin D. Vitamin D helps the body absorb dietary phosphorus and calcium. Good dietary sources of vitamin D include oily fish (e.g., trout, tuna, salmon), mushrooms, eggs, and fortified cereals and milk. Sunlight also helps in the body's production of vitamin D.
> - Limit tobacco and alcohol use. Tobacco use can lead to weak bones. Drinking more than one alcoholic drink per day for women and two for men can increase bone density loss.
> - Do weight-bearing exercises. Weight-bearing exercises, such as jogging, climbing stairs, and walking, help build strong bones and slow bone loss.

DISEASES AND DISORDERS OF THE SKELETAL SYSTEM

Disorders of the skeletal system often affect the ability to move with ease. Common signs and symptoms of skeletal disorders include:
- Inflammation
- Pain, or swelling in the joints or bones

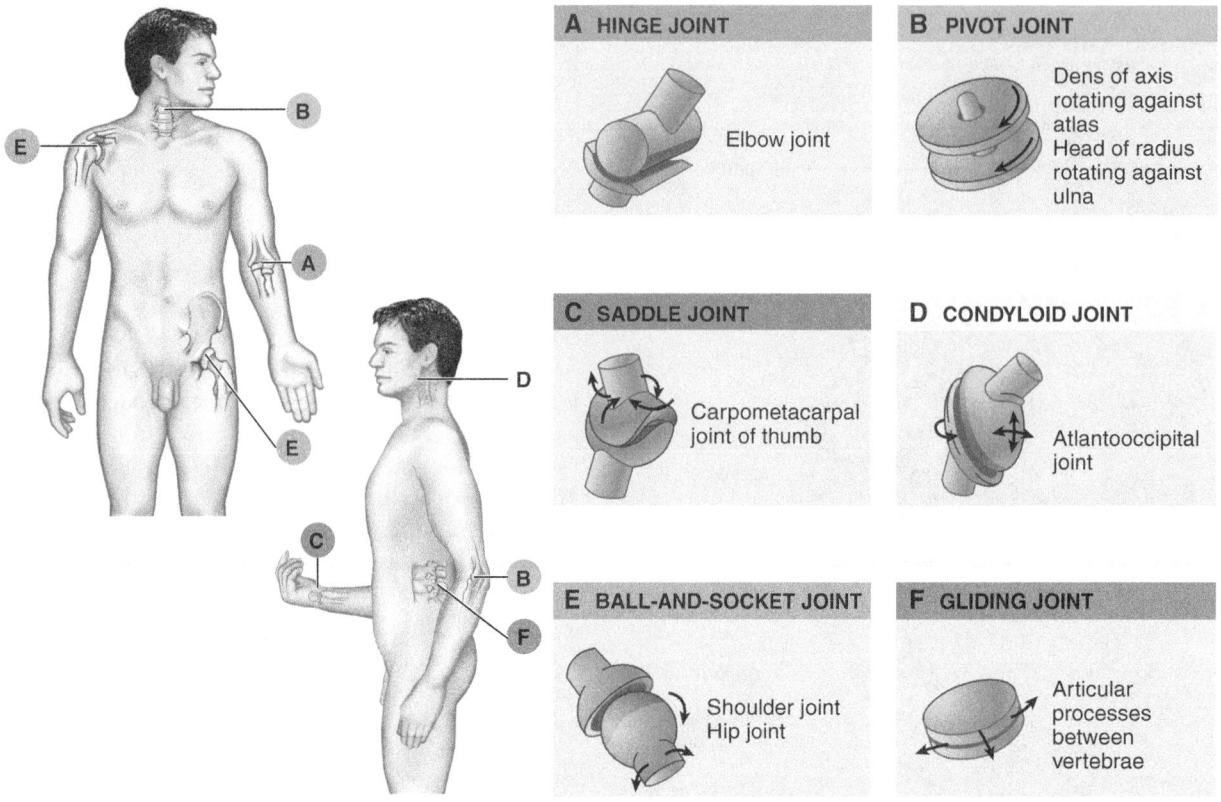

Fig. 3.9 Types of Diarthrotic Joints. (From Patton K: *Structure and function of the body,* ed 15, St. Louis, 2016, Elsevier.)

TABLE 3.1 **Types of Body Movement**		
Figure	**Type of Movement**	**Definition or Example**
ANGULAR	*Flexion* (FLEX shun)	Reducing the angle of the joint and bringing the two bones closer together.
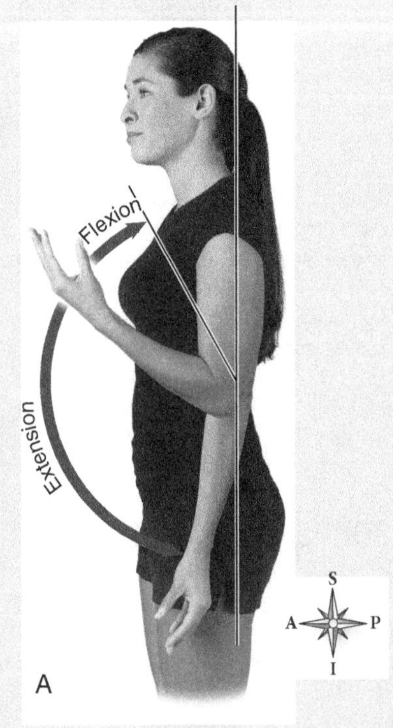	*Extension* (ecks TEN shun)	The opposite of flexion; increasing the angle or distance between two bones or parts of the body.

Flexion

Extension

A

TABLE 3.1   Types of Body Movement—cont'd

Figure	Type of Movement	Definition or Example
	Abduction (ab DUK shun)	Moving the body part away from the midline or median plane of the body.
	Adduction (ad DUK shun)	The opposite of abduction; moving the body part toward the midline of the body.
CIRCULAR	*Rotation* (roh TAY shun)	Moving a bone around its central axis; common in ball-and-socket joints.
	Circumduction (ser KUM duk shun)	Circular movement of a limb; a combination of abduction, adduction, extension, and flexion.

Continued

TABLE 3.1   Types of Body Movement—cont'd

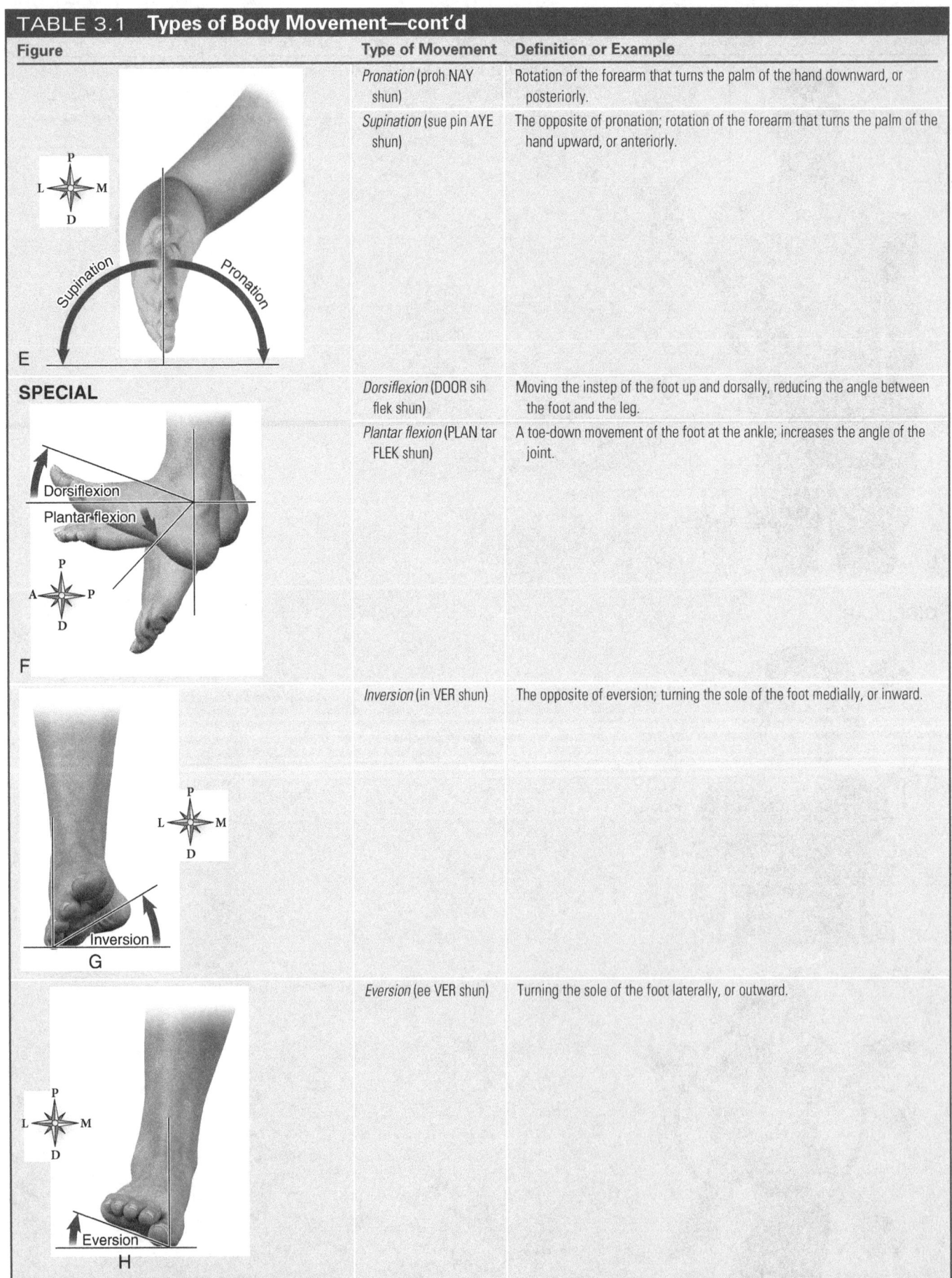

Figure	Type of Movement	Definition or Example
E	Pronation (proh NAY shun)	Rotation of the forearm that turns the palm of the hand downward, or posteriorly.
	Supination (sue pin AYE shun)	The opposite of pronation; rotation of the forearm that turns the palm of the hand upward, or anteriorly.
SPECIAL **F**	Dorsiflexion (DOOR sih flek shun)	Moving the instep of the foot up and dorsally, reducing the angle between the foot and the leg.
	Plantar flexion (PLAN tar FLEK shun)	A toe-down movement of the foot at the ankle; increases the angle of the joint.
G	Inversion (in VER shun)	The opposite of eversion; turning the sole of the foot medially, or inward.
H	Eversion (ee VER shun)	Turning the sole of the foot laterally, or outward.

Figures from Patton KT, Thibodeau GA: *The human body in health and disease,* ed 7, St. Louis, 2018, Elsevier.

- Temporary loss of function or loss of normal mobility

Common diagnostic procedures and medical laboratory tests are listed in Table 3.2. Common treatments used for skeletal disorders are described in Table 3.3.

Skeletal Disorders

Fractures. A *fracture* is a broken bone. With an *open* (or *compound*) fracture, the skin is broken above the fracture (Fig. 3.11A). With a *closed* (or *simple*) fracture, the skin is not broken and no wound is visible (see Fig. 3.11B). Fractures can also be classified by the type of damage to the bone:

- *Incomplete*: The fracture line does not go across the entire cross section of the bone.
- *Complete*: The fracture line goes across the entire cross section of the bone (see Fig. 3.11C).
- *Displaced*: The bone fragments are not in alignment.
- *Nondisplaced*: The bones fragments remain in alignment.
- *Comminuted*: The bone breaks into three or more fragments.
- *Compression*: A fracture in which the bone (e.g., vertebrae) collapses.
- *Greenstick*: The bone breaks on one side and is bent but still intact on the other side; commonly seen in children.
- *Impacted*: The bone fragments are driven into each other.
- *Linear* or *longitudinal*: The fracture line runs along the length of the bone (see Fig. 3.11D).
- *Oblique*: The fracture runs in an oblique angle across the bone.
- *Pathologic* (or *spontaneous*): The fracture is due to weakening of the bone structure by a pathologic condition.

- *Spiral*: The fracture line resembles a spiral; caused by the bone being twisted.
- *Transverse*: The fracture runs perpendicular across the bone.

Etiology. Fractures can occur from trauma, overuse, or diseases. A pathologic fracture results from an underlying disease, such as osteoporosis or cancer.

Signs and Symptoms. Signs and symptoms of a fracture include pain, swelling, bruising, numbness or tingling, deformity, and difficulty using or inability to use the affected area. Bleeding at the site of the break will also occur with compound fractures.

Diagnostic Procedures. Most commonly, the provider will order an x-ray, but a bone scan, computed tomography (CT) scan, or magnetic resonance imaging (MRI) may also be used as a diagnostic test for some types of fractures.

Treatments. Depending on the type of fracture, treatment may include:

- A cast, splint, or brace to immobilize the area.
- Surgery, if bones are not aligned. During an open reduction and internal fixation (ORIF) surgery, the surgeon *reduces* (repositions and aligns) the bones and uses *internal fixators* (special metal devices [rods, screws, plates]) to hold the bones in place during the healing process (Fig. 3.12). Sometimes, external fixators and traction are used to hold the bones in place.
- Medications, depending on the severity of the fracture. The provider may order:
  - Analgesics (an ahl JEE zik) for the pain, such as morphine, hydrocodone, and acetaminophen.
  - Anti-inflammatory drugs, such as nonsteroidal anti-inflammatory drugs (NSAIDs) and steroids.
  - Muscle relaxants

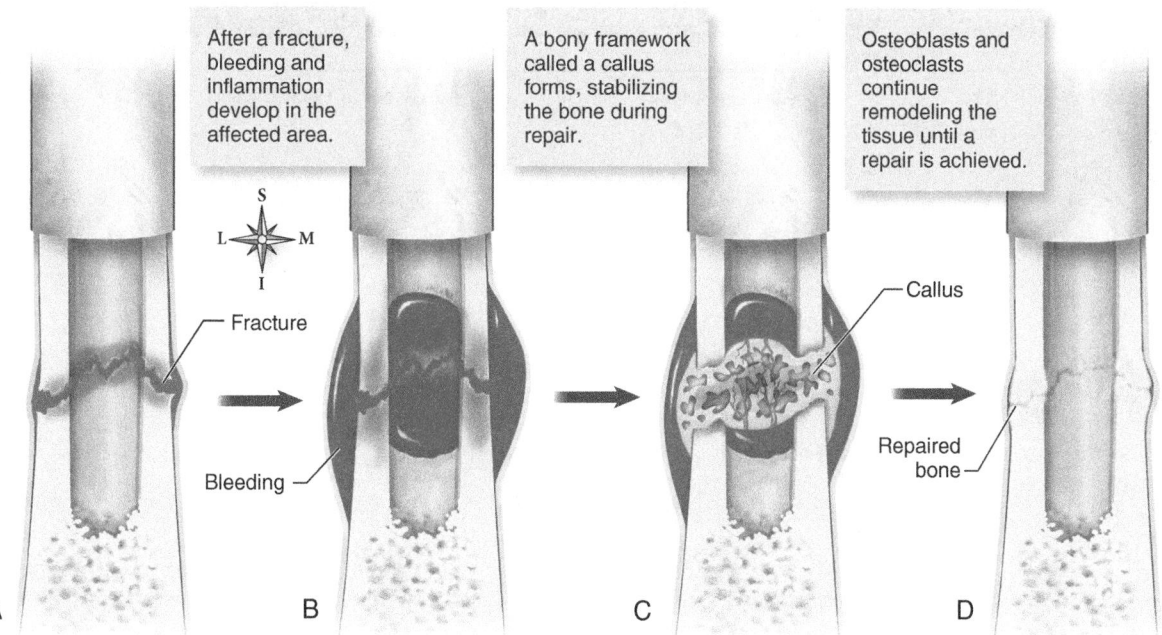

Fig. 3.10 Bone Repair. After a fracture (A), there is bleeding and inflammation around the affected area (B). Special tissue forms a bony framework called a *callus* (C) that stabilizes the bone until the repair is complete (D). (From Patton KT, Thibodeau GA: *The human body in health and disease,* ed 7, St. Louis, 2018, Elsevier.)

TABLE 3.2   Common Diagnostic Procedures Used for Skeletal System Disorders

Done by/Type of Test:	Procedure	Description
Endoscopy	Arthroscopy (ar THRAHS kuh pee)	An arthroscope is inserted into the joint and used to visualize and repair the joint. Fragments of damaged tissue may be removed, and biopsies can also be done.
Imaging procedure	Arthrography (ar THRAH gruh fee)	Provides visualization of the soft tissues in the joint (e.g., tendons, ligaments, cartilage). A series of x-rays are taken of a joint after a contrast medium (e.g., dye) is injected into the joint.
	Bone scan	Imaging test used to diagnose bone disease, tumor, or cancer. A small amount of radiotracer is injected into the vein and collects in the bones and organs. A camera slowly scans the body and takes pictures of the radiotracer that collects in the bones.
	Computed tomography (CT, CT scan)	An imaging test that takes cross-sectional pictures of the body. Used to detect fractures, tumors, and other abnormalities. Contrast medium may be used.
	Dual-energy x-ray absorptiometry (DEXA) scan (DECK suh)	A bone density test used to measure the calcium and other minerals in the bone. Central DEXA requires the scanner to pass over the spine and hip. Peripheral DEXA measures the bone density in the wrist, fingers, legs, or heels.
	Myelography (mie eh LOG rah fee)	Uses fluoroscopy and contrast medium to evaluate the spinal cord and related structures.
Other procedures	Electromyography (EMG)	Checks the nerves and muscles. A thin needle electrode is inserted through the skin into the muscle and picks up the electrical activity in the muscle.
Medical laboratory	C-reactive protein (CRP)	Blood test; some are CLIA-waived tests. CRP is produced by the liver and increases with inflammation. The CRP is a nonspecific indicator of inflammation.
	Erythrocyte sedimentation rate (ESR)	CLIA-waived blood test. Measures how quickly the red blood cells (RBCs) in a blood sample settle to the bottom of the test tube. The quicker they settle, the more it indicates inflammation in the body. The ESR is a nonspecific indicator of inflammation.
	Lyme disease blood antibodies	Blood or cerebrospinal fluid test; some are CLIA-waived tests. Also called Lyme Antibodies IgM/IgG by Western Blot. Tests looks for antibodies to *Borrelia,* which causes Lyme disease.
	Rheumatoid factor (RF) test	Blood test; some are CLIA-waived tests. Looks for RF present in the blood.

CLIA, Clinical Laboratory Improvement Amendments.

TABLE 3.3   Common Treatments Used for Skeletal System Disorders

Procedure	Description
Arthrocentesis (ar throh sen TEE sis)	Surgical procedure that involves a puncture of the joint and removal (aspiration) of fluid.
Bunionectomy (bun yun ECK tuh mee)	Surgical removal of a bunion.
Fixation device	Used to keep fractured bones stabilized and in alignment. • *External fixation (EF) device:* Screws are placed into the bone above and below the fracture. The external fixation device is attached to the screws outside the skin. • *Internal fixation (IF) device:* Rods, screws, and/or plates are surgically inserted into the bones to stabilize the bones.
Meniscectomy (men iss ECK tuh mee)	Surgical removal of a meniscus.
Prosthesis (prahs THEE sis)	An artificial body part, such as a leg, to replace a missing part.
Reduction	Alignment and immobilization of; there are two types: • *Open reduction* (OR): Requires a surgical incision for the repair. • *Closed reduction* (CR): Does not require a surgical incision.
Total or partial joint replacement / Arthroplasty (AR throh plas tee)	Surgical removal of part or all of the joint and insertion of artificial plastic or metal joint parts. *Partial joint replacement* means only part of the joint structures are replaced. With a *total joint replacement* all of the joint structures are replaced. *Minimally invasive replacement* surgery involves less cutting of the tissue. Examples: • *Patellofemoral replacement:* Type of partial knee replacement. • *Total elbow replacement:* The damaged part of the humerus and ulna are replaced with artificial components. • *Total hip replacement* (THR): The damaged femoral head and the acetabulum are replaced with artificial components. Also known as *hip arthroplasty.* • *Total knee replacement* (TKR): Replaces the knee joint. Also known as *knee arthroplasty.* • *Total shoulder replacement:* Replaces the shoulder joint. Also known as *shoulder arthroplasty.*
Traction	Treatment of a dislocation; process of pulling the bone into correct alignment.

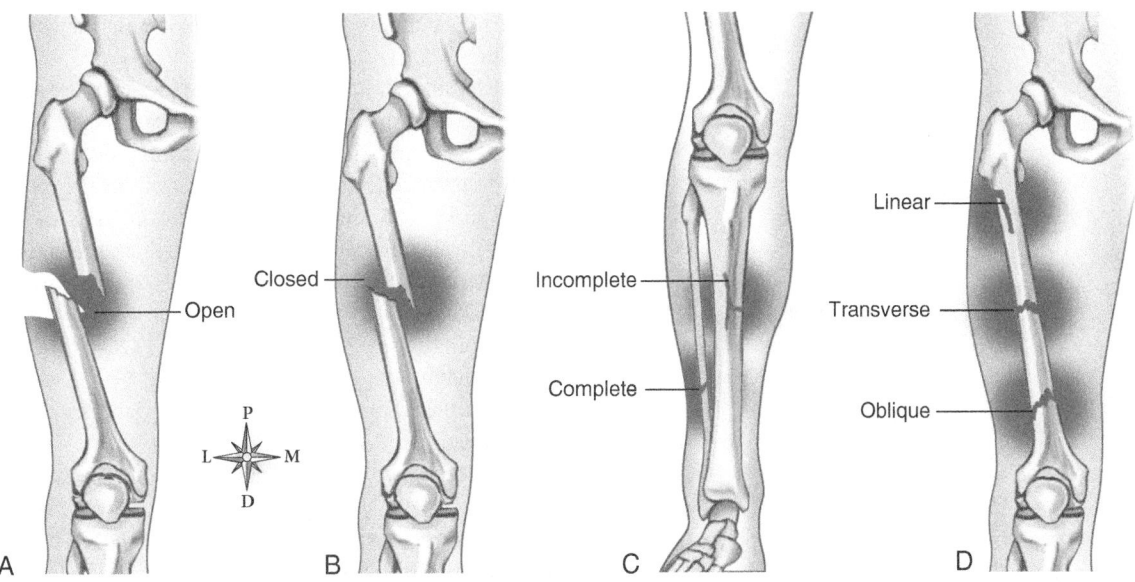

Fig. 3.11 Bone Fractures. A, Open. B, Closed. C, Incomplete and complete. D, Linear, transverse, and oblique. (From Patton KT, Thibodeau GA: *The human body in health and disease,* ed 7, St. Louis, 2018, Elsevier.)

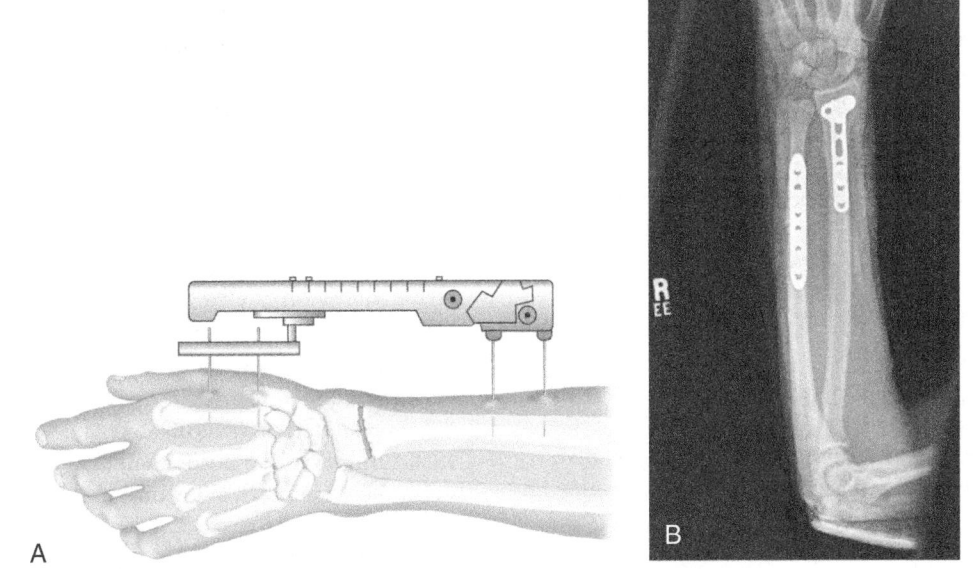

Fig. 3.12 Fixation. A, External. B, Internal. (From Kowalczyk N: *Radiographic pathology for technologists,* ed 5, St. Louis, 2009, Mosby.)

Fractures may take several weeks to months to heal. Crutches or other assistive devices may be used for lower extremity fractures. A sling is used for an upper extremity fracture. Physical therapy may be ordered once the fracture is healed to strengthen the extremity.

CRITICAL THINKING 3.3

A patient comes into the clinic hopping on one foot and holding the other in the air. She says she thinks she broke her ankle when she stepped off the curb wrong and fell. What tests will Dr. Kahn most likely order? Why?

Herniated Disk. When one of the soft disks between the vertebrae has a crack, some of the jellylike substance can leak out. This is called a *ruptured, slipped,* or *herniated* disk. The leaking jellylike substance can lead to inflammation and compression of the local nerve.

Etiology. The disks can degenerate with age. Middle-aged and older men are more at risk for a herniated disk. Typically, herniation occurs with strenuous activities, but it can also occur with lifting heavy objects, obesity, repetitive movements involving the lower back, long periods of sitting or standing, inactivity, and smoking.

Signs and Symptoms. Signs and symptoms of a lower back herniated disk include *sciatica* (pain and numbness from the hip down to the foot), back pain, and weakness. The pain usually starts slowly and gets worse with standing or sitting. A herniated disk in the neck may cause pain and numbness from the shoulder down to the fingers.

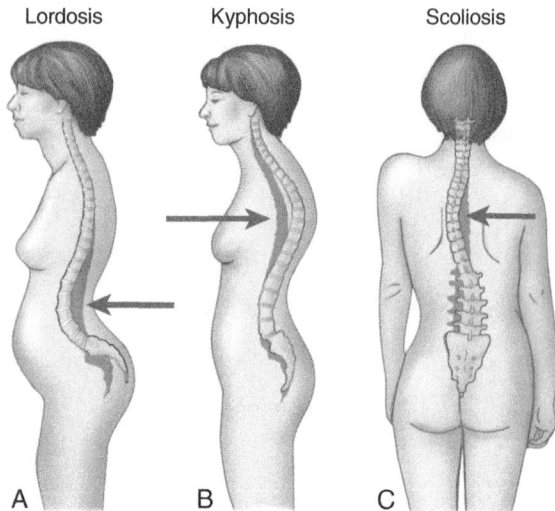

Lordosis   Kyphosis   Scoliosis

A   B   C

Fig. 3.13 Abnormal Spinal Curvatures. A, Lordosis (hyperlordosis). B, Kyphosis (hyperkyphosis). C, Scoliosis. (From Patton KT, Thibodeau GA: *The human body in health and disease,* ed 7, St. Louis, 2018, Elsevier.)

Diagnostic Procedures. The provider will check the patient's reflexes and muscle strength. The provider may order diagnostic tests (e.g., myelogram and electromyography [EMG]) and imaging procedures (e.g., spine MRI, spine CT, and spine x-ray).

Treatments. Treatments usually include:

- Medications (e.g., NSAIDs, narcotics, and muscle relaxants) to help reduce the pain, inflammation, and muscle spasms
- Rest and physical therapy
- Surgery to remove the herniation if the symptoms remain unchanged.

Usually, the condition improves in 4 to 6 weeks.

Lordosis, Kyphosis, and Scoliosis. The spine has normal curves. Abnormal curvatures of the spine deprive the body of important features related to spinal strength, balance, and posture. The three most common curvatures are:

- *Lordosis* (lor DOE sis) (swayback): An exaggerated forward curve in the lumbar region, which makes the buttock appear larger (Fig. 3.13).
- *Kyphosis* (kie FOE sis) (hunchback): An exaggerated curve in the thoracic region.
- *Scoliosis (SKOE lee oh sis)*: An abnormal side-to-side (S or C) curvature that could be in both the thoracic and lumbar regions of the back.

Etiology. Lordosis is caused by genetic and congenital conditions (e.g., muscular dystrophy, spondylolisthesis). Kyphosis can occur at any age but more commonly occurs in adults as a result of degenerative diseases of the spine, fractures, and injury. Kyphosis can also be caused by Paget disease, muscular dystrophy, scoliosis, and tumors. Many times, scoliosis occurs in children from age 10 to early teens, and the cause is unknown.

Signs and Symptoms. Abnormalities in any of the spinal curves can cause pain and fatigue in the lower back and legs. Lordosis can also cause pain that may affect mobility. Mild kyphosis may cause few symptoms, but severe kyphosis can cause back pain, stiffness, and an abnormally curved spine. Scoliosis can cause uneven shoulders and waist. One shoulder blade may be more prominent, and one hip may be higher than the other.

Diagnostic Procedures. The provider will perform a physical exam of the spine and a neurologic exam. A spinal x-ray, MRI, and CT scan are also used as diagnostic tools.

Treatments. The treatment depends on the severity of the curve and the patient's age and condition. Treatments include:

- Physical therapy to build strength and flexibility
- Medications (analgesics, NSAIDs, steroids, and muscle relaxants)
- Spinal fusion surgery
- Back brace
- Surgical placement of metal stabilizing rods maybe needed for scoliosis.

In most cases, with treatment, the prognosis is good.

Osteomalacia and Rickets. *Osteomalacia* (OS tee oh mah lae shah) is the softening of bones due to the lack of vitamin D. Vitamin D helps the body absorb calcium. Calcium is needed for strong bones. Osteomalacia occurs in adults and children; in children, this disease is called *rickets* (RIK its).

Etiology. Osteomalacia and rickets are caused by a lack of vitamin D, which can be related to an absorption issue (e.g., after gastric bypass surgery) or a lack of dietary intake. Osteomalacia can also be related to kidney failure, liver disease, and certain medications (e.g., anticonvulsants [an tee kuhn VUL sahnts]).

Signs and Symptoms. Signs and symptoms include bone fractures without related injuries, muscle weakness, and widespread bone pain, usually in the hips.

Diagnostic Procedures. The provider will order blood tests to check the vitamin D level, along with creatinine, electrolytes (e.g., calcium, phosphate), alkaline phosphatase, and parathyroid hormone levels. Bone x-rays, a bone density test, and a bone biopsy (BIE op see) may be done.

Treatments. Treatment involves oral supplements of vitamin D, calcium, and phosphorus. Sunlight for vitamin D production is also recommended. With early treatment, the prognosis for rickets in children is excellent. The prognosis for osteomalacia is good if the vitamin D deficiency is addressed.

> **VOCABULARY**
>
> **anticonvulsant** A drug used to prevent or treat seizures.
> **biopsy** Removal of tissue or cells for examination by a pathologist.

Osteoporosis. *Osteoporosis* (OS tee oh pah roe sis) is a condition that causes bones to become brittle and weak. Healthy bone is constantly being broken down and remodeled. When a person has osteoporosis, bones are being broken down more quickly than new bone can be created. This leads to weak bones that are easily fractured, especially in the wrist, hip, and spine.

Etiology. As people age, bone mass is lost faster than it can be produced, leading to osteoporosis. Increased risks for osteoporosis include menopause, family history, small body frame, white or Asian descent, hormonal imbalance, dietary deficiencies (low calcium intake), long-term corticosteroid use, celiac disease, kidney or liver disease, cancer, and some autoimmune conditions. A sedentary lifestyle, tobacco use, and excessive alcohol consumption are also risk factors for osteoporosis.

Signs and Symptoms. Early osteoporosis is asymptomatic, but as the bones become weaker, back pain, height loss, stooped posture, and fractures can occur.

Diagnostic Procedures. A bone density test is the only diagnostic tool for osteoporosis. This low-level x-ray determines the mineral content of the bone.

Treatments. Treatment for osteoporosis may include:
- Weight-bearing exercises to maintain bone density
- Modifying risk factors to prevent falls
- Appropriate calcium and vitamin D intake from food or supplements
- Medications such as bisphosphonates and hormone replacement therapy (estrogen)

Osteoporosis is a chronic condition that can be managed, but it does progress with age.

CRITICAL THINKING 3.4

Mrs. Viola Carson, a 78-year-old patient, is being seen in the office today for follow-up after hip replacement surgery. Mrs. Carson fractured her hip in a simple fall at the grocery store. Why would the physician suspect she has osteoporosis? What treatment might be recommended to prevent further fractures in this patient?

Spinal Stenosis. *Spinal stenosis* is the narrowing of the spine. The stenosis puts pressure on the nerves and spinal cord. Usually, spinal stenosis occurs in people over age 50, but it can affect younger people with spinal injuries.

Two main types of spinal stenosis are:
- Cervical stenosis, which causes narrowing of the cervical spine in the neck.
- Lumbar stenosis, which causes narrowing of the lumbar spine in the lower back.

Etiology. Causes of spinal stenosis include overgrowth of bone, herniated disks, tumors, spinal injury, and thickening of ligaments.

Signs and Symptoms. Cervical spinal stenosis causes numbness, tingling, and weakness in the extremities. Neck pain, difficulty walking, and bowel and bladder incontinence can occur. With lumbar spinal stenosis, a person can experience weakness, tingling, numbness, cramping, and pain in the legs and feet. It can also cause back pain.

Diagnostic Procedures. After an exam, the provider may order x-rays, MRI, and a CT scan. Sometimes a CT myelogram is done. With a CT myelogram, a contrast dye is injected, which outlines the spinal cord and nerves, showing abnormalities.

Treatments. Spinal stenosis can be treated with surgery, analgesics, physical therapy, and steroid injections.

Paget Disease. Paget (PAJ it) disease is also called *osteitis deformans* (ahs tee EYE tis dee FOR menz). Paget disease causes abnormal bone destruction and regrowth. The new bone is larger, but weaker, leading to deformities. Often the bones in the arms, legs, spine, skull, pelvis, and collarbones are involved.

Etiology. The etiology is unknown. It may be related to genetic factors or to a viral infection.

Signs and Symptoms. Most patients experience no symptoms. If symptoms occur, the person may experience:
- Bone pain, joint stiffness and pain, and fractures
- Deformities, including an enlarged skull and bowing of the legs
- Reduced height, kyphosis, and spinal stenosis
- Hearing loss

Diagnostic Procedures. After an examination, the provider may order a bone scan and x-rays. Laboratory tests such as alkaline phosphatase (ALP), bone-specific isoenzyme, and serum calcium may be performed.

Treatments. Not all patients with Paget disease need to be treated. Patients with deformities and other symptoms may be treated with medications to reduce bone remodeling, such as bisphosphonates and calcitonin. For lumbar spinal stenosis due to a thickened ligament, *percutaneous image-guided lumbar decompression* (PILD) can be done. For this procedure, needlelike instruments are used to remove parts of the thickened ligament, thus widening the narrowed spinal canal.

Plantar Fasciitis. The plantar fascia (FASH ee ah) is a tough fibrous tissue that connects the toes to the heel on the bottom of the feet, creating the arch of the foot. *Plantar fasciitis* (plan tur fass ee EYE tis) occurs when the plantar fascia becomes inflamed or swollen from being overstretched or overused. Plantar fasciitis is one of the most common foot issues.

Etiology. People with flat feet or high arches are at risk for plantar fasciitis. Other risk factors include running long distances, obesity, wearing shoes with poor arch support, and having a tight Achilles tendon.

Signs and Symptoms. Signs and symptoms include foot pain immediately in the morning, after standing, sitting, or intense exercise, and when climbing stairs. The pain can be on the bottom of the foot or along the sole of the foot. Mild foot swelling, redness, or stiffness can also be seen.

Diagnostic Procedures. The provider will do an examination. A foot x-ray may be ordered to rule out other issues.

Treatments. Treatment involves over-the-counter analgesics, heel and foot stretches, and good arch supports in shoes. Severe cases may require immobilization, custom-made shoe inserts, steroid injections in the heel, and surgery. Plantar fasciitis usually resolves with treatment.

VOCABULARY
fascia A tough fibrous covering of the muscles.

MEDICAL TERMINOLOGY

myel/o	bone marrow
plant/o	sole

Joint Disorders – Arthritis

Arthritis (arth RYE tis) is a term that refers to any inflammatory joint condition. More than 54 million Americans have some form of arthritis. Arthritis is the leading cause of work disabilities in the United States. About 50% of arthritic cases are in those 65 years or older, though arthritis can occur at any age.

Arthritis can be caused by autoimmunity, infection, injury, and genetic conditions. The following sections discuss common arthritic conditions, and Table 3.4 summarizes additional types of arthritis.

VOCABULARY

psoriasis A usually chronic, recurrent skin disease marked by bright red patches covered with silvery scales.

Osteoarthritis. Osteoarthritis (ahs tee oh arth RYE tis) (OA), also called *degenerative joint disease* (DJD), is the most common form of arthritis. OA can occur in any joint but most often affects the hands, hips, spine, and knees.

Etiology. Osteoarthritis occurs when the cartilage at the end of the bones wears down, causing the bones to rub together, leading to permanent damage to the joint. Risk factors include genetics, being female, obesity, age, and injury to the joint.

Signs and Symptoms. The signs and symptoms develop gradually and worsen over time. OA can cause pain, tenderness, stiffness, and swelling in joints, reducing the range of motion (Fig. 3.14A). Bone spurs may form around the affected joint.

Diagnostic Procedures. The provider will examine the affected joints and check the range of motion. X-rays, MRI, joint fluid analysis, and blood tests may be ordered to check for joint damage and rule out other types of arthritis.

Treatments. Treatment is focused on slowing the progression by maintaining a healthy weight, and limiting pain with the use of analgesics, NSAIDs, and duloxetine (Cymbalta). Additional interventions include physical therapy, occupational therapy, and cortisone injections in the joint to relieve pain. Joint replacement surgery (arthroplasty), such as a total hip or knee replacement, may also be done. The prognosis is good with surgery.

TABLE 3.4 Types of Arthritis

Disease	Description	Etiology; Signs and Symptoms	Diagnostic Tests; Treatments
Ankylosing spondylitis	Type of inflammatory arthritis affecting the back and spine, usually occurring between 17 and 35 years of age	Heredity; low back pain and stiffness, especially in the night and morning	X-rays and blood test to check for *HLA-B27* gene; medications (analgesics, NSAIDS, DMARDs, corticosteroids), and surgery
Infectious arthritis	Septic arthritis; arthritis due to a joint infection	Bacterial *(Staphylococcus aureus)*, viral, or fungal infections; pain, swelling in a joint, fever and chills	Examination, joint fluid analysis, and x-rays; antibiotics or antifungal medication, analgesics, NSAIDs
Patellofemoral arthritis	Articular cartilage on the underside of the patella wears down and becomes inflamed, making kneeling, squatting, and taking the stairs difficult	Due to dysplasia and patellar fractures; pain in the front of the knee	Examination and x-ray; medications (NSAIDs), exercise, weight loss, physical therapy
Psoriatic arthritis	Chronic autoimmune disease that can occur with psoriasis (sah RIE ah sis)	Unknown; joint pain and stiffness, fatigue, swelling of hands and feet, skin rashes, and eye problems	Examination, x-rays, and blood tests (C-reactive protein and rheumatoid factor [RF]); medications (NSAIDs, corticosteroids, and DMARDs) and light therapy

DMARDs, Disease-modifying antirheumatic drugs; *NSAIDs,* nonsteroidal anti-inflammatory drugs.

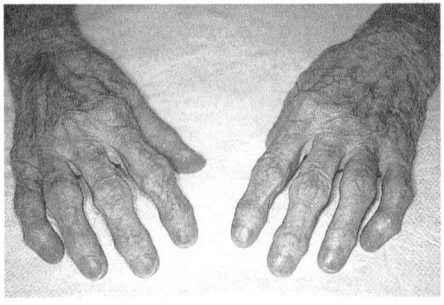 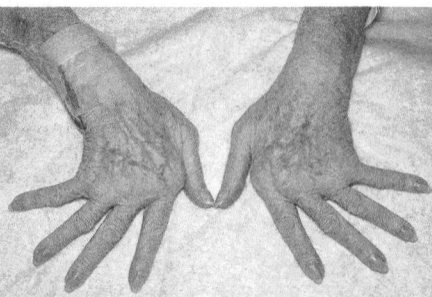 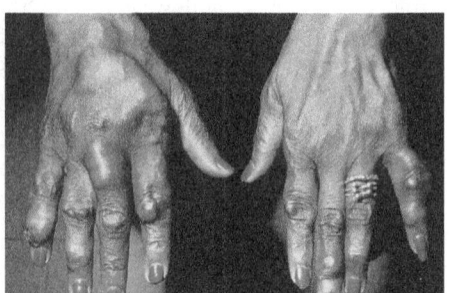

A   Osteoarthritis   B   Rheumatoid arthritis   C   Gouty arthritis

Fig. 3.14 Types of Arthritis. A, Osteoarthritis. Note the presence of nodes in the proximal interphalangeal joints (Bouchard nodes) and distal interphalangeal joints (Heberden nodes). B, Rheumatoid arthritis. Note the marked ulnar (elbowlike) deviation of the wrists. C, Gouty arthritis. Note tophi (stones) containing sodium urate crystals. (From Swartz MH: *Textbook of physical diagnosis,* ed 6, Philadelphia, 2010, Saunders.)

Rheumatoid Arthritis. Rheumatoid arthritis (ROO mah toyd arth RYE tis) (RA) is an autoimmune and inflammatory disease. RA often starts in middle age and is common in older adults. A person can have the disease for a short time, or episodes may come and go. The severe form of RA is chronic.

Etiology. With this autoimmune disease, the immune system attacks the healthy cells, causing inflammation in the joints, eyes, lungs, and mouth. Usually, it affects the wrist, finger, and knee joints. The lining of the joints becomes inflamed, causing damage to the joint tissue. Older adults and females are at most risk for RA, though women who have breastfed have a decreased risk. Other risk factors include genetics, cigarette use, and obesity.

Signs and Symptoms. Signs and symptoms of RA include pain, achiness, stiffness, swelling, and tenderness in more than one joint (see Fig. 3.14B). Weight loss, fever, weakness, and fatigue can occur. Early stages of RA can be difficult to diagnose because the symptoms are similar to those of other joint diseases.

Diagnostic Procedures. During the examination, the provider will check the reflexes and muscle strength and the joints for signs of inflammation (e.g., swelling, redness, and warmth). Imaging tests (x-rays, MRI, and ultrasound [US]) may be done, along with blood tests, including the erythrocyte sedimentation rate (ESR), C-reactive protein (CRP), rheumatoid factor (RF), and anti–cyclin citrullinated peptide (anti-CCP) antibodies.

Treatments. There is no cure for RA, but recent research has shown that early use of disease-modifying antirheumatic drugs (DMARDs) can increase the chances of remission.

VOCABULARY

remission The partial or complete disappearance of the clinical and subjective characteristics of a chronic or malignant disease.

CRITICAL THINKING 3.5

An 80-year-old male patient with arthritis comes into the office complaining of severe pain in his knees, hips, and lower back. The pain makes it impossible for him to get up onto the examination table. What should Suzanne do? Is this patient required to get onto the examination table? Why or why not?

Gout. Gout (also called *gouty arthritis*) is a common form of inflammatory arthritis. Gout can be acute or chronic, and attacks can last longer as time progresses.

Etiology. The etiology is a buildup of uric acid in the body (Fig. 3.15). Uric acid results from the breakdown of purines in foods (e.g., liver, dried peas and beans, and anchovies). The risk factors for gout include being male, a family history of gout, obesity, drinking alcohol, and eating too many purine-rich foods. Certain medications (e.g., diuretics, aspirin, niacin, and levodopa) may also increase the risk of gout.

Signs and Symptoms. The signs and symptoms of gout include swollen, red, warm, and stiff joints. The great (big) toe is the most common site for gout, though it can affect the heel, ankle, knee, elbow, wrist, and fingers (see Fig. 3.14C).

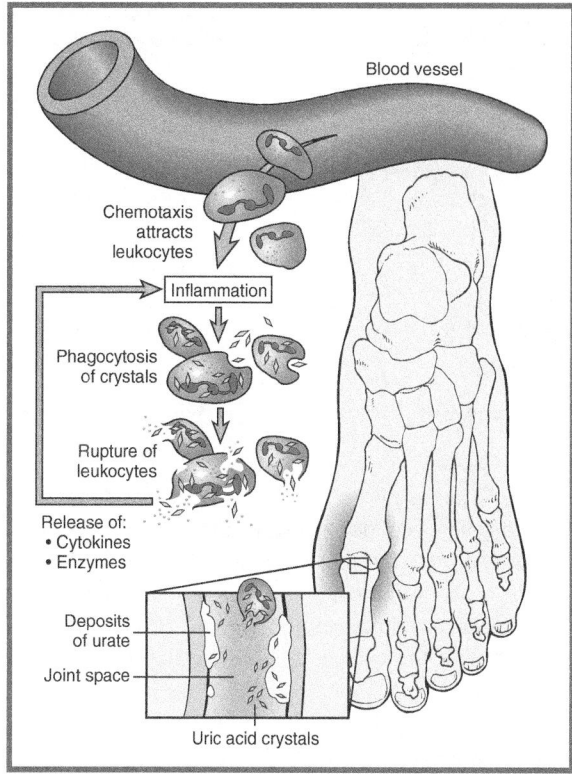

Fig. 3.15 Gout is characterized by deposits of uric acid crystals in the connective tissue. The inflammation most often affects the joint of the big toe. (From Damjanov I: *Pathology for the health-related professions,* ed 4, St. Louis, 2012, Saunders.)

Diagnostic Procedures. To diagnose gout, the provider will do a physical examination and order an x-ray and lab tests. The provider may take a sample of fluid from the inflamed joint area to look for uric acid crystals. Pseudogout has a similar presentation, but it is caused by calcium phosphate.

Treatments. Treatment includes:
- NSAIDs to reduce the pain and swelling.
- Corticosteroids (e.g., prednisone) can reduce the inflammation.
- Colchicine (KOL chi seen) (Colcrys, Gloperba) should be taken within the first 12 hours of the attack.

Full recovery may take up to 14 days. Additional treatments or to prevent future attacks by reducing the uric acid level in the blood, the person may need to take:
- Allopurinol (al oh PURE i nole) (Aloprim, Lopurin, Zyloprim)
- Febuxostat (feb UX oh stat) (Uloric)
- Probenecid (proe BEN e sid) (Probalan)
- Pegloticase (peg LOW ti kase) (Krystexxa)

Patients are also encouraged to control their weight, limit alcohol intake, and reduce their dietary intake of meats and fish rich in purines.

Juvenile Arthritis. Juvenile arthritis (JA) is a generic phrase for autoimmune, inflammatory, or rheumatic conditions that affect children under 16 years of age. Juvenile idiopathic arthritis (JIA) is the most common form of JA. Other types of JA are listed in Table 3.5.

TABLE 3.5 Types of Juvenile Arthritis	
Type	Description
Juvenile dermatomyositis (JDM) (der mah to MIE oh si tis)	Causes weakness and a rash on the eyelids and knuckles.
Juvenile systemic lupus erythematosus (LOO pus ER ah thee mah TOE sus)	Autoimmune disease that affects the kidneys, blood, skin, and joints.
Juvenile scleroderma (SKLER oh dur mah)	Causes skin to tighten and harden.
Kawasaki disease (KAH wah sah kee)	Causes rash, swollen lymph nodes, fever, inflammation of blood vessels, and heart damage.

Etiology. There is no known cause of JA. For some types of JA, there may be a genetic predisposition for the condition.

Signs and Symptoms. Signs and symptoms of JA depend on the specific condition. Most JA conditions cause pain, swelling, redness, and warmth in the joints. Some JA conditions may also cause issues with the eyes, muscles, digestive system, and the skin.

Diagnostic Procedures. The provider will perform an examination and order lab work, though no specific blood test diagnoses JA.

Treatments. The goal of the treatment is to provide the child with the best quality of life; therefore pain control and reducing inflammation are important. A combination of medications, physical therapy, and nutrition therapy may be used.

Lyme Disease and Arthritis. Lyme disease is the most common tick-borne infectious disease in the United States. Lyme disease can cause flulike symptoms and a rash (Fig. 3.16A). If the infection is not treated, about 60% of people develop Lyme arthritis.

Etiology. Lyme disease is caused by the bacterium *Borrelia burgdorferi* and rarely, *Borrelia mayonii* in the United States. Infected deer ticks and western black-legged ticks transmit the bacteria that cause Lyme disease (see Fig. 3.16B). This bacterial infection is prevalent in Wisconsin, Minnesota, California, and between Virginia and Maine. Exposure to grassy and heavily wooded areas increases the risk for coming in contact with infected ticks.

Signs and Symptoms. Early signs and symptoms of Lyme disease include flulike symptoms (fever, chills, achiness, fatigue, swollen lymph nodes, and headache) and a rash *(erythema migrans).* The rash appears about 70% to 80% of the time, usually starting 3 to 30 days after the bite. The rash begins at the bite site and slowly expands over the skin, reaching up to 12 inches or more. It can appear as a bull's-eye or target.

If left untreated, Lyme disease can cause arthritis, severe joint pain, meningitis, Bell palsy, facial palsy (affecting both sides of the face), numbness and weakness in the extremities, heart palpitations (Lyme carditis), short-term memory issues, and eye inflammation.

Diagnostic Procedures. After an examination, the provider will order an enzyme immunoassay (EIA) or immunofluorescence assay (IFA) blood test. If the results are

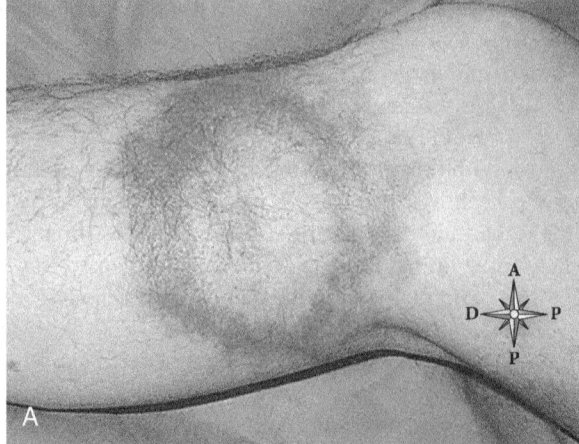
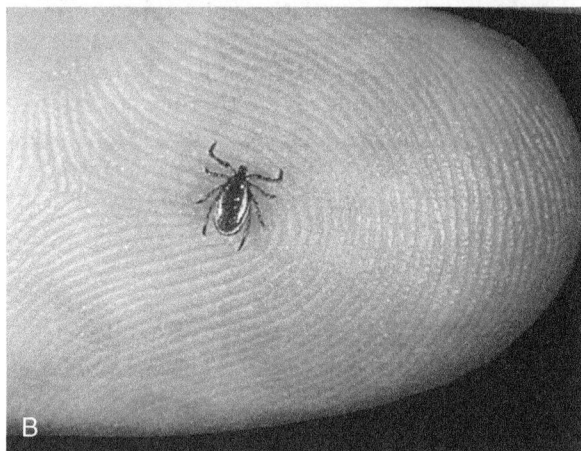

Fig. 3.16 Lyme Disease. A, Circular, expanding rash resembling a bull's-eye target caused by the spirochete bacteria *Borrelia burgdorferi.* B, Deer tick, vector for transmission of Lyme disease. (**A** from Callen JP, Paller AS, Greer KE, et al: *Color atlas of dermatology,* ed 2, Philadelphia, 2000, WB Saunders; **B** from Habif TP: *Clinical dermatology,* ed 5, St Louis, 2010, Mosby.)

positive or equivocal, further testing with IgM and/or IgG Western blot will be done. The lab test results are more reliable if a person has been infected for several weeks.

Treatments. Treatment includes antibiotics, such as:
- Amoxicillin (a mox i SIL in) (Amoxil, Moxatag)
- Cefuroxime (se fyoor OX eem) (Ceftin)
- Doxycycline (dox i SYE kleen) (Acticlate, Doryx, Oracea, Vibramycin)

Some people may have post-treatment Lyme disease syndrome, which will resolve in time. Box 3.3 provides patient education for Lyme disease prevention.

Joint Disorders – Others

Bursitis. *Bursitis* is the inflammation of the bursa. It usually affects the hip, buttock, knee, calf, and shoulder.

Etiology. Bursitis (bur SYE tis) is common after age 40. It occurs with the overuse or repetitive use of a joint. Injuries can also cause bursitis. Stress and inflammation from other conditions, such as gout and thyroid disorders, can increase the risk for bursitis.

Signs and Symptoms. Pain is the most common symptom. Joint stiffness, swelling, and redness can also occur.

Diagnostic Procedures. After an examination, the provider may order an x-ray, MRI, and ultrasound to rule out other conditions.

Treatments. Treatment consists of rest, splinting, heat and cold therapy, medications (NSAIDs, analgesics, and corticosteroid injection), and physical therapy.

CRITICAL THINKING 3.6

Suzanne has been a runner for years, but recently she was diagnosed with bursitis in her knees. Explain how Suzanne's running may have contributed to this condition.

Carpal Tunnel Syndrome. Carpal tunnel syndrome results when the median nerve becomes compressed at the wrist. The carpal tunnel is a narrow passageway, located on the palm side of the wrist, that is surrounded by bones and ligaments. This tunnel protects the median nerve to the hand and the nine tendons that bend the fingers.

Etiology. The etiology includes repetitive motions, trauma, injury to the wrist, and conditions such as thyroid disease and rheumatoid arthritis. Females are more likely to have carpal tunnel syndrome than males.

Signs and Symptoms. Signs and symptoms start gradually, with tingling, burning, or numbness of the thumb and fingers, except for the little finger. Symptoms can come and go initially but can worsen and become more persistent with time. Without treatment, a person can lose grip strength and feeling in the fingertips.

Diagnostic Procedures. The provider will examine the arm and wrist. X-rays and an electromyogram may be done.

Treatments. Treatments include limiting repetitive tasks, cold therapy, a wrist splint, NSAIDs, and corticosteroid injections. Surgery may be performed to relieve pressure on the median nerve. With treatment, the prognosis is good.

Dislocation and Subluxation. A *dislocation* (or *luxation* [luck SAY shun]) occurs when a bone has been completely displaced from the joint. A *subluxation* (sub luck SAY shun) is a partial or incomplete dislocation of the joint. The most common site of joint dislocation in children is the elbow, whereas in the adult it is the shoulder. Other joints that can be dislocated include the ankle, knee, hip, jaw, toe, or finger.

Etiology. The etiology of dislocations is related to sports and trauma (e.g., a blow or fall), which forces the joint out of position. The larger the joint, the greater the force needed for dislocation. Some people have a hereditary risk, because their ligaments are looser, making them more prone to injury.

Signs and Symptoms. Signs and symptoms include pain and swelling in the joint area and inability to move the extremity. Many times, a visual distortion in the joint area is seen.

Diagnostic Procedures. A dislocated joint is an emergency and requires immobilization and application of a cold pack as first aid. Once the provider examines the joint, an x-ray may be ordered.

Treatments. Treatment depends on the severity of the injury and the joint involved. The joint needs to be manipulated back into position. Additional complications may require surgical intervention. Once the joint is back into its normal position, the area may be immobilized in a splint or sling to heal. NSAIDs to reduce the inflammation and pain may be ordered. Once a joint has been dislocated, there is a greater risk of dislocating it in the future.

CRITICAL THINKING 3.7

A patient comes into the office from her weekly softball game. After sliding into home plate, she immediately was unable to move her right arm, and she says that she has a lot of pain in her right shoulder. What steps should Suzanne take to help this patient?

Hallux Valgus. Hallux valgus (HAL uks VAL gus), also called *bunion* (BUN yun), is a progressive condition. A bunion is an abnormal enlargement of the first metatarsophalangeal (MTP) joint of the great toe, caused by inflammation of the synovial bursa. Extra bone and a fluid-filled sac at the base of the big toe cause a bump to appear. Over time, the enlargement can cause lateral displacement of the toe.

Etiology. Bunions can be genetic. Some people have abnormalities with their feet bones that increase the likelihood of bunions. Wearing narrow-toed, high-heeled shoes can lead to bunion development. Females are more likely to have bunions than males.

Signs and Symptoms. Signs and symptoms of a bunion include:

- A hard bump at the big toe joint
- The big toe bending towards and possibly crossing over the second toe
- Pain at the big toe joint and difficulty wearing shoes

Diagnostic Procedures. After the exam, the provider will usually order a foot x-ray. Many times, the x-ray shows an abnormal angle of the big toe.

Treatments. As the bunion starts to develop, patients are encouraged to wear wide-toed shoes. Soft pads and toe spacers can be used to protect the bunion and separate the toes. The provider may recommend a *bunionectomy* to realign the toe and to remove the medial *eminence* (protrusion) of the metatarsal bone. It is important to keep a bunion from worsening. Surgery may help in some causes.

Hip Dysplasia. Hip dysplasia is an abnormality of the hip joint in which the femoral head does not fit in the acetabulum as it should. When people are born with this condition, it is called developmental *dysplasia of the hip* or *congenital hip dislocation.*

Etiology. About 1 in every 1000 infants is born with hip dysplasia. First-born children and females are more at risk for hip dysplasia. Hip dysplasia can be caused by genetics. It can also result if the baby's position in the womb puts pressure on the hip.

Signs and Symptoms. Signs and symptoms can include hip pain, a loose or unstable hip joint, limping, and unequal leg lengths. People with mild hip dysplasia may not have symptoms until teen to young adult years.

Diagnostic Procedures. Providers screen for hip dysplasia in infants by checking for it shortly after birth and during well-child exams. X-rays, ultrasound, and CT scans may also be used to confirm the diagnosis.

Treatments. The goal of treatment is to manage the pain and the protect the hip joint. A brace may be used for an infant under age 6 months. Physical therapy can help strengthen the joint and increase flexibility. In most cases, the provider will perform surgery to repair or replace the hip socket. Surgery usually corrects the dysplasia.

Patellofemoral Syndrome. Patellofemoral syndrome is also called *chondromalacia patella* and "runner's knee." It causes pain at the front of the knee around the patella. It is more common in adolescents, young adults, and women.

Etiology. Patellofemoral pain syndrome can be caused by overuse of the knee joint, muscle weakness, and trauma to the patella.

Signs and Symptoms. Dull, achy knee pain at the front of the knee is the primary symptom. The pain increases when running, kneeling, squatting, or doing stairs.

Diagnostic Procedures. After an examination, the provider might order an x-ray, CT, and MRI of the knee. Arthroscopy may also be done.

Treatments. Treatment consists of rest, avoiding climbing stairs and kneeling, and over-the-counter (OTC) analgesics. Additional treatments may include physical therapy, supportive braces, and cold therapy. For severe cases, surgical realignment procedures may be done. With treatment, the prognosis is good.

Sprain. A *sprain* is a stretched or torn ligament. A sprain can be graded to indicate the severity:

- Grade I for a stretched ligament
- Grade II for a partial tear
- Grade III for a complete tear of the ligament

Sprains of the ankle and wrist are the most common. A sprain is different from a strain, which is a stretched or torn tendon or muscle.

Etiology. Sprains occur when a person overextends or tears a ligament when stressing a joint. Sprains can occur with sport injuries, falls, and walking on uneven surfaces.

Signs and Symptoms. Signs and symptoms of sprains include pain, swelling, and difficulty moving the affected muscle. With sprains, a popping sound may be heard at the time of the injury and bruising may occur later.

Diagnostic Procedures. During the examination, the provider will check the affected area and the range of motion. X-rays and MRI may be ordered to rule out other injuries.

Treatments. Treatment includes *r*est, *i*ce (cold applications), *c*ompression (elastic wraps), and *e*levation (RICE) to help minimize the swelling. NSAIDs and analgesics may be taken. With severe sprains, a brace or splint may be used to immobilize the area. Surgery may be done to repair a torn ligament. With treatment, the prognosis is good. Stretching, warming up, and cooling down exercises are important to prevent sprains.

Additional Skeletal System Diseases and Disorders

There are many skeletal diseases and disorders. The following are some examples.

- *Adhesive capsulitis*: Also known as *frozen shoulder;* the movement in the shoulder is limited due to inflammation of the shoulder joint capsule.
- *Amputation*: The removal of a leg, foot, toes, fingers, or arm as a result of a trauma, accident, or surgery (Box 3.4).
- *Chondrosarcoma*: A rare type of cancer that begins in bones or soft tissue near the bones.
- *Collateral ligament injury*: The medial collateral ligament (MCL) runs along the inside of the knee, and the lateral collateral ligament (LCL) runs along the outside of the knee. When one or both ligaments are stretched or torn, the knee becomes unstable.
- *Contracture*: Occurs when the normal tissue is replaced with a nonstretchy, fiberlike tissue. This can affect the skin, muscles, ligaments, and tendons. The affected joint can have a limited range of motion. Contracture can be related to disorders (e.g., cerebral palsy, stroke), nerve damage, scarring, or reduced use of the joint.
- *Cruciate ligament injury*: The anterior cruciate ligament (ACL) is in the middle of the knee and works with the posterior cruciate ligament (PCL). When one or both ligaments are stretched or torn, the knee becomes unstable.
- *Cubital tunnel syndrome*: Pressure or stretching of the ulnar nerve causes numbness and tingling of the ring and small fingers, forearm pain, and hand weakness.

BOX 3.4 Amputations

Surgical amputations are done for a variety of reasons, including:

- Poor blood flow to the extremity
- Uncontrolled or worsening infection
- Severe frostbite or burn
- Tumor

Risks of amputations include blood clots, bleeding, infection, poor surgical wound healing, and phantom sensations. After a limb is removed, a person may feel that the limb is still there. This can include experiencing numbness, hot or cold sensations, and pain (called *phantom pain*) in the limb that is no longer there.

Depending on the type of amputation, many amputees use an artificial limb. Recovering from an amputation may require physical therapy, treatment with medicine, and/or counseling to help deal with sadness, anger, and frustration.

- *Dupuytren contracture*: A thickening and shortening of the palmar fascia in the hand results in the contracture of one or more fingers.
- *Ewing* (YOO ing) *sarcoma*: A rare type of cancer that starts in the bone or soft tissue near the bone. More common in children and teenagers.
- *Fibrous dysplasia*: Abnormal fibrous tissue replaces bone, leading to weak bones.
- *Hammertoe*: An abnormal bend in the middle joint of the second, third, or fourth toe.
- *Mastoiditis* (MAS toy dye tis): Infection of the mastoid bone, commonly related to middle ear infections *(acute otitis media)*.
- *Osteogenesis imperfecta* (OS tee oh jen e sis IM per fek tah): Also called *brittle bone disease;* a genetic condition that causes bones to fracture easily.
- *Osteomyelitis (*ahs tee oh mye eh LYE tis): A bacterial or fungal infection of the bone that comes from the bloodstream, surgery, or an injury. Signs and symptoms include chills and fever. The infected area can be painful, warm, red, and swollen. Antibiotics and surgery if needed to remove dead bone tissue can be done to treat the infection.
- *Osteosarcoma*: Most common bone cancer in children but can occur in adults. Usually found in large bones, although it can occur in any bone.
- *Polydactyly*: Often a genetic condition in which a person has more than five toes per foot or five fingers per hand. The extra digit is often poorly formed and is surgically removed.
- *Spina bifida occulta*: Mildest form of spina bifida; no spinal nerves are involved, but one or more vertebrae are malformed. No signs or symptoms may be present. The only indication may be an abnormal cluster of hair, a small dimple, or birthmark on the infant's back.

- *Spondylolisthesis*: A forward displacement of a vertebra over the one below it. Usually occurs in the lumbar or sacral area. Can be related to a birth defect or acute trauma.
- *Syndactyly*: The digits (fingers and toes) are fused together or are webbed together. Most commonly seen with the second and third toes.
- *Talipes (clubfoot)*: Most common congenital disorder of the legs. One foot or both feet are turned inward and downward. The calf and foot may be slightly smaller. Treatment depends on the severity and can include stretching, casting, braces, and surgery.
- *Temporomandibular joint disorder* (tem pore oh man DIB byoo lur) (TMD): Causes difficulty chewing and pain and tenderness in the jaw.
- *Torn meniscus*: The meniscus in the knee joint tears, causing pain, swelling, and locking of the knee.

LIFE SPAN CHANGES

When the skeleton is developing prior to birth, cartilage and fibrous structures are present. Over time, these structures are replaced with bone matrix and the bones change size due to the continual remodeling process of the bone cells.

During childhood, bones grow rapidly. The prime time to build bone mass or density is from childhood to young adulthood. Bone density can increase through a calcium-rich diet and regular weight-bearing exercise. Poor nutrition, inactivity, smoking, and excessive alcohol intake can reduce bone density.

The following are common skeletal system changes that occur with age:

- Bones lose calcium and other minerals, which reduces the bone mass or density. Bone density starts to decrease around age 30 to 40 in both males and females. It accelerates in women after menopause. The loss of bone density makes the bones more brittle, leading to osteoporosis and fractures.
- The disks between the vertebrae wear and tear with age. They can dehydrate and the cartilage can stiffen, causing the disk to bulge.
- Loss of height from the compression and curving of the spinal column occurs, which can cause a more stooped posture.
- Joints become stiffer and less flexible. Synovial fluid decreases and cartilage may wear away, causing degenerative changes. This can lead to inflammation, stiffness, pain, and deformities.

CLOSING COMMENTS

Working with patients with skeletal system disorders is common in primary care and orthopedics. It is important for the medical assistant to be knowledgeable about the anatomy and basic physiology of the skeletal system. The medical assistant needs to be able to pronounce and spell the names of bones, procedures, and common skeletal system disorders encountered in the ambulatory care setting. Knowing the definition and spelling of common skeletal system–related word parts will help.

The medical assistant should also understand the medication classifications used to treat skeletal system disorders (Box 3.5). Having a strong understanding of this chapter's content will help you in your future career.

BOX 3.5   **Medication Classifications**

- *Analgesics*: Relieve pain.
- *Anticonvulsants*: Used to prevent seizures; treat neuromuscular disorders and epilepsy.
- *Antigout medications:* Treat gout.
- *Anti-inflammatories*: Reduce the inflammation in the body and are used to treat injuries and inflammatory conditions, such as arthritis.
- *Corticosteroids*: Reduce the inflammation in the body and are used to treat chronic inflammatory diseases (e.g., arthritis).
- *Muscle relaxants*: Work on the central nervous system (CNS) to relax muscles, which treats conditions such as sprains.
- *Osteoporosis agents*: Promote bone mineral density and reverse the progression of osteoporosis.

Refer to Appendix D, which can be found on the Evolve website, for information on the medication classifications, including indications for use, desired effect, side effects, adverse reactions, and generic and trade names. Medical assistants should be familiar with medications that are prescribed to patients.

BEING PROFESSIONAL

Skeletal injuries and disorders are commonplace in the ambulatory care setting. Because of this, patients may ask for your advice on how to manage their health problems. Remember that as the medical assistant you should never diagnose or recommend treatment for a patient. That is the provider's responsibility. Responding professionally to inquiries and offering provider-approved educational materials and websites can be very helpful. Respectful and courteous behavior should be standard practice for medical assistants when they interact with patients and their families.

Role-play this scenario: You are a medical assistant. Mrs. Rose has a bad hip, and she asks you, "If you were me and had such bad hip pain constantly, would you go through surgery to fix it? After surgery I might have to go to a nursing home for physical therapy. I really don't want to." Respond to Mrs. Rose.

PATIENT-CENTERED CARE

An informed patient is better prepared to continue with home care. Skeletal conditions, particularly arthritis, can be so painful and debilitating that these patients may be easy prey for miracle drug promotions. It is important for you to recognize the need for patient education about the condition and to work diligently with the patient and family to encourage participation in effective care programs. When you work with the provider and the physical therapist in helping the patient, you become an important member of the healthcare team. This type of involvement leads to patient satisfaction and to personal satisfaction and a sense of achievement for the medical assistant.

CHAPTER REVIEW

The skeletal system consists of bones, joints, cartilage, tendons, and ligaments. The axial skeleton is made up of the skull, hyoid bone, vertebral column, and rib cage. The appendicular skeleton is divided into the upper and lower extremities. The bones in the upper extremities include the clavicle, scapula, humerus, radium, ulna, carpals, metacarpals, and phalanges. The bones in the lower extremities include the pelvic girdle, femur, patella, tibia, fibula, tarsals, metatarsals, and the phalanges.

The joints can be classified based on their ROM and include synarthroses (immovable), amphiarthroses (limited ROM), and diarthroses (full ROM). The diarthrotic joints can be further classified based on their unique movements. These include the hinge, pivot, saddle, condyloid, ball-and-socket, and gliding joints.

The skeletal system has an important role in the protection, movement, and support of the body. It provides a framework for the organ systems. The skeletal system develops new bone to help in the healing and growth of the bones. This system is also responsible for the regulation of the blood calcium level and hematopoiesis.

Many skeletal and joint disorders were discussed in the chapter. Common signs and symptoms of skeletal disorders include inflammation, pain and swelling in the joints and bones, and temporary loss of function. Common diagnostic procedures include arthrography, bone scan, CT scan, DEXA scan, EMG, and myelography.

The skeletal system changes with age. Prior to birth cartilage and fibrous structures are present. Over time, bone matrix replaces these structures. Bones are continually remodeled. The bone density is built during the childhood and young adult years. Around age 40, bone density starts to decrease. With age, joints become stiffer and the spinal column becomes compressed and curved. Degenerative changes can occur, that lead to inflammation, stiffness, pain, and deformities.

SCENARIO WRAP-UP

Dr. Kahn, Suzanne, and Walter wrap up the appointment. Dr. Kahn has recommended that Walter garden for shorter stretches of time, use a knee cushion when weeding, and take acetaminophen when he needs pain relief. Degenerative joint disease is manageable, and with a few changes in Walter's gardening routine, the prognosis is good.

Suzanne walks Walter out to the lobby. As she returns to the exam room, she reflects back on her 20 years as a medical assistant and is very happy with the choice she made so many years ago.

Muscular System

LEARNING OBJECTIVES

1. Describe the anatomy of the muscular system.
2. Describe the three types of muscles.
3. Describe the functions of the muscular system.
4. Explain the common diagnostic procedures and treatments for muscular system disorders.
5. Describe common muscular system disorders, including common signs and symptoms, etiology, diagnostic procedures, and treatments.
6. Compare the structure and function of the muscular system across the life span.

OUTLINE

▶ OPENING SCENARIO

Suzanne Peterson, CMA (AAMA), works with Dr. Kahn at the Walden-Martin Family Medical (WMFM) Clinic. Dr. Kahn hired Suzanne right out of school as a new graduate. Over the last 20 years she has enjoyed helping patients and the continued learning required in healthcare.

Suzanne was approached by the local medical assistant program to take a student for practicum. Today, Marissa, the medical assistant student, is starting her practicum at WMFM Clinic. Suzanne will be her mentor for the entire 6 weeks of the practicum. Suzanne is excited but a bit overwhelmed by the thought of taking a student. She remembers how nervous she was during her practicum experience. She knows she can give Marissa a lot of great experiences.

YOU WILL LEARN

1. To identify characteristics of the three types of muscles.
2. To explain the structure of the skeletal muscle.
3. To describe the location and function of major skeletal muscles.
4. To describe the four primary functions of the muscular system.

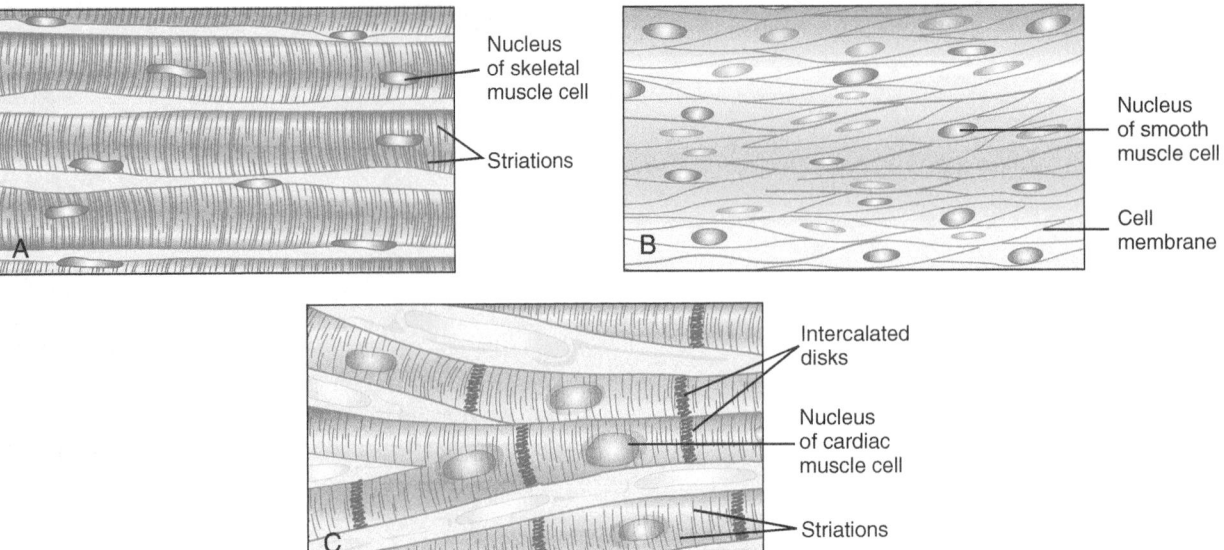

Fig. 4.1 A, Skeletal muscle. B, Smooth muscle. C, Cardiac muscle. (From Applegate E: *The anatomy and physiology learning system*, ed 4, St Louis, 2011, Saunders.)

5. To describe common muscular system disorders, including etiology, signs and symptoms, diagnostic procedures, and treatments.
6. To discuss life span changes in the muscular system.

INTRODUCTION

Patients with muscular system concerns are seen in primary care departments, such as urgent care and family practice. They are also seen in specialty care departments, including orthopedics and neurology. Patients with heart muscle concerns are seen in cardiology.

ANATOMY OF THE MUSCULAR SYSTEM

Muscles attach to bones and are found in internal organs and blood vessels. They create movement throughout the body. Not only do muscles help create movement of the arms and legs, they also assist with many internal processes, including breathing, digestion, and the circulation of blood.

Types of Muscles

Muscle tissue is composed of muscle cells (also called *muscle fibers* or *myocytes*). There are three types of muscle tissue in the body: skeletal, smooth, and cardiac. Each type has unique functions.

Skeletal Muscles. Skeletal muscles have multiple nuclei and striations that give them a striped appearance (Fig. 4.1A). Special fibers allow them to shorten (contract) and lengthen (relax), which creates movement. Skeletal muscles are voluntary, meaning we have control of them. They are found:
- Attached to the bones of the skeleton by tendons. This allows for movement of the bones at the joints and enables the body to maintain posture.

- In the upper section of the esophagus to help with swallowing.
- In the eye to allow for eye movements.
- In the urinary and digestive systems. Sphincter muscles allow for voluntary passage of urine and stool.

Smooth Muscles. Smooth muscles are nonstriated and have a single nucleus (see Fig. 4.1B). They are involuntary muscles, which means we cannot control smooth muscles. Smooth muscles contract in response to hormones and/or neurotransmitters (e.g., acetylcholine and norepinephrine).

Smooth muscles are found in:
- The hollow organ walls of the urinary, reproductive, and digestive systems. Smooth muscles in the urinary bladder, uterus, stomach, and intestines help with movement. These visceral smooth muscles can simulate each other to contract, creating a wavelike motion called *peristalsis*. This motion helps substances through tubelike organs. Peristalsis can be seen in the esophagus, intestines, and fallopian tubes.
- The respiratory system organ walls, where they regulate the airflow into the lungs.
- The walls of the blood vessels and large lymphatic vessels. The smooth muscles change the diameter of the vessels, helping the blood and lymph to circulate.
- The eyes, where they change the size of the iris and shape of the lens.
- The skin, where they cause the hair to stand erect (goose pimples).

VOCABULARY

neurotransmitters Chemicals that help a nerve cell communicate with another nerve cell or muscle.

Cardiac Muscles. Cardiac muscles are involuntary, striated muscles found in the walls of the heart (see Fig. 4.1C). Cardiac muscles can shorten and lengthen their fibers for contraction. Cardiac muscle fibers are electrically linked, forming one unit. A myocardial cell forms a strong, electrical connection to the next cells through special junctions called intercalated discs. The intercalated discs are responsible for the cell-to-cell communication that is required for coordinated muscle contraction and relaxation of the heart. The intercalated discs help the muscle fibers form one unit that contracts and relaxes all at once instead of a little at a time. The "one unit" approach is important, because the atrial chambers need to contract together, and then the ventricles also need to contract at the same time.

CRITICAL THINKING 4.1

Marissa and Suzanne had a busy morning working with Dr. Kahn in the urgent care department. Many of their morning patients had musculoskeletal symptoms. On break, Marissa decides to review the muscular system in her textbook in preparation for her national exam. She reviews the three types of muscles. Describe the three types of muscles.

Structure of Skeletal Muscles

An entire skeletal muscle is considered an organ. Each skeletal muscle consists of nerve tissue, blood vessels, muscle tissue, and connective tissue.

Skeletal muscle fibers can be very long. Besides having several nuclei, skeletal muscle cells contain other unique cellular structures:

- *Sarcolemma*, the cell membrane.
- *Sarcoplasm*, the cytoplasm in the cell.
- *Sarcoplasmic reticulum* (SR), the specialized smooth endoplasmic reticulum. Sarcoplasmic reticulum stores, releases, and retrieves calcium ions.
- *Myofibrils*, which are proteins that run the length of the cell. Myofibrils are made up of connecting *sarcomeres,* the basic functioning unit of a muscle. The sarcomere contains *myosin*, a thick myofilament, and *actin*, a thin myofilament, which create the striated appearance (Fig. 4.2).

A tough fibrous connective tissue called fascia (FASH ee ah) covers the muscle. The muscle also contains three layers of connective tissues (see Fig. 4.2):

- The *endomysium* is a thin inner layer of connective tissue that wraps around individual muscle fibers or cells. The endomysium contains extracellular fluid and nutrients to help maintain the muscle fiber.
- The *perimysium* is the middle layer of connective tissue. Individual muscle fibers are bundled together into *fascicles* (FAS ih kuls). Each fascicle is covered with perimysium. Separate fascicles can be triggered for specific movements; thus the entire muscle organ does not need to respond.
- The *epimysium*, a dense irregular connective tissue, is the outer layer. All of the fascicles are bundled together and covered with epimysium. The epimysium allows the muscle to maintain its structure during contraction yet move independently in the body.

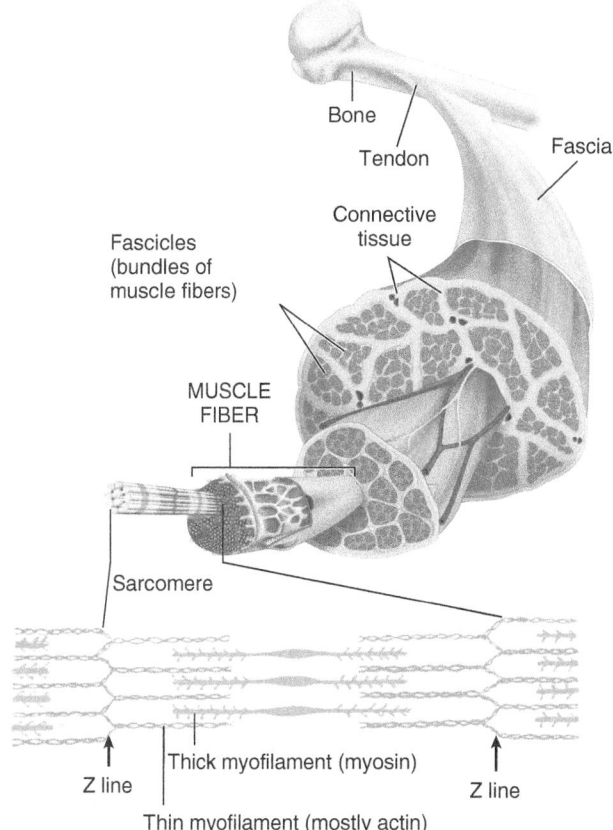

Fig. 4.2 Structure of Skeletal Muscle. A, Each muscle organ has many muscle fibers, each containing many bundles of thick and thin myofilaments. The diagrams show the overlapping thick and thin filaments arranged to form adjacent segments called *sarcomeres*. (From Patton KT, Thibodeau GA: *The human body in health and disease*, ed 7, St. Louis, 2018, Elsevier.)

The three layers of connective tissue extend beyond the muscle and mesh with either an aponeurosis (AP ah noo row sis) or a tendon (TEN dun). An *aponeurosis* is a tough, fibrous connective tissue that attaches muscles to muscles. A *tendon* attaches a muscle to a bone. *Bursae* (small sacs filled with synovial fluid) lie under the tendons or lie between some tendons and bones. The bursa helps the tendon move over the bone as the muscle contracts. Some tendons are enclosed in tendon sheaths, which are lubricated with synovial fluid.

MEDICAL TERMINOLOGY

leiomy/o	smooth muscle
muscul/o, my/o	muscle
myocardi/o	heart muscle
sarc/o	flesh
plasm/o	plasma
a-	without, no, not
endo-	in, inner, within
epi-	above, upon
peri-	surrounding, around
-osis	abnormal condition

VOCABULARY

fascia A tough fibrous covering of the muscles.

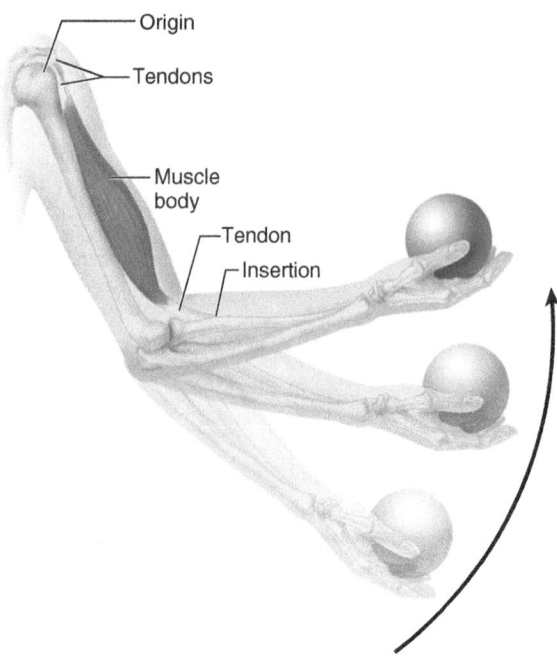

Fig. 4.3 Attachments of a Skeletal Muscle. A muscle originates at a relatively stable part of the skeleton (origin) and inserts at the skeletal part that is moved when the muscle contracts (insertion). (From Patton KT, Thibodeau GA: *The human body in health and disease,* ed 7, St. Louis, 2018, Elsevier.)

CRITICAL THINKING 4.2

Marissa has forgotten the skeletal muscle structure. The muscle contains three layers of connective tissue. Describe each of these layers.

Skeletal Muscle Movement. Most skeletal muscles attach to two bones and stretching across a joint. During a movement, one of the bones is considered to be *stationary* since it does not move. The other bone is the moveable bone. The muscle's attachment to the stationary bone is called its *origin*, and the attachment to the moveable bone is called its *insertion*. The body of the muscle sits between the origin and insertion (Fig. 4.3).

Many skeletal muscles work in pairs or groups, using antagonistic muscle movement for smooth movements. This means muscles contract while other muscles relax. The *prime mover* (or *agonist*) is the muscle responsible for the majority of the movement. The muscles that help the prime mover are called *synergists*. The synergists contract at the same time as the prime mover and stabilize the joint. This allows the prime mover muscle to work smoothly. The *antagonist* is the muscle that produces the opposite movement, relaxation. When the antagonist muscle contracts, the prime mover and its synergists produce an opposite movement.

Depending on the movement, a muscle might be a prime mover/synergist or an antagonist. An example of this is the biceps brachii and the triceps brachii. When the forearm is flexed at the elbow, the biceps brachii, the prime mover, contracts. The brachialis assists the biceps brachii, making it the synergist muscle. The antagonist for this movement is the triceps brachii, which relaxes. If you were to straighten your lower arm, the triceps brachii becomes the prime mover. The biceps brachii and the brachialis become the antagonistic muscles (Fig. 4.4).

CRITICAL THINKING 4.3

Describe the difference between a prime mover, synergists, and antagonist. Could a muscle be a prime mover for one movement and an antagonist for another? Explain.

Names of Skeletal Muscles

The names of skeletal muscles are often based on the characteristics of the muscle. Some of the characteristics include size, shape, direction of muscle fibers, number of origins, location, action, and the points of the origin and insertion (Table 4.1).

Head and Neck Muscles. The muscles of the head and neck include (Fig. 4.5):
- *Frontal*: Raises the eyebrows
- *Orbicularis oculi* (or bih kyoo LAIR is AW kyoo lie): Closes the eyes
- *Orbicularis oris* (or bih kyoo LAIR is OR is): Draws the lips together
- *Zygomaticus* (ZIE goe MAT ik us): Elevates the corners of the mouth and lips
- *Buccinator* (buk sih NAY tor): Flattens the cheeks, used for whistling and blowing, aids in chewing
- *Temporal* and *masseter* (MAS eh ter): Close the jaw

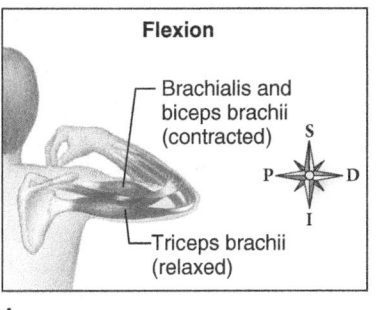
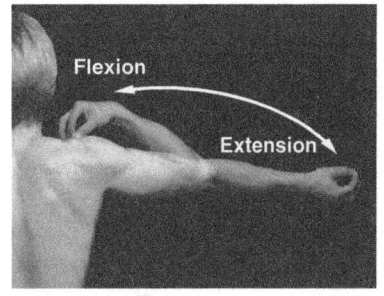
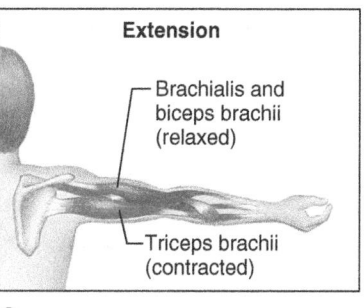

A   B   C

Fig. 4.4 Flexion and Extension of the Forearm. A and B, When the forearm is flexed at the elbow, the brachialis and biceps brachii contract while an antagonist, the triceps brachii, relaxes. B and C, When the forearm is extended, the brachialis and biceps brachii relax while the triceps brachii contracts. (From Patton KT, Thibodeau GA: *The human body in health and disease*, ed 7, St. Louis, 2018, Elsevier.)

TABLE 4.1	Naming of Skeletal Muscles	
Characteristic	**Name**	**Meaning**
Size	Brevis	Short
	Minimus	Small
	Maximus	Large
	Vastus (VAS tus)	Great, very large
	Longus (LONG gus)	Long
Shape	Rhomboid (ROM boid)	Like a rhombus
	Deltoid	Triangular
	Teres (TEE reez)	Round and long
	Latissimus (lah TIS i mus)	Wide, broad
	Trapezius (trah PEE zee us)	Like a trapezoid
Direction of muscle fibers	Rectus	Straight
	Orbicularis	Circular
	Oblique (oh BLEEK)	Diagonally
	Transverse	Across
Number of origins	Biceps	Two heads
	Triceps	Three heads
	Quadriceps	Four heads
Location	Pectoralis	Chest
	Brachii	Arm
	Gluteus	Buttock
	Supra-	Above
	Infra-	Below
	Sub-	Beneath, under
	Lateralis	Lateral
Action	Adductor	To adduct
	Abductor	To abduct
	Extensor	To extend
	Flexor	To flex
	Masseter	A chewer
	Levator	To lift
Origin and insertion	Sternocleidomastoideus	Origin on the sternum and clavicle; insertion on the mastoid process

- *Sternocleidomastoid* (ster noh kly doh MAS toyd): Rotates and flexes the head and neck
- *Trapezius* (trah PEE zee us): Extends the head and neck; moves or stabilizes the scapula

Upper Extremity Muscles. The muscles of the upper extremities include (Fig. 4.6):
- *Pectoralis major* (pek toh RAH lis): Flexes and helps adduct the upper arm
- *Latissimus dorsi* (lah TIH sih mus DOR sigh): Extends and helps adduct the upper arm
- *Deltoid* (DEL toyd): Abducts upper arm
- *Biceps brachii* (BY seps BRAY kee eye): Flexes elbow
- *Triceps brachii* (TRY seps BRAY kee eye): Extends elbow

Abdominal Muscles. The muscles of the abdomen include (Fig. 4.7):
- External oblique, internal oblique, and transversus abdominis (trans ver sus ab DAW mih nis): Compress the abdomen
- *Rectus abdominis* (REK tus AB dam i nes): Flexes the abdomen
- *Diaphragm* (DIE ah fram): Expands the chest cavity during inspiration

Lower Extremity Muscles. The muscles of the lower extremities include (see Fig. 4.6):
- *Iliopsoas* (ill ee AWP sus): Flexes the thigh or trunk
- *Sartorius* (sar TOR ee us): Flexes the thigh and rotates the leg
- *Gluteus maximus* (gloo TEE us MAK sih mus): Extends the thigh
- Adductor group (adductor longus, adductor gracilis, and adductor pectineus): Adducts the thigh
- Hamstring group (semimembranosus, semitendinosus, and biceps femoris): Flexes the knee
- Quadriceps group (rectus femoris, vastus lateralis, vastus intermedius, and vastus medialis): Extends the knee
- *Tibialis* (tib ee AL is) *anterior*: Dorsiflexes ankle
- *Gastrocnemius* (gas trawk NEE mee us) and *soleus* (SEW lee us): Plantar flexes the ankle
- Fibularis group (fibularis longus, fibularis brevis, and fibularis tertius): Everts (turns outward) and plantar flexes the ankle

MEDICAL TERMINOLOGY

brachi/o	arm
cleid/o	collarbone
delt/o	triangle
duct/o	carrying
glute/o	buttock
long/o	long
mastoid/o	mastoid process
maxim/o	large
stern/o	breastbone
ad-	towards
bi-	two
-oid	like
-or	one who

CRITICAL THINKING 4.4

The major skeletal muscle names are listed in this section. Which of these muscles have you heard about? Explain.

PHYSIOLOGY OF THE MUSCULAR SYSTEM

Muscle tissues have four characteristics in common:
- *Excitability*: Ability to react to a stimulus
- *Contractility*: Ability to shorten in response to a stimulus
- *Extensibility*: Ability to be extended in response to a stimulus
- *Elasticity*: Quality of being elastic

The muscular system has four primary functions: (1) the muscles contract, providing muscle tone and posture; (2) the muscular system is responsible for maintaining the body temperature; (3) the muscular system provides joint stability; and (4) sphincters are responsible for controlling passageways in the body. The following sections will describe these four functions in more detail.

Muscle Contractions

Before a skeletal muscle can contract, it must be stimulated by an impulse that comes from the brain or spinal cord. The impulse moves away from the brain toward the muscle via a nerve cell, called a *motor neuron*. The point of contact between the nerve ending and the muscle fiber is called a *neuromuscular*

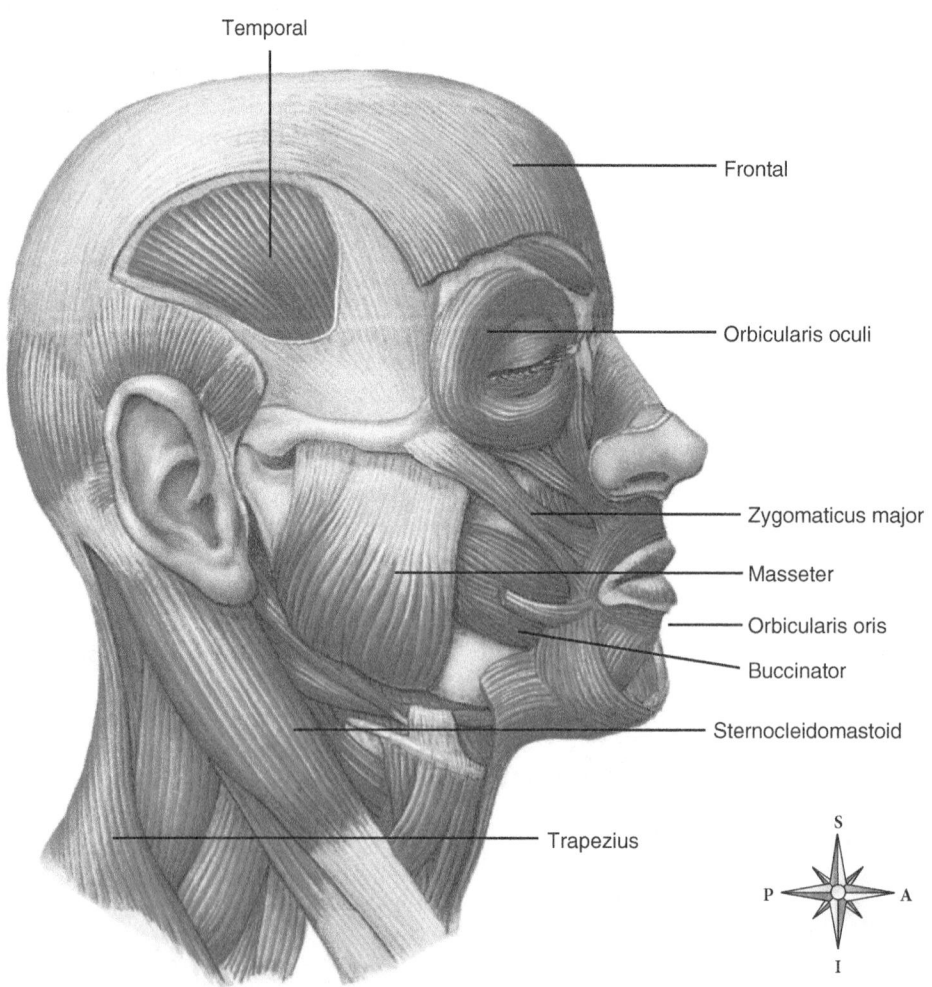

Temporal

Frontal

Orbicularis oculi

Zygomaticus major

Masseter

Orbicularis oris

Buccinator

Sternocleidomastoid

Trapezius

Fig. 4.5 Muscles of the Head and Neck. (From Patton K: *Structure and function of the body,* ed 15, St. Louis, 2016, Elsevier.)

junction (NMJ), a type of synapse (SIN aps). At the synapse, there is a very small gap called a *synaptic cleft*. Chemical messengers called *neurotransmitters* are released by the motor neuron in response to a nerve impulse.

Acetylcholine (ACh), a neurotransmitter, must travel across the synaptic cleft to continue the stimulus and generate a muscle contraction. The released ACh triggers a change in the permeability (pur mee ah BIL i tee) of the individual muscle fiber. Then, sodium ions flow into the fibers, causing calcium ions to be released from their storage area in the muscle fiber. When calcium is released, the thin actin fibers slide between the thick myosin fibers, causing the muscle to shorten, or *contract*. Muscles need calcium and energy in the form of adenosine triphosphate (ATP) to contract (Box 4.1). The muscle will relax once the ACh is inactivated by acetylcholinesterase (ah SEET l KOE leh nes teeh RASE) and the calcium ions are sent back to their storage areas of the muscle.

> **VOCABULARY**
>
> **acetylcholinesterase** An enzyme that destroys acetylcholine and counteracts its action.
> **adenosine triphosphate (ATP)** A high-energy molecule, found in every cell, that supplies large amounts of energy for various biochemical processes.
> **permeability** A quality or characteristic of a material that allows another substance to pass through it.
> **synapse** A point of communication between two cells.

CRITICAL THINKING 4.5

While Marissa reviews for her national exam, she sees the words *aerobic* and *anaerobic* discussed in different chapters. What do these terms mean?

Muscle Tone and Posture. Even when we are not actively moving, our muscles are in a state of partial contraction called *muscle tone*. Nerve impulses help maintain muscle tone so that muscles are ready to act when needed. Muscle tone is an important

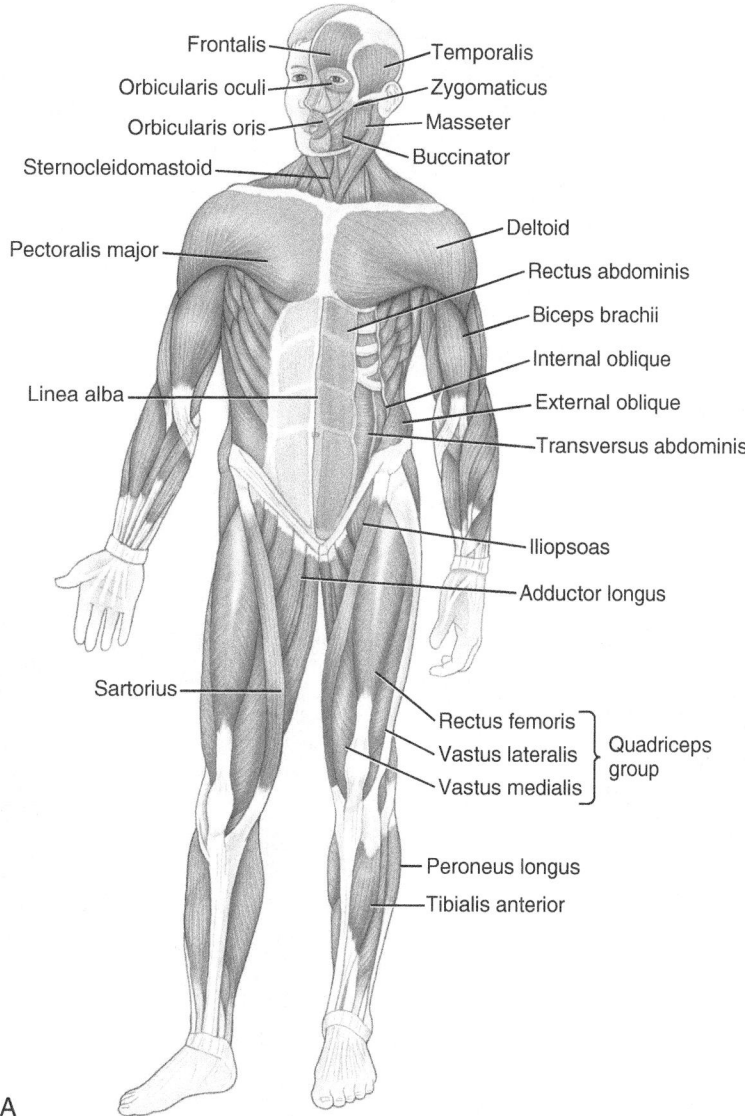

Fig. 4.6 Major Muscles of the Body. Anterior (A) and posterior (B) views. (From Shiland B: *Mastering healthcare terminology,* ed 5, St. Louis, 2016, Elsevier.)

Continued

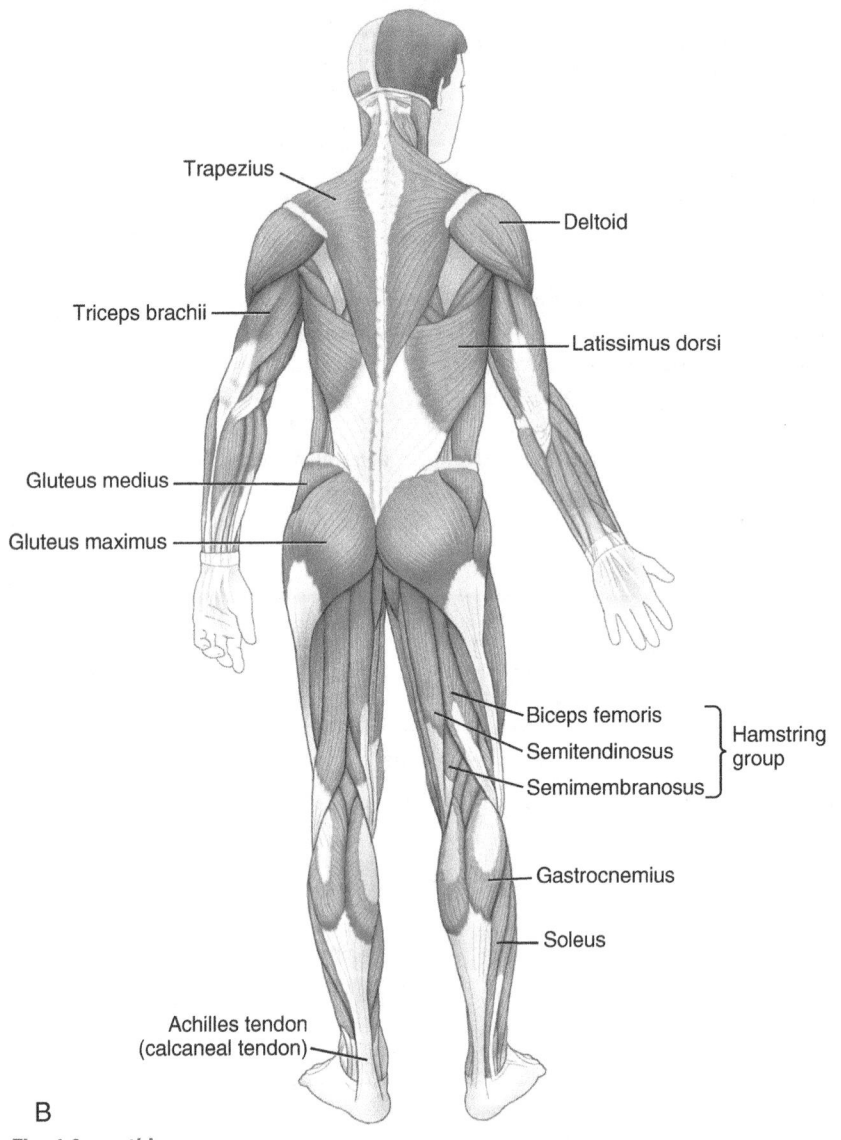

Trapezius

Deltoid

Triceps brachii

Latissimus dorsi

Gluteus medius

Gluteus maximus

Biceps femoris
Semitendinosus — Hamstring group
Semimembranosus

Gastrocnemius

Soleus

Achilles tendon
(calcaneal tendon)

B

Fig. 4.6, cont'd

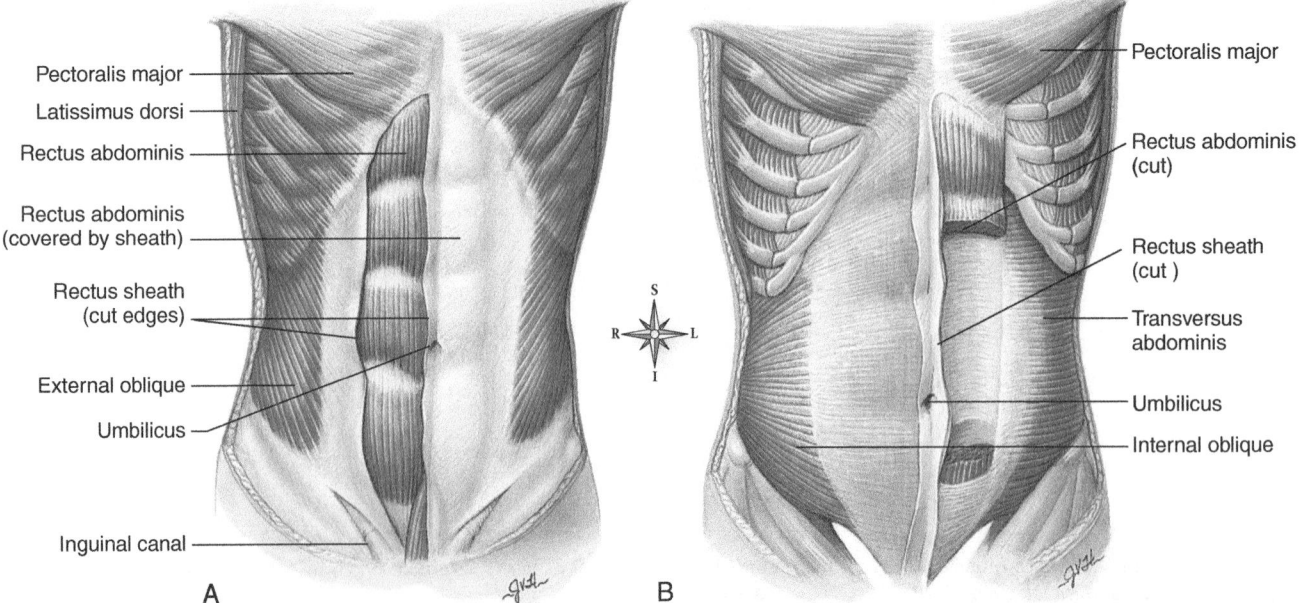

Pectoralis major

Latissimus dorsi

Rectus abdominis

Rectus abdominis
(covered by sheath)

Rectus sheath
(cut edges)

External oblique

Umbilicus

Inguinal canal

Pectoralis major

Rectus abdominis
(cut)

Rectus sheath
(cut)

Transversus
abdominis

Umbilicus

Internal oblique

A

B

Fig. 4.7 Muscles of the Trunk. (From Patton K: *Structure and function of the body,* ed 15, St. Louis, 2016, Elsevier.)

factor in proper posture. When sitting or standing, the *posture* (or the position of the body) is maintained by skeletal muscles. Muscle tone works against gravity to keep the body in a stationary position.

BOX 4.1   Muscle Fatigue

When you start exercising, your muscles feel strong. After repeating the same movements without rest, the muscles start to feel weaker, the strength decreases, and the ability to contract may be lost. This is called *muscle fatigue*.

For muscles to contract, they need APT. APT is produced through **aerobic respiration** with oxygen and glucose. If insufficient oxygen is available at the site for use, energy will be created through anaerobic respiration. A by-product of **anaerobic** respiration is lactic acid. As the lactic acid builds up in the muscle, it changes the pH of the muscle tissue. This causes the burning sensation in the muscle and leads to fatigue. As the person slows the activity, the breathing depth and rate remain at a high level. Extra oxygen is required until the lactic acid has been oxidized. The extra amount of oxygen required to rid the muscles of lactic acid is called *oxygen debt*. This is an example of **homeostasis**. The extra oxygen helps to return the energy and oxygen reserves to the normal, resting level.

Types of Muscle Contractions. Besides muscle tone and posture, four other types of muscle contractions include:

- *Twitch*: A quick, fine movement of a small area of muscles in response to a stimulus.
- *Tetanic*: Sustained and steady contraction response to a stimulus. Muscles can shorten, lengthen, or remain a constant length during a tetanic contraction. Lifting a heavy object with one hand is an example of a tetanic contraction. Tetanic contractions can occur with isotonic and isometric contractions.
- *Isotonic*: Muscle contraction that usually produces movement at a joint. The muscle usually shortens and thickens (bulges), and a task is done. Examples include walking, running, lifting weight, and twisting (Fig. 4.8).
- *Isometric*: Muscle contraction usually does not produce movement. There is no change in muscle length, but there is an increase in muscle tension. Examples include pushing against an immovable object, pushing against a wall, and pushing the palms together – there is no movement, but there is an increase in muscle tension.

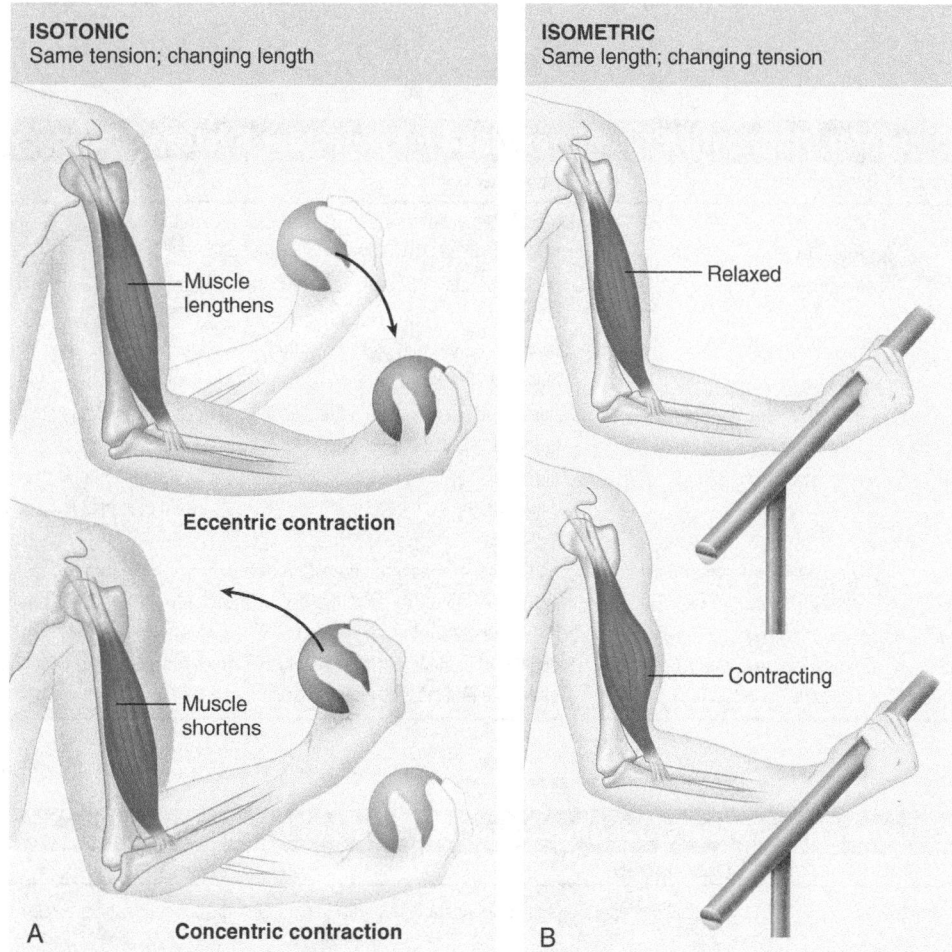

Fig. 4.8 Types of Muscle Contraction. A, In isotonic contraction the muscle changes length, producing movement either by eccentric contraction (muscle lengthens) or concentric contraction (muscle shortens). B, In isometric contraction the muscle pulls forcefully against a load but does not shorten. (From Patton KT, Thibodeau GA: *The human body in health and disease*, ed 7, St. Louis, 2018, Elsevier.)

Heat Production

A by-product of the energy (ATP) used for muscle contraction is heat production. All types of muscle contractions produce heat, with the skeletal muscles providing the most heat. About 85% of body heat comes from muscle contractions. When a person is cold, *shivering* (contractions of random skeletal muscles) produces heat. This helps maintain the body temperature.

Joint Stability

Muscles and tendons stabilize joints during movement and at rest. The tendons extend over the joint, stabilizing the joint. Joint stability depends on the strength and coordination of joint muscles. Muscle weakness can lead to joint instability.

Controlling Passageways

Sphincters are ringlike muscles that open and close body structures, regulating the flow of substances. Involuntary sphincters are found in the digestive tract, urethra, and the iris of the eye. The outer anal sphincter and urethral sphincter are voluntary and allow for a bowel movement and the passage of urine. These two sphincters are made of skeletal muscles.

DISEASES AND DISORDERS OF THE MUSCULAR SYSTEM

Disorders of the muscular system often involve other body systems, including the skeletal and nervous systems. Common signs and symptoms of muscular disorders include:
- Swelling in the joints and muscles
- *Malaise* (generalized weakness or discomfort)
- *Myalgia* (muscle pain), *myositis* (inflammation of a muscle), and muscle tenderness
- Temporary loss of function or loss of normal mobility

Common diagnostic procedures are listed on Table 4.2. Common treatments are listed on Table 4.3.

TABLE 4.2   Common Diagnostic Procedures Used for Muscular System Disorders

Done by/Type of Test:	Procedure	Description
Surgical procedure	*Biopsy* (BIE op see)	Surgical removal of tissue. A pathologist looks at the tissue sample under a microscope to check for disease, damage, or any other abnormalities.
Imaging procedure	*Myelography*	Uses fluoroscopy and contrast medium to evaluate the spinal cord and related structures.
Other procedures	*Electromyography (EMG)*	Checks the nerves and muscles. A thin needle electrode is inserted through the skin into the muscle and picks up the electrical activity in the muscle.
	Hand grip strength	Measured using a dynamometer (Fig. 4.9). Various arm and hand positions may be used for different assessments.
	Nerve conduction velocity (NCV)	Used with an EMG to test the speed of electrical signals through a nerve. Electrodes are placed on the skin. Each electrode gives off a mild electrical impulse that stimulates the nerve.
Medical laboratory	*Acetylcholine receptor (AChR) antibody test*	Blood test that measures the AChR antibodies, which are produced by the immune system. AChR antibodies mistakenly attack the protein, AChR, found on voluntary (skeletal) muscles.
	Creatine kinase (CK) or creatine phosphokinase (CPK)	Blood test that measures the CK, which is an enzyme that increases with damage or disease of the skeletal muscle, heart, or brain.

TABLE 4.3   Common Treatments Used for Muscular System Disorders

Procedure	Description
Fasciotomy (FASH ee ot ah mee)	Surgical procedure that involves opening the muscle compartment to reduce the pressure and restore blood flow
Myorrhaphy (mye ORE rah fee)	Surgical suturing of a muscle
Tenomyoplasty (ten oh MYE oh plas tee)	Surgical procedure to repair a tendon and muscle

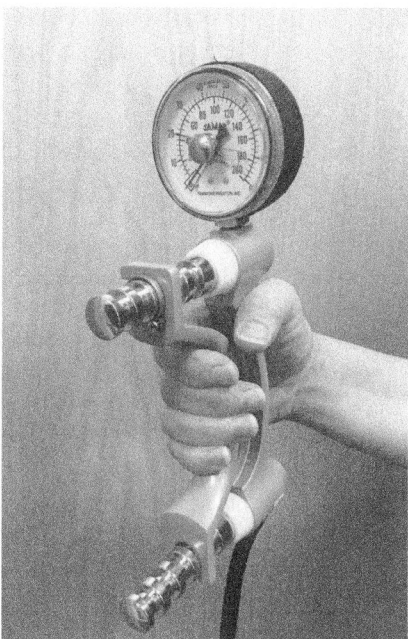

Fig. 4.9 Dynamometer.

VOCABULARY

aerobic Occurring in the presence of oxygen

anaerobic Occurring without the presence of oxygen

homeostasis The internal environment of the body that is compatible with life. A steady state that is created by all the body systems working together to provide a consistent and unvarying internal environment.

respiration A metabolic process by which cells break down substances (e.g., carbohydrates, amino acids, and fats) to produce adenosine triphosphate (ATP).

MEDICAL TERMINOLOGY

electr/o-	using electricity
myel/o	bone marrow, spinal cord
anti-	against
-algia	pain
-graphy	process of recording
-itis	inflammation

Compartment Syndrome

Compartment syndrome is a serious condition that can occur after a traumatic injury. Increased pressure is applied to muscle compartments, leading to muscle and nerve damage.

Etiology. Fascia separates groups of muscles. Inside each fascial layer is a compartment space that contains muscle tissue, nerves, and blood vessels. Swelling in the compartment space will lead to increased pressure in the area, because the fascia does not expand. Increased pressure can cause an interruption in the blood flow to the area, leading to muscle death.

Acute compartment syndrome can be caused by a fracture, bruised muscle, severe sprain, or a crushing injury. This condition can also occur if a cast or bandage is too tight. Chronic compartment syndrome is caused by repetitive activities, such as running.

Signs and Symptoms. Compartment syndrome can cause:
- Pale skin and swelling
- Decrease in sensation, numbness, tingling, and weakness
- Severe pain and inability to move the extremity

Diagnostic Procedures. After an exam, the provider may need to measure the compartment's pressure. A needle attached to a pressure meter is inserted into the compartment.

Treatments. Treatment includes immediate surgery (fasciotomy) to prevent permanent damage. To relieve the pressure, an incision is made in the fascia and muscle. With prompt treatment, the prognosis is good. If treatment is delayed, permanent muscle loss and nerve injury can occur.

Fibromyalgia

Fibromyalgia causes muscle pain, fatigue, and "tender points" on the legs, hips, back, arms, shoulders, and neck. It is estimated that 10 million people in the United States have fibromyalgia. Women develop fibromyalgia more often than men. Usually, the diagnosis occurs before age 50.

Etiology. The etiology is unknown. Research indicates that trauma, infection, or injury may change how the central nervous system (CNS) responds to pain, leading to chronic pain.

Signs and Symptoms. The signs and symptoms of fibromyalgia include widespread muscle pain, burning, aching, stiffness, or soreness. Additional symptoms include fatigue, sleep disturbances, mood and concentration problems, anxiety, headache, abdominal pain, bloating, constipation, diarrhea, bladder spasms, dizziness, numbness or tingling in the hands and feet, and tender points around the body.

Diagnostic Procedures. The provider will perform an examination and rule out other conditions. With no diagnostic tests for fibromyalgia, the provider may use these results:
- Widespread Pain Index (WPI) score, which evaluates 19 areas on the body for pain;
- Symptom Severity (SS) score, on which the patient scores specific fibromyalgia symptoms, including cognitive issues, fatigue, headache, and dizziness.

Treatments. The treatment is focused on minimizing the pain and fatigue experienced through the use of medications (e.g., pregabalin [Lyrica], duloxetine [Cymbalta], and milnacipran [Savella]), exercise, biofeedback, and acupuncture.

Ganglion Cyst

A *ganglion cyst* is a benign lump that develops in the wrist, hand, ankle, or foot. The cyst is filled with a jellylike fluid and develops along the tendons or joints.

Etiology. The cause of ganglion cysts is unknown. Women between the ages of 20 and 40 are more at risk. People with osteoarthritis or a joint or tendon injury also have a higher risk.

Signs and Symptoms. Ganglion cysts are round or oval lumps. These cysts are painless unless they put pressure on a nearby nerve. Then the person may experience tenderness, weakness, numbness, tingling, or pain in the affected area.

Diagnostic Procedures. After examining the cyst, the provider may order x-rays, an ultrasound, or magnetic resonance imaging (MRI). An *aspiration* of the fluid may also be done. During this procedure, the provider inserts a needle into the cyst and withdraws some of fluid to be analyzed. Ganglion cyst fluid is clear and thick.

Treatments. Treatment includes immobilization of the affected area. The provider may aspirate the fluid from the cyst. The cyst can also be surgically removed. With aspiration and surgical removal, the cyst might recur.

Muscle Atrophy

Muscle atrophy is the loss or wasting of muscle tissue. There are three types of muscle atrophy: physiologic, pathologic, and neurogenic.

Etiology

- *Physiologic atrophy*: When muscles are not used enough, muscle tissue is lost. People who are bedridden or have conditions that cause limited movement (e.g., casts, strokes) are at risk for muscle atrophy.
- *Pathologic atrophy*: Seen with starvation, long-term corticosteroid use, and with aging.
- *Neurogenic atrophy*: Caused when there is an injury or disease of a nerve that connects with a muscle. Amyotrophic lateral sclerosis (ALS), polio, and spinal cord injuries are examples of conditions that can lead to neurogenic atrophy. Additional causes include burns, malnutrition, muscular dystrophy, and osteoarthritis.

Signs and Symptoms. Muscle atrophy causes weakness in the extremity and a noticeably smaller arm or leg compared to the other one.

Diagnostic Procedures. After an examination, the provider may order blood tests, electromyography (EMG), muscle or nerve biopsies, nerve conduction studies, and imaging tests (e.g., x-rays, computed tomography [CT] scan, and MRI scan).

Treatments. Common treatments include exercise, physical therapy for strengthening, ultrasound therapy, a well-balanced diet, and surgery.

Muscular Dystrophy

Muscular dystrophy (MD) is a collection of over 30 inherited diseases that cause muscle weakness and muscle loss. Some of these diseases affect children, whereas others appear in middle-aged adults.

About half of the people with MD have Duchenne muscular dystrophy (DMD), which is the most common form of MD. DMD is usually diagnosed in boys between the ages of 3 and 5. This fast-progressing condition usually causes weakness in the arms and legs, leading to trouble walking. It is usually diagnosed by the age of 3. Boys are affected much more frequently than girls.

Etiology. Muscular dystrophy may be congenital or caused by a genetic mutation that disrupts the body's ability to make muscle-protecting proteins.

Signs and Symptoms. The signs, symptoms, onset, and affected muscle groups depend on the specific disease, though the main sign of MD is progressive muscle weakness. The signs and symptoms of Duchenne muscular dystrophy include frequent falls, trouble running and moving from lying to sitting position, muscle pain and stiffness, and learning disabilities.

Diagnostic Procedures. After the examination, the provider may order a creatine kinase (CK) blood test. Without trauma, high levels of CK suggest muscle disease, such as MD. Additional diagnostic tests include electromyography, genetic testing, and a muscle biopsy.

Treatments. Treatments can help improve quality of life, help people to remain mobile for as long as possible, and reduce or prevent bone and spinal complications. Treatments include corticosteroids, heart medication, range of motion and stretching exercises, braces, and assistive devices (e.g., walkers, wheelchairs). There is no cure for muscular dystrophy.

Myalgic Encephalomyelitis

Myalgic encephalomyelitis (mie AL jah en SEF ah loe mie eh lie tis) (ME), also called *chronic fatigue syndrome* (CFS), is a disabling, complex illness. People who have ME are not able to do their normal activities.

Etiology. ME is most common in people between the ages of 40 and 60, though it can affect anyone. Women are affected by it more often than men. The cause of ME is unknown, but it has been associated with viral infections.

Signs and Symptoms. Myalgic encephalomyelitis can cause:
- Greatly diminished ability to do activities that the person could do prior to the illness.
- Severe fatigue not relieved by sleep or rest.
- Sleep problems, either falling asleep or staying asleep.
- Problems with memory or thinking. Brain fog is common.
- Irregular heartbeat, shortness of breath, and orthostatic intolerance. The person may become dizzy, weak, faint, or lightheaded with standing or sitting upright.
- Digestive issues and allergies and sensitivities to foods and other products.
- Chills, night sweats, joint pain, and muscle weakness.

Diagnostic Procedures. The provider may do a complete physical and mental status examination. Blood, urine, and other tests may be ordered to rule out other conditions.

Treatments. Treatment includes management of symptoms. There is no cure for myalgic encephalomyelitis.

Myasthenia Gravis

Myasthenia gravis (mye ah STHEE nee ah GRAV us) affects the voluntary muscles, causing weakness and fatigue with activity, which improves with rest. Myasthenia gravis is most common in men over 60 and women younger than 40 years of age.

Etiology. The etiology is an autoimmune neuromuscular disease. The body produces antibodies that block the muscle cells from responding to neurotransmitters from nerve cells.

Signs and Symptoms. Myasthenia gravis causes muscle weakness, leading to issues with breathing, chewing, swallowing, talking, climbing stairs, lifting objects, and maintaining a steady gaze. Additional symptoms include drooping eyelids, facial paralysis, fatigue, hoarseness, and double vision.

Diagnostic Procedures. After a detailed neurologic examination, the provider will order imaging tests (CT or MRI), pulmonary function tests, and electromyography (EMG). With myasthenia gravis, the person will have a positive result on an acetylcholine receptor antibody blood test.

Treatments. The treatment is focused on increasing periods of remission. Lifestyle changes are encouraged, including resting, using eye patches, and avoiding stress and heat exposure, which can make symptoms worse. Medications such as neostigmine (nee oh STIG meen) (Prostigmin) and pyridostigmine (peer id oh STIG meen) (Mestinon) can help with the neuromuscular communication process. Immunosuppressants, including prednisone, azathioprine (ay za THYE oh preen) (Azasan, Imuran), cyclosporine (SYE kloe spor een) (Gengraf, Neoral, Sandimmune), and mycophenolate (mye koe FEN oh late) (CellCept, Myfortic), may also be used. There is no cure for myasthenia gravis.

VOCABULARY

autoimmune An immune response against a person's own tissues, cells, or cell parts, as in autoimmune disease, leading to the deterioration of tissue.
electrodes Adhesive patches that conduct electricity from the body to machine wires (e.g., electrocardiograph [ECG] and transcutaneous electri-cal nerve stimulation [TENS] unit).
immunosuppressant A drug used to suppress the immune system.
remission The partial or complete disappearance of the clinical and subjective characteristics of a chronic or malignant disease.

Myosistis

Myosistis is the inflammation of muscles. Types of myositis include:
- *Sporadic inclusion body myositis* (sIBM): The most common form of myositis. Affects people over 50 years of age. Symptoms gradually occur and make walking difficult.
- *Dermatomyositis* (DM): Affects people of all ages and is most common in women. Symptoms start with a rash on the face, chest, or extremities, followed by muscle weakness.
- *Polymyositis*: Affects people over 20 years of age and is most common in women. Muscle weakness in the chest, back, neck, and hips is the first symptom.

Etiology. An injury, infection, or an autoimmune disease can cause myositis.

Signs and Symptoms. Myositis can cause tripping, falling, problems breathing, difficulty swallowing, and fatigue with walking and standing.

Diagnostic Procedures. After an examination, the provider will order lab tests, imaging tests, and a muscle biopsy to diagnose myositis.

Treatments. Treatment includes corticosteroids, physical therapy, heat therapy, assistive devices, exercise, and rest. Treatment focuses on treating the symptoms. There is no cure for these diseases.

Shin Splints

Shin splints cause pain in the front of the lower leg. They are the result of inflammation of the bone tissue, tendons, and muscles around the shin (also called the *tibia*).

Etiology. The cause of shin splints is overusing the leg muscles, tendons, or shin bone. Runners, gymnasts, and dancers are most at risk for shin splints. Also, foot issues can lead to shin splints. Other risk factors of shin splints include:
- Having flat feet
- Working or exercising on a hard surface
- Wearing worn-out shoes or improper shoes

Signs and Symptoms. Signs and symptoms include sharp or dull, achy leg pain in the front of the shin. Pain may get worse with activity and better with rest.

Diagnostic Procedures. Many athletes are familiar with shin splints. The provider may order an x-ray to rule out a stress fracture.

Treatments. Treatment includes cold therapy, analgesics (an ahl JEE ziks), anti-inflammatories, arch supports, physical therapy, and doing stretching exercises. Preventing shin splints can be done by avoiding hard surfaces, wearing proper shoes, and doing warm-up exercises.

VOCABULARY
analgesics Drugs that reduce or eliminate pain.

Strain

A *strain* is a tear, partial tear, overuse, or overstretching of a muscle or tendon. A strain can occur suddenly or over time. Hamstring and back muscle strains are common.

Etiology. Acute strains occur with falling, jumping, and lifting heavy objects. Chronic strains occur with repetitive muscle movements, usually related to one's job or during a sport activity. Poor condition, fatigue, failing to do warm-up exercises, environmental conditions (e.g., ice), and poor equipment are risk factors for strains.

Signs and Symptoms. Signs and symptoms of strains include pain, swelling, and difficulty moving the affected muscle. With strains, muscle spasms may be felt.

Diagnostic Procedures. During the examination, the provider will check the affected area and the range of motion. X-rays and MRI scans may be ordered to rule out other injuries.

Treatments. Treatment includes *rest*, *ice* (cold applications), *compression* (elastic wraps), and *elevation* (RICE) to help minimize the swelling. Nonsteroidal anti-inflammatory drugs (NSAIDs) and analgesics may be taken. With severe strains, a brace or splint may be used to immobilize the area. Surgery may be done to repair a ruptured muscle. With treatment, the prognosis is good.

CRITICAL THINKING 4.7

Marissa overhears Dr. Kahn telling a patient to remember RICE for a strain. What does RICE stand for? Why is it used?

Tendinitis

Tendinitis (ten din EYE tis) is the inflammation of a tendon. Tendinitis causes severe swelling of the tendon.

Etiology. Tendinitis occurs after repeated injury to a joint, such as the wrist or ankle. Some of the most common forms are named after the sports that increase their risk:

- Tennis elbow (lateral epicondylitis): Causes pain in the forearm and wrist
- Golfer's elbow (medial epicondylitis): Causes pain in the inner forearm and numbness or tingling in the fingers
- Pitcher's shoulder, swimmer's shoulder, tennis shoulder (rotator cuff tendinitis, impingement syndrome): Causes pain and swelling in the front of the shoulder, clicking sound when raising arm, and loss of mobility
- Jumper's knee (patellar tendinitis): Pain occurs with bending or straightening of the leg

Signs and Symptoms. Tendinitis causes pain, tenderness, inflammation in the joint area, and a limited range of motion.

Diagnostic Procedures. The provider will do an examination. In most cases, x-rays and other imaging procedures are not required unless the problem continues.

Treatments. Treatment consists of rest, splinting, heat and cold therapy, medications (NSAIDs, analgesics, and corticosteroid injections), and physical therapy.

MEDICAL TERMINOLOGY

epicondyle/o	epicondyle
tendin/o, tend/o, ten/o	tendon

Tetanus

Tetanus (TET n us), also called "lockjaw," is a serious condition, that can lead to a medical emergency. Getting the tetanus vaccine can help prevent tetanus.

Etiology. Tetanus is caused by *Clostridium tetani* bacteria. The spores from the *Clostridium tetani* bacteria are found in the soil, dust, manure, and saliva. Often, the spores enter the body through an injury, such as a deep cut, puncture wound, or eye injury. Once the spores enter the body, they develop into bacteria.

Signs and Symptoms. Tetanus can cause:
- Painful muscle stiffness throughout the body
- Trouble opening the mouth and swallowing and jaw cramping
- Headache and seizures
- Fever, sweating, and vital sign changes (e.g., blood pressure and pulse)

Diagnostic Procedures. The provider performs an exam. No diagnostic tests exist to confirm tetanus.

Treatments. Treatment includes hospitalization, human tetanus immune globulin (TIG), and medications to manage the muscle spasms, tetanus vaccine, and antibiotics. The more severe the case of tetanus, the poorer the prognosis. For those that survive tetanus, recovery may take up to 4 months.

Torticollis

Torticollis occurs when the neck muscles spasm. This causes the head to tilt, lean forward or backward, or to be rotated.

Etiology. Torticollis can be genetic. In infants it can be caused by birth trauma or a spinal abnormality. In adults it can be caused by poor posture, insufficient head support while sleeping, or neck injury or infection.

Signs and Symptoms. Torticollis causes:
- Neck spasms and tremor
- Headache and neck pain
- Swelling and stiffness of neck muscles
- One shoulder possibly being higher than the other
- Limited range of motion for the head

Diagnostic Procedure. After an examination, the provider may order an x-ray or CT scan.

Treatments. Treatment for torticollis present at birth involves passive stretching of the shortened neck muscle. Depending on the cause, treatment may involve heat and cold therapy, physical

OnabotulinumtoxinA (o na BOTT you lye num tox in eh) (Botox, Botox Cosmetic) is classified as a neurotoxin. It is made from a toxin produced by *Clostridium botulinum;* the same toxin can also cause botulism. Small doses of Botox are used to treat a variety of conditions such as:

- Cervical dystonia and spasmodic torticollis
- Overactive bladder and incontinence
- *Blepharospasm* (uncontrollable blinking) and *strabismus* (misaligned eyes, "crossed eyes")
- Chronic migraines and *hyperhidrosis* (excessive sweating)
- *Spasticity* (muscle stiffness and tightness) in patients with cerebral palsy and patients who have had a stroke
- Facial wrinkles

The provider will inject a number of tiny doses of Botox into a specific muscle. The medication blocks the nerve signals that cause the muscle tightness and spasms. When used for sweating, injections of Botox can reduce the activity of the sweat glands. When injected into the bladder tissue, it reduces the bladder contractions and blocks nerve signals that indicate the bladder is full.

Botox can cause serious side effects, including visual changes, seizures, irregular heartbeat, chest pain, hives, and shortness of breath. Symptoms of overdose include weakness, difficulty moving any part of the body, and difficulty with breathing and swallowing. Symptoms of an overdose indicate a medical emergency.

therapy, Botox injections (Box 4.2), and surgery if other treatments fail.

Additional Muscular System Diseases and Disorders

Several other muscular system diseases include:

- *Botulism* (BOT choo liz um): A rare but serious disease caused by *Clostridium botulinum,* which enters the body through contaminated food (e.g., honey, home-preserved/canned foods).

The toxins cause muscle paralysis, leading to visual changes, slurred speech, and difficulty swallowing and breathing.
- *Congenital myopathies:* Rare congenital diseases that cause a lack of muscle tone and muscle weakness, cramps, and contractions, along with delayed motor skills, facial weakness, and drooping eyelids.
- *Endocrine myopathies:* Caused by abnormal thyroid gland activity; they lead to weakness, atrophy, stiffness, cramps, and slowed reflexes.
- *Myotonia congenita* (MIE oh TOE nee ah kon JEN i tah): A congenital condition that causes a delay in muscle relaxation after contraction. Early symptoms include difficulty swallowing, shortness of breath, falls, and difficulty opening the eyes. After the person starts moving, the muscles relax, and the movements become normal.
- *Sarcopenia* (sar koe PEE nee ah): Causes progressive skeletal muscle loss due to age; this causes a decrease in muscle strength.

LIFE SPAN CHANGES

Men can see muscle changes in their 20s, whereas women are usually in their 40s when changes become obvious. With age, muscle tissue is replaced more slowly and may be replaced with tough, fibrous tissue. This makes the extremities look thin and bony. Muscles have less of an ability to contract. Lean body mass decreases. With the muscle mass changes, older people experience loss of strength and endurance. They can experience fatigue and reduced activity tolerance. *Fasciculations* (fah SIK yeh LAE shuhns) (involuntary muscle tremors and fine movements) are more common with age. People who are unable to move an extremity may get muscle contractures.

CLOSING COMMENTS

Patients with muscular disorders are seen in primary care, urgent care, and specialty departments. It is important for the medical assistant to be familiar with the names and locations of muscles. Knowing how to pronounce the muscle names is critical in healthcare for communicating with the provider, peers, and patients. The medical assistant should also be knowledgeable about common muscular system symptoms, disorders, diagnostic tests, and treatments. Box 4.3 lists medication classifications commonly used to treat muscular system disorders.

- *Analgesics:* Relieve pain
- *Anticholinesterase agents:* Block the action of cholinesterase, which treats conditions such as myasthenia gravis.
- *Anti-inflammatories:* Reduce the inflammation in the body and are used to treat injuries and inflammatory conditions, such as strains and tendinitis.
- *Immunosuppressants:* Suppress the immune response and are used to treat conditions such as myasthenia gravis.

- *Muscle relaxants:* Work on the central nervous system (CNS) to relax muscles, which treats conditions such as strains and muscle injuries.

Refer to Appendix D, which can be found on the Evolve website, for information on the medication classifications, including indications for use, desired effect, side effects, adverse reactions, and generic and trade names. Medical assistants should be familiar with medications that are prescribed to patients.

PATIENT-CENTERED CARE

With muscular system disorders, a patient may experience limited mobility or have pain with moving. One of the ways to help provide patient-centered care is to provide the patient with information on safety at home. Patients using assistive devices such as crutches or canes should wear shoes with nonskid soles. Throw rugs, cords, and toys should be removed from walkways. Adaptive ideas for safely bathing and grooming are important for patients to know. Providing patients with helpful tips on home care is important for the patient's safety.

BEING PROFESSIONAL

Pain and limited mobility resulting from muscular disorders can affect a person's behavior. A patient may be short tempered or have limited patience. A medical assistant must remember to talk calmly and remain composed, even if the patient is not. Treating a patient with respect and listening to the person's concerns, helps the patient feel respected.

Role-play this scenario: You are a medical assistant. Mr. Green has had significant pain and mobility limitations with his tendinitis. He has returned for a follow-up visit. You ask him how he is feeling. He appears upset and angry. He states, "I am in pain. I cannot walk, sit, or sleep. If I do not get something to stop this pain, I am going elsewhere." Respond to Mr. Green in a respectful, professional manner.

CHAPTER REVIEW

Muscle tissue is composed of muscle fibers or myocytes. The three types of muscles include:

- Skeletal: Have multiple nuclei and striations. These voluntary muscles are found throughout the body, attached to bones, and in the digestive and urinary systems.
- Smooth: Are nonstriated and have a single nucleus. These involuntary muscles are found in many systems, including the respiratory, cardiovascular, urinary, reproductive, and digestive systems.
- Cardiac: Are involuntary, striated muscles found in the walls of the heart.

An entire skeletal muscle is considered an organ. The muscle contains three layers of connective tissue. The endomysium wraps around the muscle fiber. The perimysium covers each fascicle, which contains many muscle fibers. The epimysium covers the entire muscle organ, which is composed of many fascicles.

Skeletal muscles are often based on the characteristics of the muscle. The major skeletal muscles include:

- Head and neck: Frontal, orbicularis oculi, orbicularis oris, zygomaticus, buccinator, temporal, masseter, sternocleidomastoid, and the trapezius.
- Upper extremity: Pectoralis major, latissimus dorsi, deltoid, biceps brachii, and triceps brachii.
- Abdominal: External oblique, internal oblique, transversus abdominis, rectus abdominis, and diaphragm.

- Lower extremity: Iliopsoas, sartorius, gluteus maximus, adductor group (adductor longus, adductor gracilis, and adductor pectineus), hamstring group (semimembranosus, semitendinosus, and biceps femoris), quadriceps group (rectus femoris, vastus lateralis, vastus intermedius, and vastus medialis), tibialis anterior, gastrocnemius, soleus, and the fibularis group (fibularis longus, fibularis brevis, and fibularis tertius).

Muscle tissue has four characteristics: excitability, contractility, extensibility, and elasticity. These characteristics allow the muscle to contract, stretch, and return to its normal size. Muscles have four primary functions, including contraction, heat production, joint stability, and controlling passageways.

Many muscular disorders were discussed in the chapter. Common signs and symptoms of skeletal disorders include swelling in the joints and muscles, malaise, myalgia, myositis, and muscle tenderness. Common diagnostic procedures include EMG, hand grip strength, myelography, and nerve conduction velocity.

The muscular system changes with age. The muscle tissue is replaced more slowly. Fibrous tissue replaces muscle tissue. Muscles get fatigued easier, and the person has less strength and endurance. Activity tolerance is reduced. Fasciculations can occur with age.

SCENARIO WRAP-UP

Suzanne and Marissa had a busy afternoon in urgent care. Suzanne had Marissa shadow her while they roomed patients. She knew that Marissa would learn many things by just watching the process of obtaining a patient's history. With many of the patients having musculoskeletal concerns, Marissa quickly learned the type of information that should be obtained from patients.

Suzanne asked about the symptoms, when they started, what made them better and worse, and a history of similar symptoms. Both Suzanne and Marissa are looking forward to the next time Dr. Kahn works in urgent care.

5

Integumentary System

LEARNING OBJECTIVES

1. Discuss the anatomy of the integumentary system, including membranes, skin, and accessory structures.
2. Describe how the integumentary system helps maintain homeostasis.
3. Explain the common diagnostic procedures and treatments for integumentary system disorders.
4. Describe common integumentary system disorders, including signs and symptoms, etiology, diagnostic procedures, and treatments.
5. Compare the structure and function of the integumentary system across the life span.

OUTLINE

▶▶ OPENING SCENARIO

Mai Vang is a medical assistant who has been working at the Walden-Martin Family Medical (WMFM) Clinic for 2 years. She really wanted to work in a family practice clinic so that she could see patients of varying ages and medical conditions. Mai has noticed that skin conditions are a frequent reason for patient visits. When she was in high school, she visited her physician to get help for an acne breakout that would not go away. She remembers feeling self-conscious about the condition, so she tries to be especially sensitive to patients with skin diseases and disorders.

Today Mai's first patient after lunch is Casey Hernandez. She is coming in to see Jean Burke, the WMFM Clinic nurse practitioner (NP).

YOU WILL LEARN

1. To describe the connective tissue and epithelial membranes of the body.
2. To explain the two layers of the skin, along with the role of the dermal-epidermal junction.
3. To describe the accessory glands, including their location and functions.

4. To describe the five functions of the integumentary system that help maintain homeostasis.

5. To recognize common diagnostic procedures and treatments for integumentary system disorders.

6. To describe common integumentary system disorders, including signs and symptoms, etiology, diagnostic procedures, and treatments.

7. To discuss the structure and function of the integumentary system across the life span.

INTRODUCTION

Dermatology (der mah TAW loh jee) is the healthcare specialty that deals with most skin diseases and disorders. A *dermatologist* (der mah TAW loh jist) is a specialist involved in the diagnosis, treatment, and prevention of disorders of the integumentary (in te gyoo MEN tair ee) system.

Besides the dermatology department, patients with skin, hair, and nail concerns can be seen in primary care and also urgent care departments. Rashes, burns, nail trauma, and skin cancer are common patient concerns in these departments. The medical assistant may help the provider with the examination, diagnostic tests, and medical procedures.

ANATOMY OF THE INTEGUMENTARY SYSTEM

Another name for integument (in TE gyoo ment) is skin, which is also the prime organ of the integumentary system. The nails, hair, and skin glands are also part of the integumentary system.

Membranes

The skin is considered a membrane. A membrane is a thin, flexible layer of tissue that:

- Covers and protects the body surface
- Lines body cavities and covers organs within the body cavities
- Lines the inside surfaces of hollow digestive, respiratory, and reproductive organs
- Connects structures (e.g., bones to organs)

There are two types of membranes: connective tissue and epithelial (ep i THEE lee al) membranes.

Connective Tissue Membranes. Connective tissue membranes are composed of connective tissue. Connective tissue membranes cover organs, such as the kidneys. They also line diarthroses, or synovial (sih NOH vee al) joints, such as the knee and hip joints. Connective tissue membranes lining synovial joints are called *synovial membranes*. Synovial membranes secrete *synovial fluid* that lubricates the joint.

Epithelial Membranes. Epithelial membranes are made of epithelial tissue and connective tissue. Three types of epithelial membranes are mucous (MYOO cus), serous (SEER us), and cutaneous (kyoo TAY nee us) membranes.

Mucous Membranes. Mucous membranes, also called *mucosae* (myoo KOE see), consist of epithelial tissue that is attached to an underlying loose connective tissue. Mucous membranes line the body cavities that open to the outside. The respiratory, urinary, reproductive, and digestive system organs that open to the outside are lined with mucous membranes.

The epithelial cells secrete mucus, which keeps membranes soft and moist. Mucus is a thick, slimy substance that provides protection and aids movement of substances. Mucus is part of the immune system's first line of defense.

Serous Membranes. Serous membranes cover organs and line body cavities that do not open to the outside. With serous membranes, the epithelium secretes a thin layer of serous fluid, lubricating the membrane. When two organs move against each other, friction can occur. Friction is reduced when serous fluid lubricates the serous membranes.

Pleura (PLOOR uh) is a serous membrane found in the thoracic cavity. The pleura folds back on itself, creating a sac that surrounds the lung. The *visceral pleura* (VIH sur ul PLOOR ah) covers the lungs and adjoining structures. The *parietal pleura* (puh RYE uh tul PLOOR ah), the outer portion of the pleura, lines the thoracic cavity and covers the diaphragm (DYE uh fram) and mediastinum (mee dee uh STY num). Only the parietal pleura contains pain receptors, making it highly sensitive to pain. The right and left pleural sacs are entirely separate.

The *pleural cavity* is the space between the visceral and parietal pleurae. A small amount of pleural fluid is in the pleural cavity. When the lungs expand, moving the visceral pleura closer to the parietal pleura, friction is reduced between the tissues due to the pleural fluid.

Peritoneum (PER i tn ee hum) is the serous membrane in the abdominal cavity. The visceral peritoneum covers most of the organs in the abdomen. The parietal peritoneum lines the abdominal wall and pelvic cavity.

Cutaneous Membrane. The cutaneous membrane, or the skin, is the largest organ of the integumentary system. The skin will be discussed in depth later in the chapter.

VOCABULARY

epithelial cells Form cellular sheets that cover surfaces, both inside and outside the body. Epithelial cells are closely packed, take on different shapes, and strongly stick to each other.

diaphragm A broad, dome-shaped muscle used for breathing. It separates the thoracic and abdominopelvic cavities.

mediastinum The space in the thoracic cavity that lies between the lungs, containing the heart, trachea, and esophagus.

MEDICAL TERMINOLOGY

diaphragm/o, diaphragmat/o, phren/o	diaphragm
pleur/o	pleura
viscer/o	viscera

Skin

The skin weighs about 6 pounds and covers 18 square feet on an average adult. The skin is about 2 mm thick. The thickness and color of the skin vary over the body. There are two types of skin:

- Thick, hairless skin. This is found on the soles of the feet and the palms of the hands. This type of skin can withstand heavy use and large amounts of friction.

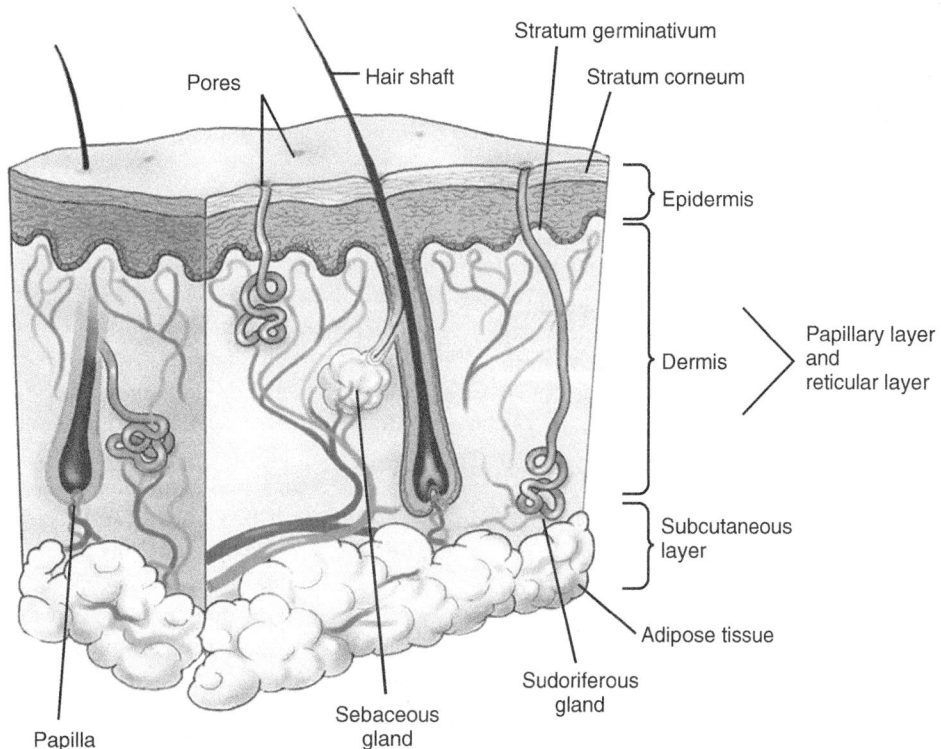

Fig. 5.1 Diagram of the Skin. (From Shiland B: *Mastering healthcare terminology,* ed 5, St. Louis, 2016, Elsevier.)

- Thin, hairy skin. This is the most common type of skin on the body.

The skin is composed of the epidermis and the dermis. These two layers cover a third fatty layer, called the *subcutaneous* (sub kyoo TAY nee us) *tissue* or the *hypodermis* (Fig. 5.1).

Epidermis. The epidermis is the outer layer of the skin (see Fig. 5.1). It is composed of several different strata of epithelial tissue. The depth of the epidermis varies around the body. The eyelid is about 0.05 mm, whereas the palms and soles are 1.5 mm.

The innermost layer of the epidermis is called the *basal cell layer* or *stratum germinativum* (STRAH tum jur mih nuh TIH vum). The basal cells multiply by mitosis. The new cells push upward. Over time, as these cells reach the surface, the cytoplasm in the cells is replaced with keratin. *Keratin* is a tough, waterproof protein. The tough outer layer of the epidermis is called the *stratum corneum* (KOR nee uhm). The cells of the outer layer continually flake off. Complete cell turnover occurs every 28 to 30 days in young adults and every 45 to 50 days in older adults.

The basal cell layer contains *melanocytes* (meh LAN oh sites), which are cells that produce melanin. *Melanin* is a pigment that gives skin its tan or brown color. It helps protect the deeper layers of the skin from the ultraviolet rays of the sun. With sun exposure, melanocytes increase the production of melanin, causing a suntan. Birthmarks, freckles, and age spots derive from patches of melanin.

Besides melanocytes, the epidermis contains Langerhans cells (involved in the immune system), sensory nerves, and Merkel (MER kul) cells. The *Merkel cells* are close to the nerve endings in the basal cell layer. These cells are involved with the sense of touch.

> **VOCABULARY**
> **strata** Naturally or artificially formed layers of material, usually multiple layers.

Dermal-Epidermal Junction. A specialized basement membrane is found at the junction where the dermis and epidermis meet. This junction is called the *dermal-epidermal junction.* The top layer of the dermis contains *dermal papillae* (pah PILL ee), which are peglike projections. These help fasten the dermis and epidermis together. Besides the dermal papillae, the dermal-epidermal junction contains a specialized gel that acts as a glue to keep the two layers of the skin connected.

A burn, irritation, friction, or abrasion can damage the dermal-epidermal junction. This can cause a blister. Damage to the dermal-epidermal junction can cause the skin to fall apart. The body can heal a small, damaged area, but a large area can lead to overwhelming infection.

> **CRITICAL THINKING 5.1**
> Yesterday Mai wore a new pair of shoes to work and developed a little blister on the heel of her right foot. What skin layers are affected by the formation of a blister? How should Mai properly care for her blister over the next few days?

Dermis. The *dermis* is the thick, underlying layer of the skin (see Fig. 5.1). It provides about 90% of the thickness of the skin. Collagen (KAW lah jen) and elastin (ee LAS tin) fibers in the dermis give the skin strength and stretch. The epidermis does not have these characteristics. The dermis is composed of vascular connective tissue arranged in two layers.

- *Papillary (pah PILL air ee) layer:* The upper, thin layer of the dermis. Much of the papillary layer is composed of fibers made from loose connective tissue, collagen, and some elastic fibers.
- *Reticular* (reh TIC koo lahr) *layer:* The lower, thicker layer, which is composed of dense collagen and elastin fibers. The reticular layer holds the *hair follicles* (FAW lih kuls), *sudoriferous* (soo doh RIF er us) *glands,* and *sebaceous* (seh BAY shus) *glands.*

The dermis contains many small blood vessels that supply the skin with nutrients and oxygen. The blood also takes away waste products and carbon dioxide and transports the vitamin D produced in the skin. Lymph and lymph vessels present in the dermis help destroy infections or invading organisms. The dermis also contains the hair follicles, sweat and oil glands, and nerve endings. The subcutaneous tissue sits below the dermis.

VOCABULARY

collagen The most abundant structural protein found in skin and other connective tissues. It provides strength and cushioning to many parts of the body.

elastin A highly elastic protein in connective tissue that allows tissues to resume their shape after stretching or contracting. It is found abundantly in the dermis of the skin.

exocrine gland A gland that secretes substances through a duct.

pores Tiny openings in the surface of the skin that allow gases, liquids, or microscopic particles to pass.

Subcutaneous Tissue. The subcutaneous tissue is not a layer of the skin. It lies below the dermis and creates a connection between the skin and the structures that are below the skin, such as muscle or bone (see Fig. 5.1). Subcutaneous tissue is made up of loose connective tissue and adipose (fat) tissue. This tissue is not rigid, but rather movable and pliable. The subcutaneous tissue can slip over underlying structures. Without subcutaneous tissue, our skin would tear with movement.

MEDICAL TERMINOLOGY

adip/o	fat
bas/o	base
cutane/o	skin
derm/o	skin
kerat/o	hard, horny
melan/o	black, dark
a-	without
epi-	above, upon
hypo-, sub-	under, below
-ar, -ous	pertaining to
-cyte	cell
-in	substance
-is	structure

Accessory Structures

Glands. The skin contains exocrine (EK suh krin) glands, which secrete substances. The *sudoriferous* glands, also called *sweat glands,* are located in the dermis (see Fig. 5.1). The role of the sudoriferous

glands is to secrete sweat through tiny pores in the surface of the skin. The sweat, or *perspiration,* on the skin helps to cold down. There are two types of sweat glands.

- *Eccrine* (EK rin) glands are most numerous and are found throughout the body. Greater numbers of these glands are found on the soles, palms, upper lip, and forehead. Eccrine glands are responsible for the highest volume of perspiration. These glands start to function around age 2, and the total number of glands is fixed throughout life. No additional glands form with age. Eccrine sweat is mostly salt water.
- *Apocrine* (AP uh krin) glands are concentrated in the axilla, breast, perineum, face, and scalp. Apocrine glands are larger than eccrine glands. They open into a hair follicle instead of onto the skin's surface. Apocrine glands start functioning at puberty. Apocrine sweat is a thick fat-rich liquid made of proteins, sugars, and ammonia.

Sebaceous (seh BAY shus) glands are found everywhere on the body except the soles and the palms. These glands secrete an oily, acidic substance called *sebum* (SEE bum). The tiny ducts of a sebaceous gland open into the hair follicle. The oil helps to lubricate hair and keep the skin soft and waterproof. The oil also inhibits the overgrowth of bacteria and fungi. Sebaceous glands produce more oil during puberty in response to the increased level of sex hormones.

CRITICAL THINKING 5.2

Mai goes to the waiting area and calls back Casey Hernandez. She introduces herself and shows Casey back to the exam room. After vital signs are completed, Mai asks Casey the reason for her visit. Casey is looking down and is a bit shy as she talks. Mai notices that the palms of Casey's hands are sweaty. What types of glands produce sweat in the integumentary system? Where are they concentrated in the body?

Hair. Hair has its roots in the dermis. The hair roots, together with their coverings, are called *hair follicles* (FALL ih kuls). The visible part of hair is called the *hair shaft.* Underneath the follicle is a nipple-shaped structure called the *papilla* (puh PIL uh). Dermal blood vessels nourish the papilla. Epithelial cells on top of the papilla are responsible for the formation of the hair shaft. When these cells die, the hair can no longer regenerate, and hair loss occurs.

The main function of hair is to assist in temperature regulation by holding heat near the body. When it is cold, hair stands on end, holding a layer of air as insulation near the body. This process is called *piloerection* (py loh ee REK shun). There is a small smooth muscle at the base of every dermal papilla that also attaches to the side of a hair follicle. This little muscle is called the *arrector pili* (ah REK tor pil ee). When the muscle contracts, piloerection occurs. This also happens when a person is scared.

Nails. Nails cover and protect the dorsal surfaces of the distal bones of the fingers and toes (Fig. 5.2). The parts of the nail include:

- *Nail body* or *nail plate,* the visible part of the nail.
- *Nail root,* which is located in a groove under the *cuticle* (KYOO tih kul) (the small fold of skin at the base of the nail).

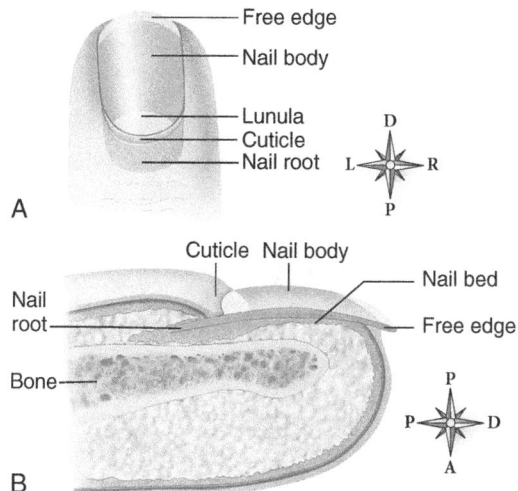

Fig. 5.2 Structure of Nails. A, Posterior view of fingernail. B, Sagittal section of fingernail and associated structures. (From Patton KT, Thibodeau GA: *The human body in health and disease*, ed 7, St. Louis, 2018, Elsevier.)

- *Nail bed*, which is the highly vascular tissue under the nail. The nail bed normally appears pink. If the nail bed appears blue or purple, it indicates that the person is oxygen deficient.
- *Lunula* (LOON yoo lah), the moonlike white area at the base of the nail.
- *Paronychium* (pair ih NICK ee um), the fold of skin near the sides of the nail.

MEDICAL TERMINOLOGY	
follicul/o	follicle
onych/o	nail
papill/o	papilla
seb/o	sebum
sebac/o	oil
sudor/i	sweat
trich/o, pil/o	hair
par-	near
-ferous	pertaining to carrying
-ium	structure

PHYSIOLOGY OF THE INTEGUMENTARY SYSTEM

The integumentary system is involved protection, temperature regulation, sensory organ activity, excretion, *synthesis,* or formation, of vitamin D, and repair of the skin. These activities help maintain homeostasis.

Protection

The most important function of the integumentary system is protecting the body from disease. The integumentary system protects the body in several ways:

- By providing a physical barrier. The skin is our first line of defense against *pathogens* (disease-causing microorganisms), toxic chemicals, and physical tears, cuts, and abrasions.
- By providing a flexible, waterproof barrier. The skin protects the internal organs from the outside environment. The keratin in our skin cells protects us from excessive fluid loss and dehydration.
- From damaging ultraviolet (UV) light, with the help of melanin in the epidermis.
- From microbial over colonization on the skin surface. *Dermcidin,* a substance found in sweat, has antibacterial and antifungal properties. Thus sweat can help deter microbes.

Skin Repair. As part of its protection role, the skin repairs itself. After an injury, such as a cut or scrape, the skin starts the repair/healing process. If bleeding occurs, a clot will form within minutes if not sooner (Fig. 5.3). This stops the bleeding. The blood clot dries and forms a scab. The scab protects the underlying tissue from pathogens. The immune system will help protect the area from pathogens during the repair process.

Cells of the stratum germinativum produce more epithelial cells. These cells rebuild the epidermis. Collagen fibers are also produced by cells in the dermis. Over time the clot dissolves, the scab falls off, and the epidermis and dermis are repaired. The new tissue forms a scar, which is denser than the original tissue. Over time the scar will fade and may completely disappear.

Temperature Regulation

The skin is a very good thermoregulator. When the skin is exposed to a cold temperature, the blood vessels constrict in the dermis. This limits the flow of warm blood to the surface of the body and prevents heat loss.

In high temperatures or with vigorous exercise, sudoriferous glands secrete perspiration. Up to 1.5 L of sweat can be produced per hour in an active person. The heat from the body transfers to the perspiration on the surface of the skin. As the perspiration evaporates from the skin surface, the body is cooled. In addition to perspiration, the body is also cooled as the arterioles in the dermis dilate. An increased amount of blood moves through the dermis. Heat in the blood can dissipate through the skin and into the surrounding environment, cooling the body. The increased blood flow causes the skin to appear red.

Sensory Organ Activity

The skin has many sensory receptors scattered throughout the dermis. Sensory receptors can feel pain, pressure, heat, and cold. This allows us to respond to the environment and make appropriate changes to keep ourselves from harm.

Excretion

The body can regulate the amount of sweat produced and the chemical content of the sweat. When we sweat, we lose water, electrolytes, and small amounts of other waste products. The integumentary system can excrete substances through the skin to help maintain the necessary chemical balance in the body as a whole.

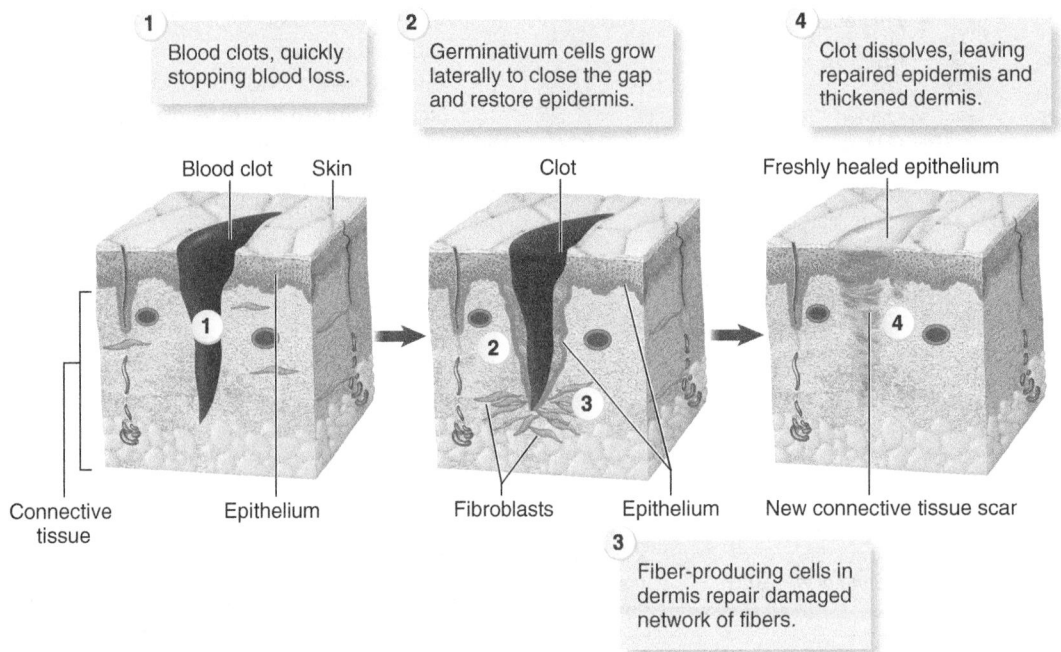

1 Blood clots, quickly stopping blood loss.

2 Germinativum cells grow laterally to close the gap and restore epidermis.

4 Clot dissolves, leaving repaired epidermis and thickened dermis.

Blood clot Skin

Clot

Freshly healed epithelium

Connective tissue

Epithelium

Fibroblasts Epithelium

New connective tissue scar

3 Fiber-producing cells in dermis repair damaged network of fibers.

Fig. 5.3 Skin Repair. A minor skin injury is followed by blood clotting and self-repair of the damaged epidermis and dermis. (From Patton KT, Thibodeau GA: *The human body in health and disease,* ed 7, St. Louis, 2018, Elsevier.)

BOX 5.1   Vitamin D Supplements

To make vitamin D, manufacturers use plant sterols found in plant cell membranes. It is comparable to cholesterol in the human body. The plant sterols must be exposed to ultraviolet energy to produce vitamin D_2. Many manufacturers just label vitamin D_2 as "vitamin D." When a person takes a vitamin D supplement, the body needs to convert it to a useable form, just as it does for vitamin D_3.

Synthesis of Vitamin D

Vitamin D is *synthesized*, or produced, in the skin. A form of cholesterol is always found in the skin. The sun's ultraviolet B (UVB) energy converts this cholesterol to vitamin D_3. Vitamin D_3 is transported by the blood to the liver and then the kidneys. The kidneys will transform the vitamin D_3 into an active, usable form of vitamin D (Box 5.1).

Vitamin D increases the intestinal absorption of phosphorus and calcium. Without vitamin D, only 10% to 15% of dietary calcium is absorbed. With vitamin D, the absorption rate can be up to 40%. Vitamin D has an important role in maintaining normal calcium and phosphorus levels in the blood. Without adequate levels of vitamin D, phosphorus and calcium levels drop. Phosphorus is used for strong bones and teeth. Calcium helps maintain strong bones, proper blood clotting, muscle function, and immunity. Low vitamin D levels may cause a person to be at

CRITICAL THINKING 5.3

As Casey is waiting for Jean Burke, NP, to come into the exam room, she takes a mirror out of her purse and looks at the acne on her face. She is hopeful that coming to see the nurse practitioner is a good idea. As a medical assistant, how could you show sensitivity to Casey on her visit today?

a higher risk for multiple sclerosis (skli ROH sis), heart disease, osteoporosis, some forms of cancer, high blood pressure, and depression.

DISEASES AND DISORDERS OF THE INTEGUMENTARY SYSTEM

Common signs and symptoms seen in patients with skin diseases and disorders include:

- Skin discoloration or redness
- Itching, weeping, or bleeding lesions
- Blisters, macules, or papules (Fig. 5.4)
- *Pustules* (superficial, elevated lesion that contains pus), *vesicles* (a circumscribed, raised lesion containing fluid), and a *wheal* (a tense, pale elevation of the skin)
- Scaly or flaky skin surface
- New or changing lesions

Common diagnostic procedures and medical laboratory tests are listed in Table 5.1. Common treatments are listed in Table 5.2.

MEDICAL TERMINOLOGY	
cry/o	extreme cold
macul/o	spot
papul/o	pimple
-ectomy	removal, excision
-ule	small

Acne Vulgaris

Acne (AK nee), also known as *acne vulgaris*, is a common inflammatory disease of the sebaceous glands and hair follicles. It causes pimples on the skin that can lead to scars. There are several types of acne.

PRIMARY LESIONS

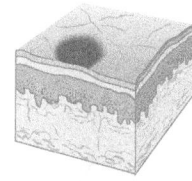

MACULE
Flat area of color change (no elevation or depression)

Example: Freckles

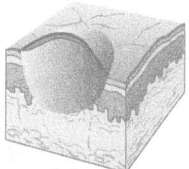

PAPULE
Solid elevation less than 0.5 cm in diameter

Example: Allergic eczema

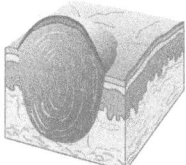

NODULE
Solid elevation 0.5 to 1 cm in diameter. Extends deeper into dermis than papule

Example: Mole

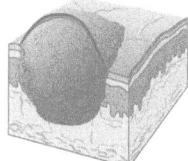

TUMOR
Solid mass—larger than 1 cm

Example: Squamous cell carcinoma

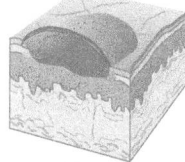

PLAQUE
Flat elevated surface found on skin or mucous membrane

Example: Thrush

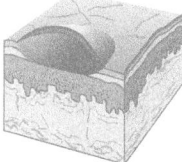

WHEAL
Type of plaque. Result is transient edema in dermis

Example: Intradermal skin test

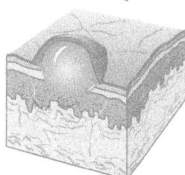

VESICLE
Small blister—fluid within or under epidermis

Example: Herpesvirus infection

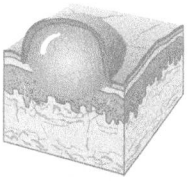

BULLA
Large blister (greater than 0.5 cm)

Example: Burn

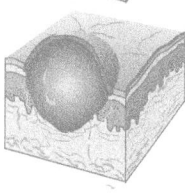

PUSTULE
Vesicle filled with pus

Example: Acne

SECONDARY LESIONS

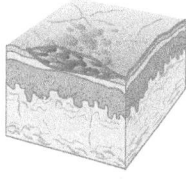

SCALES
Flakes of cornified skin layer

Example: Psoriasis

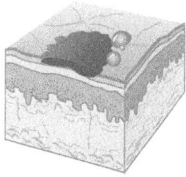

CRUST
Dried exudate on skin

Example: Impetigo

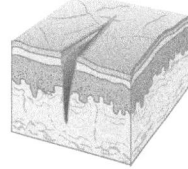

FISSURE
Cracks in skin

Example: Athlete's foot

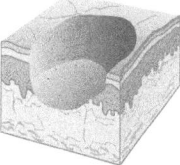

ULCER
Area of destruction of entire epidermis

Example: Decubitus (pressure sore)

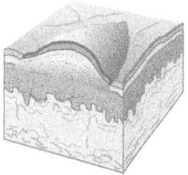

SCAR
Excess collagen production after injury

Example: Surgical healing

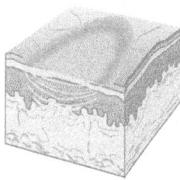

ATROPHY
Loss of some portion of the skin

Example: Paralysis

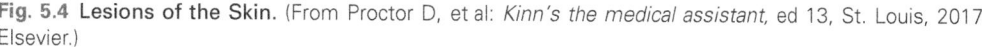

Fig. 5.4 Lesions of the Skin. (From Proctor D, et al: *Kinn's the medical assistant,* ed 13, St. Louis, 2017, Elsevier.)

TABLE 5.1   Common Diagnostic Procedures Used for Integumentary System Disorders

Procedure/Test	Description
Culture	Detects organism in body fluid or body tissue (e.g., blood, sputum, urine, wound drainage, skin).
Sensitivity testing	Determines antibiotics that would inhibit or kill bacteria.
Skin biopsy	A local anesthetic is injected into the area, and a skin sample is removed. The specimen is examined under a microscope to check for skin infections, disorders, or cancer. Three types of skin biopsies are: • An *excisional biopsy*, in which a scalpel is used to remove the sample. • A *shave biopsy*, in which a razor blade is used to remove the sample. • A *punch biopsy*, in which a cylindrical punch (tool) is used to remove the sample.
Wood light examination	A test that uses ultraviolet (UV) light to look at the skin.

TABLE 5.2   Common Treatments Used for Integumentary System Disorders

Treatment	Description
Cryosurgery (KRI oh sur jeh ree)	A treatment that involves freezing the tissue in order to destroy it. Liquid nitrogen is a common substance used for cryosurgery.
Debridement	A procedure that involves removing dead skin and tissue to help with wound healing.
Incision and drainage (I&D)	The provider will numb the area with an anesthetic and make a small incision with a scalpel. Packing gauze may be inserted into the wound to help with drainage and healing.
Laser therapy	A treatment that uses a strong beam of light to burn, destroy, or cut tissue. The term LASER stands for light amplification by stimulated emission of radiation.
Mohs surgery (mohz)	After numbing the site with an anesthetic, the provider removes a tumor and a thin layer next to the tumor. The layer is examined microscopically for cancer. If cancer exists, another layer is removed. This continues until the layer is free of cancer.
Onychectomy (ah nick ECK tuh mee)	Removal of a fingernail or toenail. A treatment used when trauma or disease affects the nail.
Rhytidectomy (RIT i DEK tah mee)	A cosmetic surgical operation that tightens sagging skin and removes wrinkles; also called a "face-lift."
Photodynamic therapy (PDT)	A treatment that uses light therapy and medications to kill cancer cells. The provider injects medication into the body, which is absorbed by cells. The cancer cells hold the medication longer than healthy cells. After a period of time, the provider directs light at the cancer cells, killing or damaging them.
Phototherapy	A treatment in which the skin is exposed to ultraviolet light; also called *light therapy*. Phototherapy helps reduce the inflammatory response in the skin.

• *Whitehead*: The follicles become blocked by oil and dead skin cells. A "whitehead" forms at the tip of the pimple.
• *Blackhead*: The follicle is blocked near the surface of the skin. When it is exposed to air, it turns black, giving the appearance of dirt in the pore.
• *Cystic acne*: Cysts form around the follicle.

Commonly, teens and young adults get acne, but anyone can at any age.

Etiology. Pimples form when the hair follicles clog up with oil and dead skin cells. Additional causes of acne include using an excessively oily product, bacteria, and androgens (AN dro jens). Androgens increase in boys and girls during puberty. These hormones cause the sebaceous glands to enlarge and secrete more sebum.

Factors that can trigger or increase acne include:
• Hormonal changes, which occur during the teen years, during pregnancy, and when using an oral contraceptive
• Medications, such as corticosteroids, testosterone, or lithium
• Dietary factors, including foods rich in carbohydrates (e.g., breads and desserts)
• Stress

Signs and Symptoms. Pimples tend to form on the face, forehead, chest, upper back, and shoulders (Fig. 5.5). These areas have the most sebaceous glands. Acne can cause:
• Pimples, whiteheads, and blackheads
• *Nodules* (solid, tender lumps under the skin)
• *Cystic lesions* (painful, pus-filled lumps under the skin)

Diagnostic Procedures. The provider will complete a history and physical, including examining the patient's skin.

Treatments. Treatments include medications and therapies.
• Medications: Retinoid-like compounds, such as tretinoin (TRET i noyn) (Retin-A), adapalene (a DAP a leen) (Differin), and tazarotene (taz AR oh teen) (Tazorac, Avage); antibiotics, salicylic acid and azelaic acid, dapsone (DAP sone), antiandrogen agents, and combined oral contraceptives.
• Therapies: Laser and photodynamic therapy, chemical peels, steroid injections, and extraction of the whiteheads and blackheads.

VOCABULARY

androgens Usually thought of as a male sex hormone, such as testosterone or androsterone, that cause the male secondary sex characteristics. Females produced a small amount of androgen in the ovaries and other organs.

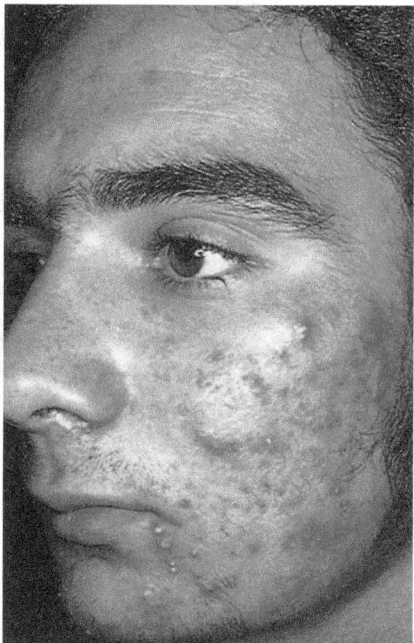

Fig. 5.5 Acne. (From Paller A, Mancini A: *Hurwitz clinical pediatric dermatology: a textbook of skin disorders in childhood and adolescence,* ed 4, Philadelphia, 2011, Saunders.)

Alopecia

Alopecia (al oh PEE sha), also called baldness, is complete or partial loss of hair from the head or other parts of the body. There are many types of alopecia. For example:

- Alopecia areata (ar ee ATE ah): An autoimmune disorder that leads to round patches of hair loss.
- Androgenetic (an dro je NET ik) alopecia: A common condition that causes progressive, diffuse, symmetric loss of hair on the head. Usually starts at age 20 to the early 30s.

Etiology. Causes of alopecia include:

- Genetics. Inherited or pattern baldness affects more men than women and can occur any time after puberty.
- Physical and emotional stress. Severe infections, childbirth, major surgery or illness, emotional stress, and crash diets can cause alopecia.
- Medications, such as oral contraceptives, antidepressants, and heart-related medications.
- Certain diseases, such as thyroid disease, autoimmune conditions, anemia, tinea capitis, ovarian tumor, adrenal gland tumor, and syphilis.
- Some types of chemotherapy and radiation therapy to the head.

Signs and Symptoms. Hair loss can occur suddenly or gradually. Depending on the type of alopecia, the hair loss can vary, possibly including:

- Gradual thinning on top of the head, which is the most common type
- Patchy or circular spots
- Sudden loosening

- Hair loss over the entire body
- Scaly patches over the scalp

Diagnostic Procedures. The provider will do a history and physical, examining the area of hair loss. Additional tests, such as blood tests and a scalp biopsy, may be done to determine the cause of the alopecia. A pull test may be done and requires the provider to pull several dozen hairs to determine the stage of the shedding process. Light microscopy may also be done to examine the hair.

Treatments. Treatments depend on the type of alopecia. Treatments may include surgery and medications, such as minoxidil (mi NOX i dill) (Rogaine) and finasteride (fin NAS teer ide) (Propecia).

Burns

Burns are classified according to the depth of the burn.

- *First-degree* or *superficial burns* damage the epidermis.
- *Second-degree* or *partial thickness burns* damage the epidermis and part of the dermis.
- *Third-degree* or *full-thickness burns* damage the epidermis, dermis, and the subcutaneous tissue.
- *Fourth-degree* or *deep full-thickness burns* damage beyond the subcutaneous tissue into the muscle and bone. (This classification is not universally accepted.)

Etiology. Heat, freezing cold temperatures, chemicals, sunlight, radiation, and electricity can cause burns to the body tissue. Hot liquids, fires, and flammable products are the most common causes of burns.

Signs and Symptoms. Signs and symptoms depend on the severity of the burn.

- *First-degree burn*: Red, painful, dry, and no blisters. A mild sunburn is an example.
- *Second-degree burn*: Red, blisters, and swollen; scars may form. Causes severe pain.
- *Third-degree burn*: Appears white or blackened and charred. Minimal pain due to the nerve destruction.
- *Fourth-degree* or *deep full-thickness burn*: No feeling in the area because the nerve endings are destroyed. Burn is leathery and dry.

Diagnostic Procedures. The provider will examine the area and determine the total body surface area burned. The rule of nines is commonly used.

Treatments. First- and second-degree burns may be treated at home. Healing may take a few weeks. Severe burns (third- and fourth-degree burns) are medical emergencies. The goal of treatment is to control pain, remove *debris* (dead tissue), prevent infection and complications, keep the patient hydrated, reduce scarring, and help regain the area's function. Treatment includes:

- Intravenous fluids to replace fluids lost and prevent shock symptoms
- Pain medication
- Occupational and physical therapy

BOX 5.2   Skin Graft

A skin graft is a section of skin that is surgically removed from one part of the body and attached or transplanted to another area. The healthy skin is removed from the donor site using a *dermatome*, which is a tool with a sharp razor blade. Donor sites are usually hidden by clothing (e.g., buttock or inner thigh). Most skin grafting procedures involve a split-thickness skin graft (STSG). This takes the epidermis and part of the dermis from the donor site. The donor site is covered with a sterile dressing for 3 to 5 days. The donor site heals quickly, but the area may have a lighter pigmentation. The graft is carefully spread on the transplanted area and held in place with a dressing, staples, or stitches.

Sometimes a full-thickness skin graft (FTSG) is required. These donor sites include the chest wall, back, or abdominal wall. A full-thickness graft includes the epidermis and the entire dermis from the donor site.

There are several types of donors. *Autograft* means the skin was from the patient. These are the most successful skin grafts and are considered permanent skin grafts. Temporary skin grafts come from human cadavers *(allograft)* or from animals *(xenograft)*, such as pigs. Temporary skin grafts are used until an autograft can be done.

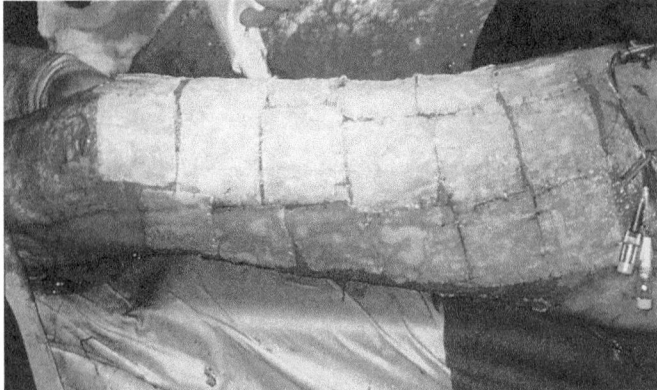

Fig. 5.6 Autograft. (From McCance KL, Huether SE: *Pathophysiology: the biologic basis for disease in adults and children,* ed 6, St. Louis, 2010, Mosby.)

- Skin grafts (Box 5.2, Fig. 5.6, and Fig. 5.7)
- Plastic surgery and *escharotomy* (es skar AH tuh mee), which is used to improve blood flow to the wound by cutting the *burn scab* (eschar). If the complete circumference of the torso (chest and back) or extremity is burned, the eschar can tighten and limit the blood circulation to the area. Burns on the torso can limit breathing.

Specialized burn centers are available around the country to provide care to patients with severe burns.

MEDICAL TERMINOLOGY	
all/o	other
xen/o	foreign
auto-	self
-tome	to cut

CRITICAL THINKING 5.4

Mai rooms Tommy Smythe, who has a second-degree burn on his right arm. Tommy asks Mai what was meant by a second-degree burn. Describe how you would explain a second-degree burn to a patient.

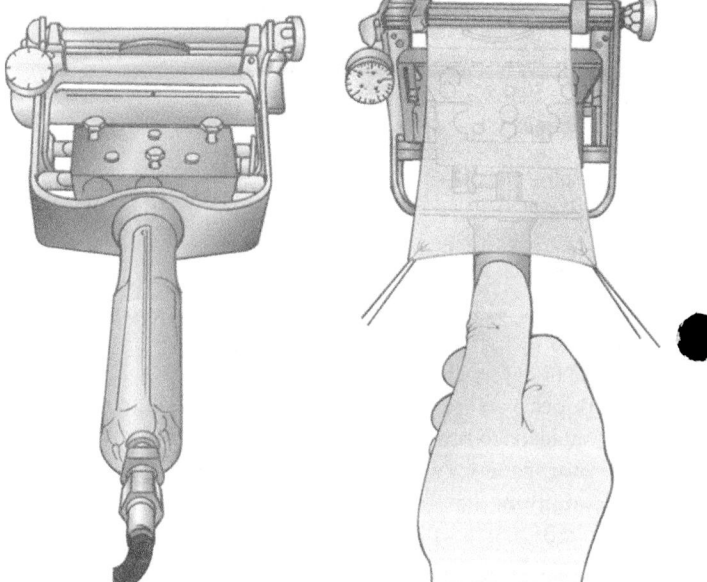

Fig. 5.7 Dermatome. (From Shiland B: *Mastering healthcare terminology,* ed 5, St. Louis, 2016, Elsevier.)

Carcinomas of the Skin

Skin cancer is an abnormal growth of skin cells. It is the most common cancer in the United States. Three of the most common skin cancers are basal cell and squamous cell carcinoma and melanoma.

Etiology. Skin cancer happens when errors occur in the cells' deoxyribonucleic acid (DNA). Ultraviolet light from the sun, tanning beds, and sun lamps can change the DNA. UV rays are an invisible kind of radiation that penetrates and changes skin cells. Skin cancer usually occurs in areas exposed to the sun. The scalp, face and lips, ears, neck, chest, legs, arms, and hands are common locations for skin cancer. Sometimes skin cancer can develop on the palms, beneath fingernails and toenails, and in the genital area.

Risk factors for skin cancer include a history of sunburns, excessive sun exposure, fair skin, moles, family and/or personal history of skin cancer, exposure to radiation, and a weakened immune system.

Signs and Symptoms. The signs and symptoms depend on the type of skin cancer.

- Squamous cell carcinoma: Firm red nodule or a flat lesion with scaly, crusted surface (Fig. 5.8A).
- Basal cell carcinoma: Waxy or pearly bump; dark lesion, scaly reddish patch, or a reoccurring bleeding sore (see Fig. 5.8B).
- Melanoma: Large brown spot with darker pigments; a mole that changes appearance (color, size, or feel); small lesion with irregular borders; may have different colors (red, white, blue, black); and itchy lesions (Box 5.3; also see Fig. 5.8C).

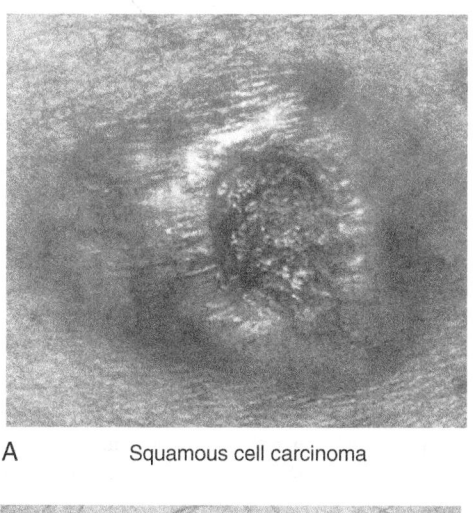

A   Squamous cell carcinoma

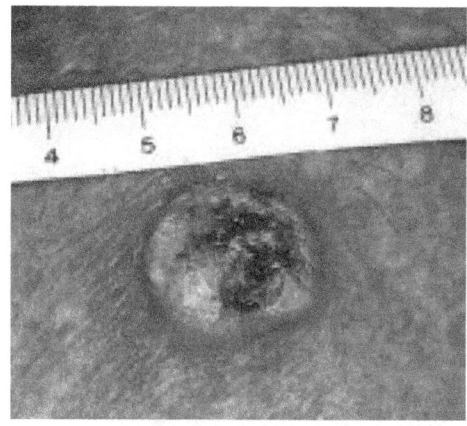

B   Basal cell carcinoma

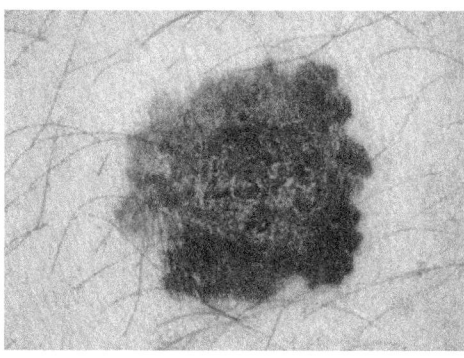

C   Malignant melanoma

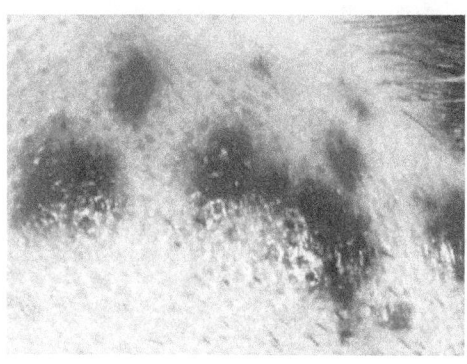

D   Kaposi sarcoma

Fig. 5.8 Examples of Skin Cancer Lesions. A, Squamous cell carcinoma. B, Basal cell carcinoma. C, Malignant melanoma. D, Kaposi sarcoma. (**A** from Goldman L, Schafer AI: *Goldman's Cecil medicine,* ed 24, Philadelphia, 2012, Saunders; **B** from Noble J, Greene HL: *Textbook of primary care medicine,* St. Louis, ed 3, Mosby, 2001; **C** from Townsend C, Beauchamp RD, Evers BM, Mattox K: *Sabiston textbook of surgery,* ed 18, Philadelphia, 2008, Saunders; **D** from Rakel R: *Textbook of family medicine,* ed 7, Philadelphia, 2007, Saunders.)

BOX 5.3   ABCDE Rule

Early warning signs of melanoma can be remembered using the ABCDE rule:
- **A**symmetry: One half of the mole does not match the other half.
- **B**order: The edges of the mole are blurred or irregular.
- **C**olor: The mole is not the same color throughout and has shades of tan, brown, black, red, white, or blue
- **D**iameter: The mole is larger than 6 mm, about the size of a pencil eraser or pea; but it could be smaller.
- **E**volving: The mole changes over time.

Diagnostic Procedures. The provider will exam the skin and obtain a skin biopsy. Excisional, shave, or punch biopsies can be done (Fig. 5.9). If skin cancer is detected, additional tests will be done to determine the stage of the skin cancer.

Treatments. Basal cell and squamous cell carcinoma are curable. Melanoma is more dangerous and can cause death. Treatments are based on the size, type, depth, and location of the cancer. Treatments may include:
- Cryosurgery, excisional surgery, or Mohs surgery (Fig. 5.10).
- Radiation therapy, chemotherapy, and photodynamic therapy (PDT).

- *Biological therapy,* which are medications that boost the body's immune system. This helps the immune system kill cancer cells.

CRITICAL THINKING 5.5

After the provider is finished seeing Tommy, Mai comes back in to wrap up the visit. Mai reads the provider's notes, which indicate that she educated Tommy on skin cancer prevention. Mai reviews the ABCDE rule with Tommy. Describe the ABCDE rule to a classmate.

Cellulitis

Cellulitis is a common bacterial infection of the skin. Cellulitis affects the dermis, subcutaneous tissue, and sometimes the muscle.

Etiology. Staphylococcal and streptococcal bacteria are the most common causes of cellulitis. Risk factors for cellulitis include injuries to the skin, insect bites, and ulcers. Other risk factors include a history of peripheral vascular disease, a suppressed immune system, and diabetes.

Signs and Symptoms. Signs and symptoms of cellulitis include:
- Fatigue, fever, chills, sweating
- Pain, tenderness, redness, warmth, and inflammation in the affected area
- Muscle and joint achiness and stiffness
- Nausea and vomiting

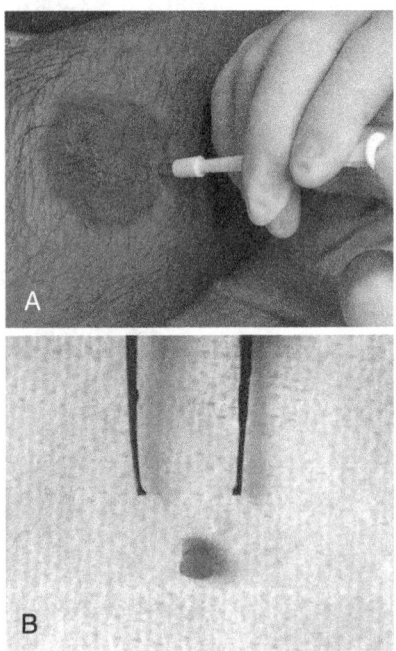

Fig. 5.9 Punch Biopsy. A, Removal of skin for diagnostic purposes. B, Specimen obtained. (From Graham-Brown R, Bourke J, Cunliffe T: *Dermatology: fundamentals of practice,* Edinburgh, 2008, Mosby.)

Diagnostic Procedures. The provider will examine the area. Often the provider will mark the edges of the redness with a pen. This helps the provider identify an increase in the redness over the next several days. Additional tests might be done, including a blood culture, complete blood count (CBC), culture of the fluid from the site, and a biopsy.

Treatments. Treatment includes antibiotic therapy, pain medication, warm compresses, and resting at home with the affected area elevated. For severe cases of cellulitis, the patient may be hospitalized and given intravenous (IV) antibiotics.

Decubitus Ulcer

Decubitus ulcers are also called *bed sores, pressure ulcers,* and *pressure sores.* Decubitus ulcers are areas of damaged skin caused by long-term pressure against the skin that limits blood flow. The ulcers are commonly found on the heels, ankles, back, elbows, and buttocks. Decubitus ulcers can cause serious and sometimes life-threatening infections (Box 5.4).

Etiology. Decubitus ulcers can be caused by friction, shearing, and continual pressure on the skin. Friction and shearing commonly occur when patients slide down in bed, which happens when the head of the bed is elevated. The pressure can lead to limited blood flow to the area and thus limited nutrients and oxygen for the tissue. Tissues become damaged and may eventually die. Just 2 hours in the same position can cause a pressure sore. Risk factors include immobility, incontinence, poor nutrition, loss of feeling, and disorders affecting blood flow (e.g., diabetes).

Signs and Symptoms. Signs and symptoms include unusual skin color, swelling, drainage, tender areas, and changes in the skin

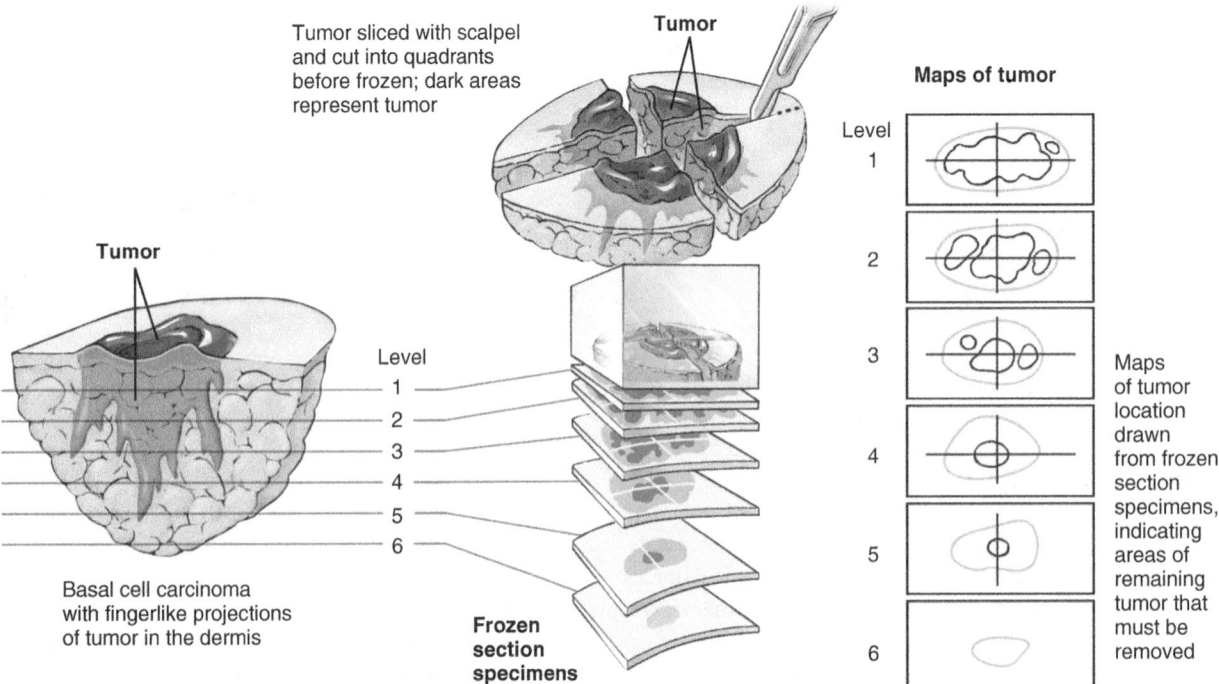

Fig. 5.10 Mohs Surgery. (From Ignatavicius DD, Workman ML: Medical-*surgical nursing: critical thinking for collaborative care,* ed 6, Philadelphia, 2011, Saunders.)

temperature. Pressure sores range from red, unbroken skin to deep injury involving muscle and bones. Overlying tissue may not always show the underlying damage from pressure sores.

Diagnostic Procedures. The provider will examine the area and determine the stage of the wound. Stage 1 is the mildest and stage 4 is the most severe (Fig. 5.11).

- Stage 1: Area is red and painful. When the area is pressed, it does not turn white.
- Stage 2: Blisters or an open sore is present. Area around the sore is irritated and red.
- Stage 3: A crater (an open, sunken hole) is present. Tissue below the skin is affected.
- Stage 4: Damage affects the muscle, bone, tendons, or joints.

Treatments. Treatment involves reducing pressure on the surrounding tissues. Wound care varies based on the severity of the ulcer. Surgery may be required to *debride* (remove the dead tissue in) the area. Pain medication prior to wound care is critical for painful wounds.

VOCABULARY

shearing Two surfaces moving in the opposite direction.

BOX 5.4 Preventing Decubitus Ulcers

- Change positions at least every 2 hours.
- Use foam or gel seat cushions in wheelchairs.
- Wear clothes that are not too tight or too loose. Make sure fabric is smooth under the body.
- Eat a high-protein diet, which includes meat, eggs, peanuts, milk, and fish.
- Increase fluid intake.
- Check the skin frequently for suspicious-looking areas.

CRITICAL THINKING 5.6

Mai's midafternoon patient, Mr. Harvey, is paralyzed below the waist from a military injury. He uses a wheelchair and has been struggling with pressure sores over the past 6 months. Describe three ways he can prevent pressure sores.

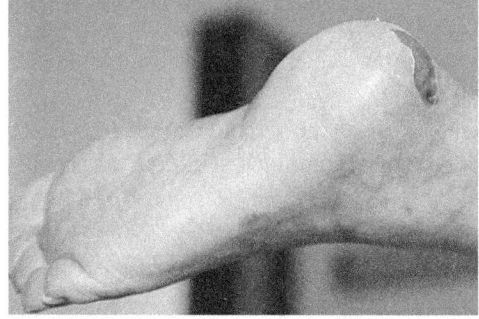

Decubitus ulcer

Fig. 5.11 Decubitus Ulcer. (From Potter P, Perry A: *Fundamentals of nursing,* ed 7, St. Louis, 2009, Mosby.)

Dermatitis

The term *dermatitis* (DER mah tie tis) means inflammation of the skin. Dermatitis is a common condition that is not contagious. There are several types of dermatitis, including atopic dermatitis, contact dermatitis, and seborrheic dermatitis.

Atopic Dermatitis. Atopic dermatitis is also called *eczema* (EK ze mah). It is a chronic condition that makes the skin red and itchy. It often starts before age 5 and may last through adulthood. There is no cure for atopic dermatitis.

Etiology. The cause is unknown, but researchers believe that genes and certain triggers are involved. An overreactive immune system plus a trigger produces the inflammation. Triggers can include dry skin, stress, and irritants (e.g., soaps, juices, cigarette smoke, and certain fabrics).

Signs and Symptoms. Signs and symptoms include dry skin, itching, scaly skin, red to brownish patches, and small bumps.

Diagnostic Procedures. The provider will obtain a medical history and perform a physical exam, assessing the skin.

Treatments. Treatments include medications and therapies.

- Medications: Corticosteroid and antibiotic creams, oral corticosteroids, and dupilumab (doo PIL ue mab) (Dupixent)
- Therapies: Wet dressings, *phototherapy* (light therapy), and counseling for emotional concerns related to the skin condition

Contact Dermatitis. Contact dermatitis occurs when the skin becomes inflamed or sore after direct contact with a substance. Two types of contact dermatitis include irritant dermatitis and allergic contact dermatitis.

Etiology. Irritant dermatitis can be caused by acid substances and alkaline materials. Common materials include dyes, long-term exposure to wet diapers, pesticides, rubber gloves, soaps, and shampoos. Allergic contact dermatitis is caused by a substance that causes an allergy. Common allergens include adhesives, antibiotics, perfumes, soaps, fabrics, plants (e.g., poison ivy, poison oak, and poison sumac), latex gloves and balloons, preservatives, and formaldehyde.

Signs and Symptoms. The signs and symptoms vary based on the type of dermatitis. The rash may have bumps, blisters, or scales. The area may be warm and tender.

Diagnostic Procedures. The provider will examine the area and get a health history. Allergy testing may be recommended. A skin biopsy or culture of the skin lesion may be done to rule out other conditions.

Treatments. Treatments depend on the cause. Washing the area to eliminate the irritant is important. Skin moisturizers, topical corticosteroids, and *antipruritic* (anti-itch) lotions can be used. *Topical* medications are applied directly to the surface of the skin.

Seborrheic Dermatitis. Seborrheic (seb o REE ik) dermatitis is a common skin disease that causes a rash. Seborrheic dermatitis can occur at any age. Cradle cap, also called *infantile seborrheic dermatitis,* occurs in infancy.

Etiology. Researchers have found that a combination of several factors causes seborrheic dermatitis. These factors include the yeast that is normally on our skin, genes, cold and dry environments, and a person's health. Medical conditions that increase the risk include Parkinson disease, acne, rosacea, alcoholism, and recovering from a stroke.

Signs and Symptoms. Seborrheic dermatitis causes scaly, greasy, or moist patches on the skin. The skin below the patches is red. The yellowish to white scales flake off. In adolescents and adults, the patches can cause itching and a burning sensation. Patches can appear on the scalp, ears, eyebrows, eyelids, upper chest and back, armpits, ear canals, and genitals.

Diagnostic Procedures. The provider will obtain a medical history and perform a physical exam, assessing the skin. A skin biopsy may be done to rule out other conditions.

Treatments. Treatments vary depending on the age of the person and the location of the patches. For cradle cap, it is recommended to use a mild baby shampoo daily and lightly brush the scalp. Treatments for adolescents and adults can include:

- Steroid creams, ointments, and shampoos
- Antifungal gels, creams, or shampoos
- Oral antifungal medications

Dermatophytosis

Dermatophytosis (der mah to fi TOE sis) is a common superficial fungal infection of the skin and nails. It is also called *ringworm* or a *tinea* (TIN ee uh) infection. Approximately 40 different types of fungi cause ringworm. Tinea infections are named based on the area of the body infected.

- *Tinea capitis* (scalp ringworm) mostly occurs in children. Tinea capitis causes scaling and patchy hair loss.
- *Tinea corporis* causes ringworm over the body, such as the arms and legs (Fig. 5.12).
- *Tinea cruris* (jock itch) causes a rash in the groin area. The rash has an itchy, spreading red border. It is more common in males.
- *Tinea pedis* (athlete's foot), the most common type, is spread by direct contact. It causes itching, blisters, and white, soft skin on the sole of the foot. The skin between the toes peels away (Fig. 5.13).
- *Tinea unguium* is also called *onychomycosis* (on ih koh my KOH sis) and *nail fungus*. Most often it affects the toenails, and usually the large toenail is the first to show signs. The nails become yellow and thicken over time and can easily break.

Etiology. Ringworm is caused by a fungus. It occurs when certain types of fungus grow and multiply on the skin or enter the skin near the nails. Many types of ringworm are contagious, meaning you can get it from touching others and from pets. Nail fungus is not contagious.

Signs and Symptoms. The skin can be red, itchy, cracked, flaking, or peeling. The person may have burning or stinging pain. A scaly ring-shaped area and blisters may also be seen.

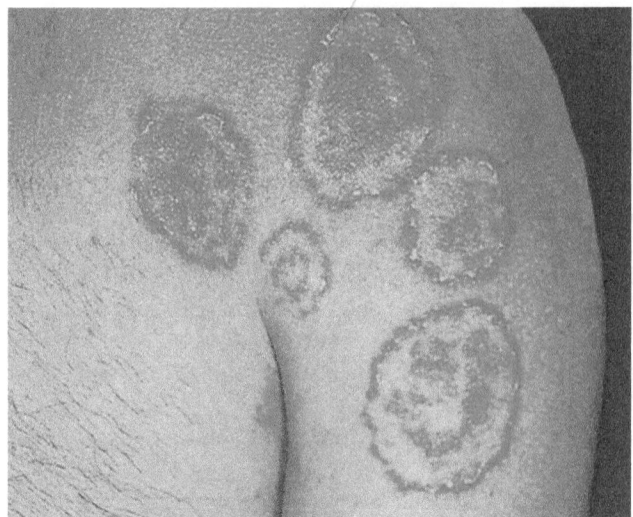

Fig. 5.12 Tinea corporis (ringworm). (From Habif TP: *Clinical dermatology*, ed 4, St. Louis, 2004, Mosby.)

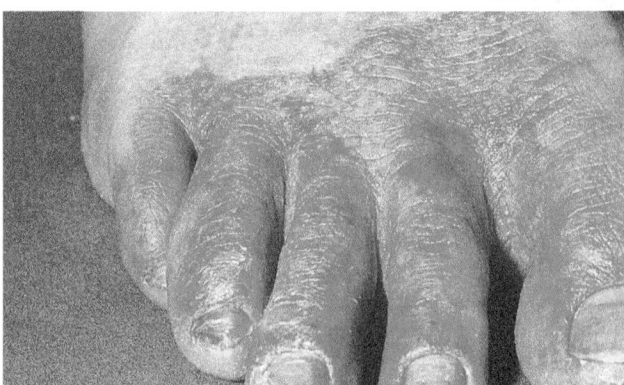

Fig. 5.13 Tinea pedis (athlete's foot). (From Gawkrodger D: *Dermatology*, ed 5, New York, 2012, Churchill Livingstone.)

Diagnostic Procedures. After obtaining the medical history, the provider will examine the area affected. A potassium hydroxide (KOH) exam, skin culture, and a skin biopsy might be done to diagnose the fungal infection.

Treatments. Treatments usually consist of antifungal medication. Depending on the type of infection, some antifungal medications are available over the counter, whereas others are prescribed. Oral antifungal medications are prescribed for toenail fungus and may require 12 weeks of treatment. It is important to keep the affected area clean and dry.

Impetigo

Impetigo is a common, highly contagious bacterial infection. Impetigo is most common in children but can also affect adults.

Etiology. Impetigo is caused by *Streptococcus, Staphylococcus,* and methicillin-resistant *Staphylococcus aureus* (MRSA).

Signs and Symptoms. Impetigo usually starts with a rash in a single spot but can spread with scratching. Blisters occur that are itchy and filled with yellow or honey-colored pus. They can ooze, pop,

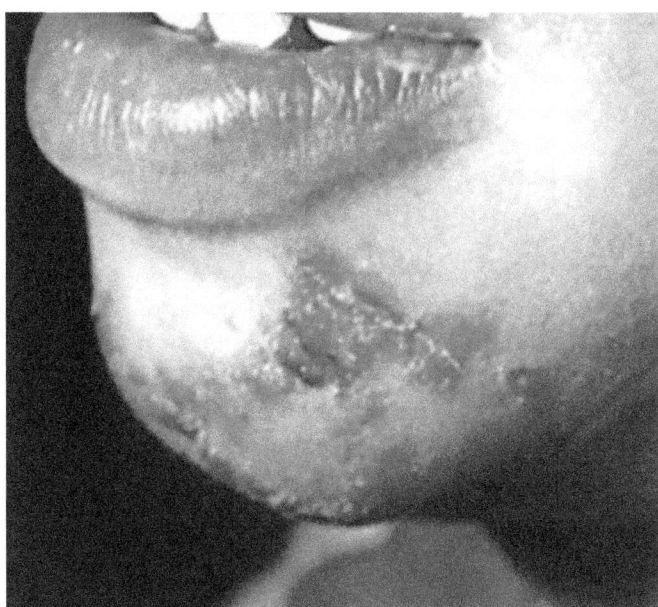

Fig. 5.14 Impetigo. (From Marks JG Jr, Miller JJ: *Lookingbill & Marks' principles of dermatology*, ed 4, London, 2006, Saunders.)

and crust over. Blisters can appear on the face, lips, arms, and legs (Fig. 5.14). Swollen lymph nodes can also be seen.

Diagnostic Procedures. The provider will do a history and physical exam. A culture of the blisters' fluid also may be done.

Treatments. Treatment includes antibacterial cream and oral antibiotics for severe infections. Home care includes washing the skin with antibacterial soap several times a day.

Kaposi Sarcoma

Kaposi sarcoma (KAP uh see sar KOH mah) (KS) is a cancer that causes abnormal tissue to grow in the skin, mucous membrane lining of the gastrointestinal tract, lymph nodes, lungs, and other organs.

Etiology. Kaposi sarcoma is caused by human herpes virus–8 (HHV-8). Many people have HHV-8, though they do not get KS. For KS to occur, the person's immune system usually has to be weakened. This can be caused by infection with the human immunodeficiency virus (HIV) and by antirejection medications taken after organ transplantation.

Signs and Symptoms. The lesions are purple, red, or brown, flat or raised spots on the skin (see Fig. 5.8D). Commonly, they are seen on the feet, legs, and face. Lesions can also be seen on the mucous membranes and in the lungs, which may cause the patient to cough up blood.

Diagnostic Procedures. After a history and physical exam, the provider may order a fecal occult blood test, chest x-ray, bronchoscopy, upper endoscopy, and colonoscopy.

Treatments. Treatment depends on the cause of the weakened immune system. Treatments may include minor surgery to remove the lesions, cryotherapy, or electrodessication (ee LEK troe DES

i kay shun), low-dose radiation, chemotherapy injections into the lesion, and applications of a vitamin A drug.

> **VOCABULARY**
> **cryotherapy** Using an extremely cold liquid or instrument to freeze and destroy abnormal tissue.
> **electrodessication** Destruction of lesions or sealing off of blood vessels using electric current.

Pediculosis and Scabies

Pediculosis (pe dik u LOW sis) (lice) and *scabies* (itch mites) are the two most common types of skin parasites. Parasitic infestations of the skin can occur at any age. They are spread in group settings, such as among families or in childcare groups, school classes, nursing homes, prisons, and dormitories.

Etiology. Pediculosis is caused by lice that populate three specific areas of the body. A person can have head lice *(Pediculus capitis)*, body lice *(Pediculus corporis)*, or pubic lice or crabs *(Pthirus pubis)*. Lice crawl but cannot fly or hop. Scabies is caused by the parasitic itch mite *Sarcoptes scabiei*. Both parasites can move from person to person through close physical contact and through sharing of inanimate objects *(fomites)*, such as combs, brushes, clothes, and bedding.

Signs and Symptoms. Signs and symptoms of scabies and pediculosis are similar and include:
- Intense itching
- A tickling feeling as parasites move hair on the skin
- Lice: Small red bumps on the skin and nits (eggs) on body, facial, or pubic hair
- Scabies: Little burrows or tunnels can be seen under the skin, frequently in areas of the skin that fold, such as between fingers and toes, around the waist, in the armpits, and on knees and elbows (Fig. 5.15)

Diagnostic Procedures. For lice, physical examination often involves the use of a magnifying lens to see the lice and nits on hair. Using a Wood light, the nits can be detected and appear pale blue (Fig. 5.16). For scabies, physical examination involves looking for the characteristic burrows under the skin. The provider may scrape the skin and exam it under the microscope to look for eggs.

Treatments. Prescription shampoo, body wash, and lotion can be used to kill parasites on the head, hair, and body. The lice and mites are generally killed quickly, but the patient must follow all instructions to make sure eggs are also killed. There may be some itching after the parasites are killed, but that does not necessarily indicate a continued infection. In addition to proper washing of the hair and body, all clothing, bedding, personal items, and furniture should be cleaned with hot, soapy water. If all the eggs are not removed, reinfections can occur.

> **CRITICAL THINKING 5.7**
> While Mai is rooming Sunny Dae, the patient states, "I think I have lice again. I am so tired of it. My two children had it last week, and I had it 3 weeks ago." Why might she have another episode of lice?

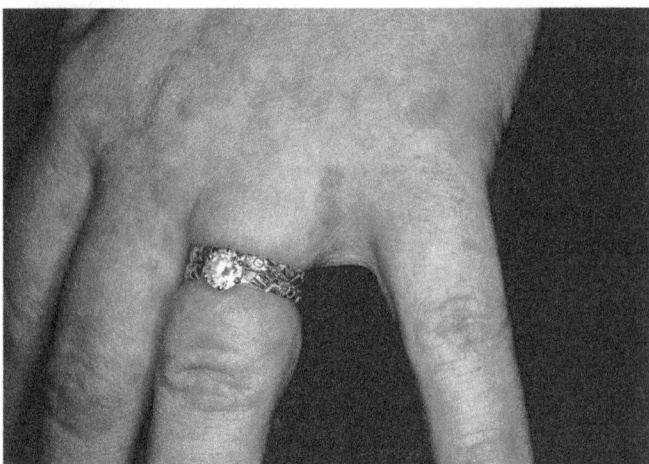

Fig. 5.15 Scabies on the Hand. (From James WD, et al: *Andrews' diseases of the skin,* ed 11, Philadelphia, 2011, Saunders.)

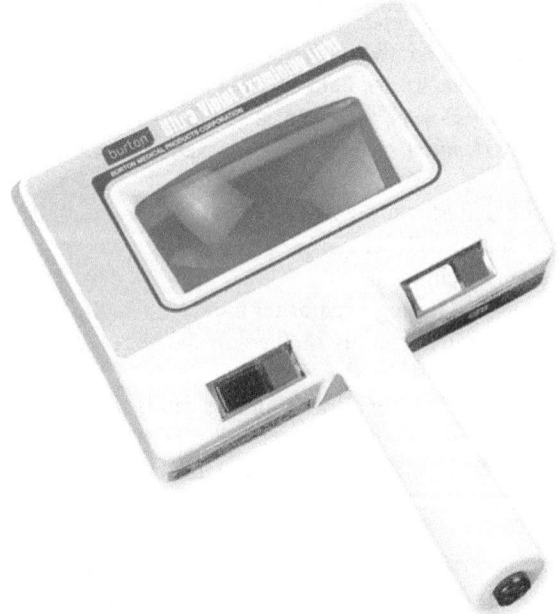

Fig. 5.16 Wood Light. (From Seidel HM, Ball JW, Dains JE, et al: *Mosby's guide to physical examination,* ed 7, St. Louis, 2011, Mosby.)

Pilonidal Cyst

Pilonidal (pie low NIE dul) cyst is an abnormal pocket in the skin that contains skin and hair debris. The cyst usually appears near the tailbone. The cyst can become infected and painful; if it does, it is called a *pilonidal abscess.*

Etiology. The cause is not clear but is thought to be related to ingrown hair near the tailbone. Risk factors include obesity, trauma to the area, and excessive coarse, curly body hair. It is more common in males.

Signs and Symptoms. Signs and symptoms include:
- Pus draining to a small pit in the skin
- Warm, tender, swollen area near the tailbone
- Fever (rare)

Diagnostic Procedures. The provider will do a history and physical exam. The area will be examined.

Treatments. For an *abscess* (infected cyst), the provider will do incision and drainage (I&D) surgery. The wound may be packed with dressing to allow it to heal from the inside out, or it may be immediately closed with *sutures* (stitches). Pilonidal cyst infections can reoccur.

Pityriasis Versicolor

Pityriasis versicolor (pit I RI ah sis vur si KUL ur), also called *tinea versicolor,* is a common fungal infection of the skin. It interferes with the normal skin pigmentation. Pityriasis versicolor frequently occurs in teens and young adults.

Etiology. The cause is an overgrowth of a common fungus found in the skin. Factors that can cause the overgrowth include hot, humid weather, oily skin, hormonal changes, and a weakened immune system.

Signs and Symptoms. Pityriasis versicolor causes lighter or darker discolored patches on the back, chest, upper arms, and neck. The patient can also experience mild itching and scaling.

Diagnostic Procedures. The provider will complete a history and physical exam. A skin biopsy may be done to rule out other conditions.

Treatments. Treatment consists of oral and topical antifungal medications.

Psoriasis

Psoriasis (sohr EYE ah sis) is a common, chronic disease that causes itchy or sore patches of thick, red skin with silvery scales. Some people who have psoriasis can also get psoriatic arthritis. There are many types of psoriasis.

Etiology. Psoriasis is an autoimmune condition. The epithelial cells regenerate faster than normal rates. Psoriasis can be triggered by infections, weather, injury, stress, drugs, and alcohol.

Signs and Symptoms. Common signs and symptoms include:
- Red patches of skin covered with thick, silvery scales
- Dry, cracked skin
- Itching, burning, or soreness
- Swollen and stiff joints

The most commonly affected areas include the lower back, elbows, knees and legs, soles, palms, face, and scalp (Fig. 5.17).

Diagnostic Procedures. After a history and an exam, the provider may perform a skin biopsy. This will provide information on the type of psoriasis and will rule out other disorders.

Treatments. Treatments include topical therapy, light therapy, and oral or injected medications.
- Topical therapy includes corticosteroids, retinoids, salicylic acid, and coal tar.

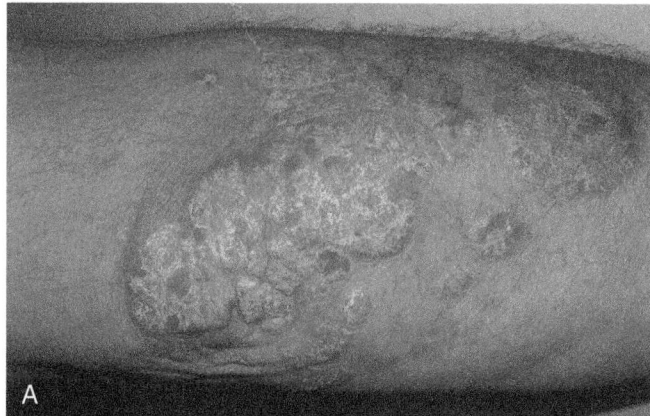

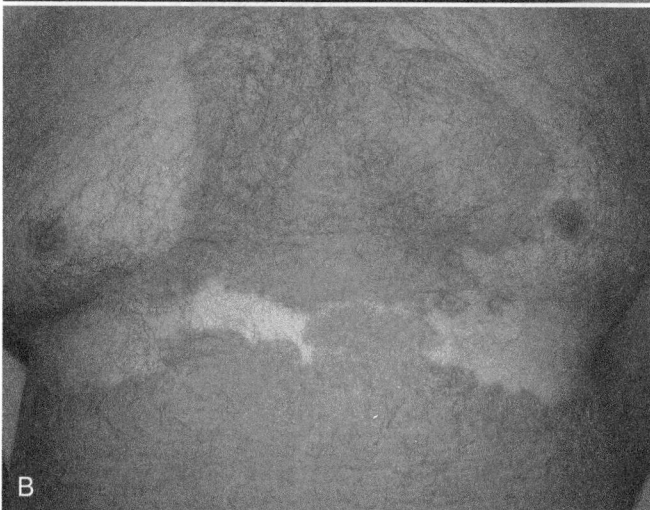

Fig. 5.17 Psoriasis. (From Marks JG Jr, Miller JJ: *Lookingbill & Marks' principles of dermatology*, ed 4, London, 2006, Saunders.)

- Light therapy is the first-line treatment for moderate to severe cases.
- Oral or injected medications include steroids, cyclosporine (SYE kloe spor een), and biologics that alter the immune system to disrupt the disease cycle.

CRITICAL THINKING 5.8

Mai's last patient of the day, Annie Burns, is being seen for a follow-up check for psoriasis. Mai notices that Annie is wearing long sleeves on a very hot day. When Mai asks Annie if she can check her blood pressure, Annie rolls up her sleeve. Her lower arm is covered with red patches with silvery scales. Why might Annie cover up her arms? How could a medical assistant show sensitivity in this situation?

Rosacea

Rosacea (roe ZAY she uh) is a chronic condition that affects the skin and sometimes the eyes. It causes redness and pimples. Rosacea more often affects females, people with fair skin, and middle-aged and older adults.

Etiology. The cause is unknown, but it might be due to a combination of genetics and environmental factors.

Signs and Symptoms. Signs and symptoms include:
- Flushing or facial redness
- Acne and small red lines under the skin
- Swollen nose and thick skin, usually on the forehead, chin, and cheeks
- Red, dry, itchy eyes and sometimes vision problems

Diagnostic Procedures. The provider will obtain a health history and perform an examination of the skin. No specific test is used to diagnose rosacea.

Treatments. Treatment is focused on controlling the signs and symptoms. Treatments consist of medication and light therapy. Medications include topical medications to reduce the facial redness, in addition to oral antibiotics and acne drugs.

Scleroderma

Scleroderma causes the buildup of scarlike tissue in the skin and elsewhere in the body. It can also damage the walls of small arteries. Some types of scleroderma affect only the skin, and others affect the entire body. The disease occurs in people ages 30 to 50 years, most often females.

Etiology. Scleroderma is an autoimmune disorder. A buildup of collagen in the skin and organs leads to the symptoms experienced.

Signs and Symptoms. Signs and symptoms include:
- Raynaud (ray NODE) phenomenon, stiffness and tightness of the skin on the fingers, forearm, hands, and face
- Hair loss, ulcers on the fingers and toes, and small white lumps of calcium below the skin
- Joint pain, stiffness, and swelling
- Difficulty swallowing, heartburn, bloating, and constipation
- Heart arrhythmias and kidney failure

Diagnostic Procedures. Besides a history and examination, the provider may order blood and urine tests (e.g., scleroderma antibody testing, complete blood count, and urinalysis). In addition, imaging tests (e.g., chest x-ray, computed tomography [CT] scan of the lungs) and an electrocardiogram (ECG) may be ordered.

Treatments. There is no specific treatment for scleroderma. The focus is to control the symptoms of the disease. Medications such as corticosteroids and immunosuppressants may be used.

VOCABULARY

Raynaud phenomenon Cramping of small arteries in the fingers and toes in cold temperatures, causing limited blood flow to the area. Skin feels cold and looks white or bluish.

Additional Integumentary System Diseases and Disorders

There are many integumentary diseases and disorders. The following are some examples.

- *Acrochordon* (ak ro KOR don): A small benign polyp that develops on the neck, axilla, and groin area. Also called a skin tag or a fibroepithelial polyp.
- *Albinism* (AL bih niz um): Inherited condition characterized by the lack of pigment in the skin, hair, or eyes.
- *Candidiasis* (kan dih DYE ah sis): A fungal infection caused by *Candida* organisms; it can occur on the skin or in the mouth, respiratory tract, and the vagina.
- *Corns* and *calluses*: Areas of thickened skin caused by pressure on the skin. Corns appear on the top or sides of the toes. Calluses form on the soles of the feet. Treatments include using padding in shoes, changing shoes, and cortisone injections.
- *Folliculitis* (foh lick yoo LYE tis): Inflammation or infection of one or more hair follicles.
- *Furuncle* (FYOOR ung kul): Also called a *boil*; a painful pus-filled nodule that forms under the skin. Caused by an infected hair follicle. A *carbuncle* is a cluster of furuncles.
- *Hemangioma* (hee man jee OH mah): A vascular tumor, which is present at birth or develops later; it forms a reddish or purplish birthmark.
- *Hidradenitis* (hye drah din EYE tis): A severe, chronic infection of the apocrine glands.
- *Hirsutism* (HER soo tih zum): Excessive growth of body or facial hair in females.
- *Hyperhidrosis* (hye pur hye DROH sis): A disorder that causes excessive sweating.
- *Nevus* (NEE vus): A congenital or acquired pigmented and raised lesion on the skin; also called a *birthmark.*
- *Peritonitis* (per i to NIE tis): An inflammation of the peritoneum.
- *Pleurisy* (PLURE i see): Inflammation of the pleura.
- *Pleural effusion*: A buildup of pleural fluid in the chest cavity, causing sharp chest pain with coughs or deep breaths, shortness of breath, and fever.
- *Vitiligo* (vit I LIE goe): An inherited disorder that causes the loss of melanocytes, producing smooth, white patches of skin (Fig. 5.18).
- *Warts*: Caused by the human papilloma virus (HPV). Common warts appear on the fingers (Fig. 5.19). Plantar warts appear on the soles of the feet. Warts can go away on their own. Freezing, surgical, and laser treatments can also be used to remove warts.

MEDICAL TERMINOLOGY	
angi/o	vessel
-oma	mass
-osis	abnormal condition

LIFE SPAN CHANGES

Often infants are born with *vernix*, a thick waxy substance, covering their skin. Vernix protects the skin from the amniotic fluid in the womb. Usually, the vernix washes off during the first bath. Infants may also have *lanugo*, a fine, soft hair on their forehead, cheeks, shoulders, back, and scalp. Usually, lanugo disappears within the first few weeks after birth.

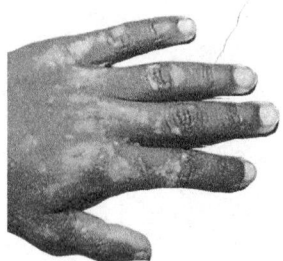

Fig. 5.18 **Vitiligo.** (From Patton KT, Thibodeau GA: *The human body in health and disease,* ed 7, St. Louis, 2018, Elsevier.)

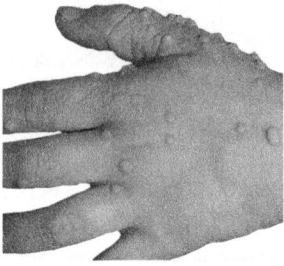

Fig. 5.19 **Warts.** (From Patton KT, Thibodeau GA: *The human body in health and disease,* ed 7, St. Louis, 2018, Elsevier.)

Premature infants have thin, transparent skin, and full-term infants have thicker skin.

Young children may have colored birthmarks or skin markings, including:

- *Congenital nevi*, which are moles or dark pigmented skin markings present at birth. Larger nevi carry a greater risk of skin cancer later in life.
- *Mongolian spots,* which are blue-gray or brown spots that usually fade by the first birthday.
- *Café-au-lait spots,* which are light tan spots and can be present at birth or develop within the first few years.
- *Port-wine stains* are red to purplish in color, because they contain blood vessels. Commonly they appear on the skin.
- *Hemangiomas,* small collections of blood vessels, may be present at birth or develop within the first few months (Fig. 5.20).
- *Stork bites,* small red patches, which are usually on the forehead, back of the neck, upper lip, or eyelids. These are caused by stretching of the blood vessels and usually disappear by 18 months of age.

Skin changes relate to environmental factors, nutrition, genetic makeup, and other factors. Sun exposure is the greatest factor in skin changes. Protecting the skin throughout the life span is important.

As a person advances into adulthood, the epidermis thins, though the number of cell layers remains unchanged. The number of melanocytes decreases. The aging skin looks thinner, paler, and translucent. Large, pigmented spots (e.g., age spots, liver spots, or lentigos) may appear on the sun-exposed areas, such as the arms. Changes in the connective tissue reduce the skin's strength and elasticity, leading to a leathery, weather-beaten appearance. This is commonly seen on the arms and faces of those who work outdoors. Older adults are more prone

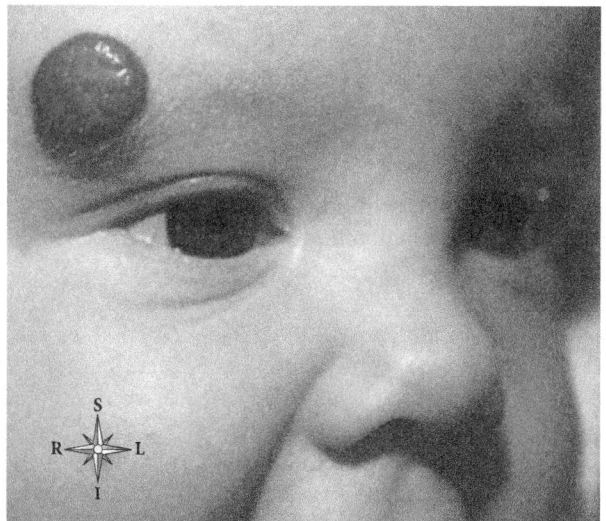

Fig. 5.20 Strawberry Hemangioma. This birthmark resembles a strawberry because of a mass of dilated dermal blood vessels. (From Habif TP: *Clinical dermatology*, ed 6, St. Louis, 2016, Mosby.)

to bruising *(senile purpura)* due to fragile blood vessels in the dermis. Sebaceous glands produce less oil, causing drier skin. The subcutaneous fat layers thin, increasing the risk for skin injury and an inability to maintain the body temperature. With sweat glands producing less sweat, this also leads to overheating and a higher risk of heat stroke.

CLOSING COMMENTS

In an ambulatory care setting, assisting patients with skin diseases and disorders is common. It is important for the medical assistant to understand the anatomy of the skin and the functions of the integumentary system as a whole. The skin has amazing qualities that allow it to repair and recover from injury and disease. Dermatology is the specialty that focuses on the skin, but medical assistants working in urgent care and primary care (e.g., pediatrics, internal medicine, and family practice) will see many skin-related diseases and disorders, too. Medical terminology related to the integumentary system will be invaluable in your career. Knowing word parts, definitions, and common abbreviations is vital when working with patients and providers. The medical assistant should also know about the etiology, signs and symptoms, diagnostic procedures, treatments, prognoses, and prevention of common integumentary diseases, disorders, and traumas. The medical assistant should also understand the medication classifications used to treat skeletal system disorders (Box 5.5).

BOX 5.5 Medication Classifications

- *Analgesics*: Relieve pain.
- *Antibiotics*: Used to treat bacterial infections, such as cellulitis and impetigo.
- *Antifungals*: Used to treat fungal infections, such as ringworm.
- *Antihistamines*: Block the action of histamines and relieve the signs of allergies, such as hives.
- *Anti-inflammatories*: Reduce the inflammation in the body and are used to treat inflammatory conditions.
- *Corticosteroids*: Used to reduce inflammations with chronic conditions, such as eczema, seborrheic dermatitis, and psoriasis.

Refer to Appendix D, which can be found on the Evolve website, for information on the medication classifications, including indications for use, desired effect, side effects, adverse reactions, and generic and trade names. Medical assistants should be familiar with medications that are prescribed to patients.

PATIENT-CENTERED CARE

Chronic skin conditions, such as psoriasis and eczema, often have a psychological and social impact on patients. Many people with these conditions feel self-conscious about their appearance and must deal with comments, stares, and questions from others. Providing patients with support during patient encounters is critical. Healthcare professionals can help patients find the right words to explain their condition to others. Learning how to describe the condition can help the patient feel less self-conscious and become more comfortable in public.

BEING PROFESSIONAL

When you work with patients, expressing empathy and compassion is important. Using nonverbal cues and positive gestures can help express empathy and compassion. It is important that the medical assistant use active listening, make appropriate eye contact, and have open body language. This includes being at the same level as the patient and smiling when applicable. Arms should not be crossed or behind the back. The medical assistant should refrain from looking at the clock and fidgeting.

Role-play this scenario: You are a medical assistant. You are rooming Mrs. Grant, who is here today for a follow up on her psoriasis. She tells you, "I have decided not to go out in public when this flares up. I hate the questions and stares from complete strangers. I find it easier just to stay home, by myself." Respond to Mrs. Grant.

CHAPTER REVIEW

The integumentary system is composed of membranes, nails, hair, and skin glands. Skin is the largest organ in the system. Two types of membranes include the connective tissue membranes and the epithelial membranes, which can be divided into mucous, serous, and cutaneous membranes.

The skin is composed of the epidermis and the dermis. These two layers cover the subcutaneous tissue or hypodermis. The epidermis is composed of layers; the stratum germinativum is the innermost layer, and the stratum corneum is the tough outer layer. The dermal-epidermal junction is between the epidermis and dermis. The dermis contains hair follicles, sudoriferous (sweat) and sebaceous (oil) glands, blood vessels, and nerve endings.

The integumentary system is involved in protection, temperature regulation, sensory organ activity, excretion, and the *synthesis* (formation) of vitamin D. The skin is a physical waterproof barrier that protects the body from pathogens and excessive fluid loss. By blood vessel dilation or constriction and sweat, the skin can help regulate the body temperature. The dermis contains sensory receptors for pain, pressure, heat, and cold. The integumentary system can excrete substances through the skin. Vitamin D_3 is produced in the skin in the presence of sunlight and is converted to a useable form of the vitamin by the kidneys.

Many integumentary disorders were discussed in the chapter. Common signs and symptoms include skin discoloration, itching, blisters, macules, papules, scaly skin surface, and lesions. Common diagnostic procedures include cultures, sensitivity testing, skin biopsies, and Wood light examination. Common treatments include cryosurgery, debridement, incision and drainage, laser therapy, Mohs surgery, onychectomy, photodynamic therapy, and phototherapy.

The integumentary system undergoes changes throughout the life span. Infants may be covered with vernix and lanugo at birth. Colored birthmarks and skin markings may be present at birth and many disappear early in life. As a person ages, the epidermis thins. More bruising can occur due to the fragile dermal blood vessels. The heat-regulating role of the integumentary system is affected by age due to the thinning of subcutaneous fat layers and the decrease sweat production.

SCENARIO WRAP-UP

Mai has thought over her past week of work. She realizes that she works with many patients who have integumentary concerns. Not only does Mai room patients and obtain their history, but she also helps the provider with diagnostic tests and treatments. Just last week Mai assisted with three minor surgeries that involved skin repairs and one toenail removal. She enjoys the variety of patients and values her understanding of the body systems and common diseases. Mai looks forward to more experiences at WMFM Clinic.

6

Nervous System

LEARNING OBJECTIVES

1. Describe the anatomy of the central and peripheral nervous systems.
2. Describe the autonomic nervous system, including its structure and function.
3. Describe the functions of the nervous system.
4. Explain the common diagnostic procedures and treatments for nervous system disorders.
5. Describe common nervous system disorders, including common signs and symptoms, etiology, diagnostic procedures, and treatments.
6. Compare the structure and function of the of the nervous system across the life span.

OUTLINE

▶ OPENING SCENARIO

Nancy Gehir, CMA (AAMA), is a medical assistant at Walden-Martin Family Medical (WMFM) Clinic. She was hired at WMFM Clinic shortly after passing her Certified Medical Assistant (CMA) exam. She has recently accepted a position to help the outreach providers. Outreach providers deliver specialty services that are not offered at WMFM Clinic.

Nancy will be assisting with the neurology providers, who come to the clinic weekly to see patients. Prior to starting with neurology, Nancy spent some time reviewing her anatomy textbook and researching common diseases. Today, she is helping Dr. Arzt and Tammy Tamar, nurse practitioner (NP).

YOU WILL LEARN

1. To describe the anatomy of the central and peripheral nervous systems.
2. To discuss the cells of the nervous system.
3. To describe the autonomic nervous system, including the sympathetic and parasympathetic nervous systems.
4. To describe the functions of the nervous system.
5. To describe common nervous system disorders, including etiology, signs and symptoms, diagnostic procedures, and treatments.
6. To discuss life span changes in the nervous system.

INTRODUCTION

Neurology is the healthcare specialty that deals with the diseases and disorders of the nervous system. A *neurologist* is a specialist involved in the diagnosis, treatment, and prevention of nervous system diseases and disorders.

Besides the neurology department, patients with nervous system concerns can be seen in primary care and also urgent care departments. The medical assistant may help the provider with the examination and screening questions.

ANATOMY OF THE NERVOUS SYSTEM

The main structures of the nervous system include the brain, spinal cord, and nerves. Various other sense organs, besides the nerves, exist throughout the body, such as the eyes. The nervous system is made up of nerve cells, or *neurons*. (Neurons are discussed in the "Physiology of the Nervous System" section.)

The nervous system is divided as follows:

- *Central nervous system* (CNS), which is composed of the brain and the spinal cord.
- *Peripheral nervous system* (PNS), which is made up of all the nervous tissue outside of the CNS, including the 12 pairs of cranial nerves and 31 pairs of spinal nerves. The PNS can be further divided into:
  - *Somatic nervous system*, which is voluntary. It collects information from and returns instructions to the skin, voluntary muscles, and joints.
  - *Autonomic nervous system* (ANS), which is involuntary. It collects information from and returns instructions to involuntary structures (e.g., involuntary muscles, glands, organs).

Central Nervous System

Brain. The brain, enclosed in the skull, is one of the most complex organs of the body. It is divided into the cerebrum, cerebellum, diencephalon, and brainstem (Fig. 6.1).

Cerebrum. The cerebrum is the largest portion of the brain and is divided into two hemispheres by a deep fissure (FISH er). The right hemisphere controls artistic functions, such as drawing, rhythm, and picture memory. The left hemisphere controls verbal functions, such as reading, writing, speaking, and mathematic calculations. The hemispheres are connected by the *corpus callosum*, a bundle of nerve tissue that facilitates communication between the two sides of the brain. If the corpus callosum only partially develops or is absent, the person is diagnosed with *corpus callosum agenesis*.

Most of the signals between the brain and body cross over. This means that the left cerebral hemisphere primarily controls the right side of the body and that the right hemisphere primarily controls the left side of the body. For instance, if a person has a stroke affecting the right hemisphere, the symptoms will be seen on the left side of the body.

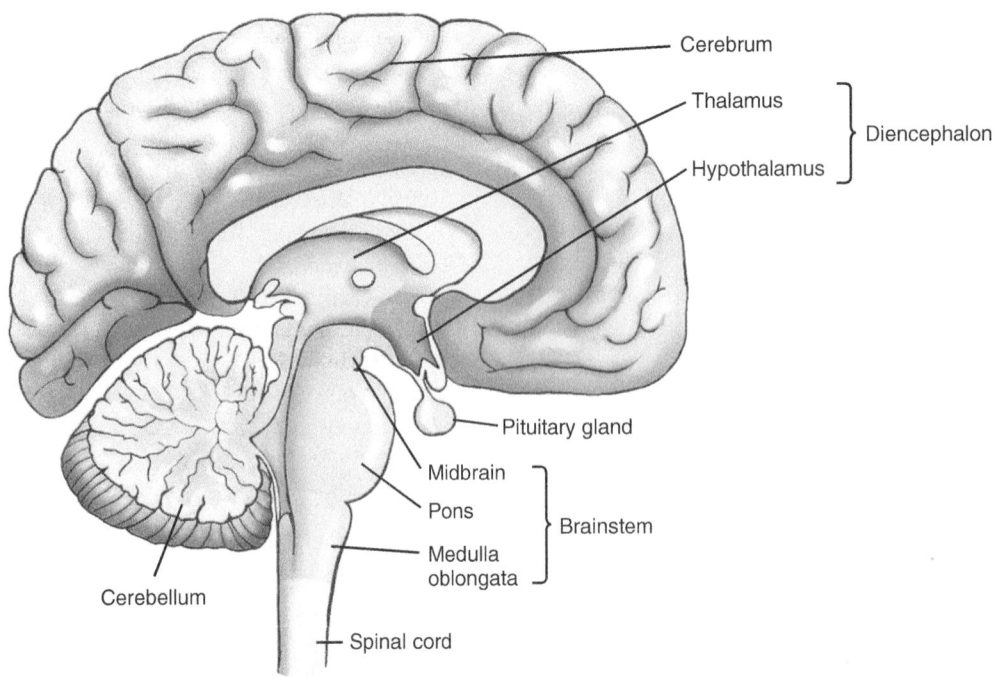

Fig. 6.1 The Brain.

Each cerebral hemisphere is further divided into four sections, called *lobes*. These are the functions of the lobes:

- *Frontal lobes*: Lie directly behind the forehead. These lobes are responsible for personality, intelligence, concentration, self-awareness, problem solving, short-term memory, planning, and judgment. In the back of the frontal lobe is a *motor area*, which controls the voluntary movements on the opposite side of the body. The *Broca area*, found on the left frontal lobe, is involved with speech (e.g., moving thoughts into words when speaking and writing) (Fig. 6.2). When damage occurs in the Broca area (e.g., stroke or head injury), aphasia (ah FAY zhah) can occur.

- *Parietal lobes*: Found behind the frontal lobes. These lobes are involved with reading and interpreting visual, auditory, motor, sensory, and memory signals, along with spatial and visual perceptions. The *sensory areas*, found near the motor area of the frontal lobe, receive information from the body regarding touch, pain, and temperature (see Fig. 6.2). Reading and math skills are also functions of the parietal lobe.

- *Occipital lobes*: Found at the back of the brain. These lobes handle images from the eyes and connect the information with stored image memories. Damage to or a lack of these lobes can cause blindness.

- *Temporal lobes*: Found in front of the occipital lobes on the right and left side of the brain. The top of each temporal lobe receives information from the ears, and the underside of the lobe forms and retrieves sound-related memories. The *Wernicke area*, found in the left temporal lobe, is important for language comprehension and speech (see Fig. 6.2). The temporal lobes are also responsible for processing memories and sensations of taste, touch, sight, and sounds. The amygdala

(ah MIG dah lah) is found in each temporal lobe and is involved with the limbic system.

The surfaces of the hemispheres are covered by gray matter, or the *cerebral cortex*. The cerebral cortex is a thin layer ranging from 1 to 4.5 mm in thickness. Most of the information processing in the brain takes place in the cerebral cortex. Gyri (JIE rie) add more surface area, thus increasing the amount of information that can be processed. Sulci (SUL sie) are also visible on the cerebral cortex.

VOCABULARY

amygdala A small mass of gray matter found in each temporal lobe of the cerebrum and involved with memories, emotions, and activating the fight-or-flight response; part of the limbic system.

aphasia Partial or complete loss of the ability to articulate ideas or understand written or spoken language.

fissure A groove that divides an organ into lobes or parts.

gray matter Nerve tissue that lacks the insulation that causes a white appearance to other nerves; thus gray matter looks gray.

gyri Folds or convolutions on the surface of the cerebral hemisphere, which increase the gray matter surface area. Gyrus (JIE rus) is the singular form.

limbic system Consists of several structures, including the amygdala, hippocampus, and hypothalamus; plays an important role in behavior, memories, and emotions.

sulci Grooves or depressions on the surface of the brain between the gyri. Sulcus (SUL kus) is the singular form.

MEDICAL TERMINOLOGY

cerebr/o	cerebrum
cerebell/o	cerebellum
cortic/o	cortex
dermat/o	skin
dur/o	dura mater
encephal/o	brain
hemat/o	blood
hydr/o	water
lob/o	lobe
medull/o	medulla
mening/o, meninge/o	meninges
phas/o	speech
somat/o	body
ventricul/o	ventricle
a-	without, no
auto-	self
-cephalus	head
-ia	condition
-oma	tumor, mass
-tome	instrument used to cut

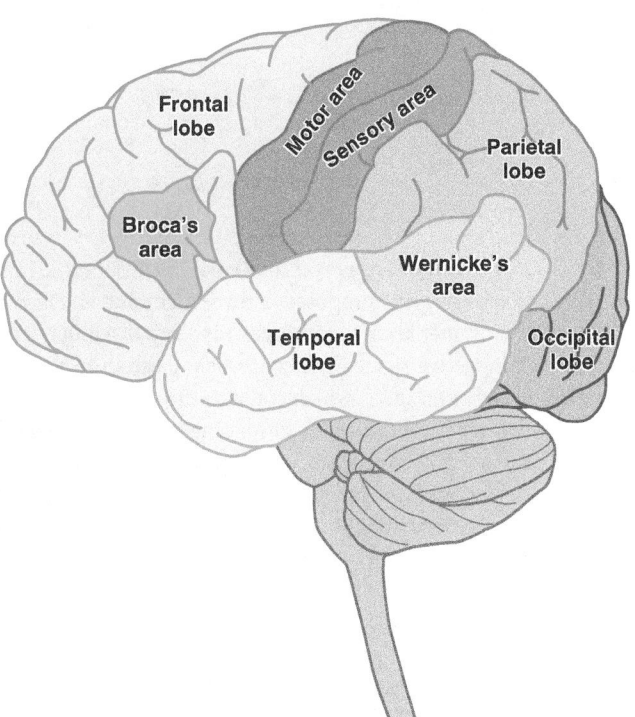

Fig. 6.2 The Lobes of the Cerebrum. (From Niedzwiecki B, et al: *Kinn's the medical assistant*, ed 14, St. Louis, 2020, Elsevier.)

Cerebellum. The cerebellum is located below the occipital lobe of the cerebrum. It is also covered by the cortex. The cerebellum gathers input from other parts of the brain and spinal cord to provide accurate timing for coordinated smooth movements. The cerebellum coordinates the equilibrium, or balance, posture, and muscle coordination. Damage to the cerebellum, as is caused by a stroke, can cause nausea, dizziness, and balance and coordination issues.

Diencephalon. The diencephalon is located just above the brainstem and is almost surrounded by the cerebral hemispheres. It serves as a relay station for sensory input neurons and other parts of the brain. It plays important roles in the functioning of the CNS, endocrine system, and the limbic system. The diencephalon is composed of the posterior pituitary gland and the pineal gland, which are part of the endocrine system. The diencephalon also includes two other parts:

- *Thalamus:* Processes information going to and from the body and the cerebrum.
- *Hypothalamus:* Controls body temperature, hunger, and thirst; part of the limbic system.

A tract of nerve cells connects the thalamus and hypothalamus to the hippocampus (hip oh KAM pus). The hippocampus works with memories, sending memories to cerebral hemispheres for storage (long-term memories) and then retrieving them when needed.

CRITICAL THINKING 6.1

Nancy has roomed Elaine. While Nancy is taking her medical history, Elaine mentions that she feels unsteady from time to time and loses her balance a few times. What part of the brain is involved in maintaining balance?

Brainstem. The brainstem connects the cerebral hemispheres to the spinal cord. It controls the flow of information from the body to the brain. The brainstem is composed of these structures:

- *Midbrain:* Connects the hemispheres of the cerebrum with the pons. It serves as a relay center for auditory, visual, and motor information. It also contains centers to regulate pupillary reflexes and eye movements.
- *Pons:* Serves as a bridge between the medulla oblongata and the cerebrum and helps to regulate respirations.
- *Medulla oblongata:* Lowest part of the brainstem. It contains vital centers of life (e.g., cardiac, respiratory, and vasomotor centers) that regulate the heart rate, respirations, and the diameter of blood vessels, which affect the blood pressure. Nonvital centers also are found in the medulla oblongata, including centers that regulate coughing, sneezing, hiccupping, vomiting, and swallowing. Some medications work to "quiet" these centers.

Spinal Cord. The spinal cord is a bundle of nervous tissue. It extends from the medulla oblongata to about the second lumbar vertebra (Fig. 6.3). The spinal cord passes through the foramen magnum (for AY men MAG num) in the skull and is protected by the vertebrae. It is covered by meninges (meh NIN jeez). The spinal cord is composed of the cell bodies of motor neurons (gray matter), and the myelin-covered axons. Thirty-one pairs of spinal nerves extend from the spinal cord. Each nerve stimulates a specific organ or area of the body. The spinal cord carries messages between the spinal nerves and the brain. This can slow with age.

VOCABULARY

axon A long extension of a nerve fiber that conducts the impulse away from the nerve cell body; white matter.

choroid plexus A network of capillaries found in the lateral ventricles and the third and fourth ventricles that secrete cerebrospinal fluid.

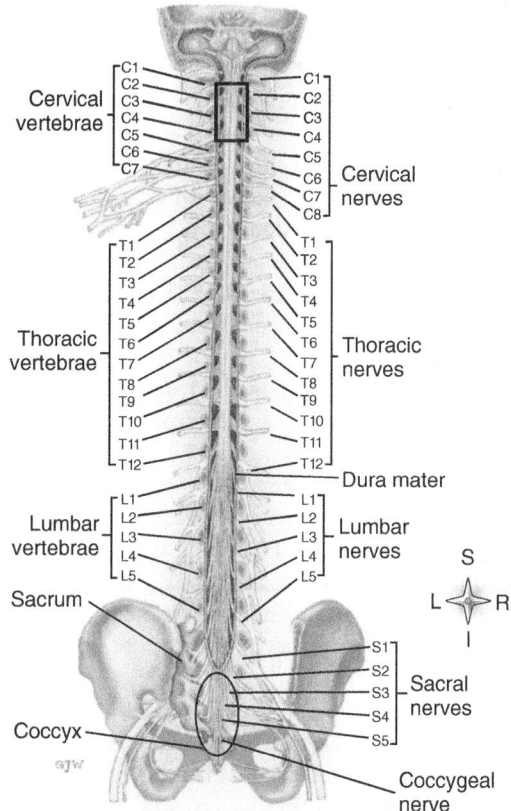

Fig. 6.3 The Spinal Cord, Showing the Spinal Nerves. (From Vidic B, Suarez FR: *Photographic atlas of the human body*, St. Louis, 1984, Mosby.)

---

foramen magnum A large opening in the base of the skull. It forms a passageway for the spinal cord.

hippocampus A ridge in the floor of the lateral ventricle; composed of gray matter. Involved with the limbic system and with creating and filing new memories.

meninges A protective covering around the brain and spinal cord.

pineal gland A small organ in the brain that secretes melatonin, a hormone that regulates the sleep/awake cycle.

tract A system of tissues (e.g., neuronal axons) and/or organs (e.g., intestines) that function together.

Meninges. Meninges are a protective covering around the brain and spinal cord. They are composed of three membranes (Fig. 6.4).

- *Dura mater:* Outer layer of meninges; made up of a tough white fibrous connective tissue. The space below the dura mater is called the *subdural space*, which contains tiny blood vessels.
- *Arachnoid mater:* Middle layer of meninges; made up of a thin layer of threadlike strands resembling a cobweb. The space below the arachnoid is called the *subarachnoid space,* and it is filled with cerebrospinal fluid (CSF) and blood vessels.
- *Pia mater:* Innermost layer of meninges; a thin, highly vascular membrane that is tightly bound to the surface of the spinal cord and brain.

The ventricular system in the brain is made up of four connected *ventricles* (spaces or cavities). CSF originates in the choroid plexus (KOR oid PLEK sus) in the ventricles. CSF is a clear fluid that resembles water, and it has three roles:

- Cushions the brain and spinal cord
- Removes waste products from cerebral metabolism
- Supplies nutrients to the nervous system tissues

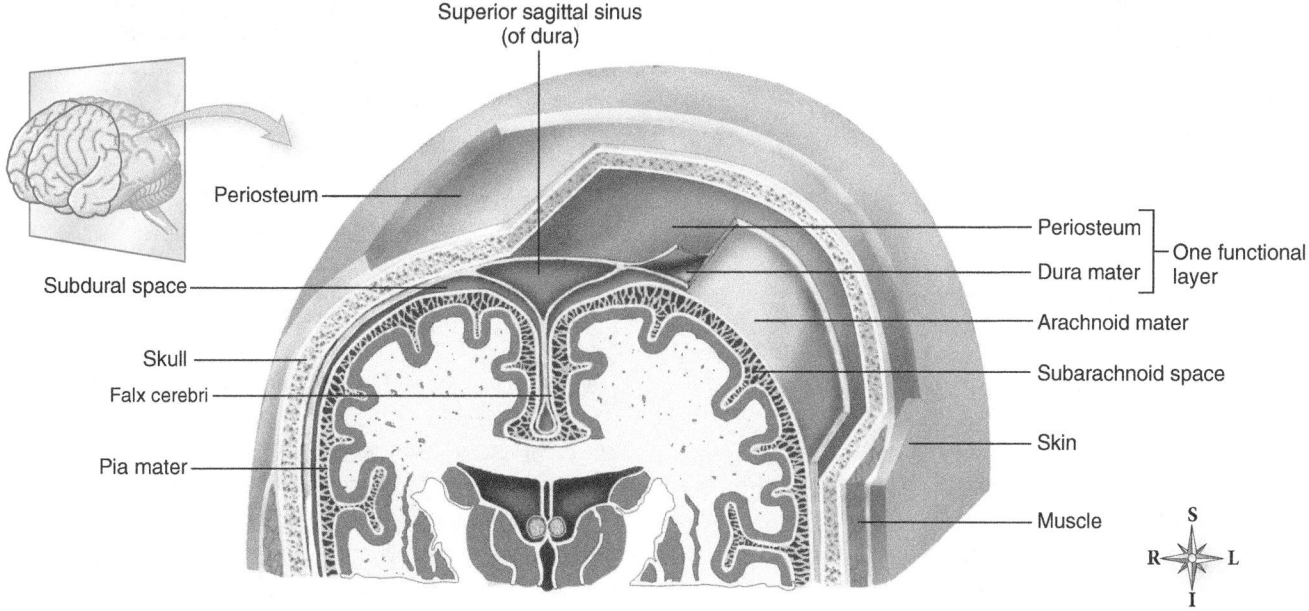

Fig. 6.4 Protective Coverings of the Brain. (Modified from Patton K, Thibodeau G: *The human body in health and disease,* ed 9, St. Louis, 2016, Mosby.)

CSF flows through the ventricles, exits into the cisterns at the base of the brain, and moves around the brain and spinal cord. Eventually, CSF is reabsorbed into the bloodstream. The balance between CSF production and absorption is critical. Excessive amounts of CSF result in abnormal widening of the ventricles, which can put pressure on the brain tissue and lead to hydrocephalus (hi droe SEF ah luhs).

VOCABULARY

afferent Pertaining to carrying toward a structure.
hydrocephalus An abnormal accumulation of cerebrospinal fluid that causes enlargement of the skull and compression of the brain.
myelin sheath A protective insulation that covers the axons and helps with the transmission of nerve impulses.

Peripheral Nervous System

The peripheral nervous system is made up of the nerves that exit the brain or spinal cord. The peripheral nerves exiting the brain directly through the skull are called *cranial nerves.* Cranial nerves originate from the underside of the brain and relay information to and from the sensory organs and muscles of the face and neck (Table 6.1). Cranial nerves have either motor function, sensory function, or both.

The *spinal nerves* exit the spinal canal through spaces between the vertebrae. Spinal nerves closely mimic the organization of the vertebrae and provide stimulation to the rest of the body. If the nerve fibers from several spinal nerves form a network, it is called a *plexus.* Spinal nerves are named by their vertebrae location (e.g., cervical, thoracic) and by number. Spinal nerves carry information to and from the brain through the spinal cord.

Dermatomes are skin surface areas supplied by a single afferent (AF er uhnt) spinal nerve. These areas are so specific, the body can be mapped by dermatomes (Fig. 6.5). Shingles, for example, appears on specific dermatomes based on which nerve the virus has infected.

CRITICAL THINKING 6.2

Using the mnemonic "On Old Olympus Towering Top A Fine Vocal German Viewed Some Hops," list the cranial nerves in order.

Cells of the Nervous System

The nervous system is made up of two types of cells:
- *Neurons:* Also called *parenchymal cells,* which carry out the work of the nervous system.
- *Neuroglia:* Also called *stromal cells* or *glia.* These cells provide a supportive function for the neurons.

Neurons. The nervous system is composed of nerve cells, or *neurons.* Neurons are composed of a cell body, dendrites, and an axon. The *dendrites* are short projections off the cell body. They pick up electrical impulses, often from other neurons, and send the signals along to the cell body. The impulse is then passed to the axon, which is a long extension off the cell body. Some axons can be over 3 feet long. The axon transmits the impulse to other dendrites, glands, or muscles.

Neuroglia. Neuroglial cells care for and support neurons throughout the body. These specialized cells perform specific functions within the nervous system. There are several types of neuroglia, including:
- *Schwann cells:* Form the myelin sheath, which covers the axons of peripheral nerves.
- *Astrocytes:* Help form the *blood-brain barrier* (BBB), which closely regulates what substances enter the brain tissue. Oxygen, water, and glucose molecules easily pass into the brain. Many chemicals and drugs are prevented from moving into brain tissue.

TABLE 6.1 Cranial Nerves

Number	Name	Function	Testing Method
I	Olfactory	Sensory function: Smell	Identifying familiar odors while the eyes are closed.
II	Optic	Sensory function: Vision	A visual acuity test may be given. A light may be shined in the eyes.
III	Oculomotor	Sensory and motor functions: Eye movement, pupil constriction and accommodation	The pupil is examined using a light. The patient may be asked to follow the light with the eyes without moving the face.
IV	Trochlear	Motor function: Eye movement	Testing to see if the eyes can follow a moving light, as described for cranial nerve III.
V	Trigeminal	Sensory and motor functions: Muscles for chewing, general sensations from the anterior half of the head, including the face and meninges	The provider may feel the face in different locations and have the patient clench the teeth.
VI	Abducens	Motor function: Eye movement	Testing to see if the eyes can follow a moving light, as described for cranial nerve III.
VII	Facial	Sensory and motor functions: Muscles used for facial expressions; tearing, salivation, and taste	Patient may be asked to identify common tastes, puff cheeks, smile, wrinkle forehead, and close eyes tightly.
VIII	Vestibulocochlear	Sensory function: Hearing and equilibrium	Assessed using a hearing acuity test.
IX	Glossopharyngeal	Sensory and motor functions: Swallowing and taste	Gag reflex is tested with a tongue blade.
X	Vagus	Sensory and motor functions: Breathing, speech, sweating, regulating heartbeat, stimulating muscles of the gastric region	Patient is asked to say "ahh," swallow, and talk (voice quality assessed). Gag reflex is tested with a tongue blade.
XI	Spinal accessory	Motor function: Shoulder and head movements	Assessed by turning the head from side to side against mild resistance and shrugging the shoulders.
XII	Hypoglossal	Motor function: Tongue movements	Assessed by sticking out and moving the tongue from side to side.

- *Microglia*: Found in the CNS. If brain tissue is inflamed or damaged, microglia engulf and destroy microorganisms or debris.
- *Oligodendrocytes:* Found in the CNS; they myelinate the CNS axons and help hold nerve fibers together.

CRITICAL THINKING 6.3

What type of cell produces the myelin sheath that surrounds some nerve axons?

MEDICAL TERMINOLOGY

astr/o	star
dendr/o	dendrite
home/o	same
neur/o	nerve
inter-	between
-cyte	cell
-glia	glue
-on	structure
-stasis	stopping, controlling

PHYSIOLOGY OF THE NERVOUS SYSTEM

The *nervous system* is a complex system that plays a major role in homeostasis (hoh mee oh STAY sis). The nervous system works in partnership with the endocrine system to help the body respond to its internal and external environments. This effort is responsible for communication and control throughout the body. There are three main functions of the nervous system:

- Collecting information about the external and internal environments (sensing)
- Processing this information and making decisions about action (interpreting)
- Directing the body to put into action the decisions made (acting)

For example, the sensory function begins with a *stimulus* (e.g., the uncomfortable pinch of a tight shoe). That information travels to the brain, where it is *interpreted*. The return message is sent to *react to the stimulus* (e.g., remove the shoe).

The basic flow of information in the nervous system includes:

- *Afferent* or *sensory neurons*, which collect stimuli received from receptors. Receptors are found throughout the body (e.g., skin, eyes, nose, tongue, and internal organs). Pain receptors are also found throughout the body. The afferent neurons carry the stimuli from the receptors to the CNS (e.g., brain and spinal cord).
- The brain and spinal cord process the information and direct the necessary response. The central nervous system contains *interneurons*, nerve cells, that connect sensory and motor neurons.
- The response from the CNS is sent via the efferent (EF er uhnt) or *motor neurons*. The efferent neurons carry the response to an organ, gland, or muscle. The efferent neurons that direct the skeletal muscles are part of the somatic nervous system. The efferent neurons that direct internal organs to contract and secrete are part of the autonomic nervous system.

VOCABULARY

efferent Pertaining to carrying away from a structure.
homeostasis The internal environment of the body that is compatible with life. A steady state that is created by all the body systems working together to provide a consistent and unvarying internal environment.

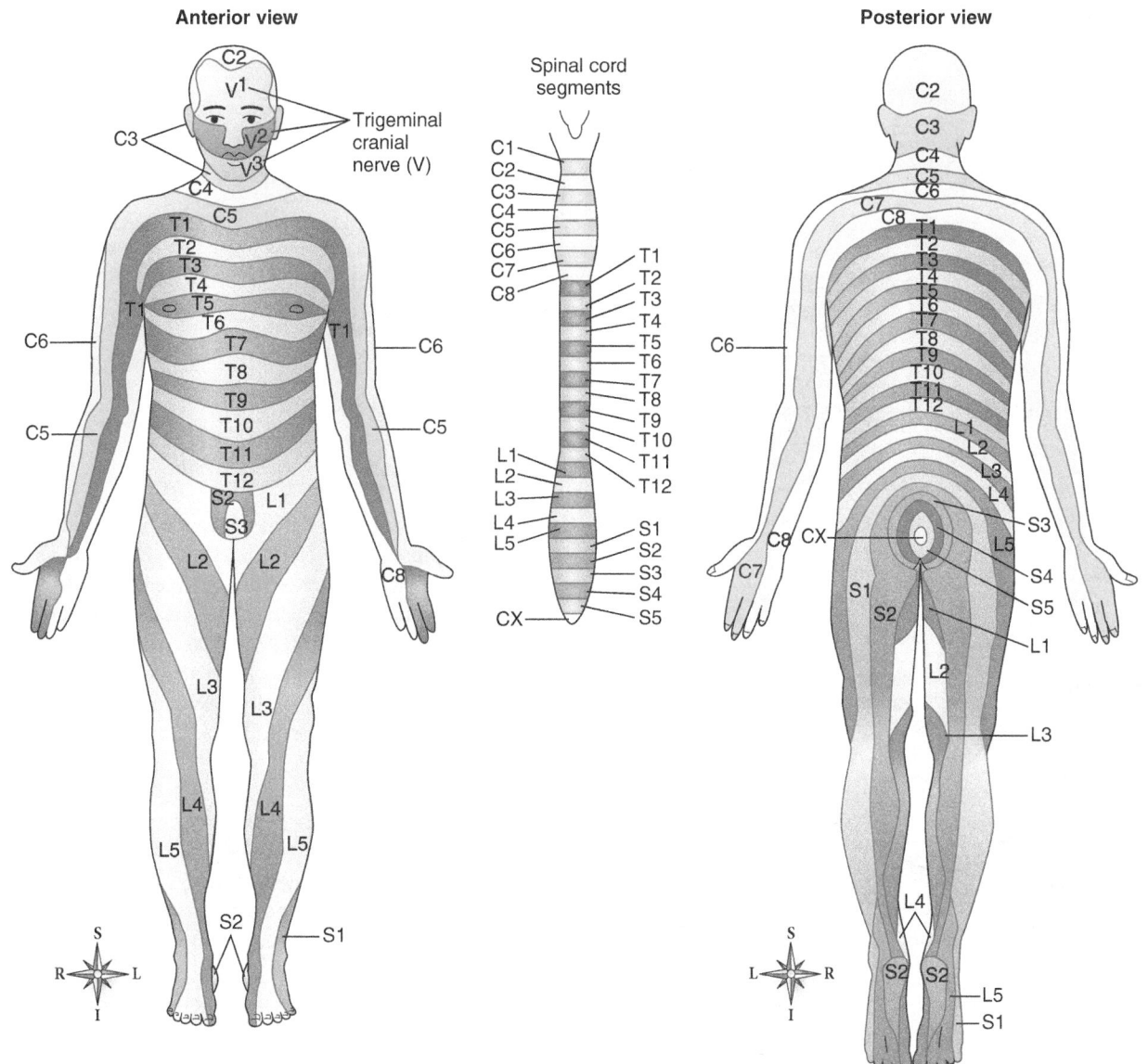

Fig. 6.5 Map of the Dermatomes. (From Patton K, Thibodeau G: *The human body in health & disease,* ed 7, St. Louis, 2018, Mosby.)

Peripheral Nervous System

The peripheral nervous system consists of voluntary and involuntary nerves. The PNS can be divided into the *somatic nervous system* (voluntary nervous system) and the *autonomic nervous system* (involuntary nervous system). The autonomic nervous system can be further divided into the sympathetic nervous system and the parasympathetic nervous system (Fig. 6.6).

Somatic Nervous System. The somatic nervous system is the part of the peripheral nervous system that sends motor impulses to the skeletal muscles. The somatic nervous system transmits signals from the CNS to the skeletal muscles and from the sense receptors (vision, hearing, and touch). It is associated with the voluntary control of body movements and is also involved with involuntary reflex arcs.

Reflex Arc. A *reflex* is an involuntary, almost instantaneous movement in response to a specific stimulus. A reflex arc is the route followed by nerve impulses in the production of a reflex act. The stimulus is picked up by the receptors. The impulse is carried by the afferent neuron to the central nervous system (brain or spinal cord). The efferent neuron carries the message from the central nervous system to the effector organ, where the response occurs.

A *three-neuron arc* consists of sensory neurons, interneurons, and motor neurons (Fig. 6.7). A *two-neuron arc* is the simplest reflex arc. It does not require the brain to cause a response. The two-neuron arc consists of just sensory neurons and motor neurons. The knee-jerk reflex, also called the *patellar reflex,* is an example of the two-neuron arc. A sharp tap on the patellar tendon below the patella results in a sudden kicking movement of the lower leg. The tap on the tendon (the

Subdivisions of the Nervous System

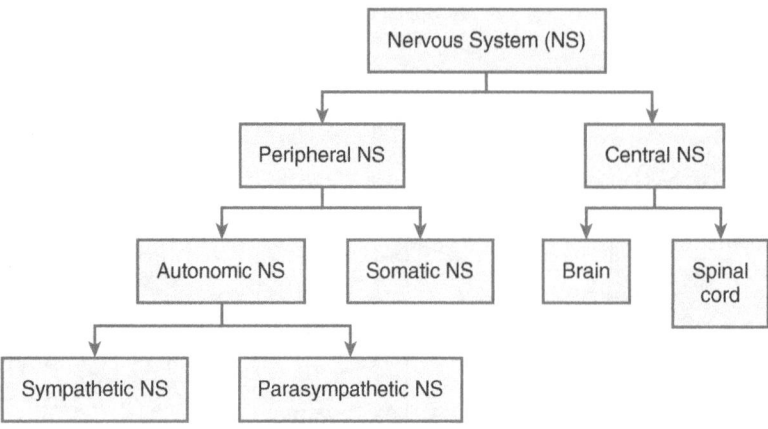

Fig. 6.6 Nervous System Flow Chart.

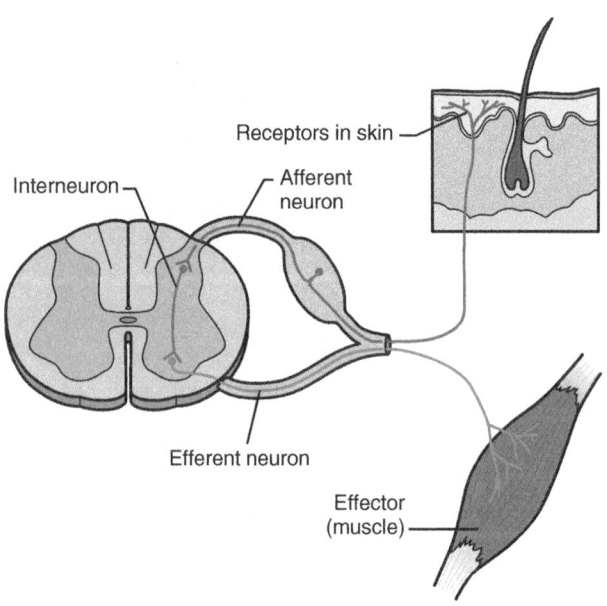

Fig. 6.7 Three-Neuron Arc.

stimulus) is picked up by receptors. The impulse is carried by the afferent neuron (part of the femoral nerve) to the spinal cord. The response from the spinal cord is sent back by the efferent neuron to the muscles thigh. The muscles contract, and the kick occurs.

Autonomic Nervous System. The autonomic nervous system consists of nerves that conduct impulses from the brainstem or spinal cord to cardiac and smooth muscle tissue and glands. The ANS controls the muscles in blood vessel walls, organs, and glands. It regulates involuntary functions such as breathing, heart rate, sweating, circulation, and digestion.

The motor portion of this system is further divided into the sympathetic nervous system and the parasympathetic nervous system. These two opposing systems help maintain homeostasis throughout the body systems (Fig. 6.8).

Sympathetic Nervous System. The *sympathetic nervous system* can produce a "fight-or-flight" response. This is the part of the nervous system that helps the individual respond to perceived

stress. It speeds up the heart rate, raises blood glucose levels, raises blood pressure, slows the digestive system, and widens the bronchioles, allowing more oxygen to enter the body quickly. It also stimulates the adrenal glands to increase their secretions.

Parasympathetic Nervous System. The *parasympathetic nervous system* does the opposite of the sympathetic nervous system. It slows the heart rate, lowers blood pressure, increases digestive functions, and reduces adrenal and sweat gland activity.

CRITICAL THINKING 6.4

It is important to know the differences between the sympathetic and parasympathetic nervous systems. List three characteristics of each and compare your list with a classmate. Do your lists agree?

Action Potential

Neurons carry information from one cell to another by creating and spreading electronic impulses. An *action potential* is a self-propagating wave of electrical impulse that travels along the surface of a neuron membrane. An action potential proceeds in the following steps:

1. A stimulus (e.g., pressure, temperature, sound wave) starts an impulse.
2. The resting nerve cell has a slightly positive charge (due to sodium ions) on the outside of the cell membrane, and a negative charge inside the cell. This state is called *polarization*.
3. When a section of the membrane is stimulated, the positively charged ions on the outside of the cell enter the nerve cell. This changes the outside charge to a negative charge. This state is called *depolarization*.
4. Almost immediately after the impulse passes, the positively charged ions move outside the nerve cells again. This returns the outside charge to a positive charge. This state is called *repolarization*.
5. Once everything changes back, the cell is at rest again, and the cycle continues.

The transfer of the action potential begins as the electrical impulse travels down an axon. It becomes a chemical impulse

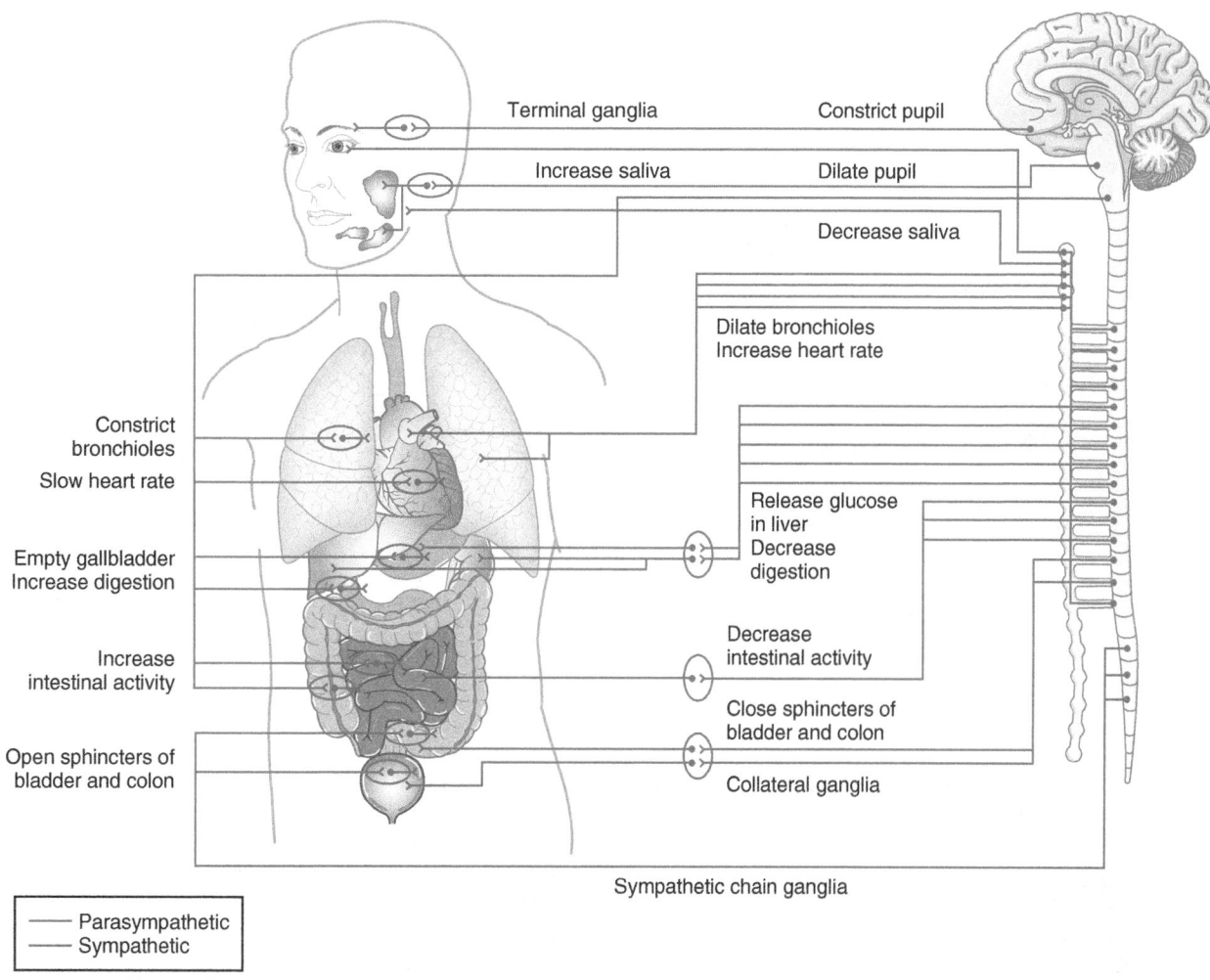

Fig. 6.8 Structure and Function of the Autonomic Nervous System. (From Applegate E: *The anatomy and physiology learning system,* ed 4, St. Louis, 2011, Saunders.)

while moving across the *synapse*, the gap between the neurons. The transfer of impulses from the end of one neuron to the dendrites of another is enhanced by chemical neurotransmitters found in the synapse (Fig. 6.9). Examples of neurotransmitters include epinephrine, norepinephrine, dopamine, serotonins, endorphins, and enkephalins.

Neurotransmitters bind to specific receptor sites on the dendrites of the next neuron or the target tissue. Messages move throughout the entire nervous system in this manner. Impulses in the neuron are electrical; the impulses become chemical as a neurotransmitter is released at each synapse. The action potentials become electrical again as they are picked up by the next dendrites of another neuron or by the target tissue. Changes in the amount of available neurotransmitters can cause different conditions.

VOCABULARY

neuralgia Sharp, spasmlike pain in a nerve or along the course of one or more nerves.

neurotransmitter A chemical that helps a nerve cell communicate with another nerve cell or muscle.

target tissue The destination, or intended tissue, in the nervous impulse (e.g., a muscle).

DISEASES AND DISORDERS OF THE NERVOUS SYSTEM

Patients with symptoms of nervous system disorders can be seen in primary care and urgent care departments. The medical assistant may need to ask screening questions and assist the provider with the examination.

Common signs and symptoms of neurologic disorders include:
- Neuralgia (noo RAL jah), *paresthesia* (feelings of prickling, burning, or numbness)
- Lack of coordination, muscle rigidity, *spasms* (involuntary muscle contractions, such as stuttering and tics), seizures, and *tremors* (rhythmic, purposeless muscle movements)
- Recurrent headache, amnesia *(memory loss)*, difficulty speaking or finding the right word, slurred speech
- Loss of sight or double vision
- Confusion, disorientation, or loss of consciousness

To check the patient's mental status, a neurologic examination (also called a *neuro exam*) may be done (Box 6.1 and Figs. 6.10 and 6.11). Based on the patient's symptoms, the provider may perform a lumbar puncture (LP) (also called a *spinal tap*) (Box 6.2 and Fig. 6.12). This is done to collect a small amount

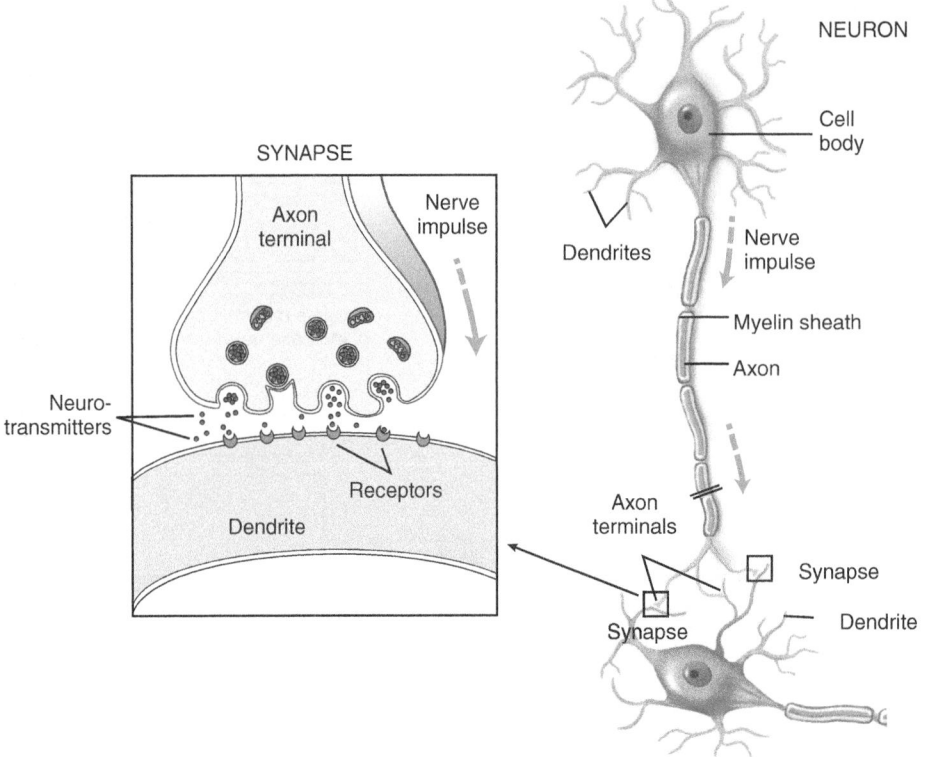

Fig. 6.9 Neuron and Synapse (Inset). (From Shiland B: *Mastering healthcare terminology,* ed 5, St. Louis, 2016, Mosby.)

BOX 6.1   Neurologic Examination

The neurologic status examination tests the patient's cognitive functions. It provides a baseline of neurologic information for the provider (Fig. 6.10).

During the examination, the provider assesses the patient's emotional status, intellectual performance, cognitive ability, and general behavior. The patient's grooming, mannerisms, and ability to communicate are carefully observed. The provider assesses the patient's appropriate use of speech, language, and writing skills. Many different areas, including the following, may be assessed.

- *Mental status:* The patient's level of awareness of person, place, and time are assessed. "Person" is assessed by asking the person's name. "Place" is assessed by asking where the patient is. "Time" is assessed with questions related to what year or day it is. If the patient provides the correct answers, providers may document "Alert and oriented," "Alert and oriented to person, place, and time," or "A&O×3."
- *Functioning of the cranial nerves:* Table 6.1 describes how the nerves are assessed.
- *Motor function, balance, and coordination:* To assess these areas, the patient needs to:
  - Push or pull against the provider's hand with each extremity
  - Walk following a line on the floor
  - Stand with the eyes closed
  - Touch the nose with the eyes closed
- *Sensory function:* The provider may test the patient's ability to feel sensations by using sharp, dull, or light touches, in addition to hot, cold, and vibrating items.
- *Reflexes (children and adults):* Using a reflex hammer, the provider will tap the extremities in different locations to check the reflexes (Fig. 6.11). If the reflex is present and normal, a small movement of the extremity will occur.

---

of CSF. The fluid is analyzed to help confirm or rule out many diseases, including meningitis (men in JYE tis), encephalitis (en seff uh LYE tis), cancer, and dementia. Table 6.2 shows the typical laboratory values for CSF. Additional common diagnostic procedures are listed in Table 6.3. Common treatments are listed in Table 6.4.

There are more than 600 neurologic diseases. The conditions discussed are grouped as neurodegenerative diseases, functional disorders, infections, structural disorders, and vascular disorders.

Neurodegenerative Disorders

Neurodegenerative diseases affect a person's ability to move, talk, and breathe. These diseases can also affect a person's balance and heart function. The etiology may be genetic, related to a medical condition (e.g., tumor, stroke), or caused by a virus or toxin. With some diseases, the etiology is unknown.

Amyotrophic Lateral Sclerosis. Amyotrophic lateral sclerosis (ALS), or Lou Gehrig disease, is a progressive neurological disorder that attacks the motor neurons in the brain and spinal cord. ALS usually affects adults between 40 and 60 years of age.

Etiology. There is no known *etiology* (cause) for ALS, though there is a genetic component to the disease in up to 10% of the cases.

Signs and Symptoms. Early signs and symptoms include mild muscle problems, including trouble walking, running, writing, swallowing *(dysphagia),* and speaking. The muscle weakness starts in the hands and feet and spreads throughout the body, leading to an inability to move the legs and arms. Eventually,

WALDEN–MARTIN
FAMILY MEDICAL CLINIC
1234 ANYSTREET | ANYTOWN, ANYSTATE 12345
PHONE 123-123-1234 | FAX 123-123-5678

Instructor: Becky Swisher

Neurological Status Exam

The Neurological Status Examination tests the individual's sense of cognitive functions and quickly allows the provider to screen for cognitive impairment and/or loss. In addition to testing language recall and motor skills, the NSE also allows you to test an individual's orientation to time, detail, and attention.

There are five sections. Each section of the test involves relating a series of questions or commands to a patient; the patient should receive one point for each correct answer. Conduct the test without interruptions in a well-lit, private exam room. Instruct the patient to listen carefully and to answer each question as accurately as possible. In the event that there is a caregiver accompanying the patient, ask the Caregiver Questions and record the responses (these are not part of the final score).

Read each question once and document the patient's response. Do not time the patient's answers or duration of the test overall; once completed, score the test immediately. To do so, add only the number of correct responses. The individual can receive a maximum score of 10 points; a score below 4 indicates cognitive impairment.

Patient Name: _____   Date of Birth: _____
Performed By: _____   Date: _____

Caregiver Questions (if available): (Yes, No, Not Aware)

Name of Caregiver: _____	Yes	No	Not Aware
• Does the patient have difficulty remembering recent events or conversions?	☐	☐	☐
• Does the patient have difficulty performing activities of daily living (bath, driving, cooking, etc.)?	☐	☐	☐
• Have you noticed changes to speech patterns?	☐	☐	☐

Patient Interview

Sequencing:

Read the following statement to the patient three consecutive times: **"Drive the red car to Washington Street."** Then ask the Patient to restate the sentence; you will ask the patient to recall the statement later in the test.

	Yes	No
The patient was able to repeat the exact statement to you	☐	☐

Total: _____

Time Orientation:

Ask the patient the following questions:

	Correct	Incorrect
• What is today's date?	☐	☐
• What season is it?	☐	☐
• What is the day of the week?	☐	☐

Total: _____

Drawing:

Give the individual a piece of paper and ask him/her to copy a design of the two intersecting shapes. One point is awarded for correctly copying the shapes. All angles on both figures must be present, and the figures must have one overlapping angle.

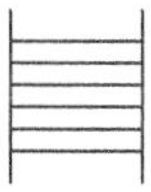

	Correct	Incorrect
	☐	☐

Total: _____

Information:

Ask the patient the following questions:

	Correct	Incorrect
• Who is president of the United States?	☐	☐
• How may stars are on the American flag?	☐	☐

Total: _____

Recall:

Ask the patient to restate the sentence that you asked him/her at the beginning of the procedure. One point is given for repeating each of the following words.

	Correct	Incorrect
• Drive	☐	☐
• Red car	☐	☐
• Washington Street	☐	☐

Total: _____

Total Exam Score: _____

Fig. 6.10 Neurologic Status Exam Form. (From Niedzwiecki B, et al: *Kinn's the medical assistant,* ed 14, St. Louis, 2020, Elsevier.)

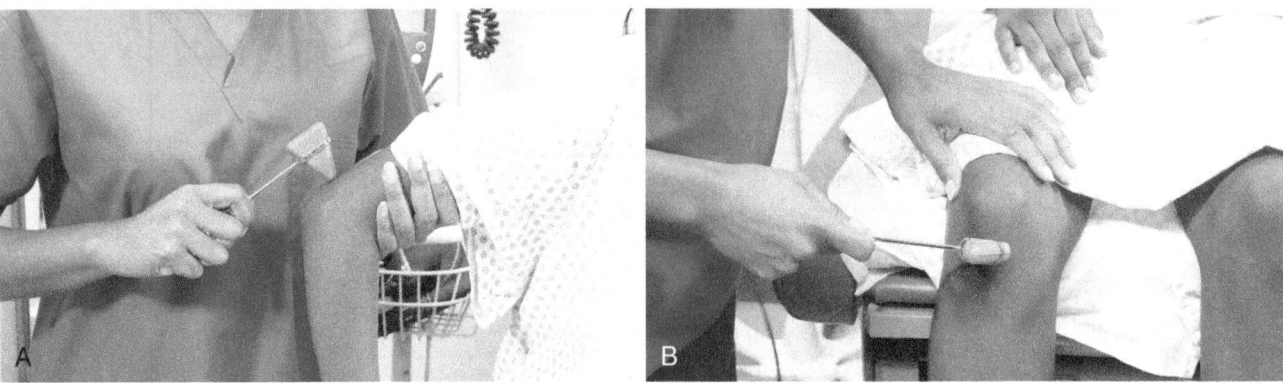

Fig. 6.11 The provider checks (A) the triceps reflex and (B) the quadriceps reflex. (From Niedzwiecki B, et al: *Kinn's the medical assistant*, ed 14, St. Louis, 2020, Elsevier.)

BOX 6.2   Lumbar Puncture

In the ambulatory care setting, the most common reason for a lumbar puncture (LP) is to collect a sample of the cerebrospinal fluid (CSF). The patient is placed in either a left side-lying position with the knees drawn up to the chest or in a sitting position leaning forward on a stable surface. For an infant or young child, the medical assistant might need to hold the child in a side-lying position during the procedure. The site is cleansed with an antiseptic, and a local anesthetic is injected to numb the area. The provider then inserts a hollow needle between the third and fourth or the fourth and fifth lumbar vertebrae and advances it into the subarachnoid space. The CSF flows out of the needle into the sterile collection tubes. Usually 1 to 2 mL of fluid is needed in each tube. When multiple tubes are required, a total of about 10 to 15 mL of CSF is typically collected. The tubes need to be numbered in the order that they are collected. The needle is then removed, and a bandage or small dressing is applied to the site.

the person has difficulty eating, speaking, and breathing. Some people experience memory issues and dementia.

Diagnostic Procedures. The provider will do an examination that will show abnormal reflexes, weakness, twitching, and difficulty moving. Tests may be done to rule out other conditions, including blood tests, computed tomography (CT), magnetic resonance imaging (MRI), electromyography, and lumbar puncture. Breathing tests may be done to assess the lung muscles.

Treatments. Riluzole (RIL yoo zole) (Rilutek) may be prescribed to slow symptoms, and other medications may be given to help with the symptoms. Physical therapy and assistive devices (e.g., wheelchair, braces) may be used. A feeding tube may help with the nutritional status. Assistance with breathing may also be needed. There is no cure for ALS.

MEDICAL TERMINOLOGY	
electr/o	electric
esthesi/o	feeling
later/o	side
my/o	muscle
phag/o	eat
troph/o	development
dys-	difficult
hypo-	deficient
para-	abnormal
-al	pertaining to
-algia	pain
-graphy	process of recording
-ic	pertaining to
-itis	inflammation

Alzheimer Disease. Alzheimer (ALTS high mer) disease (AD) is a degenerative disease of the brain. It is characterized by disorientation, memory failure, speech disturbance, and a loss of mental capacity. It is the most common cause of dementia. AD causes an increased amount of microscopic neurofibrillary tangles and amyloid plaques in the cerebral cortex and the loss of neurons.

Etiology. Usually, AD begins after age 60, and the risk increases with age. The risk also increases if family members have AD. Researchers feel that AD is caused by a

Site of needle puncture

Dura mater
Distal end of spinal cord
Third lumbar vertebra

Subarachnoid space

Fig. 6.12 Lumbar Puncture. (From Niedzwiecki B, et al: *Kinn's the medical assistant*, ed 14, St. Louis, 2020, Elsevier.)

TABLE 6.2   Typical Laboratory Values for Cerebrospinal Fluid (CSF)

	Normal CSF	Abnormal CSF and Related Conditions
Pressure (mm H₂O)	70–180	*Increased:* Increased intracranial pressure *Decreased:* Spinal cord tumor, fainting, diabetic coma, and shock
Appearance	Clear, colorless	*Cloudy:* Infection, elevated white blood cells or protein *Bloody or red:* Bleeding *Brown, orange, or yellow:* Increased protein or previous bleeding
Glucose (mg/dL)	50–80	*Increased:* Hyperglycemia (high blood glucose) *Decreased:* Hypoglycemia (low blood glucose), bacterial or fungal infection (e.g., bacterial meningitis), tuberculosis
Protein (mg/dL)	15–60	*Increased:* Blood in the CSF, diabetes, polyneuritis, injury, inflammation, infection, or tumor *Decreased:* Rapid CSF production
Blood Cells	0–5 White blood cells (WBCs) 0 Red blood cells (RBCs)	*Increase in WBCs:* Meningitis, acute infection, tumor, abscess, stroke, multiple sclerosis *Increase in RBCs:* Traumatic lumbar puncture, bleeding into the CSF

TABLE 6.3   Common Diagnostic Procedures Used for Nervous System Disorders

Procedure	Description
Cerebral angiography (an jee OH gruh fee)	Used to see how the blood flows through the brain. A person must lie on the x-ray table without moving. The head is held still. A local anesthetic is given in the groin area, and a catheter is threaded through an artery in the groin until it reaches the neck. X-ray is used to help guide the process. A dye is injected and highlights the blood flow through the brain.
Electroencephalography (EEG) (ee leck troh en seff fah LAH gruh fee)	Used to record the brain wave activity of a patient. Done to rule out or confirm seizure activity, Alzheimer disease (AD), psychosis, and narcolepsy, a sleep disorder.
Electromyography (EMG) (i LEK troe MIE OG rah fee)	Used to test the health of nerves and muscles. A fine needle with an electrode is inserted into the muscle. The electrode picks up the electrical activity from the muscle during activity and at rest. The activity is recorded.
Nerve conduction velocity (NCV) test	Usually done with EMG. Done to test the speed of electrical signals as they move through a nerve. Electrode patches are placed on the skin over nerves and give off a mild electrical impulse. The electrical activity is recorded by other electrodes.
Nerve biopsy	The removal of a small piece of the nerve for examination. After applying an analgesic, the provider makes a small surgical incision and removes a piece of the nerve from the ankle, forearm, or rib area.

TABLE 6.4   Common Treatments Used for Nervous System Disorders

Procedure	Description
Craniectomy (kray nee ECK tuh mee)	Surgical removal of a portion of the cranium.
Craniotomy (kray nee AH tuh mee)	Surgical incision into the skull.
Neurectomy (noo REK tuh mee)	Surgical removal of part or all of a nerve.
Neuroplasty (NOO roh plas tee)	Surgery of the nerve.
Ventriculoperitoneal shunt (ven trick yoo loh pair ih tuh nee uhl)	A catheter is inserted into the brain and drains extra fluid from the brain ventricles into the abdominal cavity.

activities or the names of people the person knows. AD affects thinking, reasoning, making judgments and decisions, memory, performing familiar tasks, personality, and behavior. Over time, the symptoms worsen, affecting a person's ability to speak, read, write, or remember family members. Personality changes, aggression, and wandering away from home can occur (Box 6.3).

> **VOCABULARY**
> **amyloid plaques** Masses or clumps of proteins that form between neurons and disrupt cellular function.
> **coma** A state of deep, often prolonged unconsciousness, usually the result of a head injury, neurologic disease, intoxication, or metabolic abnormalities.
> **neurofibrillary tangles** Abnormal structures composed of twisted protein fibers within nerve cells.

Diagnostic Procedures. The provider will do a medical history and physical exam. There is no specific test for AD. Neurologic tests, CT, MRI, positron emission tomography (PET), psychiatric evaluation, and cognitive and neuropsychological tests may be done. Laboratory tests are done to rule out other conditions. A lumbar puncture may be done, and the cerebrospinal fluid may be examined for biomarkers that indicate AD.

combination of lifestyle, genetics, and environmental factors that affect the brain. Some research suggests a link between herpes simplex virus type 1 and AD. The causes are not fully understood.

Signs and Symptoms. The signs and symptoms of AD begin slowly; initially, there is difficulty remembering recent

---

BOX 6.3   Dementia

Several disorders, such as a stroke or Alzheimer disease (AD), cause dementia, though dementia is not a disease. It is a name for a group of symptoms that affect the brain. Symptoms of dementia include being unable to do normal activities of living (e.g., eating, dressing, grooming), solve problems, and control emotions. To be diagnosed with dementia, a person needs to have at least two or more problems with brain function (e.g., memory, language). AD is the leading cause of dementia.

Treatments. Current treatments may only keep symptoms from getting worse for a limited time; no cure is available. Medications that help treat cognitive symptoms include:

- Cholinesterase inhibitors: Boost the acetylcholine in the brain, which is depleted with AD. Common medications include donepezil (doe NEP e zil) (Aricept), rivastigmine (ri va STIG meen) (Exelon), and galantamine (ga LAN ta meen) (Razadyne).
- Memantine (MEM an teen) (Namenda) is used for moderate to severe AD.

Huntington Disease. Huntington disease (HD), also called *Huntington chorea*, is a progressive neurodegenerative disorder. There are two forms of HD:

- Early-onset HD: Begins during childhood or in the teen years; affects a small number of people.
- Adult-onset HD: Symptoms usually start in the 30s or 40s; most common form of HD.

Usually, people with HD die within 15 to 20 years.

Etiology. HD is caused by a genetic defect. If the gene is inherited from one parent, the child has a 50% chance of getting the disease. As the gene is passed through families, the disease develops at an earlier age.

Signs and Symptoms. Behavior issues are usually seen first and include behavioral disturbances, hallucinations (hah LOO si nae shuns), moodiness, irritability, restlessness, psychosis, and paranoia. Abnormal movements can also occur and include facial grimacing, jerky movements, slow and uncontrolled movements, or a prancing gait. Dementia also occurs and affects the memory and speech.

Diagnostic Procedures. The provider will do an examination and order additional tests, including psychological testing, head CT or MRI, and a PET scan of the brain.

Treatments. There is no cure for HD. The goal of the treatment is to slow the symptoms. Medications such as dopamine blockers help to reduce abnormal movements and behaviors, and amantadine may help to control extra movements.

Multiple Sclerosis. Multiple sclerosis (MS) is an autoimmune neurodegenerative disorder that affects the brain and spinal cord. The myelin sheath is damaged, leading to slowed or blocked messages to the brain. MS often occurs between the ages of 20 to 40 and affects females more than males. The disease can be mild, but some people may not be able to write, walk, or speak. There are four types of MS:

- *Clinically isolated syndrome (CIS)*: A person has an MS-like episode but does not meet the criteria for an MS diagnosis.
- *Relapsing-remitting MS (RRMS)*: Most common form; a person experiences relapses of the neurologic symptoms, followed by periods of partial or complete remission (recovery).
- *Secondary progressive MS (SPMS)*: Follows the initial relapsing-remitting course; most people will eventually have worsening symptoms.
- *Primary progressive MS (PPMS)*: Symptoms worsen from the onset. The person does not experience early relapses or remissions.

Etiology. The etiology is unknown, though the disorder is an autoimmune disease. The immune system destroys the myelin sheath. Some risk factors include a family history, infection with the Epstein-Barr virus, and a history of thyroid disease, type 1 diabetes, or inflammatory bowel disease.

Signs and Symptoms. Signs and symptoms include tingling, numbness, or weakness in the extremities, partial or complete loss of vision, double vision, slurred speech, fatigue, and lack of coordination.

Diagnostic Procedures. The provider will perform an examination and evaluate the person's mental and language functions, along with movement and coordination. Vision and other senses will be evaluated. There are no blood tests to diagnose MS. The provider may order an MRI, cerebrospinal fluid analysis, and an evoked potential test.

Treatments. There is no cure for MS, though the goal of treatment is to slow the progression of the disease and speed up recovery time from attacks. Corticosteroid medications may be given to reduce nerve inflammation. Ocrelizumab (ok re LIZ ue mab) (Ocrevus) may be used in some cases of MS.

VOCABULARY

autoimmune An immune response against a person's own tissues, cells, or cell parts, as in autoimmune disease, leading to the deterioration of tissue.

biomarkers Detectable cellular indicators used as a marker for a substance or disease process.

evoked potential test A nerve response test that uses electrodes, which are placed on the scalp to measure brain reaction to a stimulus.

hallucination A sensory experience (e.g., a smell, sound, sight, touch, or taste) involving something that is not present.

Parkinson Disease. Parkinson disease (PD) is a progressive neurodegenerative disorder that affects movement. With PD, the dopamine-producing neurons in the brain gradually die. The dopamine levels decrease in the brain, leading to the symptoms. PD usually begins around age 60, and it is more common in males.

Etiology. The cause of PD is unknown, but genetics and environmental triggers (e.g., exposure to certain toxins) can increase the risk of the disease.

Signs and Symptoms. Signs and symptoms of PD include:

- Tremors and *pill-rolling tremors* (thumb and forefinger are rubbed back and forth)
- *Bradykinesia* (slow movement), shuffling gait, rigid muscles, impaired balance and posture, stooping, and writing changes
- Loss of automatic movements (e.g., blinking, smiling), *masked face* (facial appearance of depression or anger), and speech changes (e.g., slurring, soft voice)
- Loss of sense of smell, trouble sleeping, dizziness, and constipation
- Excessive sweating or very little sweating, and drooling

Diagnostic Procedures. There are no specific tests for PD. The provider will do a neurologic examination, and with the history of symptoms, the diagnosis can be made. Additional tests may be done to rule out other diseases.

Treatments. Medications can be used to manage the symptoms; some of these include:

- Carbidopa-levodopa (lee voe DOE pa kar bi DOE pa) (Sinemet): Used to increase the dopamine in the brain.
- Dopamine agonist: Used to mimic dopamine's effect in the brain. Examples include pramipexole (pra mi PEX ole) (Mirapex), ropinirole (roe PIN i role) (Requip), and rotigotine (roe TIG oh teen) (Neupro).
- MAO-B inhibitors: Prevent the breakdown of dopamine. Examples include safinamide (sa FIN a mide) (Xadago) and selegiline (se LE ji leen) (Eldepryl, Zelapar).

Deep brain stimulation (DBS) may also be done. This treatment requires a generator to be implanted, and electrodes from it send impulses to the brain, which decrease the symptoms.

MEDICAL TERMINOLOGY	
kinesi/o	movement
brady-	slow

Restless Legs Syndrome. Restless legs syndrome (RLS) is also known as *restless legs syndrome/Willis-Ekborn disease* (RLS/WED). RLS causes a creeping, tingling, or burning sensation in the legs when the person is lying down or sitting. Moving the legs helps reduce the sensations for a short period of time. RLS can affect a person's quality of sleep. Most people with RLS also have periodic limb movement disorder (PLMD), which causes the legs or arms to twitch or jerk uncontrollably in sleep. RLS can occur at any age and can worsen with age.

Etiology. In many situations, there is no known cause for RLS. For some people, RLS is caused by a condition (e.g., pregnancy, anemia) or by a medication. Caffeine, alcohol, and tobacco can worsen the symptoms. Researchers believe that RLS may be related to a dopamine imbalance in the brain. There also may be a genetic cause if the condition appears before age 40. Associated risk factors for RLS include peripheral neuropathy, iron deficiency, kidney failure, and spinal cord lesions.

Signs and Symptoms. The signs and symptoms include abnormal sensations in the legs and feet that begin after rest (often at night) and decrease with movement. The abnormal sensations can be described as itching, electric, aching, throbbing, pulling, crawling, or creeping. The symptoms may disappear for a while and then come back.

Diagnostic Procedures. Besides an examination, the provider may order blood tests and a sleep study.

Treatments. Treatments include exercise and massage of the legs, stress reduction activities, and decreased caffeine and tobacco use. Medication therapy may include iron for anemia and medications to increase the dopamine in the brain, including ropinirole (roe PIN i role) (Requip), pramipexole (pra mi PEX ole) (Mirapex), and rotigotine (roe TIG oh teen) (Neupro). Opioids and anticonvulsants, such as gabapentin (GA ba pen tin) (Neurontin, Horizant), pregabalin (pre GAB a lin) (Lyrica), and clonazepam (kloe NA ze pam) (Klonopin), may be used. RLS is a lifelong condition with no cure.

Other Neurodegenerative Disorders. The following are additional neurodegenerative disorders.

- *Friedreich ataxia* (ah TAK see ah): An inherited disease that causes damage to the spinal cord and nerves. Signs and symptoms are seen as early as 5 years of age. The person can experience ataxia, difficulty walking, muscle weakness, scoliosis, heart palpitations, involuntary eye movements, and speech issues. There is no cure for this disease. Treatments may include assistive devices (e.g., wheelchair), braces, physical therapy, and surgery.
- *Frontotemporal dementia* (also called *Pick disease*): A rare condition that can start by age 20. Pick bodies and cells (abnormal proteins) are found in the damaged neurons. Behavior changes, speech difficulty, and problems thinking occur and slowly get worse. There is no specific treatment, but medications may be used to help with mood swings.
- *Lewy body disease* (also called *dementia with Lewy bodies*): Lewy bodies (abnormal structures) build up in the brain. Signs and symptoms include decreased alertness, hallucinations, muscle stiffness, confusion, and loss of memory. This disease is one of the more common causes of dementia. There is no cure; treatments help with symptoms.
- *Tay-Sachs disease*: An inherited disease that progressively destroys the neurons in the brain and spinal cord. With the most common form, signs and symptoms are seen in infancy. The infant's motor skills (e.g., sitting, crawling, and rolling) are affected. As the disease progresses, the child can experience seizures, vision and hearing loss, intellectual disability, and paralysis.
- *Vascular dementia*: The second most common cause of dementia for people over age 65. This disease is caused by small strokes over time. Signs and symptoms include difficulty performing tasks, language issues, misplacing items, sleep pattern changes, hallucinations, poor judgment, and memory issues. The goal is to control symptoms because there is no treatment.

VOCABULARY
paralysis A loss of muscle function and/or sensation, causing the inability to move or use a body part.

Functional Disorders

Cluster Headaches. Cluster headaches occur in cyclical patterns or clusters. The person may awaken in the middle of the night with a headache on one side of the head.

Etiology. The etiology is unknown, but there may be an increase in the release of histamine or serotonin that causes the pain.

Signs and Symptoms. The signs and symptoms include a severe, sudden, one-sided headache with tearing of the eyes, droopy eyelid, and stuffy nose. The onset commonly occurs 2 to 3 hours after falling asleep.

Diagnostic Procedures. The provider will do a physical examination and may order an MRI to rule out other conditions.

Treatments. Often medications such as sumatriptan (Imitrex), dihydroergotamine (DHE), and analgesics (an ahl JEE ziks) may be ordered. Breathing in 100% pure oxygen may also help to reduce the headaches. The cluster of headaches may last for weeks to months and then a remission period follows.

VOCABULARY

analgesic A drug that reduces or eliminates pain.
ataxia Loss of the ability to coordinate muscular movement.
paralysis A loss of muscle function and/or sensation, causing the inability to move or use a body part.

Tension Headaches. Tension headaches are the most common type of headaches.

Etiology. Tension headaches occur when the neck and scalp muscles become tense. Stress, depression, anxiety, and head injuries may be the most common causes.

Signs and Symptoms. The person may experience a dull, aching headache and feelings of tightness and pressure in forehead area to the back of the head.

Diagnostic Procedures. After taking a history, the provider may order a CT scan or MRI.

Treatments. Usually, the patient manages the pain with home treatments, such as over-the-counter (OTC) analgesics. Muscle relaxants and antidepressants may also be used.

Migraine. Migraines are recurring headaches that can affect children through adults.

Etiology. The causes of migraines may include stress, anxiety, hormone changes, strong smells, and bright lights.

Signs and Symptoms. Many times, migraines progress through four stages:

- *Prodrome* (1 to 2 days before): May cause mood changes, food cravings, neck stiffness, increase in thirst, and constipation.
- *Aura* (may occur before or during the migraine): May cause visual, sensory, motor, or verbal disturbances. Examples include hearing noises, difficulty speaking, vision loss, and jerking.
- *Attack* (may last up to 72 hours): May cause throbbing pain on one or both sides of the head; sensitivity to light, noise, and smells; nausea and vomiting, blurred vision, and lightheadedness.
- *Postdrome* (up to 24 hours after): May cause confusion, moodiness, dizziness, weakness, and sensitivity to noise and light.

Diagnostic Procedures. The provider will do physical and neurologic examinations.

Treatments. Treatment consists of rest, fluids, and medications such as sumatriptan (Imitrex), dihydroergotamine (DHE), and analgesics.

Seizure Disorders. A *seizure* (or *convulsion*) is a sudden increase of electrical activity in one or more parts of the brain. The seizures are classified based on how the abnormal brain activity begins.
- *Generalized onset seizure* (was called generalized seizure): Affects both sides of the brain.
- *Focal onset seizure* (was called partial seizure): Affects one area of the brain.
- *Unknown onset seizure*: How it affects the brain is unknown.
  Some seizures may start as a focal onset and then spread to both sides of the brain, like clonic seizures and atonic seizures. There are many types of seizures, and the more common types are listed in Table 6.5.

Etiology. Seizures can be caused by medications, high fevers, head injuries, diseases, and illegal drugs.

Signs and Symptoms. The signs and symptoms of the different seizure classifications are listed in Table 6.5. Most seizures do not cause harm, but if they last longer than 5 minutes or if the person has repeated seizures without waking up between them, it is a medical emergency.

Diagnostic Procedures. The provider will do a neurologic exam and may order blood tests to check for conditions associated with seizures (e.g., infections). Additional tests may include neuropsychological tests, an electroencephalogram (EEG), CT, MRI, PET, and a single photon emission computed tomography (SPECT) scan.

Treatments. Depending on the type of seizure, antiseizure medication may be used.

Epilepsy. Epilepsy (EP ih lep see) is a disorder that causes recurring seizures. A person must have at least two unprovoked seizures before epilepsy is diagnosed. The type of seizure is

TABLE 6.5 Seizure Classification

New Groups	New Classification (Older Name)	Description	Symptoms
Generalized Onset	*Tonic-clonic* (Grand mal)	Loses consciousness. Tonic phase (rigid muscles) comes first, followed by clonic phase (jerking rapidly). May be incontinent of stool and urine. Lasts 1–3 minutes; sleepy and confused after seizure.	Motor: Sustained jerking *(clonic)*, weak muscles *(atonic)*, rigid muscles *(tonic)*, brief twitching *(myoclonus)*, and spasms Nonmotor: Staring spells, twitching
	Focal to bilateral tonic-clonic (Secondarily generalized)	Starts in one area of the brain and spreads to involve both sides. Usually lasts 1–3 minutes.	
	Absent (Petit mal)	Lapse of awareness of the environment; more common in children.	
	Atypical absence	Will stare but may be able to respond; begin and end gradually. May fall. Can last 5–30 seconds.	
Focal Onset	*Focal aware* (Simple partial)	Awake and alert during seizure; lasts less than 2 minutes.	Motor: Clonic, atonic, tonic, myoclonus, spasms, automatic movements (e.g., lip smacking, clapping, chewing) Nonmotor: Changes in emotions, thinking, heart palpitations, goose bumps, lack of movement
	Focal impaired awareness (Complex partial)	Confused during seizure; lasts 1–2 minutes. Aura may occur.	
	Atonic	Can begin as a focal seizure and then spread to both sides of the brain, becoming a generalized seizure. Lasts less than 15 seconds.	Loss of muscle tone, head or body may go limp; head may drop
Unknown Onset/Unknown		When seizure began is not known, or seizure was not witnessed.	Motor: Tonic-clonic, spasms Nonmotor: No movements, stares

From the Centers for Disease Control and Prevention (CDC): https://www.cdc.gov/epilepsy/communications/features/seizures.htm; and the Epilepsy Foundation: https://www.epilepsy.com/learn/types-seizures.

classified either as generalized or focal. Epilepsy can affect anyone at any age, of any ethnic background, or of either gender. Children can outgrow epilepsy.

Etiology. There are several causes of epilepsy, including genetics, brain injury, abnormal development, and illness. Many times, the cause is not known.

Signs and Symptoms. Signs and symptoms vary based on the type of seizure and can include confusion, staring, uncontrolled jerking, and loss of consciousness (see Table 6.5). *Status epilepticus*, an emergency condition, occurs when a seizure lasts longer than 10 minutes or if the person has three or more seizures without regaining consciousness between them.

Diagnostic Procedures. The provider will do a neurologic examination and may order the tests listed in the "Seizure Disorder" section.

Treatments. Treatments include antiseizure medications, a ketogenic diet (eating foods high in fats and low in carbohydrates), vagus nerve stimulation, and deep brain stimulation (from a surgically implanted generator and electrodes). If medications fail to control the seizures, surgery can be done to remove the portion of the brain causing the seizures.

Other Functional Disorders. The following are additional functional disorders.

- *Functional neurologic disorder (FND)* (also called *conversion disorder* and *functional movement disorder*): A neurologic disorder that affects the transmission of signals from the nervous system and the body. The cause is unknown. Symptoms include motor dysfunction (e.g., limb weakness, paralysis, spasms, problems walking), dysphagia, sensory dysfunction (e.g., numbness, loss of vision), syncope (SIN ko pee), and seizures.

- *Narcolepsy* (NAR koh lep see): A chronic neurologic disorder that affects the brain's ability to control the sleep-wake cycle, thus causing extreme daytime sleepiness, cataplexy (KAT ah PLEK see), hallucinations, and sleep paralysis. Narcolepsy can be genetic and also an autoimmune disease.

- *Sciatica (*sye AT ick kah): Occurs when the sciatic nerve can become compressed by a herniated disk, spinal stenosis, or a bone spur on the vertebrae. This condition causes burning or stabbing pain that radiates along the path of the sciatic nerve. The person can have pain and numbness in the lower back, hip, buttock, and leg on one side of the body.

> **VOCABULARY**
>
> **cataplexy** A sudden loss of muscle strength and tone associated with an emotional stimulus.
>
> **syncope** Loss of consciousness and postural tone caused by diminished blood flow to the brain.

- *Tourette syndrome* (tur ETT) *(TS):* A neurologic disorder that causes tics and can be seen as early as 3 years of age. *Tics* are repetitive, involuntary movements and vocalizations. *Simple motor tics* involve a small number of muscle groups and cause sudden, brief, repetitive movements, such as eye blinking, facial grimacing, shoulder shrugging, and head jerking. *Complex motor tics* involve several muscle groups and several movements (e.g., grimacing, shrugging, and jerking). *Simple vocal tics* involve sounds made by moving air through the mouth or nose, causing barking, hissing, sniffing, grunting, or throat-clearing. *Complex vocal tics* may include repeating phrases, words, or sentences. People may repeat their own phrases, another person's words, or obscene words. Tics can worsen with emotion (e.g., excitement and anxiety).

MEDICAL TERMINOLOGY	
narc/o	sleep
cata-	down
epi-	above
-lepsy	seizure

Infections

Encephalitis. Encephalitis is the inflammation of the brain. There are several types of encephalitis, including:

- *Japanese encephalitis*: Mosquito-transmitted viral infection that occurs in Asia and the western Pacific. Travelers can be vaccinated for prevention of this disease.
- *La Crosse encephalitis*: Mosquito-transmitted viral infection that occurs in the upper Midwestern, mid-Atlantic, and southeastern states.
- *Saint Louis encephalitis*: Mosquito-transmitted viral infection that occurs in the eastern and central states.

Etiology. Encephalitis can be caused by a viral or bacterial infection.

Signs and Symptoms. With a mild case, a person may have flulike symptoms. With a severe case, a person may experience a severe headache, drowsiness, vomiting, confusion, seizures, and a sudden fever. Babies may constantly cry, not eat well, and have body stiffness and bulging fontanels (fon tah NELS).

Diagnostic Procedures. After a physical and neurologic examination, the provider may order a cerebrospinal fluid analysis, which requires a lumbar puncture. Blood laboratory tests and CT may also be done.

Treatments. Severe cases require hospitalization and intravenous (IV) medications to treat the infection and reduce the brain inflammation. Milder bacterial infections require oral antibiotics. Physical, speech, and occupational therapies may be required for some patients after other symptoms have resolved.

VOCABULARY
fontanel A soft membranous gap between the incompletely formed cranial bones of an infant; also called a soft spot.

Meningitis. Meningitis is the inflammation of the meninges surrounding the brain and spinal cord.

Etiology. Viral meningitis, the most common form, is caused by a viral infection that affects the nose or mouth and travels to the brain. Bacterial meningitis, usually caused by pneumococcal or meningococcal infections, starts with a coldlike infection and can be deadly. The meningitis vaccine can help prevent certain types of bacterial infections that cause meningitis.

Meningitis can be caused by a viral, bacterial, or fungal infection. There is also a noninfectious meningitis and a cancer-related meningitis.

Signs and Symptoms. The symptoms may include a sudden high fever, severe headache, stiff neck, nausea, and vomiting. Bacterial meningitis can cause hearing loss, brain damage, and a stroke.

Diagnostic Procedures. After a physical exam and a neurologic examination, the provider will order blood tests (e.g., blood culture), imaging tests, and a lumbar puncture to obtain a cerebrospinal fluid specimen for analysis.

Treatments. With bacterial meningitis, the patient usually receives IV antibiotics to treat the infection and corticosteroids to reduce the inflammation. With viral meningitis, bed rest, fluids, and OTC analgesics are usually prescribed. Antifungal medications will be given for a fungal meningitis. The underlying cause of the meningitis also needs to be treated.

Shingles. Herpes zoster, also known as *shingles*, affects about 33% of all adults. Anyone who has had chickenpox can get shingles, including children. Typically, if a person gets shingles, it only occurs once, but there have been cases in which it has developed more than once. Vaccines are available to help prevent shingles.

Etiology. Shingles is caused by the varicella-zoster virus, the same virus that causes chickenpox. After a person has chickenpox, the virus remains inactive in the body. It can reactivate for unknown reasons and cause shingles.

Signs and Symptoms. The beginning symptoms include tingling, pain, or itchiness on one side of the body or face, usually on the torso. This can occur 1 to 5 days before a rash with fluid-filled blisters develops (Fig. 6.13). The person is

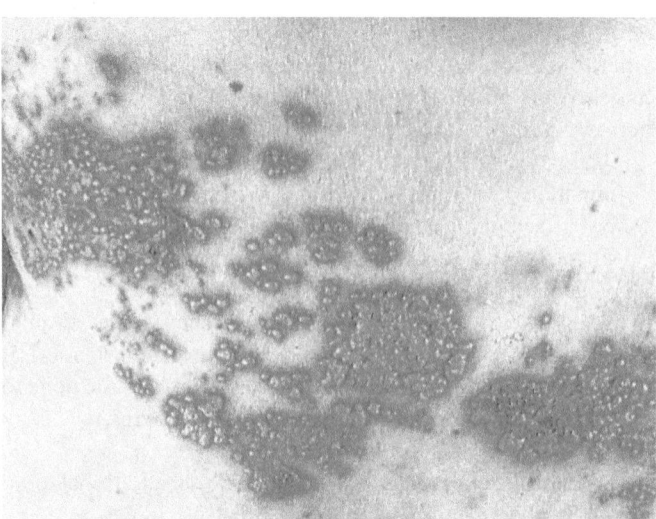

Fig. 6.13 Herpes Zoster (Shingles). (From Swartz MH: *Textbook of physical diagnosis*, ed 7, Philadelphia, 2014, Saunders.)

contagious to others who have not had chickenpox until the blisters scab over, in about 10 days. The rash clears up within 1 month. The person may also have fever, chills, headache, and nausea. Shingles can cause postherpetic neuralgia, vision loss, encephalitis, and facial paralysis.

Diagnostic Procedures. The provider will do a history and physical examination to diagnose shingles.

Treatments. There is no cure, but antiviral medications may be ordered to help reduce complications and hasten recovery. Depending on the pain, the provider may also order anticonvulsants, antidepressants, or analgesics.

Structural Disorders

Bell Palsy. Bell palsy is the most common cause of facial paralysis. The symptoms typically affect one side of the face, and the symptoms are at their worst about 48 hours after the onset.

Etiology. The exact cause is unknown. The facial nerve becomes swollen and inflamed. The risk of Bell palsy increases with pregnancy, diabetes, or with an upper respiratory viral infection.

Signs and Symptoms. The signs and symptoms include facial twitching, weakness, and paralysis; drooping of the eyelid or corner of the mouth; dry eyes or excessive tearing; and drooling, dry mouth, and a diminished ability to taste (Fig. 6.14).

Diagnostic Procedures. The provider will do a medical history and a physical examination. No other tests are usually ordered.

Treatments. Usually symptoms resolve within 2 weeks, but it may take 3 to 6 months to return to normal function. Some mild cases do not require treatment, whereas others may be treated with antiviral and corticosteroid medications. Protecting the eye from injury is important, thus eyedrops for lubrication and a patch for protection may be used.

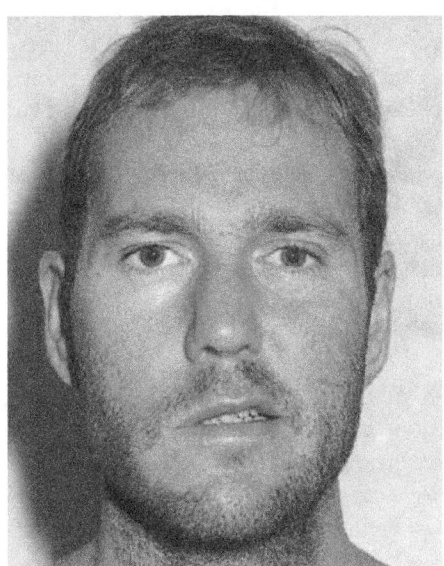

Fig. 6.14 Bell Palsy (Right Sided). (From Niedzwiecki B, et al: *Kinn's the medical assistant,* ed 14, St. Louis, 2020, Elsevier.)

Guillain-Barré Syndrome. Guillain-Barré (gee YAH buh RAY) syndrome is a rare autoimmune disorder in which the immune system attacks the peripheral nervous system.

Etiology. The etiology is unknown, but the disorder may be triggered by surgery, an infection, or vaccination.

Signs and Symptoms. Weakness and tingling start in the legs and spread through the body, making the person almost paralyzed. The disease is life-threatening, and the person may require a respirator to breathe. It may take several weeks before the symptoms improve, and recovery can take up to a few years.

Diagnostic Procedures. After the physical examination, the provider may order electromyography, nerve conduction studies, and a lumbar puncture. This disorder is difficult to diagnose.

Treatments. Treatment is aimed at relieving the symptoms and supporting breathing if needed.

Trigeminal Neuralgia. Trigeminal neuralgia (TN) is also called *tic douloureux*. TN is a chronic pain condition that affects the trigeminal nerve (cranial nerve V).

Etiology. A blood vessel or tumor pressing on the trigeminal nerve can cause trigeminal neuralgia. People with multiple sclerosis can also experience TN. This condition is more common in people over age 50 and in females than in males.

Signs and Symptoms. Pain can vary from sudden, severe, and stabbing, to constant, aching, and burning. The pain can be widespread or just in a small area. Activities such as shaving, eating, and talking can trigger intense flashes of pain. The symptoms can stop for a period of time but will come back with greater intensity.

Diagnostic Procedures. The provider will perform a physical examination and neurologic examination. An MRI may also be ordered.

Treatments. Treatment may include analgesics, anticonvulsants, and antidepressants. Surgical procedures may also be done. A *rhizotomy* (rye ZAH tuh mee) is a surgical procedure that damages nerve fibers to block pain. This procedure may cause sensory loss and facial numbness. Trigeminal neuralgia is a debilitating disorder.

Other Structural Disorders. The following are additional structural disorders.

- *Astrocytoma* (as troh sye TOH mah): A malignant tumor of nervous tissue composed of astrocytes. This type of tumor can spread widely throughout the brain, making it hard to surgically remove.
- *Medulloblastoma* (med yoo loh blass TOH mah): A fast-growing brain tumor composed of medulloblasts, seen in children and adolescents.
- *Meningioma* (meh nin jee OH mah): A common malignant tumor that begins in the meninges. The risk increases with age, and this tumor is more common in females.
- *Neuroblastoma* (noor oh blass TOH mah): A rare malignant tumor of the sympathetic nervous system, seen in young children.

MEDICAL TERMINOLOGY	
blast/o	embryonic
cyt/o	cell
rhiz/o	spinal nerve root
quadri-	four
-plegia	paralysis
-tomy	incision

Injuries

Traumatic Brain Injury. Traumatic brain injury (TBI) is an acquired brain injury. TBIs can occur as a result of falls, motor vehicle accidents, violence (e.g., shaken baby syndrome, gunshot wounds), sports injuries, and service in military combat zones. A concussion is a mild form of a TBI and is the most common type of sports injury. A *contusion* is bruising or swelling of the brain that occurs when small cerebral blood vessels bleed into brain tissue.

Etiology. TBI can occur as a result of a violent jolt or blow to the head or body, or when something pierces the skull (e.g., bullet) and injures the brain tissue (Box 6.4).

Signs and Symptoms. Symptoms of TBI may not appear for weeks after the injury. TBI can be mild, moderate, severe, or life-threatening, depending on the brain damage.

- Mild TBI symptoms include headache, neck pain, nausea, ringing in the ear, dizziness, lightheadedness, blurred vision, tiredness, dazed feeling, mood changes, and trouble concentrating or remembering. Children experience irritability and changes in eating.

BOX 6.4   Shaken Baby Syndrome

Shaken baby syndrome (SBS) is the leading cause of child abuse deaths. There are over 1300 cases a year in the United States, and about a quarter of the children die. SBS occurs when a child is violently shaken or when the head strikes against a hard surface (e.g., wall, counter, floor). Crying is the leading trigger for the violence that leads to SBS, and most babies are less than 6 months old when it occurs.

Signs and symptoms of SBS include lethargy, extreme irritability, bruises, rigidity, difficulty breathing, bulging fontanels, inability to focus the eyes or track movement, unequal pupil size, seizures, and poor feeding.

About 80% of the children who survive SBS have lifelong disabilities, including blindness, seizures, hearing loss, developmental delays (e.g., speech, learning, memory, attention), cerebral palsy, and severe mental retardation.

According to the National Center on Shaken Baby Syndrome (https://www.dontshake.org), the Period of PURPLE Crying program is an evidence-based shaken baby syndrome prevention program that helps caregivers understand crying in infants and helps to prevent SBS. The letters in PURPLE describe important information for parents and caregivers.

- **P**eak of crying: Crying may increase weekly until 2 months of age.
- **U**nexpected: The child may cry off and on, though the parent/caregiver may not know why.
- **R**esists soothing: The child may not stop crying regardless of what the parent/caregiver does.
- **P**ainlike face: The facial appearance may indicate that the child is in pain, though that may not be the situation.
- **L**ong lasting: The child can cry more than 5 hours a day.
- **E**vening: Crying may increase in the late afternoon or evening.

- Moderate or severe TBI symptoms are similar. The headache is constant and gets worse. The person may experience repeated vomiting, seizures, inability to awaken, dilation of one or both pupils, slurred speech, agitation, loss of coordination, and weakness in the extremities. Children may also be inconsolable and refuse to eat.

Diagnostic Procedures. For severe injuries, emergency personnel will use the Glasgow Coma Scale to assess the patient. In the hospital, imaging tests (CT and MRI), along with intracranial pressure monitoring, will be done. In the ambulatory care facility, the provider will obtain information on the injury and perform physical and neurologic examinations. CT or MRI may be ordered to check for skull fractures.

Treatments. For mild TBIs, treatment consists of rest and OTC analgesics. For moderate to severe TBIs, medications are given to reduce the brain swelling and prevent more damage. Surgery may be done to remove hematomas, repair skull fractures, stop bleeding in the brain, and relieve pressure (by removing a portion of the skull). Various rehabilitation specialists may be involved during the recovery phase.

VOCABULARY

concussion A type of brain injury resulting from a hit to the head or body that causes the brain to move rapidly back and forth.

Glasgow Coma Scale A scale used to measure the level of consciousness and severity of a head injury; the ability to open the eyes, verbal response, and motor response are evaluated, and the score is determined based on the findings.

hematoma A localized collection of blood, usually clotted, caused by a break in a blood vessel wall.

shaken baby syndrome Condition resulting from internal head injuries that occur when a baby or young child is violently shaken.

Spinal Cord Injury. Spinal cord injuries occur when a blow, gunshot, or stabbing fractures or dislocates the vertebrae and the bone pieces cut into the cord or press on the nerves.

Etiology. Common causes include motor vehicle accidents, falls, acts of violence, alcohol, and diseases. Spinal cord injuries can be:

- *Complete*: No signals can be sent below the level of the injury, and the person is paralyzed below the injury.
- *Incomplete*: Some signals can be sent below the injury, and thus the person has some movement and sensation below the injury.

The cause is an injury to the vertebrae. This is a medical emergency.

Signs and Symptoms. Initially, the person may experience extreme back or neck pain, incontinence of bowel or bladder, difficulty breathing, and paralysis.

- *Quadriplegia* (or *tetraplegia*): The spinal cord injury affects the arms, hands, trunk, legs, and pelvic organs (e.g., bowel, bladder, and sexual functions).
- *Paraplegia*: The spinal cord injury affects some or all of the trunk, legs, and pelvic organs.

Diagnostic Procedures. The emergency providers will perform physical and neurologic examinations. Imaging studies (x-ray, myelogram, MRI, and CT) will be done.

Treatments. Treatments include surgery, traction, corticosteroids, and rehabilitation (e.g., physical and occupational therapies).

Peripheral Neuropathy. Peripheral neuropathy occurs as a result of damage to the peripheral nervous system. Over 100 types of peripheral neuropathy have been identified, each with its own symptoms. Diabetic neuropathy is one of the most common forms.

Etiology. The cause may be inherited, acquired, or unknown (which is called *idiopathic*). Acquired peripheral neuropathy can be caused by:

- Physical injury: Related to trauma (accidents, sports-related activities, surgical procedures, and falls) or stress from repetitive activities.
- Diseases: Related to metabolic and endocrine disorders (e.g., diabetes mellitus), small vessel disease (e.g., vasculitis), autoimmune diseases (e.g., lupus, rheumatoid arthritis), kidney disorders, cancer, and infections (Lyme disease).
- Exposure to toxins: Includes medications, environmental and industrial toxins, and heavy alcohol consumption.

Signs and Symptoms. Signs and symptoms include tingling and numbness, paresthesia, weakness, increased sensitivity to stimuli, burning pain, muscle wasting, paralysis, and organ dysfunction. With diabetic neuropathy, pain and numbness are felt in both legs, with gradual progression up the legs. Eventually, the person may feel pain and numbness in the fingers, hands, and arms.

Diagnostic Procedures. The provider will do physical and neurologic examinations. Additional tests will be done, including nerve conduction velocity (NCV), electromyography (EMG), MRI, and nerve and skin biopsies.

Treatments. Treatment addresses the underlying causes and symptom management. Medications such as antidepressants, anticonvulsants, antiarrhythmics, narcotics, and nonsteroidal anti-inflammatory drugs (NSAIDs) may help ease the neuropathic pain.

CRITICAL THINKING 6.7

Nancy's last patient of the day has severe neuropathy in both her hands and feet. The patient states that she can't feel much with her hands. After rooming the patient, Nancy thinks about her own life if she could not feel much in her hands and feet. How might that affect a person's life? What complications might occur?

Congenital Disorders

Fetal Alcohol Spectrum Disorders. Fetal alcohol spectrum disorders (FASDs) are a group of conditions that occur to a person whose mother drank alcohol during the pregnancy. The physical and mental deficiencies will last for life. Some of the disorders include the following:

- *Fetal alcohol syndrome* (FAS), which is at the farthest end of the spectrum, is the most complex disorder. People can experience the signs and symptoms indicated in the following section. People with FAS have a difficult time with school and getting along with others.
- *Alcohol-related neurodevelopmental disorder* (ARND), which affects learning and behavior.
- *Alcohol-related birth defects* (ARBD), which causes problems with the heart, kidneys, bones, and hearing.

Etiology. These disorders are caused by alcohol consumption by the mother during the pregnancy. The alcohol in the mother's bloodstream crosses the placenta. Alcohol can interfere with oxygen and nutrient delivery in the growing baby. It can also harm the development of tissues and organs.

Signs and Symptoms. The signs and symptoms depend on the amount of alcohol consumed during the pregnancy and the time in pregnancy when it was consumed. Common signs and symptoms include:

- Poor memory, hyperactive behavior, difficulty with attention and math concepts
- Speech and language delays, learning and intellectual disabilities
- Poor reasoning and judgment skills
- Vision or hearing problems
- Babies may experience low body weight, sleeping and sucking problems
- Poor coordination, small head size, shorter-than-average height, abnormal facial features (e.g., smooth ridge between the nose and upper lip)
- Heart, kidney, or bone problems

Diagnostic Procedures. Knowing at delivery that the mother drank alcohol during the pregnancy can help with early diagnosis. At birth a thorough assessment will be done. The provider will assess for issues during childhood. The child will be screened for cognitive, learning, and language development delays. Health issues, along with social and behavioral problems, will also be monitored.

Treatments. There is no cure for FASDs. Early intervention can help reduce some of the effects. Not drinking alcohol during pregnancy is the only way to prevent FASDs.

Spina Bifida. Spina bifida is a neural tube defect that occurs when the spinal column does not close during the first month of pregnancy. Spina bifida can cause damage to the nerves and spinal cord. Pregnant females are encouraged to take folic acid during pregnancy to reduce the risk of spina bifida.

Etiology. The cause is unknown.

Signs and Symptoms. There are four types of spina bifida:

- *Spina bifida occulta*: Mildest form; no spinal nerves are involved, but one or more vertebrae are malformed. No signs or symptoms may be present. The only indication may be an abnormal cluster of hair, a small dimple, or birthmark on the infant's back (Fig. 6.15).
- *Closed neural tube defect*: Includes a malformation of the fat, bone, or meninges associated with the spinal cord. Symptoms range from no symptoms to incomplete paralysis with bowel and urinary dysfunction.

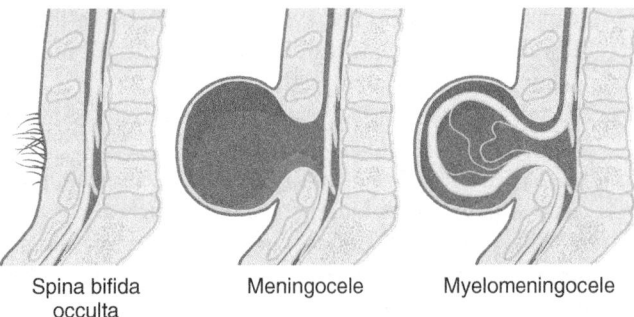

Spina bifida   Meningocele   Myelomeningocele
occulta

Fig. 6.15 **Types of Spina Bifida.** (From Niedzwiecki B, et al: *Kinn's the medical assistant,* ed 14, St. Louis, 2020, Elsevier.)

- *Meningocele*: The meninges protrude through an abnormal vertebral opening, creating a sac. The sac is filled with fluid. Symptoms range from no symptoms to complete paralysis with bowel and bladder dysfunction.
- *Myelomeningocele*: The most serious type because the spinal canal is open along several vertebrae. A sac containing fluid, part of the spinal cord, and nerves comes through the opening in the infant's back. This type can cause partial or complete paralysis below the opening. The child may have weakness or paralysis of the legs, bowel and bladder incontinence, lack of feeling in the legs, and an increase in cerebrospinal fluid.

Diagnostic Procedures. During pregnancy, the mother can take a maternal serum alpha-fetoprotein (MSAFP) test (also known as the *Triple Test* and *Quad Screen*). If abnormally high amounts of alpha-fetoprotein (AFP) are found, it suggests that the baby has a neural tube defect (e.g., spina bifida). The accuracy of the MSAFP test is not perfect. Even though abnormally high levels of AFP are found, the baby may be normal. With negative test results, there is still a small risk of spina bifida. Amniocentesis can also be done, if the MSAFP test result comes back abnormal. Most of the time, ultrasound can detect the two most severe types of spina bifida during pregnancy.

Treatments. Prenatal surgery for spina bifida can occur around 26 weeks of pregnancy. The child may have fewer disabilities if the spinal cord is repaired at that time. Surgery can also occur after birth. Additional treatments focus on the complications that occur, including leg weakness, bowel or bladder problems, and hydrocephalus (Fig. 6.16 and Box 6.5).

Other Congenital Disorders. The following are additional structural disorders.

- *Cerebral palsy* (CP): A group of nonprogressive disorders caused by abnormal brain development or brain injury, resulting in muscle weakness or problems with using the muscles. CP can affect people's ability to move and maintain their posture and balance. Signs and symptoms usually appear during infancy or the preschool years. The child can have abnormal reflexes, floppiness or rigidity of the extremities, abnormal posture, involuntary movements, and an unsteady *gait* (manner or style of walking). CP is classified by the main type of movement disorder involved: *spasticity* (stiff muscles), *dyskinesia* (uncontrollable movements), and ataxia.
- *Down syndrome* (also called *trisomy 21*): The most common chromosomal condition in the United States. It is a condition in which a person is born with an extra copy of chromosome

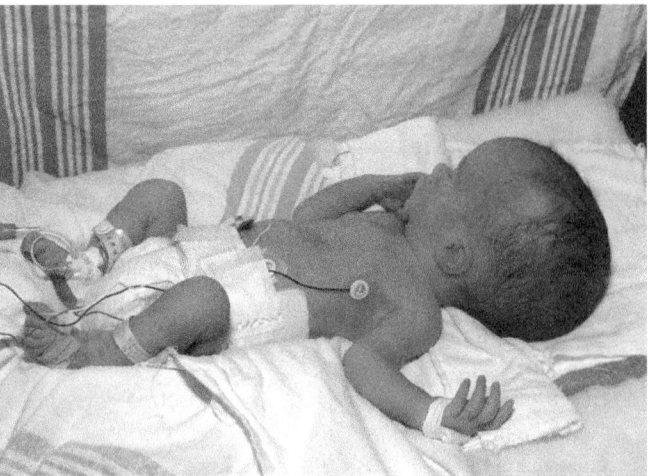

Fig. 6.16 **Hydrocephalus.** (From Kliegman R, Stanton BF, St. Geme JW, et al: *Nelson textbook of pediatrics,* ed 19, St. Louis, 2011, Saunders.)

BOX 6.5   Shunt System

Hydrocephalus can be treated with surgical placement of a shunt system. The shunt system drains the extra cerebrospinal fluid (CSF) from the ventricles in the brain into another part of the body (e.g., abdomen), where it is absorbed into the bloodstream. The ventriculoperitoneal shunt is one of the more common shunts (Fig. 6.17).

The shunt system consists of:

- An inflow *catheter* (a tube) with a pressure-sensitive valve. When the pressure reaches a certain level, the valve opens, allowing CSF to drain into the catheter.
- A valve mechanism that regulates the pressure levels. Usually, this device is implanted under the skin on the top of the head or behind the ear.
- An outflow catheter, which drains the CSF into another part of the body.

A shunt system needs to be replaced as the person ages or when it gets blocked. Increased intracranial pressure (ICP) is a sign that the shunt system is not functioning correctly. A person may experience a headache, nausea and vomiting, confusion, double vision, and decreased mental abilities with ICP.

---

21. The complications from Down syndrome range in severity and can include intellectual disabilities, dementia, heart disease, hearing and visual issues, thyroid disease, and musculoskeletal complications (e.g., poor muscle tone).

- *Tuberous sclerosis*: A rare genetic disease that causes benign tumors to grow in major organs (e.g., heart, brain, liver, and skin). Symptoms depend on the location of the tumors and may include seizures, intellectual disabilities, and kidney problems.

Vascular Disorders

Vascular disorders that affect the nervous system tend to affect the brain. These can include aneurysms (AN yeh rizms) and hemorrhages, which can lead to strokes.

VOCABULARY

aneurysm An abnormal blood-filled sac formed by a localized dilation of the wall of a vein, artery, or heart.

Cerebrovascular Accident. A cerebrovascular (seh ree broh VAS kyoo lur) accident (CVA), also called a *stroke*, is the fifth leading cause of death in the United States and a major cause of

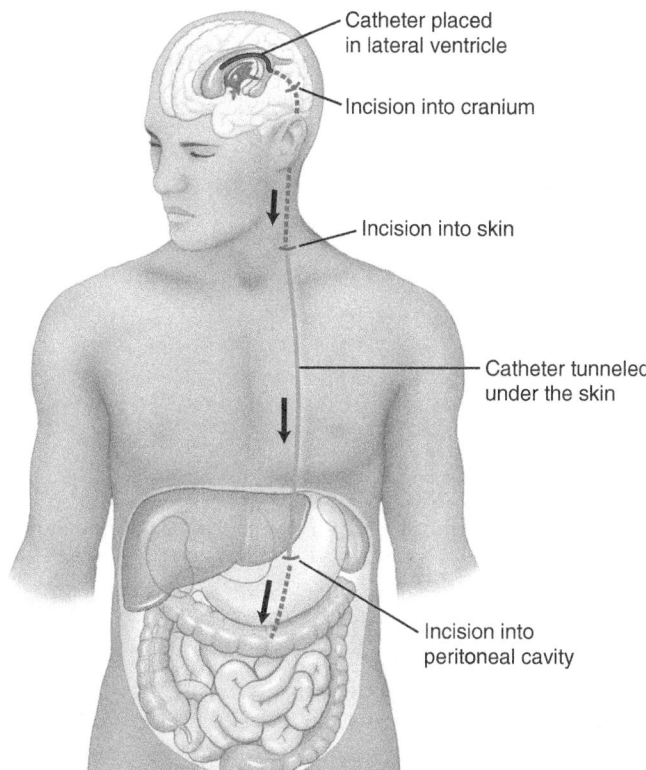

Catheter placed
in lateral ventricle

Incision into cranium

Incision into skin

Catheter tunneled
under the skin

Incision into
peritoneal cavity

Fig. 6.17 Ventriculoperitoneal Shunt. (From Shiland B: *Mastering healthcare terminology*, ed 5, St. Louis, 2015, Elsevier.)

serious disability. Strokes can occur at any age, but they usually occur in older adults. A stroke is a medical emergency.

Etiology. There are three types of strokes.

- *Ischemic stroke*: Occurs when the arterial blood flow to part of the brain is blocked. The brain cells start to die after a few minutes. This is the most common type of stroke. Two common types of ischemic strokes are:
  - *Thrombotic stroke*: A blood clot forms in an artery, blocking the blood to part of the brain.
  - *Embolic stroke*: A blood clot or other debris forms elsewhere in the body and moves into the brain arteries, blocking the blood flow.
- *Hemorrhagic stroke*: Occurs when an artery in the brain leaks or ruptures. The leaked blood puts pressure on the surrounding brain cells, causing damage. High blood pressure and aneurysms can cause hemorrhagic strokes. Two types of hemorrhagic strokes are:
  - *Intracerebral hemorrhage*: The most common type; it occurs when a cerebral aneurysm ruptures.
  - *Subarachnoid hemorrhage*: Bleeding occurs in the subarachnoid space, usually caused by small aneurysms.
- *Transient ischemic (TRANS ee ent is KEE mick) attack (TIA)*: Also called a "ministroke" because it lasts for only a few minutes. The blood supply to a part of the brain is briefly blocked. Symptoms are similar to stroke symptoms but do not last as long (e.g., 1 to 24 hours).

Risk factors for CVAs include:

- Family history of stroke
- Cardiovascular disease, hypertension, and high cholesterol
- Diabetes

- Cigarette smoking, heavy or binge drinking, and use of illicit drugs (e.g., cocaine and methamphetamines)
- Being overweight and physical inactivity

Signs and Symptoms. The symptoms of a CVA relate to the part of the brain affected. The individual may not have all the symptoms:

- Confusion or mental changes
- Speech difficulty (trouble forming words, difficult to understand, or using words that do not make sense)
- Numbness of the face, arm, or leg, usually on one side of the body
- Problem seeing in one or both eyes
- Trouble walking, lack of coordination or balance, or arm weakness
- Sudden, severe headache
- Facial drooping
- *Hemiparesis* (hem mee pah REE sis) (weakness on one side of the body) and *hemiplegia* (hem mee PLEE jee ah) (one-sided paralysis)

Diagnostic Procedures. The emergency department providers will perform physical and neurologic examinations. Blood tests and imaging tests (CT, MRI, and cerebral angiogram) will indicate the type of stroke.

Treatments. The type of stroke determines the treatment.

- Ischemic strokes are treated with clot-dissolving medications (e.g., a tissue plasminogen activator) that help the body break down the clot that is blocking the artery. The clot can also be removed by surgery if needed.
- Hemorrhagic strokes are treated with antihypertensives and surgical repair of the vessel. If the person is taking an anticoagulant or antiplatelet medication, medications to reverse the effects may be given.
- TIAs are treated with antihypertensive, anticoagulant, and antiplatelet medications. The goal is to prevent a future stroke.

Additional treatments address the life-changing complications of stroke. Physical, occupational, and speech therapies may be used to help with the disabilities.

MEDICAL TERMINOLOGY	
ischem/o	hold back
spin/o	spine
vascul/o	vessel
bi-	two
hemi-	half
-ar	pertaining to
-fida	split
-paresis	slight paralysis

CRITICAL THINKING 6.8

A patient had a stroke in the right side of her brain that affected her left arm and hand. What types of daily activities (e.g., bathing, grooming, eating) might she struggle with if she is left-hand dominant? What if she is right-hand dominant?

Hematoma. The most common cranial hematomas include:

- *Epidural hematoma*: A collection of blood between the skull and the dura mater (Fig. 6.18).

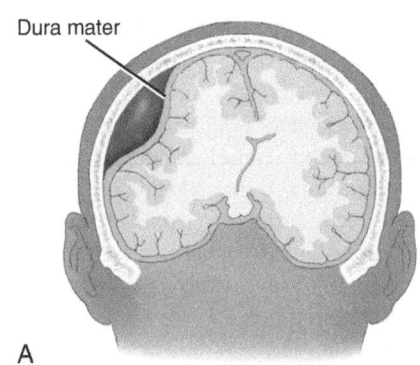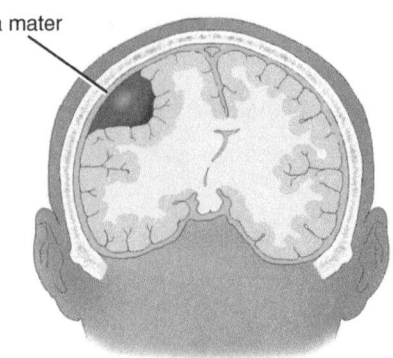

Fig. 6.18 A, Epidural hematoma. B, Subdural hematoma. (From Damjanov I: *Pathology: a color atlas*, St. Louis, 2000, Mosby.)

- *Subdural hematoma*: A collection of blood between the dura mater and the arachnoid mater, which causes pressure on the brain.
- *Intraparenchymal* (in trah PAR en ki mahl) or *intracerebral hematoma*: A collection of blood pools in the brain.

The pressure outside of the brain increases the *intracranial pressure* (ICP) (the pressure in the skull). With increased ICP, both the nervous system and blood vessel tissues are under pressure, which can be life-threatening. Thus a cranial hematoma is a medical emergency.

Etiology. Head trauma is the most common cause of hematomas. An intraparenchymal hematoma can also be caused by a leaking aneurysm, high blood pressure, or a tumor. These conditions can cause blood to leak into the brain.

Signs and Symptoms. Signs and symptoms of an epidural hematoma include:

- Confusion, dizziness, altered level of alertness or drowsiness
- Enlarged pupil, severe headache
- Loss of consciousness, followed by alertness, and then deterioration of alertness
- Nausea and vomiting
- Weakness in part of the body

Diagnostic Procedures. Imaging procedures are the best method to determine the location and size of the hematoma. Imaging procedures used include a head CT scan, MRI scan, and an angiogram for diagnosing blood vessel conditions.

Treatments. The treatment goals include controlling symptoms and minimizing permanent damage. Emergency surgery to remove the hematoma (craniotomy), surgery to reduce the ICP, and life support measures are done. Medications to prevent seizures and to help reduce the ICP are also given.

LIFE SPAN CHANGES

Infants are born with an immature nervous system. Over the first few years of life, the process of myelination continues, causing an increase in the child's brain size. As the child matures, learning and thinking processes become more complex. During adulthood, the brain function is stable.

As a person ages, the nervous system changes. The brain and spinal cord lose nerve cells. Nerve cells break down in the brain, and waste products accumulate, which can cause plaques and neurofibrillary tangles to form. Nerve impulses become slower. This causes a slower reaction time, and tasks may take longer to perform. Reflexes can also be reduced. Slowing of thought, thinking, and memory is a normal part of aging.

▉ CLOSING COMMENTS

Patients with nervous system disorders are seen in every ambulatory care environment. Knowing the signs and symptoms, along as with treatments (e.g., medications) will help the medical assistant provide the best patient care (Box 6.6).

Many nervous system disorders can affect a patient's mobility and change behaviors. It is important for the medical assistant to adapt procedures so as to respect the patient and keep the patient safe during the visit.

BOX 6.6   Medication Classifications

- *Analgesics.* Relieve pain.
- *Anesthetics.* Produce *local anesthesia* (no loss of consciousness) or *general anesthesia* (loss of consciousness).
- *Anti-Alzheimer drugs.* Used to treat AD by increasing naturally occurring substances, such as acetylcholine, in the brain.
- *Anticonvulsants.* Reduce the frequency and severity of seizures by reducing excessive stimulation of the brain.
- *Antidepressants.* Used to treat depression, anxiety, and other neurologic disorders.

- *Antimigraine drugs.* Alter circulation to the brain and are used to treat migraine headaches.
- *Corticosteroids.* Used to treat chronic inflammatory and some autoimmune diseases (e.g., multiple sclerosis).

Refer to Appendix D, which can be found on the Evolve website, for information on the medication classifications, including indications for use, desired effect, side effects, adverse reactions, and generic and trade names. Medical assistants should be familiar with medications that are prescribed to patients.

PATIENT-CENTERED CARE

Providing patient-centered care extends to the caregiver of the patient. In many situations the caregiver is the spouse or significant other of the patient; sometimes it may be an adult child. With many chronic neurologic diseases, the patient may require a caregiver to assist with daily care (e.g., toileting, bathing, grooming), meal preparation, shopping, medical appointments, and so on. As the condition worsens, more burdens fall on the caregiver. Providing 24/7 caregiving to a loved one is physically and emotionally stressful. With behavioral differences and with increasing dependency, relationship roles may change, and the stress can affect the caregiver's health.

The medical assistant needs to recognize the importance of the caregiver in the patient's life. The caregiver's concerns are important, just as are the patient's concerns. The medical assistant may need to provide the caregiver with emotional encouragement and resources for additional assistance, including in-home services, adult day care, support groups, and medical equipment.

BEING PROFESSIONAL

When you work with patients with dementia, communicating with them can be challenging. The medical assistant should remember the following:
- Speak clearly and use short sentences.
- Make eye contact.
- Give the patient time to respond. Do not pressure the person into giving a response.
- Allow patients to speak for themselves.
- Keep the tone of your voice friendly and positive. Remain calm.
- Do not patronize or ridicule the patient.

Role-play this scenario: You are a medical assistant. You are rooming Mrs. Barrows, who has been diagnosed with dementia. She is by herself today. You need to obtain her medical history and the reason for her visit. As you talk with her, she continues to state that she is here because her husband died. You know her husband is not dead. How do you respond to Mrs. Barrows?

CHAPTER REVIEW

The nervous system is composed of the central and peripheral nervous systems. The central nervous system is composed of the brain and spinal cord, which are covered by meninges. The cerebrum, cerebellum, diencephalon, and brainstem make up the brain. The peripheral nervous system is composed of the cranial nerves, which exit the brain, and the spinal nerves, which exit the spinal cord. The nervous system is composed of two types of cells: neurons and neuroglia. Neurons are composed of a cell body, dendrites, and an axon.

The peripheral nervous system consists of voluntary and involuntary nerves. The PNS can be divided into two parts:
- Somatic nervous system, which sends motor impulses to the skeletal muscles. It is associated with the voluntary control of body movements and is also involved with involuntary reflex arcs. A three-neuron arc consists of sensory neurons, interneurons, and motor neurons. A two-neuron arc, the simplest reflex arc, consists of just sensory neurons and motor neurons. The knee-jerk reflex (patellar reflex) is an example of the two-neuron arc.
- Autonomic nervous system, which consists of nerves that conduct impulses from the brainstem or spinal cord to cardiac and smooth muscle tissue and glands. It regulates involuntary function, such as breathing, heart rate, sweating, circulation, and digestion. The autonomic nervous system can be further divided into the sympathetic nervous system (the "fight-or-flight" response) and the parasympathetic nervous system.

Many nervous system disorders were discussed in the chapter. Common signs and symptoms include neuralgia, paresthesia, lack of coordination, spasms, seizures, tremors, headaches, visual changes, amnesia, difficulty speaking, confusion,

disorientation, and loss of consciousness. Common diagnostic procedures include cerebral angiography, EEG, EMG, NCV, and nerve biopsy.

The following are nervous system disorders discussed in this chapter.
- Neurodegenerative disorders: Amyotrophic lateral sclerosis, Alzheimer disease, Huntington disease, multiple sclerosis, Parkinson disease, Friedreich ataxia, frontotemporal dementia, Lewy body disease, Tay-Sachs disease, and vascular dementia.
- Functional disorders: Cluster headaches, tension headaches, migraines, seizure disorders, epilepsy, functional neurologic disorders, narcolepsy, sciatica, and Tourette syndrome.
- Infections: Encephalitis, meningitis, and shingles.
- Structural disorders: Bell palsy, Guillain-Barré syndrome, trigeminal neuralgia, astrocytoma, medulloblastoma, meningioma, and neuroblastoma.
- Injuries: Traumatic brain injury, spinal cord injury, and peripheral neuropathy.
- Congenital disorders: Fetal alcohol spectrum disorders, spina bifida, cerebral palsy, Down syndrome, and tuberous sclerosis.
- Vascular disorders: Cerebrovascular accident, including ischemic strokes, hemorrhagic strokes, and transient ischemic attacks; and epidural, subdural, and intraparenchymal hematomas.

The nervous system in infants is immature. Over childhood, the thinking and learning processes become more complex. During adulthood, the brain function is stable. As a person ages, the nervous system changes. Nerve impulses become slower, thus slowing down reaction time.

SCENARIO WRAP-UP

Nancy had a very busy day with the outreach neurologic services providers. One of the most interesting parts of Nancy's day was talking with a patient's wife. The patient had had a stroke, and

his wife shared with Nancy the different types of adaptive equipment available. Nancy learned that there were different types of walkers, shower chairs and tub benches, raised toilet seats with handles, dressing devices, grooming aids, kitchen utensils (e.g., rocker knives, cutting boards with suction cups), and specially shaped utensils. Many of the devices were designed to be used with one hand. Nancy was impressed with the variety of adaptive equipment available.

During the day, Nancy felt a little overwhelmed by the complexity of neurologic tests and all the different types of test orders. She realizes that she needs to research more about neurologic disorders and diagnostic tests before she assists the outreach providers next week. She enjoyed working with the patients and their caregivers and looks forward to getting to know them in the coming months.

7

Endocrine System

LEARNING OBJECTIVES

1. Describe the anatomical location of the major organs of the endocrine system.
2. Describe the actions of the hormones secreted from the endocrine glands.
3. Explain the common diagnostic procedures and treatments for endocrine system disorders.
4. Describe common endocrine system disorders, including common signs and symptoms, etiology, diagnostic procedures, and treatments.
5. Differentiate between type 1 and type 2 diabetes mellitus.
6. List signs and symptoms of hypoglycemia, hyperglycemia, and diabetic ketoacidosis.
7. Describe complications of diabetes.
8. Compare the structure and function of the of the endocrine system across the life span.

OUTLINE

⫸ OPENING SCENARIO

Cecilia Cukier, CMA (AAMA), has worked at Walden-Martin Family Medical (WMFM) Clinic for 3 years. She enjoys working with the primary care providers. Working with patients who have diabetes mellitus has been a special interest of hers since her medical assistant practicum in college. When a position was posted to work with the outreach endocrinology team, which came from a clinic 50 miles away, Cecilia applied for the position. She was accepted into the new position and now will be working 2 days a week with the endocrinology team, which sees WMFM Clinic patients. During the remaining 3 days, Cecilia will continue to work with the primary care team.

Cecilia is excited to start working with the endocrinology team and patients. She has decided to review the anatomy, physiology, and pathology of the endocrine system in preparation for her new duties.

YOU WILL LEARN

1. To describe the anatomy of the endocrine system.
2. To list the hormones the endocrine glands secrete.
3. To describe the functions of the endocrine system.
4. To describe common endocrine system disorders, including the etiology, signs and symptoms, diagnostic procedures, and treatments.
5. To discuss the differences between type 1 and type 2 diabetes mellitus.
6. To discuss life span changes in the endocrine system.

INTRODUCTION

Endocrinology (end oh kruh NOL uh jee) is the healthcare specialty that deals with endocrine disorders. These disorders relate to endocrine glands, hormones, and hormonal effects on the body. An *endocrinologist* (end oh kruh NOL uh jist) is a specialist involved in the diagnosis, treatment, and prevention of endocrine disorders.

Besides being seen in the endocrine department, patients with endocrine concerns are typically seen in primary care and urgent care departments. Medical assistants should have a strong understanding of common endocrinology diseases, diagnostic tests, and treatments.

ANATOMY OF THE ENDOCRINE SYSTEM

The endocrine system is composed of ductless glands throughout the body. Endocrine glands release hormones directly into the bloodstream, and the blood transports them to target cells. The hormones act as messengers to the target cells, telling the cells to alter their functions to help maintain homeostasis (hoe mee oh STAY sis) in the body. Hormones function as the body's chemical messengers, transferring information from one group of cells to another. They control metabolism, growth, mood, sexual maturity, reproduction, and water and electrolyte (ee LEK troe lite) balance. Hormone levels vary and can be affected by outside factors, such as illness and stress. Fig. 7.1 shows the endocrine glands and their locations.

The nervous system and the endocrine system can work alone or together. Working jointly, as a neuroendocrine system, they perform communication functions and maintain homeostasis. The brain sends out signals to and continually receives feedback from the endocrine system. The nervous system communicates quickly through nerve impulses and delivers rapid responses to maintain homeostasis. The endocrine system communicates slowly through hormones, which maintain homeostasis for a longer period of time. The body needs both systems working together through communication to maintain homeostasis.

Hypothalamus

The *hypothalamus* (hahy puh THAL uh muhs), located in the middle of the brain, is the major connection for the neuroendocrine system. It plays an important role in controlling the endocrine system. When the hypothalamus detects rising levels of a target organ's hormones, it sends a signal to the pituitary gland to release or prevent the pituitary hormone production.

The hypothalamus is also responsible for the production of antidiuretic hormone (ADH) and oxytocin (ok si TOE sin). These two hormones are produced by the hypothalamus and stored and secreted by the posterior lobe of the pituitary gland. They will be discussed in more detail in the next section.

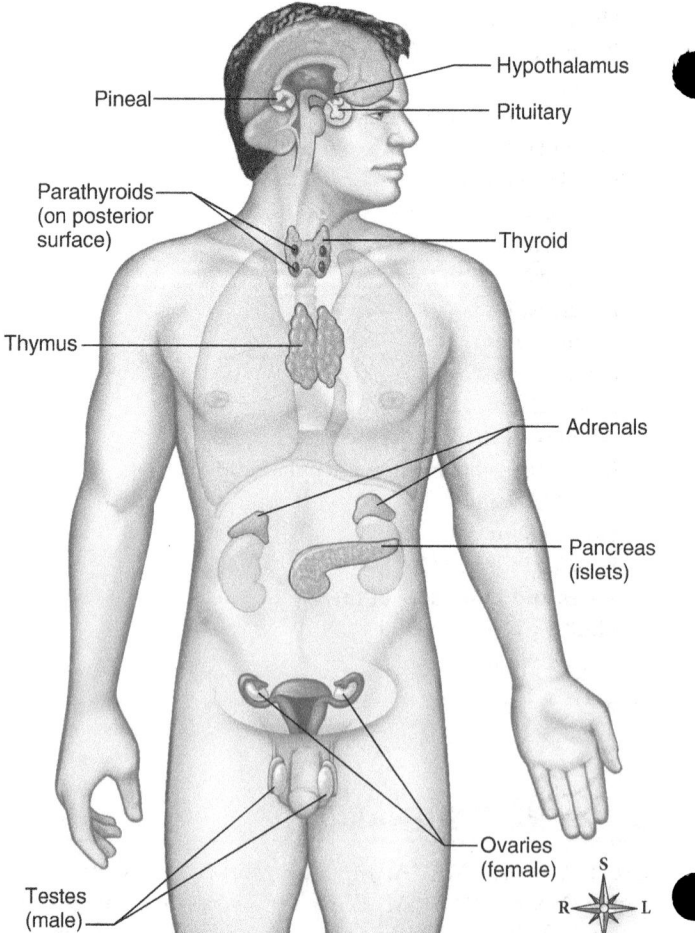

Fig. 7.1 Location of the Endocrine Glands. (From Patton KT, Thibodeau GA: *Anatomy and physiology*, ed 9, St. Louis, 2016, Mosby.)

MEDICAL TERMINOLOGY

aden/o	gland
adren/o	adrenal gland
cortic/o	cortex
crin/o	to secrete
hypophys/o, pituitar/o	pituitary gland
lob/o	lobe
pancreat/o	pancreas
parathyroid/o	parathyroid gland
ren/o	kidney
thyr/o, thyroid/o	thyroid gland
thalam/o	thalamus
thym/o	thymus gland
endo-	within
hypo-	deficient, below, less than normal, under
para-	near, beside, abnormal, apart from
-al	pertaining to
-crine	to secrete
-logy	study of
-us	structure

Pituitary Gland

The pituitary (pih TOO ih tare ree) gland is also known as the *hypophysis* (hye POFF ih sis). The pituitary gland is a pea-sized gland that is connected to the hypothalamus by the *infundibulum* (IN fun DIB you lum), a small stalk of tissue. The hormones from the pituitary control the other endocrine glands; thus the pituitary gland is called the "master gland." The pituitary gland is composed of two lobes. The anterior lobe and the posterior lobe act as separate glands, each having its own function.

Anterior Lobe of the Pituitary Gland. The anterior lobe, also known as the *adenohypophysis* (add uh noh hye POFF ih sis), produces and secretes these hormones (Fig. 7.2):

- *Adrenocorticotropic hormone* (uh DREE noh kawr ti koh TROP ik) (ACTH): Causes the adrenal cortex to produce and release steroids (e.g., cortisol).
- *Follicle-stimulating hormone* (FSH): Stimulates the development of ova (eggs) through ovulation in females and stimulates the seminiferous tubules to produce sperm in males.
- *Growth hormone* (GH): Stimulates growth of the long bones and muscles in children and teens. Growth hormone is also involved with glucose metabolism in the body. Growth hormone is also called *somatotropin* (SOE mah toe TROE pin) or *somatotropic hormone* (STH).
- *Luteinizing hormone* (LOO tee nahyz ing) (LH): In females, it simulates the ovaries to produce estrogen, ova to mature, and the production of progesterone. LH also initiates ovulation and signals the corpus luteum to develop. In men, it stimulates interstitial cells in the testes to develop and secrete testosterone. Thus in men, LH is also called *interstitial cell–stimulating hormone* (ICSH).
- *Prolactin* (proh LAK tin) (PRL): Stimulates breast tissue development and milk production toward the end of pregnancy and after childbirth.

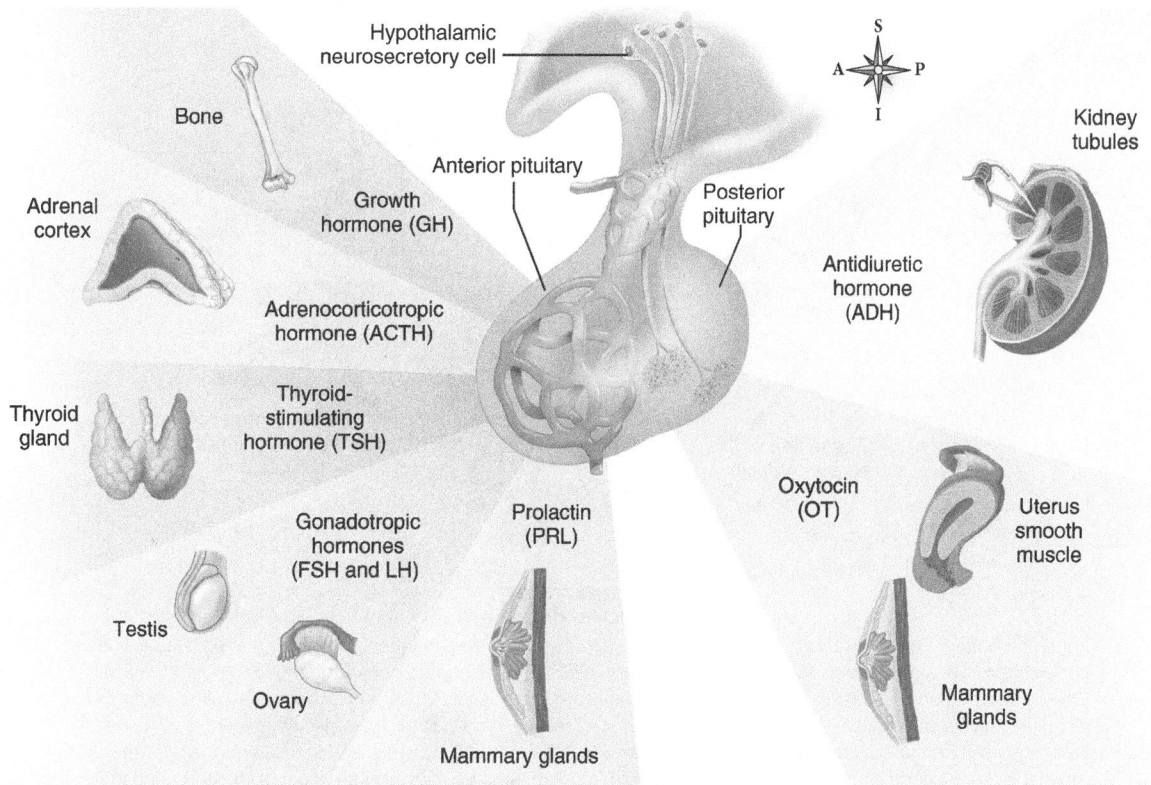

Fig. 7.2 Anterior and Posterior Pituitary Hormones and the Target Organs. (From Patton KT, Thibodeau GA: *The human body in health and disease,* ed 7, St. Louis, 2018, Elsevier.)

- *Thyroid-stimulating hormone* (TSH): Stimulates the thyroid gland to release T_3 and T_4. (More information about the thyroid will be presented later in the chapter.)

Posterior Lobe of the Pituitary Gland. The posterior lobe, also known as the *neurohypophysis* (noo roh hahy POF uh sis), is composed of nervous tissue. It does not produce hormones, but it stores hormones produced by the hypothalamus. The hormones are transported from the hypothalamus to the posterior lobe directly through the infundibulum. The posterior lobe stores the hormones until it gets a signal from the hypothalamus to release them into the bloodstream. The blood then carries the hormones to their target organ (see Fig. 7.2). The two hormones released by the posterior lobe are:

- *Antidiuretic hormone* (an tee dahy uh RET ik) (ADH): Also called *vasopressin*. Stimulates contraction of the blood vessels, raising the blood pressure. It also stimulates the kidney tubules to reabsorb water, which concentrates the urine.
- *Oxytocin* (OT): During the delivery of a child, OT is released and stimulates the uterine muscles to contract. This is an example of a positive feedback loop (Fig. 7.3). OT also helps with releasing breast milk, by stimulating the contraction of the muscles surrounding the mammary ducts.

> **CRITICAL THINKING 7.1**
>
> Cecilia is struggling to remember the hormones secreted by the posterior and anterior lobes of the pituitary gland. What might be some helpful ways to remember the hormones from this gland?

> **VOCABULARY**
>
> **positive feedback loop** A process in which a change causes a response that enhances that change.

Thyroid Gland

The thyroid gland is a butterfly-shaped gland in the neck above the collarbone. The thyroid produces, stores, and secretes:

- *Triiodothyronine* (trahy ahy oh doh THAHY ruh neen) (T_3): Regulates metabolism and increases the basal metabolic rate.

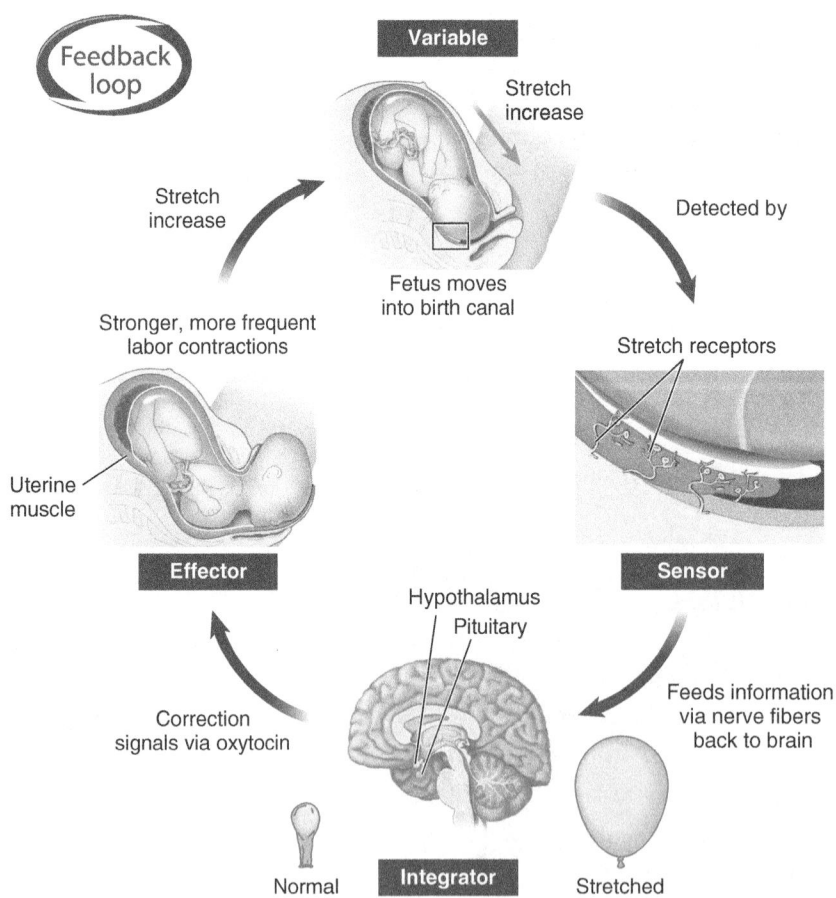

Fig. 7.3 Positive Feedback Loop. An example of positive feedback occurs when a baby is born. As the baby is pushed from the womb *(uterus)* into the birth canal *(vagina)*, stretch receptors detect the movement of the baby. Stretch information is fed back to the brain, triggering the pituitary gland to secrete a hormone called *oxytocin* (OT). OT travels through the bloodstream to the uterus, where it stimulates stronger contractions. Stronger contractions push the baby farther along the birth canal, thereby increasing stretch and stimulating the release of more OT. Uterine contractions quickly get stronger and stronger until the baby is pushed out of the body, and the positive feedback loop is broken. OT also can be injected therapeutically by a physician to stimulate labor contractions. (From Patton KT, Thibodeau GA: *The human body in health and disease*, ed 7, St. Louis, 2018, Elsevier.)

- *Thyroxine* (thahy ROK seen) (T$_4$): Regulates metabolism and increases the basal metabolic rate. It also supports the activities of growth hormone.
- *Calcitonin* (kal sih TOH nin): Regulates calcium and phosphate levels in the blood. It works against the parathyroid hormone action. Calcitonin helps lower blood calcium levels by inhibiting the osteoclast activity. By inhibiting the breakdown of bone, it helps to retain calcium in the bones. Calcitonin also works in the kidney by reducing the resorption of calcium, thus also lowering the blood calcium level.

When thyroid hormone levels decrease in the body, the hypothalamus secretes TSH-releasing hormone. This hormone "tells" the anterior lobe of the pituitary gland to produce TSH, which then stimulates the thyroid to produce hormones. Iodine from our diet is absorbed in the blood and carried to the thyroid gland. Iodine is required to produce T$_3$ and T$_4$ (Box 7.1).

VOCABULARY

basal metabolic rate The rate the body burns calories while the person is at rest.

calcium A naturally occurring element that is necessary for many body functions, including strong bones and teeth, proper blood clotting, nerve conduction, and muscle contractions.

exocrine A glandular secretion released through a duct.

Parathyroid Gland

The parathyroid glands are four pea-sized glands located on the back side of the thyroid gland. They secrete *parathyroid hormone* (PTH), which helps regulate calcium and phosphorus levels in the body. When the blood calcium level decreases, PTH is secreted, causing calcium to be released from bone. The released calcium is absorbed in the blood, which increases the blood calcium levels.

A balance needs to be maintained. If too much PTH is secreted, hyperparathyroidism occurs, causing bones to lose calcium and the blood calcium level to rise. If too little PTH is secreted, hypoparathyroidism occurs. The blood calcium level decreases, and the blood phosphorus level increases.

Adrenal Glands

The adrenal (uh DREE nul) glands are located on the top of each kidney. The outer part of the gland is the adrenal cortex (KORE tecks), and the inner part is called the *adrenal medulla* (muh DOO lah).

Adrenal Cortex. The adrenal cortex produces cortical hormones, also called *steroids*. As a group, these three hormones are called corticosteroids. They include:

- *Mineralocorticoids* (min er uh loh KAWR ti koids): Regulate the electrolytes in the body. Aldosterone, the most important

mineralocorticoid, regulates the sodium and water balance in the body through the reabsorption of sodium and water in the kidneys. As the sodium is reabsorbed into the blood, hydrogen or potassium is excreted into the urine.

- *Glucocorticoids* (gloo koh KAWR ti koids): Regulate protein, fat, and carbohydrate metabolism. They also hasten the breakdown of proteins into amino acids, which are converted to glucose in the liver. This process increases the blood glucose level. Norepinephrine and epinephrine need glucocorticoids to constrict blood vessels, which increases the blood pressure. Glucocorticoids also have anti-inflammatory properties. The main glucocorticoid secreted is cortisol (also called *hydrocortisone*). Cortisone and corticosterone are produced in lesser amounts. Stress can increase the amount of glucocorticoids secreted.
- *Gonadocorticoids* (GOE nah do KAWR ti koids): Small amounts of male sex hormones (androgens) are secreted and responsible for some of the secondary sexual characteristics (e.g., pubic and axillary hair) in both males and females during puberty.

The hypothalamus and the anterior lobe of the pituitary gland (through the secretion of ACTH) regulate the corticosteroids secreted by the adrenal cortex.

CRITICAL THINKING 7.2

The actions of mineralocorticoids and glucocorticoids confuse Cecilia. Summarize the actions of these two corticosteroids.

Adrenal Medulla. The hypothalamus, with the help of the sympathetic nervous system, stimulates the adrenal medulla to secrete these nonsteroid hormones:

- *Epinephrine* (ep i NEF rin) (adrenaline [ah dren ah lin]): Secreted in response to physical or mental stress, providing the fight-or-flight response. It increases the heart rate and strength of the contractions, blood pressure, and blood glucose level. It also relaxes the smooth muscles in the bronchioles. These changes allow more glucose and oxygenated blood to get to the cells for the fight-or-flight response.
- *Norepinephrine* (noradrenalin): Also secreted in times of stress. It increases the blood glucose level, heart rate, and the force of the heart's contractions; in addition, it causes vasoconstriction, thus raising the blood pressure.

Pancreas

The *pancreas* is located inferior and posterior to the stomach. It has both endocrine and exocrine (EK suh krin) functions. As already discussed, an endocrine gland releases hormones into the blood, whereas an exocrine gland releases secretions through ducts. The pancreas releases digestive enzymes into the small intestine through pancreatic ducts.

The pancreas contains *pancreatic islets* or *islets of Langerhans* (EYE lets of LANG gur hahnz), which produce hormones. The pancreas produces several hormones, including:

- *Glucagon* (GLOO kuh gon): Secreted by the alpha islet cells. It raises the blood glucose level two different ways. It stimulates

---

BOX 7.1   Increasing the Basal Metabolic Rate

T$_3$ and T$_4$ hormones increase the **basal metabolic rate,** which:

- Causes an increase in the body temperature and pulse rate; it also creates a stronger heartbeat.
- Helps the brain mature in children and promotes growth.
- Improves concentration and faster reflexes.
- Uses more energy (calories).

the stored glycogen in the liver to be converted into glucose. It also stimulates fatty acids and amino acids in the liver to be converted into glucose. The glucose is absorbed by the bloodstream, which increases the blood glucose level.

- *Insulin* (IN suh lin): Secreted by the beta islet cells. Normally after a meal, the blood glucose level is elevated. This triggers the pancreas to release insulin. Insulin helps move the blood glucose from the blood to the cells. This lowers the blood glucose level. This is an example of a negative feedback loop (Fig. 7.4).
- *Somatostatin* (SOE mah toe STAT in): Secreted by the delta islet cells; it regulates the other pancreatic hormones and also inhibits the secretion of growth hormone.
- *Ghrelin* (grel in) (GHRL): Secreted by the epsilon islet cells. Research has found that GHRL works in the brain to regulate

body weight, glucose metabolism, and food intake. Multiple additional actions of ghrelin have been reported in research studies, including involvement with learning, memory, intestinal peristalsis, gastric acid secretion, sleep/wake rhythm (circadian rhythms), reward-seeking behavior, and taste sensation.

> **VOCABULARY**
>
> **fatty acids** Result when fats are broken down; used by the body for energy and tissue development.
>
> **negative feedback loop** A process in which a change from the normal ranges causes a response that opposes or decreases the change, thus helping to maintain homeostasis.

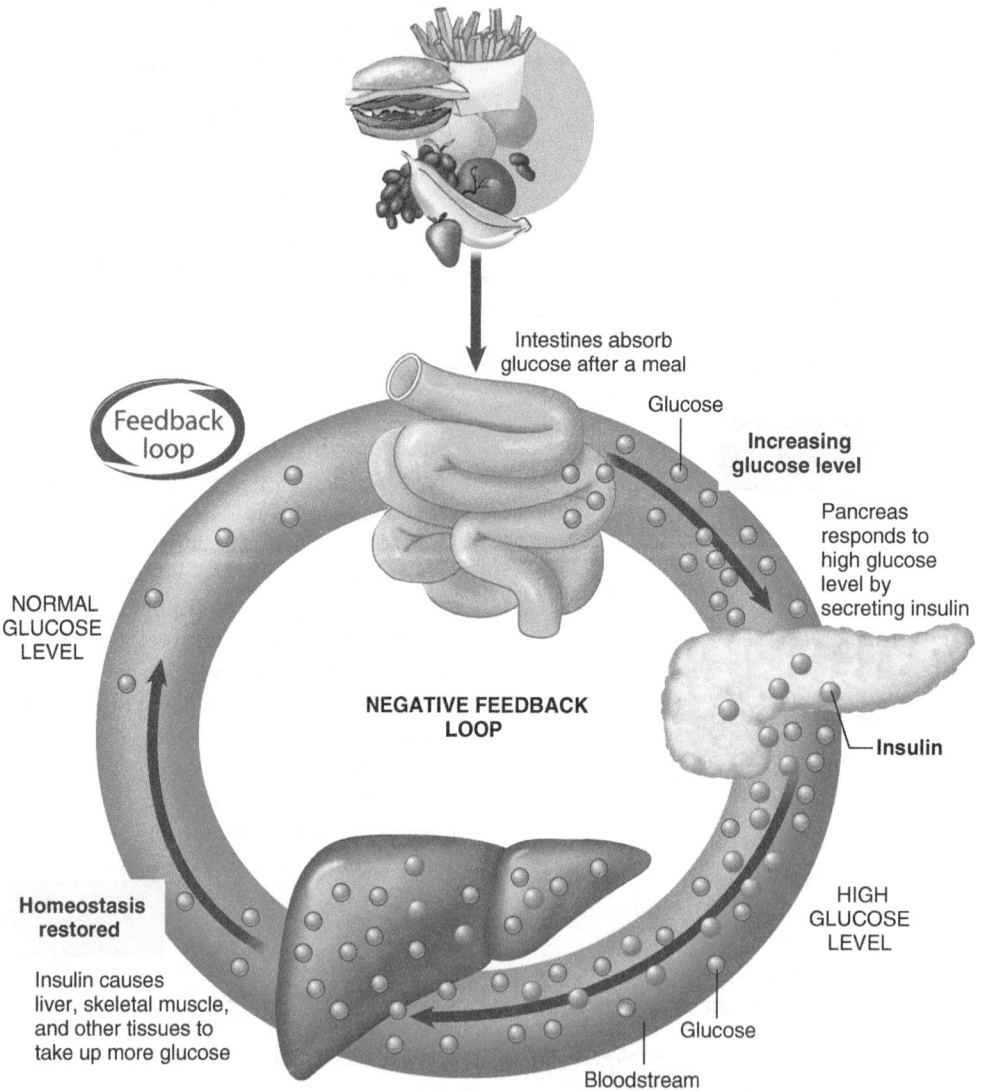

Fig. 7.4 Negative Feedback Loop. The secretion of most hormones is regulated by negative feedback mechanisms that tend to reverse any deviations from normal. In this example, an increase in blood glucose triggers the secretion of insulin. Because insulin promotes glucose uptake by cells, the blood glucose level is restored to its lower, normal level. (From Patton KT, Thibodeau GA: *The human body in health and disease*, ed 7, St. Louis, 2018, Elsevier.)

Thymus

The thymus gland is in the mediastinum (mee dee AH sti nuhm) behind the sternum (breastbone) and secretes *thymosin* (THAHY moh sin) and *thymopoietin* (THIE moe poy ee tin) hormones. These hormones stimulate the production and maturity of T cells, a type of lymphocyte (white blood cell). T cells have an important role in immunity.

Gonads

The *gonads* are considered the primary sex organs. The male gonads are the testes (TES teez), and the female gonads are the ovaries (OH vuh REES). Both types of gonads produce hormones.

- Testes: Secrete *testosterone* (tes TOS tuh rohn), which stimulates the development of male secondary sexual characteristics (e.g., voice changes, growth of facial and pubic hair). Testosterone also promotes sperm production and muscle development.
- Ovaries: Produce *estrogen* and *progesterone*. Estrogen stimulates the development of breasts and other female secondary sexual characteristics. Progesterone helps maintain a pregnancy. Both estrogen and progesterone are important in the menstrual cycle.

Pineal Gland

The pineal (PIN ee uhl) gland is located deep within the brain and secretes the hormone *melatonin* (mel uh TOH nin). Melatonin helps regulate waking and sleeping patterns and may affect seasonal reactions to the availability of sunlight.

MEDICAL TERMINOLOGY	
exo-	outward
gluc/o, glyc/o	glucose, sugar
medull/o	medulla
gonad/o	gonads

PHYSIOLOGY OF THE ENDOCRINE SYSTEM

Mechanisms of Hormone Regulation

The goal of hormone regulation is to maintain homeostasis. Nervous system stimulation, endocrine control, and feedback systems regulate hormone secretion. The following examples demonstrate these three mechanisms.

- Nervous system regulation: During a stressful event, the adrenal medulla releases adrenaline (epinephrine) in response to stimulation from the sympathetic nervous system.
- Endocrine control regulation: TSH from the anterior pituitary stimulates the thyroid to secrete T_3 and T_4. (A hormone from one gland stimulates another gland to secrete a hormone.)
- Feedback system regulation: A negative feedback loop system example: If the calcium blood level falls below normal,

the parathyroid glands are stimulated to release PTH. PTH increases blood calcium levels by stimulating the absorption of calcium from the intestines or by chemically breaking down bone to release stored calcium into the blood. The change in the blood calcium level is detected by the parathyroid gland, which then stops production of PTH. (An imbalance activates the endocrine gland, which then acts to correct the imbalance by stopping the hormone secretion process.)

Target Cells

Each hormone released into the bloodstream has specific target cells for action. The target cells have receptors that attract only certain hormones. The cell membrane only lets selected hormones pass into the cell and affect cellular action.

Hormone Action

There are two categories of hormones, nonsteroid hormones and steroid hormones. All hormones are messengers, but how they deliver their message is where they differ. Both types of hormones maintain homeostasis.

Nonsteroid hormones are made up of protein or amino acids. This type of hormone attaches to a target cell membrane. Another molecule takes the message from the nonsteroid hormone and carries it to the target cell nucleus or organelle, which then puts the message into action in the cell.

Steroid hormones are small *lipid-soluble* (fat-soluble) molecules that attach to a target cell membrane and then pass directly into the target cell. Once inside the target cell, steroid hormones travel to and enter the nucleus. They bind to a receptor site, which creates a hormone–receptor site complex. This complex communicates its message with deoxyribonucleic acid (DNA) in the nucleus, and the DNA tells the cell how to put the hormone's message into action.

VOCABULARY
diffuse To spread, scatter, disperse, or move.
mediastinum The space in the thoracic cavity that lies between the lungs, containing the heart, trachea, and esophagus.
nucleus A specialized organelle of a cell that is encased in a membrane and directs growth, metabolism, and reproduction of the cell.
organelle A structure within a cell that performs a specific function.
receptors Structures or sites on or in a cell that bind with substances such as hormones, antigens, or drugs.

Prostaglandins

Prostaglandins (pros tuh GLAN dins) (PGs), also known as *tissue hormones,* are substances found in many body tissues. PGs are produced in tissues and diffuse only a short distance to affect cells in their local area. They help regulate processes such as respiration, blood pressure, digestive system secretions, and reproductive functions. They are powerful molecules that are made locally and act locally.

DISEASES AND DISORDERS OF THE ENDOCRINE SYSTEM

Many diseases affect the endocrine system. Most of the pathology of the endocrine system is the result of either hyper- (excessive) or hypo- (deficient) hormonal secretion. Common signs and symptoms of endocrine conditions include:

- *Exophthalmia* (eck soff THAL mee ah), a noticeable protrusion of the eyeball
- *Glucosuria* (glook oh SOOR ee ah), the presence of glucose in the urine
- *Goiter* (GOY tur), the swelling of the neck and visible enlargement of the thyroid gland
- *Hirsutism* (HER soo tizm), excessive facial or body hair growth in women
- *Hypocalcemia* (hye poh kal SEE mee ah), a low blood calcium level
- *Hypoglycemia* (hye poh gly SEE mee ah), a low blood glucose (sugar) level
- *Ketoacidosis* (kee toh ass ih DOH sis), the presence of ketones in the blood that cause metabolic acidosis (a pH imbalance due to too much acid)
- *Ketonuria* (kee toh NOOR ee ah), the presence of ketones in the urine
- *Polydipsia* (pah lee DIP see ah), or excessive thirst
- *Polyphagia* (pah lee FAY jee ah), or excessive eating
- *Polyuria* (pah lee YOO ree ah), or excessive urine volume

Common diagnostic procedures are listed in Table 7.1. Common surgical treatments are listed in Table 7.2.

MEDICAL TERMINOLOGY	
acid/o	acid
calc/o	calcium
ket/o	ketone
ophthalm/o	eye
phag/o	to eat, swallow
ur/o	urine
ex-	out
hyper-	excessive
poly-	excessive
-dipsia	condition of thirst
-emia	blood condition
-ia	condition
-osis	abnormal condition
-uria	urinary condition

Pituitary Gland Diseases

Anterior pituitary gland dysfunction can lead to several disorders. Hypersecretion of growth hormone causes acromegaly and gigantism, whereas hyposecretion causes dwarfism. Hypersecretion of prolactin causes prolactinoma. Women with hyposecretion of prolactin are unable to maintain breast milk production. Hyposecretion of all the anterior pituitary hormones causes panhypopituitarism.

Posterior pituitary gland hypersecretion of ADH causes syndrome of inappropriate antidiuretic hormone (SIADH) and hyposecretion causes diabetes insipidus. The following sections discuss the more common pituitary diseases.

Acromegaly. Acromegaly (AK roh MEG uh lee) is a rare condition in which there is too much growth hormone in the body. It is seen after normal bone growth has stopped (end of puberty).

Etiology. Acromegaly is caused when the pituitary gland makes too much growth hormone. Usually a benign tumor in the pituitary gland releases too much GH.

Signs and Symptoms. Acromegaly can cause:
- Excessive sweating and body odor
- Decrease in muscle strength, carpal tunnel syndrome, and joint pain and swelling
- Large bones of the face, jaw, feet, and hands (Fig. 7.5)
- Hirsutism, high blood pressure, and weight gain
- Decreased peripheral vision, headache, hoarseness, and sleep apnea

Diagnostic Procedures. After a medical history and physical, the provider will order laboratory tests, including for blood glucose, growth hormone and growth hormone suppression, insulin-like growth factor 1, and prolactin. A magnetic resonance imaging (MRI) scan of the brain and a spinal x-ray may be ordered, along with an echocardiogram, colonoscopy, and sleep study.

Treatments. Treatment consists of surgery to remove the tumor, radiation, and medication to block the production of GH. Follow-up visits are usually required to ensure acromegaly does not come back.

Gigantism. Gigantism (jye GAN tiz um) is a rare condition in which there is too much growth hormone in the body during childhood.

Etiology. Gigantism is caused when the pituitary gland makes too much growth hormone. Usually a benign tumor of the pituitary gland releases too much GH. Gigantism can also be caused by rare genetic diseases.

Signs and Symptoms. The child will grow extremely large for his or her age (Fig. 7.6). Additional signs and symptoms include:
- Delayed puberty and irregular periods (menstruation)
- Double vision, difficulty with peripheral vision, and voice changes
- Large hands and feet, thickening of facial features, and prominent forehead and jaw
- Joint pain, weakness, and gaps between teeth
- Increased sweating and headaches

Diagnostic Procedures. After an examination, the provider will order the laboratory tests, such as:
- Insulin-like growth factor-1 (IGF-1) level, growth hormone levels, and oral glucose tolerance test (OGTT)
- Cortisol and prolactin
- Estradiol (type of estrogen) for girls and testosterone for boys
- GH suppression test and thyroid hormone

A computed tomography (CT) or MRI scan of the head may also be done.

Treatments. Surgery can cure many cases. If the tumor cannot be completely removed, medications that suppress the GH release can be given.

TABLE 7.1   Common Diagnostic Procedures Used for Endocrine System Disorders

Done by/Type of Test:	Procedure	Description
Medical assistant	Peripheral neuropathy screening	Used for assessing peripheral neuropathy symptoms.
Imagining procedure	Radioactive iodine uptake (RAIU) scan	Uses a radioactive iodine tracer to measure the uptake of iodine in the thyroid. As with the thyroid scan, the patient swallows a radioactive iodine pill. A scan is done 4 to 6 hours after the pill is taken and then again 24 hours later. Often done along with the thyroid scan.
	Thyroid scan	Uses a radioactive iodine tracer to examine the thyroid gland. The patient swallows a pill with the radioactive iodine. The scan is done 4 to 6 hours later as the iodine collects in the thyroid. Often done with the radioactive iodine uptake test.
	Thyroid ultrasound	Ultrasound of the thyroid gland. Used to check for nodules and other abnormalities in the gland.
Medical laboratory	A_{1C} test	Also called HbA_{1C} and hemoglobin A_{1C} test. Measures the average blood glucose level over the past 3 months. Some CLIA-waived tests are available. • Normal level: <5.7%, • Indicates prediabetes: 5.7–6.4% • Indicates diabetes: >6.5%
	Calcium blood test	Measures the calcium level in the blood. Total calcium test measures the calcium attached to specific proteins in the blood. Ionized calcium test measures the calcium unattached to proteins in the blood.
	Fasting blood glucose (FBG) test	Measures the glucose level in the blood after fasting. Some CLIA-waived tests are available. • Normal level: 70–99 mg/dL • Indicates prediabetes: 100–125 mg/dL • Indicates diabetes: >126 mg/dL
	Urine glucose test	Measures the amount of glucose in the urine sample. Some CLIA-waived tests are available. May also be part of a urinalysis.
	Urine ketone test	Measures the amount of ketones in the urine sample. Ketones are produced when fat is used for energy instead of glucose. Some CLIA-waived tests are available.
	Serum ketone test	Measures the level of ketones in the blood.
	Oral glucose tolerance test (OGTT)	Blood test to measure the body's response to a concentrated glucose solution. Patient fasts for 8 to 12 hours and then drinks 75 or 100 grams of glucose. Blood may be drawn and tested prior to the drink and then every 30 to 60 minutes for up to 2 to 3 hours after taking the glucose. Nonpregnant levels: • Normal level: fasting 60–100 mg/dL; 1 hr <200 mg/dL; 2 hr <140 mg/dL • Indicates prediabetes: 2 hr 140–200 mg/dL • Indicates diabetes: >200 mg/dL
	Random blood glucose test	Measures the glucose level in the blood without fasting. A glucometer (a handheld instrument) may be used at home or in the ambulatory care environment. Some CLIA-waived tests are available. • Normal level: <125 mg/dL • Indicates diabetes: >200 mg/dL
	Thyroid antibody test	Measures the thyroid antibodies in the blood. Used to diagnose autoimmune thyroid disorders.
	Thyroid function tests (TFTs)	Measures the levels of TSH, T_3, and T_4 in the blood. Used to evaluate the thyroid function. Some CLIA-waived tests are available.
	Thyroid-stimulating hormone (TSH)	Blood test that measures the thyroid-stimulating hormone. TSH stimulates the thyroid to make T_3 and T_4. When the thyroid does not, the pituitary continues to release TSH. High levels of TSH may indicate hypothyroidism. Low blood levels of TSH may indicate hyperthyroidism. Some CLIA-waived tests are available.
	Triiodothyronine (T_3) test	A blood test that measures the triiodothyronine level. Bound T_3 is attached to proteins and stored for later use. Free T_3 is the active form of T_3. Tests are available to measure free T_3 and total T_3 (bound plus unbound) in the blood.
	Thyroxine (T_4) test	A blood test that measures the thyroxine levels. As with T_3, there is bound T_4 and free T_4. Free T_4 is the thyroxine that can enter the body tissues. This test is preferred for checking thyroid function.

CLIA, Clinical Laboratory Improvement Amendments.

TABLE 7.2   Common Treatments Used for Endocrine System Disorders

Procedures	Description
Adrenalectomy (uh dree nuh LECK tuh mee)	Surgical removal of one or both of the adrenal glands
Hypophysectomy (hye poff uh SECK tuh mee)	Surgical removal of the pituitary gland
Pancreatectomy (pan kree uh TECK tuh mee)	Surgical removal of part or all of the pancreas
Parathyroidectomy (pair uh thigh roy DECK tuh mee)	Surgical removal of one or more of the parathyroid glands
Thyroidectomy (thigh roy DECK tuh mee)	Surgical removal of part or all of the thyroid gland

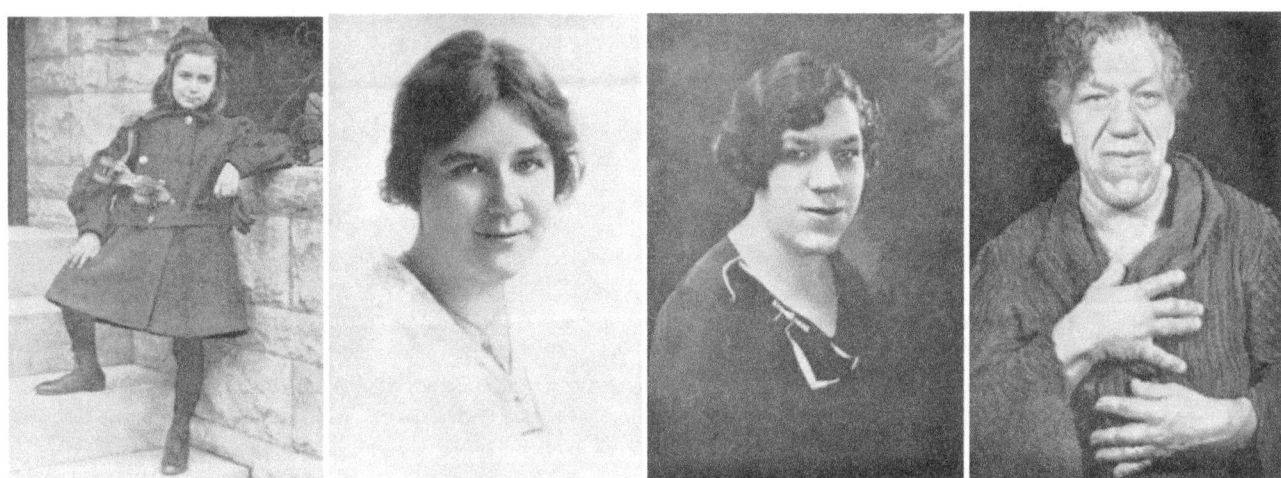

Fig. 7.5 **Acromegaly.** (From Ignatavicius DD, Workman ML: *Medical-surgical nursing: critical thinking for collaborative care*, ed 6, Philadelphia, 2011, Saunders.)

MEDICAL TERMINOLOGY

acro-	extremities
-ism	condition
-megaly	enlargement

Dwarfism. Dwarfism (dwore FIX ehm) is also known as "short stature" and "little person." The person has a short stature or an adult height of under 4 feet 10 inches (58 inches) (Fig. 7.7). Dwarfism does not affect intelligence. It can occur in families with average-height parents. Two types of dwarfism are:

- *Disproportionate dwarfism,* which occurs when some parts of the body are small, whereas others are average or above-average size.
- *Proportionate dwarfism,* which occurs when the parts of the body are proportionate. Usually medical conditions in early childhood that limit growth and development cause proportionate dwarfism.

Etiology. Most types of dwarfism are caused by a genetic mutation. There are over 300 different conditions that cause dwarfism, with achondroplasia being the most common. Achondroplasia, a genetic condition, causes the arms and legs

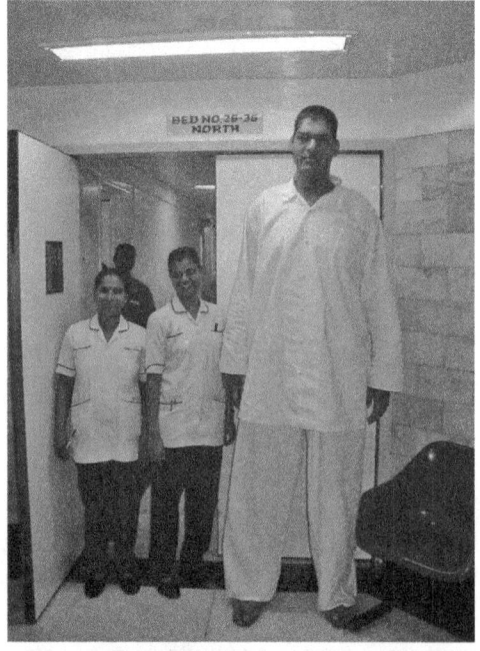

Fig. 7.6 **Gigantism.** (From Sainani GS, Joshi VR, Sainani RG: *Manual of clinical & practical medicine*, New Delhi, 2010, Elsevier India.)

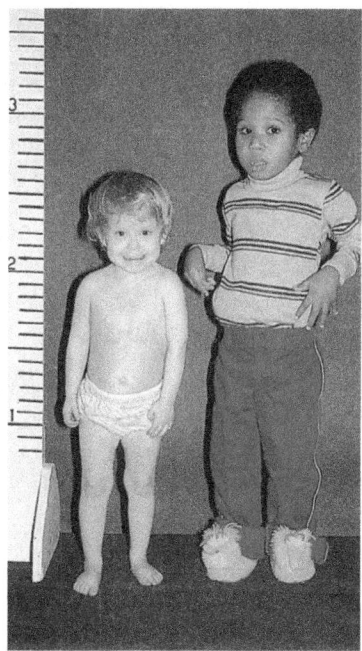

Fig. 7.7 The normal 3½-year-old boy is in the 50th percentile for height. The short 3-year-old girl exhibits the characteristic "kewpie doll" appearance, suggesting a diagnosis of growth hormone deficiency (GHD). (From Zitelli BJ, Davis HW: *Atlas of pediatric physical diagnosis*, ed 5, St. Louis, 2007, Mosby.)

to be short in comparison to the head and trunk. Metabolism problems, hormones, kidney disease, and other genetic conditions can also cause dwarfism.

Signs and Symptoms. Besides a short stature, the signs and symptoms vary based on the condition causing the dwarfism. People with disproportionate dwarfism may have:

- Short fingers, arms, and legs; limited mobility at the elbows; bowed legs; and swayed lower back
- Average-size trunk
- Disproportionately large head with a prominent forehead

People with proportionate dwarfism have a height below the third percentile on growth charts. Their growth rate is slower than expected for their age. Sexual development is delayed or absent during the teen years.

Diagnostic Procedures. Dwarfism can be diagnosed during pregnancy or early in life as the child's growth slows. Measurements and appearance, along with imaging technology (e.g., x-rays), genetic testing, and hormone tests are used.

Treatments. Treatment is focused on maximizing functioning and independence. Most treatments do not increase the stature, but rather correct problems caused by complications. For some patients, growth hormone therapy can be given to help increase stature. Daily injections may be needed for several years until the child stops growing.

Diabetes Insipidus. Diabetes insipidus (dye ah BEE teez in SIP ih dus) (DI) is caused by a hyposecretion of ADH. The hypothalamus does not produce enough of the hormone, or the posterior pituitary gland does not release a sufficient amount of it.

Etiology. There are several types of DI, and the causes vary, including genetics, a tumor, trauma, or pituitary gland surgery.

Diabetes insipidus can also occur if there is an inadequate response to ADH in the renal tubules in the nephrons, due to kidney disease or certain medications.

Signs and Symptoms. The signs and symptoms usually have an acute onset and include:

- Polydipsia, polyuria, *nocturia* (frequent urination at night), and very dilute urine
- Trouble sleeping, fussiness, and irritability
- Fever, vomiting, diarrhea, and *hypotension* (low blood pressure)
- Delayed growth and weight loss in children

Complications may occur, such as *hypernatremia* (abnormally high blood sodium level), severe dehydration, electrolyte imbalance, and hypotension.

Diagnostic Procedures. The provider will do a physical exam and may order laboratory tests, including a urinalysis and blood tests. A water deprivation test and imaging tests can also be done.

Treatments. Diabetes insipidus can be fatal if not adequately treated. Treatment focuses on the cause of the condition. Medications such as a synthetic ADH hormone (desmopressin [DDAVP]) and diuretics may be given.

Additional Pituitary Gland Diseases. Additional pituitary gland diseases include:

- *Prolactinoma (proe LAK ti NOE mah)*: A benign tumor of the pituitary gland that causes the hypersecretion of prolactin. Women have abnormal lactation and abnormal menstrual cycles. Men experience impotence.
- *Panhypopituitarism (pan hye poh pih TOO ih tur iz um)*: Caused by the hyposecretion of all anterior pituitary hormones, which results from the destruction or deficiency of the entire anterior lobe. It is most common in women. It causes hypotension, weight loss, weakness, and loss of libido.
- *Syndrome of inappropriate antidiuretic hormone* (SIADH): Caused by the hypersecretion of ADH. SIADH causes inability to produce and secrete diluted urine. Water retention, *hyponatremia* (a low blood sodium level), and weight gain are seen.

VOCABULARY

libido Sexual drive or instinct.

water deprivation test A test to measure the amount and concentration of urine produced when water is withheld from a patient for a period of time.

MEDICAL TERMINOLOGY

prolactin/o	prolactin
pan-	all
-oma	tumor, mass

CRITICAL THINKING 7.3

Cecilia is working with Landon, who was just diagnosed with diabetes insipidus. Landon's mother asks Cecilia how often he would need to take insulin. How would you address this question? Could you as a medical assistant correct the mother's misconception about diabetes insipidus?

TABLE 7.3 Thyroid Diseases

Condition	Thyroid Function	Description
Simple goiter	Hyperthyroidism or hypothyroidism	Simple enlargement of the thyroid gland, causing swelling in the neck. Usually not malignant. Can be caused by iodine deficiency, immune disorders, infections, medications, and other thyroid conditions. More common in people over age 40, women, and those with a family history of goiters. Depending on the symptoms, may be treated with potassium iodide or thyroid hormone.
Thyroid nodule	Hyperthyroidism or hypothyroidism	A growth in the thyroid gland. Can be benign or malignant. More common in women. Causes neck enlargement, pain, hoarseness, and problems swallowing. Treatment may consist of monitoring, surgery, and thyroid hormone if hypothyroidism is occurring.
Thyroiditis	Hyperthyroidism or hypothyroidism	Inflammation of the thyroid. There are several types of thyroiditis. Can be an autoimmune condition or caused by a virus, bacteria, or medication. For several types, the patient may start with hyperthyroidism symptoms and then have hypothyroidism symptoms. Treatment depends on the symptoms and type.
Thyroid carcinoma	Hyperthyroidism or hypothyroidism	The most common types of thyroid carcinoma are follicular and papillary. Both have high 5-year survival rates. Women are three times more at risk for thyroid cancer. Causes a hard, painless lump in the thyroid gland. May cause hoarseness and enlargement of the neck. Treatment depends on the type of cancer; may include surgery, chemotherapy, radiation, and thyroid hormone.
Graves disease	Hyperthyroidism	Autoimmune disease that results in hypersecretion of the thyroid hormone. Most common cause of hyperthyroidism. Causes heat intolerance, heart palpitations (pounding heart in chest), weight loss, and nervousness. Can cause Graves eye disease or Graves ophthalmopathy (e.g., bulging of the eyes [*exophthalmia*], double vision, light sensitivity, and irritation).
Cretinism	Hypothyroidism	Occurs during infancy and childhood. Leads to low metabolic rate, stunted growth and sexual development, and cognitive deficits. Treated with thyroid hormone.
Myxedema	Hypothyroidism	Occurs during adolescence and adulthood. Symptoms include menorrhagia; dry, scaly skin with no perspiration; weakness; fatigue; bloating; facial puffiness; cold intolerance; and cognition issues. Treated with thyroid hormone.
Hashimoto thyroiditis	Hypothyroidism	A chronic autoimmune disease that attacks the thyroid gland. Often occurs in middle-aged females. Occurs slowly, leading to difficulty thinking, dry skin, goiter, fatigue, hair loss, cold intolerance, mild weight gain, and irregular periods. Treatment may include thyroid medication.

Thyroid Gland Diseases

Thyroid diseases cause hypersecretion or hyposecretion of thyroid hormone. Table 7.3 describes thyroid diseases. Hyperthyroidism and hypothyroidism are described in depth in the following sections.

Hyperthyroidism. Hyperthyroidism (hye pur THIGH roy diz um) occurs when too much thyroid hormone is produced. Hyperthyroidism is more common in women, people with other thyroid conditions, and those over 60 years of age.

Etiology. The most common cause of hyperthyroidism is Graves disease, and additional causes include thyroid nodules, pituitary disorders and tumors, and thyroiditis (see Table 7.3). Risk factors include a family history of thyroid disorders and having an existing autoimmune disease.

Signs and Symptoms. Hyperthyroidism can cause:
- Fatigue, muscle weakness, sensitivity to heat, and increased sweating
- More frequent bowel movements and weight loss, even with adequate food intake and an increased appetite
- Difficulty sleeping, restlessness, irritability, nervousness, and anxiety
- Rapid heart rate, irregular heart rate, and palpitations
- Goiter and exophthalmia (Figs. 7.8 and 7.9)
- Changes in the menstrual cycle
- Thyrotoxicosis (thyroid storm), a life-threatening condition that causes elevated vital signs (e.g., temperature, pulse, respiration, and blood pressure)

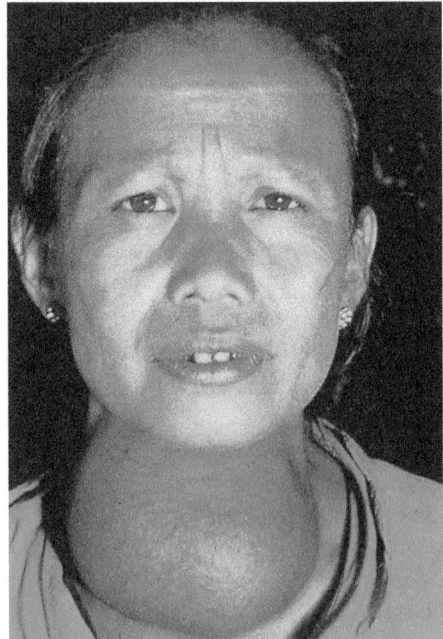

Fig. 7.8 Goiter. (From Thibodeau GA, Patton KT: *The human body in health and disease*, ed 5, St. Louis, 2010, Mosby.)

Diagnostic Procedures. After performing a physical exam, the provider may order thyroid function tests and a radioactive iodine uptake (RAIU) scan.

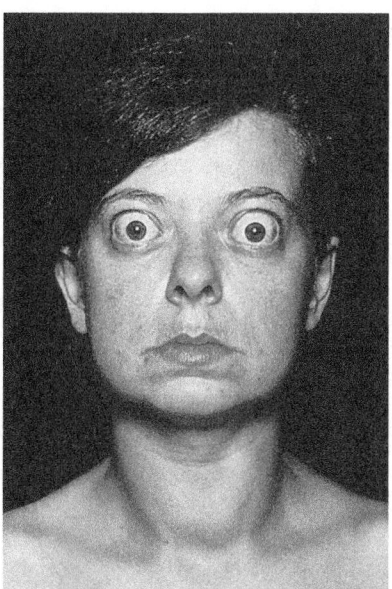

Fig. 7.9 Exophthalmos in Graves Disease. (From Seidel HM et al: *Mosby's guide to physical examination*, ed 6, St. Louis, 2006, Mosby.)

Treatments. Treatment includes radioactive iodine therapy to shrink the thyroid, antithyroid medication (e.g., methimazole [Tapazole]), and a thyroidectomy.

Hypothyroidism. Hypothyroidism occurs when too little thyroid hormone is produced.

Etiology. Hypothyroidism (hye poh THIGH roy diz um) occurs after thyroidectomy and radiation therapy. Table 7.3 describes additional conditions that cause hypothyroidism. Risk factors for hypothyroidism include having a history of an autoimmune disease, a family history of hypothyroidism, or pregnancy in the past 6 months. Another risk factor is being a female over 60 years of age.

Signs and Symptoms. The signs and symptoms relate to the metabolism slowing down and may include:
- Fatigue, muscle weakness, tenderness, aches, and stiffness
- Constipation and weight gain
- Dry skin, sensitivity to cold, and thinning hair
- Slowed heart rate, hoarseness, and depression
- Elevated blood cholesterol

Diagnostic Procedures. After the provider performs the physical exam, thyroid function tests and a thyroid ultrasound may be done.

Treatments. Treatment requires taking lifelong synthetic thyroid hormone (e.g., levothyroxine [Synthroid]).

Parathyroid Gland Diseases

Hyperparathyroidism. Hyperparathyroidism (hye pur pair uh THIGH roy diz um) is a relatively common disorder. It occurs when one or more of the four parathyroid glands oversecrete PTH. Hyperparathyroidism causes excessive bone resorption, and the calcium from the bones causes *hypercalcemia* (abnormally high blood calcium level).

Etiology. Primary hyperparathyroidism occurs as a result of an adenoma or a hyperplasia of one of the four glands, causing the increase in PTH secretion. Secondary hyperparathyroidism occurs with renal disease, which causes hypocalcemia and low vitamin D levels that trigger PTH secretion.

Signs and Symptoms. The signs and symptoms are related to hypercalcemia and include:
- Muscle pain, atrophy, and weakness
- Gastrointestinal pain, nausea, vomiting, and anorexia
- Cardiac arrhythmias, renal calculi, bone tenderness, and fractures

Diagnostic Procedures. After the physical exam, the provider may order blood tests (e.g., calcium, phosphorus) and imaging tests (e.g., x-ray studies, bone density test, radioimmunoassay studies).

Treatments. Treatment depends on the cause. Minimally invasive surgery may be done to remove a tumor or gland(s). When hyperplasia occurs, all but half of a gland can be removed. For secondary hyperparathyroidism, the underlying cause is treated. Medications may be prescribed to help increase calcium excretion by the kidneys.

Hypoparathyroidism. Hypoparathyroidism occurs when there is hyposecretion of parathyroid hormone. This reduction of PTH causes hypocalcemia to occur.

Etiology. Hypoparathyroidism (hye poh pair uh THIGH roy diz um) results from injury or damage to the parathyroid glands. Damage and destruction of the glands can result from cancer, radiation, and surgery (e.g., thyroidectomy).

Signs and Symptoms. The signs and symptoms relate to the hypocalcemia and can include:
- Numbness and tingling, spasms, and twitching in the hands and feet
- Confusion and irritability
- *Tetany* (continuous muscle spasms), laryngospasm, arrhythmias, respiratory paralysis, and death

Diagnostic Procedures. The provider will perform a physical exam and order blood tests (e.g., calcium, phosphate), an electrocardiogram, and imaging tests (e.g., radioimmunoassay studies).

Treatments. Lifelong treatment includes calcium and vitamin D supplements and a high-calcium diet.

CRITICAL THINKING 7.5

Cecilia is rooming Mr. Jones, who came with his wife, Sally. Over the past few months, he has been depressed, forgetful, and weak. At times he has experienced abdominal pain and joint pain. His primary care provider diagnosed him with hyperparathyroidism, and today he came in to see the specialist. Mr. Jones had never heard about the parathyroid gland, and he asks Cecilia about it. How would you explain the parathyroid gland to a patient?

Adrenal Gland Diseases

Addison's Disease. Addison's (ADD ih sun) disease is a malfunction of the adrenal cortex, leading to adrenal insufficiency (hyposecretion) of cortisol. Addison's disease affects adults ages 30 to 50, though it can occur at any age. Addison's disease can be acute or

CRITICAL THINKING 7.4

Cecilia is working with a patient who has been diagnosed with hypothyroidism. What are the signs and symptoms of hypothyroidism? What treatments are usually prescribed?

chronic. Acute Addison's disease may be called Addisonian crisis, a condition marked by life-threatening symptoms. A crisis can be brought on by stressful situations, infections, minor illness, or surgery.

Etiology. The causes of Addison's disease include an autoimmune reaction, tuberculosis, and damage to or disease of the adrenal glands or pituitary gland.

Signs and Symptoms. Acute Addison's disease can cause:
- Pain in the lower back, abdomen, and legs
- Severe vomiting and diarrhea, dehydration, and low blood pressure
- Loss of consciousness
- *Hyperkalemia* (an abnormally high blood potassium level) and hyponatremia

Chronic Addison's disease may occur over weeks to months. It can cause:
- Irritability, extreme fatigue, weight loss, lack of appetite, and a craving for salt
- Darkening of the skin and buccal membranes (*hyperpigmentation*)
- Hypotension, fainting, nausea, diarrhea, and vomiting
- Hypoglycemia
- Muscle pain, depression, and loss of body hair

Diagnostic Procedures. After a physical exam, the provider may order blood tests (e.g., cortisol, sodium, potassium, and ACTH), imaging tests, and an ACTH stimulation test. The ACTH stimulation test measures the blood cortisol level before and after an injection of synthetic ACTH. If the adrenal gland is damaged, cortisol levels after ACTH stimulation will still be low or absent.

Treatments. Addisonian crisis treatment requires immediate administration of an intravenous saline and dextrose solution with corticosteroids. Other treatments involve corticosteroids to replace cortisol and aldosterone and dietary changes (e.g., a diet high in carbohydrates and protein; adequate sodium and fluids).

Cushing Disease. Cushing (CUSH ing) disease is a malfunction of the cortex of the adrenal gland, causing increased levels of cortisol.

Etiology. Cushing disease can be caused by:
- A benign pituitary tumor
- An adrenal adenoma (benign adrenal cortex tumor), a tumor that secretes ACTH
- Taking long-term corticosteroids for another medical condition (e.g., organ transplantation, severe asthma, or rheumatoid arthritis)

Signs and Symptoms. Cushing disease can cause:
- High blood pressure
- Weight gain, especially in the abdomen, upper back, face (moon face), and between the shoulder blades (buffalo hump)
- Pink or purple stretch marks on the abdomen, thighs, breasts, and arms
- Fragile, thin skin that bruises easily
- Infections, slow-healing wounds, and acne
- Severe fatigue, muscle weakness, and headaches

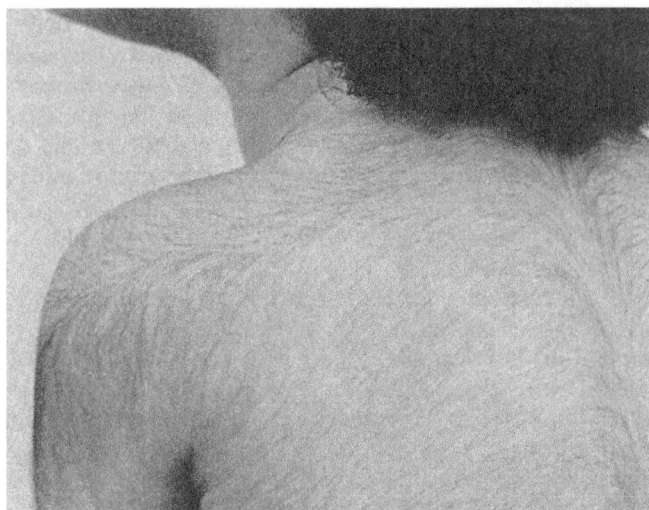

Fig. 7.10 Hirsutism. (From *Mosby's medical, nursing, and allied health dictionary,* ed 8, St. Louis, 2009, Mosby.)

- Depression, anxiety, irritability, loss of emotional control, and difficulty thinking clearly
- Slowed or impaired growth in children
- Thicker or more noticeable facial and body hair (*hirsutism* or *hypertrichosis*) in women (Fig. 7.10)
- Decreased libido and infertility in men

Diagnostic Procedures. After obtaining a medical history and performing a physical exam, the provider may order:
- Blood, saliva, and urine tests to measure cortisol levels
- An ACTH stimulation test
- Imaging tests

Treatments. Treatment is focused on the cause of the disorder and may include medications to control cortisol levels, radiation therapy to shrink the tumor, or surgery to remove the tumor.

CRITICAL THINKING 7.6

Describe the difference between Cushing disease and Addison's disease.

Additional Adrenal Gland Diseases. Additional adrenal gland diseases include:
- *Adrenocortical carcinoma*: A malignant adrenal tumor that starts in the adrenal cortex.
- *Congenital adrenal hyperplasia* (CAH): A genetic disorder that causes the body to make a decreased amount of cortisol. Usually, people with CAH also have other hormone imbalances.
- *Pheochromocytoma* (fee oh kroh moh sigh TOH muhs): A type of paraganglioma tumor that develops in the adrenal medulla and produces adrenaline, causing high blood levels of epinephrine.

Pancreatic Diseases

Diabetes Mellitus. Diabetes mellitus (DM) is the most common pancreatic disease. DM is a group of metabolic disorders characterized by an inadequate production of insulin, a resistance to insulin, or a combination of both. Table 7.4 describes

TABLE 7.4   Types of Diabetes Mellitus

	Type 1 Diabetes Mellitus	Type 2 Diabetes Mellitus	Latent Autoimmune Diabetes in Adults
Onset	Occurs at any age, though it is often diagnosed between childhood and the young adult years.	More common in older adults, but with the rise in obesity, children and younger adults are also diagnosed with it.	Usually seen in adults over 30 years of age.
Use of Insulin/ Function of the Pancreas	The pancreas produces very little or no insulin.	Insulin resistance occurs, or the pancreas does not make enough insulin to meet the body's needs, leading to hyperglycemia.	The pancreas slowly stops producing adequate insulin.
Risk Factors	Family history of type 1 diabetes mellitus (DM), genetics, age (peaks between ages 4 to 7 and then again between ages 10 to 14). Possible viral or environmental exposure.	Obesity, extra fat carried in the abdominal area, inactivity, family history of type 2 DM, race (greater risk if Native American, Asian American, Hispanic, or Black), greater risk if over 45 years of age or with a history of prediabetes, gestational diabetes, or polycystic ovarian syndrome.	May have a family history of diabetes; obesity, physical inactivity, alcohol consumption, and smoking.
Treatment	Insulin injections, regular exercise, frequent blood glucose monitoring, and dietary changes, including carbohydrate, fat, and protein counting.	Healthy eating, regular exercise, weight loss if obese, medications (e.g., antihyperglycemics, insulin), and glucose monitoring. Bariatric surgery if body mass index (BMI) is 35 or greater.	Initially managed with diet, weight loss if needed, exercise, and oral medication. Insulin injections will be needed months to years after the patient is diagnosed.

BOX 7.2   Hyperglycemia

With a fasting blood glucose test, the normal level is 70 to 99 mg/dL. *Hyperglycemia* occurs when the blood glucose level is elevated or above the normal limit. Blood glucose levels increase due to:

- Eating too many carbohydrates without enough insulin
- An infection, injury, or surgery regardless of the amount of carbohydrates eaten
- Missing an insulin injection

Usually during an illness, people with type 1 diabetes mellitus have a special diabetic management plan to follow, which may include extra insulin and increased blood glucose monitoring.

---

type 1 DM, type 2 DM, and latent autoimmune diabetes in adults (LADA, sometimes called type 1.5 DM). (Gestational diabetes will be discussed in a separate section.)

Etiology. The exact cause of DM is unknown. Type 1 DM and LADA are autoimmune conditions. The immune system destroys the beta islet cells of the pancreas. See Table 7.4 for risk factors for the different types of diabetes.

Signs and Symptoms. Signs and symptoms relate to hyperglycemia (Box 7.2). With type 1 DM, the hyperglycemia can occur suddenly, whereas with type 2 DM and LADA it can be gradual. Hyperglycemia signs and symptoms include polydipsia, polyuria, polyphagia, weight loss, fatigue, blurred vision, frequent infections, and slow-healing wounds.

Diagnostic Procedures. After a medical history and physical exam, the provider will order laboratory tests. The following diagnostic results suggest diabetes:

- Glycated hemoglobin (A_{1C}) test, 6.5% or greater on two separate samples
- Fasting blood glucose test, 126 mg/dL or greater on two separate samples
- Oral glucose tolerance test, greater than 200 mg/dL for the 2-hour level
- Random blood glucose test, no matter when the person ate last, 200 mg/dL or greater and diabetes symptoms

Treatments. See Table 7.4 for the treatments for each type of DM.

Complications. According to the Centers for Disease Control and Prevention (CDC; https://www.cdc.gov), during the past 20 years the number of people with DM has tripled. During that same time span, the top complications of DM – heart attack and stroke – have decreased because of the advances in DM education and care. The complications of diabetes mellitus develop over time. Two factors increase the risk of complications: the longer a person has DM and the more uncontrolled the blood glucose.

Diabetes affects the entire body. The following list provides a snapshot of possible complications of diabetes mellitus:

- *Cardiovascular disease*: People with DM have twice the risk of having a heart attack and stroke compared to people without diabetes mellitus. Diabetes increases the risk for coronary artery disease with *angina* (chest pain) and *atherosclerosis* (narrowing of the arteries).
- *Blindness and eye conditions*: Diabetic retinopathy (reh tin OP ah thee), glaucoma (glou KOE mah), and cataracts can lead to vision loss. Early prevention and screening can prevent blindness with diabetic retinopathy. It is recommended that people with diabetes have their eyes checked every 4 to 6 months.

VOCABULARY

cataracts Clouding of the lens, leading to decreased vision.

diabetic retinopathy Damages the blood vessels in the retina, leading to loss of vision and eventual blindness.

glaucoma Increase in the fluid pressure in the eye, which can lead to blindness if not treated.

- *Neuropathy*: One of the most common complications of DM is nerve damage affecting the digestive system, reproductive system, cardiovascular system, and the extremities. Capillaries help nourish the nerves in the body, but hyperglycemia can damage the capillary walls, thus also causing nerve damage. Damage to the nerves in the GI system can cause nausea, vomiting, constipation, or diarrhea. Men can have erectile dysfunction. A person with neuropathy can experience burning, tingling, pain, and numbness in the fingers and toes, which gradually moves up the extremities. If left untreated, a loss of feeling in the extremities may occur, which can affect functioning.

- *Poor healing of wounds*: Diabetes also makes a person more susceptible to bacterial and fungal skin infections. With the lack of feeling in the extremities, the person is more at risk for foot sores, blisters, and cuts. Left untreated, they can become infected, which increases the blood glucose levels. This affects the healing process, which may lead to amputations to stop the spread of infection.
- *Kidney disease*: Hyperglycemia also damages the tiny blood vessels (glomeruli) in the kidney, leading to chronic kidney disease (CKD). Untreated CKD leads to kidney failure, which requires dialysis or a kidney transplantation.
- *Dementia*: Type 2 diabetes increases a person's risk of dementia-related disorders (e.g., Alzheimer disease).
- *Depression*: Is common in patients with type 1 and type 2 DM.
- *Periodontal disease*: Gum infections and tooth loss can occur, which also increases hyperglycemia. It is recommended that patients with diabetes have dental cleanings and exams twice a year.

CRITICAL THINKING 7.7

Summarize the difference between type 1 and type 2 diabetes mellitus.

Gestational Diabetes. Gestational diabetes develops during pregnancy. The hyperglycemia can affect the health of the pregnancy and the baby. Usually after the pregnancy, gestational diabetes resolves, though there is a greater risk for type 2 DM.

Etiology. The exact cause is unknown, though hormones produced by the placenta impair the action of insulin, leading to hyperglycemia. Risk factors include being older than age 25, having a family history of type 2 DM, a personal history of prediabetes, being overweight, and race (greater risk if Native American, Asian, Hispanic, or Black).

Signs and Symptoms. There are no signs or symptoms of gestational diabetes.

Diagnostic Procedures. A routine oral glucose tolerance test is usually done during weeks 24 to 28 of pregnancy.

Treatments. Treatment for gestational diabetes includes eating a healthy diet, monitoring blood glucose levels, regular exercise, insulin injections, and closer follow-up for both the patient and baby.

Complications. Complications of gestational diabetes can include issues with the baby and the mother. For the baby, complications include:

- Excessive growth in utero: The extra glucose in the mother's blood passes into the baby's bloodstream, causing the baby's pancreas to make extra insulin. This causes extra weight to be added to the baby, thus increasing the likelihood the child may need to be delivered by a C-section.
- Death: If the mother does not get treated for gestational diabetes, the risk of death for the baby during pregnancy or after birth increases.

- Hypoglycemia shortly after birth: With the extra insulin production in utero, the baby may be at risk for hypoglycemia shortly after birth.
- Risk of developing obesity and type 2 DM later in life.

For the mother, complications include preeclampsia (pree ih KLAMP see ah) and C-section delivery. She is at a greater risk for gestational diabetes with future pregnancies and having type 2 DM later in life.

> **VOCABULARY**
>
> **preeclampsia** A form of toxemia during pregnancy, characterized by high blood pressure, fluid retention, and protein in the urine. May progress to eclampsia.

Diabetic Ketoacidosis. Diabetic ketoacidosis (DKA) is a life-threatening hyperglycemic condition that is more commonly seen with type 1 DM and LADA.

Etiology. DKA occurs when there is not enough insulin in the body, which helps the blood glucose move to the cells. Because the cells need energy, the body starts rapidly breaking down fats, which leads to a buildup of ketones in the blood and urine, causing ketoacidosis.

Signs and Symptoms. DKA can cause:

- Decreased alertness and headache
- Nausea, vomiting, abdominal pain, and dry mouth
- Muscle aches or stiffness, dry skin, and flushed face
- Frequent urination or thirst lasting for 1 or more days
- Fruity-smelling breath

Diagnostic Procedures. Laboratory tests include blood glucose, urine, and blood ketones. A basic metabolic panel (which includes electrolytes [e.g., sodium and potassium] levels) may also be done.

Treatments. The goals of treatment are to correct the hyperglycemic level, replace lost fluids, and correct any electrolyte imbalances. Treatment usually consists of insulin, intravenous (IV) fluids, and frequent glucose and electrolyte monitoring. Sometimes, DKA treatment can be done in an ambulatory care facility, and other times patients will be transported to the local emergency department for care.

Hypoglycemia. *Hypoglycemia* means low blood glucose (below 70 mg/dL). Hypoglycemia is commonly seen with DM but also can be seen with other conditions.

Etiology. Hypoglycemia in DM usually occurs due to a medication side effect. A person takes too much insulin or oral medication for the amount of carbohydrates consumed, thus dropping the blood glucose level.

Signs and Symptoms. Early hypoglycemia can cause:

- Irregular heart rhythm
- Pale skin, sweating, shakiness, and fatigue
- Irritability, hunger, and tingling sensation around the mouth
- Crying out while sleeping

As hypoglycemia worsens (the blood glucose level drops more), a person may experience:

- Visual disturbances and blurred vision
- Clumsy movements and seizures

- Confusion, abnormal behavior (e.g., incoherent speech, slurring words, inability to complete routine tasks), and loss of consciousness

The behavior may be similar to being intoxicated.

Treatments. Immediate treatment is required and involves increasing the blood glucose level. If people are alert and can swallow, they should follow the 15/15 rule. People should eat 15 grams of fast-acting carbohydrate, then wait 15 minutes before retesting the blood glucose level. This cycle should be followed until the blood glucose level returns to normal. At that time, the person should eat a small, balanced snack that contains both a protein and a carbohydrate if the next meal is more than 2 hours away. Examples of 15 grams of fast-acting carbohydrate include:

- 3 glucose tablets
- 4 ounces or ½ cup of fruit juice or regular soda (not diet soda)
- 6 to 7 hard candies
- 1 tablespoon of sugar

For an unconscious adult patient or child over age 6, glucagon 1 mL should be given subcutaneously or intramuscularly (IM) to treat hypoglycemia. This dose should be repeated in 15 minutes if the patient is still unconscious. Children younger than 6 years of age should receive glucagon 0.5 mL. The blood glucose should be monitored, and once the person is alert and able to swallow, additional food should be given.

CLOSING COMMENTS

An important part of becoming a professional medical assistant is to be familiar with the medical terminology and abbreviations related to the endocrine system. Many endocrine disorders require hormone therapy as treatments and frequent follow-up visits. The professional medical assistant will work closely with the providers and patients to ensure patients receive the best care possible. Knowing the signs and symptoms, along as with treatments (e.g., medications) will help the medical assistant provide the best patient care (Box 7.3).

Additional Pancreatic Diseases. Additional pancreatic diseases include:

- *Hyperinsulinism* (hye pur IN suh lin iz um): Hypersecretion of insulin; seen in some newborns of diabetic mothers. Causes severe hypoglycemia.
- *Islet cell carcinoma*: Also called *pancreatic cancer*; fourth leading cause of cancer death in the US. Treated with a Whipple procedure (pancreatoduodenectomy).
- *Prediabetes*: Condition in which the blood glucose level is higher than normal, but not high enough for a diagnosis of type 2 diabetes.

LIFE SPAN CHANGES

Changes in hormone levels vary with age. Some increase, and others decrease. Hormones that decrease with age include:

- Estrogen: In females, the declining level leads to menopause.
- Testosterone: In males, levels gradually decrease.
- Growth hormone.
- Melatonin: Older adults may experience a loss of the normal sleep/wake cycles.

Cortisol, insulin, and thyroid hormone usually remain unchanged or slightly decrease with age. Norepinephrine, epinephrine, parathyroid hormone, follicle-stimulating hormone, and luteinizing hormone may increase with age.

BOX 7.3 Medication Classifications

- Antihyperglycemics: Used to manage diabetes mellitus
- Hormone replacement: Used to maintain adequate hormone levels
  - Estrogen: Used for menopause
  - Estrogen and progestin: Used for menopause
  - Insulin: Used to treat type 1 and type 2 diabetes mellitus
  - Thyroid hormone: Used for hypothyroidism
  - Vasopressin: Used for diabetes insipidus

Refer to Appendix D, which can be found on the Evolve website, for information on the medication classifications, including indications for use, desired effect, side effects, adverse reactions, and generic and trade names. Medical assistants should be familiar with medications that are prescribed to patients.

PATIENT-CENTERED CARE

Providing patients and families with information, education, and emotional support is part of providing patient-centered care. When working with patients with endocrinology disorders, especially diabetes mellitus, the medical assistant has an important role in connecting patients with additional resources. These can include local support groups, medication discount programs, and websites, including:
- American Diabetes Association: https://www.diabetes.org
- Centers for Disease Control and Prevention: https://www.cdc.gov
- National Institutes of Health: Genetic and Rare Diseases Information Center: https://rarediseases.info.nih.gov
- US National Library of Medicine: MedlinePlus: https://medlineplus.gov

BEING PROFESSIONAL

An important part of becoming a professional medical assistant is a commitment to lifelong learning. This chapter focused on the details of diabetes mellitus because it is the most common endocrine system disease and also one of the most serious. Regardless of where you work as a medical assistant, you will end up caring for patients with diabetes and interacting with their families on some level. Diabetes researchers are constantly discovering more information about the disease: how it is diagnosed, the best treatment methods, and the pathophysiology of possible complications. You must commit to continual learning about diabetes so that you are best prepared to care for patients with this life-threatening disorder.

Role-play this scenario: You and Joan are medical assistants in a family practice setting. The department manager just announced a mandatory training session on diabetes. Joan and you are discussing it. Joan states, "Why do we need to go to these training sessions? I've worked here for 15 years and know everything I need to know about diabetes." How should you respond to Joan?

CHAPTER REVIEW

The endocrine system is composed of ductless glands that release hormones directly into the bloodstream. The blood transports the hormones to target cells. The nervous system and the endocrine system work together to maintain homeostasis. The hypothalamus is the major connection for the neuroendocrine system.

The following structures are involved with hormone production and secretion:

- Hypothalamus produces antidiuretic hormone and oxytocin.
- Anterior lobe of the pituitary gland produces and secretes adrenocorticotropic hormone, follicle-stimulating hormone, growth hormone, luteinizing hormone, prolactin, and thyroid-stimulating hormone.
- Posterior lobe of the pituitary gland releases antidiuretic hormone and oxytocin.
- Thyroid gland produces, stores, and secretes triiodothyronine, thyroxine, and calcitonin.
- Parathyroid glands secrete parathyroid hormone.
- Adrenal cortex produces mineralocorticoids, glucocorticoids, and gonadocorticoids.
- Adrenal medulla secretes epinephrine and norepinephrine.
- Pancreas produces glucagon, insulin, somatostatin, and ghrelin.
- Thymus secretes thymosin.
- Testes secrete testosterone and ovaries produce estrogen and progesterone.
- Pineal gland secretes melatonin.

The goal of hormone regulation is to maintain homeostasis. Nervous system stimulation, endocrine control, and feedback systems regulate hormone secretion.

Many endocrine system disorders were discussed in the chapter. Common signs and symptoms include glucosuria, goiter, hirsutism, hypocalcemia, hypoglycemia, ketoacidosis, ketonuria, polydipsia, polyphagia, and polyuria. Common diagnostic procedures and laboratory tests include peripheral neuropathy screening, thyroid ultrasound and scan, radioactive iodine update scan, A_{1C} test, calcium blood test, hormone tests, blood glucose tests, and urine ketone and glucose tests. Besides medications, surgery is also used as a treatment for several endocrine disorders.

Endocrine system disorders discussed in this chapter include:

- Pituitary gland diseases: Acromegaly, gigantism, dwarfism, and diabetes insipidus
- Thyroid gland diseases: Hyperthyroidism and hypothyroidism
- Parathyroid gland diseases: Hyperparathyroidism and hypoparathyroidism
- Adrenal gland diseases: Addison's disease and Cushing disease
- Pancreatic diseases and disorders: Diabetes mellitus (type 1, type 2, and LADA), gestational diabetes, diabetic ketoacidosis, and hypoglycemia

Changes in hormone levels vary with age. Estrogen, testosterone, growth hormone, and melatonin decrease with age. Norepinephrine, epinephrine, parathyroid hormone, follicle-stimulating hormone, and luteinizing hormone may increase with age.

SCENARIO WRAP-UP

Cecilia enjoyed working with the endocrinology team and patients. She was able to observe the diabetic nurse educator work with a newly diagnosed patient. The amount of information that newly diagnosed diabetic patients need to learn to manage their disease is incredible. All of the information was not given to the patient during the first visit. The nurse educator explained that over the coming weeks, the patient would get the information. During the first visit, the patient needed to learn how to administer insulin, test blood glucose levels, and learn about hypoglycemia and hyperglycemia. These topics were most critical at this stage.

Later in the day, Cecilia observed the dietitian working with a patient with type 2 DM. The patient stated he enjoyed his beer, snack foods, and sweets and really did not want to give them up. Cecilia was impressed by how the dietitian worked with the patient, so that eventually, the patient was willing to cut back on some of his "not so healthy" habits. Cecilia's experiences reinforced her belief that she had made the right decision by volunteering to work with the endocrinology team.

8

Sensory System

LEARNING OBJECTIVES

1. List the major organs of the sensory system and identify the anatomic location of major sensory system organs.
2. Describe the normal function of the sensory system.
3. Explain common diagnostic procedures and treatments for sensory system disorders.
4. Describe common sensory system disorders, including common signs and symptoms, etiology, diagnostic procedures, and treatments.
5. Compare the structure and function of the sensory system across the life span.

OUTLINE

▷▷ OPENING SCENARIO

Tom Rozsadek, CMA (AAMA), has been working at Walden-Martin Family Medical (WMFM) Clinic for about 5 years. Over that time, he has worked with a variety of patients in the family care setting. Typically, they see several patients a week for eye or ear concerns. During the summer months, more patients come in for foreign bodies in the eyes due to yard work. During the fall and winter months, eye and ear infections are common.

    While assisting the WMFM Clinic providers, Tom has observed the providers perform eye and ear assessments. Eye and ear procedures interest Tom. Every week he does several ear irrigations and uses the otoscope to check if the earwax

(cerumen) is removed. For well-child exams, Tom assists the providers by performing audiometry and vision screening tests. He enjoys performing these screening tests.

YOU WILL LEARN

1. To describe the general and special senses.
2. To discuss the anatomy of the eye, along with the normal function and physiology of the eye.
3. To describe common diseases of the eye, including the etiology, signs and symptoms, diagnostic procedures, and treatments.
4. To discuss the anatomy of the ear, along with the normal function and physiology of the ear.

5. To describe common diseases of the ear, including the etiology, signs and symptoms, diagnostic procedures, and treatments.

6. Compare the structure and function of the sensory system across the life span.

INTRODUCTION

Patients with eye or ear concerns are typically seen in primary care and urgent care settings. Patients who need routine eye exams or have an eye disease are seen in *ophthalmology* (OF thahl mol uh jee). Two types of healthcare professionals that see patients in ophthalmology include:

- An *optometrist* (op TOM I trist): A licensed healthcare professional who practices optometry. An optometrist performs eye exams and vision tests, prescribes and dispenses corrective lenses (e.g., glasses and contact lenses), and diagnoses and treats certain eye disorders.
- An *ophthalmologist* (OF thahl mol uh jist): A medical doctor who diagnoses and treats all eye diseases and disorders, performs eye surgery, and can prescribe and dispense corrective lenses.

Patients with ear concerns are often referred to otolaryngology (OH toe lar ing GOL uh jee). *Otolaryngology* (also called *otorhinolaryngology* [oh toh rahy noh lar ing GOL uh jee]) is the branch of medicine that deals with diagnosis and treatment of diseases and disorders of the ear, nose, and throat. An otolaryngologist (OH toe lar ing GOL uh jist) can also be called *otorhinolaryngologist* (oh toh rahy noh lar ing GOL uh jist). An *otolaryngologist* is a specially trained physician who medically and surgically treats diseases of the ear, nose, and throat (ENT). *Audiology* (AW dee ol oh jee) is the study of hearing disorders and their treatment. An *audiologist* (AW dee ol oh jist) is a licensed healthcare specialist in this field.

Medical assistants can work in both ophthalmology and otolaryngology. Additional training and certifications may be required in ophthalmology.

INTRODUCTION TO GENERAL AND SPECIAL SENSES

There are two categories of senses in the body, general and special senses. *General senses* include touch, pressure, temperature, and pain. General senses have receptors scattered throughout the body. They gather information through all areas of the body.

The special senses have receptors that are concentrated in one area. *Special senses* include vision, hearing, equilibrium (balance), taste, and smell. Each of the special senses has a complex organ with receptors to gather stimuli and send the information to the brain for interpretation.

Senses allow us to experience our environment and then act on our perceptions. They also give the body information that can protect us from harm. The following section discusses smell and taste, and the remainder of the chapter covers the eyes, ears, and equilibrium.

Smell and Taste

The senses of taste and smell work together. Most tastes are linked with odors. The olfactory (ol FAK tuh ree) sense is the sense of smell. The receptors for smell are in the upper part of the nasal cavity. The sense of smell is very sensitive, but it can easily become fatigued. When you enter a room, you may smell a scent or an odor, but within a few minutes you may not notice it anymore. That is *sensory fatigue*.

The gustatory (GUHS tuh tawr ee) sense is the sense of taste. A newborn child has about 10,000 taste buds on the tongue, which decrease after age 50. There are five tastes: sweet, sour, bitter, salty, and savory (umami [oo MOM ee]). Eating something sweet at the end of a meal helps the brain form a memory of a meal.

Smell- and taste-related disorders include:

- *Hyposmia* (high POSE mee ah): Reduced ability to detect odors.
- *Anosmia* (ah NOSE mee ah): Complete inability to detect odor. Congenital anosmia means the person was born without a sense of smell.
- *Parosmia* (pahr OZE mee ah): A change in the normal perception of odors, such as a pleasant smell that now smells foul.
- *Phantosmia* (fan TOES mee ah): Sensation of an odor that is not there.
- *Phantom taste perception*: A lingering, often unpleasant taste in the mouth when there is nothing in the mouth.
- *Hypogeusia* (hie poe GYOO zee ah): A reduced ability to taste sweet, sour, bitter, salty, and savory.
- *Ageusia* (ah GYOO zee ah): A condition in which a person cannot detect any tastes, which is rare.
- *Dysgeusia* (dis GYOO zee ah): A condition in which a foul, salty, rancid, or metallic taste sensation persists in the mouth.

MEDICAL TERMINOLOGY	
audi/o, acous/o	hearing
laryng/o	throat
ocul/o, ophthalm/o	eye
opt/o, optic/o	vision
orbit/o	orbit
ot/o	ear
rhin/o	nose
-ar	pertaining to
-logy	study of

ANATOMY OF THE EYE

The eye is the organ of sight. The structures of the eye can be divided into the supporting structures and the eyeball. The eyeball can be further divided by the three layers and the inner part of the eye.

Supporting Structures

Each eyeball is located in an orbit, a bony eye socket in the skull. Fatty tissue in the orbit provides a cushion for the eyeball. Holes in the orbit create pathways for blood vessels, nerves, and muscles to reach the eyeball. The ophthalmic artery brings blood to the eye, and the superior and inferior ophthalmic vein carries blood away from the eye. Many cranial nerves, including the optic, trochlear, and the oculomotor nerves, are involved with vision

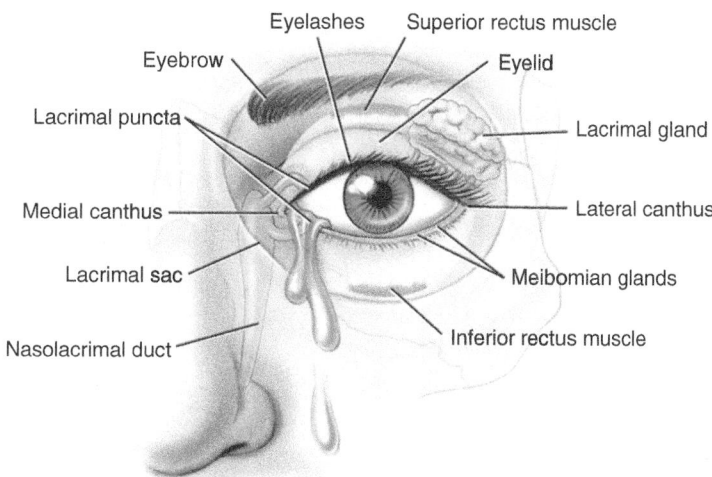

Fig. 8.1 Supporting Structures of the Eye. (From Shiland B: *Medical terminology & anatomy for ICD-10 coding*, ed 4, St. Louis, 2021, Elsevier.)

and eye movements. The extraocular muscles, such as the inferior and superior rectus muscles, control eye movements (Fig. 8.1).

The inner canthus (KAN thuhs), or *medial canthus*, is the corner of the eye near the nose. The outer canthus, or *lateral canthus*, is on the opposite side of the eye.

The eyelashes and eyebrow help prevent foreign debris (e.g., dust and dirt) from entering the eye. The eyelid covers the eye and protects it from foreign debris and from bright light.

The eyelid is lined with the *conjunctiva* (KON junk tie vah), a thin mucous membrane. The conjunctiva also spreads across the anterior surface of the eye. Two types of glands surround the eye, the meibomian glands and the lacrimal gland.

> **VOCABULARY**
> **canthus** The inner or outer corner of the eye where the upper and lower eyelids meet.
> **pupil** The opening in the center of the iris through which light enters the eye.
> **vascular** Having (blood) vessels that conduct or circulate liquids (blood).

Glands. The *meibomian* (my BOW mee an) *glands* are oil glands located along the edge of the eyelids, near the eyelashes. These glands secrete oil that helps keep tears from drying up too quickly. Dry eyes can occur if the oil production decreases.

The *lacrimal* (LAK ri mal) *gland*, also called the *tear gland*, is located within the orbit above the lateral end of the eye (see Fig. 8.1). The gland releases tears, which mix with the oil and mucus in the eye, forming a *tear film*. The tear film protects and lubricates the eye.

The tears drain into the *lacrimal puncta* (PUNGK tah), which are located on both the upper and lower eyelid. The lacrimal puncta drain into the *lacrimal sac*. The lacrimal sac drains inferiorly to the *nasolacrimal duct*, or tear duct, which carries the tears into the nasal cavity (see Fig. 8.1).

CRITICAL THINKING 8.1

When Tom was studying for the certification exam, he needed to know all of the supporting structures of the eye. Describe these supporting structures.

Eyeball

The eyeball is a spherical globe. The eyeball consists of three layers and the inner part.

Outer Layer. The outer layer is fibrous and protective. It is made up of the sclera and the cornea. The *sclera* (SKLAIR uh), also called the "white of the eye," covers almost the entire surface of the eyeball. The sclera is made up of dense collagen fibers. The visible part of the sclera is covered by the conjunctiva. The extraocular muscles attach to the sclera. These muscles pull on the sclera, enabling the eye to look in all directions.

The *cornea* (KOR nee uh) is the transparent circle over the front center of the eye. The cornea covers the iris and pupil (Fig. 8.2). (These structures will be discussed in the coming sections.) Light enters the cornea, and the cornea bends the rays, which helps with focusing.

Middle Layer. The middle layer is vascular. It is made up of the choroid (KOR oyd), iris, and ciliary (SILL ih air ee) body. The *choroid* makes up the majority of the middle layer. It contains many blood vessels, which provide oxygen and nutrients to the eye. *Melanin*, a dark pigment, is also contained in the choroid. By absorbing light, the melanin prevents light reflecting in the eye. This helps the eye to focus on the image.

The *iris* is the colored portion of the eye (see Fig. 8.2). The amount of pigment in the iris determines the person's eye color. The iris is composed of two types of muscles that regulate the size of the pupil. The papillary sphincter muscle constricts the pupil and is under the parasympathetic nervous system control. The papillary dilator muscle, under sympathetic nervous system control, dilates or opens the pupil.

The anterior portion of the choroid meets the *ciliary body*, a ring of tissue that encircles the lens. The ciliary body is an extension of the iris. The ciliary body contains smooth muscle fibers, called *ciliary muscles*. The ciliary muscles control the shape of the lens, which is flexible. The changing of the shape of the lens allows the light to be focused on the retina. This process is called *accommodation*.

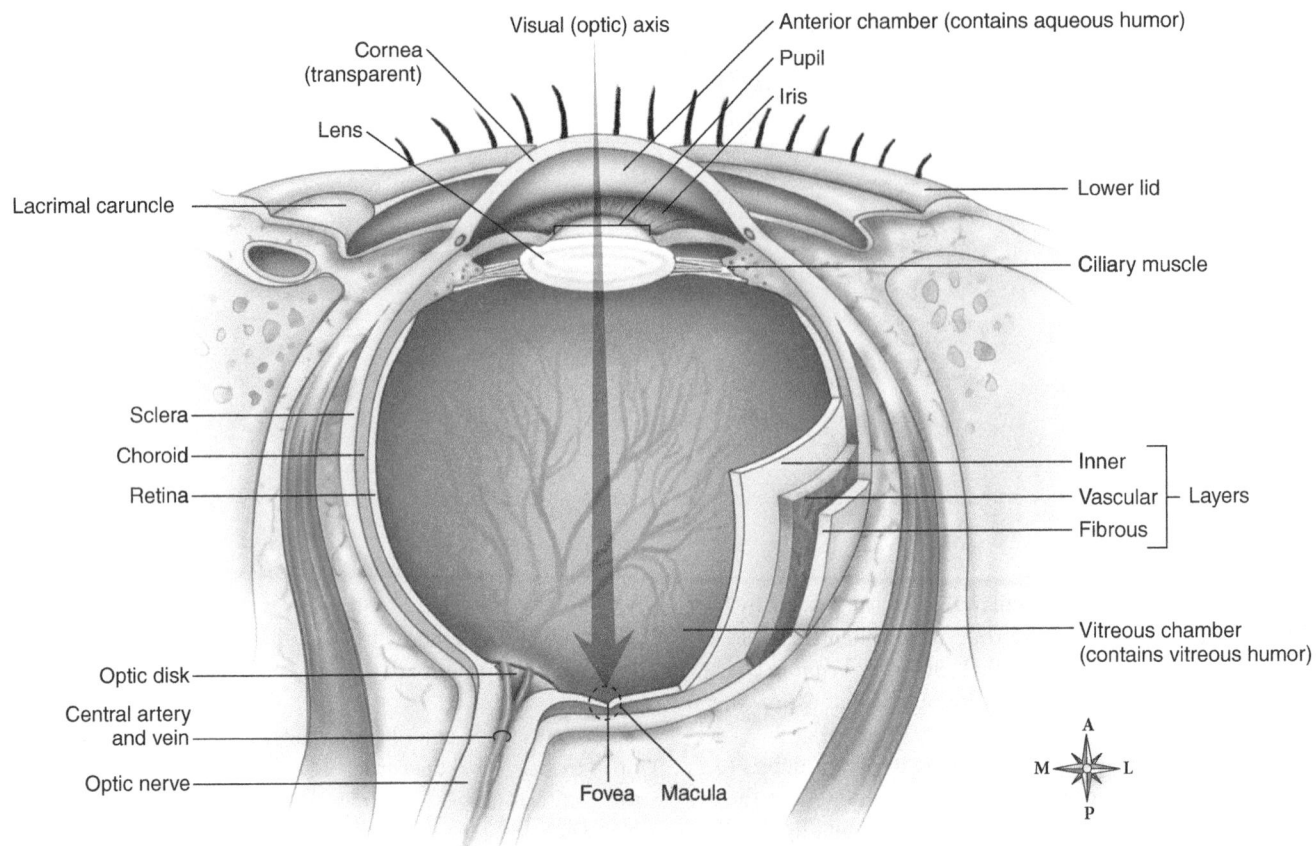

Fig. 8.2 Eye. This transverse (horizontal) section through the left eyeball is shown as if viewed from above. (From Patton KT, Thibodeau GA: *The human body in health and disease*, ed 7, St. Louis, 2018, Elsevier.)

CRITICAL THINKING 8.2

List the structures found in the outer and middle layers of the eyeball. Describe the function of each structure.

Inner Layer. The innermost layer is the nervous or sensory layer. This layer contains the *retina* (RET in uh), which is responsible for vision. The retina is a light-sensitive layer of tissue at the back of the eye. Special cells (photoreceptors) in the retina include:

- *Rods*: Provide the perception of black and white vision. They are very sensitive to low light levels. Vitamin A is an essential component of *rhodopsin* (row DOP sin), a protein found in the rods. A lack of vitamin A can lead to *night blindness.*
- *Cones*: Help to see colors in bright light. Three types of cones see red, blue, and green colors. Using the input from these cones, the brain interprets the color.

The *optical disc* is the point where the optic nerve leaves the eyeball. This area does not contain any photoreceptors and thus is called the "blind spot." The *macula lutea* (MAK u lah LOO tee uh) is a small yellow depression on the retina that is directly opposite the lens (see Fig. 8.2). This area receives and analyzes light only from the center of the visual field. Within the macula lutea is a small area called the *fovea* (FOH vee uh) *centralis*, which contains tightly packed cone cells. This is the place where the vision is the most accurate and detailed.

Inner Part of the Eye. The inner part of the eye consists of the anterior and posterior chambers, the lens, and the vitreous chamber. The *anterior chamber* is located between the iris and the cornea. The *posterior chamber* is between the iris and the lens. Capillaries of the ciliary body produce a clear fluid called *aqueous* (AY kwee us) *humor*. The aqueous humor fills both the anterior and posterior chambers. It provides nutrients to the cornea and gives shape to the anterior eye. Aqueous humor is continually being produced, circulated, and drained from the eye. Aqueous humor drains from the anterior chamber into the canals of Schlemm (shlem) and then into the anterior ciliary veins. If a blockage occurs or the drainage out of the eye slows, the intraocular (in trah AHK yoo lur) pressure (IOP) increases.

The *lens* is a transparent, biconvex structure found between the posterior chamber and the vitreous chamber. When the shape and size of the lens are adjusted, the focus can change. The lens refracts (bends) the light rays, so they focus on the retina.

The *vitreous chamber* is located at the back of the eyeball and is the largest chamber. It is filled with *vitreous* (VIT ree us) *humor* or vitreous, a clear jellylike substance. The vitreous humor fills the space between the lens and the retina. This substance is made up of mostly water. About 1% of it is a mixture of salts, sugars, proteins, and collagen. The vitreous humor helps the eye to maintain its spherical shape. The pressure of the vitreous humor helps to keep the retina in place.

VOCABULARY

biconvex Having two outward-curving surfaces on a lens.
intraocular pressure Pressure exerted against the outer layers by the content (e.g., humors) of the eyeball.

MEDICAL TERMINOLOGY

aque/o	water
blephar/o, palpebr/o	eyelid
choroid/o	choroid
conjunctiv/o	conjunctiva
corne/o, kerat/o	cornea
cycl/o	ciliary body
dacryoaden/o	lacrimal gland
ir/o, irid/o	iris
lacrim/o, dacry/o	tears
macul/o	macula lutea
nas/o	nose
ocul/o	eye
papill/o	optic disk
phak/o, phac/o	lens
pupill/o, core/o, cor/o	pupil
retin/o	retina
scler/o	sclera
vascul/o	blood vessel
vitre/o	vitreous humor
extra-	outside
-al	pertaining to
conjunctiva (singular)	conjunctivae (plural)
iris (singular)	irises, irides (plural)
lens (singular)	lenses (plural)

CRITICAL THINKING 8.3

There are two types of photoreceptors on the retina. Describe each type of receptor and indicate which detects color and which receptor functions in dim light.

PHYSIOLOGY OF THE EYE

As light passes through the dome-shaped cornea, it bends the light. Some of this light passes through the pupil. The iris controls how much light the pupil lets into the eye. After the pupil, the light passes the lens. The lens refracts (bends) the light rays, so they focus on the retina. When you view closer objects, the light rays from the objects must be bent more sharply to bring them to focus on the retina. When you view distant objects, the light rays do not require as much refraction.

The light and color impulses received by the rods and cones are transmitted to nerve cells in the retina. From there the optic nerve picks up the signals and brings them to the visual cortex in the brain. The brain uses the electrical signals to create the images seen.

CRITICAL THINKING 8.4

In your own words describe how a person sees. Start with light entering the cornea.

DISEASES AND DISORDERS OF THE EYE

Many diseases affect the eyes. Common signs and symptoms of eye disorders include:

- Crusting, redness, irritation, and itching
- Burning sensation and dry eyes
- Blurred vision, sensitivity to light, and difficulty seeing at night

Common diagnostic procedures are listed in Table 8.1. Common treatments are listed in Table 8.2.

Age-Related Macular Degeneration

Macular degeneration is an eye disorder that slowly causes difficulty seeing fine details, such as when reading. The disease destroys sharp, central vision (Fig. 8.4A, B). When macular degeneration occurs in people over age 60, it is called *age-related macular degeneration* (ARMD or AMD). Two types of AMD include:

- Dry AMD: The blood vessels under the macula become thin and brittle. *Drusen*, small yellow deposits, form.
- Wet AMD: New abnormally formed blood vessels form under the macula. These vessels leak blood and fluid, causing vision loss.

Almost all people with macular degeneration first have dry AMD.

Etiology. AMD is caused by damage to the blood vessels that supply the macula. The cause of the blood vessel damage is unknown. Females, Caucasians, and a family history of AMD are risk factors. Additional risk factors include a high-fat diet and cigarette smoking.

Signs and Symptoms. People with dry AMD usually have blurred center vision. The objects look distorted and dim, and the colors look faded. As the condition progresses, the blurred spot in the center part of the vision increases in size. Wet AMD causes straight lines to look wavy and distorted. A small dark spot in the center of the vision gets larger as the condition progresses.

Diagnostic Procedures. During the dilated eye exam, the retina, blood vessels, and optic nerve are examined. The Amsler grid can be used; if the lines are wavy, it may be a sign of AMD (Fig. 8.5). Additional tests include fluorescein angiography, fungus photography, and optical coherence tomography. The pigment in the macula can also be measured.

TABLE 8.1   Common Diagnostic Procedures Used for Eye Disorders

Procedure	Description

Standard ophthalmic exam	A general eye exam that may include:
	• *Visual acuity test:* Determines sharpness of vision. The patient identifies objects or letters from standardized eye charts. The *Snellen chart* is used to check distance vision acuity. The *Jaeger eye chart* is used to check near vision acuity.
	• *Visual field test:* Manual or automated test used to check the peripheral vision. The *visual field* refers to the total area in which objects can be seen in the peripheral (side) vision as the eyes are focused on a central point.
	• *Slit lamp exam:* Uses a slit lamp, an instrument with a microscope and a light source, to examine the structures at the front of the eye, such lens, sclera, and retina (Fig. 8.3).
	• *Tonometry:* Used to measure eye pressure. Anesthetic drops may be given prior to the test.
	   • *Goldmann applanation tonometry test:* Most common type of tonometry test. The tonometer is attached to the slit lamp. A small probe is pressed into the eye, and the pressure of the cornea pushing back on the probe is measured (see Fig. 8.3)
	   • *Pneumotonometry* (noo moe toe MON eh tree): The instrument blows a puff of air at the cornea, and the eye pressure is measured.
	   • *Tono-Pen:* A handheld instrument used to measure the eye pressure. The tip is placed on the cornea.
	• *Fundus examination:* Uses an ophthalmoscope to examine the inner structures of the eye, such as the optic nerve and macula.
	• *Refraction test:* Used to determine the correct prescription for glasses or contact lenses.
	• Retinal examination.
	• Tests to check the muscles that move the eyes.

Ishihara test	Used to check for color vision deficiency.
Amsler grid	Used to test the central vision. Can help with the diagnosis of age-related macular degeneration. The patient needs to cover one eye and focus on the dot. An abnormality occurs when the patient sees wavy lines.
Electroretinography (ee LEK trow RET i NOG rah fee)	A test to measure the electrical response to the rods and cones.
Fluorescein angiography (FA) (FLOO reh seen an jee AH gruh fee)	The pupils are dilated, and fluorescein (an orange-red dye) is injected into a vein. Within 10–15 minutes the dye travels to the blood vessels in the eye, causing them to be seen easily. As the dye passes through the retina, pictures are taken by a special camera.
Fluorescein staining	A piece of blotting paper containing the orangish dye is touched to the surface of the eye. The dye coats the surface of the cornea. A blue light is used to detect foreign bodies in the eye and damage to the cornea.
Fundus photography	A photograph is taken of the inner lining of the eye.
Gonioscopy (GOE nee OS kah pee)	After numbing the eye, the provider uses a gonioscope or a slit lamp and a contact prism lens to examine the angle of the anterior chamber of the eye.
Optical coherence tomography	Light waves are used to view the retina.
Retinoscopy (RET n OS kah pee)	A test to measure the refraction using reflected light.
Wood lamp examination	An ultraviolet (UV) light is shown onto the eye. It is used to detect corneal abrasions or scratches. More common in ambulatory care, where slit lamps are not always available.

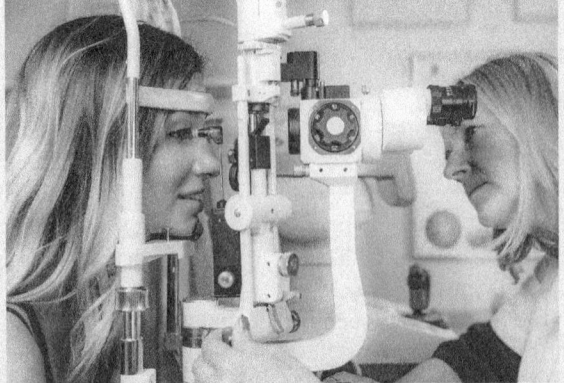

Fig. 8.3 Slit Lamp with an Applanation Tonometer Attached. (Courtesy microjen/iStock.com.)

TABLE 8.2   Common Treatments Used for Eye Disorders

Procedures	Description
Blepharoplasty (BLEFF or uh plas tee)	Surgical repair of the eyelid.
Cataract extraction	Surgical removal of the lens. Used to treat cataracts.
Keratoplasty (KAIR uh toh plas tee).	Surgical transplantation of corneal tissue from a donor or from the patient. Also called corneal transplant.
Intraocular lenses (IOLs) (in truh OK yuh ler)	Surgical implantation of an artificial lens behind the iris.
Laser in-situ keratomileusis (LASIK)	Laser surgery done to correct myopia, hyperopia, and astigmatism.
Photocoagulation (FOE toe koe AG you LAY shun)	Also known as focal laser treatment. A laser is used to stop or slow the leakage of fluid and blood in the eye.
Panretinal photocoagulation (PRP)	Also known as scatter laser treatment. A laser is used to shrink abnormal blood vessels.
Photodynamic therapy	A medication is injected into the body. Light activates the drug, which destroys leaking blood vessels.
Vitrectomy (vi TREK tah mee)	A tiny surgical incision is made in the eye, and blood and scar tissue are removed.
Iridotomy (IR I DOT ah mee)	A laser is used to open a new channel in the iris, which helps reduce the intraocular pressure.

Treatments. With advanced dry AMD, no treatments are available to restore the vision. With early AMD, vitamins, antioxidants, and zinc may help to prevent vision loss. Smoking is not recommended. With wet AMD, laser photocoagulation and photodynamic therapy can be used. Patients are encouraged to use low-vision aids, such as strong magnifying reading glasses and magnifiers.

CRITICAL THINKING 8.5

There are many types of adaptive tools available for people with age-related macular degeneration (AMD). Based on what you know about this disease, describe how wearable, handheld, and desktop video magnifiers are helpful with AMD.

Amblyopia

Amblyopia (am blee OH pee ah), also known as "lazy eye," is blurry vision in one eye due to disuse. This is the most common cause of vision problems in children.

Etiology. Amblyopia is caused when the nerve pathway from one eye to the brain does not correctly develop. When the vision is blurry, the brain may learn to ignore the image from the weaker eye. Causes of amblyopia include:

- *Strabismus* (strah BISS mus): Lack of coordination between the eyes. The most common cause of amblyopia
- Childhood cataracts
- *Hyperopia* (hye pur OH pee ah): Farsightedness

- *Myopia* (mye OH pee ah): Nearsightedness
- *Astigmatism* (ah STIG mah tiz um): Inability of the cornea to focus, causing blurred vision

Signs and Symptoms. Amblyopia can cause the eyes to turn in or out. The eyes may appear not to work together. The person may have difficulty judging depth correctly. One eye may see poorly.

Diagnostic Procedures. Amblyopia is typically diagnosed during a complete eye exam.

Treatments. Treatment is aimed at correcting the condition causing amblyopia. Surgery is required to remove cataracts. Corrective lenses are used with refractive errors (e.g., myopia and hyperopia). A patch is placed over the strong eye so to force the brain to recognize images from the poor eye.

Blepharitis

Blepharitis is irritated, inflamed, itchy, and reddened eyelids (Fig. 8.6). It most often occurs where the eyelashes grow. Blepharitis is more likely to occur with seborrheic dermatitis and rosacea.

Etiology. The exact cause of blepharitis is unknown. It may be related to an overgrowth of bacteria or a decrease in the normal oils produced by the eyelid.

Signs and Symptoms. A person may experience red, irritated eyelids and a burning sensation. Crusting, swelling, and itching of the eyelids can occur. It may feel like sand is in the eye when blinking.

Diagnostic Procedures. The provider can diagnose the condition by examining the eyelids during an eye exam.

Treatments. The patient is encouraged to clean the eyelid edges daily to remove bacteria and oil. An oral antibiotic or a topical antibiotic ointment may be ordered. Home care can include applying warm compresses to the eyes for 5 minutes at least twice daily.

Cataract

A *cataract* (KAT ur ackt) is an opacity or a clouding of the lens of the eye, resulting in light scattering (Fig. 8.7). Two types of cataracts include:

- *Adult cataract*: Develops slowly and painlessly with age. Mild clouding often occurs after age 60, and by age 75 it affects the vision.
- *Congenital cataract*: Clouding of the lens of the eye that is present at birth. Congenital cataracts are a common abnormality that causes blindness in infants.

Table 8.3 describes both types of cataracts.

Color Blindness

People with color blindness see colors differently than most people. This condition may be present at birth or can develop later in life due to a more serious condition. Three types of color blindness include:

- *Red-green color vision defects*: Most common and occur more in men. Depending on the type, red and green may look like the other or they both may look the same.

- *Blue-yellow color vision defect*: Less common type. Causes a problem telling the difference between blue and green and yellow and red.

- *Achromatopsia* (ah kroh mah TOP see ah): An inherited visual disorder caused by a partial or a complete lack of

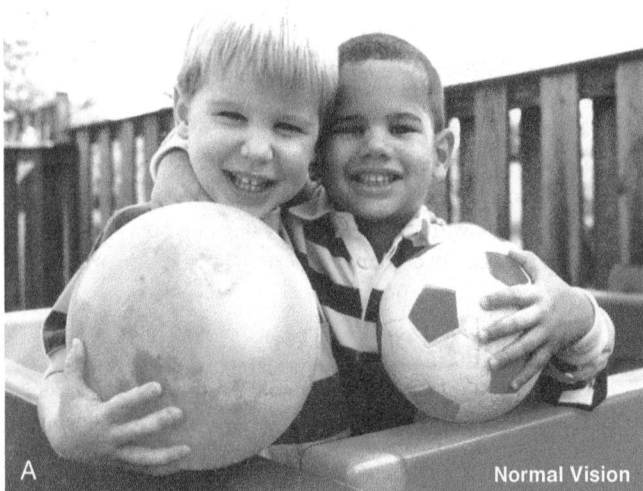
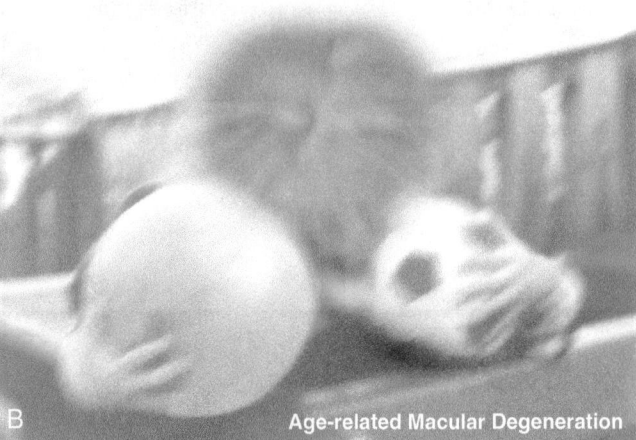
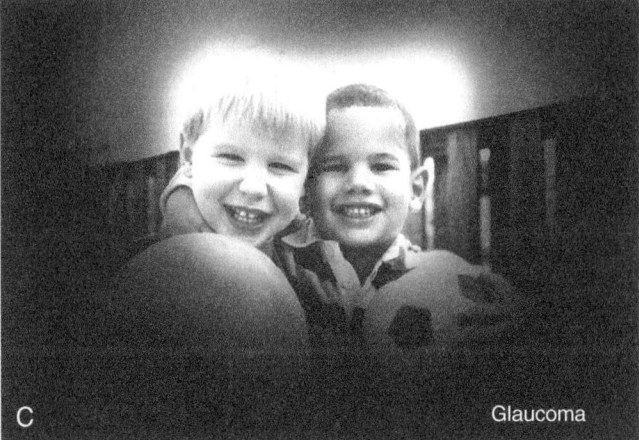

Fig. 8.4 A, Normal vision. B, Macular degeneration. C, Glaucoma. (From the National Eye Institute: *Age-related macular degeneration: what you should know,* Bethesda, MD, National Institutes of Health.)

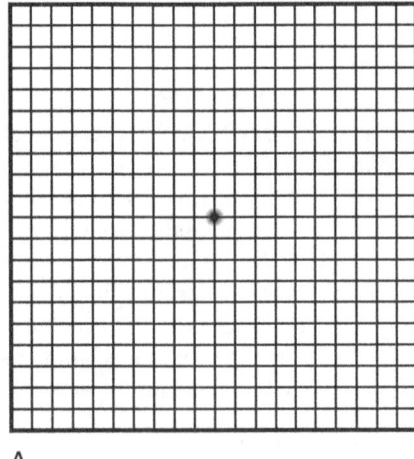
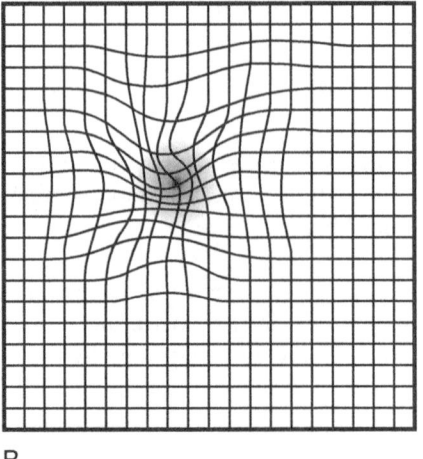

A   B

Fig. 8.5 Amsler Grid. (From Miller RG, Ashar B, Sisson SD: *The Johns Hopkins Internal Medicine Board Review* 2010-2011, ed 3, Philadelphia, 2010, Mosby.)

functioning cones in the retina. The person experiences a complete absence of color vision, decreased vision, and nystagmus.

Etiology. In many cases, color blindness is genetic. It can also occur later in life due damage to the eyes or brain from diseases such as AMD, diabetes, and multiple sclerosis. Color blindness occurs when one or more of the color cones cells are absent, nonfunctional, or detect a different color than normal. The severity of color blindness depends on the number of color cone cells present and working correctly.

Signs and Symptoms. A person with color blindness may have difficulty distinguishing between colors, how bright colors are, and

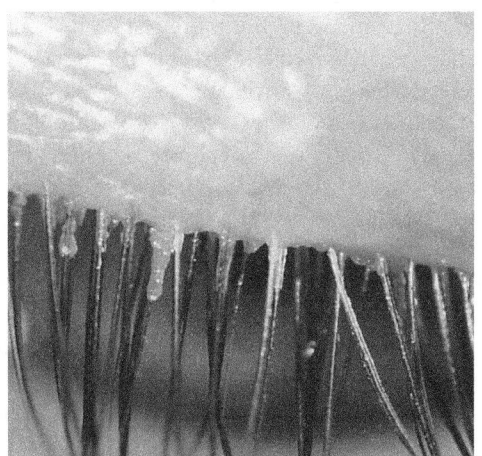

Fig. 8.6 Blepharitis. (From Zitelli BJ, Davis HW: *Atlas of pediatric physical diagnosis*, ed 6, Philadelphia, 2012, Mosby.)

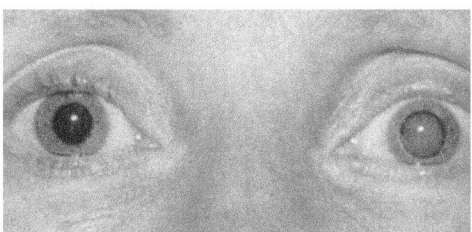

Fig. 8.7 Cataract. Notice the cloudiness of the left eye characteristic of advanced cataracts. The normal right eye is not cloudy. (From Swartz MH: *Textbook of physical diagnosis*, ed 6, Philadelphia, 2010, Saunders.)

different shades of color. Severe causes of color blindness can cause nystagmus or sensitivity to light.

Diagnostic Procedures. The Ishihara test, a color plate test, is used to diagnose color blindness.

Treatments. There is no cure for color blindness. A person usually tries to adapt to it. Special contact lenses and glasses can be used to tell the difference between colors. Visual aids, apps, and other technology can be used to help a person live with color blindness.

CRITICAL THINKING 8.6

Based on what you learned about color blindness, what objects in your everyday environment would pose a problem for someone with color blindness?

Conjunctivitis

Conjunctivitis is also known as pink eye. It causes the conjunctiva to be swollen and inflamed (Fig. 8.8). Conjunctivitis usually does not affect the vision.

Etiology. Conjunctivitis can be caused by bacterial or viral infections, allergies, an irritant (e.g., smoke, dust, and contact lenses), and dry eyes.

Signs and Symptoms. A person with conjunctivitis may experience:
- Blurred vision and sensitivity to light
- Eye pain, itching, and a gritty feeling in the eye
- Redness in the eye and increased tearing

Diagnostic Procedures. The provider will examine the eyes and may take a swab of any secretion for analysis.

Treatments. Treatment depends on the cause. Cool compresses and antihistamine eyedrops may be used for conjunctivitis related to allergies (also called *allergic conjunctivitis*). Antibiotics are used for conjunctivitis caused by bacteria. Viral conjunctivitis will go away on its own.

VOCABULARY
nystagmus Unusual involuntary rapid eye movements.

TABLE 8.3	**Types of Cataracts**	
	Adult Cataract	**Congenital Cataract**
Etiology	With age, the proteins in the lens begin to break down, causing cloudiness. A cataract can form sooner due to diabetes, eye injury, family history of cataract, long-term use of corticosteroids, and smoking.	Seen with certain birth defects, including Down syndrome and trisomy 13. Can also be inherited.
Signs and Symptoms	Sensitivity to glare, foggy vision, difficulty seeing at night, double vision, loss of color intensity, and seeing halos around lights.	Infants may not seem to be visually aware of their environment. The pupil may look gray or whitish. May have nystagmus (nye STAG mus).
Diagnostic Procedures	Standard eye exam and slit lamp examination.	Standard eye exam.
Treatments	For mild cataract: Change in eyeglass prescription, increased lighting, magnifying lenses, and sunglasses. Surgery is the only treatment for a cataract.	For mild cataract: No treatment is done. Moderate to severe cataracts are surgically removed. The infant may need to wear a contact lens after surgery.

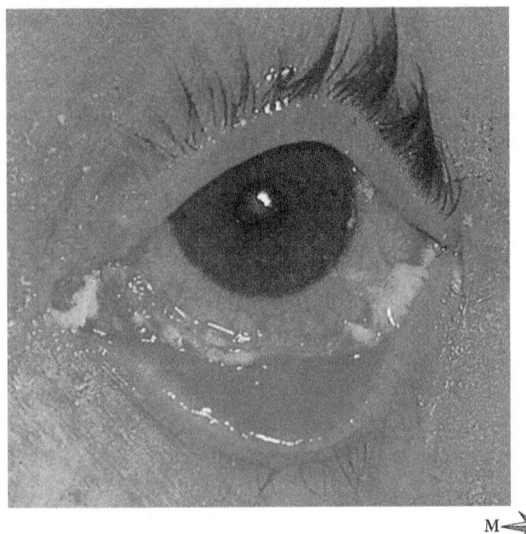

S
M —✦— L
I

Fig. 8.8 Conjunctivitis. In this case of acute bacterial infection, notice the discharge of mucous pus characteristic of this highly contagious infection of the conjunctiva. (From Newell FW: *Ophthalmology: principles and concepts*, ed 8, St Louis, 1996, Mosby.)

Diabetic Retinopathy

Diabetic retinopathy (ret ih NOP uh thee) occurs when the small blood vessels in the retina are damaged by diabetes. It is the main cause of decreased vision or blindness in American adults ages 20 to 74.

Etiology. Over time, *hyperglycemia* (too much glucose/sugar in the blood) can cause blockages in the small blood vessels in the retina. This decreases the blood flow to the retina. New blood vessels develop but are abnormal and leak easily. Risk factors for diabetic retinopathy include poor blood glucose control, type 1 or 2 diabetes mellitus, high blood pressure, high cholesterol, and tobacco use.

Signs and Symptoms. There are no symptoms initially, but the condition progresses to mild vision problems. Eventually it can cause blindness.

Diagnostic Procedures. A comprehensive dilated eye exam is used to diagnose diabetic retinopathy. A fluorescein angiography and optical coherence tomography can also be used.

Treatments. Treatment depends on the type and severity of the diabetic retinopathy. The goal is to slow or stop the progression of the disease. Photocoagulation, panretinal photocoagulation, and vitrectomy are used to control or remove the blood in the eye. Vascular endothelial growth factor inhibitor can be injected into the vitreous to help stop the growth of new blood vessels.

Glaucoma

Glaucoma (glah KOH mah) is a group of eye conditions that can damage the optic nerve by increased intraocular pressure. Glaucoma is the second most common cause of blindness in the US. The four major types of glaucoma include:

- *Open-angle glaucoma*: The most common type of glaucoma. A slow increase in intraocular pressure occurs, which damages the optic nerve.
- *Angle-closure* or *closed-angle glaucoma*: Fluid in the eye is suddenly blocked and cannot flow out of the eye. The increase in fluid causes a quick, severe rise in intraocular pressure, which is an emergency.
- *Congenital glaucoma*: Occurs in babies and is present at birth.
- *Secondary glaucoma*: Occurs due to a known cause. If the cause of open- or closed-angle glaucoma is known, the condition is considered secondary glaucoma.

Table 8.4 describes the four major types of glaucoma.

Refractive Errors

Refractive errors occur when the shape of the eye keeps the person from focusing well. The cause can be the length of the eyeball, changes in the cornea's shape, or aging of the lens. Common refractive errors include:

- *Myopia*: Also called *nearsightedness*. The light rays are focused in front of the retina instead of directly on it. The person can see clearly close up, but distant objects are blurry (Fig. 8.9A).
- *Hyperopia*: Also called *farsightedness*. The cornea does not refract light properly. The light rays are focused behind the retina instead of directly on it as with normal vision. The person can see objects in the distance clearly, but close-up objects appear blurry (see Fig. 8.9B).
- *Astigmatism*: The cornea is abnormally curved and causes the vision to be out of focus and blurred (see Fig. 8.9C).
- *Presbyopia* (prez bee OH pee uh): A natural condition of aging in which the lens of the eye loses its ability to focus and the person has a hard time seeing objects up close.

Table 8.5 describes these four common refractive errors.

Retinal Detachment

Retinal detachment occurs when the retina separates from the supporting structures (Fig. 8.10). When the retina separates, the cells no longer receive oxygen and nutrients from the blood vessels. This condition is a medical emergency. The longer it goes untreated, the greater the risk of permanent visual loss.

Etiology. The most common causes of retinal detachment include:

- *Rhegmatogenous* (reg mah TODGE uh nus) *detachment*: A tear or hole occurs in the retina, which allows eye fluid to leak out, causing the retina to pull away from the underlying tissues. This can occur with posterior vitreous detachment, trauma, or very bad nearsightedness.
- *Tractional detachment*: Scar tissue grows on the retinal surface, causing the detachment. This can occur with uncontrolled diabetes, retinal surgery, or chronic inflammation.
- *Exudative detachment*: Fluid accumulates beneath the retina, causing the detachment. Can be seen with age-related macular degeneration, injury, tumors, or inflammatory diseases.

Signs and Symptoms. When the retina becomes detached, bleeding can cloud the inside of the eye. This can cause blurred vision or

TABLE 8.4   Types of Glaucoma

	Open-Angle Glaucoma	Angle-Closure or Closed-Angle Glaucoma	Congenital Glaucoma	Secondary Glaucoma
Etiology	Can be genetic.	Can be caused by dilating eyedrops and certain medications.	Genetic; also caused when the eye does not develop normally.	Caused by corticosteroids, eye diseases, diabetes, and eye injury.
Signs and Symptoms	No symptoms until damage is severe. Loss of peripheral vision and blind spots in the vision (see Fig. 8.4C). Can lead to blindness.	May come and go or become worse. Include severe eye pain, cloudy vision, nausea, vomiting, rainbowlike halos around lights, swollen eye, and red eye.	Cloudiness in the front of the eye, enlarged eye, red eye, tearing, and sensitivity to light.	Depends on the underlying cause.
Diagnostic Procedures	Complete dilated eye exam and tonometry; additional tests include optic nerve imaging, slit lamp examination, visual acuity, and visual field measurement.			
Treatments	Eyedrops and oral medications to lower pressure; surgery.	Eyedrops and oral medications; iridotomy.	Surgery	Treat the cause of the glaucoma.

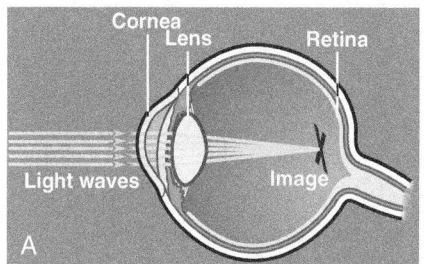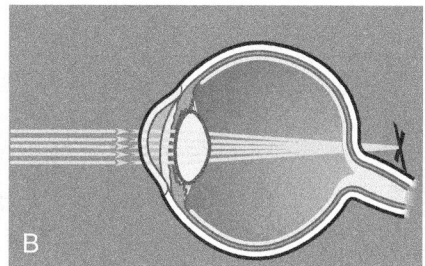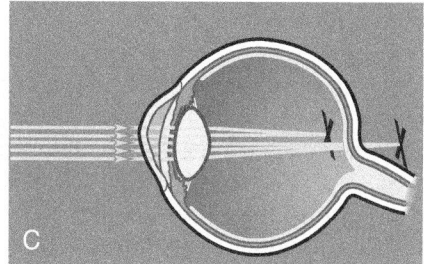

Fig. 8.9 **Refraction Errors.** A, Myopia. B, Hyperopia. C, Astigmatism. (From Herlihy B, Maebius NK: *The human body in health and illness*, ed 4, Philadelphia, 2011, Saunders.)

TABLE 8.5   Refractive Errors

	Astigmatism	Hyperopia	Myopia	Presbyopia
Etiology	Unknown; can occur after eye surgeries, such as cataract surgery.	May be caused by the eyeball being too small or the focusing power being too weak.	Caused due to a mismatch between the focusing power of the eye and the length of the eye.	The elasticity of the lens decreases with age. Condition is noticeable around age 45.
Signs and Symptoms	Difficulty seeing fine details, either close up or from a distance.	Aching eyes, blurred near vision, eye strain, and headache while reading.	Blurred distant vision; squinting, eye strain, and headache.	Decreased focusing ability for near objects, eyestrain, and headaches.
Diagnostic Procedures	Standard ophthalmic exam			
Treatments	Mild cases may not need correction. Corrective lenses will correct astigmatism. Laser surgery will eliminate it.	Corrective lenses help to shift the focus of the light image directly on the retina. Surgery is available for correcting the condition in adults.		Corrective lenses including bifocals and reading glasses; eyedrops.

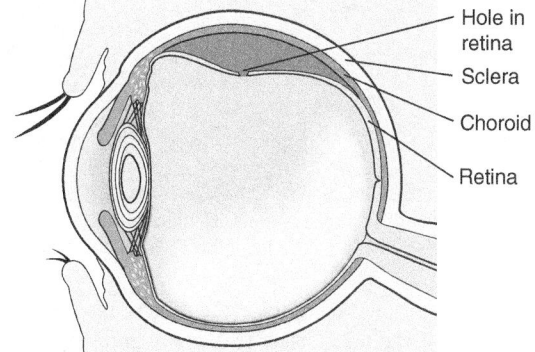

Fig. 8.10 **Retinal Detachment.** (From Frazier MS, Fuqua T: *Essentials of human disease and conditions*, ed 7, St. Louis, 2021, Elsevier.)

complete loss of vision. If the macula detaches, it affects the sharp, detailed vision. Additional symptoms include:
- Bright flashes of light *(photopsia)*, especially in the peripheral vision in one or both eyes
- Blurred vision and a gradually reduced peripheral vision
- New floaters in the eye
- A shadow or curtain seems to come over the visual field

Diagnostic Procedures. Retinal detachment is diagnosed with a retinal examination and ultrasound imaging.

Treatments. Surgery is required to repair the retinal detachment. Several techniques can be used to help secure the detached retina.

Laser surgery *(photocoagulation)* and freezing *(cryopexy)* can done. Both procedures produce a scar, which helps to secure the retina to the underlying tissues.

Additional Eye Disorders

There are many eye disorders. The following provides a brief description of some of them:

- *Blepharoptosis* (bleff ah rop TOH sis): Also called *ptosis*; drooping of an upper eyelid. Caused by normal aging, damage to the third cranial nerve, muscular weakness, and also diseases such as a stroke.
- *Blepharospasm* (BLEF ah roe spazm): Abnormal, involuntary blinking or eyelid spasm. Treated with Botox injections, surgery, and relaxation techniques.
- *Chalazion* (kuh LAY zee on): Also called *meibomian cyst*; a small bump in the eyelid caused by the blockage of one of the meibomian glands. Usually resolves within several weeks without treatment (Fig. 8.11A)
- *Corneal abrasion:* A scratch on the top layer of the eye. The cornea can be scratched from contact with other substances, such as dirt, wood or metal particles, and contact lenses.
- *Corneal ulcer:* An opened sore on the cornea often caused by a bacterial, viral, fungal, or parasitic infection. The ulcer can also be caused from a foreign body in the eye.
- *Dacryoadenitis* (dack ree oh add eh NYE tis): Inflammation of a lacrimal gland.
- *Dacryocystitis* (dack ree oh sis TYE tis): Inflammation of a lacrimal sac (Fig. 8.12).
- *Dry eyes:* The eyes do not produce enough oil and tears to stay wet. Causes burning, dry or scratch feeling, blurry vision, and red eyes. Treated with eyedrops and dietary changes (increase of vitamin A and omega-3 fatty acids). Also called *xerophthalmia* (zeer off THAL mee ah).
- *Ectropion* (ek TROW pee on): The eyelid turns outward and the inner, moist conjunctival surface is visible (Fig. 8.13A)
- *Entropion* (en TROW pee on): The margin of the eyelid curls inward and the lashes tend to rub on the eye, causing irritation and ulcerations of the cornea (see Fig. 8.13B)
- *Floaters:* Small, dark spots or threadlike strands that move around the vision in one eye. No treatment for mild cases; surgery can be done for severe cases.
- *Hordeolum* (hor DEE uh lum): Also called a *stye*; a small red, painful lump that grows on the eyelash or under the eyelid (see Fig. 8.11B). Usually caused by a bacterial infection.
- *Intraocular melanoma* (mell uh NOH mah): A disease in which malignant (cancer) cells form in the middle layer of the eye (Fig. 8.14).
- *Keratitis* (KER ah tie tis): Inflammation of the cornea, most commonly caused by contact lenses.
- *Neonatal conjunctivitis:* Also called *ophthalmia neonatorum* (off THAL mee uh nee oh nay TORE um); conjunctivitis in a newborn caused by a blocked tear duct or a bacterial or viral infection. More serious eye damage can be caused by gonorrhea, chlamydia, and genital and oral herpes.
- *Optic neuritis* (nyo RYE tis): Inflammation of the optic nerve; causes blindness.
- *Retinoblastoma* (RET noe blah STOW mah): A type of cancer that forms in the retina. Causes eye swelling or redness.

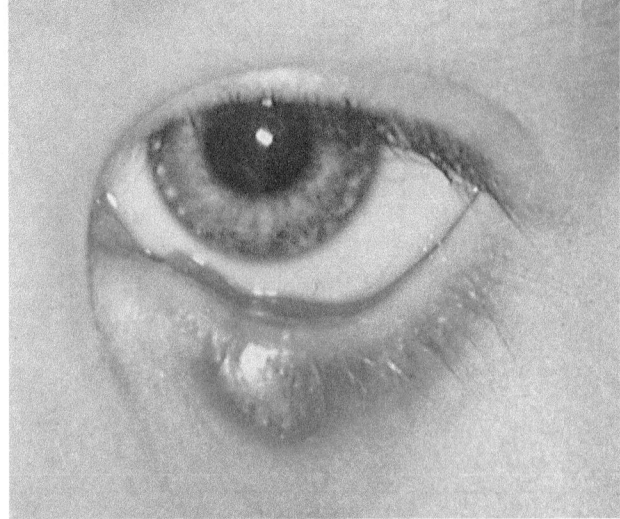

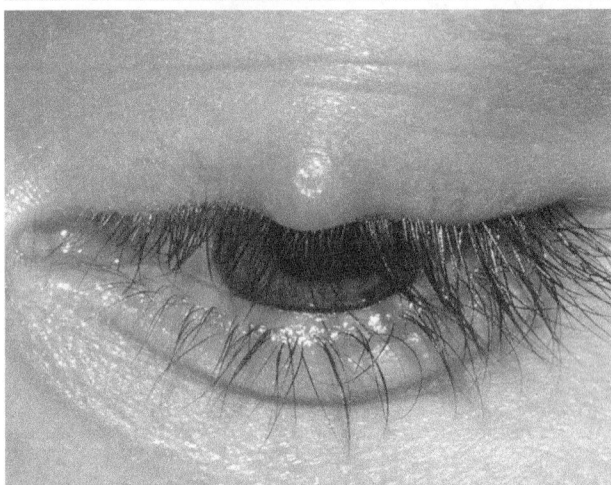

Fig. 8.11 A, Chalazion. B, Hordeolum. (**A** from Zitelli BJ, Davis HW: *Atlas of pediatric physical diagnosis,* ed 5, St. Louis, 2007, Mosby; **B** from Seidel HM, Ball JW, Dains JE, et al: *Mosby's guide to physical examination,* ed 7, St. Louis, 2011, Mosby.)

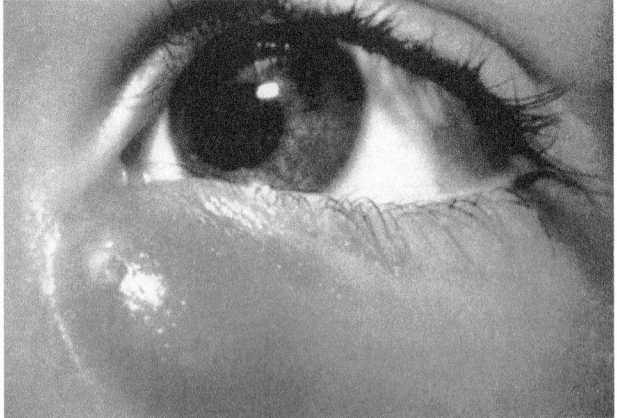

Fig. 8.12 **Dacryocystitis.** (From Marx J, Hockberger R, Walls R: *Rosen's emergency medicine,* ed 7, Philadelphia, 2010, Saunders.)

The eyes may not line up in the same directions. Treated with chemotherapy, radiation, laser treatment, and surgery.

- *Strabismus* (struh BIZ muh s): Both eyes do not line up in the same direction, thus they do not look at the same object at the same time. The lack of coordination is usually due to

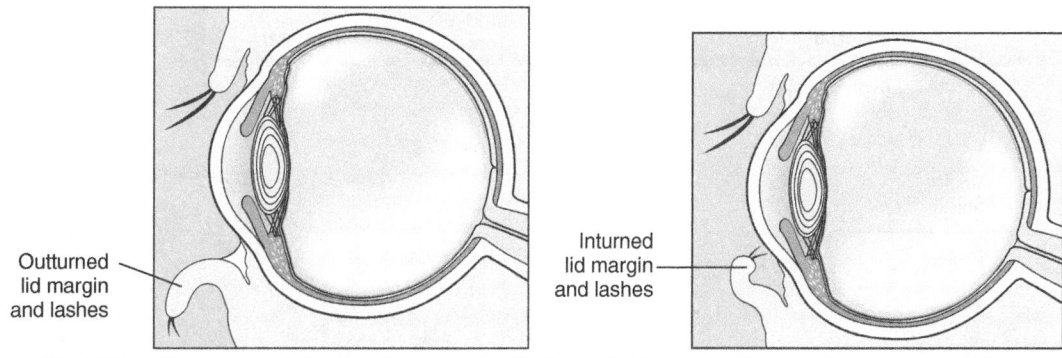

Fig. 8.13 A, Ectropion. B, Entropion. (From Frazier MS, Fuqua T: *Essentials of human disease and conditions*, ed 7, St. Louis, 2021, Elsevier.)

Outturned lid margin and lashes

Inturned lid margin and lashes

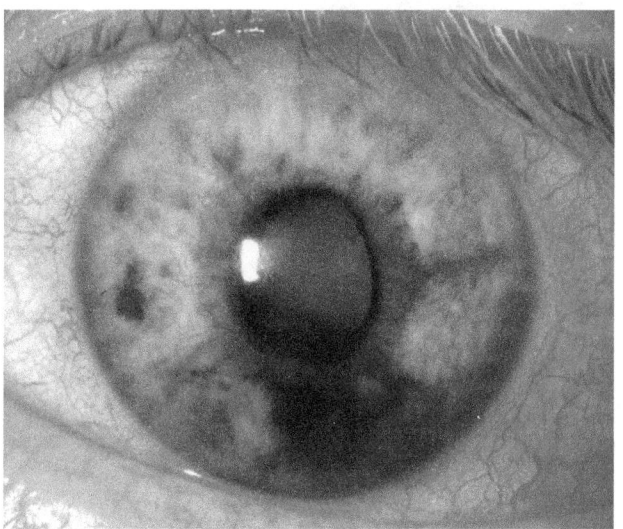

Fig. 8.14 Intraocular Melanoma. (From Nguyen Q, Rodrigues EB, Farah ME, et al: *Retinal pharmacotherapy*, London, 2010, Saunders.)

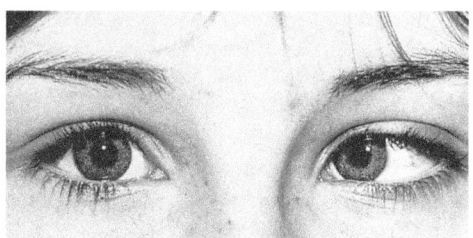

Fig. 8.15 Strabismus. This child exhibits convergent left eye strabismus. (From: Seidel H et al: *Mosby's guide to physical examination*, ed 3, St Louis, 2002, Mosby.)

ANATOMY OF THE EAR

The ear is an organ of hearing and balance. The ear is divided into the outer, middle, and inner ear (Fig. 8.16).

Outer Ear

The outer or external ear is the visible part of the ear. It consists of the:

- *Pinna* (PIN ah) or *auricle* (AW i kahl): A cartilaginous outer projecting portion of the ear that sits on the lateral aspect of the head (see Fig. 8.16). The *tragus* (TRAY gus) is the cartilaginous projection in front of the opening to the ear canal.
- *External auditory canal*: Also called the *external acoustic canal, external auditory meatus,* and the *ear canal*. It is a passageway that extends from the pinna to the *tympanic* (tim PAN ik) *membrane* (eardrum). Apocrine (AP uh krin) glands produce *cerumen* (sih ROO mun) (earwax), and small hairs line the canal. The cerumen and small hairs help capture dust and dirt. The cerumen lubricates the ear canal and also has antimicrobial properties. Usually the cerumen drains out of the ear, but it can become impacted, limiting hearing.

The tympanic membrane divides the outer ear and the middle ear. It creates a barrier that protects the middle and inner ear from foreign objects.

muscle weakness or paralysis. Most common type of strabismus is known as "crossed eyes" (Fig. 8.15).
- *Uveitis* (yoo vee EYE tis): Inflammation of the choroids, ciliary body, and iris.

MEDICAL TERMINOLOGY	
ambly/o	dull, dim
blast/o	embryonic, immature
glauc/o	gray, bluish green
my/o	to shut
nat/o	born
neur/o	nerve
uve/o	uvea
hyper-	excessive
neo-	new
presby-	old age
-ia	condition
-ic	pertaining to
-itis	inflammation
-ptosis	drooping
-oma	tumor, mass
-opia	visual condition
-um	structure

CRITICAL THINKING 8.7

Susie Jones, age 3, has an appointment with Dr. Walden because she has a cut on her ear. She fell onto a sprinkler while she was playing in the yard with her sister. The sprinkler cut her ear, and her mother brought her in to see if she might need stitches. Tom cleaned up the wound, and now Susie's mother is holding a gauze in place until Dr. Walden can see Susie. What is the name of the outer ear? What is the function of the outer ear?

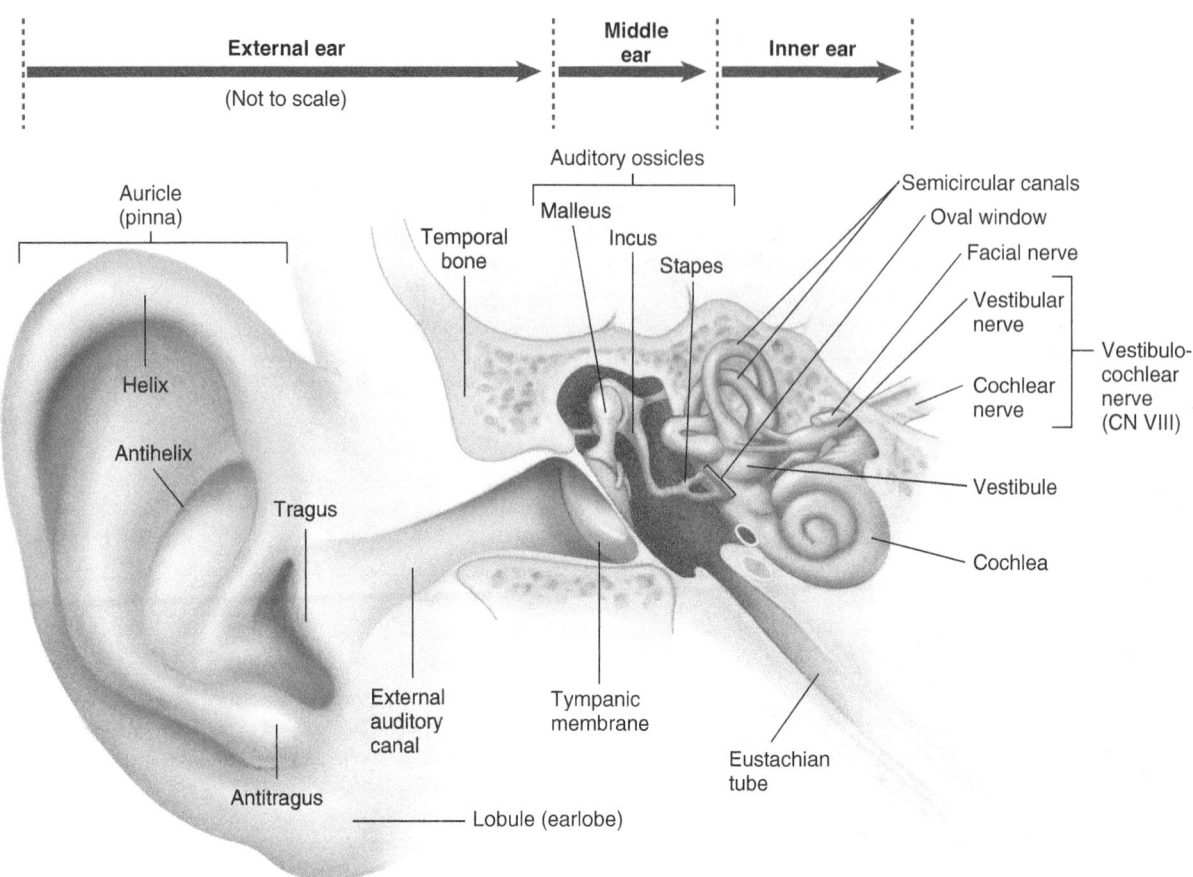

Fig. 8.16 Ear. External, Middle, and Inner Ear Structures. Structures not shown to scale. (From Patton KT, Thibodeau GA: *The human body in health and disease,* ed 7, St. Louis, 2018, Elsevier.)

Middle Ear

The middle ear, or tympanic cavity, consists of ossicles (AH sick kuls) and the eustachian (you STAY shahn) tube. The *ossicles,* three small bones, are named for their shape. They include the:

- *Malleus* (MAL ee us), or hammer, which is attached to the tympanic membrane
- *Incus* (ING kus), or anvil
- *Stapes* (STAY peez), or stirrup, which sits next to the oval window

The *eustachian* (u stay shee ahn) *tube,* or *auditory tube,* opens in the middle ear and connects to the throat. This continuous pathway from the middle ear to the throat is the reason that a throat infection can cause middle ear infection *(otitis media).* The eustachian tube helps equalize the pressure in the middle ear with the outside environment. This is needed for proper soundwave transfer.

Blockage of the eustachian tube or altitude changes, such as an airplane's ascent or descent, can cause unequal pressure between the middle ear and the outside environment. Unequal pressure can cause the tympanic membrane to remain stretched, thus limiting its ability to vibrate. The person may have fullness, pain, or discomfort in the ear. Slight to moderate hearing loss can occur. Yawning, swallowing, or chewing gum can help improve the ear symptoms.

Inner Ear

The inner ear, or *labyrinth* (LAB uh rinth), consists of three cavities in the temporal bone. The hard outer wall of the inner ear is called the *bony labyrinth,* or *osseous labyrinth* (Fig. 8.17). The three cavities in the bony labyrinth include the:

- *Vestibule* (VES tih byool), which is found near the oval window and between the semicircular canals and the cochlea. Within the vestibule, the *utricle* (YOO trick ul) and the *saccule* (SACK yool) (two saclike structures) function to establish the body's static equilibrium (ee kwuh LIB ree uh m).
- *Cochlea* (KAH klee ah), a small snail-shaped structure that contains the organ of Corti (KAWR tee), which contains hearing receptors. The cochlea is split into an upper and lower section by the *basilar membrane,* an elastic-like tissue.
- *Semicircular canals,* which consist of three curved tubular canals that contain the crista ampullaris (KRIS tah am pyoo LAIR is), which detects dynamic equilibrium.

The membranous labyrinth, which contains endolymph (EN doh limf), is suspended in the bony labyrinth. The space between the membranous and bony labyrinths is filled with perilymph (PAIR ee limf). Hair cells within the inner ear are sensory epithelial cells and function as receptors for hearing and equilibrium. The cochlea contains receptors for hearing. The vestibule and the semicircular canals contain receptors for equilibrium.

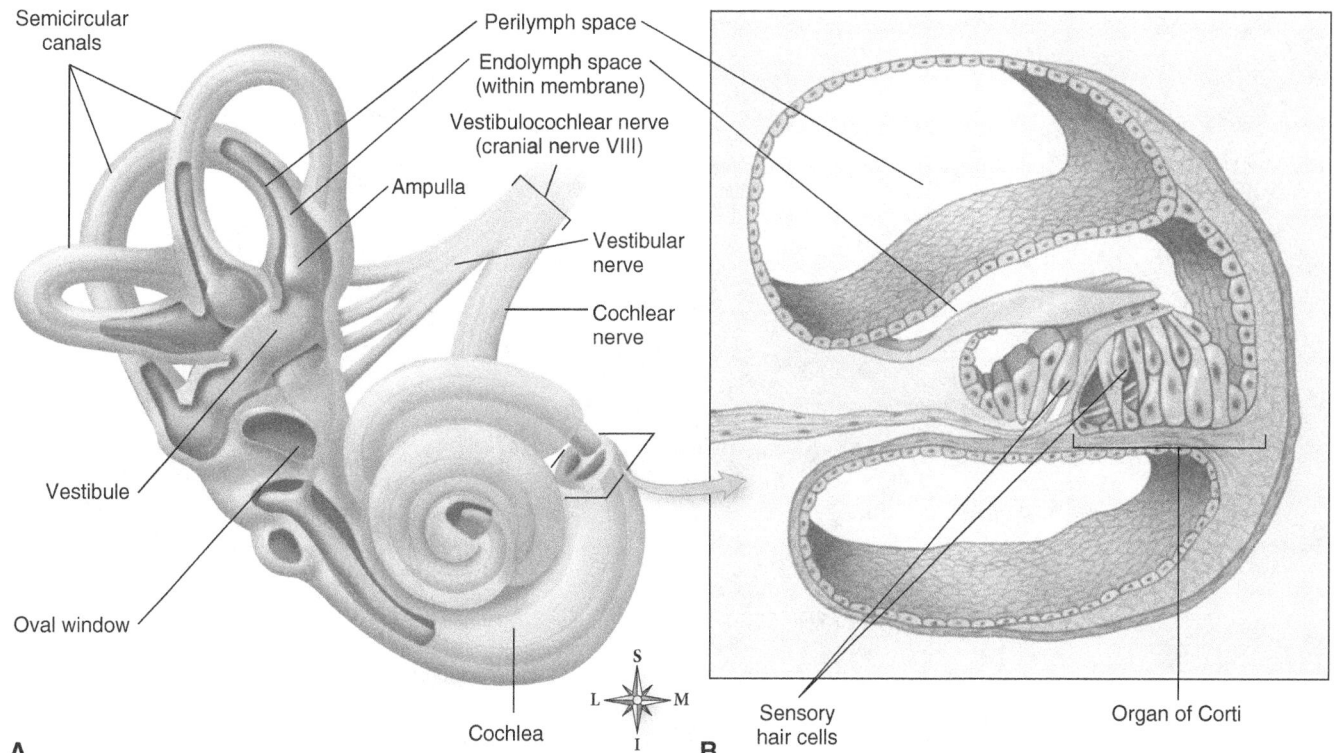

Fig. 8.17 Inner Ear. A, Within the bony labyrinth is the membranous labyrinth *(purple)*, which is surrounded by perilymph and filled with endolymph. Each ampulla in the vestibule contains a crista ampullaris that detects changes in head position and sends sensory impulses through the vestibular nerve to the brain. B, The inset shows a section of the membranous cochlea. Hair cells in the organ of Corti detect sound and send the information through the cochlear nerve. (From Patton KT, Thibodeau GA: *The human body in health and disease*, ed 7, St. Louis, 2018, Elsevier.)

The *vestibulocochlear nerve*, cranial nerve VIII, consist of two branches, the cochlear and vestibular nerves. The cochlear nerve transmits auditory information from the cochlea. The vestibular (ve STIB yeh lahr) nerve carries equilibrium information away from the semicircular canals (see Fig. 8.17).

> **VOCABULARY**
> **dynamic equilibrium** Relating to balance when moving at an angle or rotating.
> **endolymph** Fluid found in the membranous labyrinth of the inner ear.
> **organ of Corti** Organ of hearing in the inner ear that contains hair cells, sensory epithelial cells.
> **perilymph** A watery fluid found between the membranous labyrinth and the bony labyrinth in the inner ear.
> **static equilibrium** Relating to balance when moving in a straight line.

PHYSIOLOGY OF THE EAR

The ear is responsible for hearing and for balance. Hearing is a complex process in which sound waves are changed into electrical signals. The process proceeds like this:

- *Outer ear*: The pinna funnels the sound waves to the external auditory canal, which concentrates the sound waves onto the tympanic membrane. This causes the tympanic membrane to vibrate, starting a chain reaction.

- *Middle ear*: The vibrating tympanic membrane causes the malleus to move, striking the incus, which moves the stapes. The movement of the stapes causes vibrations on the oval window, which is part of the inner ear. Thus the sound waves are transmitted from the outer to the inner ear. During this process, the ossicles amplify or increase the sound wave vibrations.

- *Inner ear*: The vibrations on the oval window trigger the cochlear fluid to move, causing a wave to form along the basilar membrane (Fig. 8.18). Hair cells on the basilar membrane are responsible for helping change the vibrations into electrical signals, which are then transmitted to the cochlear nerve (a branch of the *vestibulocochlear nerve*). The impulses are carried to the temporal lobe of the cerebrum, where they are interpreted.

MEDICAL TERMINOLOGY	
audi/o, acous/o	hearing
cerumin/o	cerumen, earwax
cochle/o	cochlea
labyrinth/o	labyrinth, inner ear
ossicul/o	ossicle
ot/o, aur/o, auricul/o	ear
pharyng/o	pharynx
salping/o	eustachian tube
staped/o	stapes
tympan/o, myring/o	eardrum
vestibul/o	vestibule
-ic	pertaining to

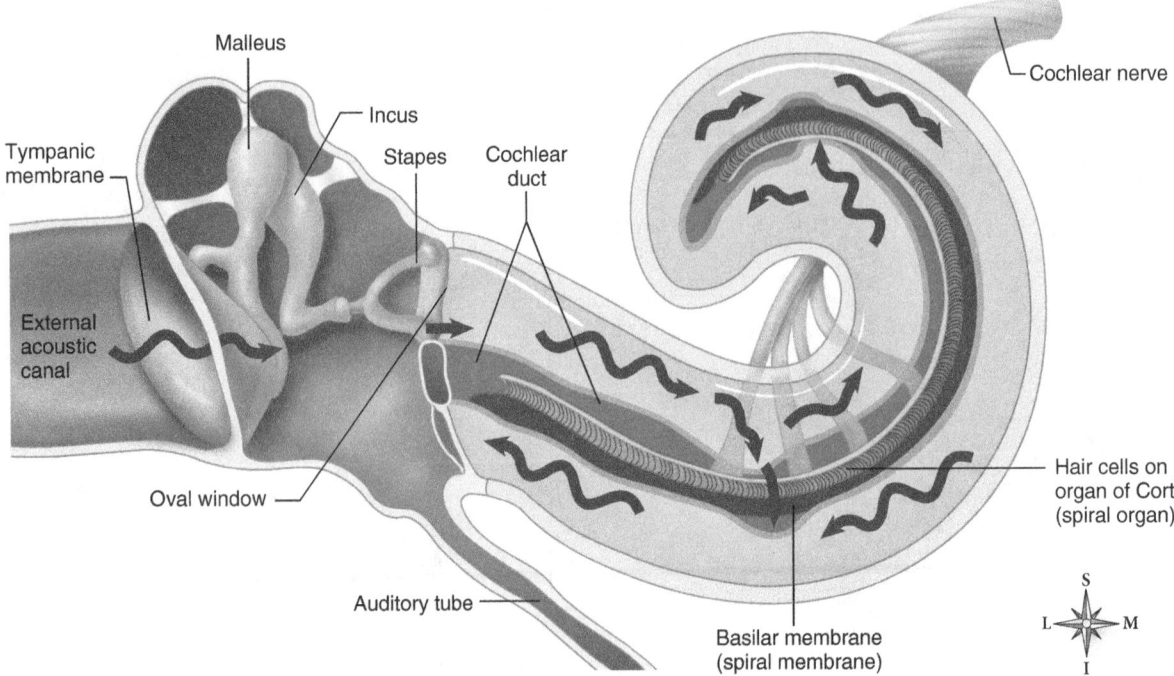

Fig. 8.18 Effect of Sound Waves in the Ear. Sound waves strike the tympanic membrane and cause it to vibrate. This vibration causes the membrane of the oval window to vibrate. Vibration of the oval window causes the perilymph in the bony labyrinth of the cochlea to move, which causes the endolymph in the membranous labyrinth of the cochlea or cochlear duct to move. This movement of endolymph stimulates hair cells on the organ of Corti (spiral organ) to generate a nerve impulse. The nerve impulse travels over the cochlear nerve, which becomes a part of cranial nerve VIII. (From Patton KT, Thibodeau GA: *The human body in health and disease*, ed 7, St. Louis, 2018, Elsevier.)

DISEASES AND DISORDERS OF THE EAR

Common signs and symptoms of ear disorders include:
- *Otalgia* (oh TAL juh): Ear pain
- *Otorrhea* (oh tuh REE ah): Discharge from the external auditory canal
- *Tinnitus* (tin EYE tis): Ringing or buzzing sound in the ear. Caused by certain medications, trauma, or disease
- *Vertigo* (VUR tih goh): A false sensation that you or your environment is spinning or moving

Common diagnostic procedures are listed in Table 8.6. Common treatments used for ear diseases are described in Table 8.7. The following sections describe in detail some of the more common ear disorders.

Benign Positional Vertigo

Benign positional vertigo, or benign paroxysmal positional vertigo (BPPV), is the most common type of vertigo. *Vertigo* causes people to feel as if they are spinning or that everything around them is spinning.

Etiology. BPPV is caused by a problem in the inner ear. *Canaliths,* small pieces of bonelike calcium, break free from the inside of the semicircular canals and float in the fluid. This sends confusing messages to the brain about the body's position. Risk factors for BPPV include a family history of BPPV, a prior head injury, and *labyrinthitis* (lab uh rinth EYE tis) (inner ear infection).

Signs and Symptoms. BPPV symptoms include:
- Vertigo, which may be triggered by moving the head and lasts a few seconds
- Loss of balance
- Nausea and vomiting
- Visual problems, such as items jumping or moving
- Hearing loss

Diagnostic Procedures. The provider will obtain a complete medical history and perform a physical exam. The provider may perform the Dix-Hallpike maneuver. If the results are not clear, additional neurologic testing will be done, including head computed tomography (CT) and magnetic resonance imaging (MRI) scans, caloric stimulation, and a hearing test.

Treatments. The provider may perform the Epley maneuver. The provider puts the head through a series of movements to reposition the canaliths in the inner ear. Antihistamines, anticholinergics, and sedative-hypnotics may also be used to relieve the spinning sensations.

Ear Infections

An infection or inflammation in each part of the ear is treated as a separate disease.
- *Otitis externa* (oh TYE tis eck STER nah): Inflammation or infection of the outer ear. Also called swimmer's ear. May be acute (sudden and short-term) or chronic (long-term).

TABLE 8.6   Common Diagnostic Procedures Used for Ear Disorders

Procedure	Description
Acoustic reflex measures	Also called *middle ear muscle reflex* (MEMR). When loud noises are heard, a muscle in the ear tightens, which causes the acoustic reflex. This test measures how well the ears respond to loud sounds.
Audiometry (ah dee AH meh tree)	Also called *pure-tone test*. The patient wears headphones and a series of tones are sent to the headphones. The test uses a variety of pitches and volumes. The patient is asked to respond when a tone is heard.
Balance disorder testing	Noninvasive tests that use technology to measure eye movement, a person's ability to balance with standing, and reactions to sound and movements.
Caloric stimulation test	Examines the eye reflexes by warming and cooling the inner ear with water.
Dix-Hallpike maneuver	The provider holds the patient's head in a specific position and has the patient lie quickly backward over the table. The provider looks for nystagmus, and the patient is asked if spinning occurs.
Electrocochleography (ECOG) (ee LEK trow kok LEE OG rah fee)	A test that measures the electrical stimulation generated in the inner ear and the nerve as a result of sound stimulation.
Electronystagmography (ENG) (ee LEK trow NIS tag mog rah fee)	A test that records the involuntary movements of the eye caused by nystagmus. Used to diagnose the cause of vertigo.
Otoscopy (oh TAH skuh pee)	An otoscope is inserted into the ear canal. Used to look at the external auditory canal and the tympanic membrane (Fig. 8.19A, B).
Speech and word recognition tests	During the test, the patient wears headphones and hears the audiologist, who will ask the patient to repeat a series of simple words, spoken at different volumes.
Tuning fork tests	A tuning fork has two prongs that make a tone when the fork vibrates. During the test, patients are asked if they can hear the sound in each ear. • *Weber test*. The vibrating tuning fork is placed at the midline of the patient's forehead. • *Rinne test*. To check bone conduction, the vibrating tuning fork is placed on the mastoid bone. To check air conduction, the vibrating tuning fork is placed in front of the ear.
Tympanometry (tim pan NAH muh tree)	A small device is inserted into the ear that pushes air against the tympanic membrane. The machine records the movement of the membrane on graphs called *tympanograms*. Used to help diagnose ear infection, cerumen buildup, or a perforated tympanic membrane.
Universal Newborn Hearing Screening (UNHS) test	A hearing screening used in newborns to assess the risk for hearing loss. Two tests are used: • *Auditory brainstem response* (ABR): Done on a sleeping child. Small electrodes are placed on the forehead and earlobe or mastoid bone. Earphones are placed on the child. As sound is played through the earphones, and the electrodes record the brain responses. • *Otoacoustic* (OH toe ah KUE stik) *emissions* (OE): A small microphone and ear-tip speakers are placed in the child's ears, and the child will hear soft sounds through the tips. A computer records the otoacoustics emissions (sounds that generate from within the ear).

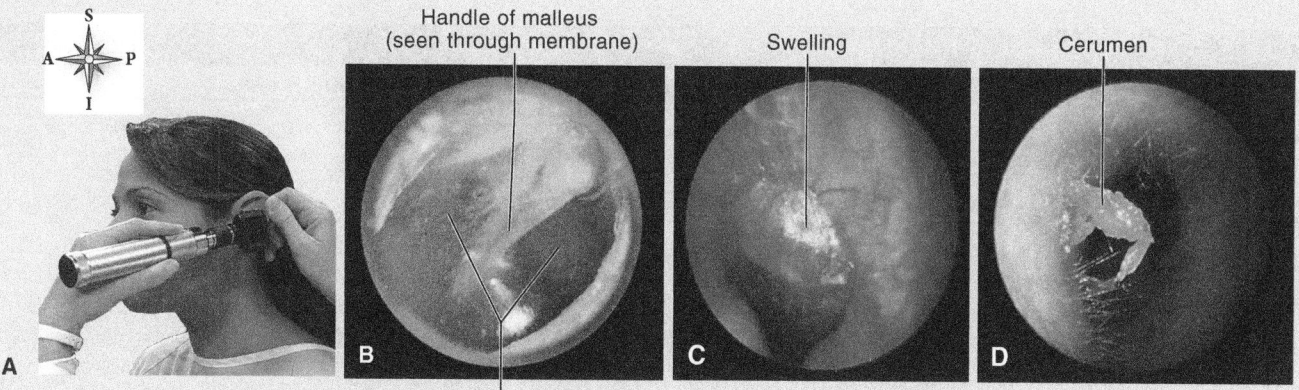

Fig. 8.19 Examining the External Ear. A, A lighted otoscope is used to view the external ear canal and tympanic membrane. B, Note the translucent pearly-gray appearance of a normal tympanic membrane (with a bit of white glare from the otoscope light in the lower right). The "handle" of the malleus can be seen attaching near the center of the inner surface of the membrane. C, Acute otitis media. Note the red, thickened, and bulging tympanic membrane. D, Cerumen (earwax) in the ear canal. (A from Ball JW, Dains JE, Flynn JA: *Seidel's guide to physical examination*, ed 8, St Louis, 2015, Mosby; B from Patton KT, Thibodeau GA: *The human body in health and disease*, ed 7, St. Louis, 2018, Elsevier; C and D from Bingham BJG, Hawke M, Kwok P: *Atlas of clinical otolaryngology*, St Louis, 1992, Mosby-Year Book.)

- *Otitis media* (OM) (oh TYE tis MEE dee ah): Inflammation or infection of the middle ear. The tympanic membrane may be red, bulging, or perforated (Fig. 8.19C). Fluid or air bubbles may be behind the ear. *Otitis media with effusion* (OME) occurs when there is thick fluid behind the eardrum but no ear infection. *Chronic suppurative otitis media* (CSOM) is a chronic ear infection that continues even when treated.
- *Otitis interna* (oh TYE tis IN ter nah): Also called *labyrinthitis*. Inflammation or irritation of the inner ear. With prompt treatment, the infection can resolve in under 2 weeks with no permanent damage. Some infections may lead to permanent partial or total hearing loss or damage to the vestibular system, causing equilibrium issues.

Table 8.8 describes these three types of ear diseases.

Hearing Loss

Hearing loss affects about 50% of those over age 75 and about 30% of those between the ages of 65 and 75. There are three types of hearing loss:

- *Conductive*: Involves outer or middle ear structures; sound waves are prevented from getting to the inner ear. Conductive hearing loss is usually mild, treatable, and temporary.
- *Sensorineural* (sen suh ree NOOR uhl): Involves inner ear and nerve damage. May show up at birth or occur later in life. Hearing loss may range from mild (inability to hear certain sounds and tones) to profound (inability to hear any sounds). Sensorineural hearing loss is usually permanent.
- *Mixed*: Combines both the conductive and sensorineural types of hearing loss.

Etiology. Causes of hearing loss include:

- Impacted cerumen: A buildup of cerumen can prevent the conduction of sound waves.
- Inner ear damage: Aging and exposure to loud noise can damage the hair cells, decreasing the electrical signals transmitted to the nerve.
- Diseases, such as meningitis, ear infections, abnormal bone growths, and tumors.

TABLE 8.7   Common Treatments Used for Ear Disorders

Procedures	Description
Balloon dilation	A balloon is inserted into the narrowed eustachian tube. The balloon is inflated and widens the eustachian tubes.
Cochlear implant (KAH klee ur)	A device implanted surgically in the ear. The sound bypasses damaged inner ear structures and directly stimulates the nerve.
Hearing aid	A device that is worn behind or in the ear. It amplifies sound and directs the sound into the external acoustic canal.
Mastoidectomy (mass toyd ECK tuh mee)	Surgical removal of the part or all of the mastoid bone.
Myringotomy (mir ring AH tuh mee)	A surgical incision is made in the tympanic membrane to relieve pressure, by allowing the drainage of pus and fluid from the middle ear. A myringotomy or tympanostomy tube can be surgically placed in the tympanic membrane, preventing fluid buildup behind the membrane.
Stapedotomy (stay pee DOT oh mee)	Surgical removal of part of the stapes. A small hole is made in the bottom of it, and a prosthetic bone is inserted.
Stapedectomy (stay puh DECK tuh mee)	Surgical removal of the stapes bone and the insertion of a prosthetic bone to restore hearing.
Tympanoplasty (TIM pan oh plas tee)	Surgical repair and rebuilding of the tympanic membrane using a skin or tissue graft from another part of the ear.

TABLE 8.8   Types of Ear Infections

	Otitis Externa	Otitis Media	Otitis Interna
Etiology	Fungal or bacterial infection caused by middle ear infection or swimming in unclean water. Chronic inflammation can occur due to an allergic reaction to something placed in the ear or chronic skin conditions.	Blockage of the eustachian tube caused by allergies, viral or bacterial infections, excess mucus and saliva during teething, infected adenoids, and tobacco smoke.	Virus, such as influenza, herpes, Epstein-Barr, and polio; bacteria.
Signs and Symptoms	Drainage from the ear, hearing loss, ear pain, itching of the ear or ear canal.	Ear pain, fullness in the ear, nasal congestion, cough, lethargy, vomiting, diarrhea, hearing loss in the affected ear, drainage from the ear, and loss of appetite.	Dizziness, vertigo, nausea, vomiting, difficulty with balance and walking, hearing loss, ear pain, and tinnitus.
Diagnostic Procedures	The provider will examine the outer ear and ear canal.	Observe the tympanic membrane using an otoscope.	Observe the tympanic membrane using an otoscope. May need to rule out other conditions, such as stroke and neurologic disorders.
Treatments	Antibiotic, corticosteroid, and acetic acid (vinegar) ear drops and analgesics.	Some cases clear up without treatment. Antibiotics can be given. Multiple infections can lead to a myringotomy and placement of ear tubes.	Antibiotics for bacterial infections, analgesics, steroids to reduce inflammation, and medications to control the nausea.

- Tympanic membrane perforation.
- Medications, such as gentamicin, sildenafil (Viagra), and some chemotherapy drugs, can cause inner ear damage. High doses of aspirin, antimalarial drugs, or loop diuretics can cause temporary tinnitus or hearing loss.

Signs and Symptoms. A person with hearing loss may experience muffling of sounds and difficulty hearing words with background noise. Television and radio volumes may need to be increased. A person may withdraw from conversations and avoid some social gatherings.

Diagnostic Procedures. During the physical exam, the provider will check for possible causes for the hearing loss, including impacted cerumen and an infection. Additional testing includes general screening tests, such as tuning fork tests and audiometer tests.

Treatments. Most types of hearing loss cannot be reversed. Treatments depend on the cause of the hearing loss; for instance, if the person has impacted cerumen, it will be removed. Some hearing loss can be treated with surgery, such as ossicle procedures (e.g., *stapedotomy*) and myringotomy. Hearing aids and cochlear implants are also used for hearing loss (Fig. 8.20).

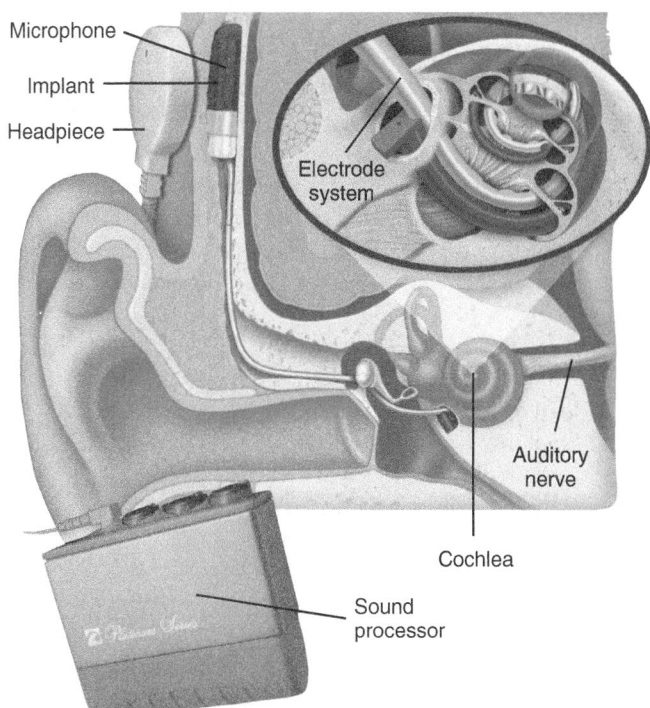

Fig. 8.20 Cochlear Implant. (From Lewis S, et al: *Medical-surgical nursing: assessment and management of clinical problems*, ed 8, St Louis, 2011, Mosby.)

CRITICAL THINKING 8.8

Based on what you learned about hearing loss, what sounds in your everyday environment would pose a problem for someone with hearing loss?

Ménière Disease

Ménière disease is a fairly common inner ear disorder that affects hearing and equilibrium. Attacks of Ménière disease can occur daily or rarely. The severity can also vary.

Etiology. The cause is unknown. In some cases, it is related to a middle or an inner ear infection or head injury. Risk factors include alcohol use, allergies, family history, smoking, and stress. A recent cold or illness or certain medications can also cause it.

Signs and Symptoms. Ménière disease usually has four main symptoms:
- Hearing loss that can occur in one or both ears. Hearing can improve between attacks but gets worse over time.
- Ear pressure.
- Tinnitus.
- Vertigo, which may also cause nausea, vomiting and sweating.

The person may also experience diarrhea, headaches, abdominal pain or discomfort, and nystagmus.

Diagnostic Procedures. The physical exam may indicate issues with hearing, balance, or eye movements. Additional tests include a caloric stimulation test, electrocochleography (ECOG), electronystagmography (ENG), and a head MRI scan.

Treatments. There is no cure, but lifestyle changes are recommended to manage the symptoms. To reduce the amount of fluids in the body, the provider may order diuretics and a low-salt diet. Patients are taught to avoid sudden movements, bright lights, and to remain still when symptoms occur. Additional treatments include a hearing aid and surgical procedures to help reduce the vertigo.

Otosclerosis

Otosclerosis is an abnormal bone growth in the middle ear causing hearing loss in one or both ears. The person has an abnormal extension of spongelike bone growths in the middle ear, which prevents the ossicles from vibrating. Otosclerosis is the most common cause of middle ear hearing loss in young adults, especially in females.

Etiology. The exact cause of otosclerosis is unknown, but it may be genetic.

Signs and Symptoms. Otosclerosis causes gradual hearing loss that worsens over time. The person may experience tinnitus and vertigo.

Diagnostic Procedures. A hearing test (e.g., audiometry) may determine the severity of the hearing loss. A temporal bone CT scan can identify other causes for the hearing loss.

Treatments. The condition may not be treated until the person has more serious hearing problems. Fluoride, calcium, and vitamin D may help slow the hearing loss. A hearing aid may help with the hearing loss. Surgery, such as a stapedectomy and stapedotomy, can cure or improve conductive hearing loss.

Presbycusis

Presbycusis (prez bee KYOO sis), or age-related hearing loss, is the slow loss of hearing that occurs when a person gets older.

Etiology. The inner ear changes as a person gets older. The hearing loss occurs when the hair cells become damaged or die. They do not regrow; thus the damage is permanent. Genes and loud noise can also cause the changes. Factors that contribute to presbycusis include:
- A family history of presbycusis
- Repeated exposure to loud noises (e.g., rock concerts, loud music with headphones)
- Smoking
- Certain disorders, such as diabetes
- Certain medications, such as chemotherapy drugs

Signs and Symptoms. The person may experience a gradual hearing loss and tinnitus. They may ask others to repeat themselves and have problems hearing in noisy areas. Certain sounds, such as "s" or "th," can be difficult to tell apart. Higher pitched voices can be difficulty to hear.

Diagnostic Procedures. The provider will do a complete examination and use an otoscope to look in the ears. A referral to the audiologist for hearing testing is common.

Treatments. There is no cure for presbycusis. Treatment is focused on improving hearing and may include hearing aids, telephone amplifiers, and cochlear implants. Sign language and speech reading (lip reading) can also be helpful.

Additional Ear Disorders

There are many ear disorders. The following list provides a brief description of some of them.
- *Acoustic neuroma* (ah KOO stik noo ROH mah): A slow-growing benign tumor of the vestibulocochlear nerve. Has been linked to the genetic disorder neurofibromatosis type 2 (NF2).
- *Ear barotrauma*: Also called *barotitis media*. A change in altitude, such as flying, driving in the mountains, or scuba diving, causes ear pain and pressure, hearing loss, and dizziness.
- *Impacted cerumen*: A gradual buildup of earwax, which can affect hearing (see Fig. 8.19D).
- *Cholesteatoma* (koh less tee ah TOH mah): A type of skin cyst located in the middle ear and the mastoid bone. Can be caused by a birth defect or chronic ear infections.
- *Mastoiditis* (mass toy DYE tis): Inflammation of the mastoid process of the temporal bone (Fig. 8.21). Typically caused by acute otitis media. The patient experiences redness and swelling behind the ear.
- *Motion sickness*: A common problem for people of all ages when traveling. The brain senses movement by getting signals from the inner ear, eyes, muscles, and joints. Conflicting signals can cause a reaction that leads to motion sickness.

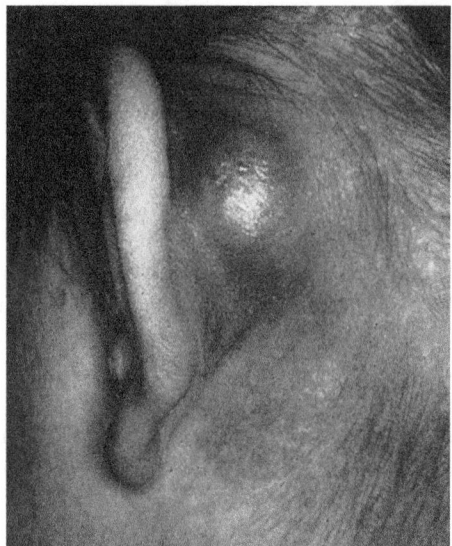

Fig. 8.21 Mastoiditis. (From Stone DR, Gorbach SL: *Atlas of infectious diseases*, Philadelphia, 2000, Saunders.)

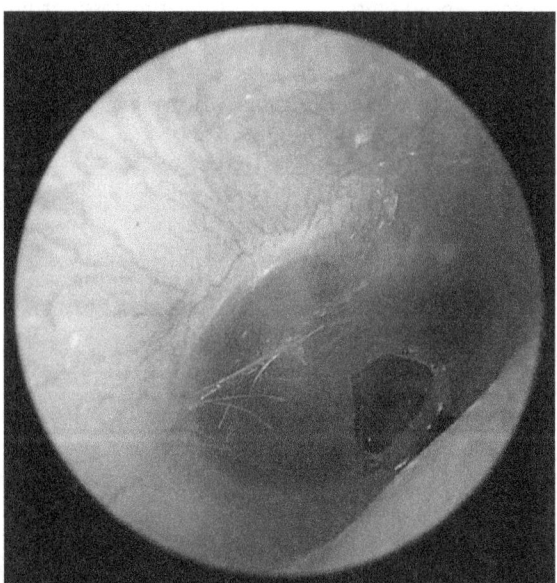

Fig. 8.22 Ruptured Tympanic Membrane. (Courtesy Michael Hawke, MD. From Zitelli BJ, Davis HW: *Atlas of pediatric physical diagnosis*, ed 5, St. Louis, 2007, Mosby.)

The person experiences nausea, a cold sweat, fatigue, and vomiting.
- *Ruptured tympanic membrane*: Also called *perforated eardrum*. Sudden pressure changes, puncturing of the tympanic membrane with an object, infections, and loud sudden noises can cause rupture of the eardrum (Fig. 8.22).

LIFE SPAN CHANGES

Touch, taste, and smell mature at birth. Babies have about 10,000 taste buds and prefer sweet tastes. Taste buds decrease after age 50 and remaining taste buds begin to shrink. By age 70, the sense of smell can also diminish.

The touch, vibration, and pain sensations decrease or change with age. By age 50, a person may have a reduced sensitivity to pain. Older people may become more sensitive to light touches because their skin is thinner.

At birth, newborns can see about 8 to 12 inches. Color vision develops between 4 to 6 months. By 2 months, babies can track moving objects up to 180 degrees. By age 3 to 4 months, infants have better eye-muscle control that allows them to track objects. Their vision increases, allowing them to tell objects apart from their backgrounds with very little contrast.

Visual changes can occur with age. The vitreous liquefies and shrinks. The vitreous separates from the retina, causing vitreous detachment, which does not require treatment. Floaters in the vision increase. Collagen and proteins in the vitreous become "stringing" and float in the vitreous, casting a shadow on the retina. Reduced peripheral vision is common in older people. Weakened eye muscles may prevent people from moving their eyes in all direction. Eye glands reduce production of tears and oil. Dry eyes can be common. Presbyopia is common. Age-related macular degeneration (AMD) and cataracts are the most common causes of blindness in older adults.

Hearing begins at birth and is mature at birth. Infants respond to changes in position and rocking. Children tend to have more middle ear infections than adults. This is attributed to the horizontal position of the eustachian tube in children. The tube does not drain as well and gets blocked easier, leading to otitis media.

Hearing changes occur with age. With age, structures in the ears change and their functions decline. Tinnitus is more common in older adults. It can be caused by impacted cerumen and certain medications that damage ear structures. The ability to hear sounds decreases, especially high-frequency sounds. Presbycusis is also common with age. A person may also have problems maintaining their balance with sitting, standing, and walking.

CLOSING COMMENTS

Patients with vision or hearing impairment face serious challenges. For these patients, the medical assistant must use good listening skills and appropriate nonverbal communication to convey empathy and understanding. Patient coaching may have to be adapted to meet the special needs of these patients. A person with a vision loss benefits from large-print forms and handouts, increased lighting, and verbal rather than written instructions to reinforce learning. For an individual with a hearing deficit, printed instructions, demonstrations of how to manage treatments, or sign language interpretation should be available to ensure accurate communication. Including family members in the patient's treatment plan and offering referrals to appropriate community or professional resources may be very beneficial to a patient with sensory loss. Important medication information should be given to both the patient and family members (Box 8.1). Each patient must be assessed individually to determine the type of adaptation that the person needs.

BOX 8.1 Medication Classifications

- *Antibiotics:* Used to treat bacterial infections.
- *Antiemetics:* Act on the hypothalamic center in the brain to reduce or prevent nausea and vomiting. Used to manage motion sickness.
- *Antifungals:* Used to treat systemic or local fungal infections.
- *Anti-inflammatories:* Used to reduce inflammation.
- *Corticosteroids:* Used to treat chronic and acute inflammatory diseases.
- *Miotics:* Allow excess fluid to drain from the eye. Used to treat glaucoma.
- *Mydriatics:* Dilate the pupil; some cause paralysis of the ciliary muscle. Used for ophthalmic procedures.

Refer to Appendix D, which can be found on the Evolve website, for information on the medication classifications, including indications for use, desired effect, side effects, adverse reactions, and generic and trade names. Medical assistants should be familiar with medications that are prescribed to patients.

PATIENT-CENTERED CARE

Diminished sight or hearing may render a patient seriously impaired. To prevent accidents and office injuries, always ask sight- or hearing-impaired patients whether they require assistance. When you escort the patient to an examination room, offer your arm and tell the patient the approximate distance you will be walking. If the patient is to have an examination that involves local anesthesia or eyedrops that dilate the pupil, be sure the patient has recovered, has sunglasses, and that someone is available to drive the patient home before allowing the person to leave the facility.

BEING PROFESSIONAL

When working with patients with hearing impairments, it is important to use these communication techniques:
- Face the person when speaking.
- Determine if the person has better hearing in one ear over the other. Position yourself so your voice is close to that side.
- Use a low-pitched voice, and speak clearly, slowly, and distinctly. Pause between sentences or phrases. Speak naturally; do not shout.
- Say the person's name before you begin a conversation.
- Keep your hands away from your face when talking.

You are rooming a patient who has a hearing impairment. The patient is coming in for blurred vision. Using critical thinking skills, role-play this scenario with a peer. Ask the patient questions to get more information about his concern. Use the communication techniques for hearing impairment.

CHAPTER REVIEW

The senses are divided into general senses and special senses. General senses include touch, pressure, temperature, and pain and receptors scattered throughout the body. The special senses have receptors that are concentrated in one area. *Special senses* include vision, hearing, equilibrium (balance), taste, and smell.

The anatomy of the eye was discussed in detail. The structures of the eye can be divided into the supporting structures and the eyeball. The eyeball can be further divided by the three layers and the inner part of the eye. The supporting structures include:

- Ophthalmic artery and the superior and inferior ophthalmic vein
- Optic, trochlear, and the oculomotor nerves
- Eyelashes, eyelashes, and the conjunctiva
- Meibomian glands and lacrimal glands

The eyeball consists of three layers and the inner part of the eye. The eyeball structures include:

- Outer layer: Sclera and cornea
- Middle layer: Choroid, iris, and ciliary body
- Inner layer: Retina, photoreceptors (rods and cones), macula lutea, and the fovea centralis
- Inner part of the eye: Anterior and posterior chambers, the lens, and the vitreous chamber

Together rods and cones detect light and convert it into neurologic impulses. The impulses travel along the optic nerve to the brain. The brain then converts the impulses to visual images.

Common signs and symptoms of eye disorders include crusting, redness, irritation, itching, burning sensation, and visual changes. Typical diagnostic tests ordered include a standard ophthalmic exam, Amsler grid, electroretinography, fluorescein angiography, fluorescein staining, fundus photography, optical coherence tomography, and retinoscopy. Many eye diseases were discussed in the chapter.

The ear is divided into the outer, middle, and inner ear. The outer ear consists of the pinna and the external auditory canal. The tympanic membrane separates the outer and inner ear. The middle ear consists of the ossicles (malleus, incus, and stapes) and the eustachian tube. The inner ear, or labyrinth, consists of three cavities in the temporal bone: vestibule, cochlea, and semicircular canals. The vestibulocochlear nerve consists of two branches, the cochlear and vestibular nerves. The cochlear nerve transmits auditory information from the cochlea. The vestibular nerve carries equilibrium information away from the semicircular canals.

Common signs and symptoms of ear disorders include otalgia, otorrhea, tinnitus, and vertigo. Many common diagnostic procedures were discussed, including audiometry, balance disorder testing, electrocochleography, electronystagmography, otoscopy, and tuning fork tests. Many ear diseases were discussed in the chapter.

Senses diminish with age. Taste buds shrink. The touch, vibration, and pain sensations change with age. The vision in babies improves over the first year of life. Visual changes occur with age, including an increase in floaters, reduced peripheral vision, and weakened eye muscles. Presbyopia is common. Age-related macular degeneration and cataracts are the most common causes of blindness in older adults.

SCENARIO WRAP-UP

As Tom works with older patients, he recognizes the need to adapt to their limitations. Often, he extends his arm and has the patient hold onto his arm; they slowly walk to the exam room. He knows that with hearing impairment, yelling is not the best way to communicate. He talks louder and towards the patient's good ear while enunciating his words. For patients with visual impairments, he ensures that there is adequate lighting in the room. He encourages patients to wear their glasses when he is reviewing forms and patient education materials. Working with those with visual and hearing impairments, Tom has learned a lot about the adaptive tools and equipment available on the market. With the providers' permission, Tom has created an educational display in the reception area focusing on adaptive equipment for visual and hearing impairments.

9

Blood, Lymphatic, and Immune Systems

LEARNING OBJECTIVES

1. Describe the composition of blood.
2. List the major organs and structures for the lymphatic and immune systems. Also identify the anatomic location of these major organs and structures.
3. Describe coagulation and hemostasis.
4. Differentiate between innate and acquired immunity and the types of acquired immunity.

5. Identify the etiology, signs and symptoms, diagnostic procedures, treatment, prognosis, and prevention of blood, lymphatic, and immune system diseases and disorders.
6. Compare the structure and function of the lymphatic and immune systems across the life span.

OUTLINE

▶▶ OPENING SCENARIO

Mia Vang, CMA (AAMA), is a medical assistant working at Walden-Martin Family Medical (WMFM) Clinic. She is working with Dr. Walden today. Mia enjoys the family practice setting. She works with a variety of patients, from infants to older adults. The patients have various conditions, which helps Mia continue to learn new diseases and treatments. Today, Dr. Walden and Mia will see both new patients and existing patients.

YOU WILL LEARN

1. To recognize and use terms related to the blood, lymphatic, and immune systems.

2. To recognize the components of the blood.
3. To locate the structures related to the lymphatic and immune systems.
4. To understand and describe the functions of the blood, lymphatic, and immune systems.
5. To recognize the etiology, signs and symptoms, diagnostic processes, and treatment of common blood, lymphatic, and immune system.
6. To discuss life span changes in the blood, lymphatic, and immune systems.

INTRODUCTION

Hematology (HEE mah TOL oh jee) is the branch of medicine that focuses on the diagnosis and treatment of diseases related to blood and blood-forming organs. A *hematologist* (hee mah TOL oh jist) is a physician who specializes in internal medicine and hematology. A hematologist treats patients with blood, bone marrow, vascular system, lymph gland, and spleen disorders.

Immunology (im yuh NOL uh jee) is the healthcare specialty that deals with many immune- and lymphatic-related diseases and disorders. An *immunologist* (im yuh NOL uh jist) is a physician involved in the diagnosis, treatment, and prevention of disorders of the immune and lymphatic systems.

The blood, lymphatic (lim FAT ik), and immune (ih MYOON) systems are three different systems. The blood carries oxygen and nutrients to the cells and carries waste from the cells. The lymphatic system returns proteins and excess interstitial fluid to the circulatory system. The immune system defends the body from microorganisms, foreign tissues, and cancerous cells.

These three systems interact closely to maintain homeostasis (hoh mee uh STEY sis). With the immune system being more functional, instead of structural, structures in other systems have roles in the immune system. Simply put, the cells, tissues, and organs that have roles in the immune system are also considered part of another body system, such as the blood and the lymphatic systems. White blood cells and lymphatic system cells, tissues, and organs also function as part of the immune system.

This chapter will begin by discussing the structures in the blood and lymphatic systems, followed by the role of the immune system. Diseases of these three systems will be discussed later in the chapter.

ANATOMY OF THE BLOOD, LYMPHATIC, AND IMMUNE SYSTEMS

Anatomy of the Blood

Blood is made up of two components:
- Liquid portion: Called *plasma* (PLAZ muh) and makes up about 55% of the total blood volume.
- Formed elements: Includes red blood cells (RBCs), white blood cells (WBCs), and platelets. The formed elements are suspended (freely float) in the plasma and make up about 45% of the total blood volume.

A milliliter of blood has approximately 4.2 million to 6 million RBCs, 4500 to 11,000 WBCs, and 150,000 to 450,000 platelets. The average 150-pound (68 kg) person has approximately 5 liters of blood circulating throughout the body. The following sections will discuss plasma, platelets, WBCs, and RBCs in more detail.

Blood Composition

Plasma. Plasma is the liquid portion of whole blood. Plasma contains 90% water. Water is the solvent for all the dissolved substances that travel in the plasma. Plasma also contains:
- *Plasma proteins*: Made in the liver and include the following:
  - *Albumin*: It is the most abundant protein in plasma, and it attracts water. It normally stays in the blood vessel; thus it helps to maintain the blood volume.
  - *Globulins*: Antibodies are a type of globulin; they protect against infections.
  - *Clotting factors*: Include fibrinogen and prothrombin, which are important in the blood clotting or coagulation process.
  - *Complements*: Enzymes (proteins) that are normally inactive in the blood. When activated they create protein rings that destroy pathogens.
- Inorganic substances and electrolytes (sodium, calcium, potassium, chloride, magnesium, bicarbonate).
- Organic substances (amino acids, glucose, fats, cholesterol, hormones).
- Waste products (urea, uric acid, ammonia, creatinine).

Organic and inorganic substances are needed for metabolism and cellular function, repair, and reproduction. Cellular metabolism waste products are dissolved in the plasma and are transported to the liver, kidneys, and lungs for excretion.

Plasma has a very narrow pH range (7.35 to 7.45), which is necessary to make sure that red blood cells can transport the optimal level of oxygen in the blood. The range also allows needed chemical reactions in the body to continue to work. Most chemical reactions in the body are pH dependent. Without a stable blood pH, homeostasis is unlikely to be maintained.

VOCABULARY

enzymes Special proteins that speed up a chemical reaction in the body.

microorganisms Any living organisms of microscopic size. Examples include bacteria, protozoa, fungi, parasites, and helminths. Some definitions include viruses, which are not alive.

solvent A liquid that can dissolve other substances.

whole blood Plasma and the formed elements of blood in a free-flowing liquid form.

Thrombocytes. Thrombocytes (THROM boh sites), also called *platelets*, have an irregular round or oval shape (Fig. 9.1). They are formed in the bone marrow from stem cells. They are just a small piece or fragment of a much larger cell called a *megakaryocyte* (meg uh KAR ee oh site) that is in the bone marrow. Platelets aid in coagulation, the process of changing a liquid to a solid. When an injury to a blood vessel occurs, platelets rush to the area and *agglutinate* (ah GLOO tih nate), or clump together. This stops or slows the bleeding, thus controlling the blood flow *(hemostasis)*.

Leukocytes. Leukocytes (LOO koh sites), also called *white blood cells* (WBCs), protect the body from invading pathogens. The two main types of WBCs are:

- *Granulocytes* (GRAN yoo loh sites): Have granules within the cytoplasm, and they also have a segmented or multilobed nucleus. There are three types of granulocytes: neutrophils (NOO troh fils), eosinophils (ee oh SIN oh fils), and basophils (BAY soh fils). Each has its own role in immunity (Table 9.1 and Fig. 9.2).
- *Agranulocytes* (a GRAN yoo loh sites): Lack granules in the cytoplasm, and they have one nucleus. Granulocytes originate in the bone marrow and mature after entering the lymphatic system. There are two types of agranulocytes, monocytes (MON oh sites) and lymphocytes (LIM foh sites) (see Table 9.1 and Fig. 9.2).

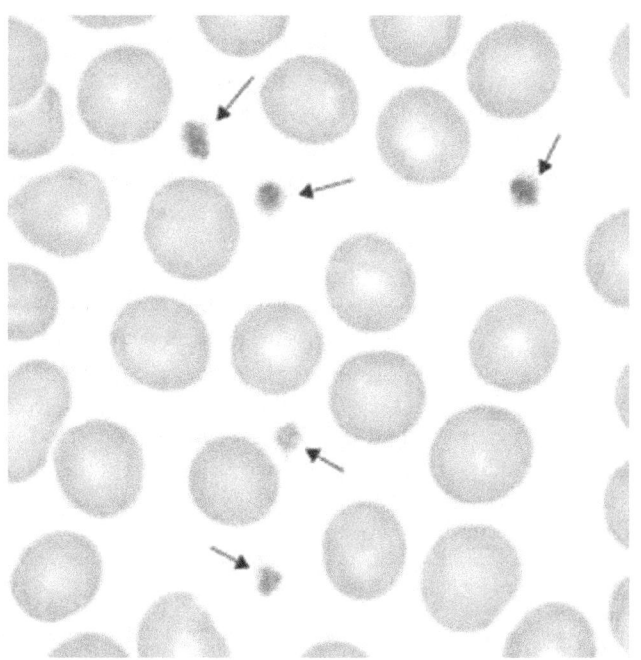

Fig. 9.1 Thrombocytes (Platelets). (From *Mosby's dictionary of medicine, nursing, & health professions,* ed 8, St. Louis, 2009, Elsevier.)

VOCABULARY

antigens Substances (usually proteins) on the surface of cells, viruses, bacteria, fungi, and nonliving substances, including drugs, chemicals, toxins, and foreign particles (e.g., wood splinters).

cytoplasm Jellylike substance that surrounds the nucleus and fills the cells. Organelles (structures in the cell) are suspended in the cytoplasm.

hematopoiesis The formation of blood cells.

stem cells Undifferentiated cells that can become specialized cells in the body.

Erythrocytes. Erythrocytes (eh RITH roh sites), or red blood cells, have the important function of transporting oxygen (O_2) and carbon dioxide (CO_2) throughout the body. *Hemoglobin* (HEE moh gloh bin) (Hgb), a molecule on the RBC, is capable of binding, transporting, and releasing oxygen and carbon dioxide. Hemoglobin is made up of protein and iron.

RBC production is stimulated by *erythropoietin,* a hormone produced in the kidneys. Hematopoiesis of RBCs takes place in red bone marrow. Stem cells produce immature RBCs that contain a nucleus. As an RBC matures, it loses its nucleus and is released into the bloodstream. RBCs are biconcave (curved inward on both sides), which allows for more surface area for the hemoglobin, thus allowing more O_2 and CO_2 to be carried (Fig. 9.3). The shape also allows more flexibility as the RBC moves through the tiny capillaries.

Red blood cells have a life span of approximately 120 days. When an RBC is no longer useful, it is broken down into iron and bilirubin in the spleen. The iron is stored mainly in the liver and is recycled into new RBCs. The bilirubin is further broken down into bile, which is excreted by the liver.

CRITICAL THINKING 9.1

Describe the three types of cells found in the blood.

Blood Types. Two major classification systems are used with blood types, the ABO system and the Rh system. In the ABO system, each person has an A, a B, an ABO, or an O blood type. In

TABLE 9.1	**Types of White Blood Cells**	
Type	**Description**	**Role**
Granulocytes		
Neutrophils	Also called *segs, polys,* or *polymorphonucleocytes* (PMNs); most abundant white blood cell (WBC)	Phagocytic (FAG uh sih tik) (protect by engulfing and destroying foreign substances); clean up the infection site and aid in the healing process.
Eosinophils	Also called *eos;* make up about 1% of the WBCs	Increase in number when the body is defending against allergens and parasites.
Basophils	Also called *basos;* make up 1% or less of the WBCs in the circulation	Respond to an allergic reaction by releasing histamine, which causes an inflammatory response; also release heparin (an anticoagulant).
Agranulocytes		
Monocytes	Also called *monos;* contain a single, large nucleus; largest phagocytic WBC; transform into macrophages when in lymphatic tissue	Very aggressive phagocytic cells that can destroy pathogens, malignant cells, and tumor cells in the body
Lymphocytes	Also called *lymphs;* two types: T lymphocytes (T cells) and B lymphocytes (B cells)	Involved in the immune response and destroy pathogens; B cells produce antibodies; T cells attack foreign substances and assist B cells

Granulocytes			Agranulocytes	
	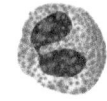	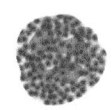	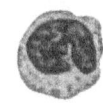	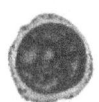
A. Neutrophil	B. Eosinophil	C. Basophil	D. Monocyte	E. Lymphocyte

Fig. 9.2 White Blood Cells. (From Proctor D, et al: *Kinn's the medical assistant,* ed 13, St. Louis, 2017, Elsevier.)

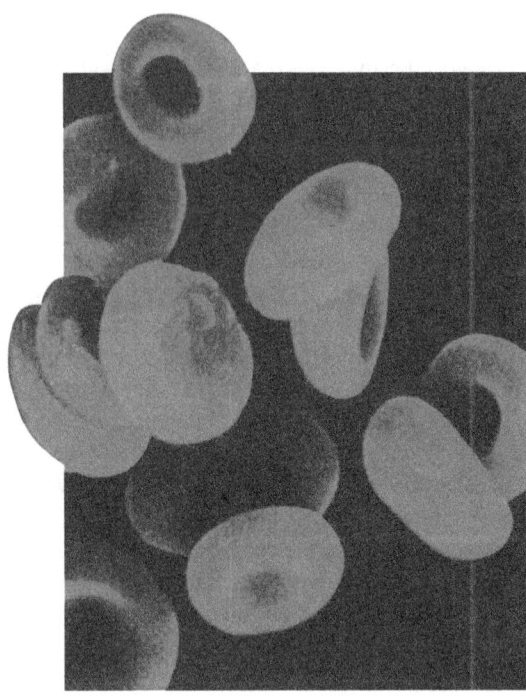

Fig. 9.3 Red Blood Cells (RBCs). Color-enhanced scanning electron micrograph shows the detailed structure of normal RBCs. Note the biconcave shape of each RBC. (From Patton KT, Thibodeau GA: *The human body in health and disease,* ed 7, St. Louis, 2018, Elsevier.)

the Rh system, a person is either Rh positive or Rh negative. For example, a person may have O-negative blood. In the ABO system, the person has type O blood and is Rh negative. These two systems will be explained in more detail in the following sections.

ABO System. In the ABO system, each blood type is unique based on the specific antigens present or absent on the surface of the RBCs and specific antibodies circulating in the plasma (Table 9.2). Antigens are foreign substances to the body, and the immune system makes specific antibodies to fight off specific antigens. When a person receives a blood transfusion, the blood given must be compatible with the person's blood. If an antibody is present in the recipient's blood, the corresponding antigen cannot be in the donor's blood. For example, type O blood contains both A and B antibodies, thus blood with A or B antigens cannot be given. The only type of blood that is compatible with type O is type O. Another example is a person with type AB blood, which contains no antibodies. These people can receive all four blood types because they have no antibodies to attack the donor blood. Type AB blood is considered the universal recipient because it does not contain any antibodies. Type O is considered the universal donor because it does not contain any antigens, and everyone can receive type O blood.

Rh System. In the Rh system, there is a collection of 47 antigens that act together as a group and are referred to as the *Rh antigen* or *Rh factor.* When the Rh antigen is present, the person is said to be Rh positive. About 85% of the population in the United States is Rh positive, and 15% is Rh negative.

Rh antibodies are different from ABO antibodies. Rh antibodies are not preformed (present before antigen exposure), as are ABO antibodies. The first time a person is exposed to the Rh antigen, the immune system produces antibodies. This process is called *sensitization.* Nothing is noticeable during the first exposure, though subsequent exposures to the Rh antigen will cause lysis (destruction) of RBCs.

Blood typing is the process of determining a person's blood type using the ABO and Rh systems. If the person receives the wrong type of blood, a *transfusion reaction* can occur, which may be a serious, life-threatening situation. For instance, if a person with type A blood is transfused with type B blood, the anti-B antibodies in the recipient's blood will attack the B antigens in the donor's blood, causing *agglutination* (blood clumping) or *lysis* (blood cell rupture).

MEDICAL TERMINOLOGY

bas/o	base
eosin/o	rose colored
erythr/o	red
granul/o	little grain
leuk/o	white
morph/o	shape
myel/o	bone marrow
neutr/o	neutral
nucle/o	nucleus
phag/o	eat, swallow
plasm/o	plasma
ser/o	serum
thromb/o	clotting, clot
vas/o	vessel
mono	one
-poly-	many
-cyte, -cyto	cell
-globin	protein substance
-lysis	breaking down
-ous	pertaining to
-phil	attraction
-poietin	forming substance
serum (singular)	sera (plural)

TABLE 9.2 Blood Types

Type	Antigens Present	Antibodies Present	Can Give Blood To	Can Receive Blood From
ABO System				
A	A antigen	B antibodies	A, AB	A, O
B	B antigen	A antibodies	B, AB	B, O
AB	A and B antigens	None	AB	AB, A, B, O
O	None	A and B antibodies	O, A, B, AB	O
Rh System				
Negative	Rh not present		Negative and positive	Negative
Positive	Rh present		Positive	Positive and negative

BOX 9.1 Lymph Vessels in the Digestive System

The lymphatic system is also involved with the absorption of fats and fat-soluble vitamins in the digestive system. The lymphatic system transports these substances to the venous circulation.

The lining of the small intestine has plicae (folds), which contain small projections called villi (VILL eye). Each villus contains a lacteal (LACK tee ul) (lymph vessel) that absorbs lipids (fats) and fat-soluble vitamins. The lymph, which is usually a clear yellowish liquid, is milky in appearance in the lacteals. This is due to the high fat content of the liquid, called chyle (kile).

Anatomy of the Lymphatic System

The blood plays an important role in the body by bringing cells needed substances and carrying waste away from cells (Box 9.1). Fluid from the blood diffuses through the capillary walls into the space between the cells. Much of the fluid moves back into the blood in the capillaries, but not all of it. The remaining fluid makes up the *interstitial* (in ter STISH uhl) *fluid*, or the fluid around the cells.

Excess interstitial fluid drains into tiny blinded-ended *lymphatic capillaries*. The fluid, now called lymph (limf), moves through the lymphatic system and eventually returns to the circulatory system. The lymph contains substances, such as proteins, that are too large to cross through the blood capillary walls. Minerals, nutrients, damaged cells, foreign particles (e.g., viruses and bacteria), and cancer cells can also be found in lymph. Returning extra fluid and proteins to the blood helps to prevent edema and to maintain normal blood volume and pressure.

Lymphatic capillaries only carry fluids away from the tissue. They are tiny blind-ended vessels found in all areas of the body except the central nervous system, bone marrow, and tissues that lack blood vessels, such as the epidermis. The capillary walls are created by overlapping simple squamous cells. This allows the fluid to drain in, but not drain out of, the capillary (Fig. 9.4).

Lymph flows from lymphatic capillaries into larger vessels called *lymphatic venules*. From there, the lymph flows into larger vessels called *lymphatic veins*. Eventually, the veins empty into either the right lymphatic duct or the thoracic duct. The *right lymphatic duct* drains lymph from the upper right quadrant of the body into the right subclavian vein (Fig. 9.5A). The *thoracic duct* drains lymph from the remaining part of the body into the left subclavian vein (Fig. 9.5B and C).

The lymph vessels contain valves that prevent the backflow of lymph. Skeletal muscle action, respiratory movement, and

CRITICAL THINKING 9.2

Describe the flow of lymph until it reaches the circulatory system.

smooth muscle contractions in vessel walls help to move lymph through the vessels.

Lymphatic Organs. Lymphatic organs contain lymphocytes and other cells (e.g., macrophages [MACK roh fay jehs]) mixed in a framework of connective tissue fibers. These cells defend against invading pathogens in the body. Lymphatic organs include lymph nodes, tonsils, spleen, and thymus.

Lymph Nodes. As lymph moves through the vessels, it is filtered in the *lymph nodes* (also called *lymph glands*). The lymph nodes are small bean-shaped structures in the lymph vessels. The lymph nodes contain immune cells (lymphocytes and macrophages). These cells help fight infection by attacking and destroying pathogens carried in the lymph.

The afferent lymphatic vessel brings lymph to the lymph node (see Fig. 9.4). In the lymph node, pathogens, cancer cells, and damaged cells are filtered from the lymph. The lymph moves out of the lymph node through the efferent lymphatic vessel. The trapped debris is destroyed by phagocytosis. As the node fills with debris, it can become enlarged or swollen. It may become less efficient filtering debris; thus debris may be able to pass through the node and along to the next node.

There are hundreds of lymph nodes throughout the body. Most are grouped in clusters. The multiple clusters of lymph nodes form an effective filtering system to prevent the debris from entering the bloodstream. Fig. 9.5A shows major lymph nodes, including the cervical (SUR vi kuhl), axillary (AK suh ler ee), inguinal (ING gwuh nuhl), and popliteal (pop lih TEE uhl) lymph nodes.

VOCABULARY

chyle A mix of lymph and triglyceride fats that creates a milky fluid, which is taken up by the lacteals from the intestine and transported to the bloodstream via the thoracic duct.

debris The remains of anything broken down or destroyed; ruins, rubble.

lymph A clear, yellowish fluid containing white blood cells in a liquid similar to plasma. The fluid comes from the tissues of the body and is moved through the lymphatic vessels and the bloodstream.

macrophages Very large monocytes that grew in size once they migrated out of the bloodstream and lived in the tissues. Engulf foreign particles, microorganisms, and cell debris.

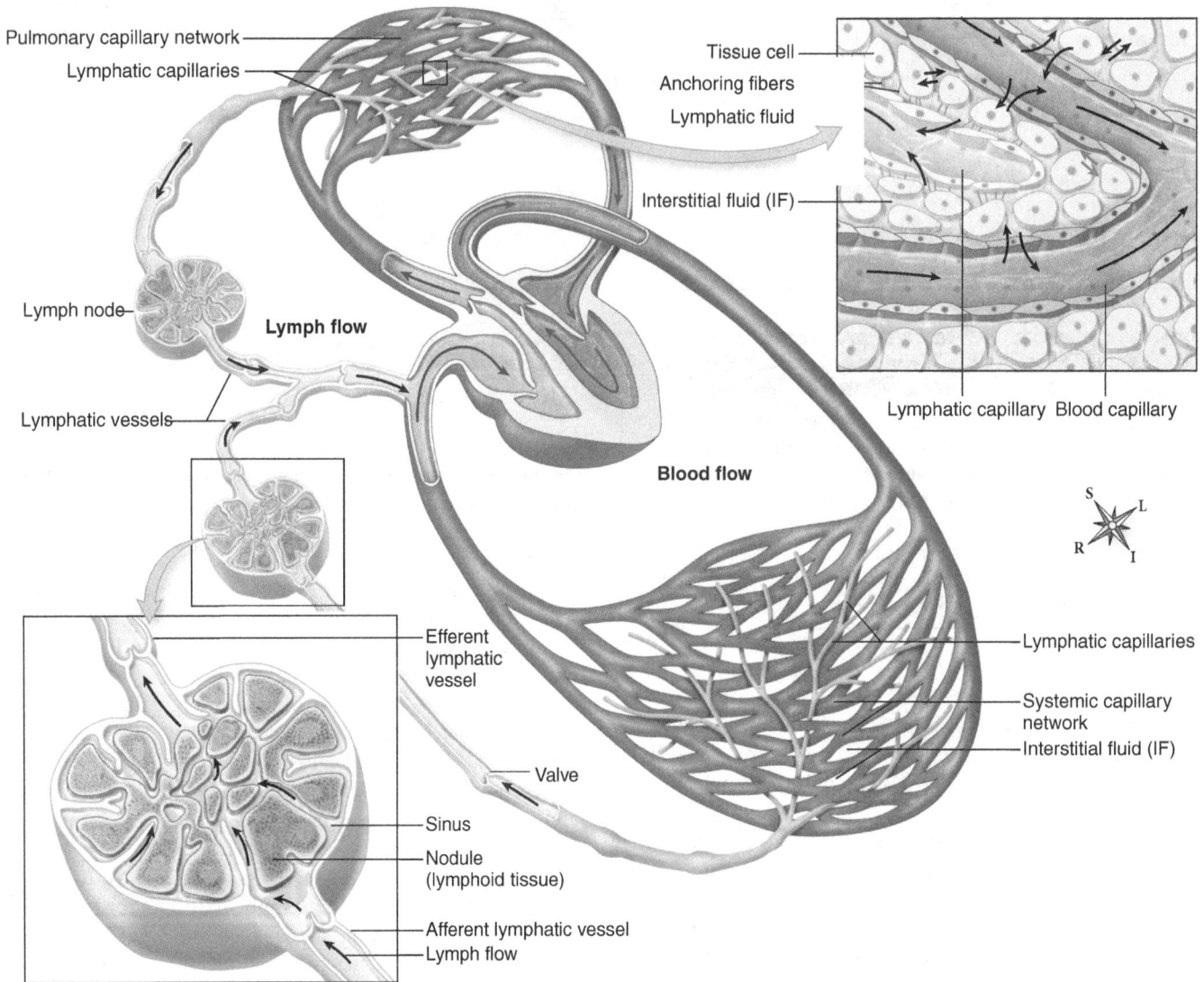

Fig. 9.4 Role of the Lymphatic System in Fluid Homeostasis. Fluid filtered from blood plasma that is not reabsorbed by blood vessels drains into lymphatic vessels. Lymphatic drainage prevents accumulation of too much tissue fluid. Lymph nodes and other lymphoid structures filter the lymphatic fluid before it is returned to the bloodstream. (From Patton KT, Thibodeau GA: *The human body in health and disease,* ed 7, St. Louis, 2018, Elsevier.)

Tonsils. Tonsils are clusters of lymphatic tissue. Three groups of tonsils are:

- *Pharyngeal tonsils* (fur IN jee ul TAHN suls): Also called *adenoids* (AD uh noyds). They are located near the nasopharynx (NAY zoh fair inks), which is the part of the throat (pharynx) behind the nasal cavity (Fig. 9.6). When these tonsils become enlarged, they can interfere with breathing.
- *Palatine tonsils* (PAL ah tyne TAHN suls): Found in the oropharynx (or oh FAIR inks), which is posterior to the mouth.
- *Lingual tonsils* (LING gwal TAHN suls): Located on the posterior aspect of the tongue.

Macrophages and lymphocytes in the tonsils provide protection against pathogens and harmful substances that may enter through the mouth and nose.

MEDICAL TERMINOLOGY	
axill/o	axilla, armpit
cervic/o	neck
inguin/o	groin
lymph/o, lymphat/o	lymph
lymphaden/o	lymph gland
lymphangi/o	lymph vessel
splen/o	spleen
thym/o	thymus
tonsill/o	tonsil
macro-	large
-itis	inflammation

Spleen. The spleen is the largest lymphatic organ. It is located in the upper left abdominal cavity, just beneath the diaphragm

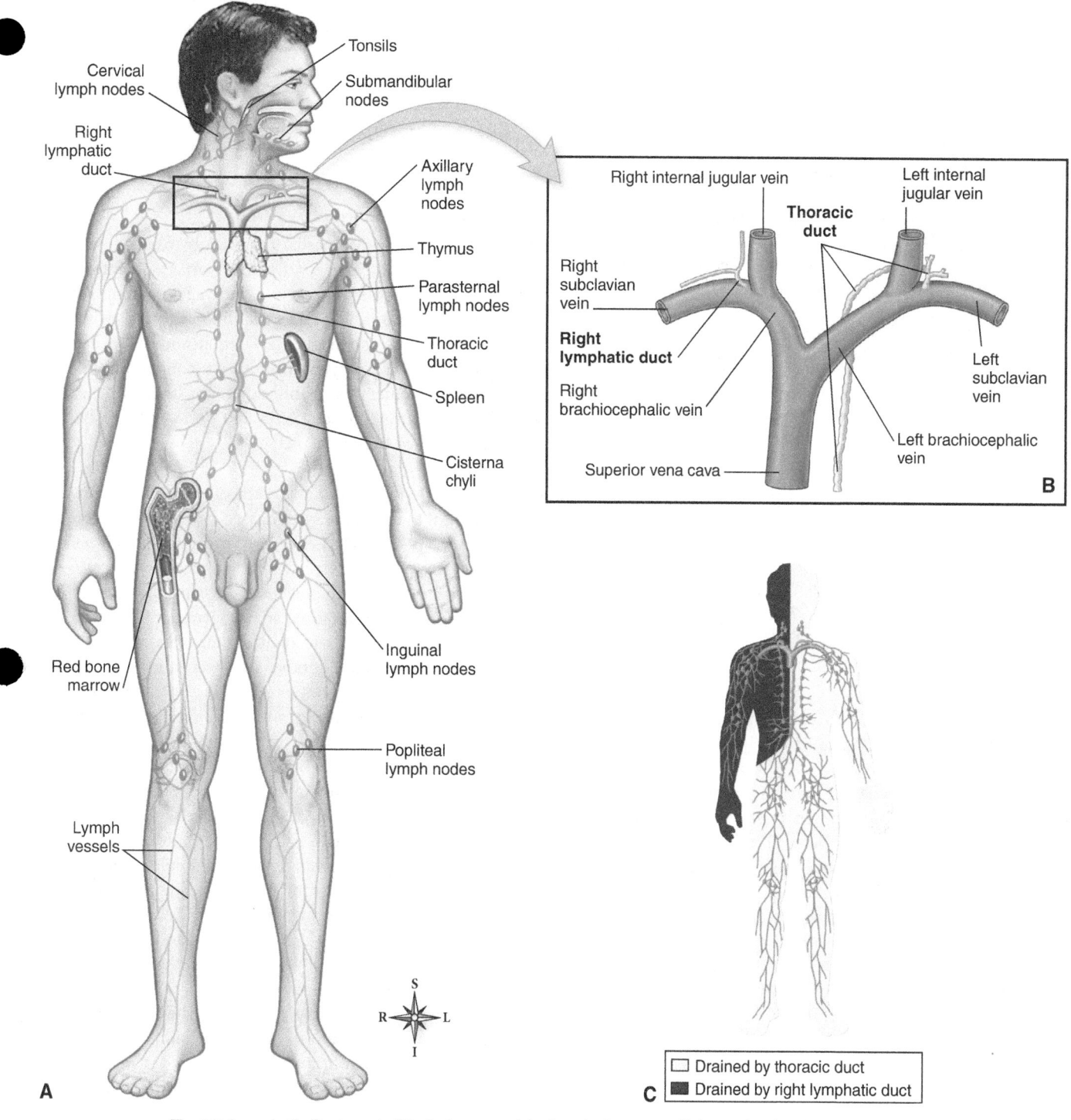

Fig. 9.5 Lymphatic System. A, Principal organs of the lymphatic system. B, Inset showing the major lymphatic ducts draining lymphatic fluid into veins, just before systemic blood is returned to the heart. C, Lymph drainage. The right lymphatic duct drains lymph from the upper right quarter of the body into the right subclavian vein at its junction with the internal jugular vein. The thoracic duct drains lymph from the rest of the body into the left subclavian vein at its junction with the internal jugular vein. (A and C from Patton KT, Thibodeau GA: *The human body in health and disease,* ed 7, St. Louis, 2018, Elsevier; **inset** from Drake RL et al: *Gray's anatomy for students,* ed 3, Philadelphia, 2015, Churchill-Livingstone.)

CRITICAL THINKING 9.3

Ryenn Ablesman is an 8-year-old girl who has been having some problems with a recurring sore throat and tonsillitis. Can you name the three types of tonsils in the nasopharynx?

and posterior to the stomach. The spleen consists of two types of pulp:

- White pulp, which is lymphatic tissue consisting mainly of lymphocytes around arteries.

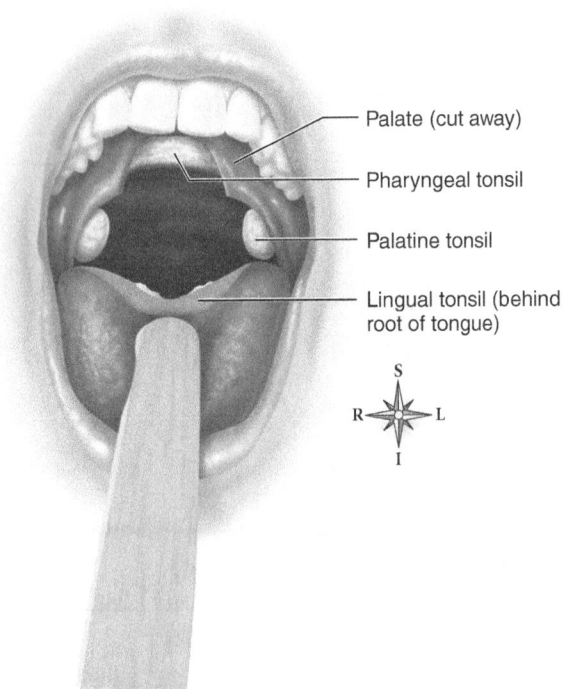

Palate (cut away)

Pharyngeal tonsil

Palatine tonsil

Lingual tonsil (behind
root of tongue)

Fig. 9.6 Location of Tonsils. Small segments of the roof and floor of
the mouth have been removed to show the protective ring of tonsils
(lymphoid tissue) around the internal opening of the nose and throat.
(From Patton KT, Thibodeau GA: *The human body in health and disease,*
ed 7, St. Louis, 2018, Elsevier.)

- Red pulp, which consists of venous sinuses filled with
  blood and cords of lymphatic cells (lymphocytes and
  macrophages).

Blood enters the spleen through the splenic artery. As it
moves through the venous sinuses, it is filtered. Blood leaves
the spleen through the splenic vein. The lymphocytes attempt
to destroy pathogens in the blood, and macrophages engulf the
resulting debris, damaged cells, and other large particles.

The sinuses in the spleen are reservoirs for blood. If a hemorrhage occurs, smooth muscles in the spleen contract, squeezing the blood into general circulation. Trauma or injury to the
spleen can cause life-threatening bleeding in the abdomen. A
splenectomy (surgical removal of the spleen) may be required to
stop the blood loss.

Thymus. The thymus has two lobes and is located anterior to
the ascending aorta and posterior to the sternum. The role of
the thymus is to produce and mature T lymphocytes (T cells).
The thymus produces *thymosin,* a hormone that stimulates the
maturation of lymphocytes in other lymphatic organs.

Mucosa-Associated Lymphoid Tissue. Lymphoid tissue is found
throughout the body. For instance, *mucosa-associated lymphoid
tissue* (MALT) is located throughout the mucosal lining in the
body. MALT initiates a response to the specific antigens that come
in contact with the mucosal surface. The Peyer patches within
the small intestine and the vermiform appendix are examples of

MALT. *Peyer patches* monitor intestinal bacteria populations and
prevent the growth of pathogenic bacteria in the intestines.

CRITICAL THINKING 9.4

Describe the lymphatic organs, including their role.

Anatomy of the Immune System

The immune system uses cells, tissues, organs, and proteins
throughout the body. These structures work as an interactive
network to identify and defend the body against antigens and
maintain homeostasis. Major structures involved with the
immune system include leukocytes, lymph nodes, tonsils, thymus, spleen, and lymphocytes. Immune system proteins include
cytokines, complements, and antibodies. The following sections
will address the immune structures and proteins that have not
yet been described in this chapter.

Lymphocytes. Lymphocytes are a type of white blood cells that
are also part of the immune system. Two main types of lymphocytes are B lymphocytes (B cells) and T lymphocytes (T cells).

B Lymphocytes. B lymphocytes are produced from stem cells
in the bone marrow. They migrate to the spleen and lymph nodes.
B cells are part of the acquired immune response, specifically
humoral immunity. B cells recognize pathogens (e.g., bacteria,
fungi, parasitic worms, and protozoans) circulating in the lymph
or blood. Once activated, they produce memory cells and also
plasma cells, which create specific antibodies in response to specific
antigens. The memory cells go to the lymph nodes and wait for
another occurrence of that specific antigen invasion. The plasma
cells create specific antibodies in response to specific antigens.

T Lymphocytes. T lymphocytes are produced and mature in the
thymus. After the T cells have matured, they enter the blood and
move to other lymphatic organs, such as the spleen and tonsils.
Four main types of T cells are involved with acquired immunity:

- *T helper cells*: Also known as *CD4+ T cells.* They help in
  B-cell activation, produce cytokines, and activate cytotoxic T cells.
- *Cytotoxic T cells*: Also known as *CD8+ cells.* They destroy
  virus-infected cells and tumor cells. They also can cause
  damage to or rejection of organ transplants. In addition,
  they can cause autoimmune diseases.
- *Memory T cells*: Rapidly multiply if an antigen is reexposed to the body.
- *Regulatory T cells*: Also known as *suppressor T cells.* They
  help shut down the immune response when the antigen
  has been destroyed. These T cells have an important role
  in suppressing autoimmune diseases.

CRITICAL THINKING 9.5

Why are memory cells so important in the immune system? Share your ideas
with the class.

Cytokines. *Cytokines* (SYE toh kynez) are small proteins secreted mainly by the T cells. Cytokines act as chemical messengers, interacting and communicating with other cells. They include interleukins, lymphokines, and cell signal molecules (e.g., tumor necrosis factor and interferons).

Complement System. *Complements* are enzymes (proteins) normally found in the blood plasma. The *complement system* is a group of about 60 proteins, 30 of which are circulating blood proteins that promote immune and inflammatory responses. The role of the complement system is to identify, destroy, and remove foreign antigens. The complement system works with the body's natural defenses. The complements work together in a cascadelike approach to activate and form protein rings that destroy bacteria and other microorganisms. They provide quick, nonspecific assistance to the immune system.

Rarely, a person may inherit a deficiency of some complement proteins. These people are prone to certain infections or autoimmune disorders.

Dendritic Cells. The dendritic cells are tree-shaped leukocytes that are formed in the bone marrow and circulate in the bloodstream. They are activated by pathogens and mature. They engulf pathogens and then migrate to the lymph nodes, where they present the antigen to T helper cells. Dendritic cells help activate T helper cells and memory cells.

Antibodies. Antibodies are proteins found in the blood or tissues. Antibodies are produced by the B lymphocytes (B cells) in the immune system. They are unique to certain antigens. Antibodies work in several different ways to rid the body of the antigens, including agglutination, dissolving antigens, and with the help of complements, rupturing cell walls.

Antibodies are also called *immunoglobulins* (IGs) and include:

- *IgG*: Mostly found in circulating blood and tissues. Crosses the placenta to the unborn baby. IgG provides the majority of antibody-based immunity.
- *IgM*: Produced early in the immune response before IgG.
- *IgA*: Found in the gastrointestinal, urinary, and respiratory systems. It is secreted in tears, saliva, and breast milk.
- *IgE*: Created in response to an allergic reaction and multicellular organisms (e.g., parasitic worms).
- *IgD*: Found in low levels in the serum. May interact with mast cells and basophils.

> **VOCABULARY**
> **genetic immunity** An inherited ability to resist certain diseases because of one's species, race, gender, or individual genetic makeup.
> **serum** The liquid portion of a clotted blood specimen. It no longer contains active clotting agents.

> **CRITICAL THINKING 9.6**
> Review the five immunoglobulins. Can you make a saying, word or rhyme that might help you remember them? Share your ideas with the class.

PHYSIOLOGY OF THE BLOOD, LYMPHATIC, AND IMMUNE SYSTEMS

Coagulation and Hemostasis

The process required to form a blood clot is complicated, with many specific chemical reactions and clotting factors involved. What follows is a simplified version of this process.

First, a damaged vessel will constrict to slow the flow of blood through the vessel. In response to the injury, platelets become sticky and clump together *(aggregation)*. Platelets then stick to the area of injury *(adhesion)*. Because of platelet aggregation and adhesion, a platelet plug is formed over the injury and platelets release clotting factors, which aid in the process of coagulation. The injured blood vessel tissue also activates clotting factors in the blood plasma. The interaction between the clotting factors works to form *fibrin*, a white, filamentous, tough protein strand that creates a netlike structure. The fibrin net traps red blood cells and more platelets to form a thrombus. This process is called *blood clotting* or *coagulation*. When the body stops the flow of blood through coagulation, the process is called *hemostasis*.

Immune System Response

The immune system is responsible for defending the body against antigens. The immune system must be able to tell the difference between foreign antigens and the body's own cells, which contain antigens (human leukocyte antigens [HLAs]). The immune system learns to see the HLA complexes as normal and thus does not react to them. The immune system has two responses to foreign antigens, the innate immune response and the acquired immune response.

Innate Immunity. Innate, or nonspecific, immunity is the defense system that a person is born with (genetic immunity). Innate immunity recognizes antigens and responds quickly to protect the body, but it lacks a memory of past exposures to antigens. The goals of the innate immune response are to contain the antigen and present the antigen to the acquired immune cells. Thus the innate response works closely with the acquired response.

The innate immunity consists of barrier mechanisms, chemical substances, and nonspecific immune responses. The first two lines of defenses in the body include nonspecific defenses (Fig. 9.7).

Barrier Mechanisms and Chemical Substances. The barrier mechanisms act to keep antigens out of the body. Barrier mechanisms include:

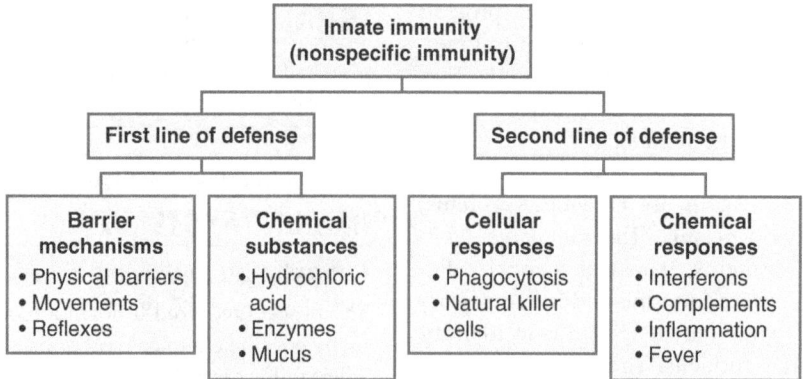

Fig. 9.7 Innate or Nonspecific Immunity.

- *Physical barriers*: Intact skin and the mucous membranes that line all organs that exit the body are natural physical barriers against pathogens. These tissues are hard to penetrate, and only a few pathogens can enter through intact skin and mucous membranes.
- *Movements*: Cilia (tiny hairs in the nose and bronchi) sweep or move particles out of the airway. Intestinal peristalsis (muscle movement in the intestines) moves pathogens out of the body (e.g., diarrhea). Sweat, urine, and tears also move pathogens out of the body or off the body surface.
- Reflexes: Coughing and sneezing help move particles and pathogens out of the airway.

Chemical substances such as hydrochloric acid in the stomach, enzymes (EN zahym) (e.g., lysozymes in tears and saliva), and mucus prevent antigens from entering the body tissues. Barrier mechanisms and chemical substances are considered the first line of defense in the body.

VOCABULARY

intact Complete or whole. Not altered; unbroken.

reflexes Movements or processes caused by a reflex response. A reflex is an automatic response; it does not require thought.

CRITICAL THINKING 9.7

What are the barrier mechanisms and chemical substances that make up the first line of defense? Write your answer down, briefly describing each one in your own words. Share your answers with your classmates.

Nonspecific Immune Responses. The second line of defense in the body involves cellular and chemical responses.

- Cellular responses:
  - *Phagocytosis* (fag oh sye TOH sis): The process by which a cell attaches to a pathogen, particle, or other cell and then ingests and destroys it (Fig. 9.8). Neutrophils and monocytes, which turn into macrophages, are aggressive phagocytic cells. Each of these stages must take place to successfully destroy the foreign invader:
    1. *Chemotaxis* (KEE moh tak sis): The movement of phagocytic cells towards a potential threat to the body in response to a chemical signal or stimulus.

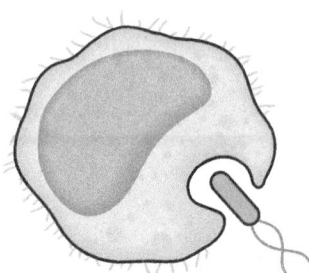

Fig. 9.8 Phagocytosis.

2. *Attachment*: After locating the potential threat, the phagocytic cell must attach to it, so it does not get away.
3. *Ingestion*: The phagocytic cell extends its cell membrane around and engulfs the potential threat.
4. *Digestion*: Enzymes in the phagocytic cell digest or destroy the potential threat.
- *Natural killer* (NK) *cells:* A type of lymphocyte that kills cells that have been infected by certain viruses and cancer cells. NK cells are derived from stem cells in the bone marrow and are concentrated in the liver and lungs.
- Chemical responses:
  - *Interferons* (in tur FEER ons): Protective proteins that disrupt viral replication and limit a virus's ability to damage cells.
  - *Complements*: Protective enzymes in the blood that activate and create protein rings that work with antibodies to destroy pathogens.
  - *Inflammation* (in fluh MEY shuhn): During this response, the blood vessels dilate (*vasodilation*) and blood carries neutrophils to the site of injury. Capillary walls become more permeable (PUR mee uh buhl), and the granular cells squeeze through to the site of infection. Once at the site of infection or injury, the neutrophils engulf the invading microorganism. The collection of WBCs, dead WBCs, bacteria, and tissue cells creates *pus* at the site of infection. The increase in blood flow to the area causes heat and *erythema* (redness). The vascular permeability causes swelling and pain. If the swelling becomes too much for the area, movement may become limited. Thus heat, redness, swelling, and pain are important signs and

symptoms of inflammation. Besides local inflammation, systemic inflammation may occur from the response of inflammation mediators (e.g., cytokines). This can cause a fever.

- Fever or *pyrexia* (pye RECK see uh): Most pathogens survive at the body temperature. When the temperature is increased, they are not able to survive. A fever also increases the action of phagocytes.

VOCABULARY

permeable A substance or structure that can be passed through, especially by liquids or gases.

replication The production of exact copies of a complex molecule, such as DNA.

CRITICAL THINKING 9.8

Mia needs to change a dressing on a patient's infected wound today. Robert Harrison has an abrasion that became infected. It is red and a little swollen, and there is pus at the margins of the wound. What is pus? Write down a definition in your own words and be ready to share it with the class.

Acquired Immunity. Acquired immunity (also called *specific* or *adaptive immunity*) is the third line of defense used by the body. Acquired immunity creates specific immunity against each pathogen. During the first exposure to the pathogen, the body fights off the antigen. The person may experience disease signs and symptoms as the body fights the antigen. If the person has a second exposure to the antigen, the immune memory kicks in and the person gets minimal or no symptoms. Acquired immunity is slow to act with the initial exposure, but with each recurring exposure, the response becomes quicker and stronger.

Two main types of immunity within the acquired immune system are humoral immunity and cell-mediated immunity (Fig. 9.9). These types of immunity will be discussed in the following sections.

Humoral Immunity. Humoral immunity, also called *antibody-mediated immunity*, involves the production of B lymphocytes (B cells) and antibodies. The humoral response is very complex. The following steps summarize the response.

1. Immature B cells bind to antigens in the body fluid. This binding action, along with interleukins or cytokines released from the T helper cells, activates B cells.
2. Activated B cells mature and multiply, producing plasma cells and memory cells.
   - Plasma cells produce antibodies rapidly and efficiently. The antibodies are specific to the antigen that activated the B cells. They are released and circulate through the body, binding to that specific antigen, which forms antibody-antigen complexes. These complexes signal neutrophils to come and destroy them. Neutrophils engulf the complexes and destroy the antigen.
   - Memory cells stay in the immune system and can recognize the same antigen if it ever invades the body again. They can quickly produce antibodies anytime in the future.

Cell-Mediated Immunity. The cell-mediated response involves T cells, which are responsible for destroying cells infected with antigens (e.g., viruses) and abnormal body cells, such as cancerous cells and transplanted tissues. Cell-mediated immunity is also a complex response. The following points summarize the response.

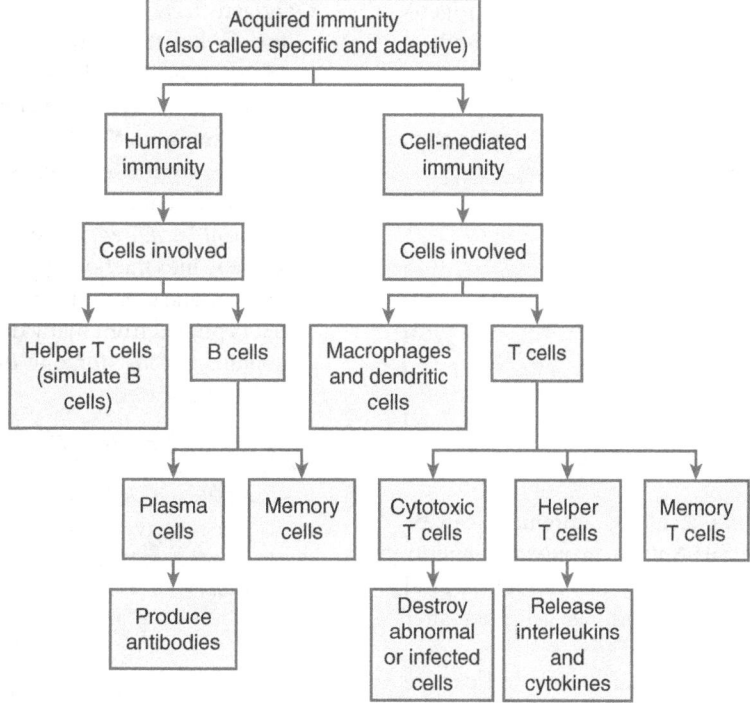

Fig. 9.9 Acquired Immunity.

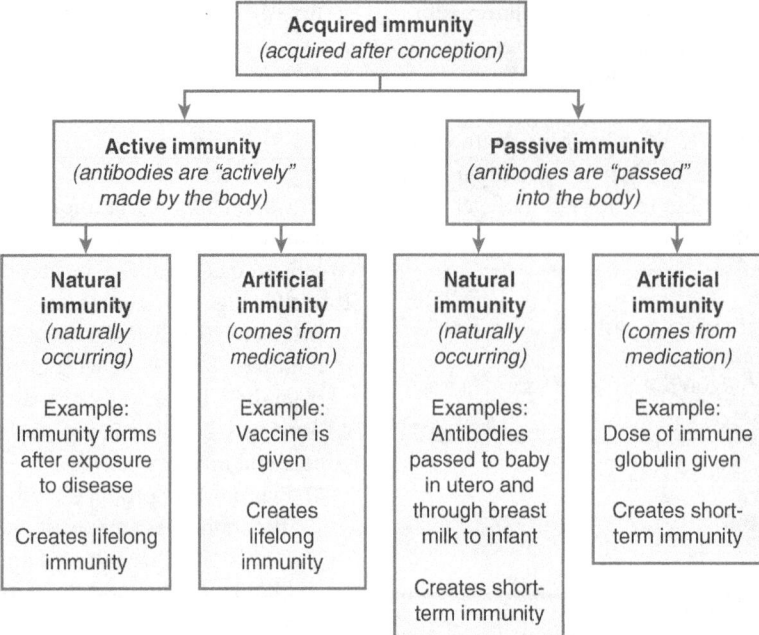

Fig. 9.10 Types of Acquired Immunity.

1. An antigen invades a host, and *chemokines* (a type of cytokines) are released from the infected cell. The chemokines initiate the immune response and warn neighboring cells of the threat.
2. A macrophage or dendritic cell engulfs and digests the infected cells. The macrophage or dendritic cell then presents the antigen to the T cells.
3. T cells bind to the antigen, and interleukin is secreted, which activates the T cells.
4. Activated T cells multiple and produce:
   - *Cytotoxic T cells*, which find cells displaying the antigen and release enzymes into the cell. The enzymes destroy the cell membrane, causing cell death. The antigens in the cell are then exposed to circulating antibodies, and the humoral response takes over to destroy the antigen.
   - *T helper cells*, which release interleukins and cytokines.
   - *Memory T cells,* which rapidly multiply if an antigen is reexposed to the body.

MEDICAL TERMINOLOGY	
humor/o	liquid
cyto-	cell
-al	pertaining to
-exia	condition
-osis	abnormal condition

Types of Acquired Immunity. Acquired immunity can be described as natural or artificial. *Natural acquired immunity* occurs "naturally" through the course of life without medical intervention. *Artificial acquired immunity* is achieved after receiving medications.

Acquired immunity can be classified as active and passive (Fig. 9.10). With *active immunity*, the body is exposed to the antigen and the body "actively" produces the antibodies. This type of immunity is slow to start working, but it can last a lifetime. With *passive immunity*, antibodies (immune globulin or immunoglobulins) are "passed" into the body and the body does not need to make them. This type of immunity works quickly, but it is short acting (weeks to about 3 months). Examples of acquired immunity include:

- *Natural acquired active immunity*: A person is exposed to a disease. and the body "actively" produces antibodies for protection.
- *Artificial acquired active immunity*: A person receives a vaccine that contains antigens for a specific disease. The antigens have been altered so that they cannot cause the disease, but the body will "actively" make antibodies to protect against the disease.
- *Natural acquired passive immunity*: Antibodies are passed from the mother to the unborn baby in utero. Another example are the antibodies that are passed in the breast milk to the baby.
- *Artificial acquired passive immunity*: Antibodies are "passed" into the body by an injection of immune globulin. Immune globulin comes from donated blood plasma that is pooled from many donors. Some types of immune globulin are just for one disease, whereas others cover multiple diseases.

CRITICAL THINKING 9.9

Rich and Jan Dallman have an appointment to see Dr. Walden today. They both want to get the shingles vaccine. Mia prepares their vaccinations and then sits down with Rich and Jan to go over the Vaccine Information Statement (VIS), which discusses the vaccine. What type of immunity is a vaccination, active or passive? Is it natural or artificial? Discuss your answers with the class.

Hypersensitivity. *Hypersensitivity* (hahy per SEN si tiv ih tee) is an exaggerated or inappropriate immune response to a specific antigen. The response causes harmful effects on the body tissue. There are four types of hypersensitivity reactions.

- *Type I* or *anaphylactic response*: Considered an immediate allergic reaction. IgE antibodies produced in response to the antigen bind with mast cells and basophils, causing histamines to be released. Histamines cause inflammatory and other allergic signs and symptoms. Type I hypersensitivity reactions can be seen with allergic rhinitis, dermatitis, and conjunctivitis. The most severe and life-threatening type I hypersensitivity reactions can cause asthma, food allergies, and anaphylaxis (an uh fuh LAK sis). Common triggers for type I hypersensitivity reactions include:
  - Drugs, such as penicillin and cephalosporins
  - Food allergies (e.g., tree nuts, peanuts, milk, eggs, and shellfish)
  - Latex, insect venom, and environmental allergies (e.g., dust mites, animal dander, pollens)
- *Type II* or *cytotoxic-mediated response*: Causes damage to the body's own tissues. IgG and IgM antibodies cause a cytotoxic response by activating the complement system and phagocytes. This can cause autoimmune conditions, such as rheumatic fever, autoimmune hemolytic anemia, Graves disease, hemolytic disease of the fetus and newborn, and idiopathic thrombocytopenic purpura (ITP).
- *Type III* or *immunocomplex reaction*: Causes inflammation and tissue damage. IgG and IgM antibodies react with antigens, forming antigen-antibody complexes. The complement system and the neutrophils become active, leading to tissue damage, such as vasculitis and glomerulonephritis. Type III hypersensitivity reactions can be seen with serum sickness, poststreptococcal glomerulonephritis, and systemic lupus erythematosus (SLE).
- *Type IV* or *cell-mediated hypersensitivity*: A delayed response caused by a cell-mediated response. This response occurs 24 to 72 hours after the exposure to the antigen. Conditions related to type IV hypersensitivity include transplant rejection, contact dermatitis, Stevens-Johnson syndrome, graft-versus-host disease, multiple sclerosis, and rheumatoid arthritis. The tuberculin skin test (TST) is also an example of this hypersensitivity response.

VOCABULARY

anaphylaxis A rapidly progressing, life-threatening allergic reaction; characterized by hives, swelling of the mouth and airway, difficulty breathing, wheezing, and loss of consciousness.

glomerulonephritis A kidney disease affecting the glomeruli of the nephron. Characterized by albumin in the urine, edema, and high blood pressure.

purpura A condition characterized by hemorrhages in the tissues, causing the appearance of purplish spots.

CRITICAL THINKING 9.10

- What type of hypersensitivity is hemolytic disease of the newborn (HDN)?
- What type of hypersensitivity is anaphylaxis?
- What type of hypersensitivity is delayed hypersensitivity?

DISEASES AND DISORDERS OF THE BLOOD, LYMPHATIC, AND IMMUNE SYSTEMS

Diseases and Disorders of the Blood

Common signs and symptoms of blood disorders include:
- Fatigue, weakness, pale skin, lightheadedness, and shortness of breath (SOB)
- Bruising and bleeding
- Fever and weight loss
- A deficiency in WBCs (*leukopenia* [LOO koe PEE nee ah]) or an elevated number of WBCs (*leukocytosis* [LOO koe sie TOE sis])
- A deficiency of RBCs (anemia) or an elevated number of RBCs (*erythrocytosis* [e RITH roe sie TOE sis])
- A deficiency of platelets (*thrombocytopenia* [THROM boh SIE to pee nee ah]) or an elevated number of platelets (*thrombocytosis* [THROM boe sie TOE sis])

Common diagnostic tests for blood diseases are similar to those used for immune and lymphatic system diseases. Table 9.3 describes the diagnostic tests. The following sections describe blood disorders.

Anemia. Anemia is a common blood disorder. It occurs when the blood does not have enough healthy red blood cells or enough hemoglobin, which carries oxygen to the rest of the body. Table 9.4 presents the types of anemia, along with their etiologies and treatments.

Signs and Symptoms. Signs and symptoms include weakness, fatigue, pale skin, arrhythmias, SOB, dizziness, lightheadedness, cold hands and feet, headache, and chest pain.

Diagnostic Procedures. A physical exam and a complete blood count (CBC) will be done. Additional tests may be done to rule out or confirm the type of anemia.

Hemophilia. Hemophilia is a genetic bleeding disorder that can lead to spontaneous bleeding. There are two types of hemophilia:
- Hemophilia A, or classic hemophilia: Caused by a lack of or decrease in clotting factor VIII.
- Hemophilia B, or Christmas disease: Caused by a lack of or decrease in clotting factor IX.

About 20,000 males in the United States live with the disorder.

Etiology. Hemophilia is caused by a mutation on a gene that provides information to make clotting factor proteins needed for making a blood clot. Because the mutation is on the X chromosome, a male with the mutation will have the disease. A female must have two X chromosomes with the mutation to have the disease. She will be a carrier of hemophilia if she just has one X chromosome with the mutation.

Signs and Symptoms. Signs and symptoms include bleeding within the joints, skin, mouth, nose, and gums. Blood can be in the urine or stool. Bleeding can occur after surgery or injury. Complications include chronic joint disease and pain, seizures, paralysis, and possibly death.

Diagnostic Procedures. If hemophilia runs in the family, the provider will test the male newborn. Blood clotting tests are performed, and if the results are abnormal, clotting factor tests (factor assays) will be done.

TABLE 9.3 Common Medical Laboratory Tests Used for Blood, Lymphatic, and Immune Disorders

Procedure	Description
Antinuclear antibody (ANA) test	Also known as *fluorescent antinuclear antibody* (FANA) and *antinuclear antibody screen*. A blood test that detects antibodies to the nucleus or parts of the nucleus of cells. Used to detect and diagnose autoimmune disorders.
Autoantibody tests	Detects antibodies that mistakenly target healthy tissue.
Complement blood test	Measures the amount of active complement proteins in the blood.
Complete blood count (CBC)	A group of tests that evaluate RBCs, WBCs, and platelets (PLTs). Includes RBC count, hemoglobin, hematocrit, RBC indices, WBC count and diff, platelet count. CLIA-waived tests are available.
Comprehensive metabolic panel (CMP)	Also known as *chemistry 14, chem 14, chemistry panel,* and *chemistry screen.* A group of 14 tests. Includes kidney and liver tests and measures glucose, calcium, proteins, and electrolytes. Some CLIA-waived tests are available.
C-reactive protein (CRP)	A blood test for a nonspecific indicator of inflammation. CRP is produced in the liver and increases with inflammation in the body. Some CLIA-waived tests are available.
Erythrocyte sedimentation rate (ESR) (eh RITH roh syte seh dih men TAY shun)	Also known as *sed rate, sedimentation rate, Westergren sedimentation rate,* and *Wintrobe sedimentation rate.* A test that measures the time required for mature RBCs to settle out of a blood sample after an anticoagulant has been added. Used to detect the presence of inflammation. Some CLIA-waived tests are available.
Hematocrit (Hct) (hee MAT oh krit)	Measure of the percentage of RBCs in a blood sample. Some CLIA-waived tests are available.
Hemoglobin (Hgb) (HEE moh gloh bin)	Measure of iron-containing pigment in RBCs. Some CLIA-waived tests are available.
Hemoglobin electrophoresis (ih lek troh fuh REE sis)	A blood test that can separate different types of hemoglobin using an electric current and gel media. Useful for diagnosing hemophilia and thalassemia.
Immunoglobulin blood test	A blood test that measures the amount of IgG, IgM, and IgA.
Mean corpuscular hemoglobin (MCH) (kor US kyoo lur)	Test to measure the average weight of hemoglobin per RBC.
Mean corpuscular hemoglobin concentration (MCHC)	Test to measure the concentration of hemoglobin in RBCs.
Monospot	Used to check for antibodies to Epstein-Barr virus in a blood sample. Used to diagnose infectious mononucleosis. Some CLIA-waived tests are available.
Partial thromboplastin time (PTT) or activated partial thromboplastin time (aPTT)	The PTT/aPTT measures the number of seconds it takes for a clot form after regents are added to the blood sample. Used to diagnose and monitor bleeding disorders and heparin anticoagulant therapy.
Prothrombin time and international normalized ration (PT/INR)	A prothrombin time (PT) measures the number of seconds it takes a clot to form after reagents are added to the blood sample. The PT is used to detect bleeding disorders or excessive clotting disorders. The INR is calculated based on the PT and used to monitor patients taking anticoagulants. CLIA-waived tests are available.
White blood cell (WBC) differential	Also known as *diff, blood differential, leukocyte differential count, peripheral differential,* and *differential count.* A measure of the different types of WBCs. Helps to identify the cause of an abnormal WBC count. Use to monitor different conditions and diagnose infections and cancers.
Urinalysis	A urine test that evaluates different components of the urine. Some CLIA-waived tests are available.

CLIA, Clinical Laboratory Improvement Amendments.

Treatments. Treatment consists of infusing commercially prepared factor concentrates as prophylaxis (prevention) or when bleeding occurs.

Idiopathic Thrombocytopenic Purpura. Idiopathic thrombocytopenic purpura is also called *immune thrombocytopenia* and *immune thrombocytopenic purpura.* ITP is a rare autoimmune disease that results in the destruction of platelets.

Etiology. The immune system produces antibodies that destroy platelets, thus causing ITP. In children, ITP sometimes occurs after a viral infection. In adults, ITP is a chronic disease that can occur after a viral infection, pregnancy, or infection with *Helicobacter pylori.*

Signs and Symptoms. This disease can cause abnormally heavy menses, petechial rash (a rash with pinpoint red spots), easy bruising, nosebleeds, or bleeding (Fig. 9.12).

Diagnostic Procedures. After the physical exam, the provider will order a CBC to check the patient's platelet level and a platelet antibodies blood test. A biopsy or bone marrow aspiration may also be done.

Treatments. Treatment for adults consists of steroids and immunosuppressant medications, high-dose immune globulin infusions, drugs to stimulate the bone marrow, and a splenectomy.

Leukemia. Leukemia is cancer of the blood-forming tissues, such as the bone marrow and the lymphatic system (Fig. 9.13). The bone marrow produces abnormal white blood cells. Leukemia is classified as either acute or chronic. The secondary classification of leukemia is the type of white blood cell affected by the disease. Table 9.5 describes different types of leukemia with the signs and symptoms.

TABLE 9.4   Types of Anemia

Type	Description	Etiology	Treatment
Aplastic anemia	Rare, life-threatening condition; the body does not produce enough red blood cells (RBCs)	Caused by infections, certain medications, exposure to toxic chemicals, and autoimmune disorders	Blood transfusions, stem cell transplantation, immunosuppressant medications, and bone marrow stimulants
Hemolytic anemia	Early destruction of RBCs occurs; bone marrow is not making enough RBCs to replace the destroyed RBCs	Autoimmune disorder, genetic RBC defect, infection, blood clots	Blood transfusions and treat the cause
Iron-deficiency anemia	Most common form; not enough iron to make RBCs	Heavy menstrual periods, intestinal disease (e.g., Crohn disease, cancer), use of aspirin, ibuprofen, or arthritis medication, ulcers; not enough dietary iron	Iron supplements or iron medications
Sickle cell anemia	Inherited disorder that causes the RBCs to form a sickle (crescent) shape, get stuck in the blood vessels, and break apart (Fig. 9.11)	Caused by a defective form of hemoglobin (hemoglobin S)	Manage and control the symptoms to prevent crises; folic acid supplements; blood transfusions, pain medications, and fluids during crisis
Thalassemia	Inherited condition causing an abnormal form or inadequate amount of hemoglobin	Genetic condition	Blood transfusions and folate supplements
Vitamin B_{12}–deficiency anemia	A low RBC count due to a lack of vitamin B_{12}	Lack of dietary B_{12}, chronic alcoholism, Crohn disease, bariatric surgery, antacids	Depends on the cause; vitamin B_{12} supplements or monthly injections of vitamin B_{12}
Pernicious anemia	A type of vitamin B_{12}–deficiency anemia	Body destroys the cells that make intrinsic factor, which absorbs dietary vitamin B_{12} in the intestine	Monthly injections of vitamin B_{12}

A   Normal red blood cells (RBCs)

B   RBCs in sickle cell disease

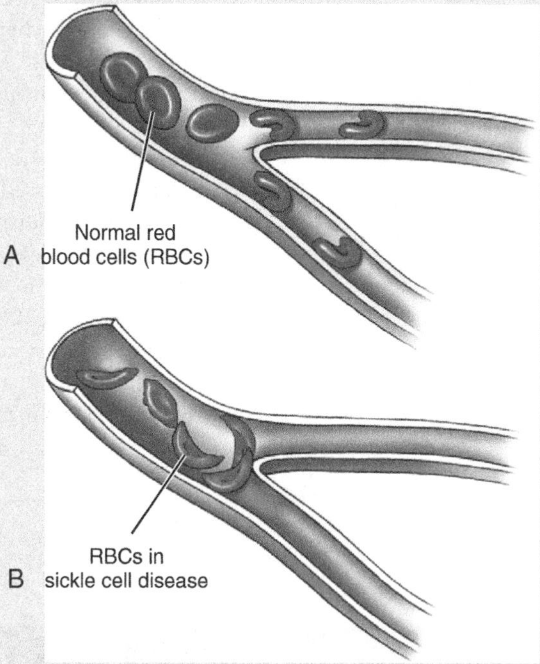

Fig. 9.11 Sickle Cells. (From Herlihy B, Maebius NK: *The human body in health and illness*, ed 4, Philadelphia, 2011, Saunders.)

Etiology. The exact cause of leukemia is unknown, but scientists believe it is a combination of genetics and environmental factors. Risk factors for leukemia include prior cancer treatments, genetic disorders, exposure to certain chemicals, family history of leukemia, and a history of smoking.

Diagnostic Procedures. After the physical examination, a CBC will be ordered. A specific type of WBC will be elevated, depending on the type of leukemia. A bone marrow biopsy may also be done.

Treatments. Treatment for acute leukemia is more aggressive and consists of chemotherapy, radiation, and in some cases a splenectomy. With chronic leukemia, as the disease worsens, the patient may receive chemotherapy and radiation. Biological therapy can also be used for leukemia. It boosts the body's natural ability to fight cancer. In addition, targeted therapy may be used, which uses substances that fight cancer cells but do not harm normal cells.

Additional Blood Disorders. The following are additional blood disorders.

- *Hemolytic disease of the fetus and newborn* (HDFN): Also called *erythroblastosis fetalis* and *hemolytic disease of the*

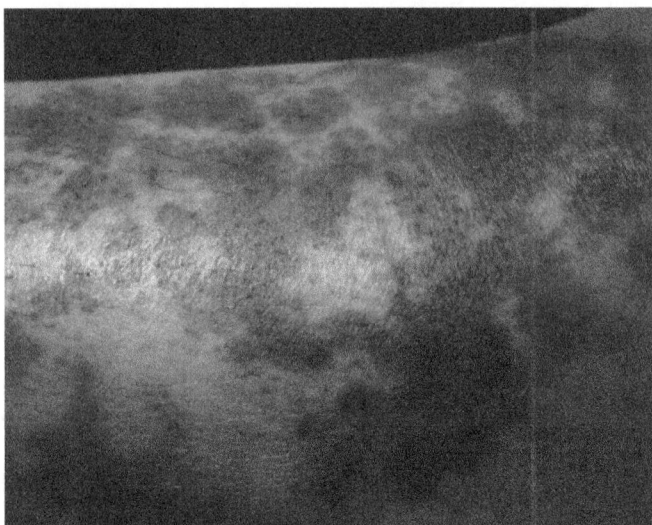

Fig. 9.12 Purpura. (From Bolognia JL: *Dermatology*, ed 2, St. Louis, 2008, Mosby.)

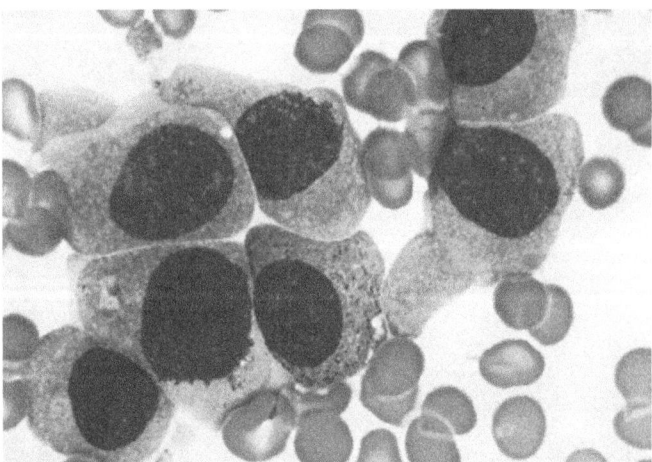

Fig. 9.13 Microscope Slide of Leukemia. (From Damjanov I: *Anderson's pathology*, ed 10, St. Louis, 2000, Mosby.)

newborn (HDN). A mismatch between the fetus and the mother involving the Rh factor can cause hemolytic disease of the newborn. The RBCs in the baby's blood to break down at a faster rate. (See Chapter 14 for more information.)

- *Polycythemia vera:* A bone marrow disorder characterized by an increased number of red blood cells in the bloodstream. The number of WBCs and platelets may also be higher than normal.
- *Von Willebrand disease:* Most common inherited bleeding disorder in the United States. Affects both males and females. An inherited condition that results when the blood lacks functioning von Willebrand factor, a protein that helps blood clot.

Diseases and Disorders of the Immune System

The immune system can cause either an underactive or overactive immune response. With an overactive immune response (autoimmune disorders), the immune system cannot tell the difference between healthy tissue and potentially harmful antigens. Thus the immune system mistakenly attacks and destroys the healthy tissue. The exact cause of most autoimmune disorders is unknown. Some experts believe viruses, bacteria, or a drug may trigger the change in the immune system. This may occur more often when a person has a family history of autoimmune disorders. Common signs and symptoms of immune system disorders include fatigue, fever, malaise (mah LAZE), joint pain, and rash.

There are over 80 autoimmune disorders. Many autoimmune disorders are discussed in other chapters:

- Skeletal system disorder: Rheumatoid arthritis (ROO mah toyd arth RYE tis) (RA) (see Chapter 3)
- Muscular system disorder: Myasthenia gravis (mye ah STHEE nee ah GRAV us) (see Chapter 4)
- Integumentary system disorder: Psoriasis (sohr EYE ah sis) (see Chapter 5)
- Nervous system disorder: Multiple sclerosis (MS) (see Chapter 6)

VOCABULARY

malaise A feeling of general discomfort

TABLE 9.5	**Types of Leukemia**	
Type	**Description**	**Signs and Symptoms**
Acute lymphocytic leukemia (ALL)	Also called *acute lymphoblastic leukemia;* most common cause of cancer in children. Causes an increase in large, immature lymphocytes (lymphoblasts).	Weakness, fever, bleeding, shortness of breath, and weight loss; bone, stomach, or rib pain; painless lumps in the underarm, neck, and stomach.
Acute myeloid leukemia (AML)	Also called *acute myelogenous leukemia*. Most common type of acute leukemia in adults. Causes an elevated level of *myeloblasts* (immature cells of the bone marrow).	Fever, shortness of breath, bleeding, bruising, tiredness, weight loss.
Chronic lymphocytic leukemia (CLL)	Second most common type of leukemia in adults. Occurs during middle age. A slow-growing cancer that causes a gradual increase in B lymphocytes. Affects the lymph nodes, liver, and spleen. Eventually the bone marrow's function declines.	May not have symptoms. If present, may have painless swelling in the lymph nodes in the neck, stomach, groin, or underarm; fatigue, rib pain, fever, infection, and weight loss.
Chronic myeloid leukemia (CML)	Also called *chronic granulocytic* or *chronic myelogenous leukemia*. A slow-growing cancer that causes an increase in myeloblasts. An elevated level of myeloblasts can cause a decrease in RBCs and platelets.	May not have symptoms. If present, may have fatigue, fever, rib pain, night sweats, and weight loss.

- Endocrine system disorders: Addison disease, Graves disease, Hashimoto thyroiditis, and type 1 diabetes (see Chapter 7)
- Cardiovascular system disorder: Pernicious (pur NIH shush) anemia (see Chapter 10)
- Digestive system disorders: Celiac disease and inflammatory bowel disease (IBD) (see Chapter 12)

Autoimmune Vasculitis. Autoimmune vasculitis causes inflammation and swelling of blood vessels. The walls of the blood vessels can thicken, narrow, scar, or weaken with this disease. Autoimmune vasculitis can affect one organ or many organs. There are several types of autoimmune vasculitis, though they are rare.

Etiology. This is an autoimmune disorder. The immune system attacks the blood vessels.

Signs and Symptoms. Signs and symptoms include:
- Fever, fatigue, weight loss, headache, and achiness
- Night sweats and numbness or weakness

The other signs and symptoms can vary, depending on the type of autoimmune vasculitis the person has.

Diagnostic Procedures. Blood tests (e.g., C-reactive protein), urine tests, and imaging tests are used to diagnose autoimmune vasculitis. Angiography and a biopsy can also be done.

Treatments. Treatment is focused on controlling the inflammation and resolving the disease triggering the condition. Corticosteroids, such as prednisone, and other medications are given to help control inflammation. Surgery may be required to treat aneurysms.

Dermatomyositis. Dermatomyositis is an autoimmune condition that causes skin changes and muscle weakness. It is most common in adults between the ages of 40 and 60.

Etiology. The cause of dermatomyositis is unknown. It may be related to genetics and environmental factors.

Signs and Symptoms. Signs and symptoms include:
- A red skin rash around the eyelids and discolored skin on the shoulders, neck, and upper back
- Red bumps around the joints, joint pain
- Muscle weakness in the arms and legs that gets worse over time and can lead to stiff joints and muscle wasting

Diagnostic Procedures. The provider will complete a history and physical exam. A microscopic examination of a skin biopsy and a muscle tissue biopsy are used to diagnose this condition.

Treatments. Treatment is focused on managing the symptoms. Medications, such as corticosteroids and immunosuppressant medications, are prescribed. Physical therapy and daily exercises can help to reduce the muscle weakness and wasting.

Acquired Immunodeficiency Syndrome. The human immunodeficiency virus (HIV) causes acquired immunodeficiency syndrome (AIDS). Having HIV is a chronic condition. The HIV attacks the blood cells, CD4 cells (T helper cells). Over time the immune system becomes so weak, due to the virus, that the person develops AIDS. The person is also at risk for life-threatening opportunistic infections and cancer, such as Kaposi sarcoma.

Etiology. The cause of AIDS is HIV. The virus is spread from person to person through certain body fluids. Contaminated blood, semen, preseminal fluid, breast milk, vaginal fluids, and rectal fluids can spread HIV to another person if they come in contact with mucous membranes or damaged tissue or are injected into the bloodstream. Most often, HIV is spread through vaginal or anal sex and through needle sharing. It can also be spread from mother to baby and through needle sticks in healthcare.

Signs and Symptoms. When people are first infected with HIV, they may have no symptoms, or they may experience:
- Fever, muscle pains, sore throat, headache
- Mouth sores, thrush, swollen lymph glands, and diarrhea

This stage of the infection can last up to several months before the person becomes asymptomatic. The asymptomatic stage can last for 10 years or longer. During this time, the infected person can spread the virus to others.

Treating HIV can help delay the onset of AIDS for 10 to 20 years. Without treatment, the onset of AIDS can occur within a few years after infection with HIV. Signs and symptoms of AIDS can include weight loss, sweats, rashes, swollen lymph glands, and fever. Opportunistic infections and cancers can also be seen.

Diagnostic Procedures. The testing regimen for HIV is a two-step process. There are several screening tests, with some using blood and others using saliva. These tests check for antibodies to the HIV virus, HIV antigen, or both. CLIA-waived kits are available for home use, but their results should be confirmed by laboratory tests. The second test is a confirmatory test, such as the enzyme-linked immunosorbent assay (ELISA) and Western blot testing.

The CD4 cell count is monitored in patients with HIV. As the HIV damage to the immune system increases, the CD4 count drops. When the CD4 count drops below 200, the person is said to have AIDS.

Treatments. Treatment consists of antiretroviral therapy (ART). ART is typically started with the person is diagnosed with the HIV infection. Providers typically encourage the patient to join a support group for information and emotional support.

> **VOCABULARY**
> **opportunistic** A microorganism that causes disease only in a person with a lowered resistance.

Sjögren Syndrome. Sjögren syndrome is an autoimmune disorder that destroys the lacrimal glands (tear glands) and the salivary glands. This disorder can also affect other parts of the body, such as the lungs and kidneys.

Primary Sjögren syndrome causes dry eyes and dry mouth without any other autoimmune disorders. Secondary Sjögren syndrome occurs with another autoimmune disorder, such as rheumatoid arthritis or scleroderma.

Etiology. The cause of Sjögren syndrome is unknown. This autoimmune disorder most often occurs in females between the ages of 40 and 50.

Signs and Symptoms. Dry eyes and dry mouth are the most common symptoms of Sjögren syndrome. The eyes may feel itchy. The person may have difficulty swallowing, thick saliva, mouth sores, dental decay, hoarseness, and a loss of taste. Additional signs and symptoms include:

- Fatigue, fever, nausea, heartburn, and swollen glands
- Joint pain and swelling, numbness. and pain due to neuropathy
- Cough, shortness of breath, and arrhythmias

Diagnostic Procedures. The provider will gather a medical history and perform a complete physical exam, including a neurologic exam. The following tests can be done:

- Blood chemistry, a complete blood count, antinuclear antibodies (ANA) test, rheumatoid factor test, and urinalysis
- Salivary gland and skin biopsies
- Imaging tests, such as ultrasound, a chest x-ray, or magnetic resonance imaging (MRI).

Treatments. The treatment is focused on relieving symptoms. Medications to treat the dry eyes and disease-modifying antirheumatic drugs (DMARDs) are used to treat other symptoms. Dental care and routine dental checkups are encouraged.

Systemic Lupus Erythematosus. Systemic lupus erythematosus is an autoimmune disease. The immune system attacks the healthy tissue in the skin, joints, kidneys, brain, and other organs. SLE is more common in females than in males and can occur at any age. African Americans and Asian Americans are more often affected than people of other races.

Etiology. The cause of SLE is not known. It might be linked to genetics, environmental factors, hormones, and certain medicines.

Signs and Symptoms. Signs and symptoms vary and can come and go. SLE can cause joint pain and joint swelling. Other symptoms include:

- Fatigue, fever, general discomfort, and chest pain when taking a deep breath
- Hair loss, weight loss, mouth sores, and swollen lymph nodes
- Sensitivity to sunlight and a butterfly rash over the cheeks and bridge of the nose (Fig. 9.14)
- Headaches, seizures, visual problems, and abdominal pain
- Inflammation of the heart muscle, valve problems, and difficulty breathing

Diagnostic Procedures. To be diagnosed with SLE, the patient must have 4 of 11 common signs of the disease. Most patients have an ANA test. Many blood and urine tests, along with imaging tests and a kidney biopsy, can be done.

Treatments. There is no cure for SLE. The goal of treatment is to control symptoms. Corticosteroids, nonsteroidal anti-inflammatory drugs (NSAIDs), hydroxychloroquine, and immunosuppressive medications can be prescribed. Patients are encouraged to avoid tobacco and drink minimal amounts of alcohol. They should stay up-to-date with immunizations.

Additional Immune System Disorders. The following are additional immune system disorders.

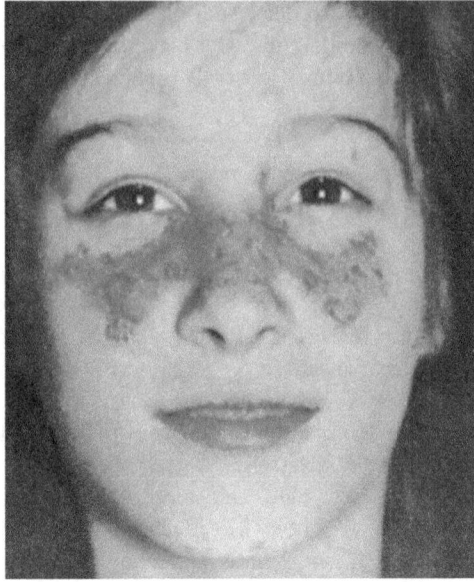

Fig. 9.14 Butterfly Rash of Systemic Lupus Erythematosus (SLE). (Modified from Kliegman RM, et al: *Nelson textbook of pediatrics,* ed 18, Philadelphia, 2007, Saunders.)

- *Graft-versus-host disease* (GVHD): A life-threatening complication that occurs after bone marrow transplantation or after certain stem cell transplants. Acute GVHD usually occurs days to up to 6 months after the transplantation. The person may experience abdominal pain, jaundice, skin rash, and an increased risk for infection. Chronic GVHD starts 3 months after the transplantation and lasts a lifetime. The person can experience fatigue, joint pain, shortness of breath, weight loss, cytopenia, and pericarditis.
- *Serum sickness*: A type of delayed allergic reaction. Usually appears 4 to 10 days after exposure to antibodies or antiserum. Can cause joint pain, fever, swelling, and nausea.
- *Stevens-Johnson syndrome/toxic epidermal necrolysis* (SJS/TEN): A severe skin reaction that can be triggered by certain medications. Begins with a fever and flulike symptoms and leads to blistering and peeling of the skin and mucous membranes in the mouth and airway. Stevens-Johnson syndrome is the less severe end of the disease spectrum, and toxic epidermal necrolysis represents the more severe end.
- *Transplant rejection*: After organ transplantation, the recipient's immune system attacks the transplanted tissue or organ. *Hyperacute rejection* occurs within a few minutes after the transplantation because the antigens are completely unmatched. The transplanted organ or tissue must be removed, or the person will die. *Acute rejection* occurs from the first week through 3 months after the transplantation. *Chronic rejection* can take place over many years. The body's immune system slowly damages the transplanted tissue or organ. To prevent transplant rejection, the person must take daily immunosuppressant drugs.

Lymphatic System Diseases and Disorders

Disorders of the lymphatic system usually involve infection, inflammation, cancer, or obstructions. Common signs and symptoms include redness and tenderness over the inflamed lymph node. The lymph node is swollen, tender, and hard. The person may have a fever and *lymphocytosis* (lim foe sie TOE sis) (high lymphocyte count). Common diagnostic tests for lymphatic disorders include:

- Blood tests, such as a WBC differential.
- *Lymphoscintigraphy* (lim foe sin TIG rah fee), a nuclear medicine imaging technique that provides images of the lymphatic system. A small amount of radioactive tracer is injected into the skin. A nuclear medicine camera is used to detect and record the distribution of the radioactive tracer. The test can identify the *sentinel lymph node* (the first node to receive the lymph drainage from a tumor).
- Sentinel lymph node biopsy.

The following sections discuss specific lymphatic disorders.

Infectious Mononucleosis. Infectious mononucleosis (also called "mono" and the "kissing disease") is a contagious disease. It is commonly seen in teens and young adults.

Etiology. Infectious mononucleosis is usually caused by the Epstein-Barr virus (EBV), although other viruses also can cause it. The virus is spread through body fluids, especially saliva. Blood from blood transfusions and semen are additional ways the virus can spread. Of those infected with EBV, about 25% will develop infectious mononucleosis. For some people, a history of an EBV infection increases their risk of developing SLE, multiple sclerosis (MS), rheumatoid arthritis (RA), juvenile idiopathic arthritis (JIA), irritable bowel disease (IBD), celiac disease, and type 1 diabetes.

Signs and Symptoms. In individuals who get infectious mononucleosis, the symptoms appear about 4 to 6 weeks after infection with EBV. Signs and symptoms can include:

- Extreme fatigue, fever, rash, sore throat, and achiness
- Swollen lymph nodes in the neck and axilla area
- Swollen liver and enlarged spleen (*splenomegaly*)

Diagnostic Procedures. Many times, infectious mononucleosis is diagnosed based on a person's medical history and the physical exam. In addition, providers may order a CBC, liver function tests, and a CLIA-waived mono test.

Treatments. Treatment usually includes keeping hydrated by drinking plenty of fluids, getting adequate rest, and taking over-the-counter medications for the discomfort and fever. Many providers will also encourage patients not to take part in any contact sports or similar activities that may increase the risk of rupturing an enlarged spleen.

CRITICAL THINKING 9.11

Mia is working with Renee Berkley, who has just been diagnosed with infectious mononucleosis. Renee tells Mia, "I heard that mononucleosis is called the 'kissing disease.' Why is that?" Thinking of what you have learned about infectious mononucleosis, how might Mia answer this question?

Lymphadenitis. *Lymphadenitis* is an infection or inflammation of the lymph nodes. Lymphadenitis can be a complication of some bacterial infections, such as streptococcal or staphylococcal infections.

Etiology. The lymph nodes become inflamed and enlarged as a response to a nearby bacterial, viral, or fungal infection, tumor, or inflammation.

Signs and Symptoms. The skin over the inflamed and enlarged lymph node might be red and tender. The lymph node can feel swollen, tender, or hard. The person may have a fever.

Diagnostic Procedures. The provider will obtain a medical history and perform a physical exam. The provider will palpate the lymph nodes and may order blood work, blood cultures, and a biopsy to diagnose the cause of the enlarged lymph node.

Treatments. Treatments include antibiotics to treat bacterial infections, analgesics for pain, and anti-inflammatory medications to reduce inflammation. Applying a cool compress to the area can help reduce inflammation and pain. Surgery may be required if an abscess has formed.

Lymphangitis. *Lymphangitis* is an infection of the lymph vessels. It can be a sign that a skin infection is getting worse. If the infection continues to spread and remains untreated, it can cause life-threatening problems.

Etiology. An acute streptococcal infection of the skin most often causes lymphangitis. Staphylococcal infections can also cause lymphangitis.

Signs and Symptoms. Signs and symptoms include:

- Fever, chills, malaise, and headache
- Muscle aches and throbbing pain in the area
- Enlarged and tender lymph node (usually in the elbow, axilla, or groin area) and red streaks in the infected area (Fig. 9.15)

Diagnostic Procedures. The provider will obtain a medical history and perform a physical exam. The provider will palpate the lymph nodes and may order blood work, blood cultures, and a biopsy to diagnose the cause of the enlarged lymph node.

Treatments. Treatments include antibiotics to treat bacterial infections, analgesics for pain, and anti-inflammatory medications to reduce inflammation. Applying a warm, moist compress to the area can help reduce inflammation and pain. Surgery may be required if an abscess has formed.

Lymphedema. *Lymphedema* is the buildup of lymph fluid in an area of the body, such as the arm or leg. The disorder can be lifelong.

Etiology. Lymphedema occurs when the lymph vessels cannot drain the lymph fluid from an area of the body. Infection, cancer, scar tissue from radiation therapy, or surgical removal of lymph nodes can cause lymphedema. It can start 6 weeks to months after surgery or radiation treatment for cancer. Inherited conditions that cause abnormal or absent lymph nodes or vessels can also cause lymphedema.

Signs and Symptoms. Signs and symptoms include:

- Swelling of the arm, fingers, leg, or toes
- Restricted range of motion due to the swelling
- Aching or a feeling of tightness or heaviness
- Hardening or thickening of the skin

Diagnostic Procedures. The provider will obtain a medical history and perform a physical exam. The provider will palpate

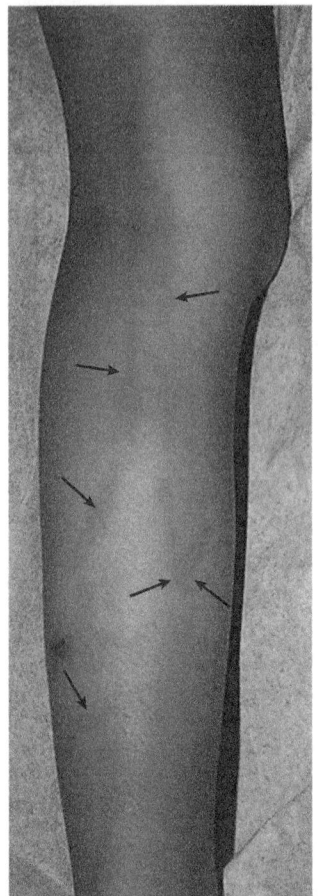

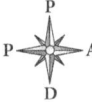

Fig. 9.15 Lymphangitis. This condition is characterized by inflamed lymphatic vessels that appear as red streaks (highlighted by *arrows*) radiating from the source of infection. (From Zitelli B, McIntire SC, Nowalk AJ: *Atlas of pediatric physical diagnosis*, ed 6, Philadelphia, 2012, Mosby)

and assess the area. If the underlying cause (e.g., surgery) for the lymphedema is not known, the provider will perform additional tests.

Treatments. Treatments include controlling the symptoms. Exercises, compression devices, skin care, and massage can help reduce the swelling. Using the extremity that has lymphedema will help. Resting the extremity above the heart level several times a day can also help to reduce the edema.

Hodgkin Lymphoma. Hodgkin lymphoma was formally called Hodgkin disease. This condition is a rare type of lymphoma, a lymphatic system cancer. It is most common in adults between 20 and 40 and older than 55 years of age.

Etiology. The cause of Hodgkin lymphoma is unknown. Risk factors include age, family history of lymphoma, and a personal history of an Epstein-Barr infection (infectious mononucleosis).

Signs and Symptoms. The first sign is often an enlarged lymph node. The disease can spread to nearby lymph nodes. As the disease progresses, it spreads to the lungs, liver, and bone marrow. Additional signs and symptoms include:
- Painless swelling of neck, axilla, or groin lymph nodes
- Fever, chills, and night sweats
- Weight loss, loss of appetite, and itchy skin

Diagnostic Procedures. The provider will obtain a medical history and perform a physical exam. Blood tests and a lymph node biopsy can be done. People diagnosed with Hodgkin lymphoma have large, abnormal cells called Reed-Sternberg cells. These cells are found in the lymph nodes.

Treatments. Treatment includes radiation therapy and chemotherapy. The sooner the disease is diagnosed, the more effective the treatment. In most causes Hodgkin lymphoma can be cured.

Non-Hodgkin Lymphoma. Non-Hodgkin lymphomas are a group of lymphatic system cancers. A T cell or B cell becomes abnormal, and more abnormal cells are created through cell division. These abnormal cells spread throughout the body. They can overwhelm the lymph nodes, causing the nodes to enlarge.

Etiology. The cause of non-Hodgkin lymphomas is unknown. Risk factors include immunosuppressive medications, HIV, Epstein-Barr infections, *H. pylori* infection, certain pesticides, and age (over 60 years old).

Signs and Symptoms. Signs and symptoms include painless swelling of lymph nodes found in the neck, axilla, and groin. Additional signs and symptoms include:
- Abdominal pain or swelling and weight loss
- Chest pain, coughing, and dyspnea
- Fatigue, fever, and night sweats

Diagnostic Procedures. Besides obtaining a medical history, the provider will perform a physical exam, checking for swollen lymph nodes. Blood and urine tests, along with imaging tests, might be done. Lymph node and bone marrow biopsies can also be done to help diagnose this condition. The lymphoma will be staged to help determine the prognosis and treatment.

Treatments. Sometimes treatment is delayed if the lymphoma is slow growing, but the patient will have regular checkups. Treatment may consist of chemotherapy, radiation therapy, bone marrow transplantation, and biological therapy to help the immune system fight the cancer.

Multiple Myeloma. Multiple myeloma is a cancer that begins in the plasma cells. The cancer cells collect in the bone marrow, where healthy blood cells are crowded out. The cancer cells produce abnormal proteins that cause complications.

Etiology. The exact cause is unknown. It is more common in African Americans, older adults, and people with a family history of multiple myeloma.

Signs and Symptoms. Signs and symptoms include:
- Back and rib pain, fractures, and numbness or weakness in the legs
- Weight loss, loss of appetite, frequent infections, and fevers
- Frequent urination, feeling very thirsty, and constipation
- Mental fogginess, confusion, fatigue, and weakness

Diagnostic Procedures. Tests used to diagnose multiple myeloma include:
- Blood tests: M proteins and beta-2-microglobulin proteins produced by myeloma cells can be found. Kidney function and blood cell counts can also be done.

- Urine tests: M proteins can also be found in the urine and are called *Bence Jones proteins* when found there.
- Imaging tests, such as x-rays, MRI, and positron emission tomography (PET).
- Bone marrow biopsy.

The disease will be staged to determine the best treatment.

Treatments. Treatment depends on how advanced the disease is and if symptoms are present. Treatment includes chemotherapy, bone marrow transplantation (also called *stem cell transplantation*), corticosteroids, radiation, and target therapy, which attacks specific cancer cells. Biological therapy can be used to help the immune system fight myeloma cells. Vaccines may also be given (Box 9.2).

Tonsillitis. Tonsillitis is the inflammation of the tonsils.

Etiology. Tonsillitis is caused from viruses and bacteria.

Signs and Symptoms. Tonsillitis can cause the following signs and symptoms:

- Sore throat and problems swallowing
- Red, swollen tonsils or a white or yellow coating on the tonsils
- Swollen neck glands and fever
- Bad breath

If the person has problems breathing, starts drooling, or severe swallowing problems, emergency care should be obtained.

Diagnostic Procedures. The provider will do a history and physical examination. A CLIA-waived rapid strep test and throat culture may be done.

Treatments. Antibiotics are used for bacterial infections, such as strep throat, depending on the cause of the tonsillitis. Home treatments including rest, drinking fluids, warm liquids, and saltwater gargles can be done. A tonsillectomy (surgical removal of the tonsils) can be done if a person has:

- Repeated tonsillitis.
- Bacterial tonsillitis does not get better with antibiotics.
- Difficulty swallowing or breathing due to enlarged tonsils.

An adenoidectomy (removal of the adenoids or pharyngeal tonsils) may also be done with a tonsillectomy.

BOX 9.2   Stem Cell Transplants and Vaccinations

When a person receives a hematopoietic or blood stem cell transplant (SCT), the patient's blood-forming stem cells are replaced with new stem cells. After the transplantation, the patient may have limited or no immunity against contagious diseases. Any immunity gained from childhood vaccinations are usually gone. It is standard practice to revaccinate these patients with the standard childhood immunizations.

Additional Lymphatic System Disorders. The following are additional lymphatic system disorders.

- *Elephantiasis:* A condition characterized by gross enlargement of an area of the body, such as the leg (Fig. 9.16).
- *Lymphatic filariasis:* Caused by a parasitic disease caused by microscopic, threadlike worms. The parasite is spread from person to person by mosquitoes in the tropics. Can cause lymphedema and elephantiasis (see Fig. 9.16).
- *Mesenteric lymphadenitis:* Lymphadenitis of the lymph nodes in the mesentery in the abdomen. Usually caused by a viral intestinal infection. Also called *mesenteric adenitis.*

LIFE SPAN CHANGES

There are only slight changes in the blood with age. Aging can reduce the total body water, which creates less fluid in the bloodstream. This decreases blood volume.

The immune system is immature in newborns until around age 2 or 3 months. The thymus is relatively large in infants and children. After puberty it begins to decrease in size. In older adults the thymus is very small.

As you grow older, the immune system functions change. The response time to infections becomes slower. There is a greater chance of an autoimmune disease developing. Fewer immune cells are available for healing. The immune system's ability to detect and destroy cell defects declines, thus the risk for cancer increases.

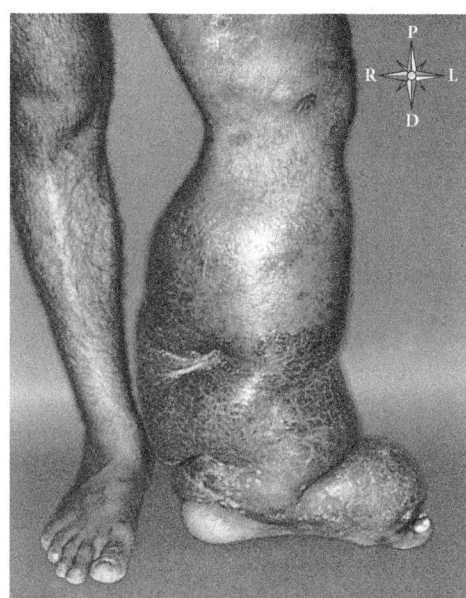

Fig. 9.16 Elephantiasis. Lymphedema caused by prolonged infestation by filarial worms produces elephant-like limbs. (From Goldstein B, editor: *Practical dermatology,* ed 2, St. Louis, 1997, Mosby.)

CLOSING COMMENTS

Patients with blood, lymphatic, or immune system disorders are seen in primary care, urgent care, and specialty departments. Being knowledgeable about the blood cells, lymphatic structures, and how the immune system functions can help the medical assistant understand the different diseases that affect these systems. It is important for the medical assistant to be familiar with the more common diseases, tests, and treatments. Box 9.3 lists medication classifications commonly used to treat blood, lymphatic, and immune system diseases.

BOX 9.3   Medication Classifications

- *Antibiotics*: Used to treat bacterial infections. Kill or inhibit bacterial growth.
- *Anticoagulants*: Prevent blood clots from forming. Decrease blood clotting ability.
- *Antihistamines*: Used to relieve allergies. Block the action of histamines, which cause allergic symptoms.
- *Anti-inflammatories:* Used to treat inflammatory diseases. Reduce inflammation.
- *Antiplatelets*: Used for post treatment of strokes, heart attack, and angina. Inhibit the function of platelets.
- *Hematopoietics:* Used to treat anemia in patients undergoing chemotherapy. Promote blood cell production.

- *Hemostatics*: Used to control acute or chronic blood clotting disorders. Act as a blood coagulant, thereby clotting blood.
- *Immunosuppressants*: Suppress the immune response and are used to treat conditions such as myasthenia gravis.
- *Tumor necrosis factor (TNF) inhibitors*: Used to treat autoimmune disorders. Block the action of TNF, thus preventing inflammation.

  Refer to Appendix D, which can be found on the Evolve website, for information on the medication classifications, including indications for use, desired effect, side effects, adverse reactions, and generic and trade names. Medical assistants should be familiar with medications that are prescribed to patients.

PATIENT-CENTERED CARE

Coaching patients with bleeding disorders is an important aspect of patient-centered care. Patients with bleeding disorders need to avoid situations in which bleeding can occur. Kneepads, elbow pads, and helmets are encouraged to prevent injuries. Contact sports such as wrestling, hockey, and football are not recommended. Patients should avoid certain pain medications that exacerbate bleeding, such as ibuprofen and aspirin. Anticoagulant medications, which prevent clotting, need to be avoided. Patients should be encouraged to wear a medical alert bracelet.

BEING PROFESSIONAL

Patients who have a weakened immune system need to take care to prevent infections. This can be done by good hand hygiene, avoiding others who are sick, and getting vaccinated.

  Role-play this scenario with a peer. Your peer is a patient with a weakened immune system. This patient does not believe that washing hands and avoiding sick people are important to the person's condition. Respond to the patient in a respectful, professional manner.

CHAPTER REVIEW

The blood carries oxygen and nutrients to the cells and carries waste from the cells. The lymphatic system returns proteins and excess interstitial fluid to the circulatory system. The immune system defends the body from microorganisms, foreign tissues, and cancerous cells. These three systems interact closely to maintain homeostasis.

The blood is made up of plasma and formed elements. The plasma contains water and plasma proteins (e.g., albumin, globulins, clotting factors, and complements), inorganic and organic substances, and electrolytes. Formed elements include RBCs, WBCs, and platelets. The lymphatic system is made up of the lymphatic vessels, lymph, lymph nodes, tonsils, spleen, and thymus. The immune system is composed of leukocytes, lymph nodes, tonsils, thymus, spleen, lymphocytes, cytokines, complements, and antibodies.

The process involved in forming a blood clot is complicated. This process is called *blood clotting* or *coagulation*. When the body stops the flow of blood through coagulation, the process is called *hemostasis*.

The immune system has two responses to foreign antigens:
- Innate immunity: Consists of barrier mechanisms, chemical substances, and nonspecific immune responses, which include cellular and chemical responses.

- Acquired immunity: Includes humoral immunity, which involves the production of B lymphocytes (B cells) and antibodies, and the cell-mediated immunity. The cell-mediated response involves T cells, which are responsible for destroying cells infected with antigens (e.g., viruses) and abnormal body cells, such as cancerous cells and transplanted tissues.

The etiology, signs and symptoms, diagnostic procedures, and treatments were discussed for the following diseases:
- Blood disorders: Anemia, hemophilia, idiopathic thrombocytopenic purpura, and leukemia.
- Immune system disorders: Autoimmune vasculitis, dermatomyositis, acquired immunodeficiency syndrome, Sjögren syndrome, and systemic lupus erythematosus.
- Lymphatic disorders: Infectious mononucleosis, lymphadenitis, lymphangitis, lymphedema, Hodgkin and non-Hodgkin lymphoma, multiple myeloma, and tonsillitis.

Over the lifetime, there are only slight changes in the blood. With aging, the total body water may decrease, causing a decrease in blood volume. The immune system is immature in newborns until around age 2 or 3 months. The thymus is relatively large in infants and children and shrinks with age. As a person ages, the immune system functions change. The response time for infections slows, and there is a greater chance of an autoimmune disease.

SCENARIO WRAP-UP

Dr. Walden and Mia had a busy day seeing patients. Mia enjoys her role as a medical assistant. Mia takes great pride in giving her patients the best care. Being in family medicine, she sees patients come back over and over. This allows her to follow their care and treatment. She feels as if her job makes an impact on her patients

and their health. She also feels it is a job in which she will continue to learn new things each and every day. When a patient is diagnosed with a disease she is not aware of, she spends time researching it. She likes to learn new tests and treatments also. Mia feels this is a job in which she will continue to grow as a professional.

10

Cardiovascular System

LEARNING OBJECTIVES

1. List the major organs of the cardiovascular system and identify the anatomic location of major cardiovascular system organs.
2. Describe the structure of the heart.
3. Describe the pulmonary, systemic, coronary, hepatic portal, and fetal circulations.
4. Describe the normal function of the cardiovascular system.
5. Explain factors that affect the blood pressure.
6. Explain the common diagnostic procedures and treatments for cardiovascular system disorders.
7. Describe common cardiovascular system disorders, including common signs and symptoms, etiology, diagnostic procedures, and treatments.
8. Compare the structure and function of the cardiovascular system across the life span.

OUTLINE

▶ OPENING SCENARIO

Rebecca White is a certified medical assistant (CMA) at Walden-Martin Family Medical (WMFM) Clinic. She was hired 8 months ago. She works with several family practice providers at the clinic. Many of the patients she works with have cardiovascular diseases. High blood pressure, or hypertension, seems to be the most common cardiovascular disease seen in her patients.

During her first few months at the clinic, Rebecca spent a lot of time learning about cardiovascular diseases, diagnostic procedures, and treatments. She found out that learning about the cardiovascular system takes time, but she is proud of how much she has learned over the months.

Rebecca's supervisor approached her and asked her to mentor a medical assistant student, Lizzy, for her practicum experience. Rebecca is excited about the opportunity, but she is a bit nervous to teach someone else about her job.

YOU WILL LEARN

1. To recognize and use terms related to the cardiovascular system.
2. To locate the cardiovascular system structures.
3. To understand and describe the process of the conduction system.
4. To understand and describe factors that affect blood pressure.
5. To recognize disease states of the cardiovascular system: the cause, signs and symptoms, diagnostic process, treatment, prognosis, and prevention.
6. To discuss life span changes related to the cardiovascular system.

INTRODUCTION

Cardiology (kar DEE ol oh jee) is the healthcare specialty that deals with cardiovascular disorders. A *cardiologist* (kar DEE ol oh jist) is a physician who specializes in internal medicine and cardiology. A cardiologist treats patients with cardiovascular system disorders.

Vascular surgeons are medical doctors who specialize in vascular diseases. They diagnose and treat artery and vein conditions in every part of the body except for the brain and the heart. *Cardiothoracic surgeons* are medical doctors who specialize in surgical procedures involving the lungs, heart, esophagus, and other organs in the chest. They can also be called *cardiac surgeons, cardiovascular surgeons,* and *general thoracic surgeons.*

Cardiology-related tests are common in the ambulatory care setting. Patients with cardiovascular diseases are seen in primary care, urgent care, and specialty departments. Patients seen for other conditions may also have cardiovascular diseases. Medical assistants may need to coach patients on cardiovascular procedures. Having a strong understanding of the cardiovascular system and common diseases is important for medical assistants.

ANATOMY OF THE CARDIOVASCULAR SYSTEM

The cardiovascular (kar dee oh VAS kyoo lur) system is also called the *circulatory* (sir kue lah TORE ee) *system.* The cardiovascular system brings oxygen (O_2), nutrients, water, and other substances (e.g., salts and hormones) to the body's cells. It also carries waste products away from the cells to be excreted. These waste products include metabolic waste and carbon dioxide (CO_2).

The cardiovascular system is a closed system that includes:
- Blood vessels, consisting of arteries, arterioles, capillaries, venules, and veins that act as pipes to carry the blood around the body.
- A heart, which pumps the blood.

- Blood, which contains the nutrients for the cells and the waste products to be excreted (see Chapter 9).

Cellular injury and death of the cells will occur if the system malfunctions and critical substances are withheld from the cells.

Blood Vessels

Blood vessels create a "pipeline" for blood to move out to the body and back to the heart. Blood vessels differ in their role, structure, and size.
- *Arteries* (AR tur reez): Strong, stretchy, thick-walled vessels that carry blood from the heart. They are made to withstand the pressure of the blood being pumped out from the heart. Arteries are involved with maintaining blood pressure (Fig. 10.1).
- *Arterioles* (ar TEER ee olez): Smaller arteries that move blood to the capillaries and are also involved with maintaining blood pressure.
- *Capillaries* (CAP ih lair eez): Thin-walled vessels that allow for exchange of oxygen, nutrients, waste products, and other substances between the blood and cells. The diameter of the capillaries is so thin that only one blood cell can pass through at a time.
- *Venules* (VEEN yools): Vessels that collect blood from capillaries and begin the return journey to the heart.
- *Veins* (vayns): Vessels that collect blood from the venules and return blood to the heart. Medium to large veins have valves, which help keep blood moving in one direction. The skeletal muscle contractions help move the blood toward the heart. Vessel walls are thinner and less rigid than arteries (Fig. 10.2 and Table 10.1). Veins hold about 70% of the blood supply at any one time.

The Heart

The heart, which is the size of a fist, is a complex muscular organ that pumps blood around the body. It is located in the mediastinum (mee dee uh STY num) of the thoracic cavity, slightly left of the midline. The *apex* (pointed tip) of the heart rests just above the diaphragm. The area of the chest wall anterior to the heart and lower thorax is referred to as the *precordium* (pree KORE dee um).

> **VOCABULARY**
> **mediastinum** The space in the thoracic cavity that lies between the lungs, containing the heart, trachea, and esophagus.

Heart Chambers. The heart has two sets of chambers. The two upper chambers are called *atria* (A tree uh). The atria are small chambers with thin walls. The right atrium receives blood from the body, and the left atrium receives blood from the lungs. The two larger lower chambers with thick muscular walls are called the right and left *ventricles* (VEN trih kuls) (Fig. 10.3). They pump blood to the body and the lungs.

The *septum* (SEP tum) is the thick muscular wall that divides the heart into right and left sections. The *interatrial* (in ter A tree uhl) *septum* separates the left and right atria, and the *interventricular* (in ter ven TRICK yoo lur) *septum* divides the right and left ventricles.

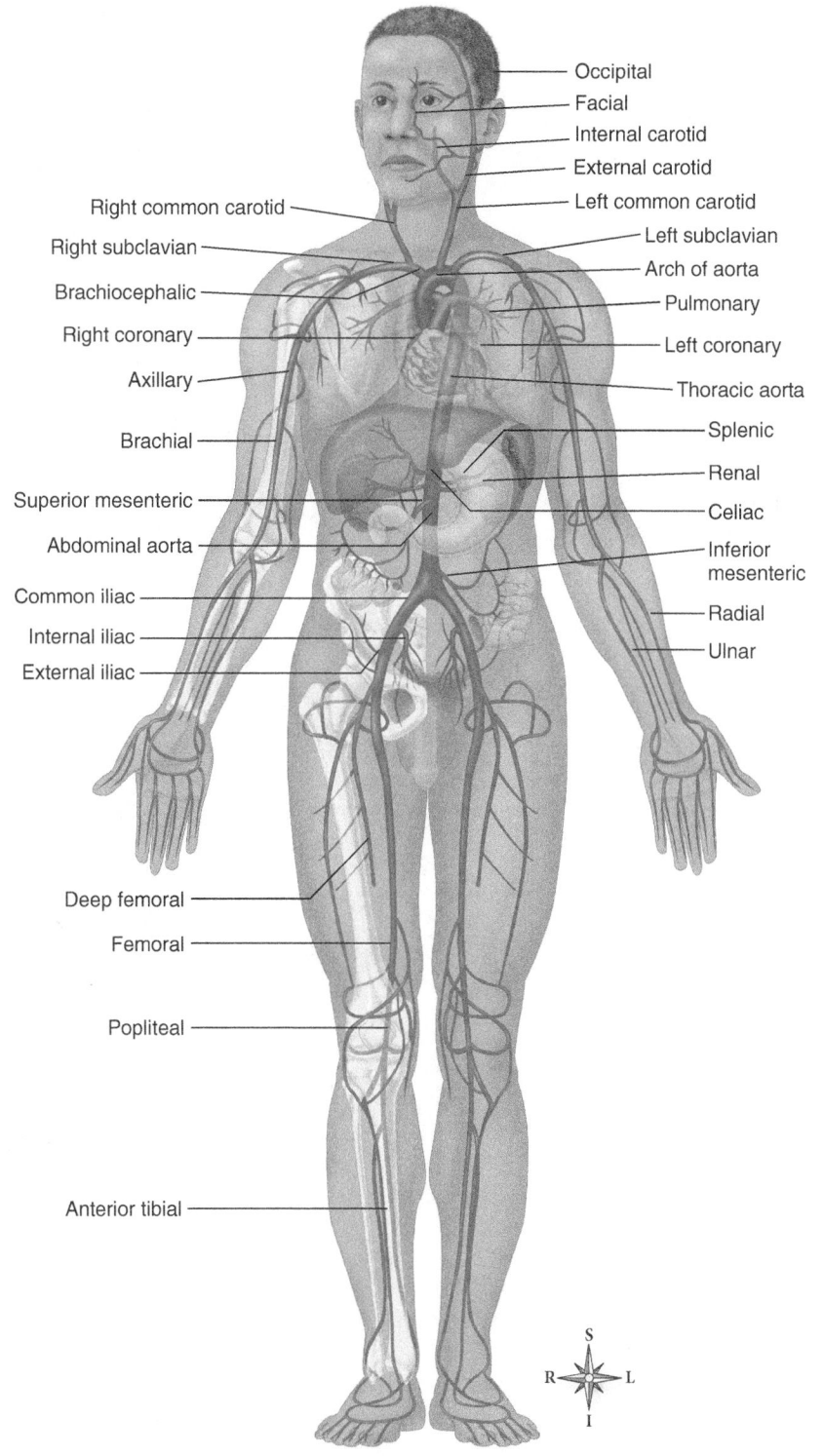

Fig. 10.1 Principal Arteries of the Body. (From Patton KT, Thibodeau GA: *The human body in health and disease*, ed 7, St. Louis, 2018, Elsevier.)

The heart wall is composed of three layers:

- *Endocardium* (en doh KAR dee um): The inner thin endothelial layer that lines the chambers and valves.
- *Myocardium* (mye oh KAR dee um): The middle and thickest layer of the heart, composed of cardiac muscles.
- *Epicardium* (eh pee KAR dee um) or *visceral* (VIS uh rul) *pericardium* (pare ee KAR dee um): The outer

layer that covers the heart. A space separates the epicardium from the *parietal* (puh RYE uh tul) *pericardium*, which loosely covers the heart like a sac. The two layers of pericardium are serous membranes. As the heart beats, the two layers rub against each other, and the moisture between the layers reduces the amount of friction.

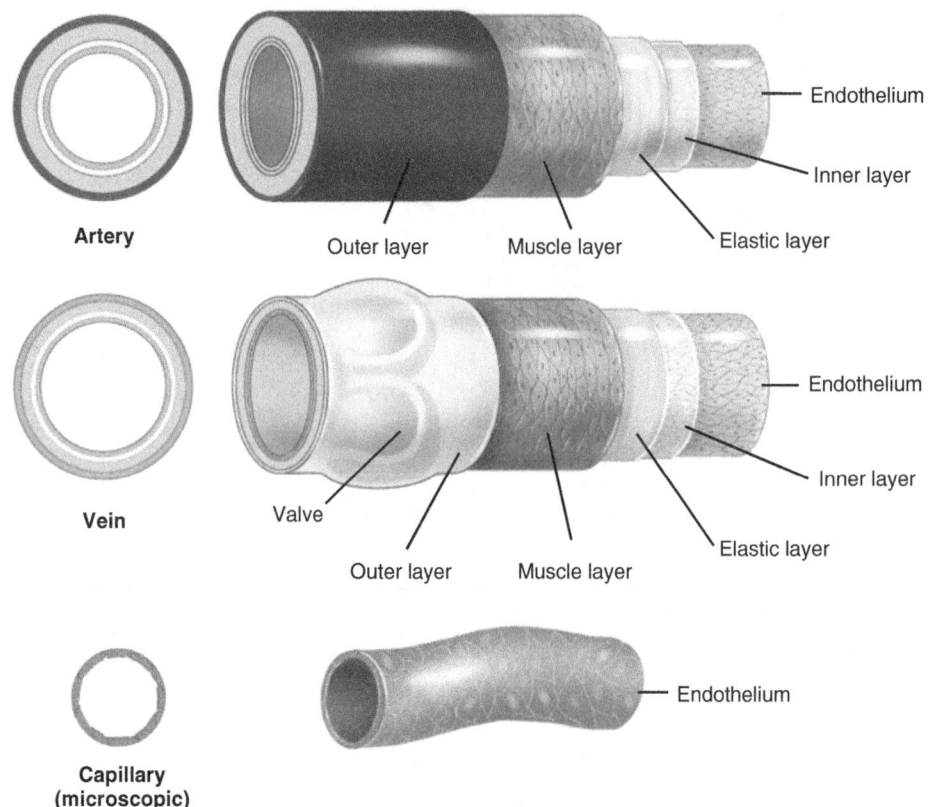

Fig. 10.2 Differences Among Arteries, Veins, and Capillaries. (From Shiland B: *Mastering healthcare terminology*, ed 5, St. Louis, 2016, Elsevier.)

MEDICAL TERMINOLOGY

apic/o	apex
arteri/o, arter/o	artery
arteriol/o	arteriole
atri/o	atrium
capillar/o	capillary
cardi/o, coron/o, cordi/o	heart
endocardi/o	endocardium
myocardi/o	myocardium
pariet/o	parietal
pericardi/o	pericardium
sept/o	septum, wall
valvul/o	valve
vascul/o, angi/o, vas/o	vessel
ven/o, phleb/o	vein
venul/o	venule
ventricul/o	ventricle
viscer/o	visceral
epi-	above, on top of
pre-	before
-ar	pertaining to
-logy	study of
-um	structure
atrium (singular)	atria (plural)
chorda tendinea (singular)	chordae tendineae (plural)
septum (singular)	septa (plural)

TABLE 10.1 Comparison of the Walls of the Arteries and Veins

Layers of the Walls	Arteries	Veins
Tunica intima (inner layer)	Contains epithelium and elasticlike fibers	Some contain valves to prevent backflow of blood
Tunica media (middle layer)	Thick layer of smooth muscles regulated by the autonomic nervous system that constricts or dilates vessels to maintain blood pressure	Contains smooth muscles; thin layer
Tunica externa (outer layer)	Made of connective tissue	Thickest layer and made of connective tissue

through or holding back an expected amount of blood. The heart has two sets of valves: atrioventricular (AV) valves and semilunar (SL) valves.

An AV valve is found between each atrium and ventricle. When opened, it allows blood to flow into the ventricle. When closed, it prevents the backflow of blood into the atrium. The AV valves open and close with the help of the papillary muscles. These muscles are attached to the valve by the *chordae tendineae* (KOR dee ten DIN ee ee), cordlike tendons. The AV valves are located as follows:

- *Bicuspid* (bye KUSS pid) or *mitral* (MYE trul) *valve*: Found between the left atrium and ventricle and made up of two cusps, or flaps (see Fig. 10.3).

Heart Valves. The heart has valves between the chambers and the arteries. The valves allow the blood to flow in one direction. Valves are *competent* if they open and close properly, letting

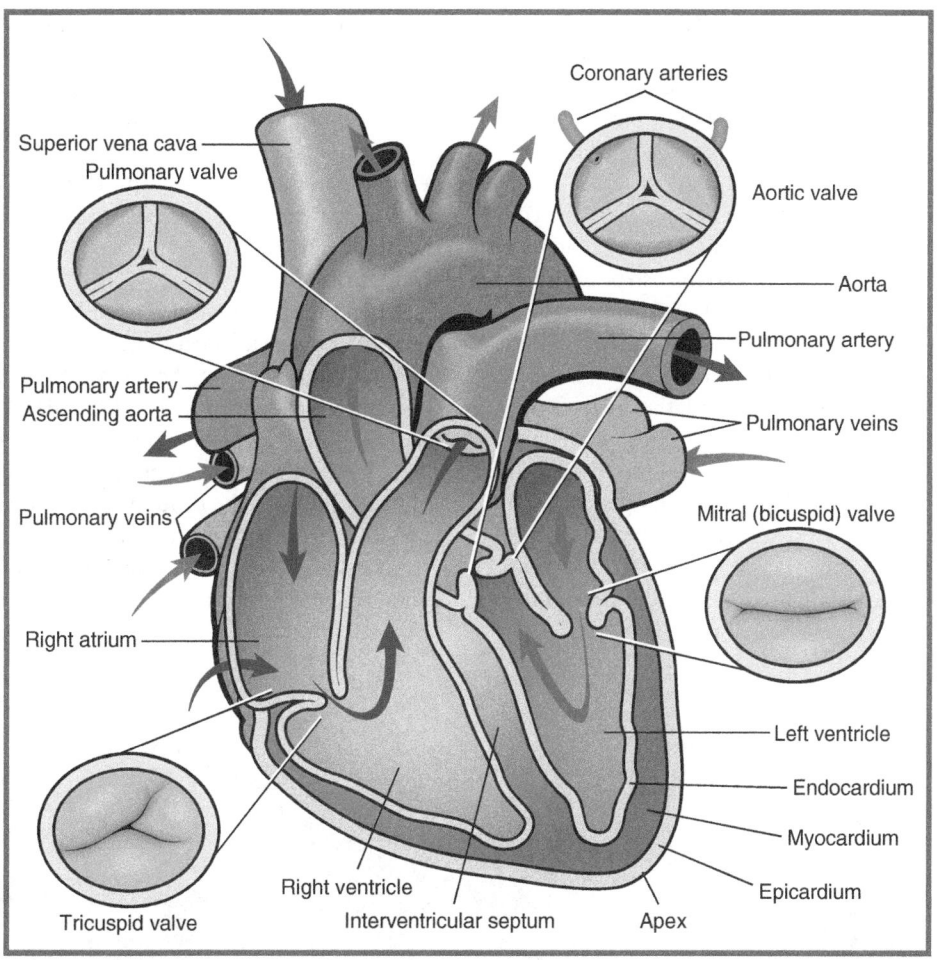

Fig. 10.3 Chambers and Valves of the Heart. (From Damjanov I: *Pathology for the health-related professions,* ed 4, St. Louis, 2012, Saunders.)

- *Tricuspid* (try KUSS pid) valve: Found between the right atrium and ventricle and made up of three cusps.

The SL valves are found between the ventricles and the arteries leading out of the heart. The SL valves allow blood to flow out of the heart and prevent the backflow of blood into the ventricles. The valves are created by flaps from the pulmonary artery and aorta (AE ore tah). The SL valves are located as follows:

- *Pulmonary valve*: Between the right ventricle and the pulmonary artery
- *Aortic* (AE ore tik) *valve*: Between the left ventricle and the aorta

Heartbeat. A provider listens to the heart sounds with a stethoscope. The normal sound is a *lub dub*. The *lub* sound occurs when the AV valves close as the ventricles contract. This is a lower pitch and a longer sound, which is followed by a pause. The *dub* sound occurs when the SL valves close. With incompetent valves, the provider might hear additional abnormal noises.

A complete heartbeat or *cardiac cycle* can be divided into the diastole (di AS toe lee) and systole (SIS toe lee) phases. During the *diastole* phase, the heart is at rest and the atria fill with blood. The *systole* phase occurs when the heart is contracting.

Blood Flow

The body has several types of blood flow pathways, or circulations. The heart, being a double pump, sends blood in two different directions, resulting in two major circulatory pathways:

- *Pulmonary circulation*: Deoxygenated (dee OCK sih juh nay tid) blood is pumped from the right side of the heart to the lungs, gas is exchanged, and oxygenated blood returns to the heart.

VOCABULARY

deoxygenated Oxygen deficient; oxygen was removed.
incompetent valves Valves that do not close completely and allow blood to leak backward into the prior chamber; also called "leaky valves."

- *Systemic circulation*: Oxygenated (OCK sih juh nay tid) blood is pumped from the left side of the heart and moves through the body. Oxygen, nutrients, and other substances are brought to the cells while the blood picks up waste products. The deoxygenated blood returns to the heart.

Because the pulmonary circulation and the systemic circulation are closely tied, they will be discussed together. The *coronary circulation* (blood flow through the heart tissues) and *fetal circulation* (blood flow of a baby in utero) will also be examined.

Pulmonary and Systemic Circulations. Pulmonary circulation begins as the blood returns from the body. The superior vena cava (VEE nuh KAY vuh) and the inferior vena cava bring deoxygenated blood from the body to the right atrium (Fig. 10.4). As the atria contract, the blood from the right atrium passes the tricuspid valve and empties into the right ventricle. When the ventricles contract, the blood in the right ventricle is pushed out past the pulmonary valve and enters the pulmonary artery trunk. The pulmonary artery trunk splits into the right and left pulmonary arteries. From there, the blood moves into the arterioles and then into the pulmonary capillaries in the lungs. The gas exchange occurs. Carbon dioxide leaves the blood and enters the lungs to be expelled. Oxygen enters the blood from the lungs. The oxygenated blood leaves the pulmonary capillaries and enters the pulmonary veins. The right and left pulmonary veins bring the blood back to the left atrium. This is the start of systemic circulation.

When the atria are full of blood, they contract. The oxygenated blood in the left atrium moves past the bicuspid, or mitral, valve and empties into the left ventricle. When the ventricles contract, the blood in the left ventricle moves out of the heart, passing the aortic valve, and empties into the aorta. From here, the blood will move through the body before it returns to the heart. Blood from the head, neck, chest, and upper extremities empties into the superior vena cava before returning to the right atrium. Blood from the lower body empties into the inferior vena cava before returning to the right atrium.

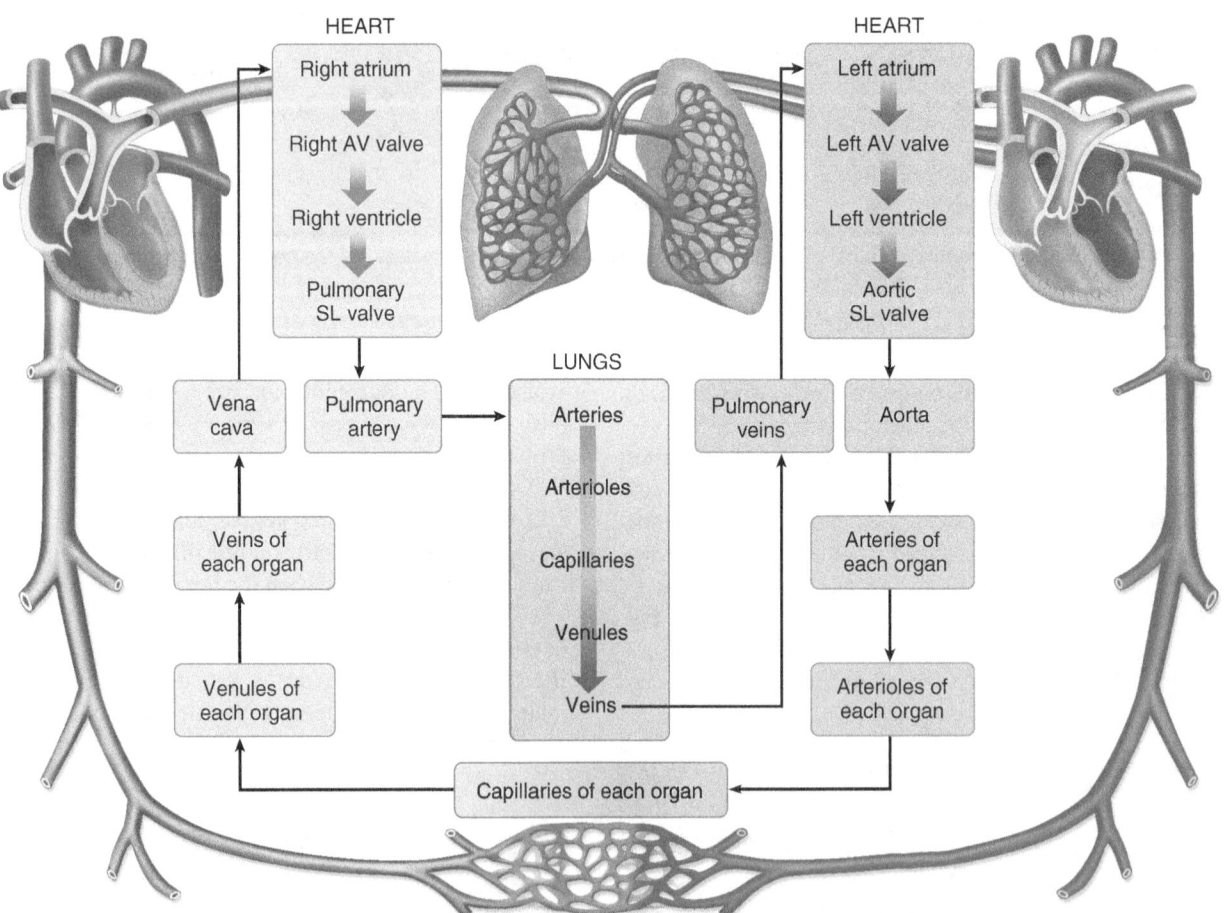

Fig. 10.4 Diagram of Blood Flow in the Cardiovascular System. Blood leaves the heart through arteries, then travels through arterioles, capillaries, venules, and veins before returning to the opposite side of the heart. *AV*, Atrioventricular; *SL*, semilunar. (From Patton KT, Thibodeau GA: *The human body in health and disease*, ed 7, St. Louis, 2018, Elsevier.)

CRITICAL THINKING 10.2

Rebecca is helping Lizzy review the blood flow through the body. She asks Lizzy to explain the blood flow through the pulmonary and systemic circulations, starting with the blood returning from the body. How should Lizzy answer her?

VOCABULARY

glucose A simple sugar that is absorbed by the intestines and found in the blood. It is used by cells for energy, and the extra is stored in the liver as glycogen.

Coronary Circulation. The heart has its own blood vessels that support the tissues. The right and left coronary (KORE ih nair ee) arteries are the first branches off the ascending aorta (Fig. 10.5). The coronary arteries bring nutrients and oxygen to the heart tissue. The blood moves from the arteries to the capillaries in the myocardium. From there, the blood moves into the coronary veins. The coronary veins remove the waste products from the heart tissue. Blood from the coronary veins drains into the coronary sinus, which opens into the right atrium.

Coronary arteries have the important role of maintaining the myocardium. If a branch of the coronary artery becomes blocked, a person will experience a heart attack. The tissue supplied by the blocked artery will be deprived of oxygen and nutrients.

Hepatic Portal Circulation. In most cases, veins leaving an abdominal organ empty blood into the inferior vena cava as it heads to the heart. Veins from the spleen, gallbladder, pancreas, stomach, and intestines take an alternative route. Veins from these organs dump the blood into the hepatic portal vein, which takes the blood to the liver. In the liver, the blood moves through capillaries as it is filtered. Eventually, the blood drains into the hepatic veins before emptying into the inferior vena cava.

The liver has a special role in filtering the blood; it also metabolizes, or breaks down, substances. The hepatic portal system has many advantages:
- The glucose absorbed can be filtered and stored in the liver as glycogen. It will later be added back to the blood when the glucose levels are low.
- Toxic substances such as alcohol and medications can be partially filtered before moving to the rest of the body.

Fetal Circulation. Prior to birth, the baby is called a *fetus*. Fetal circulation differs from what we have discussed so far in this chapter. Before birth, the baby's lungs, gastrointestinal tract, and kidneys are not functioning as they will after birth. Toward the end of pregnancy, babies "practice" breathing, as they breathe in the amniotic fluid. No gas exchange occurs. Babies also urinate, but the waste products in their blood are removed by their mothers' blood. Nutrients are passed through the blood from the mother.

During the early weeks of pregnancy, the placenta (reproductive organ) begins to grow. It attaches to the mother's uterus and connects to the growing baby via the umbilical cord. The umbilical cord contains two umbilical arteries and one umbilical vein. The arteries carry the fetal blood to the placenta. The umbilical vein carries oxygen and nutrient-rich blood to the baby. The waste, oxygen, and nutrient exchange occurs in the placenta. There is a very thin wall separating the fetal blood from the mother's blood. There is no mixing of the two different blood supplies, though substances can pass between the separating wall. Oxygen and nutrients move from the mother's bloodstream to the fetal blood. Waste products (i.e., carbon dioxide) move from fetal blood to the mother's blood.

Other structures that are unique to the growing baby in utero include:
- *Ductus venosus* (DUK tus vee NOE sus): Shifts the majority of the blood from the umbilical vein and empties it into the inferior vena cava (Fig. 10.6). This structure helps the blood bypass the immature liver. After birth, with the lack of blood flow from the umbilical vein, the ductus venosus constricts. Within 1 to 3 months after birth, it is permanently sealed.
- *Foramen ovale* (FOR ae men oh VAL ee): A small flaplike opening in the interatrial septum that allows blood to move

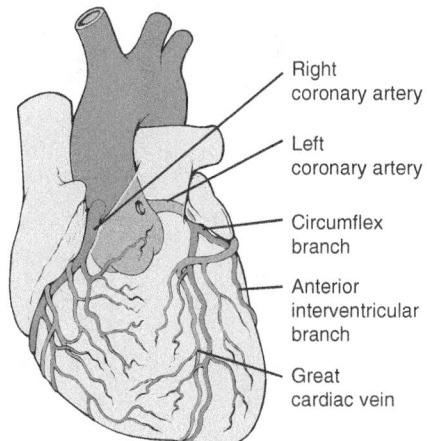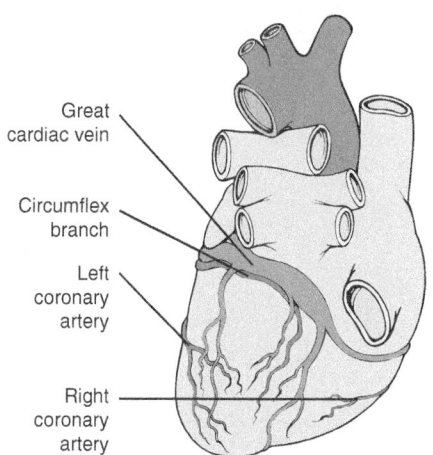

Right coronary artery

Left coronary artery

Circumflex branch

Anterior interventricular branch

Great cardiac vein

Great cardiac vein

Circumflex branch

Left coronary artery

Right coronary artery

Fig. 10.5 Coronary Arteries. (From Frazier MS, et al: *Essentials of human diseases and conditions,* ed 5, St. Louis, 2013, Saunders.)

from the right atrium to the left atrium (see Fig. 10.6). This allows most of the blood to bypass the immature lungs. After birth, the flap opening is forced closed by the pressure of the blood pumping in the heart. During infancy, the flap should seal permanently.

- *Ductus arteriosus* (DUK tus are TEER ee oh sus): A short vessel that connects the pulmonary artery with the aorta. About 90% of the blood in the pulmonary artery is redirected to the aorta, bypassing the immature lungs. Usually it closes at birth or shortly after.

At birth, when a baby takes the first breath and the umbilical cord is cut, these special structures are no longer needed. With the first breath, more pressure is created in the cardiovascular system. This helps with the closure of the foramen ovale. With the cutting of the umbilical cord, the remaining structures (ductus venosus, ductus arteriosus, and umbilical vessels) collapse.

PHYSIOLOGY OF THE CARDIOVASCULAR SYSTEM

To explore the physiology of the cardiovascular system, the action of the heart, blood vessels, and the blood components will be examined. The following sections discuss the conduction system, factors that affect blood pressure, and coagulation.

Conduction System

To understand the conduction system, it is first necessary to learn the cardiac muscle characteristics and the three states they must undergo for each impulse. After this discussion, the conduction system and the blood volume will be examined.

Cardiac Muscle. There are two kinds of cardiac cells, electrical or conduction system cells and myocardial cells. The

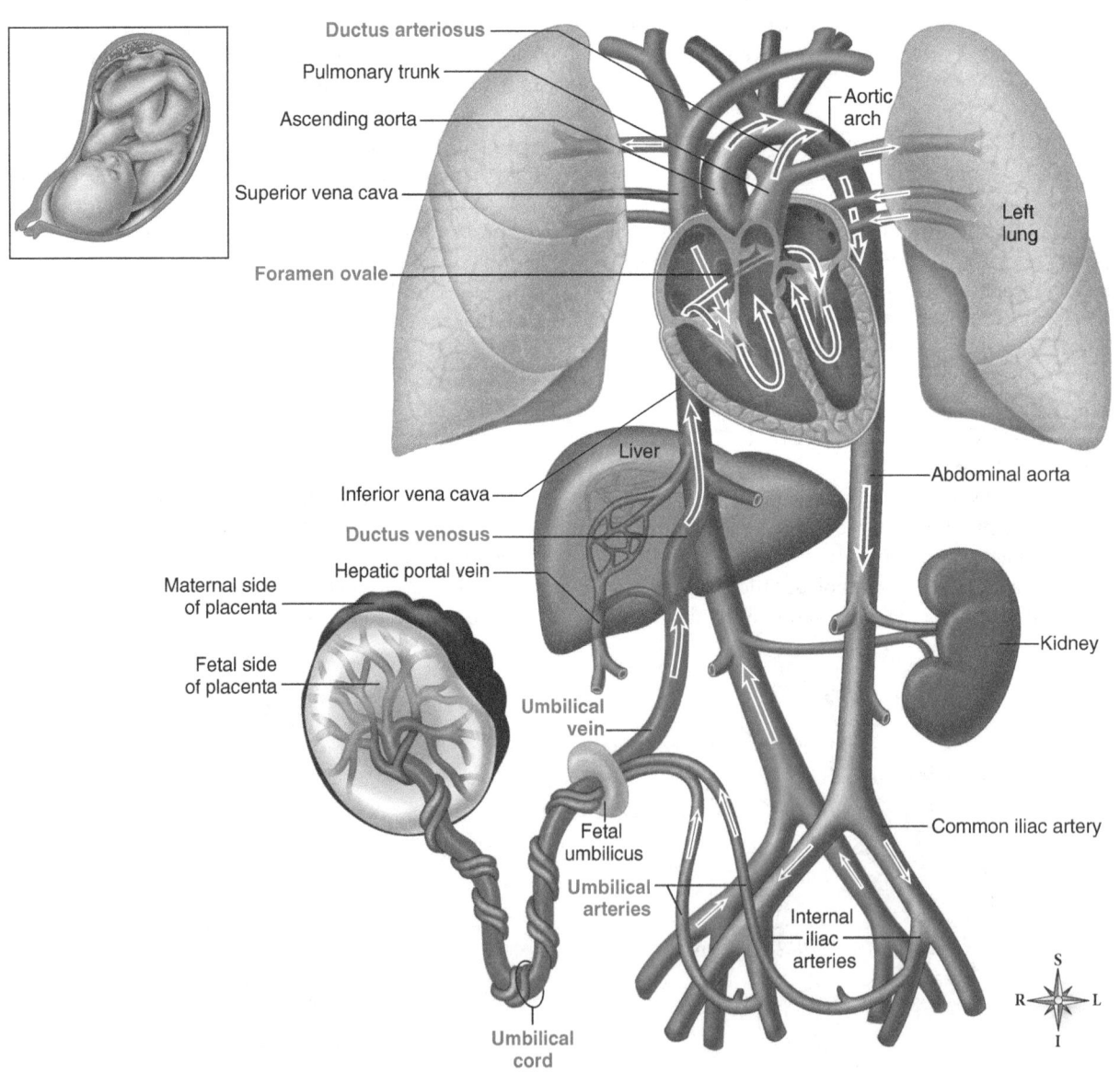

Fig. 10.6 Fetal Circulation. (From Patton KT, Thibodeau G: *The human body in health and disease,* ed 6, St. Louis, 2014, Mosby.)

electrical cells are found in the conduction system. They have three unique characteristics:

- *Automaticity*: The cells create and discharge the electrical impulse.
- *Excitability*: The cells respond to the electrical impulse.
- *Conductivity*: The cells transmit electrical impulses to other cells.

The myocardial cells are found in the myocardium. They can shorten and lengthen their fibers for contraction (called *contractility*). The fibers made from the myocardial cells can contract for prolonged periods of time without fatigue and use less adenosine triphosphate (ATP) than other muscles. These features are beneficial for the heart.

Cardiac muscle fibers are electrically linked, forming one unit. A myocardial cell forms a strong, electrical connection to the next cells through special junctions called *intercalated discs*. The intercalated discs are responsible for the cell-to-cell communication that is required for coordinated muscle contraction. The intercalated discs help the muscle fibers form one unit that contracts all at once instead of a little at a time. The "one unit" approach is important, because the atrial chambers need to contract together, and the ventricles need to contract at about the same time.

Conduction System Structures. As previously stated, the electrical cells make up the conduction system of the heart. These cells are found throughout the myocardium. They can respond to and transmit electronic impulses to neighboring cells. The conduction system is composed of five structures (Fig. 10.7):

- *Sinoatrial* (SIE noe ae tree el) (SA) *node*: Located in the posterior superior wall of the right atrium, the SA node is called the "pacemaker of the heart." This is because the electrical cells in the SA node generate the impulse that starts the heartbeat. When the SA node discharges the impulse, it travels in many directions through the heart muscle. The impulse also moves quickly across special bands of tissue called *internodal tracts*. The Bachmann bundle, a specialized internodal tract, takes the impulse to the left atrium. Other internodal tracts take the impulse quickly to the AV node. The impulse moving through the atrial chambers triggers the chambers to contract.
- *Atrioventricular* (AE tree oh ven trik yah lar) (AV) *node*: The AV node is located at the base of the interatrial septum. When the impulse reaches the AV node, it moves very slowly through it.
- *Bundle of His* (also called the *atrioventricular* [AV] *bundle*): The bundle of His is located in the upper interventricular septum. When the impulse leaves the AV node, it moves to the bundle of His.
- *Right and left bundle branches*: The bundle branches are located in the lower interventricular septum. After the impulse passes through the bundle of His, it enters the right and left bundle branches. The right bundle branch brings the impulse to the right ventricle. The left bundle branch brings the impulse to the left ventricle.
- *Purkinje* (pur KIN jee) *fibers*: The bundle branches split into many Purkinje fibers. Purkinje fibers transmit the impulse quickly and efficiently to the ventricular myocardial cells. This causes the ventricular chambers to contract.

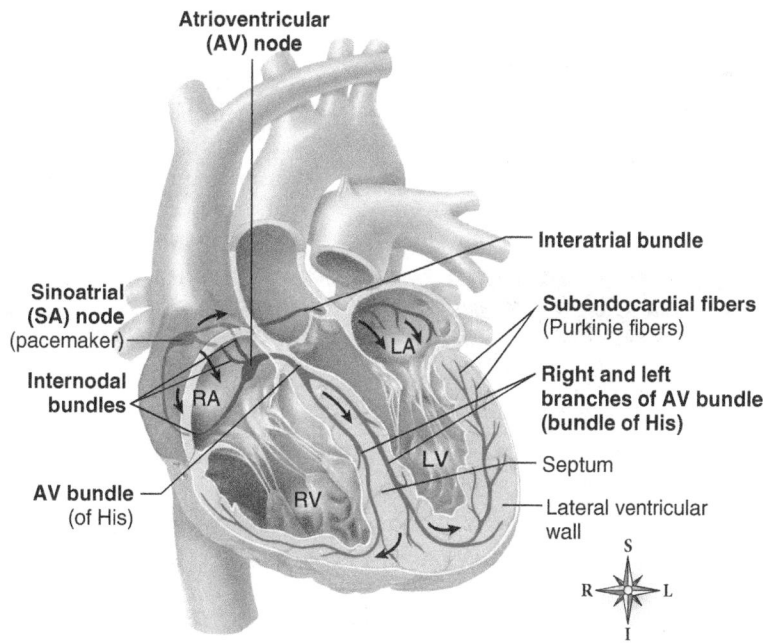

Fig. 10.7 Conduction System of the Heart. Specialized cardiac muscle cells (red) in the wall of the heart rapidly conduct an electrical impulse throughout the myocardium. The signal is initiated by the sinoatrial (SA) node (pacemaker) and spreads to the rest of the atrial myocardium and to the atrioventricular (AV) node. The AV node then initiates a signal that is conducted through the ventricular myocardium by way of the AV bundle (of His) and Purkinje fibers. Labels for parts of the heart's conduction system are highlighted in bold font. *LA,* Left atrium; *LV,* left ventricle; *RA,* right atrium; *RV,* right ventricle. (From Patton KT, Thibodeau G: *The human body in health and disease,* ed 6, St. Louis, 2014, Mosby.)

States of Cardiac Cells. The cardiac cells cycle through three states or steps in the same sequence for each impulse:

1. *Polarized state*: Before the impulse hits the cells, they are in a polarized state. There is no electrical activity during the polarized state. Think of this as the "waiting" stage.
2. *Depolarized state*: When the impulse hits the cells, the cells' charges change. This is due to the movement of the ions (e.g., sodium, potassium, and calcium) across the cells' membrane. The change of the cells' charges allows the impulse to move through the cell, causing action potential (also called *depolarization*). Electrical activity can be recorded on an electrocardiogram (ECG) when the cells are in the depolarized state. (ECGs are discussed in Chapter 48.)
3. *Repolarized state*: After the impulse passes over the cells, the ions move back to their original location. This causes the cells' charge to change. This recovery phase is called the *repolarized state*. Electrical activity (less than the depolarized state) can also be recorded on an ECG during the repolarized state.

When you are discussing the three states and the chambers affected, the chamber (atrial, ventricular) comes before the state (e.g., atrial polarization, ventricular depolarization). This terminology will be used as we examine the blood flow and the conduction system together.

Conduction System and Blood Flow. The conduction system is the electrical system in the heart. As already mentioned, it is recorded on the ECG. Electrical impulses from the conduction system cause the chambers of the heart to contract. This contraction is a mechanical action, and, as a result, blood moves through the heart. The mechanical action can be seen with echocardiography (eck oh kar dee AH gruh fee) (ECHO), which will be described later in this chapter.

Table 10.2 summarizes an impulse's path through the conduction system and the resulting mechanical action with the blood flow movement. Notice that the atrial chamber state is always one step ahead of the ventricular chambers.

Conduction System and the Nervous System. Cardiac muscle is different from other muscles in the body. The heart is controlled by the autonomic nervous system and the heart's own conduction system. When the heart rate needs to change to meet the demands of the body, the autonomic nervous system automatically kicks in.

Blood Pressure

About 1 in 3 American adults has high blood pressure. This means that many of the patients seen in an ambulatory care center may be diagnosed with high blood pressure, or *hypertension* (hye pur TEN shun). More information on hypertension will be provided later in the chapter. By contrast, low blood pressure, or *hypotension*, can be life-threatening in some cases.

The pressure of the blood is highest in the arteries and lowest in the veins. Thus we measure arterial blood pressure. *Blood pressure* (BP) can be defined as the resulting force of blood against the walls of the arteries. Two measurements are taken during the cardiac cycle (a complete heartbeat):

- *Systole* (SIS toh lee) or the *contractive phase*: Systolic pressure is measured when the heart is contracting and pumping out the blood.
- *Diastole* (dye AS toh lee) or the *relaxation phase*: Diastolic pressure is measured when the heart is resting between contractions.

TABLE 10.2	Impulse Pathway Through the Conduction System With the Triggered Mechanical Actions				
Impulse Moving Through Conduction System	**Atrial Cardiac Cells' State**	**Ventricular Cardiac Cells' State**	**MECHANICAL ACTION TRIGGERED BY IMPULSE**		
			Right Side of Heart	**Left Side of Heart**	
SA node *(pacemaker)* generates the impulse, which travels to the AV node	Atrial depolarization	Ventricular polarization	Right atrium contracts; blood passes the tricuspid valves and empties into the right ventricle	Left atrium contracts; blood passes the bicuspid valves and empties into the left ventricle	
Impulse moves slowly through AV node			Allows the atrial chambers to finish contracting		
Impulse leaves the AV node and moves to the bundle of His, to the right and left bundle branches, and to the Purkinje fibers	Atrial repolarization	Ventricular depolarization	Right ventricle contracts; blood passes the pulmonary valve before emptying into the pulmonary artery as it heads to the lungs	Left ventricle contracts; blood passes the aortic valve before emptying into the aorta as it goes to the body	
(The impulse is now done.)	Atrial polarization	Ventricular repolarization (then moves into ventricular polarization)	Right atrium fills with deoxygenated blood from the body via the inferior vena cava and the superior vena cava	Left atrium fills with oxygenated blood from the lungs via the pulmonary vein	

You will learn more about the procedure to take blood pressures in Chapter 33. This section addresses the factors that can influence blood pressure.

Blood Volume. *Blood volume,* or the amount of circulating blood, has a direct influence on blood pressure. The greater the blood volume, the more force it exerts on the arterial walls. If the blood volume is low, less force or pressure will be put on the arterial walls. Think of a garden hose attached to a faucet. If you turn on the faucet to the maximum level, there will be a lot of water pressure in the hose. If you turn on the faucet to get a trickle, there is very little water pressure in the hose.

Let us briefly examine the factors that increase and decrease blood volume. The blood volume can be raised by:
- Blood, plasma, and fluid (intravenous [IV]) transfusions
- Increased sodium intake (because water follows sodium, more water will be drawn into the bloodstream due to the elevated sodium levels)

Blood volume can decrease due to *hemorrhage* (HEM ahr ij) (bleeding), dehydration, and diuretic (DIE ah ret ik) medications. Diuretics help pull water and sodium from the blood, thus lowering blood volume.

Strength of Ventricular Contractions. The left ventricle pumps blood to the body. The greater the force of the contraction, the more blood is pumped into the arteries. This increases the blood pressure. If the left ventricular contraction is weak, less blood is pumped out of the heart and thus the blood pressure is lower. Digoxin is a medication that reduces the heart rate and strengthens the contractions of the heart.

With heart disease, tests are done to check how the left ventricle is functioning. The *stroke volume* is the amount of blood that is pushed out of the left ventricle compared with the total volume of blood that filled the ventricle. It is a measure of the ejection fraction of the cardiac output. As heart disease occurs, the stroke volume can decrease.

Resistance to Blood Flow. Any factor that increases the resistance to blood flow through the arteries will increase the blood pressure. Factors that increase resistance include the size of the *lumen* (inner opening) of the arteries, the elasticity of the arterial walls, and the *viscosity* (thickness) of the blood.

The *peripheral resistance* of blood vessels refers to the size of the lumen and the amount of blood flowing through it. The smaller the vessel's lumen, the greater the resistance to blood flow, thus increasing blood pressure. Several dynamics lead to decreased lumen size, including:
- *Plaque* (plak) (waxy substance) builds up in the arteries and hardens over time. This buildup narrows the arteries and causes higher blood pressure.
- Smoking.
- Constriction of smooth muscles, causing vasoconstriction (VAE zoe kon strik shahn). Several medications, including benazepril, lisinopril, and losartan, relax smooth muscles, thus reducing blood pressure.

Another factor that increases blood flow resistance is the loss of vessel elasticity. The inner layer of an artery contains elastic-like fibers that allow the vessel to expand and contract. Arteries dilate as the blood is pumped out of the heart and narrow between heartbeats to help maintain blood pressure. Increasing age and plaque buildup reduce the elasticity of the vessels. To understand the effect of plaque on the vessels, think of dried glue on a balloon. The dried glue prevents that section of the balloon from expanding. The plaque is like the dried glue. It prevents the walls from expanding.

Lastly, the viscosity of blood influences the resistance to blood flow. As the viscosity of the blood increases, so does the resistance, and the blood pressure rises. The thickness of blood increases when more blood cells are present (e.g., polycythemia [pol ee sie THEE mee ah], blood transfusion).

In summary, blood pressure can be influenced by blood volume, the strength of ventricular contractions, and the resistance to blood flow. Resistance can be increased by:
- Narrowed lumen (e.g., due to plaque, smoking, and vasoconstriction)
- Loss of vessel elasticity due to aging and plaque
- Increased viscosity of the blood

CRITICAL THINKING 10.5

With many of their patients having high blood pressure, Rebecca wants to make sure Lizzy understands the factors that affect blood pressure. She asks Lizzy to summarize factors that increase blood pressure. How might Lizzy respond?

VOCABULARY
polycythemia A condition caused by an abnormally large number of red blood cells (RBCs) in the blood.

DISEASES AND DISORDERS OF THE CARDIOVASCULAR SYSTEM

Many patients seen in the ambulatory care facility have cardiovascular diseases. Common signs and symptoms include:
- *Angina pectoris* (an JYE nuh PECK tore us): Chest pain
- *Bradycardia* (brad dee KAR dee ah): A pulse less than 60 beats per minute (bpm)
- *Tachycardia* (tack ee KAR dee ah): A pulse greater than 100 bpm
- *Palpitations*: Fast, strong, or irregular heartbeats
- *Bruit* (BROO ee): An abnormal blowing or swishing sound heard over the artery when a Doppler ultrasound or stethoscope is used (Fig. 10.8)
- *Cardiomegaly*: An enlargement of the heart
- *Cyanosis* (sye uh NOH sis): A bluish discoloration of the skin, lips, and nail beds
- *Pallor*: Paleness of the skin
- *Diaphoresis* (dye uh foh REE sis): Profuse sweating
- *Edema*: Swelling
- *Syncope* (SING kuh pee): Fainting or loss of consciousness and postural tone caused by diminished blood flow to the brain
- *Dyspnea* (DISP nee uh): Difficulty breathing

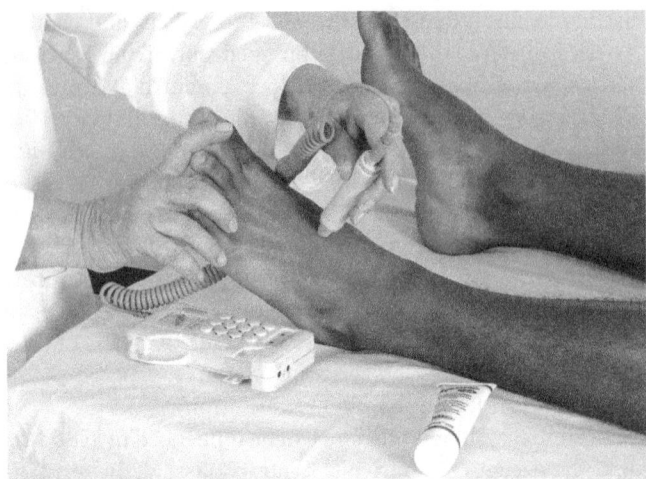

Fig. 10.8 **Using a Doppler to Check the Pulse.** (From Jarvis C: *Physical examination and health assessment*, ed 7, St. Louis, 2016, Saunders.)

- *Orthopnea* (or THOP nee uh): Dyspnea with lying flat, relieved when sitting up
- *Shortness of breath* (SOB): Breathlessness
- *Venous distension*: Enlarged veins

Common diagnostic procedures and medical laboratory tests are listed in Table 10.3. Common treatments used for cardiovascular system diseases are described in Table 10.4. The following sections describe in detail some of the cardiovascular diseases.

CRITICAL THINKING 10.6

To see if Lizzy understands the difference between an ECG and an ECHO, Rebecca asks her to describe what each test shows. What might be Lizzy's answer?

Arrhythmias

An *arrhythmia* (ah RITH mee ah) or dysrhythmia is an abnormal heart rate or rhythm.. The rhythm may be irregular, or tachycardia or bradycardia may be occurring. The most common arrhythmia is *atrial fibrillation*, which means the rate is fast and the rhythm is irregular.

Etiology. Arrhythmias are caused by an issue with the heart's conduction system, including an extra beat; the impulse is blocked, slowed, or takes a different pathway through the heart. Arrhythmias can be caused by diseases (e.g., heart failure), stress, substances (e.g., medications, caffeine), and electrolyte imbalances. Arrhythmias may be intermittent or constant.

Signs and Symptoms. Signs and symptoms of arrhythmias include:

- Fast or slow heart rate
- Irregular, skipping, or uneven heartbeats
- Lightheadedness, dizziness, shortness of breath (SOB)
- Pallor, angina, sweating

Diagnostic Procedures. The provider will listen to the heart with a stethoscope. An ECG is usually the first test done. Heart monitoring devices (e.g., the Holter monitor and an event monitor) provide ECG monitoring over days to weeks. Other tests ordered may include ECHO, coronary angiography, and an *electrophysiology study* (EPS), an in-depth study of the heart's electrical system.

Treatments. Treatment depends on the severity of the arrhythmia. Treatments may include *defibrillation* or *cardioversion*, which shocks the heart into a normal rhythm, or an implantable pacemaker to help establish a normal rate and rhythm. Antiarrhythmic medications, cardiac ablation, and an implantable cardiac defibrillator may also be used.

Atherosclerosis-Related Diseases

Atherosclerosis is a condition in which plaque or *atheromas* (ath uh ROH mahs) build up and narrow the arteries. The plaque can prevent the arteries from properly constricting and dilating. At times, small cracks in the vessel wall can occur, causing a thrombus to form over the atheroma, partially or completely occluding the vessel. If a section of the thrombus breaks away and travels in the bloodstream, this is an *embolus* (Fig. 10.14).

Etiology. The cause of atherosclerosis is unknown. Studies have shown that it can develop in childhood and gets worse with age. Risk factors for atherosclerosis include smoking, an unhealthy diet, lack of physical activity, high blood pressure, unhealthy cholesterol levels, and uncontrolled diabetes mellitus.

Signs and Symptoms. The signs and symptoms depend on which arteries are affected by the plaque. In many cases, no symptoms are felt until the artery is severely narrowed or blocked. Several diseases can result from plaque buildup. Table 10.5 presents the descriptions, signs, and symptoms of atherosclerosis-related diseases.

Diagnostic Procedures. Diagnostic procedures include blood tests to check the cholesterol, glucose, and protein levels. Additional tests include an ECG, echocardiography, chest x-ray, computed tomography (CT) scan, angiography, and stress test.

Treatments. The goals of treatment are to lower the risk of blood clot formation, prevent diseases, and widen the affected arteries. Heart-healthy lifestyle changes will be encouraged. This involves exercise, a healthy diet, building stress-coping and management skills, maintaining a healthy weight, and smoking cessation. Medications that lower cholesterol levels may be used. Percutaneous coronary intervention, coronary artery bypass grafting (CABG), or a carotid endarterectomy may also be performed.

VOCABULARY

thrombus A blood clot that blocks the flow of blood.

TABLE 10.3 Common Diagnostic Procedures Used for Cardiovascular System Disorders

Done by/Type of Test	Procedure	Description
Provider during the exam	*Heart sounds*	Provider uses a stethoscope to listen to (or auscultate) the heart sounds.
Medical assistant	*Blood pressure*	A measure of the systolic over the diastolic pressure. The instrument used is a *sphygmomanometer* (sfig MOE mah nom i tur).
Imaging procedures	*Angiocardiography* (an jee oh kar dee AH gruh fee)	Injection of a radiopaque substance during cardiac catheterization for the purpose of imaging the heart and related structures. Also called *coronary angiography* (KORE ih nair ee an jee AH gruh fee).
	Cardiac catheterization (KAR dee ack kath ih tur ih ZAY shun)	Threading of a catheter (thin tube) into the heart under fluoroscopic guidance to collect diagnostic information about structures in the heart, coronary arteries, and great vessels; also used to aid in treatment of coronary artery disease (CAD), congenital abnormalities, and heart failure.
	Digital subtraction angiography (DSA) (an jee AH gruh fee)	Digital imaging process wherein contrast images are used to "subtract" the noncontrast image of surrounding structures, leaving only a clear image of blood vessels (Fig. 10.9).
	Doppler ultrasound	An imaging test that uses sounds waves to show blood moving through blood vessels.
	Color Doppler	An ultrasound that uses a computer to change sound waves into different colors. The colors show the speed and direction of the blood flow.
	Echocardiography (ECHO) (eck oh kar dee AH gruh fee)	Use of ultrasonic waves directed through the heart to study the structure and motion of the heart (Fig. 10.10). *Transesophageal echocardiography* (TEE) images the heart through a transducer introduced into the esophagus.
	Magnetic resonance imaging (MRI)	Computerized imaging that uses radiofrequency pulses in a magnetic field to detect damaged areas and areas of blood flow.
	Multiple-gated acquisition scan (*MUGA scan*) (MOO guh)	A noninvasive method of imaging a beating heart by tagging red blood cells (RBCs) with a radioactive substance. A gamma camera captures the outline of the chambers of the heart as the blood passes through them.
	Myocardial perfusion imaging (mye oh KAR dee ul pur FYOO zhun)	Use of radionuclide to diagnose CAD, valvular or congenital heart disease, and cardiomyopathy.
	Phlebography (fleh BAH gruh fee)	X-ray imaging of a vein after the introduction of a contrast dye.
	Positron emission tomography (PET) (POZ ih tron ee MIH shun toh MAH gruh fee)	Computerized nuclear medicine procedure that uses inhaled or injected radioactive substances to help identify how much a patient will benefit from revascularization procedures.
Other tests	*Electrocardiography* (ECG, EKG) (ee leck troh kar dee AH gruf ee)	Recording of electrical impulses of the heart as wave deflections on an instrument called an *electrocardiograph*. The record, or recording, is called an *electrocardiogram*.
	Exercise stress test (EST)	Tests the electrical activity of the heart during exercise on a treadmill; may include the use of radioactive substance. Also called an *exercise electrocardiogram*.
	Holter monitor (HOLE tur)	Portable electrocardiograph that is worn to record the reaction of the heart to daily activities.
	Swan-Ganz catheter (swann ganz)	Long, thin cardiac catheter with a tiny balloon at the tip that is fed into the femoral artery near the groin and extended up to the left ventricle. Used to determine left ventricular function by measuring pulmonary capillary pressure.
Medical laboratory	*Cardiac enzymes test*	Blood test that measures the level of cardiac enzymes, which characteristically released during a heart attack (myocardial infarction); determines the amount of lactate dehydrogenase (LDH) and creatine phosphokinase (CPK) in the blood.
	Lipid profile	Blood test to measure the lipids (cholesterol and triglycerides) in the circulating blood. Some CLIA-waived tests available.
	Prothrombin time	A prothrombin time (PT) measures the number of seconds it takes a clot to form after reagents are added to the blood sample. The PT is used to detect bleeding disorders or excessive clotting disorders. CLIA-waived tests are available.

CLIA, Clinical Laboratory Improvement Amendments.

CRITICAL THINKING 10.7

Lizzy is working with Ken Thomas, a patient. He asks her about plaque in the arteries and what can happen if a person has a lot of plaque. How might Lizzy answer Ken's questions?

Blood Pressure–Related Disorders

Hypertension. *Hypertension* (hye pur TEN shun) (HTN) is high blood pressure. HTN occurs when the force of the blood pushing against the artery wall is elevated. There are three types of hypertension:

- *Primary hypertension* (or *essential hypertension*): The most common type with no identifiable cause; develops with age.
- *Secondary hypertension*: High blood pressure is caused by another disease, condition, or medication. If the disease is treated or the medication is removed, the high blood pressure resolves.
- *Malignant hypertension*: Very high blood pressure that causes organ damage.

Etiology. Hypertension has many causes:

- Genetics: Hypertension tends to run in families.
- Environmental factors: High-sodium diet, alcohol, smoking, lack of exercise, obesity, and some medications can lead to hypertension.
- Kidney fluid and salt balances: The kidney regulates the electrolyte and water balance in the body. Kidney disease can lead to increased blood volume, which leads to hypertension.
- Renin-angiotensin-aldosterone system: A complex system that makes angiotensin, which constricts blood vessels. It also makes aldosterone, which affects kidney function and leads to increased blood volume. Both can cause hypertension.
- Sympathetic nervous system: Involved with blood pressure regulation.
- Changes in blood vessels: Loss of elasticity in the walls can lead to hypertension.

Signs and Symptoms. Hypertension has no symptoms. The only sign is a high blood pressure reading. However, it can cause serious problems, including stroke, heart attack, heart failure, and kidney failure.

Diagnostic Procedures. Blood pressure is measured and recorded as two numbers. The top number is the systolic pressure, or the blood pressure during a heartbeat. The bottom number is the diastolic pressure, or the blood pressure when the heart rests. Blood pressure is measured in millimeters of mercury (mm Hg). Table 10.6 lists the stages of blood pressure.

Treatments. Treatment involves a low-salt or heart-healthy diet, maintaining a healthy weight, stopping smoking, exercise, limiting alcohol intake, and developing healthy strategies to cope with stress. Medications may also be used, including:

- Diuretics ("water pills"), which help the kidneys pull extra water and sodium from the blood, thus reducing blood volume.
- Angiotensin II receptor blockers (ARBs), angiotensin-converting enzyme (ACE) inhibitors, calcium channel blockers (CCBs), and alpha-blockers, which relax blood vessels, thus reducing blood pressure.

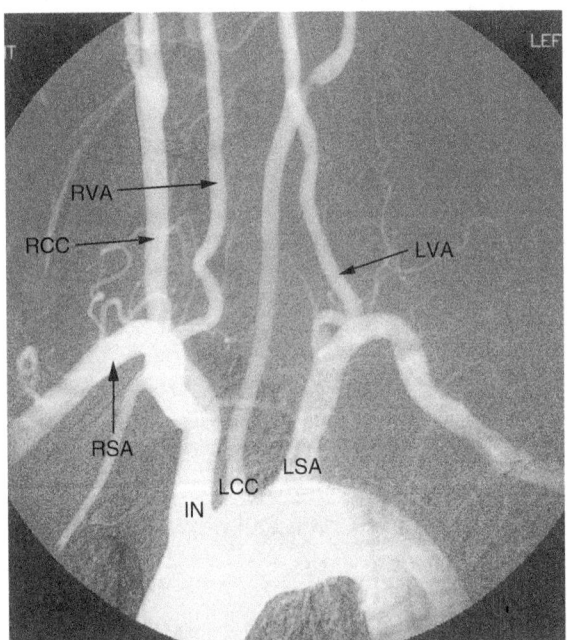

Fig. 10.9 Digital Subtraction Image of the Aorta. *IN,* Innominate (brachiocephalic) artery; *LCC,* left common carotid artery; *LSA,* left subclavian artery; *LVA,* left vertebral artery; *RCC,* right common carotid artery; *RSA,* right subclavian artery; *RVA,* right vertebral artery. (From Frank ED, Long BW, Smith BJ: *Merrill's atlas of radiographic positions and radiologic procedures,* ed 12, St. Louis, 2012, Mosby.)

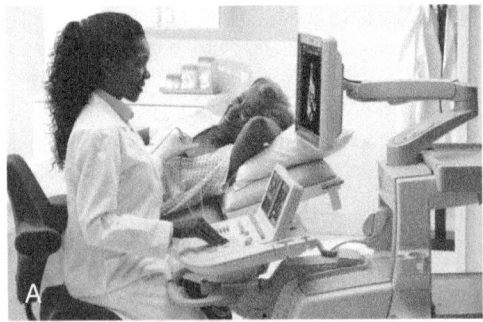
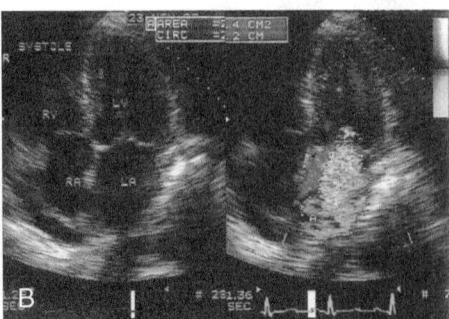

Fig. 10.10 A, Person undergoing echocardiography. B, Color Doppler image of the heart. (From Frank ED, Long BW, Smith BJ: *Merrill's atlas of radiographic positions and radiologic procedures,* ed 12, St. Louis, 2012, Mosby.)

MEDICAL TERMINOLOGY

pector/o	chest
tens/o	stretching
hyper-	excessive
pro-	forward
-ion	process of
-is	structure
-itis	inflammation
-lapse	fall

Hypotension. *Hypotension* is lower than normal blood pressure. When the blood pressure is lower than normal, the heart, brain, and other organs are not getting enough blood. A drop as little as 20 mm Hg can cause problems for some people.

Etiology. Severe hypotension can be caused by sudden loss of blood, severe infection, heart attack, or severe allergic reaction (anaphylaxis). Additional causes of hypotension include:

- Orthostatic (postural) hypotension, caused by a sudden change in body position, such as moving from sitting to standing
- Postprandial orthostatic hypotension, caused by eating
- *Neurally mediated hypotension* (NMH), which occurs when standing for a long time

- Medications, such as antianxiety drugs, antidepressants, and diuretics
- Drinking alcohol, heart failure, dehydration, and arrhythmias

Signs and Symptoms. Signs and symptoms of hypotension include:

- Blurry vision, confusion, dizziness, fainting, and light-headedness
- Nausea, vomiting, sleepiness, and weakness

Diagnostic Procedures. Besides a medical history, the provider will perform a physical exam. Laboratory tests, such as blood cultures, a complete blood count (CBC), and a urinalysis might be done. An ECG and x-rays can also be done.

Treatments. Treatment depends on the cause of hypotension. With symptoms of hypotension, the patient should sit or lie down immediately and raise the feet above heart level. Medication dosages may be adjusted. Wearing compression stockings can prevent pooling of blood in the legs, keeping more blood in the upper body.

VOCABULARY

orthostatic (postural) hypotension A temporary fall in blood pressure that occurs when a person rapidly changes from a recumbent position to a standing position.

TABLE 10.4 Common Treatments Used for Cardiovascular System Disorders

Procedure	Description
Angioplasty, balloon angioplasty (AN gee oh plas tee)	A procedure to restore blood flow through the artery. A thin tube is threaded through a blood vessel in the arm or groin and up to the narrowed or blocked coronary artery. At the narrowed artery site, a tiny balloon is inflated, which pushes the plaque outward against the wall. A *stent* (wire mesh tube) can be placed in the artery to keep the area opened (Fig. 10.11).
Atherectomy (ath uh RECK tuh mee)	A catheter with a cutter is inserted into the femoral artery and moved up to the narrowed coronary artery. The cutter rotates and removes plaque, widening the artery.
Cardiac ablation (uh BLAY shun)	Procedure that is used to scar small areas of the heart that are causing arrhythmias. *Electrodes* (small wires) are placed in the heart and detect abnormal electrical activity. When the site causing the abnormality is identified, the tissue is destroyed.
Cardiac defibrillator (dee FIB ruh lay tur)	External or implantable device that delivers an electric shock to the heart. The goal is to restore a normal sinus rhythm.
Cardiac pacemaker	Uses electrical pulses to increase or decrease the heart rate. Most pacemakers are implanted in the chest (Fig. 10.12). Prior to the surgical procedure, an external pacemaker may be used.
Cardioversion	The use of drugs or an external defibrillator to treat an arrhythmia and restore a normal sinus rhythm.
Coronary artery bypass graft (CABG)	A surgery that creates a bypass around a coronary blockage. The surgeon uses a piece of vein from the leg or artery from the chest and attaches it above and below the blockage. This creates a bypass for the blood around the blockage (Fig. 10.13).
Endarterectomy (en dar tur ECK tuh mee)	Surgical procedure used to restore the blood flow to the brain. A catheter is inserted into the carotid artery, and blood flows through the catheter while the surgeon removes the plaque from the artery.
Implantable cardioverter defibrillator (ICD)	Implantable devices that monitor and correct the heart rhythm. The ICD can deliver a shock if the rhythm is life-threatening.
Heart transplant	The removal of a patient's diseased heart and transplantation of a donor heart.
Hemorrhoidectomy (hem uh royd ECK tuh mee)	Surgical removal of hemorrhoids.
Sclerotherapy (skleh roh THAIR uh pee)	Used to treat varicose veins. The provider injects a solution or foam into the varicose vein and a scar forms, blocking the vein. The blood flow is rerouted to adjoining vessels.
Valvuloplasty (VAL vyoo loh plas tee)	A procedure to repair a narrowed heart valve. A catheter with a balloon on the tip is guided into the narrowed heart valve. The balloon is inflated and widens the valve opening. Also called *balloon valvuloplasty* and *balloon valvotomy*.
Ventricular assist device (VAD)	An implantable device that helps the heart pump blood.

Postural Orthostatic Tachycardia Syndrome. Postural orthostatic tachycardia syndrome (POTS) is estimated to affect 1 million to 3 million Americans and can occur at any age, though it commonly affects females between 15 and 50 years of age. POTS is considered a dysautonomia, an abnormal condition of the autonomic nervous system (ANS). The ANS does not control the blood pressure or heart rate when a person is standing up.

Etiology. Many times, the underlying cause of a person's POTS is unknown. Diseases that cause or are associated with POTS include autoimmune diseases, diabetes, infections (e.g., mononucleosis, Epstein-Barr virus, Lyme disease), multiple sclerosis, trauma, and vitamin deficiencies.

Signs and Symptoms. The signs and symptoms can vary but may include *hypovolemia* (low blood volume), tachycardia, and orthostatic (postural) hypotension. Other symptoms include:

- Fatigue, exercise intolerance, nausea, headaches, and poor concentration

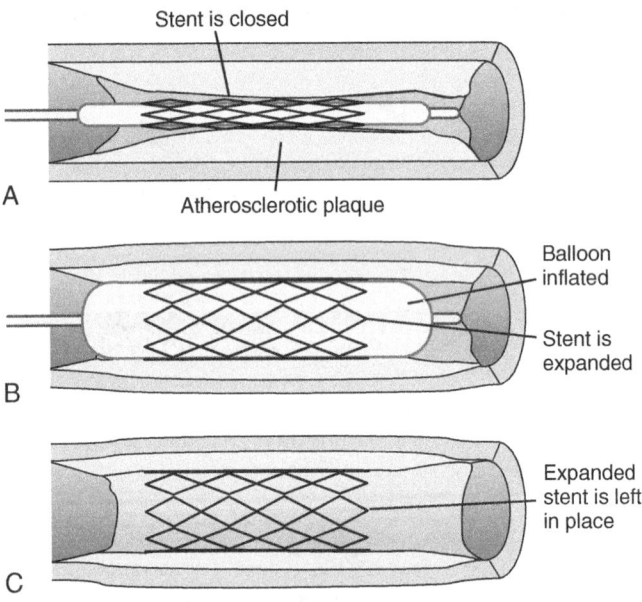

Stent is closed

A

Atherosclerotic plaque

Balloon inflated

Stent is expanded

B

Expanded stent is left in place

C

Fig. 10.11 Angioplasty with Stent Placement. (From LaFleur Brooks M: *Exploring medical language,* ed 9, St. Louis, 2014, Mosby.)

- Lightheadedness, blurred vision, syncope, heart palpitations, chest pain, and shortness of breath
- Cold or painful extremities (fingers and toes)
- Fainting with blood draws (phlebotomy) or deep breathing

With some people, the symptoms are mild and do not interfere with daily activity. Others experience significant symptoms that interfere with eating, moving, bathing, and working. About 25% of patients with POTS are disabled and cannot work.

Diagnostic Procedures. Diagnostic testing for POTS includes:

- *Tilt table test*: A patient is strapped to a table; gradually the table is tilted into the upright position and the patient is monitored for the effects of the position changes.
- *Orthostatic vital signs*: Blood pressure and heart rate are obtained as the patient reclines, sits, and stands. In many cases, the blood pressure drops and the heart rate increases.

Orthostatic (postural) hypotension occurs when there is a decrease in blood pressure within 3 minutes of standing up. The systolic blood pressure drops 20 or more mm Hg, and the diastolic blood pressure decreases 10 or more mm Hg.

Treatments. Treatment varies and may include medications to regulate the heart rate and blood pressure. Drinking plenty of fluids (2 to 3 L per day); eating a high-salt, low-carbohydrate diet; exercise; and compression stockings may also be encouraged as part of the treatment.

CRITICAL THINKING 10.8

Rebecca and Lizzy are working with a patient who has been diagnosed with postural orthostatic tachycardia syndrome (POTS). Having never heard of POTS, Rebecca asks the patient to explain the disease. The patient explains that her blood volume is low. She needs to consume a lot of sodium and water to maintain the blood volume. The patient states that she faints with blood draws. Rebecca thanks the patient for her explanation. Why is it important for medical assistants to listen to their patients about their special needs?

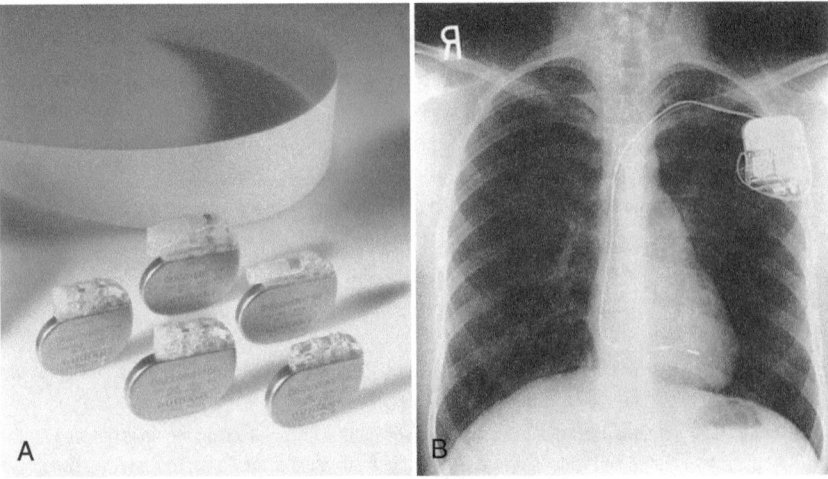

A   **B**

Fig. 10.12 A, Pacemakers. B, Chest x-ray of a patient with a permanent implanted pacemaker. (From Frank ED, Long BW, Smith BJ: *Merrill's atlas of radiographic positions and radiologic procedures,* ed 12, St. Louis, 2012, Mosby.)

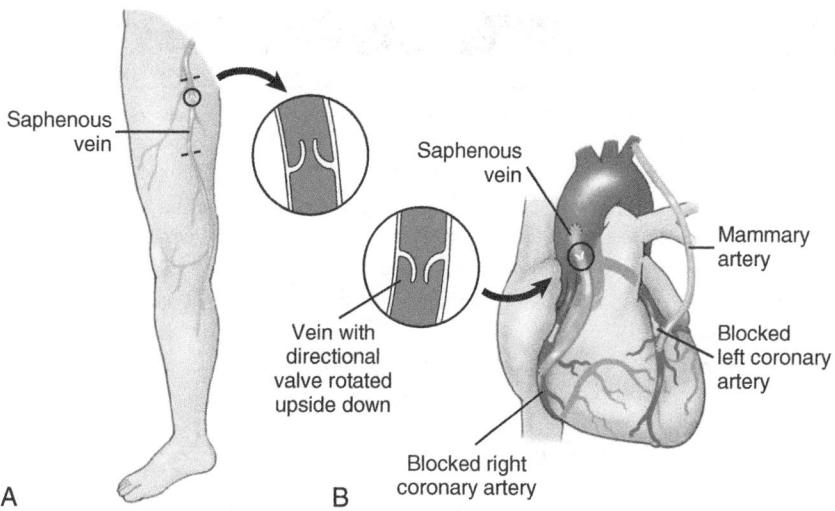

Fig. 10.13 Coronary Artery Bypass Graft (CABG). A, A section of vein is harvested from the right leg and is anastomosed to a coronary artery to bypass an occlusion of the right coronary artery. B, Bypass of the left coronary artery with a mammary artery. (From Shiland B: *Medical terminology and anatomy for ICD-10 coding*, ed 2, St. Louis, 2016, Mosby.)

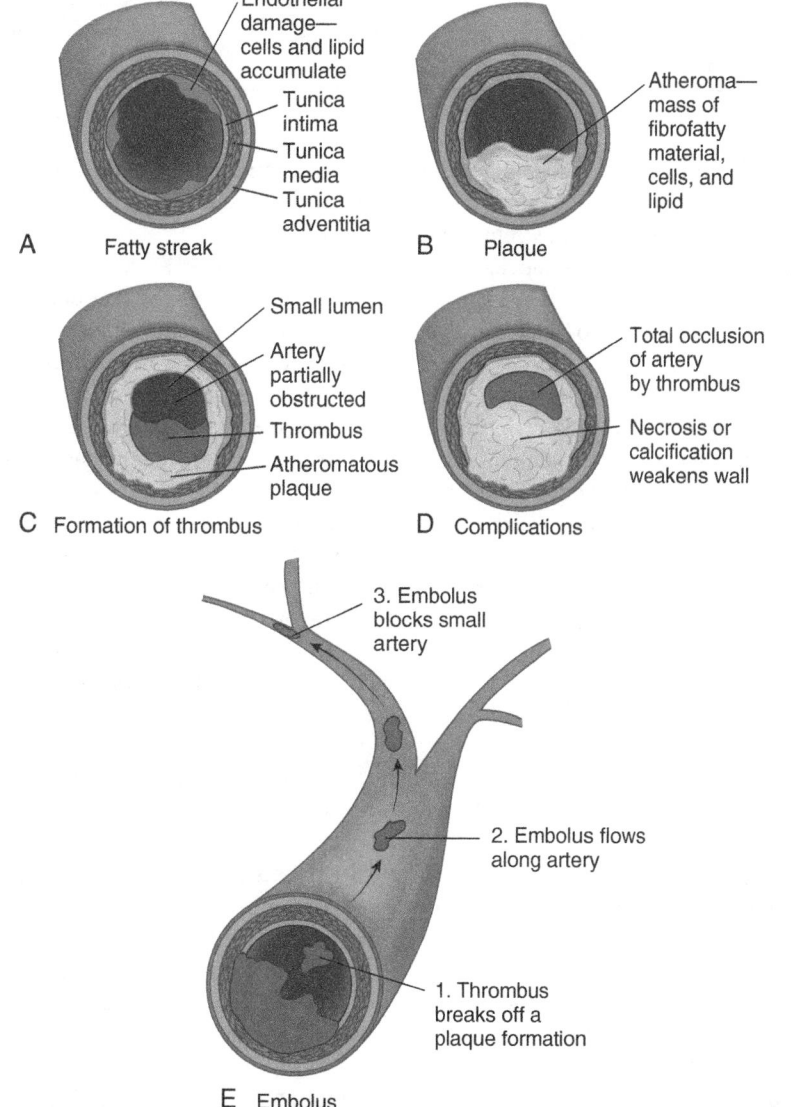

Fig. 10.14 Development of an Atheroma, Leading to Arterial Occlusion. (From Proctor D, et al: *Kinn's the medical assistant*, ed 13, St. Louis, 2017, Elsevier.)

TABLE 10.5 Atherosclerosis-Related Diseases

Disease	Description	Signs and Symptoms
Carotid artery disease	Plaque builds up in the carotid arteries and may lead to a stroke.	Sudden weakness or paralysis (inability to move), numbness, confusion, problems speaking or seeing, dizziness, and other symptoms of a stroke
Coronary heart disease (CHD) or coronary artery disease (CAD)	Plaque builds up in the coronary arteries. Can lead to *angina* (chest pain) or *myocardial infarction* (heart attack). Also known as *ischemic heart disease*.	Angina; pain in the shoulder, arm, neck, jaw or back; indigestion, shortness of breath, arrhythmias
Coronary microvascular disease (MVD)	Plaque builds up in the tiny coronary arteries, damaging the vessel walls.	Angina, shortness of breath, fatigue, lack of energy, sleep problems
Peripheral artery disease (PAD)	Plaque builds up in the large arteries of the legs, arms, and pelvis.	Numbness, pain, and life-threatening infections
Chronic kidney disease	Plaque builds up in the renal arteries and can cause kidney damage.	Tiredness, loss of appetite, nausea, swelling of hands or feet, numbness, changes in amount of urine

TABLE 10.6 Blood Pressure Stages for Adults

Categories	Systolic		Diastolic
Normal blood pressure	Less than 120 mm Hg		Less than 80 mm Hg
Elevated	120–129 mm Hg	and	Less than 80 mm Hg
Hypertension stage 1	130–139 mm Hg	or	80–89 mm Hg
Hypertension stage 2	At least 140 mm Hg	or	At least 90 mm Hg
Hypertensive crisis	More than 180 mm Hg	and/or	More than 120 mm Hg

Shock. Shock occurs when there is not enough blood and oxygen getting to the organs and tissues. It causes very low blood pressure.

Etiology. Shock usually happens with a serious injury and can be life-threatening. There are several types of shock:

- *Anaphylactic*: Severe allergic reaction; caused by exposure to an allergen (e.g., insect bites/stings, food allergy, drug allergy).
- *Cardiogenic*: Inability of the damaged heart to pump blood effectively; caused by a heart attack, arrhythmias, pulmonary embolism, or congestive heart failure.
- *Hypovolemic*: Excessive loss of blood or body fluids from internal or external hemorrhage (bleeding); severe dehydration, burns, vomiting, or diarrhea.
- *Neurogenic*: Peripheral vessels dilate due to a neurologic injury or disorder (e.g., spinal cord injury).
- *Septic*: Overwhelming infection; caused by bacteria, fungi, and rarely viruses.

Signs and Symptoms. Signs and symptoms of shock include:

- Weak, rapid pulse and rapid, shallow respirations
- Changes in the level of consciousness: confusion, lack of alertness, loss of consciousness
- Dizziness, lightheadedness, or faintness
- Sweaty, pale skin; cool hands and feet; bluish lips and fingernails
- Reduced or no urine output

Diagnostic Procedures. Shock is diagnosed based on the history, exam, and vital signs of the patient. If time allows, additional testing may be done to identify the cause.

Treatments. The goals of medical treatment include increasing the cardiac output and blood pressure with medications, blood transfusions, and IV fluids. Additional treatments address the cause of the shock.

Cardiomyopathy

With cardiomyopathy (kar dee oh mye AH puh thee), the heart muscle becomes abnormal. It may become thin and weakened, enlarged and thick, or rigid. As the disease worsens, the heart becomes less efficient at pumping blood and maintaining a normal electrical rhythm. Cardiomyopathy can lead to arrhythmias, heart failure, edema, and heart valve problems.

Etiology. There are many types of cardiomyopathy; some develop due to other diseases, and others are inherited. This disease can affect people of all ages. Major risk factors for cardiomyopathy include:

- Diabetes mellitus, metabolic diseases, or severe obesity
- Diseases that cause heart damage (e.g., heart attack, coronary heart disease)
- A family history of cardiomyopathy
- Long-term alcoholism
- Long-term hypertension (high blood pressure)

Signs and Symptoms. Some people may never have symptoms, whereas others do not experience symptoms during the early stages of the disease. As the condition worsens, a person may experience:

- Shortness of breath, especially after activity
- Swelling of the legs, feet, ankles, abdomen, and neck veins
- Fatigue

Diagnostic Procedures. The provider will obtain a history and perform a physical exam. Abnormal heart sounds and lung sounds might be heard with a stethoscope. A heart murmur may be present. Crackling in the lungs may indicate fluid in the lungs. Swelling can also be seen, as mentioned in the previous section. A chest x-ray, an ECG, ECHO, and a stress test may be ordered. Further procedures may include cardiac catheterization, coronary angiography, or myocardial biopsy.

Treatments. Treatments depend on the severity of the condition. Treatments may include healthy lifestyle changes and medications, such as antiarrhythmics, anticoagulants, diuretics, and beta-blockers, which lower the heart rate. Surgery can also be done, including a septal myectomy (removal of the thickened septal muscle), a heart transplantation, and an implanted device.

Congenital Heart Defects

There are numerous congenital heart defects. Table 10.7 describes common defects. Depending on the type and severity of the defect, the newborn baby may require immediate surgery.

Etiology. The cause of these congenital defects may be genetic, chromosomal, or unknown.

Signs and Symptoms. The signs and symptoms of the defect will depend on its type and severity. For some, there are no symptoms, and the person may not realize the condition exists until adulthood. Other defects may cause the baby to have the following conditions:

- Cyanosis, increased respiration rate, or breathing difficulties
- Difficulty feeding, tiredness with feeding, or weight loss
- Abnormal heart murmur
- Sweating with feeding or crying

Diagnostic Procedures. Some of the defects may be identified during the pregnancy. Fetal echocardiography can be used on a baby in utero to detect cardiac abnormalities. After birth, ECHO, pulse oximetry, ECG, and chest x-rays may be performed to help diagnose the defect.

Treatments. Treatment for congenital heart defects depends on the type and severity of the defect. Some holes may close on their own, whereas others may require surgery to patch them. Some defects will be monitored, but no treatment will be required. Life-threatening defects will require emergency surgery after birth and follow-up through childhood.

Congestive Heart Failure

Congestive heart failure (CHF), also called *heart failure,* occurs when the heart does not efficiently pump blood. Blood backs up behind the failing pump (side of the heart). *Systolic heart failure* occurs when the heart muscle cannot pump the blood out of the heart. *Diastolic heart failure* occurs when the chamber muscle is stiff and does not completely fill up with blood. Heart failure can affect one or both sides of the heart. Types of heart failure include:

- *Right-sided heart failure*: Fluid may back up into the body, causing swelling in the legs, feet, and abdomen.

TABLE 10.7	Congenital Heart Defects
Congenital Heart Defects	**Description**
Atrial septal defect (ASD)	A hole in the interatrial septum allows oxygen-rich blood from the left atrium to flow into the right atrium. May not have many symptoms. Hole may close on its own or with surgery.
Atrioventricular septal defect	Holes are between the right and left chambers, and the valves are malformed. Surgery is required to patch holes.
Coarctation of the aorta (koh ark TEY shun)	Narrowing of the aorta, resulting in blood back-flowing into the left ventricle, high blood pressure, and weakened pulses in the legs. Surgery or balloon angioplasty can correct the condition.
Dextrotransposition of the great arteries (d-TGA) (DECKS tro trans poh ZI shun)	The pulmonary artery and the aorta are switched. Oxygen-rich blood is pumped back to the lungs, and the deoxygenated blood is pumped back to the body. Requires emergency surgery.
Hypoplastic left heart syndrome (hi puh PLAS tik)	Structures on the left side of the heart are not correctly developed. Treated with medications and surgery to improve blood flow.
Patent foramen ovale (PFO)	Foramen ovale does not close during infancy but remains *patent* (open). May not have any symptoms and may not require treatment.
Patent ductus arteriosus (PDA)	Ductus arteriosus does not close soon after birth, causing too much blood to move into the pulmonary circulation. A heart murmur may be the only sign.
Pulmonary atresia (PULL mun airy ah TREE sha)	Pulmonary valve does not form, and blood cannot flow to the lungs. Requires immediate surgery after birth to improve blood flow to the lungs.
Tetralogy of Fallot (TOF) (te tral uh jee of Fal oh)	Consists of four major conditions: ventricular septal defect, pulmonary stenosis, defective aortic valve, and ventricular hypertrophy. Requires immediate surgery.
Ventricular septal defect (VSD)	Septal wall is not fully developed between the ventricles, causing a hole. Blood tends to flow from the left ventricle into the right ventricle, stressing the pulmonary system.

- *Left-sided heart failure*: Fluid may back up into the lungs, causing shortness of breath and abnormal lung sounds.
- *Cor pulmonale*: Right-sided heart failure caused by high blood pressure in the right ventricle and pulmonary arteries.

Etiology. Coronary artery disease (CAD) and high blood pressure are the most common causes of heart failure. Other causes include congenital problems, heart attack, faulty valves, arrhythmias, infections, and other diseases (e.g., thyroid problems).

Signs and Symptoms. Symptoms can develop slowly or suddenly, depending on the cause. Symptoms can differ based on the side of the heart that is failing. Common signs and symptoms include:

- Cough and shortness of breath with reclining or activity
- Fatigue, faintness, weakness, and loss of appetite
- Fast or irregular pulse, and palpitations
- Pitting edema in the feet and legs
- Swollen liver and abdomen, weight gain

Diagnostic Procedures. During the physical exam, the provider will listen for abnormal heart and lung sounds and check for edema (Fig. 10.15). Echocardiography, imaging tests, and blood tests may be ordered.

Treatments. Treatment includes monitoring weight; limiting dietary cholesterol, salts, and fluids; and medications (e.g., diuretics, antihypertensives, and digoxin). Surgery, a pacemaker, an implantable defibrillator, or heart transplantation may also be needed.

Deep Vein Thrombosis

Deep vein thrombosis (thrahm BOW sis) (DVT) or thrombophlebitis occurs when a thrombus forms in a vein deep in the body, usually in the legs. DVTs can occur at any age, but they most commonly occur in people over the age of 60. An embolus (EM boh lus) can occur from a DVT, which can lead to life-threatening conditions, including a pulmonary embolism (EM boh li zehm) (PE), cerebrovascular (seh ree broh VAS kyoo lur) accident (stroke), or myocardial infarction (mye oh KAR dee ul in FARCK shun) (heart attack).

Etiology. Blood clots can form when the vein's inner lining and valves are damaged by surgery, injuries, inflammation, or an immune response (Fig. 10.16). Blood clots can also occur when the blood flow is slow or if the blood has an increase in viscosity. Estrogen, birth control pills, and inherited conditions can cause an increased risk for clotting. Other risk factors for DVTs include:

- A family history of blood clots
- Medical conditions: Pregnancy or up to 6 months after delivery, pelvis and leg fractures, bed rest, polycythemia, surgery, indwelling catheter in a blood vessel, lupus, and cancer
- Certain medications (e.g., estrogen, birth control pills), smoking, and obesity

Signs and Symptoms. Signs and symptoms include leg pain, swelling, warmth, and redness.

Diagnostic Procedures. The provider will do a history and physical examination. An ultrasound may be ordered and also blood tests (e.g., D-dimer blood test, antithrombin levels, and CBC).

Treatments. Treatment includes anticoagulant medications, compression stockings, and possibly surgery to remove the clot.

VOCABULARY

embolus An air bubble, blood clot, or foreign body that travels through the bloodstream and blocks a blood vessel.

infarction Tissue death.

insufficiency Also called regurgitation or incompetence; the valve does not close completely, and blood leaks backward across the valve into the prior chamber.

pitting edema Excessive fluid in the intercellular spaces in the tissue; when external pressure (e.g., socks, finger pressure) is relieved, a depression is seen in the tissue.

stenosis Occurs when the heart valve flaps are stiff or fused together, thus narrowing the valve.

MEDICAL TERMINOLOGY

cerebr/o	cerebrum
tetra-	four
embolus (singular)	emboli (plural)
thrombus (singular)	thrombi (plural)

CRITICAL THINKING 10.9

Lizzy is preparing for a national exam. She is struggling to remember the difference between an embolus and a thrombus. What is a creative way to remember the differences between the two terms?

Heart Valve Diseases

There are many types of valvular disease. Two types of heart valve disease can occur with each of the valves: either stenosis (sten OH sis) or insufficiency (also called *regurgitation* or *incompetence*). When you name the disease, the valve is followed by "stenosis" or "insufficiency" (e.g., tricuspid stenosis, tricuspid insufficiency). With stenosis, the heart may need to work harder to push blood through the smaller opening. With insufficiency, the valve does not close completely, and blood leaks backward across the valve into the prior chamber (Fig. 10.17). The following sections will discuss more common valvular diseases.

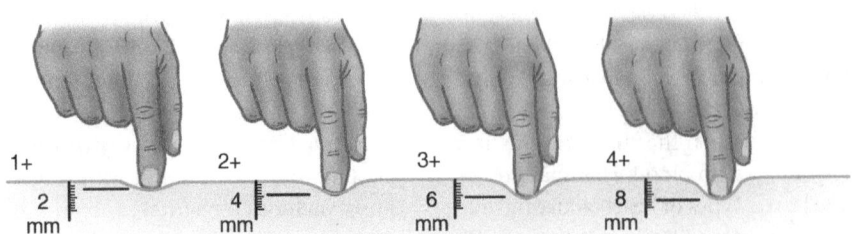

Fig. 10.15 **Providers Measure Pitting Edema From 1+ To 4+.** (From Ball J, et al: *Seidel's guide to physical examination*, St. Louis, 2019, Mosby.)

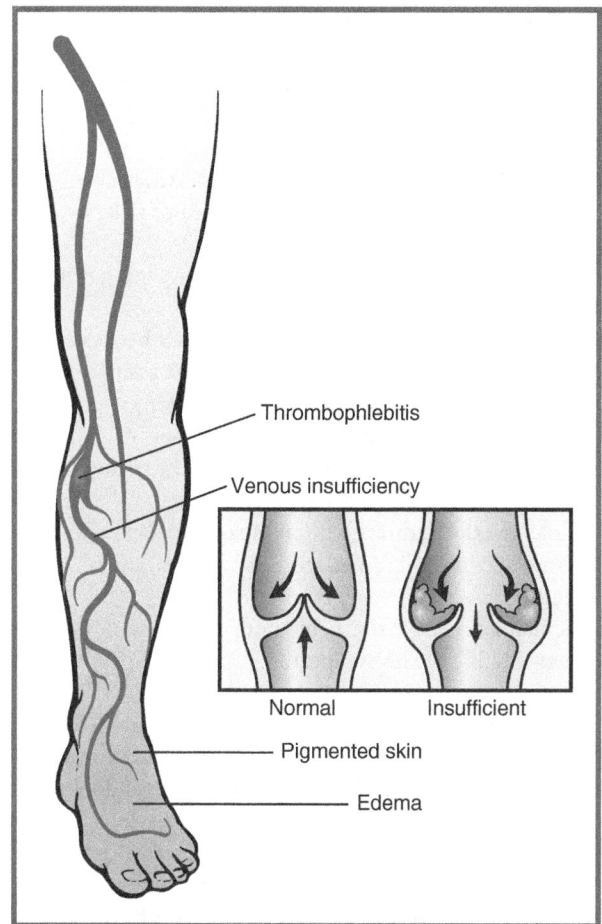

Fig. 10.16 Deep Vein Thrombosis or Thrombophlebitis. (From Damjanov I: *Pathology for the health-related professions*, ed 4, St. Louis, 2012, Saunders.)

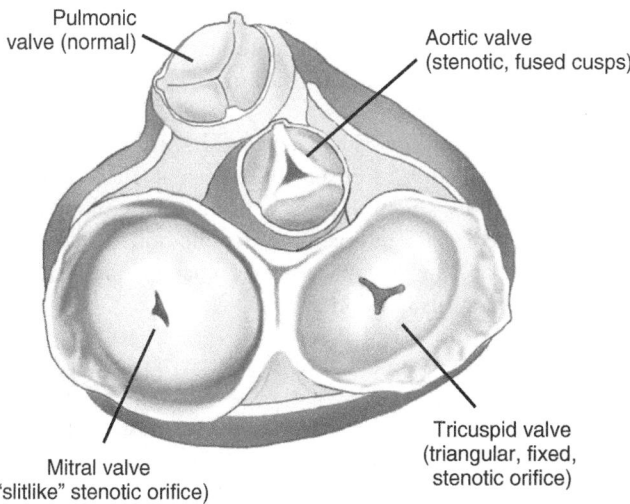

Fig. 10.17 Valvular Heart Diseases. Disorders of the aortic, mitral, and tricuspid valves. (From Shiland B: *Medical terminology and anatomy for ICD-10 coding*, ed 2, St. Louis, 2016, Mosby.)

Aortic Insufficiency. With aortic insufficiency, the aortic valve does not close tightly. The blood backs up into the left ventricle.

This is more common in males between the ages of 30 and 60.

Etiology. Many conditions cause this disease, including high blood pressure, syphilis, congenital problems, and endocarditis.

Signs and Symptoms. Signs and symptoms may not be present or may be slow to develop. They include a bounding pulse, angina, fainting, fatigue, palpitations, SOB, and swelling of the feet.

Diagnostic Procedures. Besides the physical exam, a person may have aortic angiography, ECHO, left heart catheterization, magnetic resonance imaging (MRI), and transthoracic echocardiography done to diagnose the condition.

Treatments. The treatment goal is to reduce blood pressure through medications. The patient may need surgery to replace the valve.

Mitral Valve Prolapse. Mitral valve prolapse occurs when one or both cusps of the mitral valve protrude back into the left atrium during ventricular systole.

Etiology. This condition is congenital or genetic.

Signs and Symptoms. The patient may experience palpitations, SOB, cough, fatigue, dizziness, anxiety, migraines, and chest discomfort.

Diagnostic Procedures. The provider will do a physical exam and additional tests will be ordered, including ECHO, Doppler ultrasound, chest x-ray, and an ECG.

Treatments. Treatment consists of medications (beta-blockers, diuretics, vasodilators) and surgery to repair or replace the valve.

Rheumatic Fever. Rheumatic fever is an inflammatory reaction that affects the heart valves (valvulitis) and causes swelling and scarring of the valves. Permanent damage to the valves leads to rheumatic heart disease.

Etiology. Rheumatic fever occurs 2 to 4 weeks after a strep (group A *Streptococcus*) throat infection. Antibodies made by the body to attack the streptococcal infection start attacking the body tissues (joints and heart valves), causing inflammation, swelling, and scarring.

Signs and Symptoms. The patient may have a fever, joint pain, stomach pain, weakness, SOB, *nodules* (small bumps) under the skin by the elbows and knees, and rash on the chest, abdomen, or back.

Diagnostic Procedures. After the physical exam, the provider may order blood tests, chest x-rays, ECHO, and an ECG.

Treatments. Treatment consists of antibiotics to treat the infection and nonsteroidal anti-inflammatory drugs (NSAIDs) and corticosteroids to reduce the inflammation. Surgery may be needed to repair the valve.

> **VOCABULARY**
> **valvulitis** Inflammatory condition of a valve that results in valve stenosis and obstructed blood flow; caused most commonly by rheumatic fever, bacterial endocarditis, or syphilis.

Metabolic Syndrome

Metabolic syndrome is also called *metabolic syndrome X* and *insulin resistance syndrome.* Metabolic syndrome is a group of factors that increase a person's risk for heart disease, type 2 diabetes, and stroke.

Etiology. Several causes act together. These include an inactive lifestyle, being overweight, obesity, and insulin resistance. With insulin resistance, the body cannot use insulin properly, which leads to elevated blood glucose levels. Other risk factors for metabolic syndrome include:

- Age: The risk increases with age.
- Ethnicity: Hispanic women have the greatest risk.
- Obesity: Carrying too much weight in the abdomen increases the risk.
- History of gestational diabetes, nonalcoholic fatty liver disease, polycystic ovary syndrome, or sleep apnea.
- Family history of type 2 diabetes.

Signs and Symptoms. The only signs include a large waist circumference and symptoms of diabetes if the blood glucose is elevated. These symptoms include increased thirst, frequent urination, fatigue, and blurred vision.

Diagnostic Procedures. The provider will diagnose metabolic syndrome based on the physical exam findings and the blood test results. A patient must have at least three of these risk factors to be diagnosed with metabolic syndrome:

- A large waistline: A waist measurement of 35 inches or more for females and 40 inches or more for males.
- A high triglyceride level of 150 mg/dL or higher.
- A low high-density lipoprotein (HDL) cholesterol level of less than 50 mg/dL for females and less than 40 mg/dL for males.
- High blood pressure, which is 130/85 mm/Hg or higher.
- A high fasting blood glucose level of 100 mg/dL or higher.

Treatments. Treatment is focused on a heart-healthy lifestyle. This includes a heart-healthy eating plan, limiting the saturated and trans fats eaten. It also includes managing stress, getting regular physical activity, smoking cessation, and aiming for a healthy weight.

Myocardial Infarction

Myocardial infarction (MI), also called a *heart attack,* affects more than 1 million people in the United States each year, and about half of them die as a result. With an MI, the blood flow is limited or blocked, and the heart muscle cells die due to the lack of oxygen.

Etiology. An MI can be caused by a blood clot or plaque buildup in the coronary arteries. Risk factors that can be changed include:

- Smoking, drinking alcohol, lack of exercise, obesity, and stress
- High cholesterol, high blood pressure, and uncontrolled diabetes

Factors that cannot be changed include:

- Age: Risk increases with age.
- Gender: Males have a higher risk; after menopause females have almost the same risk as males.
- Genetics: Family history increases risk.
- Race: African Americans, Mexican Americans, Native Americans, and Hawaiians have a greater risk.

Signs and Symptoms. The most common warning symptoms of MIs include:

- Angina pectoris (chest pain): May also be described as mild or severe heaviness, squeezing, pressure, or heartburn; pain may be constant or intermittent.
- Upper body discomfort or pain in one or both arms, shoulders, neck, jaw, or upper part of the abdomen.
- Shortness of breath with activity or rest.
- Cold sweat, tiredness without a reason, nausea and vomiting, dizziness, lightheadedness, arrhythmias, or palpitations.
- Females may have sharp, burning chest pain or back pain; two-thirds have no symptoms.

Diagnostic Procedures. Diagnostic tests for an MI include an ECG and blood tests (i.e., troponin, creatine kinase [CK], creatine kinase–MB [CK-MB], and serum myoglobin tests). *CK-MB* is an enzyme found in the heart muscle cell. Within hours of a heart attack, the CK-MB level increases in the blood. It peaks within 12 to 24 hours and returns to normal by 48 to 72 hours. The blood tests may be repeated over time to look for changes. Angiocardiography may be done to study the coronary blood flow and to identify blockages.

Treatments. Immediate treatment involves:

- Chewing aspirin to prevent additional clots
- Nitroglycerin to dilate the coronary arteries and help increase the oxygen to the heart muscle
- Oxygen therapy

As soon as the diagnosis is determined, thrombolytic medications (also called "clot busters") are given. These medications help the body's natural process of dissolving blood clots. Percutaneous coronary intervention may be done to open the coronary artery. Medications, lifestyle changes, and cardiac rehabilitation may also be done.

CRITICAL THINKING 10.10

Rebecca reviews the chest pain protocol with Lizzy. It states that patients with chest pain need to chew an aspirin. Nitroglycerin and oxygen must also be administered to the patient. Rebecca asks Lizzy why aspirin, nitroglycerin, and oxygen are important if a person is experiencing chest pain. How might Lizzy answer this question?

Varicose Veins

Varicose veins are swollen, twisted veins seen under the skin, usually in the legs or rectum (*hemorrhoids*). This is a common disorder.

Etiology. The cause is the one-way valves in the veins, which keep blood flowing toward the heart. If the valves become weakened or damaged, the blood backs up or pools, leading to swollen or varicose veins. Risk factors include a family history of varicose veins, prolonged standing, heavy lifting, multiple pregnancies, and advancing age.

Signs and Symptoms. Signs and symptoms include dark purple or blue twisty veins; swelling; and feelings of heaviness, fullness, aching, pain, fatigue, or cramping.

Diagnostic Procedures. The provider will examine the legs and feet (or other areas involved) during the physical exam. An ultrasound may be ordered to check the functioning of the vein valves.

Treatments. Treatment includes wearing compression stockings, exercising, losing weight, avoiding standing for long periods of time, and elevating the legs. There are many other treatments for varicose veins:
- *Sclerotherapy*: Involves an injection of a substance that closes the vein, and within a few weeks the varicose vein should fade.
- *Foam sclerotherapy*: Used for large veins and involves injecting a foam substance in the vein to close it.
- *Laser surgery*: Involves using a laser to close off small veins.
- *High ligation and vein stripping*: Involves tying off the vein and removing it through small incisions.

Additional Cardiovascular System Diseases

There are many cardiovascular diseases. The following list provides a brief description of some of them.
- *Aneurysm* (AN yoo rizz um): A bulging of the arterial wall that can burst, causing bleeding and possible death of the blood vessel wall (Fig. 10.18). Most commonly seen aneurysms occur in the aorta (aortic aneurysm). A brain aneurysm that ruptures causes a stroke.
- *Cardiac tamponade* (tam pon ADE): Blood or fluid buildup in the pericardial sac, causing pressure on the heart.
- *Endocarditis* (en doh kar DYE tis): Also called *infective endocarditis* (IE). The inner lining of the heart is inflamed. Bacterial endocarditis is most common and can damage the valves.
- *Esophageal varices* (eh sof uh JEE ul VARE ih seez): Enlarged veins in the esophagus that can rupture. Found in people with cirrhosis of the liver.
- *Pericarditis* (pair ee kar DYE tis): Inflammation of the pericardium.
- *Raynaud* (ray NODE) *disease*: Rare blood vessel disorder that affects the toes and fingers. With cold temperatures or stress, the blood vessels narrow, and blood cannot get to the surface of the skin. The toes and fingers affected turn white or blue (Fig. 10.19). When the blood flow returns, the skin is red and painful.

LIFE SPAN CHANGES

An unborn child receives oxygen and nutrients from the mother's blood through the placenta. As described earlier in this

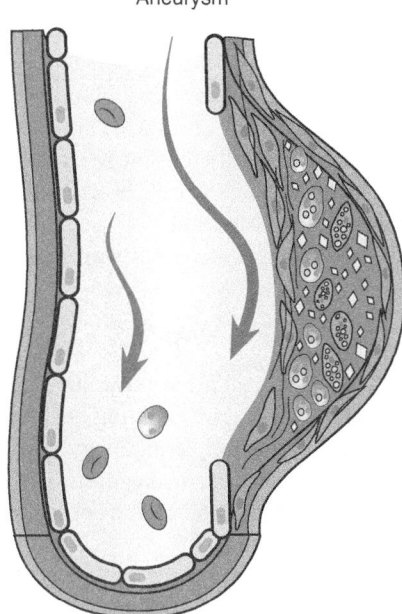

Aneurysm

Fig. 10.18 Aneurysm Caused by Weakening of the Vessel Wall. (From Damjanov I: *Pathology for the health-related professions*, ed 4, St. Louis, 2012, Saunders.)

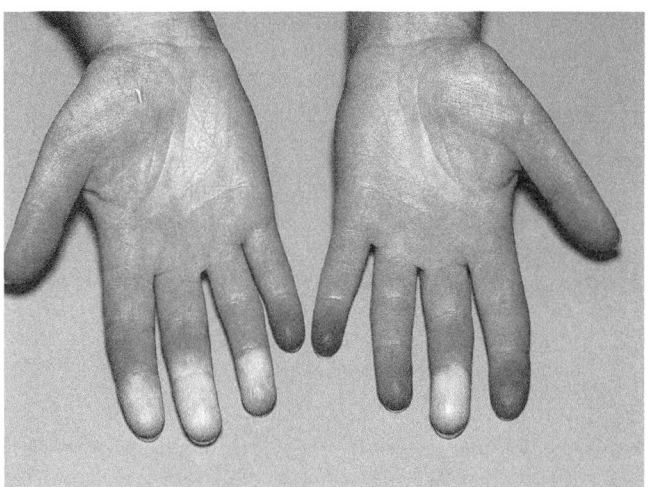

Fig. 10.19 Raynaud Disease. (From Hallett J, et al: *Comprehensive vascular and endovascular surgery*, ed 2, Philadelphia, 2009, Mosby.)

chapter, the ductus venosus, ductus arteriosus, foramen ovale, and umbilical vessels are special structures that help with fetal circulation. After birth, these structures are no longer necessary.

As a child grows and matures, the heart rate decreases. The systemic vascular resistance increases with age. This means that the resistance for blood flow increases, and thus the blood pressure increases with age.

During pregnancy, the mother's cardiovascular system undergoes changes:
- Cardiac output (amount of blood pushed out of the heart in 1 minute) increases.
- Extracellular fluid volume increases, thus the blood volume is greater.
- Total peripheral resistance decreases, thus reducing the blood pressure.

- Blood flow to various organs increases.
- As the pregnancy progresses into the third trimester, the blood pressure increases.

As a person ages, the heart and blood vessels undergo changes. Heart changes that occur include:

- SA node loses some cells; thus the heart rate can be slower.
- The left ventricle may increase in size, thus reducing the amount of blood it can hold.
- Normal ECG changes can occur with age.

- Valves can become thicker and stiffer, causing a heart murmur.
- Arterial walls become stiffer, thus increasing the blood pressure.

Baroreceptors in the carotid arteries and aorta detect changes in blood pressure and help maintain a fairly constant blood pressure with position changes. With age, the baroreceptors become less sensitive, making older people more at risk for orthostatic hypotension when changing positions.

CLOSING COMMENTS

Working with patients who have cardiovascular disorders is common in ambulatory care. It is important for the medical assistant to know medical terminology and abbreviations related to cardiovascular system diagnostic tests and procedures. Besides medical terminology and abbreviations, medical assistants need to understand:

- Basics of the cardiovascular system, including the structures and functions of the structures

- Importance of the heart's conduction system
- Factors that affect blood pressure
- Diseases that affect the cardiovascular system
- Common medications used for cardiovascular system diseases (Box 10.1)

Having this understanding will help you provide great care to your patients. It will also help you recognize the importance of different treatments ordered by the providers.

BOX 10.1 Medication Classifications

- *Antiarrhythmics:* Used to treat arrhythmias
- *Anticoagulants:* Used to prevent blood clots from forming
- *Antihypertensives:* Used to lower and control the blood pressure; several categories include:
  - *Beta-blockers:* Reduce the heart rate, the workload, and the output of the heart
  - *Alpha blockers:* Dilate arteries
  - *Angiotensin-converting enzyme (ACE) inhibitors:* Reduce angiotensin production, which causes blood vessels to dilate
  - *Angiotensin II receptor antagonists:* Block the effects of angiotensin, causing blood vessels to dilate
  - *Calcium channel blockers:* Prevent calcium from entering the heart and arteries' smooth muscles; reduce contraction force, dilate blood vessels, and reduce the heart rate
- *Antiplatelets:* Used post treatment of stroke, heart attack, or angina; work by stopping platelets from sticking together and forming a blood clot
- *Cholesterol-lowering agents:* Reduce low-density lipoprotein (LDL) and triglycerides; increase high-density lipoprotein (HDL)
- *Diuretics:* Increase urinary output and lower blood pressure
- *Hematopoietics:* Treat anemia in patients undergoing chemotherapy
- *Hemostatics:* Control acute or chronic blood-clotting disorders; promote formation of absorbable, artificial clots

Refer to Appendix D, which can be found on the Evolve website, for information on the medication classifications, including indications for use, desired effect, side effects, adverse reactions, and generic and trade names. Medical assistants should be familiar with medications that are prescribed to patients.

PATIENT-CENTERED CARE

Two important aspects of patient-centered care are information and education. Many of the more common cardiovascular diseases require patients to be on medication for treatment. It is important that patients know the following:
- Name of the medication
- Reason for the medication
- Side effects/adverse reactions to report to the provider

When a patient is put on a new medication, providing information on the medication is important. The medical assistant should review the information with the patient. Also, giving the patient a handout to take home and a phone number to call if questions arise promote patient-centered care.

BEING PROFESSIONAL

Critical thinking is a crucial part of professional behavior. The ability to question patients logically and comprehensively about possible cardiac signs and symptoms can greatly contribute to high-quality care. The provider relies on the medical assistant for initial information about the patient. Given the seriousness of cardiac conditions, medical assistants must use their knowledge about the topic to gather and analyze the patient's comments so that the provider is better prepared to make an accurate diagnosis and develop an effective treatment plan.

You are rooming a patient who is being seen for a heart concern. The patient tells you he has a funny feeling in his chest. He gives you no other symptoms nor does he explain when it started. Using critical thinking skills, role-play this scenario with a peer. Ask the patient questions to get more information about his concern.

CHAPTER REVIEW

The cardiovascular system consists of blood vessels, the heart, and blood. The cardiovascular system brings O_2, nutrients, water, and other substances (e.g., salts and hormones) to the body's cells. It also carries waste products (e.g., metabolic waste, CO_2) away from the cells to be excreted. The heart has two sets of chambers (atria and ventricles) and two sets of valves. The AV valves are between the atria and ventricles. The SL valves are between the ventricles and the arteries leading out of the heart.

The pulmonary circulation takes deoxygenated blood from the right side of the heart to the lungs. Blood returns from the lungs and empties into the left atrium. Blood from the left side of the heart is pumped to the body, which is the systemic circulation. The coronary circulation provides oxygen and nutrients to the heart muscle. The hepatic portal circulation allows blood from the spleen, gallbladder, pancreas, stomach, and intestines to be taken directly to the liver, where it is filtered. The filtered blood then is returned to the inferior vena cava. The last circulation system is fetal circulation, which is found in unborn babies. This system allows oxygen and nutrients to move from the mother's bloodstream to the baby's blood. Fetal circulation is no longer needed at birth.

The conduction system is the heart's electrical system. It is composed of the SA node (the pacemaker), the AV node, the bundle of His, right and left bundle branches, and the Purkinje fibers. An electrical impulse is required for the heart muscle to contract. With each cardiac cycle, blood is moved from the atria to the ventricles and then out of the heart.

Blood pressure is influenced by several factors, including blood volume, the strength of ventricular contractions, and the resistance to blood flow. The size of the lumen of the arteries, the elasticity of the arterial walls, and the viscosity of the blood affect the resistance to blood flow. The higher the resistance, the higher the blood pressure.

Many cardiovascular diseases were discussed in the chapter. A common etiology includes unhealthy habits (high-cholesterol diets, high-sodium diets, lack of exercise, smoking, and being overweight), congenital problems, and infection. Common signs and symptoms of cardiovascular diseases affect the heart rate and rhythm and the respiration status. Many symptoms can be related to the lack of adequate blood flow to tissues. Typical diagnostic tests ordered include blood pressure reading, ECG, many imaging procedures, and several blood tests. Several CLIA-waived tests are available for diagnosing and monitoring cardiovascular diseases. These include cholesterol testing and prothrombin testing.

The cardiovascular system changes with age. After birth, the fetal circulation structures are no longer used. Older adults have changes in their heart and blood vessels. Cardiovascular diseases are more common with advanced age.

SCENARIO WRAP-UP

As the weeks followed, Lizzy became more independent in practicum. She was very excited to interview for a medical assistant position in a cardiology department in a nearby city. During her last day with Rebecca, they celebrated her completion of practicum. Lizzy shared that she was offered the medical assistant position, which she accepted.

In the weeks that followed Lizzy's last day, Rebecca thought about all the information she had shared with Lizzy. She realized that she, too, had learned a lot from the practicum experience and found that she really enjoyed mentoring students. Rebecca plans to talk with her supervisor about future opportunities to mentor students in the department.

Respiratory System

LEARNING OBJECTIVES

1. List the major organs of the respiratory system and identify the anatomic location of major respiratory system organs.
2. Describe the normal function of the respiratory system.
3. Explain the common diagnostic procedures and treatments for respiratory disorders.
4. Describe common respiratory system disorders, including common signs and symptoms, etiology, diagnostic procedures, and treatments.
5. Identify Clinical Laboratory Improvement Amendments–waived tests associated with common respiratory system disorders.
6. Compare the structure and function of the respiratory system across the life span.

OUTLINE

OPENING SCENARIO

Renee Thomas, a certified medical assistant (CMA) through the American Association of Medical Assistants (AAMA), was hired 6 months ago. She assists the specialists who hold outreach clinics at Walden-Martin Family Medical (WMFM) Clinic. On Tuesdays, the pulmonologist from a local larger city comes for a pulmonary outreach clinic. The pulmonologist brings his own equipment and one medical assistant, John.

Renee's job is to help the pulmonology medicine team because she knows the WMFM Clinic and the local community resources. Renee studied the anatomy and physiology of the respiratory system during her medical assistant training. She learned about common diseases, but she found that she has a lot more to learn. Besides obtaining patients' vital signs and medical histories, Renee does a pulse oximetry measurement on most of her patients. She has observed John performing a spirometry test, which she will learn to do in the future.

In her work with the pulmonologist and John, Renee sees patients with many interesting respiratory diseases. She continues to learn from her work with the specialist and the patients.

YOU WILL LEARN

1. To recognize and use terms related to the respiratory system.
2. To locate the upper and lower respiratory system structures.
3. To understand and describe the ventilation process.
4. To recognize disease states of the upper and lower respiratory tract. This includes the causes, signs and symptoms, diagnostic processes, treatment, prognosis, and prevention.

INTRODUCTION

Pulmonology (PULL mum hal ah jeep) is the healthcare specialty that deals with respiratory disorders. A *pulmonologist* (PULL mum hal ah jest) is a specialist involved in the diagnosis, treatment, and prevention of disorders of the respiratory system.

Pulmonary procedures and treatments are common in the ambulatory care area. Besides the pulmonary department, patients with respiratory concerns are typically seen in primary care and urgent care departments. Medical assistants measure peak flow rates, perform spirometry, and assist with pulmonary treatments. Nebulizer treatments and oxygen therapy are the most frequent pulmonary treatments in ambulatory care.

ANATOMY OF THE RESPIRATORY SYSTEM

The respiratory system is divided into the upper respiratory tract and the lower respiratory tract. The upper respiratory tract structures are considered passageways for the air, whereas the lower respiratory tract structures are involved in gas exchange.

Upper Respiratory Tract

The upper respiratory tract is composed of structures from the nose to the larynx. These organs are located outside the chest cavity. The main functions of the upper respiratory tract include:
- Warming and cleaning the inspired air
- Serving as a passageway for air
- Providing the sense of smell

Air can enter through the mouth or the two *nares* (nostrils) in the nose. The nasal septum (SEP tum) separates the nares. The air then moves into the nasal cavity. The surface capillaries, mucous membrane, and *cilia* (SEE lee ah) (small hairs) found in the nasal cavity clean, warm, and moisten the air. The cilia continually move in a wavelike motion to push mucus and debris out of the respiratory tract. Receptors for smell are in the nasal cavity. The nasal cavity is connected to four pairs of parana-sal sinuses (pair uh NAY zul SYE nus suhs). The four pairs of

paranasal sinuses are named for the bones they are found in: maxillary, frontal, sphenoid, and ethmoid.

Air continues to travel into the *pharynx* (throat) (Fig. 11.1), which is divided into three sections:
- *Nasopharynx* (NAY zoh fair inks): Located behind the nasal cavity. The *eustachian* (yoo STAY shun) *tube* connects the middle ear to the nasopharynx and equalizes the pressure in the ear with the air pressure outside the body.
- *Oropharynx* (or oh FAIR inks): Located behind the mouth and part of the respiratory and digestive systems.
- *Laryngopharynx* (luh ring goh FAIR inks): Located between the epiglottis and the esophagus. The *epiglottis* (eh pee GLOT is), a flap of cartilage at the larynx opening, closes off the trachea (TRAY kee uh) when food is swallowed. As air passes back out through the opening, the *larynx* (vocal cords) vibrates to produce speech. The vocal cords are paired bands of cartilaginous (kahr ti LAJ i nus) tissue.

VOCABULARY

paranasal sinuses Hollow, air-filled cavities in the skull and facial bones. They lighten the weight of the skull and increase the tone, or resonance, of speech.

MEDICAL TERMINOLOGY

epiglott/o	epiglottis
salping/o	eustachian tube
laryng/o	larynx
or/o	mouth
muc/o	mucus
nas/o, rhin/o	nose
pharyng/o	pharynx
sinus/o, sin/o	sinus

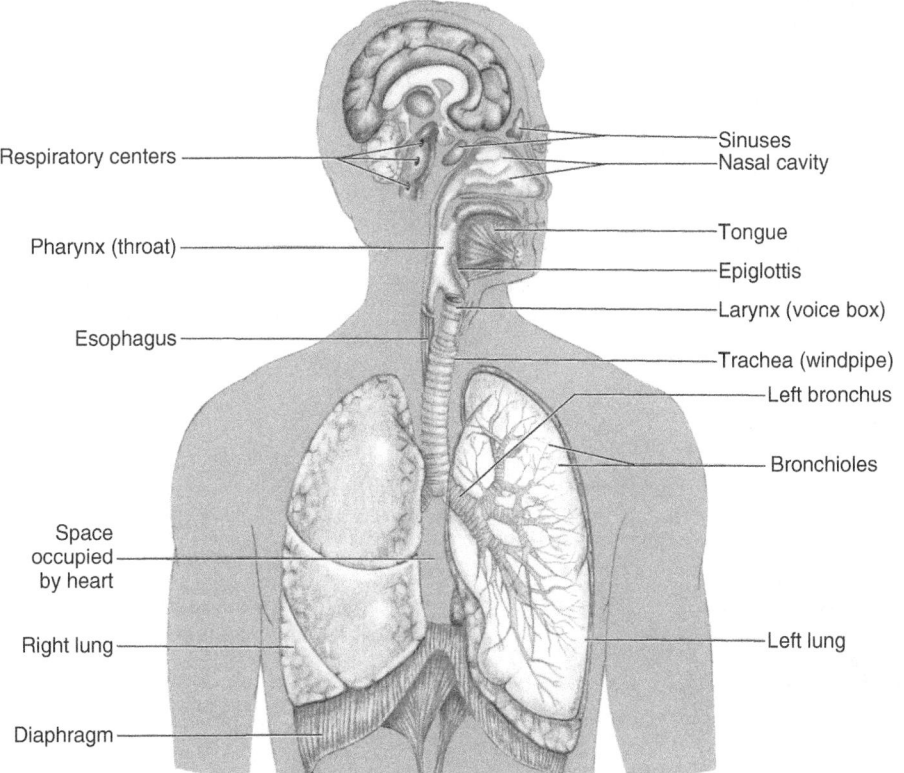

Fig. 11.1 Anatomic Structures of the Respiratory System. (Modified from Solomon EP: *Introduction to human anatomy and physiology,* ed 3, St. Louis, 2009, Saunders.)

Lower Respiratory Tract

The lower respiratory tract consists of the trachea, bronchial tubes, and lungs (see Fig. 11.1). These structures are lined with mucous membranes and cilia. The *trachea* (windpipe) lies in the space between the lungs, called the mediastinum (mee dee uh STY num). Air travels from the larynx through the trachea, and then the trachea branches into the right and left bronchi (BRONG kie). The right bronchus is wider than the left bronchus.

The bronchi divide into smaller branches, called *bronchioles* (BRONG kee ohls). These bronchioles end in microscopic ducts capped by air sacs, called *alveoli* (al VEE oh lye). Each thin-walled alveolus is in contact with a blood capillary. This contact between the two structures allows the exchange of gases. It is at this point that oxygen (O_2) from the inspired air moves across the one-cell membrane into the blood cells. Carbon dioxide (CO_2) moves in the other direction, from the blood into the air to be expired. Each alveolus is coated with a substance called surfactant (sur FACK tunt), which keeps it from collapsing. Without surfactant, the alveoli stick together during *exhalation* (breathing out) and deflate. *Inhalation* (breathing in) becomes more difficult, and less O_2 is able to move into the bloodstream. This condition is life-threatening. Babies born before 37 to 39 weeks of gestation are at risk for not having enough surfactant. If time permits before delivery, steroids can be given to the mother to help mature the baby's lungs.

The bronchial tree and alveoli are the major structures in the right and left lungs. The lungs are soft and spongy because of the air sacs that make up most of their mass. They hang in the right and left sides of the chest, separated by the pericardial sac, which contains the heart. Each lung is composed of sections called *lobes*. The right lung consists of three lobes, whereas the left has only two lobes (Fig. 11.2).

Because each lobe has its own bronchus and blood supply, the removal of one lobe *(lobectomy)* results in little or no damage to the rest of the lung. The left lung is longer and narrower. It has a distinct indentation in its center, known as the *cardiac notch*. This is where the left ventricle of the heart is located and where an apical pulse is heard.

Pleura (PLOOR uh) is a thin serous membrane found in the thoracic cavity. The pleura folds back on itself, creating a sac that surrounds the lung. The *visceral pleura* (VIH sur ul PLOOR ah)

covers the lungs and adjoining structures. The *parietal pleura* (puh RYE uh tul PLOOR ah), the outer portion of the pleura, lines the thoracic cavity and covers the diaphragm (DYE uh fram) and mediastinum. Only the parietal pleura contains pain receptors, making it highly sensitive to pain. The right and left pleural sacs are entirely separate.

The *pleural cavity* is the space between the visceral and parietal pleurae. A small amount of pleural fluid is in the pleural cavity. When the lungs expand, moving the visceral pleura closer to the parietal pleura, friction is reduced between the tissues due to the pleural fluid.

The muscles responsible for normal, quiet respiration are the diaphragm and the intercostal (in tur KOS tul) muscles. On inspiration, the diaphragm is pulled down and flattened as it contracts, and the intercostal muscles expand, pulling air into the lungs. On expiration, the diaphragm relaxes and moves upward, pushing air out of the lungs.

VOCABULARY

diaphragm A broad, dome-shaped muscle used for breathing. It separates the thoracic and abdominopelvic cavities.

expiration Exhaling; movement of waste gases from the alveoli into the atmosphere.

inspiration Inhaling; movement of O_2 from the atmosphere into the alveoli.

intercostal muscles Muscles located between the ribs that help with quiet respiration.

mediastinum The space in the thoracic cavity that lies between the lungs, containing the heart, trachea, and esophagus.

surfactant A mixture of protein and fats that lines the alveoli and prevents the tissues from sticking together and collapsing during exhalation.

CRITICAL THINKING 11.1

Renee works with patients of all ages in the pulmonary outreach clinic. Today Pedro Gomez, an elementary school student, comes in with his mother. He is there for a checkup on his asthma. As Renee is rooming him, Pedro mentions that he is learning about the respiratory system in school. He asks Renee to tell him all the structures, from the nose to the lungs, in order. Renee agrees to his request. What does she say? (What would be your answer to Pedro's request?)

MEDICAL TERMINOLOGY

alveol/o	alveolus
bronch/o, bronchi/o	bronchus
bronchiol/o	bronchiole
capn/o	carbon dioxide
diaphragm/o, diaphragmat/o, phren/o	diaphragm
lob/o, lobul/o	lobe
mediastin/o	mediastinum
pariet/o	wall
pleur/o	pleura
pneumon/o, pulmon/o, pneum/o	lung
thorac/o, steth/o, pector/o	chest
trache/o	trachea
viscer/o	viscera
alveolus (singular)	alveoli (plural)
bronchus (singular)	bronchi (plural)
pleura (singular)	pleurae (plural)

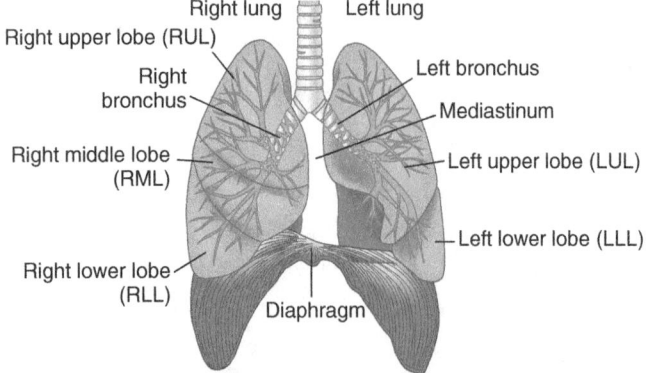

Fig. 11.2 Lobes of the Lung. (From Niedzwiecki B, et al: *Kinn's the medical assistant*, ed 14, St. Louis, 2020, Elsevier.)

Right lung — Left lung
Right upper lobe (RUL)
Right bronchus
Left bronchus
Right middle lobe (RML)
Mediastinum
Left upper lobe (LUL)
Left lower lobe (LLL)
Right lower lobe (RLL)
Diaphragm

Bronchioles and Alveoli

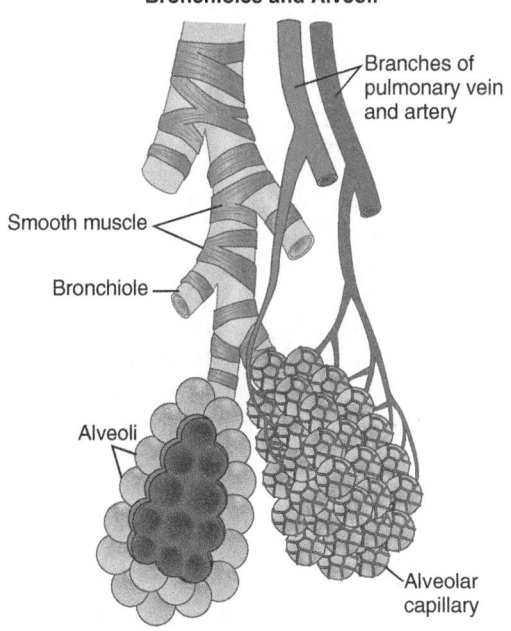

Branches of
pulmonary vein
and artery

Smooth muscle

Bronchiole

Alveoli

Alveolar
capillary

Fig. 11.3 Alveoli With Their Capillary Network. (From Niedzwiecki B, et al: *Kinn's the medical assistant*, ed 14, St. Louis, 2020, Elsevier.)

PHYSIOLOGY OF THE RESPIRATORY SYSTEM

The two primary functions of the respiratory system are to exchange O_2 from the atmosphere for CO_2 waste and to maintain the acid-base balance in the body. Both functions involve *ventilation* (breathing), which is the movement of gases between the lungs and the environment. Ventilation includes the process of inspiration and expiration.

Two types of respiration occur during the ventilation process.
- *External respiration* occurs when oxygenated air moves into the alveoli. Surrounding each alveolus is a pulmonary capillary network (Fig. 11.3). The alveoli and the pulmonary capillaries are made of single-celled walls. This allows the O_2 to move easily across the alveoli and capillaries into the blood. CO_2 and other wastes are forced out of the capillaries and move into the alveoli.
- *Internal respiration* occurs when O_2 is exchanged for CO_2 between the cells in the body and the blood.

Inspiration

A healthy person breathes when the blood CO_2 level increases. A person with chronic obstructive pulmonary disease (COPD) has a constantly elevated blood CO_2 level. At some point, the body no longer uses the elevated blood CO_2 level as a trigger to breathe. A secondary system kicks in, and breathing is triggered by a decreased blood O_2 level.

When the breathing trigger is activated, it signals the medulla oblongata (the respiratory center) in the brainstem. The respiratory center causes a stimulus (i.e., signal) to be carried by the phrenic nerve to the diaphragm. When the diaphragm receives the signal, it flattens out and pulls downward. At the same moment, the intercostal muscles between the ribs contract, causing the ribs to move outward. The movement enlarges the chest cavity and causes the lungs to expand, increasing their volume. The greater the contraction, the deeper the inhalation and the greater the air volume.

When individuals are experiencing respiratory distress, they are unable to move enough air into the lungs. To help move additional air into their lungs, they use accessory muscles. To identify whether a person is using the accessory muscles, expose the chest and look for chest retractions with breathing. With intercostal retractions, the chest tissue in between the ribs is indrawn or pulled in during breathing. Upper airway obstructions can cause:
- *Suprasternal retractions*, sucking in of the skin just above the sternum
- *Supraclavicular retractions*, sucking in of the skin just above the clavicle

Lower airway obstructions can cause:
- *Substernal retractions*, sucking in of the abdomen just below the sternum
- *Subcostal retractions*, sucking in of the abdomen just below the ribs

Using accessory muscles to breathe can tire a person. This can lead to respiratory arrest, a medical emergency. Typically, this occurs quicker in infants and young children.

CRITICAL THINKING 11.2

The pulmonologist asks Renee to review the signs of respiratory distress with the mother of an asthmatic patient. Discuss what Renee should review with the mother.

VOCABULARY
accessory muscles Muscles in the neck, abdomen, and back that assist in breathing.
respiratory arrest Stoppage of breathing.

Expiration

The second half of ventilation is *expiration*. Once inspiration is complete, the diaphragm and intercostal muscles relax, which causes the diaphragm to move upward into the thoracic cavity and the ribs to move inward. This movement reduces the lung capacity and forces air out of the lungs. Typically, expiration requires very little energy. However, with some conditions (e.g., asthma and emphysema), the person has difficulty getting air out of the lungs. The accessory muscles are needed to help with complete exhalation.

Acid-Base Balance

The body attempts to keep the pH between 7.35 and 7.45. The respiratory system has an important role in acid-base balance. It regulates the amount of CO_2 in the blood. CO_2 in the blood can combine with water to form the buffer bicarbonate. If a person *hyperventilates* (breathes rapidly), the CO_2 and bicarbonate levels in the blood decrease. This causes the pH of the body to rise, resulting in *respiratory alkalosis* (al kah LOW sis). This condition can be seen in patients with anxiety or an acute asthma attack. If hypoventilation occurs, the CO_2 in the blood increases (*hypercapnia* [hie per KAP nee ah]), and *respiratory acidosis* can occur. Respiratory alkalosis and respiratory acidosis are both life-threatening disorders if the underlying causes are not corrected.

DISEASES AND DISORDERS OF THE RESPIRATORY SYSTEM

Common signs and symptoms of respiratory disorders include:
- Abnormal breathing rate changes.
  - *Apnea* (AP nee ah): Temporary absence of breathing.
  - *Bradypnea* (brad IP nee ah): Abnormally slow breathing.
  - *Cheyne-Stokes* (shayne stokes) *respiration*: An increase in the depth and rate of breathing, followed by a decrease in breathing, and then a period of apnea.
  - *Hyperpnea*: An increase in the depth of breathing; the rate may also be increased.
  - *Hyperventilation*: Abnormal increase in breathing.
  - *Orthopnea* (or THOP nee ah): Difficulty breathing unless in an upright position (e.g., sitting or standing).
  - *Tachypnea* (tack ip NEE ah): Rapid, shallow breathing.
- Changes in the oxygen amount in the blood and tissues.
  - *Cyanosis* (sye uh NOH sis): Lack of oxygen in the blood, causing a bluish color in the skin, nail beds, and lips.
  - *Hypoxemia* (hye pock SEE mee ah): Insufficient oxygen in the blood.
  - *Hypoxia* (hye pock SEE ah): Decrease in oxygen in the tissues.
- Abnormal lung sounds heard using a stethoscope, which is placed over the lung field.
  - *Pleural rub* or *pleuritic rub*: An auscultatory sound caused by the rubbing together of the visceral and costal pleurae.
  - *Rales*: Inspiratory auscultatory sounds resembling crackles or popping sounds caused by fluid in the airway or alveoli. Can be described as moist, dry, fine, or coarse.
  - *Rhonchi* (RON kye): Auscultatory sounds resembling snoring. Occurs when airflow is partially blocked through the large airways.
  - *Stridor* (STRY dur): High-pitched inspiratory sound due to a blockage in the upper airway; can be heard with or without a stethoscope.
  - *Wheezing* (WHEE zeeng): High-pitched sound produced by a narrowed airway; can be heard with or without a stethoscope.
- *Dyspnea* (DISP nee ah): Difficulty with breathing.
- *Shortness of breath* (SOB): Breathlessness.
- *Hemoptysis* (hi MOP ti sis): Expectorate (eks PEK tor ate) of blood or blood-streaked sputum (SPYOO tumm).
- *Hiccup* (HIK up): Sound produced by the spasmodic involuntary contraction of the diaphragm that causes an uncontrolled breathing in of air followed by the rapid closure of the glottis.
- *Epistaxis*: Nosebleed.
- *Rhinorrhea* (rye noh REE ah): Nasal discharge.

Common diagnostic procedures and medical laboratory tests are listed in Table 11.1. Common treatments used for respiratory disorders are described in Table 11.2.

VOCABULARY

expectorate To cough up and spit out mucus from the lower respiratory tract.
sputum Mucous secretion coughed up from the lungs and expectorated through the mouth.

TABLE 11.1   Common Diagnostic Procedures for Respiratory System Disorders

Performed by/Test Type	Procedure	Description
Provider during the exam	Lung sounds	The provider uses a stethoscope to listen to (or auscultates) the lung sounds as the patient inhales and exhales.
Medical assistant	Peak flow monitor	A handheld device that measures the exhaled air. It can also be used at home.
	Pulse oximetry (ok SIM e tree)	A noninvasive test used to measure the oxygen saturation level in blood.
	Spirometry test (spi ROM e tree)	Measures the volume of inhaled and exhaled air, and the time required for each.
Endoscopy	Bronchoscopy (bron KOS ko pee)	The insertion of an instrument (bronchoscope) through the mouth to visualize the trachea and bronchi.
Imaging procedures	Chest x-rays (CXRs)	Images taken from several directions, which provide a good outline of the heart and lungs. Abnormal air "pockets," fluid, and tumors can be seen on chest x-rays.
	Computed tomography (CT)	An imaging technique that can provide more information than chest x-rays.
	Magnetic resonance imaging (MRI)	An imaging technique that can provide more information than chest x-rays.
	Lung ventilation/ perfusion scan (VQ scan)	A procedure in which a radioisotope substance is inhaled and also injected; then a special x-ray scanner creates a picture of the blood flow and airflow in the lungs.
	Pulmonary angiography (an jee AH gruh fee)	A procedure in which a catheter is inserted into the pulmonary blood vessels. Dye is injected, and x-ray pictures show the blood flow through the pulmonary vessels
Medical laboratory	CLIA-waived tests	• *Legionella* Urinary Antigen Test – for legionnaires disease • Mono test – for infectious mononucleosis • Influenza A & B test – for influenza • Rapid strep A test – for strep throat • RSV test – for respiratory syncytial virus pneumonia
	Arterial blood gas (ABG)	A test in which a blood specimen is collected from the artery in the wrist, and the pH of the blood, carbon dioxide (CO_2) and oxygen (O_2) content are measured.
	Sputum cytology (sye TALL uh jee)	A test in which sputum is collected and examined under a microscope for abnormal cells.
	Sputum culture	A test in which sputum is collected and analyzed in the lab for bacterial growth over a period of days.

CLIA, Clinical Laboratory Improvement Amendments.

TABLE 11.2   Common Treatments Used for Respiratory System Disorders

Procedure	Description
Endotracheal (ET) intubation (EN doe TRAY kee al)	An ET tube is inserted into the trachea and provides an airway.
Laryngectomy (lair in JEK tuh mee)	Partial or complete surgical removal of the larynx; typically used as a treatment for cancer of the larynx.
Metered-dose inhaler (MDI)	Provides aerosol medication that is breathed into the lungs. A *spacer* is a long tube that is attached to the mouthpiece of an MDI.
Nebulizer treatment	A small machine is used to turn liquid medication into a fine spray that can be inhaled.
Oxygen therapy	Supplemental oxygen is provided via a nasal canula or a mask in ambulatory care. Can also be used at home.
Rhinoplasty (RYE noh plas tee)	Surgical repair of the nose.
Septoplasty (SEP toh plas tee)	Surgical repair of the nasal septum.
Thoracocentesis (thor ak koh sen TEE sis)	The surgical puncture using a hollow needle and the aspiration (as pi RAY shun) of the fluid from the pleural cavity. Also called *thoracentesis* (thor ah sen TEE sis).
Thoracotomy (thor uh KOT uh mee)	Surgical incision of the chest wall.
Tracheostomy (tray kee OS tuh mee)	Creation of an opening *(stoma)* into the trachea.
Tracheotomy (tray kee AH tuh mee)	A surgical incision of the trachea, usually to gain access to the airway.

MEDICAL TERMINOLOGY

cyan/o	blue
hemo/o	blood
orth/o	straight
ox/o	oxygen
a-	without
brady-	slow
dys-	difficult
endo-	within
hyper-	excessive
hypo-	deficient
tachy-	fast
-al	pertaining to
-ia	condition
-ectomy	removal, excision
-emia	blood condition
-osis	abnormal condition
-plasty	surgical repair
-pnea	breathing
-ptysis	spitting
-rrhea	discharge
-stomy	new opening
-tomy	incision

Chronic Respiratory Diseases

Allergic Rhinitis. When a person is allergic to dust, animal dander, pollen, or foods, allergic rhinitis can occur. When the reaction is due to a pollen allergy, the person is said to have hay fever, seasonal allergies, or allergic rhinitis.

Etiology. The cause of allergic rhinitis can be traced to an allergen that triggers an allergy in the person. When the allergen is breathed in, histamines in the body cause allergy symptoms to occur.

Signs and Symptoms. Allergic rhinitis can cause:
- Itchy nose, mouth, eyes, and throat
- Problems smelling and runny nose
- Sneezing and watery eyes

Later symptoms may include:
- Nasal congestion, coughing, decreased sense of smell, and sore throat
- Dark circles, puffiness under the eyes, fatigue, and headache

Diagnostic Procedures. The provider will perform a physical exam and ask about the patient's allergy history. Allergy testing, a complete blood count (CBC), and other allergy-related tests (e.g., the IgE radioallergosorbent test [RAST] test) may be done.

Treatments. Treatment consists of avoiding the allergen or reducing exposure. A nasal wash may be recommended to remove mucus from the nose. Medications such as antihistamines, decongestants, and corticosteroids may also be ordered. Depending on the severity, the provider may also refer the patient to an allergy department for evaluation. Allergy shots *(immunotherapy)* are sometimes recommended.

VOCABULARY

aspiration The process of removing fluids or gases from the body using a suction device. Inhalation of a liquid (e.g., blood and vomitus) or a foreign object into the respiratory tract.

corticosteroids A group of steroid hormones produced in the body or given as a medication. Some have metabolic functions, and others reduce tissue inflammation. Glucocorticoids and mineralocorticoids are two types.

decongestant A drug that is used for nasal congestion.

Asthma. Asthma (AZ muh) is a chronic disease that affects the airway. Bronchospasms and airway swelling narrow the passageway. Mucus in the lungs clogs the airway (Fig. 11.4). Getting air into and out of the lungs becomes harder. The frequency of asthma episodes can vary. Severe asthma attacks are life-threatening and require immediate emergency care.

Etiology. Many different things can trigger an asthma episode. Common triggers include:
- Allergens including foods (e.g., tree nuts), medications, and environmental substances such as pollen, mold spores, pet dander, tobacco smoke, dust mites, cockroaches, wood smoke, and latex.
- Environmental causes such as chemical gases or fumes, dust, high humidity, and cold, dry air
- Strong emotional states
- Strenuous physical exercise

Signs and Symptoms. Asthma symptoms can vary in type and frequency. Typical symptoms include:
- Shortness of breath or breathlessness
- Chest tightness or pain
- Coughing or wheezing attacks
- Early morning or nighttime coughing

During asthma symptoms

Normal airway

Airways

Muscle

Airway wall

Narrowed airway (limited air flow)

Tightened muscles constrict airway

Inflamed/ thickened airway wall

Lungs

Muscle

Airway wall

Muscle

Mucus

A

B

C

Fig. 11.4 Inflammation and Bronchospasm. (From Proctor D, et al: *Kinn's the medical assistant,* ed 13, St. Louis, 2017, Elsevier.)

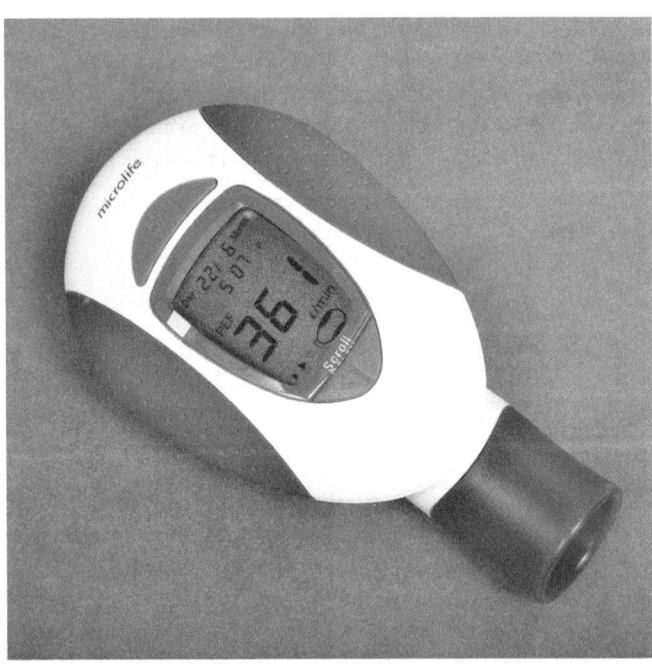

Fig. 11.5 Digital Peak Flow Meter. (From Proctor D, et al: *Kinn's the medical assistant,* ed 13, St. Louis, 2017, Elsevier.)

TABLE 11.3	**Asthma Action Plan**	
Zone	**Symptoms**	**Action to Take**
Green Zone – Doing Well	No asthma symptoms; peak flow is more than 80% of normal peak flow	Take prescribed long-term control medications
Yellow Zone – Asthma is getting worse	Asthma symptoms are present, or waking at night, or can't do usual activities, or peak flow is 50%–79% of normal peak flow.	Add quick-relief medication to the Green Zone medication. Continue to monitor. Contact provider if not improving.
Red Zone – Medical Alert	Very short of breath, or quick-relief medications have not helped, or peak flow is less than 50% of best peak flow.	Take short-acting beta agonist medication and/or oral steroid. Contact the provider immediately.

Adapted from National Institutes of Health. Asthma Action Plan. https://www.nhlbi.nih.gov/files/docs/public/lung/asthma_actplan.pdf.

Diagnostic Procedures. The provider may order peak flow monitoring, pulse oximetry, and spirometry tests for diagnostic testing. Peak flow monitoring measures the amount of air exhaled. Peak flow monitoring can be used with at-home management of asthma (Fig. 11.5). The provider can set up an Asthma Action Plan to accompany the peak flow readings (Table 11.3).

Treatments. Treatment for asthma is based on the severity of the disease. Asthma medications can be taken orally or inhaled. Inhaled medications are usually taken via a metered-dose inhaler with a spacer or a nebulizer (Fig. 11.6). Long-term control medications are usually taken daily and may include:

- Inhaled corticosteroids: fluticasone, budesonide, beclomethasone, and mometasone
- Leukotriene modifiers: montelukast, zafirlukast, and zileuton
- Long-acting beta agonists: salmeterol and formoterol

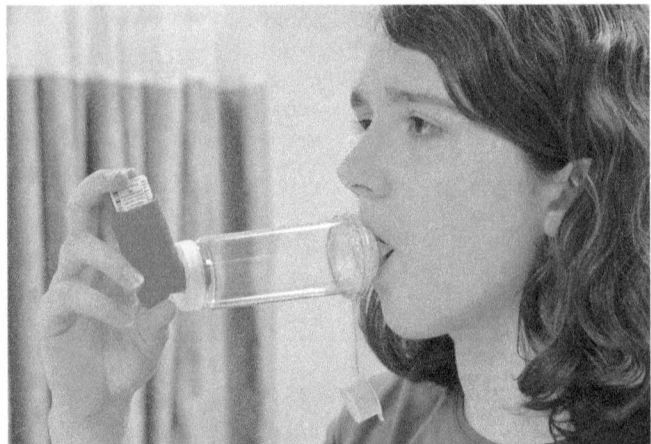

Fig. 11.6 Using a Metered-Dose Inhaler with Spacer. (From Niedzwiecki B, et al: *Kinn's the medical assistant,* ed 14, St. Louis, 2020, Elsevier.)

- Combination inhalers: fluticasone-salmeterol, budesonide-formoterol, and formoterol-mometasone

Quick-relief medications are usually taken during the asthma episode, because they provide rapid, short-term relief. Quick-relief medications include short-acting beta agonists supplied by metered-dose inhalers (MDIs), such as albuterol and leval-

buterol. If the quick-relief medications do not reduce the episode, immediate emergency care is required.

Chronic Obstructive Pulmonary Disease. More than 11 million Americans have COPD. It is the third leading cause of death in the United States. But this condition is both treatable and preventable. COPD develops slowly, making it hard for the affected person to breathe. It includes two conditions:

- *Emphysema* (em fi SEE mah): Thinning and eventual destruction of the alveoli. This usually accompanies chronic bronchitis.
- *Chronic bronchitis* (bron KIE tis): Inflammation of the bronchial tubes, excessive production of mucus, and diminished activity of the cilia.

Etiology. The main cause of COPD is smoking tobacco. Other causes include secondhand smoke, air pollution, dust, and chemical fumes. COPD can also be caused by an alpha-1 antitrypsin (AAT) deficiency (Box 11.1).

Signs and Symptoms. The symptoms of COPD often appear after damage has already been done to the lungs. With chronic bronchitis, a long-term, daily productive cough is seen. Additional symptoms of COPD include shortness of breath, chest tightness, breathlessness, wheezing, cyanosis of the lips and nail beds, and clubbing (Fig. 11.7). The patient may experience a lack of energy and fatigue. Frequent respiratory infections are common.

Diagnostic Procedures. Typical diagnostic tests include lung function tests (i.e., spirometry and pulse oximetry), chest x-ray, and chest computed tomography (CT) scan (Fig. 11.8 and Fig. 11.9).

An arterial blood gas test may be done to identify the severity of the COPD.

Treatments. Because there is no cure for COPD, the goal of treatment is to slow the disease progression. Patients typically use bronchodilators and a bronchodilator-corticosteroid

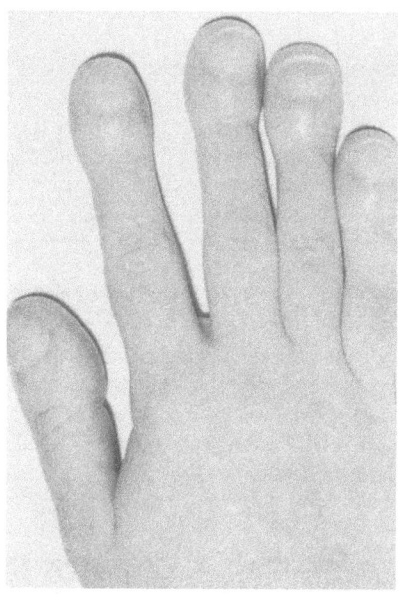

Fig. 11.7 Clubbing. (From Frowen P, et al: *Neale's disorders of the foot,* ed 8, Oxford, 2010, Churchill Livingstone.)

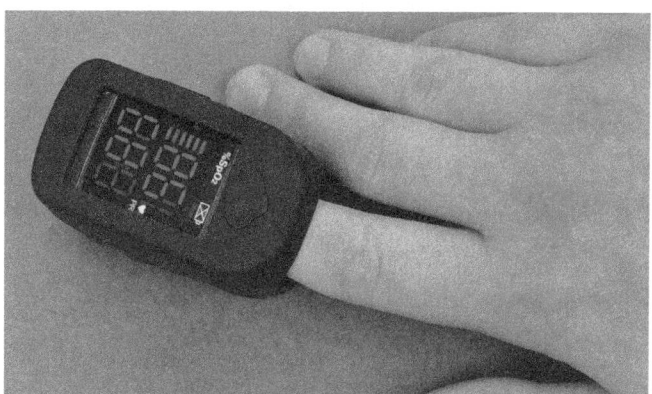

Fig. 11.8 Pulse Oximeter. (From Proctor D, et al: *Kinn's the medical assistant,* ed 13, St. Louis, 2017, Elsevier.)

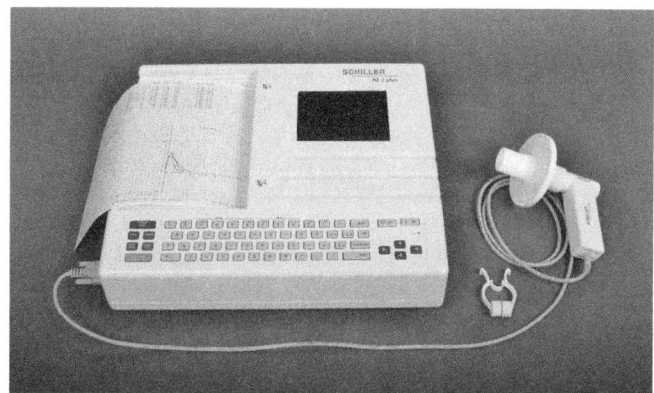

Fig. 11.9 Spirometer. (From Proctor D, et al: *Kinn's the medical assistant,* ed 13, St. Louis, 2017, Elsevier.)

combination to reduce the inflammation. Patients may use low-level oxygen therapy. Adequate nutrition, vaccinations, and smoking cessation are also important in the treatment plan. (Box 11.2) With severe COPD, surgical options may be considered, such as lung volume reduction surgery (removal of damaged lung tissue) and lung transplantation.

VOCABULARY

bronchodilator A drug that relaxes smooth muscle contractions in the bronchioles to improve lung ventilation.

clubbing Abnormal enlargement of the distal phalanges (fingers and toes) associated with chronic tissue hypoxia due to cyanotic heart disease or advanced chronic pulmonary disease.

productive cough A cough that produces phlegm or mucus.

CRITICAL THINKING 11.4

Renee sees many patients with chronic obstructive pulmonary disease (COPD) who are using oxygen constantly. She realizes that the amount of oxygen is much lower than the amount providers order for patients without COPD. Confused, she asks John why patients with COPD use smaller amounts of supplemental oxygen. How would you answer this question?

Cystic Fibrosis. Cystic fibrosis (SIS tik fie BROE sis) (CF) is a life-threatening, congenital disease. Mucus builds up in the lungs, pancreas, and other organs. The mucus blocks the airways and increases the risk of infections. In the pancreas, the mucus interrupts the release of digestive enzymes used to break down food.

More than 30,000 people in the United States have cystic fibrosis. Half of them are age 18 or younger. All states require newborn screening tests for cystic fibrosis. With improvements in treatments, people with CF can live, work, and play with a much greater quality of life than in the past.

Etiology. CF is a genetic disease. Each parent gives one copy of a specific gene to the child. As a result, the child gets two copies of a specific gene. If one of the copies is defective, the person will be a carrier of that disease. If both copies are defective, the person will have the disease.

Signs and Symptoms. CF can cause:

- Higher than normal levels of salt in the sweat and electrolyte imbalances
- A persistent cough that produces a thick, sticky sputum
- Breathlessness, shortness of breath, wheezing, and frequent lung infections
- Poor growth and weight gain

BOX 11.2 Health Risks Associated With Smoking and Smokeless Tobacco

Tobacco smoke contains more than 7000 chemicals. Of these, 250 are harmful, and at least 69 can cause cancer. It is estimated that one in five deaths are related to smoking. According to the Centers for Disease Control and Prevention (CDC), smokers are more likely to develop heart disease, lung cancer, and strokes. Smoking can cause the following effects:

- *Respiratory system:* Pneumonia, chronic obstructive pulmonary disease (COPD), tuberculosis, asthma, and cancer of the trachea, bronchus, and lung
- *Nervous system:* Stroke
- *Cardiovascular system:* Aortic aneurysm, early abdominal aortic atherosclerosis in young adults, coronary heart disease, atherosclerotic peripheral vascular disease, and acute myeloid leukemia
- *Sensory system:* Blindness, cataracts, and age-related macular degeneration
- *Digestive system:* Orofacial clefts (congenital defect from maternal smoking) and periodontitis; oropharynx, larynx, esophagus, stomach, liver, and colorectal cancers
- *Endocrine system:* Type 2 diabetes mellitus and pancreatic cancer
- *Musculoskeletal system:* Hip fractures and rheumatoid arthritis
- *Urinary system:* Cancer of the bladder, kidney, and ureters
- *Immune system:* Immune function issues
- *Reproductive system:* In females, reproductive effects (e.g., reduced fertility), ectopic pregnancy, and cervical cancer; in males, erectile dysfunction

Passive or *secondhand smoke*, which stays in the air and can be breathed in by others, causes lung cancer, strokes, low-birth-weight babies, and heart disease. Exposure to secondhand smoke increases a person's risk for lung cancer by 20%. Children exposed to secondhand smoke have an increased risk of sudden infant death syndrome (SIDS), ear infections, bronchitis, pneumonia, colds, and asthma. Secondhand smoke causes more than 53,000 deaths a year in the United States.

Thirdhand smoke is the residue or chemicals from the smoke that gets on skin, clothing, furniture, carpets, and so on. This can be harmful to little children and animals that spend time on the floor. Besides breathing in the residue, these chemicals can be ingested. They can transfer from the carpet, clothing, and so on to hands and then into the person's mouth.

The CDC reports that at least 28 cancer-causing chemicals have been found in smokeless tobacco (e.g., chew and dip). Smokeless tobacco can cause cancer of the mouth, pancreas, and esophagus.

E-cigarettes, which are used for vaping, are also considered tobacco products because they usually contain nicotine. E-cigarettes (also called *e-cigs, vape pens, mods,* or *e-hookahs*) are battery-operated devices that heat liquids to form an aerosol, which is then inhaled. The liquids typically contain nicotine, flavorings, and other additives. E-cigs can also be used for marijuana and other drugs. An e-cig may look like a cigarette, pipe, whiteout, marker, lipstick, pen, or USB (flash) drive. Compared to cigarettes, e-cigs are safer, but they still can be harmful. The aerosol can contain nicotine, heavy metals (e.g., lead), volatile organic compounds, and cancer-causing substances. One example of a health risk comes from diacetyl, which is found in many e-cigarette flavors. It has been known to cause bronchiolitis obliterans, commonly called "popcorn lung." Diacetyl was an ingredient in microwave popcorn and food flavorings until it was linked to hundreds of cases of bronchiolitis obliterans. Like COPD, this disease can cause wheezing, persistent cough, shortness of breath, and death. The alveoli become scarred, and the airway becomes narrowed.

According to the CDC, advantages of giving up the use of tobacco products include the following:

- Blood pressure and heart rate begin to return to normal.
- Within a few hours, carbon monoxide levels in the blood decline.
- Within a few weeks, circulation improves and abnormal respiratory symptoms (e.g., cough, wheezing) decrease.
- One year after quitting, the cardiovascular risks decrease sharply.
- Two to 5 years after quitting, the risk for stroke returns to a nonsmoker's level.
- Five years after quitting, the risk of cancer of the esophagus, bladder, throat, and mouth is cut in half.
- Ten years after quitting, the lung cancer risk decreases by 50%.

Local resources and prescriptive medications are available if a person wants to quit using these products. Websites (e.g., https://smokefree.gov) and quit lines are also available (e.g., National Cancer Institute Smoking Quitline: 1-877-44U-QUIT).

- Intestinal blockage, severe constipation, and foul-smelling, greasy stools

Diagnostic Procedures. To diagnose CF one of the following can be done:

- Two positive sweat tests (the tests must be performed on different days)
- Genetic testing, to detect two defective genes (for CF), and one positive sweat test

Treatments. There is no cure for CF. Treatment centers on reducing the complications and symptoms. Treatment can include:

- Antibiotics for lung infections and anti-inflammatory medications to reduce the swelling in the lungs.
- Bronchodilators and mucus-thinning medication can help clear the lungs of mucus.
- Oral pancreatic enzymes are used to help with digestion.
- Chest physical therapy, vest therapy (vibrating vest), and O_2 therapy.
- Surgical options for CF complications include lung transplantation and bowel surgery for obstructions.

Laryngeal Cancer. Laryngeal cancer is throat cancer, and it affects the vocal cords and larynx (voice box). In most cases, laryngeal cancer develops in adults older than 50 years, and males are more likely to get it than females.

Etiology. The causes of laryngeal cancer include tobacco and alcohol use.

Signs and Symptoms. Laryngeal cancer can cause:

- A constant sore throat and painful swallowing
- Ear pain and a lump in the neck or throat
- Hoarseness

Diagnostic Procedures. After a physical exam, the provider may order a biopsy with laryngoscopy or endoscopy, a CT scan, magnetic resonance imaging (MRI), a positron emission tomography (PET) scan, bone scan, and barium swallow (or upper gastrointestinal series).

Treatments. Treatment consists of surgery, chemotherapy, and radiation therapy.

Lung Cancer. There are two main types of lung cancer, non–small cell and small cell. Non–small cell lung cancer is more prevalent. Lung cancer is the leading cause of cancer-related deaths in the United States.

Etiology. The leading cause of lung cancer is cigarette smoking. The longer a person has smoked and the more a person has smoked, the more likely it is that the individual will contract lung cancer. High exposure levels of asbestos, radiation, and pollution can also increase a person's risk for lung cancer.

Signs and Symptoms. Lung cancer can cause:

- A chronic, worsening cough with hemoptysis and constant chest pain
- Wheezing, breathlessness, shortness of breath, clubbing, and more frequent respiratory infections
- Fatigue, loss of appetite, weight loss, and swelling of the face and hands

Diagnostic Procedures. Chest x-rays and CT scans, sputum cytology, bronchoscopy, and lung tissue biopsy are used to diagnose lung cancer.

Treatments. Treatment for lung cancer is based on the person's health, the stage of the disease, and the person's preferences. Treatments can include chemotherapy, radiation therapy, targeted drug therapy, and surgery. Common surgical options for lung cancer include:

- *Wedge resection*: Removal of a small portion of the lung tissue. It includes the tumor and the healthy tissue on the edge of the tumor.
- *Segmental resection*: Removal of a larger portion or segment of the lung
- *Lobectomy* (low BEK tah mee): Removal of a lobe of the lung
- *Pneumonectomy* (NOO mah NEK tah mee): Removal of the entire lung

Sleep Apnea. Sleep apnea occurs when a person stops breathing or the breathing becomes very shallow. Breathing pauses may last a few seconds to minutes and may occur 30 or more times an hour.

Etiology. The cause of sleep apnea depends on the type.

- *Obstructive sleep apnea* (OSA): The most common type of sleep apnea; it causes breathing to pause during sleep. OSA results from a blockage or narrowing of the airway when the throat muscles relax. It can be caused by excessive weight, a thicker neck circumference, a narrowed airway, smoking, and nasal congestions. Males are twice as likely to have it, and age increases the risk.
- *Central sleep apnea*: The breathing stops repeatedly during sleep. The brain temporarily stops sending signals to the muscles that control breathing. This condition can be caused by brainstem injuries (including infections and stroke), congestive heart disease, and narcotic analgesics.
- *Complex sleep apnea syndrome*: Occurs when a person has both obstructive sleep apnea and central sleep apnea.

Signs and Symptoms. The most common signs and symptoms of these conditions include loud snoring, breathing cessation during sleep, dry mouth, sore throat, morning headache, difficulty staying asleep, excessive daytime sleepiness, irritability, and attention problems.

Diagnostic Procedures. After an examination, the provider may refer the patient to a sleep specialist or order a sleep study.

Treatments. Treatments may include weight loss or stopping the use of alcohol or medications that may be causing the condition. Continuous positive airway pressure (CPAP) therapy is the most common treatment for OSA (Fig. 11.10). It uses mild air pressure to keep the airway opened.

Acute Respiratory Diseases

There are many acute respiratory diseases. Tables 11.4 and 11.5 list several acute upper and lower respiratory diseases. In addition, the following sections describe commonly seen acute respiratory diseases.

> **VOCABULARY**
> **analgesics** A drug that reduces or eliminates pain.
> **antipyretics** A drug that is used to reduce a fever.
> **pharyngitis** Inflammation or infection of the pharynx, usually causing the symptoms of a sore throat.

Acute Bronchitis. Acute bronchitis is an inflammation of the lining of the bronchial tubes. The bronchial tubes become irritated and swollen, narrowing the airway. Excessive mucus is produced, leading to increased coughing.

Etiology. Acute bronchitis is usually caused by a lower respiratory viral infection. Viral conditions, such as the common cold, influenza, and pertussis (whooping cough), can also cause acute bronchitis. In rare cases a bacterial infection causes the disease. In addition, breathing in irritants or inhaling food or vomit can cause acute bronchitis.

Signs and Symptoms. Acute bronchitis can cause:
- A dry, hacking cough that can turn into a productive cough
- A low-grade fever
- Fatigue and weakness

Diagnostic Procedures. After obtaining a medical history and performing an examination, the provider may order a chest x-ray. Pulse oximetry may also be performed.

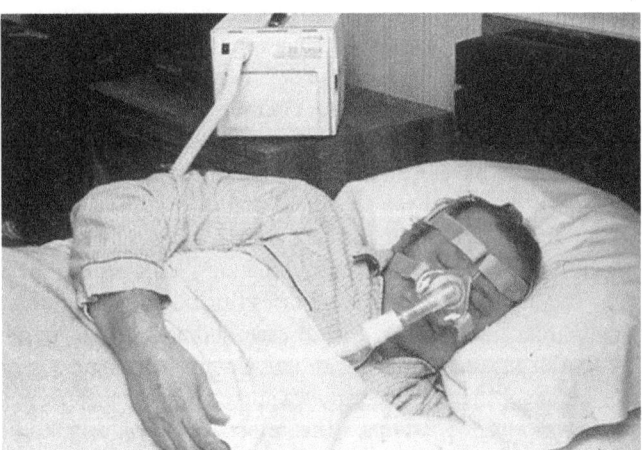

Fig. 11.10 Patient with a Continuous Positive Airway Pressure (CPAP) Machine. (Courtesy Respironics, Murrysville, PA.)

Treatments. In most cases, acute bronchitis is viral, so no antibiotics are prescribed. At-home treatments include using cough drops and a humidifier to soothe a dry throat. Patients are encouraged to drink plenty of fluids and get adequate rest. Over-the-counter (OTC) medications are used for fevers and body aches. Patients are encouraged to stop smoking and using e-cigarettes.

CRITICAL THINKING 11.5

Renee is working with a patient who needs to have a pulse oximetry measurement. The patient asks Renee what this test shows. Thinking back to what you have learned already in this chapter, how should Renee answer the patient?

COVID-19. COVID-19 is also called coronavirus disease 2019 and SARS-CoV-2. This disease originated in China in 2019 and created a world-wide pandemic. In 2021, the FDA approved Comirnaty (koe MIR na tee), a vaccine to prevent COVID-19. Because this is a new disease, new information is being learned all the time.

Etiology. COVID-19 is caused by the severe acute respiratory syndrome coronavirus 2 (SARS-CoV-2). Coronaviruses are a group of viruses that cause several illnesses including the common cold and severe acute respiratory syndrome (SARS).

Factors that put people at a higher risk of serious illness with COVID-19 are:
- Age over 65
- Lung disease, such as COPD, asthma, and cystic fibrosis
- Weakened immune system, from cancer treatments, transplants (e.g., bone marrow, solid organ), and chronic diseases
- Type 1 or type 2 diabetes mellitus
- Chronic kidney disease, liver disease, and sickle cell disease
- High blood pressure and heart disease
- Severe obesity
- Nervous system conditions

TABLE 11.4	Upper Respiratory System Diseases			
Disease	**Epiglottitis** (eh pee glah TYE tis)	**Laryngitis** (lair in JYE tis)	**Sinusitis** (sye nuh SYE tis)	**Strep Throat**
Description	Life-threatening inflammation of the epiglottis	Inflammation of the voice box (larynx)	Inflammation of the sinuses	Highly contagious bacterial infection of the throat.
Etiology	*Hib, Streptococcus pneumoniae,* or viruses	Overuse, irritation, or infection	Structural abnormalities or a cold may cause mucus to pool and pathogens to grow	Group A streptococcal bacteria are highly contagious.
Signs and Symptoms	High fever, pharyngitis (fair in JYE tis), stridor, cyanosis, drooling, difficulty breathing and swallowing, hoarseness	Hoarseness, weakened (or loss of) voice, tickling sensation, sore or dry throat, dry cough	Fever, weakness, fatigue, nasal and sinus congestion, cough, bad breath, or loss of smell	Rash, nausea and vomiting, fever, headache, painful swallowing, sore throat, tiny red spots at the back of the throat, or white pus patches.
Diagnostic Procedures	History and physical exam, blood/throat cultures, CBC, neck x-ray	History and physical exam; for chronic problems, laryngoscopy, biopsy	History and physical exam, x-rays	History and physical, rapid antigen test (CLIA waived), throat culture.
Treatment	Hospitalization, humidified oxygen, antibiotics, corticosteroids	Antibiotics, corticosteroids, increase fluid intake, rest voice, breathe moist air	Antibiotics, decongestants, analgesics (an ahl JEE ziks), heating pads, saline nasal sprays, vaporizers	Antibiotics, antipyretics (an tie pie RET ik), stay home until on antibiotics for 24 hours, analgesics

CBC, Complete blood count; *CLIA,* Clinical Laboratory Improvement Amendments; *Hib, Haemophilus influenzae* type b.

TABLE 11.5 Lower Respiratory System Diseases

Disease	Croup	Influenza (in floo EN zah)	Pertussis (pur TUSS is)	Pleurisy (PLOOR ih see)	Pneumothorax (noo moh THOR acks)
Description	Inflammation of the trachea and larynx	Acute viral infection; also called *flu*	Bacterial infection; also called *whooping cough*	Infection of the pleura	Air or gas in the pleural space, causing the lung to collapse (atelectasis [atl EK tah sis])
Etiology	Variety of viruses, including influenza	Influenza viruses	*Bordetella pertussis* (bacteria)	Bacteria, fungus, parasites, or viruses; also caused by inhaled toxins	Rupturing of a small blister on the lung's surface; trauma
Signs and Symptoms	Harsh, barklike cough; hoarseness, fever, and inspiratory stridor	Fever, cough, sore throat, muscle aches, headaches, and fatigue	Early stage: runny nose, low-grade fever, mild cough, apnea in babies; later stage: fits of many, rapid coughs, followed by a whooping sound, vomiting, and exhaustion	Stabbing pain (especially with inspiration), cough, fever, chills, and dyspnea	Sudden, sharp pleuritic pain that increases with movement, breathing, or coughing; shortness of breath, cyanosis, rapid pulse, and respiratory distress
Diagnostic Procedures	History and physical exam, cultures to identify causative organism; neck and chest x-ray	History and physical exam, nasopharyngeal swab, and rapid influenza diagnostic tests (CLIA waived)	History and physical exam, nasopharyngeal specimen culture, PCR (rapid test)	History and physical exam, pleural friction rub is heard over the lung field, chest x-ray, ultrasound, CT scan	History and physical exam, decreased breath sounds heard over the collapsed lung field, chest x-ray, CT scan, pulse oximetry, and arterial blood gases
Treatment	Antipyretics, humidifier, bed rest, increase fluid intake, and sitting may help child breathe easier; in severe cases, hospitalization with antibiotic and oxygen therapy	Bed rest, increased fluids, antiviral medications, and analgesics	Antibiotics, stay home, good hand washing, and humidifier	Analgesics, anti-inflammatory agents, bed rest, thoracentesis (thor ack sen TEE sis)	Treatment depends on cause of collapse; bed rest and monitoring of vital signs, chest tube, surgical procedures to remove a portion of the pleura (*pleurectomy* [plure EK to mee])

CLIA, Clinical Laboratory Improvement Amendments; *CT,* computed tomography; *PCR,* polymerase chain reaction.

Signs and Symptoms. The severity of the signs and symptoms can vary and can appear 2 to 14 days after exposure to the virus. COVID-19 can cause:
- Fever, chills, muscle aches, and fatigue
- New loss of taste or smell, headache
- Rhinorrhea, sore throat, cough, shortness of breath, and chest pain
- Nausea, vomiting, and diarrhea
- Emergency warning signs: dyspnea, persistent chest pressure or pain, new confusion, inability to wake or stay awake, and cyanosis

Diagnostic Procedures. A viral test is performed to diagnose a current infection. A nasal or throat specimen is obtained, and one of two viral tests can be used to check for SARS-CoV-2, the virus that causes COVID-19. Nucleic acid amplification tests (NAATs) detect the virus's genetic material. NAATs are more accurate but takes longer to process than the antigen test. Antigen tests detect viral proteins and are less sensitive, thus the test result may need to be confirmed with an NAAT. The antibody (serology) test is used to test for COVID-19 antibodies, indicating a past infection.

Treatments. Treatments depend on the severity of the illness. Home care treatments include analgesics, cough medication, rest, and fluid intake. Quarantining helps to minimize the spread of the disease. Severe cases can lead to hospitalization and oxygen therapy. Many clinical studies are under way, and additional treatments are being researched.

Most people return to normal health, but some people can have symptoms for weeks to months after the acute illness. Common long-term symptoms include fatigue, shortness of breath, cough, joint pain, and chest pain. Additional symptoms include:
- Heart palpitations and inflammation of the heart muscle
- Lung function abnormalities and acute kidney injury
- Difficulty with thinking and concentration, memory problems, sleep issues, headache, and smell and taste problems
- Muscle pain, intermittent fever, rash, and hair loss
- Depression, anxiety, and changes in mood

Pneumonia. Pneumonia (noo MOAN yah) is an infection of the lungs. It may affect one or both lungs. The alveoli fill with fluid or pus. Young children, adults over 65 years of age, people who smoke, and those with chronic illnesses are at more risk for pneumonia. The severity of pneumonia can range from mild to life-threatening. In the United States, about 1 million people have pneumonia a year, and about 50,000 people die from the disease. Adults are at most risk. Globally, it is the leading infectious disease killer of children under age 5.

Etiology. Pneumonia can be caused by bacteria, viruses, and fungi (Table 11.6). If a person has viral pneumonia, there is also a risk of getting bacterial pneumonia. Various chemicals can also cause pneumonia. Aspirating fluid or a foreign material into the lungs can also cause pneumonia.

TABLE 11.6 Examples of Pathogens That Cause Pneumonia

Type of Pathogen	Pathogen	Description
Bacteria	Streptococcus pneumoniae	Children under 2 years of age and adults 65 years or older are at most risk; pneumococcal vaccines are used for prevention.
	Haemophilus influenzae	Haemophilus influenza type b (Hib) vaccine is used as a prevention.
	Legionella pneumophila	Causes legionnaires disease and Pontiac fever.
	Mycoplasma pneumoniae	Called "walking pneumonia."
	Chlamydia pneumoniae	Most common in school-aged children.
	Chlamydia psittaci	Causes psittacosis; transmitted by infected pet birds and poultry.
Virus	Influenza virus	Prevention includes the yearly influenza vaccine.
	Respiratory syncytial virus (RSV)	Most common cause of pneumonia in children under 1 year of age.
Fungi	Pneumocystis jirovecii	More common in people with weakened immune systems.

Signs and Symptoms. Signs and symptoms of pneumonia vary based on the severity and type of pneumonia. Typically, pneumonia causes:

- High fever and chills
- Productive cough, shortness of breath, and chest pain with coughing or breathing
- Decreased appetite and fatigue
- Confusion in older adults

Diagnostic Procedures. Providers will listen to a patient's lungs for abnormal sounds. Chest x-rays, a CBC, a sputum culture, and pulse oximetry are typical diagnostic procedures used to check for pneumonia.

Treatments. Treatment for pneumonia is based on the type of pneumonia a person has. Antibiotics are used for bacterial pneumonia, and antiviral medications are used for viral pneumonia. Patients are encouraged to drink plenty of fluids and get rest. OTC antipyretics and analgesics (e.g., ibuprofen and acetaminophen) may be recommended.

CRITICAL THINKING 11.6

Renee is rooming Carl Bowden. He is here today for a recheck appointment. He was diagnosed 10 days ago with pneumonia. As Renee is gathering Carl's history, he tells her that he has smoked two packs a day for the past 30 years. He also states that he has had pneumonia six times over the past 2 years. He asks Renee if smoking might have something to do with that. Thinking back to the respiratory structures and functions you have learned about in this chapter; how would you answer his question?

Pulmonary Embolism. Pulmonary embolism (PE) is a condition in which one of the pulmonary arteries is blocked. PE is a medical emergency and can be life-threatening. Due to the blockage, blood flow may be interrupted to that section of the lung. This can lead to pulmonary hypertension. Oxygen can be limited to other body organs.

Etiology. Often PE is a complication of deep vein thrombosis (DVT). Blood clots form in the veins, usually in the legs. Some of the clots break off and travel through the bloodstream. Eventually, the clot blocks a pulmonary artery. Risk factors for PE include:

- Current or past DVT
- Being bedridden, having surgery
- Breaking a bone
- Pregnancy
- Chronic illness (stroke, hypertension, chronic heart disease, obesity)
- Smoking
- Use of birth control pills or hormone therapy pills

Signs and Symptoms. Pulmonary embolism can cause:

- Problems breathing, unexplained shortness of breath, and rapid breathing
- Chest pain, coughing or coughing up blood, and arrhythmias
- Lightheadedness and fainting

Diagnostic Procedures. Besides a medical history and physical examination, the provider may order the following diagnostic procedures:

- Ultrasound: to detect DVT in the legs
- CT scan with contrast: to detect PE or DVT
- Lung ventilation/perfusion scan (VQ scan)
- Pulmonary angiography
- Chest x-ray and chest MRI scan
- Echocardiography and electrocardiogram (ECG)

Treatments. The goals of treatment include preventing more clots or larger clots from forming. Treatment includes:

- *Anticoagulants*: "Blood thinners" (e.g., warfarin [Coumadin] and heparin) to prevent clots from forming.
- *Thrombolytics*: Medications that break up the clot. These are used in emergencies. Thrombolytics can be delivered by a catheter to the site of the clot.
- *Compression stockings*: To help prevent blood from pooling and clotting in the legs.

VOCABULARY

pulmonary hypertension High blood pressure that affects the pulmonary system (pulmonary arteries and the right side of the heart).
thoracentesis Aspiration of a fluid from the pleural cavity.

Pulmonary Tuberculosis. Pulmonary tuberculosis (too bur kyoo LOH sis) (TB) is caused by bacteria that can affect the lungs. There are two TB-related conditions: latent TB infection and TB disease.

Etiology. Tuberculosis is caused by *Mycobacterium tuberculosis,* which is spread through the air. Individuals at risk for TB include:

- Anyone who has lived in a country where TB is prevalent
- Anyone in frequent close contact with someone with TB disease
- Those working in healthcare a homeless shelter, or a prison
- Those living in a nursing home, prison, or homeless shelter

- People who have latent TB infection and a weakened immune system, because TB can become active under these conditions

Signs and Symptoms. There are differences regarding the spread and the signs/symptoms of the two TB-related conditions.

- With latent TB infection, a person cannot spread TB bacteria to others and there are no signs or symptoms.
- With TB disease, a person can spread the disease by coughing, sneezing, singing, or talking. TB disease can cause a bad cough that lasts 3 or more weeks, pain in the chest, blood in the sputum, weakness, no appetite, weight loss, chills, fever, and night sweats.

Diagnostic Procedures. Initially, the person is tested with either a Mantoux tuberculin skin test (TST) (also known as a purified protein derivative [PPD] test) or a TB blood test (e.g., QuantiFERON-TB Gold [QFT], T-SPOT.TB). If the test is positive, then the person will have additional testing (e.g., chest x-ray and sputum smear/culture) to determine if it is latent TB infection or TB disease. With latent TB infection, the chest x-ray is normal, and the sputum smear/culture is negative. With TB disease, the chest x-ray is abnormal, and the sputum smear/culture is positive.

Treatments. Treatments include:

- For latent TB infections, isoniazid or rifapentine may be prescribed. The goal is to prevent TB disease; a weakened immune system can increase the risk of TB disease.
- For TB disease, isoniazid, rifampin, ethambutol, or pyrazinamide may be prescribed. With treatment, TB disease symptoms tend to diminish within 2 to 3 weeks, but medication treatment may last for 6 to 9 months.

CRITICAL THINKING 11.7

Renee is confused about the two different types of tuberculosis (TB). She asks John to summarize the difference between latent TB infection and TB disease. How would you summarize the differences?

Respiratory Syncytial Virus. Respiratory syncytial (sin SISH uhl) virus (RSV) produces upper respiratory "cold" symptoms in healthy older children and adults. For young children and adults with medical problems, it can cause pneumonia and severe breathing problems.

Etiology. RSV spreads by coughing or sneezing. The virus can survive for several hours on infected surfaces. Typical outbreaks of RSV occur in winter and early spring.

Signs and Symptoms. RSV can cause nasal congestion, low-grade fevers, a runny nose, and a mild cough. Complications can include a barking cough from swelling near the vocal cords, high fevers, wheezing, apnea, cyanosis, and difficulty breathing.

Diagnostic Procedures. During the physical exam, the provider listens to the lungs, checking for wheezing and other abnormal lung sounds. Additional diagnostic procedures include pulse oximetry, chest x-rays, and laboratory tests (e.g., a CLIA-waived RSV test), viral cultures of the respiratory secretions from the nose).

Treatments. Treatment consists of over-the-counter medication (e.g., acetaminophen [Tylenol]) for the fever and plenty of fluids to prevent dehydration. People with severe cases of RSV are hospitalized. Supplemental oxygen, albuterol breathing treatments, and inhaled epinephrine may be given.

Additional Respiratory System Diseases

There are many respiratory diseases. The following list provides a brief description of several of them.

- *Acute respiratory distress syndrome*: A life-threatening condition that prevents enough oxygen from getting into the blood. Fluid buildup in the lungs reduces the lungs' ability to expand and causes hypoxemia.
- *Anthracosis* (AN thrah KOE sis): A loss of lung capacity caused by an accumulation of coal dust in the lungs; also called black lung disease.
- *Atelectasis* (AT l EK tah sis): A partial or complete collapse of the lung, which prevents normal oxygen absorption. Can be caused from lung disease, surgery, or a blockage.
- *Bronchiectasis* (brong kee ECK tuh sis): An infection or other conditions that cause damage to the airway, leading to bronchial dilation and scarring.
- *Bronchiolitis* (brong kee oh LYE tis): A common viral infection in young children and infants. The bronchioles become inflamed, and mucus builds up in the airway, affecting breathing.
- *Bronchopulmonary dysplasia* (BPD): Chronic respiratory condition that affects premature infants or infants who are on a *ventilator* (breathing machine). Infants require high concentrations of oxygen and assisted ventilation. They may have lung damage and are at greater risk for repeated respiratory infections.
- *Deviated septum*: A shifting of the nasal septum from the midline.
- *Diphtheria* (diff THEER ee ah): A bacterial respiratory infection characterized by sore throat, fever, and headache.
- *Hemothorax*: A condition that results in a collection of blood in the space between the chest wall and the lung (the pleural cavity). Caused by chest trauma, blood clotting defect, thoracic surgery, lung cancer, and tuberculosis.
- *Histoplasmosis* (his toe plaz MOE sis): Fungal disease of the lungs, caused by inhalation of *Histoplasma capsulatum. H. capsulatum* is found in soil and dust contaminated with bird or bat droppings.
- *Influenza A (H1N1) infection*: Results from transmission of the novel influenza A (H1N1) virus to humans, causing influenza symptoms, diarrhea, and vomiting. Also called swine flu.
- *Legionnaires'* (LEE juh nares) *disease*: A serious, life-threatening type of pneumonia caused from breathing in mist or swallowing water containing *Legionella pneumophila* bacteria. Can come from water in hot tubs, showers, or air conditioning units. Also called legionellosis.
- *Nasal polyps*: Soft, sac-like growths on the lining of the nose or sinuses. Can obstruct the airway and block drainage from the sinuses.
- *Nasopharyngeal carcinoma*: Malignant tumors in the pharynx, which can be related to diet or to the Epstein-Barr virus. They cause a mass in the neck, nasal obstruction, epistaxis, and serous otitis media (middle ear infection).
- *Neonatal respiratory distress syndrome* (RDS): Often seen in premature babies born before 37 to 39 weeks of gestation.

They lack enough surfactant in their lungs, which leads to respiratory distress. Infants are given warm, moist oxygen and may be put on a ventilator.

- *Pleural effusion* (PLOOR ul eh FYOO zhun): An abnormal, excessive buildup of fluid between the layers of tissue that line the lungs and chest cavity.
- *Pulmonary abscess*: Localized collection of infectious material in the lungs.
- *Pulmonary edema*: Accumulation of fluid in the lung tissue, caused by the inability of the heart to pump blood. It is often present in congestive heart failure.
- *Pulmonary fibrosis*: Scarring of lung tissue, causing the tissues to get stiff and thick. Breathing can be difficult, and the person can have hypoxemia.
- *Pulmonary hypertension* (PH): The blood pressure is high in the pulmonary arteries, which affects the blood flow in the lungs. The blood vessels become hard and narrow, causing hypoxemia. PH may be related to genetics or other conditions, such as heart or lung disease.
- *Pyothorax* (pye oh THOR acks): Pus in the pleural cavity. Also called empyema.
- *Rhinomycosis* (RYE noe my KOE sis): Fungal infection of the nasal mucous membranes.
- *Sarcoidosis* (sar koi DOE sis): Condition that causes lesions to form in the lungs and chest lymph nodes. It can lead to chronic illness and organ damage. Its origin is unknown.
- *Severe acute respiratory syndrome* (SARS): Viral respiratory disorder, caused by a coronavirus. It usually results in pneumonia.
- *Silicosis* (sil ih KOH sis): Loss of lung capacity, caused by an accumulation of glass dust in the lungs.

- *Upper respiratory tract infection*: Inflammation and/or infection of the upper respiratory structures. Known as the common cold.

LIFE SPAN CHANGES

An infant has a narrow airway, with a shorter and softer trachea. If the neck is overextended, the airway can collapse. Infants tend to breathe through their noses, which means nasal congestion can make breathing difficult. Infants are abdominal breathers and have immature respiratory muscles, meaning fatigue with breathing difficulties can set in quickly. With a disproportionately larger tongue and epiglottis, infants and young children are at risk for airway obstruction.

At around age 20 to 25, the lungs reach maturity. By age 35, lung function starts to decline. People who smoke can increase the aging of their lungs. As a person ages, the following respiratory system changes occur:

- Chest wall and thoracic spine deformities cause increased work of breathing.
- The diaphragm grows weaker, leading to a decreased ability to inhale and exhale.
- Weakness in respiratory muscles causes the coughing reflex to be less effective.
- A decrease in tissue elasticity leads to an inability to keep the airway completely open.
- Alveoli lose their shape, which causes air to be trapped in the lungs. This leads to a decrease in gas exchange and lung capacity.

CLOSING COMMENTS

Many times, with pulmonary disorders and treatments, patients may become dizzy. This can affect their balance or even cause them to faint. If a patient has a recent history of fainting, or "passing out," it is important for the medical assistant to keep the patient safe in the ambulatory care environment. Some ways to assist patients and prevent falls include:

- Assist the patient as needed when stepping on and off the scale.
- Assist the patient on and off the exam table.
- Do not leave the patient on the exam table unattended.
- Ask the patient if they would like a wheelchair.

Many lawsuits have been brought forward involving situations in which patients were injured from falls in the ambulatory care environment. Several cases have involved medical assistants not helping patients on and off equipment such as scales or having patients wait unattended on exam tables. Remember, safety is one of the most important concerns when caring for patients.

BOX 11.3 Medication Classifications

- *Antihistamines:* Counteract the effects of histamine.
- *Antivirals:* Inhibit the growth or reduce the spread of viral cells.
- *Antitussives:* Inhibit the cough center.
- *Bronchodilators:* Relax the smooth muscles of the bronchi.
- *Corticosteroids (oral, nasal, and inhaled):* Reduce airway inflammation and bronchial resistance.
- *Decongestants:* Relieve local congestion in the nasal and sinus tissues.
- *Expectorants:* Thin the secretions in the bronchial tubes to make it easier to cough up the mucus.
- *Leukotriene receptor antagonists:* Block the action of substances that cause asthma and allergic rhinitis.

  Refer to Appendix D, which can be found on the Evolve website, for information on the medication classifications, including indications for use, desired effect, side effects, adverse reactions, and generic and trade names. Medical assistants should be familiar with medications that are prescribed to patients.

PATIENT-CENTERED CARE

To provide patient-centered care, medical assistants need to:

- Provide patients with clear instructions on the pulmonary procedure being done
- Perform the procedure correctly, so the patient's results are accurate
- Be sensitive to patients' concerns and feelings regarding pulmonary diseases

BEING PROFESSIONAL

Part of being professional is one's appearance and grooming. When working with patients, it is essential that medical assistants have no odors on their bodies. Perfume, cologne, or scented lotions can trigger an allergic reaction in a patient. Patients with asthma can have flare-ups when they are around different scents, such as perfume, cologne, or scented lotions.

Medical assistants who smoke cigarettes need to be especially concerned with the odor. Research has shown that tobacco smoke contains more than 7000 chemicals, of which 250 are harmful. When the olfactory (sense of smell) system is exposed to these chemicals, reversible or permanent injuries can occur. The injury relates to the length of time the person has smoked and the tobacco toxicity. Ultimately, smoking tobacco can lead to a decrease in odor

sensibility and recognition. This means people who smoke may not be able to smell the cigarette smoke on their clothing or body, yet it may be noticeable to others.

Many patients who have a chronic illness, such as cancer or chronic obstructive pulmonary disease (COPD), have quit smoking tobacco products. It is important that the healthcare professionals who care for these patients (and all other patients) do not smell of cigarette smoke.

Role-play this scenario: You and Jane are medical assistants in a family practice setting. You are a smoker. After rooming a patient, Jane comes to you and tells you quietly that you smell of cigarette smoke. How should you respond to Jane? What should you do?

CHAPTER REVIEW

The upper respiratory tract is composed the nose, pharynx, and the larynx. These organs are located outside of the chest cavity. The main functions of the upper respiratory tract include warming and cleaning the inspired air, serving as a passageway for air, and providing the sense of smell.

The lower respiratory tract consists of the trachea, bronchial tubes, and lungs. The trachea (windpipe) lies in the space between the lungs, called the *mediastinum*. Air travels from the larynx through the trachea, and then the trachea branches into the right and left bronchi. The bronchi divide into smaller branches, called *bronchioles*. These bronchioles end in microscopic ducts capped by air sacs, called *alveoli*, which are involved with gas exchange.

The two primary functions of the respiratory system are to exchange O_2 from the atmosphere for CO_2 waste and to maintain the acid-base balance in the body. Both functions involve ventilation (breathing), which is the movement of gases between the lungs and the environment. Ventilation includes the process of inspiration (air moving into the lungs) and expiration (air moving

out of the lungs). Two types of respiration occur during the ventilation process, external respiration and internal respiration.

The chronic respiratory diseases discussed in this chapter include allergic rhinitis, asthma, chronic obstructive pulmonary disease (i.e., chronic bronchitis and emphysema), cystic fibrosis, laryngeal cancer, lung cancer, types of pneumoconiosis, and sleep apnea.

Acute respiratory conditions explained include acute bronchitis, COVID-19, croup, epiglottitis, influenza, laryngitis, pertussis, pleurisy, pneumonia, pneumothorax, pulmonary embolism, pulmonary tuberculosis, respiratory syncytial virus, sinusitis, and strep throat.

An infant has a narrow airway, with a shorter and softer trachea and tends to breathe through the nose. Infants are abdominal breathers and have immature respiratory muscles, meaning fatigue with breathing difficulties can set in quickly. As a person ages, the diaphragm grows weaker. The respiratory muscles become weaker, and there is a decrease in tissue elasticity. The alveoli lose their shape.

SCENARIO WRAP-UP

As Renee works with John, she realizes she has a lot more to learn. Pulmonary disease is common. Renee decides to research the diseases she encounters every week. She feels that to be professional, it is important to be up-to-date on the latest information. She likes to be confident in her skills and knowledge. This helps when patients have questions about diseases, procedures, or treatments.

Renee looks forward to her weekly pulmonary experiences. She is confident in rooming patients, performing pulse oximetry, and gathering sputum specimens. She is excited about learning how to do peak flow and spirometry tests in the coming weeks.

12

Digestive System

LEARNING OBJECTIVES

1. Describe the anatomical location of the major organs of the digestive system.
2. Describe the four processes that occur in the digestive system and discuss the chemical digestion of carbohydrates, proteins, and fats.
3. Explain the common diagnostic procedures and treatments for digestive system disorders.
4. Describe common digestive system disorders, including common signs and symptoms, etiology, diagnostic procedures, and treatments.
5. Identify CLIA-waived tests associated with common digestive system disorders.
6. Compare the structure and function of the of the digestive system across the life span.

OUTLINE

▶▶ OPENING SCENARIO

Keith Williams, CMA (AAMA), has been newly hired as a medical assistant at the Walden-Martin Family Medical (WMFM) Clinic. He just graduated from the local community college last semester after returning to school to study for a second career.

Now, at age 49, he has accepted a job at WMFM Clinic. He has been asked by his supervisor to assist the gastroenterology outreach team, which comes to WMFM Clinic twice a week.

Keith is excited about his new duties yet realizes that he needs to review the digestive system and related diseases. He decides to spend the next week reviewing the anatomy, physiology, and pathology related to the digestive system, along with the diagnostic procedures and commonly ordered treatments.

YOU WILL LEARN

1. To describe the anatomy of the digestive system, including the gastrointestinal tract and accessory structures.
2. To describe the four digestive system processes.
3. To explain the chemical digestion of carbohydrates, proteins, and fats.
4. To describe common digestive system disorders, including etiology, signs and symptoms, diagnostic procedures, and treatments.
5. To discuss life span changes in the digestive system.

INTRODUCTION

Gastroenterology (gas troh en tuh ROL uh jee) is the healthcare specialty that deals with most digestive diseases and disorders. A *gastroenterologist* (gas troh en tuh ROL uh jist) is a specialist involved in the diagnosis, treatment, and prevention of disorders of the digestive organs and liver. A *proctologist* (prok TOL uh jist) is a subspecialist who treats disorders of the rectum and anus. *Hepatology* (hep ah TOL uh jee) is a subspecialty that deals with liver disorders. A *hepatologist* (hep ah TOL uh jist) is a specialist who focuses only on the liver.

Gastrointestinal system disorders are common in the ambulatory care facility. Besides the gastroenterology department, patients with digestive concerns are seen in primary care, pediatrics, internal medicine, and urgent care settings.

ANATOMY OF THE DIGESTIVE SYSTEM

The digestive system is also called the *gastrointestinal (GI) system*. It is made up of these structures:

- Gastrointestinal tract: Also called the *digestive tract* and the *alimentary* (al in MEN tair ee) *canal*. It consists of a large, muscular tube that, with the help of hormones and enzymes, digests food. The GI tract starts at the mouth and extends to the anus. It includes the mouth, pharynx (throat), esophagus, stomach, small intestine, and large intestine.
- Accessory organs: The salivary glands, gallbladder, liver, and pancreas are considered the major accessory organs. These structures secrete fluids into the GI tract, aiding in digestion.

The following sections will discuss the GI tract structures and the accessory organs.

CRITICAL THINKING 12.1

As Keith starts to review the anatomy of the digestive system, he tries to remember the major and accessory organs. List the major organs and accessory organs of the digestive system.

Gastrointestinal Tract Structures

Mouth. The cheeks, lips, tongue, hard palate (PAL it), and soft palate form the mouth (also called the *oral cavity* or *buccal cavity*).

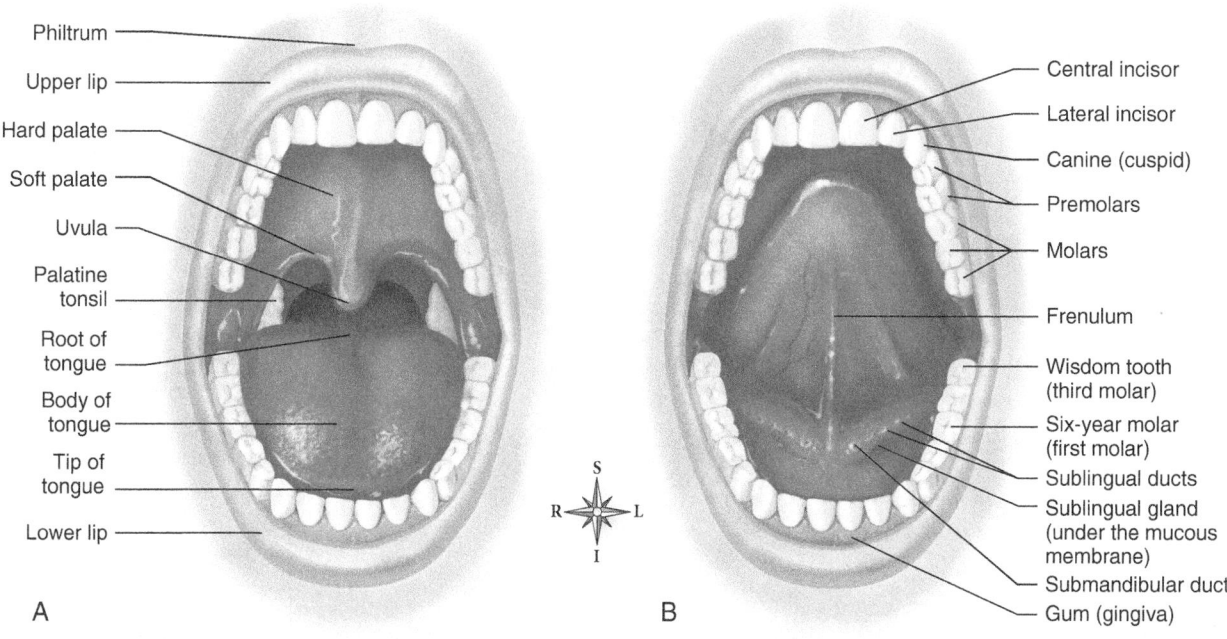

Fig. 12.1 Mouth. A, Mouth cavity showing hard and soft palates, tongue surface, and uvula. B, Undersurface of tongue showing frenulum, sublingual gland, and opening of sublingual duct. *GI,* Gastrointestinal. (From Patton KT, Thibodeau GA: *The human body in health and disease,* ed 7, St. Louis, 2018, Elsevier.)

The roof of the mouth is created by the anterior hard palate and the posterior soft palate. The uvula (YOO vyoo lah) is a fleshy structure that hangs above the throat, at the back of the soft palate (Fig. 12.1). Adults have 32 permanent teeth that are set in the gums (also called *gingivae* [JIN jeh vee]). Saliva from the salivary glands helps to lubricate the food, making it easier to swallow. The salivary glands will be discussed later in the chapter.

Pharynx. When food or liquid is swallowed, it moves into the pharynx (FAIR inks), or throat. The pharynx is divided into three sections:

- Nasopharynx (nay soh FAIR inks): Located behind the nasal cavity
- Oropharynx (oh roh FAIR inks): Located behind the mouth; part of the respiratory and digestive systems
- Laryngopharynx (lah RING goe FAIR inks): Located between the epiglottis (ep i GLOT is) and the esophagus

Esophagus. The esophagus (eh SAH fah gus) connects the pharynx to the stomach (Fig. 12.2). This muscular tube runs behind the trachea and the heart. The esophagus is lined with a mucous membrane that secretes mucus, helping the mass of

food, or bolus, pass into the stomach. Peristalsis (payr i STAHL sis), or the muscular contractions of the esophagus, helps to move the food into the stomach.

A sphincter (SFINK tur) is located at the top and bottom of the esophagus. When the upper esophageal sphincter (UES) constricts, it prevents air from entering the esophagus. The lower esophageal sphincter (LES), or the cardiac sphincter, is located between the esophagus and the stomach. When the LES constricts, it prevents the stomach contents from moving up the esophagus. When a person swallows, the LES relaxes, allowing the bolus to move into the stomach.

VOCABULARY

epiglottis Lid-like structure over the glottis that prevents food and liquids from entering the trachea when swallowing occurs.

mucous membrane A mucus-producing membrane that lines tracts and structures of the body (e.g., GI tract, respiratory tract); also called mucosa.

peristalsis Wavelike movement from alternate circulate contraction and relaxation of a tubular structure (e.g., intestine), which propels the content forward.

sphincter A circular muscle that either constricts and closes the opening or relaxes and allows substances to pass through the opening.

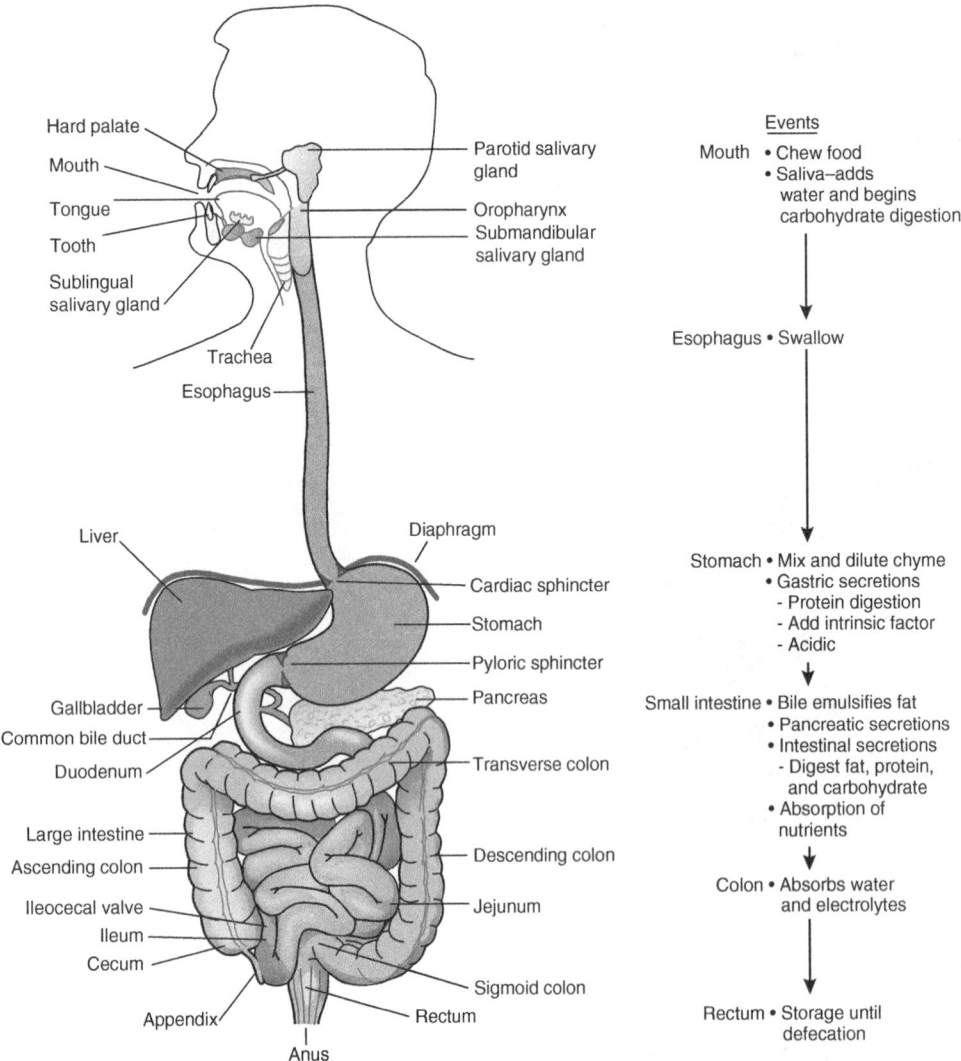

Fig. 12.2 The Anatomy of the Digestive System and Associated Events. (From VanMeter KC, Hubert RJ: *Gould's pathophysiology for the health professions*, ed 5, Philadelphia, 2015, Saunders.)

MEDICAL TERMINOLOGY

cheil/o, labi/o	lips
bol/o	bolus
bucc/o	cheek
corpor/o	body, corporis
dent/i, odont/o	teeth
esophag/o	esophagus
fund/o	fundus
gastr/o	stomach
gingiv/o	gums
gloss/o, lingu/o	tongue
laryng/o	voice box, larynx
mucos/o, myx/o	mucus, mucosa
nas/o	nose
or/o, stomat/o, stom/o	mouth, oral cavity
palat/o	palate
pharyng/o	throat, pharynx
pylor/o	pylorus
sial/o	saliva
sialaden/o	salivary glands
peri-	surrounding
-al	pertaining to
-stalsis	contraction

Stomach. The stomach serves as a reservoir for food. The stomach is divided into three sections:

- *Fundus* (FUN dus): Top of the stomach, sits just below the diaphragm
- *Body*: Main part of the stomach
- *Pylorus* (pye LORE us): Bottom of the stomach, between the body and the small intestine

The stomach wall contains rugae (ROO gah), which when unfolded allow for greater expansion of the stomach size.

Tiny glands in the mucous membrane lining of the stomach produce digestive enzymes, intrinsic factor, hydrochloric acid, mucus, and bicarbonate. These make up the gastric juice. Gastric juice is continually being made, but the amounts made at certain times vary. Certain things trigger more gastric juice to be made, including thoughts of eating, the smell of food, and the presence of food in the mouth and stomach. The smooth muscles in the stomach provide churning and mixing action, which helps combine the gastric juice with the food ingested, creating a mixture called *chyme* (kime). A continuous coating of mucus protects the stomach and the rest of the digestive system from the acidic nature of chyme and the gastric juices.

Besides being a food reservoir and secreting gastric juices, the stomach has additional roles, which include:

- Producing *gastrin* (GAS trin), a hormone that regulates the digestive functions
- Producing *ghrelin* (GREL in), which increases the appetite
- Protecting the body by killing disease-causing bacteria in food
- Absorbing alcohol, some water, certain drugs, and some fatty acids

The pyloric sphincter is located between the pylorus and the small intestine and regulates the passage of food into the small intestine (Fig. 12.3). When the pyloric sphincter relaxes, the chyme empties out of the stomach and into the small intestine.

> ## VOCABULARY
> **intrinsic factor** Secreted by the parietal cells of the stomach; necessary for the absorption of vitamin B_{12} to prevent pernicious anemia.
> **rugae** Folds in the wall of an organ; when an organ (e.g., stomach, bladder, uterus) fills or needs to expand, the rugae unfold.

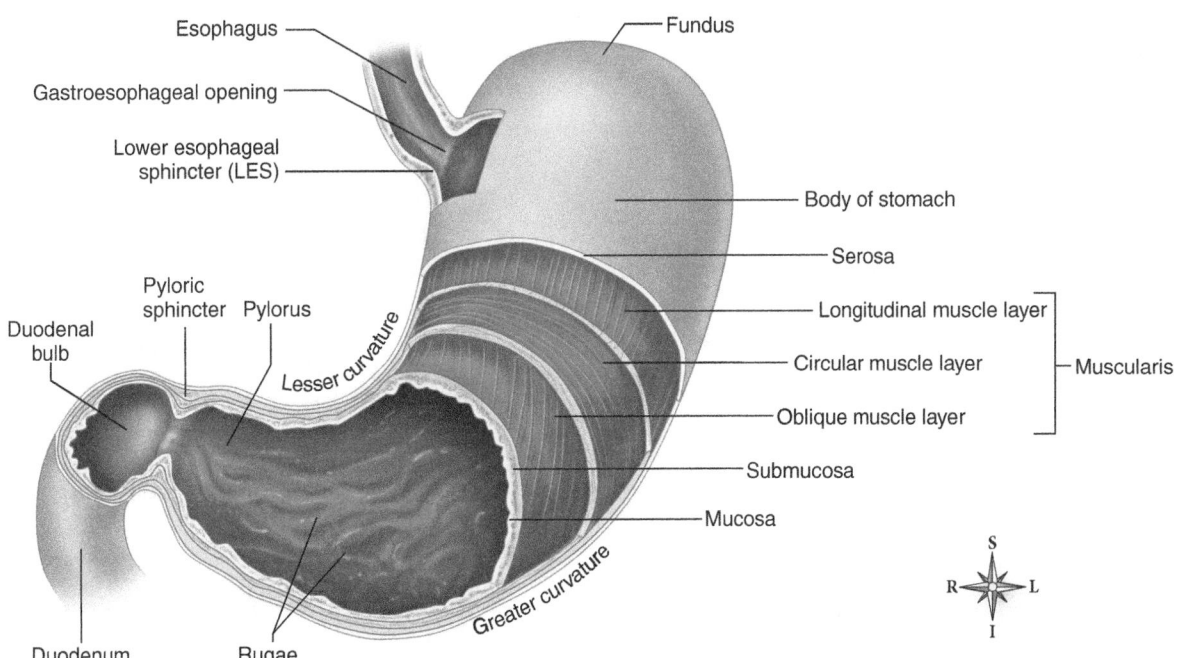

Fig. 12.3 Stomach. A portion of the anterior wall has been cut away to reveal the three muscle layers of the stomach wall. Notice that the mucosa lining the stomach forms folds called *rugae*. (From Patton KT, Thibodeau GA: *The human body in health and disease*, ed 7, St. Louis, 2018, Elsevier.)

Small Intestine. The small intestine has about a 1-inch lumen and is about 20 feet long. It loops around and fills most of the abdominal cavity. The small intestine is made up of three parts:

- *Duodenum* (doo AH deh num): Smallest part of the small intestine; connected to the stomach by the pyloric sphincter.
- *Jejunum* (jeh JOO num): Second largest part of the small intestine; connected to the duodenum and the ileum.

- *Ileum* (ILL ee um): Largest part of the small intestine; connects to the jejunum and the large intestine. It joins the cecum at the ileocecal valve.

The lining of the small intestine has *plicae* (PLY kah) (folds), which contain small projections called *villi* (VILL eye). The villi are covered by *microvilli* (epithelial cells that have a brushlike shape). The villi and microvilli increase the surface area of the small intestine and make absorption of nutrients more efficient. Each villus contains a *lacteal* (LACK tee ul) (lymph vessel) that absorbs lipids (fats) and fat-soluble vitamins. The blood capillary absorbs glucose and amino acids (Fig. 12.4).

Each of the three sections of the small intestine has important roles.

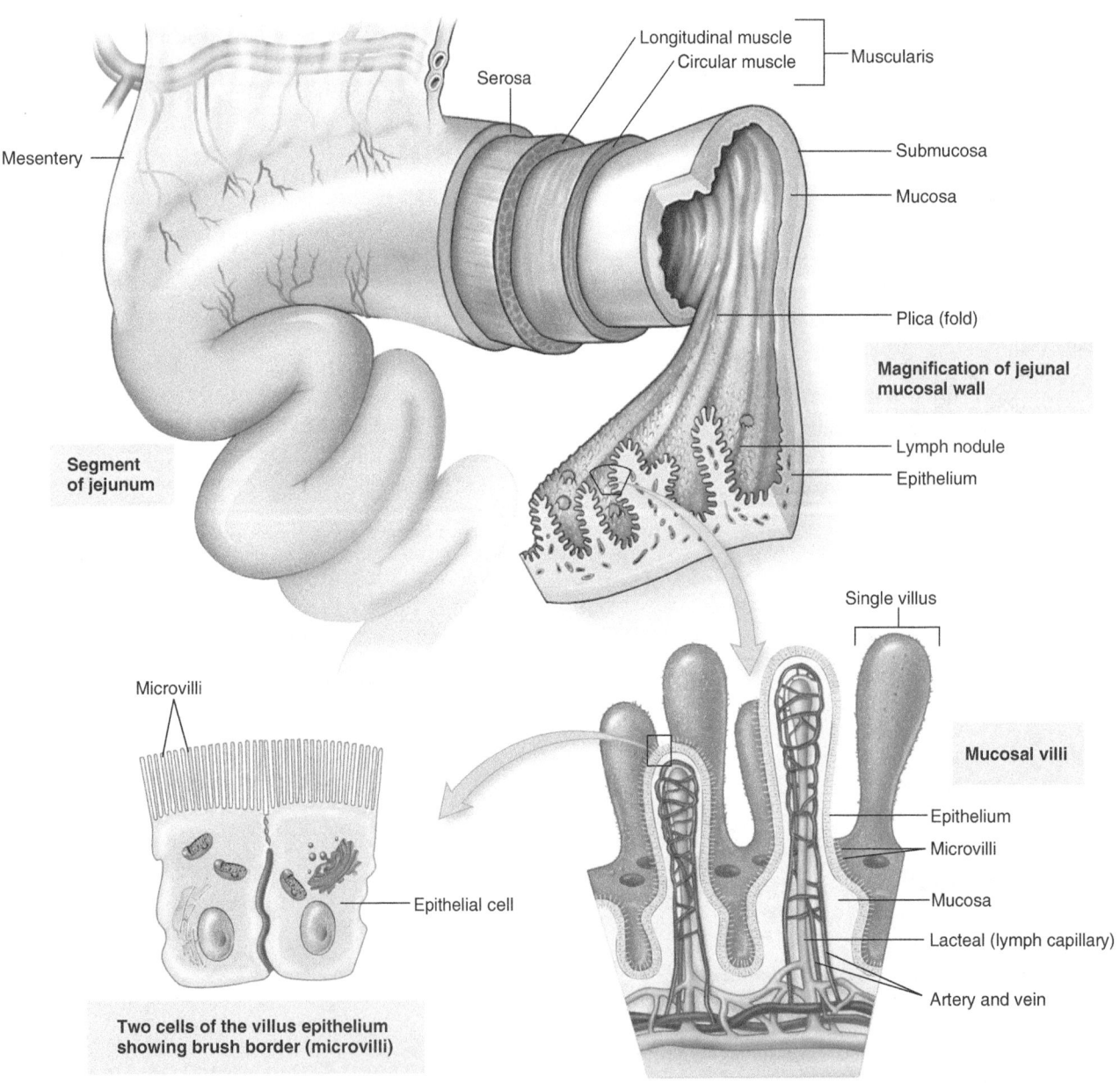

Fig. 12.4 Small Intestine. Note the four tissue coats or layers and the presence of villi and microvilli, which increases the area available for absorption. (From Patton KT, Thibodeau GA: *The human body in health and disease,* ed 7, St. Louis, 2018, Elsevier.)

- *Duodenum:* Receives chyme from the stomach. Pancreatic enzymes, bile from the liver, and bicarbonate mix with the chyme. Pancreatic enzymes break down chyme. Bile helps break down and absorb fat. Bicarbonate neutralizes the acid from the stomach.
- *Jejunum:* Contains larger villi, thus absorption is the primary function of this section. Sugars, fatty acids, and amino acids are absorbed.
- *Ileum:* Limited absorption occurs in this section. Bile acids and vitamin B_{12} are most often absorbed for reuse in the body.

Chyme from the stomach empties into the duodenum. Peristalsis moves the chyme through the duodenum, jejunum, and the ileum. The ileocecal (ILL ee oh SEE kul) valve is found between the ileum (of the small intestine) and the cecum (of the large intestine). The ileocecal valve controls the passage of chyme into the cecum and prevents the backflow of chyme into the small intestine.

> **VOCABULARY**
> **lumen** The cavity, channel, or open space within a tube or tubular organ.

MEDICAL TERMINOLOGY

abdomin/o, lapar/o, celi/o	abdomen
duoden/o	duodenum
enter/o	small intestine
ile/o	ileum
intestin/o	intestines
jejun/o	jejunum
lip/o, lipid/o	fat, lipid
lumin/o	lumen
plic/o	fold, plica
vill/o	villus

Large Intestine. The large intestine or colon has about a 3-inch lumen and is about 5 feet long. The large intestine is made up of these six sections:

- *Cecum* (SEE kum): A 2- to 3-inch pouch or tubelike structure in the lower right abdomen that is considered the first section of the large intestine. The main roles of the cecum include receiving chyme from the small intestine and absorbing fluids and salts. Mucus is also mixed with the chyme in the cecum. Attached to the cecum is the vermiform appendix (VUR mih form ah PEN dicks). The function of the appendix is not entirely known, though research suggests that it harbors "good bacteria," which will repopulate the intestines after an illness.
- *Ascending colon:* The second part of the large intestine, which extends vertically from the cecum to just below the liver (see Fig. 12.2).
- *Transverse colon:* Extends horizontally from the ascending colon to the descending colon.
- *Descending colon:* Extends vertically on the left side of the abdomen from the transverse colon to the sigmoid colon.
- *Sigmoid colon:* Forms an S-shaped curve; attaches to the descending colon and the rectum.

- *Rectum:* Stores the stool until defecation, or a bowel movement (BM), occurs and the stool is released through the anus.

The watery waste products move from the small intestine into the large intestine. The primary functions of the large intestine include:

- Reabsorption of water and electrolytes: The large intestine has no villi for nutrient absorption but can reabsorb water and electrolytes (e.g., sodium and potassium). The longer a stool is in the colon, the more water is absorbed. The quicker a stool passes through the large intestine, the more water it contains.
- Making vitamin K: The bacteria in the large intestine make vitamin K, which is used for blood coagulation, bone mineralization, and cardiovascular health (Box 12.1).
- Eliminating waste products from the body.

> **CRITICAL THINKING 12.3**
>
> Keith is reviewing the anatomy of the GI tract. List the sections of the small and large intestines in order.

MEDICAL TERMINOLOGY

appendic/o, append/o	appendix
an/o	anus
cec/o	cecum
col/o, colon/o	large intestine, colon
proct/o	rectum and anus
rect/o	rectum, straight
sigmoid/o	sigmoid colon

Accessory Organs

Accessory organs have a role in digestive activities, though they are not part of the digestive tract. Accessory organs include the salivary glands, liver, gallbladder, and the pancreas. Each of these accessory organs will be discussed in the following sections.

Salivary Glands. Three pairs of salivary glands are found in the mouth. The *parotid glands* are near the ear in the cheeks. The *submandibular glands* are on the floor of the mouth, and the *sublingual glands* are under the tongue. These glands produce and secrete saliva, which mixes with the food eaten. Saliva not only moistens the food, it aids in the breakdown and swallowing of food. Saliva contains salivary amylase, an enzyme, which will be discussed later in the chapter.

Liver. The liver is one of the largest organs in the body and is located just below the diaphragm, in the right hypochondriac and epigastric regions (see Fig. 12.2). The liver is divided into two major lobes and two smaller lobes.

The hepatic artery brings oxygenated blood to the liver. The hepatic portal vein brings blood from the digestive tract, which can contain nutrients, medications, alcohol, and toxic substances. These substances are filtered from the blood and are processed, stored, changed, detoxified, and returned to the blood or eliminated in the stool. Besides these roles, the liver has additional important functions:

- Producing plasma proteins (e.g., albumin and blood clotting factors).
- Breaking down old or damaged blood cells.
- Breaking down proteins and fats and producing energy.
- Producing up to a liter of bile a day. Bile contains bilirubin (a breakdown product of red blood cells), bile acids or salts, cholesterol, water, and salts (e.g., sodium, potassium) and metals (e.g., copper). Bile is stored in the gallbladder until it is secreted into the duodenum. Bile breaks down fats into fatty acids.
- Removing extra minerals (e.g., iron and copper), vitamins (B$_{12}$, A, D, and K), and glucose from the blood and stores them in the liver. The liver releases them into the blood when needed. (For instance, the liver stores extra glucose as glycogen. When the blood glucose level decreases, the liver breaks down the glycogen and releases the glucose into the blood.)
- Manufacturing triglycerides and cholesterol.

CRITICAL THINKING 12.4

Keith is amazed at all of the activities that occur in the liver. List at least four roles of the liver.

Gallbladder. The gallbladder (GB) is found in a small area on the underside of the liver (see Fig. 12.2). The gallbladder stores and concentrates bile. The bile is made by the liver, and then it flows through the common bile duct to smaller ducts before going into the gallbladder, where it is stored. When a person eats, the gallbladder contracts and squeezes the bile through the bile duct and then into the common bile duct, before emptying into the duodenum. If gallbladder emptying is delayed (as in pregnancy), gallstone formation can occur.

Pancreas. The pancreas is a gland found behind the stomach and in front of the spine (see Fig. 12.2). It is about 6 to 10 inches long. The pancreas has two main roles:

- Exocrine function: About 95% of the pancreas is made up of exocrine tissue that produces digestive enzymes. These enzymes are released into the duodenum.
- Endocrine function: About 5% of the pancreas is made up of endocrine cells, called *islets of Langerhans,* which make hormones (e.g., insulin) that regulate blood sugar and pancreatic secretions. (See Chapter 7 for additional details.)

The pancreatic enzymes created in the exocrine tissue include trypsin, chymotrypsin, amylase, and lipase. When food enters the stomach, pancreatic enzymes and sodium bicarbonate are released into the main pancreatic duct. This duct joins the common bile duct to form the ampulla (am PUL ah) of Vater (also called the *hepatopancreatic duct* or *ampulla*), which is located at the duodenum.

VOCABULARY

endocrine A glandular secretion that is released into the blood or lymph directly (does not go through a duct).

exocrine A glandular secretion released through a duct.

MEDICAL TERMINOLOGY

adnex/o	accessory
bil/i, chol/e	bile
choledoch/o	common bile duct
cholecyst/o	gallbladder
cholesterol/o	cholesterol
fec/a	feces
hepat/o	liver
lob/o	lobe
pancreat/o	pancreas
endo-	within
exo-	outside
hypo-	below
-crine	to secrete
-kinin	movement substance

PHYSIOLOGY OF THE DIGESTIVE SYSTEM

The role of the digestive system is to provide nutrients to the cells of the body. Four processes occur in the digestive system:

- *Ingestion:* The intake of food and liquids into the body
- *Digestion:* The breakdown of food into chemical substances
- *Absorption:* The passage of substances and liquids through the lining of the GI tract into the body fluids and tissues
- *Excretion:* The elimination of indigestible materials and waste products of metabolism

The following sections will focus on digestion, absorption, and elimination processes in the body.

CRITICAL THINKING 12.5

Summarize the four processes that occur in the digestive system.

Digestion

Once food is ingested, it must be digested for absorption to occur. Two digestive processes happen to break down food into chemical substances:

- *Mechanical digestion:* The breakdown of food into smaller particles. This process starts in the mouth as the food is being chewed. The smooth muscles in the stomach provide the churning and mixing action, which also aids in the breakdown of the food.
- *Chemical digestion:* The smaller particles of food are broken down into small molecules that can be absorbed.

Chemical Digestion. Chemical digestion starts in the mouth. During *mastication* (MAS ti KAE shun) (the process of chewing), saliva moistens and aids in the breakdown and swallowing (*deglutition* [dee glue TISH uhn]) of food. Saliva contains an enzyme called *salivary amylase,* which starts to break down complex carbohydrates.

In the stomach, hydrochloric acid softens and breaks down proteins and other foods. The pH of hydrochloric acid also kills many pathogens (e.g., bacteria) that are consumed. Pepsin, an enzyme found in the gastric juices, breaks down proteins into amino acids.

Hydrochloric acid, amino acids, or fatty acids in the stomach or duodenum stimulate the small intestine to secrete cholecystokinin (CCK), a hormone. CCK causes the gallbladder to contract and release bile into the duodenum through the common bile duct. Bile from the liver is also secreted in the duodenum and emulsifies (ee MUL sih fyez) fats. CCK also increases secretion of pancreatic juices, which contain the following enzymes:

- *Trypsin* and chymotrypsin: Break down proteins into amino acids
- *Amylase:* Breaks down carbohydrates into sugars
- *Lipase:* Breaks down fats into fatty acids and glycerol

Pancreatic juices also contain sodium bicarbonate, which helps to neutralize the acidity of the chyme in the duodenum.

In the small intestine, *brush-border enzymes* (sucrase, lactase, and maltase) are found in the microvilli. These enzymes help with the final breakdown of carbohydrates, including:

- *Sucrase:* Breaks down sucrose (or cane sugar) into glucose and fructose.
- *Lactase:* Breaks down lactose (found in milk) into galactose and glucose.
- *Maltase:* Breaks down maltose (from starches) into glucose.

CRITICAL THINKING 12.6

Summarize the chemical digestion of carbohydrates, proteins, and fats.

Absorption and Excretion

Once chemical digestion is complete, small nutrient molecules move from the small intestines into the bloodstream through the process of absorption. As mentioned earlier, the villi and microvilli in the small intestine increase the surface area, which makes absorption of nutrients more efficient. The lacteal in the villus absorbs lipids, and the capillary absorbs glucose and amino acids. Chemical digestion and nutrient absorption are completed by the time chyme leaves the small intestine.

As chyme moves through the large intestine, water and electrolytes are reabsorbed to prevent dehydration. The consistency of chyme changes to a soft-formed solid, called *feces,* which is excreted. The composition of feces is water, bacteria, undigested carbohydrates, fiber, and some protein and fat.

DISEASES AND DISORDERS OF THE DIGESTIVE SYSTEM

Many patients seen in ambulatory care facilities have digestive system diseases. Common signs and symptoms include:

- Constipation, diarrhea, *hematochezia* (bloody stool), and *melena* (black, tarry stools)
- *Pyrosis* (heartburn), *dyspepsia* (indigestion), *dysphagia* (difficulty swallowing), and *flatus* (gas)
- *Halitosis* (bad-smelling breath)
- Nausea, vomiting, and *hematemesis* (vomiting of blood)
- *Jaundice* (yellowing of the skin and whites of the eyes caused by elevated bilirubin levels)

Tables 12.1 and 12.2 provide common diagnostic procedures and treatments used for digestive disorders. The following sections discuss digestive disorders.

VOCABULARY

cholecystitis Inflammation of the gallbladder.

emulsifies When a substance suspends tiny droplets of one liquid in a second liquid. By creating an emulsion, you can mix two liquids that usually do not mix well, such as oil and water.

enema Fluid introduced into the rectum for a therapeutic or diagnostic purpose.

occult Hidden or unseen.

Disorders of the Mouth

Orofacial Clefts. Orofacial clefts are one of the most common birth defects in the United States. Orofacial clefts include the following congenital disorders:

- *Cleft lip:* An opening in the upper lip caused by the lip tissues not completely joining before birth.
- *Cleft palate:* The tissue that makes up the palate (roof of the mouth) does not completely join before birth. The hard palate makes up the front section and the soft palate makes up the back section. Cleft palate can affect one or both palates.

Children can have a cleft lip, a cleft palate, or both (Fig. 12.5). Children with clefts can have problems with feeding, speaking, hearing, and ear infections.

Etiology. In most cases the etiology is unknown, but researchers believe it involves genetics and environmental factors. Research studies have shown that women who smoke, have diabetes, or use certain medications (e.g., valproic acid)

TABLE 12.1 Common Diagnostic Procedures Used for Digestive Disorders

Done by/ Type of Test:	Procedure	Description
Provider during the exam	Digital rectal examination (DRE)	Done during the physical exam. The provider inserts a gloved, lubricated finger into the rectum to feel for abnormalities in the prostate, bladder, and so on.
	Anoscopy (ae NOS kah pee)	Done during the physical exam. A short speculum is used for examining the anal canal and lower rectum.
Endoscopy	Capsule endoscopy	Pill-sized video camera is swallowed, which allows examination of the small intestine. Used to detect bleeding, polyps, inflammatory bowel disease, ulcers, and tumors in the small intestine.
	Colonoscopy	An endoscope is inserted through the anus. Used to visualize the large intestine. Polyps can be removed during the procedure.
	Endoscopic retrograde cholangiopancreatography (ERCP)	An endoscope is inserted into the mouth and passed through the stomach and duodenum, before it is inserted into the bile ducts. Used to treat stones, tumors, or narrowed areas of the ducts. Can obtain biopsies with this procedure.
	Endoscopic ultrasound (EUS)	An endoscope is inserted either into the mouth or rectum. Sound waves are sent out the end of the tube and bounce off the organs. Ultrasound pictures are created on the computer that receives these waves. A thin needle can be passed through the endoscope to take a sample or biopsy.
	Esophagogastroduodenoscopy (EGD) (also called an upper endoscopy)	An endoscope is inserted into the mouth and passed through the stomach and duodenum. Biopsies can be taken.
	Flexible sigmoidoscopy	A sigmoidoscope is inserted into the rectum, sigmoid colon, and descending colon. Used to diagnose inflammatory diseases, ulcers, polyps, and cancer.
	Proctoscopy (prok TOS ko pee)	Inspection of the rectum with a proctoscope.
	Upper gastrointestinal (UGI) endoscopy	Fiberoptic view of the esophagus and stomach. Used to diagnose GERD, ulcers, cancer, Barrett esophagus, celiac disease, strictures, and blockages.
Imaging procedure	Abdominal computed tomography (CT) scan	Used to help detect diseases of the digestive system.
	Abdominal Ultrasound (US)	Used to produce a picture of the abdominal organs (e.g., liver, gallbladder, bile ducts, and pancreas). Used to diagnose liver disease, gallstones, pancreatic tumor, abscess, or inflammation.
	Computed tomography (CT) colonography, or virtual colonoscopy	A small tube is inserted into the rectum. The lower colon is inflated with gas. CT images are taken of the colon and rectum.
	Gallbladder radionuclide scan	Nuclear scan of the liver, gallbladder, and bile ducts. Used to diagnose cholecystitis, bile duct obstructions, and liver disorders. Also known as cholescintigraphy, hepatobiliary iminodiacetic acid (HIDA) scan, and hepatobiliary scintigraphy.
	Lower gastrointestinal (LGI) series, or barium enema	X-ray evaluation of large intestine after instillation of a barium sulfate enema. Used to diagnose colorectal cancer or inflammatory disease of the colon. It can also detect polyps, diverticula, or obstructions.
	Upper gastrointestinal (UGI) series (also called a barium swallow)	X-ray evaluation of the esophagus, stomach, and duodenum after the patient drinks barium sulfate. Used to diagnose swallowing issues, esophageal disorders (e.g., varices and strictures), hiatal hernia, ulcers, tumors, and GERD.
Medical laboratory	Comprehensive metabolic panel	Includes glucose, electrolytes, liver function, and kidney function tests. Some CLIA-waived tests are available.
	C-reactive protein (CRP)	The CRP increases with inflammation in the body. May be used as an inflammation marker test for IBD. Some CLIA-waived tests are available.
	Fecal immunochemical test (FIT)	Also called the immunochemical fecal occult blood test (iFOBT). Stool test that detects human hemoglobin from the large intestine.
	Guaiac fecal occult blood test (gFOBT)	A test that detects occult blood in a stool smear; a CLIA-waived test.
	Helicobacter pylori testing	Includes blood test, breath test, and stool tests, all of which can be used to detect H. pylori. Some CLIA-waived tests are available.
	Hepatitis virus panel	Series of blood tests used to detect current or past infection with hepatitis A, B, and C.
	Liver function tests	Also called hepatic function panel and liver panel. Measures proteins, enzymes, and other substances. Examples of tests included in this panel include albumin, total protein, liver enzymes (alanine transaminase [ALT], aspartate transaminase [AST], alkaline phosphatase [ALP], and gamma-glutamyl transpeptidase [GGT]), bilirubin, and prothrombin time. Some CLIA-waived tests available.
	Multitargeted stool DNA test (MT-sDNA)	Stool test that screens for DNA markers (cancer and precancerous cells) and the presence of occult hemoglobin.
	Ova and parasite examination (O&P)	A microscopic exam that looks for parasites and eggs (ova) in a stool specimen.
	Stool culture	Also called fecal culture. A stool exam to test for the presence of pathogenic bacteria in the feces.
	Total bilirubin	A blood test or urine test used to measure the level of bilirubin. Some CLIA-waived tests available.

CLIA, Clinical Laboratory Improvement Amendments; DNA, deoxyribonucleic acid; GERD, gastroesophageal reflux disease; IBD, irritable bowel disease.

TABLE 12.2   Common Treatments Used for Digestive Disorders

Procedure	Description
Appendectomy (ap en DEK tha mee)	Surgical removal of the appendix
Cholecystectomy (koh lee sis TECK tuh mee)	Surgical removal of the gallbladder
Colectomy (koe LEK toe mee)	Surgical removal of the colon
Colostomy (koh LOSS tuh mee)	Surgical redirection of the bowel to a **stoma** (STOH mah)
Gastrectomy (gass TRECK tuh mee)	Surgical removal of part of the stomach *(subtotal gastrectomy)* or all of the stomach *(total gastrectomy)*
Ileostomy (il ee OS tah mee)	The end of the ileum is brought to the surface of the abdomen through a stoma, allowing waste to drain from the body
Hemorrhoidectomy (heh moh roy DECK tuh mee)	Surgical removal of hemorrhoids
Herniorrhaphy (hur nee OR rah fee)	Surgical repair of a hernia
Laparoscopic surgery (lap uh roh SCAH pick)	Surgical procedure using a laparoscope. Several small incisions are made in the abdominal wall
Laryngectomy (LAR ehn JEK tah mee)	Surgical removal of all or part of the larynx (voice box)
Pancreatectomy (PAN kree ah TEK tah mee)	Surgical removal of part or all of the pancreas
Pharyngectomy (far in JEK tah mee)	Surgical removal of all or part of the pharynx (throat)
Proctocolectomy (PROK toe koe LEK to mee)	Surgical removal of the rectum and part or all of the colon
Proctocolectomy with ileal pouch–anal **anastomosis** *(IPAA)* (ah nas tih MOH sis)	Requires multiple surgeries; a proctocolectomy is done, but the anus and anal sphincter muscles remain. A pouch is created with the ileum when it is connected to the anus
Pyloromyotomy (pye lor oh mye AH tuh mee)	Often a laparoscopy surgery done to cut through part of the pyloric muscle of the pyloric valve

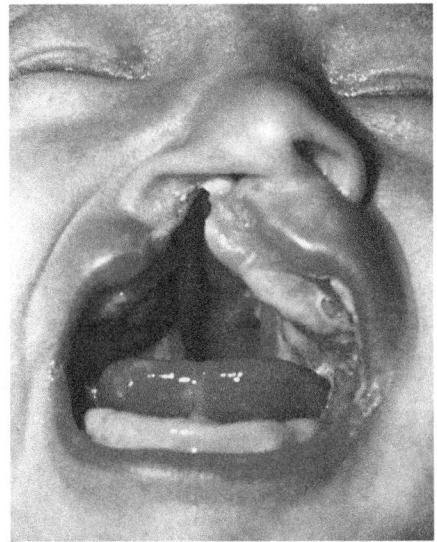

Fig. 12.5 Cleft Lip and Cleft Palate. (Zitelli BJ, Davis HW: *Atlas of pediatric physical diagnosis*, ed 4, St. Louis, 2002, Mosby.)

during pregnancy have an increased risk of having a baby with an orofacial cleft.

Signs and Symptoms. The signs of an orofacial cleft are visible at birth. The child may have a split in the lip or the roof of the mouth. The cleft can affect one or both sides of the face.

Diagnostic Procedures. The provider will identify the cleft right after birth. Sometimes the cleft is detected during a prenatal ultrasound.

Treatments. Treatment involves surgery to improve the child's ability to eat, speak, and hear. A team of specialists is involved with the treatment of the related complications.

Additional Disorders of the Mouth. Additional disorders of the mouth include:
- *Cavities:* Also called *tooth decay* or *dental caries;* plaque on the tooth creates the decay.
- *Gingivitis:* An inflammatory disease of the gums that causes redness, swelling, and bleeding. Part of the early stages of periodontal disease; caused by plaque depositing on the tooth for a short amount of time.
- *Herpetic stomatitis:* Inflammation of the mouth caused by the herpes simplex virus (also known as a *fever blister* or a *cold sore*).
- *Leukoplakia:* A condition of white patches on the lips and buccal mucosa often associated with tobacco use.
- *Periodontal disease:* Infection and inflammation in the mouth that destroys the gums, periodontal ligaments, and bone that support the teeth.
- *Thrush:* A yeast infection of the mouth and tongue. Risk factors include older age, infants, poor health, a compromised immune system (e.g., infection with the human immunodeficiency virus [HIV], acquired immunodeficiency syndrome [AIDS], chemotherapy), and taking antibiotics.

VOCABULARY

anastomosis The surgical connection of separate or severed tubular hollow organs to form a continuous channel.

stoma A temporary or permanent surgically created opening used for drainage (i.e., urine, stool).

plaque Sticky substance made of mucus, food particles, and bacteria that builds up on the exposed part of the tooth.

Disorders of the Esophagus and Stomach

Gastroesophageal Reflux Disease. Gastroesophageal reflux (GER) occurs when the stomach contents back up into the esophagus, causing acid reflux or heartburn. Gastroesophageal

BOX 12.2   Gastroesophageal Reflux Disease (GERD) in Infants

Infants can have gastroesophageal reflux (GER) and GERD. The cause of GER and GERD in infants is an immature (not fully developed) lower esophageal sphincter. The sphincter becomes weak or relaxed, and stomach contents back up into the esophagus.

The main symptom of GERD in infants is spitting up more than normal. Additional symptoms include:

- Arching of the back during or right after feedings
- Colic, coughing, trouble breathing, wheezing, gagging, and projectile or forceful vomiting
- Poor feeding and refusal to feed
- Poor growth and weight gain; malnutrition

Treatment for GERD focuses on feeding changes and medications. Rice cereal may be added to the milk. Holding the baby upright for 30 minutes after feeding and avoiding overfeeding the child may be encouraged. H2 blockers or proton-pump inhibitors may be given to reduce acid production. Surgery may be recommended in severe cases. Most infant GERD resolves by 9 to 18 months of age.

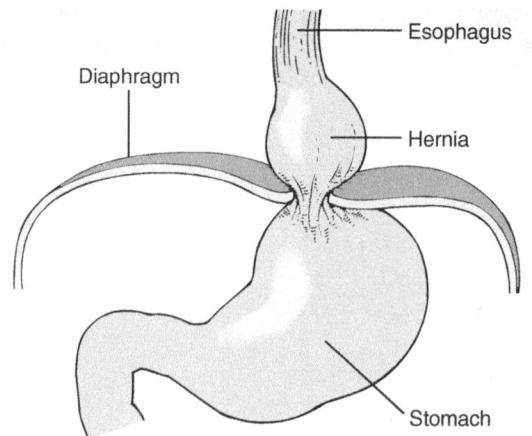

Fig. 12.6 Hiatal Hernia. (Frazier MS, Drzymkowski JW: *Essentials of human diseases and conditions*, ed 4, Philadelphia, 2008, Saunders.)

reflux disease (GERD) is more serious and longer lasting than GER. GERD can occur in adults and infants. The presentation in infants is different from that in adults.

Etiology. The cause of GERD is a weakened or an abnormal lower esophageal sphincter. The sphincter may relax when it should not, causing stomach contents to back up into the esophagus. The risk for GERD and GER in adults increases with pregnancy, being overweight, certain medications, and smoking.

Signs and Symptoms. The most common symptom of GERD in adults is heartburn. Other common GERD symptoms in adults include bad breath, nausea, vomiting, chest pain, upper abdominal pain, respiratory problems, and erosion of the teeth.

Diagnostic Procedures. A provider will do a history and physical examination. Diagnostic procedures include an upper endoscopy, esophageal manometry, ambulatory acid probe test, and an upper digestive system x-ray.

Treatments. Treatment is based on the severity of the symptoms and can include lifestyle changes, medications, or surgery. Usually, patients are encouraged to reduce their intake of the foods and drinks that make the symptoms worse (Box 12.2).

CRITICAL THINKING 12.7

What are the similarities and differences between GERD in adults and infants?

Hiatal Hernia. A hiatal hernia occurs when a section of the upper stomach pushes through an opening of the diaphragm into the chest (Fig. 12.6).

Etiology. The cause is unknown. The risk of hiatal hernias increases with age, obesity, and smoking. Often people over 50 years of age experience this condition.

Signs and Symptoms. The signs and symptoms include chest pain, heartburn, and difficulty swallowing.

Diagnostic Procedures. The provider will order an upper GI (UGI) series (also called a *barium swallow*) and an esophagogastroduodenoscopy (EGD) done to help diagnose the condition.

Treatments. The goal of treatment is to relieve symptoms and prevent complications. Treatment includes medications for acid reflux and surgery to repair the hernia. The person should avoid alcohol and use medications with care.

Peptic Ulcer. Peptic ulcers are also known as duodenal, gastric, and stomach ulcers. A peptic ulcer is a sore or breakdown in the lining of the stomach or duodenum. Gastric ulcers occur in the stomach, and duodenal ulcers occur in the first section of the small intestine.

Etiology. The most common etiology for peptic ulcers is infection of the stomach by *Helicobacter pylori (H. pylori)* bacteria. The risk for peptic ulcers may increase with drinking too much alcohol, regular use of aspirin or nonsteroidal anti-inflammatory drugs (NSAIDs) (e.g., ibuprofen and naproxen), using cigarettes and chewing tobacco, radiation treatments, and stress. Zollinger-Ellison syndrome can also cause peptic ulcers.

Signs and Symptoms. Signs and symptoms include upper abdominal pain at night or when the stomach is empty (1 to 3 hours after a meal). Additional symptoms include nausea, melena, chest pain, fatigue, vomiting and hematemesis, and weight loss.

Diagnostic Procedures. After a physical exam, the provider may order upper GI (UGI) endoscopy or a UGI series to visibly examine the lining of the esophagus, stomach, and duodenum (Fig. 12.7). Testing for *H. pylori* requires a biopsy of the stomach lining or a urea breath test. A stool occult blood test and a hemoglobin test may also be done.

Treatments. Treatment is based on the reasons for the ulcer. If *H. pylori* bacteria are present, the patient may need to take medication, such as antibiotics and an H_2 blocker or a proton-pump inhibitor (PPI) (e.g., omeprazole [Prilosec], lansoprazole [Prevacid], or esomeprazole [Nexium]). Additional ulcer treatment may include a lining protectant, such as sucralfate.

VOCABULARY

Zollinger-Ellison syndrome Rare condition that causes tumors to form in the pancreas or duodenum. Tumors secrete large amounts of gastrin, which causes an increase in acid production.

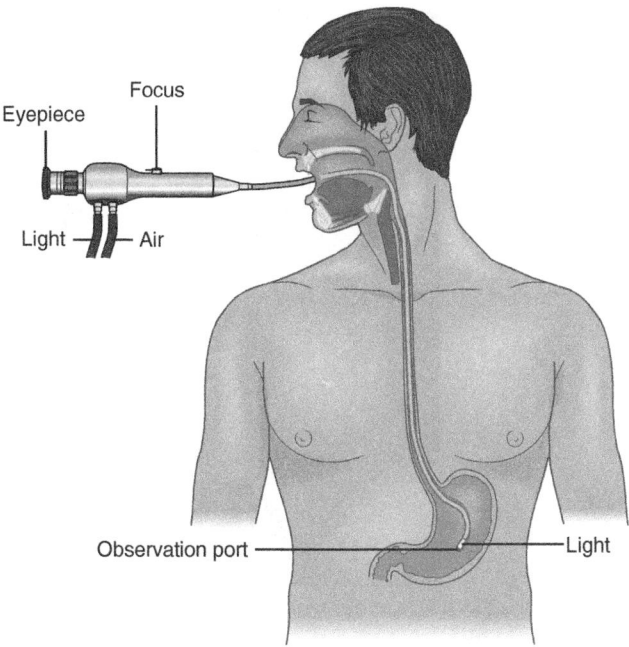

Eyepiece
Focus
Light — Air
Observation port — Light

Fig. 12.7 Upper Gastrointestinal Endoscopy. (From Niedzwiecki B, et al: *Kinn's the medical assistant,* ed 14, St. Louis, 2020, Elsevier.)

Pyloric Stenosis. Pyloric stenosis is the narrowing of the pylorus, the muscular opening between the stomach and the small intestine. It occurs more often in males than females and in infants younger than 6 months.

Etiology. The exact etiology is unknown, but there is a genetic link. Other risk factors include taking certain antibiotics, hyperacidity in the duodenum, and conditions such as type 1 diabetes mellitus.

Signs and Symptoms. Vomiting is the most common sign. It can occur after feedings, may be *projectile* (forceful), and usually starts around 3 weeks of age. Other signs and symptoms include weight loss, constant hunger, dehydration, burping, abdominal pain, and a wavelike motion of the abdomen just before vomiting. Upon physical exam, the provider may feel an olive-sized mass in the upper abdomen.

Diagnostic Procedures. The provider will order an abdominal ultrasound and possibly a UGI series to detect the stenosis, in addition to blood tests to identify electrolyte imbalances.

Treatments. Treatment depends on the severity of the stenosis and may include surgery to widen the pylorus (*pyloromyotomy*). If surgery cannot be done, an endoscope is inserted in the upper GI tract and a balloon is inflated to widen the pylorus. Medications or a feeding tube may also be used to relax the pylorus.

Additional Disorders of the Esophagus and Stomach. The following are additional disorders of the esophagus.

- *Achalasia:* The lower esophageal sphincter does not relax. Also, the esophageal peristalsis is reduced. Both factors delay the emptying of the food from the esophagus.
- *Barrett esophagus:* Caused by GERD; the lining of the esophagus changes to resemble the lining of the intestines; this can lead to a potentially fatal condition called *esophageal adenocarcinoma.*

- *Esophageal atresia:* The esophagus ends in a blind pouch and does not connect to the stomach.
- *Esophageal varices:* Enlarged veins in the esophagus, usually associated with severe liver disease; the veins can leak or rupture, causing life-threatening bleeding.

Additional disorders of the stomach include:

- *Cyclic vomiting syndrome* (CVS): Causes sudden, repeated episodes of severe nausea and vomiting. Vomiting episodes usually occur at the same time each day and last for about the same amount of time.
- *Dumping syndrome:* Rapid gastric emptying; occurs when foods (most commonly carbohydrates) empty too quickly into the duodenum. Can occur after bypass surgery or other types of bariatric surgeries for weight loss.
- *Gastritis:* Inflammation of the stomach lining; caused by bacteria, pain relievers, and alcohol.
- *Gastroparesis:* Stomach motility is slowed, causing delayed gastric emptying. Can be caused by certain medications (e.g., opioids, antidepressants, and antihypertensives).
- *Hypochlorhydria:* Deficiency in the hydrochloric acid in the stomach, which can lead to improper digestion, lack of nutrient absorption, infections, and other health issues.

MEDICAL TERMINOLOGY	
femor/o	femur
hiat/o	an opening
inguin/o	groin
umbilic/o	umbilicus
a-	without
-eal, -ic	pertaining to
-itis	inflammation
-tresia	condition of an opening

Disorders of the Intestines

Acute Appendicitis. Appendicitis is an inflammation of the appendix. Commonly, it occurs between the ages of 10 and 30, though it can occur at any age.

Etiology. The etiology is a blockage in the appendix, which can increase pressure, affect blood flow, and cause inflammation. If the blockage is not treated, the appendix can burst and cause *peritonitis* (inflammation of the peritoneum), a life-threatening condition.

Signs and Symptoms. The pain usually begins near the umbilicus and then moves to the lower right side of the abdomen. Rebound pain can occur with peritonitis. Additional signs and symptoms include low fever, abdominal bloating, anorexia, nausea, vomiting, constipation, diarrhea, and inability to pass gas.

Diagnostic Procedures. After the physical exam, blood and urine laboratory tests will be performed to rule out other conditions. A complete blood count (CBC) will show an elevated white blood cell count. Imaging tests (e.g., x-ray, computed tomography [CT] scan, and abdominal ultrasound [US]) will be done to confirm appendicitis or rule out other conditions.

Treatments. Treatments consist of antibiotics and an appendectomy. Laparoscopic surgery will result in a few small incisions. If a laparotomy is done, the incision may be 2 to 4 inches long. If the appendix bursts and an abscess forms, surgery may be delayed while the abscess is drained.

Celiac Disease. Celiac disease, also called *gluten-sensitive enteropathy* or *celiac sprue,* is a digestive and an autoimmune disorder. When people with this disease eat foods with gluten, their immune system damages their small intestine. Gluten, a protein, is found in barley, rye, wheat, spelt, and triticale. It can also be found in other products, including vitamins and supplements, toothpastes, lip balm, and hair and skin products.

Etiology. Celiac disease is a genetic, autoimmune disorder.

Signs and Symptoms. The signs and symptoms of celiac disease can vary, depending on the age of the person. For example:

- Young children: Abdominal pain, vomiting, diarrhea, bloating, and constipation; irritability, emotional withdrawal, or very dependent behavior; failure to gain weight and grow; and obesity
- Teenagers: Diarrhea, constipation, delayed puberty, hair loss, slowed growth, and short height
- Adults: Diarrhea, constipation, fatigue, bone or joint pain, depression, anxiety, irritability, missed menstrual periods, anemia, and osteoporosis

Celiac disease can also cause lactose intolerance, anemia, dermatitis herpetiformis (an itchy, blistering skin condition), and canker sores in the mouth.

Diagnostic Procedures. The provider will perform a history and physical exam. Blood tests and an intestinal biopsy may be ordered.

Treatments. Treatment consists of a gluten-free diet. Foods that are safe to eat include rice, oats, corn, quinoa, millet, and buckwheat.

Diverticulitis. *Diverticula* are small marble-sized pouches that form in the large intestine (Fig. 12.8). The pouches protrude through the weakened walls of the large intestine. These pouches are common after age 40 and usually do not cause symptoms unless they become inflamed or infected. When the diverticula become inflamed or infected, the condition is called *diverticulitis.*

Etiology. When a diverticulum tears, inflammation and infection can occur. Risk factors include aging, obesity, smoking cigarettes, lack of exercise, low-fiber diet, and a high saturated fat diet. Medications such as steroids, opioids, and NSAIDs can also increase the risk.

Signs and Symptoms. Signs and symptoms of diverticulitis include constant lower left abdomen pain and tenderness, nausea, vomiting, diarrhea, constipation, and fever.

Diagnostic Procedures. After a physical exam, the provider will order imaging and medical laboratory tests. Blood and urine tests are used to rule out infection, pregnancy, and liver disease. A CT scan can identify the inflamed pouches, thus confirming the diagnosis.

Treatments. Treatment depends on the symptoms. Antibiotics, over-the-counter (OTC) analgesics, and a liquid

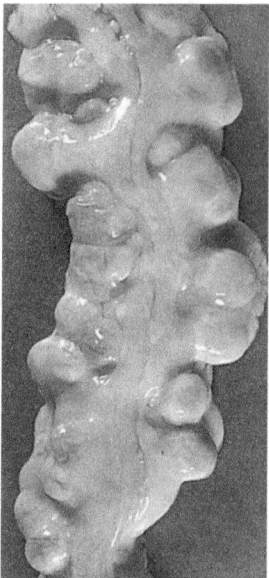

Fig. 12.8 Diverticulitis. (From Damjanov I: *Pathology: a color atlas,* St. Louis, 2000, Mosby.)

diet may be recommended. With severe attacks, intravenous (IV) antibiotics are given and drainage of abscesses, if present, is done. A primary bowel resection or a bowel resection with a colostomy (koh LOS tuh mee) may be done.

VOCABULARY

colostomy A surgical procedure in which the large intestine is brought though the abdominal wall, creating either a temporary or a permanent opening (stoma) to allow stool to pass out of the body.
rebound pain Pain felt when the pressure on the abdomen is released.
resection Surgical removal of all or part of an organ.

Food-Borne Illnesses. Eating or drinking contaminated food can result in a food-borne illness. Typically, food-borne disorders are acute illnesses, which occur suddenly and last for a short time. Most people recover without treatments, though sometimes more serious complications can occur.

Etiology. Many different types of bacteria, viruses, parasites, and chemicals can contaminate food, including:

- *Salmonella:* Found in raw or undercooked meat, poultry, and seafoods. It can also be found in dairy products, eggshells, and inside eggs.
- *Shigella:* Bacterium that spreads to others from one infected person who does not wash their hands after using the bathroom.
- *Escherichia coli (E. coli):* Found in raw or undercooked hamburger, unpasteurized milk and fruit juices, and fresh produce.
- *Listeria monocytogenes:* Found in raw and undercooked meats, unpasteurized milk, deli meats, soft cheeses, and hot dogs.

- *Clostridium botulinum:* Found in improperly canned foods and smoked and salted fish.
- *Norovirus:* Found in foods prepared by infectious food handlers. Can cause inflammation of the intestines and stomach.
- *Hepatitis A:* A virus spread through food or drinks contaminated with a small amount of stool from an infected person.
- *Trichinella spiralis:* A roundworm parasite found in raw or undercooked pork or wild game.

Signs and Symptoms. Common signs and symptoms include vomiting, diarrhea, abdominal pain, chills, and fever. Symptoms may last for a few hours to a few days. Complications can lead to dehydration, hemolytic uremic syndrome, and other disorders, such as reactive arthritis and irritable bowel syndrome.

Diagnostic Procedures. After a physical exam, the provider may order a stool culture and blood work.

Treatments. Treatment consists of replacing lost fluids and electrolytes. Over-the-counter antidiarrheal medications such as loperamide (Imodium) and bismuth subsalicylate (Pepto-Bismol, Kaopectate) can help decrease diarrhea in adults. These medications should not be used if the person has bloody diarrhea, which could be a sign of a parasitic or bacterial infection.

Hemorrhoids. Hemorrhoids are swollen and inflamed veins. External hemorrhoids are located around the anus, and internal hemorrhoids affect the lining of the anus and the lower rectum. About 50% of those over 50 years of age have hemorrhoids.

Etiology. Hemorrhoids can be caused by straining during a bowel movement and by pregnancy, aging, chronic constipation, and diarrhea.

Signs and Symptoms. The most common symptom of internal hemorrhoids is bright red bleeding, which usually goes away within a few days. Anal itching can occur with external hemorrhoids.

Diagnostic Procedures. During the physical exam, the provider will check the anal area and perform a digital rectal exam. An anoscope, a proctoscope, or a sigmoidoscope may be used to examine the lower part of the large intestine and rectum.

Treatments. Home treatment includes a high-fiber diet, topical treatments (e.g., hydrocortisone, analgesic), sitz baths (soaking in a warm bath), cold packs, oral analgesics, and keeping the area clean.

Inguinal Hernia. An inguinal hernia occurs when tissue (e.g., part of the intestine) protrudes through a weak spot in the abdominal muscles (Fig. 12.9 and Box 12.3). Sometimes people can gently push the hernia back into the abdomen, but other times the hernia may become trapped (incarcerated), and blood flow may be cut off to the tissue (strangulation), causing tissue death. This can be a life-threatening complication if it is not treated.

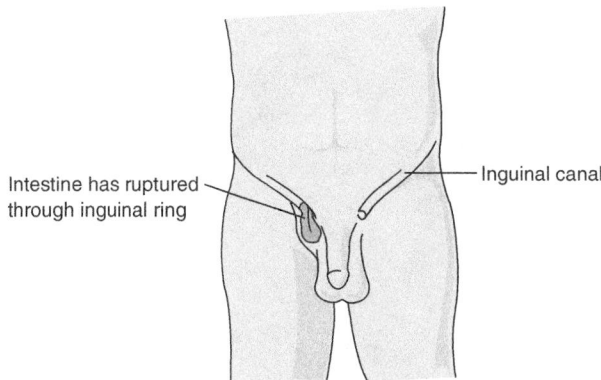

Fig. 12.9 Inguinal Hernia. (From Niedzwiecki B, et al: *Kinn's the medical assistant,* ed 14, St. Louis, 2020, Elsevier.)

BOX 12.3 Hernia

A hernia is a common disorder that occurs when part of an internal organ (e.g., intestine) bulges through a weak area in the muscles. The hiatal hernia was already discussed in a prior section. Other types include:

- *Femoral hernia:* A bulge below the groin, in the upper thigh. More common in women.
- *Inguinal hernia:* Most common type of hernia. A bulge forms in the groin and may extend into the scrotum.
- *Umbilical hernia:* The muscle around the umbilicus does not close at birth and a bulge forms.

VOCABULARY

hemolytic uremic syndrome Kidney disorder that can occur after a digestive infection with Escherichia coli, shigella, or salmonella; red blood cells are destroyed and block the kidneys' filtering system, causing acute kidney failure.

incarcerated Confined or trapped.

strangulation Constriction of a tubular structure, such as an intestine or vessel, leading to a lack of blood supply to the tissues.

Etiology. For some inguinal hernias, the etiology is unknown. Other times straining, strenuous activities, pregnancy, or chronic coughing may cause it.

Signs and Symptoms. Signs and symptoms include bulging on the side of the pubic bone, burning or aching at the bulge, and groin heaviness, pain, or pressure.

Diagnostic Procedures. The provider will do a physical examination. The patient may be asked to stand and cough, which makes the inguinal hernia more prominent. A CT or magnetic resonance imaging (MRI) scan may be ordered if the hernia is not felt.

Treatments. For a small hernia that is asymptomatic, the provider may just wait and monitor it. Painful or enlarged hernias are treated with surgery (either an open hernia repair or a laparoscopic repair).

Inflammatory Bowel Disease. Inflammatory bowel disease (IBD), an autoimmune disorder, includes two chronic conditions that cause inflammation of the digestive tract:

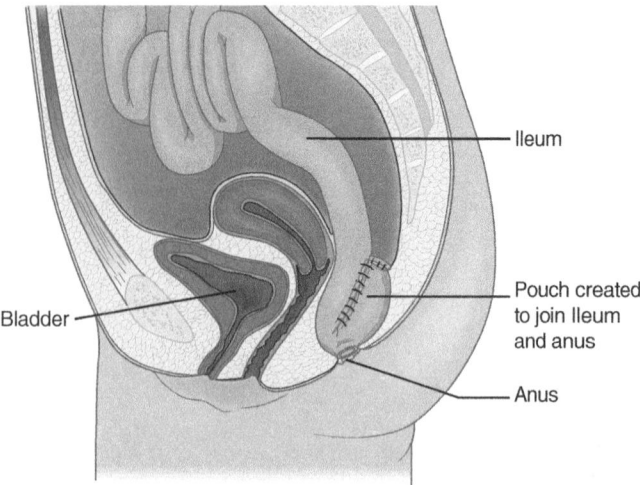

Fig. 12.10 **Ileal Pouch–Anal Anastomosis (IPAA).** (From Niedzwiecki B, et al: *Kinn's the medical assistant,* ed 14, St. Louis, 2020, Elsevier.)

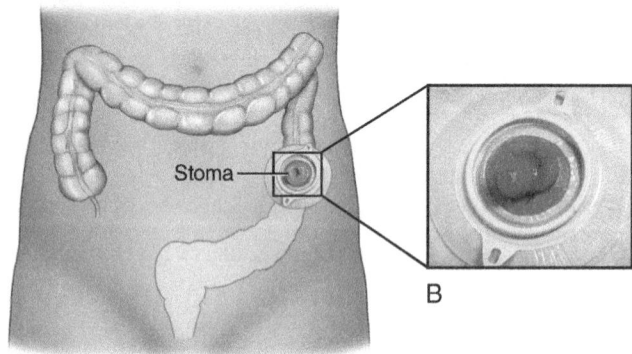

Fig. 12.11 A, Colostomy. B, Inset shows the stoma. (Potter PA, Perry AG: *Fundamentals of nursing,* ed 7, St. Louis, 2011, Mosby.)

- *Ulcerative colitis:* Usually starts in the rectum and spreads into the large intestine. Damaged areas are in patches along the intestine. The inflammation may affect many layers of the GI tract wall.
- *Crohn disease:* Can affect any part of the GI tract, but most often affects the ileum. Damage appears in patches next to healthy tissue. The inflammation affects several layers of the GI tract walls.

Etiology. The etiology of IBD is unknown, but it is the result of a defective immune system. IBD has a genetic component, and environmental triggers cause inflammation of the digestive tract.

Signs and Symptoms. Common signs and symptoms of IBD include persistent diarrhea, abdominal pain, blood in the stool, weight loss, and fatigue.

Diagnostic Procedures. After the medical history and physical exam, the provider will order imaging tests and endoscopy exams. Stool samples are tested to rule out other conditions.

Treatments. Treatment consists of corticosteroids, immuno-modulators, and biologics. Severe IBD may require surgery to remove the damaged GI tract. Common surgical procedures include colectomy, proctocolectomy, proctocolectomy with ileal

pouch–anal anastomosis (IPAA), and ileostomy (Figs. 12.10 and 12.11).

Intestinal Obstructions. Intestinal obstructions are also called *bowel obstructions.* The obstruction can be either partial or complete and prevents stool or food from moving through the intestine. A complete intestinal obstruction is a medical emergency.

Etiology. The obstruction can be related to a mechanical cause, such as adhesions, hernias, volvulus, impacted feces, and cancers. A non-mechanical obstruction, also called *ileus* or *paralytic ileus,* occurs because peristalsis stops. A paralytic ileus can be caused from infections, certain medications (e.g., narcotics), electrolyte imbalance, decrease intestinal blood flow, or abdominal surgery.

Signs and Symptoms. Signs and symptoms include severe abdominal pain, cramping, bloating, nausea, vomiting, swelling of the abdomen, loud bowel sounds, inability to pass flatus (gas), and constipation.

Diagnostic Procedures. Tests to diagnose an intestinal obstruction can include an abdominal CT scan, an abdominal x-ray, an LGI series, and a UGI series.

Treatments. Treatment includes hospitalization and a *nasogastric tube* (a tube passed from the nose to the stomach), which is used to relieve abdominal contents and swelling. A bowel resection surgery may be required if the obstruction continues. A temporary or permanent colostomy may be done (see Fig. 12.11A).

Irritable Bowel Syndrome. Irritable bowel syndrome (IBS) is a disorder of the large intestine, though it does not cause harm to the colon. IBS is a common disorder, affecting females twice as often as males. People younger than age 45 often have IBS.

Etiology. There is no known cause of IBS. Factors that may lead to IBs include changes in peristalsis, severe infection, early life stress, and changes in the intestinal microbes. Stress can increase the symptoms of IBS.

Signs and Symptoms. The signs and symptoms include abdominal cramping, bloating, constipation, and diarrhea. Sometimes people go back and forth between diarrhea and constipation.

Diagnostic Procedures. There is no specific test for IBS. The provider may do a colonoscopy, an upper endoscopy, x-ray, and/or CT scan to rule out other diseases.

Treatments. Treatment for IBS includes dietary changes, stress management, medications, and probiotics.

Additional Disorders of the Intestines. The following list presents additional intestinal disorders.

- *Anal fissure:* A small tear in the anal mucosa that causes pain.
- *Anorectal abscess:* A collection of pus in the anal and rectal area, caused from a blocked gland, an anal fissure, trauma, or a sexually transmitted infection (STI). Deep rectal abscesses can be caused by intestinal disorders such as Crohn disease.

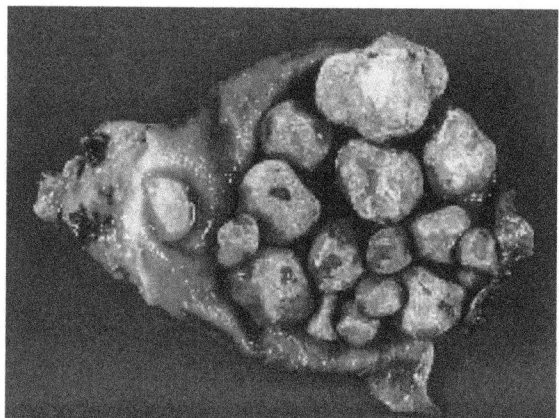

Fig. 12.12 Cholelithiasis (gallstones). (From Damjanov I: *Pathology: a color atlas*, St. Louis, 2000, Mosby.)

- *Bowel incontinence:* Accidental passage of a stool; also called *accidental bowel leakage.*
- *Fistula:* An abnormal connection between body parts, commonly developing between different organs, such as the bowel and vagina. Can be caused by injuries, infections, complications from surgery, and diseases such as Crohn disease and ulcerative colitis.
- *Gastroenteritis:* Inflammation of the intestinal lining; caused by a virus, bacteria, or parasites. Viral gastroenteritis is a very common illness.
- *Hirschsprung disease:* Congenital disorder caused by malformed intestinal nerves; also called congenital megacolon. Leads to severe constipation and intestinal obstructions.
- *Intestinal ischemia* and *infarction:* Occur when there is a partial or complete blockage in the arteries supplying the intestines. Can cause damage or death to the intestinal tissues.
- *Intestinal volvulus:* Occurs when the intestine twists around itself and the supporting mesentery, leading to an obstruction.
- *Intussusception:* Occurs when part of the intestine slides onto another portion of the intestine. It can cause an intestinal blockage. The blood supply may be constricted, leading to intestinal tissue death.
- *Small intestinal bacterial overgrowth* (SBO): Caused when a large number of bacteria grow in the small intestine, which may use up important nutrients needed by the body, leading to malnourishment.

Disorders of the Accessory Organs

Cholelithiasis. Cholelithiasis (or gallstones) occur when the substances in the bile harden and form stones (Fig. 12.12). The stones can be small, like a piece of rice, or large, like a walnut. Cholesterol gallstones are the most common type and usually contain undissolved cholesterol. Pigment gallstones are darker black and occur when the bile contains too much bilirubin.

Etiology. It is unclear why gallstones form, but it may be related to the bile containing too much cholesterol or bilirubin. They may also form if the gallbladder does not empty completely, causing the bile to become concentrated. Females, Native Americans, Mexican Americans, and people over age 40 are at higher risk for gallstones. Additional risk factors include:

- Eating a high-fat, high-cholesterol, or low-fiber diet

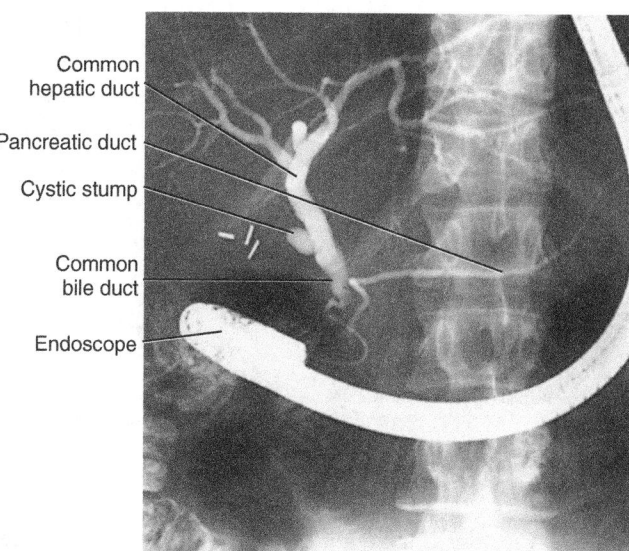

Fig. 12.13 Endoscopic Retrograde Cholangiopancreatography (ERCP). (From Frank ED, Long BW, Smith BJ: Merrill's *atlas of radiographic positions and radiologic procedures*, ed 12, St. Louis, 2012, Mosby.)

- Being overweight or obese; losing weight very quickly
- Having diabetes, leukemia, sickle cell anemia, or liver disease
- Having a family history of gallstones
- Taking estrogen-containing medication

Signs and Symptoms. If signs and symptoms are present, they may include nausea, vomiting, and referred pain. The person may have pain in the upper back, right shoulder, upper right abdomen, or below the sternum. Many of these symptoms are similar to a heart attack, thus they can be scary for the patient.

Diagnostic Procedures. After a physical exam, a gallbladder radionuclide scan, MRI, or endoscopic retrograde cholangiopancreatography (ERCP) may be done.

Treatments. Treatment is based on the intensity of the symptoms. A cholecystectomy may be done. Gallstones can be removed during the ERCP (Fig. 12.13). Patients who cannot undergo surgery may take medications to dissolve the gallstone, though it may take months or years to work.

VOCABULARY

referred pain Pain that is felt at a site in the body at a distance from the cause (e.g., the injury or diseased part).

CRITICAL THINKING 12.8

Keith is rooming a female patient who works as an office assistant. She has had upper back and right shoulder pain, nausea, and vomiting for 2 days. The patient states that she has lost 50 pounds in the past 3 months. She is on oral contraceptives and acetaminophen for pain as needed. After examining her, Dr. Martin wants her to have an MRI for possible gallstones. What risk factors does this patient have for gallstones? What signs and symptoms does she have that are related to gallstones?

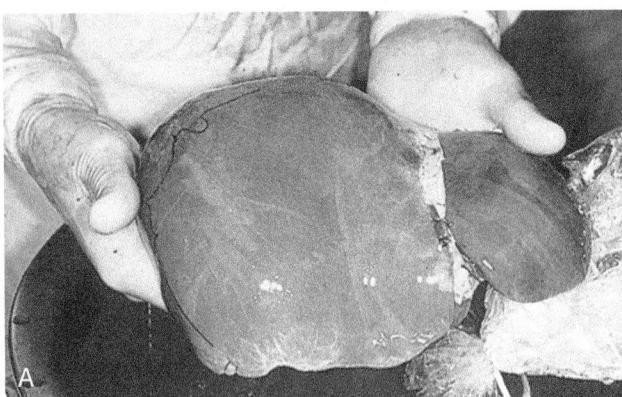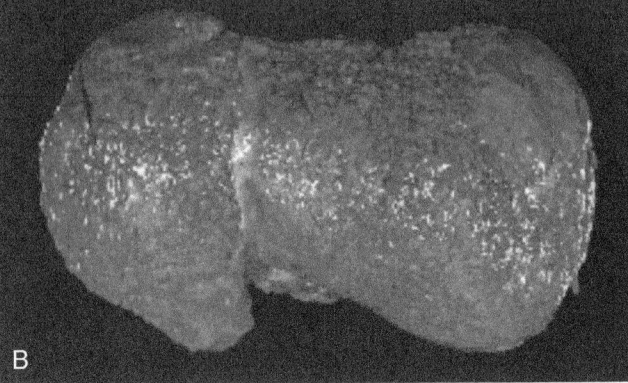

Fig. 12.14 A, Normal liver. B, Cirrhosis of the liver. (**A** from Mahan LK, Escott-Stump S: *Krause's food and nutrition therapy*, ed 12, Philadelphia, 2008, Saunders/Elsevier. **B** from Damjanov I: *Pathology: a color atlas*, St. Louis, 2000, Mosby.)

Cirrhosis. Cirrhosis is a chronic liver disease. The liver cells are damaged and are replaced with scar tissue (Fig. 12.14). The scar tissue reduces the liver's ability to function, and over time the liver fails.

Etiology. Diseases such as alcoholic liver disease, nonalcoholic fatty liver disease, and chronic hepatitis B and C cause cirrhosis.

Signs and Symptoms. The signs and symptoms of cirrhosis may not appear until the liver is significantly damaged. Cirrhosis can cause nosebleeds, abdominal swelling, hypertension, kidney failure, jaundice, severe itching, gallstones, varices in the stomach and esophagus, and increased sensitivity to medications. Cirrhosis, like other liver diseases, can cause ascites, a buildup of fluid in the space between the organs and the abdominal lining.

Diagnostic Procedures. Besides a medical history and physical exam, liver function tests, imaging tests, and a liver biopsy may be done.

Treatments. There is no cure for cirrhosis. Treatment of the underlying disease causing the cirrhosis can help to slow liver destruction.

Hepatitis. Hepatitis is an inflammation of the liver. It can affect the functioning of the liver. Depending on the type, hepatitis can be an acute and/or chronic infection. There are different types of hepatitis including alcoholic, toxic, autoimmune, and viral. With viral hepatitis, there are five main types: A, B, C, D, and E. In the United States, hepatitis A, B, and C are the most common. Vaccines to prevent hepatitis A and B are available.

Etiology. Hepatitis is caused by alcohol use, toxins, certain medications and conditions, and viruses.

- *Alcoholic hepatitis*: Caused by heavy alcohol use.
- *Toxic hepatitis*: Caused from certain chemicals, medications, supplements, or poisons.
- *Autoimmune hepatitis*: A chronic type of hepatitis caused by the body's immune system attacking the liver.
- *Viral hepatitis*: Hepatitis A virus (HAV) and hepatitis E virus (HEV) are spread from ingestion of food or drink contaminated by infected fecal matter. Hepatitis B virus (HBV), hepatitis C virus (HCV), and hepatitis D virus (HDV) are spread through contact with blood, semen, and other body fluids from an infected person. These viruses can also be passed from an infected mother to her baby during birth.

Signs and Symptoms. The signs and symptoms include fatigue, nausea, vomiting, anorexia, abdominal pain, clay-colored stools, dark urine, low-grade fever, joint pain, jaundice, and intense itching.

Diagnostic Procedures. Besides a medical history and physical exam, the provider will order blood tests to diagnose hepatitis. Imaging tests may also be ordered. Screening for hepatitis C is recommended for adults ages 18 to 79.

Treatments. Treatment depends on the type of hepatitis. Chronic hepatitis may cause liver failure or liver cancer, and a liver transplant may be needed. Treatment for hepatitis A and E include bed rest and fluids. Supportive care is given with hepatitis D. Hepatitis B and C are treated with rest, interferon, and antiviral medications. Antiviral medications for hepatitis B include adefovir (a DEF o veer), entecavir (en TE ka veer), lamivudine (la MI vyoo deen), telbivudine (tel BIV ue deen), and tenofovir (te NOE fo veer).

CRITICAL THINKING 12.9

Summarize how hepatitis A, B, C, D, and E are transmitted. What prevention strategies can be taken to prevent the transmission of each type?

Jaundice in the Newborn. Jaundice in newborns can be life-threatening. Jaundice is a condition caused by high levels of bilirubin in the blood. Bilirubin is a yellow to orange pigment that results when heme (from red blood cells) is broken down.

Etiology. The cause of jaundice in newborns is *hyperbilirubinemia* (excess bilirubin). During the first days of life, red blood cells are produced and broken down at a faster rate compared to adults. In infants the bilirubin can build up in the blood because the liver is not mature enough to get rid of it. Additional disorders that may cause jaundice in newborns include hemorrhage, infection, incompatibility between the mother's blood and the baby's blood, liver malfunction, red blood cell abnormality, and an enzyme deficiency. The risk for jaundice also increases with premature birth, significant bruising during birth, and breastfeeding.

Signs and Symptoms. Signs and symptoms of jaundice include yellowish coloring to the skin and sclera, listlessness, poor feeding and weight gain, and high-pitched cries.

High levels of bilirubin can lead to severe complications in newborns. Acute bilirubin encephalopathy occurs when the bilirubin passes into the baby's brain. Signs and symptoms include listlessness, difficulty waking, high-pitched crying, fever, backward arching of the neck and back, poor sucking, and poor feeding. *Kernicterus* occurs if the acute encephalopathy causes permanent brain damage. Signs of kernicterus include involuntary and uncontrolled movements, a permanent upward gaze, and hearing loss.

Diagnostic Procedures. The provider will do a physical exam and then order a blood test to measure the bilirubin level.

Treatments. Treatment may consist of these measures:

- *Phototherapy:* The infant is placed under a lamp that emits blue-green spectrum light, which changes the structure of the bilirubin molecule. The change allows the bilirubin to be excreted in the urine and stool. Light therapy can also be done using a light-emitting mattress or pad. The baby wears only a diaper and protective eye patches.
- *Intravenous immunoglobulin* (IVIg): Used for blood incompatibility–related jaundice. The immunoglobulin reduces the levels of antibodies and may reduce the jaundice.
- *Exchange transfusion of blood:* Used for severe jaundice.

Nonalcoholic Fatty Liver Disease. Nonalcoholic fatty liver disease (NAFLD) causes a buildup of fat in the liver, unrelated to drinking alcohol.

Etiology. The cause of NAFLD is unclear. The risks for NAFLD include obesity, prediabetes, type 2 diabetes, high cholesterol and triglycerides, and high blood pressure. Additional risks include rapid weight loss, gastric bypass surgery, bowel disease, and medications (e.g., calcium channel blockers and some chemotherapy drugs).

Signs and Symptoms. A person with NAFLD may experience fatigue and upper right abdominal pain. If the person has liver damage, then weakness, loss of appetite, nausea, jaundice, itching, leg and abdominal swelling, GI bleeding, and mental confusion may be experienced.

Diagnostic Procedures. Often NAFLD is found during routine blood tests. The provider may order additional laboratory tests, including a CBC, prothrombin time, and blood albumin level. US, MRI, a CT scan, and a liver biopsy may also be done.

Treatments. Treatment is focused on healthy choices, including losing weight, healthy eating, being physically active, and not drinking alcohol.

Pancreatitis. Pancreatitis is an inflammation of the pancreas. The digestive enzymes start to break down the pancreas. If treated, acute pancreatitis may last a few days, but chronic pancreatitis gets worse over time and permanent damage occurs.

Etiology. Gallstones commonly cause acute pancreatitis, and patients may have severe upper abdominal pain radiating to the back, a rapid pulse, nausea, and vomiting. Heavy alcohol use, cystic fibrosis, some inherited and autoimmune diseases, and certain medications can lead to chronic pancreatitis.

Signs and Symptoms. Signs and symptoms of chronic pancreatitis include nausea, vomiting, weight loss, and oily stools.

Diagnostic Procedures. Besides a medical history and physical exam, lab and imaging tests are used to diagnose pancreatitis.

Treatments. Treatment includes hospitalization, IV fluids, analgesics, antibiotics, and nutritional support (e.g., low-fat diet, enteral feeding).

Additional Disorders of the Accessory Organs. The following conditions are related to the accessory organs.

- *Acute cholecystitis:* A sudden inflammation and swelling of the gallbladder, which causes severe abdominal pain. Can be caused when a gallstone blocks the cystic duct, causing irritation and pressure in the gallbladder.
- *Mumps:* Caused by a viral infection, which leads to painful swelling of the salivary glands.
- *Primary biliary cirrhosis:* Chronic liver disease causing the bile ducts to be inflamed and damaged, leading to the buildup of bile in the liver.
- *Hemochromatosis:* Causes too much iron to build up in the body, especially in the liver, heart, and pancreas, which damages the organs and causes a bronze or gray skin color.
- *Sialoliths:* The buildup of crystallized saliva deposits blocks the flow of saliva, causing pain and swelling; also called *salivary stones*.
- *Sialadenitis:* A bacterial infection of a salivary gland, usually related to blockage of the duct. Can cause a painful lump in the gland, severe pain, high fever, and a foul-tasting pus in the mouth.

MEDICAL TERMINOLOGY	
cirrh/o	orange-yellow
lith/o	stones
-iasis	presence of
-osis	abnormal condition

Cancers of the Gastrointestinal System

Oral Cavity, Pharyngeal, and Laryngeal Cancers. Oral cavity, pharyngeal, and laryngeal cancers can form in any of the tissues in the mouth and throat. Males are more likely than females to have oral cavity or pharyngeal cancer.

Etiology. Using alcohol and tobacco products (e.g., cigarettes, betel quid, and gutka) can increase the risk of these cancers. A personal history of oral or throat cancer, human papillomavirus (HPV) infection, or Epstein-Barr virus can also increase the risk.

Signs and Symptoms. The signs and symptoms depend on the type of cancer:

- *Oral cancer:* White or red patches, bleeding, or a continuous sore in the mouth, loose teeth, pain with swallowing, earache, and lump in the neck
- *Throat cancer* (pharyngeal and laryngeal cancers): Continuous sore throat, lump in the neck, ear pain, ringing in the ear, and problems swallowing

Diagnostic Procedures. Besides a history and physical exam, the provider may order a biopsy of the mouth lesion. A UGI

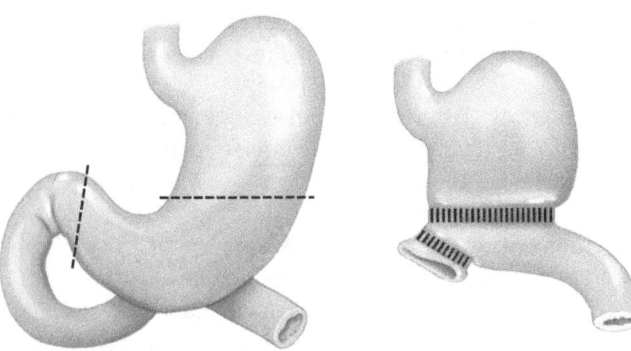

Fig. 12.15 Anastomosis. Part of the stomach has been cut out, and the duodenum has been anastomosed to the remaining stomach. (From Frank ED, Long BW, Smith BJ: *Merrill's atlas of radiographic positions and radiologic procedures,* ed 12, St. Louis, 2012, Mosby.)

endoscopy and imaging tests, such as CT scans, are used for throat cancer.

Treatments. Treatment consists of:
- Surgical removal of the tumor, a laryngectomy, or a pharyngectomy
- *Targeted therapy,* which uses medications that attack only the cancer cells
- Radiation therapy and chemotherapy

Stomach Cancer. About 65% of stomach cancer cases occur in adults over age 65. Diagnosing stomach cancer in its early stages can be difficult because the symptoms (e.g., indigestion and stomach discomfort) can be caused by many other conditions.

Etiology. Males have a greater risk of stomach cancer. A personal history of *H. pylori* infection or stomach inflammation is also a risk factor, along with a family history of stomach cancer. The risk of stomach cancer increases with cigarette smoking and often consuming smoked, pickled, or salted foods.

Signs and Symptoms. Besides indigestion and stomach discomfort, other signs and symptoms include bloody stools, vomiting, weight loss, jaundice, and difficulty swallowing.

Diagnostic Procedures. Besides a history and physical exam, the provider will order UGI endoscopy and imaging tests (e.g., CT scan and UGI series).

Treatments. Treatment consists of:
- Surgical removal of the tumor, subtotal gastrectomy (with an anastomosis), or a total gastrectomy (Fig. 12.15)
- Radiation therapy, chemotherapy, and targeted drug therapies

Pancreatic Cancer. Pancreatic cancer is difficult to diagnose in its early stages because the symptoms are vague and may go unnoticed. This type of cancer spreads quickly, and because the condition usually is diagnosed in the later stages of the disease, it can be difficult to treat.

Etiology. Risk factors for pancreatic cancer include smoking, long-term diabetes mellitus, chronic pancreatitis, and certain hereditary disorders.

Signs and Symptoms. Signs and symptoms include jaundice, abdominal and back pain, weight loss, and fatigue.

Diagnostic Procedures. Besides a history and physical exam, the provider will order an endoscopic ultrasound and imaging tests (e.g., CT scan, MRI, positron emission tomography [PET]). Blood tests and biopsies may also be done.

Treatments. Treatment consists of:
- Surgical removal of the tumor; part or total pancreatectomy
- Radiation therapy and chemotherapy

Liver Cancer. Liver cancer can either be *primary* (the initial site) or *metastatic* (spread to the liver from the initial site elsewhere in the body). Primary liver cancer may be difficult to treat if it is diagnosed in an advanced stage.

Etiology. Risk factors for primary liver cancer include a personal history of hepatitis B or C, cirrhosis, obesity, diabetes, hemochromatosis, and heavy alcohol use.

Signs and Symptoms. Signs and symptoms include jaundice, right abdominal pain, and a lump in the right abdomen. The symptoms may not appear until the cancer is in an advanced stage.

Diagnostic Procedures. Besides a history and physical exam, the provider will order blood tests, imaging tests (e.g., CT scan, MRI, and US), and biopsy.

Treatments. Treatment consists of:
- Surgical removal of the tumor or liver transplantation
- Localized treatments, including heating or freezing cancer cells, injecting alcohol or chemotherapy into the tumor, or placing radiation beads into the liver
- Radiation therapy, chemotherapy, targeted drug therapies, and immunotherapy

Small Intestinal Cancer. Small intestinal or small bowel cancer can also be called *duodenal, ileal,* and *jejunal cancer.* Adenocarcinoma is the most common form of small intestine cancer.

Etiology. Risk factors for small intestine cancer include eating a high-fat diet or having a personal history of Crohn disease, colonic polyps, or celiac disease.

Signs and Symptoms. Signs and symptoms include abdominal pain, weight loss, bloody stools, and a lump in the abdomen.

Diagnostic Procedures. Besides a history and physical exam, the provider will order blood tests, imaging tests (e.g., CT scan, MRI, PET, LGI series, and US), and endoscopic procedures (e.g., upper endoscopy and capsule endoscopy).

Treatments. Treatment consists of surgery, chemotherapy, targeted drug therapies, and immunotherapy.

VOCABULARY

polyp A growth or mass protruding from a mucous membrane (e.g., nose, bladder, intestine).

Colorectal Cancer. Colorectal cancer is also called *colon cancer* and *rectal cancer.* It affects both males and females. Screening is recommended to start at age 45 for those with an average risk.

Etiology. Risk factors for colorectal cancer include being over 50 years of age, smoking tobacco, and eating a high-fat diet. A family history of colorectal cancer, ulcerative colitis, or Crohn disease also increases the risk.

Signs and Symptoms. A person with colorectal cancer may experience diarrhea, constipation, bloody stools, cramps, bloating, flatus (gas), nausea, vomiting, fatigue, or weight loss.

Diagnostic Procedures. Besides a history and physical exam, the provider will order colonoscopy and biopsy. A carcinoembryonic antigen (CEA) blood test may also be done. CEA is sometimes produced by colon cancers.

Treatments. Treatment consists of:
- Surgical removal of the tumor or polyp (*polypectomy*) or colectomy
- Radiation therapy, chemotherapy, targeted drug therapies, and immunotherapy

LIFE SPAN CHANGES

At birth, the baby's digestive system is not fully mature. The infant does not have teeth to help break down food. Salivary secretions (which start starch breakdown) are insufficient until about 6 months of age. Pancreatic amylase levels may not be sufficient until 12 to 18 months of age. Bile salts and lipase levels are not sufficient until 6 to 9 months of age.

During pregnancy, progesterone (a hormone) causes the smooth muscles to relax. This causes less peristalsis in the digestive system, thus slowing digestion. Gallbladder emptying may be delayed, leading to gallstone formation. Morning sickness, constipation, and heartburn can result from digestive system changes.

With age, the stomach cannot accommodate as much food because of decreased elasticity. The stomach empties more slowly. The lactase levels decrease with age, leading to lactose intolerance (milk products). Bacterial overgrowth (excessive growth of certain intestinal bacteria) is more common with age and leads to bloating, weight loss, and pain. Bacterial overgrowth can also lead to reduced absorption of certain nutrients (e.g., iron, calcium, and vitamin B_{12}). With aging, constipation is more common and can be caused by many factors, including:

- Slowing of fecal contents through the large intestine, allowing for more water absorption
- Increased use of drugs that can cause constipation
- Decreased physical activity and fluid intake

Age-related changes can be seen with the accessory organs. A decrease of salivary flow is not related to age, although it is common in older adults. It is related to diseases, medications, and head and neck radiation therapy (used for cancers). The pancreas decreases in weight as some tissue is replaced with scar tissue, although these changes do not affect the organ's ability to produce digestive enzymes and sodium bicarbonate. With age, the liver gets smaller and blood flow decreases. Liver function test results, however, are unchanged. Metabolism of many substances decreases, which affects drug metabolism; thus older adults may experience dose-related side effects. The production and flow of bile decreases with age, leading to more gallstones.

BOX 12.4 Medication Classifications

- *Antacids:* Used to treat gastric hyperacidity
- *Antidiarrheal:* Used to treat diarrhea
- *Antiemetics:* Used to prevent and relieve nausea, vomiting, and motion sickness
- *Laxatives:* Used to increase and hasten bowel evacuation
- *Proton-pump inhibitors:* Used to treat gastroesophageal reflux disease (GERD) and ulcers

Refer to Appendix D, which can be found on the Evolve website, for information on the medication classifications, including indications for use, desired effect, side effects, adverse reactions, and generic and trade names. Medical assistants should be familiar with medications that are prescribed to patients.

CLOSING COMMENTS

The digestive system is an interesting system to learn. Learning common diseases, related signs and symptoms, diagnostic tests, and treatments will help medical assistants provide patient care in many ambulatory care environments. Box 12.4 provides a list of medication classifications commonly used with digestive disorders.

PATIENT-CENTERED CARE

When a patient is scheduled for a diagnostic test, the medical assistant must make sure the patient is instructed on the test. Patients need to know basic information on date, time, and where to go for the procedure. They also need to understand why the test has been ordered and what to expect during the procedure. The medical assistant needs to discuss any preparation required for the test.

After the medical assistant coaches a patient on a topic, it is important to evaluate the patient's learning. The patient should be encouraged to "teach back" the preparation instructions or information so that the medical assistant can evaluate whether the patient has an accurate understanding of the directions. Any errors or misunderstandings can be clarified. The patient should have a copy of the directions or information to take home.

BEING PROFESSIONAL

Diagnostic procedures and treatment protocols, especially medications, are constantly changing. The professional medical assistant must be committed to lifelong learning to keep up with the rapid changes in the medical field. Maintaining a current understanding of the human body, the disease process, and how specific digestive system diseases are diagnosed and treated requires a willingness to learn and adapt over time. This commitment to lifelong learning is a crucial part of becoming a professional medical assistant.

Role-play this scenario: You are a medical assistant. You are working with Shelly, who has been a medical assistant in the same department for 20 years. She tells you she knows everything there is about the diseases she encounters. She complains about the continuing education required to keep her certification. How do you respond to Shelly?

CHAPTER REVIEW

The digestive system consists of the gastrointestinal tract and the accessory organs. The gastrointestinal tract is a large, muscular tube that, with the help of hormones and enzymes, digests food. It includes the mouth, pharynx, esophagus, stomach, small intestine, and large intestine. The major accessory organs include the salivary glands, gallbladder, liver, and pancreas. These structures secrete fluids into the GI tract, aiding in digestion.

Four processes occur in the GI system:
- Ingestion: The intake of food and liquids into the body
- Digestion: The breakdown of food into chemical substances
- Absorption: The passage of substances and liquids through the lining of the GI tract into the body fluids and tissues
- Excretion: The elimination of indigestible materials and waste products of metabolism

Saliva contains an enzyme called *salivary amylase*, which starts to break down complex carbohydrates into sugars. In the stomach and duodenum, hydrochloric acid softens and starts breaking down proteins. Pepsin, in the stomach, breaks down proteins into polypeptides. Pancreatic enzymes (trypsin and chymotrypsin) break down proteins into amino acids. Bile emulsifies fats, and lipase breaks down fats into fatty acids and glycerol. In the small intestine, brush-border enzymes help with the final breakdown of carbohydrates.

Common signs and symptoms include constipation, diarrhea, hematochezia, melena, pyrosis, dyspepsia, flatus, halitosis, nausea, vomiting, hematemesis, and jaundice. The etiologies of GI disorders vary; some examples include blockages, cell mutation, other disorders, genetics, and infections. CLIA-waived tests are available for the comprehensive metabolic panel, C-reactive protein (CRP), guaiac fecal occult blood test (gFOBT), *H. pylori* testing, liver function tests, and total bilirubin.

Digestive disorders include:
- Mouth: Orofacial clefts (cleft lips and cleft palates), cavities, gingivitis, periodontal disease, and thrush
- Esophagus and stomach: Gastroesophageal reflux disease, hiatal hernia, peptic ulcers, pyloric stenosis, cyclic vomiting syndrome, dumping syndrome, gastritis, gastroparesis, and hypochlorhydria
- Intestines: Acute appendicitis, celiac disease, diverticulitis, food-borne illnesses, hemorrhoids, hernias (including inguinal hernias), inflammatory bowel disease, intestinal obstructions, irritable bowel syndrome, bowel incontinence, gastroenteritis, Hirschsprung disease, intestinal ischemia and infarction, intestinal volvulus, intussusception, and small intestinal bacterial overgrowth
- Accessory organs: Cholelithiasis, cirrhosis, hepatitis, jaundice in newborns, nonalcoholic fatty liver disease, pancreatitis, primary biliary cirrhosis, hemochromatosis, sialoliths, and sialadenitis
- Cancers: Cancer of the oral cavity, pharyngeal and laryngeal cancers, stomach cancer, pancreatic cancer, liver cancer, small intestinal cancer, and colorectal cancer

Changes in the GI system occur during the first years of life. During pregnancy, progesterone causes the smooth muscles to relax, which affects the digestive system. With age, the stomach empties more slowly. Aging does not affect nutrient absorption. Constipation is more common with aging.

SCENARIO WRAP-UP

Keith has learned a lot from the gastroenterology outreach team. He was able to shadow at the hospital to see several diagnostic procedures. Keith realizes that he will be continually learning with the team. He looks forward to learning more about digestive diseases, diagnostic procedures, and treatments. With everything he has seen to this point, he feels excited about his medical assistant career.

13

Urinary System

LEARNING OBJECTIVES

1. Discuss the anatomy of the urinary system, which will include listing the major organs of the urinary system and identifying the anatomic location of major urinary system organs.
2. Describe the normal functions of the urinary system.
3. Describe common urinary system disorders, including common signs and symptoms, etiology, diagnostic procedures, and treatments.
4. Compare the structure and function of the urinary system across the life span.

OUTLINE

OPENING SCENARIO

Hannah Yang, CMA (AAMA), was hired 4 months ago as a certified medical assistant. She assists the specialists who hold outreach clinics at Walden-Martin Family Medical (WMFM) Clinic. She has been training with the urology staff that comes for the outreach clinics four times a month.

Hannah's role with the urology staff is to help room patients and assist the staff. To prepare for working with the specialist, Hannah spent some time reviewing her medical assistant textbook. She had forgotten the process of urine formation. She had to brush up on the way the urinary system affects the homeostasis of the body. Hannah knows that the urinary system is important and that if a person's kidneys are not functioning, the individual will need to go on dialysis.

As part of her orientation to this specialty, she was able to spend 4 hours at the local dialysis clinic. There, the "regular" patients enjoyed telling her their experiences. Their experiences and the information from the dialysis technicians helped Hannah understand what patients go through with kidney disease.

By assisting the urologist, Dr. Ubert Riney, and his team, Hannah has learned a great deal. However, she knows she has more to learn about this specialty.

YOU WILL LEARN

1. To recognize and use terms related to the urinary system.
2. To locate the urinary system structures.

3. To understand and describe the process required to make urine.
4. To recognize disease states of the urinary system, including their etiology, signs and symptoms, diagnostic procedures, treatment, prognosis, and prevention.

INTRODUCTION

Urology (yoo ROL ah jee) is the healthcare specialty that deals with most urinary disorders. A *urologist* (yoo ROL ah jist) is a specialist involved in the diagnosis, treatment, and prevention of disorders of the urinary system. *Nephrology* (ne FROL o jee) is the healthcare subspecialty that focuses on kidney function and disorders. A *nephrologist* (ne FROL o jist) diagnoses and treats kidney conditions.

Besides the urology department, patients with urinary concerns are typically seen in primary care, urgent care, and even specialty departments. Medical assistants should have a strong understanding of the common urinary signs, symptoms, diseases, diagnostic tests, and treatments.

ANATOMY OF THE URINARY SYSTEM

The urinary system is composed of two kidneys, two ureters, a urinary bladder, and a urethra (Fig. 13.1). The kidneys filter the blood and eliminate waste through the passage of urine. The *ureters* (YOOR eh turs) move urine from the kidneys to the bladder. The urinary bladder stores the urine until it is excreted. The *urethra* (yoo REE thrah) is the tube that conducts the urine out of the bladder.

Kidneys

The kidneys are bean-shaped organs with an indentation, called the *hilum* (HYE lum). The hilum is the location on the kidney where the ureter and renal vein leave the kidney and the renal artery (AR tur ree) enters. The kidneys are about the size of a fist and are located posterior to the peritoneum (PER i tn ee hum) and against the muscles of the back. They are roughly between the T12 and L3 vertebrae. The left kidney is situated about 1 inch (2 cm) higher than the right because of the location of the liver.

The kidneys remove unwanted substances from the blood and form urine for excretion. Blood is delivered to the two kidneys by the renal arteries, which branch off of the abdominal aorta (Fig. 13.2). Blood flows from the renal arteries into afferent (AF fur ent) arterioles (ar TEER ee olez) (smaller arteries) and then through a network of capillaries (CAP ih lair eez) called the *glomeruli* (gloh MER yoo lie). Filtration of the blood occurs in the glomerulus (gloh MER yoo lus). Blood from the glomerulus moves into the efferent (EF fur ent) arterioles and then into the peritubular (PER i too bu lar) capillaries. As the blood leaves the kidneys, it moves from the peritubular capillaries to the venules (VEN yuhls) and then empties into the renal veins. The renal veins take the blood

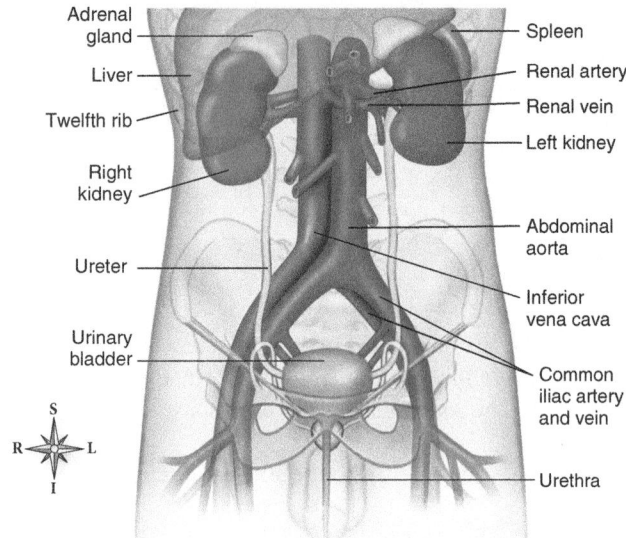

Fig. 13.1 Urinary System. Anterior view of urinary organs. (From Patton KT, Thibodeau GA: *The human body in health and disease*, ed 7, St. Louis, 2018, Elsevier.)

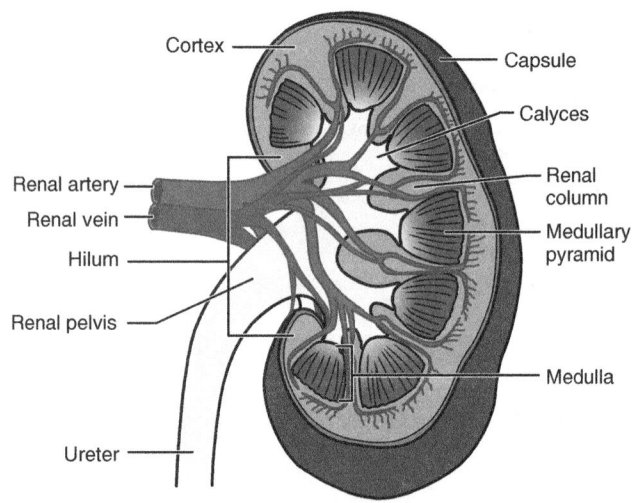

Fig. 13.2 Cross Section of a Kidney.

out of the kidneys. Blood from the renal veins flows into the inferior vena cava as it heads to the heart to become oxygenated again (Fig. 13.3).

VOCABULARY

afferent Pertaining to carrying toward a structure.
arterioles Small arteries.
efferent Pertaining to carrying away from a structure.
filtrate Fluid and substances that are filtered out of the blood in the Bowman capsule.
peritoneum A serous membrane lining of the abdominal cavity, which folds inward to enclose the viscera (internal organs).
peritubular capillaries Blood capillaries surrounding the proximal and distal convoluted tubules in the kidneys.
venules Very small veins.

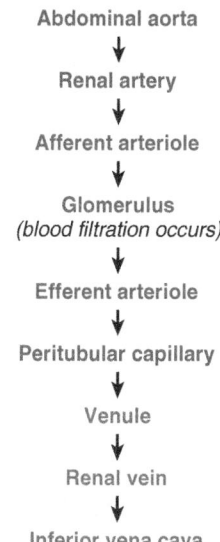

Abdominal aorta
↓
Renal artery
↓
Afferent arteriole
↓
Glomerulus
(blood filtration occurs)
↓
Efferent arteriole
↓
Peritubular capillary
↓
Venule
↓
Renal vein
↓
Inferior vena cava

Fig. 13.3 Blood Flow to and from the Kidney.

MEDICAL TERMINOLOGY

calic/o, cali/o, calyc/o	calyx
cortic/o	cortex
cysto/o, vesic/o	bladder
fer/o	to carry
glomerul/o	glomerulus
hil/o	hilum
medull/o	medulla
pyel/o	pelvis
trigon/o	trigone
ureter/o	ureter
urethr/o	urethra
ven/o	vein
af-	toward
ef-	away from
peri-	surrounding
-ent	pertaining to
-ule	small
calyx (singular)	calyces (plural)
cortex (singular)	cortices (plural)
glomerulus (singular)	glomeruli (plural)
medulla (singular)	medullae (plural)

If a kidney were sliced open, you would see the following:
- *Capsule*: The fibrous outer covering of the kidney
- *Cortex* (KORE tecks): The outer portion of the kidney
- *Renal column*: Extensions of the cortex that dip down between the medullary pyramids
- *Medulla* (muh DOO lah): The inner portion that extends from the end of the cortex to the calyces
- *Medullary* (me dah ler EE) *pyramid*: A cone-shaped structure located in the medulla and containing straight tubular structures and blood vessels
- *Minor* and *major calyces* (KAL ih seez) and the renal pelvis are extensions of the ureter inside of the kidney

Each kidney contains tissue with millions of microscopic units called *nephrons* (NEFF rons). Nephrons are the functional units of the kidneys. They are located in the cortex and extend into the medulla. Each nephron is a very long tube or tubule. One end of the nephron is the *renal corpuscle* (KORE pus sul), and the remaining section of the nephron is the *renal tubule*. The renal corpuscle consists of the following:
- *Bowman capsule*: A cup-shaped structure of the nephron that surrounds the glomerulus
- *Glomerulus*: A cluster of capillaries inside of the Bowman capsule

The afferent arteriole brings blood into the glomerulus, and the efferent arteriole takes blood away from the glomerulus. The diameter of the afferent arteriole is much larger than the diameter of the efferent arteriole. The importance of the narrowed diameter will be discussed in the "Physiology of the Urinary System" section of this chapter.

The renal tubule is a long, thin, twisted tube that brings the filtrate (which will become urine) from the Bowman capsule to the renal pelvis. During the passage of filtrate from the Bowman capsule to the renal pelvis, water and electrolytes move between the urine and the blood to maintain homeostasis. The formation of urine will be discussed in the "Physiology of the Urinary System" section. The renal tubule is made up of the following:
- *Proximal (convoluted) tubule* (PCT): The first section of the renal tubule that is attached to the Bowman capsule.
- *Henle loop*: Follows the PCT and includes a straight descending section, a loop, and then a straight ascending section.
- *Distal (convoluted) tubule* (DCT): Follows after the ascending section of the Henle loop.
- *Collecting duct* (CD): Multiple distal tubules join and form this straight collecting duct, which empties into the calyx.

To summarize, the nephron begins on one end with the Bowman capsule, which is filled with the capillaries. The proximal tubule is the next section of the nephron. It is followed by the Henle loop, then the distal tubule, and finally the collecting duct. Many collecting ducts empty into one calyx. Many calyces merge into the renal pelvis, which is an extension of the ureter inside of the kidney. The Bowman capsule, proximal tubules, and distal tubes are in the cortex. The Henle loop and the collecting ducts are in the medulla of the kidney.

CRITICAL THINKING 13.1

Hannah is working with Mrs. Green, a urology patient. Mrs. Green has kidney disease and asks Hannah what the kidneys do. How should Hannah explain the role of the kidneys to Mrs. Green?

Ureters

The bilateral ureters are thin, muscular tubes approximately 10 inches long. The tube's muscular layer creates peristaltic waves that help move the urine to the bladder. The ureters' walls are made of transitional epithelium, which allows the ureters to stretch to accommodate urine flow. Many nerve endings are also in the walls. A stone in the ureter can cause severe pain.

The point where the ureter enters the bladder is called the *ureterovesical* (you REE ter oh ves i kal) *junction*. The ureters enter the bladder at an angle. This creates a flap over the end of the ureter. The flap serves as a valve. Urine can empty into the bladder, but it cannot back up from the bladder and reenter the ureter. This mechanism also prevents bacteria from moving from the bladder up to the kidneys.

Bladder

The urinary bladder is a hollow organ in the pelvic cavity. It serves as a holding tank for urine. Urine enters the bladder through the ureters and leaves the bladder through the urethra. The triangular area in the bladder between the ureters' entrance and the urethral outlet is called the *trigone* (TRY gohn).

Transitional epithelium creates the inner lining of the bladder. When the bladder is empty, it flattens and the walls overlap in folds, also known as rugae (ROO gee). This creates a wrinkled appearance. As the bladder starts to fill with urine, the rugae and transitional epithelium allow for greater bladder volume. Think of a balloon that was blown up and then emptied of air. The balloon is smaller and wrinkly in appearance. When inflated, the wrinkles are gone, and it can accommodate a large volume of air. The same thing happens with the bladder and urine.

The bladder is also composed of smooth muscle fibers that make up the *detrusor* (de TROO ser) *muscle*. The detrusor muscle relaxes when the bladder fills. It contracts to push urine out of the bladder and into the urethra. Normally, the bladder holds about 1.5 to 2 cups (360 to 480 mL) of urine during the day and doubles that amount at night. As the bladder fills to about 150 mL, stretch receptors in the detrusor send a message to the central nervous system. As more urine enters the bladder, the urge to urinate increases. After urination or *micturition*, residual urine remains (usually less than 50 mL) in the bladder.

> **VOCABULARY**
> **residual urine** Urine that remains in the bladder after micturition or urination.
> **rugae** Folds in the walls of some organs; when the organ (e.g., stomach, bladder, uterus) fills or needs to expand, the rugae unfold.
> **stretch receptor** A sensory nerve ending that responds to a stretch stimulus.
> **transitional epithelium** A type of cell found in the lining of hollow organs; it has the ability to stretch with the contraction and distention of the organ.

Urethra

The urethra (yoo REE thrah) is a mucous membrane–lined tube that drains urine out of the bladder. In males, the internal urethral sphincter (SFINK tur) is located at the bladder end (or proximal end) of the urethra. The sphincter is made of smooth involuntary muscles. The external sphincter is located in different places in males and in females (Table 13.1). The external sphincter is made of skeletal muscles and is a voluntary muscle. A voluntary muscle provides you the ability to control when you urinate. The distal end of the urethra is called the *urinary meatus* (mee ATE us). The urinary meatus is the final point before the urine leaves the body.

TABLE 13.1 Difference in the Urethra Between the Genders

	Female	Male
Length	1–1.5 inches	8 inches
Function	Urination	Urination and ejaculation
Location of Internal Sphincter	None	At the proximal end (bladder end) of the urethra; may prevent semen from moving into the bladder
Location of External Sphincter	Extends up to the bladder, encircles the vagina and urethra	Under the prostate gland

The *prostate* is a walnut-sized gland found below the bladder in males. It surrounds part of the urethra. This gland produces fluid for semen. The prostate is considered a reproductive organ, but it also is part of the urinary system. As males get older, the prostate grows. This condition is known as *benign prostatic hyperplasia* (BPH). When the prostate increases in size, it can obstruct the urethra, blocking the urine flow.

> **CRITICAL THINKING 13.2**
>
> Hannah is working with Katrina, the urology medical assistant. Hannah asks Katrina what the major differences are between the male and female urinary systems. How would Katrina respond to Hannah's question?

PHYSIOLOGY OF THE URINARY SYSTEM

The urinary system has several important roles that help regulate homeostasis in the body, including:

- Maintaining fluid volume. The urinary system increases fluid loss in urine when fluid volume is high. It reduces the fluid loss when the fluid volume is low (e.g., with dehydration).
- Maintaining the normal composition of body fluids. The urinary system can increase or decrease the loss of certain electrolytes in the urine as it regulates the normal makeup of the body fluids. This helps to keep the pH of the blood within normal limits.
- Maintaining an adequate blood pressure. Renin, an enzyme, is secreted in the urinary system and is involved with increasing the blood pressure.
- Controlling the red blood cell production. Erythropoietin (eh rith roh POY ee tin) is secreted by the urinary system, which is involved with red blood cell production.
- Activating vitamin D. The kidneys are involved with the final step of vitamin D activation. Vitamin D is important in the absorption of calcium and phosphorus.

Many of these roles are performed during the formation of urine. The body rids itself of unneeded substances produced during the metabolic process. The process of urine formation includes three steps: filtration, reabsorption, and secretion. Each step will be described in more detail in the coming sections.

Filtration

Filtration is the first step in urine formation. It is a continual process that involves the renal corpuscle. If you recall, the renal corpuscle consists of a cup-shaped structure (Bowman capsule) that surrounds the network of capillaries (glomerulus).

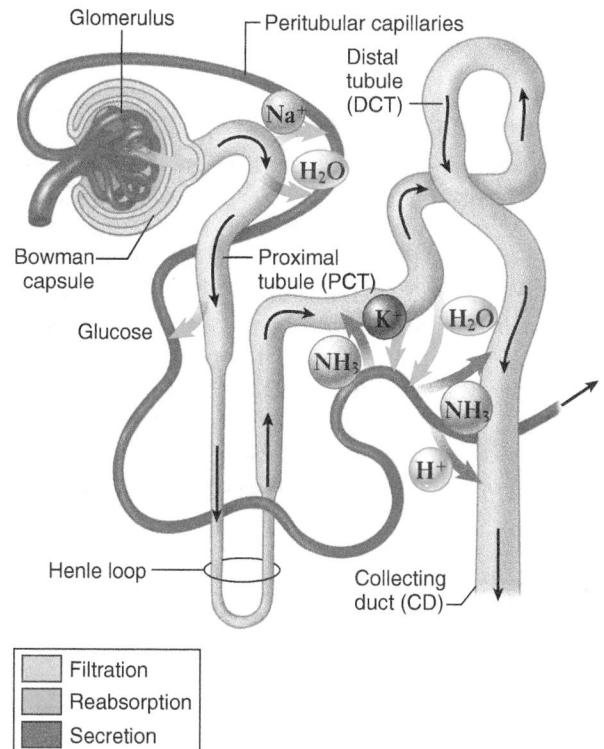

Fig. 13.4 Formation of Urine. Diagram shows examples of steps in urine formation in successive parts of a nephron: filtration, reabsorption, and secretion. (From Patton KT, Thibodeau G: *The human body in health and disease*, ed 6, St. Louis, 2014, Mosby.)

The blood is brought to the kidneys by the renal arteries. The arteries branch into smaller vessels that transport the blood throughout the kidney. As the blood gets to the nephron, an afferent arteriole brings the blood into the glomerulus, and an efferent arteriole takes the blood away. Eventually the blood moves into the renal vein and out of the kidney.

Let us focus on what occurs in the glomerulus. The diameter of the afferent arteriole is larger than the efferent arteriole's diameter. This means the blood moves into the glomerulus faster than it leaves. The pressure inside the glomerulus is high, with the quantity of blood moving into the glomerulus. This forces water and dissolved substances through the one-celled wall of the capillary and into the Bowman capsule. The substance in the Bowman capsule is known as *filtrate*. (Think of a garden hose that is wide at one part and then narrowed at another. The pressure builds up behind the narrowed section. Water can leak from any weakened areas in the wall. This is similar to what occurs in the glomerulus.)

Several dissolved substances can move through the capillary wall:

- Electrolytes (i.e., sodium, chloride, and potassium)
- Waste products (i.e., urea, metabolites [muh TAB uh lites])
- Other substances (i.e., amino acids and glucose)

White blood cells, red blood cells, and plasma proteins are too large to pass through the capillary wall. With normal kidney function, they remain in the capillary.

If the blood pressure falls (i.e., with hemorrhaging), the pressure in the glomerulus is not high enough to cause movement of the fluids, so little to no filtrate is created and the person will have little to no urine output.

Reabsorption

Reabsorption means substances move from the filtrate back into the blood in the peritubular capillaries. As the filtrate moves out of the Bowman capsule and into the proximal tubule, the reabsorption process starts. Water (H_2O) and solutes (e.g., sodium [Na+] ions and glucose) move back into the blood (Fig. 13.4). Table 13.2 presents the list of solutes that move back into the blood.

TABLE 13.2	Movement of Substances Between the Blood and Filtrate in the Nephron				
Nephron Sections Processes	**Renal Corpuscle**	**Proximal Tubule**	**Henle Loop**	**Distal Tubule**	**Collecting Duct**
Filtration *(moves from blood to create filtrate)*	Water, electrolyte ions (sodium, chloride, potassium), urea, glucose, and amino acids	—	—	—	—
Reabsorption *(moves from filtrate to blood)*	—	Water, glucose, amino acids, urea, and electrolyte ions (sodium, chloride, phosphate)	Water and electrolytes ions (chloride, sodium)	Electrolytes ions (chloride, sodium) and water (only in the presence of antidiuretic hormone [ADH])	Electrolytes ions (sodium), urea, water (only in the presence of ADH)
Secretion *(moves from blood to filtrate)*	—	—	Urea	Ammonium, potassium, hydrogen, some drugs	Ammonium, potassium, hydrogen, some drugs

In the Henle loop, the reabsorption process is a bit different. The Henle loop dips down into the medulla and then moves back up. The countercurrent flow occurs as the filtrate flows down and then moves back up. During this time, the chloride (Cl⁻) and sodium ions move out of the filtrate and into the interstitial (in ter STISH uh l) fluid and blood. This creates a salty interstitial fluid, which then helps pull water from the distal tubule filtrate. Water, chloride, and sodium are reabsorbed back into the blood as the filtrate passes through the distal tubule.

In the distal tubules, some sodium and chloride ions are reabsorbed from the filtrate. The walls of the distal tubules do not allow water to move out of the filtrate without special help. This help is *antidiuretic hormone* (ADH). ADH is a hormone produced by the posterior pituitary gland. This hormone increases the water permeability of the walls of the distal tubule and collecting duct. With the help of ADH, water moves out of the filtrate into the bloodstream. Without ADH a person would pass vast quantities of urine. This condition is called *diabetes insipidus.*

Besides ADH, another hormone, called *aldosterone*, works on the urinary system. Aldosterone is secreted by the adrenal cortex. This hormone increases the movement of sodium out of the filtrate in the distal tubule and collecting duct. (See Table 13.2 for the complete list of substances reabsorbed in the distal tubule and collecting duct.)

To maintain homeostasis, the kidneys retain (or reabsorb) what the body needs. Substances in excessive concentrations and metabolism waste products remain in the filtrate. The filtrate becomes more concentrated as water is reabsorbed back into the bloodstream. The kidneys create about 48 gallons (about 182 L) of filtrate a day. By the time reabsorption occurs, they produce only 1 to 2 quarts (about 0.9 to 1.9 L) of urine a day.

VOCABULARY

antihypertensive A substance (i.e., medication) that reduces high blood pressure.

interstitial Between the cells.

permeability A quality or characteristic of a material that allows another substance to pass through it.

CRITICAL THINKING 13.3

Hannah is confused about diabetes insipidus. She always thought diabetes related to insulin and blood glucose. She does not recall learning about diabetes insipidus in school. She asks Katrina to explain how diabetes insipidus affects the urinary system. How might Katrina respond to Hannah's question?

Secretion

Secretion means that substances move from the blood to the filtrate. This allows the body to maintain homeostasis and move unneeded substances back into the filtrate. Urea moves back to the filtrate in the Henle loop. As the filtrate moves through the distal tubule and collecting duct, more adjustments are made. Ammonia (NH₃), certain drugs, hydrogen (H⁺), and potassium

---

BOX 13.1   Antihypertensive Medications and the Renin-Angiotensin-Aldosterone System (RAAS)

Many antihypertensive (an tie hie per TEN siv) medications affect the RAAS at various points in the hope of lowering the blood pressure. Sometimes it takes more than one medication to lower a person's blood pressure to a safe level.

(K⁺) move from the blood into the filtrate. The movement of potassium into the filtrate can be caused by aldosterone. After the filtrate or urine leaves the collecting ducts, no more adjustments are made. The urine then flows to the calyces and to the ureter before going through the rest of the urinary system structures.

Renin and Blood Pressure

As mentioned before, the kidneys have an important role in maintaining blood pressure. The *juxtaglomerular* (JUKS tah glo MER you lar) *cells* are smooth muscle cells in the afferent arterioles. These cells make and secrete the enzyme *renin.* When the arterial blood pressure decreases or when there is a decrease in sodium, renin is released. Secreting renin is one of the first steps in the complex renin-angiotensin-aldosterone system (RAAS). Ultimately when renin is secreted, a series of events occur. The outcome affects the blood plasma volume and the constriction of blood vessels. An increase in the blood plasma volume or the constriction of blood vessels can increase blood pressure (Box 13.1).

Erythropoietin

As the blood is moving through the kidneys, specialized kidney cells can detect low oxygen levels in the blood. When this occurs, a hormone called *erythropoietin* is released from the kidney cells. Erythropoietin travels to the bone marrow and stimulates the marrow to make more red blood cells.

Vitamin D

Vitamin D assists with calcium absorption and helps maintain calcium and phosphorus levels. These minerals are important for strong bones. We get vitamin D from exposure to sunlight and also from the consumption of supplements and food. The kidneys must convert vitamin D to an active form so that the body can use it.

DISEASES AND DISORDERS OF THE URINARY SYSTEM

Urologic diseases are conditions that affect one or more of the urinary system structures. Common urinary signs and symptoms include:

- *Dysuria* (dis YOOR ee ah): Painful or difficult urination
- *Nocturia* (nock TOOR ee ah): Urination at night
- *Polyuria* (pah lee YOOR ee ah): Excessive excretion of urine, may be accompanied by *polydipsia* (excessive thirst)
- *Frequency*: Urination at short periods without an increase in the daily volume of urine output

TABLE 13.3 Common Diagnostic Procedures Used for Urinary System Disorders

Done by/Type of Test:	Procedure	Description
Provider during the exam	Digital rectal examination (DRE)	Done during the physical examination. The provider inserts a gloved, lubricated finger into the rectum to feel for abnormalities in the prostate, bladder, ovaries, or uterus. For urinary tract issues, the DRE may be done to check if the prostate gland is swollen and obstructing the urinary tract structures.
Endoscopy	Cystoscopy and ureteroscopy	An endoscope is inserted into the urethra and used to look at the urinary system.
Imaging procedures	Computed tomography (CT) scan	Images can show urinary tract obstructions. (See Chapter 2 for more information.)
	Dimercaptosuccinic acid (DMSA) scan	A renal scan that uses the radioisotope, technetium-99m DSMA scan to evaluate the kidneys. Function, shape, position, size, and scarring can be observed. The radioisotope is injected, and a gamma camera is used to take pictures of the kidney.
	Intravenous pyelogram (IVP)	Iodine contrast is given intravenous (IV). Then x-ray images will be taken to see how the kidneys filter the contrast from the blood. The test can provide information on the functioning of the kidneys, bladder, and ureters.
	Postvoid residual (PVR) urine test	Measures the amount of urine in the bladder after urination. A straight catheter can be inserted to drain the remaining urine so the volume can be measured, but this procedure can increase the risk of urinary tract infections (UTIs). A portable ultrasound unit can also be used as a noninvasive test. The scan identifies the urine left, and the unit automatically calculates the volume of residual urine.
	Ultrasound (US)	Images can show urinary tract obstructions. (See Chapter 2 for more information.)
	Voiding cystourethrogram (VCUG)	A minimally invasive test that involves fluoroscopy to visualize the urinary tract and bladder. Images are taken while the bladder is full and during urination. Contrast medium is used to help visualize the urinary structures on the x-ray image.
Medical laboratory	Blood urea nitrogen (BUN) test	Urea is a waste product in the blood that is filtered out by the kidneys. If the kidney function is abnormal, the blood level of urea will be increased.
	Creatinine and creatinine clearance tests	Creatinine is a waste product from normal muscle breakdown. Creatinine is filtered out of the blood by the kidneys. The blood creatinine level indicates kidney function. The creatinine clearance rate shows how the kidneys filter creatinine from the blood.
	Urinalysis (UA)	A urine sample is collected in a special container. The urine is analyzed in the lab for abnormal levels of substances. Some of the substances that may be found in urine include blood, ketones, bilirubin, glucose, protein, and nitrites. The urinalysis is a CLIA-waived test, including glucose and ketones.
	Urine culture	A urine sample is collected in a special container. The urine is analyzed in the lab for bacterial growth over a period of days (usually 1–3 days). Specific bacteria grown in the sample will be listed on the urine culture report.
	Urine culture and sensitivity (C&S)	A urine culture is done as discussed previously. The sensitivity results indicate if the pathogen is susceptible or resistant to specific antibiotics.

CLIA, Clinical Laboratory Improvement Amendments.

- *Urgency*: The sudden, almost uncontrollable need to urinate
- *Urinary incontinence* (in KON tih nense): Inability to hold urine
- *Urinary retention*: Inability to release urine
- *Calculi* (KAL kyuh lie): Stones formed in the kidneys, gallbladder, and other parts of the body
- *Hydronephrosis* (hie droh nuh FROH sis): A backup of urine that causes dilation of the ureters and calyces; can increase pressure on the nephron units
- *Azotemia* (AZ oh TEE mee ah): An abnormal increase in nitrogenous waste products in the blood; also called uremia
- Abnormal substances found in the urine, which include:
  - Albumin, which is called *albuminuria* (al byoo mih NOOR ee ah)
  - Bacteria, which is called *bacteriuria* (back tur ee YOOR ee ah)
- Excessive nitrogenous compounds, called *azoturia* (a zoh TOOR ee ah)
- Glucose (sugar), called *glycosuria* (gly kohs YOOR ee ah)
- Blood, which is called *hematuria* (hee mah TOOR ee ah)
- Pus, called *pyuria* (pye YOOR ee ah)

Common diagnostic procedures are listed on Table 13.3. Common treatments are listed on Table 13.4.

Urinary diseases can include infections, stones, kidney problems, cancer, and bladder control problems. A urinary tract infection (UTI) is an infection in one or more of the urinary tract structures. Specific infections will be discussed in the following section, along with other diseases.

VOCABULARY

intravenous (IV) Through a vein; fluids and medications can be given through a vein.

TABLE 13.4   Common Treatments Used for Urinary System Disorders

Procedure	Description
Catheterization	The insertion of a catheter (KATH uh tur) to drain urine from the bladder. An *indwelling catheter* remains in, and a *straight catheter* is removed after the procedure.
Dialysis (die AL I sis)	A technique in which filtration through a semipermeable membrane is used to remove metabolic wastes and extra fluid from the blood.
Extracorporeal shock wave lithotripsy (ESWL)	Nonsurgical approach using shock waves to break up stones in the ureters and kidneys.
Kidney transplantation	Surgical transplantation of an entire kidney from a donor to a recipient.
Nephrectomy (neh FRECK tuh mee)	Surgical removal of a kidney. Types of surgical procedures include: • *Partial nephrectomy.* Removal of the cancer and surrounding tissue; kidney remains functional; used when the other kidney has been damaged or removed • *Simple nephrectomy.* Removal of the kidney • *Radical nephrectomy.* Removal of the kidney, adrenal gland, surrounding tissue, and local lymph nodes
Nephrolithotomy (nef roe lih THOT uh mee)	A surgical incision of the kidney to remove a stone. The surgeon makes a small incision on the lower back to reach the kidney, and a nephroscope is inserted with other instruments to remove the stone. With *percutaneous nephrolithotripsy* (PNL), the stones are crushed and removed using suction.
Nephroureterectomy (nef roe you REE ter ek to mee)	Removal of the kidney and ureter.
Segmental resection of the ureter	Removal of the diseased section of the ureter; ureter is then reconnected.

VOCABULARY

catheter A hollow, flexible tube that can be inserted into a vessel, organ, or cavity of the body to withdraw or instill fluid, monitor information, and visualize a vessel or cavity.

MEDICAL TERMINOLOGY

albumin/o	protein
azot/o	nitrogen
bacteri/o	bacteria
glycos/o	sugar, glucose
hemat/o	blood
noct/i	night
olig/o	scanty, few
py/o	pus
ur/o	urine
di-	through, complete
dys-	painful, abnormal
en-	in
poly-	excessive, frequent
-emia	blood condition
-esis	state of
-uria	urinary condition

CRITICAL THINKING 13.4

Hannah is confused about the terms *azotemia* and *azoturia*. How might she remember which term relates to blood and which relates to urine?

Cancer

Bladder Cancer. Bladder cancer, cancer of the urinary bladder, is the sixth most common cancer in the United States. Bladder cancer tends to affect four times more males than females. This type of cancer tends to recur, so follow-up testing is critical. There are several types of bladder cancer:

- *Transitional cell carcinoma* or *urothelial carcinoma* is the most common cause; it involves the transitional (epithelium) cells that change and stretch as the bladder fills with urine.
- *Squamous cell carcinoma* occurs with frequent infections, especially parasitic infections; it is rare in the United States.
- *Adenocarcinoma* involves the cells that make and release fluids (e.g., mucus) in the bladder wall; it also is rare in the United States.

Etiology. The cause of bladder cancer is the mutation of bladder cells. Risk factors for developing bladder cancer include:

- Smoking: Due to the harmful chemicals excreted in the urine
- Chemical exposure: Arsenic and chemicals used in the manufacturing process of different products (e.g., paint, rubber, dyes)
- Family history of the disease
- Chronic bladder infections and inflammation
- Aging: Rarely seen in people younger than age 40
- Caucasian race: Greatest risk compared with other races
- Male gender: Greater risk than females
- Medications: Certain chemotherapy products and diabetes mellitus drugs

Signs and Symptoms. Bladder cancer causes:

- Hematuria
- Frequency and urgency to urinate
- Dysuria, pelvic pain, and low back pain

Diagnostic Procedures. Urine testing, cystoscopy, and biopsy are procedures used to diagnose bladder cancer (Fig. 13.5). Imaging tests, such as computed tomography (CT), magnetic resonance imaging (MRI), and positron emission tomography (PET), are used to identify whether the cancer has spread.

Treatments. Treatments used for bladder cancer include surgery, radiation therapy, and chemotherapy. *Biologic therapy* or *immunotherapy* is also a treatment option. Biologic therapy can be useful because it increases the body's ability to help fight the cancer.

Kidney Cancer. Kidney cancer or primary kidney cancer occurs when a cancer starts in the kidney. There are three main types of primary kidney cancer:

- *Renal cell carcinoma* (RCC) (or renal adenocarcinoma): Most common type in adults; forms in the lining of the kidney tubules.
- *Wilms tumor*: Accounts for about 95% kidney cancer in children, usually diagnosed when the person is younger than 5 years; occurs in the kidney tissue; improved treatments have increased the survival rate.
- *Transitional cell cancer*: Occurs in adults; forms in the ureter and renal pelvis.

Etiology. The cause of kidney cancer is not clear. A mutation occurs in the kidney cells. This can lead to the development of a tumor. Table 13.5 presents the etiology and risk factors for the three common types of kidney cancer.

Signs and Symptoms. With kidney cancer, pain and hematuria can be key symptoms. See Table 13.5 for the symptoms of the three types of kidney cancer.

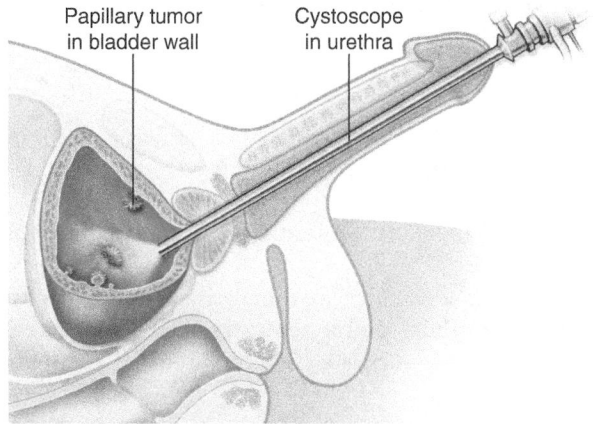

Fig. 13.5 Cystoscope in Male Bladder. (From Patton KT, Thibodeau GA: *The human body in health and disease*, ed 7, St. Louis, 2018, Elsevier.)

Diagnostic Procedures. Diagnostic procedures for the three types of kidney cancer are similar (see Table 13.5). During the exam, the provider may identify a kidney mass. Urinalysis and blood work may be done to check for hematuria and evaluate the person's overall health. Once kidney cancer has been diagnosed, imaging tests are done to check for cancer in other parts of the body.

Treatments. Treatment for kidney cancer can involve surgery. A person can live with just a part of one kidney functioning. If the person does not have any kidney function, dialysis is required. Kidney transplantation could also be a treatment option. Radiation and chemotherapy are additional treatment options with kidney cancer.

If surgery is not an option, an *arterial embolization* can be done. A catheter is inserted through an incision. It is passed into the main blood vessel of the kidney. A special gelatin sponge is inserted through the catheter into the blood vessel. This creates a blockage, which then cuts the blood flow to the cancerous area. Cancer cells rely on blood flow for oxygen and nutrients.

Biologic therapy and targeted therapy are also treatment options. Biologic therapy, as already described, boosts the body's natural ability to fight off cancer. Targeted therapy requires the use of drugs that attack cancer cells only. The normal cells remain unharmed, and the medications cause the tumor to shrink.

VOCABULARY

aniridia A condition in which the iris in the eye is partially formed or fails to form.

hypospadias A condition in which the urethral opening is on the underside of the penis.

intermittent Occurring in intervals.

undescended testicles A condition in which one or both testicles do not descend into the scrotum.

TABLE 13.5	**Common Types of Kidney Cancer**		
	Renal Cell Carcinoma	**Transitional Cell Cancer**	**Wilms Tumor**
Other Names	Renal adenocarcinoma	—	Nephroblastoma
Etiology and Risk Factors	Etiology is unclear. Risk factors: Misuse of some pain medications, obesity, high blood pressure, smoking, inherited conditions.	Etiology is unclear. Risk factors: Misuse of some pain medications, smoking cigarettes, exposure to certain dyes and industrial chemicals.	Etiology is unclear. Risk factors: Family history of the disease, African American descent, congenital abnormalities, including aniridia (ane eye RID ee ah), hypospadias (hie poe SPA de as), and undescended testicles.
Signs and Symptoms	Hematuria, lump in abdomen, side and back pain (below the ribs), loss of appetite, weight loss, anemia, intermittent fever.	Hematuria, back pain, extreme fatigue, weight loss, dysuria.	Hematuria, fever, and abdominal pain, mass and swelling.
Diagnostic Procedures	Physical exam, CBC, blood chemistry tests, UA, liver function tests, CT, MRI, US, biopsy.	Physical exam, CBC, blood chemistry tests, UA, ureteroscopy, IVP, CT, US, MRI, biopsy.	Physical exam, CBC, blood chemistry tests, UA, US, CT, MRI.
Treatment	Nephrectomy, radiation, chemotherapy, biologic therapy, targeted therapy.	Segmental resection of the ureter, nephroureterectomy, chemotherapy, radiation.	Nephrectomy, radiation, chemotherapy.

CBC, Complete blood count; *CT,* computed tomography; *IVP,* intravenous pyelogram; *MRI,* magnetic resonance imaging; *UA,* urinalysis; *US,* ultrasonography.

Acute Cystitis

Acute cystitis (si STIE tis) is an inflammation of the bladder.

Etiology. In many cases, inflammation is related to a bacterial infection. One of the most common causes is *Escherichia coli (E. coli)*. Due to their shorter urethra, females are more at risk than males to get infections. Risk factors for cystitis include:

- Indwelling or straight catheter and urinary tract procedure
- Pregnancy, menopause
- Urinary retention and obstructions (bladder, urethra, or due to an enlarged prostate gland)
- Bowel incontinence
- Diabetes

Besides bacteria, inflammation can be caused by medications, radiation therapy, spermicidal jellies, and long-term catheterization.

Signs and Symptoms. Acute cystitis can cause:

- Low-grade fever
- Nocturia, dysuria, urgency, frequency, and urinary retention
- Cloudy, bloody, and strong/foul-smelling urine
- Low abdominal pressure and cramping
- Confusion and mental changes in older adults

Diagnostic Procedures. Usually the provider will order a urinalysis and a urine culture and sensitivity. The urinalysis will provide information fairly quickly that will help diagnose cystitis. It may take up to 3 days for the culture and sensitivity to identify the organism and then provide information on the best medications to treat the infection. If the urinalysis and culture come back negative for an infection, the provider may do additional tests (e.g., cystoscopy) to try to identify the cause of the symptoms.

Treatments. For bacterial cystitis, antibiotics are used to treat the infection. After the patient starts the antibiotic, the symptoms should improve within a few days. If a patient has a history of repeated infections, the provider may refer the patient to a urologist for more testing. Hospital-acquired bladder infections are usually resistant to the common antibiotics used to treat UTIs. Stronger antibiotics may be given.

Home care treatments may include:

- Drinking plenty of liquids and avoiding coffee, alcohol, and soft drinks
- Taking an analgesic, having a sitz bath, or using a heating pad to reduce the discomfort

To reduce the risk of UTIs, keeping hydrated and urinating frequently are recommended. Women can reduce the risk of UTIs by:

- Wiping from front to back, which prevents bacteria in the anal area from spreading to the urethra
- Taking showers instead of baths
- Urinating after intercourse

CRITICAL THINKING 13.5

Hannah is working with Dr. Riney. He ordered an antibiotic for Mrs. Williams, who has a UTI. When the urine culture and sensitivity (C&S) report comes back to the department, he asks Hannah to call Mrs. Williams about a change in the antibiotic. Why might the provider change the antibiotic once the urine C&S report becomes available?

Glomerulonephritis

Several diseases affect kidney functioning by their effects on the glomeruli. *Glomerulonephritis* (gloe MER yuh loe nah FRIE tis) is inflammation of the glomeruli. Damage to the glomeruli can cause protein and red blood cells to leak into the urine. Glomerulonephritis usually has an abrupt onset.

Etiology. The cause is often unknown. It can follow a streptococcal infection.

Signs and Symptoms. Glomerulonephritis can cause:

- Changes in the urine, such as hematuria, cola-colored urine, proteinuria, and oliguria
- Headache
- Pain over the kidney region
- Puffy eyes, fatigue, and low-grade fever

Diagnostic Procedures. After the physical exam, the provider may order:

- Laboratory tests, such as urinalysis, blood urea nitrogen (BUN), creatinine, and erythrocyte sedimentation rate (ESR)
- Imagining tests, such as a CT scan, x-ray, and ultrasound
- Renal biopsy

Treatments. Treatment is based on the cause of the illness. Possible treatments may include:

- Antihypertensive and diuretic medications and antibiotics if bacterial related
- Bed rest
- Dietary restrictions, such as protein, salt, and potassium

Kidney Failure

Chronic Kidney Disease. Chronic kidney disease is also called *chronic kidney failure*. With this condition, the kidney function is gradually lost. During the early stage of chronic kidney disease, there may be few symptoms. As the kidney function diminishes, more symptoms occur.

Etiology. Diseases that can lead to chronic kidney disease include:

- Type 1 or type 2 diabetes mellitus
- Hypertension (HTN) (high blood pressure)
- Glomerulonephritis
- Interstitial nephritis (inflammation of the kidney tubules)
- Polycystic kidney disease
- Prolonged obstructions or recurrent kidney infections
- Vesicoureteral (ves ih koe yoo REE tur ul) reflux

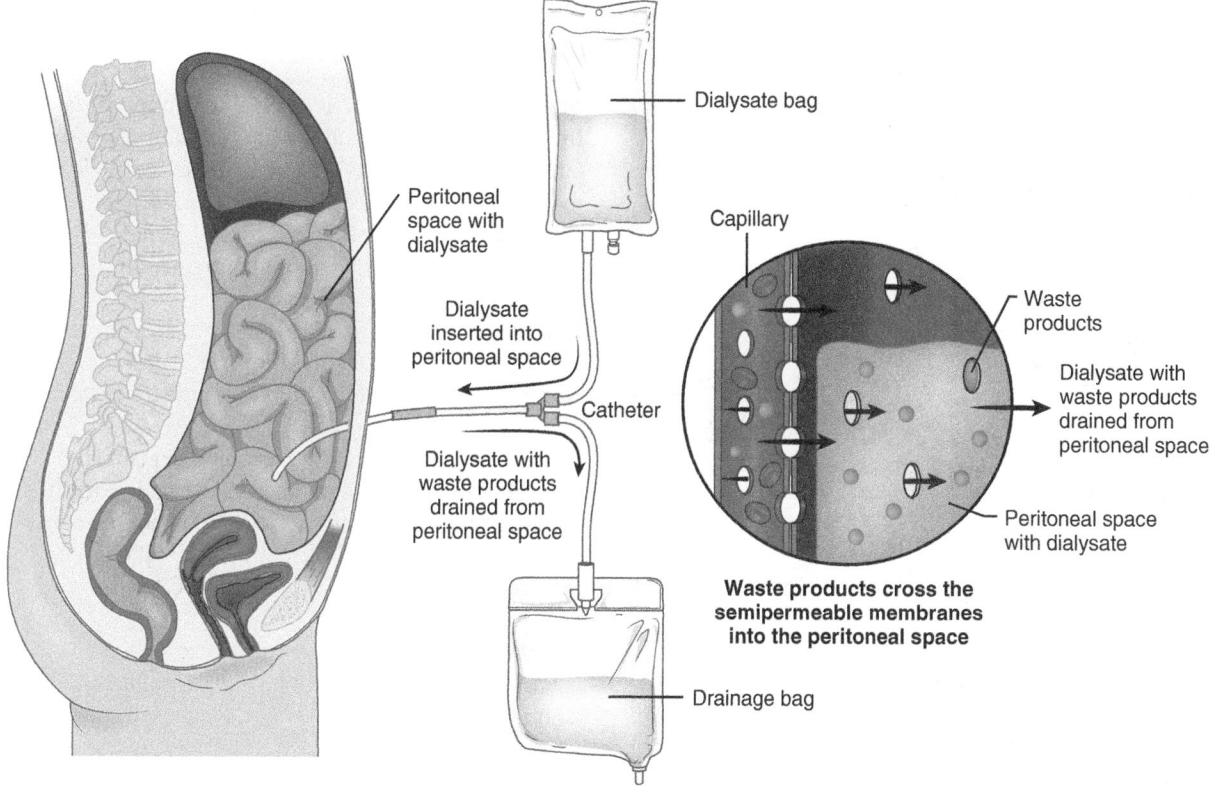

Fig. 13.6 Peritoneal Dialysis. (From Proctor D, et al: *Kinn's the medical assistant*, ed 13, St. Louis, 2017, Elsevier.)

Signs and Symptoms. Signs and symptoms may be minimal at first. As the kidney function diminishes, the person may experience:

- Nausea, vomiting, loss of appetite, weakness, and fatigue
- Sleep issues and a reduction in mental sharpness
- Muscle cramps, twitching, and itching *(pruritus)*
- Decreased amounts of urine
- Hypertension

Diagnostic Procedures. After a history and examination, the provider may order urine and blood tests to assess the kidney function. Imaging test may be done to assess the kidney size, shape, and structure. A kidney biopsy can also be done.

Treatments. For chronic kidney disease there is no cure. Treatment is focused on slowing the progression of the disease and reducing complications. Underlying conditions, such as hypertension and diabetes, are also treated.

End-Stage Renal Disease. End-stage renal disease (ESRD), also called *end-stage kidney disease* and *kidney failure*, is advanced-stage chronic kidney disease. ESRD occurs when the kidneys are no longer filtering waste from the blood. Dangerous levels of electrolytes, waste products, and fluids build up in the bloodstream.

More than 660,000 Americans have kidney failure. Over 44% of those patients are between the ages of 45 and 64. The top two causes of ESRD are diabetes mellitus and hypertension.

Etiology. End-stage kidney disease is a complication of several diseases:

- Diabetes mellitus with poor glucose control
- Hypertension
- Glomerulonephritis
- Polycystic kidney disease
- Prolonged obstructions or recurrent kidney infections
- Vesicoureteral reflux

Additional factors that can increase a person's risk for ESRD include tobacco use, African American descent, gender (male), and being age 45 years or older.

Signs and Symptoms. The kidneys can slowly stop functioning over the course of 10 to 20 years before ESRD occurs. The signs and symptoms are the same as for chronic kidney disease.

Diagnostic Procedures. Besides performing a physical exam, providers will order blood work and a bone density test. The blood work usually includes a complete blood count (CBC), electrolytes (e.g., potassium, sodium, calcium, and magnesium), albumin, and parathyroid hormone. The patient's blood pressure will be monitored closely.

Treatments. ESRD is often treated with dialysis or kidney transplantation. Dialysis works like a kidney by filtering out the waste products, extra fluids, and electrolytes. There are two different types of dialysis:

- *Peritoneal dialysis:* A catheter is surgically placed in the abdomen. The patient can then infuse a special sterile solution through the catheter into the abdomen. The peritoneal membrane is used as a natural filter, and waste from the blood moves into the infused solution. After a few hours, the patient drains the fluid out of the abdomen via the catheter (Fig. 13.6). New fluid is then infused into the abdomen. There may be four to six exchanges of fluid a day. This type of

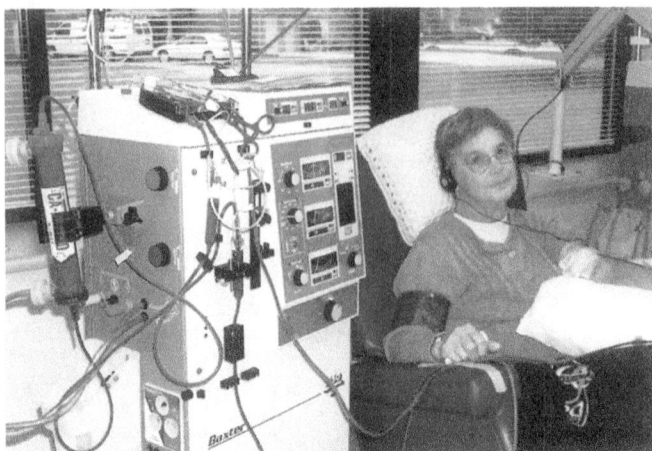

Fig. 13.7 Hemodialysis Machine. (From Ignatavicius DD, Workman ML: *Medical-surgical nursing: critical thinking for collaborative care*, ed 6, Philadelphia, 2011, Saunders.)

dialysis allows the person to work, travel, or sleep during the process.

- *Hemodialysis*: A vascular access (i.e., catheter, arteriovenous [ahr teer ee oh VEE nuhs] graft, arteriovenous fistula) is placed. Using the vascular access, the patient is hooked up to a dialysis machine. The person's blood flows through the special filter inside of the machine (Fig. 13.7). The filter cleans the blood of waste products and extra fluids. Typically, patients need to have hemodialysis three times a week at the dialysis center.

Besides dialysis and kidney transplantation, other treatments include:

- Dietary modifications, such as low protein, limiting fluids, and electrolyte supplements
- Antihypertensive medication and supplements (i.e., iron and vitamin D)

CRITICAL THINKING 13.6

With Hannah's experience in the dialysis unit, she has learned that many people need to do hemodialysis three times a week for several hours each day. How might this affect a patient's lifestyle?

Nephrotic Syndrome

Nephrotic (nah FROT ik) syndrome consists of a collection of symptoms that indicate kidney damage. The syndrome is caused by other disorders that eventually lead to kidney tissue destruction.

Etiology. Nephrotic syndrome occurs more often in males than in females. It can affect children, usually 2 to 6 years of age, and adults. Minimal change disease is the most common cause of nephrotic syndrome in children. Membranous glomerulonephritis is the most common cause in adults. Nephrotic syndrome can also occur as the result of cancer, chronic disease (e.g., diabetes, systemic lupus erythematosus),

infections, immune and genetic disorders, and with certain drugs.

Signs and Symptoms. The most common sign is swelling of the face, extremities, and abdomen. Additional symptoms can include poor appetite, weight gain, seizures, skin sores, and foamy-appearing urine. Blood and urine tests show proteinuria, hyperlipidemia (hie per lip i DEE mee ah), and hypoalbuminemia (hie poh al byoo mi NEE mee ah).

Diagnostic Procedures. Providers will do a physical exam, laboratory testing, and a kidney biopsy. Laboratory work includes:
- Blood testing: Albumin, blood chemistry tests, BUN, creatinine
- Urine testing: Creatinine clearance, urinalysis

Additional testing may be ordered to identify the specific cause of nephrotic syndrome. Infection with the human immunodeficiency virus (HIV), hepatitis, and syphilis are just a few of the diseases that could lead to nephrotic syndrome.

Treatments. The treatment goals are to reduce symptoms, delay kidney damage, and prevent additional complications. Common treatments include:
- Antihypertensive medications to keep the blood pressure in the normal range.
- Vitamin D supplements.
- Corticosteroids, anticoagulants (an tee koe AG UE lants), antihyperlipidemics (an tie hie per lip i DEE mik), and diuretics.
- Dietary modifications, such as low-fat, low-cholesterol, low-salt, and low-protein diets.

VOCABULARY

arteriovenous fistula An abnormal joining of an artery and a vein.

arteriovenous graft A synthetic tube that connects an artery to a vein; also called AV graft.

anticoagulant A substance (i.e., medication or chemical) that prevents clotting of blood.

antihyperlipidemic A substance (i.e., medication) that lowers the lipid levels in the blood.

corticosteroids A group of steroid hormones produced in the body or given as a medication; some have metabolic functions, and others reduce tissue inflammation. Glucocorticoids and mineralocorticoids are two types.

diuretic A substance (i.e., medication) that increases the amount of urine produced.

hyperlipidemia An elevated level of lipids in the blood.

hypoalbuminemia A decreased level of albumin (protein) in the blood.

vascular access A surgical procedure that creates a vein to remove and return blood during the hemodialysis procedure.

Neurogenic Bladder

The central nervous system, nerves that supply the bladder, and muscles work together for bladder control. Damage or disorders that affect the bladder nerves or the central nervous system can cause neurogenic bladder. A person with neurogenic bladder lacks bladder control. The bladder can be overactive or underactive.

The bladder muscles contract uncontrollably with an overactive bladder. This causes urgency and frequency with urination and an inability to control urination. With an underactive bladder, the bladder fills but the person does not have the urge to go. Overfill incontinence (or urine leakage) can occur when the bladder is full.

Etiology. The central nervous system disorders that can cause neurogenic bladder include:
- Birth defects (e.g., spina bifida) and cerebral palsy
- Alzheimer disease and brain or spinal cord tumors
- Multiple sclerosis (MS)
- Parkinson disease
- Stroke and spinal cord injury

Damage and disorders of the bladder nerves can be caused by diabetes, syphilis, heavy alcohol use, neuropathy (nu ROP a thee), and nerve damage from pelvic surgery, herniated disk, or spinal canal stenosis.

Signs and Symptoms. Neurogenic bladder can cause overactive or underactive bladder activity. With an overactive bladder, a person experiences loss of bladder control. Urgency and frequency to urinate are common.

With an underactive bladder, the bladder fills but the person does not have the urge to go. Incontinence or urine leakage can occur with a full bladder. Problems starting to urinate or completely emptying the bladder can also be experienced.

Diagnostic Procedures. Procedures used to help diagnose neurogenic bladder include:
- Postvoid residual volume
- Blood tests to check kidney functioning (i.e., serum creatinine)
- Renal ultrasonography and cystoscopy

Treatments. Treatment is aimed at managing the symptoms of neurogenic bladder. Possible treatments consist of:
- Medications, such as antimuscarinics (AN tee mus kah RIN ik), anticholinergics (AN tee kol i NER jik), botulinum toxin, gamma aminobutyric acid (GABA) supplements, and antiepileptics
- Surgical procedures, including an artificial urinary sphincter, an implanted electronic device to stimulate bladder nerves, and a urinary stoma (STOH mah) (urostomy [yoo ROS te mee])
- Kegel exercises (Box 13.2) and a urinary catheter

> **VOCABULARY**
>
> **neuropathy** A nervous system disorder of the peripheral nerves that causes discomfort, numbness, and weakness, especially in the extremities.
>
> **stoma** A temporary or permanent surgically created opening used for drainage (i.e., urine, stool).
>
> **urostomy** A surgically created opening on the abdominal wall used to drain urine.

> **BOX 13.2 Kegel Exercises**
>
> Kegel exercises are used to strengthen the pelvic floor muscles. Both males and females can do them. To use the right muscles, pretend you have to urinate but hold it. The muscles you tighten to stop urination help tighten the pelvic floor muscles. Muscles in the vagina (for females), rectum, and bladder should tighten. The muscles in the thighs, buttock, and abdomen should not be tightened. Kegel exercises should be done three times a day.
>
> To perform Kegel exercises:
> 1. Empty your bladder.
> 2. You can be sitting or lying down during the exercises.
> 3. Tighten the pelvic floor muscles ("hold the urine"). Tighten as you count to 8.
> 4. Relax the muscles as you count to 10.
> 5. Repeat this sequence 10 times.

> **CRITICAL THINKING 13.7**
>
> Dr. Riney asks Hannah to coach Mrs. Smith on doing Kegel exercises. How might Hannah explain the process of doing Kegels to Mrs. Smith?

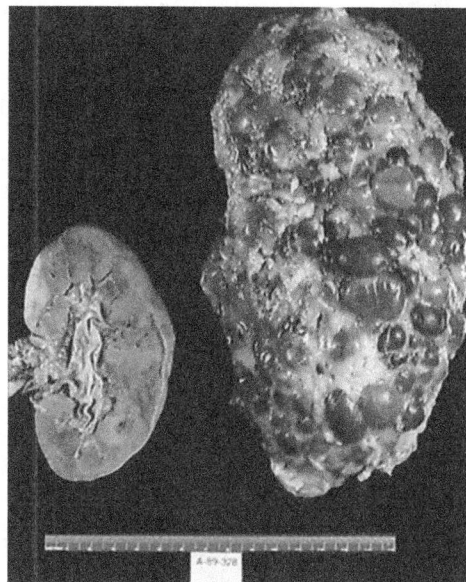

Fig. 13.8 Comparison of a Polycystic Kidney *(Right)* with a Normal Kidney *(Left)*. (From Lewis SM: *Medical-surgical nursing: assessment and management of clinical problems,* ed 8, St. Louis, 2011, Mosby.)

Polycystic Kidney Disease

Polycystic (POL ee sis tik) kidney disease (PKD) is an inherited condition. Cysts form in the kidneys, causing the kidneys to become enlarged (Fig. 13.8). A cyst-filled kidney could weigh up to 30 pounds.

Etiology. There are two types of PKD:
- *Autosomal* (aw toe SOE mal) *dominant*: If the gene is inherited from one parent, the child will get the disease. Often the parent also has the disease. This is the most common form of PKD and also the most common inherited kidney disorder. It is typically identified between the ages of 30 and 50, though it can occur in childhood.

- *Autosomal recessive*: To get the disease a person must get a copy of the defective gene from both parents.

People with PKD may also have cysts in their liver and pancreas. Aneurysms and diverticula of the colon may also be associated with PKD. Males can have cysts in their testes and tend to have more kidney failure. Women with PKD, hypertension, and who have had three or more pregnancies are also more at risk for kidney failure.

Signs and Symptoms. PKD can cause:
- Pain in the flank, abdomen, and joints
- Nocturia and hematuria
- Drowsiness and nail abnormalities
- Pain or tenderness over the liver and an enlarged liver
- Heart murmur and hypertension

Diagnostic Procedures. The provider may order a CT, MRI, and ultrasound (US) may be ordered to check the cysts on the kidneys.

Treatments. PKD is a chronic condition that slowly gets worse. The treatment goals are to control symptoms and prevent complications. Treatment often includes antihypertensive medications, diuretics, and a low-salt diet. PKD can increase the risk of urinary tract infections due to blockages. UTIs should be treated quickly with antibiotics. Surgery to remove one or both kidneys may be required. The patient may also need dialysis or kidney transplantation.

With the chronic nature of this condition, it is important for patients to get support. Sometimes support groups can help the patient and family cope with the disease process.

Pyelonephritis

Pyelonephritis (PIE ah loe ni frie tis) is a urinary tract infection of one or both of the kidneys. Prompt treatment is required to prevent kidney damage and septicemia (sep tih SEE mee ah). The bacteria can spread to the bloodstream, causing an overwhelming infection that can be life-threatening.

Etiology. Like other UTIs, pyelonephritis is caused by a bacterium or virus. The pathogen can move from the bladder to the kidneys, or it can be carried by the bloodstream to the kidneys. An increased risk of pyelonephritis may be seen with structural defects, urinary reflux, obstruction, and bladder infection.

Signs and Symptoms. Pyelonephritis can cause:
- Fever and chills
- Nausea and vomiting
- Dysuria and frequency
- Low back, side (flank), and groin pain
- Blood in urine and foul-smelling urine

The only symptom sometimes seen in infants and young children is the fever. For older adults, confusion and speech difficulties may be present, but other symptoms may not be experienced.

Diagnostic Procedures. After the patient's history has been taken and the physical examination has concluded, the provider

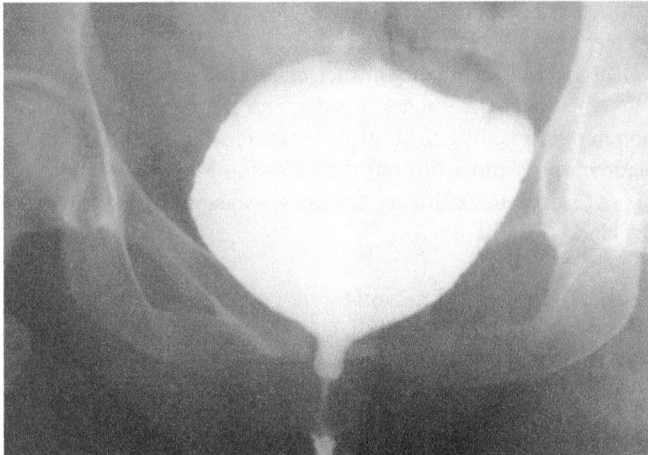

Fig. 13.9 Female Voiding Cystourethrogram (VCUG). (From Bontrager KL: *Textbook of radiographic positioning and related anatomy*, ed 7, St. Louis, 2009, Mosby.)

will usually order a urinalysis, urine culture, blood culture, and blood work. For the most accurate results, all cultures need to be obtained before the patient starts on antibiotics. Additional tests may include a US, CT scan, voiding cystourethrogram (VCUG), digital rectal exam (DRE), and a dimercaptosuccinic acid (DMSA) scan (Fig. 13.9).

Treatments. Initially the provider will treat the infection with a broad-spectrum antibiotic. When the blood and urine culture results are known, the provider may have the patient take an antibiotic that is known to kill the pathogen. For severely ill patients, hospitalization, intravenous fluids and antibiotics, and close observation may be required. Repeat cultures may be taken after the antibiotics have been completed to ensure that the infection is gone.

MEDICAL TERMINOLOGY	
septic/o	infection
bacterium (singular)	bacteria (plural)

Renal Calculi

Renal calculi or kidney stones are mineral pebbles that form in the kidney. Small stones may not cause issues. If they grow larger or move into the ureters or renal pelvis, symptoms can occur (Fig. 13.10). If a stone blocks the flow of urine, infection can develop from the backflow of urine. This blockage also can result in hydronephrosis (Fig. 13.11).

Etiology. Renal calculi can occur when high levels of certain minerals collect in the kidney. Common minerals include calcium, oxalate, and uric acid. Calculi can also form if fluid intake is low and the filtrate becomes highly concentrated. The tendency to develop kidney stones runs in families.

Signs and Symptoms. With small stones, the person may not experience symptoms as the stone passes through the urinary tract. With larger stones or stones that cause blockages, symptoms will be experienced. Kidney stones can cause:

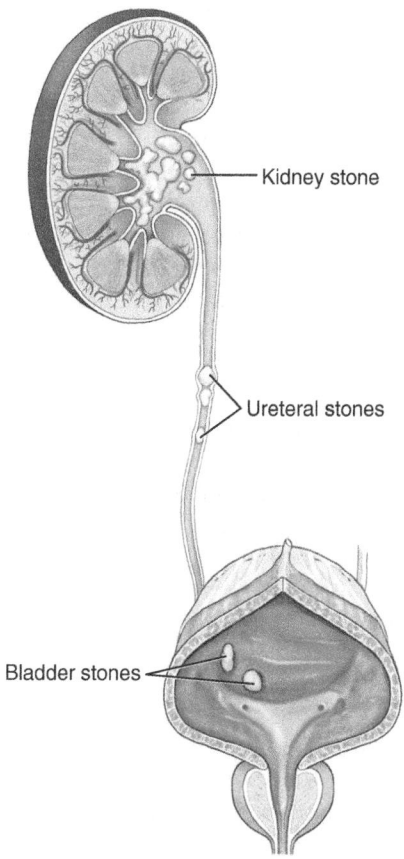

Fig. 13.10 Locations of Ureteral Calculi. (From Shiland B: *Mastering healthcare terminology,* ed 5, St. Louis, 2016, Elsevier.)

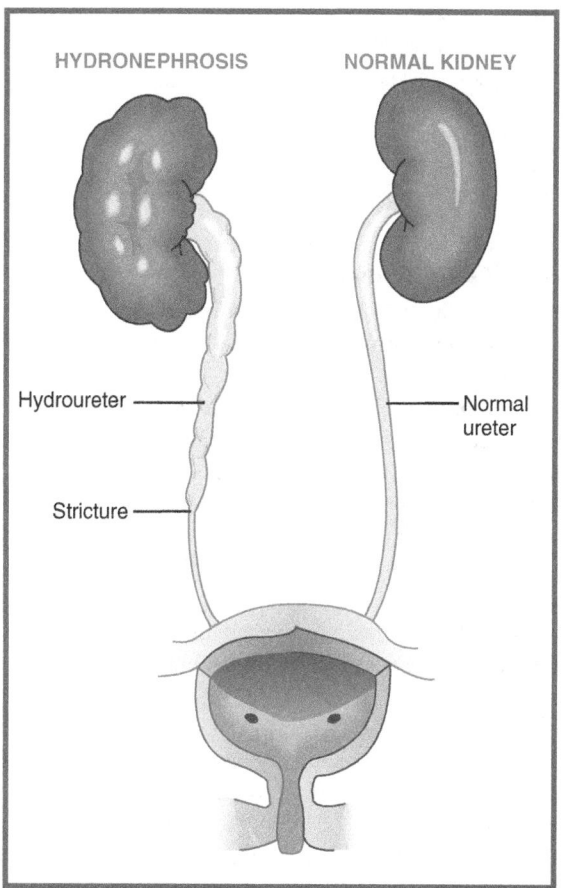

Fig. 13.11 Hydronephrosis. (From Proctor D, et al: *Kinn's the medical assistant,* ed 13, St. Louis, 2017, Elsevier.)

- Severe constant pain on either side of the lower back
- Cloudy, foul-smelling, or bloody urine
- Dysuria
- Nausea and vomiting
- Fever and chills

Diagnostic Procedures. After the medical history has been taken and the physical exam concluded, urine, blood, and imaging tests are used to diagnose renal calculi. Common tests include:

- A urinalysis, which can detect blood and minerals in the urine. White blood cells and bacteria can indicate an infection.
- Blood tests, which can indicate high levels of certain minerals that might be causing the stones.
- An abdominal x-ray, which may be able to show stones, although not all stones are visible, depending on the size and type of stone.
- A CT scan, which is usually done without contrast, although contrast can be used. The CT scan can show the location and size of the stone.

Treatments. Treatment of renal calculi depends on the size, type, and location of the stones. Small stones may pass on their own. Analgesics may be encouraged for the pain and discomfort. Extra fluids are encouraged to flush the stone out. Typically, patients are asked to strain their urine. Kidney stone

strainers should be supplied. If the patient finds a stone, it should be placed in a specimen container and brought to the lab to be analyzed.

If stones are too large to pass or are causing complications, providers will recommend other treatments. *Extracorporeal shock wave lithotripsy* (ESWL) can break up stones in the ureters and kidneys, so they pass without a problem. Ureteroscopy is a common technique to remove stones. The ureteroscope is threaded up through the bladder and ureter. If the provider sees a stone, it can be removed during the procedure. Sometimes ESWL and ureteroscopy are both done. The stone is broken up before it is removed.

For patients who cannot have ESWL or ureteroscopy due to the stone size or other medical conditions, a nephrolithotomy or percutaneous nephrolithotripsy is done.

To prevent future stones, dietary changes are recommended. Based on the type of stones experienced, a dietitian can help identify foods to limit. For the following stones, these dietary changes are recommended:

- Calcium oxalate stones: Reduce sodium, oxalate, and animal protein; consume adequate calcium; oxalate-rich foods include rhubarb, beets, spinach, wheat bran, potato chips, French fries, and nuts.
- Calcium phosphate stones: Reduce sodium and animal protein; consume adequate calcium.
- Uric acid stone: Reduce animal protein.

CRITICAL THINKING 13.8

Hannah receives a call from Zach Backstrom. He states that he has a kidney stone, and he wonders if he really needs to strain his urine and have it analyzed in the lab. What might be the benefits to Zach if he continues to strain his urine for the stones?

Urinary Incontinence

Urinary incontinence (UI) is the loss of bladder control causing an accidental loss of urine. There are several types of urinary incontinence:

- *Stress incontinence*: Leakage of urine from stress on the bladder; caused by obesity, pregnancy, laughing, running, sneezing, coughing, or lifting heavy objects.
- *Urge incontinence*: Also called *overactive bladder*; strong sudden urge (urgency) before the accidental loss of urine.
- *Overflow incontinence*: Most often affects males; the person has difficulty emptying the bladder.
- *Functional incontinence*: Caused by a mental or physical disease; leakage occurs before the person can reach the toilet.
- *Mixed incontinence*: Typically affects females; leakage of urine due to overactive bladder and stress incontinence.
- *Total incontinence*: Severest type; constant urine leakage.
- *Enuresis* (en yoor EE sis): Also known as "bed wetting." Usually seen in children; bladder fills during the night and child does not get up to urinate

Etiology. UI can occur for many reasons, including:
- Damage to the nerves that control the bladder
- Weak or overactive bladder muscles
- Diseases that make moving difficult
- Urethral blockages (i.e., from an enlarged prostate)
- Increase in urine volume: diuretics, alcohol, caffeine, and sweeteners can increase the urine volume
- UTI and constipation

Additional conditions that can lead to persistent incontinence include:
- Pregnancy, childbirth, and menopause: Hormone changes, extra pressure on the bladder, and weakened supportive tissues can lead to UI.
- Pelvic surgery: May cause weakening of the pelvic floor muscles.
- Prostate diseases: Can cause enlargement of the prostate that leads to urinary obstruction.
- Aging: With age, the bladder capacity for storing urine decreases.
- Obstructions: Any conditions that cause an obstruction in the urinary flow.
- Neurologic disorders: Can limit the nerve signals from the brain to the bladder.

Signs and Symptoms. Symptoms include accidental leakage of urine. Based on the type of urinary incontinence, the person may have urgency, constant dribbling, and an inability to empty the bladder completely.

Diagnostic Procedures. Procedures used to diagnose incontinence include:
- Urinalysis to check for abnormalities.
- A bladder diary. The patient records the amount drank, urinated, number of incontinence episodes, and frequency and urgency feelings.
- Postvoid residual measurement.
- *Urodynamic testing*, which consists of filling the bladder with water via a catheter while the bladder pressure is measured.
- Cystoscopy, cystogram, and pelvic ultrasound.

Treatments. Treatments can vary based on the type of incontinence. Behavior techniques recommended include:
- Bladder training (timed delay in urination after feeling the urge)
- Double voiding (attempting to empty the bladder more completely)
- Scheduling toilet trips
- Managing fluids and diet to regain control
- Maintaining a healthy weight
- Practicing Kegel exercises
- Avoiding caffeine and alcohol

Medications can be used as part of the treatment. Anticholinergics, mirabegron, alpha-blockers, Botox, and topical estrogen can be used for incontinence. Surgical procedures can be performed to treat certain types of incontinence.

Medical devices can also be used as treatment, including:
- *Urethral insert*: A disposable device is inserted into the urethra before activities that trigger incontinence.
- *Pessary*: A stiff ring is inserted into the vagina that holds up the bladder; used for incontinence due to prolapsed bladder.
- *Nerve stimulator*: An implanted device delivers electrical pulses to the nerves that control the bladder.

Additional Urinary System Diseases

There are several urinary system diseases.

- *Acute tubular necrosis*: Rapid destruction of the tubular sections of the nephrons due to blood flow impairment or toxins.
- *Bladder outlet obstruction* (BOO): Blockage at the opening of the bladder or in the urethra.
- *Hydronephrosis*: Distention of the renal pelvis and calyces due to urinary tract obstruction; caused by a congenital defect or renal calculi.
- *Interstitial cystitis* (IC): Causes recurring bladder and pelvic region pain and discomfort, frequency, and urgency. Also called *painful bladder syndrome* (PBS).
- *Membranous glomerulonephritis*: Inflammation occurs in the kidney due to glomerular changes, and large amounts of protein are excreted in the urine. The exact etiology is unknown.
- *Minimal change disease*: Damage occurs to the glomeruli, though the cause is unknown.
- *Nocturnal enuresis*: Bladder fills up during the night and the child is in too deep of a sleep to get up to urinate; can run in families. Also called *bed wetting*.
- *Prune belly syndrome* (PBS): Group of genetic birth defects usually occurring in boys; involves enlarged ureters and

bladder, hydronephrosis (kidney swelling), poor development of the abdominal muscles, undescended testicles, and wrinkled skin over the abdomen.

- *Reflux nephropathy*: Urine backflows from the bladder, causing kidney damage. Can be due to a ureter defect, obstruction, or swelling.
- *Ureterocele*: End of ureter is malformed and bulges, creating an ureterocele, and may obstruct the ureter or bladder.
- *Ureteropelvic junction* (UPJ) *obstruction*: Blockage where the ureter joins the kidney, causing kidney swelling.
- *Urethritis*: Inflammation of the urethra due to bacteria, viruses, injury, or chemical sensitivity.
- *Vesicoureteral* (ves ih koe yoo REE tur ul) *reflux* (VUR): Urine backs up into the ureter from the bladder due to a malformed or missing valve over the end of the ureter.

LIFE SPAN CHANGES

At about 10 to 12 weeks after conception, the kidneys start producing urine. While the baby is in utero, the mother's placenta performs most of the kidneys' function until the last few weeks before birth. When babies are born, they have the same number of nephrons as an adult. The nephrons are immature and mature by age 2. A baby's kidneys do not retain water like adult kidneys do. Thus babies can lose water quickly, especially when they are hot or if they have diarrhea. During childhood, the bladder continues to grow. Bladder control is learned usually between the ages of 2 and 3.

During the adult years, males are more likely to develop kidney stones. This may be attributed to the amount of food they eat. They need to drink more water than females to clear the waste products from the body. Male kidneys also have an increased ability to concentrate urine, a risk factor for kidney stones. Females are at more risk for urinary tract infections than are males. This is attributed to the anatomic differences. Most UTIs are caused by *Escherichia coli,* which is found near the vagina and rectum. The closeness of the urethra to these structures and the shortness of the urethra increase the risk of UTIs.

During pregnancy, the filtration rate increases in females. The number of nephrons remains the same, but the filtration surface increases. This increase allows the kidneys to filter more blood, which is useful with the increased blood flow during pregnancy. In late pregnancy, the bladder may be twice as big. The anatomic and physiologic changes that occur during pregnancy put females at more risk for pyelonephritis at that time.

In older adults, the kidney tissue and number of nephrons are reduced up to 20%. The renal arteries can harden. This causes the kidneys to filter blood more slowly. The kidneys become less able to regulate water balance. Older adults are at more risk of dehydration when the weather is hot or if they have diarrhea. The bladder wall becomes less stretchy with age. The bladder cannot hold as much urine as before. Bladder muscles weaken. The urethra may be obstructed by an enlarged prostate gland or a prolapse of the bladder or vagina. Older adults are at more risk for chronic kidney disease, UTIs, and incontinence.

CLOSING COMMENTS

For medical assistants working in the ambulatory care field, assisting patients with urinary disorders is common. It is important for the medical assistant to be familiar with the pronunciation and spelling of medical terminology. Many healthcare providers will use common abbreviations when documenting or talking with other healthcare professionals. It is critical that you know what the abbreviations stand for so that miscommunication does not occur.

Remember, patients may not be aware of what an abbreviation or a medical term means. It is very important that, when working with patients, medical assistants explain the meaning of commonly used terminology and abbreviations. If patients can understand what is being discussed, they will be more comfortable and adhere to the treatment plan. In addition to medical terminology and abbreviations, medical assistants need to understand:

- The basics of the urinary system (e.g., urinary structures)
- The important roles that the urinary system plays to maintain the homeostasis of the body
- The diseases that affect the urinary system

Having this understanding will help you provide great care to your patients. It will also help you recognize the importance of the different treatments ordered by providers.

Box 13.3 lists medication classifications commonly used to treat urinary system disorders.

BOX 13.3 Medication Classifications

- *Alpha-blockers*: Relax bladder neck and prostate muscles, make it easier to empty the bladder; used to treat urge or overflow incontinence
- *Anticholinergics* (AN tee kol i NER jik): Stimulate the bladder to contract, which helps urination; used to treat overactive bladder and urge incontinence
- *Antimuscarinics* (AN tee mus kah RIN ik): Relax bladder muscles and reduce bladder contractions
- *Beta-3 adrenergic agonists*: Relax the bladder muscles to prevent urgent, frequent, or uncontrolled urination; used to treat urge incontinence

Refer to Appendix D, which can be found on the Evolve website, for information on the medication classifications, including indications for use, desired effect, side effects, adverse reactions, and generic and trade names. Medical assistants should be familiar with medications that are prescribed to patients.

PATIENT-CENTERED CARE

Respecting a patient's preference is a key element of patient-centered care. When a medical assistant gathers a medical history on a patient regarding a male reproductive or a urology concern, the patient may hesitate to give information. These topics are sensitive, and the patient may only want to discuss concerns with the provider. Telling the patient, "If you would rather share the information with the provider, I will let them know" can show sensitivity. It is important for the medical assistant to respect the patient's wishes and help put the patient at ease.

BEING PROFESSIONAL

A urology practice manages many sensitive patient issues that require strict adherence to confidentiality guidelines. The Health Insurance Portability and Accountability Act of 1996 (HIPAA) protects the patient's confidential information, not just the paper or electronic records of that information. This means that verbal disclosure of a patient's information is limited to only the personnel who have the right to that information according to individual state laws.

Role-play this scenario: You and Sam are medical assistants. You have just finished rooming Mr. Brown, who is a frequent patient in the urology department. Sam asks you why Mr. Brown is being seeing today. Respond to Sam in a respectful, professional manner, yet protecting the patient's confidential information.

CHAPTER REVIEW

The urinary system is composed of two kidneys, two ureters, a bladder, and a urethra. The role of the urinary system is to filter the blood and eliminate the waste through urine. The urine moves down the ureters from the kidneys. The bladder stores the urine until it is excreted from the body via the urethra.

Through complex processes the kidney can save or excrete substances, including electrolytes and water. This helps the body maintain homeostasis. The nephrons in the kidney are responsible for filtering the blood and maintaining homeostasis. One end of the nephron is the renal corpuscle, and the rest of the nephron is the tubule. The renal corpuscle includes the glomerulus, which is inside the Bowman capsule. The pressure of the blood in the glomerulus helps push the substances past the thin walls and into the Bowman capsule. This is the filtration process.

From there, the filtrate moves through the proximal tubule and the Henle loop. During this time, the reabsorption process occurs as substances move from the filtrate back to the blood. Water, glucose, amino acids, urea, and electrolytes (i.e., sodium, chloride, and phosphate) move to the blood. The secretion process also starts as urea moves from the blood to the filtrate to maintain homeostasis. This occurs in the Henle loop. As the filtrate moves farther along the tubule, through the distal tubule and collecting duct, the reabsorption and secretion processes continue. Antidiuretic hormone helps more water to be reabsorbed in these structures. Sodium and chloride are also reabsorbed. The body rids itself of extra substances (e.g., ammonium, potassium, and hydrogen) as the final secretion processes occur. Once the filtrate moves past the collecting ducts, it enters the calyces and renal pelvis. These are extensions of the ureter inside the kidney. The urine then goes into the ureter, bladder, and urethra before it is excreted from the body.

Urinary diseases were also discussed in this chapter. Common etiologies include age, genetics, and congenital abnormalities, in addition to viral, bacterial, and other diseases. Common signs and symptoms of urinary disease include pain, nocturia, dysuria, hematuria, frequency, and urgency. Typical diagnostic tests ordered include a digital rectal examination, cystoscopy, ureteroscopy, CT, dimercaptosuccinic acid (DMSA) scan, IVP, postvoid residual urine test, US, voiding cystourethrogram, BUN test, urinalysis, and urine culture. The urinalysis is a CLIA-waived test.

The urinary system changes with age. The kidneys start to function 10 to 12 weeks after conception and mature by age 2. Adult males are more prone to kidney stones, and females are at more risk for UTIs. In older adults, the kidneys become less able to regulate water balance. The bladder muscles weaken, and the urethra can be obstructed by other organs (e.g., the prostate).

SCENARIO WRAP-UP

When Hannah started working with the urology team, she realized she knew very little about the urinary system. She had studied it during her medical assistant program, but she never appreciated what it might be like if her kidneys did not work. She was familiar with kidney cancer and UTIs, but she was amazed at all of the other urinary diseases. As she learned more, she realized that hypertension (high blood pressure) could lead to kidney disease. She also figured out that kidney disease could lead to hypertension.

Looking back over the last weeks, Hannah realized that one of her favorite experiences was working with Mr. Rodgers. He had been on dialysis for the past 5 years and never had a vacation. He wanted to see his new grandson, who lived on the East Coast. Hannah found a dialysis unit in the city where he was going to stay. She was able to get him scheduled for 2 weeks' worth of dialysis during his stay. She still can recall Mr. Rodgers' excitement when he realized he could do dialysis while on vacation. He started talking about other trips he was dreaming of taking.

Hannah is excited to continue her work with the urology team. She has learned so much in the short time she has worked with the patients.

Reproductive System

LEARNING OBJECTIVES

1. Identify the anatomic location of the major organs of the male reproductive systems.
2. Describe the normal function of the male reproductive systems.
3. Describe common male reproductive system disorders, including common signs and symptoms, etiology, diagnostic procedures, and treatments.
4. Identify the anatomic location of the major organs of the female reproductive systems.
5. Describe the normal function of the female reproductive systems.
6. Describe the changes that occur with pregnancy and intrauterine development.
7. Describe common female reproductive system disorders, including common signs and symptoms, etiology, diagnostic procedures, and treatments.
8. Describe disorders related to pregnancy, including common signs and symptoms, etiology, diagnostic procedures, and treatments.
9. Describe sexually transmitted infections, including common signs and symptoms, etiology, diagnostic procedures, and treatments.
10. Compare the structure and function of the male and female reproductive systems across the life span.

OUTLINE

⟫ OPENING SCENARIO

Marie Rodríguez, CMA (AAMA), has been working at Walden-Martin Family Medical (WMFM) Clinic. She was hired at WMFM Clinic shortly after passing her CMA exam 4 years ago. She has recently accepted a position helping the obstetrics/gynecology (OB/GYN) outreach providers. Marie will still work with the family medicine providers when the outreach providers are not at the clinic.

As a medical assistant over the last 4 years, Marie has worked with patients who have had reproductive disorders. Both male and female patients with reproductive system concerns are commonly seen in family medicine. Marie anticipates that her new position will allow her to learn more about pregnancy, pregnancy disorders, and infertility. She is excited to expand her knowledge in these areas. As she learns her new position, she has an opportunity to shadow with the medical assistants who assist the OB/GYN providers.

YOU WILL LEARN

1. To recognize and use terms related to the male and female reproductive systems and pregnancy.
2. To locate the male and female reproductive system structures.
3. To recognize disease states of the reproductive system, in addition to their causes, signs and symptoms, diagnostic processes, treatment, prognoses, and prevention.
4. To recognize disease states related to pregnancy and also their causes, signs and symptoms, diagnostic processes, treatment, prognoses, and prevention.

INTRODUCTION

Obstetrics (awb STE triks) is the branch of medicine that deals with pregnancy, labor, and the postpartum period. *Gynecology* (gy neh KAW loh jee) is the study of the female reproductive system. Providers who treat patients with reproductive conditions include:

- *Urologists* (yoor AW loh jist): Medical doctors who specialize in male reproductive disorders, along with female and male urinary system disorders.
- *Obstetricians* (awb steh TRIH shun): Medical doctors who treat women during pregnancy, deliver infants, and follow women through the postpartum period.
- *Gynecologists* (gy neh KAW loh jist): Medical doctors who diagnose and treat female reproductive system diseases. Often times, a provider practices both obstetrics and gynecology and is known as an OB/GYN provider.
- *Nurse midwives* or *certified nurse midwives* (CNMs): Healthcare providers who assist women through pregnancy, labor, and delivery.
- *Doula* (DOO lah): A woman who assists another woman during labor and delivery. She may also provide support to the family after childbirth.

Male and Female Reproductive Systems

The male reproductive system is responsible for producing, transporting, and sustaining sperm cells. The female reproductive system is responsible for producing, transporting, and sustaining egg cells. It also needs to nurture the developing offspring. Both male and female reproductive systems produce hormones.

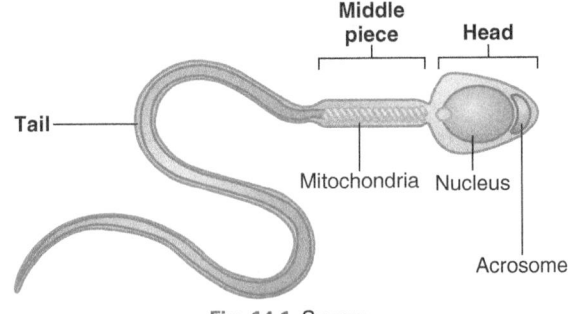

Fig. 14.1 Sperm.

The egg and sperm cells are called *sex cells* or gametes (GAM eets). Each of these sex cells contributes half of the genes of the new offspring. The gametes are produced in organs called gonads (GOH nads). Gonads are considered primary or *essential sex organs*. They are also responsible for producing hormones. The other organs in the reproductive systems are secondary or *accessory organs*.

The anatomy, physiology, and disorders of the male reproductive system will be discussed in the following sections. The discussion of the female reproductive system and pregnancy will follow.

> **VOCABULARY**
> **gamete** A mature sexual reproductive cell; spermatozoon or ovum.
> **gonad** Organs that produce sex cells in both males and females.

ANATOMY OF THE MALE REPRODUCTIVE SYSTEMS

The primary reproductive organs in the male are the testes (TESS teez). Each testis is oval and measures about 1.6 inches (4 cm) long and 1 inch (2.5 cm) wide. The testes are surrounded by a white, fibrous capsule and are suspended together in a sac outside the body called the *scrotum* (SKROH tum). Testes produce the gametes called spermatozoa (spur mat ah ZOH ah). Spermatozoa are made up of three parts (Fig. 14.1):

- *Head*: Contains the chromosomes in the nucleus; the acrosome covers the head of the sperm and contains enzymes to help penetrate the ovum.
- *Midpiece*: Contains mitochondria, which produce energy for movement.
- *Tail* or *flagellum* (flah JEL um): Used for movement.

The formation of sperm is called *spermatogenesis* (spur mat toh JEN ih sis). The spermatozoa are formed in a series of tightly coiled tiny tubes in each testis called the *seminiferous tubules* (sem ih NIFF ur us TOO byools). From the seminiferous tubules, the formed spermatozoa travel to the *epididymis* (eh pih DID ih mis), where they mature and are stored. The epididymis is a coiled tube that is almost 20 feet (6 meters) long and rests on top of and behind each testis.

From the epididymis, the spermatozoa move into the *vas deferens* (vas DEH fur ens) or *ductus deferens* (DUCK tus DEH fur ens) (Fig. 14.2). Each vas deferens is a muscular tunnel about 18 inches (45 cm) long that connects to the base of the epididymis

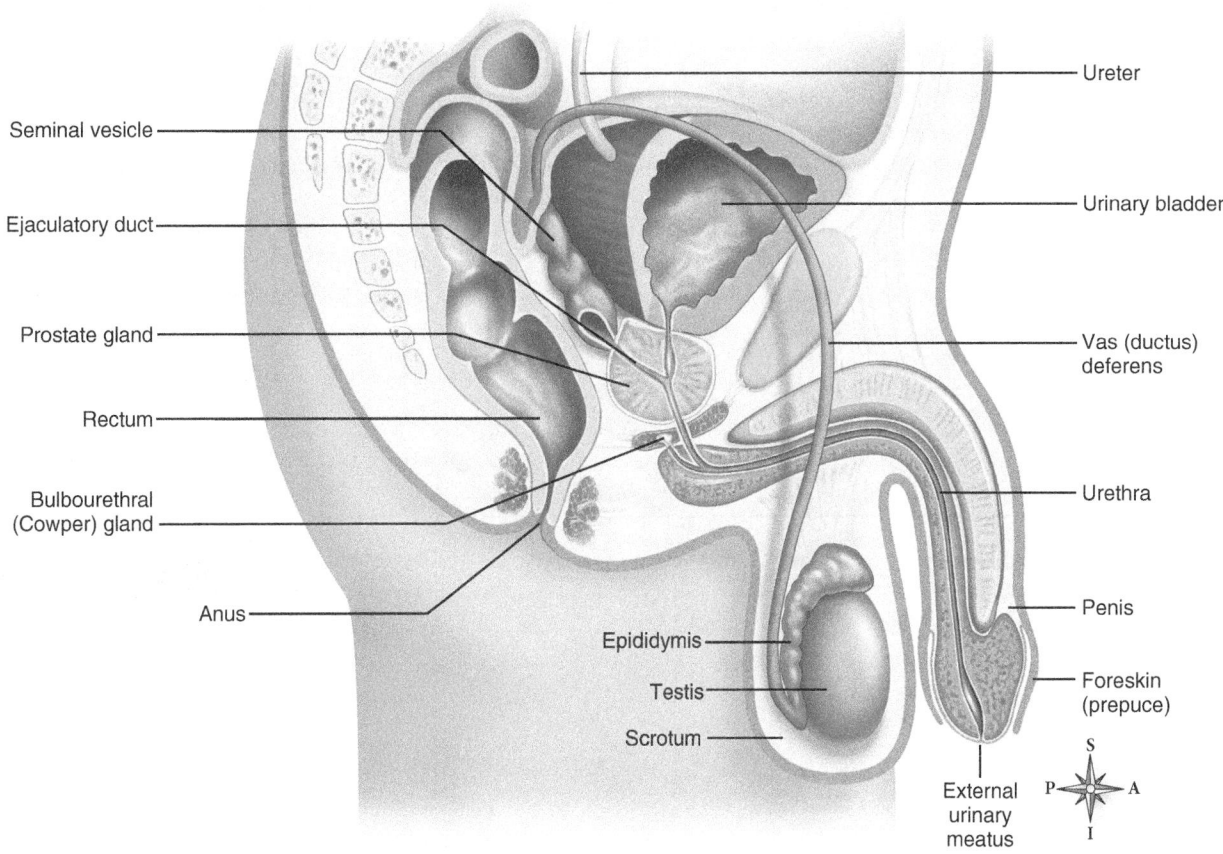

Fig. 14.2 Male Reproductive System. Sagittal section of pelvis showing locations of male reproductive organs. (From Patton KT, Thibodeau GA: *The human body in health and disease*, ed 7, St. Louis, 2018, Elsevier.)

and passes along the side of the testis. The vas deferens travels into the pelvic cavity to just behind the bladder. Spermatozoa can stay in the vasa deferentia for several months in an inactive state.

The *prostate* (PROS tate) *gland* is the size of a walnut and is found below the bladder in males. It surrounds part of the urethra. The prostate is considered a reproductive organ, but it also affects the urinary system. When the prostate increases in size (as with benign prostatic hyperplasia [BPH]), it can obstruct the urethra, blocking the urine flow.

The prostate gland, *seminal vesicles* (SEM ih nul VESS ih kuls), and *Cowper glands* (or bulbourethral glands) provide fluid either to nourish or to aid in motility and lubrication. The sperm and the fluid together make up a substance called *semen.* The ejaculatory (ee JACK yoo lah tore ee) duct begins where the seminal vesicles join the vas deferens, and this "tube" joins the urethra. The urethra is found within the penis and transports the semen to the outside of the body. The urethra also transports urine to the outside of the body. The semen exits the body through the tip of the penis, the *glans penis.* At birth, the glans penis is surrounded by a fold of skin called the *prepuce* or *foreskin,* which can be removed by circumcision.

MEDICAL TERMINOLOGY

epididym/o	epididymis
gonad/o	gonad
gynec/o	female
phall/o	penis
semin/i	semen
scrot/o	scrotum
spermat/o	spermatozoon
test/o, testicul/o, orchi/o, orchid/o, orch/o	testis, testicle
vas/o	vas deferens, ductus deferens
vesicul/o	seminal vesicles
-ferous	pertaining to carrying
-genesis	production
-logist	one who specializes in the study of
spermatozoon (singular)	spermatozoa (plural)
testis (singular)	testes (plural)
vas deferens (singular)	vasa deferentia (plural)

VOCABULARY
spermatozoa Mature male reproductive cells.
testes Male gonads; also called testicles.

CRITICAL THINKING 14.1

Describe the process of spermatogenesis, including all of the structures needed from the formation of the sperm until it leaves the body in semen.

TABLE 14.1   Common Diagnostic Procedures Used for Male Reproductive Disorders

Done by/Type of Test	Procedure	Description
Provider during the exam	Digital rectal examination (DRE)	Done during the physical exam. The provider inserts a gloved, lubricated finger into the rectum to feel for abnormalities in the prostate, bladder, and so on.
	Testicular exam	Done during the physical exam. The provider will check the penis, scrotum, and testicles for lumps, swelling, and other abnormalities.
Surgical procedure	Biopsy	Used to remove samples from the testicles, prostate, and other organs.
Imaging procedures	Ultrasound (US)	• *Scrotal/testicular ultrasound:* Used to examine the testicles and supporting structures. • *Transrectal ultrasound:* Used to exam the prostate, ejaculatory ducts, and seminal vesicles.
	Magnetic resonance imaging (MRI)	Used to evaluate structural abnormalities and tumors in the male reproductive system.
Medical laboratory	Hormone testing	Blood tests to measure the levels of testosterone and other hormones.
	Prostate-specific antigen (PSA)	Blood test used as a screening tool for prostate cancer.
	Semen analysis	Measures the number of sperm present. Provides information on any abnormalities in *motility* (movement) and *morphology* (shape) of the sperm.

TABLE 14.2   Common Treatments Used for Male Reproductive Disorders

Procedure	Description
Circumcision (sur kum SIH zhun)	Surgical removal of the foreskin (or *prepuce*) of the penis.
Laser therapy	A high-energy laser is used to destroy overgrown tissues, such as prostate tissue.
Prostatectomy (pras tah TEK tah mee)	Removal of the prostate. With a *radical prostatectomy*, the prostate and nearby lymph nodes and nearby tissue including the seminal vesicles are removed.
Orchidectomy (or kih DECK tuh mee)	Removal of the testicle.
Orchiopexy (or kee oh PECK see)	Surgical procedure for an undescended testicle (cryptorchidism). The testicle is brought down and implanted in the scrotum.
Transurethral resection of the prostate (TURP) surgery	A lighted scope is inserted into the urethra, and all but the outer part of the prostate is removed.
Vasectomy (vas SECK tuh mee)	A surgical procedure in which the vasa deferentia are cut, tied, and cauterized for the purpose of male sterilization.

PHYSIOLOGY OF THE MALE REPRODUCTIVE SYSTEMS

At puberty, the interstitial cells in the testicles begin to produce testosterone (tess TOS tuh rohn). Testosterone is responsible for maintaining reproductive structures and for the development of sperm cells. Testosterone also helps with the development of secondary sex characteristics, which include the deep voice, broad shoulders, narrow hips, and additional body hair.

In addition to testosterone, *follicle-stimulating hormone* (FSH), which is secreted by the pituitary gland, promotes the formation of spermatozoa. The pituitary gland also produces *luteinizing hormone* (LOO tee nahyz ing) (LH), which stimulates the interstitial cells to produce testosterone.

Under the influence of these hormones, sperm cells develop and move into the epididymis to mature. As described in the anatomy section, eventually the sperm reach the urethra and travel through the shaft, or body, of the penis. The penis is composed of three columns of highly vascular erectile tissue. There are two columns of *corpora cavernosa* and one of *corpus spongiosum* that fill with blood through the dorsal veins during sexual arousal. During ejaculation, the sperm exit through the glans penis.

VOCABULARY

interstitial cells Testosterone-secreting cells of the testes that are found in the spaces between the seminiferous tubules.

puberty The stage of life in which males and females become functionally capable of sexual reproduction.

testosterone Male sex hormone produced by the interstitial cells in the testes.

DISEASES AND DISORDERS OF THE MALE REPRODUCTIVE SYSTEM

Common male reproductive disorder signs and symptoms include redness, swelling, or lumps in the organs. Changes in the urinary stream or issues during sexual intercourse *(copulation)* can also be seen.

Tables 14.1 and 14.2 provided common diagnostic procedures and treatments used for male reproductive disorders. The following sections discuss male reproductive disorders.

Benign Prostatic Hyperplasia

Benign prostatic hyperplasia, also called an enlarged prostate, is a nonmalignant condition. This condition is seen in about half of men over the age of 50 and in more than 90% of men in their 70s and 80s.

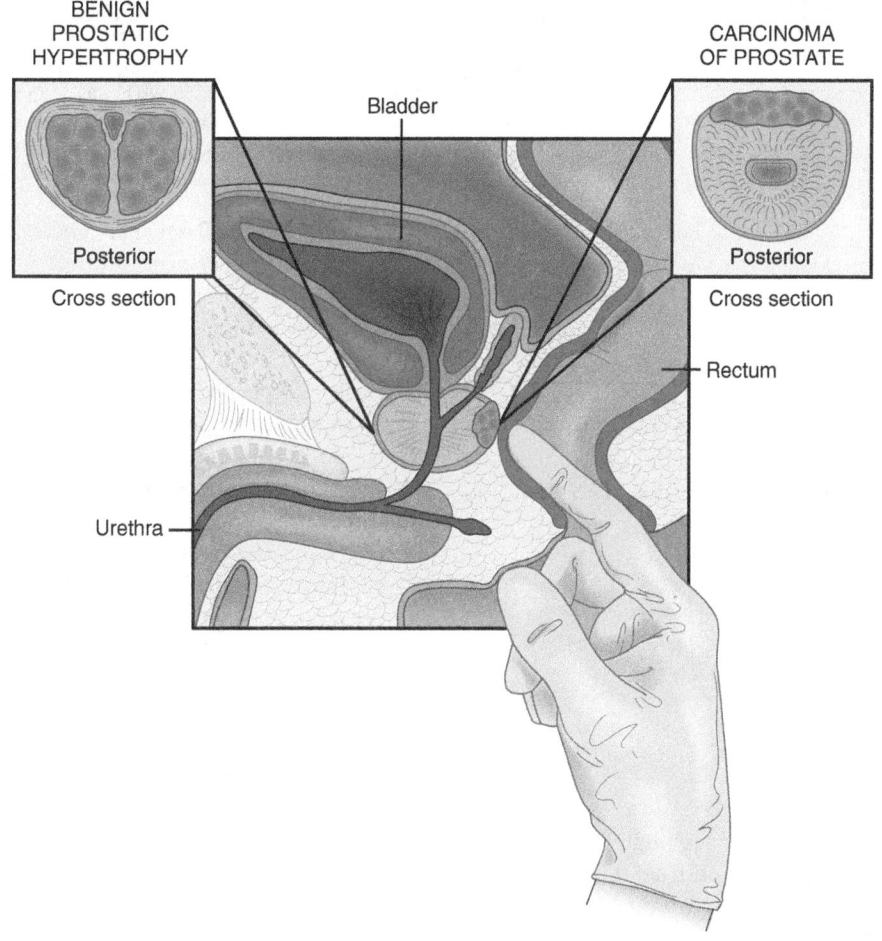

BENIGN PROSTATIC HYPERTROPHY

Posterior

Cross section

CARCINOMA OF PROSTATE

Posterior

Cross section

Bladder

Rectum

Urethra

Fig. 14.3 Digital Rectal Exam (DRE).

Etiology. As men age, the cells of the prostate gland that surround the urethra can start to reproduce more rapidly, causing the organ to enlarge *(hyperplasia)*. The enlarged prostate compresses the urethra, leading to the signs and symptoms.

Signs and Symptoms. With BPH, men can have:
- Urinary urgency and frequency
- Difficulty starting urination, urine retention, and dribbling
- Hematuria and repeated urinary tract infections (UTIs)

> **VOCABULARY**
> **frequency** Urination at short periods without an increase in the daily volume of urine output.
> **urgency** The sudden, almost uncontrollable need to urinate.

Diagnostic Procedures. During the physical exam, the provider will do a digital rectal exam (DRE) by inserting a gloved finger into the rectum to palpate the prostate (Fig. 14.3). Additional tests to diagnose BPH include:
- Blood tests, such as prostate-specific antigen (PSA) and tests of kidney function (Box 14.1)
- Urinalysis, transrectal biopsy, and urodynamic tests
- Transrectal biopsy and a cystoscopy

> **BOX 14.1 Prostate-Specific Antigen Blood Test**
>
> The prostate-specific antigen (PSA) blood test is used as a screening tool for prostate cancer. Both normal and cancerous prostate cells make the protein PSA. Often PSA levels increase in the blood with prostate cancer, prostatitis, and benign prostatic hypertrophy (BPH). It is recommended for males to have a baseline PSA test at the age of 40. If the patient has an increased risk, the provider may decide to get a baseline PSA test earlier than age 40. The provider then checks the PSA level over time by comparing it to the baseline level. The higher the PSA level, the more likely it is that the patient has prostate cancer. However, because the PSA level can be elevated with other disorders, one abnormal screening value is not enough to diagnose cancer. The reliability of the PSA blood test is debated, but it is the only screening tool available at this time.

Treatments. Treatments may focus on lifestyle changes, including bladder training, avoiding caffeine and alcohol, and preventing constipation. Laser therapy and *transurethral resection of the prostate* (TURP) *surgery* are also used. Medications can be used alone or in combination with other treatments. Medications typically used include:
- *Alpha-blockers*: Relax the smooth muscles of the prostate and the bladder neck to improve urine flow and reduce the blockage. Examples include terazosin (ter AY zoe sin), doxazosin (dox AY zoe sin) (Cardura), tamsulosin (tam SOO loe sin) (Flomax), alfuzosin (al FYOO zoe sin) (Uroxatral), and silodosin (sye lo DOE sin) (Rapaflo).

- *5-Alpha reductase inhibitors*: Prevent growth of or shrinks the prostate. Examples include finasteride (fi NAS teer ide) (Proscar, Propecia) and dutasteride (doo TAS teer ide) (Avodart).

CRITICAL THINKING 14.2

Marie is working with Mr. Endl, who has BPH. He asks Marie why the BPH affects his urine flow. How should she respond to Mr. Endl?

Cancer

Prostate Cancer. Prostate cancer is the most common cancer among males, and the survival rate is very high. With prostate cancer, the gland can increase in size, obstruct the urethra, and cause additional urinary complications. About 1 in 8 men will be diagnosed with prostate cancer.

Etiology. Cells in the prostate gland mutate, causing the cancer. The risk for prostate cancer is increased in men over 60 years of age, African Americans, or those with a family history of the disease. Having a brother or father with the disease doubles the risk. The risk for the aggressive form of prostate cancer is increased in men who are tall, obese, lack exercise, have a family history of the disease, are African American, consume a high intake of calcium, and have been exposed to Agent Orange (Box 14.2).

Signs and Symptoms. Prostate cancer tends to be a silent disease in the early stages. It is not until the cancer grows large enough to obstruct the urethra that symptoms are noticeable. With advanced prostate cancer, signs and symptoms include:

- Problems with urination: slow, weak stream; frequency, nocturia
- Hematuria, blood in the semen
- Difficulty getting an erection
- Hip pain, back pain
- Loss of bladder or bowel control

Diagnostic Procedures. The provider completes a DRE during the examination, and a PSA blood test is done. If the DRE is abnormal or the PSA blood test level has increased from the baseline, a needle biopsy of the prostate may be done. If cancer is detected, additional imaging tests will be ordered to determine the extent of the cancer.

Treatments. Treatment will be based on the type of prostate cancer. With nonaggressive cancers, the provider may suggest frequent checks to monitor the cancer growth. For aggressive prostate cancers, a prostatectomy and radiation may be done.

CRITICAL THINKING 14.3

Marie is rooming Sam Fox, a 40-year-old father of three children. He is 6 feet tall. When Marie obtains a family history on Sam, she learns that his father, a Vietnam veteran, was just diagnosed with aggressive prostate cancer. What risk factors does Sam have for prostate cancer?

Testicular Cancer. Testicular cancer is rare and highly treatable. About 1 in 250 males will get testicular cancer. It is the most common cancer in males between 15 and 35 years of age. Males between these ages are recommended to do a monthly testicular self-exam (TSE) to help identify abnormalities. The TSE will be explained in Chapter 41.

Etiology. Many causes of testicular cancer are unknown. It is more common in men who had abnormal testicle development, an undescended testicle, and a family history of the cancer.

Signs and Symptoms. Men may experience:

- Swelling or a lump in the testicle
- A heavy sensation in the scrotum
- Pain in a testicle, the scrotum, abdomen, and groin

Diagnostic Procedures. To determine if a lump is testicular cancer, a provider may order:

- Ultrasound and a computed tomography (CT) scan
- Biopsy of testicular tissue
- Blood tests to check the testicular cancer markers (alpha fetoprotein [AFP], beta human chorionic gonadotropin [beta-hCG], and lactate dehydrogenase [LDH])

Treatments. Treatment consists of a radical inguinal orchiectomy, radiation therapy, and chemotherapy.

Erectile Dysfunction

Erectile dysfunction (ED), also called *impotence,* occurs when a male has trouble keeping or getting an erection. ED is an ongoing issue that can impact relations, affect the male's self-confidence, and cause stress.

Etiology. Common conditions that lead to ED include heart disease, hypertension, tobacco use, alcoholism, diabetes, metabolic syndrome, Parkinson disease, prior pelvic surgeries and treatments, obesity, depression, and stress. Male arousal involves hormones, emotions, muscles, blood vessels, nerves, and the brain; thus any change in these may lead to ED.

Signs and Symptoms. The sign of ED is trouble keeping or getting an erection firm enough for intercourse.

Diagnostic Procedures. After the physical exam, the provider may order tests to identify the cause of ED.

Treatments. Treatment consists of a healthy lifestyle. Oral erectile dysfunction medications can also be prescribed, such as:

- Avanafil (a VAN a fil) (Stendra)
- Sildenafil (sil DEN a fil) (Viagra, Revatio)
- Tadalafil (tah DA la fil) (Adcirca, Cialis)
- Vardenafil (var DEN a fil) (Levitra, Staxyn)

Male Infertility

Infertility is defined as not getting pregnant after 1 year or longer of unprotected sex. In about one-third of couples dealing with infertility issues, the cause is male infertility.

Etiology. In about half of the male infertility cases, the cause is unknown. Known causes of infertility include infections, undescended testicles, inherited disorder, dilated veins around the testicle *(varicocele)*, hormone imbalances, and blockages preventing sperm movement. Sperm production can be affected by heat, chemicals, and toxins (e.g., heavy metals, industrial chemicals). Stress, depression, and using drugs, alcohol, and nicotine can also cause infertility.

Signs and Symptoms. The main sign is not being able to conceive a child. Other signs and symptoms can include problems with sexual function, testicular swelling or pain, recurring respiratory infections, an inability to smell, low sperm counts, and decreased body and facial hair.

Diagnostic Procedures. The provider will do a complete medical history and physical exam. Additional diagnostic testing includes a semen analysis, hormone testing, testicular biopsy, and scrotal and transrectal ultrasounds.

Treatments. Treatments depend on the cause of infertility. Treatments may include surgery, antibiotics to treat an infection, hormone treatments, and assisted reproductive technology (ART), such as in vitro fertilization.

> **VOCABULARY**
>
> **in vitro fertilization** An assisted reproductive technology procedure that involves removing mature eggs from the ovaries and fertilizing the eggs with sperm outside of the body. The fertilized eggs are then transferred to the uterus.

Additional Male Reproductive Disorders

There are many male reproductive disorders. The following list provides a brief description of additional conditions.
- Penile disorders:
  - *Balanitis* (bale n EYE tis): Inflammation of the head and foreskin of the penis.
  - *Peyronie's* (pay roe NEES) disease: Thick scar tissue develops in the penis, causing it to bend.
  - *Priapism* (PRY ah piz um): Painful erection that does not go away.
  - *Penile cancer:* A rare form of cancer that is highly curable in the early stages.
- Disorders of the testicle, epididymis, breast, and other structures:
  - *Epididymitis* (ep ih did ih MYE tis): Inflammation of the epididymis; often caused by a bacterial infection that starts in the bladder, prostate, or urethra.
  - *Gynecomastia* (gye neh koh MASS tee ah): An enlargement of breast tissue in males caused by an estrogen and testosterone imbalance.

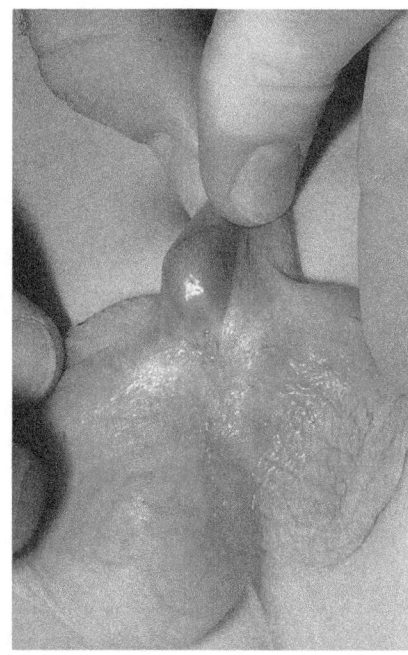

Fig. 14.4 Cryptorchidism in Left Testicle of a Neonate. (From Zitelli BJ, Davis HW: *Atlas of pediatric physical diagnosis*, ed 5, St Louis, 2007, Mosby/Elsevier.)

- *Orchitis* (or KYE tis): Inflammation of one or both of the testicles, usually caused by bacteria or viruses (e.g., mumps).
- *Prostatitis* (pros tah TYE tis): An inflammation of the prostate that can obstruct urinary flow; usually caused by bacteria and treated with antibiotics.
- *Spermatocele* (sper MAT oh sele): A cystlike mass filled with fluid and dead sperm cells; located in the epididymis.
- *Testicular torsion:* Twisting of the spermatic cord, causing the blood supply to be blocked off from the testicles; may occur after an injury to the area.
- *Varicocele* (veh sick yoo LYE tis): Enlargement of the veins in the scrotum; may cause low sperm production and quality, leading to infertility.
- Congenital disorders:
  - *Anorchism* (AN or kih zum): The absence of one or both testes at birth.
  - *Chordee* (KORE dee): Downward curve of the penis due to a congenital condition, such as hypospadias.
  - *Cryptorchidism* (kript OR kid iz um): Also called undescended testicle; the testicle fails to descend into the scrotum (Fig. 14.4). Treatment for this condition consists of gonadotropic hormones and surgery (orchiopexy).
  - *Epispadias* (eh pee SPAY dee ahs): Congenital malformation causing the urethra to open on top of the penis.
  - *Hypospadias* (hye poh SPAY dee ahs): Congenital malformation causing the urethra to open on the underside of the penis.
  - *Hydrocele* (HYE droh seel): Fluid-filled sac in the scrotum, common in newborn infants, that may go away in a few months; often caused by an inguinal hernia.
  - *Phimosis* (fih MOH sis): Tightening of the penile foreskin that may result in the closure of the urethral opening; also, the foreskin may not retract.

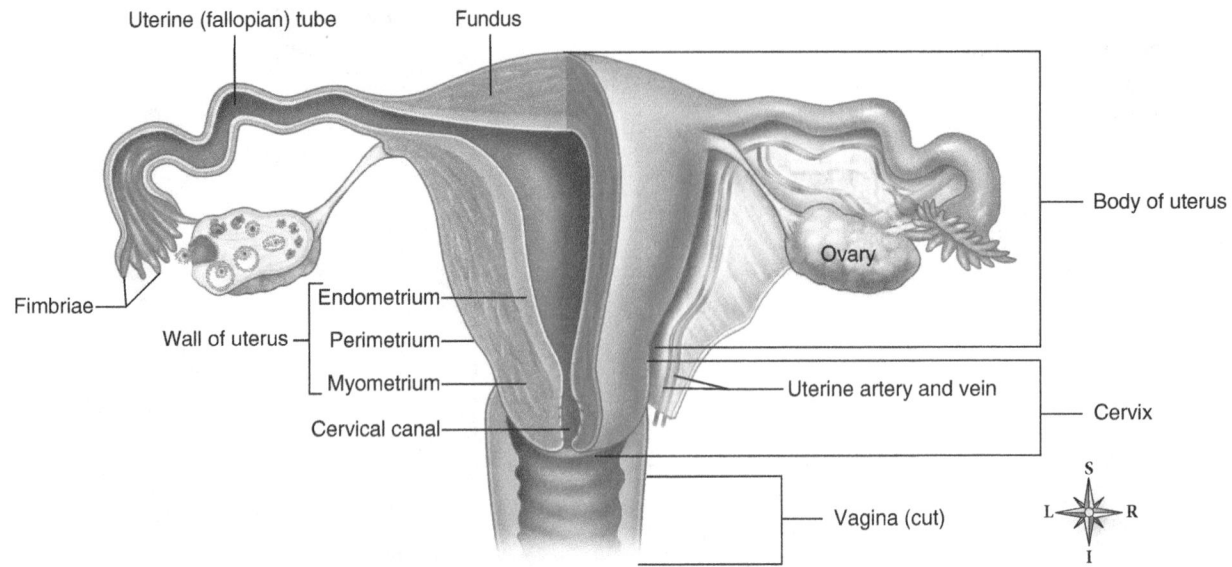

Fig. 14.5 Uterus. Sectioned view shows muscle layers of the uterus and its relationship to the ovaries and vagina. (From Patton KT, Thibodeau GA: *The human body in health and disease*, ed 7, St. Louis, 2018, Elsevier.)

ANATOMY OF THE FEMALE REPRODUCTIVE SYSTEMS

The primary reproductive organs in females are the gonads, two ovaries (OH vuh reez). The ovaries produce *oocytes* (OH o site), also called *ova, eggs,* or *female sex cells*. The ovaries are the size and shape of almonds. An ovary sits on each side of the uterus (YOO ter us), and they are held in place by peritoneal ligaments (Fig. 14.5). A *fallopian* (fuh LOH pee un) *tube* (also called *oviduct* and *uterine tube*) is located near each ovary. One end of the fallopian tube is funnel shaped with *fimbriae*, fingerlike extensions, along the edges. The funnel-shaped end of the fallopian tube sits above the ovary but is not connected to the ovary. The other end of the fallopian tube is attached to and opens into the uterus. Each fallopian tube is about 4 inches (10 cm) in length.

The uterus is a muscular organ about the size and shape of a pear. During pregnancy, the uterus grows in size to accommodate the growing fetus and fluid. After childbirth, the uterus is larger, but it decreases in size after *menopause* (the end of menstruation). The uterus is composed of:

- *Perimetrium* (pair ih MEE tree um), the outer layer
- *Myometrium* (mye oh MEE tree um), the middle layer, which is the muscle layer
- *Endometrium* (end oh MEE tree um), the inner layer, which is the lining of the uterus

The middle portion of the uterus is called the *body* or *corpus*. The *fundus* is the rounded protrusion at the top of the body where the fallopian tubes attach. The portion below the body is a narrow neck section called the *cervix*.

The *vagina*, sometimes referred to as the *birth canal*, extends from the cervix to the external genitalia. The vagina is a muscular tube about 4 inches in length. It is lined with mucous membrane and mainly composed of smooth muscle. The vagina sits between the rectum and the urinary bladder.

External Genitalia

The external genitalia, also called *vulva* (VUL vah) or *pudendum* (pyue DEN dum), are accessory structures external to the vagina. The vulva consists of the vaginal opening or orifice (ORE ih fis). The *hymen* (HIE men) is a membrane covering the orifice. Additional external genitalia structures include:

- *Labia majora* (LAY bee ah muah JOR ah): The larger fold of skin surrounding the opening.
- *Labia minor* (LAY bee ah min NOR uh): The smaller fold of skin surrounding the opening.
- *Mons pubis* (mon PYOO bis): A pad of fatty tissue over the symphysis pubis, which gets covered with hair at puberty.
- *Clitoris* (KLIT uh ris): The sensitive, erectile tissue.
- *Bartholin* (BAR toh lin) *glands* (or the greater vestibular glands) and the *skene glands* (or the lesser vestibular glands): These glands secrete mucous lubricant during sexual intercourse.
- *Perineum* (pair ih NEE um): Located between the vaginal opening and the anus (Fig. 14.6).

Breasts

The breasts, which contain the mammary glands, overlie the pectoralis major muscles on the chest. Externally the circular pigmented area called the *areola* surrounds the nipple (also called the *mammary papilla*). The nipples are sensitive to touch. They contain smooth muscles that contract, causing the nipple to become erect when simulated.

About 15 to 20 lobes of glandular tissue radiate around the nipple inside of the breast. Each lobe consists of lobules that contain the milk-secreting glandular cells arranged in grapelike clusters, called *alveoli*. Contractile cells surrounding the alveoli help to push the milk into the ductule, which drains into a small lactiferous ducts. Each lobe has its own lactiferous duct, which widens into a *lactiferous sinus* just before the nipple. The sinus stores the milk until the baby nurses. Multiple narrow ducts take the milk from the lactiferous sinuses to the surface of the nipple.

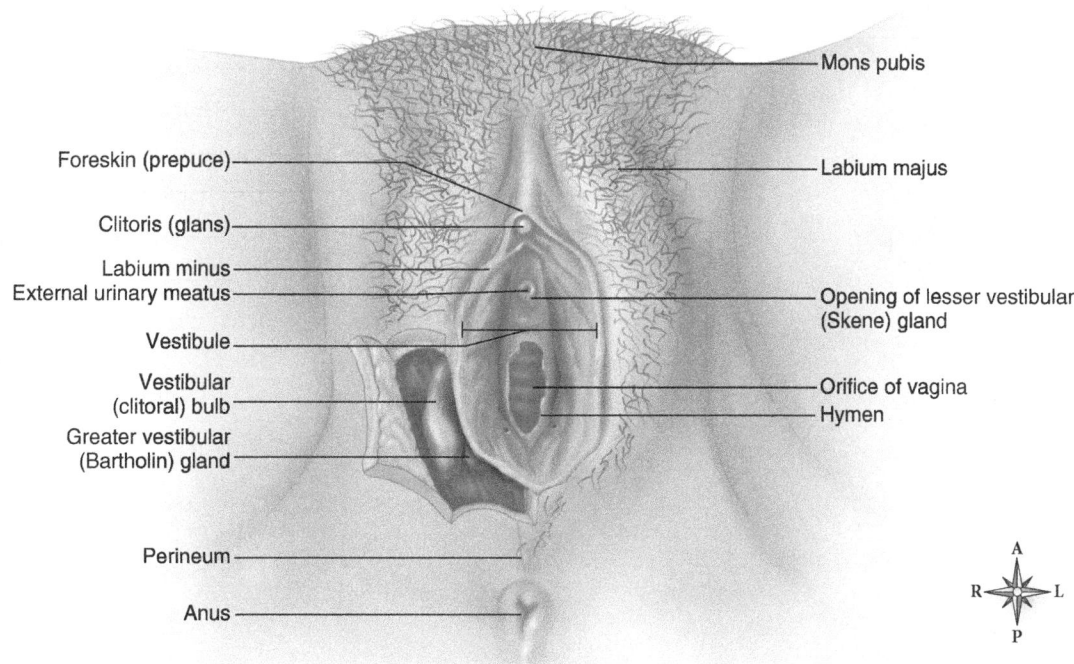

Fig. 14.6 Vulva. External Female Genitals and Related Structures, shown from an Inferior View. (From Patton KT, Thibodeau GA: *The human body in health and disease*, ed 7, St. Louis, 2018, Elsevier.)

Connective tissue, including Cooper or suspensory ligaments, help support the breast (Fig. 14.7, and Box 14.3).

At puberty estrogen stimulates breast tissue development. Estrogen also causes the accumulation of adipose tissue in the breasts. Progesterone stimulates the development of the duct system. During pregnancy, estrogen and progesterone help with further development of the mammary glands. Prolactin stimulates milk production within the glandular tissue. Oxytocin stimulates the small contractile cells of the alveoli, and milk is pushed into the ducts. This is called the "milk let-down" process.

MEDICAL TERMINOLOGY	
bartholin/o	Bartholin gland
cervic/o	cervix
clitorid/o	clitoris
endometri/o	endometrium
fund/o	fundus
hymen/o	hymen
hyster/o, metri/o, metr/o, uter/o	uterus
labi/o	labia
lact/o, galact/o	milk
mamm/o, mast/o	breast
myometri/o	myometrium
o/o, ov/o, ov/i, ovul/o	ovum, egg
oophor/o, ovari/o	ovary
papill/o, thel/e	nipple
perimetri/o	perimetrium
perine/o	perineum
salping/o	fallopian tube
vulv/o, episi/o	vulva
-ation	process of

PHYSIOLOGY OF THE FEMALE REPRODUCTIVE SYSTEM

At birth, a newborn girl has about 500,000 to 700,000 ovarian follicles, each containing an oocyte. Between birth and puberty, the follicles change and the number decreases. Over the female's reproductive years, only about 500 follicles become mature follicles.

Starting at puberty, the ovaries secrete estrogen and progesterone. Estrogen is responsible for:
- Development and maintenance of the female secondary sex characteristics. This includes the development of pubic hair and breasts.
- Development of the female curves.
- Stimulation of the uterine epithelial cell lining to grow and regulation of the menstrual cycle.

Menstrual Cycle

The first *menses* (menstrual period) is called the *menarche* (meh NAR kee). During the menstrual cycle, changes occur in the ovaries, uterus, and breasts due to hormones. In most females the menstrual cycle occurs on a regular basis, usually every 21 to 28 days. The menstrual cycle consists of the menses, proliferative phase, ovulation, and secretory phase.

The menstrual cycle starts on the first day of the menstrual flow (Fig. 14.8). The menses lasts for 4 to 5 days. During this time, part of the uterine lining sloughs off. The bleeding comes from the torn blood vessels. During the menses phase, the hypothalamus secretes gonadotropin-releasing hormone (GnRH). The GnRH stimulates the anterior pituitary gland to release

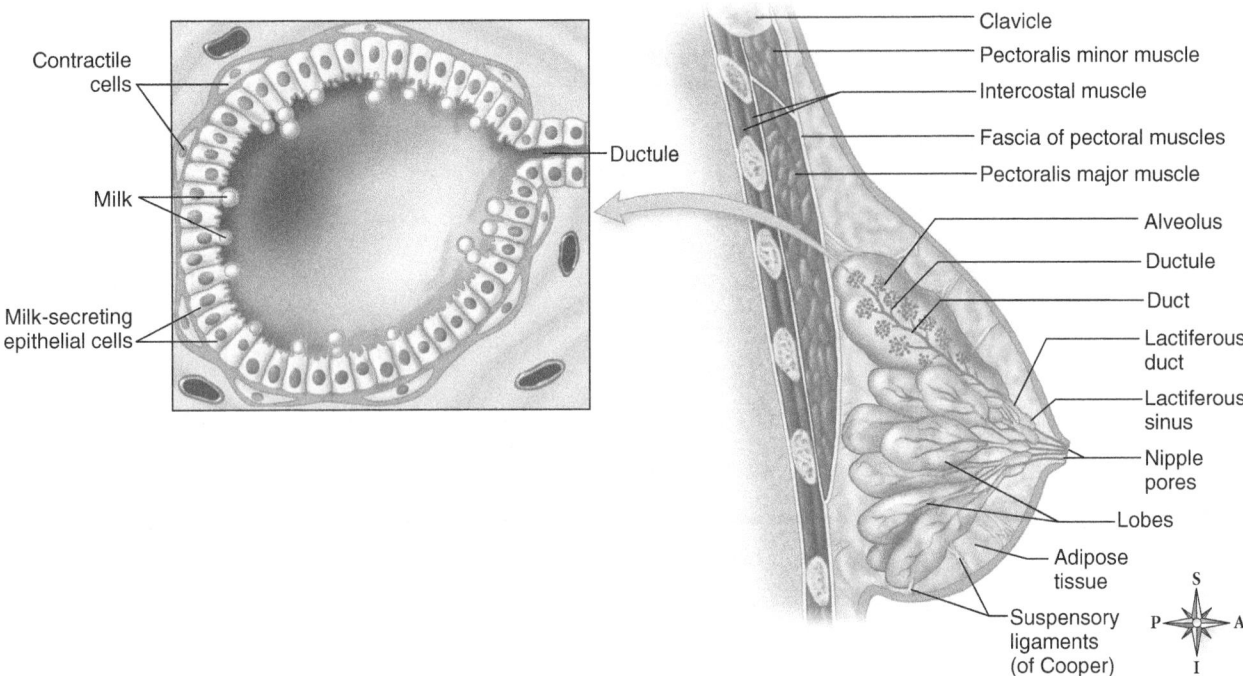

Fig. 14.7 Female Breast. Sagittal section shows the gland fixed to the overlying skin and the pectoral muscles by the suspensory ligaments (of Cooper). Each lobule of secretory tissue is drained by a lactiferous duct that opens through the nipple. The inset *(left)* shows one of the milk-producing alveoli of the mammary gland. (From Patton KT, Thibodeau GA: *The human body in health and disease*, ed 7, St. Louis, 2018, Elsevier.)

BOX 14.3   Fibrocystic Breasts

Fibrocystic breast, once thought a disease, is a common condition that women experience around their periods. More than half of women experience fibrocystic breast sometime in their lifetime. The breast tissue thickens, and fluid-filled cysts develop in one or both breasts. This can make the breasts swollen, lumpy, or painful. Self-care recommendations include taking over-the-counter pain medications, applying heat or ice to the breast, and wearing a well-fitting bra.

FSH and LH. FSH stimulates several of the immature follicles in the ovaries to grow. LH helps the follicles and ovum mature.

The proliferative phase starts on the last day of the menstrual flow and lasts until ovulation. During this phase, FSH and LH continue to help the follicles mature. The maturing follicles secrete estrogen. Estrogen secretion increases to its highest level during this phase. Estrogen causes the uterine lining to grow and thicken to prepare for pregnancy. The combination of GnRH and estrogen further promotes the secretion of LH.

A surge of LH stimulates ovulation. *Ovulation* occurs when the mature follicle (also called *graafian follicle*) at the surface of the ovary ruptures. A mature ovum is released from the follicle into the peritoneal cavity, in hopes of moving into the fallopian tube. Usually, only one follicle makes it to the point of ovulation. The remaining maturing follicles break down and are reabsorbed.

The secretory phase starts at the beginning of ovulation and lasts until the first day of the menses. After ovulation and with the help of LH, the remaining part of the follicle in the ovary is transformed into a *corpus luteum*. The corpus luteum (a Latin

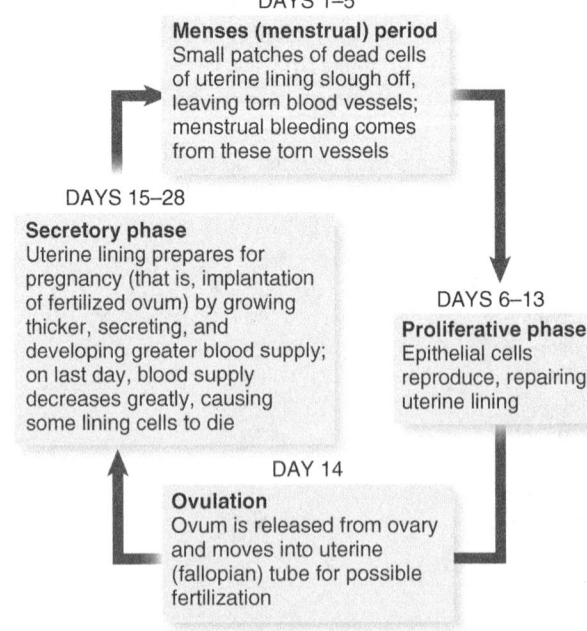

Fig. 14.8 Twenty-Eight-Day Menstrual Cycle. (From Patton KT, Thibodeau GA: *The human body in health and disease*, ed 7, St. Louis, 2018, Elsevier.)

phrase for "yellow body") secretes progesterone and some estrogen. These two hormones help support and thicken the uterine lining. If fertilization does not occur, the corpus luteum functions for about 10 days before it starts breaking down. The sharp decrease in progesterone and estrogen causes the uterine lining

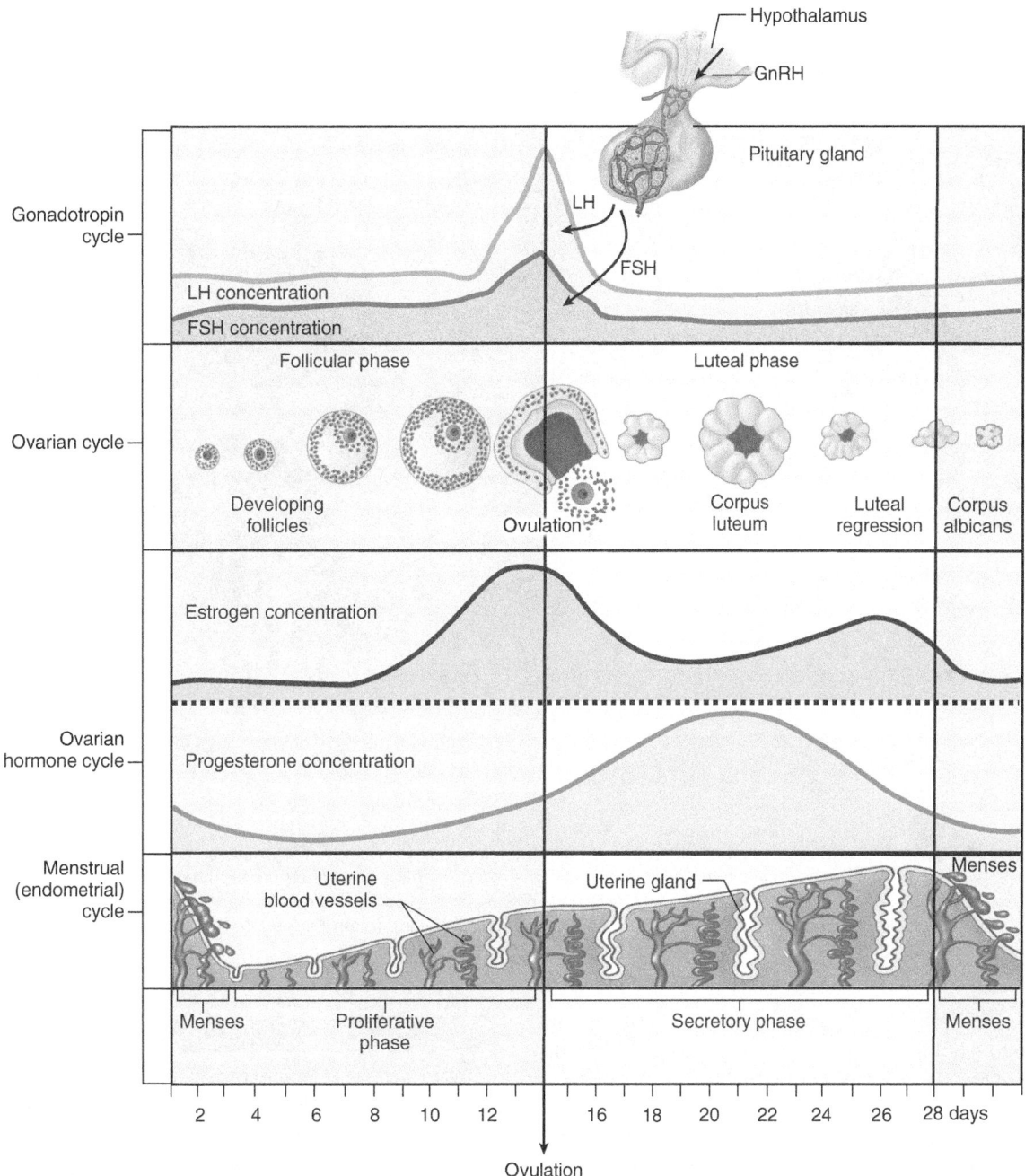

Fig. 14.9 Female Reproductive Cycle. Diagram illustrates the interrelationship of pituitary, ovarian, and uterine functions throughout a typical 28-day cycle. A sharp increase in luteinizing hormone (LH) levels causes ovulation, whereas menstruation (sloughing off of the endometrial lining) is initiated by lower levels of progesterone. (From Kumar V, Abbas AK, Fausto N: *Robbins and Cotran pathologic basis of disease*, ed 8, Philadelphia, 2010, Saunders.)

to break down. This ends the secretory phase and causes the next menses (Fig. 14.9).

If fertilization occurs, the corpus luteum continues to secrete progesterone and estrogen until the placenta develops enough to secrete these two hormones. The progesterone levels continue to rise. This helps the uterus support the developing baby.

Pregnancy

Pregnancy, also called *gestation* (jes TAY shun), is the time between fertilization (conception) to birth. The gestational age of the growing baby is measured in weeks from the first

day of the mother's last menstrual cycle (LMP). The pregnancy is divided into trimesters. During the first 2 weeks of "pregnancy," the body is preparing for pregnancy and there is no pregnancy yet.

The intrauterine development is divided into the pre-embryonic, embryonic, and fetal periods. The following sections will discuss the growth of the offspring based on age from conception.

VOCABULARY

conception Formation of a viable zygote by the union of the ovum from the female and the sperm from the male; also called *fertilization*.

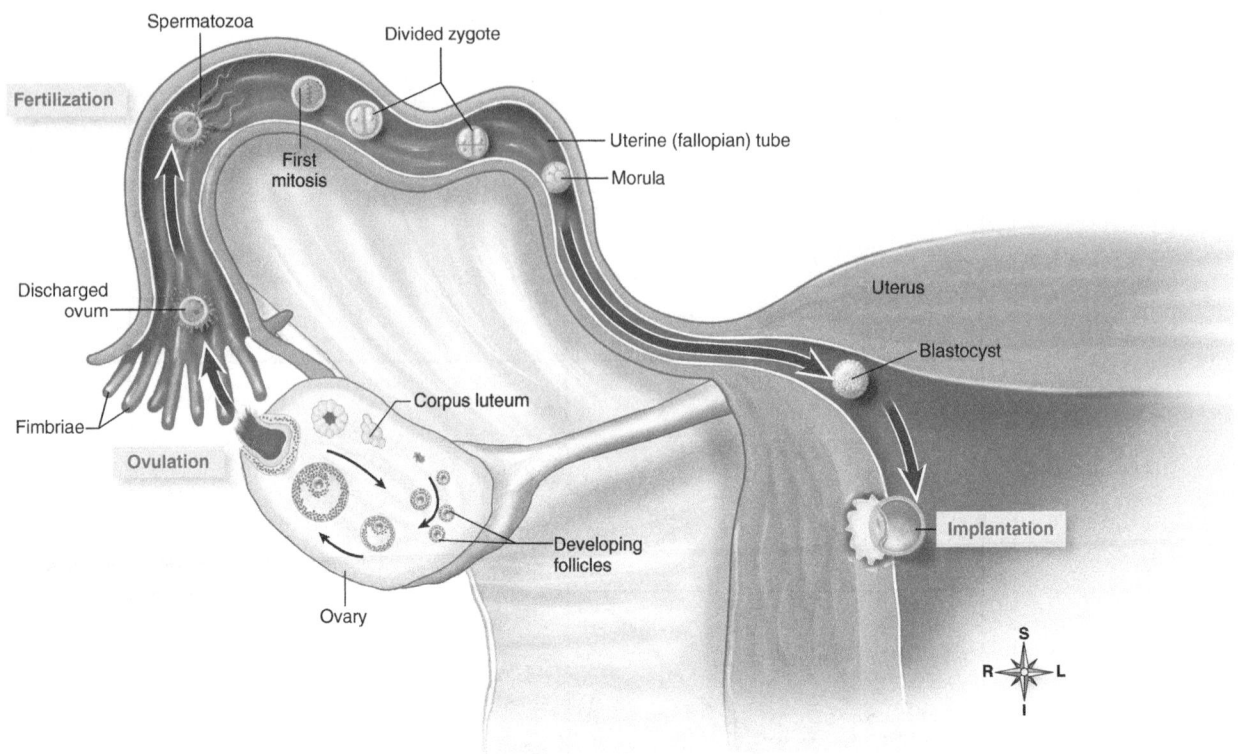

Fig. 14.10 Fertilization and Implantation. At ovulation, an ovum is released from the ovary and begins its journey through the uterine tube. While in the tube, the ovum is fertilized by a sperm to form the single-celled zygote. After a few days of rapid mitotic division, a ball of cells, called a *morula,* is formed. After the morula develops into a hollow ball, called a *blastocyst,* implantation occurs. (From Patton KT, Thibodeau GA: *The human body in health and disease,* ed 7, St. Louis, 2018, Elsevier.)

Pre-embryonic Period. The pre-embryonic period lasts from conception to day 14. At ovulation, the egg is released into the peritoneal cavity (Fig. 14.10). During ovulation, the fimbriae increase their sweeping motion, creating currents in the peritoneal fluid. This helps to propel the egg into the fallopian tube. The egg moves through the fallopian tube with the help of:

- The peristaltic action of the smooth muscles in the wall of the fallopian tube
- The rhythmic beating of the cilia, which line the fallopian tube

The eggs that do not make it into the fallopian tube remain in the pelvic cavity and are reabsorbed.

After intercourse, sperm cells move up the fallopian tubes. The sperm will penetrate the membrane around the egg (Box 14.4). When the egg and sperm unite, *fertilization* occurs. The fertilized ovum, the *zygote* (ZYE gote), continues to divide as it moves down the fallopian tube. Within 3 days a solid ball of cells forms, called a *morula* (MAWR oo luh). By the time the morula moves into the uterus, the cells have developed into a hollow ball called a *blastocyst* (BLAS tuh sist).

The blastocyst implants itself into the endometrium 6 to 10 days after conception. The *trophoblast,* the outer cell layer

> **BOX 14.4 Fertilization**
>
> The egg is able to be fertilized up to 24 hours after ovulation. Sperm retain their fertilization ability for about 24 to 72 hours after ejaculation. A few may be viable until day 5. This means the female is fertile from 3 to 5 days before and up to 24 hours after ovulation.

of the blastocyst, will form the placenta (plah SEN tah), chorion (KORE ee on), and amnion (AM nee on). The blastocyst cavity forms between the trophoblast and *embryoblast.* The embryoblast, the inner cell mass of the blastocyst, will form into the *embryo* (EM bree oh). The embryoblast has three primary germ layers that will develop into structures and systems:

- *Ectoderm*: The outer layer, forms into the skin, nails, glands, central and peripheral nervous system
- *Mesoderm*: The middle layer, develops into the skeletal, muscular, and cardiovascular systems and some of the urinary and reproductive structures
- *Endoderm*: The inner layer, forms the respiratory and digestive systems, and the urethra, bladder, and vagina

The blastocyst produces hCG hormone, which signals the

TABLE 14.3 Hormones During Pregnancy

Hormone	Description
Estrogen	Initially secreted in limited amounts by the corpus luteum in response to human chorionic gonadotropin (hCG), then the placenta secretes it. Estrogen helps maintain the pregnancy and enlarges the milk ducts to prepare the breast for milk production.
Progesterone	Initially secreted by the corpus luteum in response to hCG and then secreted by the placenta around week 10. Stimulates the thickening of the uterine lining. Relaxes smooth muscles in the uterus.
Human chorionic gonadotropin (hCG) (kore ee AH nick goh nad doh TROH pin)	Produced by the blastocyst; it signals the corpus luteum to produce more estrogen and progesterone. HCG levels double every 2 days during the first 10 weeks of the pregnancy.
Human placental lactogen (hPL)	Secreted by the placenta. Simulates the milk glands in the breast to produce milk.
Prolactin (PRL) (proh LAK tin)	Secreted by the anterior pituitary gland. Promotes the growth of breast tissue; simulates and sustains breast milk production.
Oxytocin (ok si TOE sin)	Created in the hypothalamus; stored and released by the posterior pituitary. Causes uterine contractions and helps with releasing breast milk by stimulating the contraction of the muscles surrounding the mammary ducts.
Relaxin (ree LAK sin)	Secreted by the corpus luteum and then secreted by the placenta. Relaxes muscles and loosens joints and ligaments, especially in the pelvic area, to help with delivery. Also inhibits uterine contractions.

corpus luteum to produce more estrogen and progesterone (Table 14.3). The high levels of estrogen and progesterone stop the menstrual cycle, inhibiting the release of FSH and LH.

CRITICAL THINKING 14.4

Combination oral contraceptive pills contain estrogen and progestin (a synthetic form of progesterone). Explain how these two hormones interfere with ovulation.

Multiple Births. A *multiple pregnancy* refers to the birth of more than one infant from the same pregnancy. Often babies from a multiple pregnancy are born prematurely. With *identical twins*, the embryonic tissue splits from the same zygote (Fig. 14.11). This means identical twins are genetically the same.

Fraternal twins result from two separate fertilized eggs. More than one ovum is released during a single menstrual cycle. Having fraternal twins can be genetic or related to ART (e.g., fertility drugs and in vitro fertilization).

Embryonic Period. The embryonic period is between day 15 to about week 8 after fertilization (or weeks 5 to 10 of pregnancy). During this phase, the offspring is called an *embryo*. Many changes occur during the embryonic phase:

- *Placenta*: The chorion arises from the trophoblast. The chorionic villi on the surface of the chorion develop into the placenta. Throughout the pregnancy, the highly vascular placenta assists with the exchange of nutrients, gases (e.g., oxygen), and waste products between the mother and embryo. The placenta also secretes high levels of estrogen and progesterone. The placement of the placenta can change as the uterus changes in pregnancy.
- *Umbilical* (um BILL ih kul) *cord*: This cord connects the embryo to the placenta. The umbilical cord contains two umbilical arteries that carry deoxygenated blood and wastes from the embryo to the placenta. It also contains one umbilical vein that carries oxygenated blood and nutrients from the placenta to the embryo. When a baby in utero has a *two-vessel*

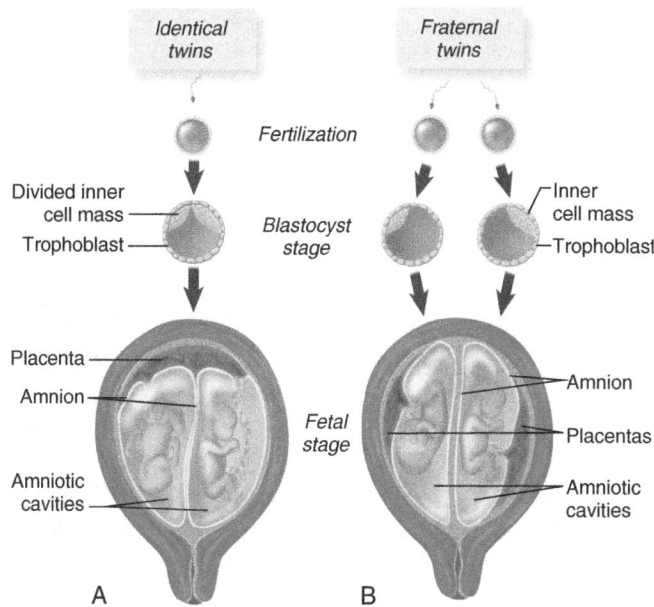

Fig. 14.11 Multiple Births. A, Identical (monozygotic) twins develop when embryonic tissue from a single zygote splits to form two individuals. Notice that the placenta and the part of the amnion separating the amniotic cavities are shared by the twins. B, Fraternal (dizygotic) twins develop when two ova are fertilized at about the same time, producing two separate zygotes. Notice that each fraternal twin has its own placenta and amnion. (From Patton KT, Thibodeau GA: *The human body in health and disease*, ed 7, St. Louis, 2018, Elsevier.)

umbilical cord (just one umbilical artery), other congenital or chromosomal abnormalities may also be present.
- *Amnion and amniotic fluid*: The amnion (AM nee on) is a tough, thin protective membrane that forms a sac around the embryo. Amniotic fluid surrounds the embryo inside of the amnion (Box 14.5).
- *Yolk sac*: The yolk sac develops from a blastocyst cavity and is involved in the development of the preliminary circulatory system.

- *Structures*: By week 5 of pregnancy, all the major organs have started to develop, including the brain, spinal cord, and heart. During weeks 6 and 7, the arm and leg buds start to grow, and the heart starts beating. Between weeks 8 to 10, the arms, legs, hands, and feet continue to grow. The lungs, toes, eyelids, ears, and facial features are forming.

BOX 14.5   Amniotic Fluid

Amniotic fluid is a clear, slightly yellowish liquid that surrounds the unborn baby. The amount of amniotic fluid increases over the course of the pregnancy and can be 1 liter by the end of pregnancy. Initially, the fluid comes from the maternal blood supply through diffusion. By week 11, the fetus urinates, which increases the volume. The amniotic fluid constantly circulates as the baby swallows and "inhales" it, then releases it through urine and breathing.

Amniotic fluid serves several roles, including:

- Helping to maintain a constant body temperature and protecting from heat loss
- Cushioning the growing baby and preventing pressure on the umbilical cord
- Promoting lung development (the baby practices breathing by breathing in the amniotic fluid)
- Helping the developing baby to move, which allows for proper bone growth
- Acting as an infection barrier

The amniotic fluid can be green or brown in color towards the end of pregnancy. The color change indicates that the baby in utero had a bowel movement (*meconium*). This can be a sign that the baby was in distress or simply the baby passed the first stool in utero.

Fetal Period. The time span from week 11 of pregnancy to the birth (around week 39 to 42) is considered the *fetal period*. The offspring is now called a *fetus* (FEE tus). The fetus continues to grow (Fig. 14.12).

- Week 11 to 18: Fingernails and toenails are present. The liver makes red blood cells. The baby in utero can make sucking motions, a fist, stretch, move, and reacts to touch. *Lanugo* (la NUE goe), a fine soft hair, starts to cover the skin and helps to hold the vernix (VER niks) caseosa (KAE see OH sah) on the skin. The *vernix caseosa* is a thick white substance made of sebum and epithelia cells that provides a waterproof protective covering on the skin.
- Week 19 to 26: The baby can hear, becomes more active, and can swallow. *Quickening* is the first baby movements felt by the mother. *Meconium* (me KOE nee uhm), the first bowel movement, is made in the intestinal tract. The bone marrow begins to make blood cells, and the lower airway develops. The eyebrows, eyelashes, footprints, fingerprints, and alveoli (in the lungs) are formed. The baby will startle with loud noise.
- Week 27 to 34: The nervous, skeletal, and muscular systems continue to grow and develop. The respiratory system produces surfactant that helps the alveoli fill with air. The eyelids open and close.
- Weeks 35 to 37: The baby continues to grow and put on weight. The average weight is about 5.5 pounds. The bones and muscles are fully developed. The baby has sleeping patterns.

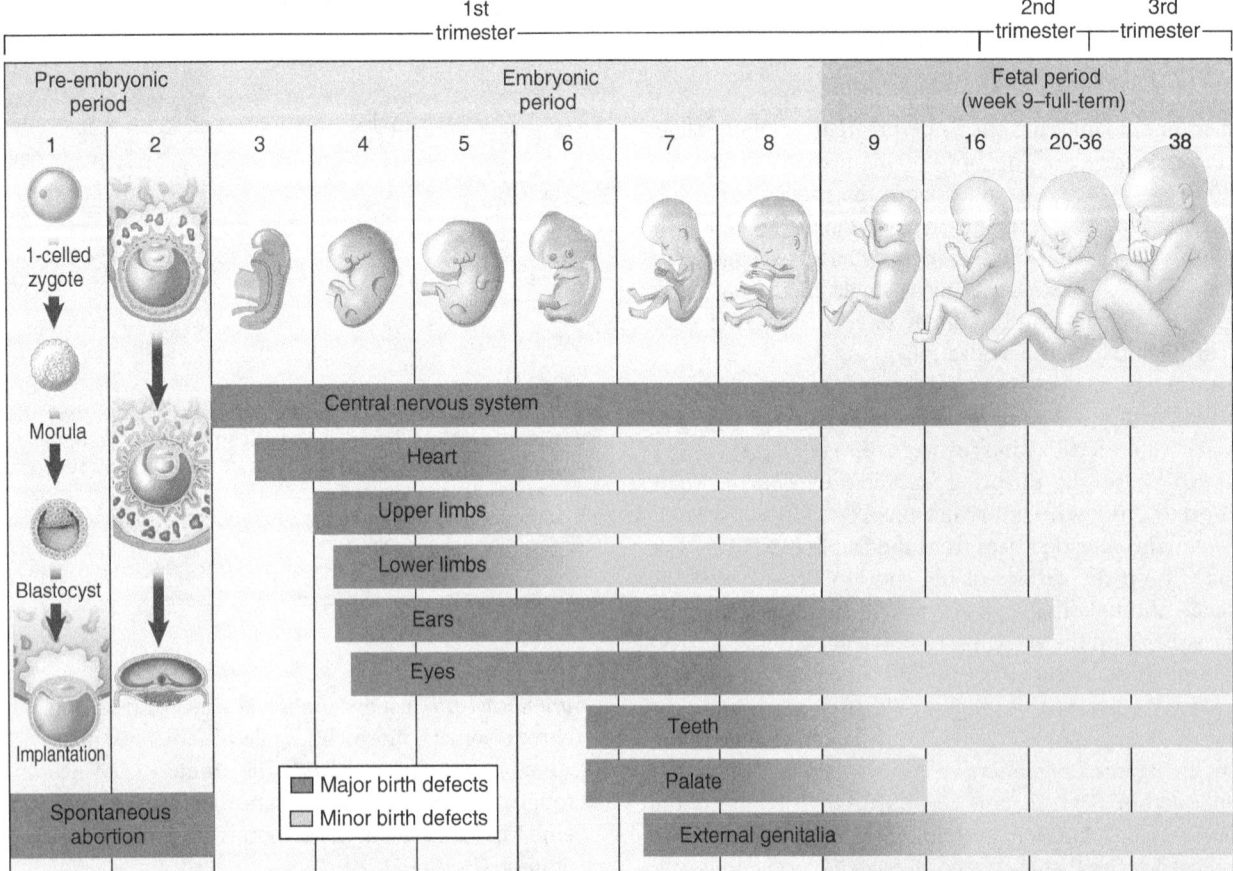

Fig. 14.12 Critical Periods of Neonatal Development. The *red areas* show when teratogens are most likely to cause major birth defects, and the *yellow areas* show when minor defects are more likely to arise. *Numbers* refer to weeks of gestation. (From Patton KT, Thibodeau GA: *The human body in health and disease*, ed 7, St. Louis, 2018, Elsevier.)

- Week 38 to 40: The lanugo may only remain on the upper arms and shoulders. Small breast buds are present. Hair on the head is thicker.
- The delivery of the infant is called *parturition* (par tur RIH shun). A vaginal delivery is most common. The alternative to a vaginal delivery is a cesarean section (CS, C-section). With a *cesarean section*, the infant is delivered through an abdominal incision. *Vaginal birth after cesarean section* (VBAC) describes the delivery of an infant vaginally following a previous C-section.

MEDICAL TERMINOLOGY	
amni/o, amnion/o	amnion
chori/o, chorion/o	chorion
fet/o	fetus
men/o, menstru/o	menstruation
nat/o	birth, born
part/o	parturition
placent/o	placenta
umbilic/o, omphal/o	umbilicus
-amnios	amnion
-arche	beginning
-para, -partum, -tocia	parturition (delivery)
-gravida	pregnancy

DISEASES AND DISORDERS OF THE FEMALE REPRODUCTIVE SYSTEM

Common female reproductive disorder signs and symptoms include:

- Changes in the menses: *amenorrhea* (lack of menstrual flow), *dysmenorrhea* (painful menstrual flow), *menorrhagia* (abnormally heavy menstrual flow), and *oligomenorrhea* (abnormally light or infrequent menstrual flow)
- Painful intercourse
- Pain, discomfort, and redness
- Lumps in the breasts

Tables 14.4 and 14.5 provided common diagnostic procedures and treatments used for female reproductive disorders. The following sections discuss female reproductive disorders.

Cancer

Breast Cancer. Breast cancer is the second most common cancer in women. About 1 in 8 women will be diagnosed with it. There are several types of breast cancer. Breast cancer can also occur in males, though it is considered rare.

Etiology. Breast cells begin to grow abnormally, accumulate, and form a mass. For some, breast cancer can be inherited. A number of inherited mutated genes can increase the risk of breast cancer. There are many risk factors for breast cancer, including:

- Environmental and lifestyle factors, such as drinking alcohol, obesity, and radiation exposure
- A personal or family history of breast conditions
- Menarche (me NAHR kee) before age 12 or menopause at an older age
- Having never been pregnant or having the first baby after age 30
- Taking estrogen and progesterone therapy to treat menopause symptoms

Signs and Symptoms. Signs and symptoms of breast cancer include:

- Breast or nipple pain
- Changes in the shape or size of the breast; thickening or swelling of a portion of the breast
- Skin changes, including redness, scaling, irritation, and dimpling
- Nipple changes, including redness or scaling, turning inward, or discharge other than breast milk.
- Lump in the breast or armpit (axilla).

Diagnostic Procedures. Mammograms and breast magnetic resonance imaging (MRI) are used to screen women who are at high risk for getting breast cancer. Clinical breast exams by providers and breast self-awareness are also important for finding breast cancer early. Breast ultrasound, mammograms, MRI, and a biopsy are used to diagnose breast cancer. If breast cancer is diagnosed, the staging will be determined.

Treatments. Treatments include surgery to remove the cancer tissue. Chemotherapy and radiation are used to shrink or kill the cancer cells. Hormonal therapy can be used to block cancer cells from getting the hormones they need to grow. Biological therapy may also be used to assist the body's immune system to fight the cancer cells. Reconstructive surgery is an option once the patient has healed.

> **VOCABULARY**
> **menarche** Time of the first menstrual period.
> **sentinel lymph node** First lymph node to which cancer cells are most likely to spread from the primary tumor.

Other Cancers. Cancers affecting the female reproductive organs include:

- *Cervical cancer:* Cancer of the cervix; several types exist.
- *Endometrial cancer:* Cancer of the lining of the uterus; also called *uterine cancer.*
- *Ovarian cancer:* Cancer of the ovary or ovaries. Usually, ovarian cancer is advanced before it is detected.
- *Vaginal cancer:* Cancer of the vagina; a rare form of cancer.
- *Vulvar cancer:* Cancer of the vulva; a rare form of cancer.

Table 14.6 provides additional information on the more common forms of cancer.

Endometriosis

Endometriosis (en doe mee tree OH sis) causes endometrial-like tissue to grow outside of the uterus. The tissue can grow outside the ovaries, fallopian tubes, and on the tissue lining

TABLE 14.4   Common Diagnostic Procedures Used for Female Reproductive Disorders

Done by/Type of Test:	Procedure	Description
Provider during the exam	Papanicolaou (Pap) test	During a pelvic exam, the provider scrapes cells from the cervix. These are examined in the lab for abnormalities, including cancer and precancerous cells.
Surgical procedure	Biopsy	• *Cone biopsy (conization)*: Deeper layers of cervical cells are removed under general anesthesia. • *Loop electrosurgical excision procedure (LEEP)*: Uses a thin, low-voltage electrified wire to obtain the tissue sample. Usually done under local anesthesia. • *Endocervical curettage*: A curette (spoon-shaped instrument) or thin brush is used to collect the cervical tissue sample. • *Endometrial biopsy*: Endometrial cells are removed; usually does not require anesthesia. • *Punch biopsy*: A punch tool removes a small sample of cervical tissue. • *Sentinel lymph node biopsy (SLNB)*: Surgical procedure in which the sentinel lymph node is identified, removed, and examined to determine the extent of the cancer.
Endoscopy	Colposcopy	A colposcope is inserted into the vagina to visualize the cervix and vagina. Biopsies can be obtained using punch biopsy or endocervical curettage.
	Hysteroscopy	A hysteroscope is inserted into the vagina and cervix. Allows the provider to examine the uterus and endometrium.
Imagining procedure	Ultrasound (US)	• *Breast US*: Used to visualize breast tissue. • *Pelvic (transabdominal) US*: Used to examine organs in the pelvis. • *Transvaginal US*: Transducer is inserted into the vagina. Used to examine the uterus, ovaries, fallopian tubes, cervix, and pelvic area.
	Hysterosalpingography (HSG) (his tur oh sal pin GAH gruh fee)	An x-ray done with a contrast medium to exam the uterus and fallopian tubes.
	Mammography (mam MOG gruh fee)	Used to detect abnormalities in the breast tissue. A mammogram is the record produced by the mammography.
Medical laboratory	Estrogen	Many types of estrogen. Estrogens can be tested in blood, saliva, or urine. Common tests include: • *Estrone* (E1): Main female hormone made after menopause. • *Estradiol* (E2): Main female hormone made by nonpregnant women; used to diagnose menstrual and infertility problems.
	Hormone testing	Blood tests to assess hormone levels.
	Human papillomavirus (HPV) DNA test	Involves testing cervical cells obtained during a Pap test for HPV infections.
	Progesterone blood test	Used to find the cause of infertility and identify ovulation.

the pelvis. The tissue grows and then breaks down and bleeds with each menstrual cycle. Scar tissue and adhesions can develop.

Etiology. The cause is unclear. Risk factors include having never given birth, early menarche, late-onset menopause, short menstrual cycles, low body mass index, family history of the condition, and higher than normal estrogen levels.

Signs and Symptoms. Endometriosis can cause:
• Dysmenorrhea and excessive bleeding
• Pain with intercourse, bowel movements, and urination
• Fatigue, diarrhea or constipation, bloating, and infertility

Diagnostic Procedures. The provider will obtain a medical history and perform a pelvic examination. Imaging tests such as an ultrasound and an MRI may be done. A laparoscopy might be done to detect endometrial tissue outside of the uterus.

Treatments. Treatment depends on the severity of the condition. Pain medications, supplemental hormone therapy, fertility treatments, and surgical options (e.g., hysterectomy and oophorectomy) may be chosen.

> **VOCABULARY**
> **adhesions** Bands of scar tissue that can bind anatomic structures together.

Female Infertility

Female infertility is more common than male infertility, which was discussed in a prior section of this chapter.

Etiology. Female infertility can be caused by:
• Autoimmune disorders, thyroid disease, cancer, diabetes, clotting disorders, and hormone imbalances
• Uterine and cervical polyps, congenital reproductive disorders, ovarian cysts, and polycystic ovary syndrome (PCOS)

- Eating disorders, poor nutrition, smoking, drinking too much alcohol, exercising too much, and being overweight or underweight
- Tubal ligation or failure of tubal ligation reversal

TABLE 14.5 Common Treatments Used for Female Reproductive Disorders

Procedure	Description
Dilation and curettage (D&C) (dye LAY shun kyoor ih TAHZH)	Surgical procedure involving cervical dilation (widening) and scraping of the lining of the uterus with a curette (curettage).
Hysterectomy (hiss tur RECK tuh mee)	Removal (resection) of the uterus. Can be done laparoscopically, vaginally, or through an abdominal incision. *Total abdominal hysterectomy with a bilateral salpingo-oophorectomy* (TAH-BSO) involves the removal of the uterus, both ovaries as well as both fallopian tubes.
Hysteropexy (HISS tur oh peck see)	Fixation of a displaced uterus.
Lumpectomy	Surgical removal of a breast tumor and a small amount of the surrounding tissue.
Mammoplasty (MAM oh plas tee)	Surgical repair of the breast. Can be done for cosmetic repair, such as breast reduction or augmentation.
Mastectomy (mass TECK tuh mee)	Removal of the breast.
Oophorectomy (oo ah fore ECK tuh mee)	Resection of an ovary.
Salpingectomy (sal pin JECK tuh mee)	Resection of a fallopian tube. With a *salpingo-oophorectomy* the fallopian tubes and ovaries are removed.

Signs and Symptoms. The sign of infertility is not getting pregnant.

Diagnostic Procedures. The provider will obtain a medical history and perform a physical examination. Blood tests, such as progesterone, thyroid, and FSH levels, may be checked. The provider may also order a pelvic ultrasound and a hysterosalpingography.

Treatments. Treatment depends on the cause of infertility. It may involve education and counseling about the condition. Fertility treatments may be used, along with medications that help with the growth and release of eggs from the ovaries. About 1 in 5 women get pregnant without treatment, and most get pregnant with treatment.

CRITICAL THINKING 14.6

During her orientation, Marie was able to work with the medical assistant who assisted the outreach fertility provider. Marie overheard the struggles that several female patients experienced trying to get pregnant. If either a male or a female patient expressed struggles regarding fertility, how might you respond?

Ovarian Cyst

An *ovarian cyst* is a fluid-filled sac that forms on or inside of an ovary. Many women have ovarian cysts at one time or another. The majority of ovarian cysts disappear without treatment in a few months. Cysts after menopause have a higher risk for being cancer.

Etiology. Ovarian cysts that develop as a result of the monthly menses are called *functional cysts*. Functional cysts are harmless,

TABLE 14.6 Female Reproductive Organ Cancers

	Cervical Cancer	Endometrial Cancer	Ovarian Cancer
Etiology	Unclear, but human papilloma virus (HPV) plays a role. Risk factors include multiple sexual partners, early sexual activity, smoking, and sexually transmitted infections (STIs).	Unclear. Risk factors include changes in the hormone level, early menarche or late onset of menopause, older age, obesity, history of taking tamoxifen for breast cancer, and inherited colon cancer syndrome.	Unclear. Risk factors include older age (50–60), inherited gene mutations, long-term use of estrogen replacement therapy, early menarche or late onset menopause, and family history of ovarian cancer.
Signs and Symptoms	Absent early on. Advanced cancer can cause bleeding and abnormal vaginal discharge.	Pelvic pain, bleeding between menses, and vaginal bleeding after menopause.	Abdominal swelling and bloating, feeling full soon after eating, weight loss, urinary frequency, pelvic area discomfort, and bowel changes.
Diagnostic Procedures	The Pap test and HPV DNA test are used for screening. A colposcopy with a punch biopsy or endocervical curettage may be done. For additional information, the provider may do LEEP or cone biopsy to obtain deeper cervical cell layers. Imaging tests may be done for staging the cancer.	Pelvic exam, transvaginal ultrasound, hysteroscopy, and an endometrial biopsy. Imaging tests may be ordered to stage the cancer.	Pelvic exam, imaging tests (ultrasound, computed tomography [CT] scan of the abdomen and pelvis), blood tests (e.g., cancer antigen 125 test), and surgery.
Treatments	Surgery (excision of the cancer, removal of the cervix, or a hysterectomy) may be done, along with chemotherapy, radiation, targeted drug therapy (targeting the cancer cells), and immunotherapy.	Surgery (hysterectomy and salpingo-oophorectomy) may be done, along with chemotherapy, radiation, targeted drug therapy, and immunotherapy.	Surgery to remove one or both ovaries, surgical removal of other reproductive organs, chemotherapy, and targeted drug therapy.

usually painless, and often disappear within 2 to 3 months. Other types of cysts can occur, including endometriomas, which are caused by endometriosis. Risk factors for developing ovarian cysts include hormonal problems, pregnancy, prior history of cysts, endometriosis, and severe pelvic infection.

Signs and Symptoms. Most cysts have no signs and symptoms. Larger cysts can rupture and bleed, cause twisting (torsion) of the ovary, and interfere with the ovarian blood supply. With these cysts, a person may experience:

- Sudden and severe pelvic pain with nausea and vomiting (occurs with torsion)
- Constant achy pelvic pain, pain with menses, or pain with intercourse
- Bloating and a feeling of fullness in the abdomen

Diagnostic Procedures. In addition to a pelvic exam, imaging tests (e.g., ultrasound, CT scan, and MRI) and hormone level tests are used to diagnose ovarian cysts.

Treatments. No treatment is needed for functional ovarian cysts. Other cysts may need to be surgically removed.

Pelvic Floor Disorders

The *pelvic floor* is a group of muscles and tissues that holds the uterus, bladder, bowel, and other pelvic organs in place. Pelvic floor disorders (PFDs) include urinary and fecal incontinence and pelvic prolapse. With pelvic prolapse, one or more of the pelvic organs press into the vagina or bulge out ("drop out") of the vagina. Types of pelvic prolapse include:

- *Cystocele*, also called *prolapsed, anterior prolapse,* or *dropped bladder.* The bladder bulges into the vagina or through the vaginal opening (Fig. 14.13).
- *Enterocele* (en the roe SEEL), the bulging of the small intestine into the upper part of the vagina.
- *Rectocele*, which occurs when the rectum bulges into or out of the vagina.
- *Uterine prolapse*, also called *dropped uterus.* The uterus bulges into or out of the vagina.
- *Vaginal vault prolapse*, occurs when the top of the uterus drops down, creating a bulge.

Etiology. Pelvic floor disorders are caused by pelvic floor injuries, resulting from pregnancy, vaginal childbirth, menopause, aging, and prior pelvic surgery. Pelvic floor disorders can be genetic.

Signs and Symptoms. Pelvic floor disorders can cause:

- Feeling a bulge in the vagina or seeing something coming out of the vagina
- Discomfort, fullness, or aching in the pelvis
- Pelvic pressure that gets worse with coughing, standing, or as the day progresses
- Urinary incontinence and difficulty having a bowel movement (stool)
- Problems inserting tampons

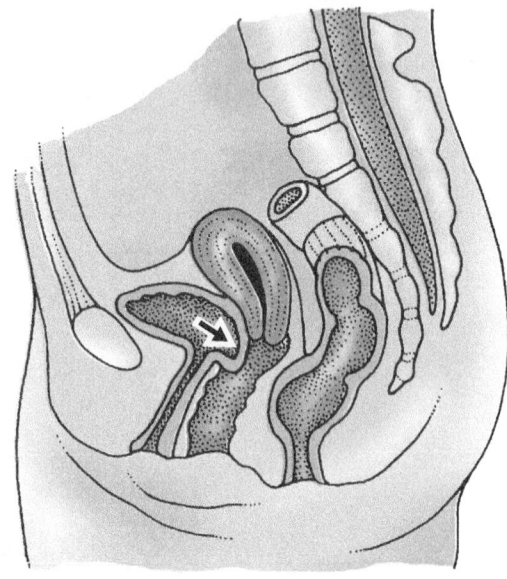

Fig. 14.13 Anterior Prolapse. The urinary bladder is displaced downward *(arrow)*, which causes bulging of the anterior vaginal wall. (From Ignatavicius DD, Workman ML: *Medical-surgical nursing: critical thinking for collaborative care,* ed 6, Philadelphia, 2011, Saunders.)

Diagnostic Procedures. The provider will obtain a medical history and perform a pelvic exam. Additional tests that might be done include:

- Cystoscopy, urinalysis, and urodynamics for ladder control problems
- Colonoscopy, sigmoidoscopy, and dynamic defecography for bowel control problems

Treatments. Treatments depend on the type of disorder and include:

- Nonsurgical: Bladder training, pelvic floor muscle training (PFMT), medications, and a *vaginal pessary*, which fits into the vagina and provides support to the structures.
- Surgical: Hysterectomy for uterine prolapse; sacral colpopexy (a surgical mesh strap is used to suspend the vagina in its original position); suspension surgery (vagina is stitched to ligaments); a midurethral sling for urinary incontinence; and anal sphincter muscle repair surgery.
- Lifestyle changes: Weight loss, high-fiber foods, and limiting caffeinated and alcoholic beverages.

Pelvic Inflammatory Disease

Pelvic inflammatory disease (PID) is an infection and inflammation of the reproductive organs. PID can lead to organ scarring, infertility, ectopic pregnancy, and abscesses. It is the most common preventable cause of infertility in the US.

Etiology. The most common causes of PID are gonorrhea and chlamydia. Other bacteria can also cause PID. Bacteria move from the vagina or cervix to the upper reproductive structures. A female is at a higher risk of PID if she douches, is sexually active with more than one partner, and is younger than age 25.

Signs and Symptoms. A female may not have any symptoms, or PID can cause:
- Lower abdominal pain, mild pelvic pain, and pain with intercourse
- Increased vaginal discharge and irregular menstrual bleeding
- Fever
- Frequent urination
- Abdominal, pelvic organ, and uterine tenderness

Diagnostic Procedures. During the pelvic exam, the provider may obtain vaginal discharge specimens to diagnose infections or sexually transmitted infections (STIs). Additional testing may include blood and urine tests for pregnancy, STIs, and the human immunodeficiency virus (HIV). An ultrasound, endometrial biopsy, and laparoscopy may also be done.

Treatments. Treatment includes antibiotics. The partner should also be examined and tested to prevent reinfection. Sexual intercourse should be avoided until the treatment is completed.

VOCABULARY
laparoscopy A procedure used to visually examine the abdomen.

Polycystic Ovary Syndrome

Polycystic ovary syndrome (PCOS) is a hormonal disorder that causes cysts to grow on the ovaries.

Etiology. The exact cause of PCOS is unknown. Genetics, excessive androgen and insulin, and low-grade inflammation may be factors.

Signs and Symptoms. Signs and symptoms can occur around the first menses and include:
- Irregular menstrual period, pelvic pain, and infertility
- Excessive facial and body hair, severe acne, and male-pattern baldness, caused by excess androgen
- Oily skin, patches of thickened skin, and weight gain

Diagnostic Procedures. The provider will obtain a medical history and perform a physical exam, along with a pelvic exam. Androgen, glucose, cholesterol, and triglyceride blood levels may be checked. A transvaginal ultrasound may also be done.

Treatments. There is no treatment for PCOS. The goal is to control the symptoms with a low-calorie diet, exercise, and medications, such as oral contraceptive and progestin medications. Surgery and in vitro fertilization (IVF) can be used to help treat symptoms.

Premenstrual Syndrome

Premenstrual syndrome (PMS) refers to a wide range of symptoms. The symptoms usually start during the second half of the menstrual cycle and end 1 to 2 days after the menstrual period starts. The symptoms get worst during the late 30s until menopause.

Etiology. The exact cause of PMS is unknown. PMS may be related to psychological, biological, social, and cultural factors.

Signs and Symptoms. PMS can cause a wide range of symptoms, including:
- Bloating, constipation, diarrhea, and food cravings
- Confusion, trouble concentrating, forgetfulness, anxiety, irritableness, sadness, and mood swings
- Sleep problems, breast tenderness, headaches, and less tolerance for lights and noise

Diagnostic Procedures. After obtaining a medical history and performing a physical and pelvic examination, the provider may order tests to rule out other conditions. A symptom calendar can help the provider confirm the diagnosis of PMS. The symptom calendar could include symptoms experienced, the severity of the symptoms, and the length of time they were experienced.

Treatments. The goal is to manage the PMS symptoms. These lifestyle approaches may include:
- Limiting sugary, caffeine, and alcoholic beverages and drinking plenty of water and juice
- Eating a balanced diet (small frequent meals can be helpful)
- Taking nutritional supplements, such as vitamin B_6, calcium, and magnesium
- Getting regular aerobic exercise
  Over-the-counter analgesics and oral contraceptives can help reduce PMS symptoms.

Vaginitis

Vaginitis is an infection or inflammation of the vagina. Vaginitis is a common disorder in women during their reproductive years. There are different types of vaginitis, with different causes, symptoms, and treatments. Vaginitis occurs when there is a change in the balance of bacteria or yeast normally found in your vagina. Vaginitis can occur from an allergy or a sensitivity to products such as vaginal sprays, douches, spermicides, and soaps. Table 14.7 describes bacterial vaginitis and candidiasis.

Additional Female Reproductive Disorders

The following list provides a brief description of additional conditions.
- *Bartholin's cyst* or *abscess*: Caused from a blockage of the Bartholin's gland. Fluid backs up in the gland, resulting in a painless swollen area on the side of the vaginal opening.
- *Cervical dysplasia*: Abnormal changes in the cells on the surface of the cervix; considered precancerous.
- *Cervicitis*: Swollen or inflamed tissues of the cervix, typically caused by STIs.
- *Uterine fibroids*: Most common benign tumors in women of childbearing age. These muscular tumors grow in the wall of the uterus.
- *Paget disease of the breast*: A rare type of cancer that involves the skin of the nipple and areola.

TABLE 14.7   Types of Vaginitis

	Bacterial Vaginosis (BV)	Candidiasis
Etiology	Caused by an overgrowth of one of several bacteria that are naturally found in the vagina. Overgrowth can occur from taking antibiotics, douching, using an intrauterine device (IUD), and sexual intercourse (e.g., multiple partners, unprotected sex).	Fungus *Candida albicans*; overgrowth of yeast can occur from taking antibiotics, pregnancy, uncontrolled diabetes, and corticosteroid medications.
Signs and Symptoms	Thin, gray, green, or white vaginal discharge; foul-smelling "fishy" vaginal odor; vaginal itching; and burning during urination.	Vaginal rash, pain, soreness, itching and irritation; burning during intercourse or while urinating; redness and swelling of the vulva; thick, white, odor-free vaginal discharge with cottage cheese appearance, watery vaginal discharge.
Diagnostic Procedures	Medical history, pelvic exam, testing of vaginal pH, and microscopy study of vaginal secretions.	Medical history, pelvic exam, and testing of vaginal secretions
Treatments	Medications including metronidazole (me troe NI da zole) and clindamycin (kin da MYE sin)	Antifungal medication, such as miconazole (mi KON a zole), terconazole (ter KON a zole), and fluconazole (floo KON na zole).

- *Primary ovarian insufficiency* (POI): Also called *premature ovarian failure*; the ovaries stop working before age 40, causing reduced fertility and irregular menses.
- *Uterine fibroids*: Most common benign tumors in women of childbearing age. These muscular tumors (*myomas*) grow in the wall of the uterus.

DISEASES AND DISORDERS RELATED TO PREGNANCY

Table 14.8 provides common diagnostic procedures used to monitor and detect pregnancy disorders. The following sections discuss pregnancy disorders.

Ectopic Pregnancy

An ectopic pregnancy occurs when the fertilized egg implants and grows outside of the uterus. In many cases the implantation occurs in the fallopian tube, but other sites include the ovary, abdomen, or cervix. An ectopic pregnancy can be life-threatening for the mother.

Etiology. An ectopic pregnancy can occur when the movement of the fertilized egg is slowed or blocked as it moves through the fallopian tubes. This can be caused by fallopian tube abnormalities, scarring from prior surgeries or infections, and endometriosis. Risk factors for having an ectopic pregnancy include:

- A prior history of an ectopic pregnancy
- Being over 35 years of age
- Having an STI
- Having multiple sexual partners
- Getting pregnant with an intrauterine device (IUD) in place

Signs and Symptoms. An ectopic pregnancy can cause abnormal vaginal bleeding, mild cramping, and pain in the pelvic area. If the implantation site ruptures and bleeds, the female may experience:

- Fainting and low blood pressure
- Pain in the shoulder or neck from blood pooling and irritating certain nerves
- Severe, sharp, sudden lower abdominal pain

Diagnostic Procedures. The healthcare provider will do a pelvic exam. A pregnancy test and a vaginal ultrasound will confirm the ectopic pregnancy.

Treatments. If the ectopic pregnancy has not ruptured, treatment involves surgery or medication to end the pregnancy. It is a medical emergency if it has ruptured.

> **CRITICAL THINKING 14.7**
>
> Explain why an ectopic pregnancy is a medical emergency.

Hemolytic Disease of the Fetus and Newborn

Hemolytic disease of the fetus and newborn (HDFN) is also called *erythroblastosis fetalis* and *hemolytic disease of the newborn* (HDN). HDFN causes the red blood cells (RBCs) in the baby's blood to break down at a faster rate. This disease can affect newborns and unborn babies (fetuses) (Fig. 14.14).

Etiology. HDFN can occur if the mother and baby have different blood types (e.g., A, B, AB, or O) or Rh factors. Most often it occurs when a Rh-negative mother has a baby with Rh-positive blood and the baby's red blood cells cross into the mother's blood. The Rh-negative mother's immune system develops antibodies against the Rh-positive red blood cells. The mother is now Rh sensitized.

The Rh-negative mother's risk for HDFN is greater if she has had a Rh-positive baby and hasn't received treatment or if the mother is Rh sensitized due to an injury or test during a pregnancy with an Rh-positive baby.

Signs and Symptoms. Rh sensitivity is usually not a problem with a first (Rh-positive) pregnancy. Most complications occur in future pregnancies of Rh-positive babies. During a subsequent pregnancy, the mother's antibodies cross the placenta and fight the Rh-positive cells in the baby's blood.

During pregnancy, the baby may have an enlarged liver, spleen, or heart. *Hydrops fetalis* may occur, causing extra fluid to

TABLE 14.8   Common Diagnostic Procedures Used for Pregnancies

Done by/Type of Test:	Procedure	Description
Provider during the exam	Doppler fetal heart rate	Used to listen to the fetal heartbeat.
Surgical procedure	Amniocentesis (am nee oh sen TEE sis)	An ultrasound is done to show the position of the baby in utero while a needle is inserted and a sample of amniotic fluid is withdrawn. The fluid is analyzed for genetic testing, fetal lung maturity, paternity testing, pathogens (to diagnose an infection), and as treatment of polyhydramnios.
	Chorionic villus sampling (CVS)	Removal of a small part of the chorionic villi either through transcervical or transabdominal (through a small incision in the abdominal wall). The tissue is analyzed for chromosomal abnormalities.
Imagining procedure	Contraction stress test (CST)	Oxytocin (Pitocin) is given to the mother, which causes uterine contractions. The baby's heart rate during uterine contractions is monitored using a fetal heart rate monitor. A decreased heart rate during the contraction can indicate an issue.
	Nonstress test (NST)	The baby's heart rate is monitored using a fetal heart rate monitor. The mother is at rest or moving.
	Ultrasound (US)	• Biophysical profile (BPP): An NST with an ultrasound exam. The baby's movement, body tone, and breathing are examined, along with the amniotic fluid. • Fetal US or pregnancy US: Used to examine the mother's reproductive structures, along with the baby in utero. • Modified biophysical profile (MBPP): An NST with an ultrasound exam. The amniotic fluid is examined.
Medical laboratory	Alpha fetoprotein (AFP) test	Maternal blood test. May indicate fetal abnormalities.
	Estriol (E3) test	An estrogen hormone that increases during pregnancy; used to monitor high-risk pregnancies and help diagnose certain birth defects (e.g., Down syndrome) during pregnancy. Part of the prenatal or triple screen test.
	Pregnancy test	Urine or blood test used to examine for the presence of hCG. Some are CLIA-waived tests.
	Progesterone blood test	Used to monitor pregnancy and diagnose ectopic pregnancy.

CIA, Clinical Laboratory Improvement Amendments; hCG, human chorionic gonadotropin.

accumulate in the stomach, lungs, or scalp. The amniotic fluid may be yellow from bilirubin, a by-product of the RBCs breaking down. HDFN can cause miscarriages.

Besides having enlarged organs and hydrops fetalis, a newborn may look pale from anemia and have jaundice from the excess bilirubin. Jaundice causes the yellow coloring of the skin and whites of the eyes.

Diagnostic Procedures. To prevent this disorder, it is standard practice for the pregnant mother's blood to be tested (typed) early in pregnancy, if the blood type is unknown. Testing is also done to check for Rh-positive antibodies in the mother's blood. During pregnancy additional testing might be done, including:
- An ultrasound exam to check for enlarged organs in the baby
- Amniocentesis to check for bilirubin in the amniotic fluid
- Percutaneous umbilical cord blood sampling to test for antibodies, bilirubin, and anemia

After birth, the newborn will have blood work to determine the blood group, Rh factor, bilirubin level, and red blood cell count.

Treatments. Newborns with HDFN are treated with blood transfusions and intravenous fluids for anemia and low blood pressure. Phototherapy and exchange (blood) transfusions are used to treat the high levels of bilirubin in the blood.

Prevention. Mothers with Rh-negative blood receive an injection of RhoGAM around week 28 of pregnancy. After the baby

is born, the cord blood is tested. If the baby has Rh-positive blood, the mother receives another injection of RhoGAM within 72 hours of delivery.

MICRhoGram (a smaller dose of RhoGAM) should be given to Rh-negative women 72 hours after a threatened or actual termination of pregnancy (spontaneous [miscarriage] or induced) through week 12 of the pregnancy. For threatened or actual exposure to Rh-positive blood (e.g., through an invasive procedure, trauma, ectopic pregnancy, or pregnancy termination), Rh-negative women should receive RhoGAM within 72 hours. RhoGAM and MICRhoGAM are Rho (D) human immune globulin, a blood product that prevents Rh immunization by binding to Rh-positive cells that sneak into the bloodstream, making them invisible to the mother's immune system.

Hyperemesis Gravidarum

Morning sickness causes nausea and vomiting during pregnancy. It can occur at any time of the day. Morning sickness usually decreases after the first trimester, but not always. Severe morning sickness can progress into *hyperemesis gravidarum*. With hyperemesis gravidarum, the extreme nausea and vomiting causes dehydration, electrolyte imbalance, and weight loss.

Etiology. The exact cause of hyperemesis gravidarum is unknown.

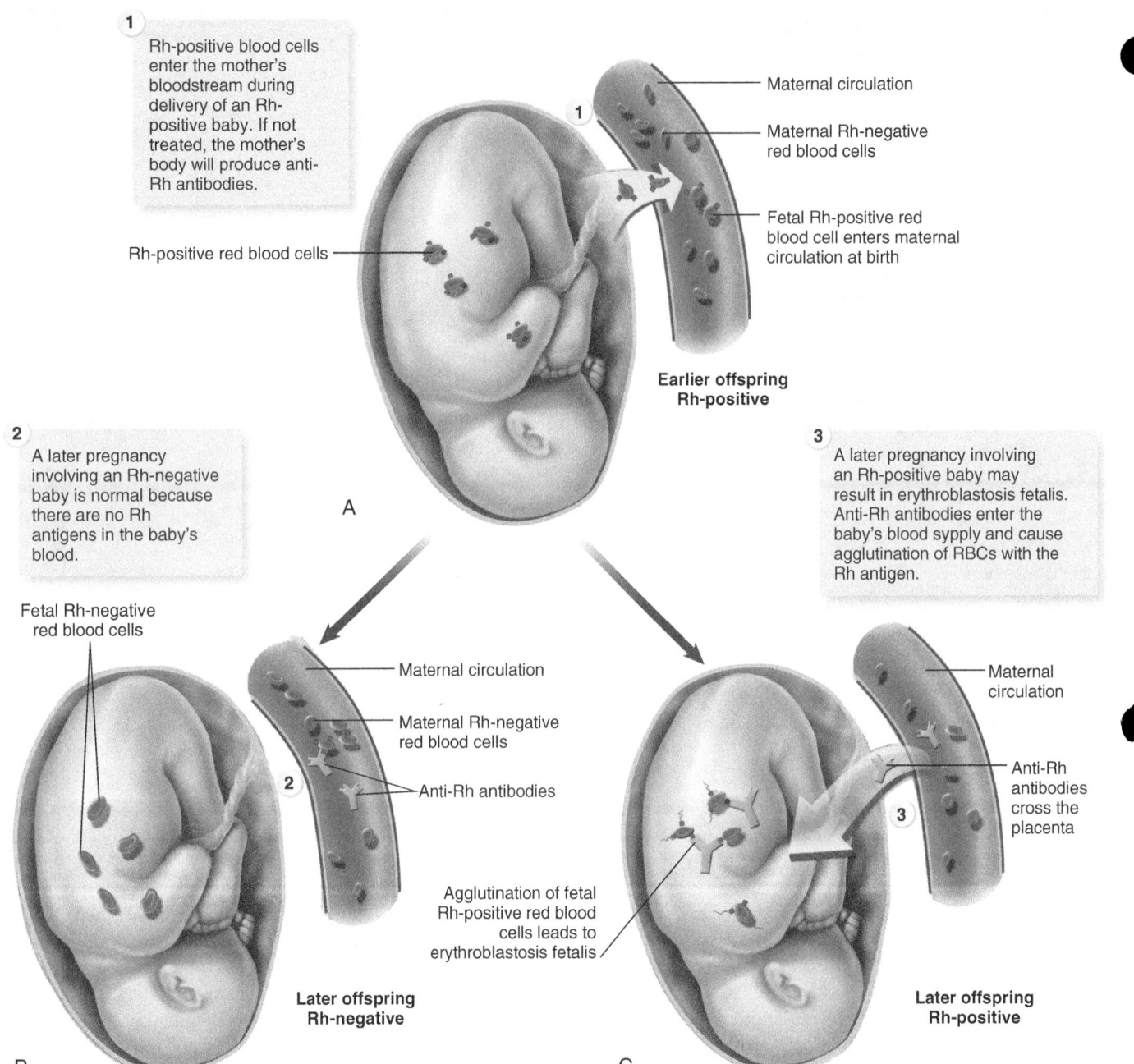

1 Rh-positive blood cells enter the mother's bloodstream during delivery of an Rh-positive baby. If not treated, the mother's body will produce anti-Rh antibodies.

Rh-positive red blood cells

Maternal circulation

Maternal Rh-negative red blood cells

Fetal Rh-positive red blood cell enters maternal circulation at birth

Earlier offspring Rh-positive

A

2 A later pregnancy involving an Rh-negative baby is normal because there are no Rh antigens in the baby's blood.

Fetal Rh-negative red blood cells

Maternal circulation

Maternal Rh-negative red blood cells

Anti-Rh antibodies

Later offspring Rh-negative

B

3 A later pregnancy involving an Rh-positive baby may result in erythroblastosis fetalis. Anti-Rh antibodies enter the baby's blood sypply and cause agglutination of RBCs with the Rh antigen.

Maternal circulation

Anti-Rh antibodies cross the placenta

Agglutination of fetal Rh-positive red blood cells leads to erythroblastosis fetalis

Later offspring Rh-positive

C

Fig. 14.14 Hemolytic Disease of the Fetus and Newborn. Under certain conditions, anti-Rh antibodies may enter the offspring's blood supply and cause red blood cell (RBC) agglutination (clumping) and destruction. (From Patton KT, Thibodeau GA: *The human body in health and disease*, ed 7, St. Louis, 2018, Elsevier.)

Signs and Symptoms. Hyperemesis gravidarum causes:
- Severe, persistent nausea and vomiting during pregnancy and an inability to take in adequate nutrition or liquids
- Salivation more than normal
- Dehydration (e.g., dark urine, lightheadedness, weakness, and fainting)
- Constipation and weight loss

Diagnostic Procedures. During the prenatal visit, the patient's weight and blood pressure are obtained. Blood and urine tests may be ordered to check for signs of dehydration.

A pregnancy ultrasound may be done to check for multiple births or hydatidiform mole (which is explained later in this chapter).

Treatments. The goal of treatment is to ensure the mother gets adequate fluids and nutrition. To avoid the nausea and vomiting, it is recommended to avoid triggers, such as certain smells, noise, lights, and toothpaste. Eating dry, bland foods and small frequent meals can help. Antinausea medications, intravenous fluids, and feeding tubes may also be part of the treatment plan.

Mastitis

Mastitis is an inflammation of breast tissue. It most commonly affects females who are breastfeeding, though it can occur without breastfeeding.

Etiology. Mastitis can be caused by a blocked milk duct. The backed-up milk can lead to an infection. Bacteria, such as *Staphylococcus aureus*, can enter through the milk duct opening or a crack in the nipple.

Signs and Symptoms. Mastitis causes breast enlargement, swelling, tenderness, redness, and pain. Fever and flulike symptoms can also be experienced, along with itching and nipple discharge.

Diagnostic Procedures. The provider will obtain a medical history and perform a physical exam. A breast ultrasound exam may be done to check for abscesses. If the infection returns, the provider may also recommend a breast biopsy, MRI, ultrasound, and a mammogram.

Treatments. Treatments include antibiotics, over-the-counter pain relievers, and applications of moist heat on the infected tissue.

Placenta Previa

With placenta previa (pluh SEN tuh PREH vee uh), the placenta grows at the lower part of the uterus covering the cervical opening. If it covers part of the cervical opening, it is called *partial placenta previa. Complete placenta previa* means it covers the entire cervical opening.

Etiology. The exact cause is unknown. The risk can increase with:
- A history of placenta previa or the presence of uterine scars from prior procedures
- Being 35 years of age or older, having prior pregnancies, or carrying more than one baby
- Smoking and using cocaine

Signs and Symptoms. The main sign is sudden vaginal bleeding during the second half of pregnancy. Some women may have contractions or cramping. If the bleeding is severe, it can be life-threatening.

Diagnostic Procedures. A pregnancy ultrasound exam is used to diagnose the condition.

Treatments. Treatment depends on the severity of the bleeding and current length of the pregnancy. After 36 weeks, usually the baby can be delivered by C-section. A vaginal delivery may cause severe life-threatening bleeding. Severe bleeding may require blood transfusions and steroid shots to help mature the baby's lungs. For less severe bleeding, reducing activities and bed rest may be recommended. Sex, tampons, and douching need to be avoided.

Placental Abruption

Placental abruption or *abruptio placentae* occurs when the placenta separates from the uterus before the baby is born.

Etiology. The exact cause is unknown. The risk can increase with:
- A history of placental abruption, chronic or sudden hypertension, heart disease, abdominal trauma, or uterine fibroids
- Smoking and using alcohol and/or cocaine
- Being over 40 years of age and being Caucasian or African American

Signs and Symptoms. Vaginal bleeding and contractions are the most common sign and symptom. The severity of bleeding depends on the amount of detachment.

Diagnostic Procedures. The provider will do a physical exam to detect the source of bleeding and an ultrasound might be done. The fetal heart rate is also checked. Electronic fetal monitoring to assess how the baby handles the contractions and a pregnancy ultrasound exam may also be done.

Treatments. For small placental abruptions, bed rest for a few days may be recommended. Larger placental abruptions involve hospitalization for monitoring of the bleeding and the baby's well-being. Blood transfusions may be required.

CRITICAL THINKING 14.8

Describe the difference between placenta previa and placental abruption.

Preeclampsia and Eclampsia

Preeclampsia occurs after week 20 of pregnancy. It occurs in about 3% to 7% of pregnancies. Preeclampsia can progress to severe preeclampsia and then eclampsia. If the female with preeclampsia has a new onset of seizures or coma, the condition is called *eclampsia*.

Etiology. The cause of preeclampsia is unknown. Risk factors for preeclampsia include:
- A first pregnancy or a multiple pregnancy, such as having twins
- A past history or family history of preeclampsia
- Obesity
- Being older than age 35 and being African American
- A history of diabetes, high blood pressure, or kidney disease

Signs and Symptoms. Preeclampsia causes edema in the hands, face, or around the eyes, and a sudden weight gain of 2 or more pounds within 2 days. Severe preeclampsia causes:
- Trouble breathing, headache that intensifies or does not go away
- Right shoulder or abdominal pain
- Decreased urination
- Seizures or changes in mental function
- Nausea, vomiting, and visual changes (e.g., flashing lights, spots)

- Lightheadedness or feeling faint
- A blood pressure higher than 140/90 mm Hg (hypertension)
- Low platelet counts, proteinuria, and elevated blood liver enzymes and creatine levels

Diagnostic Procedures. The provider will do a physical exam, including blood pressure and weight. Blood and urine tests will be done. To assess the baby's health, an ultrasound exam, non-stress test, and other tests will be done.

Treatments. Preeclampsia resolves upon delivery of the infant. If it is too early for delivery of the baby, management of the disease is critical. Blood pressure medications and frequent follow-up visits are recommended. Hospitalization may be required until delivery to help monitor the mother's blood pressure and prevent seizures and other complications.

CRITICAL THINKING 14.9

Describe the difference between preeclampsia and eclampsia.

Additional Pregnancy-Related Disorders

The following list provides a brief description of additional conditions.

- *Gestational diabetes*: Develops during pregnancy. The hyperglycemia can affect the health of the pregnancy and the baby. (See Chapter 7 for additional information.)
- *Miscarriage*: Also called *spontaneous abortion*; an unexpected loss of pregnancy before week 20 of pregnancy.
- *Molar pregnancy* or *hydatidiform mole* (HM): Rare growth that forms in the uterus at the beginning of the pregnancy due to the abnormal fertilization of the egg. With a *partial molar pregnancy*, there is an abnormal placenta and some fetal development. With a *complete molar pregnancy*, there is an abnormal placenta and no fetal tissue.
- *Oligohydramnios*: A condition of too little amniotic fluid. Can occur with late pregnancies, ruptured membranes, placental dysfunction, or fetal abnormalities.
- *Pica*: Eating of non-food materials, such as paper, ice, clay, or dirt. Seen in children and during pregnancy. May be caused from a lack of certain nutrients that produce unusual cravings.
- *Polyhydramnios*: A condition of too much amniotic fluid. Can occur with multiple pregnancies (e.g., twins), congenital anomalies, or gestational diabetes.
- *Postpartum depression*: Occurs after giving birth. The person has feelings of extreme sadness, exhaustion, and anxiety. These feelings interfere with daily life and caring for the new baby.
- *Preterm labor*: Labor that starts before 37 completed weeks of pregnancy; can lead to premature birth.
- *Stillbirth*: Loss of a pregnancy due to natural causes after week 20.
- *Toxoplasmosis*: Caused by the parasite *Toxoplasma gondii*, commonly found in cat litter. Can cause damage to the brain, eyes, and other organs of the baby in utero whose mother becomes infected for the first time during pregnancy.

- *Zika*: A virus spread by mosquitoes, blood transfusions, and sexual contact. A pregnant mother who is infected can pass the virus to her baby in utero. Symptoms if present include fever, rash, joint pain, and conjunctivitis. For babies in utero, it can cause microcephaly (abnormal smallness of the head) and other problems.

SEXUALLY TRANSMITTED INFECTIONS

Sexually transmitted infections are passed from one person to another through sexual activity, including vaginal, oral, and anal sex. There are more than 20 STIs caused by bacteria, parasites, and viruses. Millions of new STIs occur yearly in the US, with the human papillomavirus (HPV) infection being the most common.

STIs affect both males and females. Some STIs cause no or very mild symptoms. Females usually have more severe health problems. An STI in a pregnant woman can cause a serious health concern for the baby. (Tables 14.9 and 14.10).

- *Chlamydia*: Can be passed to the baby during a vaginal delivery. It can cause pneumonia and a serious eye infection in the newborn. (Table 14.9).
- *Gonorrhea*: Can be passed to the baby during a vaginal delivery. It can cause blindness, joint infections, and a life-threatening infection in the newborn (Fig. 14.15).
- *Syphilis*: Can be passed to the baby through the placenta or during birth. It may cause a rash, deafness, teeth deformities, and nasal deformities. Most states require syphilis screening during pregnancy. Nontreponemal tests (e.g., rapid plasma reagin [RPR], venereal disease research laboratory [VDRL]) can be used for screening. People with a reactive nontreponemal test always need a treponemal test to confirm the syphilis diagnosis. Some examples of treponemal tests include fluorescent treponemal antibody absorption test (FTA-ABS), chemiluminescence immunoassays, immunoblots, and rapid treponemal assays.
- *Genital herpes*: Can be passed to the baby during pregnancy or childbirth. The baby may get a life-threatening herpes infection (Table 14.10 and Fig. 14.16).
- *HIV/acquired immunodeficiency syndrome* (AIDS): HIV can be passed to the baby during pregnancy, childbirth, or breastfeeding. (HIV and AIDS are discussed in more depth in Chapter 9.)

STI testing is typically done during the first prenatal visit and can be repeated later in the pregnancy if the patient is considered high risk for STI or HIV.

STIs are preventable. The most effective way to avoid STIs is to abstain from sex. Other ways to reduce the risk of STIs include:

- Having a long-term mutually monogamous relationship. Neither partner is infected, and the couple only has intercourse with each other.
- Getting tested for STIs before having intercourse with a new partner.
- Getting vaccinated to prevent HPV.
- Refraining from substances (e.g., alcohol, drugs) that can impair reasoning and increase sexual risks.
- Using protection, such as condoms and dental dams.
- Limiting the number of sex partners.

TABLE 14.9 Common Bacterial Sexually Transmitted Infections (STIs)

Disease	Chlamydia (klah MID ee ah)	Gonorrhea (gaw noh REE ah)	Syphilis (SIF ih lis)
Description	Most frequent bacterial STI in the US; common STI in women age 25 or younger	A very common STI, especially in people between ages 15 and 24.	A common STI, which is becoming more prevalent.
Complications	If left untreated in females, can cause infertility.	*Females:* Pelvic inflammatory diseases (PIDs), infertility and increased risk of ectopic pregnancy. *Males:* Epididymitis and infertility. If untreated, can lead to disseminated gonococcal infection, which is life-threatening.	Without treatment can severely damage brain, heart, eyes, liver, and joints, and can be life-threatening.
Etiology	*Chlamydia trachomatis* bacterium	Neisseria gonorrhoeae bacterium can infect the cervix, uterus, and fallopian tubes in females and the urethra, mouth, throat, eyes, and rectum in males and females.	Treponema pallidum bacterium; transmitted by direct contact with a sore called a chancre (SHANG kur).
Signs and Symptoms	*Males:* Penile discharge, burning with urination and testicular pain and swelling. *Females:* Abnormal vaginal discharge, bleeding between menses and after sex, painful intercourse, and a burning feeling on urination. *Both:* Rectal pain, bleeding, and discharge.	*Males:* May have no symptoms; white, yellow, or green urethral discharge, dysuria, testicular pain. *Females:* May have no symptoms, dysuria, vaginal discharge, bleeding between menses. *Both:* Anal discharge, itching, and soreness, painful bowel movements, bleeding; pink or red eye, mucous discharge or crusting on eyelashes, swollen lids, foreign body sensation, decreased vision.	A *chancre* is a firm, round painless lesion, which usually appears first. Then a rash over the body, oral and genital wartlike sores, loss of hair, muscle aches, sore throat, fever, and swollen lymph nodes.
Diagnostic Procedures	Testing of urine or discharge. Tests include nucleic acid amplification testing (NAAT); culture can also be done.	Testing of urethral (males), or endocervical or vaginal (females), or urine specimens using NAAT; culture can also be done.	Treponemal (blood) test, such as immunoblots and rapid treponemal assays, which detect antibodies that are specific for syphilis.
Treatments	Treated with antibiotics; usually resolves within 2 weeks.	Due to the rise of antimicrobial resistance in gonorrhea, dual therapy (two medications) is recommended.	Treated with antibiotics, such as Penicillin G injection and doxycycline (dox i SYE kleen).

TABLE 14.10 Viral and Parasitic Sexually Transmitted Infections (STIs)

Disease	Genital Herpes	Human Papillomavirus (HPV)	Trichomoniasis (trik oh moh NY ah sis)
Description	Common viral STI. Herpes simplex virus type 2 is more common in women.	Most common STI, with over 79 million Americans in their teens to early 20s having it. Over 40 strains of HPV.	Very common STI caused by a parasite.
Etiology	Transmitted through contact with herpes simplex virus type 1 (HSV-1) or type 2 (HSV-2) in herpes lesions, mucosal surfaces, and genital or oral secretions.	Transmitted even if infected person has no symptoms.	A protozoan parasite, *Trichomonas vaginalis*, spreads from infected person to uninfected person during sex.
Signs and Symptoms	No symptoms; recurring herpes lesions (small blisters) in genital or rectal area, or mouth. May have genital pain or tingling, shooting pain in legs or hips before eruption of herpetic lesions. Can cause aseptic meningitis.	Depend on the type of HPV. Genital warts (raised or flat or shaped like a cauliflower) in the genital area or mouth. May have bleeding with intercourse and itching. A few types of genital HPV cause cervical cancer. Vulval, penile, and anal cancer, along with oropharyngeal cancer, can also occur.	About 70% of infected people have no symptoms. *Males:* Penile discharge, itching or irritation and burning after ejaculation or urination. *Females:* Genital itching, burning, redness, or soreness; discomfort with urination. Clear, white-, yellow-, or green-colored vaginal discharge with a fishy smell.
Diagnostic Procedures	Swab of lesion is taken and tested by nucleic acid amplification testing (NAAT) or viral culture.	If genital warts are present, usually diagnosed upon appearance. HPV tests for women age 30 years or older used as cervical cancer screening. Abnormal Pap test results may be an indication.	Microscopic examination of a wet mount preparation of vaginal discharge (females) or urine (males); NAAT, rapid antigen test.
Treatments	Herpes is not curable; treatment focuses on management of symptoms. Antiviral medications can prevent or shorten outbreaks.	HPV is not curable, and warts may return after treatment. Warts can be treated with medications, electrocautery, surgical excision, and cryotherapy. HPV vaccines protect against cervical cancer and genital warts.	Metronidazole (me troe NI da zole) (Flagyl) or tinidazole (tye NI da zole) (Tindamax); retesting encouraged 2 weeks to 3 months after treatment.

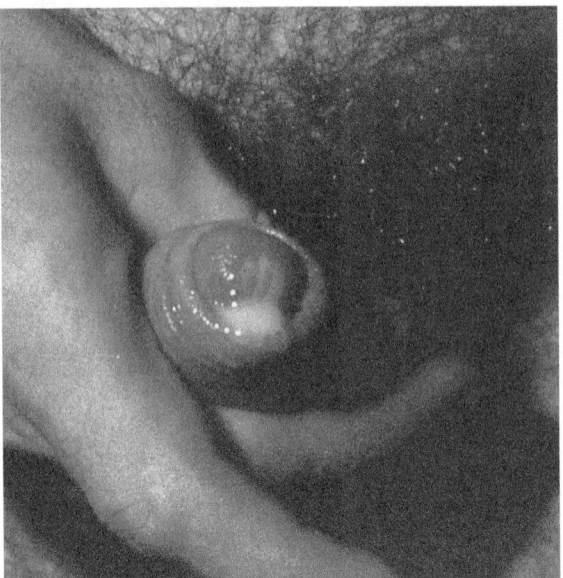

Fig. 14.15 Gonorrhea in a Male Patient. (From *Mosby's medical nursing and allied health dictionary*, ed 8, St. Louis, 2009, Mosby.)

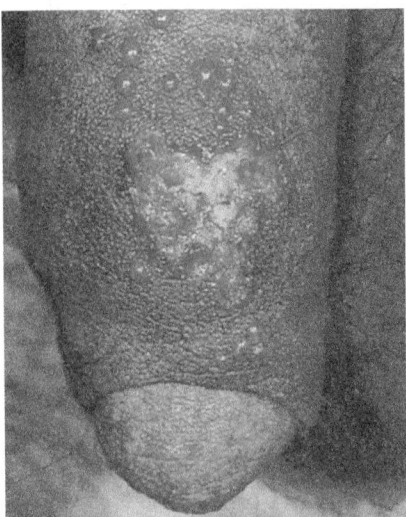

Fig. 14.16 Genital Herpes. (From *Mosby's medical nursing and allied health dictionary*, ed 8, St. Louis, 2009, Mosby.)

Treatment usually requires abstinence from intercourse during this time. The partner must also be treated at the same time to prevent the couple from reinfecting each other. Having an STI does not protect the person from becoming infected again.

LIFE SPAN CHANGES

Changes in the Male Reproductive System

The testicle develops in the abdomen and starts its descent into the scrotum in utero around the seventh month. At puberty, the testicles start producing testosterone, which is responsible for the development of sperm and the secondary sex characteristics (e.g., deep voice, broad shoulders, narrow hips, and additional body hair).

As a male gets older, gradual aging changes begin. Changes occur in the testicular tissue, sperm production, and erectile function. The testicular tissue mass decreases. Testosterone levels gradually decrease and may cause issues with erections. The testes continue to create sperm, but at a slower rate. Benign prostatic hyperplasia can occur, leading to issues with urine retention, ejaculation, and a slowed urine stream.

Changes in the Female Reproductive System

From birth to puberty, the number of ovarian follicles decreases. At puberty, the ovaries secrete estrogen and progesterone. Estrogen is responsible for the secondary sex characteristics (e.g., pubic hair and breast development).

Perimenopause is the time before menopause, or when the menstrual periods permanently stop. Perimenopause may occur several years before menopause. Signs of perimenopause include:

- More frequent periods, followed by occasional missed periods
- Shorter or longer periods
- Changes in the menstrual flow

Over time, the periods become less frequent, until they stop completely. Being without menstrual periods for 1 year, means the female is in *menopause*. If contraceptives are being used, they should be used until the female is free from menstrual periods for a year. Most women experience menopause around age 50, though it can occur at any age. Additional information on menopause is provided in Chapter 36.

CLOSING COMMENTS

Patients with reproductive disorders are seen in primary care, urgent care, OB/GYN, and urology departments. The female and male reproductive systems are complex. Knowing the structures and how the systems function are crucial. Having a strong understanding of the related medical terminology, common signs and symptoms, diagnostic procedures, and treatments is important for medical assistants (Box 14.6). Having this knowledge not only helps the medical assistant provide the best patient care, but also allows the medical assistant to communicate professionally with others.

PATIENT-CENTERED CARE

Providing patient-centered care means the patient's and family's preferences are respected. It also includes their values, cultural traditions, and socioeconomic condition. Patients and their families are part of the care team and play an important role in deciding their care.

As in other departments, delivering patient-centered care in an OB/GYN department is important. Whether patients are pregnant, experiencing infertility, or being seen for a gynecologic concern, it is important to remember that their wishes need to be respected. Patients should be educated on their condition so they can help make decisions about their care.

BOX 14.6   Medication Classifications

- *Antibiotics*: To treat bacterial infections.
- *Contraceptives*: Used to prevent pregnancy.
- *Erectile dysfunction agents*: Used to facilitate an erection in patients with erectile dysfunction (impotence) and symptoms of benign prostatic hypertrophy (enlarged prostate).
- *Hormone replacements*: Used to maintain adequate hormone levels.

  Refer to Appendix D, which can be found on the Evolve website, for information on the medication classifications, including indications for use, desired effect, side effects, adverse reactions, and generic and trade names. Medical assistants should be familiar with medications that are prescribed to patients.

BEING PROFESSIONAL

When working with pregnant teenagers, the medical assistant must remember to be respectful and nonjudgmental. The medical assistant must also use age-related communication strategies, such as:
- Providing privacy and independence
- Encouraging responsible decision making
- Encouraging discussion and questions

  Role-play this scenario: You are a medical assistant. You are rooming Tonya Green, who is pregnant with her first child. She is 15 years old. Tonya shares with you that she is nervous about having a baby. She states that her old friends are no longer talking with her, so she found new friends. These new friends like to smoke and drink. They want her to do the same. How do you respond to Tonya?

CHAPTER REVIEW

The male reproductive system is responsible for producing, transporting, and sustaining sperm cells. The male reproductive system consists of a pair of testes and a network of excretory ducts (epididymis, vas deferens, and ejaculatory ducts), seminal vesicles, the prostate gland, the Cowper glands, urethra, and the penis. At puberty, testosterone is produced, which helps with the development of the secondary sex characteristics. FSH promotes the formation of sperm. LH stimulates the production of testosterone.

Common male reproductive disorders were discussed. Common etiologies include age and cell mutations, in addition to viral, bacterial, and other diseases. Common signs and symptoms include redness, swelling, or lumps in the organs. Changes in the urinary stream or issues during intercourse can also be seen. Diagnostic tests and procedures done include digital rectal examinations, testicular exams, biopsies, ultrasounds, MRIs, hormone testing, prostate-specific antigen blood test, STI tests, and semen analysis. Treatments consist of surgical procedures, laser therapy, and medications.

The female reproductive system is responsible for producing, transporting, and sustaining egg cells. It also needs to nurture the developing offspring. The female reproductive system consists of the ovaries, fallopian tubes, uterus, vagina, external genitalia, and breasts. At puberty, the ovaries secrete estrogen and progesterone. Estrogen is responsible for the secondary sex characteristics. The first menses is called the *menarche*. During the menstrual cycle, changes occur in the ovaries, uterus, and breasts due to hormones. The menstrual cycle consists of menses, proliferative phase, ovulation, and secretory phase.

Gestation is the time between fertilization to birth. The development of the baby in utero is divided into the pre-embryonic, embryonic, and fetal periods. The pre-embryonic period lasts from conception to day 14. During this time, fertilization and implantation occur. The embryonic period starts day 15 to about week 8 after fertilization. At this point, the offspring is called an *embryo*. The placenta, umbilical cord, amnion, amniotic fluid, and yolk sac develop. All the essential organs begin to grow. From week 9 to the end of the pregnancy is considered the fetal period. The offspring is now called a *fetus*.

Common female reproductive and pregnancy disorders were discussed. Common etiologies include age, genetics, past medical history, and cell mutations, in addition to viral, bacterial, and other diseases. Common signs and symptoms include changes in the menses, painful intercourse, pain, discomfort, redness, and breast lumps. Changes in the urinary stream or issues during intercourse can also be seen. Diagnostic tests and procedures done include a Pap test biopsy, colposcopy, hysteroscopy, ultrasound, hysterosalpingography, and a mammography. Medical laboratory tests include hormone testing, STI tests, and HPV DNA tests. Pregnancy-specific tests include a Doppler fetal heart rate, amniocentesis, chorionic villus sampling, nonstress and stress tests, hormone levels, and a pregnancy test. Treatments consist of surgical procedures and medications.

As males age, gradual changes begin. Changes occur in the testicular tissue, sperm production, and erectile function. As females age, they experience perimenopause prior to menopause. Menopause may occur several years later.

SCENARIO WRAP-UP

Marie is enjoying her new job. As she works with the outreach providers, she is learning about many conditions that she did not see in family medicine. She is especially enjoying the obstetric patients. Because they come back for repeated prenatal appointments, she is beginning to get to know the patients. That is one of her favorite parts of the job.

Today was her first experience arranging a patient's admission for labor and delivery. It was exciting to know the patient was reaching the end of her pregnancy. Marie hopes to arrange a shadow opportunity at the local hospital to learn more about the labor and delivery process. She feels that seeing the entire process will help her provide better patient care to the obstetric patients.

15

Behavioral Health

LEARNING OBJECTIVES

1. Explore the differences between types of common behavioral health professionals.
2. Explain the common diagnostic procedures and treatments for behavioral health and substance use disorders.
3. Differentiate among common behavioral health disorders, including the etiology, signs, symptoms, diagnostic procedures, and treatments.
4. Discuss substance use disorders and other addictions.
5. List commonly used substances and describe a "standard" drink of alcohol.

OUTLINE

▶▶ OPENING SCENARIO

Mike Brewer, CMA (AAMA), is a medical assistant at Walden-Martin Family Medical (WMFM) Clinic. He has been with the clinic for 2 years. Mike currently assists outreach providers, who come to WMFM Clinic to provide services for patients. Recently, Mike has been working with the outreach behavioral health providers. During his medical assistant training, Mike learned about different behavioral health disorders but never felt he wanted to go into that specialty. Over the past 2 years at WMFM Clinic, he has realized that no matter what position he holds, he works with patients who have behavioral health disorders, depression being the most common. He is looking forward to learning more about behavioral health disorders as he continues to help the outreach providers.

YOU WILL LEARN

1. To describe different healthcare professionals who work in behavioral health.
2. To discuss common diagnostic procedures and treatments for behavioral health and substance use disorders.
3. To describe common behavioral health disorders, including the etiology, signs, symptoms, diagnostic procedures, and treatments.
4. To discuss substance use disorders.
5. To explain a "standard" drink of alcohol.

INTRODUCTION

Many times, healthcare students hear about mental health and quickly decide whether or not they are interested in that specialty.

In today's healthcare environment, many healthcare professionals, including medical assistants, are involved with mental health and substance use issues, regardless of where they work. The number of people in the United States with a mental health or substance use disorder has been increasing over the years. It is estimated that 1 in 5 adults in the United States have a mental health condition. Over 81,000 people died from a drug overdose in the United States in a 12-month period ending in May 2020. Over 70% of those deaths were related to a prescription or illicit opioid.

According to the Centers for Disease Control and Prevention (CDC), *mental health* encompasses our psychological, emotional, and social welfare. Our mental health influences how we behave, feel, think, handle stress, interact with others, and make choices. Over the years, the field of mental health has changed and grown. *Psychiatry* is the healthcare specialty that studies the brain and its effects on the body. Today, the phrase "*behavioral health*" is used to refer to mental health, substance use, and associated physical disorders.

This chapter begins by describing behavioral health specialists and locations where patients are treated. Information on specific behavioral health disorders will follow.

BEHAVIORAL HEALTH PROFESSIONALS

Psychotherapist (SIE koe THER ah pist) is a general term for a healthcare professional who treats people with behavioral health conditions. This term is used for psychiatrists (sie KIE ah trists), psychologists (sie KOL oh jist), social workers, and so on. In behavioral health departments, there are people with many different credentials. Having a basic understanding of behavioral health professionals is important. The following are some of the more common behavioral health professionals:

- *Psychiatrist*: Trained as a medical doctor and has had 4 years of residency training in psychiatry, usually in a hospital setting. A psychiatrist assesses the mental and physical conditions related to psychological disorders. A psychiatrist treats patients with psychological disorders and can prescribe medications.
- *Psychologist*: Studied personality development, psychological problems, and how to diagnose mental and emotional disorders; must obtain a PhD or PsyD doctoral degree. Primarily focuses on providing psychotherapy (sie KOE ther ah pee) and performing psychological testing. Most psychologists cannot prescribe medications.
- *Social worker*: Has a similar educational background as a psychologist but cannot provide psychological testing. The social worker provides psychotherapy. Depending on the state licensure, social workers may have different titles: Licensed Clinical Social Worker (LCSW), Licensed Independent Clinical Social Worker (LICSW), and Licensed Social Worker (LSW).
- *Cognitive behavioral therapist*: Specializes in cognitive behavioral therapy and helping people change the way they think and behave in order to help manage their condition (e.g., depression, relationship issues).
- *Psychiatric nurse*: A registered nurse who has advanced training (e.g., master's or doctoral degree) in assessing and treating behavioral health issues.
- *Substance use (or addiction) therapist* or *counselor:* Has specialized training to treat patients with substance use disorders and other addictions.
- *Behavioral health therapist* or *counselor:* Trained to treat patients with behavioral health disorders (e.g., depression, anxiety).

In many states, most of these healthcare professionals need a license to practice. There are some exceptions. Some states allow unlicensed behavioral health professionals to provide treatment to patients, but their billing capacity is limited. State laws dictate the licensing and credential requirements for behavioral health professionals.

Patients with behavioral health conditions may be seen in community mental health clinics or in private practice clinics. When patients are a threat to themselves or others, they may be admitted to hospitals until their behavioral health conditions stabilize. Specialty inpatient settings for eating disorders and addictions are also available.

VOCABULARY

psychotherapy The treatment of behavioral health disorders through the use of psychological techniques, which encourage communication of conflicts and insights into the person's problems. The goals of this treatment include symptom relief, changes in behavior leading to improved social and vocational function, and personality growth.

MEDICAL TERMINOLOGY

iatr/o	treatment
psych/o, thym/o, phren/o	mind
-logist	one who specializes in the study of
-iatrist	one who specializes in treatment

CRITICAL THINKING 15.1

Mike is asked by a patient to explain the difference between a psychiatrist and a psychologist. If you were asked this question, how would you respond?

DIAGNOSTIC AND STATISTICAL MANUAL OF MENTAL DISORDERS

The *Diagnostic and Statistical Manual of Mental Disorders* (DSM) is used by behavioral health professionals in the United States and other countries. The first DSM was published in 1952, and subsequent versions have been published since then; the latest is the DSM-5. The DSM provides descriptions, signs, symptoms, and other criteria for diagnosing behavioral health disorders. It provides a common language that is used in the behavioral health environment.

The DSM-5 contains the International Classification of Disease (ICD) codes required for insurance reimbursement and for monitoring morbidity (more BID i tee) and mortality (more TAL I tee) statistics. In other words, the ICD codes allow researchers to gather information on how often the disorder occurs and how many deaths are attributed to the disease.

CRITICAL THINKING 15.2

Where have you seen or heard morbidity and mortality statistics? Explain your answer.

BEHAVIORAL HEALTH DISORDERS

Behavioral health disorders are conditions that cause changes in the mood, behavior, or thoughts of an individual. These disorders can affect how a person functions on a day-to-day basis, at work, school, and at home.

Biological factors (e.g., genetics), life experiences, and a family history of behavioral health problems can contribute to behavioral health problems. It is important for a person to seek help immediately if signs of behavioral health disorders exist.

Common signs and symptoms of behavioral health disorders include:

- Withdrawing from others, isolating oneself
- Eating or sleeping too little or too much
- Having no or low amounts of energy
- Feeling helpless, hopeless, numb, or as if nothing matters
- Having unexplained pains and aches
- Smoking, drinking alcohol, or using drugs more than usual
- Feeling unusually forgetful, on edge, angry, worried, scared, confused, or upset
- Having persistent thoughts or memories "stuck" in your head
- Thinking of harming oneself or others
- Inability to function or do your daily activities
- Hearing voices or believing things that are not true

Behavioral health providers will perform mental status testing and other psychological tests. Box 15.1 provides additional information on mental status testing. There are many psychological tests used to help diagnose behavioral health disorders. Table 15.1 provides examples of psychological testing.

Many behavior health disorders are treated with psychotherapy. Psychotherapy is commonly referred to as "talk therapy." It is a general term used for a variety of treatment techniques that help a person identify and change troubling behaviors, thoughts, or emotions. Behavioral health therapists are trained in several types of psychotherapy. Based on the person and the disorder being treated, the therapist may use one or more types of psychotherapy (Table 15.2).

BOX 15.1   Mental Status Testing

Mental status testing (also called *neurocognitive testing*) assesses a person's ability to think. Providers are able to identify cognitive impairments. The testing involves the provider asking the patient a series of questions. Common tests include the Mini-Mental State Examination (MMSE), Folstein test, and the Montreal Cognitive Assessment.

The provider assesses cognitive functioning by examining the following aspects.

- *Short- and long-term memory.* Questions relate to recent and past events. The person may be asked to remember something and in 5 minutes will need to recall what was remembered.
- *Attention span and concentration.* Can the person complete a thought and solve problems? The provider may ask the patient to count by fives or sevens.
- Orientation: Does the person know his or her name, age, and job? Does the person know the day, time, date, and season?
- *Language and communication skills:* Questions will examine the person's ability to form clear ideas. The patient may be asked to read or write a sentence.
- *Judgment and intelligence.* The person is given a scenario and asked to solve it.
- The provider's general observations are formed by assessing the following: *Physical appearance, behavior, and motor activity.* The provider checks the appropriateness of clothing, grooming, posture, facial expression, and eye contact. Does the stated age match the apparent physical appearance? Is the person friendly, withdrawn, shy, hostile, irritable, relaxed, or cooperative?
- *Mood and affect.* The provider asks the patient to give information on his or her emotional state or mood. The provider observes the patient's emotional state through body movements and facial expressions. The provider observes the person's affect or external expression of emotion. The provider uses the body language and the facial features to detect expressions of emotion. The following are types of affect:
  - Restricted or constricted affect: A small reduction in the intensity of the affect.
  - Blunted affect: A severe reduction in the intensity of the affect; much less emotion is shown compared to the restricted affect.
  - Flat affect: A lack of emotional expression in both the face and the body language.
  - Labile affect: Rapidly changing emotions that are unrelated to external events.
  - Inappropriate affect: The emotional expressions are incongruent with the situation or the person's verbal message.

Anxiety Disorders

Having periodic anxiety about a problem or an important decision is normal. With an anxiety disorder, the anxious feeling is a constant companion and it gets worse with time. The anxiety interferes with daily living, for instance, school, work, and relationships.

The risk factors for anxiety disorders include shyness in childhood, being divorced or widowed, exposure to stressful life events, a family history of anxiety disorder, and a parental history of behavioral health disorder. The following sections will discuss the different types of anxiety disorders.

Generalized Anxiety Disorder. With generalized anxiety disorder (GAD), a person has many different worries. The person finds it difficult to control the anxiety. GAD is a common disorder that can affect a person at any age. GAD occurs more often in females than in males.

Etiology. The cause of GAD is unknown, but genetics may be a factor. Stress also contributes to the development of GAD.

TABLE 15.1 Psychological Testing

Test	Description
Wechsler Adult Intelligence Scale (WAIS)	Measures the verbal intelligence quotient (IQ), performance IQ, and full-scale IQ. It is used for people 16 years of age or older. Other versions of the Wechsler can be used for younger children.
Boehm Test of Basic Concepts	Used to test a child's understanding of basic positional concepts. Using pictures, the child must select the correct one when given cues such as "over," "least," and "left."
Bender Visual Motor Gestalt Test	Used to evaluate a person's visual-motor maturity. It is used to screen for developmental delays and can be used to assess for neurologic issues and brain damage. This test is used for people age 5 years or older.
Adaptive Behavior Assessment System	Used to test developmental and intellectual disabilities.
Draw-a-Person (DAP) Test	An analysis to measure nonverbal intelligence and to screen for behavioral or emotional disorders in children.
Minnesota Multiphasic Personality Inventory (MMPI)	A widely used and researched personality assessment. It is used to diagnose behavioral health disorders, to screen for certain high-risk jobs, and as part of criminal defense and custody issues in legal cases.
Thematic Apperception Test (TAT)	A test in which patients are asked to make up stories about the pictures on cards they are shown. This may provide information about a patient's thoughts, attitudes, and emotional responses.

TABLE 15.2 Types of Psychotherapy

Types of Psychotherapy	Description
Cognitive behavioral therapy (CBT)	A scientifically proven treatment that produces changes in behavior by helping the person face fears, role-play situations, and learn problem-solving skills to cope with difficult issues. It is used for many behavioral health disorders, including depression, anxiety disorders, substance use disorders, and eating disorders.
Dialectical behavioral therapy (DBT)	This evidence-based CBT approach is used for individuals who are diagnosed with personality disorders, are suicidal, or engage in self-harm behaviors. DBT focuses behavioral change, problem solving, and regulation of emotions in a manner that is socially acceptable.
Exposure therapy	A type of CBT that is used to help people process their traumatic experiences or feared situations. The person revisits and recounts the memories, which gradually helps the person emotionally process the experience or situation. The person may start by thinking about the object or situation, then progress to looking at pictures of it, then to getting near it, and then to touching it or experiencing it for short periods of time.
Eye movement desensitization and reprocessing (EMDR)	Used to process and resolve traumatic memories (e.g., post-traumatic stress disorder [PTSD]). During the therapy, the person concentrates on the memory while focusing on controlled stimuli (e.g., eye movements or sounds). The patient discusses any new thoughts that occur and continues until the memory is no longer distressing.
Interpersonal psychotherapy (IPT)	Used to treat behavioral health disorders, such as eating disorders and major depression, by helping the person understand the relationship between symptoms and social interactions, thus improving social skills and functioning.
Play therapy	Used for children who are experiencing behavioral, emotional, social, or relational disorders. Using play and the therapeutic relationship, the child is able to express feelings and thoughts.
Psychodynamic therapy	Used to treat depression, addictions, social anxiety disorder, and eating disorders. It focuses on helping the patient recognize, express, and overcome negative feelings and repressed emotions, so that the person's interpersonal experiences and relationships improve.

Signs and Symptoms. The main symptom of GAD is excessive worrying for over 6 months about multiple issues without a clear reason. Other signs and symptoms of GAD include restlessness, fatigue, irritability, difficulty concentrating, difficulty stopping or controlling the anxiety, muscle tension, and sleep problems.

Diagnostic Procedures. There is no test to diagnose GAD. A physical exam and laboratory tests may be done to rule out other conditions. The provider will ask questions regarding the symptoms of GAD prior to making the diagnosis.

Treatments. The goal of treatment is to help the person feel and function better. Treatment includes psychotherapy. The most effective and common type of talk therapy is cognitive behavioral therapy (CBT). With CBT, a person learns to identify stressors, gain control of panic-causing thoughts, and manage stress, and also to relax. Medications such as antidepressants and sedative-hypnotics may be prescribed.

Obsessive-Compulsive and Related Disorders. Obsessive-compulsive disorder (OCD) causes a person to have frequent, upsetting thoughts *(obsessions)*. Examples of obsessions include fear of germs or of being hurt. Then, to control the thoughts, the person has an overwhelming urge to repeat certain behaviors *(compulsion)*. Examples of compulsions include hand washing, counting, rechecking things (e.g., locked doors), or cleaning. The obsessions and compulsions affect the person's daily life.

Etiology. The cause of OCD is not completely understood, but it may relate to changes in brain function, genetics, and environmental factors. Risk factors include a family history of OCD, other behavioral health disorders (e.g., depression, substance use), and/or a traumatic event.

Signs and Symptoms. OCD can cause:

- Fear of touching items others touched.
- Items need to be in a certain position, organized, and orderly.
- Doubts about locking the door or turning off an appliance, causing continual rechecking.
- Avoidance of events that trigger the obsessions.
- Frequent hand washing, even to the point that the skin is raw.
- Silently repeating a prayer or phrase.

The symptoms start gradually and may increase in severity over time.

Diagnostic Procedures. The provider will do a physical exam, laboratory tests (e.g., blood work, thyroid tests), and a psychological evaluation.

Treatments. Treatment consists of psychotherapy (e.g., cognitive behavioral therapy, and exposure and response prevention) and antidepressants.

Hoarding Disorder. Hoarding disorder (HD) is the persistent difficulty of getting rid of personal possessions. People with HD feel they need to save items and are distressed at the thought of discarding them or having them touched or moved without their permission. Sometimes the thoughts center around "hurting the feelings" of the item if it is discarded. Others hold onto their possessions, because they may come in handy someday, or, if discarded, the memories attached to the object may be lost. As a result, people with HD have cluttered living areas that can become a significant public health burden and safety issue. It is estimated that up to 5% of the population has HD.

Etiology. The cause of hoarding disorder is unknown. Risk factors include being indecisive, family history of hoarding disorder, and stressful life events.

Signs and Symptoms. HD can cause:

- Excessively acquiring items that are not needed
- Difficulty throwing out items
- Feeling the need to save items
- Personality characteristics of indecisiveness, perfectionist, avoidance, and procrastination

Diagnostic Procedures. The behavioral health provider will perform a psychological evaluation. The provider may also review pictures of the patient's living conditions and talk with family members.

Treatments. Treatment consists of cognitive behavioral therapy. Medications may be ordered if the patient has anxiety or depression.

CRITICAL THINKING 15.3

List three safety issues related to hoarding and share them with your class.

Panic Disorder. Panic disorder causes recurrent unexpected *panic attacks*, or sudden feelings of terror without real dangers being present. A person experiencing a panic attack is very frightened and feels a loss of control.

Etiology. The cause of panic disorders is unknown, but genetics, major stress, sensitivity to stress, and certain changes in brain function may play a factor.

Signs and Symptoms. Panic attacks can cause:

- A sense of impending doom
- A rapid and pounding heart rate and chest pain
- Sweating, trembling, chills, and hot flashes
- Abdominal cramping and nausea
- Dizziness, lightheadedness, and numbness

The signs and symptoms can mimic those of a heart attack, which can also increase the person's anxiety.

Diagnostic Procedures. After a physical exam and laboratory tests to rule out other conditions, the provider will do a psychological evaluation. The DSM-5 criteria for panic disorder include:

- Having frequent, unexpected panic attacks.
- One attack that is followed by 1 month or more of constant worry about having another attack.
- The panic attack is not related to substance use, medications, or other medical or behavioral health conditions.

Treatments. Treatment for panic disorder is similar to that for GAD; psychotherapy and medications can be helpful.

Phobia. A *phobia* is a type of anxiety disorder in which a person has a strong, irrational fear of something that causes little to no danger. There are many types of phobias (Table 15.3). Phobias typically start in childhood and continue into adulthood.

Etiology. Phobias can be caused by negative experiences, genetics, changes in brain function, and the environment.

Signs and Symptoms. A phobia can cause panic, persistent and unreasonable fear, an increase in the heart rate, shortness of breath (SOB), trembling, and a strong desire to get away. A phobia can interfere with a person's daily life.

Diagnostic Procedures. The provider will do a physical exam and gather a medical history.

Treatments. Often treatment includes psychotherapy, exposure therapy, and medication.

Social Anxiety Disorder. With social anxiety disorder, people have a persistent and irrational fear of social situations. People avoid situations in which they feel others will judge them. Some of the more common avoidances include:

- Attending social gatherings and eating and drinking in public

---

TABLE 15.3   Examples of Phobias

Types		Fear of...
acrophobia	(ak roe FOE bee ah)	heights
agoraphobia	(AG ore ah FOE bee ah)	open spaces
algophobia	(AL goe FOE bee ah)	pain
aquaphobia	(AK wah FOE bee ah)	water
arachnophobia	(Ah RAK neh FOE bee ah)	spiders
belonephobia	(BEL oh neh FOE bee ah)	needles, pins, and other sharp-pointed objects
brontophobia	(BRON toe FOE bee ah)	thunder
cancerophobia	(KAN ser oh FOE bee ah)	cancer
claustrophobia	(KLAW stro FOE bee ah)	closed spaces
cyberphobia	(SIE ber FOE bee ah)	computers
hemophobia	(HEE mah FOE bee ah)	blood or injury
kleptophobia	(KLEP toe FOE bee ah)	stealing or becoming a thief
nosophobia	(NOS oh FOE bee ah)	disease
ochlophobia	(OK lah FOE bee ah)	crowds

- Meeting new people and public speaking
- Using public restrooms

This disorder affects a person's ability to go to school, function at work, and have relationships. The disorder may begin in a person's teenage years. Males and females are equally affected by this disorder.

Etiology. The cause of social anxiety disorder may be related to overprotective parents or limited social opportunities. Other possible causes include genetics, learning behaviors early on in life, and an overactive amygdala (ah MIG dah lah), in the brain, which increases the fear response.

Signs and Symptoms. Social anxiety disorder causes blushing, an increased heart rate, trembling, sweating, nausea, dizziness, lightheadedness, SOB, and muscle tension. Elevated afternoon cortisol levels have also been reported.

Diagnostic Procedures. After a physical exam and laboratory tests to rule out other conditions, the provider will do a psychological evaluation. The DSM-5 criteria for social anxiety disorder include:

- Persistent, intense anxiety or fear related to social situations in which one perceives others will be judgmental
- Avoidance of such social situations
- Excessive anxiety that interferes with daily life
- Fear or anxiety that is not related to substance use or a medical or behavioral health disorder

Treatments. Treatment for social anxiety disorder includes psychotherapy and medications, such as:

- Antidepressants: Selective serotonin reuptake inhibitors (SSRIs) and serotonin and norepinephrine reuptake inhibitors (SNRIs)
- Antianxiety medications, including benzodiazepines
- Beta-blockers

> **VOCABULARY**
> **amygdala** A small mass of gray matter found in each temporal lobe of the cerebrum and involved with memories, emotions, and activating the fight-or-flight response; part of the limbic system.
> **delusion** Unshakable belief in something untrue; may be accompanied by hallucinations and/or paranoia.
> **hallucination** A sensory experience (e.g., a smell, sound, sight, touch, or taste) involving something that is not present.

Autism Spectrum Disorder

Autism spectrum disorder (ASD) is a developmental disorder with symptoms that appear by age 2. The child has difficulty interacting and communicating with others. The communication issues and behaviors, such as repetitive behaviors and limited interests, affect the person's ability to function at school and at home. There can be a wide range of symptoms and severity; thus it is known as a "spectrum" disorder. Prior diagnoses, such as Asperger syndrome, are now included in ASD.

Etiology. The exact cause of ASD is unknown, but research suggests that a person's genetics, with environmental influences, can affect development, leading to ASD. Risk factors for ASD include having a family member with ASD, older parents, certain genetic conditions, and a low birth weight.

Signs and Symptoms. Autism spectrum disorder can cause:

- *Social communication and interaction behavior issues*: Little to no eye contact, not listening to others, failing to respond when being called, difficulty with holding a conversation, talks at length about a favorite topic without realizing others are not interested, body language does not match the verbal message, and having a singsong or flat, robotlike tone of voice.
- *Restrictive and repetitive behaviors*: Repeating certain behaviors or words, intense interest in certain topics (e.g., numbers, details, facts), getting upset with routine changes, and more or less sensitivity to light, noise, clothing, or temperature.

Often people with ASD have sleeping issues. They may be strong auditory and visual learners, who excel in art, music, science, or math. They may remember information for long periods of time and can learn information in detail.

Diagnostic Procedures. The American Academy of Pediatrics recommends that children be screened for developmental delays during the 9-month, 18-month, and 24- or 30-month well-child visit. ASD screening tools are available. Children suspected of having ASD are referred for additional evaluation by a healthcare team specializing in diagnosing ASD.

Treatments. Treatment may consist of medication and behavioral, educational, and psychological therapies. These therapies focus on teaching the person life skills to live independently, including social, communication, and language skills.

Depression and Other Mood Disorders

Depression is the second leading behavioral health condition. The symptoms affect how a person acts, thinks, feels, and handles their daily life. Depression must be present for at least 2 weeks for a diagnosis to be given. Table 15.4 describes some types of depression. Depression can happen at any age.

TABLE 15.4	Types of Depression
Types	**Description**
Persistent depressive disorder	Also called *dysthymia*; depression that lasts for at least 2 years.
Postpartum depression	Occurs after giving birth. The person has feelings of extreme sadness, exhaustion, and anxiety. These feelings interfere with daily life and caring for the new baby.
Psychotic depression	Episodes of psychosis occur with severe depression. The person experiences delusions (de LOO zhuns) and hallucinations (hah loo si NAY shuns).
Seasonal affective disorder	Depression occurs during the winter months when there is less sunlight. The depression usually lifts in the spring. During the winter, the person may experience increased sleepiness, weight gain, and social withdrawal.

Etiology. The cause of depression is not known, but many factors may be involved, including changes in the brain and the functioning of neurotransmitters, hormone changes, and genetics. Risk factors include age (from teens to 30-year-olds), female, low self-esteem, stressful event, family history (of depression, bipolar disorder, alcoholism, or suicide), substance use, chronic medical or behavioral health illness, and certain medications.

Signs and Symptoms. Depression can cause:
- Feeling sad, very tired, hopeless, irritable, anxious, or guilt
- Loss of interest in favorite activities (e.g., hobbies)
- Pain, headaches, cramps, digestive issues, anorexia, and overeating
- Thoughts of death or suicide

Diagnostic Procedures. The provider will do a physical exam, possibly laboratory tests (e.g., complete blood count, thyroid function tests), and radiology tests (Fig. 15.1). A psychiatric evaluation will also be completed to gather more information on the patient's symptoms, thoughts, feelings, and behaviors.

Treatments. Psychotherapy and antidepressant medications are the most common treatments for depression.

CRITICAL THINKING 15.4

Mike rooms Mrs. Johnson, who states she has not been sleeping well since her husband died 10 days ago. She states she has not been feeling hungry and is always tired. If you encountered a patient like Mrs. Johnson, how would you respond?

Bipolar Disorder. Bipolar disorder causes people to go from mania (MAY nee ah) to depression. They cycle through highs and lows in their moods, with periods of normal moods. Bipolar disorder usually starts in the late teens to early adult years and lasts a lifetime.

Etiology. The cause of bipolar disorder is unclear. There is a genetic link to the disorder, and abnormal brain structure and function may also be related.

Signs and Symptoms. Bipolar disorder causes:
- *Mania and hypomania*: Euphoria (yoo FOR ee ah) and energetic feelings, decreased need for sleep, distractibility, poor decision making, and exaggerated sense of well-being
- *Major depression episode*: Insomnia or sleeping too much, fatigue, feelings of worthlessness, suicidal thoughts, feelings of no pleasure, and weight gain or loss
- Moods affect relationships, school or job performance, and even cause suicide.

Diagnostic Procedures. The provider will do a physical exam and a psychiatric assessment. Patients may be asked to chart their moods.

Treatments. Treatments include lifelong treatments, psychotherapy, and support groups. Medications can also be prescribed and include anticonvulsants and mood stabilizers, antidepressants, anxiolytics, and antipsychotics.

VOCABULARY

euphoria An exaggerated sense of physical and mental well-being.
mania Abnormally elated mental state; the person may have feelings of euphoria, lack of inhibitions, sleeplessness, talkativeness, risk-taking behaviors, and irritability.

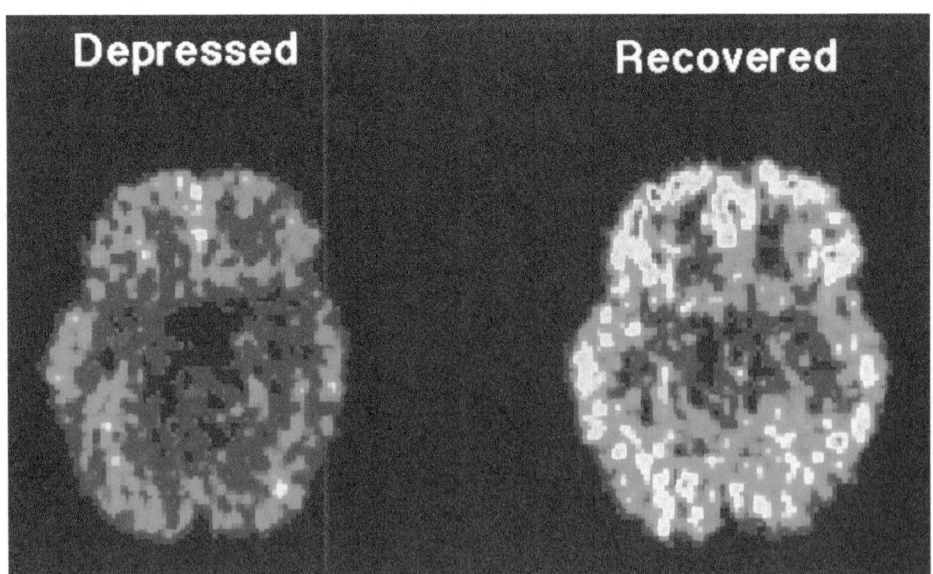

Fig. 15.1 Positron emission tomography (PET) scans of an individual's brain when depressed *(left)* and after recovery through treatment with medication *(right)*. Several brain areas, particularly the prefrontal cortex (at top), show diminished activity (darker colors) during depression. (From Fortinash KM: *Psychiatric mental health nursing*, ed 4, St. Louis, 2008, Mosby.)

MEDICAL TERMINOLOGY	
pol/o	pole
phor/o	to carry, to bear
somn/o	sleep
bi-	two
dys-	abnormal
eu-	good, well
hypo-	decreased
-ar	pertaining to
-ia	condition
-mania	condition of madness
-phobia	condition of fear
-thymia	condition of the mind

Behavioral Disorders

Behavioral disorders in children involve a pattern of disruptive behaviors that cause issues at home, in school, and in social situations. According to the diagnostic criteria, the disruptive behaviors must have lasted at least 6 months. Behavioral disorders may involve defiant behavior, impulsiveness, hyperactivity, inattention, drug use, and criminal activity. Behavioral disorders include:

- Attention deficit hyperactivity disorder (ADHD)
- Oppositional defiant disorder (ODD)
- Conduct disorder (CD).

ODD and CD are also considered disruptive behavior disorders. Disruptive behavior disorder involves uncooperative or hostile action patterns of behavior. The person may have temper tantrums, argue, demonstrate cruel and defiant behaviors, and fight with others. People with disruptive behavioral disorders have problems controlling their emotions and actions, leading to issues at school and home.

Attention Deficit Hyperactivity Disorder.
ADHD is a chronic condition that affects children and can continue into adulthood. With ADHD, a person is not able to focus or able to control behaviors, may be overactive, or any combination of these characteristics. Often ADHD and ADD (attention deficit disorder) are used interchangeably, but the correct term is ADHD. Typically, symptoms begin before age 12, yet some have seen it in the toddler years. This disorder is more prevalent in males than in females.

Etiology. The cause of ADHD is unknown, but possible factors include genetics, environmental factors (e.g., lead exposure), and developmental factors. Many conditions can co-exist with ADHD, including learning disabilities, anxiety, depression, bipolar disorder, and Tourette syndrome.

Signs and Symptoms. ADHD causes:

- *Inattention*: Fails to pay close attention, has problems staying focused, appears not to listen, has difficulty following directions, has trouble with organizational skills, and is easily distracted.
- *Hyperactivity and impulsivity*: Fidgets, constantly moving, talking too much, difficulty waiting for their turn, and problems doing quiet activities.

Males may be more hyperactive, whereas females may be quietly inattentive. According to the diagnostic criteria, the symptoms can range from mild to severe and must last for at least 6 months, affecting school and home life. There are three subtypes of ADHD based on the symptoms: predominantly inattentive, predominantly hyperactive-impulsive, and combined (a mix of both).

Diagnostic Procedures. There is no specific test for ADHD. The provider will do a physical exam, including vision and hearing, and ask questions of the parents and teachers.

Treatments. Treatments for ADHD include behavioral therapy to help manage the symptoms and provide coping skills. Medications can also be prescribed, including:

- Stimulants: Methylphenidate (METH il FEN i date) (Ritalin LA, Concerta, Methylin) and amphetamine (am FET a meen) (Adzenys ER, Dyanavel XR, Evekeo). Stimulants provide a calming effect by increasing the dopamine in the brain, which helps with attention and motivation.
- Nonstimulants: Atomoxetine (AT oh mox e teen) (Strattera), guanfacine (GWAHN fa seen) (Intuniv, Tenex), and clonidine (KLOE ni deen) (Catapres, Kapvay).

Conduct Disorder.
With conduct disorder (CD), the person demonstrates disruptive and violent behaviors. The person hurts others and destroys property. Children with CD can have behavior problems that last into adulthood. Symptoms usually start during the preteen and teen years, though they can be seen in preschool. The disorder is more common in males.

Etiology. There is no single cause for CD. Having a parent with a behavioral disorder; exposure to neglect, abuse, or violence; and having a high emotional reactivity can be risk factors.

Signs and Symptoms. Conduct disorder causes:

- Aggression toward animals and people: Includes bullying, threatening, starting fights, using weapons, forcing others into sexual activity, stealing from others, and physical cruelty to people or animals.
- Destruction of property, such as setting fires.
- Deceit or theft: Includes lying to get things, breaking in and stealing items, and shoplifting.
- Serious violations of rules: Includes running away from home overnight at least twice, or once without returning for a long time, and truancy.

Diagnostic Procedures. There is no specific test for CD, so the provider will do a complete medical history.

Treatments. Treatment is based on the individual's need and addresses co-existing diseases. Common intervention programs include parent training, behavioral family therapy, and skills-based interventions, in addition to anger management and coping skills.

Oppositional Defiant Disorder.
With oppositional defiant disorder (ODD), the child or teen demonstrates ongoing hostility to parents, friends, and teachers. ODD usually is diagnosed during preschool or childhood.

Etiology. There is no single cause for ODD. Having a parent with a behavioral disorder; exposure to neglect, abuse, or violence; and having a high emotional reactivity can be risk factors. Depression and anxiety can co-exist with ODD.

Signs and Symptoms. Oppositional defiant disorder can cause ongoing hostility, defying rules, holding grudges, and rebel-like behaviors. These symptoms interfere with school and home life. Three types of ODD are:

- *Angry and irritable mood*: Annoyed by others easily, loses one's temper, and has rage outbursts.
- *Argumentative and defiant behaviors*: Argues with those in authority, defies rules, purposely annoys others, and blames others.
- *Vindictiveness*: Being cruel, nasty, vengeful, and mean.

Diagnostic Procedures. There is no specific test for ODD, so the provider will do a complete medical history.

Treatments. Treatment is based on the individual's need and addresses co-existing diseases. Common intervention programs include parent training, behavioral family therapy, and skills-based interventions, which teach the patient how to reduce behavior problems and learn how to appropriately interact with peers. Anger management and coping skills are also part of the intervention.

Dissociative Disorders

Dissociative disorders cause a person to involuntarily escape from reality. A person may have a disconnection between memories, thoughts, actions, identity, and surroundings. Dissociative disorder can cause a variety of conditions, such as amnesia (am NEE zhah) and alternative identities. Table 15.5 describes types of dissociative disorders.

Etiology. Dissociative disorders develop as a coping mechanism due to trauma (e.g., abuse, war, and natural disasters). A risk factor includes experiencing long-term sexual, physical, or emotional abuse during childhood.

Signs and Symptoms. Dissociative disorders can cause:
- Amnesia and an unclear sense of identity
- A sense of being detached from oneself
- A distorted or unreal perception of others

TABLE 15.5	Types of Dissociative Disorders
Types	**Description**
Dissociative amnesia	Memory loss without an explained medical condition. No recollection of self, events, and familiar people. May involve confused wandering away from home (dissociative fugue). May last for hours to years.
Dissociative identity disorder	Formerly known as multiple personality disorder. People may feel two or more people "in their head" as if they have alternative identities. Each identity may have a name, history, and unique personality.
Depersonalization-derealization disorder	Episodic or long-term sense of detachment with depersonalization and derealization. People feel they are an outside observer of their thoughts, actions, and sensations. They also feel as if they are detached from their surroundings.

- Significant stress and inability to cope
- Behavioral health issues, such as depression and anxiety

Diagnostic Procedures. The provider will do a physical exam and a psychiatric evaluation.

Treatments. Treatment consists of psychotherapy and medications (e.g., antidepressants, antianxiety drugs, and antipsychotics).

VOCABULARY

amnesia Memory loss.
depersonalization Alternative perception of the self; a person's own reality is lost. People feel they are not in control of their own actions or speech.
derealization Loss of sensation of the reality of one's surroundings.

Eating Disorders

Eating disorders affect both genders, but the occurrence of eating disorders in females is 2.5 times greater than it is in males. Eating disorders typically appear during the teen years or young adulthood, but they can start earlier or later in life.

Eating disorders are real, treatable illnesses. They typically co-exist with other illnesses, including substance use, anxiety disorders, and depression. Eating disorders, especially anorexia, can be life-threatening without treatment.

Anorexia Nervosa. Anorexia nervosa causes people to lose more weight than is healthy. Individuals with this disorder have an intense fear of gaining weight (Fig. 15.2). Often it starts during the preteen to teen years. It is more prevalent in females.

Etiology. The etiology is unknown. Genetics, hormones, and social attitudes may play a role in the development of anorexia nervosa. Risk factors for anorexia nervosa include:
- A history of anxiety disorder or eating problems as a child
- Worry about weight and shape of the body and a negative self-image
- An exaggerated focus on rules and trying to be perfect

Signs and Symptoms. Signs and symptoms of anorexia nervosa include:
- Being underweight, an intense fear of gaining weight, and a very distorted body image
- Severely limiting the amount of food eaten and refusing to eat around others
- Exercising all the time
- Going to the bathroom right after meals, vomiting secretly after eating
- Using diuretics, laxatives, or diet pills
- Blotchy or yellow dry skin covered with fine hair and a dry mouth
- Confused, poor memory or judgment, slow thinking, depression
- Extreme sensitivity to cold
- Osteoporosis, wasting away of muscle, and loss of body fat

Diagnostic Procedures. The provider will order extensive laboratory tests to look at thyroid, liver, and kidney function. An electrocardiogram and bone density test may also be ordered. Many healthcare facilities have patients with eating disorders

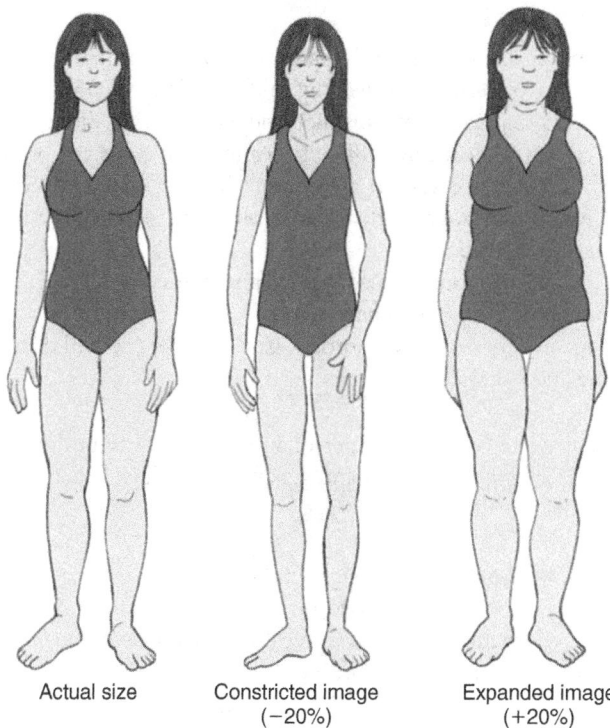

Actual size   Constricted image   Expanded image
                        (−20%)   (+20%)

Fig. 15.2 The perception of body shape and size can be evaluated with the use of special computer drawing programs. These programs allow a subject to distort (increase or decrease) the width of an actual picture of a person's body by as much as 20%. Individuals with anorexia consistently adjusted their own body picture to a size 20% larger than its true form. This suggests that they have a major problem with the perception of self-image. (From Stuart GW, Laraia MT: *Principles and practice of psychiatric nursing,* ed 9, St Louis, 2009, Mosby.)

get on the scale backward, so they cannot see the weight (Fig. 15.3).

Treatments. Treatment focuses on helping these patients recognizing they have an illness. Many types of treatments are available, including psychotherapy (e.g., cognitive behavioral therapy, group therapy, and family therapy) and support groups. Compliance with treatment is difficult, and it is common for the disease to return.

CRITICAL THINKING 15.5

Mike weighs Alexis White, who is being treated for anorexia. He has her step backwards on the scale and does not allow her to see the weight. She asks him repeatedly to tell her the weight. If you encountered a patient like Alexis, how would you handle the situation?

MEDICAL TERMINOLOGY	
orex/o	appetite
an-	without

Binge Eating Disorder. Binge eating disorder, also called *compulsive overeating,* is the most common eating disorder in the

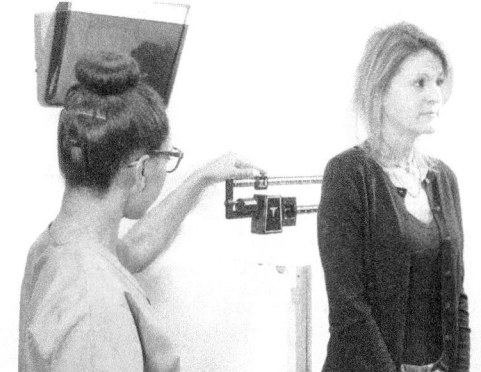

Fig. 15.3 Weighing a Patient Backward.

United States. It occurs when people regularly eat unusually large amounts of food in a short amount of time. They feel out of control, unable to manage what or how much they eat. A person may have binge eating disorder if this behavior occurs weekly for 3 months. It affects young women and middle-aged men.

Etiology. The exact cause is unknown. Genetics, depression, stress, unhealthy dieting, and changes in brain chemicals may be factors in the condition.

Signs and Symptoms. Signs and symptoms of binge eating disorder include:
- Eating very quickly and eating until uncomfortably full
- Eating when not hungry
- Eating huge amounts of food over a very short period of time
- Eating in secret
- Feeling disgusted, ashamed, or depressed about one's eating patterns
- Frequent dieting

Diagnostic Procedures. A physical exam and a psychological evaluation will be done. Blood and urine tests (e.g., cholesterol, blood glucose) may be done to evaluate the consequences of binge eating.

Treatments. Treatment may consist of behavioral weight-loss programs and psychotherapy (e.g., cognitive behavioral therapy, interpersonal psychotherapy, and dialectical behavior therapy). Medications may also be used, including lisdexamfetamine (lis dex am FET a meen) (Vyvanse), topiramate (toe PYRE a mate) (Topamax), and antidepressants.

Bulimia Nervosa. Bulimia nervosa, or bulimia, causes overeating that leads to purging and can be a life-threatening disorder. To prevent weight gain, self-induced vomiting, laxative use, weight-loss supplements, and enemas may be used. Bulimia may also occur with anorexia nervosa. More females than males have bulimia. It is more common in teens and young women.

Etiology. The etiology is unknown. Genetics, hormones, and social attitudes may play a role in the development of bulimia.

Signs and Symptoms. Signs and symptoms of bulimia nervosa include:
- Broken blood vessels in the eyes (this occurs from the strain of vomiting)
- Dry mouth and a pouchlike look to the cheeks
- Rashes and pimples

- Small cuts and calluses on the tops of fingers (from inducing vomiting)
- Dehydration and electrolyte imbalance

Other people may notice:

- Excessive exercising.
- Eating large amounts of food or buying large amounts of food that disappear right away
- Trips to the bathroom after meals
- Discarded boxes from laxatives, diet pills, and emetics to induce vomiting, or diuretics

Diagnostic Procedures. The provider will do a physical exam and urine and blood tests.

Treatments. Treatment is usually on an outpatient basis unless the individual has a co-existing diagnosis. Support groups, counseling, and medications can be helpful.

Other Eating Disorders. Additional eating disorders include:

- *Pica*: Eating of nonfood materials such as paper, ice, clay, or dirt. Seen in children and during pregnancy. May be caused from a lack of certain nutrients that produce unusual cravings.
- *Rumination disorder*: A condition in which a person regurgitates food from the stomach and rechews the food.
- *Avoidant/restrictive food intake disorder* (ARFID): Similar to anorexia since it limits the amount of food consumed, but with ARIF the person is not stressed about his or her body shape or size. The child does not consume enough calories to grow and develop. Previously called selective eating disorder.

CRITICAL THINKING 15.6

Describe the three types of eating disorders in your own words.

Personality Disorders

Personality disorders include a group of conditions that involve long-term patterns of unhealthy and inflexible thoughts and behaviors that affect relationships and work. Personality disorders cause people to have difficulty dealing with stress and problems. Personality disorders are grouped by clusters (Table 15.6):

- Cluster A personality disorders: Cause odd, eccentric thinking and behaviors
- Cluster B personality disorders: Cause dramatic, overly emotional thinking and behaviors
- Cluster C personality disorders: Cause anxiety, fearful thinking and behaviors

Etiology. The etiology of personality disorders is unknown, but childhood experiences and genetics may play a role in the disorders.

Signs and Symptoms. The signs and symptoms can range from mild to severe and vary based on the type of disorder. People with a personality disorder may feel they do not have a problem and blame others for their problems.

Diagnostic Procedures. The provider will do a physical exam and a psychiatric evaluation.

Treatments. Treatments involve psychotherapy and medications (e.g., antidepressants, mood stabilizers, antipsychotic medications, and antianxiety medications).

Post-traumatic Stress Disorder

Post-traumatic stress disorder (PTSD) is a condition that occurs after a person experiences or witnesses a traumatic or terrifying event. The symptoms of PTSD can vary over time

---

TABLE 15.6   Types of Personality Disorders

Cluster	Types	Description
Cluster A personality disorders	*Paranoid personality disorder*	Unjustified beliefs that others are trying to do harm to the person. Very suspicious, untrusting, angry, and hostile. May feel that their partner is unfaithful.
	Schizoid personality disorder	Avoidance of social activities and interacting with other people. The person may be seen as a loner and may not show emotion.
	Schizotypal personality disorder	Odd, peculiar, and unusual behaviors; flat or inappropriate emotional responses; belief in special powers, excessive social anxiety, and suspicious or paranoid thoughts.
Cluster B personality disorders	*Antisocial personality disorder*	No regard for others; persistent lying, and impulsive and aggressive behaviors.
	Borderline personality disorder	Intense relationships, distorted self-image, impulsivity, and extreme emotions (e.g., intense fear of abandonment, anger, mood swings). Usually begins in early adulthood and may get better with age.
	Histrionic personality disorder	Seeks constant attention. Very dramatic, emotional, and opinionated.
	Narcissistic personality disorder	Inflated ego, an excessive need for attention, lacks empathy for others, has troubled relationships and a very fragile self-esteem.
Cluster C personality disorders	*Avoidance personality disorder*	Too sensitive to criticism; feels inadequate; avoids interpersonal contact or is extremely shy/withdrawn during social activities.
	Dependent personality disorder	Very clinging and dependent on another person. Fears being left alone. Lacks self-confidence.
	Obsessive-compulsive personality disorder	Preoccupied with rules, organization/orderliness, and details. Wants to control everything (e.g., tasks, situations, people, events).

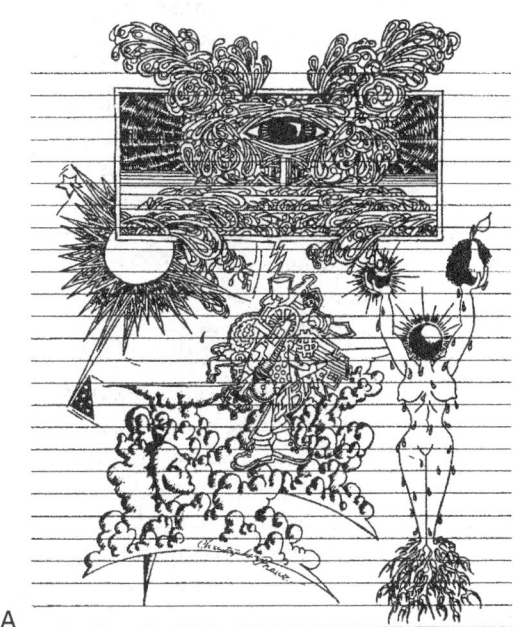
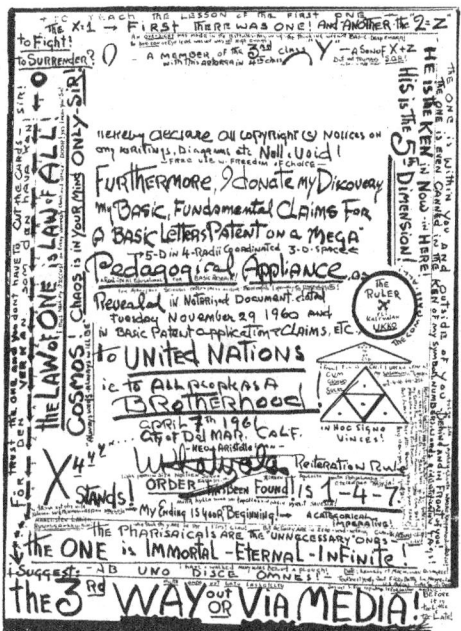

Fig. 15.4 A, Drawing by a delusional patient with schizophrenia. B, This drawing by a patient with schizophrenia demonstrates thought disorder. (From Stuart GW, Laraia MT: *Principles and practice of psychiatric nursing,* ed 9, St Louis, 2009, Mosby.)

and from person to person. Anyone can develop PTSD, from children, to war veterans, to people who have experienced the death of a loved one, physical or sexual assault, an accident, or a natural disaster. Females are more likely to have PTSD than males.

Etiology. The cause of PTSD is experiencing a stressful, terrifying event. It is unknown why some develop the disorder and others do not.

Signs and Symptoms. PTSD signs and symptoms include:
- *Intrusive memories*: Reliving the trauma (flashbacks); nightmares and recurrent distressful memories
- *Negative changes*: Negative thoughts, hopelessness, and difficulty maintaining close relationships
- *Changes in reactions*: Being easily frightened, self-destructive activities (drinking, drugs), trouble concentrating and sleeping, and aggressive behaviors
- *Avoidance*: Avoiding places, people and things that remind one of the situation; not talking about the event

Diagnostic Procedures. The provider will do a physical exam and a psychological evaluation.

Treatments. Treatment is focused on regaining a sense of control. Psychotherapy, including cognitive therapy, eye movement desensitization and reprocessing (EMDR), and exposure therapy, may be prescribed. Antidepressants and antianxiety medications may be prescribed.

Schizophrenia

Schizophrenia causes disruptions in thought processes, perceptions, emotional responsiveness, and social interactions

(Fig. 15.4). Schizophrenia is usually diagnosed in the late teen years to the early 30s. The symptoms tend to occur earlier for males than females. Schizophrenia is a debilitating disorder, and about half of those with it also have another mental or behavioral health disorder.

Etiology. The cause of schizophrenia is unknown, but as with many other conditions, it is believed that a combination of brain chemistry, environmental factors, and genetics plays a role in the development of the disease.

Signs and Symptoms. Schizophrenia can cause:
- Delusions, hallucinations, and disorganized thinking and speech
- Abnormal motor behavior and lack of response (no eye contact, lack of facial expression)
- Neglect of personal hygiene
- Teens are more likely to withdraw and have insomnia

Diagnostic Procedures. The provider will do a physical exam and may order a magnetic resonance imaging (MRI) or computed tomography (CT) scan to rule out other conditions. A psychiatric evaluation will be done.

Treatments. Treatment is lifelong and includes psychosocial therapy and antipsychotic medications. Hospitalization is required if the person experiences severe and/or life-threatening symptoms.

MEDICAL TERMINOLOGY	
schiz/o	split
-phrenia	condition of the mind

CRITICAL THINKING 15.7

Mike rooms Mr. James, who states he is seeing little green men coming out of the wall. If you encountered a patient like Mr. James, how would you respond?

Substance Use Disorders and Other Addictions

Substance Use Disorders. In the DSM-5, substance use disorder includes both substance use and substance dependence. Substance use disorder is measured from mild to severe. Each substance is addressed as a separate disorder. These substances include alcohol; cannabis; hallucinogens; opioids; inhalants; sedatives, hypnotics, and anxiolytics; tobacco; and stimulants. Caffeine is not included in the use disorder, though it may be in a future revision because there is sufficient evidence to support such a condition.

Substance use disorder occurs when a person uses alcohol or other substances (drugs) that lead to school, work, or home issues. Many people with substance use disorders also have other behavioral health conditions, including depression, anxiety, attention deficit disorder, and post-traumatic stress disorder. Table 15.7 describes commonly used drugs.

Etiology. The exact cause of substance use disorders is unknown, but genetics, drug action, peer pressure, anxiety, depression, emotional distress, and stress can all be factors.

Signs and Symptoms. Substance use disorders can cause:
- Confusion, violence, and hostility
- Making excuses to use drugs, lack of control over use, and need for regular/daily use
- Continuing drug use even when work, family, and health are affected
- Missing work or school
- Secretive behaviors related to drugs
- Neglecting to eat or to care for one's appearance

Diagnostic Procedures. To diagnose substance use, urine and blood drug tests (toxicology screens) are done.

Treatments. Treatment starts by recognizing the problem. Substances may either be slowly withdrawn or stopped abruptly. Hospitalization or residential treatment programs address

TABLE 15.7   Commonly Used Drugs

Drug	Street Names	Common Form/Ways Taken	Possible Health Effects	Withdrawal Symptoms
Ayahuasca	Aya, Yage, Hoasca	Brewed as tea/swallowed	Strong hallucinations, increases in heart rate (HR), hypertension (HTN), gastric burning.	Unknown
Central nervous system depressants	*(Barbiturates, pentobarbital)* Barbs, Red Birds, Yellow Jackets, Yellows *(Benzodiazepines)* Candy, Downers, Sleeping pills, Tranks *(Sleep medications)* Mexican Valium, R2, Roche, Roofies, Roofinol, Rope, Rophies	Pill, capsule, liquid/swallowed, injected Pill, capsule, liquid/swallowed, snorted Pill, capsule, liquid/swallowed, snorted	Drowsiness, slurred speech, poor concentration, confusion, dizziness, problems with movement and memory, lowered blood pressure (BP), slowed breathing.	Must be discussed with a healthcare provider; barbiturate withdrawal can cause a serious abstinence syndrome that may even include seizures.
Cocaine	Blow, Bump, C, Candy, Charlie, Coke, Crack, Flake, Rock, Snow, Toot	White powder, whitish rock crystal/swallowed, snorted, smoked	Enlarged pupils, increased HR, HTN, abdominal pain, euphoria, increased energy, violent behavior, panic attacks, paranoia, stroke, seizure, coma.	Depression, tiredness, increased appetite, insomnia, vivid unpleasant dreams, slowed thinking and movement, restlessness.
Dimethyltryptamine	DMT, Dimitri	White or yellow crystalline powder/smoked, injected	Intense visual hallucinations, depersonalization, and altered perception, HTN, increased HR, agitation, seizures, dilated pupils.	Unknown
Gamma hydroxybutyrate (GHB)	Home Boy, G, Georgia, Goop, Grievous Bodily Harm, Liquid Ecstasy, Liquid X, Soap, Scoop	Colorless, liquid, white powder/ swallowed, often combined with alcohol and other beverages	Euphoria, drowsiness, vomiting, confusion, memory loss, unconsciousness, slowed HR, seizures, coma, death.	Insomnia, anxiety, tremors, sweating, increased HR and BP, psychotic thoughts.
Heroin	Brown Sugar, China White, Dope, H, Horse, Junk, Skag, Skunk, Smack, White Horse	White or brownish powder, or black sticky substance known as "black tar heroin"/injected, smoked, snorted	Euphoria, slowed HR, constipation and stomach cramps, liver or kidney disease, pneumonia.	Restlessness, muscle and bone pain, insomnia, diarrhea, vomiting, cold flashes with goose bumps ("cold turkey").
Inhalants	Poppers, Snappers, Whippets, Laughing gas	Paint thinners, lighter fluid, permanent markers, glue, spray paint, and other types of aerosol products/Inhaled through the nose or mouth	Confusion, slurred speech, lack of coordination, hallucination, headaches, heart failure, seizures, coma, death, liver and kidney damage.	Nausea, tremors, irritability, problems sleeping, and mood changes

TABLE 15.7 Commonly Used Drugs—cont'd

Drug	Street Names	Common Form/Ways Taken	Possible Health Effects	Withdrawal Symptoms
Ketamine	*(Anesthetic in veterinary practice)* Cat Valium, K, Special K, Vitamin K	Liquid, white powder/injected, snorted, smoked, swallowed	Problems with attention, learning, and memory; hallucinations, sedation, HTN, very slowed breathing; kidney problems.	Unknown
Khat	Abyssinian tea, African salad, Catha, Chat, Kat, Oat	Fresh or dried leaves/chewed or brewed as a tea	Euphoria, increased alertness, depression, loss of appetite, fine tremors, heart attack.	Depression, nightmares, hypotension, decreased energy
Kratom	Herbal speedball, Biak-biak, Ketum, Kahuam, Ithang, Thom	Fresh or dried leaves, liquid, gum/chewed, eaten with other foods, smoked	Increased energy, alertness, sedation, euphoria, decreased pain, hallucinations.	Muscle aches, insomnia, hostility, jerky movements, aggression
Lysergic acid diethylamide (LSD)	Acid, Blotter, Blue Heaven, Cubes, Microdot, Yellow Sunshine	Tablet; capsule; clear liquid; small, tainted decorated absorbent paper squares/swallowed, absorbed through mouth tissues	Rapid emotional swings; HTN, increased HR, tremors, enlarged pupils, visual disturbances, paranoia, mood swings.	Unknown
Marijuana (Cannabis)	Blunt, Bud, Dope, Ganja, Grass, Green, Herb, Joint, Mary Jane, Pot, Reefer, Sinsemilla, Skunk, Smoke, Trees, Weed; Hashish: Boom, Gangster, Hash, Hemp	Greenish gray mixture of dried, shredded leaves, stems, seeds, and/or flowers; resin (hashish) or sticky, black liquid (hash oil)/smoked, eaten (mixed in food or brewed as tea)	Enhanced sensory perception and euphoria, drowsiness, slowed reaction time; problems with balance and coordination; HTN, anxiety, chronic cough.	Irritability, trouble sleeping, decreased appetite, anxiety
MDMA (Ecstasy/Molly)	Adam, Clarity, Eve, Lover's Speed, Peace, Uppers	Colorful tablets, capsules, powder, liquid/swallowed, snorted	Lowered inhibitions, increase in heart rate and blood pressure, kidney failure, death.	Fatigue, loss of appetite, depression, problems concentrating
Mescaline (Peyote)	Buttons, Cactus, Mesc	Fresh or dried buttons, capsule/swallowed	Enhanced perception and feeling, euphoria, hallucinations, HTN, sweating, problems with movement.	Unknown
Methamphetamine	Crank, Chalk, Crystal, Fire, Glass, Go Fast, Ice, Meth, Speed	White powder or pill, shiny blue-white rocks/swallowed, snorted, smoked, injected	Increased wakefulness, increase HR, HTN, paranoia, hallucinations, delusions, dental problems.	Depression, anxiety, tiredness
Dextromethorphan (over-the-counter DM products)	Robotripping, Robo, Triple C	Syrup, capsule/swallowed	Slurred speech, increase HR, HTN, dizziness.	Unknown
Loperamide (Imodium)	None	Table, capsule, liquid/swallowed	High doses cause euphoria, lessen drug craving, kidney failure, loss of consciousness.	Severe anxiety, vomiting, and diarrhea
Phencyclidine (PCP, or "angel dust")	Angel Dust, Boat, Hog, Love Boat, Peace Pill	White or colored powder, tablet, or capsule; clear liquid/injected, snorted, swallowed, smoked	Delusions, hallucinations, paranoia, anxiety, HTN, sweating, drooling, loss of balance, seizures, coma, and death.	Headaches, increased appetite, sleepiness, depression
Prescription opioids	Captain, Cody, Lean, Schoolboy, Purple (multiple names depending on medication)	Varies: tablet, capsule, liquid/swallowed, injected, snorted	Pain relief, drowsiness, euphoria, slowed breathing, death.	Restlessness, pain, insomnia, cold flashes with goose bumps ("cold turkey"), leg movements
Prescription stimulants	(Amphetamine – Adderall) Bennies, Black Beauties, Crosses, Hearts, Speed, Uppers	Tablet, capsule/swallowed, snorted, smoked, injected	Increased alertness, attention, and energy; HTN, increase in HR; arrhythmias, paranoia, seizures.	Depression, tiredness, sleep problems
	(Methylphenidate – Concerta, Ritalin) JIF, MPH, R-ball, Skippy, The Smart Dog, Vitamin R	Liquid, tablet, chewable, tablet, capsule/swallowed, snorted, smoked, injected, chewed		
Psilocybin	Little Smoke, Magic Mushrooms, Purple Passion, Shrooms	Fresh or dried mushrooms with long, slender stems topped by caps with dark gills/swallowed	Hallucinations, altered perceptions, inability to tell fantasy from reality, panic, problems with movement, enlarged pupils, drowsiness.	Unknown

Continued

TABLE 15.7   Commonly Used Drugs—cont'd

Drug	Street Names	Common Form/Ways Taken	Possible Health Effects	Withdrawal Symptoms
Rohypnol (Flunitrazepam) *(Similar to Xanax and Valium)* Date rape drug, Mind Eraser, Mexican Valium, Roach (multiple names)		Tablet/swallowed	Drowsiness, amnesia; impaired reaction time, motor coordination, mental functioning, and judgment; confusion; slurred speech.	Headache, extreme anxiety, restlessness, confusion, irritability; hallucinations; delirium; convulsions; seizures; or shock
Salvia	Magic mint, Maria Pastoria, Sally-D, Shepherdess's Herb	Fresh or dried leaves/smoked, chewed, brewed as tea	Intense hallucination, altered perceptions, mood swings, sweating.	Unknown
Tobacco	Multiple brands	Cigarettes, cigars, bidis, hookahs, smokeless tobacco (snuff, spit tobacco, chew)/smoked, snorted, chewed, vaporized	Increased HR, HTN, risk of lung and oral cancer, chronic bronchitis; emphysema; heart disease; leukemia; cataracts; pneumonia.	Irritability, attention and sleep problems, depression, increased appetite

From the National Institute of Drug Abuse: https://www.drugabuse.gov/drug-topics.

withdrawal symptoms and behaviors. Medications may be given for some withdrawal symptoms. Support groups are helpful.

VOCABULARY

coma A state of deep, often prolonged unconsciousness, usually the result of a head injury, neurologic disease, intoxication, or metabolic abnormalities.

paranoia An unfounded or excessive suspicion of the motives of others.

Alcohol Use Disorder. Alcohol use disorder (AUD) is a chronic relapsing brain disease that includes a compulsion to use alcohol, loss of control over alcohol intake, and a negative emotional state when abstaining from alcohol. Many people are not aware of what a standard drink means (Box 15.2). According to the National Institute on Alcohol Abuse and Alcoholism (https://www.niaaa.nih.gov/), in 2019 about 15 million people in the US have AUD, including 414,000 children under age 18. AUD can range from mild to severe. AUD can include periods of alcohol intoxication and symptoms of withdrawal.

Etiology. Psychological, genetic, social, and environmental factors can play a role in how alcohol affects one's body and behavior.

Signs and Symptoms. Alcohol intoxication signs include inappropriate behavior, unstable moods, impaired judgment, slurred speech, impaired memory, poor coordination, and blackouts. Signs and symptoms of AUD include:

- Being unable to limit the amount of alcohol consumed
- Wanting to cut back on drinking or making unsuccessful attempts to do so
- Spending significant time obtaining alcohol, drinking, and recovering
- Having the effects of alcohol affect one's work, school, or home life
- Being unable to stop drinking even if it is causing problems in one's life
- Using alcohol in situations in which it is not safe (e.g., driving, boating, swimming)
- Feeling as if one needs more alcohol to get the same effect

---

BOX 15.2   Standard Drink

One "standard" drink is about 14 grams of pure alcohol. This can be found in:
- 12 fluid ounces (oz) of regular beer (about 5% alcohol)
- 8–9 fluid oz of malt liquor (about 7% alcohol)
- 5 fluid oz of table wine (about 12% alcohol)
- 1.5 fluid oz of distilled spirits (gin, rum, tequila, vodka, and whiskey) (about 40% alcohol)

From the National Institute of Alcohol Abuse and Alcoholism: https://www.niaaa.nih.gov/what-standard-drink.

- Drinking to avoid withdrawal symptoms

The effects of alcohol on the body include:

- Changes in mood and behavior; makes it harder to think clearly and move with coordination
- High blood pressure, stroke, *arrhythmias* (irregular heartbeat), and cardiomyopathy
- Liver inflammation, fatty liver, alcoholic hepatitis, fibrosis, and cirrhosis
- Pancreatitis
- Cancer of the mouth, esophagus, throat, liver, and breast
- A weakened immune system

Diagnostic Procedures. The provider will do a physical exam, urine and blood tests, imaging tests, and a psychological evaluation.

Treatments. Treatment includes medically managed detoxification and withdrawal in an inpatient setting. Sedating medications may be required to help manage the withdrawal symptoms, which can last 2 to 7 days. Treatment also consists of psychological counseling, behavior change techniques, support groups, lifelong support, and medications, including:

- Naltrexone (nal TREX one) (ReVia, Vivitrol), which blocks the "feel good" part of alcohol and reduces the urge to drink
- Acamprosate (a KAM pro sate) (Campral), which helps reduce the cravings
- Disulfiram (dye SUL fi ram) (Antabuse), which helps prevent drinking by causing flushing, nausea, vomiting, and headaches if alcohol is consumed

Other Addictions. In the DSM-5, addictive disorders are addressed with substance use–related disorders. Research has shown similarities in the biology of addictions to that of substance use disorders. Comparing gambling disorder with substance use disorder shows that they share the following:

- An urge or craving state prior to using or gambling.
- The activity reduces anxiety and results in a positive mood state ("a high").
- Co-existence of other types of substance use disorders. For instance, many with gambling addictions also have a substance use disorder. Many with one type of substance use disorder also have another type.
- Similar abnormal functioning in the brain's cortex has been found in both.

There are several addictions recognized by the behavioral health professionals. The following are examples of addictions, though they are not all currently recognized as disorders in the ICD and DSM-5.

- *Exercise addiction*: This is a compulsive disorder that causes people to feel the uncontrollable need to exercise excessively; it can lead to illness or injury. This addiction can co-exist with anorexia nervosa or bulimia nervosa.
- *Gambling addiction*: With this disorder, people cannot control their gambling, and it affects their financial, social, recreational, familial, and occupational functioning. With gambling, dopamine is released in the brain (about 10 times the normal amount), causing a "feel good" sensation.
- *Gaming addiction*: With this serious disorder, a person excessively plays video games, which disturbs normal life activities, including school, work, and hygiene.
- *Internet addiction*: With this disorder, people have tremendous anxiety if they are forced to be without the internet (e.g., their phones, tablets, computers). They have excessive preoccupation or behaviors related to computer use and internet access. Excessive internet usage has been associated with other behavioral health and psychosocial conditions, including social isolation, impaired social skills, ADHD, depression, and suicidal ideation.
- *Shopping addiction*: It is known by many names, including compulsive spending or compulsive buying disorder. The person has an intense preoccupation with buying and shopping and an uncontrollable urge to do these activities, even if negative consequences exist. It is estimated about 6% of the adults in the US have a shopping addiction.

In future editions of the ICD and DSM, more addictions may be added. Currently, gambling is the only addictive disorder listed in the DSM-5.

Suicidal Behavior

Suicide is death caused by a self-inflicted injury with an intent to die as a result of the behavior. A *suicide attempt* is a nonfatal, self-directed, potentially harmful behavior with an intent to die as a result of the behavior. An injury may not be caused by the attempt. *Suicidal ideation* refers to thinking about, considering, or planning suicide.

In 2018, suicide was the tenth leading cause of death in the United States. More than 1.4 million Americans attempt suicide, and on average, 132 die by suicide each day. Suicide is the second leading cause of death between age 10 and 34, and the fourth leading cause of death between ages 35 and 54.

Etiology. The three most common methods of suicide are firearms, suffocation, and poisoning. Certain factors increase the risk of suicide. Ninety percent of those who die by suicide have a mental disorder at the time, including depression, bipolar disorder, and schizophrenia. Additional risk factors include previous suicide attempts, a family history of suicide, substance use, incarceration, a low level of job satisfaction, and being the victim of bullying. Those who have the highest risk for suicide include males, people over age 45, Caucasians, American Indians, and Alaskan Natives. Veterans and other military personnel also have a higher risk of suicide. People with suicidal ideation are often overwhelmed with hopelessness and sadness.

Signs and Symptoms. Warning signs and symptoms of suicidal behavior include:

- Looking for a way to kill oneself
- Talking about killing oneself or wanting to die; feelings of hopelessness, feeling trapped or in unbearable pain; having no reason to live or being a burden on others
- Increased use of drugs or alcohol
- Socially withdrawn and isolated; agitation, feelings of rage, anxiousness, and behaving recklessly
- Sleeping too much or too little
- Extreme mood swings

If someone is showing some of these signs or symptoms, it is important to get help for the person. The National Suicide Prevention Lifeline is 1-800-273-TALK (8255).

Diagnostic Procedures. The provider will do a physical exam and possibly lab tests to rule out other conditions. The provider will ask the patient in-depth questions about these factors:

- Mental and physical health conditions
- Alcohol and drug use
- Medication use

Treatments. Protective factors help prevent suicidal thoughts and behaviors. The following are considered protective factors: effective clinical care for behavioral health conditions and for physical and substance use disorders; easy access to care; family and community support; support from ongoing medical and behavioral healthcare relationships; and skills in problem solving, conflict resolution, and nonviolent ways of handling disputes.

Treatment for suicide attempts includes treating any behavioral health disorders. Medications and psychotherapy (e.g., cognitive behavior therapy) may also be used.

LIFE SPAN CHANGES

Behavioral health problems are very common. Research has shown that 1 out of 7 children in the United States from ages 2 to 8 have been diagnosed with a mental, developmental, or behavioral disorder. Many times, the related factors included poverty, neighborhood concerns, parents with behavioral health issues, and childcare problems that affected the parent's job. Other studies have found that about half of all behavioral health disorders affect a person before the age of 14, and 75% of disorders begin before age 24. Less than 20% of children with a diagnosed behavioral health problem receive the treatment they need.

Behavioral health disorders in children cause changes in the way children learn, behave, or handle their emotions. This can cause problems getting through their days. Common disorders in childhood include anxiety, depression, oppositional defiant disorder, conduct disorder, ADHD, OCD, and PTSD. Substance use and suicides are occurring in growing numbers.

The National Alliance on Mental Illness (https://www.nami.org) states that about 1 in 5 adults experience a behavioral health disorder every year. About 4% of the adult population in the US lives with a serious mental health condition (e.g., bipolar disorder, major depression, and schizophrenia). In 2018, about 20.3 million adults in the United States had a substance use disorder. With older adults who have been diagnosed with heart disease, diabetes, and a stroke, research has shown that depression is more prevalent. Depression can complicate treatment and change a person's quality of life.

CLOSING COMMENTS

Whether you work in primary care, such as pediatrics, or specialty care, such as neurology, you will care for patients who have behavioral health and substance use disorders. Understanding the signs, symptoms, and treatments of common behavioral health and substance use disorders will help you provide better patient care. Having this understanding will help the medical assistant remember that certain behaviors may be related to disorders. Medical assistants should be knowledgeable about the medication classifications used to treat behavioral health and substance use disorders (Box 15.3).

BOX 15.3 Medication Classifications

- *Antianxiety.* Used to reduce anxiety, produce calmness and sedation, and release muscle tension.
- *Anticonvulsants* and *mood stabilizers.* Used to treat mania and mixed episodes (mania and depression) with bipolar disorder.
- *Antidepressants.* Used to treat depression, anxiety, and other behavioral health disorders.
- *Antipsychotics.* Used to treat schizophrenia and bipolar disorder, by altering chemical actions in the brain.
- *Sedative-hypnotics.* Used to treat insomnia, by slowing activity in the brain to allow sleep.
- *Stimulants.* Stimulate the brain and body, making the messages move faster between the brain and the body. The person becomes more alert and physically active. Used to treat attention deficit hyperactivity disorder (ADHD).

Refer to Appendix D, which can be found on the Evolve website, for information on the medication classifications, including indications for use, desired effect, side effects, adverse reactions, and generic and trade names. Medical assistants should be familiar with medications that are prescribed to patients.tga

---

PATIENT-CENTERED CARE

In behavioral health, providing patient-centered care not only includes the patient but may also include the family. Behavioral health professionals need to develop a strong professional, therapeutic relationship with patients. This relationship provides the emotional support that helps patients feel accepted, so they share their concerns, thoughts, and feelings with behavioral health professionals.

Often families play an important part in the management and treatment of behavioral health disorders. Some of these disorders may come from issues related to family relationships. Other times, the family needs to provide emotional support to help assist the patient through treatment. Depending on the situation and the patient, family members may be brought into the therapy to ultimately help the patient through the situation or effectively manage the disorder.

BEING PROFESSIONAL

Medical assistants working outside the behavioral health department will often come in contact with patients who have behavioral health disorders. It is important for medical assistants to remain professional in their nonverbal and verbal communication. If patients make inappropriate or nonsensical statements, seem "off" in their affect, or demonstrate other unusual behaviors, the medical assistant should relay the information to the provider.

Inappropriate comments to the patient or about the patient to others is unprofessional and should not happen. Remember, all information about the patient is confidential.

Role-play this scenario: You are a medical assistant and Amanda is a receptionist in the same department. You have just finished rooming Jim Smith, who has schizophrenia. Today, he made no eye contact with you. He lacked facial expression. His clothes were dirty, and there was a strong urine smell on his person. Amanda states to you, "Wow, he looked like he hasn't had a bath in a month. What is going on with him?" Respond to Amanda.

CHAPTER REVIEW

Common behavioral health professionals include psychiatrists, psychologists, social workers, cognitive behavioral therapists (CBTs), psychiatric nurses, substance use (or addiction) therapists or counselors, and mental health therapists or counselors. In many states, most of these healthcare professionals need a license to practice, and they all have different degrees of training and specialties.

Behavioral health disorders are conditions that cause changes in the mood, behavior, or thoughts of an individual. Common diagnostic procedures for behavioral health disorders include:
- Mental status testing, which assesses a person's ability to think
- Psychological testing, which examines intellectual functioning, academic achievement, psychological process, adaptive behavior, personality, and attitudes

Psychotherapy is used to treat many of the behavioral health and substance use disorders. Patients with behavioral health disorders are prescribed a variety of medications. Psychotherapy is a general term used for a variety of treatment techniques that help a person identify and change troubling behaviors, thoughts, or emotions.

This chapter discussed anxiety disorders, including generalized anxiety disorder, OCD, panic disorder, phobias, and social anxiety disorder. Autism spectrum disorder, depression, behavioral disorder, dissociative disorder, eating disorders, personality disorders, post-traumatic stress disorder, schizophrenia, and suicidal behaviors were discussed. Substance use disorder, including drugs and alcohol, was discussed.

In the DSM-5, substance use disorder includes both substance abuse and substance dependence. Substance use disorder is measured from mild to severe. Alcohol use disorder is a chronic relapsing brain disease that includes a compulsion to use alcohol, loss of control over alcohol intake, and a negative emotional state when abstaining from alcohol. Other addictions include exercise, gambling, gaming, internet, and shopping. Currently, gambling is the only addictive disorder listed in the DSM-5.

Commonly used substances, along with their street names, common forms, and ways to take the drug, in addition to possible health effects and withdrawal symptoms, were discussed. Common substances abused include ayahuasca, CNS depressants, cocaine, DMT, GHB, heroin, inhalants, ketamine, khat, kratom, LSD, marijuana, MDMA, mescaline, methamphetamine, dextromethorphan, loperamide, PCP, prescription opioids and stimulants, psilocybin, rohypnol, salvia, and tobacco.

One "standard" drink is about 14 grams of pure alcohol. This can be found in 12 fluid ounces (oz) of regular beer, 8 to 9 fluid oz of malt liquor, 5 fluid oz of table wine, and 1.5 fluid oz of distilled spirits (e.g., gin, rum, tequila, vodka, and whiskey).

SCENARIO WRAP-UP

Mike has learned a lot about the policies and procedures used by the behavioral health staff. At first, he was uncomfortable working with patients who were experiencing signs and symptoms of behavioral health disorders. To his surprise he found working with patients in behavioral health very interesting and rewarding. Having learned about these conditions in school, he was nervous, not knowing how he would deal with such situations. Mike was professional and felt he provided excellent patient-centered care. Mike realizes he still has a lot more to learn, because there are over 200 mental health disorders and many substance use disorders. He looks forward to spending more time with the behavioral health staff.

16

Healthcare and the Professional Medical Assistant

LEARNING OBJECTIVE

1. Discuss customer service and patient-centered care in the ambulatory care facility.
2. Describe the medical assistant's role and how it is affected by the current trends in healthcare, such as care coordination, home visits, scribing, and telemedicine.
3. Discuss what tasks can be delegated to the medical assistant.
4. Describe the characteristics and appearance of a professional medical assistant.
5. Describe professional characteristics important to the medical assistant as a team member.
6. Explain the healthcare system, including acute, ambulatory, and extended care, along with population health.
7. Describe types of provider practices.

OUTLINE

 OPENING SCENARIO

Christi Michelson is a newly hired medical assistant at Walden-Martin Family Medicine (WMFM) Clinic. She graduated from the local community college last month. She is currently in her probationary period at WMFM Clinic. Christi has orientation for 1 month, and her probationary period will last for 3 months. Over the next 3 months, she must pass a national certification exam. At the end of 3 months, she will have an evaluation. If the evaluation is positive, she will continue in her position.

Christi is very excited with her first healthcare job. In the past, she has worked as a waitress and a salesclerk. These jobs have helped her learn customer service skills, which she is now using in her current position. Christi is finding that the professionalism at WMFM Clinic is much different than at her previous jobs. She now has a dress code that she must follow. Christi is learning the clinic's customer service policies and procedures. She was surprised to learn that her customers include not only the patients, but also her co-workers. Christi is excited to continue learning more skills to help her provide the best patient care possible.

YOU WILL LEARN

1. To describe the medical assistant's role.
2. To discuss the medical assistant's role with regard to the current healthcare trends.
3. To recognize characteristics of professional medical assistants.
4. To discuss the healthcare system, including the patient-centered medical home.
5. To identify types of provider practices.

INTRODUCTION

A medical assistant is a multiskilled healthcare professional. A healthcare professional:

- Has high ethical standards
- Displays integrity
- Completes work accurately and in a timely fashion

It is important for successful professionals to show professionalism. *Professionalism* is having a courteous, conscientious, and respectful approach. This approach is used during all interactions and situations in the workplace. Our patients and co-workers expect professional behavior. Patients base much of their trust and confidence in those who show professionalism.

In this chapter, we will start by describing customer service and its importance to the healthcare facility. Customer service closely relates to professional behaviors and to patient-centered care. One must be professional to provide patient-centered care. We will explore professional characteristics as they relate to patients and team members. We will also examine the healthcare environment, including the healthcare system and types of practices.

> ### VOCABULARY
> **ambulatory care** Medical services provided by healthcare professionals in an outpatient setting, without admission to the facility.
> **conscientious** Meticulous, careful.
> **integrity** Adhering to ethical standards or right conduct standards.

Customer Service

In healthcare today, many of our patients have the ability to choose where they go to seek care. Healthcare is a business. The ambulatory care facility needs to attract and retain patients to remain open and for you to have a job. Two of the quickest ways to lose patients are to treat them poorly and to act in an unprofessional manner. Happy patients will tend to tell others about their experiences. Great customer service leads to a successful healthcare facility and allows growth.

To understand customer service, we first need to know who our customers are. A *customer* is one who purchases goods or services. A customer can also be a person whom you deal with in the work environment. By that definition, we can see that patients are our customers. They choose our ambulatory care facility to seek healthcare services. They (or their insurance companies) pay for the services provided. Patients are considered *external customers*, or people we do business with who are "outside" (i.e., not employed by) the healthcare facility. Other external customers include medical equipment and supply vendors and pharmaceutical representatives.

The second part of the customer definition relates to *internal customers*, or people whom you deal with in the work environment. These are individuals we interact with inside the facility. They include our co-workers, employees in other departments, and the administrative staff. Both internal and external customers are important for the success of the healthcare facility.

Customer service is whatever we do for our customers to improve their experience at our healthcare facility. People may have different ideas about how they should be treated during their interactions. Our goal is to provide *customer satisfaction*, or a sense of contentment with the interaction. Typically, the more we get to know the customer, the better we can provide customer service. This might not always be possible. For instance, a new patient comes for an appointment. If you are at the reception desk, you do not have a lot of time to get to know the patient. The most important things for you to do are:

- Be considerate and treat the patient as you would want to be treated
- Look and act professional

Customer service with patients strongly relates to patient-centered care.

> ### CRITICAL THINKING 16.1
> During Christi's orientation, she learned about customer service and customer satisfaction. In your own words, how would you define both of these phrases?

Patient-Centered Care

Patient-centered care, also called *person-centered care,* is partnering with patients and their families. It requires understanding of and respect for the patient's unique needs, diversity, values, preferences, and right to make healthcare decisions and choices. The patient and the family have a say in the decision making process of planning care and treatment.

Research has linked patient-centered care with increased adherence (ad HEER enns) to the plan of care, decreased utilization of healthcare services, improved quality of care, and improved customer satisfaction. There are many ways healthcare professionals can provide patient-centered care, such as:

- Ask the patient about the person's needs and preferences. The healthcare professionals must work to meet these.

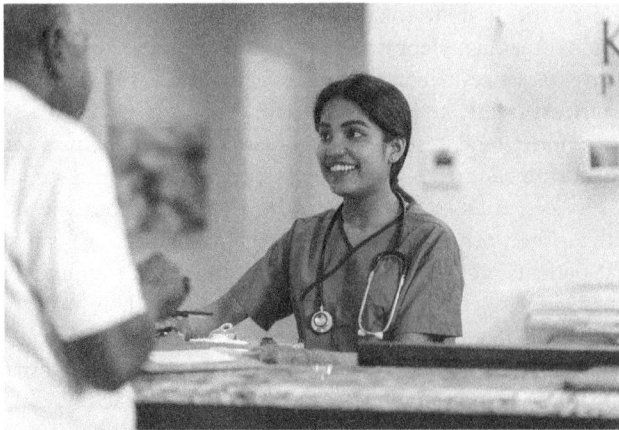

Fig. 16.1 A medical assistant may do both administrative and clinical duties. (FatCamera/iStock.com.)

- Involve the patient and family in planning and decision making on the patient's care.
- Involve a support person and, if needed, an interpreter during visits to the ambulatory care facility.
- Use language that is clear and understandable to the patient.
- Show the patient and family respect.
- Ensure the patient and family members have a way to provide feedback to the healthcare providers and facility.

As you read subsequent chapters, patient-centered care tips will be provided. It is important to use these tips as you interact with patients.

MEDICAL ASSISTANT'S ROLE

Medical assistants are cross-trained to perform administrative and clinical duties. Job duties vary by specialty, facility size, and state law. The majority of medical assistants work in ambulatory care facilities. Some may focus solely on administrative or clinical duties, whereas others do both. Common administrative duties include:

- Answering telephones, taking messages, scheduling appointments, greeting patients, and updating patient records in the computer software (Fig. 16.1).
- Updating patients' health records, filing paper records, and scanning and uploading documents to electronic health records.
- Coding visit charges, completing insurance forms, and billing and bookkeeping activities.
- Handling correspondence.
- Scheduling procedures and assisting with arranging hospital admissions.
  Common clinical duties include:
- Obtaining medical histories, vital signs, heights, and weights (Fig. 16.2).
- Reconciling patient medication lists and researching refill requests.
- Preparing patients for and assisting providers during exams.

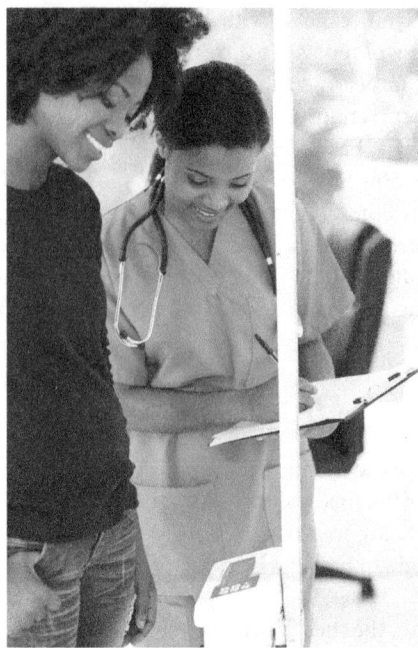

Fig. 16.2 A Medical Assistant Obtaining and Documenting a Patient's Weight. (michaeljung/iStock.com.)

- Preparing and administering oral and injectable medications as ordered by the provider.
- Collecting and preparing laboratory specimens, including performing phlebotomy.
- Performing basic laboratory tests (also called CLIA-waived tests).
- Instructing patients on diets, wound care, and other procedures.
- Providing wound care, including dressing changes, and removing sutures and staples.
- Preparing refilled prescriptions and transmitting refills as directed by the provider.
- Entering providers' orders for laboratory tests and procedures (also known as *computerized provider order entry* [CPOE]).
- Documenting in the patient's health record.
- Obtaining electrocardiograms (ECGs).
- Serving as a liaison (lee AE zon) between the provider and patient, including communicating test results to the patient as indicated by the provider.

VOCABULARY

adherence The act of sticking to something.

liaison To interact and communicate between different groups.

reconcile To compare (an account or log) so that it is consistent or compatible with another.

Growing Trends in Healthcare

Care Coordination. *Care coordination* provides personalized patient- and family-centered care in a team-based environment.

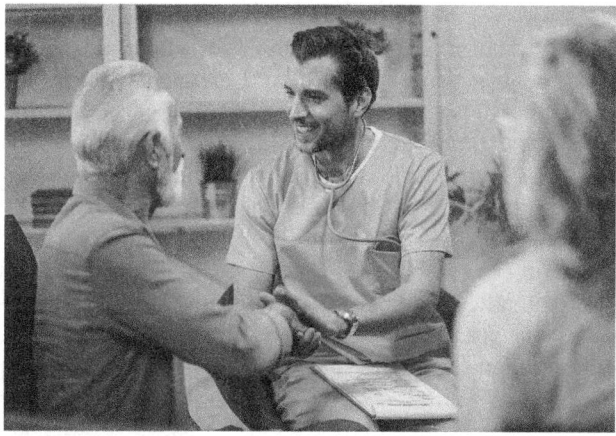

Fig. 16.3 During home visits, the medical assistant can obtain the patient's medical history and medication information for the provider. (Drazen Zigic/iStock.com.)

Care coordination can reduce cost, increase efficiency, and provide greater patient care. The care coordinator communicates between the patient and the healthcare team. Care coordinators ensure patients get timely care and do not fall through the cracks. In the ambulatory care setting, medical assistants can be hired as care coordinators. Care coordination can be set up in different ways in both primary and specialty care areas.

A patient navigator (also called a *patient advocate*) has been described as a type of care coordinator. Patient navigators typically guide chronically ill patients through the healthcare system. They identify patients' financial, cultural, physical, and emotional barriers. Then, they work closely with the healthcare team and the patients to ensure barriers are eliminated and patients get timely care.

> **VOCABULARY**
> **patient navigator** A person who identifies patients' barriers, works closely with the healthcare team and patients, and guides the patients through the healthcare system; may also be called a patient advocate.

Home Visits. Provider home visits are a growing trend in healthcare. It is estimated that over 2 million patients are homebound. For many, going to the healthcare facility for routine medical care is difficult to almost impossible. Providers who make home visits help homebound patients get routine medical care. This has reduced hospital admissions and also increased patient satisfaction. Common duties of a medical assistant who accompanies a provider on home visits include:

- Preparing and maintaining supplies and equipment for home visits
- Obtaining vital signs and medical histories (Fig. 16.3)
- Preparing patients for and assisting providers during exams
- Obtaining and packaging specimens for delivery to the lab; performing phlebotomy
- Documenting in the electronic health record

Scribes. A scribe enters provider-dictated information into the electronic health record (EHR) during the patient's visit. As the provider talks with the patient, the scribe documents the medical history, physical exam findings, patient education, diagnoses, prescriptions, and plan of care in the EHR. Having a scribe document the information allows the provider to focus more on the patient. This increases the patient's satisfaction during the visit and also increases the provider's efficiency. Besides documenting during the patient visit, the scribe may be responsible for preparing referral letters and other correspondence as directed by the provider. It is common for medical assistants to be hired as scribes.

Telemedicine. *Telemedicine* is the use of telecommunications technology to allow healthcare providers to evaluate, diagnose, and treat patients at a distance. There are many types of telecommunications technology available for telemedicine. Common duties of a medical assistant in telemedicine include:

- Scheduling, confirming, and coordinating telemedicine visits
- Coaching the patient in how to use the technology if needed
- Obtaining patients' medical history, including current medications and medication refill needs
- Providing patient education
- Ensuring the patient's record contains the test results needed by the provider
- Coordinating patient care as ordered by the provider

Working From Home. Medical assistants may have jobs where they can work from home. An important aspect of working from home is having a workspace dedicated to your job. The space should be well-lit, free from distraction, and as private as possible. If possible, the space should be separate and only used for work. This will help create a work-life balance.

The workspace should have a desk and an adjustable chair. Adjust the chair so you are comfortable and in an ergonomically correct position. (See Chapter 24 for more information on computer workstation ergonomics.) A computer with internet access is usually required. Position the computer screen on the desk so it is at eye level.

Many jobs require the use of web-based video software for virtual patient visits or meetings. If using such software, it is important to:

- Use a neutral background behind your desk, such as such as an empty wall or an appropriate picture, such as a landscape.
- Dress professionally.
- Use professional etiquette during the visit or meeting.

Delegation

Physicians can delegate tasks to the medical assistant. State laws may also indicate other types of healthcare providers and professionals who can delegate tasks to the medical assistant. Tasks must be within the medical assistant's scope of practice. In many states, the scope of practice is dictated by the state law.

Medical assistants cannot be delegated tasks that are outside of their scope of practice. Such tasks would include authorizing prescriptions, diagnosing and treating patients, and performing minor surgery. A medical assistant can perform a delegated task if:

- The task is allowed by state law.
- The task is within the medical assistant's scope of practice.
- He or she is knowledgeable and competent with the task.

VOCABULARY

scope of practice Defines the procedures, actions, and processes that individuals in a specific occupation are permitted to perform.

PROFESSIONALISM

Medical assistants represent the healthcare facility. They are viewed as an extension of the provider and the facility. How they act is a direct reflection on the facility and provider. If a medical assistant is rude to a patient, the patient will think that the provider is rude. The perceived quality of care will be negative. Medical assistants must always display professionalism. This includes their attitude, appearance, behavior, and communication. (Communication and personal boundaries with communication are discussed in Chapter 17 yet are considered an important part of professionalism.) Regardless of the situation, they must always act professionally.

Professional Behaviors of Medical Assistants

Medical assistants must demonstrate professional behaviors, which may also be called characteristics or traits. You will start developing these traits while in school. You will put them into practice during practicum. They will follow you into your first job. If a student is unprofessional during practicum, it will be difficult to get a job. That behavior may be *detrimental* (harmful) to the medical assistant's professional career.

Courtesy and Respect. Courtesy, respect, and dignity often come together when professionalism is discussed. *Courtesy* is having good manners or being polite. Courteous behavior is polite, open, and welcoming. *Respect* means to show consideration of or appreciation for another person. *Dignity* (DIG ni tee) is the inherent worth or state of being worthy of respect.

We show our patients dignity by treating all patients the way we would want to be treated. It does not matter if the patient has bad body odor or is dressed in tattered clothes. The patient is a person worthy of respect. Patients expect to be treated as individuals who matter. They want to be respected and not be treated as an annoyance or a medical condition. How can the medical assistant treat others with courtesy and respect?

- Make patients feel welcome and respected. A pleasant greeting and eye contact should be the first things patients experience. Thanking patients at the end of the visit is also important.
- Display positive nonverbal behaviors. Use a calm tone of voice, eye contact when appropriate, and provide privacy for patients. Maintain patient confidentiality.
- Learn about other cultures in your area. When working with patients from those cultures, make sure to avoid gestures, words, and behaviors that could be perceived as disrespectful.

- Always use proper grammar, without slang words. Explain medical treatments and conditions in simple lay language. If you need to use a medical word, explain it to the patient.

Empathy and Compassion. It is important that professional medical assistants demonstrate empathy and compassion to their patients. Empathy, sympathy, and compassion can easily be confused. *Empathy* (EM pah thee) is the ability to understand another's perspective, experiences, or motivations. We can share another's emotional state. Empathy differs from sympathy. *Sympathy* is feeling sorrow or concern for what the other person has gone through. *Compassion* means we have a deep awareness of the suffering of another and wish to ease it.

Tact and Diplomacy. Tact and diplomacy are extremely valuable traits in healthcare professionals. Being *tactful* means being acutely sensitive to what is proper and appropriate when interacting with others. A tactful person has the ability to speak or act without offending others. Being *diplomatic* means using tact and sensitivity when interacting with others. The medical assistant must be sensitive to the needs of others. How can a medical assistant use these traits when communicating with others?

- Consistently be polite and honest during your communication. Show sensitivity to others through your communication and behaviors.
- Recognize the needs and rights of others. Attempt to reach a mutually beneficial resolution to the problem.
- Assess your personal response to the situation. Your personal beliefs and biases should not prevent you from interacting diplomatically and tactfully with others.

CRITICAL THINKING 16.2

During Christi's orientation, she learned about the importance of courtesy, respect, empathy, compassion, tact, and diplomacy. Select three of these words and share with a peer examples of how a medical assistant could display these traits.

Respect for Individual Diversity. Medical assistants work with diverse populations. Your patients will come from different backgrounds. Diversity describes the differences and similarities in identity, perspective, and points of view among people. Diversity is discussed in Chapter 17.

It is important to be open and nonjudgmental when working with patients and co-workers who are different from ourselves. Be aware and accepting of other cultural differences. Be aware of your own cultural values. What preconceived ideas do you have about other diverse groups? How might your biases affect the care you provide to those in different groups?

It is important to educate yourself about other groups. Get to know their customs and practices. Culture can affect healthcare. It can influence how people describe their symptoms, when healthcare is sought, and how treatment plans are followed. For instance, people in some cultures eat traditional foods high in sodium. This could be an issue if a person has high blood pressure or kidney disease. Understanding and accepting

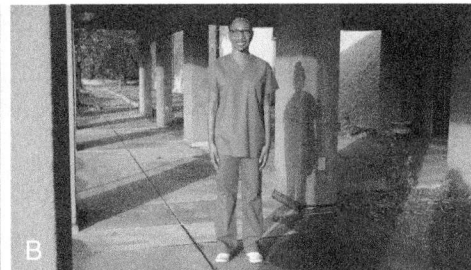

Fig. 16.4 A professional appearance is important for a medical assistant. A, Business attire. B, Scrubs.

the differences represented by your patients will help you provide the best care possible for them.

Honesty, Dependability, and Responsibility. To be *honest* means to be sincere and upright. *Dependable* is the same as trustworthy. *Responsible* is defined as being trusted or depended upon. These are three traits that are valuable for employers to have in employees. Professional medical assistants should be honest, dependable, and responsible. When given a task, they should complete it accurately, on time, and to the best of their ability. If they make an error, they should be upfront about it. Patient safety is the number one priority. Any mistake in patient care needs to be reported immediately to the provider and to the supervisor. Dependability and honesty are critical components in earning the trust and respect of others. How can medical assistants perform their duties using these three characteristics?
- Be honest and straightforward when interacting with others.
- Accept responsibility for your mistakes. Determine how to prevent them in the future.
- Follow through on your promises.
- Complete your work to the best of your abilities. Complete it on time.

CRITICAL THINKING 16.3

During Christi's orientation, she shadowed Grace, another medical assistant. Grace has a personality that always makes the patients comfortable. She follows up with patients and does what she promised to do. Christi could see how much the provider trusted Grace. What kind of traits did Grace demonstrate to Christi?

Professional Appearance

Most ambulatory healthcare facilities have dress codes for employees. Medical assistants are usually required to wear scrubs, along with the facility's nametag (and a photo) clearly visible (Fig. 16.4). Table 16.1 provides a typical dress code. Dress codes will vary by facility. Some communities are more conservative and thus the dress codes reflect this.

Typically, healthcare facilities include terms such as "modest" and "business attire" in describing their dress codes. The rule of thumb is to make sure the employee does not expose too much at the neckline, the abdomen, and below the waist when bending and raising the arms. Business attire is not casual clothes. Casual clothes include jeans, T-shirts, shorts, exercise/sports clothing, and so on. Business attire is considered dressier, more professional, than casual clothes.

CRITICAL THINKING 16.4

Rosie, a business office employee at the clinic, is allowed to dress in business attire. She interacts with patients who have questions about their bill. Describe how Rosie should dress.

Professionalism as a Team Member

A *team* is a group of people organized for work or a specific purpose. In the healthcare setting, usually the team consists of the employees working in the same department. A broader definition could include all the employees at the facility. A *team member* is loyal to the group and works well with the other people in the group (Fig. 16.5). As a member, the medical assistant must help the team function. To do this, it is important to know the roles of the different team members. Tables 16.2 and 16.3 describe various healthcare professionals found in ambulatory care facilities. Box 16.1 describes interprofessional collaborative practice.

To be a valuable team member, it is important to have several qualities. Work ethic, punctuality, cooperation, and the willingness to help are important traits in a team member. It takes all members working together to make an effective and productive team. When a member "drops the ball," others must step in and do extra work (Box 16.2).

Work Ethic and Punctuality. A *work ethic* is composed of sets of values based on hard work and diligence. The medical assistant should always display initiative (i NISH eh tiv) and be reliable. People with a good worth ethic arrive on time, are rarely absent, and always perform to the best of their ability. Co-workers become frustrated if another employee consistently arrives late or is absent. This forces the co-workers to take on additional duties, and it may prevent them from completing their own work. One missing employee can disrupt the entire day. Phones may not be answered promptly. Patients may have to wait longer for appointments. Lunch breaks may be shortened to allow all the work to be done. All employees should know and follow the attendance policies of the facility as outlined in the policies and procedures manual.

Most new hires have a probationary period that may last 30 to 90 days. Excessive absences or *tardiness* (being late) will negatively affect the employee. It may be grounds for *termination* (job loss). If the medical assistant must be absent or tardy, the supervisor must be notified prior to the start time. Make sure to follow the office policy. All employees must be *punctual*

TABLE 16.1   Typical Dress Code

Dress Code	Professional	Unprofessional	Comments
Uniform: Scrubs and white shoes	• Scrubs must be clean, pressed (ironed), and fit properly. • Scrub pants must be hemmed to the appropriate length. • Closed-toed shoes must be white and clean.	• Dirty, wrinkled, ripped scrubs • Scrub pants dragging on the floor • Scruffy, dirty shoes • Open shoes (sandals), fabric shoes	• Shoes need to protect your feet. Cloth and open-toed shoes provide very little protection. • Pants dragging on floors pick up and transfer bacteria.
Hair	• Natural colors; clean and styled • Long hair must be tied back.	• Unnatural colors; dirty, messy hair • Hair in face or hanging down	• Hair hanging in front can interfere with patient care, spread bacteria, and get caught in equipment.
Fingernails	• Cut short, unpolished	• Long, polished, artificial nails	• Bacteria can multiply and grow under long, artificial, and/or polished nails.
Cosmetics and body odors	• Professional makeup • No odors on the body	• Overuse of makeup • Wearing perfume, cologne, etc. • Smelling like a cigarette • Body odor (from not bathing)	• Too much makeup can look unprofessional. • Smells like perfumes, colognes, or cigarettes can trigger allergies in others. • Offensive body odor is unprofessional because we are in patients' intimate/personal space.
Jewelry	• Wedding band (no stones) • One pair of earrings (studs) • Watch	• Rings with stones • Multiple earrings on each ear • Necklaces, bracelets • Lanyards	• Bacteria can accumulate in rings and bracelets. • Necklaces and lanyards can be choking hazards if grabbed by a patient.
Tattoos and body piercings	• Tattoos and body piercings must follow the healthcare facility's policy.	• Not following the healthcare facility's policy	• In conservative communities, body piercings and tattoos may be perceived as unprofessional.
Professional dress (street clothes) for special events	• Blouse, top, or sweater • Dress pants • Dress or skirt (to the top of the knee) • Dress shoes	• Low-cut tops; sheer tops • Jeans, ripped pants, exercise clothes • Flip-flops, tennis shoes • Mini skirts	• Clothes should look professional; should not be ripped or casual in appearance.

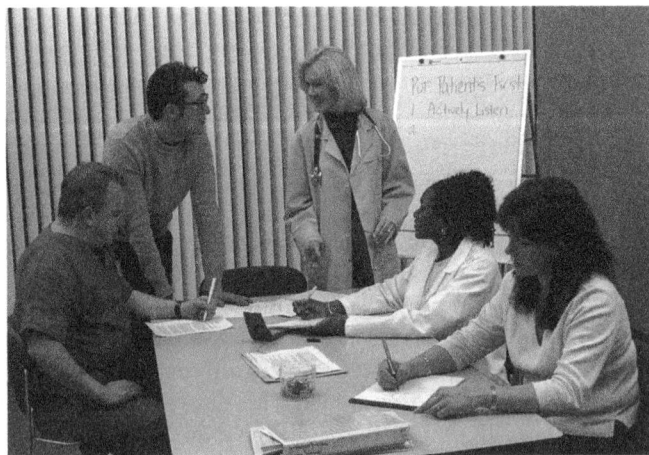

Fig. 16.5 Teamwork is a vital part of the medical profession. All staff members must work together to care for the patient and perform required duties in the healthcare facility. (From Proctor D, Niedzwiecki B: *Kinn's the medical assistant*, ed 13, St. Louis, 2017, Elsevier.)

(on time) every day. Providers and patients alike expect this reliability.

VOCABULARY

initiative The ability to start a task and energetically complete it.
reliable Dependable, able to be trusted.

CRITICAL THINKING 16.5

Christi tends to arrive at the clinic with about 1 minute to spare. She realizes that she needs to change her habits and arrive about 10 minutes before her start time. This would give her a little "cushion" if traffic is slow. If you were Christi, what strategies could you use to make sure to get to the healthcare facility 10 minutes before the start time?

Cooperation and Willingness to Help. Each team member must be willing to cooperate and help others on the team. It is not uncommon that one team member might be very busy or handling an emergency. Other team members must be willing to step up and lend a helping hand. For instance, a medical assistant may be tied up caring for a very sick patient. Other patients who have appointments are waiting to be seen. One of the other team members needs to help room the patients (e.g., take their vital signs and histories for the provider). This is how the department can provide exceptional customer service. Team members watch out for each other. If someone is getting behind, others help out.

Through cooperation, the team is more productive. Team members have greater job satisfaction. When members cooperate and work together, there is a great sense of communication and understanding in a team. Most importantly, the patients are cared for, and great customer service is provided.

TABLE 16.2 Ambulatory Allied Health Occupations

Title (Credential)	Job Description
Diagnostic cardiac sonographer or vascular technologist (DCS, DVT)	Trained and certified to perform noninvasive tests (e.g., echocardiographs and electrocardiographs) to help diagnose cardiac and vascular diseases.
Diagnostic medical sonographer (RDMS)	Trained and certified to use medical ultrasound, which can aid the diagnosis of a variety of conditions and diseases; also monitors fetal development.
Electroneurodiagnostic technologist (REEG-T)	Records and studies the electrical activity of the brain and nervous system.
Health information management professional (RHIA, RHIT)	Provides expert assistance in the management of health information.
Medical assistant (CMA [AAMA], RMA, CCMA, CMAA)	Performs both administrative and clinical procedures and duties; a multiskilled health professional.
Nuclear medicine technologist (RT)	Performs nuclear diagnostic tests, which helps in the diagnosis of diseases.
Certified ophthalmic assistant (COA); Certified ophthalmic technician (COT)	Assists an ophthalmologist in providing eye care.
Pharmacy technician (CPhT)	Supervised by a pharmacist; assists in preparing medications based on prescriptions.
Surgical technologist (ST, CST)	Helps prepare patients for surgery and assists surgeon during the surgery.

TABLE 16.3 Licensed Healthcare Professionals

Title (Credential)	Job Description
Audiologist (CCC-A)	Assesses individuals with hearing loss, balance issues, and neural problems.
Certified nurse midwife (CMN)	Advanced practice registered nurse (RN prepared with a master's or post master's education level and certification) who provides prenatal, labor/delivery, and gynecologic care.
Certified nurse practitioner or nurse practitioner (CNP, NP)	Advanced practice registered nurse who provides direct patient care and can diagnose and treat patients, including prescribe medications.
Certified registered nurse anesthetist (CRNA)	Advanced practice registered nurse who provides anesthesia care during surgical procedures.
Clinical nurse specialist (CNS)	Advanced practice registered nurse who often works with other providers to manage the care of patients; educates and supports interprofessional staff.
Doctor of osteopathic medicine (DO)	Licensed physician whose training emphasized a whole-person approach to care and treatment. Received special training in the musculoskeletal system.
Licensed practical or vocational nurse (LPN, LVN)	A nurse who has been trained to assess and care for patients in a variety of environments; has less education than a registered nurse.
Medical doctor (MD)	Licensed physician.
Medical technologist (MT)	Performs tests on blood, body fluids, and other types of specimens to assist the provider in arriving at a diagnosis.
Occupational therapist (OT)	Assists patients with physical disabilities to learn daily skills so they can be as independent as possible
Physical therapist (PT)	Assists patients in regaining mobility and strength.
Physician assistant (PA)	Provides direct patient care services under the supervision of a licensed physician; can diagnose and treat patients (write prescriptions).
Radiology technician (RT)	Performs medical imaging procedures (e.g., computed tomography [CT], magnetic resonance imaging [MRI], x-rays).
Registered dietitian (RD)	Trained in nutrition; provides a dietary education to patients.
Registered nurse (RN)	A nurse who has been trained to assess and care for patients in a variety of environments.
Respiratory therapist (RT)	Performs diagnostic tests that measure lung capacity.
Speech-language therapist (SLP)	Often called a "speech therapist." Evaluates and treats patients for disorders with speaking, forming words, cognition-communication, feeding, and swallowing.

"Interprofessional collaborative" means healthcare professionals from a variety of different disciplines work together to provide the highest level of care for patients, their families, and community. Interprofessional collaboratives can improve patient care, reduce errors and repeated tests, reduce costs, and improve the relationship between healthcare professionals.

In 2009, six healthcare education associations from different disciplines worked together to promote interprofessional collaboration in the colleges. They created four core competencies that addressed values and ethics, roles and responsibilities, interprofessional communication, and teamwork. When team members work with other healthcare professionals, it is important that they:

- Have shared values. Respect each other and the expertise each brings to the team.
- Know their role and the roles of all other team members. Between the team members, they address patients' health concerns and those of the community.
- Professionally communicate with each other, patients, families, and community members.
- Function as an effective team to promote the health of patients and the community.

For additional information on the four core competencies, visit Interprofessional Education Collaborative at https://www.ipecollaborative.org/.

BOX 16.2   **Huddles at the Start of the Day**

Huddles are becoming more popular at the start of the day in ambulatory care. The purpose of huddles is to communicate important information to all team members, from the administrative staff to the clinical staff and providers. Huddles are quick meetings that help communicate the care needs of the patients being seen that day.

Prior to the huddle, a medical assistant reviews the patients' records, identifying missing information, preventive care required, and chronic disease management needs. These details are shared at the huddle. This information helps the providers, medical assistants, and other team members to be aware of the patients' needs. If the provider is busy, the medical assistant can work with the patient to obtain missing information and arrange preventive care.

Huddles help the staff members support each other. They also provide supervisors an opportunity to communicate quick messages on staffing issues, policy changes, and upcoming events.

Prioritizing and Time Management Skills. Prioritizing duties and using time management skills are critical for the success of medical assistants. *Prioritizing* means to arrange and complete duties in the order of most importance. *Time management strategies* are methods that maximize personal efficiencies and prioritize tasks. This means that we are to use our time efficiently and concentrate on the most important duties first. To do this, we must first prioritize our duties. We must arrange our schedules to ensure that these duties can be performed. The first way to improve time management is to plan the tasks that need to be done that day. Take 10 minutes to write down the tasks for the day. This helps ensure the tasks get done. Make sure to reference the list throughout the day to keep on track. Do not schedule too much to do each day, so that it is impossible to get everything done. Keep the list manageable. You need to build in some extra time in case

of emergencies or urgent issues that come up. The key to managing time is prioritizing.

When prioritizing your tasks, use a code system to indicate when they need to be done. For instance:

- Use an "M" for tasks that *must* be done that day.
- Use an "S" for tasks that *should* be done that day.
- Use a "C" for tasks that *could* be done if time permits.

Once the tasks have been divided into these categories, they can be further classified in each section. For instance, if category *M* has six tasks, they can be numbered in the order they should be performed. The same process is completed with the tasks in categories *S* and *C*. As the tasks are completed, they are checked off. At the end of each day, create a new "to do" list for the next day so that nothing important is forgotten.

CRITICAL THINKING 16.6

Christi needs to practice her time management skills. Using the system described, make your "to do" list. Use M, S, and C to categorize your activities.

Responding to Criticism. As we work, we are evaluated by others. It may be informal or formal for a job evaluation. We learn from others' feedback on our performance. This criticism can be hard to take. It threatens our confidence and self-esteem. We need to realize the value of the feedback. It will help us improve our skills and refine our professional skills. When a person gives us feedback or criticism, it is important to take it as a professional. Becoming defensive or blaming others is not professional. This type of behavior will be a negative reflection on you.

Problem Solving and Chain of Command. When you are working as part of a team, it is important to understand how to solve differences with other members. Typically, it is best to talk with the person with whom you are having an issue. Try not to use statements that accuse the other person. Refrain from using sentences that start with "You are..." Try to remove the emotion from the situation if you can. Use more "I feel..." statements. If your attempt to resolve the situation is unsuccessful, then it is usually recommended that you talk with the supervisor.

If the issue is related to theft, confidentiality, or harassment, you may need to follow the chain of command in the healthcare facility. Usually, you need to start with your supervisor or the person to whom you report. Then the next step is the supervisor of your supervisor, and so on. Most employee handbooks discuss the facility's chain of command.

Continuing Education

As a professional medical assistant, it is important to stay current (up-to-date) with the newest medications, treatments, and diagnostic tests. Education beyond your medical assistant degree is considered continuing education. Most healthcare professionals need to do continuing education to renew their certification or license. There are many opportunities for continuing education. These include:

- Reading professional journals and reputable health websites

TABLE 16.4 Credentialing Agencies for Medical Assistants

Agency/Website	Credential	Recertification Methods
American Association of Medical Assistants (AAMA) http://www.aama-ntl.org	Certified Medical Assistant (CMA [AAMA])	Recertify every 5 years either by exam or by earning 60 continuing education points. Specific points must be achieved in the three content areas. At least 30 points must be from AAMA-approved continuing education units (CEUs).
American Medical Technologists (AMT) https://www.americanmedtech.org	Registered Medical Assistant (RMA)	Recertify every 3 years either by exam or by completing specific activities.
National Healthcareer Association (NHA) https://www.nhanow.com	Clinical Medical Assistant (CCMA) Medical Administrative Assistant (CMAA)	Recertify every 2 years either by exam or by earning continuing education credits.
National Center for Competency Testing (NCCT) https://www.ncctinc.com	Medical Assistant (NCMA)	Recertify every year either by exam or by completing 14 contact hours of continuing education.
American Medical Certification Association (AMCA) https://www.amcaexams.com	Clinical Medical Assistant Certification (CMAC)	Recertify every 2 years either by exam or by earning continuing education credits.

- On-the-job educational conferences
- Local, state, and national medical assistant conferences

Typically, additional continuing education opportunities exist if a medical assistant is a member of an organization. Two popular medical assistant professional organizations are:

- American Association of Medical Assistants (AAMA) (https://www.aama-ntl.org/)
- American Medical Technologists (AMT) (https://www.americanmedtech.org)

Achieving a Credential. Medical assistants have several options if they choose to become credentialed. Being a credentialed medical assistant has certain benefits:

- Credentialed medical assistants have had to pass a national standardized exam. Passing the exam indicates that they have the knowledge to perform the medical assistant's duties.
- Some employers require the credential prior to hiring or within a few months after hiring.
- Some employers will pay more if a person has achieved a medical assistant credential.

There are several national agencies that will provide credentials to medical assistants upon successful completion of their exam. Table 16.4 presents some of the more common medical assistant credentials. It is important for graduating medical assistants to research whether credentials are preferred or required by the local employers. It is also important to identify which credential is most wanted by local employers. Your instructors are also excellent resources if you have additional questions on credentials for medical assistants.

Barriers to Professionalism

At times it is not easy to be a professional. Sometimes patients and co-workers try our patience. It can be difficult to maintain a professional attitude in these cases. Some of the obstructions to professional behavior are discussed in this section.

Personal Problems and "Baggage." We all have a personal life. Sometimes things happen in our lives before we go to work.

It is important that we push these issues aside and focus on our job. If we carry this "baggage" to work, it can interfere with our ability to do our job. We may be tempted to make personal calls, check emails, and so on. This takes time away from our job, and our focus is not on our job. If the "baggage" is so important and concerning, the medical assistant needs to speak with the supervisor. It might not be appropriate to be working if one cannot concentrate on the job at hand. The patient must be the prime concern of all the employees in the healthcare facility.

Gossip. *Gossip* is casual or idle chat (rumors) about other people and their business. Many times, the "discussion" is based on someone's opinion and not fact. Most people enjoy working in an environment in which employees cooperate and get along with each other. Rumors and gossip can cause problems with employee morale. They can affect how a team functions. A medical assistant should refuse to participate in the rumor mill (Fig. 16.6). Attempting to be cordial and friendly to everyone at work is important. Supervisors regard those who gossip or spread rumors as unprofessional and untrustworthy. You should always avoid passing along work-related rumors to patients and family members.

Personal Communication. Making personal phone calls and checking personal emails should not be done during work time. Only emergency calls can be taken. Many healthcare facilities require cell phones to be silenced and out of sight during the workday. Because most phones have cameras, facility administrators are concerned about unlawful pictures being taken. Many healthcare computer networks block certain nonhealthcare websites (e.g., social media sites). Table 16.5 describes acceptable and unacceptable activities for digital communication devices and online activities.

CRITICAL THINKING 16.7

Christi loves her phone. But she learned very quickly that her phone was to be turned off and put away during work hours. Explain why having cell phones out and turned on can create issues in the healthcare facility.

Healthcare Environment

Part of being professional is understanding how your job fits into the department, the healthcare facility, and the healthcare system in general. A medical assistant should be knowledgeable about the healthcare system. By calling the local hospital to arrange a test for a patient or helping make a referral to a home healthcare agency, the medical assistant interacts with other parts of the healthcare system.

Healthcare System. The *healthcare system* is an organized plan of healthcare services for the public. Healthcare services are provided in many different locations throughout the community. For instance, a diabetic patient may have a leg ulcer. He is seen in the emergency department at the local hospital and then hospitalized. As an inpatient, he undergoes surgery, recovers, and is discharged home. Upon discharge, the doctor orders home healthcare, outpatient physical therapy, and a follow-up visit at the clinic. To help manage his diabetes, the patient is regularly followed by the chronic care management team. This patient received many different types of healthcare service. This section will explain the different healthcare services available in many communities.

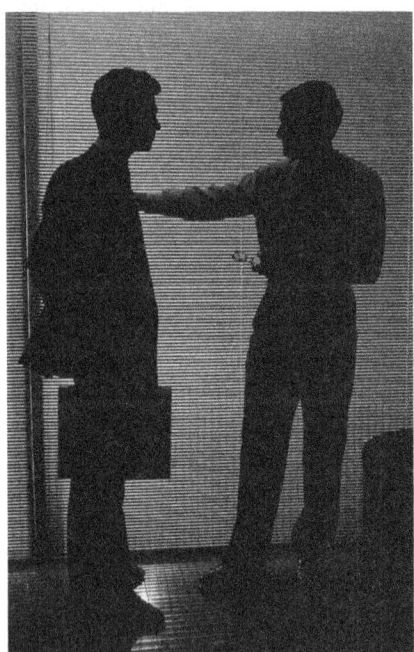

Fig. 16.6 Gossip and rumors have no place in the medical profession. Avoid employees who participate in this type of activity. (From Proctor D, Niedzwiecki B: *Kinn's the medical assistant*, ed 13, St. Louis, 2017, Elsevier.)

> **VOCABULARY**
>
> **inpatient** A person who is admitted to a healthcare facility that requires at least one overnight stay.
>
> **outpatient** A person who receives healthcare services at a healthcare facility but is not admitted for an overnight stay.

Acute Care. *Acute care* delivery of healthcare services includes the hospital, inpatient surgery, and the emergency department. Patients may opt to go or may be brought to the emergency department. Providers may refer patients to the emergency department based on their symptoms. In the emergency department, patients are treated and discharged or admitted to the hospital (called an *emergency admit*).

Patients may also be directly admitted to the hospital without going to the emergency department.

- *Direct admit*: A patient who is admitted to the hospital by the provider without being seen in the emergency department. In most cases, the patient is seen in an ambulatory care facility and needs to be hospitalized.
- *Scheduled admit*: A patient who is admitted to the hospital for a scheduled surgery or procedure.

In both of these situations, the medical assistant is involved with the admission. The medical assistant must relay information to the hospital staff, obtain information for the patient, and then provide the patient with the information.

Ambulatory Care. *Ambulatory care* refers to medical services provided by healthcare professionals in an outpatient setting, without admission to the facility. Common ambulatory care settings include medical offices and clinics, urgent cares, ambulatory surgical centers, hospital outpatient departments, and dialysis centers. These are all settings that may employ medical assistants.

Table 16.6 lists specialties that can be found in ambulatory care facilities. In ambulatory care, physicians, physician assistants, and nurse practitioners are the *healthcare providers*, who examine, diagnose, and treat patients.

Healthcare providers who work in pediatrics, internal medicine, family medicine, and obstetrics and gynecology can also be referred to as *primary care providers*. A *primary care provider* (PCP) is a provider who manages a patient's healthcare.

TABLE 16.5	Using Digital Communication Devices and Online Activities in Healthcare Facilities	
	Acceptable, Professional	**Unacceptable, Unprofessional**
Phone calls/text messages	• Emergency calls only • Turn off or silence ringer • Make personal calls only on break time	• Frequent checking for calls received • Making personal calls • Having phone out and visible when working with patients • Taking pictures
Personal emails and social media	• Do not open, read, or post	• Sending and reading personal emails • Viewing or posting social media postings
Online	• Work-related web-related activity	• Shopping, gaming, nonwork websites

TABLE 16.6 Medical Specialties

Specialty	Practitioner's Title	Description of Practitioner
Allergy	**Allergist** (AL ahr jist)	A physician who specializes in the diagnosis and treatment of diseases or conditions caused by allergies.
Anesthesiology	**Anesthesiologist** (AN is thee zee ol ah jist)	A physician who provides pain relief and pain management during surgical procedures; also treats patients with chronic pain.
Bariatric medicine	**Bariatric medicine physician**	A physician who treats overweight and obese patients through lifestyle changes and weight loss strategies.
Cardiology	**Cardiologist** (kar DEE ol oh jist)	A physician who specializes in internal medicine and cardiology; treats patients with cardiovascular system disorders.
Colon and rectal surgery	**Colorectal surgeon**	A surgeon who specializes in the diagnosis and treatment of intestinal conditions.
Dermatology	**Dermatologist** (DUR mah tol ah jee)	A physician who specializes in skin disorders.
Emergency medicine	**Emergency physician**	A specially trained physician who assesses and treats patients in emergency conditions (emergency departments).
Endocrinology	**Endocrinologist** (en doh kruh NOL uh jist)	A physician who specializes in internal medicine and endocrinology; treats patients with endocrine system disorders.
Family medicine	**Family practice physician**	A physician who provides comprehensive primary care for infants through the elderly.
Gastroenterology	**Gastroenterologist** (gas troh en tuh ROL uh jist)	A physician who specializes in internal medicine and gastroenterology; treats patients with digestive system disorders.
General surgery	**Surgeon** (SUR jen)	A physician who performs surgical procedures to correct deformities and injuries or treat diseases.
Genetics	**Medical geneticist** (juh NET i sist)	A physician specially trained to treat patients with genetically linked diseases.
Geriatrics	**Geriatrician** (JER ee ah TRISH ahn)	A physician specially trained to care for and treat the elderly.
Hematology	**Hematologist** (hee mah TOL oh jist)	A physician who specializes in internal medicine and hematology; treats patients with blood, bone marrow, vascular system, lymph gland, and spleen disorders.
Internal medicine	**Internist** (in TUR nist)	A physician who provides comprehensive primary care to adults.
Internal medicine–pediatrics	**Internist** and **pediatrician**	A physician who is an internist and a pediatrician. Provides comprehensive primary care to infants through adults. Also called "med-peds" (med peeds) doctors.
Nephrology	**Nephrologist** (neh FROL oh jist)	A physician who specializes in internal medicine and nephrology; treats patients with kidney and urinary system disorders.
Neurology	**Neurologist** (noo ROL uh jist)	Specially trained physician who treats patients with nervous systems conditions.
Neurosurgery	**Neurosurgeon** (NOOR oh sur jen)	Specially trained surgeon who provides surgical care for patients with nervous systems conditions.
Nuclear medicine	**Nuclear radiologist**	A specially trained physician who uses radioactive materials to diagnose and treat disease.
Obstetrics and gynecology	**Obstetrician/gynecologist** (OB stri trish uhn)/(GIE ni KOL uh jist)	An obstetrician is a physician who provides care to females during and immediately after pregnancy. A gynecologist is a physician who provides reproductive care to females.
Occupational medicine	**Occupational and environmental physician/Occupational medicine physician**	A physician who diagnoses and treats work-related injuries. Environmental medicine addresses the environmental chemicals and physical stressors that affect workers.
Oncology	**Oncologist** (on kol oh jist)	A physician who diagnoses and treats cancer. Radiation oncologists specialize in using high-energy radiation therapy for treating cancer.
Ophthalmology	**Ophthalmologist** (OF thahl mol uh jist)	A specially trained physician who diagnoses, treats, and provides comprehensive care for the eye and its supporting structures. Can also offer vision services, including corrective lenses.
Orthopedics	**Orthopedic surgeon** (ORE thoe PEE dik)	A specially trained physician who medically, surgically, and physically treats musculoskeletal disorders.
Otolaryngology	**Otolaryngologist** (Oh toe lar ing GOL uh jist)	A specially trained physician who medically and surgically treats diseases of the ear, nose, and throat (ENT).
Pathology	**Pathologist** (pa THOL uh jee)	Physicians who study the cause and development of disease.

Continued

TABLE 16.6   Medical Specialties—cont'd

Specialty	Practitioner's Title	Description of Practitioner
Pediatrics	**Pediatrician** (PEE dee ah trish ahn)	A physician who provides comprehensive primary care to children.
Physical medicine and rehabilitation	**Physiatrist** (FIZ ee at rist)	A physician who specializes in physical medicine, which includes treating patients with musculoskeletal disabilities.
Plastic surgery	**Plastic surgeon**	A specially trained surgeon who performs reconstructive cosmetic surgery.
Podiatry	**Podiatrist** (poe DIE ah trist)	A Doctor of Podiatric Medicine (DPM), also called a *podiatric physician* or *surgeon*. Specially trained to diagnose and treat conditions affecting the foot and ankle.
Psychiatry/Behavioral medicine	**Psychiatrist** (si KIE ah trist)	A physician who specializes in the diagnosis and treatment of people with mental, emotional, or behavioral disorders.
Pulmonary	**Pulmonologist** (PULL mun ahl ah jist)	A physician who specializes in internal medicine and pulmonary conditions; treats patients with lung and airway diseases.
Radiology/Diagnostic Radiology	**Radiologist** (RAE de ol uh ist)	A physician who specializes in the diagnosis and treatment of conditions using medical imaging procedures (e.g., computed tomography [CT], magnetic resonance imaging [MRI], x-rays).
Rheumatology	**Rheumatologist** (roo muh TOL uh jist)	A physician who specializes in internal medicine and rheumatology; treats patients with diseases of the joints, muscles, bones, and tendons.
Thoracic surgery	**Thoracic surgeon** (thah RAS ik)	A surgeon who specializes in the operative treatment of the chest and chest wall, lungs, heart, heart valves, and respiratory passages.
Urology	**Urologist** (yoo ROL ah jist)	A physician who specializes in the treatment of urinary tract diseases and male reproductive disorders.

A primary care provider performs routine physicals, screening, and immunizations; treats minor illnesses; and manages chronic disease conditions.

Ambulatory care facilities may use different healthcare delivery models. For instance, primary care departments may use the patient-centered medical home model. The Veterans Administration (VA) ambulatory care facilities use the patient-aligned care team (PACT) approach.

Patient-Centered Medical Home. Many healthcare facilities are adopting the patient-centered medical home (PCMH) model of healthcare. Using the PCMH care delivery model, the primary care provider coordinates the patient's treatment and necessary care. The goal of the PCMH is to improve patient care and reduce costs. The patient is the key player on the PCMH team. This is a model that responds to each patient's unique needs and preferences.

The PCMH team may vary by healthcare facilities but might include:

- Primary care providers, who diagnose and manage the treatment of patients. The physician works with complex patients. Physician assistants, certified nurse practitioners, and certified nurse midwives work with less complex patients.
- Medical assistant(s), who follow provider-directed protocols to administer immunizations, order labs, coach patients, provide care coordination, and assist the providers.
- Registered nurse, who provides case management, supervision, and triage (tree AHZH).
- Pharmacist, who reviews and monitors medications patients are taking.
- Behavioral health specialist, who assists with substance use and behavioral health issues.
- Receptionist, who schedules appointments, takes messages, and prepares the health record for patient visits.

Patients are actively involved in their own healthcare when the PCHM model is used. In fact, patient-centered care is part of the PCHM model. Steps are taken to ensure that patients receive the care and services they need from their healthcare team.

> **VOCABULARY**
>
> **triage** To sort out and classify the injured; used in the military and emergency settings to determine the priority of a patient to be treated.

Patient-Aligned Care Team. The VA has designed PACT, a model of care that focuses on personalized care to meet the individual veteran's healthcare goals. Veterans work with healthcare professionals to plan for their whole-person care, which includes lifelong health, wellness, and disease prevention. The key components of PACT are:

- Partnership between the healthcare team and the veteran
- Access to care using diverse methods, including ambulatory care visits, online services, and education seminars
- Coordinated care among the healthcare team members
- Team-based care, with the veteran as the center of the team

Medical assistants are employed at VA ambulatory care facilities and participate in the PACT model.

Extended Care. *Extended care* provides care to patients in a nonhospital setting. There are many types of extended care services.

- *Skilled nursing facility* (SNF): Provides patients with a wide range of health and personal cares. Patients receive continuous nursing care. Some facilities offer rehabilitation services, including physical, speech, and occupational therapies.
- *Home healthcare:* Provides patients with convenient, less expensive care in their homes. Frequent skilled home

healthcare services include wound care, medication administration, and monitoring of serious illnesses.

- *Hospice care*: Provides end-of-life care through a team of healthcare professionals and volunteers. The hospice team provides medical, psychological, and spiritual support to the patient and family. Usually, a hospice patient is expected to live 6 months or less. Hospice care can be provided in the hospital, skilled nursing facility, or the patient's home.
- *Respite care*: Provides short-term relief for primary caregivers. Respite care is available for children with chronic conditions, older adults, and those who are disabled and dependent on others. Respite care may include medication management and personal hygiene cares.

Population Health. *Population health* is focused on improving the health outcomes of a population while controlling the cost of healthcare. Many healthcare agencies are now investing resources into population health. These facilities are ensuring that patient health outcomes are being met, while keeping the overall cost of healthcare down. Population health services focus on:

- *Health promotion and disease prevention strategies.* These strategies include weight loss and substance use cessation programs, prenatal care, and vaccinations.
- *Chronic disease management.* The population health teams work with patients who have cancer, hypertension, and asthma. They help patients manage symptoms and maintain their health. Care coordination and coaching are helpful strategies with chronic disease management.
- *Screening and early detection programs.* These programs may include screenings for cancer, substance use, and diabetes.

Medical assistants are being used to help with population health strategies. For example:

- *Health record reviews* include identifying patients who need vaccines, wellness exams, and prevention screenings. These patients are notified and encouraged to obtain these services to maintain and improve their health.
- *Care coordination* provides personalized patient- and family-centered care in a team-based environment. It ensures the patient's needs and preferences for healthcare services are met. The care coordinator communicates between the patient and healthcare team. Care coordinators ensure patients get timely care and do not fall through the cracks.
- *Coaching* provides patients with skills, knowledge, support, and confidence to manage their disease between provider visits.

Types of Practices

Providers work in a variety of practices. Depending on the practice type, providers may have management, administrative, and financial responsibilities. Usually, with these practice types, providers have more independence and decision making abilities. With other practice types, providers are employed by a healthcare agency and the additional responsibilities are done by other staff members.

Solo Practice. *Solo practice* is also called *private practice* or *independent practice*. One provider owns and manages the practice. This gives the provider the most flexibility. The provider is also responsible for all practice policies and guidelines, hiring, finances, office hours, after-hours (patient) coverage, and legal issues.

Group Practice. A *group practice* involves two or more providers practicing in the same facility. This type of healthcare practice may involve a single specialty or a multispecialty model.

- *Single specialty*: The providers all practice in the same field or see the same types of patients. For example, a group practice may be composed of pediatricians who see children.
- *Multispecialty*: The providers practice in different fields or see different types of patients. For instance, the group practice may consist of pediatricians, family practice providers, and internal medicine providers.

With group practices, the office hours, after-hours coverage, resources (e.g., supplies and equipment), and staff are all shared. Associations and partnerships are types of group practices.

Association. An *association* is a legal agreement between the providers on how the expenses are shared. The expenses may include rent, supplies, equipment, and staff. The associates may share after-hours coverage, resources, and staff. They do not share income or the legal and financial risk of the practice. In this way, an association is like a solo practice. Each provider is solely responsible for the financial and legal aspects of their own practice.

Partnership. A *partnership* is two or more doctors who co-own the practice. Each partner has equal rights and responsibilities for managing the practice. They equally share the income and are equally responsible for the legal and financial risks of the practice.

Employed Provider Practice. With employed provider practices, the provider is hired as an employee. There are several practice models that hire providers.

- Hospitals may purchase existing solo or group practices. The providers are then hired as employees of the hospital.
- *Integrated delivery system* (IDS) involves multiple types of providers, specialties, clinics, and at least one hospital.
- Healthcare corporations own and manage clinics that hire providers.

With employed provider practices, the facilities provide management and support personnel, along with resources and staff. The provider gets benefits and income as an employee, without the concerns of "managing the business."

Alternative and Complementary Providers

The use of healthcare practices outside of the conventional or Western healthcare is common in the United States. The words "complementary" and "alternative" are often used interchangeably, but there is a difference. If the healthcare practices are used together with conventional medicine, they are *complementary*. *Alternative* healthcare practices are used in place of conventional medicine.

The following types of providers are explained in more detail in Chapter 43.

- *Acupressurist*: A therapist who performs acupressure, by applying firm pressure on specific points on the body.
- *Acupuncturist*: A therapist who performs acupuncture, by inserting fine needles into acupuncture points (specific sites on the body) (Fig. 16.7).
- *Chiropractic doctors*: Help correct spinal alignment problems and thereby alleviate pain, improve function, and support the body's natural ability to heal itself.
- *Massage therapists*: Are specially trained to apply pressure to a person's skin and muscles, which can reduce stress, pain, and muscle tension.

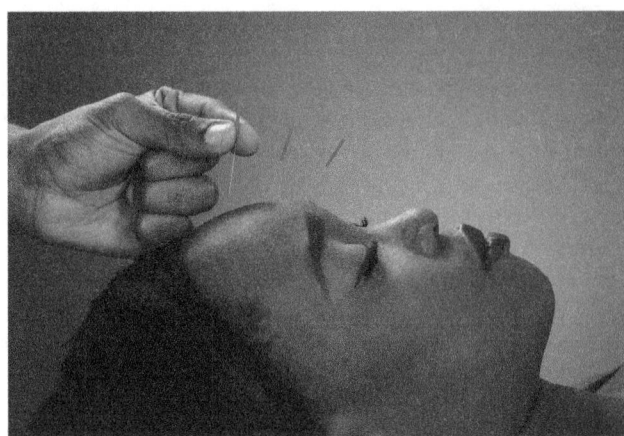

Fig. 16.7 Acupuncture. (AndreyPopov/iStock.com.)

CLOSING COMMENTS

When a medical assistant is working with a patient, it is important that the medical assistant practices **GIVE**:

G: Greet the patient.

I: Identify yourself. Give your name and your position. For instance, "I am Christi, Dr. Walden's medical assistant."

V: Verify the patient's identity. Ask the patient (or parent/guardian) for the patient's full name and date of birth. If the last name has many spellings locally, some facilities encourage medical assistants to have the patient spell the last name. This ensures they have the correct patient. The medical assistant needs to verify the patient's name and date of birth with the health record.

E: Explain what you will be doing. Make sure to use language that the patient understands. Answer any questions the patient or family may have.

Using GIVE shows respect for the patient and provides the person the needed information of who you are and what is going to happen. It also helps to ensure you have the correct patient. Throughout this textbook, GIVE is incorporated into the procedures. By practicing GIVE in the classroom, you will learn to incorporate it during your patient interactions in practicum.

PATIENT-CENTERED CARE

For patient-centered care to occur, healthcare professionals must work together as a team and the patient must be included. To provide patient-centered care, medical assistants need to:

- Remember that patients, family members, and co-workers are all customers.
- Be professional in behavior and appearance.
- Consider cultural differences when working with patients and their families.
- Use GIVE during patient interactions.

BEING PROFESSIONAL

Medical assistants can only perform tasks that are within their scope of practice. If a provider delegates a task outside of the medical assistant scope of practice, the medical assistant cannot legally perform the task. The medical assistant must talk with the provider and professionally refuse to perform such a task.

Role-play this scenario: Your peer will play the provider, and you are the medical assistant. A patient has a laceration, and the provider determines sutures are needed. The provider has you set up the supplies and equipment for the minor surgery. Before beginning, the provider tells you to administer the anesthetic and suture the laceration. You know this is beyond your scope of practice. Respond professionally and respectfully to the provider.

CHAPTER REVIEW

A medical assistant is a multiskilled healthcare professional who works with internal and external customers. The goal is to provide customer satisfaction, or a sense of contentment with interactions with customers, especially patients. Patient-centered care is partnering with the patient and the family. It requires understanding and respect for the patient's unique needs, diversity, values, preferences, and right to make healthcare decisions and choices. Patient-centered care strongly relates to customer service.

The job duties for medical assistants vary based on the specialty, facility size, and state law. Medical assistants may have clinical duties, administrative duties, or both. With the current healthcare trends, the medical assistant may be involved with care coordination, patient home visits, scribing, and telemedicine.

Medical assistants represent the healthcare facility and are viewed as an extension of the provider and facility. Medical assistants must always display professionalism. This includes their attitudes, appearance, behavior, and communication. Professional characteristics of a medical assistant include courtesy, respect, empathy, compassion, tact, diplomacy, respect for individual diversity, honesty, dependability, and responsibility. Being part of the healthcare team means the medical assistant must help the team function. To do this, the medical assistant should:

- Display initiative
- Be reliable, cooperative, and willing to help
- Prioritize duties and use time management skills
- Respond to criticism appropriately
- Know how to problem-solve and use the chain of command when needed

Barriers to professionalism include bringing personal problems to work, gossiping, and the inappropriate use of personal communication during work hours (e.g., social media and phone calls).

Part of being professional is understanding how your job fits into the department, the healthcare facility, and the healthcare system in general. A medical assistant should be knowledgeable about the healthcare system, which is composed of acute care, ambulatory care, extended care, and population health. There are a variety of practices, including solo, group, associations, partnership, and employed provider practices.

SCENARIO WRAP-UP

The more Christi learns about her new job and the WMFM Clinic and providers, the more she is happy with her job. Last week she was able to work with another medical assistant and a provider as they made home visits. Christi never thought about how bedridden patients received healthcare. After her experience, she was proud to be part of the home visiting team and looks forward to many more home visits in the future.

This week Christi learned that the WMFM Clinic providers are considering using the patient-centered care model and

scribing. A team of providers and medical assistants is researching and discussing the advantages and disadvantages of having the medical assistants scribe for the providers. Christi enjoys computers and hopes to have an opportunity to scribe for a provider. She knows she will learn a great deal being in the examination room with the provider. She will be able to help patients when they have questions regarding their plan of care after the visit.

17

Applied Interpersonal Communication

LEARNING OBJECTIVES

1. Describe examples of cultural, social, and ethnic diversity, and explain how to demonstrate respect for individual diversity, including gender, race, religion, age, economic status, and appearance.
2. Discuss types of nonverbal communication, including positive and negative nonverbal communication.
3. Describe the communication cycle and types of verbal communication.
4. Describe the behaviors seen in passive, aggressive, passive-aggressive, manipulative, and assertive communicators.
5. Describe therapeutic communication and active listening.

6. Describe barriers to communication, including how Erikson's psychosocial development stages and Kübler-Ross's stages of grief and dying relate to communication and behavior.
7. Describe personal boundaries with professional verbal communication.
8. Discuss how Maslow's hierarchy of needs relates to communication and behavior.
9. Discuss defense mechanisms and differentiate between adaptive and maladaptive coping mechanisms.

OUTLINE

⯮ OPENING SCENARIO

Christi Michelson is a newly hired medical assistant at Walden-Martin Family Medicine (WMFM) Clinic. She is very excited about her first healthcare job but is noticing differences from her past jobs as a waitress and a salesclerk. Those jobs helped her learn customer service skills, but she is realizing there is much more to communication than what she has experienced in past jobs. During her medical assistant program, she learned a lot of information about nonverbal and verbal communication. As a medical assistant she is finding herself using that knowledge more than in past jobs.

YOU WILL LEARN

1. To recognize different types of diversity and how to demonstrate respect for individual diversity.
2. To describe types of nonverbal communication.
3. To explain the communication cycle and the different types of communicators.
4. To describe therapeutic communication and active listening, along with identifying barriers to communication.
5. To describe the importance of Erikson's psychosocial developmental stages, Kübler-Ross's stages of grief and dying, and

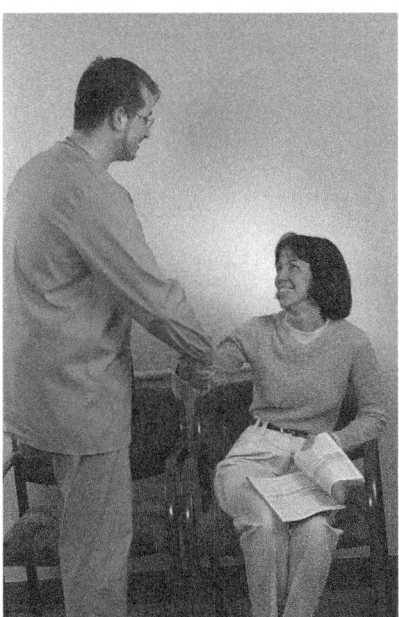

Fig. 17.1 First impressions are critical in gaining the patient's trust. (From Niedzwiecki B, et al: *Kinn's the medical assistant,* ed 14, St Louis, 2020, Elsevier.)

Maslow's hierarchy of needs as they relate to communication and behavior.

INTRODUCTION

Communication is the exchange of information, feelings, and thoughts between two or more people using spoken words or other methods. What we say and how we say something directly affects how the other person perceives the message. We need to communicate effectively, or in a manner that is clear, concise, and easy to understand. This helps the message to be understood by the other person.

First Impressions

The opinions formed in the early moments of meeting someone remain in our thoughts long after the first words have been spoken. The first impression involves much more than just physical appearance or dress. It includes attitude, compassion, and therapeutic communication skills that clearly help the patient and family members realize that the medical assistant is interested in who they are and what they need (Fig. 17.1).

Delivering quality patient care is the primary objective of the professional medical assistant. Patients are the reason the facility exists. Each patient should be welcomed warmly by name and with a polite greeting. The medical assistant should smile and introduce himself or herself to the patient. A smile should show not only on the face, but in the voice and the eyes. This small effort helps put the patient at ease in the healthcare environment.

To provide high-quality patient care, we must communicate effectively with the patient and provide a warm, caring environment. Positive reactions and interactions with the patient are vital. Because medical care by nature is extremely personal, a medical assistant must always remember that each patient is an individual with certain anxieties. Their anxieties often cause people to act and react in different ways; therefore effective verbal communication and nonverbal communication with each patient are absolutely essential.

Healthcare professionals accept the responsibility of developing helping relationships with their patients. The interpersonal nature of the patient–medical assistant relationship carries with it a certain amount of responsibility to forget one's self-interest and focus on the patient's needs. A medical assistant can elicit either a positive or a negative response to patient care simply by the way they treat and interact with patients. A medical assistant is usually the first person with whom the patient communicates; therefore the medical assistant plays a vital role in initiating therapeutic patient interactions.

> **VOCABULARY**
> **compassion** Having a deep awareness of the suffering of another and the wish to ease it.
> **nonverbal communication** A type of communication that occurs through body language and expressive behaviors rather than with verbal or written words.

DIVERSITY AND COMMUNICATION

Medical assistants work with diverse populations. Your patients will come from different backgrounds. *Diversity* describes the differences and similarities in identity, perspective, and points of view among people. Not only does a medical assistant need to respect diversity, it is also important to understand how it impacts the communication process. Your patients and co-workers will come from backgrounds that are different from your own. Their traditions, customs, beliefs, and values affect how they communicate with others. Knowing more about the diversity around you will help you become a better healthcare professional.

There are several types of diversity that a medical assistant should be aware of, including:

- *Nationality*, which pertains to the country where the person was born and holds citizenship. For example: John was born in Mexico and moved to the United States. He became a US citizen.
- *Race*, a group of people who have the same physical characteristics, such as skin color. For example: Even though John was born in Mexico, his mother is Mongolian, and his father is Caucasian.
- *Culture*, which is the general customs, norms, values, and beliefs held by a group of people. For example: John has adapted to the US culture. He likes to be on time for appointments. Even though he grew up in a large family (six children), he is comfortable with having two or three children. John values honesty, timeliness, punctuality, and motivation.
- *Ethnicity*, a group of people who share a common ancestry, culture, religion, traditions, nationality, language, and so on. For example: John states he is Mexican. Growing up he learned his family's Mexican traditions. He plans to share these with his children someday. He values his family and respects his grandparents and parents.
- *Social factors* are all the ways a person is different from others (e.g., lifestyle, religion, tastes, and preferences). For example:

TABLE 17.1   Individual Diversity Factors

Factor	Discussion
Language	Some people are fluent in more than one language. For others, English is not their primary language. It is important to be sensitive to and respectful of language differences. Using resources (e.g., translated materials, an interpreter) can also show respect to patients.
Age	There are many stereotypes about age. For instance, the older generation may not be college educated but may have "street smarts." The younger generation may be more comfortable with computers and digital devices. It is important not to stereotype a person because of age. Ask, never assume anything!
Religion	There is a wide range of belief systems in this country. There are also different degrees of religious observations in the workplace. Some patients may refuse certain medical treatments based on their religion. Be sensitive to patients who refuse medical care or want to involve their shaman or healer in their care.
Economic status	Our patients may be from a variety of economic backgrounds. Some patients may be very wealthy and can afford to pay for healthcare without insurance. Other patients may rely on food banks and charities to get by. Be sensitive and respectful if your patient doesn't have the financial means to pay for healthcare services. Help the patient seek resources for medications, transportation, and food.
Gender	There are many stereotypes attributed to gender. We need to make sure we do not stereotype our patients and peers. Some of our patients may identify as a gender other than their birth sex. We need to respect their choices and be sensitive to any issues that arise.
Appearance	Our patients' appearances can greatly vary. If you work in a farming community, patients may come to appointments in their work clothes and smell of the barn. With the popularity of piercings, tattoos, and hair dye, we can see a variety of differences in our patients. We need to move beyond the patient's appearance and provide exceptional patient care.

John does not drink alcohol or smoke. He exercises in the gym each day. He likes to visit art museums and learn about history.

Besides these five types, we also have individual diversity. Factors that relate to individual diversity include language, age, religion, economic status, gender, and appearance. Many times, certain stereotypes, biases, and beliefs are attached to these factors (Table 17.1). Healthcare professionals need to identify personal biases, stereotypes, and beliefs that will prevent effective communication with patients, family, and co-workers. Taking steps to overcome these negative beliefs will help healthcare professionals show respect for and maintain the dignity (DIG ni tee) of others (Box 17.1).

VOCABULARY

dignity The inherent worth or state of being worthy of respect.
poised Having a composed and self-assured manner.
respect Showing consideration or appreciation for another person.

BOX 17.1   Demonstrating Respect

Healthcare professionals need to show respect to others. This can be achieved with a smile, a pleasant greeting, and appropriate eye contact, if appropriate, when first meeting the person. During the interaction, it is important to be courteous, sincere, polite, welcoming, and professional. Using a calm tone of voice, appropriate eye contact, and proper grammar without slang or generational terms also shows respect.

Being respectful also means maintaining the person's dignity, or in other words, treating others as we would want to be treated. People expect to be treated as individuals who matter. By treating others as though they matter, you are also showing them the respect they deserve.

NONVERBAL COMMUNICATION

As mentioned in the opening section, communication occurs by what we say and how we say it. These two forms of communication—verbal and nonverbal—affect how the other person perceives the message. Experts agree that nonverbal communication greatly exceeds verbal communication. In other words, we communicate more by our body language and expressive behaviors than through our words.

Think of a time when you were talking with a person, and that person did something that left a greater impression on you than the verbal message did. Nonverbal communication is powerful. It is important that the verbal message matches the perceived nonverbal message.

With therapeutic communication, we use nonverbal communication to show respect, acceptance, and understanding. We want to appear positive and open with others. We can do this through our nonverbal communication, which involves nonverbal behaviors, communication delivery factors, our appearance, and respecting cultural differences and spatial distance.

Nonverbal Behavior

Our nonverbal behaviors can be judged by others as positive and open or negative and closed. When our behaviors are judged as negative and closed, they can be interpreted by others in ways we may not intend. Table 17.2 discusses positive and open behaviors that should be used by the medical assistant. It also describes common interpretations of negative and closed behavior. Box 17.2 discusses the importance of nonverbal communication while wearing a mask.

CRITICAL THINKING 17.1

Think about your nonverbal behaviors. If you are wearing a mask, how can a person tell you are smiling?

Communication Delivery Factors

Communication delivery factors relate to how we deliver our verbal message. For instance, do we speak fast, using a high-pitched, loud voice as we deliver our verbal message? The communication delivery factors used help create the context of the message. Table 17.3 provides a list of delivery factors and the

TABLE 17.2 Positive and Negative Nonverbal Behaviors

Nonverbal Behaviors	Positive and Open	Negative and Closed (Common interpretations)
Position	Be at the level of the other person, angled toward the other person	Being at a higher level (looking down on the person); leaning backward (disinterest); direct face to face (confrontational, intimate)
Arms, shoulders, and hands	Arms at the sides, shoulders relaxed	Arms are crossed in front of the body (discomfort, defensive, disagree); hands behind back (secretive, mistrustful); clenched fists (anger, aggressive); pointing at a person (accusatory). Hands on hips (ready for aggressive activity); hands in the pockets (insecurity and lack of confidence)
Posture	Poised	Poor or slumped posture (poor self-worth, lack of confidence, unwillingness, lack of interest, less knowledgeable, unreliable); stiff, immobile (uncomfortable)
Facial expression	Smile	Rolling eyes, yawning (boredom); frowning (sadness, disagree, anger)
Gestures	Small gestures	Overuse of hands (nervousness, excitement)
Touch	Light touch on hand, appropriate touch	Inappropriate touching or hugging (makes the person feel uncomfortable or violated)
Eye contact	Movement of eyes, blinking	Staring at the person (makes it awkward); avoiding eye contact (low self-esteem, low confidence, and dishonesty)
Eyebrows	Raised eyebrows indicate surprise and openness	Lowered eyebrows (displeasure); one raised eyebrow (cynicism or doubtful)
Mannerisms	Focus on the person, nod when appropriate to acknowledge the patient	Fidgeting (nervous, impatient); looking at a watch, phone, or clock (bored, anxious, impatient)

BOX 17.2 Nonverbal Communication When Wearing a Mask

A genuine smile can make others smile. Research as shown that when people are shown a smile and told to frown, they smile instead. Many times, our first message to a person is a smile. A smile is a greeting and a way to acknowledge another person. We smile to be polite and to appear approachable.

When we need to wear a mask, our smiles are covered. With our facial expressions limited, our eyes and body language must deliver the message that our smile would give. We need to ensure that our nonverbal behaviors are positive and open.

professional expectations for which medical assistants should strive.

CRITICAL THINKING 17.2

While working at the reception desk, Christi needs to demonstrate positive and open nonverbal behaviors. Describe the positive and open nonverbal behaviors she should be demonstrating.

Our Appearance

How we dress can send a message to others. For instance, a medical assistant who has a dirty uniform and messy hair may send a negative message to others. Chapter 16 discussed the importance of a professional appearance for medical assistants.

Respecting Cultural Differences

The meaning of nonverbal behaviors can greatly vary among cultural groups. What is acceptable to one group may be considered offensive to others. As you work with patients from diverse groups, make sure to learn cultural differences in communication. It will reduce the likelihood of offending the other person. It also will help make the patient's experience a positive one. Table 17.4 provides some examples of cultural differences with nonverbal behaviors.

If you are interacting with a person from another cultural group and you are unfamiliar with it, try following these tips:

- Follow the other person's lead in terms of nonverbal behaviors and personal space.
- Use gestures cautiously. Do not point with one finger (Fig. 17.2).
- Refrain from touching a child's head.
- Remember that facial expressions can be misinterpreted (e.g., grimacing with pain may not be acceptable in some cultures, whereas other cultures "encourage" it).
- Lack of eye contact may be related to nervousness or the culture. It is not due to fear or dishonesty.

CRITICAL THINKING 17.3

Christi had heard that people from the Hmong and Vietnamese cultures do not like others commenting on their children. They fear the words might be overheard by a spirit who might try to harm the children. Christi mentions this to a co-worker. The co-worker does not believe in this. Do they need to worry about this belief when working with patients from the Hmong and Vietnamese culture? Explain your answer.

Respecting Spatial Distance

Spatial distance, or the space between one person and another, is also considered to be part of nonverbal communication. The distance between ourselves and another person can vary based on our familiarity with that person. There are different types of spaces, including:

TABLE 17.3   Nonverbal Communication Delivery Factors

Nonverbal Delivery Factors	Definition	Professional Expectations
Rate	Refers to the speed at which the speaker talks	Use a moderate rate. If the rate is too fast, the message may be missed. If the rate is too slow, it may be perceived as more negative by the receiver.
Clarity	Refers to the quality of the voice	Use a clear voice when talking with others. Muffled, mumbling, or unclear speech can create inaccuracies with the message.
Volume	Refers to the loudness of the speaker's voice	Use a moderate volume. If too loud, it may be perceived as yelling, and if too soft, the message may be missed. In healthcare, we need to keep information confidential. So, using a loud voice can violate the patient's privacy.
Pitch	Refers to the highness and lowness of the voice	Using a varying pitch, or *inflections*, helps a person to emphasize important points. It is important to have a rhythm in your voice to help the receiver understand what is important.
Tone	Refers to the emotion in the voice	Use an accepting or a neutral tone in healthcare. An angry tone can cause the receiver to misinterpret the message and/or also become angry.
Pauses	Refers to a period of not talking	Using pauses helps the receiver absorb the message. Limit verbalized pauses (e.g., "ah," "umm," and "er").
Intonation	Refers to the melodic pattern or the pitch variation	With statements, we usually use a medium intonation and finish the sentence on a lower pitch. Finishing the statement on a higher pitch usually indicates a question. Using correct intonation will help the correct message to be received.
Vocabulary	Refers to the word choice used	Using precise words helps the message to be correctly received. Incorrect use of words may create a negative impression of the speaker. It is important to use words that the receiver understands. If medical terminology, slang, or generational terms are used, the message may not be understood.
Grammatical structure	Refers to the sentence structure	Using incorrect grammatical sentence structure can create a negative impression of the speaker.
Pronunciation	Refers to how the word is said	Using the correct pronunciation will help ensure the correct message will be received. Incorrect pronunciation of a word (e.g., medication name) may lead to inaccuracies with the message.

TABLE 17.4   Cultural Differences in Nonverbal Behaviors

Nonverbal Behaviors	Cultural Differences
Eye contact	*Hispanics, Asians, Native Americans, and Middle Easterners:* Eye contact is considered rude and offensive. *Females:* May avoid eye contact with males so it is not perceived as a sign of sexual interest.
Touch	*Asians and Middle Easterners:* The head is a sacred part of the body; it is considered offensive to pat the head. *Middle Easterners:* Left hand is reserved for bodily hygiene; it is inappropriate to use that hand to touch others or transfer objects. *Muslims:* Inappropriate to touch a person of the opposite gender. *Latin Americans and Eastern Europeans:* Very comfortable with touching others, even new acquaintances.
Gestures	*Many cultures:* Using the "come here" finger/hand gesture is used with dogs and considered offensive. Pointing with one finger is considered very rude. *Asians and Indians:* Use the whole hand to point at something or someone. *Venezuelans:* Use their lips to point; finger pointing is impolite.
Winking	*Latin Americans:* Consider winking a romantic or a sexual invitation. *Nigerians:* Wink at children to indicate they should leave the room. *Chinese:* Consider winking rude.
Posture	*Many cultures:* Consider poor posture disrespectful.
Personal space	*Latin Americans and Middle Easterners:* Stand quite close to those they do not know. *Muslim males (even providers):* Cannot be too close to females.

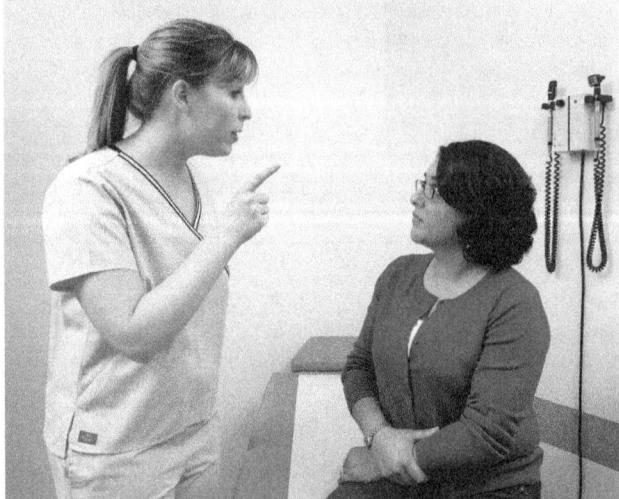

Fig. 17.2 Pointing often is an accusatory gesture and causes discomfort. (From Niedzwiecki B, et al: *Kinn's the medical assistant*, ed 14, St. Louis, 2020, Elsevier.)

- *Intimate space* or *personal space* (distance of 0 to 1.5 feet): In our personal lives, we allow close family and friends into this space. In healthcare medical assistants are in the patients' personal space for procedures such as electrocardiograms, wound care, and obtaining vital signs.
- *Casual person space* (distance of 1.5 feet to 4 feet): In our personal lives, this space is used for conversations with friends. In healthcare, the medical assistant uses this space when talking with the patient. This may include taking a medical history or coaching a patient on home care.

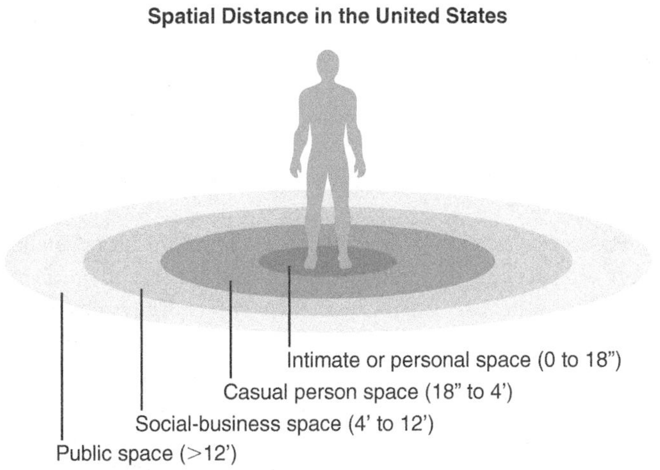

Spatial Distance in the United States

Intimate or personal space (0 to 18")
Casual person space (18" to 4')
Social-business space (4' to 12')
Public space (>12')

Fig. 17.3 Spatial Distance. (From Niedzwiecki B, et al: *Kinn's the medical assistant*, ed 14, St. Louis, 2020, Elsevier.)

BOX 17.3 Reading Others' Nonverbal Communication

Besides using nonverbal communication to convey acceptance and respect, we also read others' nonverbal communication. This provides us feedback on what is being said and how the person feels. The following are examples of how nonverbal behaviors are interpreted.

- *Self-confident*: The person appears confident and self-assured, has good posture, and makes appropriate eye contact.
- *Insecure*: The person is quiet, courteous, and has good listening skills, but tends to focus more on others than on oneself.
- *Arrogant*: The person has increased personal space, appears to bore easily, and is a poor listener.
- *Embarrassed*: The person has a nervous giggle and tends to avoid eye contact with others.
- *Fearful*: The person has wide-open eyes, looks around, grasps their hands, and has a rigid posture.
- *Resentful*: The person hunches the shoulders, crosses the arms, and mutters or whispers.

- *Social-business space* (distance of 4 to 12 feet): In our personal lives, this is the acceptable space for business transactions and socializing with acquaintances. In healthcare, the medical assistant uses this space when completing business tasks, such as answering billing questions and checking in a patient at the reception desk.
- *Public space* (distance greater than 12 feet): In our personal lives, this space is used for activities in public. In healthcare, this is the acceptable space with group events (Fig. 17.3).

Research has shown that some cultural groups have different acceptable casual person space. For instance, Middle Eastern cultures have about 1 foot, whereas North American and Western European cultures have about 1.5 feet. The Japanese culture has about 3 feet. You may have already experienced this when you were talking with friends. Some friends get closer to you than others. When a person is closer to us than we feel is acceptable for our culture, we may become uncomfortable.

We all have a personal space, or "bubble," around us. We may be uncomfortable and on guard if someone we do not know well gets into our personal space. We may take a step back or move back in a chair to increase the space between us and the other person. If someone is communicating from too far away, we may also feel uncomfortable.

It is important to realize that as healthcare professionals, we move into the personal or intimate space of patients many times while providing care. We need to respect this space. We need to be aware of our grooming, our appearance, and our habits. When working with others, we need to watch for clues regarding the person's comfort level with distance. A person who needs more space may move backward. Leaning, shifting, or moving forward shows the person wants to reduce the distance. It is important to recognize this nonverbal communication (Box 17.3).

CRITICAL THINKING 17.4

Think about the diverse cultures in your area. What differences have you observed in the nonverbal communication between these groups?

VERBAL COMMUNICATION

Verbal communication can be defined as words used either orally or in written form. Medical assistants use verbal communication all the time. This section will examine the communication process and then discuss the two forms of verbal communication, written communication and oral communication.

Communication Cycle

The *communication cycle* is a way to describe the sender-receiver process. A breakdown of any part of the cycle can lead to a message being misunderstood. The communication cycle proceeds as follows:

1. Sender creates the MESSAGE: The person with a message is called the *sender*. The sender must organize their thoughts and communicate a clear, concise, easy to understand message.
2. Receiver DECODES the message: The person getting the message is the *receiver*. This person must decode or translate the message based on personal factors and subjective perceptions. If the message was correctly translated within the context of the message sent, then it matches the message the sender sent. If the message was incorrectly translated, then the receiver develops a different perception of the message than what the sender intended.
3. Receiver creates FEEDBACK: The receiver then provides feedback based on the perceived message.
4. Sender DECODES feedback: The sender gets the feedback message. Again, the feedback must be decoded correctly for the communication to be accurate (Fig. 17.4).

As indicated in Fig. 17.4, the verbal communication cycle exists with written and oral messages. We will examine both types of verbal communication.

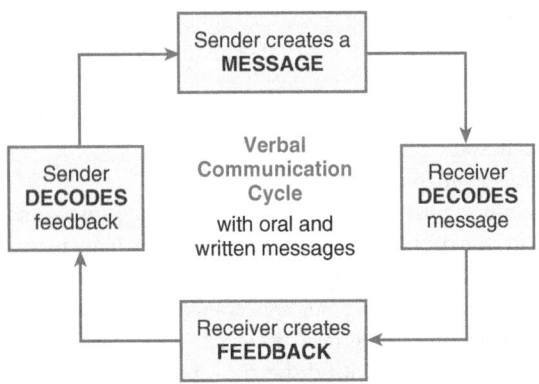

Fig. 17.4 Verbal Communication Cycle.

BOX 17.4   Tips for Composing Written Communication

All Forms of Written Communication
- Draft the message and then read what you have written. Make sure the message is clear, concise, easy to understand, and provides the message you intended.
- Check the grammar, spelling, capitalization, punctuation, and sentence structure.
- Make sure to address the message to the correct receiver.

Professional Emails
- Add a few meaningful words in the subject line.
- Start with a courteous greeting.
- Write out all words. Do not use slang and use acronyms only when necessary.
- Write in complete sentences. Capitalize the first letter of the first word and end the statement with the correct punctuation.
- Do not use all-capital letters. It is viewed as shouting at the receiver.

Written Communication

Written communication is a type of verbal communication in which we create written messages for the receiver. Written communication includes:
- Written messages (e.g., written phone messages and texts)
- Letters and emails
- Online information and media (e.g., informational flyers)

It is important that we consider how we state our written message. We want the receiver to get the message we intended on sending. Box 17.4 provides tips for composing written communication. Chapter 25 provides additional information on composing professional letters and emails.

Oral Communication

Oral communication is a type of verbal communication in which we talk with others and we listen to others. In the ambulatory care environment, oral communication occurs in person, over the phone, and using remote devices (e.g., webcams).

Styles of Oral Communication. Besides the types of communication, we need to discuss the styles of communication. How a person communicates affects their interaction with another person. There are five main styles of communication: passive, aggressive, passive-aggressive, manipulative, and assertive.

It is important that healthcare professionals understand each type. We should also evaluate our own communication style. You should ask yourself, what style do you use? Identifying how you communicate is an important part of your professionalism journey.

Passive Communication. Passive communicators avoid expressing feelings or opinions. They fail to exert themselves and allow others to infringe on their rights. They may have a "victim mentality." They may feel depressed, resentful, or anxious because life seems out of their control.

Passive communicators may use these nonverbal communication behaviors:
- Speaking in a soft voice with their head down and no eye contact
- Fidgeting and hesitating
- Being self-conscious and belittling their contribution

Others may feel exasperated and frustrated with passive communicators. They may also feel that they can take advantage of the person.

When dealing with passive communicators, be assertive. Use a firm approach. Medical assistants must also ensure they take the time to reassure the person and welcome their suggestions and contributions.

Aggressive Communication. Aggressive communicators try to dominate others. They have low frustration tolerance, and they criticize and attack others. Aggressive communicators have poor listening skills and use "you" statements. This can cause them to be alienated from or feared by others.

Aggressive communicators may use these nonverbal communication behaviors:
- Speaking in a low voice
- Using big, sharp, and fast gestures
- Glaring and frowning
- Invading others' personal space intentionally

Others may feel hurt, fearful, afraid, humiliated, and resentful with aggressive communicators. They may lose respect for the person.

When dealing with aggressive communicators, never become aggressive and always remain calm. Do not take the person's aggression personally. Attempt to see their point of view, which will help you communicate yours.

Passive-Aggressive Communication. Passive-aggressive communicators deny problems. They do not confront problems or people. Passive-aggressive communicators appear to be cooperative but plan subtle sabotage or disruptions. They may become alienated from others and feel powerless.

Passive-aggressive communicators may use these nonverbal communication behaviors:
- Speaking in a sugary sweet voice
- Looking sweet and innocent
- Moving into others' personal space and touching others to pretend to be warm and friendly

Others may feel confused, angry, and hurt by the "two-faced" personality of the person.

When dealing with passive-aggressive communicators, try to refrain from drawing negative conclusions immediately. Medical assistants can use various ways to handle this approach, based on the situation. Some approaches include using humor and trying to have a positive discussion.

Manipulative Communication. Manipulative communicators are cunning and try to control others. They use others to get what they want. Manipulative communicators create situations in which others feel sorry for them or guilty.

Manipulative communicators may use these nonverbal communication behaviors:

- Speaking in a high-pitched voice
- Being demeaning or condescending when talking with others

Others may feel angry, resentful, guilty, and frustrated with being manipulated.

When dealing with manipulative communicators, avoid being manipulated. Respectfully maintain your position.

Assertive Communication. Assertive communicators clearly state their needs and wants. They use "I" statements and listen without interrupting. They are relaxed, use good eye contact, feel connected with others, and stand up for their rights. Assertive communicators feel in control of their lives and are mature enough to address issues.

Assertive communicators may use these nonverbal communication behaviors:

- Speaking using a medium pitch, speed, and volume of voice
- Having good eye contact (when appropriate)
- Using positive and open nonverbal behaviors
- Being respectful of others

Others feel that they can trust the individual.

When dealing with assertive communicators, know the person can handle criticism and accept compliments. A healthcare professional needs to communicate in an assertive manner. This is the healthy form of communication. It leads to better team dynamics.

CRITICAL THINKING 17.5

Think of the circle of people with whom you interact. What type of communicators are they? How do they make you feel when you communicate with them? What would be the best way to communicate with them?

Therapeutic Communication

As mentioned before, therapeutic communication is a process of communicating with patients and family members in healthcare. It is an interactive relationship that conveys acceptance and respect without judgment or blame. It encourages healthcare professionals to build rapport with patients. When that bond develops and grows, patients are more comfortable with expressing their feelings, ideas, and concerns. Thus therapeutic communication techniques are helpful in building the relationship with the patient. Active listening and other therapeutic communication techniques will be described in the following sections.

Active Listening. Active listening is the most important therapeutic communication technique. This skill takes time to master. Active listening means we fully concentrate on what is being said and how it is said. This is different from passively hearing what the speaker is saying and being distracted by our own thoughts.

When a person is actively listening, the speaker can easily see it. The listener shows interest by verbal messages, such as "Yes." The listener also shows interest through nonverbal messages. As discussed earlier, nonverbal messages include eye contact, nodding your head, body position, touch, and facial expressions. Characteristics of a good listener include:

- Remaining nonjudgmental and neutral
- Refraining from interrupting with a comment or question
- Allowing for periods of silence
- Smiling and nodding your head to show you are listening to the message
- Using appropriate eye contact so the speaker is not intimidated
- Leaning slightly forward or sideways toward the speaker
- Avoiding distractions (e.g., fidgeting, looking at the clock, doodling) (Box 17.5)

Showing interest at this level will encourage the speaker to be more at ease (Fig. 17.5). Communication between the two people will be more open, honest, and clear.

Open-Ended and Closed Questions or Statements. When you gather information from a patient, it is helpful to use a combination of open-ended and closed questions or statements. An open-ended question or statement asks for general information or states the topic to be discussed, but only in general terms. Use this communication tool to begin a conversation with a patient, to introduce a new section of questions, or whenever the person introduces a new topic. It is a very effective method of gathering more details from the patient about their problem. Examples of open-ended questions include:

- "What is the reason for your appointment with Dr. Walden?"

BOX 17.5   Nontherapeutic Techniques

The following are examples of nontherapeutic techniques that must be avoided when communicating with patients.

- Overloading the patient with questions. Allow them to answer a question before asking another question.
- Judging the patient's words or actions.
- Being unresponsive to the patient's cues or failing to give feedback to the patient. Make sure to respond to a patient if they are talking with you. Never turn your back and walk away when they are talking with you.
- Making false reassurance and promises, such as "The provider will make you better" or "It's going to be okay." Such statements can give the patient false hope and in some cases it could cause legal issues.
- Not focusing on the patient.
- Giving advice, such as "If I were you…" or "I would do…" Giving advice regarding treatments can also cause legal issues in some causes.
- Laughing nervously or at inappropriate times.
- Arguing with the patient or family members.

- "How have you been getting along?"
- "You mentioned having problems with your insurance. Can you tell me more about that?"

This type of question or statement encourages patients to respond in a manner they find comfortable. It allows patients to express themselves fully and provide comprehensive information about their chief complaint.

Closed (also called *direct*) questions ask for specific information. In many cases, this form of questioning limits the patient's answer to one or two words, including yes and no. Use this form of question when you need confirmation of specific facts, such as when asking about demographic information. Examples of closed questions include:

- "What is the name of your insurance carrier?"
- "What is your birth date?"
- "Do you want your prescription sent to the clinic pharmacy?"

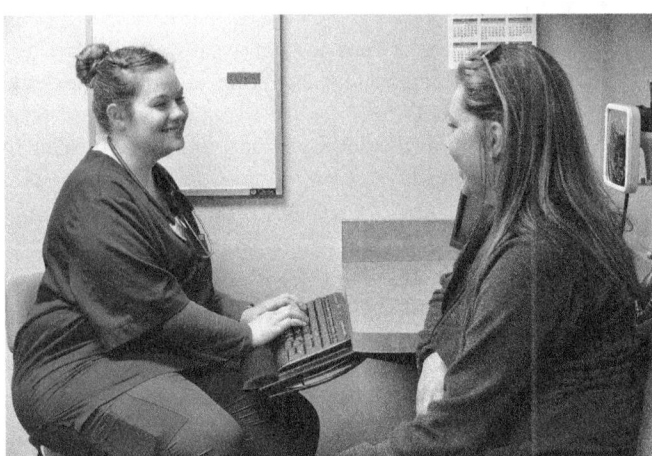

Fig. 17.5 Nonverbal communication (e.g., eye contact and a smile) is important when working with patients. (From Proctor D, Niedzwiecki B: *Kinn's the medical assistant*, ed 13, St. Louis, 2017, Elsevier.)

Other Therapeutic Communication Techniques. When you are working with patients and family members, several therapeutic communication techniques can be used. We need to make sure patients know we are listening. We also need to check that we understand the message correctly. Assuming what someone means or feels can lead to misunderstanding. Therapeutic communication techniques are detailed in Table 17.5.

Procedures 17.1 through 17.4, at the end of the chapter, provide examples of role-playing to practice communicating with patients.

> **VOCABULARY**
> **empathy** The ability to understand another's perspective, experiences, or motivations.
> **rapport** A relationship of harmony and accord between the patient and the healthcare professional.

BARRIERS TO EFFECTIVE COMMUNICATION

Effective communication is critical for compassionate, quality patient care. Medical assistants must understand barriers that prevent patients from understanding communication or communicating clearly with others (Box 17.6). Taking steps to overcome these barriers will help promote effective communication. Table 17.6 discusses common barriers and ways to overcome barriers. The following sections will provide additional information on communication barriers related to speech disorders, anger, age, and disease status.

Speech Disorders

Speech disorders can be caused by damage to the vocal cords, brain, tongue, and mouth. Conditions that can cause speech disorders include cancer (oral, laryngeal), amyotrophic lateral sclerosis (ALS), stroke, dementia, Huntington disease, attention deficit hyperactivity disorder (ADHD), autism, and traumatic brain injury.

TABLE 17.5	**Therapeutic Communication Techniques**	
Technique	**Definition**	**Feedback to the Speaker**
Clarification	Allows the listener to get additional information by explaining a specific statement or topic.	Use statements such as, "Can you clarify..." and "Do you mean..."
Exploring	Allows the listener to get additional information about a certain topic.	Use a phrase such as, "Tell me more about..."
General leads	Allows the listener to get additional information and prompts the speaker.	Use a phrase such as, "You were saying..."
Neutral	Encourages the speaker to continue and conveys you are interested and listening to the message.	Use phrases such as, "Uh huh," "I see," and "That is very interesting."
Reflection	Putting words to the person's emotional reaction, which acknowledges the person's feelings. Also helps to check what the person is feeling instead of just assuming. Shows empathy (EM pah thee) and helps build rapport (ra PORE).	Reflect what you think was said. For example: "It sounds like you are feeling scared..." or "I understand you are having trouble with..." or "You feel that..."
Restating or paraphrasing	Rewording or rephrasing a statement to check the meaning and interpretation. Also shows you are listening and understanding the speaker.	Do not repeat the person's exact words. Use phrases such as, "What I'm hearing is..." or "It sounds like you are saying..." Refrain from using "I know what you mean."
Silence	Allows time to gather thoughts and answer questions.	Can be uncomfortable to some people. Allows time to think about what was said.
Summarizing	Allows the listener to recap and review what was said.	Using a statement such as, "If I understand how you feel about this situation..."

Common speech disorders include:

- *Aphasia*, being unable to understand what is being said or to use the right words to express thoughts
- *Apraxia of speech*, difficulty coordinating mouth movements for speech
- *Dysarthria*, slurred speech
- *Cognitive-communication disorder*, which includes issues such as memory, attention, organization, processing speed, and problem solving

Depending on the speech disorder, the medical assistant may need to speak more slowly. In all cases, it is important to give the patient extra time to answer. Do not pressure the patient or overload the patient with questions.

Anger

As discussed in Table 17.6, anger is a barrier to communication. Medical assistants can encounter angry patients, family members, or co-workers (Fig. 17.6). It is critical to know how to handle and defuse the situation. It is important for the person to feel heard and for the medical assistant to remain safe and follow through on any promises made.

If the angry person is in a public area and the medical assistant feels safe, the person should be invited to a more private location. It is important to allow the person to talk out their anger. The medical assistant should present a calm attitude, speak in a low tone of voice, and take notes if needed. The medical assistant should demonstrate empathy by using active listening skills and therapeutic communication techniques (Box 17.7). If the medical assistant responds in anger or becomes argumentative, the situation will intensify, and the person's anger may increase.

BOX 17.6 Oral Communication When Wearing a Mask

Wearing masks can make communication more challenging for people who have speech or hearing impairments. Masks can muffle sounds, prevent lip reading, and cover many facial expressions. When wearing a mask in the healthcare setting, it is important to:

- Make sure to face the person with whom you are speaking. Make sure nothing is blocking your view.
- Speak a little louder and a little more slowly.
- Make sure your verbal message matches your body language.
- Ask the person if they understood you. If the person is struggling to understand you, write down the information or say the information in a different way.
- Know what the facility's policy is for working with people who lip-read. Are you able to remove your mask when you communicate with the person?

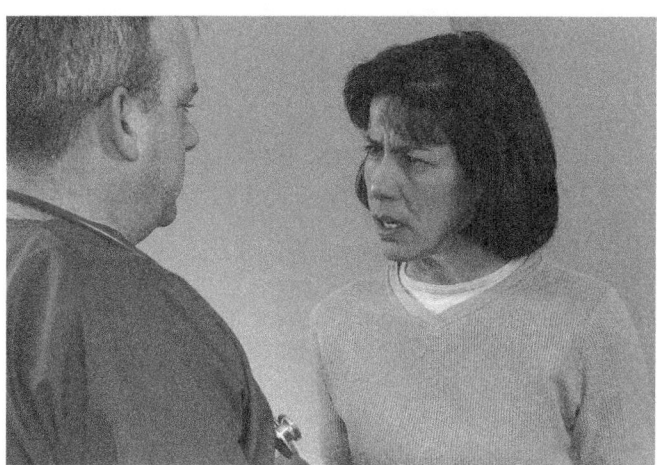

Fig. 17.6 Remain calm, even if a patient becomes verbally aggressive. Attempt to calm the person by listening and expressing empathy whenever possible. (From Proctor D, Niedzwiecki B: *Kinn's the medical assistant*, ed 13, St. Louis, 2017, Elsevier.)

TABLE 17.6 Barriers to Communication and Ways to Overcome Barriers

Type of Barrier	Patient Barriers	Ways to Overcome Barriers
Environmental distractions	Noise, lack of privacy, temperature	Provide privacy for patients. Talk with patients in a quiet room with the door closed. Make sure the room temperature is comfortable.
Internal distractions	Hunger, pain, anger, tiredness	Help make the patient comfortable. Provide food and drink if available. Administer pain medications as ordered.
Visually impaired	Unable to see written communication	Use audio recordings, screen magnifiers, large-print materials, and screen reader software.
Hearing impaired	Unable to hear verbal communication	Use print materials and written instructions. Use videos with captions. Have text telephones (TTYs) available. Use a sign language interpreter.
Intellectual disability	Unable to understand what is being said, may be functioning at a lower age level	Use "functioning age" – appropriate language and materials. Provide information also to the guardian/caregiver.
Speech disorders	Difficulty speaking or finding the right word	Give the patient time and do not rush the patient.
Illiterate	Unable to read or write	Use pictures and models. Draw pictures and use simple language.
Non-English speaking	English is not the patient's primary language; lack of understanding of medical terminology	Use interpreters and translated materials. Limit medical terminology and define medical terms that must be used. Use culturally appropriate materials and visuals (pictures, graphs, and models).
Emotional distractions (angry, distraught, anxious)	Fear and anxiety related to being judged by the healthcare professional; inability to explain personal feelings; angry or distraught patients may not hear what is said or may not be able to communicate effectively	Provide a warm, caring environment. Make sure your body language (nonverbal behaviors) is consistent with having an open, caring manner. Gain the person's trust. Keep your voice at a normal level; raising your voice can increase the person's anger.

BOX 17.7   Empathy

Healthcare professionals who are empathetic provide better patient care. Showing patients respect and dignity through empathetic care builds trust with patients, which increases their satisfaction and adherence to the treatment plan. It is critical when providing patient-centered care. Without empathy, the patients may remain anxious, feel disconnected with their care, lose trust in their healthcare team, and may have less positive health outcomes. Strategies to provide empathetic care include:

- Making sure to listen to your patient and understanding their experiences, perspective, and concerns.
- Using positive nonverbal behaviors. For instance, position yourself at the same level as the patient. Make appropriate eye contact. Nod your head and lean in as you communicate with the patient.
- Using therapeutic communication techniques (e.g., reflection, paraphrasing, and clarification) as you interact with the patient. Show your support.
- Interpreting the patient's nonverbal behaviors and clarifying any messages that differ with the verbal message received.
- Being welcoming and showing your patients dignity and respect.

During the interaction with the angry person, the medical assistant must remain safe. There should be a policy in place for dealing with angry individuals. Policies should include the following guidelines:

- Notify the facility's administrator of all difficult patients or ask for help from co-workers.
- Keep yourself at a distance from the person (e.g., try to separate yourself from the person by a desk or another piece of furniture).
- If you are in a room with the angry person, position yourself so you are the closest person to the door.
- Have another employee remain close by.
- Know under what circumstances you should contact the police or building security for assistance.

VOCABULARY
adherence The act of sticking to something.

Developmental Stage

A person's developmental stage may be a barrier to communication. Communicating with a 3-year-old child is different from communicating with an 80-year-old adult. A medical assistant must understand developmental stages to know how to interact with people of different ages. Piaget's Cognitive Development Stages provides information on a child's developmental stage. If a medical assistant does not consider a person's developmental stage when communicating, a barrier can occur. Piaget's developmental stages include:

- *Sensory Motor* (age 0-2 years): Unable to process medical information.
- *Preoperational* (age 2-7 years): Does not comprehend cause and effect or the impact in the future. Children in this stage do not understand how their actions affect their health.
- *Concrete operations* (age 7-11 years): Children in this stage can begin to understand healthcare information, such as disease. They understand concrete examples versus hypothetical situations.
- *Formal operations* (12 years and older): Children in this stage can understand illness, how it occurs, and how they can control it. Typically, they understand messages at the same level as adults. Children in this stage are capable of logical reasoning.

Besides Piaget's stages, Erikson's stages are also important to understand.

Erik Erikson, a psychoanalyst, described the emotional, physical, and psychological stages of human development. He stated

TABLE 17.7   Erikson's Stages of Psychosocial Development

Developmental Stage	Age Range	Goals of Stage	Communication Tips
Trust versus Mistrust	Infancy: 0–1.5 years old	Must develop trust, with the ability to mistrust should the need arise.	Use calm, soothing voice, hold child securely. Loud voices and noises can startle the child.
Autonomy versus Shame and Doubt	Toddler: 1.5–3 years old	Must explore and manipulate things in their "world" to develop autonomy and self-esteem.	Use simple language. Allow the child to touch and explore objects. Allow the child to play and make choices.
Initiative versus Guilt	Preschooler: 3–6 years old	Encouraged to try new activities. Must assume responsibilities and learn new skills. Will make the child feel purposeful and increase self-esteem.	Use short, simple sentences. Encourage questions. Use imitation, play, and role-playing.
Industry versus Inferiority	School age: 6–12 years old	Must seek to finish tasks. Recognition for accomplishments is important.	Use engaging simple tools to communicate information (videos, gaming software, pamphlets). Encourage discussion and questions.
Identity versus Role Confusion	Adolescence: 12–18 years old	To know who you are as a person and how you fit into the world around you. Creates a meaningful self-image.	Provide privacy and independence. Encourage responsible decision making. Encourage discussion and questions.
Intimacy versus Isolation	Young adult: 18–25 years old	Can vary. Develops friendships; takes on commitments.	Identify motivating factors and use them as needed during communication. Realize person may be juggling a lot of obligations.
Generativity versus Stagnation	Middle adulthood: 25–60 years old	Achieve a balance between the concern for the next generation (having a family) and being self-absorbed.	
Ego Integrity versus Despair	Late adulthood: 60 years and older	Reflect on one's life and come to terms with it, instead of regretting the past.	Communicate with dignity and respect. Limit slang and "generational" terms. Use simpler language. Speak clearly. Allow the patient time to respond.

that a person in each stage had a specific developmental task to complete. Understanding the task or goal of each stage helps healthcare professionals communicate more effectively with patients. Table 17.7 presents the developmental stages, goals of each stage, and communication tips for healthcare professionals.

When medical assistants work with aging patients, it is important to keep the following suggestions in mind for effective communication.

- Address the patient by Mr., Mrs., Ms., or Miss unless the patient has given you permission to use their first name.
- Introduce yourself and explain the purpose of a procedure before performing it.
- Face the aging person and softly touch the individual to get their attention before beginning to speak.
- Use expanded speech by lowering the pitch or tone of your voice and speaking firmly, making sure to enunciate each word clearly.
- Use gestures and demonstrations to clarify communication.
- Print out instructions in block print using a larger font size to be sure aging individuals can read the information.
- If the message must be repeated, paraphrase or find other words to say the same thing.
- Observe the patient's nonverbal behavior for cues indicating whether the person understands.
- Provide adequate lighting without glare.
- Allow patients time to process information and take care of themselves unless they ask for assistance.
- Conduct communication in a quiet room without distractions.
- Involve family members as needed for continuity of care.
- When leaving a telephone message, remember to speak slowly and clearly and repeat the message in the same manner. It is difficult to interpret a message, and even more difficult to write it down, if the message was delivered in a hurried manner.
- Use referrals and community resources for support.

CRITICAL THINKING 17.6

What communication tips should Christi use when communicating with:
- A 2-year-old child?
- A 13-year-old teen?
- A 30-year-old adult?
- An 80-year-old adult?

Disease Status

A person's disease status also can affect communication. For instance, think about these scenarios:

- Jim has just been notified by his provider that he may only have 3 months to live. Jim had been healthy until the past few weeks, when he started to feel very ill.
- Rose has just been informed that she has type 2 diabetes mellitus. She needs to take medication, change her diet, and exercise.

If you were Jim or Rose, how would you feel? Could you understand and remember a lot of new information after hearing the diagnosis? Could you even converse normally with others, or would you be "blown away"? Would you deny the diagnosis?

Elisabeth Kübler-Ross studied people's reactions to dying. She found that people experienced similar stages as they came to terms with the situation. Over the years, these stages have been applied to grief. They can relate to patients who are informed of a chronic or terminal illness. Family and friends of the ill person can also experience these stages. Not everyone progresses through the stages at the same time, nor does everyone get to the final stage. The stages of grief and dying include:

- *Denial.* The person refuses to accept the fact (e.g., diagnosis or prognosis). This is a defense mechanism that allows the person to ignore what is happening.
- *Anger.* This can be directed at oneself or others.
- *Bargaining.* The person attempts to bargain with the higher power the person believes in (e.g., God).
- *Depression.* The person feels sad, fearful, and uncertain. The person may not participate in normal activities and may distance oneself from others.
- *Acceptance.* The person has come to terms with the situation.

When you are communicating with those with a terminal or chronic illness, it is important to understand that they are working through these stages. Remember, the emotions they display may not be related to you. The emotions may be related to the grief with which they are dealing. For instance, a terminally ill patient yells at the receptionist. He is upset about his wait time, although it was under 5 minutes. His emotions may relate more to his stage of grieving than to his wait time. It is important that we provide a supportive, accepting environment. We should be empathetic to these patients.

COMMUNICATING IN THE WORKPLACE

Positive communication in the workplace is important. Keeping workplace relationships strong and healthy is an essential element of well-functioning teams. When working with other staff members and the manager, the medical assistant should practice these guidelines:

- Be a good listener.
- Remember to use open and positive nonverbal communication. Watch the nonverbal communication of others. Many times, you will be able to determine how they are feeling by their nonverbal communication.
- Be polite, respectful, and friendly. Have a flexible, open mind.
- Make sure your message is clear and concise.
- Be confident.
- Appropriately accept positive and negative feedback. Be able to give constructive feedback to others.

Speaking With Providers

Speaking with providers can be intimidating, especially for a new medical assistant graduate. If you need to talk with the provider about a patient issue, start by writing down the information. Read back the information and ensure you have all of the facts. Follow these guidelines:

- Make sure you are in an area where patients cannot overhear your conversation.
- Speak confidently, clearly, and concisely.
- Start with the patient's name and age if appropriate.
- Discuss the situation in an organized manner.

- If the situation is related to a series of events, start with what occurred first, then second, and so on.
- If the provider gives you information or an order, write it down. Then read it back to the provider to ensure it is correct.

PERSONAL AND PROFESSIONAL BOUNDARIES WITH COMMUNICATION

Personal boundaries (also called *self-boundaries*) are the limits that people use to protect themselves. These limits include mental, emotional, physical, and social factors. In healthcare, having personal boundaries protects the healthcare professional from getting too involved with a patient's life. Getting too close to patients and their families can blur the objectivity the healthcare professional needs to have to provide the best patient care. Thus personal boundaries also protect patients and their families (Procedure 17.5).

Professional boundaries are usually part of facility's policies and professional associations code of ethics. Professional boundaries include legal, ethical, and facility guidelines that protect patients and healthcare professionals. Using professional communication and only having a professional relationship will help establish and maintain professional boundaries.

Professional Communication

Have you ever talked to a person who shared too much personal information? How did you feel? How did that affect your relationship with the other person? As a healthcare professional, it is important to remember our personal boundaries with communication. When we are talking with family and friends, the topics of our conversations can vary greatly. We can discuss many different things. When we are in the healthcare environment, we need to remember that certain topics are inappropriate. Discussions regarding relationships, politics, religion, and other such topics are not appropriate for the workplace.

Besides what we talk about, we also need to consider the phrases or words we use. Many people swear or use words that are insulting or degrading to others. Some people routinely use religious names (e.g., God) when they are surprised or upset. For some people, religious names have sacred meaning. When you say these names in their presence, it can be offensive. We need to ensure our language is professional.

Professional Relationship

The relationship between the medical assistant and the patient needs to be professional. It cannot be a dual relationship, in which the medical assistant also becomes a friend to the patient. When working with patients, we need to keep our lives private. It is not appropriate for the medical assistant to:

- Share personal issues, struggles, life stories, or other personal intimate information
- Contact the patient outside of the work environment
- Befriend the patient on social media
- Engage in a flirty or romantic conversation or relationship with the patient
- Gossip and share what happened in the workplace with patients and others

These behaviors cross the line between a professional relationship and a personal relationship. It is important for medical assistants to keep a professional relationship with patients and their families.

Lastly, the medical assistant should remember spatial distancing. If a patient starts to back away, the medical assistant should clue into the action. The medical assistant maybe too close to the person, and the person may feel uncomfortable.

UNDERSTANDING BEHAVIOR

Throughout this chapter, we have discussed verbal and nonverbal communication. As healthcare professionals, it is important we understand why our patients and peers behave the way they do. Why do they make the choices they make? What is important to them? Many times, their behaviors relate to their needs, defense mechanisms, and coping mechanisms. By understanding these factors, we can interact more effectively with others.

VOCABULARY

coping mechanisms Behavioral and psychological strategies used to deal with or minimize stressful events.

defense mechanisms Unconscious mental processes that protect people from anxiety, loss, conflict, or shame.

Maslow's Hierarchy of Needs

In 1943 psychologist Abraham Maslow proposed a hierarchy (HIE era r kee) of needs. This is a motivational theory that depicts five levels of needs. Years later, he expanded the theory to include eight levels of needs. Maslow believed that our human needs can be categorized into these eight levels. Each level must be satisfied before we can move up to the next level. These levels are often depicted as a triangle (Fig. 17.7).

The "*Deficiency*" needs consist of the four bottom levels. They are considered the coping behaviors. We must fulfill these needs to cope with life and survival. We all have similar needs, but when they are not met, it motivates us to get them met. Fulfillment of these needs leads to instant short-term gratification. For example, when we are thirsty, we find water to drink. We are satisfied for the moment but will be thirsty a short time later.

The top four levels are "*Growth*" needs. These levels relate to making ourselves a better person or being all that we can be. Achieving these levels brings long-lasting happiness. The happiness is more meaningful than the gratification achieved from meeting the lower level needs.

The following are Maslow's eight needs, starting at the bottom and working toward.

1. *Physiologic needs*: These include air, food, drink, shelter, warmth, oxygen, sleep, and so on. We need these things to survive. For instance, when we are hungry, we look for food.
2. *Safety needs*: These include protection from the elements, security, law, order, stability, and so forth. These needs relate to keeping us safe and secure. Unmet safety needs can lead to fear, stress, and anxiety. Some examples of meeting safety needs include:
   - Staying in a job that one really dislikes for the security of the paycheck
   - Staying in an abusive relationship because it is familiar
   - Getting the brakes on your car fixed

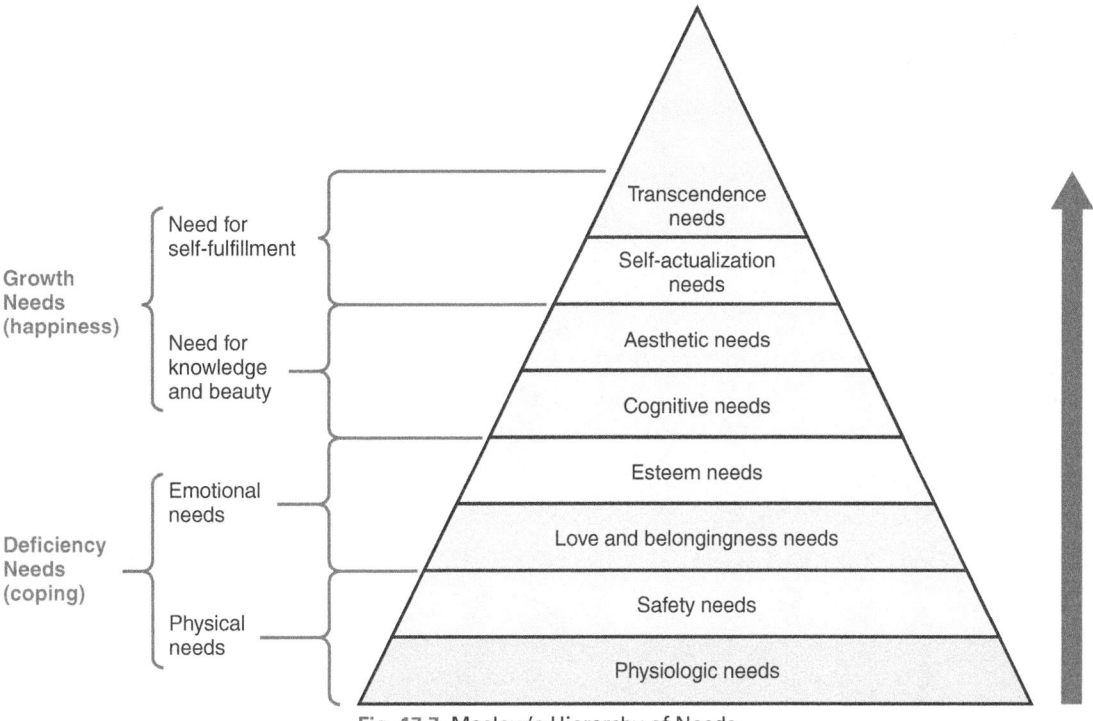

Fig. 17.7 Maslow's Hierarchy of Needs.

3. *Love and belongingness needs*: These include friendship, intimacy, acceptance in a group, and receiving and giving affection and love. We need to be accepted by others. Unmet needs in this level can lead to feelings of isolation, loneliness, and depression. A person may feel anxious about going out in social situations if this need is not met.
4. *Esteem needs*: These include our self-esteem, achievement, mastery of skills, independence, status, prestige, and so on. Our needs relate to our reputation and what we think of ourselves. It is important to remember the saying, "People who matter do not judge, people who judge do not matter." The only thing we have total control over is what we think of ourselves. Some examples of how people attempt to meet this level include:
   - Buying the latest electronic devices to "show off" to others
   - Fishing for compliments
   - Cutting down others to make oneself feel better
   - Focusing on the positives about oneself
   - Setting yourself a challenge and meeting it
5. *Cognitive needs*: These include knowledge, curiosity, understanding, and exploration. We are driven to learn more about something.
6. *Aesthetic needs*: We appreciate and search for beauty, balance, symmetry, form, and so on. Some people find true happiness when they create music, paint a picture, take a picture, or explore nature. Think of how relaxing it is to be at a beach, enjoying the sound of the water and the feeling of nature.
7. *Self-actualization needs*: We need to realize our potential, seek self-fulfillment, and experience personal growth.
8. *Transcendence needs*: We meet these by helping others achieve their very best, or self-actualization. This requires that we give of our time and talent to help others meet their needs.

Maslow believed that only a few people ever achieve the top levels of the hierarchy. He believed that when people did something bad (e.g., steal, put others down), they were motivated to meet their own needs. The method used to meet needs could be unhealthy or dysfunctional. It is important for medical assistants to realize that people meet their own needs in different ways. Their ways may be different and wrong by our standards. We still need to respect our patients and provide the best possible care.

A medical assistant can help patients meet their deficiency needs in the following ways:

- *Physiologic needs*: Provide community resources for basic needs.
- *Safety needs*: Provide domestic abuse hotline numbers and other community resources.
- *Love and belongingness needs*: Be positive and respectful. Have a caring manner when working with patients. Try to make a patient feel important.
- *Esteem needs*: Encourage independence and provide sincere compliments.

> **VOCABULARY**
> **hierarchy** Things arranged in order and rank.

Defense Mechanisms

Defense mechanisms are unconscious mental processes that protect people from anxiety, loss, conflict, or shame. We use defense mechanisms and so do our patients and peers. People use defense mechanisms to protect themselves from situations or information they cannot manage psychologically.

Defense mechanisms may hide a variety of thoughts or feelings, including anger, fear, sadness, despair, and

TABLE 17.8 Common Defense Mechanisms

Defense Mechanism	Description	Example
Denial	The person completely rejects the information.	"I couldn't possibly have kidney cancer. You must be mistaken."
Repression	The person simply forgets something that is bad or hurtful.	"I wasn't driving the car that killed my best friend."
Regression	The person reverts to an old, usually immature behavior to express their feelings.	Perhaps instead of discussing the diagnosis and the need for treatment, the person just storms out of the room and slams the door.
Displacement	The person transfers the emotion toward one person to another person or thing.	After being reprimanded by a supervisor, the person goes home and screams at the children.
Projection	The person accuses someone else of having the feelings that they have.	A patient is angry about the diagnosis. They may say, "You do not have to lose your temper about this," even though the medical assistant's demeanor is completely professional.
Suppression	The person is consciously aware of the information or feeling but refuses to admit it.	"I do not think the test is accurate. My ECGs are always normal."
Splitting	The person views another person as all bad or all good and not a mixture of good and bad traits.	An abused patient may say, "She is a good wife and mother."
Reaction formation	The person expresses feelings as the opposite of what the individual really feels.	A patient is angry at the medical assistant for insisting that a biopsy be scheduled. The person expresses the opposite emotion: "I appreciate your trying to help me, but I just can't come to the clinic that day."
Rationalization	The person comes up with various explanations to justify a response.	"I think the results are wrong. I didn't follow the directions for the tests like I should have, and besides, there's no history of leukemia in my family."

helplessness. Dealing with a patient who uses defense mechanisms can be very difficult. If medical assistants are aware of a patient's needs for psychological protection, they may be able to find a way to provide excellent care for the patient. There are many types of defense mechanisms. Table 17.8 describes several of the more common behaviors using patient and peer situations.

Coping Mechanisms

Stress is a condition that causes physical and/or emotional tension. Stress can be positive (e.g., learning a new job) or negative (e.g., dealing with a love one's terminal illness). We use coping mechanisms when we are stressed. Coping mechanisms are behavioral and psychological strategies used to deal with or minimize stressful events. Two types are adaptive and maladaptive coping mechanisms.

Adaptive or *healthy coping mechanisms* improve our functioning level and reduce our stress level. Examples of these adaptive coping mechanisms include:

- Eating healthy, well-balanced meals
- Exercising
- Drinking water
- Getting plenty of sleep
- Taking breaks when you feel stressed
- Talking and sharing with others
- Getting help when you need it

Maladaptive coping mechanism are also called *nonadaptive* or *unhealthy coping mechanisms*. They reduce the feelings

associated with stress for a short time. Maladaptive coping mechanisms do not decrease the actual stressor and can lead to future problems. Examples of maladaptive coping mechanisms include:

- Hostility, aggression, manipulation
- Recognition seeking
- Passive-aggressive behavior
- Compliance, dependence
- Social withdrawal, isolation
- Denial, fantasy
- Drugs and alcohol use
- Gambling, shopping, risk-taking behaviors

Understanding the different types of coping mechanisms is important in our own lives and in our role as a healthcare professional. We may have times when we are stressed and tend to use more maladaptive coping mechanisms. It is important for our health and well-being to use more adaptive strategies. Patients, family members, and co-workers are not immune to stress. They will also be using different coping mechanisms. Our role is to encourage the use of healthy coping mechanisms and provide resources for these strategies.

CRITICAL THINKING 17.7

Christi is starting to exercise after work each night. She has found that it helps her deal with the stress of the day. What coping mechanisms do you use when you are stressed? Are they adaptive or maladaptive coping mechanisms?

CLOSING COMMENTS

Overcoming communication barriers is more than just providing great patient care. Healthcare providers are legally required to provide ways to overcome communication barriers. This legal requirement comes from the following:

- *Civil Rights Act*: All providers who accept federal funds for the healthcare provided must ensure equal access to services.

- *Americans with Disabilities Act (ADA)*: All healthcare providers must provide free effective communication to patients (and companions) with disabilities.
- *Americans with Disabilities Act Amendments Act (ADAAA)*: Expanded the definition of disabilities established in the ADA.

Ways that providers can meet their federal obligations for accommodating patients with communication disabilities include:

- Providing informational and educational materials that have been translated into the primary languages of the patients seen in the ambulatory care facility.
- Providing large-print materials.
- Writing out instructions.
- Providing a qualified medical interpreter free of charge to the patient. This can be done by having an interpreter available to the patient or by using online interpretation services during the visit. The interpreter may be present for the visit, available over the phone, or via videoconferencing. Types of interpreters used in healthcare include:
  - o *Sign language interpreter*, who uses American Sign Language or Signed English.
  - o *Oral interpreter*, who silently mouths speech to the hearing-impaired patient and uses gestures.
  - o *Cued-speech interpreter*, who does the same as an oral interpreter but also uses a hand code to stand for each speech sound.
  - o *Qualified medical interpreter*, who interprets between the healthcare provider and the non-English-speaking or limited English-speaking patient. (Using a family member to interpret can be risky because the message may be changed. There is no guarantee the family member is translating exactly what the provider states.)

PATIENT-CENTERED CARE

Patient-centered care is focused on creating a relationship with the patient and making the patient feel respected, involved, and knowledgeable about the plan of care. The patient has a role in decision making, and ultimately, the goal is for better health outcomes for the person.

To create this relationship, the healthcare team, which includes the medical assistant, must use therapeutic communication. This process of communication helps build a respectful, empathetic, comfortable, and accepting relationship with the patient. It also gives the patient the self-confidence to express their feelings, ideas, questions, and concerns. In turn, the healthcare team members can gather the information, answer questions, and share the patient's concerns and feelings with other members.

BEING PROFESSIONAL

Medical assistants need to be assertive in the healthcare setting. Tips for being assertive include:
- Be assertive when you need to; not every situation requires it.
- Use appropriate eye contact.
- Use a medium pitch, speed, and volume of voice.
- Be respectful of others.
- Clearly state your needs; use "I" statements.
- Listen to others.
- Accept compliments graciously and learn to handle criticism professionally.

Role-play this scenario: You and Sam are medical assistants and each of you works with a different provider. Sam is taking a few online courses this semester. You see Sam working on schoolwork during the workday. Sam asks you several times a day to room patients, while they are working on schoolwork. You are feeling overwhelmed. Respond to Sam as you would address this situation.

CHAPTER REVIEW

First impressions are very important. They include more than just the first words that are exchanged. We must communicate effectively, both verbally and nonverbally, with patients, family members, and co-workers.

Medical assistants work with diverse populations. Types of diversity include nationality, race, culture, ethnicity, and social factors. Factors that relate to individual diversity include language, age, religion, economic status, gender, and appearance. Healthcare professionals need to identify personal biases, stereotypes, and beliefs that will prevent effective communication with patients, family, and co-workers.

Communication is the exchange of information, feelings, and thoughts between two or more people using spoken words or other methods. Nonverbal communication includes body language and expressive behaviors. More communication occurs nonverbally than verbally. Nonverbal communication occurs through our position, posture, facial expressions, gestures, touch, eye contact, and mannerisms. Nonverbal communication also occurs through the quality of our vocal expression. For instance, nonverbal communication includes the rate, clarity, volume, pitch, tone, intonation, and vocabulary we use when speaking.

The communication cycle is a way to describe the communication process. It involves both a sender and a receiver, in addition to the message and feedback. Oral and written communications are forms of verbal communication. Styles of verbal communication include passive, aggressive, passive-aggressive, manipulative, and assertive styles. Healthcare professionals should use the assertive communication style.

Therapeutic communication is a process of communicating with patients and family members in healthcare. It is an interactive relationship that conveys acceptance and respect without judging or blaming. Active listening is the most important therapeutic communication technique. Active listening means we fully concentrate on what is being said and how it is said.

When you gather information from a patient, it is helpful to use a combination of open-ended and closed questions or statements.

Barriers to effective communication include speech disorders, anger, age, and disease status. Additional barriers to communication, along with ways to overcome the barriers, include:

- Environmental distractions: Provide patients with privacy.
- Internal distractions: Help make patients comfortable.
- Visually impaired: Use audio recordings, large-print materials, and screen reader software.
- Hearing impaired: Use print materials, videos with captions, and sign language interpreters.
- Non-English speaking: Use interpreters and translated materials.
- Emotional distractions: Provide a warm, caring environment.

Erik Erikson described the emotional, physical, and psychological stages of human development. He stated that a person in each stage had a specific developmental task to complete. Understanding the task or goal of each stage helps healthcare professionals communicate more effectively with patients.

Elisabeth Kübler-Ross studied people's reactions to dying. She found that people went through similar stages: denial, anger, bargaining, depression, and acceptance. These stages have been applied to grief and relate to patients who have a chronic or terminal illness. Not everyone progresses through the stages at the same time, nor does everyone get to the final stage.

Maslow described what motivates people. His theory helps describe behaviors of individuals as they cope with the world or strive for happiness. Maslow believed that our human needs can be categorized into eight levels. The "Deficiency" needs consist of the four bottom levels, and they are considered the coping behaviors. We must fulfill these needs to cope with life and survival, but fulfillment only leads to instant, short-term gratification. The top four levels are "Growth" needs, which relate to making ourselves a better person. Achieving these levels brings long-lasting happiness.

Defense mechanisms are unconscious mental processes that patients and peers use to protect themselves from situations or information they cannot manage psychologically. Coping mechanisms are behavioral and psychological strategies used to deal with or minimize stressful events. Adaptive (healthy) coping mechanisms improve our functioning level and reduce our stress level. Maladaptive (nonadaptive or unhealthy) coping mechanisms reduce the feelings associated with stress for a short time, but they do not reduce the actual stressor and can lead to future problems.

SCENARIO WRAP-UP

Christi is enjoying her new job. Learning how to interact with patients, peers, and providers is an essential part of her job. She is already starting to read up on the Hmong and Mexican cultures, because a high percentage of her patients come from those two backgrounds. She has learned important facts about the cultures that helps her understand characteristics she has seen in some of her patients. Christi enjoys learning about new cultures.

Christi realizes she has met people who communicate in different ways, and she is learning how to respond to them in the professional environment. Some days are stressful, but she is trying to eat healthy meals, get enough sleep, and use healthy coping skills.

PROCEDURE 17.1 Use Feedback Techniques and Demonstrate Respect for Individual Diversity: Gender and Appearance

Tasks

Use feedback techniques (e.g., reflection, restatement, and clarification) to obtain patient information. Respond to nonverbal communication. Communicate respectfully with patients with individual diversity related to gender and appearance. Demonstrate empathy, active listening, and nonverbal communication.

Background

When working with a transgender patient, ask the patient privately which pronouns the person prefers. Make sure to add this information to the patient's health record for future reference.

Scenario

You are rooming Crystal Green. You can see that she has expertly applied her makeup, has long red fingernails, long blond hair, and is wearing at least 3-inch heels. You are surprised to see that her birth sex is male. This is the first time you have roomed a transgender patient. You are uncomfortable in this situation because you have strong personal beliefs that birth sex should be maintained throughout a person's life.

Directions

Using the scenario, role-play with a peer the rooming process (obtain the patient's chief complaint [main reason for the visit], her allergies, her pregnancy history, and her current medications). The partner (patient) should make up any information required.

Equipment and Supplies

- Patient health record
- Rooming form (optional)
- Pen

Procedural Steps

1. Greet the patient. Identify yourself. Verify the patient's identity with full name and date of birth. Explain the procedure in a manner that is understood by the patient. Answer any questions the patient may have on the procedure.

   Purpose: It is important to identify the patient in two different ways to ensure that you have the correct patient. Explaining the procedure can make the patient feel more comfortable and helps to reduce anxiety.

2. Demonstrate respect for the patient. Be sincere, courteous, polite, and welcoming. Maintain the patient's dignity. Demonstrate professional, nonjudgmental verbal and nonverbal communication. Ask appropriate questions as information is obtained.

   Purpose: It is important to provide a respectful and welcoming environment to all patients, regardless of individual diversity.

3. Using appropriate closed and open-ended questions and statements, obtain the patient's chief complaint (main reason for the visit) and history of present illness, allergies, pregnancy history, medical history, and current medications. Document the information in the health record or rooming form.

   Purpose: Medical assistants need to gather the patient's information prior to the provider seeing the patient.

4. Use feedback techniques, including reflection, restatements, and clarification, as information is obtained.

   Purpose: Feedback techniques help to ensure the information is correct.

5. Respond to the patient's nonverbal communication by using feedback techniques (e.g., reflection). If the patient's nonverbal communication is interpreted differently than the patient's oral statements, clarify the information with the patient.

   Purpose: Feedback techniques help to ensure the receiver's interpretation of the nonverbal and verbal communication is correct.

6. Use active listening skills. Remain neutral and refrain from interrupting. Allow for periods of silence. Smile and nod your head to show interest. Use appropriate eye contact. Focus on the patient and avoid distractions (e.g., looking at the clock, fidgeting).

   Purpose: Demonstrating active listening skills creates a trusting, welcoming environment for the patient. It helps build a trusting, caring relationship with the patient.

7. Use professional, positive nonverbal communication behaviors. Use a clear voice with a moderate rate and volume. Use a varying pitch and an accepting or a neutral tone. Use words the patient can understand. Correctly pronounce the words. Be at the same eye level as the patient. Smile and have a poised posture. Use a light touch on the hand if appropriate. Maintain proper eye contact.

   Purpose: Demonstrating active listening skills and positive nonverbal communication behaviors creates a trusting, welcoming environment for the patient. It helps build a trusting, caring relationship with the patient.

8. Demonstrate empathy by listening to the patients and learning about their experiences and concerns. Use therapeutic communication techniques and positive nonverbal behaviors, including appropriate eye contact. Position yourself at the same level as the patient. Show your support and respect.

   Purpose: Being empathetic will help build a trusting relationship with the patient.

PROCEDURE 17.2 Use Feedback Techniques and Demonstrate Respect for Individual Diversity: Race

Tasks

Use feedback techniques (e.g., reflection, restatement, and clarification) to obtain patient information. Respond to nonverbal communication. Communicate respectfully with patients with individual diversity related to race. Demonstrate empathy, active listening, and nonverbal communication.

Background

When working with an interpreter, allow time for the person to translate the information to the patient. Also, focus on the patient and do not look at the interpreter when speaking to the patient.

Scenario

You are rooming Maria Hernandez. She is always late for her appointments, and today she was 20 minutes late. She also does not speak English, and you need to use a Spanish interpreter for the visit. You are uncomfortable in this situation because you have not worked with an interpreter before. You are also feeling rushed because she was late for her appointment.

Directions

Role-play the scenario with two peers. One peer is the patient and the other peer is the translator. While acting as the translator, the information can be repeated in English. You need to obtain a brief medical history on this patient (e.g., chief complaint, allergies, and current medications). The peer (patient) should make up any information required.

Equipment and Supplies

- Patient health record
- Rooming form (optional)
- Pen

Procedural Steps

1. Greet the patient. Identify yourself. Verify the patient's identity with full name and date of birth. Explain the procedure in a manner that is understood by the patient. Answer any questions the patient may have on the procedure.

   Purpose: It is important to identify the patient in two different ways to ensure that you have the correct patient. Explaining the procedure can make the patient feel more comfortable and helps to reduce anxiety.

2. Demonstrate respect for the patient. Focus on the patient, not on the interpreter. Pause to give the interpreter and patient time to answer. Be sincere, courteous, polite, and welcoming. Maintain the patient's dignity. Demonstrate professional, nonjudgmental verbal and nonverbal communication. Ask appropriate questions as information is obtained.

   Purpose: It is important to provide a respectful and welcoming environment to all patients, regardless of individual diversity.

3. Using appropriate closed and open-ended questions and statements, obtain the patient's chief complaint (main reason for the visit) and history of present illness, allergies, pregnancy history, medical history, and current medications. Document the information in the health record or rooming form.

   Purpose: Medical assistants need to gather the patient's information prior to the provider seeing the patient.

4. Use feedback techniques, including reflection, restatements, and clarification as information is obtained.

   Purpose: Feedback techniques help to ensure the information is correct.

5. Respond to the patient's nonverbal communication by using feedback techniques (e.g., reflection). If the patient's nonverbal communication is interpreted differently than the patient's oral statements, clarify the information with the patient.

   Purpose: Feedback techniques help to ensure the receiver's interpretation of the nonverbal and verbal communication is correct.

6. Use active listening skills. Remain neutral and refrain from interrupting. Allow for periods of silence. Smile and nod your head to show interest. Use appropriate eye contact. Focus on the patient and avoid distractions (e.g., looking at the clock, fidgeting).

   Purpose: Demonstrating active listening skills creates a trusting, welcoming environment for the patient. It helps build a trusting, caring relationship with the patient.

7. Use professional, positive nonverbal communication behaviors. Use a clear voice with a moderate rate and volume. Use a varying pitch and an accepting or a neutral tone. Use words the patient can understand. Correctly pronounce the words. Be at the same position as the patient. Smile and have a poised posture. Use a light touch on the hand if appropriate. Maintain proper eye contact.

   Purpose: Demonstrating active listening skills and positive nonverbal communication behaviors creates a trusting, welcoming environment for the patient. It helps build a trusting, caring relationship with the patient.

8. Demonstrate empathy by listening to the patients and learning about their experiences and concerns. Use therapeutic communication techniques and positive nonverbal behaviors, including appropriate eye contact. Position yourself at the same level as the patient. Show your support and respect.

   Purpose: Being empathetic will help build a trusting relationship with the patient.

PROCEDURE 17.3 Demonstrate Respect for Individual Diversity: Religion and Appearance

Tasks

Respond to nonverbal communication. Communicate respectfully with patients with individual diversity related to religion and appearance. Demonstrate empathy, active listening, and nonverbal communication.

Background

The Sikh (sickh) religion was founded in northern India. Sikhs believe in one god, the equality of males and females, justice, and community service. Turbans and kachera (kah SHEH rruh) are worn at all times for religious reasons. Turbans or scarves cover the uncut hair. If the turban or scarf needs to be removed, an alternative head covering should be provided. A turban or scarf should be treated with respect. Placing it on the floor or near shoes would be a sign of disrespect. Kachera are undershorts/undergarments, and at least one leg is to remain in the kachera at all times.

Scenario

You are preparing a patient for an examination. The patient is Sikh. The provider always wants the patient to completely undress, wear a gown, and be seated on the exam table before she comes into the room. You are uncomfortable in this situation because you have never worked with a patient who is Sikh.

Directions

Role-play the scenario with a peer. Instruct the peer (patient) how to prepare for the examination.

Equipment and Supplies
- Gown and drape sheet (optional)
- Exam table (optional)

Procedural Steps

1. Greet the patient. Identify yourself. Verify the patient's identity with full name and date of birth. Explain the procedure (undressing) in a manner that is understood by the patient. Answer any questions the patient may have on the procedure.

Purpose: It is important to identify the patient in two different ways to ensure that you have the correct patient. Explaining the procedure can make the patient feel more comfortable and helps to reduce anxiety.

2. Demonstrate respect for the patient. Be sincere, courteous, polite, and welcoming. Maintain the patient's dignity. Demonstrate professional, nonjudgmental verbal and nonverbal communication.

Purpose: It is important to provide a respectful and welcoming environment to all patients, regardless of individual diversity.

3. Respond to the patient's nonverbal communication by using feedback techniques (e.g., reflection). If the patient's nonverbal communication is interpreted differently than the patient's oral statements, clarify the information with the patient.

Purpose: Feedback techniques help to ensure the receiver's interpretation of the nonverbal and verbal communication is correct.

4. Use active listening skills. Remain neutral and refrain from interrupting. Smile and nod your head to show interest. Use appropriate eye contact. Focus on the patient and avoid distractions (e.g., looking at the clock, fidgeting).

Purpose: Demonstrating active listening skills creates a trusting, welcoming environment for the patient. It helps build a trusting, caring relationship with the patient.

5. Use professional, positive nonverbal communication behaviors. Use a clear voice with a moderate rate and volume. Use a varying pitch and an accepting or a neutral tone. Use words the patient can understand. Correctly pronounce the words. Be at the same eye level as the patient. Smile and have a poised posture. Use a light touch on the hand if appropriate. Maintain proper eye contact.

Purpose: Demonstrating active listening skills and positive nonverbal communication behaviors creates a trusting, welcoming environment for the patient. It helps build a trusting, caring relationship with the patient.

6. Demonstrate empathy by listening to the patients and learning about their experiences and concerns. Use therapeutic communication techniques and positive nonverbal behaviors, including appropriate eye contact. Position yourself at the same level as the patient. Show your support and respect.

Purpose: Being empathetic will help build a trusting relationship with the patient.

PROCEDURE 17.4 Use Feedback Techniques and Demonstrate Respect for Individual Diversity: Age, Economic Status, and Appearance

Tasks

Use feedback techniques (e.g., reflection, restatement, and clarification) to obtain patient information. Respond to nonverbal communication. Communicate respectfully with patients with individual diversity related to age, economic status, and appearance. Demonstrate empathy, active listening, and nonverbal communication.

Scenario

You are rooming Mr. Abraham Black (79 years old), who has recently been diagnosed with dementia. He likes to talk about things that happened long before you were born, and you are not interested in those events. He also has a hard time hearing your questions, and you frequently repeat questions. Mr. Black has poor personal hygiene. His clothes are dirty and torn. He has an unpleasant body odor. Mr. Black tells you he cannot afford to eat if he buys his medications. He does not believe in government programs and refuses to take "handouts." You have worked with Mr. Black in the past and have heard this all before, numerous times. You would prefer to work with the younger generation and with patients who have better hygiene.

Directions

Using the scenario, role-play the rooming process with a peer (patient). Obtain the patient's chief complaint, allergies, and current medications. The patient should make up any information required.

Equipment and Supplies
- Patient health record
- Rooming form (optional)
- Pen

Procedural Steps

1. Greet the patient. Identify yourself. Verify the patient's identity with full name and date of birth. Explain the procedure in a manner that is understood by the patient. Answer any questions the patient may have on the procedure.

Purpose: It is important to identify the patient in two different ways to ensure that you have the correct patient. Explaining the procedure can make the patient feel more comfortable and helps to reduce anxiety.

2. Demonstrate respect for the patient. Be sincere, courteous, polite, and welcoming. Maintain the patient's dignity. Demonstrate professional,

PROCEDURE 17.4   Use Feedback Techniques and Demonstrate Respect for Individual Diversity: Age, Economic Status, and Appearance—continued

nonjudgmental verbal and nonverbal communication. Ask appropriate questions as information is obtained.

Purpose: It is important to provide a respectful and welcoming environment to all patients, regardless of individual diversity.

3. Using appropriate closed and open-ended questions and statements, obtain the patient's chief complaint (main reason for the visit), history of present illness, allergies, medical history, and current medications. Document the information in the health record or rooming form.

Purpose: Medical assistants need to gather the patient's information prior to the provider seeing the patient.

4. Use feedback techniques, including reflection, restatement, and clarification, as information is obtained.

Purpose: Feedback techniques help to ensure the information is correct.

5. Respond to the patient's nonverbal communication by using feedback techniques (e.g., reflection). If the patient's nonverbal communication is interpreted differently than the patient's oral statements, clarify the information with the patient.

Purpose: Feedback techniques help to ensure the receiver's interpretation of the nonverbal and verbal communication is correct.

6. Use active listening skills. Remain neutral and refrain from interrupting. Allow for periods of silence. Smile and nod your head to show interest. Use appropriate eye contact. Focus on the patient and avoid distractions (e.g., looking at the clock, fidgeting).

Purpose: Demonstrating active listening skills creates a trusting, welcoming environment for the patient. It helps build a trusting, caring relationship with the patient.

7. Use professional, positive nonverbal communication behaviors. Use a clear voice with a moderate rate and volume. Use a varying pitch and an accepting or neutral tone. Use words the patient can understand. Correctly pronounce the words. Be at the same eye level as the patient. Smile and have a poised posture. Use a light touch on the hand if appropriate. Maintain proper eye contact.

Purpose: Demonstrating active listening skills and positive nonverbal communication behaviors creates a trusting, welcoming environment for the patient. It helps build a trusting, caring relationship with the patient.

8. Demonstrate empathy by listening to the patients and learning about their experiences and concerns. Use therapeutic communication techniques and positive nonverbal behaviors, including good eye contact. Position yourself at the same level as the patient. Show your support and respect.

Purpose: Being empathetic will help build a trusting relationship with the patient.

PROCEDURE 17.5   Demonstrate Appropriate Self-Boundaries

Tasks

Use respectful and tactful communication while demonstrating the principles of self-boundaries.

Background

For the medical assistant to have a professional therapeutic relationship with a patient, the medical assistant must guard against crossing self-boundaries, which is also called professional boundaries. The relationship between the medical assistant and the patient needs to be professional. It cannot be a dual relationship, where the medical assistant also becomes a friend to the patient. This means the medical assistant cannot share personal intimate information, contact the patient outside of the work environment, befriend the patient on social media, or engage in a flirty or romantic relationship with the patient.

Scenario 1

You are rooming Morgan, who frequently sees the provider you work for. You have gotten to know Morgan over the time you have worked for the provider. Today, Morgan asks you for your personal phone number and social media information.

Scenario 2

You are rooming Sam, who you have gotten to know well over the time you have worked for your provider. Sam is outgoing, enjoys talking, and has many of the same interests as you do. You have just split up with your significant other and have been feeling a bit down. Sam asks you if you would be available for coffee sometime.

Directions

Role-play the scenarios with a peer. Your peer will play the patient in the scenario and you are the medical assistant.

18

Legal Basics

LEARNING OBJECTIVES

1. Discuss the balance of power in the United States and describe the four types of laws.
2. Compare criminal and civil law as they apply to the practicing medical assistant.
3. Differentiate between intentional torts and negligent (unintentional) tort.
4. Differentiate between the standard of care and the scope of practice for a medical assistant.
5. Define terms related to a civil lawsuit and describe the 4 Ds of negligence.
6. Discuss types of professional liability insurance.
7. Explain the five elements required for a contract to be legally binding.
8. Describe the reasons and the steps for terminating the patient-provider relationship.
9. Differentiate between implied consent, expressed consent, and informed consent.
10. Summarize patient's rights and responsibilities.
11. Discuss licensure, certification, registration, and accreditation.

OUTLINE

▶ OPENING SCENARIO

Daniela Garcia was just hired as a part-time float receptionist at Walden-Martin Family Medical (WMFM) Clinic. As a float receptionist, she will be working with many different co-workers and providers. Besides working, Daniela is enrolled in a medical assistant program at the local community college. She is just starting a law and ethics course. The first part of the course explains legal concepts.

Daniela learned about the government in high school, but she has never been in a courtroom, nor witnessed court proceedings. Learning about legal concepts is very different from her other courses. Many of her classmates did not realize that medical assistants need to learn about legal concepts and laws. Daniela hopes that she can relate what she does in the clinic to what she is learning in her course. She finds concepts are easier to remember if she can apply them to real-life situations.

Bella, a newly certified medical assistant (CMA), has offered to help Daniela study for her law course. Bella stated that she enjoyed learning about law and its importance in healthcare. Daniela is considering asking her for help on their breaks. Studying with another person also helps her retain and understand the concepts.

YOU WILL LEARN

1. To describe the different sources of law.
2. To explain the differences between criminal and civil law.
3. To describe intentional torts and negligent torts.
4. To explain the requirements for a legal contract.

5. To describe expressed, implied, and informed consent.
6. To describe the difference between the provider's and the medical assistant's scope of practice and practice requirements.

INTRODUCTION

In the United States, the number of lawsuits has increased over the years. Working in a litigious (LI ti jehs) society requires that we know how to protect ourselves against lawsuits. This is the reason that medical assistants need to learn about the law. To avoid the risk of lawsuits, medical assistants need to practice within the guidelines of the law.

VOCABULARY
litigious Prone to lawsuits.

SOURCES OF LAW

Law is a custom or practice of a community. It is a rule of conduct or action prescribed or formally recognized as enforceable by a controlling authority. Law is the system by which society gives order to our lives.

The United States has both federal and state laws. The US Constitution is the supreme law of the United States. Each state has a constitution that is the supreme law of that state. State laws cannot conflict with the US Constitution. In the following sections, we will examine the makeup of the federal and state governments and the sources of law.

Balance of Power

The federal government was designed to allow for a balance of power. The three branches of government share power so that no one branch is more powerful than any other. Table 18.1 describes the three branches of the federal government. The states also have three branches of government.

When members of Congress or the state houses want new legislation, a bill is brought forward. After much debate, the bill will either die or be passed and become an act or statute. The act or statute is now part of the laws for the state or country. (The terms "act" and "statute" are used interchangeably. Most of the time you will hear the word "act" in the name of a specific law; statute is used more to refer to the contents of the actual law.) On the local level, an *ordinance* is a piece of legislation passed by a municipality or local government. A city ordinance to ban smoking from restaurants is an example of local legislation.

Types of Laws

There are four types of laws:
- *Constitutional law*: Derived from the federal and state constitutions, which give power to federal and state governments. Examples of constitutional law include prohibiting slavery (based on an 1865 constitutional amendment) and the power to tax.

TABLE 18.1	**Branches of the Federal and State Governments**	
Branch	**Federal Government**	**State Government**
Legislative	Made up of: • Two houses of Congress (Senate and House of Representatives). Members of the houses are elected by eligible voters from the state they represent. Roles: • Makes new federal laws • Can impeach the President or remove judges from office for misconduct • Must approve: All appointments for judges, budget spending, and treaties • Can override the President's veto of a bill by a ⅔ vote	Made up of: • Most states have two houses, although the names can differ. Officials are elected. Roles: • Introduce legislation to become new state laws • Can impeach state officials for misconduct • Must approve state budget • Can override the governor's veto and amend the state constitution
Executive	Made up of: • President of the United States administers this branch Roles: • Can issue *executive orders* that become law without the approval of Congress • Creates a budget • Appoints judges • Carries out laws • Makes treaties with other nations • Can veto bills from Congress	Made up of: • Headed by the elected governor; each state has a different executive organizational structure. Roles: • Creates a budget • Carries out laws • Can veto bills from state houses • Issues executive orders • Appoints state court judges (in most states)
Judicial	Made up of: • Supreme Court, which has nine justices Roles: • Interpret laws according to the US Constitution • Determine if laws from Congress and executive actions are constitutional	Made up of: • State supreme court Roles: • Interpret laws according to the state constitution • Hear cases from lower courts • Determine if state laws are constitutional

- *Case law*: Derived from legal precedents and common law. Common law originated in England and was used by the colonists. An example would include the right of criminal defendants to have an attorney even if they cannot afford one, which was a ruling from the Supreme Court (*Gideon v. Wainwright* 372 U.S. 335 [1963]).
- *Regulatory* and *administrative law*: Concerns the procedures, regulations, and rules of federal, state, and local governmental administrative agencies. Examples include zoning boards, licensing agencies, the Social Security Administration, and unemployment commissions.
- *Statutory law*: Refers to the laws enacted by the state and federal legislatures. An example is the speed limits set by the state legislature.

CRIMINAL AND CIVIL LAW

Laws can be divided into two main categories:
- *Substantive law*: Laws that determine rights and obligations of people derived from common law and statutes. Substantive laws include criminal, civil, military, and international law.
- *Procedural law*: Laws that all parties (courts, officers, and lawyers) must follow when investigating and prosecuting unlawful acts. With criminal law, procedural law ensures that a person receives due process under the US Constitution.

The following sections will explain criminal and civil law in depth as they relate to healthcare.

Criminal Law

Criminal laws are statutes that define actions or *omissions* (lack of actions) that threaten and/or harm public safety and welfare. These actions or omissions are prohibited by the government and are called *crimes*. Criminal law can be summarized as crimes against the state (or government). When criminal cases are brought to court, the plaintiff (PLAIN tif) is the government. The defendant (dih FEN dant) is the person or party charged with the offense.

Criminal offenses can vary in severity from traffic violations to murders. In most states criminal offenses are classified as misdemeanors (mis di MEE ners) and felonies (FEL uh nees), which both appear on a person's criminal record.

Misdemeanors are lesser criminal offenses and include assault, battery, false imprisonment, perjury, shoplifting, and most cases of operating while intoxicated (OWI) and operating under the influence (OUI). A misdemeanor is punishable by a substantial fine and possible jail time under 1 year. (*Jails* are usually operated by local law enforcement and are used for short-term stays.)

A *felony* is a serious criminal offense and is classified by degree, with first degree being the most serious. Examples of felonies include murder, robbery, rape, sodomy, larceny, manslaughter, kidnapping, embezzlement, arson, mayhem, burglary, and treason. Felonies are punishable by substantial fines and prison time of more than 1 year. (Prisons are usually operated by the state or federal government and are for long-term

stays.) A felony conviction may prevent a person from voting and owning firearms (guns). A felon may have difficulty obtaining a job, especially in healthcare.

VOCABULARY

common law Unwritten laws that come from judicial decisions based on societal traditions and customs.

defendant An individual or a business against whom a lawsuit is filed.

liability The state of being liable or responsible for something.

negligence Failure to act as a reasonably prudent person would under similar circumstances; such conduct falls below the standards of behavior established by law for the protection of others against unreasonable risk of harm.

plaintiff An individual or a party who brings a lawsuit to court.

precedent A prior court decision that serves as a model for similar legal cases in the future.

tort A civil wrongdoing that causes harm to a person or property; excludes breach of contract.

CRITICAL THINKING 18.1

Bella and Daniela are reviewing criminal law concepts during lunch break. Bella asks Daniela how criminal law would apply to medical assistants. How might Daniela respond? Discuss your response with a peer.

Civil Law

Civil laws protect and define private rights. An individual or institution can sue another person, institution (business), or the government in a civil matter (Table 18.2). Civil laws govern disputes related to contracts, property, family law, and personal injury. Common civil disputes involve contract issues, divorce, child custody, product liability (LIE ah bil i tee), and accidents. There are many branches of civil law, including:

- *Tort law*: Applies when one person, business, or the government does a wrongdoing to an individual that causes injury or property damage. Includes intentional tort (torte), negligence (NEG li juhns), and *strict liability* (strict duty to ensure safety of manufactured products).
- *Contract law*: Applies to agreements between two or more individuals or parties.
- *Property law*: Applies to personal property (e.g., copyrights, stocks, animals, physical goods) and real property (e.g., land, mineral rights).
- *Family law*: Applies to marriage, divorce, annulment, child custody and support, birth, and adoption.

The following sections will address tort law and contract law.

TORT LAW

Tort law enforces rules that we have in our society. If these rules are violated, then an individual can sue another individual, institution (business), or government. Two types of torts will be discussed: intentional torts and negligent torts (unintentional torts).

Intentional Torts

With an *intentional tort*, the plaintiff must prove the defendant had specific intent to perform the action that caused the injury. The focus is not on whether the harm was intended, but if the

TABLE 18.2 Criminal Law Compared to Civil Law

	Criminal Law	Civil Law
Plaintiff	State or federal government	Victim (individual or institution) of the wrongdoing
Defendant	Person or party accused of the criminal complaint or charge	Wrongdoer (also called *tortfeasor* [TORTE fee zahr] with tort law); could be a business, individual, or the government
Wrong act against	Wrongful act against the government (state or federal)	Wrongful acts against an individual or an institution (business)
Offense/wrong called	Crime	Tort, breach of contract (depends on the type of civil law)
Attorney	Defendant entitled to an attorney. The state must provide an attorney if the defendant cannot afford one	Defendant must pay for the attorney or defend oneself.
Court	Tried in criminal court system; almost always involves a trial by jury	Tried in a civil court system; may not involve a jury. Cases are typically decided by the judge.
Standard of proof	Must prove beyond a reasonable doubt	The preponderance of evidence (more than likely it occurred)
Consequence	Substantial fine and prison time	*Damages*, *injunction* (in JUNGK shahn), *declaratory judgment*
Healthcare example	A medical assistant determines a patient should have a specific medication and gives the patient the medication without a provider's order, thus practicing medicine.	A medical assistant changes a sterile dressing per a provider's order but does the procedure incorrectly. The wound develops an infection, and the patient subsequently dies.

action was intended. Many intentional torts are also criminal in nature. The defendant may be prosecuted in both a civil court and a criminal court for the action. Common intentional torts include:

- *Assault*: Intentional threat to do harm or acting in a manner that causes another to fear bodily harm. Example: A medical assistant threatens a child to behave by stating, "I will give you a 'shot' if you do not behave."
- *Battery*: Intentional harmful or offensive contact with another that was unconsented. This includes unauthorized administration of medical care in a nonemergent situation. Only proof of unconsented contact is required; proof of harm is not required. Example: A medical assistant gives a child a vaccination without consent from the parent or guardian.
- *False imprisonment*: Intentional restraint of another individual without consent or reason. Example: A medical assistant uses restraints to keep a patient in a wheelchair without significant reason.
- *Fraud*: Deceiving (lying to) a person or party for monetary gain. Example: A medical assistant bills an insurance company for services not provided to the patient.
- *Defamation*: Intentionally saying something false about another person, which causes harm (Box 18.1). Written defamation is *libel*. Spoken defamation is *slander*. Example: A medical assistant posts lies about a co-worker on a social media site that could cause harm to that person.
- *Invasion of privacy*: Disclosing private facts without the consent of the individual, or intrusion into a person's personal life. Example: A medical assistant tells a family member or friend about a patient who was seen in the department, which is breaching confidentiality.

CRITICAL THINKING 18.2

Bella and Daniela are reviewing civil law concepts after work. Bella asks Daniela how civil law would apply to medical assistants. How might Daniela respond? Discuss your response with a peer.

BOX 18.1 Legal Example: Defamation Suit

According to the complaint: In 2013 in Fairfax, Virginia, the plaintiff was to have a colonoscopy. He was told he could be groggy afterward and was concerned about recalling post-procedure instructions. Prior to the procedure, he set his mobile phone to record the post-procedure instructions. His clothing and phone ended up in the operating suite with him during the procedure. His phone recorded the entire procedure. While the plaintiff was unconscious, the doctors and medical assistant joked that he had syphilis and tuberculosis that caused a penile rash. The defendants mocked the patient for a variety of reasons and then discussed how to avoid the patient when he woke up. The medical assistant attempted to mislead the plaintiff. She indicated falsely that the physician spoke to him after surgery, but the patient must not have remembered. The plaintiff and his wife discovered the recording on their way home.

The jury awarded the plaintiff $50,000 in compensatory damages for defamation for the provider's remarks about each disease. He was also awarded $200,000 for overall medical malpractice and $200,000 in punitive damages.

From *D.B. v Ingham et al.*, 2013-16811, (2015, Fairfax Circuit Court).

VOCABULARY

damages A monetary settlement the defendant pays the plaintiff in a civil case for loss or injury. Also, one of the 4 Ds of negligence, meaning the patient suffers a legally recognized injury.

declaratory judgment A court judgment that defines the legal rights of the parties involved.

injunction A court order by which an individual or institution is required to perform or refrain from performing a certain act.

tortfeasor The individual or entity who committed the tort, either intentionally or as a result of negligence.

Negligent Torts

Negligent torts, or *unintentional torts*, are more common in healthcare because they are unintentional. The harm that is caused by negligence is the result of a person's carelessness. *Negligence* results when a person's conduct falls below the standard of behavior expected of a reasonable person in the same situation.

The *reasonable person standard* applies reasonable behavior as an objective test to measure another's actions or lack of actions. The accused person's actions or lack of actions are measured against what a reasonable person would or would not do in the same situation. The accused person is negligent if their actions or lack of actions do not measure up to the reasonable person standard. Negligent acts can be classified as:

- *Malfeasance* (mal FEE zahns): Performance of an unlawful, wrongful act. For instance, a medical assistant determines that a patient needs pain medication and gives a large dose without a provider's order. The patient dies from the overdose. (It is illegal for the medical assistant to practice medicine [prescribe the medication], and the dose was incorrect.)
- *Misfeasance* (mis FEE zahns): Improper performance of a lawful act, that causes damage or injury. For instance, a medical assistant gives an injection ordered by the provider. The injection is given in the wrong location, and the patient has lifelong pain.
- *Nonfeasance* (non FEE zahns): Failure to act when one had a legal duty to act. For instance, after a patient is given an injection, the patient starts to have an adverse reaction. The medical assistant fails to act and notify the provider. The medical assistant sends the patient home, and the patient later dies.

Malpractice (mal PRAK tis) is a type of negligence that applies to professionals. Medical malpractice occurs when a healthcare professional's performance falls below the professional minimum standard of care and thus causes harm to the plaintiff (Box 18.2). *Standard of care* refers to the level and type of care an ordinary, prudent healthcare professional, having the same training and experience in a similar practice, would have provided under a similar situation.

The standard of care takes into account the accused person's skills and knowledge. It also considers the environment. For instance, the care provided by Dr. Walden, a family practice doctor practicing in a midsize Midwestern city, would be compared to a family practice doctor who practiced in a similar-sized city in the same geographic location. It would be unfair to compare Dr. Walden's family practice to a large family practice located on the East Coast. The resources available to the providers could be different.

Medical assistants need to be aware of the standard of care. If medical assistants identify themselves as nurses to patients, they may be held to the standard of care (including the educational level) of a nurse. If medical assistants practice beyond their scope of practice, they may be held to the higher standard of care. Also, medical assistants who are nationally certified may be held to a higher level than those who are not certified. It is important for credentialed medical assistants to pursue continuing education to keep updated and current in their practice. Scope of practice will be discussed later in the chapter.

CRITICAL THINKING 18.3

Bella asks Daniela to describe negligence and malpractice in her own words. How might Daniela respond?

CRITICAL THINKING 18.4

Daniela asks Bella why medical assistants cannot call themselves nurses. How might Bella address this question? How might scope of practice relate to the question?

VOCABULARY

defense A strategy used by the defendant to avoid liability in a lawsuit.
malpractice A type of negligence in which a licensed professional fails to provide the standard of care, causing harm to a person.
scope of practice Range of responsibilities and practice guidelines that determine the boundaries within which a healthcare worker practices.

Defenses to Liability. When the defendant's attorney accepts a case, a defense (di FENS) is planned for the lawsuit. There are three main defenses used for lawsuits: denial, technical, and affirmative. Denial defense is used when none of the facts are true. If even just one fact is true, then the denial defense cannot be used. The following sections will describe technical and affirmative defenses.

Technical Defenses. When attorneys review cases, they look for ways to have the cases dismissed based on a legal technicality. Four technical defenses will be discussed: statute of limitations, Good Samaritan law, release of tortfeasor, and res judicata.

The *statute of limitations* is the length of time legal action can be taken after an event has occurred. When the time has expired, the court will reject the claim or lawsuit. The statute of limitations for medical malpractice is usually 2 to 5 years, but it varies from state to state. In most states the "clock" starts when the patient "reasonably should have known" the malpractice occurred. For instance, if a patient awoke after surgery to find that the operation had been performed on the wrong leg, the clock would start then. In some cases, patients do not realize the malpractice occurred for months or years after the event. For instance, something was left in the patient's body during surgery, and it was discovered on an x-ray 3 years later. According to the Discovery Rule, the malpractice needs to be discovered (the patient "reasonably should have known") before the "clock starts" on the statute of limitations. The statute of limitations for children greatly varies; some states use age 8, whereas others use age 18.

The *Good Samaritan laws* vary in each state, with some states providing protection if the provider acts "in good faith." For

---

BOX 18.2   Legal Example: Malpractice Case

In October 2007, in Syracuse, New York, Tina Holstein (31 years old) delivered her third child at Community General Hospital. After the delivery, she began vomiting, and the nurse administered an intramuscular (IM) injection. Ms. Holstein sued the hospital and the nurse who administered the injection, alleging malpractice. She claimed she had permanent injury of her sciatic nerve because the nurse failed to properly administer the IM injection. The case against the nurse was dropped, but the jury found the hospital liable for the injury. Ms. Holstein was awarded $1.69 million.

From *Holstein v. Community General Hospital Greater Syracuse,* 17 N.Y.3d 948 (2011). https://www.leagle.com/decision/innyco20111122672

Good Samaritan protection, a person must provide care in a true emergency. The care must be provided outside of a place with necessary medical equipment (e.g., outside of a hospital or ambulatory care facility). The person providing the care cannot bill the patient for the emergency care provided.

The *release of tortfeasor* defense is used when the plaintiff had signed a release and received monetary compensation. The release indicated that the plaintiff would give up all rights to sue the defendant *(tortfeasor)* in the future, in exchange for a monetary compensation. If this signed release existed and the plaintiff decided to sue the defendant at a later time, the defendant's attorney could use the release of tortfeasor defense.

The final technical defense is res judicata (RAZE JOO di kah tah), which is Latin for "a thing decided." If a case has already been decided by the court, the plaintiff cannot bring a similar suit against the defendant in the future. The defendant's attorney would use the res judicata defense.

VOCABULARY

res judicata Latin for "a thing decided." Once a case has been decided by the court, it cannot be litigated again.

Affirmative Defenses. When attorneys review cases, if the denial defense and the technical defense cannot be used, then they attempt to use the affirmative defense. An *affirmative defense* means the defendant admits to wrongdoing, but their attorney introduces facts that support the defendant's conduct. If the defense is successful, it will reduce the defendant's legal liability. The following are common affirmative defenses:

- *Contributory negligence*: The plaintiff's actions or lack of actions caused the injury. In other words, had the plaintiff used ordinary care, the injury would not have occurred. The plaintiff's carelessness (e.g., ignoring warnings or safety rules, inattention) caused the injury. (In many states contributory negligence has been replaced by comparative negligence).
- *Comparative negligence*: The plaintiff's action or lack of action caused the injury to a certain percent. The damages to the plaintiff are calculated based on the percent the defendant was responsible.
- *Assumption of risk*: The defendant can show evidence that the plaintiff had actual, subjective knowledge of the risks involved and the plaintiff consented to proceed with the activity (Box 18.3). Informed consent is critical for this defense. (Informed consent will be discussed later in the chapter.)
- *Limited or no harm*: The defendant claims the plaintiff suffered no or little harm; much less than what the plaintiff claims.
- *Intervening cause*: The defendant acknowledges the plaintiff suffered injuries due to defendant's negligence, but the injury was made worse by the plaintiff's actions following the situation.

CRITICAL THINKING 18.5

Daniela is studying affirmative defenses. She asks Bella if she has any study tips for remembering the different affirmative defenses. How might Bella answer? Share your answer with a peer.

BOX 18.3   Legal Example: Assumption of Risk

The plaintiff was being treated for bronchitis. Following his clinic visit, a coughing episode caused him to black out and hit his head at home. Upon his return to the clinic a few weeks later for a follow-up visit on the bronchitis, a medical assistant took the plaintiff into the examination room. The medical assistant instructed the plaintiff to sit on the exam table while his vital signs were obtained. The plaintiff mentioned to the medical assistant that he had fainted twice as a result of coughing episodes. After the medical assistant left to get the physician, the plaintiff had a coughing episode, fainted, and fell to the floor. He sustained injuries because of the fall.

The plaintiff sued the clinic and the medical assistant, alleging that the medical assistant was negligent for failing to move him to another location upon learning about his fainting episodes. The defendants moved for a summary judgment. They stated that an assumption of risk defense applied. The plaintiff could have chosen to sit on one of the two chairs present in the room, but he did not. The court agreed. The plaintiff appealed, and the Georgia Court of Appeals unanimously sided with the trial court's ruling. The defendants proved the plaintiff had knowledge of the danger, understood the risks associated with the danger, and exposed himself to the danger. The plaintiff lost the case.

From *Watson v. Regional First Care, Inc.,* No. A15A1708, Ga. App. (February 19, 2016). https://www.leagle.com/decision/ingaco20160219174

Proving Malpractice. When a plaintiff sues the defendant, the defendant can attempt to settle outside of court or go to trial. *Alternative dispute resolution* (ADR) is the process of settling disputes outside of litigation. This process is usually cheaper and quicker than going to trial. Two types of alternative dispute resolution are arbitration (AHR bi trae shuhn) and mediation (MEE dee ae shuhn). Both ADR procedures involve a neutral third party who hears both sides. With mediation, the mediator facilitates an agreement that is acceptable to both parties. With arbitration, the arbitrator listens to both sides and makes the final decision, which is *legally binding* (or a legal obligation).

With civil litigation, either party or the judge can move for a summary judgment. A *summary judgment* is a process that can be used if there are no disputes about the facts in the case. This process speeds up cases. It allows a judgment to be made based on the facts. With a summary judgment, there is no trial.

If the disputing parties decide to take the lawsuit to court, a specific process must be followed (Fig. 18.1 and Box 18.4). When a medical negligence suit is brought to court, four elements must be proven for malpractice to be found. These elements are the 4 Ds of negligence: duty, dereliction, damages, and direct cause. Let's examine the 4 Ds of negligence.

- *Duty of care*: The healthcare professional has a legal obligation to the patient. Many times, the duty of care comes from the provider-patient relationship. This will be examined in more depth later in the chapter.
- *Dereliction* (DER uh lik shuhn): The healthcare professional *breaches* (violates) the duty of care to the patient. In other words, the professional did not follow through with the duty to the patient.
- *Damages*: The patient suffers a legally recognized injury. Examples of such an injury include physical pain, mental anguish, additional medical bills, and loss of work/earning capacity.
- *Direct cause*: The breach of duty of care (the negligent act or lack of action) directly causes the patient's injury.

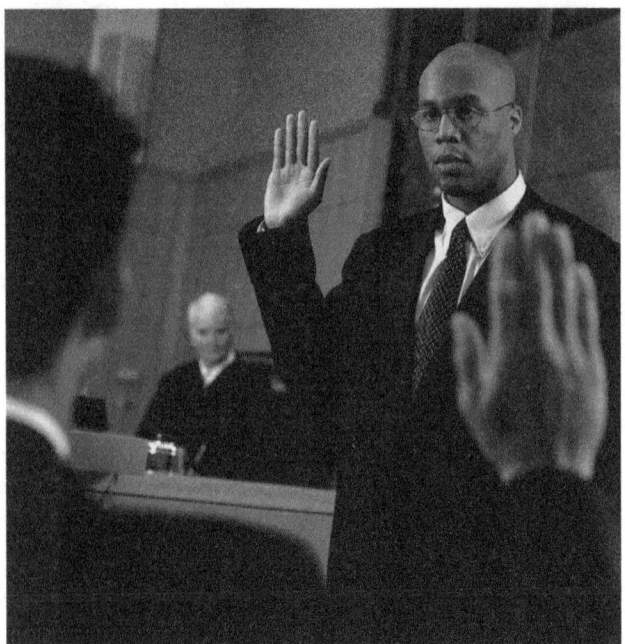

Fig. 18.1 Witnesses must be credible and must tell the truth on the stand in court to avoid charges of perjury. (From Proctor D, Niedzwiecki B: *Kinn's the medical assistant*, ed 13, St. Louis, 2017, Elsevier.)

BOX 18.4   Stages of a Civil Lawsuit

1. Prefiling phase: The situation occurs, and the patient seeks the advice of a civil attorney. After reviewing the person's story, the medical record, and other documents, the attorney accepts the case.

2. Initial pleading phase:
   - The plaintiff's attorney files a complaint with the clerk of the court. The complaint includes the patient's version of the situation and the *damages* (amount of money) sought from the defendant.
   - The clerk of the court issues a summons to the defendant. The summons outlines the complaint and damages and states a deadline for a response.
   - The defense attorney files an answer or motion with the court. The answer provides the courts with the defendant's version of the situation. (If the deadline is missed, the defendant may be responsible for the damages.)

3. Discovery phase:
   - Both sides exchange information and gather evidence to support their side in court.
   - A subpoena (suh PEE nuh) is issued for the healthcare professionals involved in the case. They may be required to go to court or to attend a deposition (dep ah ZISH uhn). They may also be required to complete an interrogatory (IN tah rog ah TOOR ee). Failure to comply with a deposition or subpoena will result in a *contempt of court* charge. The person may be fined or imprisoned.
   - A subpoena duces tecum (suh PEE nuh DOO seez TEE kuhm) may also be issued.

4. Post-discovery phase:
   - The judge may meet with both attorneys to discuss the case.
   - The plaintiff may drop the case if not enough evidence was available to make the case.
   - The defendant may settle the lawsuit by "making a deal" so it does not move to trial.

5. Trial phase: If the case is to be heard by a jury, the jury is selected. Expert witnesses and fact witnesses are questioned and cross-examined by the opposing attorney. Closing arguments are made, and the jury retires to make a decision. The verdict is read to the court, and the judge enters the judgment.

6. Appeals phase: Post-trial motions are filed. An appeal to a higher court may be made.

The plaintiff's attorney is responsible for proving each of these four elements. In many cases, medical experts are hired by attorneys to be expert witnesses. These expert witnesses help establish the standard of care and some of the 4 Ds. If one of the elements is not proven, malpractice will not be found. For instance, if the provider performed below the standard of care, but the patient did not suffer any harm, malpractice cannot be found.

In a case in which there was obvious negligence, the doctrine of res ipsa loquitur (RASE ipsah low kwah tuhr) may apply. Res ipsa loquitur is Latin for "the thing speaks for itself." The res ipsa loquitur doctrine may be used for:

- Cases that involve an object being left in the patient's body during surgery
- Cases that involve an operation on the wrong extremity

The evidence shows that the plaintiff did not cause the injury. The defendant caused the injury as a result of negligence. The defendant breached the duty to the plaintiff.

VOCABULARY

arbitration The process in which conflicting parties in a dispute submit their differences to a court-appointed person (arbitrator), who submits a legally binding decision.

deposition A sworn testimony made before a court-appointed officer; it is used in the discovery process and may be used in the trial.

expert witnesses People who are educated and knowledgeable in the area of concern; they testify in court and provide an expert opinion on the topic of concern.

fact witnesses People who observed the situation and testify in court about the facts of the case.

interrogatory Written or oral questions that must be answered under oath.

mediation The process of facilitating conflicting parties to make an agreement, settlement, or compromise.

res ipsa loquitur A Latin term meaning "the thing speaks for itself." A legal concept under which the plaintiff's burden to prove malpractice is minimal since the jury can clearly understand the details of the injury. For example, a surgical instrument was left in the body during surgery.

subpoena A court order requiring a person to appear in court at a specific time to testify in a legal case.

subpoena duces tecum A legal document commanding a person to bring a piece of evidence (e.g., the plaintiff's health record) to court.

CRITICAL THINKING 18.6

Daniela struggles with remembering the 4 Ds of negligence. Be creative and work with a peer. How might a person remember the 4 Ds of negligence?

CRITICAL THINKING 18.7

Bella is helping Daniela study for a law exam. She asks Daniela to describe the differences between the following sets of terms. How might Daniela respond?
- Subpoena and subpoena duces tecum
- Fact witness and expert witness

Damages. The defendant may need to pay damages when the plaintiff wins a civil suit. *Damages* are a monetary settlement. There are several types of damages:
- *Punitive damages*: Very large payment meant to punish the defendant.

- *Nominal damages*: Very small settlement because the plaintiff's injury was slight.
- *Compensatory damages*: A settlement for losses suffered. Losses can be related to loss of income, property damage, and medical care.
- *General damages*: A settlement for emotional pain and anguish, loss of future earning power, and so on. Often sought with compensatory damages.
- *Special damages*: A settlement for a specific dollar amount that directly relates to medical bills.

Professional Liability Insurance. Many people are familiar with car insurance and homeowner's insurance. When a person becomes a professional, the risk of being sued increases. Having insurance (to protect oneself in case of civil damages) is important. Providers, nurses, and in some cases medical assistants, purchase annual insurance policies. Ambulatory healthcare facilities also must carry insurance. It is important for medical assistants to understand the types of insurance available.

The person or company purchasing the insurance policy is called the *insured* (first party). The insured pays a specific amount of money to the insurance company (second party). This payment is called a *premium*. The insurance company is the *insurer*. The insurer agrees to compensate the insured for specific losses covered in the insurance contract or policy. When the *insurer* (insurance company) pays the plaintiff, the plaintiff is known as the *third party*.

Liability insurance provides protection from claims of injuries or damage to people or property. It can be referred to as third-party coverage because it covers claims from a party other than the insured. Different types of liability insurance include:

- *Professional liability insurance*: A type of liability coverage used by professionals to protect themselves against liability suits incurred because of errors and omissions while performing their professional services.
  - *Medical malpractice insurance*: A type of professional liability insurance. Protects healthcare professionals, including medical assistants, from liability related to wrongful practices resulting in injury, expense, and property damages. It also covers the cost of defending lawsuits.
- *General liability* or *commercial liability insurance*: A type of liability coverage purchased by companies. It protects businesses from lawsuits for property loss and bodily injury from nonemployees.
- *Personal injury insurance*: A type of liability coverage that protects against claims related to harm other than bodily injury. Coverage can be for invasion of privacy, slander, imprisonment, and so on.

When a professional purchases a policy, it is important to understand the types of policies.

- *Claims-made policy*: An insurance policy that covers claims made during the policy year. For example, if a provider has a claims-made policy for the current year, any claims that come in this year will be covered.
- *Occurrence policy*: An insurance policy that covers claims for wrongful acts that occurred during the policy year. For example, if a provider has an occurrence policy for the current year, any wrongful acts that occur this year will be covered when the claims are filed in future years.
- *Nose coverage*: A limited-term policy purchased from the new carrier the provider is joining. The policy covers the provider between the end of the prior policy and the start of next policy. Nose coverage can also be referred to as *retroactive* or *prior acts coverage*.
- *Tail coverage*: A limited-term policy purchased from the insurance carrier that the provider is leaving. The policy covers the provider until the new policy starts. A person would need only nose or tail coverage, not both.

CONTRACTS

Most people are aware of contracts. We sign contracts for cell phone plans, rental properties, and payment plans. We also have contracts in healthcare. The healthcare facility's business manager signs contracts for equipment and building rental, service agreements, and so on. The most common contract is the provider-patient contract.

A *contract* is an agreement between two parties. For a contract to be legally binding, five elements must be present:

- *Offer*: Made by one party. Example: A family practice physician advertises complete physicals for $150.
- *Acceptance*: A second party agrees to the offer. Example: After seeing the advertisement, a patient calls to make an appointment.
- *Consideration*: Each party exchanges something of value. Example: The physician gives a physical exam, and the patient pays $150.
- *Legal subject matter*: The consideration must be legal. Example: The board-certified physician can legally perform physical exams. The payment is legal tender (money).
- *Competency* and *capacity*: A person entering a contract must have the legal capacity to be held liable for the contract obligation. If one or both parties is underage (a minor) or shows signs of incompetence (in KOM pi tahns), intoxication, or acting under the influence of drugs, this would invalidate a contract. An emancipated (i MANS i pa ted) minor can enter into contracts (Box 18.5). Example: Both the physician and the patient are adults with the capacity to understand the contract.

BOX 18.5 Emancipated Minors

Conditions for Emancipation

Must be at least 16 years of age in most states and usually must meet one of the following:

- Married
- In the US military
- Living on their own and managing their own money

Benefits of Emancipation

- Can be a party in a contract (e.g., rent housing, purchase agreements)
- Can sue
- Can keep earned income and apply for public benefits
- May make all healthcare decisions regarding oneself

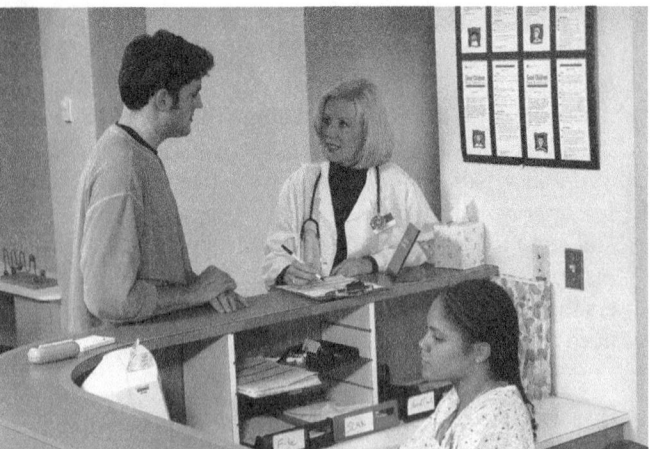

Fig. 18.2 The provider-patient relationship is built on a strong foundation of trust, but it also is a contractual relationship. (From Proctor D, Niedzwiecki B: *Kinn's the medical assistant,* ed 13, St. Louis, 2017, Elsevier.)

A contract can be either an implied contract or an expressed contract.

- *Implied contract*: The parties have agreed to the terms of the contract through their actions and behaviors. The provider-patient relationship is an implied contract (Fig. 18.2).
- *Expressed contract*: The parties have specifically stated the terms of the contract in writing, orally, or both. A service contract for office equipment maintenance is an expressed contract.

Specific types of contracts must be in writing to avoid fraud. These types of contracts are outlined in each state's statute of frauds. *Statutes of fraud* vary slightly, but all indicate that contracts need to be in writing and signed by both parties. Contracts that need to be in writing include:

- Contracts that are property related, such as real estate sales, real estate leases for longer than 1 year, and transfer of property upon the owner's death
- Agreements to pay another's debt
- Contracts that last longer than 1 year or last longer than the life of an individual
- Contracts over a certain amount of money (varies by state)

VOCABULARY

emancipated minor A minor who has been granted emancipation by the court; the minor can assume the rights and responsibilities of adulthood.

incompetence The state of being incompetent or lacking the ability to manage personal affairs due to mental deficiency; an appointed guardian or conservator manages the person's affairs.

liable Legally responsible or obligated.

minor One who has not reached adulthood; usually age 18 or 21, depending on the jurisdiction.

patient abandonment A form of medical malpractice, also called negligent termination; the provider ends the provider-patient relationship without reasonable or adequate notification.

respondeat superior Latin for "let the master answer"; a legal doctrine by which the employer/provider is legally responsible for the wrongful actions or lack of actions of employees if done within the scope of employment.

Provider-Patient Relationship

The contract that is established between the provider and the patient is legally binding. The patient accepts the provider's offer when a patient makes an appointment to see the provider. This means the provider has a duty to see, diagnose, and treat the patient. The patient has the responsibility to follow the provider's recommendations and pay the bill.

As indicated earlier, duty to the patient is one of the 4 Ds in proving malpractice. The duty to the patient is established during the initial visit of the patient. From that time onward, the provider has a duty to the patient. Both parties can terminate the contract or relationship. A patient can terminate the contract at any time. The patient may no longer need the provider's services. The patient may decide to use another provider.

Reasons providers can terminate the patient relationship or contract include:

- Retirement or moving
- Patient is not paying for the services provided
- Patient is not following or is noncompliant with the provider's treatment plan
- Patient's behavior (e.g., rude, abusive, drug seeking, and not showing up for appointments)

The provider must follow the legal process to terminate the contract. A provider can be charged with **patient abandonment** if they simply stop providing care to the patient. To prevent abandonment allegations, the provider must follow the correct legal steps to terminate the provider-patient relationship:

- Provider must notify the patient in writing of the withdrawal of care.
- A date must be indicated for the termination. There must be an adequate period of coverage to allow the patient to find another provider. Fifteen to 30 days is usually recommended.
- The termination letter should be sent as a certified letter with return receipt requested.
- A copy of the letter and the return receipt need to be placed or scanned into the patient's health record.
- Scheduling staff should be notified of the termination date so no appointments are made after that date.

There are many situations in which allegations of patient abandonment may occur:

- Failing to follow up with the patient. If a patient calls or emails the provider or facility, follow-up with the patient must be made in a reasonable period of time.
- Failing to have another provider cover the practice during vacations or when the facility is closed.
- Discharging a patient without proper instructions.

The medical assistant has an important role in ensuring that the patient is not abandoned. Typically, the medical assistant is responsible for answering patient calls and emails in a timely manner. Documentation in the patient health record must reflect all communication with the patient.

If the medical assistant does not follow up with the patient, allegations of abandonment can be brought against the medical assistant and the provider. **Respondeat superior** (re SPON dee at soo PIR ee ahr) is a common law doctrine that means "let the master answer." The doctrine means that the employer/provider is liable for actions that the employee did or did not do within the scope of employment. This means that the medical assistant's actions affect the employer and the provider. The medical assistant's actions or lack of actions can lead to malpractice allegations for the provider.

Breach of Contract

A *breach of contract* occurs when the terms of the contract are not fulfilled by one party without a legitimate legal reason. The breach can occur when the terms are not met by the stated deadline. It can also happen when the terms are not met or performed. An allegation of a breach of contract can lead to a lawsuit. The injured party attempts to force the contract terms to be met or to receive compensation for financial loss caused by the breach.

In the healthcare field, a breach of contract can occur with the provider-patient relationship. Breach of contract may occur with improper termination and abandonment situations. Breach of contract may also occur with the business side of the facility, including:

- Business contracts (e.g., leases for equipment)
- Payment contracts with patients

CONSENT

Consent means one party voluntarily agrees with another party's proposition or plan. In healthcare, several types of consent are used.

- *Implied consent*: Consent that is inferred based on signs, actions, or conduct of the patient rather than oral communication (using words). For instance, the medical assistant asks a patient if he can obtain a blood pressure reading. The patient removes her arm from her jacket sleeve and extends it toward the medical assistant.
- *Expressed consent*: Consent that is given either by the spoken or written word. For example, the medical assistant asks the patient's preference for which arm should be used for an injection. The patient states she wants the injection in her upper right arm. The medical assistant gave the patient a choice, and the patient expressed her consent by stating her choice.
- *Informed consent*: A legal process that ensures the patient or guardian understands the treatment and gives consent for the treatment. With informed consent, the provider must educate the patient on the treatment before the patient signs the consent form. More information on the informed consent doctrine is given in the following section.

- Surgical procedures; may include minor surgery done in ambulatory care facilities
- Complex procedures and tests (e.g., endoscopy, biopsy, exercise or nuclear stress test)
- Administration of high-risk medications and most vaccines
- Participation in a research study
- Cancer treatment (e.g., radiation, chemotherapy)
- Some medical laboratory testing

The provider, not the medical assistant, has a duty to provide information to the patient or guardian. The provider must educate the patient on the treatment options. Once the information has been given, the patient or guardian makes an informed decision regarding treatment.

Informed consent requirements may vary slightly from state to state. The requirements are usually described in the state's medical practice act. For an informed consent to occur, seven elements must be present:

1. The patient or guardian is competent to understand and decide.
2. The patient or guardian voluntarily decides to agree to or refuse the treatment.
3. The patient or guardian understands the diagnosis and reason for treatment.
4. The patient or guardian understands the proposed treatment and the risks of the treatment.
5. The patient or guardian understands the alternative treatments available and the risks of the treatments.
6. The patient or guardian understands the risks if treatment is delayed or not done.
7. The patient or guardian signs a treatment consent form.

Adults of sound mind can give informed consent. Married minors, minor parents, emancipated minors, and mature minors can also give informed consent (Box 18.6). Patients who cannot legally give informed consent include:

- Patients under the influence of alcohol or drugs
- Patients medicated with a preoperative medication that may affect their understanding (e.g., a sedative)
- A minor
- A patient who is mentally incompetent
- A patient who speaks little or no English. (An interpreter must be used for the patient to give informed consent. The interpreter will translate the information from the provider, questions from the patient, and the information on the consent form. It is important to document in the health record that an interpreter was used.)

CRITICAL THINKING 18.8

Daniela is studying consents. How might you define implied, expressed, and informed consents in your own words?

Doctrine of Informed Consent

With many medical procedures and treatments, informed consent is required, including:

BOX 18.6 Mature Minor

Many states address the mature minor doctrine in their statutes. The definition of a mature minor and restrictions vary from state to state. Differences can be based on:

- A specific age, such as 14 or 16 (or no age may be specified), when one can be considered a mature minor
- The availability of the parent
- The medical concern or treatment

In special situations, such as abortion, sterilization procedures, and human immunodeficiency virus (HIV) testing, each state has specific restrictions. Box 18.7 lists possible state restrictions for abortions. Currently, with abortions, the father of the fetus has no rights. No state requires the father to give consent or to be told about the abortion. For sterilization procedures, states may have waiting periods between signing the consent form and the procedure. The patient may have to be an adult (as defined by the state). For HIV testing, the Centers for Disease Control and Prevention (CDC) recommends that a general consent for medical care form be completed prior to HIV testing. Most states have specific language in the statutes regarding consent and counseling for HIV testing.

In many states, the patient's written consent is required to take a video or picture of the patient. Pictures are taken to show before and after images. These pictures are added to the patient's electronic health record.

The medical assistant may need to prepare the informed consent form (Box 18.8). The following box lists information that should be on the informed consent form. The medical assistant may also need to sign the form as a witness to the signature of the patient. It is important to ask patients before they sign the form if the provider discussed the treatment and if they have any questions. If patients have questions, let the provider know. After all the questions have been answered, then the informed consent form can be signed. Do not have the patient sign if they:

- Do not understand the treatment
- Cannot legally give consent
- Have questions

CRITICAL THINKING 18.9

Daniela is trying to distinguish between a mature minor and an emancipated minor. How would you describe each? What rights would each have in terms of healthcare?

VOCABULARY

mature minor A person under the age of adulthood who demonstrates the maturity to make a personal healthcare decision and can give informed consent for treatment.

PATIENT'S RIGHTS AND RESPONSIBILITIES

Congress has attempted to create laws effecting a patient's "bill of rights" related to patient care and services, but none of the proposed bills has passed. The Affordable Care Act's Patient's Bill of Rights focuses on rights related to insurance. With no federal laws to follow, the American Hospital Association created a patient's bill of rights for its members. In 2003 the American Hospital Association created the Patient Care Partnership. This document helps patients understand the expectations for patients and the patients' rights and responsibilities (Fig. 18.3). Ambulatory care facilities may use this document or have a similar titled document that explains these topics to patients.

A medical assistant is likely to encounter a situation in which a choice of treatments is given to a patient (see Procedure 18.1). It is important that the provider discuss the treatment choices with the patient. If the medical assistant is involved, it is important to find out if the patient has any questions. Questions need to be answered before a decision is made. It is important to be respectful and professional during the discussion. Do not attempt to sway the patient in one direction. If the patient selects the treatment that was not the provider's top choice, it is important to respect the patient's decision. The medical assistant should relay the information to the provider.

A medical assistant should know how to handle the situation if a patient refuses a procedure or treatment (see Procedure 18.1). It is important to follow the facility's policy and procedure in such a situation. Most times the following applies when a patient refuses treatment or procedures:

- Show sensitivity to the patient's rights by being respectful and professional. Remember, it is the right of the patient to refuse.
- Ask the patient if they have questions regarding the procedure. If so, let the provider know.
- Notify the provider of the refusal.
- Document the refusal in the health record. Make sure to include which provider was notified.

BOX 18.7 Types of State Restrictions for Abortions

- Must be performed by a licensed physician
- Mandated counseling on the possible link between abortion and breast cancer, the fetal development, and/or long-term mental health consequences
- Required waiting period (often 24 hours) between the counseling and performing an abortion
- Parental involvement for pregnant minor
- Must be performed in a hospital after a certain gestational age
- Gestational limits (abortion is prohibited after a certain point in the pregnancy)

BOX 18.8 Information on the Informed Consent Form

- Patient's name, date of birth, and health record number
- Name of hospital or facility
- Name of provider(s) performing treatment(s)
- Risks and benefits of the treatment(s)
- Alternative treatment(s) and risks
- Risk if treatment(s) is delayed or not done
- Statement indicating the treatment was explained to the patient or guardian
- Signature of patient or guardian
- Signature and name of person who explained the treatment options
- Signature of the witness
- Date and time consent form was completed

WALDEN-MARTIN
FAMILY MEDICAL CLINIC
1234 ANYSTREET I ANYTOWN, ANYSTATE 12345
PHONE 123-123-1234 I FAX 123-123-5678

Patient Bill of Rights
RIGHTS

1. **Medical Care and Dental Care.** The right to quality care consistent with available resources and accepted standards. The right to refuse treatment to the extent permitted by law and Government regulations, and to be informed of refusal consequences. When concerned about care received, the right to request review of care adequacy.

2. **Respectful Treatment.** The right to considerate and respectful care, with recognition of personal dignity.

3. **Privacy and Confidentiality.** The right, within law and military regulations, to privacy and confidentiality concerning medical care.

4. **Identity.** The right to know, at all times, the identity, professional status, and professional credentials of healthcare personnel, as well as the name of the healthcare provider primarily responsible for his or her care.

5. **Explanation of Care.** The right to an explanation concerning diagnosis, treatment, procedures, and prognosis of illness in terms the patient can understand. When it is not medically advisable to give such information to the patient, information should be provided to appropriate family members or, in their absence, another appropriate person.

6. **Informed Consent.** The right to be advised in non-clinical terms of information (significant complications, risks, benefits, and alternative treatments) needed to make knowledgeable decisions on treatment consent or refusal.

7. **Research Projects.** The right to be advised if the facility proposes to perform research associated with care. The right to refuse to participate in any research projects.

8. **Safe Environment.** The right to care and treatment in a safe environment.

9. **Medical Treatment Facility (MTF) or Dental Treatment Facility (DTF) Rules and Regulations.** The right to be informed of facility conduct rules and regulations. The patient should be informed about smoking rules and should expect compliance with those rules from other individuals. Patients are entitled to information about the MTF or DTF mechanism for the initiation, review, and resolution of patient complaints.

RESPONSIBILITIES

1. **Providing Information.** The responsibility to provide, to the best of his or her knowledge, accurate and complete information about complaints, past illness, hospitalizations, medications, and other matters relating to his or her health. A patient has the responsibility to let his or her primary healthcare provider know whether he or she understands the treatment and what is expected of him or her.

2. **Respect and Consideration.** The responsibility for being considerate of the rights of other patients and MTF and DTF healthcare personnel and for assistance in the control of noise, smoking, and the number of visitors. The patient is responsible for being respectful of the property of other persons and of the facility.

3. **Compliance with Medical Care.** The responsibility for complying with medical and nursing treatment plans, including follow-up care, recommended by healthcare providers. This includes keeping appointments on time and notifying the MTF or DTF when appointments cannot be kept.

4. **Medical Records.** The responsibility for ensuring that medical records are promptly returned to the medical facility for appropriate filing and maintenance when records are transported by the patients for the purpose of medical appointment or consultation, etc. All medical records documenting care provided by any MTF or DTF are the property of the U.S. Government.

5. **MTF and DTF Rules and Regulations.** The responsibility for following the MTF and DTF rules and regulations affecting patient care conduct. Regulations regarding smoking should be followed by all patients.

6. **Reporting of Patient Complaints.** The responsibility for helping the MTF or DTF commander provide the best possible care to all beneficiaries. Patients' recommendations, questions, or complaints should be reported to the patient contact representative.

Fig. 18.3 Patient's Bill of Rights.

CRITICAL THINKING 18.10

Bella is working with Daniela on the Patient's Bill of Rights. Bella asks Daniela to summarize these rights. What might Daniela say?

PRACTICE REQUIREMENTS

Many healthcare professionals are required to complete an educational program before they can work in healthcare. Upon completion, they usually must pass an exam before practicing. This section will discuss the practice requirements and scope of practice of physicians, advanced practice professionals, and other healthcare professionals (Table 18.3).

Practice Acts and State Boards

The Tenth Amendment of the US Constitution empowers each state to establish laws that protect the health and safety of that state's citizens. Each state has passed laws and regulations that govern the practice of medicine. These laws and regulations are in a state statute called the *Medical Practice Act*. The Medical Practice Act also outlines the responsibility of the state medical board.

Each state's medical board issues licenses to practice medicine. The board also investigates complaints and disciplines members who violate the law. The state medical board creates policies related to the practice of medicine. Other healthcare professionals (i.e., nurses) have Practice Acts and state boards with similar roles.

MEDICAL TERMINOLOGY	
oste/o	bone
nat/o	birth, born
pre-	before
post-	after
-al	pertaining to
-partum	delivery
-pathy	disease process

TABLE 18.3   Physicians, Advanced Practice Professionals, and Other Healthcare Professionals

Title	Scope of Practice	Education	Credential and License
Physicians			
Doctor of Medicine (MD)	Trained in all areas of medicine to diagnose, treat, and prescribe medications; more focus on symptoms experienced by patient.	Beyond a bachelor's degree, must complete 4 years of medical school and 2–4 years of residency. Additional years of training may be required for specialties.	Must pass all three parts of the United States Medical Licensing Examination (USMLE). Must obtain state license to practice.
Doctor of Osteopathy (DO)	Trained in all areas of medicine, like MD. Specially trained in the nervous and musculoskeletal systems and their influence on health and disease.		
Advanced Practice Professionals			
Physician Assistant (PA)	Diagnoses and treats illnesses and prescribes medication; may specialize. Supervised by physician.	Must complete a 3-year PA program beyond a bachelor's degree.	Physician Assistant– Certified (PA-C) after passing the national exam. Must obtain state license to practice.
Clinical Nurse Specialist (CNS)	Diagnoses and treats patients. Many work in hospital and community settings.	Must complete a master's degree beyond registered nurse (RN) training; an advanced practiced registered nurse (APRN).	Must pass the national certification exam. Must obtain state license to practice.
Nurse Practitioner (NP)	Diagnoses and treats patients and prescribes medication; may specialize. Depending on state law, can be more independent than a PA.		
Certified Nurse Midwife (CNM)	Provides prenatal and postpartum care; delivers babies.		
Certified Registered Nurse Anesthetist (CRNA)	Gives anesthesia and related care to patients in surgery and for outpatient procedures.		
Other Healthcare Professionals			
Registered Nurse (RN)	Works in a wide range of positions, including clinical and administrative; performs more advanced assessments, patient care, and treatments than LPNs.	Have 2–4 years of education.	Must pass a licensure exam to practice.
Licensed Practical Nurse (LPN)	Works in long-term care, ambulatory care, and hospital settings; performs basic patient assessments, patient care, and treatments.	Have 1 year of education.	Must pass a licensure exam to practice.
Medical Assistant (MA)	Primarily works in ambulatory care settings. Performs administrative, clinical, and CLIA-waived laboratory testing under the supervision of a provider.	Varies from about 8 to 24 months; may get a diploma or an associate degree.	National certification exam is optional.

CLIA, Clinical Laboratory Improvement Amendments.

Licensure. Many healthcare professionals must have a state license before they begin their practice. The licensure (LIE sen shur) process allows the state board to ensure that the healthcare professional meets the educational and training requirements. Passing the state licensing exam is a requirement for the license. Once a person gets a license, it needs to be renewed, about every 1 to 2 years. Besides the renewal fee, many state boards require evidence of continuing education.

If a healthcare professional is already licensed in one state, there are different methods of obtaining a license in additional states, including:

- *Licensing exam*: Passing the state's licensing exam and meeting the requirements.

- *Endorsement* (en DOORS ment): A state board grants a license to a person who is currently licensed in another state that has the same or stricter standards.
- *Reciprocity* (RES i pros i tee): A state has a written agreement with another state to recognize licenses issued by that state without additional review of the person's credentials.

In 2015 the Interstate Medical Licensure Compact was created. This compact helped create a streamlined pathway for physicians to get licensure in multiple states. With the changes in healthcare, more rural care is provided by telemedicine (TEL i med i sin), and more physicians are becoming locum tenens (LOE kuhm TEE nenz). With these changes, the need for licensure from multiple states has increased. To be eligible for licensure through the compact's process, physicians need to meet several requirements. Eligible physicians can select the compact member states where they would like to practice. Once the verification process has been completed, the physician will get a full, unrestricted license to practice medicine in those states.

VOCABULARY

licensure A mandatory process established by state law that ensures a person has met the legal standards for practicing an occupation in that state.

locum tenens Latin for "to substitute for"; the term refers to physicians or advanced practice professionals who temporarily contract to provide healthcare services when a facility has a vacancy, vacation, or a leave of absence.

telemedicine The use of telecommunication technology to provide healthcare services to patients at a distance; it is usually used in rural communities.

Scope of Practice. The *scope of practice* for an occupation defines the procedures, actions, and processes that individuals are permitted to perform. A state board determines the scope of practice for that state's specific occupations. In some cases, the medical state board oversees the scope of practice of other healthcare occupations. If healthcare professionals practice beyond their scope of practice, they risk being sued for malpractice (Box 18.9).

The scope of practice for physicians is similar across the states. Physicians diagnose, treat, prevent, or monitor disease conditions. The scope of practice differs between specialties. For instance, a family practice physician cannot perform heart surgery.

For medical assistants, the scope of practice laws vary by state. Typical duties of a medical assistant include:

BOX 18.9 Legal Example: Scope of Practice

An obstetrician-gynecologist performed a procedure on a patient in her office. A few days after the procedure, the patient had increased pain that radiated along her side to her back. The patient called the office and spoke to a medical assistant. She mentioned the increase in pain, bleeding, and changes in her bowel movements. The medical assistant thought she had a urinary tract infection, so she asked the patient if she had any of the typical symptoms. The medical assistant did not talk to the provider about the patient's pain or bleeding because she did not think the complaints were serious enough. The medical assistant did not ask more questions about the pain or bleeding. The medical assistant told the patient her symptoms could be normal and advised her to take 800 mg of ibuprofen. (The medical assistant had been instructed by the providers to advise patients to take ibuprofen, 800 mg, every 8 hours as needed, for any sort of abdominal or back pain.) Later the patient was admitted to the intensive care unit, had to undergo a hysterectomy, and later died. Two months after the procedure, the patient's antibiotic prescription was found at the front desk. (The front desk staff had failed to give the patient the prescription after the procedure.)

The plaintiff sued for damages for the doctor's professional negligence (malpractice) and the clinic for the medical assistant's and front desk staff's negligence. After a 16-day trial, the jury returned a verdict for the defense. The plaintiff appealed. The appeals court ruled that the complaint was ordinary negligence and not medical malpractice. The appeals court also stated that the plaintiff could sue the clinic and medical assistant. The jury would have to decide if the medical assistant had practiced medicine without a license.

From *Wong v. Chappell*, No. 333 Ga. App. 422, (2015). https://www.leagle.com/decision/ingaco20150713164.

- Obtaining and recording the patient's history and personal information
- Obtaining and recording vital signs (blood pressure, pulse, respiration rate), height, and weight
- Assisting the provider during physical exams
- Administering oral, injectable, and inhaled medications as directed by provider and as permitted by state law
- Obtaining blood samples for laboratory tests
- Performing CLIA-waived laboratory tests
- Scheduling patients for appointments
- Performing receptionist duties
- Billing patients for services

Some states allow medical assistants to perform injections. Some states do not allow medical assistants to give certain types of injectable medications or to calculate the medication amount. It is important for you to know the legal scope of practice in your state (see Procedure 18.2 and Box 18.9).

Disciplinary Action. The state boards have an obligation to the public to protect consumers. To do this, state boards take disciplinary action against licensed professionals for felony convictions and unprofessional, improper, or incompetent practice. Examples of unprofessional conduct by physicians include:

- Substance and alcohol abuse
- Neglect of a patient
- Sexual misconduct
- Not meeting the accepted standard of care
- Dishonesty when obtaining a license or failing to meet the continuing education requirement
- Conviction of a felony or fraud
- Inadequate record keeping
- Delegating others to practice medicine

The following are some of the disciplinary actions state boards can take against healthcare professionals:

- *License revoked*: License is terminated, and the person can no longer practice in that occupation in the state.
- *License suspended*: Person cannot practice in that occupation for a specific period of time.
- *License surrendered*: Person voluntarily gives up license.
- *Probation*: Person's license is monitored for a specific period of time.
- *Reprimand*: Person is sent a warning or letter of concern.

Certification and Registration

For some healthcare professional occupations, certification or registry is available. *Certification* (ser ti fi KAE shun) is a voluntary process indicating that a person has met predetermined criteria. The certification is granted by a nongovernmental agency, such as a national association. Most certifications require educational preparation and passing the certification exam. Medical assistants can obtain a certification. For advanced practice professionals, many state boards require certification before the professional can apply for a license. Ongoing certification requirements vary by state. In many states, the ongoing certification is voluntary.

Some healthcare occupations have registration. People working in a specific occupation have their name entered into an official registry. To become registered, a person must meet requirements. These may include educational training, passing a registry exam, participating in continuing education, and conditions of that registry.

Accreditation

Accreditation (ah KRED i tae shun) differs from licensure and certification. *Accreditation* is a recognition granted by a specific organization to educational, healthcare, or managed care organizations that have demonstrated compliance with standards. Common accreditation organizations include:

- *The Joint Commission*: Accredits ambulatory care facilities, hospitals, behavioral healthcare facilities, home healthcare agencies, and laboratory services.
- *National Committee for Quality Assurance* (NCQA): Accredits health plans (i.e., managed care plans).

- *College of American Pathologists* (CAP) Laboratory Accreditation Program: Accredits medical laboratories.
- *Commission on Accreditation of Allied Health Education Programs* (CAAHEP): Accredits specific allied health programs, including medical assisting.
- *Accrediting Bureau of Health Education Schools* (ABHES): Accredits both schools and specific allied health programs, including medical assisting.

There are advantages to being accredited. Students from accredited medical assisting programs can take specific certification examinations. Agencies that have Joint Commission accreditation gain the community's confidence in the quality and safety of the care provided. The accreditation is recognized by insurance companies and may reduce liability insurance costs.

CLOSING COMMENTS

Learning about concepts of law is important for all healthcare professionals. The medical assistant is trained to perform administrative, patient care, and laboratory skills that are CLIA waived (i.e., permitted for medical assistants by the Clinical Laboratory Improvement Amendments). With this wide range of duties, it is critical that the medical assistant always remember to work within the boundaries of the law and their scope of practice.

Areas that can be problematic for medical assistants and may lead to lawsuits include:

- Not following up with patients who call the ambulatory care facility

- Not getting consent before giving a child a vaccination
- Not documenting phone calls, procedures, and treatments
- Identifying oneself as another type of healthcare professional (e.g., a nurse)
- Giving advice to patients without the permission of healthcare providers

With the increase in lawsuits through the years, healthcare professionals must practice within their scope of practice and ensure that patients have no grounds for lawsuits.

PATIENT-CENTERED CARE

One of the elements of patient-centered care is respect for patients' preferences. The medical assistant may not understand why a patient refuses a test, procedure, or treatment. Some patients do not share their thoughts on such matters. Other patients may cite a personal belief or a religious belief. As a medical assistant, you might not agree with the patient's ideas or beliefs. To provide exceptional customer service, a medical assistant must be sensitive to the patient's rights. This means the medical assistant must be respectful of the patient's right to refuse and must notify the provider. It is not appropriate for the medical assistant to:

- Pressure the patient into changing the refusal
- Gossip with peers about the patient's refusal
- Make fun of the patient

Providing patient-centered care means the medical assistant respects patients and their right to refuse.

BEING PROFESSIONAL

As explained in the chapter, patients have the right to refuse treatments and tests. The medical assistant needs to respect the patient's wishes.

Role-play this scenario: You are a medical assistant. Your peer will play Mrs. Ella Jones, a new patient to the practice. Mrs. Jones comes in for her 28-week pregnancy check. After examining her, the provider orders RhoGAM, because she is an Rh-negative mother. (RhoGAM is a blood product made from purified plasma. It is given to Rh-negative mothers during and after pregnancy to prevent Rh incompatibility.) You prepare the medication and go to the exam room. You explain to Mrs. Jones what the provider ordered. She asks, " Is RhoGAM a blood product?" She is a Jehovah's Witness and cannot accept blood products. Respond to Mrs. Jones.

CHAPTER REVIEW

This chapter discussed the balance of power in the state and federal governments. Types of law, including criminal and civil laws, were explained. The plaintiff in criminal cases is the government. Criminal offenses are classified as misdemeanors and felonies. The plaintiff in civil cases is an individual. The plaintiff can sue the government, businesses, and individuals. When the plaintiff wins a civil suit, damages may be awarded. Intentional torts and negligent torts can occur in healthcare. It is important that all healthcare professionals

make sure their actions and behaviors do not lead to intentional or negligent torts.

In healthcare cases, the defense lawyer may use different defenses. Using a legal defense, a legal technicality (e.g., the statute of limitations) can lead to dismissal of a case. Denial and affirmative defenses may also be used.

The court process was discussed, along with the two types of alternative dispute resolution. Arbitration leads to a binding decision, whereas mediation does not.

In malpractice cases, the 4 Ds of negligence need to be proven: duty of care, dereliction, damages, and direct cause. If one of these is not proven, malpractice has not occurred. Professional liability insurance can be purchased by providers (and other healthcare professionals) to help protect against lawsuit settlements.

The provider has a unique relationship with patients. This provider-patient relationship is a contract. It is important that the staff's and the provider's actions do not lead to a breach of contract.

The following consents were discussed:
- *Implied consent*: Consent that is inferred based on signs, actions, or conduct of the patient rather than oral communication (using words).
- *Expressed consent*: Consent that is given either by the spoken or written word.

- *Informed consent*: A legal process that ensures that the patient or guardian understands the treatment and gives consent for the treatment.

The licensure process allows a state board to ensure that a healthcare professional meets the education and training requirements. Providers and other licensed healthcare professionals have several options for obtaining a secondary license to practice in another state.

The scope of practice for an occupation defines the procedures, actions, and processes that individuals in that occupation are permitted to perform. A state board determines the scope of practice for that state's specific occupation.

The state boards can take disciplinary actions against licensed professionals for felony convictions and unprofessional, improper, or incompetent practice.

SCENARIO WRAP-UP

Daniela enjoyed working with Bella as she studied for her midterm exam in her law class. She found that Bella had unique ways of remembering and explaining concepts. These methods helped Daniela. Daniela knew it was important for her to understand the concepts because they might appear on her national certification test.

Daniela now understands the legal importance of answering patients' calls and returning them. She knows this is important to prevent abandonment suits from patients. Daniela encourages her peers to return calls in a timely manner and has talked with her supervisor about strategies to make the reception desk more efficient.

Thanks to Bella's help, Daniela also realizes the importance of the Patient's Bill of Rights to patients and to every healthcare professional. These rights must be upheld and respected. Medical assistants and other healthcare professionals must be sensitive when patients refuse tests, treatments, and procedures. Daniela is looking forward to studying more about the healthcare laws and learning how they affect her job.

PROCEDURE 18.1   Apply the Patient's Bill of Rights

Tasks
Apply the Patient's Bill of Rights in scenarios related to choice of treatment, consent for treatment, and refusal of treatment. Demonstrate sensitivity to the patients' rights.

Scenario 1 (Choice of Treatment):
Julia Berkley (DOB 07/05/1992) saw Dr. Angela Perez during her entire pregnancy. Julia is experiencing some complications. Dr. Perez explained the choices Julia had for delivery. She stated that, with the complications, a cesarean delivery (C-section) may be the best option. Because you are working with Dr. Perez, you prepare the consent form for the C-section. You go into the exam room to have Julia sign the consent form. As you discuss the form, Julia tells you that she is fearful of a C-section and wants a vaginal delivery.

Scenario 2 (Consent for Treatment):
Ken Thomas (DOB 10/25/1961) sees Jean Burke, NP, before leaving on a week-long trip out of the country. He is leaving in 3 days and wants a hepatitis A vaccine injection. The area he is traveling to has a high risk for hepatitis A. Jean Burke orders immunoglobulin for Ken, which will provide immediate protection against hepatitis A. You prepare the injection and enter the exam room. As you are telling Ken about the side effects of the medication, he asks, "What is immunoglobulin?" You reply that it is a sterile medication made of antibodies from blood. Ken states that he is a Jehovah's Witness and cannot receive blood products.

Scenario 3 (Refusal of Treatment):
Aaron Jackson (DOB 10/17/2011) is brought in by his mother for his well-child checkup. His records indicate that he is due for his first varicella vaccine injection. You bring the Varicella (Chickenpox) Vaccine VIS (vaccine information statement) and the Vaccine Authorization form to the exam room. As you start to discuss the vaccine, Aaron's mother, Patricia, interrupts you and tells you she is not interested in having Aaron get his chickenpox vaccination.

Equipment and Supplies
- Patient health records
- Patient's Bill of Rights
- General Procedure Consent form
- Varicella (Chickenpox) VIS (available at https://www.cdc.gov)
- Vaccine Authorization form

Procedural Steps
1. Review the Patient's Bill of Rights. Apply the Patient's Bill of Rights as you role-play each of the three scenarios.
   Purpose: A medical assistant needs to be knowledgeable about the facility's Patient's Bill of Rights.
2. Using Scenario 1, role-play the situation with a peer. You are the medical assistant. Demonstrate how a medical assistant should handle the situation. Apply the Patient's Bill of Rights to the situation by remembering the rights of the patient.
a. Show sensitivity to the patient by being respectful and professional. Be open and accepting in your verbal and nonverbal body language.
   Purpose: Being open and accepting shows the patient sensitivity and respect. The medical assistant should never show any mannerisms that would pressure the patient into making a choice that is not what the person wants.
b. Ask the patient if she has any questions about the procedure. Let the provider know if the patient has questions.

PROCEDURE 18.1 Apply the Patient's Bill of Rights—cont'd

Purpose: All patient questions need to be addressed before the patient can make an informed decision on the treatment.

c. Ask the patient what she would like to do. Based on her answer, follow up as necessary.

Purpose: If the patient wants a C-section, then the consent form should be completed. If the patient wants a vaginal delivery, then no consent form will be needed unless indicated by state laws.

d. Using the patient's health record, document the patient's decision and the name of the provider notified.

Purpose: Documenting the patient's refusal of treatment is important legally. It is also important that the medical assistant document that the provider was informed of the decision.

3. Using Scenario 2, role-play the situation with a peer. You are the medical assistant. Demonstrate how a medical assistant should handle the situation. Apply the Patient's Bill of Rights to the situation by remembering the rights of the patient.

a. Show sensitivity to the patient regarding his right to refuse. Be respectful and professional. Be open and accepting in your verbal and nonverbal body language. Be accepting of his beliefs and his refusal.

Purpose: Being open and accepting shows the patient sensitivity and respect. The medical assistant should never show any mannerisms that would pressure the patient into making a choice that is not what the person wants. The patient has a right to make decisions that follow his religious beliefs.

b. When the patient refuses the medication, be respectful in your body language and words. Notify the provider.

Purpose: It is important to be respectful of the patient's decision and notify the provider of the refusal.

c. Using the patient's health record, document the patient's decision and the name of the provider notified.

Purpose: Documenting the patient's refusal of treatment is important legally. It is also important that the medical assistant document that the provider was informed of the decision.

4. Using Scenario 3, role-play the situation with a peer. You are the medical assistant. Demonstrate how a medical assistant should handle the situation. Apply the Patient's Bill of Rights to the situation by remembering the rights of the patient.

a. Show sensitivity to the mother of the patient by being respectful and professional. Be open and accepting in your verbal and nonverbal body language.

WALDEN-MARTIN
FAMILY MEDICAL CLINIC
1234 ANYSTREET I ANYTOWN, ANYSTATE 12345
PHONE 123-123-1234 I FAX 123-123-5678

General Procedure Consent

Patient Name: _____   Date: _____

The Doctor has discussed with you your condition and the recommended surgical or medical procedures to be performed. This discussion was intended to ensure that you had the opportunity to receive the information necessary to make a reasoned and informed decision whether or not to consent to the procedure. This document is written confirmation of the discussion and contains some of the more significant medical information discussed.

1. Based on this discussion, I understand the following condition may exist in my case:

2. I understand the procedure proposed for treating or diagnosing my condition is:

3. I have been informed of the purpose and reasonable expected benefits of the proposed procedure, the possibility of success or failure, major problems of recuperation, the reasonably anticipated consequences if the procedure is not performed, and the available alternatives.

4. I understand that all surgical and therapeutic procedures involve some risks including pain, scarring, bleeding, and infection.

5. I am aware that in the practice of medicine, other unexpected risks or complications not discussed may or may not further acknowledge that no guarantees or promises have been made to me concerning the results of any procedures. Although the benefits are judged to outweigh the risks, should any complications occur, any one of them could be permanent. I hereby voluntarily give my authority and consent to the doctor to perform the proposed procedure described above.

6. I have been given the opportunity to ask questions about my condition, alternative forms or treatment, risk treatment, the procedure to be used, and the risks and hazards involved. I believe I have sufficient information to give this informed consent.

I understand I have read and fully understand the contents of this form, that the disclosure referred to above were made to me and that all blanks and statements requiring insertion or completion were filled in before I signed my name below.

Patient Signature: _____   Date: _____

If a patient is a minor or unable to give consent,
Signature of person authorized to consent for patient: _____

Relationship to Patient: _____

General Procedure Consent Form.

Continued

PROCEDURE 18.1 Apply the Patient's Bill of Rights—cont'd

Purpose: Being open and accepting shows the family member and the patient sensitivity and respect. The medical assistant should never show any mannerisms that would pressure the patient or guardian into making a choice that is not what the person wants.

b. Ask the mother if she has any questions about the vaccine. Let the provider know if the mother has questions.

Purpose: All patient and parent/guardian questions need to be addressed before an informed decision can be made on the treatment.

c. Ask the mother what she would like to do. Based on her answer, follow up as necessary.

Purpose: If the parent/guardian consents to the vaccination, the Vaccine Authorization form must be completed. If the parent/guardian refuses, the provider needs to be notified.

d. Using the health record, document the patient's decision and the name of the provider notified.

Purpose: Documenting the patient's refusal of treatment is important legally. It is also important that the medical assistant document that the provider was informed of the decision.

WALDEN-MARTIN
FAMILY MEDICAL CLINIC
1234 ANYSTREET | ANYTOWN, ANYSTATE 12345
PHONE 123-123-1234 | FAX 123-123-5678

Vaccine Authorization

Last Name:	First Name:
Date of Birth:	Sex: Male Female

Please answer the following questions:

1. Are you sick or do you have a high fever today? (if yes, you should not receive vaccine)	Yes	No	Unknown
2. Are you allergic to chicken, eggs, or egg products?	Yes	No	Unknown
3. Have you ever has an allergic reaction to an injection?	Yes	No	Unknown
4. Are you pregnant, or think you may be?	Yes	No	Unknown
5. Do you have a blood clotting disorder or are you taking blood thinning medication?	Yes	No	Unknown

CONSENT AND RELEASE STATEMENT

I, THE UNDERSIGNED, WISH TO RECEIVE A ——————— VACCINE. I CONSENT TO THE VACCINATION BEING GIVEN TO ME. I HAVE READ THE PROVIDED INFORMATION OR HAVE HAD SUCH EXPLAINED TO ME. I UNDERSTAND THE RISKS AND BENEFITS OF THIS VACCINE. I HAVE HAD AN OPPORTUNITY TO ASK QUESTIONS WHICH HAVE BEEN ANSWERED TO MY SATISFACTION. I HEREBY REQUEST THAT THE VACCINE BE GIVEN TO ME OR TO THE PERSON NAMED ABOVE FOR WHOM I AM AUTHORIZED TO MAKE THIS REQUEST.

Signature:	Date:

Vaccine Authorization Form.

PROCEDURE 18.2   Locate the Medical Assistant's Legal Scope of Practice

Tasks

Search online to locate the legal scope of practice for a medical assistant practicing in your state. Summarize the scope of practice.

Equipment and Supplies

- Computer
- Printer with word processing software
- Internet access

Procedural Steps

1. Using the internet, search for the medical assistant's scope of practice in your state. Read the scope of practice for your state.

   Purpose: Scope of practice information is available online.

2. Using the word processing software, create a short paper summarizing the medical assistant's scope of practice. Address the following points:

   a. Can medical assistants give injections? If so, what type of injections?

   b. Can medical assistants give oral, topical, and/or inhaled medications?

   c. Can medical assistants calculate drug dosages?

   d. What is the medical assistant's role with prescriptions?

   e. Describe additional duties that a medical assistant can legally perform in your state.

   f. Include the website address(es) you used for this paper.

   Note: If your instructor does not provide you with different guidelines for the paper, follow these. Create at least a one-page paper, using double line spacing, a 10- or 12-point font, and 1-inch margins.

   Purpose: Summarizing the scope of practice will help identify the duties a medical assistant can legally perform in your state.

3. After completing the paper, proofread the paper. Use correct spelling, punctuation, sentence structure, and capitalization. Make any changes required. Based on your instructor's directions, submit the paper to the instructor.

   Purpose: Proofreading helps to identify mistakes.

19

Healthcare Laws

LEARNING OBJECTIVES

1. Describe components of the Health Information Portability and Accountability Act (HIPAA); apply HIPAA rules in regard to privacy and the release of information.
2. Describe the Health Information Technology for Economic and Clinical Health (HITECH) Act.
3. Describe the Genetic Information Nondiscrimination Act of 2008 (GINA), in addition to drug laws such as the Food, Drug, and Cosmetic Act and the Controlled Substances Act.
4. Describe the Patient Protection and Affordable Care Act, the Clinical Laboratory Improvement Amendments (CLIA), the Occupational Safety and Health Act, and the Needlestick Safety and Prevention Act.
5. Discuss Good Samaritan Laws.
6. Define the Patient Self-Determination Act, Uniform Determination of Death Act (UDDA), Uniform Anatomical Gift Act (UAGA), and the National Organ Transplant Act (NOTA).
7. Describe compliance with public health statutes related to communicable diseases and perform such compliance.
8. Describe compliance with public health statutes related to wounds of violence, abuse, neglect, and exploitation.
9. Describe compliance with reporting vaccination issues.
10. Discuss how compliance programs work, examine common compliance concerns in healthcare, follow protocol in reporting an illegal activity, and correctly complete an incident report

OUTLINE

▷ OPENING SCENARIO

Daniela Garcia was recently hired as a part-time float receptionist at Walden-Martin Family Medical (WMFM) Clinic. She works with many co-workers and providers. Daniela is attending the medical assistant program at the local community college. She is currently taking a law and ethics course. She has learned about basic law concepts. She is now learning about healthcare laws. Bella, a newly certified medical assistant (CMA), has offered to help Daniela study for her law course. Bella stated that she enjoyed learning about law and its importance in healthcare.

Many of Daniela's friends find law and ethics to be less exciting than other courses. Daniela disagrees with them. She sees the value in learning about laws that affect healthcare. She realizes it will make her a better medical assistant.

The WMFM Clinic administration created policies and procedures to follow federal and state laws. Daniela has already started to see how compliance with laws affects what she does as a receptionist. She understands the importance of following the clinic's policies and procedures. Daniela realizes that by not complying with laws, she would put her job in jeopardy. It could also raise many issues for the facility, including fines from governmental agencies. Daniela is excited to continue learning about healthcare laws.

YOU WILL LEARN

1. To describe the Health Insurance and Portability and Accountability Act, related terminology, the Privacy Rule, and the Security Rule.
2. To explain the impact of the Health Information Technology for Economic and Clinical Health Act.
3. To describe additional healthcare laws and regulations that affect ambulatory care.
4. To explain the provider's role and compliance with public health statutes.
5. To describe compliance programs, including financial, employment, and environmental safety concerns.

INTRODUCTION

In this chapter, we discuss federal and state laws that impact healthcare. Typically, a few people are the "experts" on healthcare laws in an ambulatory care setting. They work with management to create policies and procedures that follow the laws.

- *Policies* are written principles that provide goals for the employees and the facility. For instance, a policy statement may indicate that patient confidentiality is protected at all times.
- *Procedures* are step-by-step directions. They provide a consistent and repetitive approach to accomplish a goal. For instance, there might be a procedure on how to update patient information while protecting the patient's privacy.

Following the laws is important. Not only does it safeguard patients, it also protects employees and the facility. Facilities that do not comply with laws can be fined and have additional penalties imposed by governmental agencies. Therefore medical assistants need to be knowledgeable about healthcare laws.

PRIVACY AND CONFIDENTIALITY

Privacy (PRI vah see) means being free from unwanted intrusion. Privacy was one of the principles on which our country was built. The word privacy does not appear in the Constitution, but privacy elements appear in the amendments. An *invasion of privacy* is the disclosing of private facts without the consent of the individual. An invasion of privacy is an intentional tort.

Confidentiality (KON fi den shee ahl i tee) is a legally protected right of patients. Healthcare professionals have the duty not to disclose medical, financial, and insurance information unless authorized by the patient. Information is shared during the provider-patient relationship, so creating a trusting relationship is critical (Fig. 19.1). The patient shares sensitive, personal information with the provider, which

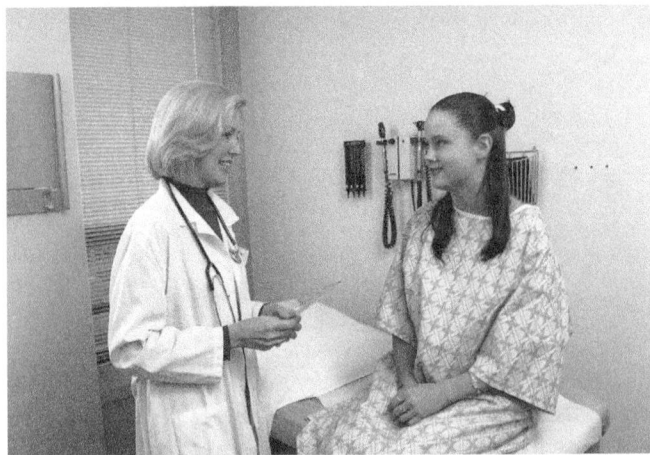

Fig. 19.1 Patient confidentiality is the most important trust that exists between the patient and the provider. (From Proctor D, et al: *Kinn's the Medical Assistant*, ed 13, St. Louis, 2017, Elsevier.)

needs to remain confidential. It cannot be discussed outside of the provider-patient relationship.

All states have laws regarding confidentiality. If the state law is stricter than the federal law, then the state law takes precedence (PRES i duhns). This concept is known as *state preemption*. We will examine the federal laws that relate to privacy and confidentiality in the following sections.

> **VOCABULARY**
> **precedence** The top priority.

Health Insurance Portability and Accountability Act

With the anticipated changes in healthcare technology (e.g., the electronic health record [EHR]), Congress passed the Health Insurance Portability and Accountability Act of 1996 (HIPAA). The US Department of Health and Human Services (HHS) is the agency responsible for developing the specific requirements of the law. The HHS Office for Civil Rights (OCR) enforces HIPAA.

Before HIPAA, the billing and payment processes were slow. Nationwide, insurance companies used many different coding systems. The coding systems were used to provide information on disease and treatments for payment purposes. It took months for facilities to receive insurance payments for services provided to patients. Paper transactions and paper checks were commonly used.

One of the goals of HIPAA was to simplify the electronic exchange of information. All health plans, claims clearinghouses, and healthcare facilities needed to be consistent with their electronic exchange of information. This meant they all needed to use the same coding systems. They also needed to follow the same requirements for the electronic exchange of information. Today, this is called *administrative simplification*. The goal is to reduce the clerical burden and increase electronic transaction adoption.

With the increased electronic transactions, HIPAA also contained provisions for the privacy and security of the patients' information. Primary provisions of the law were stated in four standards:

- *Standard 1 related to transactions and code sets*: HHS adopted standard transactions for the electronic exchange of administrative healthcare information. This included insurance claims, payment, and insurance eligibility information. The goal was to speed up the process of identifying insurance benefits, submitting insurance claims, and receiving payment. Standard 1 also included mandating universal coding systems. Processes become more efficient with everyone using the same coding systems.
  - The Current Procedural Terminology (CPT) is used to code procedures and services.
  - The International Classification of Diseases (ICD) is used to code diseases and disorders.
- *Standard 2 related to the Privacy Rule*: Healthcare facilities, insurance companies, and others need to protect written, electronic, and oral patient health information.
- *Standard 3 related to the Security Rule*: Healthcare facilities, insurance companies, and others need to protect patient information that is electronically stored and transmitted.
- *Standard 4 related to unique identifiers*:
  - National Provider Identifier (NPI): Each covered healthcare provider has a unique identification number that is used for financial and administrative transactions. The NPI is a 10-digit number.
  - Health Plan Identifier (HPI): Each health plan has a unique identifier.
  - Employer Identification Number (EIN): Each employer has a unique identifier issued by the Internal Revenue Service.

In addition to these provisions, HIPAA focused on insurance portability. HIPAA allows extra opportunities to enroll in health insurance plans. For instance, a person can request special enrollment if there is a loss in coverage from another policy. HIPAA prohibited enrollment discrimination based on a person's health history or genetics.

> **VOCABULARY**
>
> **claims clearinghouse** An organization that accepts the claim data from the provider, reformats the data to meet the specifications outlined by the insurance plan, and submits the claim.
>
> **coding system** A system designed to use characters (i.e., numbers and letters) to represent something, such as a medical procedure or a disease.
>
> **electronic health record (EHR)** An electronic record that conforms to nationally recognized standards and contains health-related information about a specific patient. It can be created, managed, and consulted by authorized clinicians and staff from more than one healthcare organization.
>
> **electronic transaction** The electronic exchange of information between two agencies to accomplish financial or administrative healthcare activities.

HIPAA-Related Terminology. HIPAA has many unique terms. The following are some of those terms.

- *Covered entities*: Healthcare providers, health (insurance) plans, and claims clearinghouses that transmit protected health information electronically. Examples of covered entities include:
  - Providers (e.g., medical doctors, doctors of osteopathic medicine, nurse practitioners, physician assistants)
  - Dentists, chiropractors, and psychologists
  - Nursing homes, pharmacies, and ambulatory care facilities (e.g., clinics)
  - Health insurance companies, government insurance programs (Medicare, Medicaid), and health maintenance organizations (HMOs)
  - Claims clearinghouses and billing services
- *Protected health information* (PHI): Individually identifiable health information stored or transmitted by covered entities or business associates. Includes verbal, paper, or electronic information.
- *Business associate*: A person or business that provides a service to a covered entity that involves access to PHI. Examples include legal, billing, and management services; accreditation agencies; consulting firms; and claims processing organizations.
- *Permission*: A reason for releasing or disclosing patient information under HIPAA.
- *De-identify*: To remove all direct patient identifiers from the PHI. In other words, this is the process for removing anything that can link the information back to a specific person. Examples of direct patient identifiers include:
  - Personal demographic information (name, date of birth, address, phone number, Social Security number)
  - Payment and insurance information
- *Limited data set*: PHI that has had all of the direct patient identifiers removed. This would include the name, contact information, Social Security number, and so on. The only information left would be health information. Examples of limited data set information include:
  - Physical or mental health conditions
  - Test results
  - Medications currently taken
  - Allergies

> **CRITICAL THINKING 19.1**
>
> Daniela is working with Bella, a medical assistant who has been helping her with the law course. They are reviewing HIPAA. Bella asks Daniela to describe the four HIPAA standards. How might Daniela respond?

Privacy Rule. The HIPAA Privacy Rule has created national standards that protect health records and other patient information. The Privacy Rule's main purpose is to define and limit the situations in which a patient's information can be used or disclosed. The rule also describes patients' rights over their information. Patients have the right to:

- Examine their health information
- Obtain a copy of their health records
- Request corrections to be made if information is incorrect

Covered entities must comply with the Privacy Rule. They must safeguard all patient information. Covered entities must ensure that business associates also keep PHI private. A written agreement detailing how the business associate will safeguard the PHI must be signed. Covered entities cannot give PHI to business associates until the agreement has been signed (Box 19.1).

BOX 19.2 **Patients and Their Health Information**

It is understood that the contents of the health record belong to the patient. The physical part of the record belongs to the facility or provider. Patients own the contents and can request a copy of their own record at any time. There are state laws that regulate the release. In most cases, the patient can get a copy and can be told of their health information immediately. The following examples illustrate cases in which patients cannot get their information immediately.

- When a provider is treating a patient for emotional or mental conditions, the provider can exercise professional judgment to determine if the records should be released to the patient. This is known as the *doctrine of professional discretion*. The provider may feel that if the patient saw the records, more harm than good would result. For instance, you are obtaining a weight on a patient with an eating disorder. The provider's policy is that you do not share the weight with the patient. The provider makes the decision if the weight is shared. For some patients, a weight gain may harm their current success.
- Another situation in which patients cannot get health information immediately when requested relates to diagnostic tests. In the ambulatory care setting, patients have diagnostic tests done all the time. The provider must review the results before they are given to the patient. After reviewing the results, the provider instructs the medical assistant what to tell the patient. The medical assistant contacts the patient and discusses what the provider stated. After the call, the medical assistant documents the call in the patient's health record.

Only PHI required for the job of the business associates can be given.

The Privacy Rule lists *permissions*, or reasons that the health information can be released. The following permissions do not require written authorization from the patient to release PHI.

- *To the individual*: A covered entity can disclose PHI to the patient. If you want a copy of your health record, you can get it without completing a written authorization (record release form) (Box 19.2).
- *Treatment, payment, and healthcare operations* (TPO): Treatment relates to when the covered entity discloses PHI when coordinating or managing healthcare. For instance, you do not need to sign a written authorization for your provider to send a prescription to a pharmacy. Payment relates to activities related to payment or reimbursement for services. For instance, if you were not paying your bill, the healthcare facility might turn your account over to a collection agency.

They would not need a written authorization from you to disclose your information. Healthcare operations relates to the financial, legal, quality improvement, and administrative activities that healthcare facilities need to do to run and support their business.

- *Uses and disclosures with opportunity to agree or object*: The patient can give informal permission when asked outright or can be given an opportunity to agree or object. For example, a patient comes into the exam room with a friend. You ask the patient if they want the friend to remain. The patient can say yes or no.
- *Incidental use and disclosure*: We need to take reasonable precautions so patient information is not overheard or seen by others. The Privacy Rule does not require that we get written authorization for incidental disclosures. For instance, you take precautions, but you are overheard discussing patient PHI on the phone. There is no need for you to get a written authorization from the patient on the phone for the incidental disclosure.
- *Public interest and benefit activities*: PHI can be released when required by law, law enforcement, and for public health activities. PHI can also be released for research, organ and tissue donation, and for workers' compensation. Funeral directors, coroners, and medical examiners can also obtain PHI.
- *Limited data set*: The direct patient identifiers are removed from the PHI. The remaining information can be used for research, public health purposes, and healthcare operations.

The only permission that requires written authorization from patients is disclosing the PHI to a third party. Examples of this type of disclosure may include when the patient wants another person to be told information or when the patient wants the records transferred to another facility. This may include a life insurance company, an employer for a pre-employment health requirement, another healthcare facility, or the patient's lawyer. In both situations, the patient must sign a form allowing the information to be released. In some agencies, a *disclosure authorization form* (also called an *authorization to disclose form*) must be completed before information can be shared with another person. The patient must complete a *record release form* before the records can be transferred. The form names can differ from facility to facility. To make things more interesting, some facilities combine the forms into one document and may call it a release of information authorization, or something similar.

The forms typically require the patient to indicate the information to be released/disclosed. The form must include the patient's name and the date of the request. The person or facility disclosing the information and receiving the information must be indicated. The form must include an expiration date. These forms also include a statement to notify patients of their right to revoke the release.

✳ **STUDY TIP**

Remember that permission is a reason for release. In HIPAA, it does not mean the patient gives permission for the release.

WALDEN-MARTIN
FAMILY MEDICAL CLINIC
1234 ANYSTREET I ANYTOWN, ANYSTATE 12345
PHONE 123-123-1234 I FAX 123-123-5678

Disclosure Authorization

Full Name: _____   Date of Birth: _____

I hereby authorize _____ to use or disclose my protected health information related to

_____

to _____

Representative's Address:

Purpose:

- I understand that I may inspect or copy the protected health information described by this authorization.
- I understand that, at any time, this authorization may be revoked, when the office that receives this authorization receives a written revocation, although that revocation will not be effective as to the disclosure of records whose release I have previously authorized, or where other action has been taken in reliance on an authorization I have signed. I understand that my healthcare and the payment for my healthcare will not be affected if I refuse to sign this form.
- I understand that information used or disclosed, pursuant to this authorization, could be subject to re-disclosure by the recipient and, if so, may not be subject to federal or state law protecting its confidentiality.

Signature of individual or Representative: _____

Date: _____

Authority or Relationship to Individual, if Representative: _____

This authorization will expire on: _____   If no date or event is stated, the expiration date will be six

years from the date of this authorization.

The subject of this authorization shall receive a copy of this authorization, when signed.

Fig. 19.2 Disclosure Authorization Form.

Disclosure Authorization Process. When patients request their information to be given to another person (e.g., family member, friend), the medical assistants can help. They can assist patients in completing the disclosure authorization form (Fig. 19.2). Once completed, this form must be added to the patient health record.

When a person calls requesting information on a current patient, the medical assistant should first ask the caller's name. The medical assistant must check to see if the caller is listed on the patient's disclosure authorization form (see Procedure 19.1). If that caller's name appears, then, per the facility's policy, the medical assistant can release information about the patient. If the caller's name is not on the form, the medical assistant

- cannot release the patient's information.
- cannot even acknowledge that that person is a patient of the facility.

Applying HIPAA rules is important when protecting a patient's privacy.

In some facilities, the patient supplies a code word or number. This is entered into the patient record. The patient gives this code to family members. When they call the staff and give the code, the staff member can provide an update on the patient. It is understood that the patient gives consent to anyone who received the code. This helps to settle the issue of who is really calling requesting information. The code system may be seen more in the ambulatory surgical departments.

Records Release Process. Patients must complete, date, and sign a (medical) records release form for their records to be transferred to another facility (Fig. 19.3; also see Procedure 19.2). No records, including images and videos, can be released without the completed form. Release forms may specifically address the release of videos and images. With these forms, patients must indicate they want these to be released. If that is not done, then the videos and images are not released.

Parts of the patient record are held at a higher level of confidentiality. Many release forms require the patient to indicate if psychotherapy notes, substance abuse information,

WALDEN-MARTIN
FAMILY MEDICAL CLINIC
1234 ANYSTREET I ANYTOWN, ANYSTATE 12345
PHONE 123-123-1234 I FAX 123-123-5678

Medical Records Release _____

Patient Name: _____	Date of Birth: _____
SSN: _____	Phone: _____
Address:	

I, _____ authorize _____
to disclose/release the following information (check all applicable):

☐ All Records   ☐ Abstract/Summary

☐ Laboratory/pathology records   ☐ Pharmacy/prescription records

☐ X-ray/radiology records   ☐ Other

☐ Billing records

Note: If these records contain any information from previous providers or information about HIV/AIDS status, cancer diagnosis, drug alcohol abuse, or sexually transmitted disease, you are hereby authorizing disclosure of this information. A copy of this signed authorization must be given to the individual.

These records are for services provided on the following _____
date(s):

Please send the records listed above to (use additional sheets if necessary):

Name: _____	Phone: _____
Address:	Fax: _____

The information may be used/disclosed for each of the following purposes:

☐ At patient's request   ☐ For employment purposes

☐ For patient's healthcare   ☐ Other

☐ For payment/insurance

This authorization shall expire no later _____ or upon the following event _____ , and may not
than:
be valid for greater than one year from the date of signature for medical records.

I understand that after the custodian of records discloses my health information, it may no longer be protected by federal privacy laws. I understand that this authorization is voluntary and I may refuse to sign this authorization which will not affect my ability to obtain treatment; receive payment; or eligibility for benefits unless allowed by law. By signing below I represent and warrant that I have authority to sign this document and authorize the use or disclosure of protected health information and that there are no claims or orders that would prohibit, limit, or otherwise restrict my ability to authorize the use or disclosure of this protected health information.

_____	_____
Patient signature (or patient's personal representative)	Date
_____	_____
Printed name of patient representative	Representative's authority to sign for patient (i.e. parent, guardian, power of attorney, executor)

Fig. 19.3 Medical Records Release Form.

Drug and alcohol substance abuse and HIV content in patient records also are held at a higher level of confidentiality (Box 19.3). There are many federal and state laws that relate to the privacy of these records. The federal statute called Confidentiality of Alcohol and Drug Abuse Patient Records, enforced by a division of HHS, is one example. This law restricts the release and use of patient records that include substance use diagnoses and services. State preemption applies with these privacy laws.

CRITICAL THINKING 19.2

Daniela and Bella are reviewing HIPAA concepts. They start to discuss local news and a case in which a medical assistant snapped a picture of a patient record and posted it to a popular social media site. Bella asks Daniela what this act violated. How would you answer this question? Why are employee cell phones a risk in the healthcare setting?

and human immunodeficiency virus (HIV) information should be released. Such information may not be automatically released with the other records due to federal and state legislation.

Under HIPAA, psychotherapy notes are treated with higher levels of confidentiality. *Psychotherapy notes* include the patient-provider details from mental health treatment either from private, group, or family therapy. Psychotherapy notes include what the patient stated during the session and the provider's analysis of the patient's statements and the situation. Psychotherapy notes need to be stored separately from the patient paper health record. If the health record is electronic, the access to the psychotherapy notes is limited to those healthcare professionals who work in the mental health area. Additional information from the visit is not held at a higher level of confidentiality and includes prescriptions, session times, types and frequency of treatments, and results of clinical tests.

Security Rule. HIPAA's Security Rule addresses the national standards used to protect electronic protected health information (ePHI). This rule covers the records that are created, used, received, and maintained by the covered entities. Safeguards important to ensure the security of the ePHI include:

- *Administrative safeguards*: The security officer is responsible for creating and carrying out security policies and procedures. Potential risks to the ePHI must be identified. Steps must be taken to prevent any issues. Cyber attackers pose a huge risk to network security.
- *Physical safeguards*: Facility, workstation, and device security must be implemented. A security officer must create procedures for the proper use of workstations and ePHI.
- *Technical safeguards*: Only authorized employees should have access to ePHI (Box 19.4). Safeguards include audits to track activities of users with the ePHI and encryption of data on mobile devices (Box 19.5). They also include safeguards to prevent improper alteration, destruction, or transmission of ePHI.

BOX 19.4   Legal Example: HIPAA Settlement for Unsecure ePHI

In 2014 Touchstone Medical Imaging notified the Office for Civil Rights (OCR) that one of its servers allowed uncontrolled access to electronic protected health information (ePHI). During the OCR's investigation, it was found that over 300,000 patients' names, birth dates, Social Security numbers, and addresses were exposed on the internet. OCR also found that Touchstone failed to have business associate agreements in place for its internet technology (IT) support vendor and third-party data center provider. As a result, Touchstone paid $3 million in a monetary settlement, along with undertaking a corrective action plan.

Resolution agreement at https://www.hhs.gov/sites/default/files/tennessee-diagnostic-medical-imaging-services-ra-cap.pdf.

BOX 19.5   Legal Example: HIPAA Settlement for Lack of Encryption of Mobile Devices

The University of Rochester Medical Center (URMC) filed breach reports with the Office for Civil Rights (OCR) in 2013 and 2017 due to a loss of an unencrypted flash drive and theft of an unencrypted laptop. OCR's investigation found URMC failed to implement multiple security measures to protect electronic protected health information (ePHI). URMC had a prior OCR investigation regarding a lost unencrypted flash drive in 2010. As a result, URMC paid $3 million in a monetary settlement, along with undertaking a corrective action plan.

Resolution agreement at https://www.hhs.gov/sites/default/files/urmc-ra-cap-508.pdf.

BOX 19.6   Legal Example: HIPAA Settlement for Inappropriate PHI Access

In 2012 Memorial Healthcare System (MHS) submitted a breach report to the Department of Health and Human Services (HHS) indicating that two of its employees inappropriately accessed protected health information (PHI), potentially affecting 80,000 patients. Several months later MHS notified HHS of another 12 users that inappropriately accessed PHI, which potentially affected another 105,646 individuals. As a result, some of the PHI was sold and fraudulent tax returns were filed. In 2017 MHS paid the HHS $5.5 million to settle the potential violations and agreed to implement a corrective action plan.

Resolution agreement retrieved from https://www.hhs.gov/sites/default/files/memorial-ra-cap.pdf.

Chapter 24 provides additional information on network security procedures. It is important for the medical assistant to follow the facility's electronic security procedures. Many facilities have policies to keep passwords confidential. Downloading personal documents puts the computer network at risk and thus is not allowed. *Audit trails* monitor who is looking at which patient's chart (Box 19.6). If the medical assistant is not working with a specific patient, then the patient record should not be accessed. Violating this rule will cause the medical assistant to breach the patient's confidentiality and security. Many healthcare professionals, from providers to medical assistants, have breached confidentiality. They have lost their jobs and licenses or certifications. Many have also been fined.

Health Information Technology for Economic and Clinical Health Act

One of the issues with HIPAA was the limited enforcement and penalties. In 2009, as part of the American Recovery and Reinvestment Act, the Health Information Technology for Economic and Clinical Health (HITECH) Act was passed. HITECH is enforced by the OCR. The HITECH Act contains provisions that increased the enforcement of the privacy and security of electronic transmission and health information. HITECH modified HIPAA in the following ways:

- Made business associates directly liable for compliance with HIPAA.
- Prohibited the sale of PHI without the patient's authorization.
- Created a tiered violation category that included unknowing, reasonable cause, willful neglect–corrected, and willful neglect–uncorrected. Violation penalties range from $100 for each "unknowing" violation to $1.5 million per calendar year. The greater the violation, the greater the penalty amount. Individuals, healthcare agencies, and business associations could be penalized and fined.
- Breach notification requirements were increased. Individuals must be notified of the breach via mail or email. If the facility does not have up-to-date contact information for 10 or more patients, then a notice must be posted on the company's website for at least 90 days. If more than 500 individuals were affected, then the media and the OCR secretary must be notified. A list of breaches reported is published on the OCR website (https://ocrportal.hhs.gov/ocr/breach/breach_report.jsf).

It is important for the medical assistant to be aware of the importance of keeping the PHI secure. Any breaches or loss/theft of computer equipment must be reported immediately to the facility's security officer.

CRITICAL THINKING 19.3

Daniela and Bella are reviewing HITECH. Daniela asks Bella why it is important for large breaches to be posted on the OCR website. How would you answer this question as an employee? How would you answer as a patient of a facility that had a posting on the OCR website?

VOCABULARY

breach Disclosure of protected health information without a reason or permission, which compromises the security or privacy of the information.

Genetic Information Nondiscrimination Act

The Genetic Information Nondiscrimination Act (GINA) became law in 2008. It modified HIPAA and increased the protection for individuals. GINA prohibits genetic discrimination in health coverage and employment.

ADDITIONAL HEALTHCARE LAWS AND REGULATIONS

This section presents additional laws that affect healthcare. Throughout the textbook, these laws and others will be discussed in more depth. This chapter introduces the more common laws that impact ambulatory healthcare.

Drug Laws

Food, Drug, and Cosmetic Act. In 1906, the Food and Drug Act became law. It prohibited the misbranding of food and drugs. It was replaced in 1938 by the Food, Drug, and Cosmetic Act, which is still enforced today. The US Food and Drug Administration (FDA) enforces the act. The FDA is responsible for the safety, effectiveness, security, and quality of drugs, cosmetics, and food. Some of the areas overseen by the FDA include human and veterinary drugs, vaccines, biological products (e.g., blood components), medical devices, food, cosmetics, dietary supplies, and products that give off radiation. When you see recalls of food, cosmetics, or medications, the FDA is involved with the process.

The FDA website (https://www.fda.gov) provides useful information for the healthcare facility. The website is the resource for information and recalls on the areas overseen by the FDA. Many times, the medical assistant is responsible for maintaining the stock medications and equipment in the department. Any medications or medical devices recalled need to be removed immediately and not used. The providers should be notified of recalls.

Controlled Substances Act. The Controlled Substances Act (part of the Comprehensive Drug Abuse Prevention and Control Act of 1970) is a federal law. The US Drug Enforcement Agency (DEA) enforces the law. The DEA oversees the manufacturing, importation, possession, use, and distribution of certain drugs and chemicals. The DEA handles both illegal and legal drugs. The Controlled Substances Act has five schedules of medications. These schedules are arranged from greatest to least abuse potential (Table 19.1). State statutes also address procedures related to scheduled medications. Some scheduled medication prescriptions are handled differently, which will be discussed in Chapter 44. It is important for the medical assistant to be aware of the schedule of medications.

Each provider prescribing scheduled medications needs to have a unique DEA number. The DEA number needs to be renewed every 3 years. The medical assistant may need to assist the provider in renewing or obtaining a DEA number. This can be done at the DEA website (https://www.deadiversion.usdoj.gov/).

Insurance Law

Patient Protection and Affordable Care Act. The Patient Protection and Affordable Care Act is commonly known as the Affordable Care Act. This federal statute was signed into law in 2010. The goal of the law was to provide Americans with affordable health insurance. It also attempted to reform the healthcare system and reduce healthcare spending. A few of the reforms include:

- Insurance coverage of preventive services and immunizations.
- People with preexisting health conditions cannot be dropped or charged more for insurance.
- Dependents can stay on their parent's insurance plan until age 26.
- Large businesses have to provide insurance to full-time workers. Small businesses are eligible for tax credits to help offer insurance coverage to their employees.
- The Physician Payments Sunshine Act (PPSA), part of the law, increases the transparency between providers, teaching hospitals, and manufacturers of medical products (e.g., drugs and medical devices). The manufacturers must report any payments and transfers of value (e.g., gifts, meals) to the Open Payments Program of the Centers for Medicare and Medicaid Services (CMS).

Medical Laboratory Regulations

Clinical Laboratory Improvement Amendments. Congress passed the Clinical Laboratory Improvement Amendments (CLIA) in 1988. CLIA establishes quality standards and regulates laboratory testing. The quality standards focus on accuracy, reliability, and timeliness of test results. The following federal agencies are involved with administering CLIA.

TABLE 19.1	Schedules of Drugs, Substances, or Chemicals	
Schedule	**Psychological and Physical Dependence**	**Examples**
I	Highest potential for abuse; drugs with no currently accepted medical use	Heroin, lysergic acid diethylamide (LSD), ecstasy
II/IIN (C–II)	High level of abuse and can lead to severe psychological or physical dependence	*Schedule II narcotics:* Oxycodone (OxyContin, Percocet), fentanyl (Duragesic), codeine, morphine *Schedule IIN stimulants:* Amphetamine (Adderall), methamphetamine (Desoxyn), methylphenidate (Concerta, Ritalin LA)
III/III N (C–III)	Moderate to low physical dependence or high psychological dependence	*Schedule III narcotics:* Acetaminophen with codeine (Tylenol #3 or #4), buprenorphine *Schedule III N non-narcotics:* Ketamine, anabolic steroids (e.g., Depo-Testosterone)
IV (C–IV)	Low potential for abuse relative to substances in schedule III	*Schedule IV:* Alprazolam (Xanax), clonazepam (Klonopin), diazepam (Valium), lorazepam (Ativan)
V (C–V)	Lowest potential for abuse relative to substances listed in schedule IV; contains limited quantities of certain narcotics	*Schedule V substances:* Robitussin AC, ezogabine (Potiga)

- *Food and Drug Administration:* Oversees the medical laboratory tests. Categorizes the tests based on their complexity: waived, moderate, or high complexity. High-complexity laboratories can perform more tests than waived-complexity laboratories.
- *Centers for Medicare and Medicaid Services:* Inspects laboratories and issues certificates. Enforces compliance with regulations.
- *Centers for Disease Control and Prevention* (CDC): Develops standards and laboratory practice guidelines. Develops professional information and resources mostly related to health and disease topics (https://www.cdc.gov/). (The CDC, a division of HHS, focuses on disease control and prevention, environmental health, and health promotion; thus its overall mission is to improve the health of the people.)

All agencies providing clinical laboratory services, including ambulatory care laboratories, must meet the CLIA requirements. The laboratories must have a CLIA certificate to operate and must be certified by the state. Smaller ambulatory care laboratories have one of the following certificates:

- *Certificate of Waiver:* Allows the facility to perform CLIA-waived tests, which are simple and accurate with little risk for error if done correctly. A urine pregnancy test is a waived test.
- *Certificate for Provider-Performed Microscopy Procedures* (PPMP): Allows the provider to perform only specific microscopy procedures and waived tests.

Additional certificates are obtained by larger laboratories. These laboratories perform more complex tests.

Workplace Safety Laws

Occupational Safety and Health Act. The Occupational Safety and Health Act of 1970 (OSH Act) is enforced by the Occupational Safety and Health Administration (OSHA). Based on this act, OSHA sets workplace standards and conducts inspections to ensure employee safety. Employers must comply with all of OSHA's regulations. Table 19.2 addresses the OSHA standards in healthcare.

> **VOCABULARY**
> **egress** Leaving a place; exit route.

> **CRITICAL THINKING 19.4**
>
> Daniela is reading about OSHA. She thinks back to what she has heard about OSHA in other businesses. What have you heard about OSHA in other businesses? Is OSHA's role in that company similar to its role in healthcare? Explain.

Needlestick Safety and Prevention Act. The Needlestick Safety and Prevention Act was signed into law in 2000. The goal of the act was to reduce the risk of healthcare workers' exposure to bloodborne diseases. The act required OSHA to update its Bloodborne Pathogens Standard. The revised standards apply to all employees with anticipated occupational exposure to blood or other potentially infectious materials (OPIM). The impact of this act includes the following:

- Healthcare workers must use safer medical devices. For example, many needles can be capped with a special safety device after use (Fig. 19.4).

TABLE 19.2 OSHA Standards Related to Healthcare

Standard	Summary	Examples of Workplace Application
Bloodborne pathogens	Protects healthcare workers against the hazards caused by bloodborne pathogens.	Exposure control plans, Universal Precautions, safety needles, personal protective equipment, hepatitis B vaccination, and record keeping.
Hazard communication	Requires employers to provide information about the chemical hazards in the workplace. The General Duty Clause states that any equipment that can pose a health danger must be considered a hazard.	All chemicals are labeled. A Safety Data Sheet (SDS) must be available for each chemical in the workplace. Employees must be trained in how to handle the chemical hazards in the workplace.
Occupational exposure to hazardous chemicals in laboratories	Also called the "laboratory standard." Specifies the requirements of a Chemical Hygiene Plan (CHP).	The CHP is a written program that includes the policies, procedures, and responsibilities that protect employees from hazardous chemicals. The CHP describes the appropriate handling of chemicals in the laboratory.
Ionizing radiation	Addresses the protections needed when working with ionizing radiation (i.e., x-rays).	Signs posted where x-rays are taken. Employees wear personal radiation monitors to detect radiation amounts. X-ray rooms are built with protected areas for the employee. X-ray exposure is limited if the employee is pregnant.
Nonionizing radiation	Addresses the protections needed in place when working with nonionizing radiation (i.e., lasers).	Signs need to be posted on the door of a room where lasers are being used. Appropriate eye protection must be worn at all times by both the patient and the employees. Goal is to prevent blindness, retinal burns, and eye damage due to the radiation.
Means of egress (E gress)	Addresses the exit routes in a building.	Employers are responsible for having appropriate building exit routes. Routes are posted. Exits are unlocked and clear in case of emergency.

OSHA, Occupational Safety and Health Administration.

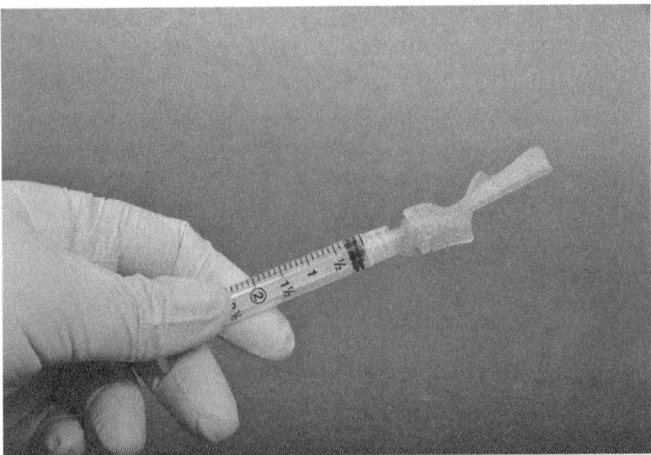

Fig. 19.4 A Safety Needle Device. (From Proctor D, et al: *Kinn's the Medical Assistant,* ed 13, St. Louis, 2017, Elsevier.)

- The facility's Exposure Control Plan must include a sharps injury log documenting all instances of injuries from sharps (e.g., used needles, blades).
- Used needles, blades, and other sharps must be put in sharps disposal containers.
- Personal protective equipment (PPE) (i.e., gloves, mask, and gown) must be worn if there is a risk of blood or body fluid exposure.

Good Samaritan Laws

Good Samaritan laws are state laws that provide legal protection for those assisting an injured person during an emergency. If possible, the injured person needs to agree to the help. The person responding must meet the following criteria:

- Not be paid for the care given
- Act reasonably, exercising the same standard of care (for their profession) within the limitations of the emergency
- Not act negligently or recklessly; such action makes the responder liable for damages

The Good Samaritan law does not mean you cannot be sued. In some states, healthcare professionals who do not assist another person in an emergency can be held liable. It is important to be aware of your state's Good Samaritan law and find out if medical assistants have an obligation to stop and provide first aid.

> ### CRITICAL THINKING 19.5
>
> Daniela is reviewing Good Samaritan laws. How might she describe these laws in terms of importance during an emergency situation?

Laws for End-of-Life Issues

A medical assistant should be aware of laws that relate to end-of-life issues. The following is a brief summary of acts that relate to advance directives, organ donation, and determining death.

- *Patient Self-Determination Act:* Requires most healthcare institutions to inform patients of their right to make decisions and the facility's policies respecting advance directives.
- *Uniform Determination of Death Act* (UDDA): Served as a guide for state lawmakers to create their own laws that define death.

- *Uniform Anatomical Gift Act* (UAGA): Purpose of the act was to make organ donation easier for people.
- *National Organ Transplant Act* (NOTA): Established the Organ Procurement and Transplant Network (OPTN) and also established a national registry for organ matching. These acts will be discussed in depth in Chapter 20.

COMPLIANCE REPORTING

Healthcare agencies and employees are required to comply with all federal and state laws and regulations. There are several areas of compliance on which the healthcare facility must focus. Administrators must have policies and procedures in place for employees to report issues. Reports need to be followed up. Documentation may need to be done for federal or state agencies regarding compliance issues. Healthcare providers also need to report specific diseases, injuries, and issues with vaccines. We will focus on compliance that occurs in ambulatory care facilities.

Compliance With Public Health Statutes

Public health statutes exist in each state to help promote the health of the residents. According to these statutes, healthcare providers have a responsibility to report specific information to various authorities, including:

- Births and deaths
- Specific diseases
- Sexually transmitted infections (STIs)
- Specific injuries related to violence
- Abuse, neglect, and exploitation (eks ploi TAY shuhn)

These topics will be examined more closely in the following sections.

Per the HIPAA permission "public interest and benefit activities," PHI can be released when required by law, law enforcement, and for public health activities. For the mandatory reporting situations based on state statutes, the provider can release PHI without the patient's authorization.

> **VOCABULARY**
>
> **advance directives** Written instructions about healthcare decisions in case a person is unable to make them.
> **abuse** An action that purposely harms another person.
> **neglect** Failure to provide proper attention or care to another person.
> **exploitation** The act of using another person for one's own advantage.

Reportable Diseases. Reportable diseases are communicable diseases that have a significant public health impact. When a provider diagnoses a reportable disease, the state's public health department must be notified. This notification process is called *disease reporting.* Each state has statutes that address disease reporting. Lists of reportable diseases and reporting requirements are typically available on the state's public health department website. The following are examples of reporting levels and reporting procedures, though each state may be slightly different.

TABLE 19.3 Types of Child Neglect and Abuse

Child Maltreatment		Description
Neglect	Physical	Failure to provide adequate nutrition, clothing, shelter, and hygiene. Child has poor growth and hygiene and may hide food for later.
	Educational	Failure to enroll child in school or to home-school child. Child may have a poor school attendance record.
	Medical	Failure to provide needed care for injury, impairment, or illness. Child may have untreated injuries. May see developmental delays from lack of therapy to help with impairment.
Abuse	Physical	Bruises, fractures, or burns that are unexplained or do not match the explanation given; untreated dental or medical problems.
	Sexual	Sexual behaviors inappropriate for child's age; sexually transmitted infections, genital pain and bruising, bleeding.
	Emotional	Delayed emotional development, loss of self-confidence, social withdrawal, headaches, depression, poor school performance.

- *Urgent reporting*: For diseases such as hepatitis A, food or water disease outbreaks, pertussis (whooping cough), measles, plague, and tuberculosis. Reporting must be done immediately, usually by phone or fax.
- *Less urgent reporting*: For diseases such as sexually transmitted infections; hepatitis B, C, D, and E; legionellosis, Lyme disease, mumps, bacterial meningitis, malaria, tetanus, varicella (chickenpox), and toxic shock syndrome. Reporting may be done electronically, by mail or fax. The provider usually has up to 3 days to file the report.
- *Highly confidential reporting*: For diseases such as acquired immunodeficiency syndrome (AIDS) and HIV infection. The provider may need to mail the paperwork to increase confidentiality.

Disease reporting procedures and regulations may vary by state. The medical assistant should be aware of the state's disease reporting process. The provider may ask the medical assistant to contact the public health department regarding a new reportable disease case (see Procedure 19.3).

VOCABULARY

communicable diseases Diseases spread from person to person by either direct contact or indirect contact (e.g., insects).

privileged communication Communication that cannot be disclosed without authorization of the person involved; includes provider-patient and lawyer-client communications.

CRITICAL THINKING 19.6

Daniela is learning about public health statutes and reporting obligations of providers. Why is it important for the public health services to be notified about specific diseases?

Wounds of Violence. Most state statutes require healthcare providers to report cases of violence. Statutes vary from state to state. Typically, reportable cases include wounds caused by gunshots and stabbings; specific types of burns; and nonaccidental wounds caused by a knife, an axe, or a sharp-pointed instrument. The medical assistant should be aware of the state's statutes for reporting wounds of violence. In some cases, the medical assistant may need to assist the provider in preparing documents for law enforcement for such cases.

CRITICAL THINKING 19.7

Daniela is learning about public health statutes and the reporting obligations of providers. Why is it important for law enforcement to be notified about cases of violence?

Child Abuse, Neglect, and Exploitation. The Federal Child Abuse Prevention and Treatment Act (CAPTA) aided the states as state statutes were drafted. The act was updated by the CAPTA Reauthorization Act of 2010. This updated act defined child abuse and neglect as follows:

- Any recent act or failure to act on the part of a parent or caretaker that results in death, serious physical or emotional harm, sexual abuse, or exploitation; or
- An act or failure to act that presents an imminent risk of serious harm

These definitions set the minimum standard for describing child abuse and neglect. States typically address child maltreatment in both civil and criminal statutes.

All states and territories require child maltreatment to be reported. Most states mandate specific professionals to report any child maltreatment, including school personnel, social workers, healthcare providers, nurses, mental health professionals, childcare providers, medical examiners or coroners, and law enforcement officers. Some states require anyone who suspects child abuse or neglect to report the situation (Table 19.3). Mandatory reporters need to provide the facts. They do not have to prove that abuse or neglect occurred. Most state statutes do not consider abuse and neglect information as privileged communication between the patient and the provider. This allows the provider to report the information (and thus protect the maltreated child). The medical assistant should be aware of the state statutes regarding child maltreatment. The Child Welfare Information Gateway website (https://www.childwelfare.gov/) can be used as a resource for state reporting information.

The Unborn Victims of Violence Act was signed into law by Congress in 2004. Prior to this act, babies in utero (also called *fetuses*) harmed or killed due to violence were not considered victims. This act considers babies in utero who are harmed or killed during certain acts of violence to be victims, and charges could be brought forth.

CRITICAL THINKING 19.8

Daniela is learning about child abuse and neglect. How might she describe the difference between abuse and neglect? Why is this information important for medical assistants to know?

Adult Abuse, Neglect, and Exploitation. In 1965 the Older Americans Act was signed into law. The purpose of the act was to maintain the rights and dignity of the older person. It also created the Administration on Aging. Since then, several federal laws have been passed to help fund federal programs.

Abuse, neglect, and exploitation of older adults and depen-dent adults are dealt with in state statutes. All states have the following:

- Adult or elder protective services statutes that provide reporting and investigating procedures for elder abuse in the state.
- Statutes that establish a Long-Term Care Ombudsman Program that advocates for the safety and rights of long-term care facility residents.
- General criminal statutes on fraud, sexual assault, battery, and other abuses that can relate to elder abuse.

Some states require financial institutions (banks) to report suspected financial abuse or exploitation of older adults.

The state statute will dictate who are mandated reporters, when to report, and how to report the situation. Many ambu-latory healthcare facilities are screening older adults to identify those who do not feel safe in their living conditions. If the med-ical assistant suspects abuse, neglect, or exploitation of an older person, it is important to bring it to the provider's attention. Typically, the provider is a mandated reporter under state law. If the provider suspects neglect, abuse, or exploitation, then a report needs to be filed.

State statutes on domestic violence and abuse vary. In some cases, the reporting for injuries caused by violence covers some domestic abuse situations. Some states have mandatory reporting for domestic violence. It is recommended that pro-viders talk to the victim of the domestic violence. They should inform the person when it must be reported. In states where domestic violence is not a mandatory reporting situation, pro-viders can encourage the victim to report the situation. Safe houses are also available in many areas for victims. Having information on local resources for domestic abuse is import-ant in the ambulatory care setting. Providing the information in restrooms is very common. Typically, that might be the only location where the abuser does not follow the victim. It is important to remember that both males and females can be victims of domestic abuse.

VOCABULARY

dependent adults People between the ages of 18 and 64 who have a mental or physical impairment that prevents them from doing normal activities or from protecting themselves.
retaliation Getting back at others for something they did to you.
retribution Punishment inflicted on someone as vengeance for a wrong or criminal act; the act of taking revenge.

Reporting Vaccination Issues

When a healthcare provider orders a vaccine to be given to a child, the medical assistant must provide the parent or guardian with a Vaccine Information Statement (VIS). This document reviews the reasons for and the risks of the vaccine. Prior to giving the vaccine, the medical assistant must have the parent or guardian sign a consent form allowing the administration of the immunization.

If a patient is having an unusual side effect from a vaccine, the provider might need to file a report with the Vaccine Adverse Event Reporting System (VAERS). Patients and families can also file a report. VAERS is a national surveillance program that monitors vaccine safety. It collects information on unusual vac-cine side effects. VAERS is co-sponsored by the CDC and FDA.

In 1986 the National Childhood Vaccine Injury Act was passed. It created the National Vaccine Injury Compensation Program (VICP). This program provides compensation for children injured by childhood vaccines. The VICP lifts the bur-den of lawsuits from vaccine manufacturers and healthcare pro-viders. The VIS contains information about VICP for patients' families.

Compliance Programs

A compliance program or corporate compliance is a program within a business that detects and prevents violations of state and federal laws. An effective compliance program helps pro-tect the organization from fines and lawsuits. Most compliance programs have reporting mechanisms (i.e., a toll-free number or website) where employees can report suspected violations, suspected illegal activity, fraud, abuse, safety issues, and non-compliance issues. It is important for employees to be able to report issues without fear of retaliation (re TAL ee shahn) and retribution (RET rah byou shahn). Many times, reports can be submitted anonymously.

If a medical assistant needs to report a situation, it is import-ant to follow the healthcare facility's policies and procedures. Different reporting pathways are seen in ambulatory care settings:

- If the facility has a compliance reporting procedure: A report can be filed through the compliance reporting mechanisms available to the employee.
- If the facility does not have a compliance reporting proce-dure: The employee may need to report the situation using the chain of command. This means the employee must report the issue to the supervisor. If the supervisor was involved with the situation, then the employee must report the issue to the supervisor's supervisor.

- For employment or conflict-of-interest issues: Some agencies require the employee to contact the human resources supervisor.

In the following sections, we will examine the more common compliance concerns in healthcare.

Financial Concerns. Financial concerns relate to financial and property theft, identity theft, conflict of interest, and fraud. Theft can be of drugs, equipment, supplies, or money. *Identity theft* occurs when someone sells or uses another person's personal information for financial gain. In healthcare, medical identity theft occurs. When a person poses as another person during a healthcare visit, this is considered medical identity theft, because the wrong person's insurance is getting billed for the services. To prevent medical identity theft, many agencies are:

- Requiring photo identification during the check-in process for visits and services
- Taking the patient's picture, which is uploaded to the electronic health record for future reference

Conflict of interest relates to any financial interest, personal or professional activity, or obligation that affects a person's objectivity when performing the job. For instance, a provider owns stock in a pharmaceutical company. This provider then prescribes medications made by that company. The provider is benefiting from patients purchasing medications from that company.

Fraud is a deceitful action that causes another to give up something of value. Healthcare fraud is prevalent. In 2019 Medicare fraud was estimated to be about $28.91 billion. Examples of healthcare fraud include the following:

- Providers and agencies bill for services that were not provided.
- Information is falsified for payment.
- Services are overcharged.
- Medical identification theft occurs.

The list of fraud examples is long. The Office of Inspector General of the HHS oversees fighting fraud and abuse in governmental programs. The following are federal laws that address fraud in healthcare.

- *Anti-Kickback Statute* (AKS): Since 1972, this federal statute has prohibited intentionally receiving or giving anything of value to get referrals or generate federal healthcare program business.
- *False Claims Act* (FCA): Originally signed into law during the American Civil War in 1863 and revised in 2010. It prohibits a person from submitting false or fraudulent Medicare or Medicaid claims for payment. Under this act, a person can bring a civil suit on behalf of the government when they find others sending false claims to the government for payment. The individual can receive part of the settlement.
- *Stark Law* (also called the *Physician Self-Referral Law*): Became law in 1989 and became effective in 1992. Several revisions have been made since then. It prohibits a healthcare provider from referring a Medicare patient for services to a facility with which the provider or the provider's immediate family has a financial relationship.

- *Healthcare Fraud Statute*: Originated in 1996 and revised in 2010. It prohibits intentionally defrauding any healthcare benefit program (Box 19.7).

A medical assistant should be aware of the laws related to fraud and conflict of interest. If violations or illegal activities are noticed in the workplace, the medical assistant should follow the reporting procedures outlined in the facility's compliance program (see Procedure 19.4). Conflicts of interest need to be reported immediately to the human resources supervisor or to your supervisor.

CRITICAL THINKING 19.9

Daniela and Bella are studying compliance. They start to discuss the importance of declaring a conflict of interest. Describe why being upfront and notifying administration/human resources about a conflict of interest is important in healthcare.

Employment Concerns. Employment concerns relate to discrimination (di SKRIM eh nae shahn), harassment (HAR ahs ment), retaliation and retribution, and unfair employment practices. In many states, most medical assistant positions are considered *employment-at-will*. This means that the employer can end employment at any time for any reason. Many states recognize this concept. It also means the employee can quit at any time for any reason, though giving a 2-week notice is considered professional. Most jobs are considered employment-at-will.

Employers cannot fire an employee for an illegal reason. The employer needs to have a just cause, or legal reason, for firing an employee. Legal reasons could include terminations due to cutbacks in staffing or an employee's behavioral issues. A terminated employee may have an opportunity to sue if wrongful termination occurred (Box 19.8). *Wrongful termination* means that the employer did not have just cause for firing the employee. For instance, an employee reported that fraud was occurring in the billing department at the facility. The facility then is under investigation for the fraud. The supervisor fires the whistleblower. Federal and state laws protect the whistleblower from retaliation and retribution (Box 19.9).

VOCABULARY

discrimination Unfair treatment of another person based on the person's age, gender (sex), ethnicity, sexual orientation, disability, marital status, or other selective factors.

harassment Continued, unwanted, and annoying actions done to another person.

whistleblower A person (usually an employee) who reports a violation of the law within an organization. The person reports the information to the public or to a person in authority.

Federal Laws Related to Discrimination. Many federal laws regulate issues regarding employment. The following are laws that address discrimination in the workplace.

A lawsuit alleged that Berkeley Heart Lab, Inc., paid kickbacks to physicians and patients to use the company for blood testing. The kickbacks were disguised as "processing and handling" fees. Patients received kickbacks in the form of waived copayments, which they were legally required to pay for the services provided. The government also alleged that unnecessary cardiovascular tests were being charged to Medicare and TRICARE programs. Quest acquired Berkeley in 2011 and ended the practice of kickbacks. In 2017 Quest Diagnostics, Inc., agreed to pay $6 million to resolve a lawsuit by the United States.

From *United States ex rel. Mayes v. Berkeley HeartLab Inc.*, et al., Case No. 9:11-cv-01593-RMG (D.S.C.) Consolidated with U.S. EX REL. LUTZ v. BERKELEY HEARTLAB, INC.

BOX 19.8 **Legal Example: Wrongful Termination and Invasion of Privacy**

The plaintiff was a security guard at Children's Hospital. He was involved in an accident while on the job. He was examined at the emergency department, given a painkiller, and released. There was no record of intoxication or impairment. The next day, while recovering at home, he was called to the hospital to submit to a drug test. The test was positive for hydrocodone, and the hospital terminated him based on its drug-free workplace policy. He had been an employee for 18 years and had a clean record with no work-related accidents or drug abuse issues. The plaintiff sued the hospital for wrongful termination, invasion of privacy, and defamation. The case went through mediation, and the hospital offered $40,000 to settle. With no resolution, the case was brought to trial. After deliberation, the 12-member jury came back with a 12–0 decision for the plaintiff. He was awarded $385,050 for past and future economic loss and $650,000 for past and future emotional distress. The total verdict for the plaintiff was $1,035,050.

From *Mckinley Nou v. Children's Hospital Central California*, (October 16, 2014) Fresno Superior Court, Case Number: 12-CECG-02169.

BOX 19.9 **Legal Example: Whistleblower Retaliation**

According to a complaint, psychologist Melody Jo Samuelson was hired by Napa State Hospital in California. For 2 years she received good reviews, and then she testified in a case in which she alleged that a patient had been improperly assessed as competent to stand trial. In court she indicated the hospital did not use adequate methods to analyze patients. She complained that the hospital immediately retaliated against her, and she was fired from her job. She appealed her firing and filed a whistleblower retaliation complaint. She was reinstated, but the retaliation continued, she stated. She claimed anxiety and depression as a result of the situation. She was awarded $1 million.

From *Samuelson v. California Department of Mental Health*, et. al., No. 26-57631 (N.D.Cal. Feb. 20, 2014).

- *National Labor Relations Act*: Also called the Wagner Act of 1935. It gave the right to most workers to organize or join a union.
- *Title VII of the Civil Rights Act of 1964* (Title VII): Prohibits employment discrimination based on color, race, gender, religion, or national origin.
- *Age Discrimination in Employment Act of 1967* (ADEA): Revised several times. It protects applicants and employees 40 years and older from discrimination and includes

hiring, promotion, termination, and compensation practices.
- *Rehabilitation Act of 1973*: Prohibits discrimination in employment practices based on physical or mental disabilities. This act applies to federal employers or employers that are federal contractors (provide services to the federal government).
- *Pregnancy Discrimination Act of 1978*: Amended Title VII of the Civil Rights Act of 1964. This act prohibits gender discrimination based on pregnancy.
- *Title I* and *Title V of the Americans with Disabilities Act of 1990* (ADA): Prohibits employment discrimination against qualified persons with disabilities.
- *Genetic Information Nondiscrimination Act of 2008*: Prohibits employment discrimination based on the person's genetic information.
- *Civil Rights Act of 1991*: Provides punitive damages in cases of intentional employment discrimination.

Federal Laws Related to Hours, Wages, and Leave. The following federal laws address hours, pay, and leave in the workplace.
- *Federal Insurance Contributions Act of 1935* (FICA): Created a payroll tax that requires a deduction from a person's paycheck. The withheld amount and an employer contribution fund the Social Security program and a portion of Medicare.
- *Fair Labor Standards Act of 1938*: Prohibits child labor and also provides overtime pay and a minimum wage.
- *Equal Pay Act of 1963* (EPA): Protects against gender-based wage discrimination; requires equal pay for both males and females who are performing the same job at the same organization.
- *Employee Retirement Income Security Act of 1974* (ERISA): Sets minimum standards for pension and health plans in private industry and protects individuals in these plans.
- *Family Medical Leave Act* (FMLA) *of 1991*: Provides unpaid leave time for maternity, adoption, or caring for ill family members.

State laws also protect employees in different areas. For instance, state workers' compensation laws protect employees who are injured on the job. An employee may collect money to cover lost wages, medical expenses, and retraining.

A medical assistant should be aware of the employment laws. If violations are noticed in the workplace, the medical assistant should follow the reporting procedures outlined in the facility's compliance program. If no program exists, then it is important to discuss the issues with the person responsible for the human resources duties.

Interview Concerns. To prevent legal issues related to hiring practices, healthcare facilities need to stay away from specific topics during the interview process. Asking questions related to these topics can put the facility at risk for discrimination lawsuits. Examples of illegal and legal questions include:
- Birthplace, ancestry, or national origin: Legal to ask, "Are you eligible to work in this state?" Illegal to ask, "When did you move to the United States?"
- Marital status, children, or pregnancy: Legal to ask, "Are you able to work an 8 a.m. to 5 p.m. schedule?" Illegal to ask, "Who will look after your child when he is born?"

- Health or medical history, or physical disability: Legal to ask, "Can you perform the essential job functions of a medical assistant with or without reasonable accommodations?" Illegal to ask, "What medications are you on?"
- Religion or religious days observed: Legal to ask, "Can you work on the weekends?" Illegal to ask, "Where do you attend church services?"
- Age, race, ethnicity, gender, or color: Legal to ask, "Are you 18 or older?" Illegal to ask, "How old are you?"
- Criminal records: Legal to ask, "Have you ever been convicted of a crime?" Illegal to ask, "Have you ever been arrested?"

Discrimination Concerns. People with disabilities have a right to accessible healthcare. The Americans with Disabilities Act (ADA) prohibits discrimination against individuals with disabilities in everyday activities, including getting healthcare. The Rehabilitation Act of 1973 prohibits discrimination against individuals with disabilities in services that receive federal financial assistance, including healthcare services. These laws require that healthcare agencies make their services accessible to people with disabilities. The following are examples of how these laws affect ambulatory care facilities.

- Patients in wheelchairs: These patients need to be moved to exam tables when the exam requires the patient to be lying down. Lifts and low exam tables are available to help in these situations. Patients with disabilities cannot be denied care on the grounds that accessible medical equipment is not available.
- Patients with disabilities: If a patient has an interpreter or a companion, it is important that the healthcare provider focus on the patient.
- Exam table location: Patients must have a minimum of 30 inches by 48 inches of clear space adjacent to the exam table and the accessible route out of the room. This allows individuals in wheelchairs to approach the table and be able to transfer onto it. An adjustable-height exam table should be available.
- Accessible scales: Special wheelchair scales and in-floor scales (built into the floor) are needed for patients with limited or no mobility.

The ADA Amendments Act of 2008 is also known as the ADA Amendment Act and the ADAAA. The original ADA narrowly defined disability. The ADA Amendment Act expanded the meaning and interpretation of the definition of disability. People with cancer, diabetes, attention deficit hyperactivity disorder, learning disabilities, and epilepsy are now included. This should ensure that individuals with disabilities receive protection under the law.

Environmental Safety Concerns. Compliance reporting also relates to environmental safety violations. Offenses can be violations of local, state, or federal regulations. The unsafe activities or practices may cause hazardous conditions that affect the health or safety of employees, patients, and others. Recall that OSHA is involved with creating a safe environment for employees. Any situation that risks the safety of employees or patients must be reported immediately.

The Occupational Safety and Health Act of 1970 gives employees the right to file a complaint with OSHA. Employees can request an OSHA inspection if they believe their workplace has safety hazards. The employee filing the report does not need to be knowledgeable about the OSHA regulations. OSHA will keep the reporting person's information confidential.

To report a safety and health issue, the employee can file an electronic form, fax or mail a report to the local OSHA office, or call the local OSHA office. Specific information and forms are available at the OSHA website (https://www.osha.gov).

Incident Reports and Risk Management. When a person is injured or equipment malfunctions, most ambulatory care facilities require an incident report to be completed. An incident report is an internal document that needs to be completed whenever an unexpected event occurs (Fig. 19.5). The purposes of the incident report are to gather information about the situation in case of a future lawsuit and to communicate issues for risk management procedures. The medical assistant should remember these points about incident reports:

- Complete an incident report for patient complaints, medication errors, medical device malfunctions, and any injury.
- Complete the incident report clearly and accurately in pen or electronically.
- List the facts. Do not speculate or draw conclusions.
- Make sure to complete it by the end of the day the situation occurred.
- Do not mention the incident report in the patient health record. If it is mentioned, a lawyer may request a copy of the report.

Usually, the incident report is given to the supervisor to review before it is sent to the risk management team. *Risk management* involves techniques used to reduce or eliminate accidental loss to the healthcare facility. It involves identifying, assessing, and controlling risks. Risks can relate to financial issues, legal liabilities, accidents, and electronic data security threats.

Patient Safety Concerns. Patient safety concerns are of utmost importance in healthcare facilities. Even with careful practices, patients can be harmed. A patient can fall. The wrong medication may be given to the patient. The wrong procedure may be done. All issues of safety can lead to potential liability for injuries that result.

If a medical assistant is involved in a situation in which a person is harmed, it is important to do the following:
- Immediately notify the provider. This is especially important if the wrong medication was given to the patient. The provider must identify what steps need to be taken.
- Arrange to have the person seen by a provider immediately. The provider can assess the extent of the injuries and provide the required treatment. Information on the injuries and treatment will then be documented in the health record should future litigation occur.
- Complete the incident report (see Procedure 4.5). The employee witnessing the situation should be the person completing the report if possible. The incident report communicates what occurred and provides information if future litigation occurs.

WALDEN-MARTIN
FAMILY MEDICAL CLINIC
1234 ANYSTREET | ANYTOWN, ANYSTATE 12345
PHONE 123-123-1234 | FAX 123-123-5678

Incident Report

Date: _____   Time: _____

Incident Type: ☐ Staff   ☐ Patient   ☐ Visitor   ☐ Equipment/Property

Witness: ☐ Staff   ☐ Patient   ☐ Visitor

Department: _____   Exact Location: _____

Medical Team: _____

Patient Reason for Visit: _____   Medication Incident: ☐ Yes ☐ No

Incident Description: [   ]   Immediate Actions and Outcome: [   ]

Contributing Factors: [   ]   Prevention: [   ]

Next of kin / guardian notified / patient?   ☐ Yes   ☐ No   ☐ N/A   Medical staff notified?   ☐ Yes   ☐ No   ☐ N/A

Reported By: _____   Position: _____

Contact Phone Number: _____

Other Persons Involved: _____   Position: _____

Contact Phone Number: _____

Medical Report (Document patient's assessment and list investigations and treatments):

_____

Provider: _____   Designation: _____

Provider Signature: _____   Date/Time: _____

Fig. 19.5 Incident Report Form.

- Notify the department supervisor. The supervisor can follow up with the patient. Many agencies do not charge the injured patient for the services provided. If the wrong medication is given, many agencies do not charge for the medication and services provided.
- Notify state or federal governmental agencies regarding the injury. Some states have medical error reporting systems in place. OSHA requires agencies to record all work-related needlestick injuries and cuts from sharp objects that are contaminated with another person's blood or other potentially infectious material. The case must be reported on the OSHA 300 Log (available at https://www.osha.gov/).

CLOSING COMMENTS

When you are working with older patients, questions on record release and disclosure authorization forms can be common. Years ago, such forms did not exist. Today patients may feel they have to complete forms for everything. Make sure to take time to explain why it is important to have the forms completed. Remember that some of the older patients may have difficulty reading the forms. Some may not be able to hear as well as they once did. Take time and communicate clearly and slowly with older patients. If appropriate, use simple phrases when answering their questions. If possible, help complete whatever information you can. Be patient and respectful during your interactions with patients.

PATIENT-CENTERED CARE

In a patient-centered care environment, the patient is the focus. When a medical assistant does a procedure incorrectly or makes a medication error, it is very important that they immediately notify the provider and the supervisor. The provider will evaluate the situation and make a judgment on what needs to be done for the care and safety of the patient. The supervisor will help manage the situation by talking with the patient, ensuring everything is done for the patient, and eliminating charges related to the error. Being upfront and honest about the error to the provider, supervisor, and patient (per agency policy) is most important for the patient's health and safety.

BEING PROFESSIONAL

Many ambulatory care facilities do not allow medical assistants to carry personal cell phones. Limiting cell phones can reduce the chance of employees recording or taking a picture of a patient and posting something patient related on social media sites. These situations are breaches of confidentiality and can lead to HIPAA violations and settlements. Besides OCR concerns, the facility may be sued by the patient. It is important to remember to maintain patient confidentiality. What you see and hear in the clinic remains there!

Role-play the following scenario with a peer: You and Sam are medical assistants. During a quiet time in the department, Sam records herself at the workstation and posts it to a social media site. You are in the video for a few seconds. Other medical assistants are talking with patients on the phone at this time. Address your concerns professionally with Sam. What else should you do?

CHAPTER REVIEW

Throughout this chapter, we discussed laws related to privacy and confidentiality. HIPAA is a complex law that influences healthcare. The medical assistant has an important role in complying with the Privacy Rule and the Security Rule. It is important to keep PHI confidential. Medical assistants can only access health records of patients with whom they are working. Browsing random patient records or looking up a family member's health information are HIPAA violations.

Additional laws that affect healthcare were also discussed. The FDA enforces the Food, Drug, and Cosmetic Act. It ensures that medications on the market are safe for the public. The DEA enforces the Controlled Substances Act. The Occupational Safety and Health Act and OSHA focus on keeping the workplace safe for employees. Acts related to end-of-life issues encourage organ donation and advance directives.

Compliance reporting is important for providers. They need to ensure that specific communicable diseases are reported to the public health department. Wounds of violence need to be reported to law enforcement agencies. Healthcare providers are mandatory reporters for child abuse, neglect, and exploitation. The reporting laws vary for adults, but in many states elder abuse needs to be reported.

Many healthcare agencies have developed compliance programs. Employees are asked to report suspicious behaviors. In turn, many times the facility then needs to file reports with governmental agencies for noncompliance issues. The medical assistant has important duties in the healthcare setting that help the provider fulfill obligated responsibilities. The medical assistant as an employee also has a responsibility to comply with laws and report suspicious behaviors. Knowing the healthcare laws is important for a medical assistant.

SCENARIO WRAP-UP

Daniela has learned a lot about healthcare-related laws. Not only did she learn about laws that healthcare professionals must follow, but she also learned about employment laws. One of Daniela's assignments for her course was to identify three risks of HIPAA violations. Daniela and Bella talked about the assignment and the risks in their department.

Unattended computers that were open to the electronic health record were a problem. This is especially a risk in the patient examination rooms because each room is equipped with a personal computer for documenting. Daniela also mentioned conversations about patients in the medical assistants' station.

Sometimes she hears medical assistants discussing a patient who came in. She feels uncomfortable about those conversations and ensures she does not take part in them.

Cell phones in the workplace and frequent use of social media sites during work hours can be risks. Bella mentioned that she has heard several stories of employees being terminated. The employees posted patient-related photos and information on social media sites. Bella and Daniela work hard to prevent HIPAA violations. They do not ever want to be named in a lawsuit for such violations.

PROCEDURE 19.1 Protect a Patient's Privacy

Tasks
Apply HIPAA rules and protect a patient's privacy. Demonstrate sensitivity to a patient and their rights.

Scenario
Ken Thomas (date of birth [DOB] 10/25/19XX) saw Jean Burke, NP (nurse practitioner), this past week. He was diagnosed with acute leukemia after several tests. You work with Ms. Burke, and you were involved with arranging Ken's tests. Today, Ken's adult child, Alex Thomas, calls you. Alex wants to know what is going on with Ken. You look at Ken's health record and see that Alex is not on the disclosure authorization form. Per the facility's policy, for information to be given to a patient's family, a disclosure authorization form must be completed.

Later Ken calls and asks why you did not update Alex on his condition. He sounds upset while he is talking with you.

Directions
Role-play the scenario with a peer. You are the medical assistant in the scenario. Your peer will play Alex and then Ken.

Equipment and Supplies
- Patient health record
- Disclosure authorization form (electronic or paper) (see Fig. 19.2)

Procedural Steps
1. You realized that Alex is not on the disclosure authorization form. Inform Alex that his name is not on a disclosure authorization form. Discuss the purpose of the disclosure authorization form. Be professional and respectful as you apply HIPAA rules to the situation.

   Purpose: As a professional, you need to follow the law and yet be professional and respectful. The patient must sign a disclosure authorization form and indicate who can be given information. If a person wants information but is not listed on the form, legally the medical assistant cannot give any information.

2. Explain to Alex how you would be able to give him information. Encourage Alex to talk with his father about the situation.

   Purpose: The medical assistant can only give information if the person's name is on the disclosure authorization form.

Scenario update: Your peer will now play the part of Ken, the patient.

3. When Ken calls, be professional and respectful as you hear his complaints. Keep your voice even and do not raise the volume. Inform Ken that you understand his frustration. Be sensitive to his feelings and his rights. Explain why you could not give information to Alex.

   Purpose: Having the patient understand that you could not legally give the information to Alex is important. Speaking in a sensitive, respectful tone may help Ken feel less frustrated with the situation.

4. Discuss with Ken how you could prepare the disclosure authorization form. Make plans for how Ken would sign the form.

   Purpose: Helping to come up with a solution to achieve the patient's wishes is important to solving Ken's frustration.

5. Document the phone calls with Alex and Ken. Describe the facts and the plan to complete the disclosure authorization form.

   Purpose: All phone calls with patients or related to patients should be documented. This provides an ongoing log of what occurs with the patient and can be helpful in a court of law should something come up.

PROCEDURE 19.2 Complete a Release of Records Form for a Release of Information

Tasks
Apply HIPAA rules and complete a release of records form for a release of information.

Scenario
Aaron Jackson was seen at Walden Hospital for a high fever. You need to help Aaron's mother complete a records release form so his record from the emergency department visit can be sent to the clinic. She needs to request all records from the visit on the first of this month. The clinic information is on the form. The release will expire in 1 month.

Aaron's Information	Walden Hospital's Information
Date of birth: 10/17/20XX	**Address:**
Social Security number: 164-72-4618	Walden Hospital
Address:	123 Healing Way
555 McArthur Avenue	Anywhere, AL 12345-1234
Anytown, AL 12345-1234	**Phone:** (123) 814-4563
Phone: (123) 814-7844	**Fax:** (123) 814-6544
Mother: Patricia Jackson	

Directions
You will complete the medical record release form. You will role play the scenario with a peer. You will be the medical assistant and the peer will be the mother.

Equipment and Supplies
- Records release form (electronic or paper) (see Fig. 19.3)
- Patient health record

Procedural Steps
1. Using the medical records release form, insert the patient information (see Fig. 19.3). Add the patient's name, DOB, and Social Security number (SSN). Include the current address and phone number that is found in the patient record. If an electronic form is used, select the correct patient and the fields will auto-populate.

   Purpose: The patient's information is required on the form. The patient's name, DOB, and SSN are direct identifiers, which will also help the hospital identify the correct patient.

2. Complete the parts of the form that specify who authorizes the release and who is to release the information.

   Purpose: Depending on state law and the facility's policy, the mother's name or the child's name may be the party authorizing the release. The hospital is the party that will release the information.

3. Check the box(es) of the information that needs to be released. If required, write in what other records need to be released.

   Purpose: Depending on state law and the facility's policy, the "Other" location might be where substance abuse and human immunodeficiency virus (HIV) records can be specifically requested. Other forms have a specific section for the release of substance abuse and HIV records.

4. Add the date of the visit. Add the name and contact information for the facility where the records need to be sent.

Purpose: The release form needs to indicate where the records are being sent.

5. Indicate how the released information will be used.

Purpose: This information tells the releasing facility how the information will be used. In this situation, the provider is requesting the information for healthcare purposes.

6. Indicate when the authorization should expire. Proofread the form for accuracy. If using an electronic form, save the form to the patient's health record. Print the form so the mother can sign.

Purpose: In some situations, this may be an ongoing release. For example, the patient may get weekly blood tests at a local clinic, and the results need to be sent to the patient's specialist.

7. During a role-play with the patient's mother, explain what the provider is requesting. Ensure she can understand and read English. Have the mother read the form.

Purpose: For the release to be legal, the mother must understand what she is signing. If she does not understand English, you will need to have a translator available to help in this situation.

8. Ask the mother if she has any questions. Answer any questions, and then explain where she needs to sign if she agrees with the documentation.

Purpose: By answering questions, you can help her understand the release process. It is important to make sure she is in agreement with the form before she signs. After the mother has signed, the form will be faxed to the hospital. The signed form should be filed in the patient record or scanned and uploaded into the electronic health record.

PROCEDURE 19.3   Perform Disease Reporting

Tasks

Research the state's disease reporting public health statutes and complete the disease reporting paperwork based on public health statutes. Document the activity in the patient's health record.

Scenario

Jean Burke, NP, received the test results for Ken Thomas. He tested positive for gonorrhea. She wants you to file the report with the public health department. Here is the information from his health record and the clinic. For any missing information, follow the instructor's directions (or, if no directions are provided for this exercise, make up the information).

Patient Information	Provider and Lab Information	Health Record Information
Ken Thomas	**Provider:**	**Diagnosis:** Gonorrhea
398 Larkin Avenue	Jean Burke, NP	**Symptoms:** Started 5
Anytown, AL 12345-1234	Walden-Martin Family	days ago, greenish
Anycounty k.thomas@	Medical Clinic	discharge from penis,
anytown.mail	1234 Anystreet	burning with urination
Phone: (123) 784-1118	Anytown, AL 12345-	**Test:** Urine specimen
DOB: 10/25/19XX	1234	was collected yester-
Race: Multiple races	**Phone:** (123) 123-1234	day; gonorrhea nucleic
Ethnicity: Unknown	**Fax:** (123) 123-5678	acid amplification
Marital status: Single,	**Lab:**	test (NAAT) test done
living with Sandy	Walden-Martin Family	yesterday, results are
Brown, who was not	Medical Clinic Lab	positive
treated		**Treatment:** Patient
		treated today with
		ceftriaxone 250 mg
		intramuscular (IM)
		single dose and azi-
		thromycin 1 g orally
		single dose

Equipment and Supplies

- Computer with internet access and printer
- Patient record (see table with information)
- Black pen

Procedural Steps

1. Using the internet, search for the disease reporting procedure in your state's public health department or similar facility. Read the procedure.

Purpose: A medical assistant needs to be aware of the disease reporting procedure for the state.

2. Identify which form is required based on the patient's diagnosis. Print the form.

Purpose: Some department of health services agencies may have several forms available on their websites. It is important to use the correct form. Gonorrhea is a sexually transmitted infection.

3. Use a black pen to complete the form. Neatly complete the patient's demographic information section using the information from the health record.

Purpose: All forms require the patient's name and contact information.

4. Complete the diagnosis, symptoms, testing, and treatment information.

Purpose: The public health department needs information on the diagnosis, symptoms, test results, and the treatment provided.

5. Complete the rest of the form. Review the form for accuracy. Make any changes required before submitting the form to the instructor.

Purpose: The form must be accurate and complete before it is sent to the public health department.

6. Document in the patient health record that the disease reporting paperwork was completed and submitted.

Purpose: All activities related to the patient must be documented in the patient's health record.

07/25/20XX 11:05 a.m. The state's disease reporting paperwork for the Gonorrhea diagnosis (on 07/25/20XX) was completed and submitted as requested by Jean Burke, NP. _____ Bella Dickens, CMA (AAMA)

PROCEDURE 19.4   Report Illegal Activity

Task
Report an illegal activity in the healthcare setting following proper protocol.

Scenario
You witness a co-worker, Sally Brown, taking medical samples from the supply cabinet. You see her sticking them into her purse. She sees you and states, "This was the same medication I had to pay $200 for the last time I was sick. I don't see why we need to pay for medications when we have samples that we give free to patients. We should be able to use them also." You know the facility's professional policy prohibits taking medical samples from the sample cabinet for personal reasons.

Facility's Compliance Reporting Protocol
Walden-Martin Family Medical Clinic's Compliance Program has a phone number and email address for employees to report suspected violations, suspected illegal activity, fraud, abuse, theft, and workplace safety concerns. Concerns can be left on the voice mail or emailed without fear of retribution or retaliation. Please include as many details as possible, including dates, names, and the situation.

   Any employee who seeks retribution or retaliation against another employee for reporting an offense needs to be aware of criminal penalties for such actions.

Equipment and Supplies
- Computer with email and internet access or phone
- Instructor's email address or voice mail phone number
- Pen and paper
- Facility's compliance reporting protocol (see the previous section)

Procedural Steps
1. Read the facility's corporate compliance reporting protocol.
   Purpose: Prior to reporting an illegal action, the medical assistant needs to identify the facility's protocol or the reporting chain of command. (Chain of command usually begins with your supervisor, then the supervisor of your supervisor, and so on. It is recommended you start with the lowest level that you feel comfortable with.)
2. Using the paper and pen, write down the facts of what you witnessed.
   Purpose: Writing down the facts soon after the situation will help you to remember the details.
3. Using the paper and pen, compose the message you want to email or leave on the voice mail for the compliance office.
   Purpose: Composing a message will help you organize your thoughts and leave an accurate message.
4. Proofread the message and make any changes required. Make sure to include the date, names of people involved, and the details of the situation.
   Purpose: It is important to have an accurate, complete message for the compliance office. Proofreading helps to ensure the message is accurate.
5. Using your email or phone, send a message to the corporate compliance office. Use the email address or phone number provided by your instructor.
   Purpose: To complete the reporting process, the medical assistant must contact the corporate compliance office or the required supervisor if following the chain of command.

PROCEDURE 19.5   Complete an Incident Report

Task
Complete an incident report form for a medication error.

Scenario
Johnny Parker (DOB 06/15/20XX) sees Jean Burke, NP, for a well-child visit. Johnny is off schedule with his hepatitis B vaccine series, and today he is to get his last hepatitis B booster. You (a medical assistant) prepare the medication and give the injection in his right deltoid muscle. Later in the day you realize that hepatitis B has been out of stock for 1 week. You must have given a hepatitis A booster to Johnny. You realize that you failed to read the label three times during preparation of the medication. You report the mistake to Jean Burke, NP, and your supervisor. Your supervisor calls Lisa Parker, Johnny's mother. They will come back next week for the hepatitis B vaccine. You need to complete the incident report.

Equipment and Supplies
- Incident report form (see Fig. 19.5) and black pen or computer with an internet connection and SimChart for the Medical Office (SCMO)

Procedural Steps
1. *SCMO method:* Access SCMO and enter the Simulation Playground. If a popup window appears, select "Return to previous session with saved patient information" and click Start. On the Calendar screen, click on the Form Repository icon. Click on Office Forms on the left Info Panel and select Incident Report. For both methods: Accurately complete the information from the date down to the reason for the patient's visit.

   Purpose: It is important to have accurate information regarding the date, time, location, incident type, and the reason for the visit. Giving the background information will help the reader understand what occurred.
2. *For both methods:* Specify the incident description, immediate action and outcome, and contributing factors, and fill in the prevention boxes. Provide as much detail as possible. Be honest and concise with your facts.
   Purpose: It is important to give a clear, concise, and honest description of what occurred. It is hard to admit fault, but doing so shows your professionalism in the situation.
3. *For both methods:* Complete the reported by, position, and contact phone number sections. Your information should be in these fields. (For this exercise, make up a contact phone number.)
   Purpose: It is important to have accurate information in these fields so that if people have questions, they can contact you.
4. *For both methods:* Complete the other persons involved, position, and contact phone number sections. Jean Burke's information should be in these fields. (Make up her contact phone number.)
   Purpose: Having additional people listed on the form helps if questions arise about the situation. The rest of the form, from the Medical Report field to the end, needs to be completed by the provider.
5. *For both methods:* Review the form for accuracy. Make any changes required before submitting the form to the instructor. (*For the SCMO method:* Save or print the form based on your instructor's directions.)
   Purpose: It is important to proofread the form to ensure it is accurate and complete.

20

Healthcare Ethics

LEARNING OBJECTIVES

1. Do the following related to ethics:
   - Define ethics and morals.
   - Differentiate between personal and professional ethics.
   - Identify the effect of personal morals on professional performance.
   - Develop a plan for separation of personal and professional ethics.
   - Recognize the impact personal ethics and morals have on the delivery of healthcare.
2. List and describe the four ethical principles in healthcare.
3. Demonstrate appropriate responses to ethical issues involving genetics.
4. Demonstrate appropriate responses to ethical issues involving reproductive issues.
5. Demonstrate appropriate responses to ethical issues involving childhood issues.
6. Demonstrate appropriate responses to ethical issues involving medical research trials.
7. Demonstrate appropriate responses to ethical issues involving end-of-life issues and discuss the theory of Elisabeth Kübler-Ross.
8. Demonstrate appropriate responses to ethical issues involving organ donation; discuss the Patient Self Determination Act and the Uniform Anatomical Gift Act, and define terms related to organ donation (e.g., advance directives, living will, medical durable power of attorney, and healthcare proxy).

OUTLINE

⟫ OPENING SCENARIO

Daniela Garcia has just been hired as a part-time float receptionist at Walden-Martin Family Medical (WMFM) Clinic. As a float receptionist, she will be working with many co-workers and providers. Besides working, Daniela is also attending the local community college for medical assisting. She is currently taking a law and ethics course.

Daniela has completed the law part of the course. She is starting the ethics unit. Daniela grew up in a conservative family. They lived in a very small town in the Midwest. She has since relocated and finds that some of the beliefs she held as a teen are now changing as she encounters more life challenges. As she studies various topics, she has also found that what she believed to be true when she was younger is not actually true. Daniela is very interested in continuing to learn about ethics.

YOU WILL LEARN

1. To describe personal and professional ethics.
2. To create a plan to separate personal and professional ethics.
3. To state the four principles of healthcare ethics.
4. To examine ethical issues related to genetics, reproductive, childhood, end-of-life, and organ donation issues.

INTRODUCTION

As you move into healthcare, you may be faced with situations in which you do not agree with a person's decision. As a healthcare professional, you need to respect a patient's decision whether or not you agree with it.

This chapter examines ethics (ETH iks). Ethical issues are different from legal issues. What may be legal may not be ethical. Personal ethics and its impact on professional performance will be discussed. Professional ethics differs from personal ethics. This topic is explored, along with how to handle the differences. Common ethical issues in healthcare are examined. End-of-life issues, including advance directives, are also discussed.

VOCABULARY

ethics Rules of conduct that differentiate between acceptable and unacceptable behavior.

morals Internal principles that distinguish between right and wrong.

personal ethics An individual's code of conduct.

PERSONAL AND PROFESSIONAL ETHICS

Personal Ethics

Personal ethics includes an individual's honesty, fairness, commitment, integrity, and accountability. It also includes doing what one considers to be correct.

Our morals (MORE ahls) tell us what is right and wrong. Our moral compass develops as we grow. Our first lessons on right and wrong come from those we live with. Our socialization and background shape our morals. For instance, if your parents instilled in you the importance of always being on time, you may grow up feeling that a person should always be on time. You may feel others are in error if they are late for an event. As we grow, our morals may change if our beliefs change. Our morals affect how we conduct ourselves or, in other words, our personal ethics.

Our personal morals affect our professional performance. If people believe in being on time, this characteristic will transfer to the work environment. Employees will be on time for work. Being timely when rooming patients will be important to employees. Having patients wait for long periods of time in the reception area will be challenging to accept. Personal ethics that

align with professional characteristics will positively affect one's professional performance.

Our personal morals may also negatively affect our professional performance. Let's say a person grew up without grandparents or older adults in the family. That person may view older people as not being as knowledgeable as the younger generations. If a medical assistant had this belief, imagine how that might affect their professional performance. That person may not respect older adults and may view them as being useless, unimportant, or irrelevant individuals. This will affect how the medical assistant would treat an older patient. As professionals, we cannot let our personal morals negatively affect the care that we provide to patients.

CRITICAL THINKING 20.1

Daniela was working on her ethics assignment on break at the clinic. She thought about her personal ethics. She decided that some of her personal ethics would benefit her in a job. She realizes that some of her personal morals may negatively affect the care she provides to patients. She realizes that she needs to explore these morals and make some personal decisions. Think about your personal ethics and morals. What will positively influence your professional performance? What personal morals will negatively affect your professional performance?

Professional Ethics

Professional ethics are codes of conduct stated by an employer or a professional association (Table 20.1). Many employers state how employees need to conduct themselves in the workplace. This information can usually be found in the employee handbook.

Many healthcare professional associations have published professional ethics for their members. These are called *codes of ethics*. A code of ethics is a set of rules about good and bad behavior. If a member or employee violates a professional ethic, the association or agency will discipline the person. We will examine the codes for physicians and medical assistants.

Code of Ethics for Physicians. One of the most famous and oldest codes of ethics is the Hippocratic oath. The original oath has been around for longer than 2000 years. Some of its concepts include treating the patient, not the disease, and maintaining the patient's confidentiality. Hippocrates, often called the father of medicine, is credited for the oath. The oath is a code of ethics for physicians. Over the years, the code has been modernized (Fig. 20.1).

In 1847 the American Medical Association (AMA) adopted its Code of Medical Ethics. The code lists the values that physicians commit themselves to as they practice medicine. The AMA's current Code of Medical Ethics is available on its website (https://www.ama-assn.org/). The code is a living document. This means that as medicine and technology change, the code is updated by the members. The following are key themes in the code.

- Physicians should provide competent care and continue learning.

TABLE 20.1	Differences Between Personal and Professional Ethics	
	Personal Ethics	**Professional Ethics**
Definition	Individual's code of conduct	Codes of conduct stated by an employer or a professional association
Ability to change	Individuals can change their own personal ethics	Individuals cannot change these codes and must comply; codes can only be changed by employer or professional association
Accountability	On the individual	On the members and organization

I swear to fulfill, to the best of my ability and judgment, this covenant:

I will respect the hard-won scientific gains of those physicians in whose steps I walk, and gladly share such knowledge as is mine with those who are to follow.

I will apply, for the benefit of the sick, all measures [that] are required, avoiding those twin traps of overtreatment and therapeutic nihilism.

I will remember that there is art to medicine as well as science, and that warmth, sympathy, and understanding may outweigh the surgeon's knife or the chemist's drug.

I will not be ashamed to say "I know not," nor will I fail to call in my colleagues when the skills of another are needed for a patient's recovery.

I will respect the privacy of my patients, for their problems are not disclosed to me that the world may know. Most especially must I tread with care in matters of life and death. If it is given me to save a life, all thanks. But it may also be within my power to take a life; this awesome responsibility must be faced with great humbleness and awareness of my own frailty. Above all, I must not play at God.

I will remember that I do not treat a fever chart, a cancerous growth, but a sick human being, whose illness may affect the person's family and economic stability. My responsibility includes these related problems, if I am to care adequately for the sick.

I will prevent disease whenever I can, for prevention is preferable to cure.

I will remember that I remain a member of society, with special obligations to all my fellow human beings, those sound of mind and body as well as the infirm.

If I do not violate this oath, may I enjoy life and art, respected while I live and remembered with affection thereafter. May I always act so as to preserve the finest traditions of my calling and may I long experience the joy of healing those who seek my help.

Written in 1964 by Louis Lasagna, Academic Dean of the School of Medicine at Tufts University, and used in many medical schools today.

Fig. 20.1 **Modern Version of the Hippocratic Oath.** (From Proctor D, et al: *Kinn's the medical assistant,* ed 13, St. Louis, 2017, Elsevier.)

- Physicians should respect human dignity and human rights.
- Physicians should follow the laws, be professional, and uphold the standards of the medical profession.
- Physicians should contribute to the welfare of the community.

The Council of Ethical and Judicial Affairs (CEJA) is one of the councils within the AMA. The CEJA analyzes ethical issues in healthcare and develops ethical policies and recommendations. These recommendations, along with the Code of Medical Ethics, are used by physicians to guide their practice. The CEJA prompts AMA members to adhere to the Code of Medical Ethics.

Code of Ethics for Medical Assistants. The American Association of Medical Assistants (AAMA) developed a code of ethics that provides the principles of ethical and moral conduct for the profession (Box 20.1).

BOX 20.1 Medical Assisting Code of Ethics

Members of the AAMA dedicated to the conscientious pursuit of their profession, and thus desiring to merit the high regard of the entire medical profession and the respect of the general public which they serve, do pledge themselves to strive always to:

A. Render service with full respect for the dignity of humanity.
B. Respect confidential information obtained through employment unless legally authorized or required by responsible performance of duty to divulge such information.
C. Uphold the honor and high principles of the profession and accept its disciplines.
D. Seek to continually improve the knowledge and skills of medical assistants for the benefit of patients and professional colleagues.
E. Participate in additional service activities aimed toward improving the health and well-being of the community.

From the American Association of Medical Assistants: Medical assisting code of ethics. https://www.aama-ntl.org/about/overview#. WSDywmjytPY.

The AAMA has also written a Medical Assisting Creed, which can be used as a guideline for medical assistants facing complex ethical and moral issues in the course of their work. The Medical Assisting Creed supports the code of ethics by asking members to abide by ethical statements of belief:

- I believe in the principles and purposes of the profession of medical assisting.
- I endeavor to be more effective.
- I aspire to render greater service.
- I protect the confidence entrusted to me.
- I am dedicated to the care and well-being of all people.
- I am loyal to my employer.
- I am true to the ethics of my profession.
- I am strengthened by compassion, courage, and faith.

The Medical Assisting Creed supports the code of ethics. The above creed can be found on the AAMA's website (https://www.aama-ntl.org/about/overview#.WSDywmjytPY).

It is important for the medical assistant to follow the code and the creed. The care provided to others must reflect respect for that person. The medical assistant is legally and ethically obligated to keep patient information confidential. Continual learning is critical. The medical assistant must provide the best care possible and uphold the standards of the profession.

> ### CRITICAL THINKING 20.2
>
> Daniela read the AMA Code of Medical Ethics and the AAMA Medical Assisting Code of Ethics. She notices some similarities between the codes. What similarities do you notice between the two codes?

Separation Plan

Sometimes an individual's personal ethics clashes with professional ethics. It is important to take steps to separate one's personal ethics from professional ethics.

Let's examine a few situations that might affect a medical assistant. Imagine if a medical assistant has personal beliefs that vaccines are not needed and harm individuals. This medical assistant obtains a job in a pediatric department. She is required to give vaccines numerous times a day. In this situation, her personal ethics would clash with her professional ethics. She would be professionally obligated to give the vaccines to patients. She could not share her antivaccine beliefs with patients. Due to the clash of ethics, it might be a stressful job for her.

In another situation, a medical assistant believes that everything that can be done should be done when someone is dying. Professional ethics mandate that each person has a right to make end-of-life decisions. Legally and ethically, the medical assistant must follow what the patient decides. The medical assistant cannot put pressure on the patient to change their decisions.

Creating a Plan. As you complete your medical assisting courses, it is important to evaluate whether your personal ethics conflict with the medical assistant code of ethics.

- Are there groups of people with whom you have issues? Maybe you do not believe in their behaviors, actions, or ideas based on your morals.
- Do you have preconceived ideas about people with differing ethnicities, sexual preferences, or specific diseases?

If you identified conflicts, how might you provide respectful care to these patients? Honestly, think about your biases. How would you approach a situation if it involved your bias? Remember, the professional code of ethics supersedes your personal code. You need to follow the professional ethics of your agency and profession (see Procedure 20.1).

Before medical assistants start applying for positions, it is important that they evaluate whether personal ethics will clash with the professional ethics of an agency. If a person does not believe in vaccinations, then working in a department that gives vaccinations would not be a good job choice. If a person does not believe in elective abortions, then working in an agency that does elective abortions would not be a good choice.

> ### CRITICAL THINKING 20.3
>
> Daniela decided to create a plan to separate her personal ethics from her professional ethics. Think about your personal ethics. What steps might you take to change your personal morals so that they better align with your professional ethics? What might you do to deal with the personal ethics that conflict with the professional ethics?

PRINCIPLES OF HEALTHCARE ETHICS

Healthcare professionals have an ethical duty to their patients. Four ethical principles summarize this ethical duty. These principles are autonomy, nonmaleficence, beneficence, and justice. Technically all four of these principles should have equal weight in ethical decisions. Many times, autonomy overshadows the other three principles.

Besides healthcare professionals, bioethicists (BYE oh eth i sists) also use the principles of healthcare ethics. They apply these principles when they evaluate medical technology and procedures. Are the new technology advances ethical? Are these procedures ethical?

We will examine the four ethical principles. Ethical actions to meet the principles will be discussed for both the provider and the medical assistant.

> **VOCABULARY**
> **bioethicists** People who study the ethical effect of biomedical advances (e.g., drugs and genetic engineering).

Autonomy

Autonomy is the freedom to determine one's own actions and decisions. Patients have the right to make their own healthcare decisions. Providers need to tell patients of the risks and benefits of different procedures (informed consent). After being told what may be most successful, the patients can make their own decisions. The patient's decision-making process should be free from pressure or interference from others. Healthcare professionals must respect and honor the patient's decision.

The medical assistant must protect patients' privacy. It is important to respect the uniqueness, dignity, and decisions of others. This includes patients, families, and co-workers. A medical assistant must demonstrate these professional behaviors, which will also maintain their own dignity and self-respect:

- Help to make others around you look good without minimizing yourself. Do this by being supportive and helpful to your team members.
- Refrain from being negative and whining.
- Be assertive, not aggressive, when standing up for your rights (e.g., adequate work environment, hours, and pay).
- Collaborate and cooperate with co-workers. Do not be afraid to stand up for what is right and fair.
- Avoid bringing personal issues into the workplace.

CRITICAL THINKING 20.4

When Daniela learned about the autonomy principle and the role of the medical assistant, it reminded her of healthcare laws that she had learned about earlier. What healthcare laws address autonomy and the healthcare professional's role?

Nonmaleficence

Nonmaleficence means to do no harm. Healthcare professionals are obligated to not inflict intentional harm on patients. By providing the appropriate standard of care, we can reduce the risk of negligence. It is important to provide competent care to patients for both legal and ethical reasons.

The medical assistant must demonstrate professionalism by preventing harm to others – this means to intervene when a patient is at risk (e.g., falling). It is important to make sure the environment is both physically and psychologically safe for others and that safety hazards are reported and corrected. For instance, malfunctioning equipment must never be used until fixed. Hazardous chemicals and sharps (needles) must be unavailable to patients. The medical assistant must also provide safe and competent care to all patients.

Beneficence

Beneficence refers to the moral obligation to act for the good or benefit of others. For healthcare professionals, this means promoting health in patients and assisting patients to recover from illness. Promoting health and disease prevention are professional behaviors for medical assistants. With the current focus on prevention of diseases, medical assistants help providers by identifying the immunizations and screening tests their patients need.

Justice

Justice means to treat patients fairly and give them care that is due and appropriate. This means that patients in similar situations should receive the same services and treatments.

Professional behaviors of the medical assistant include providing equal respect and courtesy to all people. Regardless of the person's skin color, sexual preference, nationality, religion, and health history, every person must be treated respectfully. It is important that medical assistants think about their biases. Do you really feel everyone is equal? Is there any group of individuals whose ideas you do not agree with? Understanding one's

biases is important. If we do not identify our biases, there is a tendency to treat others differently. As healthcare professionals, we are obligated to treat everyone equally and with respect (see Procedure 20.2).

ETHICAL ISSUES

There are many ethical issues in healthcare. As technology and medicine evolve, additional ethical issues arise. We will examine common ethical issues, and the CEJA's recommendations will also be explained.

Genetics Issues

Each person is made up of 46 chromosomes (KROE mah somes), 23 from each parent. Genes are the basic units of heredity, or the instructions on how our bodies should develop and function. Genes provide the differences among us and the similarities in families. From genes we get our physical appearance, in addition to our susceptibility to disease. During the process of conception and subsequent cell division, an extra chromosome (or a change in the chromosome structure) may occur, resulting in a genetic disease or disorder. The following are types of genetic diseases:

- *Monogenic disorders*: A defective gene is inherited from one or both parents. Huntington disease, cystic fibrosis, and sickle cell anemia are examples of monogenic disorders.
- *Chromosomal disorders*: An abnormal number of chromosomes or a change in the chromosomal structure causes diseases such as Klinefelter syndrome and Turner syndrome.

With advances in technology we can now test for many genetic disorders, sometimes even on a baby in utero (e.g., fetus). There has also been a lot of research in the areas of cloning, genetic engineering, and gene therapy. Along with these advancements come ethical issues and questions. We will explore cloning and genetic engineering advancements and related ethical issues.

VOCABULARY

chromosomes Rod-shaped structures found in the cell's nucleus; they contain genetic information.

Cloning. *Cloning* is the process of creating a genetically identical biological entity. A clone is the copy, which has the same genetic makeup as the original entity. Researchers have cloned genes, cells, tissues, and organisms. Dolly, a sheep, was the first mammal cloned. Since then at least eight different mammals have been cloned, including horses, pigs, dogs, and cats. Advocates for human cloning discuss the need for organ transplants. Opponents of human cloning address the rights of the clone.

Genetic Engineering. *Genetic engineering* is the manipulation of genetic material in cells to change hereditary traits or to produce a specific result. Genetic engineering is used in many areas, including agriculture and medicine. For instance, a lot of corn and soybeans are genetically modified to resist disease and insects. These foods may be labeled as genetically modified organisms (GMOs). In medicine, insulin, human growth hormone, and other drugs are genetically engineered. We will focus on genetic engineering in medicine.

A *genome* is the entire genetic makeup of an organism. The Human Genome Project, a 13-year international project, mapped the human genome. The entire human genome contains about 30,000 genes. The goal of the project was to gain information that will eventually lead to the prevention and treatment of many diseases. Genomic medicine resulted from the Human Genome Project. Genomic medicine is an emerging branch of medicine involved with using patients' genomic information as part of their clinical care. Genetic testing, pharmacogenetics, and stem cell transplants are important advances in genomic medicine. Gene therapy is currently being researched.

Genetic Testing. Genetic testing can identify issues with a person's chromosomes, genes, or proteins. More than 1000 genetic tests are available. The following are some of the types of genetic testing.

- *Newborn screening*: All states have newborn screening procedures to identify genetic disorders that can be treated early in life.
- *Diagnostic testing*: Used to diagnose a specific genetic or chromosomal condition. Testing can occur prior to birth or after. Not all genetic conditions have diagnostic tests.
- *Carrier testing*: Used to determine if a person is carrying one copy of a gene mutation. Two copies of a gene mutation (one from each parent) can result in a genetic disorder in a child.
- *Prenatal testing*: Used to detect genetic or chromosomal issues with a fetus (unborn baby).
- *Preimplantation testing*: Used to detect genetic issues in embryos (EM bree ohs) that were created using assistive reproductive technology, which will be explained later in the chapter.
- *Predictive and presymptomatic testing*: Used to detect gene mutations associated with specific disorders that occur after birth. Usually done when a patient has a family member with a genetic disorder and the patient wants to see if they also have it.
- *Forensic testing*: Used to identify crime or catastrophe victims, identify or rule out crime suspects, or establish biologic relationships between people (e.g., paternity).

Per the CEJA, the impact of genetics on diseases is complex. Understanding genetic counseling and helping the patient to understand the results require special skill from the provider. Genetic testing is most important when it makes a meaningful impact on the person's health. The provider ordering genetic testing should have the appropriate knowledge and expertise to counsel the patient on the findings and implications. Providers must keep genetic testing information confidential.

Pharmacogenetics. *Pharmacogenomics* is a branch of pharmacology that studies the genetic factors that influence a person's response to a medication. Based on a person's genome, pharmacogenomics can determine if a specific therapy will be effective. More than 100 medications approved by the US Food and Drug Administration (FDA) already have pharmacogenomics information available. Some of these medications include analgesics, antivirals, cardiovascular drugs, and anticancer drugs.

Stem Cell Transplants. Stem cells can differentiate, or develop into specialized cells (e.g., muscle, blood, or brain cells). They can self-renew or make copies of themselves. The new cell can remain as a stem cell or turn into a specialized cell. Depending on where the stem cells are located, they may be constantly repairing and replacing damaged tissue (e.g., intestinal tract). In other locations, such as the heart, they only divide in special situations.

There are two main categories of stem cells: adult and embryonic. Table 20.2 describes both types of stem cells. Stem cell research has been going on since the 1960s. New technology has helped advance the research. Many researchers are excited about the potential of stem cells. Cord blood stem cell transplants have been used to treat more than 75 diseases, including cancers, anemias, metabolic disorders, and immune system disorders.

Though both types of stem cell research have ethical issues, embryonic stem cell research has greater ethical issues. Harvesting stem cells from an embryo would mean destroying the embryo. For those believing life begins at the moment of conception, this means a life is lost.

Gene Therapy. Gene therapy is currently an experimental technique that uses genes to prevent or treat diseases. With this procedure, a gene is inserted into a patient's cell. The hopes are that the new gene might:

- Replace a mutated gene
- Prevent the mutated gene from functioning
- Help fight the disease

Gene or genome editing is a specific gene therapy. This technique can remove, add, or alter sections of the gene. With new technology emerging in this area, ethical issues have also arisen. Genome editing of somatic (soe MAT ik) cells would only affect the individual. This treatment has already been used and is considered ethical. Genome editing of germline cells can cause issues that may affect future generations. Genome editing of germline cells raises ethical concerns and is illegal in the United States.

CRITICAL THINKING 20.5

When Daniela learned about genetic testing, she remembered hearing about how people could trace their relatives. She also had heard about forensic testing while watching crime drama shows. What types of genetic testing are you familiar with?

VOCABULARY

embryo A developing organism from the moment of conception through the eighth week of development.

germline cells Sperm and egg cells.

somatic cells Nonreproductive cells; they do not include sperm and egg cells.

TABLE 20.2   Types of Stem Cells

	Adult Stem Cells	Embryonic Stem Cells
Derived from	Found in infants through adults; found in many organs and tissues, including the brain, bone marrow, blood, skin, heart, teeth, testis, liver, blood vessel, and skeletal muscles. Umbilical cord blood also contains adult stem cells.	Taken from a 4- to 5-day-old human embryo
What types of cells can they become?	Variation thought to be limited; could become cell types similar to their tissue of origin. Scientists have found a way to "reprogram" some types of adult stem cells so they act like embryonic cells.	Can become all cell types
Advantages	Thought to cause fewer rejection issues with transplants if a person's own stem cells are used.	Easy to grow in a laboratory setting
Ethical issue	Risks involved with adult stem cell use are still being evaluated.	For those believing life begins at the moment of conception, removing stem cells from an embryo would mean killing a person

Reproductive Issues

Assistive Reproductive Technology. Infertility is the inability to get pregnant after 1 year of unprotected intercourse (sex). Infertility can affect both males and females. There are many causes of infertility. With advances in technology, assistive reproductive technology (ART) has allowed many couples to have children. Assisted reproductive technology includes all procedures that involve the handling of the eggs, sperm, or embryos. Common types of ART include:

- *In vitro fertilization*: Involves removing mature eggs from the ovaries and fertilizing the eggs with sperm outside of the body. The fertilized eggs are then transferred to the uterus.
- *Intrauterine insemination* (IUI): Also called *artificial insemination*. Specially prepared sperm is placed into a woman's uterus using a long, narrow tube (e.g., a straw). The woman's partner's sperm or a donor's sperm can be used.
- *Surrogacy*: A woman carries and gives birth for another couple. A legal contract should be in place to protect all parties. *Traditional surrogacy* or *partial surrogacy* occurs when the egg is from a surrogate (SUR ah git) and the sperm is from the father. *Gestational surrogacy* or *full surrogacy* occurs when the sperm and egg come from the intended parents or are donated, and the surrogate is not related to the baby.

One of the complications of ART is multiple births. An ethical issue can arise if the success of the pregnancy may be hindered by the number of babies in utero. If this situation occurs, the provider must inform the patient of the risks with multiple births.

CEJA's opinions are that providers who offer assisted reproductive services should provide accurate advertising of their services. They need to provide all information, including success rates and costs, so patients can make an informed decision. Prospective donors need to be tested for infectious disease agents and genetic disease. Donors need to provide informed consent.

Gamete Donation. Gamete (egg or sperm) donation allows others who are unable to have children to do so. Many ethical issues surround gamete donation, including:

- The privacy of the donors
- The rights of the child born from the donated gamete
- The relationship of the child and the donor
- The number of donations from a single donor (the more children born from the donor's gamete, the greater the risk of the children mating and conceiving children together)
- The health of the donors and the children born from the donations
- The regulations on gamete storage
- The compensation for gamete donation (many countries do not allow payment for gamete donation; however, the US does allow it)

CEJA's opinions are that providers who participate in the gamete donation process must inform the prospective donors about the risk of the donation, the testing involved, and if the donor will receive the test results. Donors should be tested for infectious diseases and genetic disorders. The donor should be notified that all information will be kept indefinitely. The provider should discuss the storage of the gametes, compensation, and that the state law governs the relationship between the gamete donor and the child born from the gamete.

CEJA's opinions are that providers should not allow people to donate if they have infectious diseases. The provider should also gather the donor's preferences on the use of the gametes, whether for research or reproduction. The provider should find out the donor's preferences regarding release of identifying information to any child resulting from the donor. Donors should also limit the number of pregnancies resulting from a single gamete donor.

Egg Freezing. Egg freezing, or *egg banking*, is the cryopreservation (KRIE oh pri zur vae shun) of oocytes (OO eh site), which is done to preserve the female's fertility. Egg freezing is done for a variety of reasons, such as:

- A woman has been diagnosed with cancer and may become infertile with the cancer treatments.
- A woman wants to delay childbearing.
- A woman objects to freezing embryos.

The egg retrieval process requires the patient to undergo about 9 to 10 days of hormone injections to stimulate the

---

VOCABULARY

cryopreservation To preserve by freezing at low temperatures.

oocyte An immature ovum (egg).

surrogate A person who acts on behalf of another person or takes the place of another person. Examples include a surrogate mother or a healthcare agent.

ovaries and assist in the ripening of multiple eggs. Once the egg retrieval is completed, the eggs are frozen until they are needed. Usually 10 to 20 eggs are retrieved.

With the freezing process, the eggs are dehydrated and the water is replaced with a fluid that prevents ice from forming and destroying the egg. The eggs can be flash frozen or frozen using a slow process. When the patient wants to become pregnant, some of the eggs are thawed. They are fertilized and then transferred to the patient's uterus.

Ethical issues surrounding egg freezing include:

- Safety of the procedure for both the patient and any future children that result from the eggs
- Marketing practices that focus on healthy women
- Pressures from companies for women to focus on their career, freeze their eggs, and consider childbearing at a later time
- Disposition decisions, including egg-sharing options, for unused or unwanted eggs

CEJA has not indicated a recommendation on egg freezing. CEJA has provided a recommendation for cryopreservation of embryos, which is similar. Physicians who provide clinical services that include cryopreservation of embryos must discuss with the parties involved how the embryos will be used, thawed, or disposed of. A physician must not be involved with the sale of stored embryos.

Elective Abortion. *Elective abortion* is the deliberate termination of a pregnancy. Elective abortions can be done through medications and medical procedures. Elective abortions raise many ethical questions and concerns. Some feel that women have the right to determine what occurs with their bodies and babies have no rights until they are born. Others feel that from the moment of conception, babies have rights.

The advancement of technology has affected elective abortions. With greater technology, complex testing and treatments can occur. Surgery on babies in utero can treat health issues that in the past caused death or elected abortions. Advanced testing can diagnose issues sooner. For instance, imaging tests provide clearer pictures of babies in utero. In cases in which diagnostic tests indicate major abnormalities, providers discuss the worst-case scenarios with the parents and include termination as part of informed consent. Per the CEJA's opinion, providers are not prohibited from performing an elective abortion in situations in which it does not violate the law.

Childhood Issues

In most cases, parents of minor children must authorize or decline treatment. In some cases, the state may need to provide the parental authority. *Parens patriae* is Latin for "father of the country." This doctrine gives the courts the power to make decisions for people who cannot make their own decisions. Many times, this doctrine is used for children or adults who are incompetent. It can be used when the parent or parents refuse healthcare for the child. The court may take over the parental rights and make decisions for the child.

There have been situations in which parents refuse procedures or treatments for their children based on religious or personal beliefs. One of the more common situations in ambulatory care is the refusal of vaccinations (see Procedure 20.2). It is important for the medical assistant to respect the Patient's Bill of Rights. If the patient provides a reason for the refusal, the medical assistant should let the provider know. The provider should also be told of the refusal, so other procedures or treatments can be discussed if needed.

CEJA's opinion is that providers are encouraged to seek consultation with ethics committees in the following situations:

- The parent or guardian refuses treatment for a reversible life-threatening condition.
- There are disagreements about the minor's best interest.

The provider should only ask the courts to resolve the disagreement as the last option.

VOCABULARY

ethics committee A group composed of members from a variety of disciplines that analyze ethical issues.

Adoption. Federal and state laws govern adoption. In healthcare, we run into adoption fairly often. Our patients may be adopted and do not know their family medical history. We need to be understanding of their situation. We may also work with pregnant women who are planning to give up their babies. Again, these are situations in which medical assistants need to be sensitive and understanding. The following are different types of adoption.

- *Adopting through an agency*: Private and public adoption agencies are regulated by the state and must be licensed to place children with adoptive parents. Public agencies usually place abandoned, orphaned, or abused children who are wards of the state.
- *Adopting independently*: The birth parents and the adoptive parents have an arrangement. Some states do not allow this type of adoption.
- *Adopting through identification*: Adoptive parents and birth parents work with an adoption agency to complete the adoption process.
- *Adopting internationally*: Adoptive parents work with an international adoption agency to adopt a child from another country. International adoption agencies must be certified by the US State Department.
- *Relative adoptions*: Relatives of a child adopt the child.
- *Closed adoptions*: There is no contact between the adoptive parents and the birth parents.
- *Open adoptions*: Adoptive parents meet and may stay in contact with the birth parents.

Safe Haven Infant Protection Laws. Safe haven infant protection laws allow a person to give up an unwanted infant anonymously. The goal is to protect unwanted babies from abuse or death. The person is not prosecuted if

- the infant is not abused.
- the infant is left at a designated location, as indicated by the state law.

- the infant is within the age limit, as indicated by the state law.

The designated locations vary by state. They may include hospitals, emergency departments, fire and police stations, and child welfare agencies. The age of the child varies. A few states allow children up to 1 year of age. Opponents of the safe haven laws voice concerns for fathers' rights and the lack of family medical history obtained. Supporters state that these laws save babies by providing a safe drop-off location and no questions asked.

Confidential Healthcare for Minors. Providers have an ethical duty to promote decision making in minor patients to the degree of the child's ability. Providers have a responsibility to protect the confidentiality of minor patients, within certain limits. We see this in the ambulatory care setting when parents wait in the reception area while minor children (usually teens) have their physical exams. Many providers feel that the minor's answers to questions on safety, sex, drugs, and alcohol may be more truthful without the presence of parents.

In some states, laws permit unemancipated minors to request and receive confidential services. These services must relate to contraception, pregnancy testing, prenatal care, and delivery services. Additional services can include prevention and treatment of sexually transmitted infections (STIs), substance use disorders, and mental illness. When the law does not grant minors decision-making authority for healthcare, CEJA's opinion is that providers should:

- Involve the parent or guardian in situations in which it is necessary to prevent harm to the patient or others
- Involve the parent or guardian if the provider does not feel it will affect the patient's health
- Explore reasons the minor does not want the involvement of the parent or guardian
- Inform the minor that parents may learn of the treatment through insurance statements.
- Protect the confidentiality of the information from the minor, keeping within ethical and legal standards

---

CRITICAL THINKING 20.6

On break one afternoon, Daniela talks to Jan, a medical assistant. She asks Jan how she handles parents who want to find out confidential information about their children. How might you professionally and respectfully handle a phone call from a parent who is requesting confidential information on their child?

Research Trials

Many of the larger ambulatory healthcare facilities are involved with teaching nurse practitioner and physician assistant students and residents to become future healthcare providers. Typically, these facilities also are involved with research trials. These trials may relate to a treatment for a disease, such as a new surgical procedure or a new medication. Many healthcare disciplines use evidence-based practice that originated from research trials. Research on patient volunteers is critical

to find new ways of treating and managing diseases and caring for patients.

VOCABULARY

evidence-based practice Healthcare practice that incorporates the most current and valid research results, thus providing the best patient care.

discipline A branch of knowledge, learning, or instruction; for instance, medicine, nursing, social work, and physical therapy.

resident A physician who has graduated from medical school and is finishing specialized clinical training.

Potentially, research trials place some people at risk of harm for the good of others. This could cause the exploitation of patient volunteers and is an ethical concern. Many ethical guidelines exist at local and national levels to protect patient volunteers. These guidelines were initiated based on past abuses. The following are some of the most influential guidelines and codes of ethics that guide clinical research.

- *Nuremberg Code*: Originated in 1947 after the Nuremberg trials, in which Nazi doctors were convicted of crimes committed during human experiments on concentration camp prisoners. The code outlined what was legal when conducting human experiments. Several of the points included the need for voluntary consent, the results must be for the good of society, and the experiments must be based on prior knowledge and should avoid all unnecessary physical and mental suffering.
- *Belmont Report*: Written in 1976 by the National Commission for the Protection of Human Subjects of Biomedical and Behavioral Research. The report identifies basic ethical principles and guidelines regarding human subject research (Box 20.2).
- *Declaration of Helsinki*: A landmark document regarding research ethics developed by the World Medical Association in 1964 and revised many times. This document addressed the importance of human research, the obligations of the physicians involved, the importance of informed consent, and the protection of the participants.

According to the National Institutes of Health (NIH) Clinical Center (https://clinicalcenter.nih.gov/recruit/ethics.html), seven main principles are involved with ethical research:

BOX 20.2 Tuskegee Study

In 1932 the Public Health Service, working with the Tuskegee Institute, researched the natural history of syphilis. They hoped to justify treatment programs for African Americans. The study involved 399 black men with syphilis and 201 without it. The original 6-month study ended 40 years later when the Associated Press ran a story about the research study, and the public outcry led to an advisory panel investigation.

For this research study, the men had agreed freely to be examined and treated, but no informed consent was used. In compensation for the study, the men received free medical exams, free meals, and burial insurance. The men were told they were getting treated, but they did not receive proper treatment to cure syphilis even though penicillin was available in 1947.

In 1974, a $10 million settlement was reached for the study participants and their surviving family members. The settlement also included health benefits for the participants and their family members.

- *Social and clinical value*: It should contribute to the knowledge base of either understanding health or preventing, treating, and caring for people with a specific disease.
- *Scientific validity*: The methods used should be valid and feasible, and the study must have clear scientific objectives.
- *Fair subject selection*: The subjects recruited should be based on the goals of the study.
- *Favorable risk-benefit ratio*: Everything must be done to minimize the risk to the research subjects and to maximize the benefits. The benefits should outweigh the risks.
- *Independent review*: The study should be reviewed by an independent review panel with no vested interest to ensure that the study is ethical and to minimize potential conflicts of interest.
- *Informed consent*: To be ethical, the participants need to be informed of the purpose, methods, risks, benefits, and alternatives to the research. They need to understand the information and make a voluntary decision to participate.
- *Respect for potential and enrolled subjects*: Individuals have a right to change their minds at any time. Their information must be kept confidential, and they must be informed of information that may change their assessment of the risks and benefits of participating in the project.

Often medical assistants who are working at larger facilities may be involved with research projects. They may need to identify patients who match the project's criteria. Medical assistants may help with data collection. It is important for the medical assistant to know that all information must be kept confidential. All participants have a right to change their minds regarding their participation. Typically, the research guidelines or documents will have contact information provided if the medical assistant has questions or concerns regarding the project.

End-of-Life Issues

With the changes in healthcare and technology, more treatment options exist today to prolong a person's life. Ventilators assist the breathing process, and feeding tubes provide nutrition. Medications and defibrillators can help restart the heart. Legislation exists at the state and federal levels to help address death and dying issues. There are also many ethical questions that surround end-of-life issues.

It may sound like end-of-life issues are only addressed in the hospital. End-of-life issues also affect ambulatory care. Medical assistants may accompany providers in skilled nursing facility (nursing home) visits. Medical assistants provide ambulatory care to patients who have terminal illnesses. It is not uncommon for the medical assistant to process a referral for hospice care for a patient. The medical assistant should know the differences between palliative medicine and hospice care.

Palliative means to help relieve the symptoms of a serious illness. Palliative medicine is a subspecialty. The providers offer palliative care to patients who are seriously ill, regardless of age. The disease may be curable, chronic, or life-threatening. Palliative care focuses on the entire person. It does not provide a cure, just helps to reduce the symptoms.

Hospice is a type of palliative care for people who have about 6 months or less to live. The goal of hospice care is to allow patients who are dying to have dignity, comfort, and peace. Hospice programs not only work with the patient, but also the family. Hospice care can be provided in the hospital, skilled nursing facility, hospice center, and at home.

Working with patients who have a terminal illness can be emotionally challenging. It is important for the medical assistant to remember that patients and families go through the grieving process. The stages of grief and dying, as defined by Dr. Elisabeth Kübler-Ross, include:

- *Denial*: Person refuses to accept the diagnosis or prognosis. Defense mechanism that protects people from being overwhelmed. Disbelief and numbness may occur.
- *Anger*: Person's anger can be directed at self or others. May blame others.
- *Bargaining*: Person attempts to bargain with the higher power the person believes in (e.g., God).
- *Depression*: Person feels sadness, fear, and uncertainty. Crying and depression may occur. Person may not participate in normal activities; distances self from others.
- *Acceptance*: Person has come to terms with the situation.

Not everyone goes through all five stages, and people may not go through the stages in the order listed. Some people may switch back and forth between the stages. Various behaviors may be seen during the grieving process, such as:

- Sadness, loneliness, social isolation, crying, and difficulty concentrating
- Anger, guilt, denial, and confusion
- Fatigue, numbness, and appetite changes
- Sleep changes and nightmares

Patient Self-Determination Act. The Patient Self-Determination Act (PSDA) became law in 1990. This act requires most healthcare institutions at the time of admission to:

- Provide patients with a written document of their rights to make decisions and the facility's policies respecting advance directives
- Ask patients if they have advance directives and document the response in the health record

Healthcare agencies must provide advance directive training to their staff. Staff members cannot discriminate against patients who have or do not have advance directives.

Per the CEJA, providers should:

- Discuss advance care planning with all patients, regardless of health status or age
- Explain advance directives and document in the health record information about advance care planning
- Review advance care planning periodically with patients

If patients present advance directive paperwork, the medical assistant needs to ensure it gets into the health record. It is not uncommon for medical assistants to provide advance directive information to patients. The medical assistant must also be familiar with the different types of advance directives.

Advance Directives. Advance directives are written instructions about healthcare decisions should a person be unable to make them. Advance directives are not just for older adults to complete. It is important for everyone to consider completing advance directives. Once completed, advance directives can be modified in the future. It is important that local healthcare agencies have a copy of the person's advance directive paperwork.

Per the CEJA, providers should:

- Identify if patients have advance directives, including a healthcare proxy.
- Respect the wishes of the patient's surrogate and help the surrogate understand the patient's wishes in the advance directives.
- Seek assistance from the ethics committee if a patient lacks advance directives and is unable to communicate.

Today most states have a multiple-page document for people to complete. The document can be found online or at healthcare agencies. The document may be called *advance directives*, *durable power of attorney for healthcare*, or something similar. It replaces multiple documents of the past. Generally, the advance directives document contains sections for the different types of advance directives, including:

- *Living will*: Provides instructions about life-sustaining medical treatment to be administered or withheld when the patient has a terminal condition.
- *Medical durable power of attorney*: May be known by other names. Similar to a living will but includes all healthcare decisions. It lasts as long as the person is not able to make decisions. This document names a healthcare proxy and can include healthcare wishes. It can be used when the situation is not terminal.
- *Healthcare proxy*: Also called *healthcare agent* or *surrogate*. A competent adult can appoint a person (called a *proxy* or *agent*) to make healthcare decisions in the event they are unable to do so.
- *Organ donation*: Indicates if a person wants to donate organs.
- *Do not resuscitate* (DNR): Can be part of the living will. Indicates if the person refuses cardiopulmonary resuscitation (CPR) if they stop breathing or have no pulse.

The document can also include additional topics, such as:

- Life-sustaining treatments (e.g., drugs, machines, medical procedures, feeding tubes)
- Desires if permanently unconscious
- Desires with terminal condition
- Mental health treatment
- Admission to nursing home
- Unconscious and pregnant
- Pain relief
- Additional desires

Remember, each state has its own advance directives form for state residents to complete

Physician Orders for Life-Sustaining Treatment.

Physician Orders for Life-Sustaining Treatment (POLST) can be known by similar names across the United States. It is promoted to work with advance directives. When a person is diagnosed with advanced illness or frailty, having a POLST may be recommended. The POLST is a one-page order sheet completed and signed by the physician. It indicates the care a person should receive. The POLST should be based on the advance directives and the person's wishes.

For some people, the POLST is concerning. The POLST can supersede a person's advance directives. Keep in mind that the POLST is a limited document, and some forms state that the healthcare staff should follow the orders listed before contacting the provider. Opponents to the POLST encourage patients to refuse it. They state that the provider should be contacted when the patient's condition changes and that the advance directives in its entirety can be followed, not the summarized version listed in the POLST.

Uniform Determination of Death Act.

The Uniform Determination of Death Act (UDDA) was drafted in 1981. It served as a guide for state lawmakers to create their own laws. The act provided a definition of death. A person may legally be declared dead if one of the following two events occurs:

- Irreversible cessation of circulatory and respiratory functions
- Irreversible cessation of all functions of the entire brain, including the brainstem

This act provided an accepted definition of death. Most states have adopted the exact wording of the UDDA. Some states have added additional regulations to their laws.

> **VOCABULARY**
> **cessation** Bringing to an end.

Withholding or Withdrawing Life-Sustaining Treatment.

Withholding or withdrawing treatments that extend the life of a person can be emotional for the patient and family. This situation can also be ethically challenging for healthcare providers. It is important to remember that patients have the right to decline medical intervention. They can also determine when the intervention should be stopped. If the patient cannot make these decisions, it is up to the patient's surrogate.

Per the CEJA's opinion, providers should identify the patient's wishes early in the treatment. Should providers have questions regarding life-sustaining treatments, they should review the patient's advance directives, support the decisions of the patient or surrogate, and seek advice from an ethics committee.

Euthanasia.

Euthanasia is the act of killing a person who is suffering from an incurable disease. It can also be called "mercy killing" because it is ending the patient's suffering. Types of euthanasia include:

- *Active euthanasia*: Killing the person using an active means (e.g., an injection).
- *Passive euthanasia*: Withholding a lifesaving treatment (e.g., feeding tube) and letting the person die.
- *Voluntary euthanasia*: The patient consents to the action.
- *Involuntary euthanasia*: The patient does not consent to the action. Patients may be unconscious or unable to communicate their wishes.
- *Self-administered euthanasia*: The patient kills himself or herself.
- *Other-administered euthanasia*: Another person kills the patient.

- *Assisted suicide/assisted euthanasia*: The patient kills himself or herself with the assistance of another person (e.g., physician-assisted suicide).

Death with dignity laws are also called *physician-assisted dying* and *aid-in-dying laws*. These laws allow providers to make available the means for a patient to end their life. The means can be sleeping pills in lethal doses or some other medication that affects the breathing or heartbeat. The provider is also aware that the patient wants to commit suicide. Most states make physician-assisted euthanasia illegal. Only 10 states have legalized physician-assisted suicide. Most laws indicate a minimum age of 18, 6 months or less expected to live, and a required number of requests for the provider's assistance.

Proponents state that terminally ill patients have a right to end their suffering when they want to. Opponents state that providers have a moral responsibility to keep their patients alive. Per the CEJA's opinion, physician-assisted suicide is against the fundamental nature of the healer role of the provider. Providers must respond to the patient's needs at the end of life. They should respect the patient's autonomy and provide effective communication and emotional support. Providers need to make the patient comfortable and provide adequate pain medications.

Organ Donation Issues

According to organdonor.gov, more than 107,000 people are on the national transplant list. Six people are added to the national transplant waiting list every hour. The gap between available organs and those needing organs is increasing. More people need organs than are available. On average, 17 people die each day while waiting for a transplant. There continues to be a great need for organ and tissue donations.

According to Donate Life America (https://www.donatelife.net/), one organ donor can save eight lives. A cornea donation can restore the sight of two people. Donating tissue can heal the lives of 75 people. The following organs and tissue can be donated:

- Organs: Kidney, liver, lung, heart, pancreas, and intestines
- Tissue: Hands, faces, heart valves, skin, bones, tendons, bone marrow, cord blood stem cells, blood, platelets, corneas, and eyes

Living donations are becoming more common; that is, people donate organs or partial organs while living. For example, they can donate a kidney, a lobe of a lung, or a partial liver, intestine, or pancreas. Living tissue donations include skin after surgeries (e.g., abdominoplasty), bone after knee and hip replacement surgeries, bone marrow, umbilical cord blood, amnion, and blood. Both blood and bone marrow can be donated more than once. There are different types of living donations, including:

- *Directed donation*: The donor specifically names the person to receive the donation. Usually, this is a family member or someone the donor has heard about.
- *Nondirected donation*: The donor does not know the person nor is related to the person. The match is made based on the medical compatibility of the person and the donor. Both parties have the option to choose to meet the other person. If both agree and if the transplant center's policy permits it, they can meet.

- *Paired donation*: This involves at least two pairs of living kidney donors. The transplant candidates do not match the donor they know but match the other donor, thus the organs are swapped or traded.

If a person wishes to be a potential donor at death, registering in your state is the first step. Registration is available online or through your local motor vehicle department. (For more information, go to the website https://www.organdonor.gov.) It is also important to let your family know of your wishes. Some advance directive forms also have areas where you can include your wishes.

With organ donation, justice and medical utility are factors that are balanced. Justice refers to the fair consideration of the patient's situation and medical needs. Medical utility relates to trying to increase the number of transplants performed and the survival time of patients and organs. Many factors are considered when organs are matched to patients. When an organ becomes available, patients on the waiting list are screened for blood type, height, weight, and other medical factors. The computer uses national policies to determine the order of the candidates who would be a match for the donor's organs. The right-size organ and the geographic location of the donor organ and the candidate must be considered. Children do better with pediatric donor organs. Each organ has specific factors that are also considered in the allocation. For instance, waiting time, survival benefit, and medical needs may be considered. The following sections will examine laws and ethical recommendations related to organ donation.

Cord Blood Banking. Cord blood is found in the blood vessels of the placenta and umbilical cord. It is collected after the umbilical cord has been cut at birth. Cord blood is considered a biological product regulated by the FDA. Currently, cord blood is only used for hematopoietic stem cell transplantation procedures. Such a procedure is used for patients with leukemias and lymphomas. The cord blood has a source of stem cells that form into blood cells. If a cancer patient is given transplanted stem cells from cord blood, healthy blood cells regrow after chemotherapy has killed both cancer and healthy cells.

Collected cord blood can be frozen and stored for years. Parents may opt to store their baby's cord blood in a private bank so it can be used in the future by the child or a close relative. Private cord banks charge fees for collection and storage. Parents could also donate the cord blood to a public bank so it can be used for a patient who needs the hematopoietic stem cell transplant.

Uniform Anatomical Gift Act. The Uniform Anatomical Gift Act (UAGA) was enacted in 1968. All 50 states have adopted this law. The purpose of the act was to make it easier for people to donate organs. This act has been revised several times over the years. States enacted the UAGA, but differences existed between states. In 2006 the UAGA was revised to provide uniformity in organ and tissue donations across the nation. The 2006 revisions:

- clarified who can make donation decisions for the patient.

- strengthened language on protecting the patient's decision on donating or not donating organs.
- established standards for donor registries, which will help match donors to recipients.

The CEJA addressed organ donation. It is the opinion of the CEJA that providers should:

- avoid conflicts of interest and ensure that no members of the transplant team are involved with pronouncing the patient dead.
- ensure the death is pronounced using accepted clinical and ethical standards.
- ensure the transplantation procedures are performed by knowledgeable providers.
- ensure the prospective recipient of the donor is fully informed about the procedure.

National Organ Transplant Act. The National Organ Transplant Act (NOTA) was passed by Congress in 1984. The act established the Organ Procurement and Transplant Network (OPTN) to be run by contract by the Secretary of Health and Human Services. The act established a national registry for organ matching. NOTA also made it a criminal action to exchange organs for transplantation for something of value (e.g., money).

Xenotransplantation. With the lack of available organs and tissues, researchers are studying the use of nonhuman tissue and organs. *Xenotransplantation* is any procedure in which nonhuman cells, tissues, or organs are implanted or infused into a person.

Currently, pigs are the animals of choice for xenotransplants. Their organs are about the same size as humans, and they breed quickly. Pig heart valves are already being used to treat human heart valve issues.

CLOSING COMMENTS

When medical assistants are working with patients who are on the organ transplant waiting list, it is important for them to coach each patient on the process and encourage the patient to get emotional support. Once the patient is on the list, the transplant center will confirm the registration. If the person is removed from the list for any reason, the transplant center sends a written letter to the patient. The length of the wait is based on how sick the person is, the availability of organs that match, and the number of donors in the local area. With the organ allocation being based on many factors, a person's wait may vary. Sadly, some people's conditions deteriorate, and they are removed from the list and never get an organ.

Waiting for an organ transplant can cause a wide range of emotions. Once on the list the person is hopeful, but as the wait lengthens, the stress can increase. The same is true for the patient's family. It is important for the patient and family to get support during this time. Local or online support groups may be helpful.

PATIENT-CENTERED CARE

One of the key elements to providing patient-centered care is respecting the patient's decision and preferences. When working with ethical situations, it is important for the medical assistant to remember the Patient's Bill of Rights. Patients have the right to refuse treatment. They have the right to make their own decisions. Their decisions may not be our decisions in that situation, but we need to do what they want. It is important to respect patients and ensure their dignity during beginning-of-life issues through end-of-life issues.

BEING PROFESSIONAL

All healthcare professionals need to provide ethical, respectful care to all patients. Professional ethics guide healthcare employees on how to be ethical in their role. A medical assistant should be aware of the medical assisting code of ethics and the healthcare facility's professional ethics. The medical assistant needs to practice these professional ethics in every patient situation.

Role-play this scenario: You and Sam are medical assistants. Sam complains to you about all of the advance directive paperwork she has been handling for her provider. Sam states that he does not believe in having an advance directive. How do you respond to Sam?

CHAPTER REVIEW

Ethics are rules of conduct that differentiate between acceptable and unacceptable behavior. Morals are internal principles that distinguish between right and wrong.

Personal ethics are individual choices and are affected by one's morals. Professional ethics are created by associations for members to follow. They are also created by employers for employees to follow. Our personal morals affect our professional performance in other positive or negative ways. The chapter provided examples of both effects on our professional performance. As professionals, we cannot let our personal morals negatively affect the care that we provide to patients. It is important that medical assistants recognize the impact personal ethics and morals have on the delivery of healthcare.

There are four ethical principles in healthcare:

- Autonomy: The freedom to determine one's own actions and decisions
- Nonmaleficence: To do no harm
- Beneficence: To do good
- Justice: To treat patients fairly and give them what is due to them

These four principles need to be considered equally when one is evaluating ethical issues. The medical assistant has related responsibilities for each of these principles.

The chapter discussed ethical issues and CEJA's opinion for providers on the following ethical issues.

- Cloning, genetic engineering, genetic testing, pharmacogenetics, stem cell transplantation, and gene therapy. Many advances have occurred in genetics, and with them many ethical issues have surfaced.
- Different types of assistive reproductive technology. Gamete donation and egg freezing were also addressed, along with elective abortion.
- Adoptions, safe haven infant protection laws, and confidential healthcare.
- Abuse and influential guidelines and codes of ethics for clinical research. Seven main principles are involved with ethical research, and these include social and clinical value, scientific validity, fair subject selection, favorable risk-benefit ratio, independent review, informed consent, and respect for potential and enrolled subjects.
- End-of-life issues, such as advance directives, withholding or withdrawing life-sustaining treatment, and euthanasia. The five stages of grief and dying were discussed; these are:
- Denial: Person refuses to accept the diagnosis or prognosis.
- Anger: Person's anger can be directed at self or others.
- Bargaining: Person attempts to bargain with the higher power the person believes in.

- Depression: Person feels sadness, fear, and uncertainty.
- Acceptance: Person has come to terms with the situation.

Not everyone goes through all five stages, and people may not go through the stages in the order listed. Some people may switch back and forth between the stages.

Organ donation topics, including the need for organ and tissue donors, what can be donated, and the emotional wait for an organ, were discussed. The ethical issues related to organ donation and the CEJA's opinion were explained. It is important for potential donors to talk with their family members about their wishes.

The Patient Self-Determination Act (PSDA) requires most healthcare institutions at the time of admission to:

- Provide patients with a written document of their rights to make decisions and the facility's policies respecting advance directives.
- Ask patients if they have advance directives and document the response in the health record.

The Uniform Anatomical Gift Act (UAGA) was enacted in 1968, and all 50 states have adopted this law. The purpose of the act was to make it easier for people to donate organs. This act has been revised several times over the years.

SCENARIO WRAP-UP

Daniela has completed the ethics unit in her law and ethics course. She is excited to be done with the course. What she has learned in the ethics unit has helped her consider why she believes what she believes. She is realizing that some of her values and morals were built on information that was old or inaccurate. She needs to do some research to verify the information. Daniela feels that as she continues to learn and gain experience, her moral compass may change in the future. She hopes that this will help her to provide the best possible care to her patients.

PROCEDURE 20.1   Develop an Ethics Separation Plan

Task
To develop a plan for separating personal and professional ethics.

Scenario
You are working at WMFM Clinic. Your provider sees many children, including teens. New state laws allow confidential healthcare for minors. The agency has now adopted policies and procedures to allow providers to see teens 16 years or older without parental consent. The teens can be seen for sexually transmitted infections (STIs) and reproductive issues (including birth control). All health records related to these visits are confidential, meaning parents cannot be told about their child's visit.

 Your personal belief is that parents should always be allowed to know what is occurring with their children. They are responsible for the child until age 18, and they pay the bills. You also believe that children under 18 are too young to be in an intimate relationship with others. This type of relationship should be only for adults in a committed relationship. You do not believe in birth control.

Equipment and Supplies
- Paper and pen
- Medical Assisting Code of Ethics (see Box 20.1)

Procedural Steps
1. Read the code of ethics for medical assistants. Write down key themes or phrases.
   Purpose: Medical assistants need to follow the code of ethics for the medical assistant professional.
2. Using the scenario, write down the professional ethics involved in the situation.
   Purpose: Medical assistants need to follow the laws and the agency's policies and procedures. The procedures indicate how the healthcare professional needs to perform duties.
3. Using the scenario, write down the personal ethics involved in the situation.
   Purpose: Medical assistants need to identify their personal ethics. They need to be honest when analyzing how they think and feel about different scenarios that may occur in healthcare. Understanding one's biases is the first step in ensuring that respectful, ethical care is provided to all patients.
4. Compare the lists. Identify the personal ethics that conflict with the code of ethics and the professional ethics of the agency.
   Purpose: Medical assistants must identify areas where their personal ethics conflict with the code of ethics and the professional ethics of the agency. Medical assistants need to follow professional ethics. Personal ethics should not supersede professional ethics.

PROCEDURE 20.1   Develop an Ethics Separation Plan—cont'd

5. For each area of conflict, create a plan for how you will separate your personal and professional ethics. Remember, as a professional, you need to follow the professional ethics of the agency and the profession. Address how you will handle the situation and what would be your options if you were in the situation.

   Purpose: Medical assistants must create a plan and be aware of how they will handle situations that conflict with their personal ethics. This might

mean they need to find another job. They may need to rethink their biases. Learning more about a bias can help a person identify errors in their thinking.

6. Describe how the personal ethics and morals in this scenario would impact the patient care.

   Purpose: It is important that medical assistants recognize the impact personal ethics and morals have on the delivery of healthcare.

PROCEDURE 20.2   Demonstrate Professional Responses to Ethical Issues

Tasks

Identify ethical issues and demonstrate appropriate and professional responses. Recognize the impact personal ethics and morals have on the delivery of healthcare.

Scenario 1

You are working at WMFM Clinic. You are responsible for collecting payments from patients. Mr. Smythe, who is visually impaired, paid for his visit in cash. He gives you $500 for a $402 bill. You make change and give him a receipt. At the end of the day, you notice that you have $60 more than what you should have, and some of the bills were mixed up in the cashbox. You realize you gave Mr. Smythe the incorrect amount of money.

Scenario 2

You are setting up a laceration repair tray for Dr. Martin to use. As you are preparing the sterile equipment, one of the instruments becomes contaminated. You know Dr. Martin urgently needs the tray. You do nothing about the contamination, which you realize can cause an infection. You finish setting up the tray.

Directions:

You will role play both scenarios with a peer. You will be the medical assistant for both scenarios. Your peer will be supervisor for the first scenario and the provider for the second scenario.

Equipment and Supplies

- Paper and pen

Procedural Steps

1. Read both scenarios. Identify and write down the ethical issues involved.

   Purpose: It is important to identify the issues as the first step in responding to ethical situations.

2. With a peer, role-play scenario 1. Demonstrate a professional and appropriate ethical response to this situation.

   a. Explain the situation to the supervisor.

   b. Describe how you felt the error occurred and who received the incorrect change.

   c. Explain how you would like to handle the situation and correct the error.

   Purpose: It is important that the medical assistant act professionally and ethically when a mistake is discovered.

3. With a peer, role-play scenario 2. During the role play, demonstrate a professional and appropriate ethical response to this situation.

   Purpose: It is important that the medical assistant act ethically and notify the provider when an error is made.

4. In a written response, discuss the potential implication to the patient's health related to not reporting or correcting the error in scenario 2.

   Purpose: It is important that the medical assistant realize how unethical actions affect patient care.

21

Health Record

LEARNING OBJECTIVES

1. Discuss the importance of the health record to the patient and the healthcare team.
2. Describe the two types of health records.
3. Explain the ownership of the physical health record and its contents.
4. Describe the contents of the health record and give examples of information found in each section.
5. Differentiate between source-oriented medical records and problem-oriented medical records.
6. Describe organizational methods for progress notes, including SOAP and CHEDDAR.
7. Explain guidelines for documenting in the health record.
8. Describe how to make corrections in the paper health record.
9. Describe filing equipment and supplies needed for paper health records.
10. Discuss how to use the alphabetical and numerical filing methods.
11. Explain the filing process for paper health records.
12. Describe the features of the electronic health record and the practice management software.
13. Summarize the importance of the HIPAA Privacy Rule and Security Rule.
14. Describe storage, retention, and destruction of health records.

OUTLINE

⟩⟩ OPENING SCENARIO

Susan Beezler has just begun her career in the medical assisting profession. In the morning, she attends medical assisting school, and in the afternoon, she works part-time for Walden-Martin Family Medical (WMFM) Clinic as a record assistant. Susan is eager to learn about healthcare and looks forward to taking on more responsibility at the office.

Dr. David Kahn is a new provider who has recently joined WMFM Clinic. Dr. Kahn has enjoyed working with Susan and feels that her energy will be just what his patients need. He has taken a professional interest in Susan and often lets her assist him with patients when her other duties allow.

Susan knows that although she is a beginner in the office, she will gain trust from her supervisors and patients if she projects a teachable attitude. The office has recently converted to an electronic records system but is also still using paper health records. Susan uses the information she learned in school about both types of health records. She cheerfully performs filing and even does some transcription for Dr. Kahn. The other staff members are pleased with her willingness to perform the most mundane tasks.

Susan enjoys sharing her experiences with her classmates. She is the only student currently working in the medical field, and the others ask her lots of questions about the "real world" of medical assisting. She is careful not to breach patient confidentiality; she discusses situations only in general terms, never mentioning any patients' names.

Susan feels a great sense of pride in knowing that she is already a member of the healthcare team and can contribute to the lives of her patients.

YOU WILL LEARN

1. To describe the two types of health records and the ownership of health records.
2. To determine information found in the different sections of the health record.
3. To document and correct errors in the health record.
4. To apply the indexing rules for alphabetical and numerical filing systems.
5. To understand the impact of the Health Information Technology for Economic and Clinical Health (HITECH) Act on health records.
6. To back up an electronic health record using different methods.
7. To apply the correct procedures for destroying records.

INTRODUCTION

Health records are important legal documents in healthcare. According to the American Health Information Management Association (AHIMA) (https://www.ahima.org/), the health record serves multiple purposes. The health record:

- *Provides the documentation regarding a person's health.* This documentation shows the support for the healthcare plan of care.
- *Helps to provide the best possible medical care for the patient.* The provider uses information from the patient, the physical examination, and test results to diagnose the condition, determine a treatment plan, and the patient's prognosis (prog NOH sis). The health record provides a complete history of all the care given to the patient. During future interactions, other healthcare providers can review the documentation and provide continuity of care. By reviewing the documentation, each provider knows the services provided and can continue the care, even from one facility to another, such as the hospital to the ambulatory care facility.
- *Supports reimbursement claims.* The health record provides the necessary documentation for the reimbursement claims sent to the third-party payers (e.g., insurance companies).
- *Gives legal protection for those who provided care to the patient.* The health record is a legal document that provides information on all the patient interactions with the healthcare facility. An accurate health record provides the proof needed for a legal defense in a medical malpractice case. Remember, if it is not documented, it did not happen.
- *Provides statistical information that is helpful to researchers.* The patient's record provides information on the effectiveness of certain kinds of treatment (e.g., medications) or to determine the incidence (IN si duh ns) of a given disease. The effects of various treatments and procedures can be tracked and statistics gathered from patients' records. When tracking statistical information, the direct patient identifiers are removed.

VOCABULARY

continuity of care The smooth continuation of care from one provider to another. This allows the patient to receive the most benefit and with no interruption or duplication of care.

direct patient identifiers Used to link the information back to a specific person and can include payment, insurance, and personal demographic information

incidence How often something happens.

prognosis The likely outcome of a disease, including the chance of recovery.

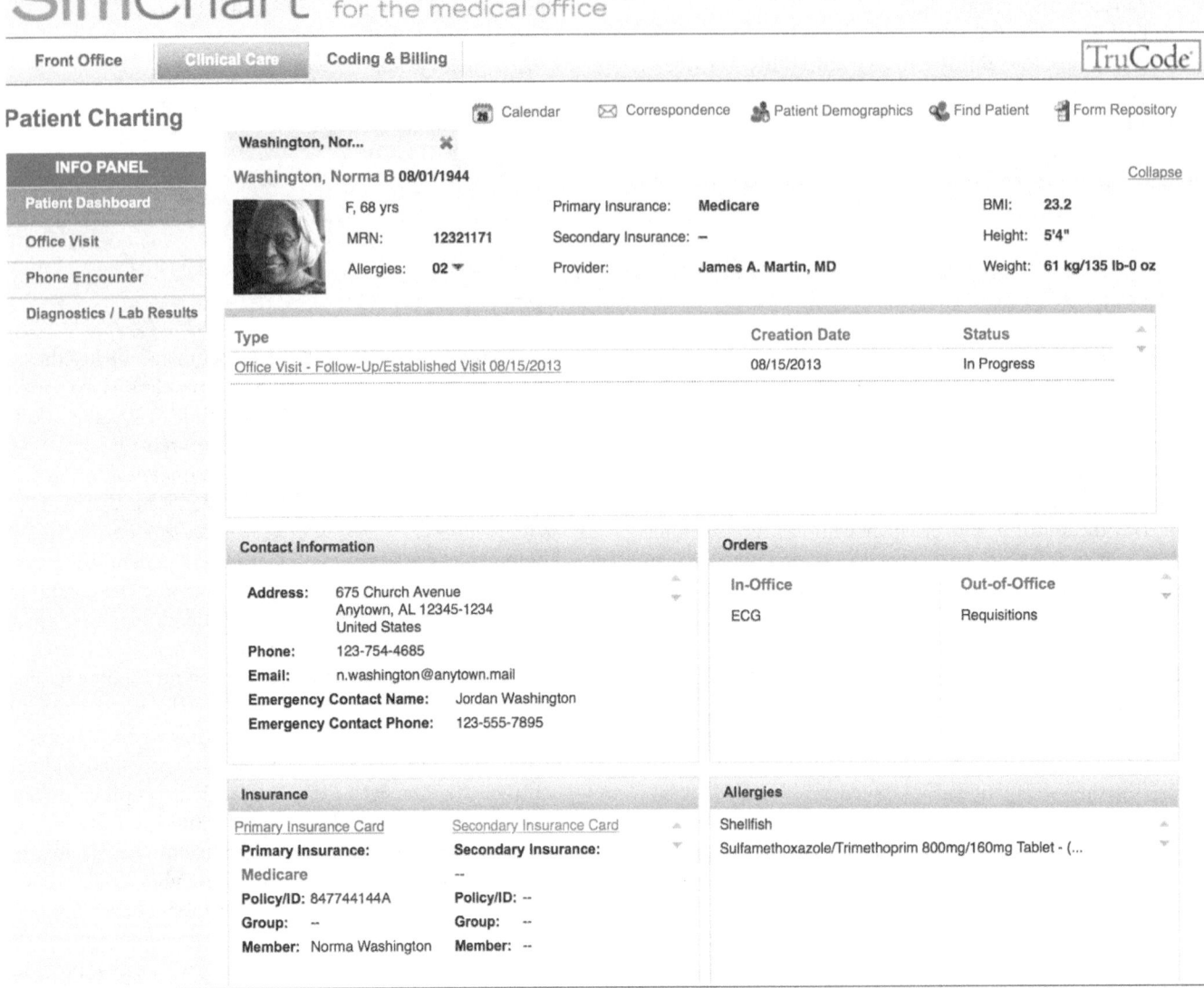

Fig. 21.1 The electronic health record (EHR) can perform numerous tasks, in addition to displaying personal information about the patient. This allows the provider and medical assistants to interact with patients and provide better service.

TYPES OF HEALTH RECORDS

There are two types of health records, paper and electronic. Paper health records have been shown to be much less efficient than an electronic health record (EHR). The paper-based record is good for patient care documentation, but it is not nearly as useful in other capacities (Fig. 21.1). An EHR can include practice management capabilities that allow for patient scheduling and the generation of reports needed for research and quality control. Box 21.1 provides the benefits and limitations of both formats. (Additional information on both formats will be provided later in the chapter.)

Most healthcare facilities have switched to the EHR format. The US federal government has also offered financial incentives for providers to implement EHRs. Although most providers are using EHRs, some still use paper records and others use a combination of electronic and paper. When a provider or facility makes the switch to an EHR, they may decide to keep the patient's paper health record and just use the EHR for all future patient interactions. Some providers may decide to scan the past 3 to 5 years of the paper record into the EHR. Whatever the scenario, it is important for the medical assistant to understand both systems and to be able to perform well with either one.

VOCABULARY

electronic health record (EHR) An electronic record that conforms to nationally recognized standards and contains health-related information about a specific patient. It can be created, managed, and consulted by authorized clinicians and staff from more than one healthcare organization.

quality control A process to ensure the reliability of test results, often using manufactured samples with known values.

BOX 21.1 Limitations and Benefits of Health Record Formats

Paper Health Records

Benefits
- No "downtime"; always able to use the paper health records

Limitations
- Less efficient; only one person can use it at a time
- Filing errors
- Challenging when gathering data for research and quality control
- Illegible handwriting makes documentation difficult to read
- Storage takes a lot of physical space

Electronic Health Records

Benefits
- Easy storage of patient information
- Accessibility to multiple users at the same time
- Fewer errors because notes are typed
- Can link clinical information for billing purposes
- More efficient claims submission process
- Data usually stored offsite and can be retrieved if facility is destroyed

Limitations
- Does not function during downtimes (e.g., computer issues, power outages). Facility must have procedures for paper documentation during downtimes. Downtime activities are then added to the (EHR) when it is functioning.
- Expense of computer equipment and software
- Training time for staff

CRITICAL THINKING 21.1

Jennifer, the office manager, has noticed that Susan seems overwhelmed in the training classes for the EHR system used by the clinic. During a break, Jennifer asks Susan whether she is having any specific problems with the training classes. She also asks for Susan's input on the system. Susan says that she just prefers clinical work and that her typing skills are a little "rusty." She is determined to do her best to learn the system and asks if she could have extra practice time. How might Jennifer respond to Susan's comments? What can Susan do to overcome her issues with the EHR system?

Ownership of the Health Record

Patients often assume that because the information in the health record is about them, ownership of the record is rightfully theirs. However, the owner of the physical health record (e.g., paper or electronic) is the provider or healthcare facility. The patient owns the information within the health record. Thus the patient has the right to access the information within the record, but does not own the physical record or other documents in the record. The patient has a vested interest and therefore has the right to demand confidentiality of all information placed in the record.

The actual paper health record should never leave the healthcare facility where it originated. Even the provider should refrain from taking the record from the office to the hospital or extended care facility. If information from the record is needed, copies can be made, and progress notes can be written on site

vested Granted or endowed with a particular authority, right, or property; to have a special interest in.

and placed into the original record later. Patients' paper records should be kept in a locked room or locked filing cabinets when the office is closed. EHRs must be protected from unauthorized access. (More will be discussed later in the chapter.)

CRITICAL THINKING 21.2

Some of Dr. Khan's patients are concerned that computer-based health records may not be completely private. They are worried that unauthorized individuals could access their information on the computer and do them harm. Should patients be allowed to decide whether their records are kept on computer or on paper? Why or why not?

CONTENTS OF THE HEALTH RECORD

Regardless of the type of health record, paper or electronic, both will contain the same information. This section will discuss the contents of the health record.

Personal Demographics

During or prior to the first visit, patients will provide their demographic information. Many times, patients need to complete a patient information form (Fig. 21.2). The following information is gathered from the form.

- Patient's full name
- Names of parents/guardians if the patient is a child or legally incompetent
- Patient's sex
- Date of birth
- Marital status
- Name of spouse if married
- Home address, telephone number, and email address
- Occupation
- Name of employer
- Business address and telephone number
- Employment information for spouse
- Healthcare insurance information
- Source of referral
- Social Security number

Past Medical History

The patient's past medical history (PMH) or past history (PH) includes:
- Previous illnesses/injuries, including usual childhood diseases (UCD), dental conditions, and behavioral health conditions
- Previous hospitalizations and surgeries
- Medications and immunizations
- Allergies
- Gynecologic and obstetric history (for women)

The dates that these occurred will need to be documented, in addition to any complications that may have arisen. The provider needs to be aware of this information because it could affect the patient's current condition. The patient may give this information along with the family, social, and occupational histories either verbally to the provider or medical assistant or in written/electronic format. The medical assistant may need to review the histories for completeness before the provider sees the patient.

Immunization and Medication Records. The immunization record may show all the vaccines the patient has received or just the vaccines given in that specific ambulatory care facility. Many

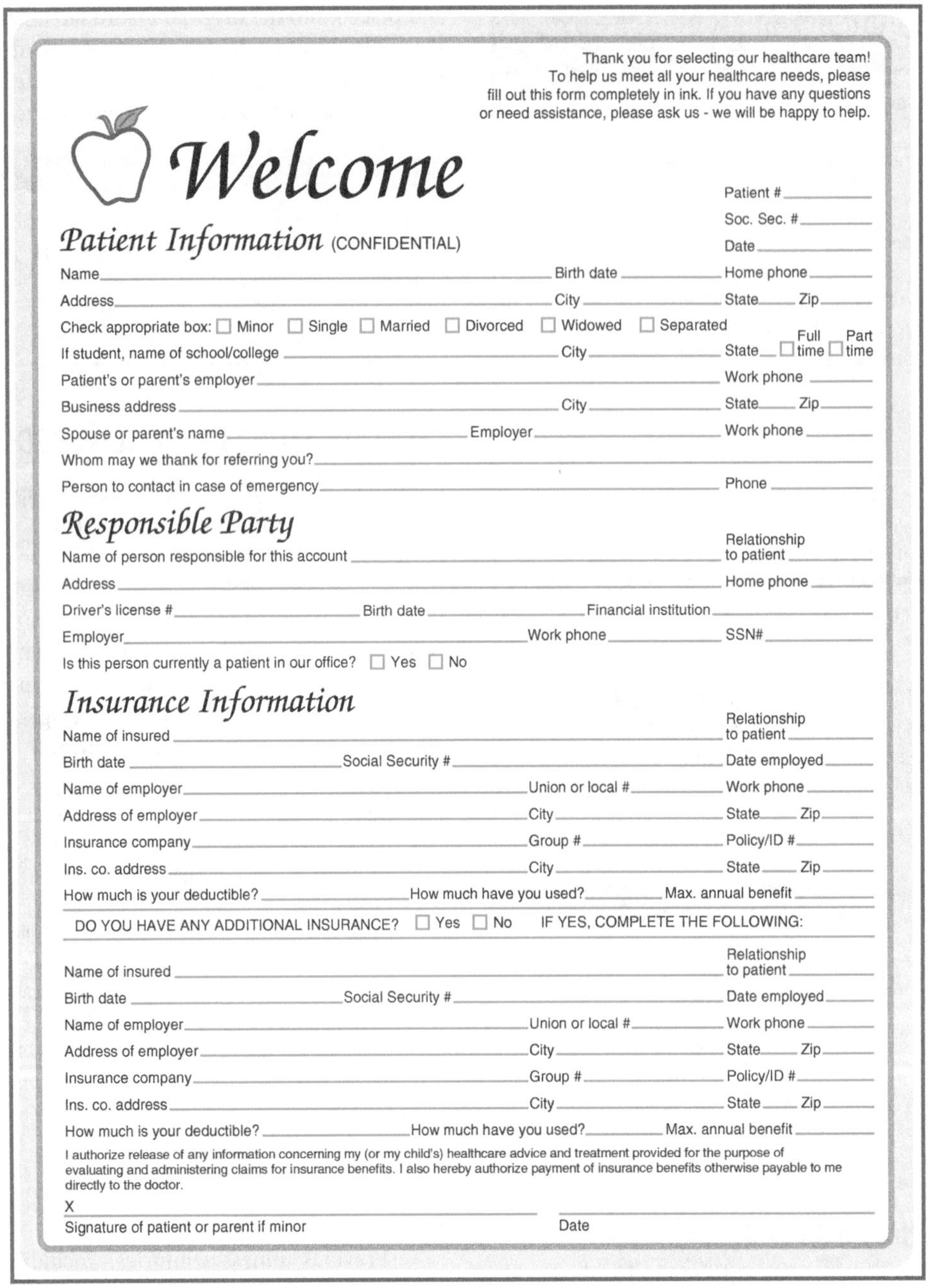

Thank you for selecting our healthcare team!
To help us meet all your healthcare needs, please
fill out this form completely in ink. If you have any questions
or need assistance, please ask us - we will be happy to help.

Welcome

Patient # _____

Soc. Sec. # _____

Date _____

Patient Information (CONFIDENTIAL)

Name _____ Birth date _____ Home phone _____

Address _____ City _____ State _____ Zip _____

Check appropriate box: ☐ Minor ☐ Single ☐ Married ☐ Divorced ☐ Widowed ☐ Separated

If student, name of school/college _____ City _____ State ___ ☐ Full time ☐ Part time

Patient's or parent's employer _____ Work phone _____

Business address _____ City _____ State _____ Zip _____

Spouse or parent's name _____ Employer _____ Work phone _____

Whom may we thank for referring you? _____

Person to contact in case of emergency _____ Phone _____

Responsible Party

Name of person responsible for this account _____ Relationship to patient _____

Address _____ Home phone _____

Driver's license # _____ Birth date _____ Financial institution _____

Employer _____ Work phone _____ SSN# _____

Is this person currently a patient in our office? ☐ Yes ☐ No

Insurance Information

Name of insured _____ Relationship to patient _____

Birth date _____ Social Security # _____ Date employed _____

Name of employer _____ Union or local # _____ Work phone _____

Address of employer _____ City _____ State _____ Zip _____

Insurance company _____ Group # _____ Policy/ID # _____

Ins. co. address _____ City _____ State _____ Zip _____

How much is your deductible? _____ How much have you used? _____ Max. annual benefit _____

DO YOU HAVE ANY ADDITIONAL INSURANCE? ☐ Yes ☐ No   IF YES, COMPLETE THE FOLLOWING:

Name of insured _____ Relationship to patient _____

Birth date _____ Social Security # _____ Date employed _____

Name of employer _____ Union or local # _____ Work phone _____

Address of employer _____ City _____ State _____ Zip _____

Insurance company _____ Group # _____ Policy/ID # _____

Ins. co. address _____ City _____ State _____ Zip _____

How much is your deductible? _____ How much have you used? _____ Max. annual benefit _____

I authorize release of any information concerning my (or my child's) healthcare advice and treatment provided for the purpose of evaluating and administering claims for insurance benefits. I also hereby authorize payment of insurance benefits otherwise payable to me directly to the doctor.

X _____   _____

Signature of patient or parent if minor   Date

Fig. 21.2 The patient information form provides all of the information the medical assistant needs to construct the patient's record.

states have statewide immunization record software that can be accessed by healthcare facilities and can be used to update the facility's record.

The medication record indicates all the medications a patient takes. This includes prescribed and over-the-counter (OTC) medications, herbal supplements, minerals, and vitamins. The name, *dose* (amount), *frequency* (how often it is taken), *route* (how it gets into the body), and reason for taking it are documented.

Allergies. An *allergy* is an immune reaction to a substance that is usually not harmful. Allergies can range from minor to severe. *Anaphylaxis* (an uh fuh LAK sis) is a severe reaction that can be life-threatening.

Medication, food, and environmental allergies need to be documented in the patient's health record. Besides indicating the substance that causes the allergy, the health record needs to document the patient's reactions. Allergies should be reviewed with the patient during each visit or clinical interaction. Allergy stickers are placed on the front of the paper health record to indicate the allergies (Fig. 21.3). EHRs have a section to document allergies. These allergies can trigger alerts to the user during specific EHR activities.

Family History

The patient's family history (FH) includes information about the health of the grandparents, parents, and siblings. The FH includes:

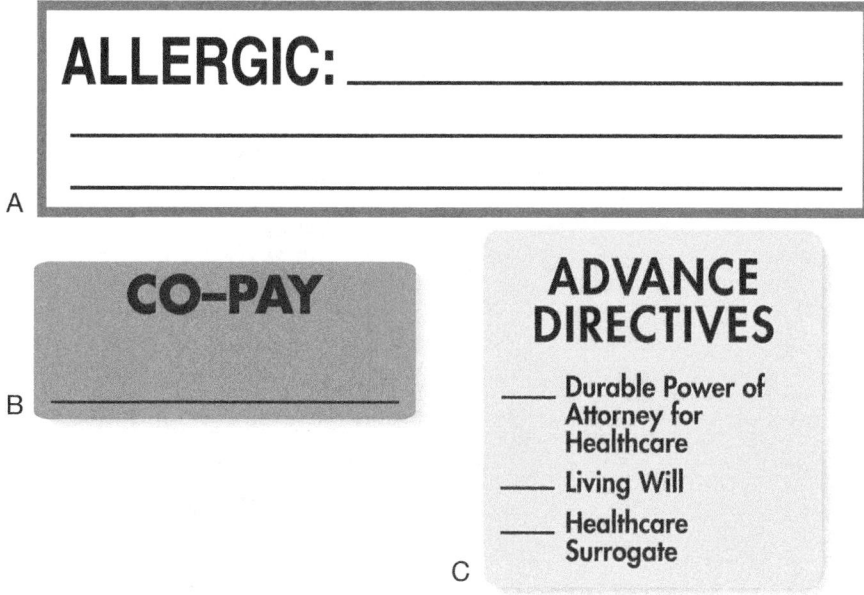

ALLERGIC: _____

A

CO-PAY

B _____

ADVANCE DIRECTIVES

____ Durable Power of Attorney for Healthcare

____ Living Will

____ Healthcare Surrogate

C

Fig. 21.3 Record Stickers. Information on stickers on the outside of the record allows the provider and medical staff to see important information about the patient quickly. (Courtesy Bibbero Systems, an InHealth Company, Petaluma, CA (800) 242-2376, https://www.bibbero.com.)

- Age and health status of living family members
- Hereditary and familial diseases
- Age and causes of death for deceased family members

> **VOCABULARY**
> **hereditary** Passed from parents to offspring through the genes.

Social and Occupational History

The social history (SH) includes information about the patient's personal habits and lifestyle. The SH includes:

- Living situation
- Marital status
- Sleep patterns
- Diet
- Hobbies
- Education

- Tobacco/nicotine use (e.g., cigarettes, cigars, e-cigs, chew, snuff, snus, dissolvable tobacco)
- Alcohol use
- Drug use
- Sexual history and preference
- Education

The occupational history (OH) contains information on the person's employment. All these factors can have an impact on a patient's overall health and also help to highlight risk factors.

> **CRITICAL THINKING 21.3**
>
> While taking a patient's medical history, Susan asks about his social history. She asks whether he drinks alcohol. The patient immediately becomes defensive and accuses Susan of getting too personal about his affairs. How might Susan explain her reasons for asking these questions? What options are available if the patient refuses to discuss his social history with Susan? Could this opposition to questions about the social history raise suspicion in Susan's mind? What might she suspect?

Chief Complaint and History of Present Illness

The chief complaint (CC) is the main reason for the patient's visit. It is usually documented using the patient's own words. When you are documenting the patient's own words, it is important to use quotation marks ("").

The history of present illness (HPI) is a concise account of the current illness. This should be a chronologic description of the patient's symptoms from when they started to the present time. The HPI elaborates on the chief complaint. (See Chapter 34 for more information on taking the HPI.)

Physical Examination

New patients complete a general health history questionnaire (also called a *review of systems* [ROS]) either in paper or electronic form prior to seeing the provider (Fig. 21.4). The patient must answer questions or indicate any concerns for each body system. In some facilities, the medical assistant completes the form while asking the patient questions. The provider will use the form to ask the patient additional questions about the person's concerns. The ROS form provides a baseline for the provider. During the physical examination, the provider will examine each body system. The provider's findings are included in the progress notes.

> **VOCABULARY**
> **baseline** An observation or value that represents the normal or beginning level of a measurable quality; used for comparison.

Progress Notes

Progress notes are written by the providers caring for and treating the patient. The notes provide an ongoing record of:

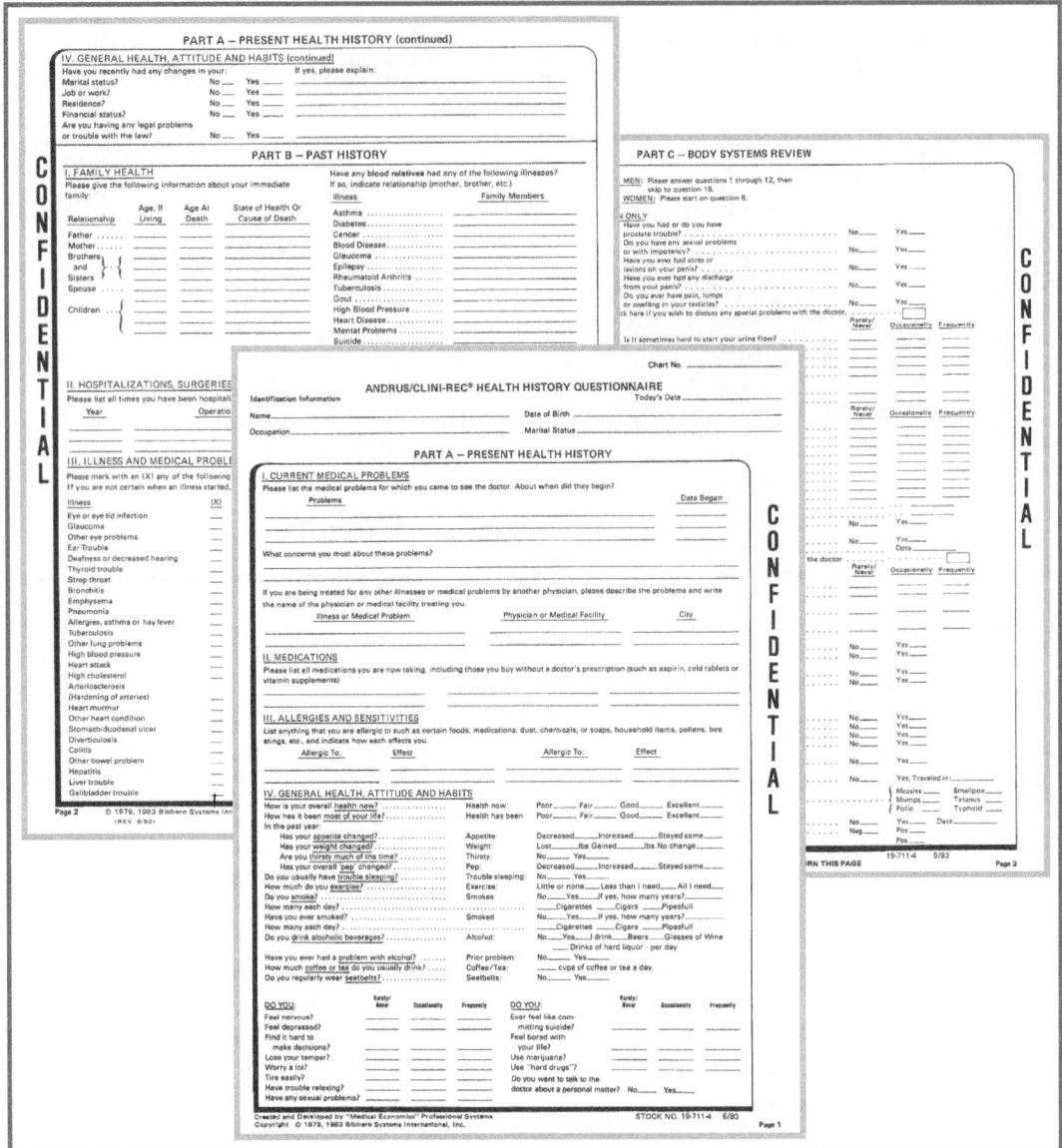

Fig. 21.4 Self-Administered General Health History Questionnaire. The patient should complete lengthy questionnaires before being seen by the provider. Either the questionnaire can be mailed to the patient in advance, or the patient can be asked to come in early to complete the paperwork. (Courtesy Bibbero Systems, an InHealth Company, Petaluma, CA (800) 242-2376, https://www.bibbero.com.)

- Signs, symptoms, feelings, and concerns reported by the patient
- Clinical findings from the physical examination and laboratory and diagnostic tests
- Provider's impression and diagnosis
- Treatment plan

Additional information on progress notes will be discussed later in the chapter.

> **VOCABULARY**
>
> **sign** Something that is measured or observed by others; also called *objective data.* Examples of signs include redness, swelling or edema, blood pressure, and pulse.
>
> **symptom** Something that is only perceived by the patient; also called *subjective data.* Examples include pain, headache, dizziness, and nausea.

Laboratory and Diagnostic Imaging Reports

The health record contains the results from the laboratory and diagnostic imaging tests performed. Laboratory ("lab") results include tests done on blood, body fluids (e.g., urine, sputum), and other tissues or substances taken from the body.

Diagnostic imaging tests provide information on the structures and activities in the body. Examples of diagnostic tests include x-rays, computed tomography (CT) scans, nuclear medicine scans, Magnetic resonance imaging (MRI) scans, and ultrasounds (US). Laboratory and diagnostic imaging tests help providers diagnose diseases or conditions.

Consultation Reports

A *medical consult* occurs when a patient is referred to another healthcare provider for an examination and treatment. Many times, the medical consult occurs in a specialty department, such as cardiology or neurology. The consultation report from the visit is sent to the referring provider and placed in the patient's health record. All paper reports must be scanned and uploaded into the EHR.

Hospital Documents

Hospital documents are dictated by the *attending physician*, or the physician responsible for the patient's care in the hospital. This physician can be the patient's regular provider or a different physician, such as a hospitalist or surgeon. Hospital documents that are typically provided to ambulatory care facilities include:

- *Discharge summary*: Created at the time the patient is discharged from the hospital. A discharge summary includes the reason for hospitalization, significant findings during the stay, treatments and procedures provided, discharge instructions given, and the patient's discharge condition.
- *Operative report*: Created after a surgical procedure is performed. The operative report indicates a diagnosis, the date and type of procedure, names of all providers involved with the procedure, summary of the patient's history, description of the procedure, and follow-up care.
- *Emergency department report*: Summarizes the patient's visit to the emergency department and includes the reason, significant findings, treatments and procedures provided, and discharge instructions.

Miscellaneous Documents

The patient's health record also contains the following:

- *Correspondence*: Letters or emails related to the patient's care.
- *Release of information forms*: Patients must complete, date, and sign a (medical) records release form for their records to be transferred to another facility. No records, including images and videos, can be released without the completed form. Patients can *rescind* (cancel) the release at any time.
- *Disclosure authorization forms*: When patients request their information to be given to another person (e.g., family member, friend), they need to complete and sign a disclosure authorization form. (See Chapter 19 for more information.)
- *Notice of Privacy Practices (NPP)*: The healthcare facility is legally obligated to give each patient a notice that explains how the health information may be used and shared. The Health Information Portability and Accountability Act (HIPAA) requires that patients state in writing that they received the NPP document. The healthcare facility may ask the patient to sign a paper or electronic document. This form is then kept in the patient's health record. If the patient refuses to sign, the provider can still use and disclose the health information as permitted by HIPAA. The refusal needs to be documented in the patient's health record.
- *Consent for treatment and authorization form*: Varies by facility; gives providers permission to treat the patient. Allows the facility to bill and collect payments from the patient's insurance provider.
- *Consent forms*: Prior to certain procedures and tests, the patient must be informed of the risks and benefits of the procedure. A signed consent form is required before the procedure or test can be performed. All consent forms signed by the patient must be maintained in the health record. (See Chapter 18 for more information on informed consents.)

- *Images/copies*: Digital images or copies of the insurance card and the patient's photo identification are included in the health record.
- *Advance directives*: These are written instructions about healthcare decisions should a person be unable to make them. The completed form is kept in the health record. (See Chapter 20 for more information on advance directives.)
- *Health records*: Past health records from other facilities are also included in the health record. This can include records from home health agencies and physical therapy clinics.

ORGANIZATION OF HEALTH RECORDS

Source-Oriented Medical Records

The traditional patient record is a source-oriented medical record (SOMR), also called a *source-oriented record* (SOR). Observations and data are filed according to their source. For example, the provider's progress notes are in one section, laboratory and diagnostic imaging results are in other sections, and so on. Each section is organized in reverse chronologic order.

VOCABULARY

hospitalist A provider who oversees the general medical care of hospitalized patients; may include physicians, nurse practitioners, and physician assistants.

reverse chronologic order A system of organization in which the most recent item is on top and oldest item is last.

Problem-Oriented Medical Records

The problem-oriented medical record (POMR), also called a *problem-oriented record* (POR), is a method of recording data in a problem-solving system. The POMR is patient centered and allows the providers to have a holistic view of the patient. The POMR is especially helpful in clinics, group practices, and hospitals, where more than one person must be able to find essential information in the record.

This system is divided into four components:

- *Database*: Includes the chief complaint, history of present illness, physical examination, and laboratory and diagnostic imaging reports.
- *Problem list*: Each problem the patient has that requires management or workup is given a number and title. The problem list can include social, psychological, and physical problems (Fig. 21.5).
- *Plan*: For each problem, a diagnosis and treatment plan are indicated. Each plan is titled and numbered, which correlates to the problem number.
- *Progress notes*: Includes structured notes that are numbered to correspond with each problem number.

SOAP Notes and CHEDDAR Format. SOAP notes or SOAP documentation evolved from the POMR. SOAP is an acronym for the following:

MASTER PROBLEM LIST
For use of this form, see AR 40-66; the proponent agency is the Office of The Surgeon General

MAJOR PROBLEMS

PROBLEM NUMBER	DATE ONSET	DATE ENTERED	PROBLEM	DATE RESOLVED
1.				
2.				
3.				
4.				
5.				
6.				
7.				
8.				
9.				
10.				
11.				
12.				

TEMPORARY (MINOR) PROBLEMS

PROBLEM LETTER	PROBLEM	DATES OF OCCURRENCES				
A.						
B.						
C.						
D.						
E.						
F.						
G.						
H.						

PATIENT'S IDENTIFICATION (Use mechanical imprint if available; for typed or written entries give: Name, SSN, Unit, Sex, Birthdate, and Duty Phone)	SUMMARY OF PROBLEMS, ALLERGIES, MEDICATIONS, SURGERIES AND TRAUMAS:
	NOTE: DO NOT DISCARD FROM CHART

Fig. 21.5 A Problem List Designed for a Problem-Oriented Medical Record (POMR). (From Proctor D, et al: *Kinn's the medical assistant,* ed 13, St. Louis, 2017, Elsevier.)

- *Subjective data*: Obtained from the patient. Includes the chief complaint, history of present illness, patient's history (medical, family, social, and occupational), review of systems, current medications, and allergies.
- *Objective data*: Clinical evidence or observations from the provider. Includes vital signs, measurements, physical exam findings, and laboratory and diagnostic test results.
- *Assessment*: Based on all the evidence provided in the patient's history, the physical examination, and any supplementary tests, the provider indicates the problem number and diagnosis. If some doubt remains, the diagnosis may be labeled as a provisional diagnosis. A *differential diagnosis* is the process of weighing the probability of one disease

causing the patient's illness against the probability that other diseases are causative.
- *Plan*: Includes the provider's suggested treatments, such as therapy, medications, procedures, specialist referrals, and patient education needed.

The SOAP documentation forces a rational approach to the patient's problems and assists in forming a logical, orderly plan of patient care (Fig. 21.6). Variations of SOAP notes are seen in ambulatory care, including:

> **VOCABULARY**
> **provisional diagnosis** A temporary diagnosis made before all test results have been received.

- SOAPE: Adds Evaluation to SOAP. The evaluation section addresses how the plan is working.
- SOAPIE: Adds Intervention and Evaluation. The intervention section addresses what was done.
- SOAPER: Adds Education and Response. The education notation shows that the patient was educated about the condition or given patient education material. The response section is used to record an assessment of the patient's understanding of and possible compliance with the treatment plan.

The CHEDDAR format can be used in place of the SOAP notes. CHEDDAR is an acronym for:

Chief complaint
History
Examination
Details of problem and complaints
Drugs or dosages
Assessment
Return visit or referral

CRITICAL THINKING 21.4

Susan learned about SOAP notes in school and is eager to use it in her new job. Dr. Kahn is seeing a patient who reports to Susan that she has had nausea and vomiting for the past 3 days. Susan obtains a weight of 132.5 pounds, temperature (T) 101.2°F tympanically, pulse (P) 94 beats/min, respiration (R) 14 breaths/min, and blood pressure (BP) 122/84 mm Hg in the right arm. What information would be documented in the Subjective field? What information would be documented in the Objective field? Who would document information in the Assessment field?

Fig. 21.6 SOAP Notes. SOAP notes keep information organized and in a logical sequence. An actual progress note would include the provider's or medical assistant's signature or initials after this entry. (Courtesy Bibbero Systems, an InHealth Company, Petaluma, CA (800) 242-2376, https://www.bibbero.com.)

DOCUMENTING IN THE HEALTH RECORD

All patient visits, no-shows, telephone calls, correspondence, and electronic communication (e.g., email and patient portal) need to be documented. Follow these guidelines when documenting in the health record:

- Check the name on the record prior to documenting.
- Document immediately after the procedure is done; never prior to performing the procedure.
- Documentation should be in the order in which the steps were completed.
- Be accurate, specific, and concise. Phrases instead of complete sentences can be used. Do not include judgmental statements.
- Use only facility-approved abbreviations.
- When using the patient's own words, use quotation marks (" ") around the patient's words.
- Use punctuation, such as periods to indicate the end of a thought.
- Do not use "I" in the documentation, because it is understood the person signing the note did it.
- Read the documentation, checking the accuracy of the spelling, punctuation, and facts.
- If a documentation error occurs, do not hide the error. If the error could, in any way, affect the patient's health and well-being, it must be brought to the provider's attention immediately. When an error is discovered in an entry at a later date or if information was erroneous left out of a prior documentation, regardless of the record format, an *addendum* containing the correct information is added to the record.

The addendum provides updated or additional information. The medical assistant should start an addendum with the current date and time. It should reference the original entry that needs revision and also provide the reason for the addition or clarification. If a provider was updated on the change, that should be included. The addendum should be signed by the medical assistant.

> **VOCABULARY**
> **concise** Using as few words as possible to express the message.
> **no-show** A patient who fails to keep an appointment without giving advance notice.
> **patient portal** A secure online website that gives patients 24-hour access to personal health information using a username and password.

Paper Health Record

When you are documenting in a paper health record, begin a new entry on the next blank line. The entry will always start with the date in the MM/DD/YYYY format. The date will be followed by the time. This may be written in 12-hour clock or military time. If 12-hour clock time is used, it must be followed by a.m. or p.m. (e.g., 2:00 p.m.). If military time is used, it consists only of a four-digit number (e.g., 1400) (Box 21.2).

Additional guidelines for documenting in the paper health record, include:

- Write legibly.
- Always use ink. Black ink is preferred, because it copies best when records are duplicated.
- Make sure the patient's name and medical record number are on each page of documentation.
- Sign the documentation as indicated by the facility. The signature usually includes the signer's first name or initial, last name, and title.

When a correction needs to be made in the paper health record, the medical assistant must follow the facility's policies and procedures. Erasing, using correction fluid, or any other type of obliteration (uh blit uh REY shun) is never acceptable. To correct a handwritten entry:

1. Draw a single line through the error.
2. Insert the correction above, immediately after the error, or in the margin. The correction needs to be in a spot where it can be read clearly.
3. Write "error."
4. Add the date and your signature and title (Fig. 21.7). (Some facilities will just require your initials instead of your signature.)

> **VOCABULARY**
> **obliteration** Removal or destruction of all traces; do away with; destroy completely.

Electronic Health Record

Documentation in an EHR involves using radio buttons, drop-down menus, and free-text boxes. The radio buttons and drop-down menus allow for standardization of the content in the EHR. The free-text boxes allow for the documentation of the unique circumstances found with each patient (Fig. 21.8). It is important to carefully review the choices made with the radio buttons and drop-down menus. Information documented using the free-text boxes should be proofread before the record is submitted.

> **BOX 21.2 Military Time**
>
> Military time or 24-hour clock uses four numbers. The first two digits show the hour, and the last two digits reflect the minutes. Military time starts with midnight, which is referred to as 0000 or 2400. Before 1 p.m., the hours are the same as the 12-hour clock time. After 1 p.m., add the hour to the 12. For example, 6 p.m. would be 1800 and 10 p.m. would be 2200.

Each EHR user gets a unique user identification. When a medical assistant documents in the EHR, the person's name is attached to the documentation. It is important to never give your unique user identification to another person. Make sure you are logged out of the EHR before others use your computer device. If you are not logged out, any activity or documentation by another person will appear to be yours.

When correcting errors in the EHR, the medical assistant must follow the facility's policies and procedures. The corrected content will be seen. An audit trail can show documentation deletions and revisions. It will also indicate the date, time, and person making the changes to the health record.

Dictation and Transcription

With the increased use of EHRs and voice recognition software, there is a decreased need for transcription. If dictation is still done in the healthcare facility, the administrative medical assistant may find that transcribing the dictation is a job they will sometimes perform. Transcription can be done from handwritten notes or, more likely, from machine dictation. Smooth operation of the facility may depend on the timely, accurate performance of assigned responsibilities, such as record documentation and the preparation of special reports. Accuracy and speed are the primary requirements, along with a strong grasp of medical terminology, anatomy, and physiology.

Dictation may be done using a machine transcription unit or a portable transcription unit. Many healthcare facilities use a system that is accessed by telephone. The provider calls the system using passwords or access codes and records the information for the health record while speaking into the telephone. Later, employees transcribe the information into the health record. The provider must acknowledge and initial all transcripts before they are placed in the health record.

> **VOCABULARY**
> **audit trail** Record of computer activity used to monitor users' actions within software, including additions, deletions, and viewing of electronic records.
> **dictation** To say something aloud for another person to write down.
> **transcription** To make a written copy of dictated material.
> **unique user identification** Each employee is assigned a unique name or number for identifying and tracking user identify.

Voice Recognition Software. Some healthcare facilities use voice recognition software for transcription. When first installed, the software requires the user to say several sentences

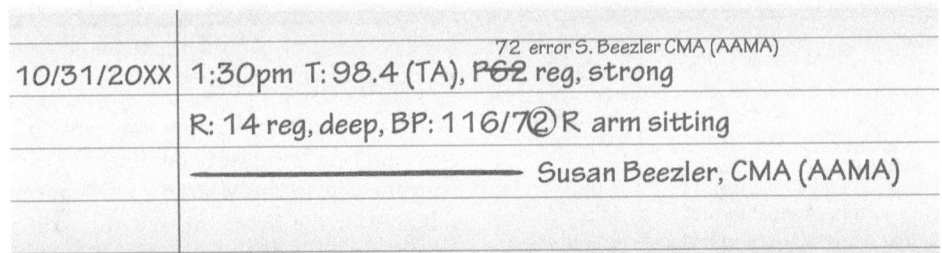

Fig. 21.7 Corrections to health records must be done in a legible manner and must be clearly understood. Always initial and date corrections to paper health records.

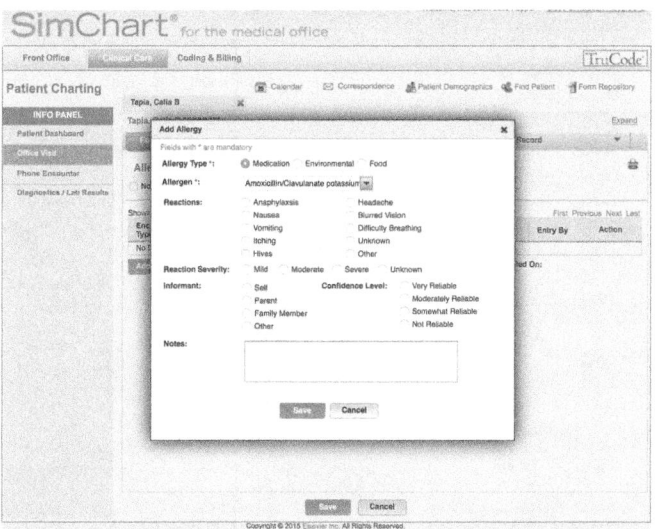

Fig. 21.8 Documentation in an (EHR) is done using radio buttons, drop-down menus, and free-text boxes.

into the unit so that it "learns" to recognize the user's voice. The system can be used to dictate progress notes, letters, emails, and any document that needs to be created.

The provider will need to approve these documents before they are permanently attached to the patient's record. Some systems have an authentication component that allows a type of electronic signature, such as those needed for hospital record dictation.

PAPER HEALTH RECORD MANAGEMENT SYSTEM

The paper health record management system should provide an easy method of retrieving information. The files should be organized in an orderly fashion. An efficient method of adding documents to the record must be established so that the provider always has the most up-to-date information. Above all, the health records management system must work for the individual facility.

Filing Equipment

When filing equipment is selected, the available space must be considered, along with the potential volume of records. With patient records, filing equipment that locks and is fireproof is an important feature for the safety and security of the records. Cost is also an important consideration. There are several types of filing cabinets or shelving units available, depending on the needs of the ambulatory care facility:

- *Drawer files*: Depending on the file cabinet, the drawers are either vertical (like a regular file cabinet) or lateral. Lateral drawers need to be completely pulled out to file. The lateral drawers vary in length. These file cabinets are usually fireproof and have a locking mechanism to safeguard paper health records. When you are working with file cabinets, open one drawer at a time to prevent the file cabinet from tipping.
- *Horizontal shelf files*: Also called an *open file with fixed shelves*. Resembles a bookcase that accommodates paper health records. Some have doors that can be pulled over the paper health records and locked.

- *Rotary circular files*: Resembles a bookcase that rotates in a circle. The double-sided shelving system stores large volumes of paper health records.
- *Electronic lateral files*: Also called *vertical carousel filing*. Vertically arranged drawers or shelves that revolve in a circle vertically, bringing the selected drawer or shelf to the user.
- *Mobile shelving system*: Resembles a double-sided bookcase and is mounted on tracks in the floor. The shelving units remain close together except for two that create an aisle. When the user needs to access records in a different location, the units are moved using a button or handle and an aisle is created to access the paper health record. The mobile shelf system uses less floor space than stationary shelving units.
- *Card files*: Used for patient ledgers, patient index, telephone numbers, and so on. The steel box or tray comes in a variety of sizes, depending on the size of the file.

Many of these filing systems have steel file divider supports that separate groups of paper health records. These dividers help the paper health records stand upright.

Filing Supplies

When the medical assistant is using or creating a patient's paper health record, several filing supplies are needed (see Procedure 21.1):

- *Divider guides*: Guides are used to separate groups of paper health records, making searching of records easier. Made of pressboard or heavy plastic and have a protruding tab. Many styles are available.
- *Out guides*: Placed in the filing shelf or drawer, replacing a paper health record that is removed. Made of heavyweight cardboard or plastic. Some have a large pocket to hold documents for the missing paper health record (Fig. 21.9).
- *File folders*: Patient records are secured in folders with fasteners. The fasteners are usually on the top or side of the folder. Tab locations can vary on the folder. Folders come in a range of colors.
- *File folder dividers*: Tabbed dividers are used to separate the sections of the paper health record.
- *Labels*: Several types of labels can be used on a patient's folder. Labels are used for the patient's name and to indicate allergies and advance directives. Based on the filing system used, alphabetical and/or numerical labels are used. Labels are available in almost any size, shape, or color to meet the individual needs of any facility.

VOCABULARY

alphabetical filing Any system that arranges names or topics according to the sequence of the letters in the alphabet.

Filing Systems

The three basic filing systems used in healthcare facilities are alphabetical filing by name, numerical filing, and subject filing. Patient records are filed either alphabetically by name

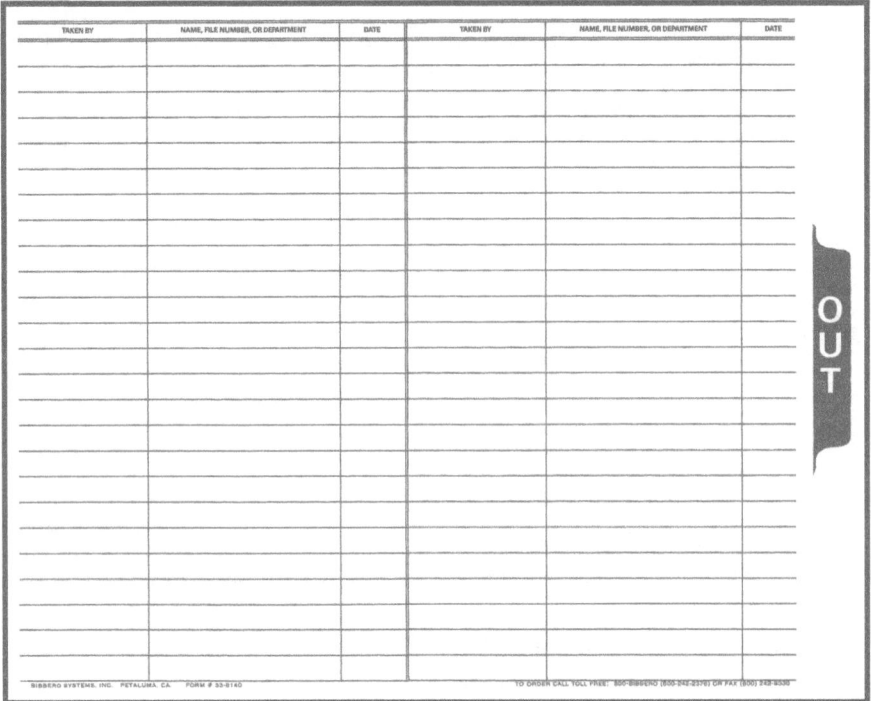

Fig. 21.9 Out guides allow tracking of a file not in its proper location by providing information on the location of the file. (Courtesy Bibbero Systems, an InHealth Company, Petaluma, CA (800) 242-2376, https://www. bibbero.com.)

or by one of several numerical methods. Subject filing is used for business records, correspondence, and educational materials.

A filing system can be either a direct or an indirect filing system. There are advantages and disadvantages to both systems. With a direct filing system, a person only needs to know the name to find the desired file, which is an advantage. Disadvantages of the direct filing system include:

- The correct spelling of the name must be known.
- As the number of files increases, more space is needed for each section of the alphabet. This results in periodic shifting of folders to allow for expansion.
- As the files expand, more time is required for filing or retrieving each folder because of the greater number of folders involved in the search. The time can be greatly reduced by color coding.

The alphabetical filing system is an example of a direct filing system.

With an indirect filing system, a person must use an alphabetical cross-reference source to find a file. A disadvantage of this filing system is the added time required to use the cross-reference source. Advantages of an indirect filing system include:

- It allows unlimited expansion without periodic shifting of folders, and shelves are usually evenly filed.
- It provides additional confidentiality to the record.
- It saves time in retrieving and filing records quickly. One knows immediately that the number 978 falls between 977 and 979. By contrast, an alphabetical system, even with color coding, requires a longer search to locate the exact spot.

The numerical filing system is an example of an indirect filing system.

> **VOCABULARY**
> **direct filing system** A filing system in which materials can be located without consulting another source of reference.
> **indirect filing system** A filing system in which an alphabetical cross-reference source must be used to determine the code assigned to the record.

Alphabetical Filing. Alphabetical filing is the oldest method for filing. It uses indexing rules, which are standard and based on current business practices. The Association of Records Managers and Administrators (ARMA) takes an active part in updating these rules. Some establishments adopt variations of these basic rules to accommodate their needs. The indexing rules are used to file paper health records and other business folders.

The indexing rules use *units,* or parts of the name, when filing. Names of individuals are split into units. Additional tips to remember include:

- When alphabetizing, there is no difference between uppercase and lowercase letters. For example, McNally and Mcnally are considered the same.
- Punctuation in the name is omitted (e.g., periods, commas, apostrophe).

Indexing Individual Names. When indexing patient names, use the following rules:

1. *Unit order:* The *surname* (last name) is the first unit. The *given name* (first name) or initial is the second unit. The middle name or initial is the third unit.

Name	Unit 1	Unit 2	Unit 3
Sam Tom Brown	BROWN	SAM	TOM

2. *Same names*: The names are filed alphabetically starting with the last name. If two or more first unit names are the same, move to the second unit names to determine the filing position. If two or more second unit names are the same, move to the third unit names and so on.
3. *Initial*: An initial is filed before a name starting with the same letter.
4. *No name*: Units that have no names are filed before a unit with an initial or a name. Remember "nothing comes before something."

Name	Unit 1	Unit 2	Unit 3
Sam Tom Brown	BROWN	SAM	TOM
Betsy Good	GOOD	BETSY	
Betsy Sue Good	GOOD	BETSY	SUE
Earl T. Good	GOOD	EARL	T
Earl W. Good	GOOD	EARL	W
Earl Will Good	GOOD	EARL	WILL

5. *Hyphenated name*: When a name is hyphenated, it is one unit. This rule applies to hyphenated names regardless if it is the first, middle or surname. The hyphen is not included in the unit.
6. *Prefix*: There are many prefixes used in surnames. Examples of surname prefixes include d', D', de, la, La, Le, M', Mac, Mc, O', Saint, St., Van, Van de, Von, and Von der. Prefixes are considered part of the name. Ignore the space or apostrophe.

Name	Unit 1	Unit 2	Unit 3
Sue A. Ko-Smit	KOSMIT	SUE	A
Mary G. L'Auburn	LAUBURN	MARY	G
Ka-Lu McMee	MCMEE	KALU	C
Amy Van Hoof	VANHOOF	AMY	

7. *Initials as names*: Often we hear names such as J.P. and A.J. These initials are considered separate indexing units.
8. *Abbreviated names and nicknames*: Abbreviated names and nicknames are indexed as they are. They are not spelled out when indexed.

Name	Unit 1	Unit 2	Unit 3
A.J. Smith	SMITH	A	J
Buddy Smith	SMITH	BUDDY	
Jer. A. Smith	SMITH	JER	A
Jos. Smith	SMITH	JOS	

9. *Title*: Comes before a person's name. A person's title is the last indexing unit when the complete name is given, such as Mrs. Mary Stone. When a title comes before an incomplete name (e.g., Father Tim), the title is the first unit. Examples of titles include Miss, Mr., Mrs., Prof., Dr., Father, Sister, King, and Capt.
10. *Suffix*: Comes after a person's name. It may indicate seniority (e.g., Jr., Sr, and II). A suffix can also be a professional or academic designation such as RMA, CMA, MD, and PhD. A suffix is the last indexing. If a person has both a title and suffix, the title is the last unit.

Name	Unit 1	Unit 2	Unit 3	Unit 4	Unit 5
Father Thomas	FATHER	THOMAS			
Mr. J.P. Garcia	GARCIA	J	P	MR	
Sister Mary Rose Garcia	GARCIA	MARY	ROSE	SISTER	
Rose A. Garcia, RMA	GARCIA	ROSE	A	RMA	
Mr. Thomas A. Garcia, Sr.	GARCIA	THOMAS	A	SR	MR

11. *Undistinguishable name*: When indexing a foreign name in which you cannot distinguish between the first and last names, index each part of the name in the order in which it is written. If you can make the distinction, use the last name as the first indexing unit.
12. *Name change*: When people change their name, the paper health record is filed using the new name. For example, when a woman marries, she might hyphenate her name, or she may also change her last name to her spouse's last name. The filing location may change due to the new name.
13. *Addresses*: When two names are identical, their names are indexed first followed by their addresses. When the address is used for indexing, the city is the first unit, the state is the second unit, the street is the third unit, and the street number is the last indexing unit. Street numbers are indexed from the lowest to the highest numbers.

Indexing Business Names. When indexing business names, follow these rules:
1. Index the business name in the order it is written. Articles (e.g., a, the) are disregarded with indexing.
2. When business names begin with "The", "The" is the last indexing unit.
3. When a business name is hyphenated, it is considered to be one unit.
4. Single letters in business names:
   - If written without spaces, these are considered one unit. For example, with ABC Supplies, ABC would be the first unit.
   - If followed by spaces, they are considered separate indexing units. For example, with J R Supplies, J would be the first unit and R would be the second unit.
   - If used as an acronym, it is indexed as one unit regardless of spaces and punctuation.
5. Abbreviated names, such as Inc., Corp., and Co., are indexed as they are. They are not spelled out when indexed.
6. Numbers are considered one unit. They are filed in numerical order from lowest to highest before alphabetical characters.
7. If a symbol is part of the business, the symbol is indexed as if it were spelled out. For example, "&" would be indexed as "and" and "#" would be indexed as "number."

Numerical Filing. Numerical filing for paper health records is commonly used in large ambulatory care facilities and hospitals (see Procedure 21.2). Each patient is assigned a unique medical record number. The paper health record is labeled with the medical record number and filed by the number. To find the patient's paper health record, a person would need a cross-referenced list of patient names with their medical record numbers. Today, most of these lists are available on the facility's computer system.

Several types of numerical filing systems can be used:

- *Consecutive numerical filing*: Also called a *straight numerical system*. Patients are given consecutive numbers as they start using the practice. This system can be expanded as the patient numbers grow. Paper health records are filed from lowest number to highest number. For example, records would be filed in this order: 00001, 00002, and 00003.
- *Terminal digit filing*: Patients are assigned consecutive numbers, but the digits in the number are separated into groups of two or three numbers. This makes filing and locating the paper health record quicker and easier. The groups of digits are read, starting from right to left. The group to the far right is the first unit. The numbers are filed from the lowest to the highest number. All files ending in the same number are grouped together and then further organized by the middle digits.

Medical Record Number	Unit 1	Unit 2	Unit 3
454-001-000	000	001	454
415-002-000	000	002	415
890-074-001	001	074	890
234-987-002	002	987	234
238-987-002	002	987	238

- *Middle-digit filing*: The digits are grouped as in the terminal digit system. When filing is done by the middle-digit system, the first unit is the middle group of numbers. The second unit is the group to the left and the last group is the third unit.

Medical Record Number	Unit 1	Unit 2	Unit 3
454-001-000	001	454	000
415-002-000	002	415	000
890-074-001	074	890	001

CRITICAL THINKING 21.5

Susan is unsure whether alphabetical or numerical filing is best in the health-care facility. What are some advantages and disadvantages of each method?

Subject Filing. Subject filing is a process of arranging and filing records based on the content or subject matter. It can use an alphabetical, a numerical, or an alphanumerical (e.g., A 1-3, B 1-1, B 1-2, and so on) system. Subject filing may be used to arrange patient education materials. For instance, the material may be in folders labeled with different diseases or tests.

Color Coding. When a color-coding system is used, both filing and finding files are easier. Errors in filing are minimized. The use of color visually restricts the area of search for a specific

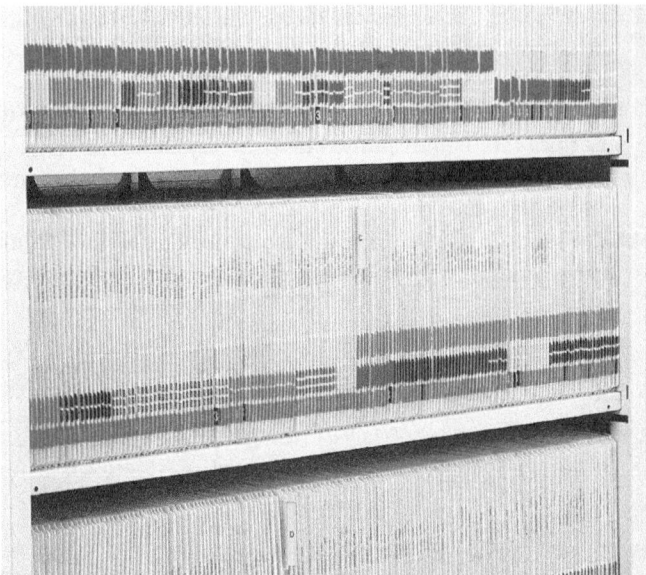

Fig. 21.10 With color coding of patients' records, a misplaced file is easily spotted. (Courtesy Bibbero Systems, an InHealth Company, Petaluma, CA (800) 242-2376, https://www.bibbero.com.)

record. A misfiled record is easily spotted even from a distance of several feet (Fig. 21.10). Colored folders or colored adhesive labels or both are used in color-coding filing. Color-coding filing can be used with other types of filing, including alphabetical filing and terminal digit filing.

In color coding, a specific color is selected to identify each letter of the alphabet or number. For instance, a specific color may be used for all paper health records beginning with the same letter (Box 21.3). The selection of the colors and the division of the colors varies by facility.

Tickler File. A tickler file is used to remind a person when a certain matter must be done. The tickler file is always in a chronologic arrangement, such as arranged by days of the months or months of the year. A tickler file in a sense is a reminder system to the medical assistant. Tickler files are electronic and can be found in practice management software or on apps for personal use. A tickler file can also be a small box of index cards and 43 dividers – 31 for the days of the month and 12 for the months.

A medical assistant would use a tickler file to remember to do a task. For instance, a provider ordered laboratory work for a patient to be done 6 months from now. Or the medical assistant must order supplies on the last Tuesday of the month. Notes would be added to the tickler file to remind the medical assistant to do these tasks. Reviewing the notes in the tickler file marked for the current day should be checked first thing each day.

VOCABULARY

alphanumerical Describes systems made up of combinations of letters and numbers.

tickler file A chronologic file used as a reminder that something must be dealt with on a certain date.

Color can work in many other ways for the efficient healthcare facility. Small tabs in a variety of colors can be used to identify certain types of insured patients and other specific information. For example, a red tab over the edge of the folder may identify a patient on Medicare; a blue tab may identify a Medicaid patient; a green tab may identify a workers' compensation patient. Matching tabs may be attached to the insured's ledger card. In a partnership practice, a different color folder or label may identify each provider's patients. Color also can be used to differentiate dates – one color for each month or year. Everyone using the paper health records should be familiar with the color coding.

CRITICAL THINKING 21.6

Susan is responsible for checking the tickler file daily. What types of documents and duties might she find inside this file?

Filing Process

When a medical assistant has a stack of documents to add to paper health records, it is recommended that they organize the records by patient. To be most efficient, they should group the records in the order patients appear in the filing area. This is determined by the filing system used.

When adding papers to the patient's paper health record, the medical assistant must follow these steps:

1. *Inspect the document*: All laboratory and diagnostic imaging test results need to be reviewed by the provider before they are added to the patient's paper health record. Many providers initial the document to indicate they reviewed the results. If the document does not contain an indication that the provider reviewed the results, the document should not be filed.
2. *Prepare the document*: Remove any staples or paper clips. If the document is smaller than the standard paper size, it should be mounted on sheets that have adhesive strips. Small records can easily be lost or misplaced. Mounting them on regular-sized paper prevents this from happening. For documents without holes for the prongs, punch holes in the proper locations.
3. *Index and code documents*: Identify where the document should be filed. Check that each document is dated and contains the person's name.
4. *Sort documents*: Multiple documents for the same patient should be organized per the facility's procedures.
5. *Verify placement*: When placing records in a patient's paper health record, verify the name on the document(s) with the health record. Each type of document should be placed behind the correct tab. The documents in a tabbed section should be organized per the facility's policy, usually with the newest on top.
6. *Replace the paper health record*: Once the documents have been organized within the patient's paper health record, the record needs to be placed in the correct location. Usually, an out guide is placed when a record is removed from the drawer or shelf. When you replace the paper health record, remove the out guide.

ELECTRONIC HEALTH RECORDS

Terminology

The acronyms EHR and EMR (for electronic medical record) have been used interchangeably for many years. The Office of the National Coordinator for Health Information Technology (ONC) has established definitions for EHR and EMR that are easy to understand.

- *Electronic health record* (EHR): An electronic record of health-related information about a patient. Conforms to nationally recognized interoperability standards. The EHR can be created, managed, and consulted by authorized clinicians and staff from more than one healthcare organizations.
- *Electronic medical record* (EMR): An electronic record of health-related information about a patient and is considered an electronic version of a paper record. The EMR is created, gathered, managed, and consulted by authorized clinicians and staff within a single healthcare organization.

There is a significant push toward having all electronic records meet the definition of an EHR. There are many advantages to having an electronic record system that can be accessed from more than one healthcare organization. The continuity of patient care is much more easily established when all providers have access to the same records regardless of what organization they are working for. There would be less running of duplicate tests and procedures, which would help reduce the cost of providing healthcare.

A *personal health record* (PHR) is defined by the ONC as an electronic record of health-related information about an individual that conforms to nationally recognized interoperability standards and that can be drawn from multiple sources but is managed, shared, and controlled by the individual. There are several ways that a PHR can be created. Some health insurance companies offer PHRs for those they insure. Some employers offer it as a service for their employees. Some healthcare facilities offer it to their patients. It is important to remember that the patient maintains a PHR. The information from an EHR does not automatically transfer to a PHR.

Patient portals allow patients to access their actual EHRs. Many patient portal systems also allow the patient to:
- view laboratory results, medication lists, and immunization records
- communicate with the provider
- complete forms online
- request prescription refills
- schedule appointments

By establishing effective patient portals, healthcare facilities can meet some of the Promoting Interoperability Program (formerly Meaningful Use) requirements.

VOCABULARY

interoperability The ability to work with other systems.
Promoting Interoperability Program Formerly known as Meaningful Use requirements. Requirements established by the Centers for Medicare and Medicaid Services (CMS) as part of the Electronic Health Records (EHR) Incentives Program. The program provides financial incentives for healthcare organizations that "meaningfully used" their certified EHR technology. The requirements include implementing security measures to ensure the privacy of patients' EHRs.

The Health Insurance Portability and Accountability Act (HIPAA) uses the term protected health information (PHI), which is any information about health status, the provision of healthcare, or payment for healthcare that can be linked to an individual patient. HIPAA requires that all PHI be protected. This applies to the EHRs, EMRs, PHRs, and patient portals.

> **VOCABULARY**
> **protected health information (PHI)** Individually identifiable health information stored or transmitted by covered entities or business associates; includes verbal, paper, or electronic information.

HITECH

The Health Information Technology for Economic and Clinical Health (HITECH) Act provides financial incentives for the meaningful use (Promoting Interoperability Program) of certified EHR technology to achieve health and efficiency goals. It was part of the American Recovery and Reinvestment Act to promote the adoption and meaningful use of health information technology. Remember, HIPAA was created in large part to simplify administrative processes through the use of electronic devices.

Promoting Interoperability Program requirements means that providers must show that they are using EHR technology in ways that can be measured significantly in quality and quantity. If providers meet the requirements, they will qualify for incentive payments. Three main requirements include:

- Use of certified EHR technology in a meaningful manner, such as e-prescribing
- Use of certified EHR technology for electronic exchange of health information to improve the quality of healthcare
- Use of certified EHR technology to submit clinical quality reports, procedure and diagnosis codes, surveys, and other measures

Providers can expect reductions in the amounts they are paid from Medicare and Medicaid if they are not in compliance. Remember, the computer system in the medical office must be more than a tool for data recall to be considered an EHR system; the provider must use the system for tasks, at a minimum, such as electronic prescribing (e-prescribing) and computerized physician/provider order entry (CPOE).

> **VOCABULARY**
> **compliance** Meeting the standards and regulations of the practice's established policies and procedures. Can also mean cooperation.
> **computerized physician/provider order entry (CPOE)** The process of entering medication orders or other provider instructions into the electronic health record.
> **e-prescribing** The use of electronic software to communicate with pharmacies and send prescribing information. It takes the place of writing a prescription by hand and giving it to a patient; most new or refill prescriptions can be submitted electronically, cutting down on fraud and errors.
> **interface** An interconnection between systems.

> **CRITICAL THINKING 21.7**
>
> Some of the patients who visit Dr. Kahn and Dr. Martin have expressed concern that EHRs may not be private enough and that their health information will be "floating around on the internet." They are worried that unauthorized individuals could somehow access their information on the computer and do them harm. How might Susan alleviate the patients' fears about their records being available on the internet? What disadvantages with regard to confidentiality are associated with the EHR?

Features of Electronic Health Records and Practice Management Software

Many ambulatory healthcare facilities use EHR software that interfaces seamlessly with practice management software (PMS). It can be difficult to identify what features are part of the EHR and what are part of the PMS. Information on schedules, patients, and charges for services automatically flow bidirectionally.

The EHR handles all the clinical information, and its main purpose is record keeping for clinical care. Common features in the EHRs can include:

- Immunization documentation, which can also be sent to the state's immunization site.
- Mobile access, which allows providers to access the EHR offsite, 24/7.
- Clinical decision supports, which helps providers manage conditions.
- e-Prescribing, which can be included in the EHR or can be a separate software tool added to the EHR and which allows the providers to send prescriptions to pharmacies.
- Basic scheduler for patient appointments (Fig. 21.11).
- Laboratory order integration, which means providers can order tests and the results are visible in the EHR.

Some EHRs have tools that are also found in the PMS.

The PMS is used to run the day-to-day business side of the facility. PMS tools can be used for scheduling appointments, new patient registration, billing, coding, and managing finances. Some of the more useful features of many practice management software programs include:

- Claims denial management and electronic claims submission
- Financial and management reporting
- Registration tool for new patients (see Procedure 21.3)
- Scheduler for patient appointments and procedures
- Medical coding or encoder
- Insurance eligibility verification

See Chapter 24 for more details on the features of PMS.

Medical Assistant's Role

The medical assistant uses the EHR to enter the patient's vital signs, measurements, allergies, medications, chief complaint, and history at the beginning of the visit. If the patient requires medications or vaccines, the medical assistant must update the patient's medication or immunization record in the EHR. Any ordered procedures performed and patient coaching must also be documented in the EHRs. If the patient requires a referral, follow-up visits, or additional tests, the medical assistant will use the EHR/PMS to arrange these.

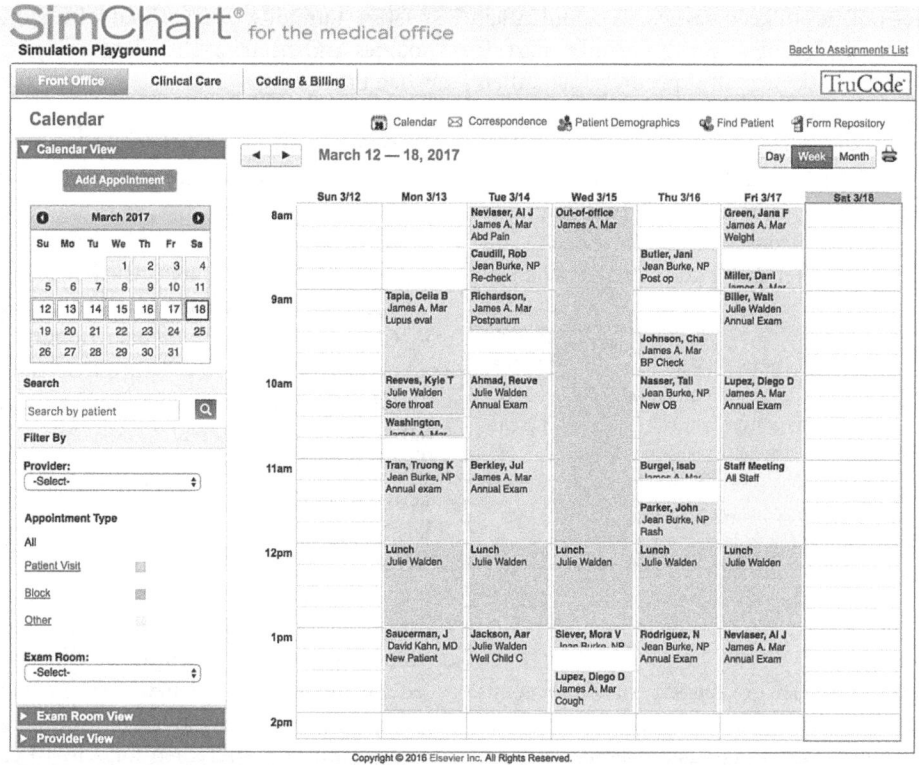

Fig. 21.11 The electronic health record (EHR) may include a scheduling system that can be changed to manage the needs of the provider and office staff.

The medical assistant also uses the EHR to review patient information, such as the last date of a preventive test or medications ordered when a patient needs a refill. The medical assistant must also scan paper documents and upload them to the patient's chart (see Procedure 21.4). When organizing the scanned records in the EHR, the medical assistant must ensure the records are placed in the correct locations to avoid any confusion or duplication of tests.

Because many patients use the patient portal to communicate with their providers, medical assistants may also be responsible for responding to the patient or forwarding the patient's concerns to the provider.

HEALTH INSURANCE PORTABILITY AND ACCOUNTABILITY ACT

Privacy Rule

The HIPAA Privacy Rule has created national standards that protect health records and other patient information. The Privacy Rule's main purpose is to define and limit the situations in which a patient's information can be used or disclosed. The rule also describes patients' rights over their information. Patients have the right to:

- examine their health information.
- obtain a copy of their health records.
- request corrections to be made if information is incorrect.

Covered entities must comply with the Privacy Rule. They must safeguard all patient information.

The HIPAA Privacy Rule lists permissions, or reasons that the health information can be released. The disclosure authorization

process and the records release process protect the confidentiality of the patient's PHI. Chapter 19 provides additional information on permissions, the disclosure authorization process, and the records release process. The medical assistant must be familiar with and follow the facility's policies and procedures when disclosing and releasing a patient's health information.

> **VOCABULARY**
>
> **covered entities** Healthcare providers, health (insurance) plans, and claims clearinghouses that transmit protected health information electronically.
> **permission** A reason for releasing or disclosing patient information under HIPAA.

Security Rule

HIPAA's Security Rule addresses the national standards used to protect electronic protected health information (ePHI). This rule covers the records that are created, used, received, and maintained by the covered entities. Safeguards important to ensure the security of the ePHI include:

- *Administrative safeguards*: The security officer is responsible for creating and carrying out security policies and procedures.
- *Physical safeguards*: Facility, workstation, and device security must be implemented. A security officer must create procedures for the proper use of workstations and ePHI.
- *Technical safeguards*: Only authorized employees should have access to ePHI. Safeguards include audits to track activities of users, encryption of mobile devices, and safeguards to prevent improper alteration, destruction, or transmission of ePHI.

Many facilities have policies to keep passwords confidential. Audit trails monitor who is looking at which patient's chart. If the medical assistant is not working with a specific patient, then they should not access the patient's record. Violating this rule will cause the medical assistant to breach the patient's confidentiality (see Procedure 21.5). Many healthcare professionals, from providers to medical assistants, have breached confidentiality. They have lost their jobs and licenses or certifications. Many have also been fined. (See Chapter 24 for additional details.)

CRITICAL THINKING 21.8

Jennifer walks behind Susan's desk and notices that she is looking at the progress notes on a patient who was recently arrested and indicted for child abuse. The case has been in the newspaper and on television consistently for several weeks. Jennifer asks Susan why she has accessed that record. Susan hesitates and then says she must have entered the wrong patient ID number. Does Susan's explanation sound convincing? Why is Jennifer concerned about Susan looking at the patient's record? Just because the individual is a patient at the clinic, does that mean any employee has the right to look at the patient's EHR?

Backup Systems for the EHR. Part of the Security Rule's focus is to safeguard patient health records. HIPAA requires that the facility adopt a backup and recovery plan that includes daily offsite software backup for the EHR system. Depending on the size of the facility, the network may be backed up once or several times a day. *Backing up* is a process in which the network files are copied either using an external hard drive, a server, or an online backup system.

To protect the data from a disaster in the healthcare facility, it is important to store the backup files offsite. When computer data is compromised, either by errors, natural causes (e.g., floods, storm damage), or human causes (e.g., fires, hackers, and malware), the data can be restored using the offsite backup copy.

Many healthcare facilities contract with cloud backup services, which copy the network data on a routine basis to protect against data loss. Cloud backup services are like cloud storage services in regard to the ability to access the data anytime and anywhere. When computer data is compromised, it can be restored using the backup copy.

In the event that the EHR system is not functioning, the ambulatory care facility must transition to paper records. Policies and procedures should indicate the process of using paper records and how the paper records become a part of the EHR. The facility should always have a supply of the most commonly used forms in a paper format available for use in such instances. When the EHR system resumes functioning, these paper forms can be scanned into the patients' EHRs or the information can be keyed into the system.

STORAGE, RETENTION, AND DESTRUCTION OF HEALTH RECORDS

Storage of Paper Health Records

Paper health records should be stored in an area accessible to only a limited number of employees. The area should be secure. The temperature should be between 65° and 70°F and at 55%

relative humidity. They should be stored away from water sources and heaters. The filing equipment should be locked when the facility is closed.

Retention and Destruction of Health Records

In ambulatory healthcare facilities, patient health records are classified as active, inactive, or closed.

- *Active*: Records used on a routine basis.
- *Inactive*: Records rarely used but kept for reference. Will become active with the next patient visit or interaction.
- *Closed:* Records of patients who have died, moved away, or otherwise terminated their relationship with the provider.

Purging is the act of separating the inactive records from the active charts, which creates more space. Purging is an ongoing process. The facility will determine when records move from active to inactive status. It can vary by facility. For instance, a large multispecialty facility may state that records become inactive after a year from the last visit. Other facilities may specify 6 or 18 months, depending on the type of facility. Ambulatory care facilities should have a retention schedule in place. The destruction of health records must be done in accordance with federal and state laws. Patient health records involved with legal action or an open investigation cannot be destroyed. Typically, closed records are retained for 7 to 10 years after the patient's last interaction. Records are retained based on state statute. In many cases, closed records of minors are usually retained a number of years after the age of majority, which is specified in the state statutes. Closed Medicaid and Medicare patient records are retained for 10 years.

VOCABULARY

age of majority The age at which the law recognizes a person to be an adult; it varies by state.

retention schedule A method or plan for retaining or keeping health records and for their movement from active to inactive to closed.

In the past, patient health records were transferred to optical disks, microfilm, or microfiche. As technology changed over the years, many facilities have not had the ability to move these records to other media. As a result, patient health records may be stored in many ways. When the retention plan indicates records should be destroyed, the facility should give patients a chance to get a copy of their records. The facility must maintain a permanent log of all records destroyed.

Paper Health Records. Most medical facilities use a year sticker on the file folder that indicates the last year the patient visited the clinic. If the file has a sticker showing that the patient's last visit was in 2021, and the patient presents to the clinic on January 5, 2023, a 2023 sticker should be placed over the one that indicates 2021. These stickers often are included with color-coded filing systems. The medical assistant can easily look at a group of files and see which ones need to be changed to inactive or closed status. If onsite storage is limited, inactive and closed paper health records may be stored in an offsite location. Most ambulatory healthcare facilities cannot retain paper health records indefinitely due to storage limits, budgets, and legal constraints. Paper health records are typically destroyed by burning or shredding

Electronic Health Records. An EHR system can be set up to automatically move the inactive records to another server so that processing time will not be slowed down, but the records are still readily accessible if the patient returns to the healthcare facility. Closed EHRs are also separated from the active records and are typically stored elsewhere. They may be placed on CDs, computer hard drives, or maintained in inactive cloud space by the EHR vendor.

CLOSING COMMENTS

Just as in every aspect of the medical profession, advances in health records management are occurring rapidly, allowing providers and other caregivers to perform their duties more efficiently and accurately. A medical assistant must constantly be willing to learn and to adapt to changes arising from legislation and technologic advances. Computers have become generally accepted as a means of recording health information.

A primary goal of all healthcare facilities is to provide efficient, high-quality patient care. The EHR system can help the staff reach that goal. In the future, every provider's office, hospital, pharmacy, and healthcare facility may be able to access information in minutes, which will improve patient care and save lives. Stay abreast of news and articles related to EHR systems. The healthcare industry is one of constant growth and learning, and today's information technology provides the medical assistant with endless opportunities to make that growth rewarding and applicable to their current position.

PATIENT-CENTERED CARE

It is important for the medical assistant to provide patient-centered care to the patient. When using the electronic health record (EHR), medical assistants must make sure that their nonverbal communication sends the right message to the patient. Eye contact is essential (Fig. 21.12). If the medical assistant constantly looks at the electronic device, the patient feels left out of the process. Tips for using the EHR with a patient include:
- Make eye contact with the patient while asking questions.
- Look at the screen only when needed to enter information.

- Do not shield the device from the patient's view when entering information. This can give the impression you are hiding something from the patient. Although patients may not understand anything they see on the screen, they will feel more at ease if their information is not hidden from them.
- Sit next to or at an angle to the patient to support the impression that those in the healthcare facility and the patient are partners in the healthcare plan.

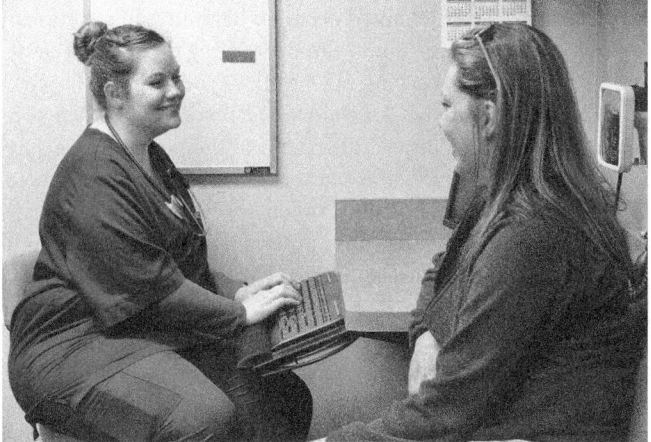

Fig. 21.12 The medical assistant must make eye contact with the patient when using an (EHR). (From Proctor D, et al: *Kinn's the medical assistant,* ed 13, St. Louis, 2017, Elsevier.)

BEING PROFESSIONAL

Patients worry about the security of their information, particularly about who can access it. Lawsuits are often filed when patients discover that an unauthorized person has accessed their protected health information. The medical assistant should listen to a patient's concerns and explain the safety procedures that apply to the electronic health record (EHR) in language the patient can understand.

The medical assistant should expect hesitation and even reluctance from patients who are concerned about the privacy of their health information. Patients are concerned about lack of control over who views their records. Be prepared to answer their questions about the safety of their records as related to the EHR. The medical assistant must know how the EHR is protected and what security measures are in place to be able to reassure the patients that their records are protected at all times.

Role-play this scenario with a peer: You will play the medical assistant, and your peer will play the patient. You are using an EHR, and the patient states that he are uncomfortable with this information being available for others to see. "Any hacker can break into your network and get my information," the patient states. Respond to the patient in a respectful and professional manner.

CHAPTER REVIEW

The patient's health record provides documentation regarding the person's health. Besides communicating the patient's information between providers, the record supports reimbursement claims and provides legal protection to those caring for the patient. Patient health records can be either paper or electronic. The provider or healthcare facility own the physical health record, and the patient owns the content.

A patient's health record contains the following:
- Personal demographics, such as the patient's name, date of birth, contact information, employer, Social Security number, and insurance information

- Past medical history (including allergies, immunizations, and medications); family, social, and occupational history
- Chief complaint and history of present illness
- Physical examination and progress notes
- Laboratory and diagnostic imaging results
- Consultation reports, hospital documents, and miscellaneous documents, such as release of information forms and disclosure authorization forms

Health records can be organized in different ways, including by source-oriented and problem-oriented systems. Four components of the POMR include the database, problem list, plan, and progress notes. POMR has evolved to SOAP notes and the CHEDDAR format. Subjective data is obtained from the patient, whereas objective data comes from clinical evidence or observations from the provider.

When the paper health record system is used, filing equipment and supplies, such as labels, folders, and dividers, are used. Filing methods that can be used with paper records include:

- Alphabetical filing: The patient's name or business name is split into units that are used for filing. Multiple indexing rules provide the order for filing the records.
- Numerical filing: Commonly used in large ambulatory care facilities. Consecutive numerical filing, terminal digit filing, and middle-digit filing are types of numerical filing systems.

When the medical assistant files records, the document must be inspected, prepared, indexed and coded, and sorted. Verify the name on the health record with the document. Make sure the document is filed correctly before the record is filed.

The EHR, EMR, PHR, and patient portals are electronic records of health-related information. By establishing effective patient portals, healthcare facilities can meet some of the Promoting Interoperability Program (formerly Meaningful Use) requirements. The EHR handles all clinical information, and the PMS contain tools to run the day-to-day business side of the facility. The medical assistant interacts with the EHR by entering patient information, uploading scanned documents, and obtaining information from the EHR.

HIPAA's Privacy Rule lists permissions or reasons that the patient's health information can be released. The disclosure authorization process and the records release process protect the confidentiality of the patient's PHI. HIPAA's Security Rule addresses the national standards used to protect ePHI. Administrative, physical, and technical safeguards are used to protect ePHI.

Patient health records are either active, inactive, or closed. Closed records are retained for 7 to 10 years after the last interaction or a number of years after the age of majority. Patients should have an opportunity to get a copy of their records before they are destroyed. Paper health records are typically destroyed by burning or shredding.

SCENARIO WRAP-UP

Susan looks forward to attending her medical assisting classes each day and works diligently to perform to the best of her ability in the classroom. She strives to do well on each procedure check-off and each examination she completes. Her instructors provide excellent feedback and appreciate her contributions to the class.

Susan has the attitude that everything she is allowed to do in the healthcare facility is a learning tool. She regularly asks for additional responsibilities and is always ready to assist a co-worker. Dr. Kahn has recognized that she has the desire to learn, and he gives her many opportunities to glean more knowledge through the everyday activities in the office.

Although she is new to the medical profession, Susan learns quickly and thinks logically. She knows the rules and regulations on patient confidentiality and is always careful about the information she provides to those who request it. She is never hesitant about asking her office manager for guidance if she is unsure about any aspect of her duties. Susan is understanding and respectful when patients are concerned about their privacy. Her confidence and warm personality play a role in the trust she earns from the patients at the clinic.

Susan is willing to admit when she has made an error and has sought advice from Dr. Kahn and her office manager when an error needed correction. Although filing is not one of her favorite duties, she can be counted on to do her best while completing this important task. She realizes that filing is critical because the documents in the patient's health record direct the care provided to the patient. An abnormal laboratory report that is missing can make a crucial difference in the patient's care. She takes pride in her work, and she is efficient and accurate where health records are concerned. When she is faced with a new task, she considers it a learning experience and asks for help if she is not completely sure about the way to handle a situation.

Susan's co-workers are supportive and always willing to help her as she learns to be the best medical assistant she can be. Her future as a professional medical assistant certainly holds opportunity and chances for advancement. Just as important, patients trust her. She has alleviated patients' concerns about EHRs by taking the time to explain privacy policies and exactly what information will be accessible to third parties. This trust also gives patients the confidence to reveal personal information and to know that it will be held in the strictest confidence, not just by Susan, but by each employee in the provider's office.

PROCEDURE 21.1   Create and Organize a Patient's Paper Health Record

Tasks

Create a paper health record for a new patient. Organize health record documents in a paper health record.

Equipment and Supplies

- End tab file folder with prongs on the left and right-hand side of the folder
- Completed patient information (registration) form
- Divider sheets with different color labels (4)
- Progress note sheet (1)
- Name label
- Color-coding labels (first two letters of last name and first letter of first name)
- Year label
- Allergy label
- Black pen or computer with word processing software to process labels
- Red pen (for allergies, optional)
- Health record documents (i.e., prior records, laboratory reports)
- Hole punch

Procedural Steps

1. Obtain the patient's first and last names.
   Purpose: To customize the record for the patient, the first and last names will be required.
2. Neatly write or word-process the patient's name on the name label. Left-justify the last name, followed by a comma, the first name, middle initial, and a period (e.g., Smith, Mary J.).
   Purpose: The label should be easy to read. The last name always comes before the first name.
3. Affix the name label to the bottom left side of the record tab. When you hold the record by the main fold in your left hand, the writing should be easy to read. (For directional purposes, assume the record main fold is on the left and the tab is at the bottom.)
   Purpose: Placing the labels in correct position will make it easier to find the information needed.
4. Put the color-coding labels on the bottom right edge of the folder. Start by placing the first letter of the last name at the farthest right edge. Working left, place the second letter of the last name, then the first letter of the first name, and lastly the year label. The year label should be close to the name label.
   Purpose: When the folders are in the file cabinet, they are sorted by the colored labels, starting with the top label (first letter of the last name), followed by the second and remaining labels.

5. Place the allergy label on the front of the folder. If allergies are known, clearly write the allergy on the label in red ink.
   Purpose: Allergies need to be clearly identified on medical records.
6. Place the divider labels on the record divider sheets, if they come separately. Ensure the labels on the divider sheets are staggered so they do not overlap. Print the name of the section on the front and back of the label. The print should be easy to read when the record is held by the main fold. (Suggested names for dividers: Progress Notes, Laboratory, Correspondence, and Miscellaneous.)
   Purpose: Placing divider labels on the divider sheets in a staggered pattern allows the provider to easily see all sections of the health record.
7. Using the prongs on the left-hand side of the folder, secure the registration form.
   Purpose: The registration form should be in an easy-to-find location in the record.
8. Using the prongs on the right-hand side of the folder, secure the index dividers with a progress note sheet under the progress note tab.
   Purpose: The provider will need the progress note sheet to document data regarding the visit.

Scenario update: The patient authorized his/her prior provider to send health records to your agency. You need to organize these records within the paper health record.

9. Verify the name and the date of birth on the health records and ensure they match the information on the health record.
   Purpose: Before organizing and filing documents in a patient's health record, it is critical to ensure the health record is for the correct patient.
10. Remove any staples or paperclips. If the document is smaller than the standard paper size, it should be mounted on sheets that have adhesive strips. For the documents without holes for the prongs, punch holes in the proper location.
    Purpose: The documents need to be prepared before filing them in the health record.
11. Identify where the document should be filed. Open the prongs on the right side of the folder, and carefully remove the record to the point at which the documents need to be inserted.
    Purpose: Documents need to be placed in the correct location in the record so the provider can easily find information.
12. Insert the papers into the record, and then reassemble the remaining part of the record. Continue to do this until all the documents are filed within health record.

PROCEDURE 21.2   File Patient Health Records

Task

File patient health records or organize patient names or medical record numbers using two different filing systems: the alphabetical system and the numerical system.

Equipment and Supplies

- Paper health records using the alphabetical filing system or a list of patients' names
- Paper health records using the numerical filing system or a list of health record numbers
- File boxes or file cabinet (optional)

Procedural Steps

1. Using the indexing rules for alphabetical filing, place the records to be filed or names in alphabetical order.

Purpose: Placing the records in alphabetical order before filing in the box or cabinet will make the filing process more efficient.
2. Using the file box or file cabinet, locate the correct spot for the first file. Place the health record in the correct location. Continue these filing steps until all the health records are filed.
   Purpose: It is important to place the record in the correct spot so that others can locate the record.
3. Using numerical guidelines, place the records to be filed in numeric order.
   Purpose: Placing the records in numerical order before filing in the box or cabinet will make the filing process more efficient.
4. Using the file box or file cabinet, locate the correct spot for the first file. Place the health record in the correct location. Continue these filing steps until all the health records are filed
   Purpose: It is important to place the record in the correct spot so that others can locate the record.

Continued

PROCEDURE 21.2   File Patient Health Records–cont'd

Alternative: Procedural Steps for Filing Using Lists of Patients' Names and Medical Record Numbers

1. Using a list of patients' names, break the names into units using the indexing rules.
2. Place the names in alphabetical order based on the indexing rules. Write the names in a list.

3. Using a list of health record numbers, break the numbers into indexing units, using the terminal digit filing system.
4. Write the health record numbers in numeric order using the terminal digit filing system.

PROCEDURE 21.3   Register a New Patient Using the Practice Management Software

Task

Register a new patient using the practice management software, accurately enter patient billing information, prepare a Notice of Privacy Practices (NPP) form and a disclosure authorization form for the new patient, and document this in the electronic health record (EHR).

Equipment and Supplies

- Computer with SimChart for the Medical Office or practice management and EHR software
- Completed patient information (registration) form and insurance card
- Scanner or digital copy of the disclosure authorization form

Procedural Steps

1. Obtain the new patient's completed information (registration) form. Log into the practice management software.
   Purpose: The registration form will provide the information needed to create the new record in the practice management system.
2. Using the patient's last and first names and date of birth, search the database for the patient.
   Purpose: To help ensure the integrity of the practice management and EHR systems, a search for the new patient's name must always be done before registering that person. This prevents a double record from being created if the patient had been entered into the database at an earlier time.
3. If the database does not contain the patient's name, add a new patient and enter the patient's demographics from the completed registration form and insurance card.

Purpose: This will create the patient's record in the practice management system.

4. Verify that the information entered is correct and that all fields are completed before saving the data.
   Purpose: Errors during the registration process can affect the communication with the patient (e.g., if a wrong address or email is entered) or can affect billing (e.g., if the incorrect insurance information is added). Accuracy is extremely important when entering the patient's information.
   Note: The software will generate a health record number for the patient.
5. Using the EHR software, prepare and print a copy of the NPP and a disclosure authorization form for the new patient. The disclosure authorization form should indicate that the information will be disclosed to the patient's insurance company.
   Purpose: Before the medical office can release patient information to the insurance company, the patient has to give consent in writing.
   Scenario update: The patient received both documents and signed the disclosure authorization form.
6. Using the EHR, document that the patient received a copy of the NPP and signed the disclosure authorization form. Scan the disclosure authorization form and the insurance card. Upload both images to the EHR.
   Purpose: Documentation in the health record provides a legal record of what was done or communicated to the patient.
7. Log out of the software upon completion of the procedure.
   Purpose: Logging into and out of the software helps to protect the integrity of the data saved in the software and prevents unauthorized people from viewing the information.

PROCEDURE 21.4   Upload Documents to the Electronic Health Record

Task

Scan paper records and upload digital files to the electronic health record (EHR).

Equipment and Supplies

- Scanner
- Computer with SimChart for the Medical Office or EHR software
- Patient's laboratory and radiology reports

Scenario

A new patient brings in a laboratory report and a radiology report that he would like to have added to his EHR. You need to scan in the original documents and upload them to the EHR.

Procedural Steps

1. Obtain the patient's name and date of birth if not on the reports.
   Purpose: You will need the patient's name and date of birth to find the patient's EHR.
2. Using a scanner that is connected to the computer, scan each document, creating an individual digital image for each one.

Purpose: The reports should be scanned separately and not combined to create one file. Each type of report must be uploaded separately to the correct location in the EHR.

3. Locate the files of the two scanned images in the computer drive. Open the files to ensure the images are clear.
   Purpose: When scanning and uploading documents to the EHR, it is crucial that the image of the document is clear and can be easily read by the provider. If the image is blurred, rescan the document.
4. In the EHR, search for the patient, using the patient's last and first names. Verify the patient's date of birth.
   Purpose: Before uploading to or documenting in the EHR, it is critical to verify that the correct record has been opened.
5. Locate the window to upload diagnostic/laboratory results and add a new result. Enter the date of the test. Select the correct type of result. Browse for the image file of the laboratory file and attach it. Save the information. Select the option to add a new result and repeat the steps to upload the second report. Verify that both documents were uploaded correctly.
   Purpose: Errors during the upload may affect the ability to see the files. Verifying at the time of the upload will help ensure providers can see the results in the future.

PROCEDURE 21.5 Protect the Integrity of the Medical Record

Task

Protect the integrity of the medical record.

Scenario

You are mentoring a medical assistant student, who is in practicum. You notice the student routinely does not sign out of the electronic health record before leaving the desk. The facility's policy is to sign out or lock the computer before leaving it.

Directions

Role-play this scenario with a peer, who plays the student. You, the medical assistant, must explain to the student the facility's policy. Also address the hazards of not protecting the medical record. If the student does not change their behavior, you will need to address the situation with the department supervisor.

Procedural Steps

1. Professionally and respectfully discuss the situation with the student.
2. Inform the student about the facility's policy and the hazards of not protecting the electronic health record.
3. Provide the student with strategies to protect the electronic health record.
4. Inform the student what will occur if she does not protect the electronic record.

22

Telephone Techniques

LEARNING OBJECTIVES

1. Identify the features found on a multiple-line telephone system and explain the uses of each feature.
2. Describe the elements of professional telephone etiquette.
3. Describe how to answer, greet, and identify the caller.
4. Discuss the methods used for taking messages and the elements of a message.
5. Discuss types of incoming calls and how a medical assistant should manage each type of call.
6. Describe how a medical assistant should manage calls from the telecommunication relay service and patients with limited English proficiency.
7. Explain how to manage difficult calls, including angry callers.
8. Discuss typical outgoing calls and also how to use directory assistance.
9. Describe how to leave a Health Insurance Portability and Accountability Act–appropriate voice message for a patient.

OUTLINE

▶▶ OPENING SCENARIO

Amy Baker RMA, a recent graduate of a medical assisting program, has begun her first position as a receptionist at Walden-Martin Family Medical (WMFM) Clinic. Amy is determined to perform to the best of her abilities. However, she has never held a job in a professional office. She knows that she needs to practice all of the skills she learned in school to be an effective receptionist.

Amy spends a lot of time on the phone. She knows that she must speak clearly and distinctly over the phone. She takes messages using the practice management and electronic health record software and then follows up with the providers and staff. Amy also has had her first experience with the

TABLE 22.1 Additional Multiline Telephone System Features

Feature	Description
Caller ID and caller ID with name	With caller ID, the caller's number is displayed on the phone display unit. With caller ID with name, the caller's name with the number are displayed.
Mute control	When the icon or button is pressed, the handset is muted. The other person cannot hear anything.
Volume control	Allows the volume of the speakerphone, handset, and ringer to be adjusted.
Fax machine integration	Allows fax machines to be connected to the multiline phone system.
Personal directory	The facility's personal phonebook can be accessed on the phone display unit. The directory provides the name of the employee and the extension number.
Speed dial directory	A small number of frequently used or emergency numbers can be preprogrammed into the directory. Using the speed dial feature is quicker than entering the number each time.
All page/ intercom	Paging lets a person speak to all phones at the same time. Some phone systems are connected to an overhead intercom system, which can be used to make emergency announcements throughout the facility.
Texting	Allows text messages to be sent to a mobile phone. Can be helpful to use for appointment reminders for small numbers of patients. Other types of patient communication may not be appropriate for texting and also need to be recorded in the health record.
Call waiting	Allows the medical assistant to see if a call is waiting on or on hold on another line.
Hold music	Allows music to be played in the background when a person is placed on hold.

telecommunications relay service. A patient who has a severe hearing impairment called to schedule an appointment. Amy is excited to learn her new job. She knows that she will continue to learn and use her skills in this job.

YOU WILL LEARN

1. To recognize the features of a multiple-line telephone system.
2. To answer phone calls, screen calls, and take messages.
3. To manage various types of incoming and outgoing calls.
4. To leave Health Insurance Portability and Accountability Act (HIPAA)-appropriate voice messages for patients.

INTRODUCTION

The phone is an important tool for the medical assistant's job. Incoming calls may be from patients or patients' families, healthcare professionals, or suppliers. The medical assistant may use the phone to contact patients, handle clinic business matters, or talk with other healthcare professionals.

Regardless of the reason for the phone use, the medical assistant's ability to communicate in a professional manner is important. This chapter will start by explaining telephone

features, professional telephone techniques, and how a medical assistant should handle incoming and outgoing calls.

TELEPHONE SYSTEMS

Multiline Telephone Systems

Ambulatory care facilities have many telephones, with each having its own extension numbers. For business to occur, multiline telephone systems are needed for incoming and outgoing calls. A multiline telephone system allows multiple people to use the telephone system at the same time. The system includes:

- *External lines* to communicate with people outside of the facility
- *Internal lines* to communicate with people within the facility

Features. Multiline telephone systems can have many different features that can be beneficial to the ambulatory care facility. These features allow healthcare professional to perform a number of different tasks. Common features include speakerphone, conference calls, call forwarding, call transfer, and voice mail. Additional features are listed in Table 22.1.

Conference Call. The *conference call* feature allows more than two people to be on the call, each using a different phone. To conference a call, the person calls one person and then places that person on hold and continues to call the remaining people, continuing the sequence until all parties are on the call. The telephone user guide is a helpful resource when one is first learning to assemble conference calls.

Conference calls can be used for meetings or to discuss a situation when more than two people need to be in on the conversation. Because it can be difficult to determine who is speaking on conference calls, it can be helpful to announce yourself before you add your thoughts. For instance, "This is Jean, I believe…"

Call Forwarding. The *call forwarding* feature allows the user of one phone to automatically send calls to another number. For instance, when medical assistants are away from the phone, it is important to forward incoming calls to the medical assistant who is covering for them. This allows callers to receive timely assistance. Call forwarding can also be used if the facility is closed. The calls can be forwarded to the answering service.

> **VOCABULARY**
> **answering service** A commercial service that answers telephone calls for its clients.

> **CRITICAL THINKING 22.1**
> Review the features of a multiline phone. What are the top three most useful features for the healthcare facility? Why?

Call Transfer. The *call transfer* feature allows the extension to transfer a call to an internal extension or to an external number. The medical assistant should be familiar with the transfer process:

- Get the caller's name and a telephone number where he can be reached if the call gets disconnected.
- Get the caller's permission before placing her on hold to start the transfer process.
- Call the number to which the call is being transferred.
- Inform the new person of the caller being transferred and the situation. If the caller on hold is a patient, it is helpful to give the date of birth or the health record number. This allows the person to access the patient's information quickly without re-asking the patient for the information. Connect the caller to the new person and introduce the two parties.
- If the new person is unavailable but should be free soon, give the caller the choice to hold or to leave a message. No longer than 1 minute should pass before you check back with the caller. When you return to the call, you can use a statement such as "Thank you for waiting. Would you like to continue to hold, or should I take a message?"
- If the new person is unavailable, ask the caller if they want to be connected to the person's voice mail.

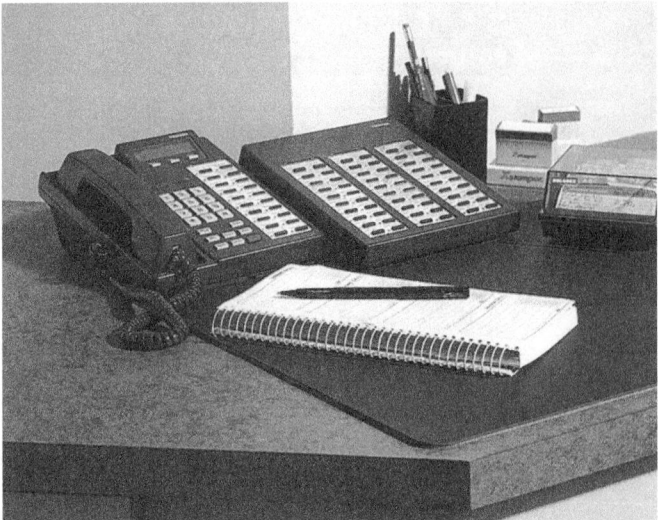

Fig. 22.1 Multiple-line telephones allow numerous calls to come into the office at once. Each call deserves the same kind of attention and care from the medical assistant. (From Proctor D, et al: *Kinn's the medical assistant*, ed 13, St. Louis, 2017, Elsevier.)

CRITICAL THINKING 22.2

Why is it important to transfer the patient to the correct person? What impression might the patient have if they are transferred repeatedly during a phone call?

Hold. The *hold* feature allows the medical assistant to place the other person on hold. A person should be on hold for no longer than 1 minute before the medical assistant checks back with the person. Usually, the person placed on hold can listen to music or messages from the ambulatory care facility. The medical assistant may use the hold feature for a variety of reasons. Regardless of the situation, the medical assistant must always ask permission to place the person on hold. If the person is unable to hold, the medical assistant can ask for a phone number to call the person back. Calling the person back should be done as soon as possible.

Voice Mail. The *voice mail* feature allows the caller to hear a message before leaving a message. The message is then stored and can be accessed at a later time. It is important for the medical assistant to create a facility-appropriate message. Many facilities will require the message to include what to do in an emergency.

Responding to voice messages left is an important aspect of a medical assistant's job. A *message waiting indicator* feature indicates that a message was left at the extension. When a message is left, many phone display units will flash a red LED light.

VOCABULARY

emergency An unexpected, life-threatening situation that requires immediate action.

Auto-Attendant. *Auto-attendant*, or automated attendant, is a voice menu system. When an incoming call is received, the system greets the caller and provides a directory of extensions. For instance, "dial or say 1 for a receptionist." The caller can dial or say the number and is then transferred to

that extension. Most menus allow the option of reaching a telephone operator should it be needed. An auto-attendant helps reduce the caller's wait time and increases the efficiency of the phone system.

CRITICAL THINKING 22.3

What are the advantages and disadvantages of using an auto-attendant for the healthcare facility and for the patient?

Automated Call Distribution System. The *automated call distribution* (ACD) *system,* or call queuing, places inbound calls in a queue or waiting line. When a person is done with one call, the next call in line can be picked up. This system is useful when the department has more than one receptionist. Incoming calls stack up, and the first one is directed to the first receptionist available.

CRITICAL THINKING 22.4

What is the advantage to the caller when a facility uses the automated call distribution system?

Telephone Equipment. An employee's telephone equipment depends on the person's job. For instance, a provider may have a smart phone. A receptionist needs a desk telephone. This section will focus on the desk telephone.

Desk telephones in the ambulatory care facility may be single-line or multiline telephones. Single-line telephones have only one line for both incoming and outgoing calls. If a person is on the telephone, the line will be "busy" to other callers. With multiline telephones, the phone is connected to two or more lines (Fig. 22.1). With many telephones, the button for the line flashes when a call comes in. To answer that call, the medical

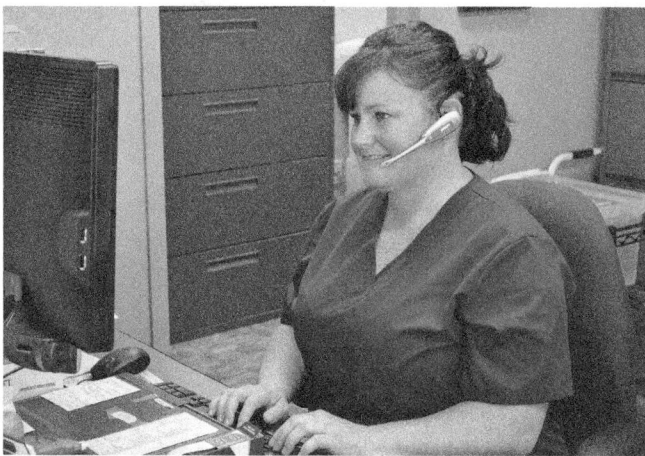

Fig. 22.2 A headset allows the medical assistant to keep the hands free. (From Proctor D, et al: *Kinn's the medical assistant,* ed 13, St. Louis, 2017, Elsevier.)

assistant must select the button for the line, and at that point the light stops flashing and remains solid.

A desk telephone typically consists of a handset and a base. Many desk telephones have a corded *telephone handset,* also called a *receiver.* The telephone handset can be replaced with a corded or wireless headset for employees who use the telephone frequently (Fig. 22.2). The headset improves the person's ergonomics (ur guh NOM iks) and helps prevent neck strain. Also, using a headset frees the person's hands to use the computer or take a message. Bluetooth, a type of short-range wireless technology, allows the employee to be more mobile while on the telephone. Sometimes the Bluetooth unit is not visible to others, and they may start a conversation with you. You should politely indicate that you are on the telephone and you will respond to the person when you can. Some healthcare facilities have a light system that indicates to patients that you are on the phone and signs that indicate you will be with them when the call is complete.

The desk telephone base varies between models. The most common features are:

- *Dial pad* or *keypad*: Usually has 12 buttons, including 0–9 and *and # buttons.
- *Function buttons* or *feature keys*: Can serve a variety of functions, including hold, call transfer, call forwarding, and call conferencing.
- *Display*: Also known as a liquid crystal display (LCD). The LCD displays can vary by the phone but may display the time, date, number dialed, and caller ID information.
- *LED lights*: Usually red but may also be other colors. May flash in different rhythms to indicate different things, including a waiting call and the line in use.
- *Speakerphone*: Has a separate speaker and microphone from the handset, along with a "speaker" button or icon. When the "speaker" button or icon is pushed, the handset can be hung up. A speakerphone is useful when two or more people need to talk with the caller using the same phone. When using a speakerphone, the medical assistant should:
  - Inform the caller that they will be placed on a speakerphone.

- Notify the caller of everyone on the call.
- Make sure the call takes place in an area where the conversation cannot be overheard. The door or reception window should be closed before the caller is placed on speaker.

VOCABULARY

ergonomics An applied science concerned with designing and arranging things, needed to do your job, in an efficient and safe way.

headset A combination earphone and microphone that is attached to the telephone by a cord or is wireless.

CRITICAL THINKING 22.5

Amy hears an employee using the speakerphone function to talk about a patient with another employee. How should she handle this situation? To whom, if anyone, should Amy report this activity? What problems might arise if this type of conversation is overheard?

Cell Phones. Cell phones are common for both personal and business communication. In the ambulatory care setting, providers and supervisors commonly use smart cell phones. The internet connectivity allows providers to access patient health records and practice guidelines when away from their personal computer. Sometimes the cell phones may have limited service in hospitals, and thus providers may also carry a pager (Box 22.1). A provider's cell number is never to be given to a patient without the provider's permission.

Cloud-Based Phone Systems

A cloud-based phone system is also called a *voice over internet protocol* (VoIP) system. VoIP is technology that allows making or receiving telephone calls over the internet. The VoIP does not require physical telephone lines but does require a device with internet connectivity (Box 22.2).

Features. Cloud-based phone systems used in healthcare settings must be compliant with HIPAA, which means patients' information must remain secure. VoIP systems include the features from multiline telephone systems. Additional features are available with VoIP systems, including:

- *Online faxing*: Faxes can be sent and received via the computer.
- *Voice mail to email*: Voicemails are sent to the person's email and can be accessible through the email system.
- *Call recording*: Calls can be recorded and usually are used for training. If this feature is used, the caller needs to be

BOX 22.3   Phonetic Alphabet

A	Alpha	N	November
B	Bravo	O	Oscar
C	Charlie	P	Papa
D	Delta	Q	Quebec
E	Echo	R	Romeo
F	Foxtrot	S	Sierra
G	Golf	T	Tango
H	Hotel	U	Uniform
I	India	V	Victor
J	Juliet	W	Whiskey
K	Kilo	X	X-ray
L	Lima	Y	Yankee
M	Mike	Z	Zulu

informed that the call may be recorded and for what reason (e.g., training purposes).

- *Call analytics*: Reports can be generated to provide data on missed calls, average wait times, call volumes, and so on. Supervisors can identify days and times where call volumes are high and calls are being missed. This information can be useful for staffing purposes.

Equipment. VoIP systems require an internet connection, which includes a router and modem. A variety of phones can be used, including:

- Internet protocol (IP) phones
- Traditional (analog) telephones with analog telephone adaptors (ATA)
- Soft phone, which turns the personal computer (PC) into a phone. A PC headset or a PC handset can be used. A PC handset resembles a telephone handset, but it connects to the computer through the USB or a sound card.

PROFESSIONAL TELEPHONE ETIQUETTE

Typically, a patient's first contact with the ambulatory care facility is by a phone call. This contact creates the patient's first impression of the facility. Each time a medical assistant uses the telephone, they are representing the healthcare facility. By using professional telephone techniques, the medical assistant can make a positive, professional impression on the other person. Being impolite, distracted, or unprofessional in any way can send a negative message.

Elements of Professional Telephone Etiquette

Being professional over the phone is a critical part of the medical assistant's job. Whether answering a call or placing a call, the medical assistant must demonstrate professionalism in all situations. Professionalism means the medical assistant is articulate, confident, tactful, empathetic, courteous, and respectful. Active listening and being prepared are important. The following sections will discuss these elements of professional telephone etiquette in more detail.

Articulate. Medical assistants must articulate their message over the phone to the other person. It is also important to be aware of nonverbal communication that occurs during a telephone conversation. Be aware of your tone of voice. Is it helping to send the message that you want to send? Your callers can tell if you are preoccupied and not focused on the current conversation. You should vary the pitch of your voice and avoid speaking in a monotone.

Enunciation (in nuhn see EY shuh n) is crucial when speaking on the telephone. You should speak clearly and concisely so that the other person can understand what you are saying. Many letters of the alphabet sound similar on the telephone, such as J and G, F or C with S, and M and N. You may need to clarify with the caller by saying, "That is B as in bravo" (Box 22.3). The medical assistant should remember these key points:

- Speak clearly and concisely. Make sure to pronounce each syllable.
- If nervous, slow down your speech and concentrate on your words. Avoid talking too much.
- Avoid the use of filler words and phrases, such as "um," "uh," "like," and "you know."
- Do not trail off on your sentences, because that can be perceived as if you are saying, "or whatever."
- Repeat important information, such as "Your appointment is scheduled for October 2nd at 8 a.m. with Dr. Walden."
- Refrain from medical jargon when speaking with patients because this makes the message more difficult for them to understand. For example, if you are giving a male patient preprocedural instructions, advise him that he must not eat or drink anything for 12 hours before the procedure; do not tell him he should "stay NPO" (nothing by mouth).
- Never eat, chew gum, or drink when on the telephone.

VOCABULARY

articulate To pronounce distinctly, concisely, and carefully; enunciate.

enunciation The use of articulate, clear sounds when speaking.

jargon The vocabulary of a particular profession as opposed to common, everyday terms.

monotone A succession of syllables, words, or sentences spoken in an unvaried key or pitch.

pitch The depth of a tone or sound; a distinctive quality of sound.

Amy tends to speak quickly in her normal conversations. How will she need to adjust when answering phones in the healthcare facility? She also is a friendly person and enjoys talking on the phone. What precautions should she take so that this does not become an issue on the job?

Confident and Tactful. When using the telephone, the medical assistant must be confident and tactful. *Confidence* is the belief in one's own abilities. By demonstrating confidence on the phone, the medical assistant shows respect and friendliness to the other person. Confidence can be shown through smiling, even though the other person cannot see you. By smiling you sound warmer, friendlier, and more confident, which helps to create a positive impression on the caller. If the medical assistant is nervous, anxious, or has a lack of self-assurance, being confident can be difficult. This can cause the person to use a higher tone of voice when on the phone. The listener may perceive this as the medical assistant not being competent, mature, or dependable. It is important to use a normal tone of voice and pretend you are confident. Confidence will come with practice.

Another important element of telephone etiquette is tactfulness. *Tactfulness* is being acutely sensitive to what is proper and appropriate when interacting with others. A tactful person has the ability to speak or act without offending others.

Empathetic, Courteous, and Respectful. Being empathetic, courteous, and respectful are three additional elements of professional telephone etiquette. A medical assistant should demonstrate empathy (EM pah thee). *Empathy* is the ability to understand another's perspective, experiences, or motivations. We can share another's emotional state. The medical assistant should consistently be polite, sensitive, and honest during the communication. *Courtesy* is having good manners or being polite. Courteous behavior is polite, open, and welcoming. *Respect* means to show consideration or appreciation for another person. The medical assistant can be courteous and respectful by asking permission prior to placing a person on hold and saying "thank you" at the end of the call. The medical assistant should also use the person's name during the conversation if it does not compromise patient confidentiality. When finishing the call, the medical assistant should let the caller hang up first.

Active Listening. The medical assistant can demonstrate active listening by listening carefully to the other person. It is important to allow the person to complete their sentences. Do not cut the person off by talking at the same time as the person. Restate what the speaker said to make sure that you received and interpreted the intended message.

For example, you receive a telephone call from a distraught mother. Using active listening skills, you pick up on the nonverbal cues, such as her tone of voice and rate of speech. You can tell she is upset. The mother states that her child has been very sick for the past several days, and nothing she has done has helped with the fever her child has had for 2 days. Your response should be to restate what you heard: the child has been ill with a fever for the past 2 days, and nothing she has tried has brought the fever down. This gives the caller the opportunity to correct any misinformation or to confirm that the information is correct. If it is correct, you should follow the healthcare facility's procedures for handling this situation; most likely, you will schedule an appointment for that same day.

Confidentiality

All communication in a healthcare facility must maintain patient confidentiality. When using the telephone, you must be aware of what is going on around you and who may be able to overhear your conversation. If patient-sensitive information will be discussed, place the call in an area where others cannot hear, especially other patients. Be careful when using a speakerphone because the sound can travel farther than you might think. Someone might overhear private medical information. This is a violation of HIPAA.

PROFESSIONAL TELEPHONE GUIDELINES

Answering Promptly

Telephone contact is often the first interaction with a patient. If the person's call is not answered promptly, this can create a negative impression before the person even talks to someone. It is important that a call be answered within three rings. If the medical assistant is on another call, the following steps should be taken:

- Ask the person you are talking with if you can place him on hold for a moment. Make sure to wait for the response before placing the person on hold.
- Answer the second call. Identify the reason for the call. If it is not an emergency, ask that person if you may place her on hold. If the person refuses, ask to call the person back.
- Return to the first caller and thank the person for holding.

Giving a Proper Greeting

When answering incoming telephone calls, medical assistants should:

- Identify the facility.
- State their name.
- Follow with an offer of help.

For example, you could begin by saying, "Good morning, Walden-Martin Family Medical Clinic. This is Amy. How may I help you?" Medical assistants must always follow the policy of the healthcare facility when answering incoming calls. Speaking slowly and smoothly, with good enunciation, ensures that your callers understand whom they have reached.

Identifying the Caller

If the caller does not offer a name, the medical assistant should ask, "May I ask who is calling?" If a patient is calling, the medical assistant must also find out the person's date of birth. The medical assistant should write down the caller's information or pull the caller's information up on the computer.

Occasionally callers refuse to identify themselves to the medical assistant and insist that they speak with the provider. Sometimes the caller may be a salesperson, and knows that if this is disclosed to you, the call will not be transferred to the provider. Strategies to take if the caller insists on talking with the provider include:

- State you cannot connect the caller to the provider without knowing who the caller is. You need to be clear and professional.
- State the provider is busy with patients and offer to take a message.
- Encourage the patient to write the provider a letter and mark it Personal. Most people do not want to wait for a response to a letter and will then give you their name so that you can take a message.

Taking Messages

Telephone messages in the ambulatory care facility used to be handwritten on paper. Deciphering handwriting and keeping track of paper message slips were challenges. Many ambulatory care facilities are now using message software, which may communicate with the electronic health record (EHR) if needed.

When answering calls, the medical assistant must be prepared to take messages. The medical assistant should have the following available:

- For paper messages: A paper message logbook, a clock, and pens
- For electronic messages: Access to a computer, pens, and scratch paper (optional)
- Facility's telephone screening guidelines
- Lists of commonly used telephone numbers, such as:
  - Extensions in the facility
  - Emergency numbers and poison control
  - Frequently used community resources to which patients are referred

Paper Messages. Many types of message pads or books are available (Fig. 22.3). Many are pressure sensitive, making a copy of the message and serving as a telephone call log. The original is given to the intended recipient of the message, and the medical assistant will have a copy to use for follow-up. Legible handwriting is a must when taking a manual, handwritten message.

With paper messages, the ambulatory care facility must have a policy on how long to keep the phone message logs. The length of time relates to the state's statute of limitations for medical professional liability cases. Phone messages can be used in lawsuits.

For messages that relate to patients, a copy of the message should be added to the patient's health record. If the health record is electronic, this may mean scanning in a copy of the paper message and attaching it to the EHR.

> **VOCABULARY**
> **statute of limitations** The length of time legal action can be taken after an event has occurred.

Electronic Messaging Systems. Ambulatory care facilities use software for communicating between providers and staff. Nonpatient telephone messages can be sent through this

software. For patient messages, most facilities use their EHR system to record telephone messages (Fig. 22.4). The EHR automatically saves a copy of the message to the patient's health record and sends the message to the provider. The provider can either call the patient directly or give the medical assistant directions to respond to the patient. The electronic system may also be able to:

- Flag a message
- Indicate its urgency or that it requires a call back
- Note that a prescription refill has been requested

Elements of a Message. Telephone messages are an important part of patient care (see Procedures 22.1 and 22.2). The patient relies on the medical assistant to deliver the message to a provider or the appropriate person, who can make a decision. This response is then communicated back to the patient without interrupting the flow of patients through the healthcare facility. You should be sure to let the caller know when to expect a call back; for example, explain that the provider usually returns calls between 3 and 4 p.m.

Whether the message is taken in a handwritten or an electronic format, the information needed for a complete message is the same:

1. Name of the person calling
2. Name of the person to whom the call is directed
3. Caller's daytime, evening, or cell phone number
4. Reason for the call, including the telephone number of the caller's pharmacy if a medication is requested

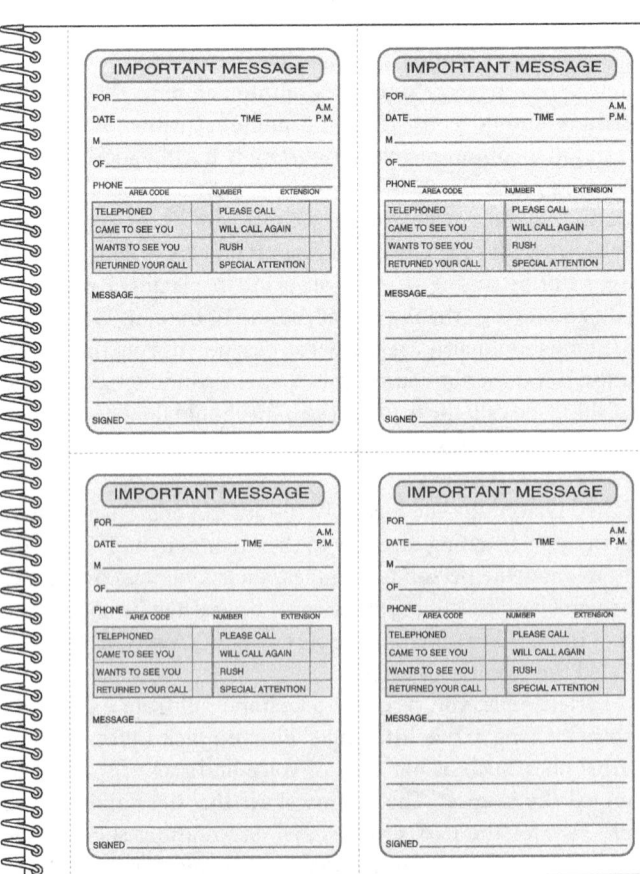

Fig. 22.3 Telephone Message Forms.

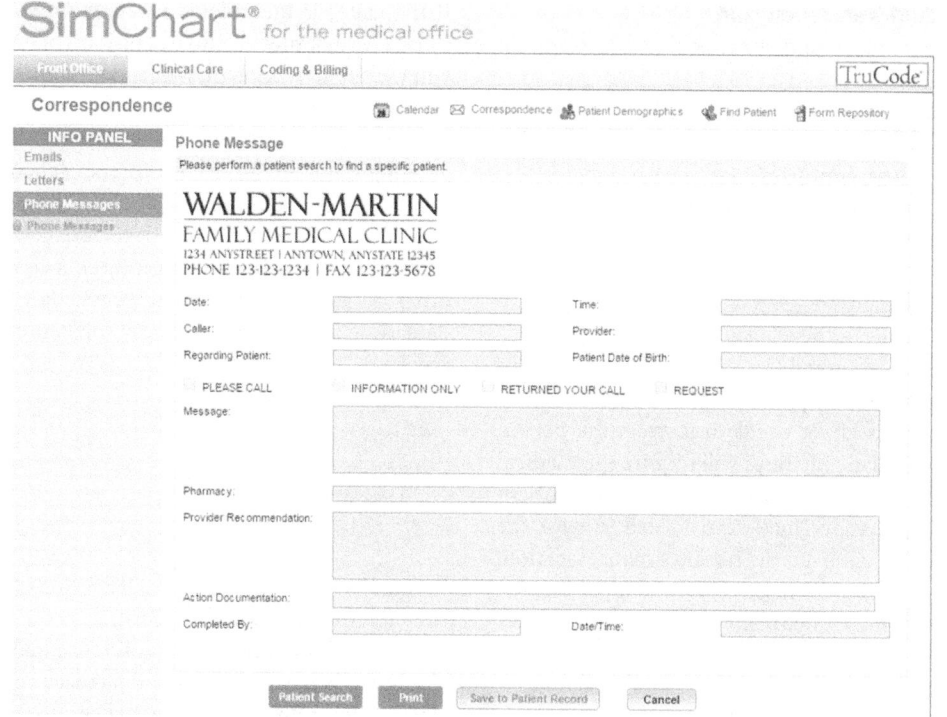

Fig. 22.4 Telephone Message Screen in an Electronic Health Record System. (From SimChart for the Medical Office, St. Louis, 2015, Elsevier.)

5. Action to be taken
6. Date and time of the call
7. Initials of the person who took the call

Following Up with Messages. The message process is not complete until the necessary action has been taken. The medical assistant needs to monitor the status of the message. Usually, the paper message logbook can be marked to indicate a message that requires action. If an electronic system is used, the medical assistant should periodically check for a response from the provider.

Typically, action on messages includes calling the patient back and relaying the provider's message or contacting the pharmacy. The medical assistant must document the action taken in the patient's health record. For risk-management purposes, the healthcare facility should have a policy on the documentation of telephone messages and the specific information that must be included. Medical assistants should become familiar with that policy.

SCREENING INCOMING CALLS

Most healthcare facilities expect the medical assistant answering the telephone to *screen* the calls. You must determine if a call should be routed to the provider, the triage (tree AHZH) area, or the billing office, or if you can assist the caller. The provider, office manager, and staff members who will be answering the telephone should work together to develop policies for screening calls. The following sections discuss the screening of incoming calls.

Calls Related to Patients

Emergencies. If a call is an emergency, policies for handling emergency calls apply. Some facilities use triage to handle emergency phone calls. The medical assistant must immediately transfer the emergency call to the triage area. In the triage area, a licensed professional staff person (e.g., registered nurse) obtains an accurate assessment of the patient's concerns and symptoms.

When a facility does not have triage personnel, policies and procedures will indicate if the provider needs to be contacted immediately or if the medical assistant must handle the phone call. The facility's written policies and procedures should indicate:

- Specific examples of questions to ask the patient
- Responses for minor problems
- Specified types of calls that require an appointment, to be transferred to the provider for more evaluation, or instructions to call 911

It is important that medical assistants receive training and clear direction on how to handle emergency situations. If the medical assistant has any questions or concerns, the provider or manager should be contacted immediately.

Typical types of concerns that usually require immediate medical attention from the emergency medical services (EMS) include:

- Allergic reactions that cause breathing issues or swelling in the face, throat, or mouth

- Breathing difficulties and chest pain
- Moderate to severe burns and human bites or deep animal bites
- Seizures or loss of consciousness
- Stroke symptoms, such as facial drooping, arm or leg weakness, vision loss, confusion, and speech difficulties
- Profuse (heavy) bleeding and trauma (e.g., car accidents, stabbing or gunshot wounds, falls, or injuries to the head, neck or back)
- Severe abdominal pain
- Poisoning, chemicals in the eye, or smoke inhalation
- Suicidal or homicidal thoughts

If a person calls on behalf of a patient experiencing a medical emergency, the medical assistant needs to instruct the person to call 911 immediately. Many facilities will require the medical assistant to remain on the line with the patient if the patient is alone. Another staff member may need to call 911 for the patient. The 911 dispatch will need the patient's name, location, and a description of what is occurring.

The medical assistant must document the call in the patient's health record. Documentation usually includes the date, time, person calling, patient concerns, and action the medical assistant took, including notifying the provider.

Patient Concerns and Requests for Appointments. Unlike emergencies, which are life-threatening, urgent calls require prompt attention, but are not life threatening. Typical urgent concerns include:

- Minor burns and cuts (with limited bleeding)
- Fever, influenza, cough, ear pain, and sore throat
- Mild to moderate breathing difficulties
- Urinary tract infection symptoms
- Digestive system symptoms such as vomiting, diarrhea, and dehydration
- Orthopedic concerns, such as sprains, strains, and minor broken bones (e.g., fingers, toes, and arms)

Facility policies and procedures should help the medical assistant identify the urgency of patient concerns.

When a patient has a concern that needs to be addressed by the provider, the medical assistant will need to gather additional information for the provider (see Procedures 22.1 and 22.2). For instance, the medical assistant may need to ask:

- What symptoms does the patient have? When did they start?
- What makes the symptoms better or worse?
- What remedies has the patient tried? What has worked? What has not worked?

As you learn more about signs and symptoms of diseases, you will be able to ask additional questions to better assist the provider. For instance, if the patient complains of painful urination, you should ask about pain in the back or blood in the urine.

When the patient needs a return call either from the medical assistant or provider, it is important that the medical assistant:

- get a phone number at which to reach the patient.
- give the patient an approximate time frame for the return call. This helps the patient anticipate the response time.

If the caller is unavailable when the provider usually returns calls, ask what time would be convenient and let the caller know you will try to work with that time frame.

As stated in a prior section of the chapter, patient phone calls need to be documented in the patient's health record. When a patient makes an appointment, scheduling the appointment provides the documentation. The appointment book is a legal record, or if an electronic scheduling system is used, a report of the patient's appointments can be created. For any other patient calls, the medical assistant must document the date, time, interaction, and action taken in the patient's health record.

VOCABULARY

urgent An acute situation that requires immediate attention but is not life-threatening.

Requests for Prescription Refills. Prescription refill requests will either come from the pharmacy or from patients. It could be that there were no refills on the original prescription or that all the refills have been used. Pharmacy refill requests are usually electronically generated emails to the provider (or provider's medical assistant).

Patients may contact the facility by telephone, email, or through the patient portal. Patients must provide the following information when requesting a prescription refill:

- Medication name
- Dosage
- How much medication (e.g., tablets) is taken daily
- Any issues with the medication
- Whether the patient wants to use a pharmacy mail-order service or pick up the prescription at the pharmacy
- Pharmacy address and phone number

Prescription refill requests should be documented in the patient's health record.

It is important for a medical assistant to be familiar with the common medication names and the abbreviations used in a prescription. Using the correct spelling of the medication is very important. See Appendix C for abbreviations and Appendix D for the most common medications and their spelling; both appendixes can be found on the Evolve website.

VOCABULARY

patient portal A secure online website that gives patients 24-hour access to personal health information using a username and password.
STAT The medical abbreviation for the Latin *term statum*, meaning immediately; at this moment.

CRITICAL THINKING 22.7

A patient calls the healthcare facility to report that she has been taking her prescribed antibiotic for 3 days and still does not feel any better. She says she might even feel worse. She asks Amy if she should stop taking the pills. How should Amy respond to this patient? What actions should Amy take in response to this telephone call? What should Amy document in the patient's record?

Progress Reports. Providers sometimes ask patients to call with an update on their condition a few days after an appointment. The medical assistant can take such calls and relay the information to the provider (see Procedure 22.2). Assure the patient that you will inform the provider of the call. The report should be documented in the health record. The provider should always be informed immediately about unsatisfactory progress reports, and they should give instructions for the patient to follow in those situations. The provider may discuss this directly with the patient, or the medical assistant may be instructed to relay the information. All instructions given should also be documented in the health record.

Radiology and Laboratory Reports. With radiology and laboratory reports, two different types of calls can be received:

- those from a healthcare facility regarding test and procedure results
- those from a patient

Radiology procedures and laboratory tests may be done in the healthcare facility. If the facility uses an EHR, the results are added to the patient's health record and can be viewed by the medical assistant and the provider. If the radiology procedure or laboratory test is done at an outside facility, the results are usually mailed to the provider. If the test has been marked STAT, reports may be telephoned, faxed, or emailed to the provider's office and an original report delivered by mail. If laboratory test results are in the critical range, the laboratory facility procedures usually require the personnel to contact the provider by phone.

When receiving calls from radiology and laboratory facilities, the medical assistant will need to write down the results for the provider. The medical assistant should listen carefully, write down the patient information and the test results, and then read everything back to the caller to ensure accuracy. These results must be immediately given to the provider. Having blank laboratory results forms available by the phone can be helpful when taking such calls. Usually the blank forms include a list of common laboratory tests with their normal values.

Radiology and laboratory results must be reviewed by the provider before a patient can be notified of the results. The provider decides whether the medical assistant can relay the results or the provider needs to speak to the patient directly. If the results are unfavorable, the provider should be the one to inform the patient and give further instructions. Some healthcare facilities have policies that allow medical assistants to give negative test results to patients.

When a patient calls for laboratory test or radiology procedure results, the medical assistant should follow these guidelines:

- *Follow the facility's policy on identifying the patient.* Some healthcare facilities give a special code to the patient, which is documented in the health record. Knowledge of this code gives the person access to the information. Other facilities may require the patient's date of birth (DOB) or other information that is known only to the patient and has been shared with the healthcare facility. You should always use at least two different methods of identifying patients before providing any information.
- *Refer the patient to the provider if the person has questions.* The medical assistant needs good communication skills to

relay information such as test results without crossing the line of practicing medicine without a license.

- *Take a message for the provider.* If the provider has not shared what to tell the patient, the medical assistant should take a message and obtain the caller's name, DOB, and a call-back number. Then the medical assistant should follow up with the provider and review the health record.
- *Document conversations with the patient.* When the medical assistant relays the results to the patient, the medical assistant must document the conversation in the patient's health record.
- *Follow the federal and state regulations regarding the release of information to people other than the patient.*

Inquiries About Bills and Fees. Calls regarding bills and fees are handled differently between facilities. Many healthcare facilities have a person or department that handles billing patients for services. Calls regarding patient bills and fees for services should be transferred to those who handle patient accounts.

If the healthcare facility uses an external billing service, the medical assistant will need to follow the facility's procedures, which may include providing the caller with that agency's telephone number. When necessary, document the patient's call in the EHR or in the physical record, such as noting that the patient promised to pay on a certain date.

If the clinic is small, the medical assistant might be responsible for handling patient accounts and billing. The medical assistant should politely ask the patient to hold while the account is accessed. When returning to the call, the medical assistant should thank the patient for waiting and ask the person to explain the concern. The medical assistant should carefully explain the charges. If an error has occurred, apologize and say that a corrected statement will be sent out at once

If the medical assistant is involved with providing a patient with a quote for potential services, it is important to remember that many services depend on the patient's condition. The medical assistant may need to talk with the provider or the office manager before giving the patient a quote, especially with more complex services.

Insurance Questions. It is common for patients to have questions regarding their insurance coverage and how it impacts their bills. In most healthcare facilities, a person or a department usually handles insurance concerns. When a medical assistant receives a call regarding an insurance question, the call should be transferred to that person or department.

Patients may call the office to inquire whether the provider is a participating provider with their insurance plan or managed care organization. A list of the insurance plans with which the provider has a contract should be readily available to the medical assistant who answers the telephone. This is important because insurance benefits vary widely for patients based on whether they see a participating provider or a nonparticipating provider. A claim may even be denied if the provider is not a participant for the patient's insurance company.

Requests for Referrals. Often patients will request referrals from their primary care providers(PCPs). Many times, this is required by their health plans, especially by point of service (POS) and health maintenance organization (HMO) plans. A referral is needed to see a specialist or other providers in the same network or outside the network. Health plans may require a written referral from the provider or may allow a call from the healthcare facility. The patient may need to have a preauthorization completed for the health plan before the referral visit can be scheduled.

When a medical assistant receives a request for a referral, the medical assistant should ask if a preauthorization is also needed. The medical assistant should take a message and obtain the name of the patient, DOB, reason for the referral, name of the referral provider if given, and any additional information required. The information should be given to the provider, and the medical assistant may be required to help with the referral paperwork. All referrals should be documented in the patient's health record.

VOCABULARY

participating provider A physician or other healthcare provider who enters into a contract with a specific insurance company or program and by doing so agrees to abide by certain rules and regulations set forth by that particular insurance company.

preauthorization A process that requires the provider to submit documentation to the payer to show the service or treatment is medically needed, and the payer determines if the service or treatment is medically necessary and covered under the insurance plan. Also called *prior authorization*.

primary care provider (PCPs) A general practice or nonspecialist provider or physician responsible for the care of a patient for some health maintenance organizations. Also called a *gatekeeper*.

referral An insurance term used when a primary care provider wants to send a patient to a specialist.

Handling Special Situations

Using Telecommunications Relay Service. Telecommunications Relay Service (TRS) is a telephone service that allows people with hearing or speech impairments to place and receive telephone calls. TRS is available in all 50 states. TRS uses communication assistants (CAs) to facilitate telephone calls between people with hearing or speech impairment and other people. The call can be initiated by either party. When people with a disability place the call, they use a teletypewriter (TTY) or another text input device to call the TRS relay center. The person gives the CA the phone number of the party they want to call. The CA calls the other party and communicates the messages between the two parties. The CA relays the text of the calling party in voice to the party called. Then the CA converts the voice message from party called to the calling party.

Dialing 711 connects the caller to certain forms of TRS anywhere in the US. There are several types of TRS available, including:

- *Text-to-Voice TTY-based TRS*: A person uses the TTY to call the CA at the relay center and the CA is involved with the call as described.

- *Voice Carry Over*: A person with a hearing impairment speaks directly to the called party, and the CA texts what the called party states.
- *Captioned Telephone Service*: A special telephone that has a text screen is used to display captions of what the other party is saying. A person with a hearing disability but who has some residual hearing may use this service. The CA repeats what the called party says, and speech recognition technology transcribes the CA's voice into captions, which are then transmitted to the users text screen.
- *Video Relay Service (VRS)*: A internet-based service that allows people whose primary language is American Sign Language (ASL) to communicate to the CA in ASL using video conferencing equipment. The CA speaks what is signed to the called party and signs the called party's response back to the caller. The availability of this service may be limited across the country.

When you receive a call using the TRS, keep these guidelines in mind:

- A TYY call may start with a beep or data line sound or an electronic announcement stating, "Hearing impaired caller." Calls that use the relay service may start with, "Hello. This is the relay service…" Do not hang up. The call is from a person with a hearing or speech disability.
- One person should speak at a time.
- Always introduce yourself at the start of the call.
- Be concise and use simple terms if possible.
- Remember to allow extra time for the CA to type or relay the responses between the two parties.

Patients With Limited English Proficiency. As part of the Affordable Care Act (ACA), patients who have limited English proficiency (LEP) are entitled to an interpreter or language assistant services at no extra charge. These services are provided if needed during a patient's visit. Phone calls to the healthcare facility can be challenging for these patients. Larger facilities have employed medical interpreters who not only assist during visits but also help when patients who have LEP call. Some clinics hire bilingual (bahy LING gwuh l) medical assistants to help with phone calls and visits. Healthcare facilities also use online or over the phone interpretation services. Many services allow for 3-way calls.

When a medical assistant is working with an interpreter over the phone, it is important to remember these guidelines:

- Speak to the patient. Use first person as you would during a normal conversation. For instance, say, "What can I help you with?" instead of, "Ask him what I can do for him."
- After you speak one or two sentences, pause to let the interpreter translate your message.
- You may need to explain some terms in more detail to the interpreter. Some concepts or words do not directly translate into all languages.
- Treat the LEP patient as you would other patients. Provide them with the same details and same level of service as you do for other patients.

VOCABULARY
bilingual The ability to communicate effectively in two languages.

Handling Difficult Phone Conversations

Patients Who Refuse to Discuss Symptoms. Sometimes patients have symptoms that they are embarrassed about. They may ask to speak only to the provider. The medical assistant should let the patient know that it will help the provider to know what the patient's concern is before returning the call. It is important to remain courteous to all patients. If the patient refuses to discuss any symptoms, follow the healthcare facility's procedures, which may include suggesting that the patient make an appointment with the provider to discuss the problem in person.

Complaints. Four magic words often calm the angry patient: "Let me help you." This reassures the patient that someone is willing to talk about the problem. However, if you are unable to calm down the patient easily, the provider or office manager may prefer to talk to the patient directly.

When callers complain, do not attempt to blame someone else, and never argue with the patient. Find the source of the problem, and then present options to the caller as to how the situation can be resolved. Remember to treat callers in the same manner that you would wish to be treated. A complaint may seem small and insignificant to the office staff, but it may be a serious issue to the patient. Provide good customer service to patients, and complaints will be few and far between.

Angry Callers. Those who call the healthcare facility for help are almost never at their best. When feeling ill, people often are short tempered and even display poor manners. When dealing with an angry patient over the phone, the medical assistant should keep these guidelines in mind:

- Do not get defensive or angry. Remain calm. Allow the person to express himself or herself.
- Listen to the patient. Summarizing or restating what the patient expresses helps the patient know you are hearing what is being said.
- Use a lower tone of voice to help calm the angry caller.
- Identify what the patient would like to see happen.
- Never "pass the buck" by saying, "That's not my job" or "I am not the person who filed that insurance claim." No matter whose fault the problem is, it is best to deal with it and find a solution instead of placing blame.
- Present a solution or ask the patient's permission to transfer them to a person who can assist with the problem. If you transfer the patient, provide the patient's information and concerns before you connect the patient.
- If medical assistants promise to act, they must keep their word.

CRITICAL THINKING 22.8

An angry caller raises his voice at Amy over an issue that happened before she began to work at WMFM Clinic. She suggests that he speak with the office manager, but he refuses and continues to berate Amy. What choices does Amy have in this situation? Should she simply hang up on the patient? How can the call be handled diplomatically?

Requests for Information From Third Parties. When patients request their information to be given to another person (e.g., family member, friend), patients must complete a disclosure authorization form. (For more information on disclosure forms see Chapter 19.)

When a person calls requesting information on a current patient, the medical assistant should first ask the caller's name. The medical assistant must check to see if the caller is listed on the patient's disclosure authorization form. If that caller's name appears, then, per the facility's policy, the medical assistant can release information about the patient. If the caller's name is not on the form, the medical assistant

- cannot release the patient's information and
- cannot even acknowledge that that person is a patient of the facility.

Applying HIPAA rules is important when protecting a patient's privacy.

Calls for Providers

Healthcare facility policies often state that calls from other providers are put through immediately. If that is not possible, assure the caller that the provider will return the call as soon as possible. Some providers may also ask that calls be put through immediately for certain family members. If the provider does not want to take the call, the medical assistant must tactfully tell the caller that the provider cannot be disturbed at this time.

Screening policies should also address how calls should be handled when the provider is out of the office. If the provider is to be out of the office for an extended period (e.g., for a conference or vacation), another provider is usually designated to handle calls. It should be explained that the provider is out of the office, but another provider is taking the calls. If the call is not an emergency, take a message, and the designated provider can return the call.

Non-Patient–Related Calls

Not all calls concern patients. Calls may come from the accountant about banking procedures, office supplies, or office maintenance. Most of these calls can be handled by the medical assistant or referred to the appropriate person. For some of these calls, the medical assistant may need to gather additional information and return the call.

Pharmaceutical representatives and salespeople will often call and ask to speak to the provider. A message should be taken that includes what product they want to discuss with the provider. The provider may decide to return these calls or may ask that an appointment be scheduled to talk about the new product. It is also possible that the provider will ask the office manager to talk to the salesperson.

Calls From Staff Members' Families or Friends

Personal calls can tie up the telephone lines. Sometimes a call is necessary in emergencies, but staff members should never monopolize the telephone for personal business and conversations. Patient emergency calls could be coming through, and the lines must be clear. Keep personal calls to an absolute minimum.

TYPICAL OUTGOING CALLS

Most outgoing calls in the healthcare facility are in response to incoming calls. The same rules for courtesy and diction apply to calls made from the healthcare facility to patients, other individuals, and businesses. Remember to treat those on the other end of the call as you would wish to be treated. Do not forget that you represent the provider and must behave in a professional manner at all times.

It is helpful to plan outgoing calls in advance. For instance, if the medical assistant is placing an order for office supplies, a list should be made that includes the product, the item number, the price, and the quantity needed. Questions about the various products ordered should be noted so that they can be asked while the medical assistant is on the telephone with the supplier. If the medical assistant is calling a patient, it is important to have the person's health record and the information that needs to be given to the patient.

Considerations

Time Zones. When making outgoing calls, the medical assistant must keep time zones in mind, especially when calling patients.

If you are trying to contact a patient who is spending the winter somewhere else, you should place that call at an appropriate time for the patient. If you are trying to get information from an insurance company, you should call when someone is available to answer your questions. The continental United States is divided into four time zones: Pacific, Mountain, Central, and Eastern (Fig. 22.5). Hawaii and Alaska are in two other time zones. When it is noon Pacific time, it is 3 p.m. Eastern time. If you will be calling from San Francisco to a business or professional office in New York, plan to make the call no later than 1 p.m. When it is 2 p.m. on the West Coast, it is 5 p.m. on the East Coast.

Long-Distance Calls. Long-distance calls are simple to place, usually inexpensive, and efficient. When information is needed in a hurry, using the telephone is much quicker than written communication. There can be an additional charge for long-distance calls, depending on the phone plan. Check with the office manager or the telephone service provider to determine what those charges might be. Some VoIP systems, such as Skype or magicJack, allow the user to call long distance, and sometimes even internationally, through the computer with no long-distance charges.

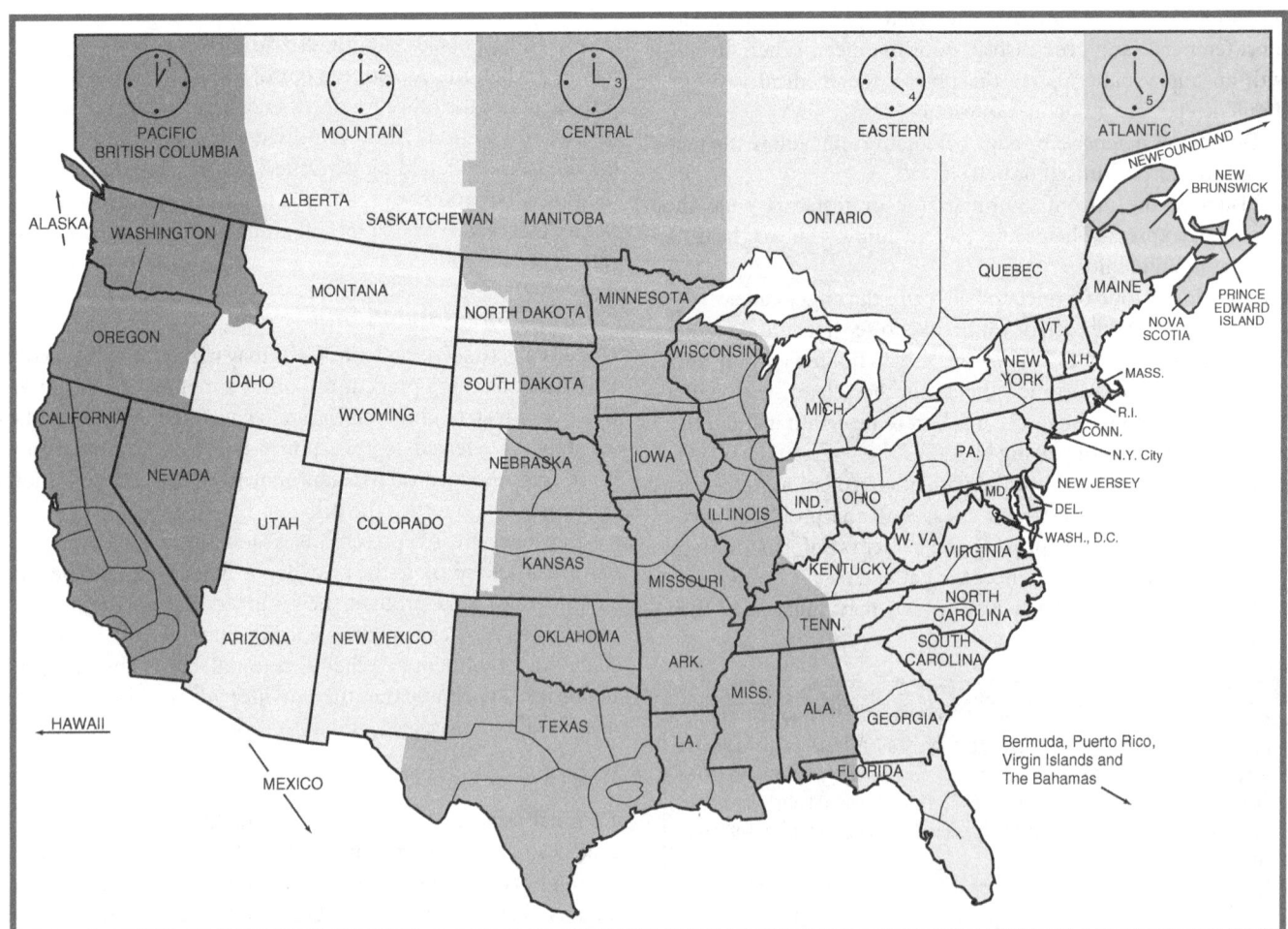

Fig. 22.5 Time Zones Across the United States. When Pacific Time is 1 p.m., Alaska Daylight Time is noon and Hawaii Standard Time is 10 a.m. (From Proctor D, et al: Kinn's *the medical assistant,* ed 13, St. Louis, 2017, Elsevier.)

Finding Telephone Numbers. When a medical assistant needs to find a phone number, several options are available.

- *Toll-free directory assistance*: Calls that use the area code "800" or "888" are toll-free numbers, which means you can call these numbers for free. To reach the toll-free directory assistance, dial 1-800-555-1212 or 1-888-555-1212.
- *Local and long-distance directory assistance*: For local directory assistance, call 1-411. To reach long-distance directory assistance, dial 1, followed by the area code of the party you want to call, and then dial 555-1212. Often directory assistance is an automated service. You will need to give the city and the name of the person you are calling. Usually, a fee is charged to the telephone bill for using directory assistance.
- *Operator-assisted dialing*: These calls can include collect or person-to-person calls. An operator surcharge may apply.
- *Telephone directory*: This is also called a *phone book*. Governmental offices usually have their own section. The yellow pages provide a listing of businesses, which can also be accessed online at https://www.yellowpages.com/. Finding an individual's phone number is more challenging with the use of cell phones. Many people are not listed in the phone book. Online websites can be used, such as https://www.whitepages.com/.
- *Web search*: A web search for the business or provider needed may give you the information.

Calling Patients

When contacting patients, the medical assistant must use the method requested by the patient. For example, if the patient requests to be contacted by email, the medical assistant must email the patient. If the patient requests to be called at a specific phone number or to have a message left or not left, these instructions need to be followed per HIPAA.

When you call a patient, it is important that you ask for the patient or parent/guardian. If the person is not available, leave a vague message and ask for the patient to return the call.

If the patient is available, verify the speaker as discussed earlier in the chapter. The medical assistant must introduce himself or herself and give the name of the healthcare facility. If calling with instructions from a certain provider, the medical assistant must indicate the provider. During the conversation, the medical assistant must relay the instructions from the provider. If the patient has questions that are outside the medical assistant's scope of practice or the medical assistant does not know the answer, the question must be referred to the provider. All calls to patients must be documented in the patients' health records.

If the medical assistant must leave a voice message for the patient, it is important to follow the healthcare facility's policies and procedures (see Procedure 22.3). Do not disclose medical conditions or private health information. Most facilities limit the information disclosed in the voice message to safeguard the patient's privacy. The amount of information left can vary; for example:

- Leave only the name of the healthcare facility and the phone number. Use caution if the clinic's name may disclose a condition, such as "Anytown Pregnancy Center." A better option might be to state, "This is Amy from Dr. Smith's office."
- Ask the individual to return the call.
- Leave very basic information regarding an appointment reminder.
- Leave a very generic message, such as, "Your test was negative." Leaving a more detailed message, such as, "The gonorrhea test was positive," is inappropriate and can violate a patient's privacy.

Politely finish the voice message.

ANSWERING SERVICES

If an emergency arises, patients expect to be able to contact their provider. This means that the telephone in the healthcare facility must be answered at all times, day and night, weekends, and holidays. During normal office hours, the medical assistant is available to answer the telephone. After office hours, most healthcare facilities use an answering service or an answering machine that directs the caller to the answering service if there is an urgent issue.

With an answering service, an actual person answers the call, which can be comforting for patients. The staff at the answering service can act as a buffer for the provider after hours by screening the calls. By following the criteria given by the healthcare facility, they can make the following determinations:

- Whether the provider (or on-call person) should be contacted
- If the patient should be directed to the hospital emergency department
- If a message can be taken and relayed to the healthcare facility in the morning

It is common courtesy to call the answering service in the morning to let the staff know that you will be answering the calls and also to retrieve any messages taken. You should also call the answering service when you are leaving for the day. Answering services also can be used to cover the telephone if all staff members need to be away from the telephone at the same time.

CLOSING COMMENTS

We have talked on telephones and cell phones in our own lives, and most of us have used at least some of the special features on our phones. It is important to recognize that the way we present ourselves on the phone in our professional lives is different from the style of communication we use in our personal lives. The way we speak in our personal lives may not be appropriate in the healthcare facility. We must maintain a professional tone in communications with our patients and other contacts. For example, slang should not be used; "Hello" by itself is not a proper way to answer a business telephone; and we must take care how we use medical terminology when on the telephone (jargon should not be used when speaking with patients). The goal is always to present a positive professional image of the healthcare facility we represent.

PATIENT-CENTERED CARE

When answering the telephone in a healthcare facility, the medical assistant has many opportunities to provide patient-centered care. The medical assistant should respect the patient's preference. This includes using the patient's preferred name. It also includes using the preferred phone number for returning calls and leaving voice messages.

The medical assistant can also provide patient-centered care by actively listening to the patient's concerns and taking accurate and complete messages for the provider. The medical assistant's role in the front office/reception area is critical to the patient-centered care approach.

BEING PROFESSIONAL

As a medical assistant interacts with patients over the telephone, often the medical assistant promises to talk with the provider or to follow up on the patient's concern. Professionally, it is critical that the medical assistant keeps their promise to the patient. Following up as promised is not only professional, but also a legal obligation of healthcare professionals. Failure to follow up or call patients back may lead to legal consequences for the provider and facility.

Role-play this scenario with a peer: You both are medical assistants. Your peer promised to call Mrs. Smith back before the end of the day and let her know about her medication refill. It is now the end of the day, and your peer needs to leave. They tell you, "I don't have time to call her. She will talk forever, and I need to get home. I will call her tomorrow and make up an excuse." Respond to your peer in a professional and respectful manner.

CHAPTER REVIEW

A multiline telephone system allows multiple people to use the telephone system at the same time. Multiline telephone systems can have many different features that can be beneficial to the ambulatory care facility. Common features include speakerphone, conference calls, call forwarding, call transfer, and voice mails. VoIP systems have additional features, including online faxing, voice mail to email, call recording, and call analytics. These features can be helpful in the healthcare facility.

Each time a medical assistant uses the telephone, they represent the healthcare facility. Whether answering a call or placing a call, the medical assistant must demonstrate professionalism in all situations. Professionalism means the medical assistant is articulate, confident, tactful, empathetic, courteous, and respectful. Active listening and being prepared are important. By using professional telephone techniques, the medical assistant can make a positive, professional impression on the other person.

The medical assistant should answer a call promptly. When answering incoming telephone calls, the medical assistant should identify the facility, state their name, and offer to help the caller. If a message must be taken, the medical assistant can take paper messages or electronic messages. The EHR automatically saves a copy of the message to the patient's health record and sends the message to the provider. A complete message should include the caller's name, the name of the person who needs to get the message, the caller's phone number, reason for the call, action to be taken, date and time of the call, and the initials of the person who took the call. The medical assistant should follow up on messages taken.

With incoming calls, the medical assistant must screen the calls. Emergency calls must be sent to the triage area, or the medical assistant must follow the facility's policies and procedures. For nonemergent calls, the medical assistant must gather information for the provider about the patient's concern. With prescription refill calls, the medical assistant must gather the following information: the medication name, dosage, the amount of medication taken in a day, any issues, and where to send the prescription. Incoming calls regarding questions on bills and fees should be transferred to the person or department that handles patient accounts. Calls related to insurance questions must be transferred to the person or department that handles insurance. Messages for referral and preauthorization requests must be sent to the provider.

The healthcare facility may also receive calls that use the Telecommunications Relay Service when a patient has a hearing or speech impairment. Dialing 711 connects the caller to certain forms of TRS anywhere in the US. There are several types of TRS available, including text-to-voice TTY-based, voice carry over, captioned telephone service, and video relay service.

The medical assistant should know how to handle difficult calls, including patients who refuse to discuss symptoms, complaints, angry callers, and requests for information from a third party. The medical assistant must remember to maintain the confidentiality of patients and remain professional during difficult calls.

When a medical assistant needs to place an outgoing call, resources are available in print form or online to help find individual and business phone numbers. When calling patients, the medical assistant must verify the identity of the person speaking. When leaving a voice message, the medical assistant must leave a HIPAA-appropriate message to safeguard the patient's privacy.

SCENARIO WRAP-UP

Amy is quickly becoming a part of the team at WMFM Clinic and is developing into a well-liked asset to the staff. She has learned to slow down when speaking on the phone and to adjust her volume and pitch, depending on the patient with whom she is speaking. Although she tends to be talkative, she is balancing just the right amount of friendly chatter with the business at hand. She does this by offering a pleasant greeting to callers, getting to the point of the call, then being cordial before ending the call. By expressing her concern and asking how she can be of help to the patients, Amy shows them that she sincerely cares about their problems. She is careful about her tone of voice, realizing that patients may take her comments the wrong way if she does not treat them in a cordial manner.

Amy takes care when she speaks to patients and others on the phone so that she does not breach confidentiality in any way. She has become comfortable with the way she is expected to answer the telephone. The pace of her speech and the wording are now a habit. Amy is determined to maintain a professional relationship with all the people related to her work environment. She is now adept at handling calls from angry patients and can maintain control with even the most aggressive callers. She leaves callers on hold for a minimum of time and reassures them frequently that she is tending to their situation. By treating callers as she would want to be treated, Amy reduces frustration, and she feels that the office is more efficient at handling the large volume of calls that comes in each day. Amy contributes to the efficiency of the healthcare facility by constantly refining her knowledge about her job.

PROCEDURE 22.1   Use Critical Thinking When Performing Patient Screening

Tasks

Demonstrate professional telephone techniques. Incorporate critical thinking skills when performing patient assessment. Take an accurate telephone message and document the patient's history and chief complaint. Document in the patient's health record.

Scenario

You are a medical assistant at Walden-Martin Family Medical (WMFM) Clinic. A patient calls and states that she has had nausea, vomiting, diarrhea, and abdominal pain for 3 days. You need to gather the patient's information before talking with the provider, per the facility's policy.

Directions

Role-play the scenario with a peer, who is the patient. Your peer can make up any needed information. Your instructor is the provider.

Equipment and Supplies

- Telephone
- Computer with electronic health record (EHR) and messaging software, or message pad, pen, and patient's health record
- Notepad (optional)

Procedural Steps

1. Demonstrate telephone techniques by answering the telephone by the third ring. Speak distinctly with a pleasant tone and expression, at a moderate rate, and with sufficient volume for the person to understand every word.
   Purpose: To convey interest in the caller by answering promptly. Proper enunciation will help the patient to understand.
2. Greet the caller. Identify the office or provider and yourself. Offer to help the caller.
   Purpose: To assure the caller that the correct number has been reached and to identify the staff member.
3. Verify the caller's identity and date of birth. If using an electronic health record, bring the patient's health record to the computer's active screen. Note the patient's phone number in case you are disconnected.
   Purpose: To confirm the origin of the call.
4. Screen the call if necessary. Determine the needs of the caller.

Purpose: To determine whether the caller has an emergency and needs immediate attention or referral to a hospital emergency department.
5. Upon learning the patient's complaint, use critical thinking skills and ask appropriate questions to obtain information about the patient's condition for the provider. Identify the onset, frequency, and duration of the complaint. If related to pain, identify the exact location, quality (e.g., sharp, dull, stabbing), and rating (using a 0–10 pain scale). Identify significant history and factors that increase or decrease the complaint.
   Purpose: Gathering relevant information helps the provider form an opinion on the patient's care.
6. Using a message pad or the computer, take the phone message (either on paper or by data entry into the computer) and obtain the following information:
   - Name of the person to whom the call is directed
   - Name of the person calling
   - Caller's telephone number
   - Reason for the call
   - Action to be taken
   - Date and time of the call
   - Initials of the person taking the call
   Purpose: To obtain accurate information, which allows the staff member or provider to address the caller's issues quickly and efficiently.
7. Apply active listening skills and repeat the information back to the caller after recording the message.
   Purpose: To verify that all the information was recorded accurately.
   Scenario update: You know the provider is available, and the patient is willing to be put on hold as you talk with the provider.
8. Discuss the patient's information with the provider. Present the information in an accurate, logical method.
   Purpose: Presenting the patient's information in a logical manner helps eliminate confusion and misunderstanding.
9. Upon returning to the phone, give the patient the information from the provider. Conclude the phone call.
10. Document the patient interaction, including the patient's medical history, the provider notified, and the information relayed to the patient.
    Purpose: Legally it is important to document all patient interactions.

PROCEDURE 22.2 Demonstrate Professional Telephone Techniques and Document a Telephone Message

Tasks

Demonstrate professional telephone techniques. Take an accurate telephone message and follow up on the requests made by the caller. Document in the patient's health record.

Scenario

Norma Washington, DOB 8/1/19XX, an established patient of Dr. Martin, has called to report her blood pressure readings that she has been taking at home. Dr. Martin had made a recent change in her medication and wanted her to monitor her blood pressure at home for 3 days and call in with the results. She has taken her blood pressure in the morning and in the evening for the past 3 days, with the following results:

- Day 1: 144/92 in the am, 156/94 in the pm
- Day 2: 136/84 in the am, 142/86 in the pm
- Day 3: 132/80 in the am, 138/82 in the pm

Directions

Role-play this with a peer. The instructor will be the provider. You are a medical assistant at Walden-Martin Family Medical (WMFM) Clinic.

Equipment and Supplies

- Telephone
- Computer with electronic health record (EHR) and messaging software or message pad, pen, and patient's health record
- Notepad (optional)

Procedural Steps

1. Demonstrate telephone techniques by answering the telephone by the third ring. Speak distinctly with a pleasant tone and expression, at a moderate rate, and with sufficient volume for the person to understand every word.
   Purpose: To convey interest in the caller by answering promptly. Proper enunciation will help the patient to understand.
2. Greet the caller. Identify the office or provider and yourself. Offer to help the caller.

Purpose: To assure the caller that the correct number has been reached and to identify the staff member.

3. Verify the caller's identity and date of birth. If using an electronic health record, bring the patient's health record to the computer's active screen. Note the patient's phone number in case you are disconnected.
   Purpose: To confirm the origin of the call.
4. Screen the call if necessary. Determine the needs of the caller.
   Purpose: To determine whether the caller has an emergency and needs immediate attention or referral to a hospital emergency department.
5. Using a message pad or the computer, take the phone message (either on paper or by data entry into the computer) and obtain the following information:
   - Name of the person to whom the call is directed
   - Name of the person calling
   - Caller's telephone number
   - Reason for the call
   - Action to be taken
   - Date and time of the call
   - Initials of the person taking the call

   Purpose: To have accurate information, which allows the staff member or provider to address the caller's issues quickly and efficiently.
6. Apply active listening skills and repeat the information back to the caller after recording the message.
   Purpose: To verify that all the information was recorded accurately.
7. End the call and wait for the caller to hang up first.
8. If not using an EHR, document the telephone call with all pertinent information in the patient's health record. Deliver the phone message to the appropriate person and follow up as needed. Once the patient's concerns have been addressed, file the phone message in the patient's health record.
   Purpose: To make sure important issues are addressed in a timely manner.

PROCEDURE 22.3 Leave a Voice Message for a Patient

Tasks

Demonstrate professional telephone techniques. Leave a HIPAA-appropriate voice message for a patient. Document in the patient's health record.

Scenario

You are a medical assistant at Walden-Martin Family Medical (WMFM) Clinic. Jean Burke, NP, asks you to call Talibah Nasser (DOB 07/09/19XX) and let her know that her chlamydia test was negative. She would like to see Talibah in 3 months for a repeat Pap test. You call Talibah and have to leave a voice message.

Directions

Call the patient (your instructor) and leave a voice message.

Equipment and Supplies

- Telephone
- Patient (instructor) phone number
- Computer with electronic health record (EHR) and messaging software or message pad, pen, and patient's health record
- Notepad (optional)

Procedural Steps

1. Demonstrate telephone techniques by speaking distinctly with a pleasant tone and expression, at a moderate rate, and with sufficient volume for the person to understand every word.
   Purpose: Proper enunciation will help the patient to understand the message.
2. Identify the office or provider and yourself.
   Purpose: When leaving voice mail, some information must be provided so the person knows who called.
3. Provide a call-back number.
4. Leave a HIPAA-appropriate voice message.
   Purpose: The message should not violate the patient's privacy if it is overheard. Do not disclose medical conditions or private health information.
5. Politely finish the voice message.
   Purpose: Being polite and professional is important for excellent customer service.
6. Document in the patient's health record that the message was left.
   Purpose: To ensure that the patient's health record is kept up-to-date.

Scheduling and Reception

OPENING SCENARIO

Catalina McDowell CMA (AAMA), a recent graduate of a medical assisting program, has begun her first position as a receptionist at Walden-Martin Family Medical (WMFM) Clinic. Catalina is determined to perform to the best of her abilities. However, she has never held a job in a professional office. She knows that she needs to practice all of the skills she learned in school to be an effective receptionist.

WMFM Clinic is customer service oriented and wants its patients to feel cared for and special. Catalina is anxious to build trust with the patients and to offer them help with the problems they encounter that fall within her realm of responsibility.

When scheduling appointments, Catalina wants to ensure that the healthcare facility remains on schedule throughout the day with minimal wait time for the patients and providers. She leaves a little time in the morning and afternoon for emergency appointments. The healthcare facility uses an automatic call routing system to contact patients to confirm appointments in advance, which increases the show rate.

Catalina will strive to be the type of employee who has a willingness to learn, an ability to adapt, and a heart full of compassion for the patient. She is a team player who sincerely wants to cooperate with other staff members who might need her help.

All of the providers at WMFM Clinic are pleased that they have found such an eager person to add to the staff, and they will assist and guide Catalina as she learns how to make the patients feel like part of the clinic's family. Catalina's self-esteem has increased because she feels she is making a great contribution to healthcare.

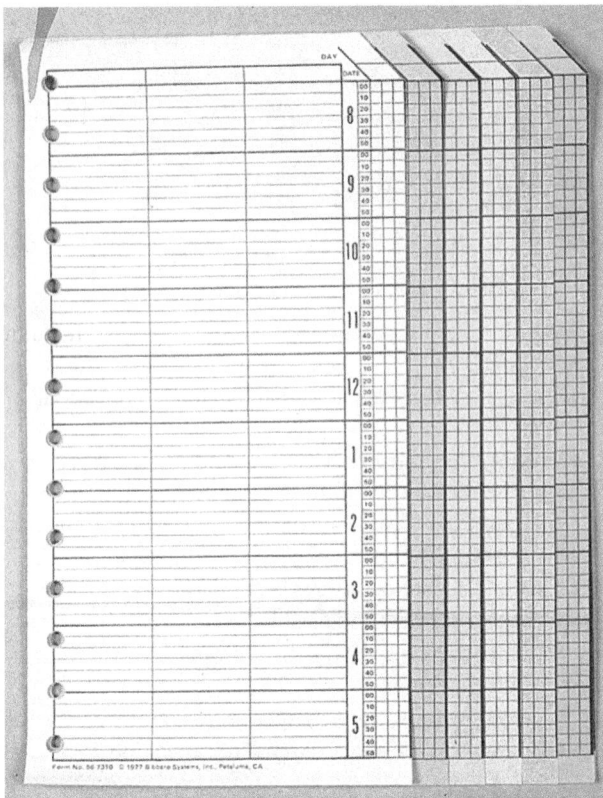

Fig. 23.1 Color-coded appointment book pages help the medical assistant flip to the right day of the right week quickly. Appointments for multiple providers can be color coded in the book. (From Proctor D, et al: *Kinn's the medical assistant,* ed 13, St. Louis, 2017, Elsevier.)

YOU WILL LEARN

1. To set up the appointment matrix.
2. To differentiate among the various types of appointment scheduling.
3. To schedule patient appointments and procedures.
4. To recognize patient processing procedures for new and established patients.
5. To work with angry and talkative patients and with children.

INTRODUCTION

The provider's time is the most valuable asset of a medical practice. The person responsible for scheduling this time must understand the practice, be familiar with the working habits and preferences of the provider (or providers), and have clear guidelines for time management in the practice.

Appointment scheduling is the process that determines which patients the provider sees, the dates and times of appointments, and how much time is allotted to each patient based on the complaint and the provider's availability. Time management involves the realization that unforeseen interruptions and delays always occur and must be handled appropriately. In addition, the medical assistant must assign the appropriate appointment time length for the complaint, along with ensuring that the appointments are scheduled so that there are minimal gaps in the schedule. Most healthcare providers find that efficient appointment scheduling is one of the most important factors in the success of the practice. Scheduling can be done in a number of ways, and each facility must find the way that suits it best.

SCHEDULING SYSTEMS

The two most common appointment scheduling systems are:
- Paper-based scheduling
- Computerized scheduling

Each has advantages and disadvantages. The healthcare facility should weigh the benefits and choose the method that best suits the provider and the staff.

Paper-Based Scheduling System

The paper-based scheduling system (also called *appointment book scheduling*) uses appointment books for scheduling. Office suppliers carry a variety of appointment book styles. Variations can include:
- A day, week, or month on one page
- Color coding, such as a different color for each day of the week (Fig. 23.1)
- Number of columns for providers
- Blank or preprinted with dates
- Time increments, such as 10 or 15 minutes
- Size

- The paper-based scheduling system works when the computerized scheduling system is down or during power outages. Disadvantages include storage for old appointment books, difficulty finding a patient's future appointment, less efficiency identifying opened appointments, and difficulty reading the writing in the appointment book.

Computerized Scheduling System

Many ambulatory care facilities have moved to computerized scheduling. Some electronic health records come with a basic scheduling program included. Other facilities use practice management software that includes a scheduling program. The complexity of the computer scheduling programs varies. Some are basic, whereas others perform additional tasks such as sending appointment reminders. The search features on some scheduling systems allow the medical assistant to add the length and type of appointment, along with the patient's day or time preferences. The search results show available time slots, which helps make the process more efficient.

A computerized scheduling system also has the ability to search for future appointments. For example, when a patient calls and asks about a previously scheduled appointment, the system can search by their name to find the time and date. Computerized scheduling allows multiple users to access the schedule at the same time, minimizing the wait time for patients.

Another advantage of computerized schedules is the reports that can be generated. A hard copy of the provider's daily schedule can be created showing patients' names, telephone numbers, and reasons for the visits. Some healthcare facilities print these out, and others use them on screen.

With computerized scheduling, the healthcare facility must have procedures to follow when the technology is down. These procedures should be reviewed periodically to ensure all scheduling staff members know the process.

Self-Scheduling. Self-scheduling allows the patient to schedule an appointment online using the patient portal or facility's website. Patients can schedule at any time of the day or night, without the assistance of the ambulatory care staff. The popularity of self-scheduling has increased because the process is fast and convenient for patients. Studies have estimated that it takes 4 to 8 minutes to schedule a patient over the phone. When self-scheduling is an option, facilities save time and resources. Patient satisfaction increases. Lastly, experts state that patients are more likely to come to the appointment when they self-schedule.

Self-scheduling software varies in complexity and may include these features:
- Can send notifications when the patient is due for prevention screenings and examinations
- Can send notifications to remind and confirm future appointments
- Allows the patient to complete and submit forms and medical history questionnaires from a mobile device

When setting up a self-scheduling system, the healthcare facility should clearly indicate the different types of appointments.

This will help the patient select the correct appointment time, which will then give the provider the required time to see the patient. Being clear with patients can create successful self-scheduling.

It is important for the medical assistant to realize that not all patients will use the self-scheduling system. Some patients do not have access to the internet. Others may not be comfortable using it or putting their information online. The ambulatory care facility should allow patients to schedule appointments over the phone.

CRITICAL THINKING 23.1

The software used by the WMFM Clinic allows patients to self-schedule. Catalina has heard about patient self-scheduling and would like to try this method in the office, but Dr. Martin is concerned that his patients will miss the personal contact and is not sold on the idea. What can Catalina say to convince Dr. Martin to try this new, timesaving method of scheduling? What challenges might the use of this system bring?

VOCABULARY

demographics Statistical data of a population. In healthcare this includes the patient's name, address, date of birth, employment, and other details.

parameters A rule that controls how something should be done; guidelines or boundaries.

patient portal A secure online website that gives patients 24-hour access to personal health information using a username and password.

practice management software A type of software that allows the user to enter demographic information, schedule appointments, maintain lists of insurance payers, perform billing tasks, and generate reports.

ESTABLISHING THE APPOINTMENT SCHEDULE

Developing a schedule that meets the needs of both the providers and the patients is key to keeping the office running smoothly and efficiently. The scheduling team, along with the provider, should come up with scheduling parameters (puh RAM it ers) that both meet the needs of patients and also keep the providers' preferences and habits in mind.

Patient Needs

Consider the demographics of the patients when determining office hours and appointment times. The staff should answer these questions:
- Is the office in a busy metropolitan area or a rural community?
- What types of patients are seen? Are they of a specific age or gender? Do they have common diagnoses? Is the provider a general practitioner?
- Do most of the patients served need evening and weekend appointments?

Knowing when the providers need to be available for patients is one of the factors to be considered when creating the patient schedule.

Provider Preferences and Habits

Consider the preferences and habits of the providers in the practice before establishing and implementing a scheduling plan. Ask these questions:

- Is the provider careful about being in the facility when patient appointments are scheduled to begin?
- Is the provider typically late in the morning after rounds at the hospital?
- Does the provider move easily from one patient to another?
- Does the provider require a "break time" after a few patients?
- Would the provider rather see fewer patients and spend more time with each one or schedule more patients each day?

All of these preferences and habits become an integral (IN ti gruh l) part of the scheduling process. Keep in mind that the provider cannot spend every moment of the day with patients. The provider also has telephone calls to make and receive, reports to examine and dictate, meetings to attend, mail to answer, and many other business responsibilities. An experienced staff can handle many but not all of these tasks.

CRITICAL THINKING 23.2

Catalina has noticed that Dr. Walden is taking a little longer with patients than normal and that she is consistently running behind schedule by approximately 5 to 15 minutes. How can Catalina help fix this situation?

Discuss ways of approaching a provider when they are the cause of the delays in the schedule. What opening remarks can the medical assistant use to start the discussion in a positive way?

VOCABULARY
integral Essential; an indispensable part of a whole.

Creating the Appointment Matrix

Setting up the appointment matrix (see Procedure 23.1) involves blocking out the times when the provider is not available to see patients, such as lunchtime, hospital rounds, conferences, meetings, and vacation (Fig. 23.2). The appointment matrix keeps appointments from being scheduled at times when the provider or the facilities are not available. In a paper-based appointment book, the matrix is usually established for 6 months at a time. In a computerized system, the matrix can be set up indefinitely.

To set up the appointment book, the medical assistant will need a black pen, pencil, highlighters, calendar, and the providers' preferences and schedules. Using a black pen, the medical assistant writes in the providers' names and their unavailable times are crossed out with an X. Use a pencil when saving time blocks for same-day appointments. The pencil can be erased as the blocks are filled.

When computerized scheduling software is set up, the providers' unavailable times are entered, which blocks these times from appointments.

Establishing Guidelines for Appointment Scheduling.

Another important step when working with the schedule matrix is to consider the required time for each type of appointment. For newly established practices or new providers, management and/or the providers determine the length of time required. For established practices, these times have already been determined and usually are in the policies and procedures manuals. Most ambulatory care facilities use 10- to 15-minute time intervals for appointments. Some types of appointments are more complex and require additional time. Depending on the type of practice, the appointment types and time can vary. Typically, primary care appointment types include:

- *Follow-up or recheck*: Usually scheduled for 10 to 15 minutes. Used when a patient needs to see the provider after a condition should have been resolved or to monitor an ongoing condition, such as hypertension.
- *Urgent visit*: Usually scheduled for 15 to 20 minutes. The patient has an urgent concern that needs to be addressed by the provider.
- *Wellness examination, school exams,* and *sports physicals*: Usually scheduled for 20 to 30 minutes. The provider will do a physical examination, and immunizations might be needed. Specific paperwork may need to be completed.
- *Pelvic exam, Pap smear,* and *minor surgery*: Usually scheduled for 20 to 30 minutes. These visits may require special rooms and equipment.
- *Complete physical examination*: Usually scheduled for 30 to 60 minutes. A yearly visit that entails a review of the patient's medical history and medications, a visual exam, and a complete physical examination. Disease management treatment plans will be revised/reviewed. Preventive screenings will be done or scheduled.
- *New patient visit*: Usually scheduled for 30 to 60 minutes. The provider will review any medical records provided, obtain a complete medical history, and perform a physical exam.
- *Telemedicine visit* or *virtual check-in*: Usually scheduled for 15 to 20 minutes. Provides a time in which the patient and provider can communicate.

It is important for the medical assistant to select the correct type of appointment for the patient's concern (Box 23.1).

When using the paper scheduling system, the medical assistant should keep a list of appointment types and required times near the appointment book to reference when needed. When a computerized scheduling system is used, the appointment types and required times can be customized for the different providers or set the same for all providers.

Besides the length of the appointment type, the availability of facilities (e.g., procedure room) and/or equipment needed must be considered. For example, if the healthcare facility has only one electrocardiograph, do not book two electrocardiograms (ECGs) at the same time. As the medical assistant gains proficiency (pruh FISH uh n see) in scheduling, it becomes easier to match patients' needs with the available facilities. Major equipment frequently used, or a certain room with such equipment, may need its own scheduling column in the appointment book or software system.

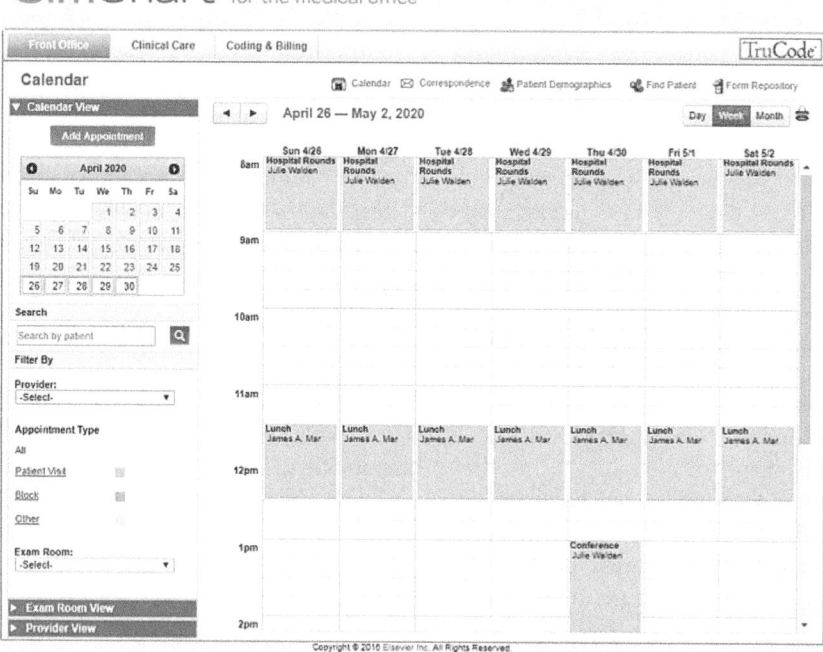

Fig. 23.2 Schedule Matrix Showing Provider Availability. (From SimChart for the Medical Office, St. Louis, 2015, Elsevier.)

With providers focusing on patients, they do not always watch the time spent in the room. Some providers have the clinical medical assistant signal near the end of the appointment time. This might include sending a message to the provider's pager or phone. When the device vibrates, the provider knows that the appointment time is almost ended. The clinical medical assistant and the administrative medical assistant must work together to keep the healthcare facility running smoothly and efficiently.

VOCABULARY

interval Space of time between events.

matrix The environment where something is created or takes shape; a base on which to build.

proficiency Skilled as a result of training or practice.

Adding Patient Appointments

When creating an appointment using the paper scheduling system, the administrative medical assistant includes the following in the appointment book:

- *Patient's full name*: The medical assistant should make sure the name is spelled correctly.
- *Telephone number*: Obtain a number that can be used to reach the person prior to the appointment if needed.
- *Purpose of the visit*: Provide a brief description of the patient's concern. Do not violate the privacy of the patient by describing too much. Also be aware of sensitive concerns, such as sexually transmitted infections. Facilities may have

guidelines on what to enter as a brief description. Use only facility-approved abbreviations.

Based on the appointment type, the medical assistant needs to block the required amount of time.

When scheduling a patient's appointment using the computerized scheduling system, the medical assistant must obtain the patient's name and date of birth. If the patient is an established patient with the facility, the name will appear in the database. The medical assistant will select it and proceed to schedule the appointment, entering the reason for the visit and selecting the appointment type and time. If the patient is a new patient to the facility, the medical assistant will need to enter the patient's demographics into the system. It is critical that the spelling of the patient's name and the date of birth are correct.

Legality of the Appointment Scheduling System

Both paper-based appointment books and computerized scheduling records can be used as a legal record. They must be accurate and provide correct information about the patients at the healthcare facility. Patients are expected to follow the provider's orders; this includes keeping appointments. The medical assistant must document in the patient's health record if the person is a no-show or cancels an appointment and does not reschedule. No documentation is required if the patient cancels, reschedules, and keeps an appointment.

Because the appointment book is a legal document, it is recommended to write the patient's information in black ink. If the patient cancels the appointment, the medical assistant should cross out the patient's information with a single line. The reason should be indicated next to the patient's name, for instance "cancelled, rescheduled." Erasing, using correction fluid, or any other type of obliteration (uh blit uh REY shun) is never acceptable. Even though using ink is recommended, some facilities allow the medical assistant to write the appointment information in pencil. At the end of the day, they have to rewrite over the top of the pencil entry using ink to create the permanent record.

Computerized scheduling systems can also be used to track patient appointments. Most computerized scheduling systems allow the user to indicate if the patient has checked in, canceled, or missed the scheduled appointment. When a patient misses or cancels an appointment, it should be documented in the electronic patient record for legal purposes.

The appointment book and computerized records need to be kept for the required number of years per the state's statute of limitations. When the appointment book is discarded, it should be burnt or shredded to maintain patient confidentiality.

VOCABULARY

no-show Failure to keep an appointment without giving advance notice.
obliteration To remove or destroy all traces of; do away with.

TYPES OF APPOINTMENT SCHEDULING

Different types of appointment scheduling are used to meet the various needs of the healthcare facility, the providers, and the patients. Some offices use a combination of methods to create the right mix of activity during the day and to ensure that the day runs smoothly and efficiently. The medical assistant should become proficient at managing appointments. The following sections present several methods of appointment scheduling.

No matter what appointment scheduling method is used, the medical assistant should make it a policy to leave some open time during each day's schedule. This is so that if a patient calls with a special problem that is not an immediate emergency, time will be available to book the patient for at least a brief visit. Mondays and Fridays generally are the most hectic days of the week. Keeping a time slot available in the morning and the afternoon specifically for emergencies also is a wise practice. A busy provider always fills these open slots, and having them in the schedule causes the least disruption during the day. Depending on the facility's policy, sometimes time is set aside in the morning and afternoon for the provider to get caught up and handle patient documentation, such as prescription refills.

Time-Specified (Stream) Scheduling

Time-specified scheduling is also called *fixed, stream, or single-booking scheduling*. With time-specified or stream scheduling, patients are given a specific time for their appointment.

This method keeps a steady flow of patients moving through the office. This is the most common type of scheduling used in healthcare facilities. Studies have shown that providers can see more patients with less pressure when patient appointments are scheduled for a specific time slot. With time-specified scheduling, the medical assistant must book the correct amount of time required for each appointment type. Keeping time slots available for urgent visits, as previously stated, is important.

Wave Scheduling

Wave scheduling is an attempt to create flexibility within each hour. Wave scheduling assumes that the actual time needed for all the patients seen will average out over the course of the day. With wave scheduling, three patients are given the same appointment time. They are then seen in the order of their arrival. This way, one person's late arrival does not disrupt the entire schedule.

Modified Wave Scheduling

The wave schedule can be modified in several ways. For example, one method is to have two patients scheduled to come in at 10 a.m. and a third at 10:30 a.m. This hourly cycle is repeated throughout the day. In another version, patients are scheduled to arrive at given intervals during the first half of the hour, and none are scheduled to arrive during the second half of the hour. This would allow time for urgent or walk-in patients to be seen.

Double-Booking

Double-booking means to schedule an extra patient to come in during a time slot that is already booked. Double-booking is usually used for acutely ill or injured patients. Some facilities require that double-bookings be approved by the provider. Other facilities limit the number of double-booked patients a provider sees in a day. Double-booking works out best if one patient needs laboratory work or another procedure done before seeing the provider. The provider can see one patient while the other one is being prepared. Double-booking can be used with other scheduling types.

Open Booking

Open booking is also called *open office hours* and *open access*. With this method, the facility is open at given hours. The patients are told that they can come in at any time. This type of system is often used in an urgent care setting. Patients are seen in the order in which they arrive, although patients with urgent conditions may be given priority.

The open office hours system can have many disadvantages. The office may already be crowded when the provider arrives, resulting in an extremely long wait for some patients. Patients may arrive in waves throughout the day, which causes parts of the day to be very busy and other parts to be slow. This makes accomplishing other office duties difficult. Without planning, the facilities and staff can be overburdened.

Group (Cluster) Scheduling

Group scheduling is also called *cluster* or *category scheduling*. Patients with similar appointment types are seen on specific days. For instance, an internist might reserve all morning appointments for complete physical examinations, or a pediatrician might keep that time for well-baby visits. A surgeon might devote 1 day each week to seeing only referral patients. Obstetricians often schedule pregnant patients on different days from gynecology patients. In applying a grouping system of appointments, the medical assistant may find it helpful to color-code the sections of the appointment book reserved for specific procedures.

Advance Scheduling

With advance scheduling, a patient may schedule an appointment weeks to months out. For example, a parent may schedule a well-child exam for 6 months from now. Most paper scheduling systems can book patients up to 6 months out. With computerized systems, some facilities allow scheduling to be booked out 1 year. A disadvantage to advance scheduling is that the provider may not be available, and the appointment may need to be rescheduled. Advance scheduling can be used with most other scheduling types.

SCHEDULING APPOINTMENTS

In Person Scheduling

Most return appointments for established patients are scheduled when the patient is leaving the healthcare facility. A good policy is to have all patients stop by the appointment desk to check out before leaving in case any information is needed from the patient or any outside scheduling must be done. The patient's health record can be reviewed to see whether the provider ordered any laboratory tests or procedures, and these can be scheduled and discussed with the patient. When making a return appointment, follow the same procedures as for scheduling any appointment by phone, offering the patient choices in the day and time slots. If a certain time the patient specifically requests is not available, offer two other choices. Always give the patient an appointment card and any necessary instructions, along with a bright smile. Never forget to provide excellent customer service.

If the patient needs to make a series of appointments, it is best to schedule the appointments on the same day of the week and at the same time. This will help the patient remember them more easily.

VOCABULARY

established patient A patient who has been treated by the healthcare provider within the past 3 years.

Telephone Scheduling

A pleasant manner and a willingness to help are just as important on the telephone as when meeting patients face to face. This is especially true when making appointments. The telephone contact may be the patient's first impression of the facility. Often the way the appointment scheduling process is handled makes more of an impression than the convenience of the appointment time.

Be especially considerate if the time requested for an appointment is not available. Briefly explain why and offer a different date and time. Comply with the patient's wishes as much as possible, and do not show annoyance if the patient does not understand the scheduling process. Most people, however, understand the need for a well-managed office and are willing to cooperate.

Many offices offer the patient a choice when scheduling the appointment and let the patient decide which option is best for them. For example, the following dialog might take place during the scheduling call.

Medical assistant:	"Mrs. Thomas, Dr. Stern is available to see you in the office next Tuesday or Wednesday, January 6 or 7. Which day is better for you?"
Patient:	"I will be working on Wednesday, so I would like to come in on Tuesday."
Medical assistant:	"Do you prefer a morning or afternoon appointment?"
Patient:	"The afternoon is best for me."
Medical assistant:	"Great. Would 1:30 or 3:30 be a better time?"
Patient:	"I can be there at 1:30."
Medical assistant:	"Then Dr. Stern will see you at 1:30 next Tuesday, January 6. Thank you for calling, Mrs. Thomas. We'll see you then!"

These small courtesies give patients the feeling that they control their time. Always repeat the time to reinforce the appointment. Do not hesitate to ask the patient if they have a pen ready to jot down the time and date. While repeating the information to the patient, check the appointment book or computer screen to ensure that it was posted correctly. When appointments are scheduled over the telephone, it is not possible to give the patient a reminder card for the appointment. Be sure to ask if the patient would like a telephone, email, or text message reminder of the appointment.

Besides the basic conversation described, the healthcare facility may also have the administrative medical assistant provide information for fasting for certain laboratory tests if applicable. Some ambulatory care facilities require the administrative medical assistants to update patient information during the scheduling process. This may include the patient's address, phone number, and current insurance (see Procedure 23.2). It is important to remember that others can overhear what is said by the medical assistant. It is often recommended to have the patient state the information without having the medical assistant saying the information.

Scheduling Appointments for New Patients. Arranging the first appointment for a new patient requires time and attention to detail (see Procedure 23.3). This encounter provides the first impression of the healthcare facility and may set the tone for all subsequent visits. Tact, courtesy, and professionalism are extremely important. For example, the patient may be required to be fasting for certain laboratory tests to be performed. Patient demographic information should be collected during the conversation, including the type of insurance the patient has. Some insurance carriers restrict which providers can be used.

After the necessary information has been collected, offer the patient the first available appointment. Whenever possible, offer a choice between two dates and times. Additional information to share with the patient:

- Need to arrive 15 minutes before the scheduled appointment time. This allows for the completion of any necessary paperwork.
- Directions to the facility or offer the physical address for those who use a GPS or an internet direction website.
- Any special parking conveniences available and whether the healthcare facility provides a token or parking validation.
- Options for the first payment. Inform the patient if payment is expected at the time of service.
- If a questionnaire will be mailed or if the patient will need to complete an online questionnaire.

Before ending the conversation, repeat the appointment date and time, and thank the patient for calling.

Many healthcare facilities have new patient packets, which may include:

- A brochure on the healthcare facility
- A health history form
- The Notice of Privacy Practices (NPP)
- A release of information form to obtain past records
- A consent for treatment and authorization form, which gives providers permission to treat the patient and allows the facility to bill and collect payments from the patient's insurance provider

This information can be sent to the patient prior to the appointment or given to the patient when they arrive.

If the patient was referred by another provider, the medical assistant may need to call the referring provider's office to obtain additional information before the patient's appointment. Any information obtained should be given to the provider before the patient is seen for the visit. Remember to send a thank you note to anyone who refers a patient to the facility.

Often, the medical assistant will need to conduct preauthorization or precertification to determine whether a patient is eligible for treatment or for certain procedures. The office manager must make certain that these procedures are being done and should assign these duties to a specific person. More about preauthorization and precertification is presented in Chapter 27.

VOCABULARY

Notice of Privacy Practices (NPP) A written document describing the healthcare facility's privacy practices. The patient must be provided with the NPP and must sign an acknowledgment of receipt.

preauthorization A process that requires the provider to submit documentation to the payer to show the service or treatment is medically needed and the payer determines if the service or treatment is medically necessary and covered under the insurance plan. Also called prior authorization.

precertification The process of determining if a procedure or service is covered by the insurance plan and what the reimbursement is for that procedure or service.

Scheduling Urgency. The medical assistant should work with the provider and office manager to determine types of patient concerns that should be seen that day and those that can be scheduled within a few days. The list will vary by provider and facility. Some providers may consider the following concerns to be urgent and may have the patient seen on that day:

- Fever of 101°F or higher
- Light sensitivity or migraine
- Sinus pain or pressure
- Productive cough
- Burning or discomfort with urination
- Sore throat for over 3 days or white patches in the mouth or throat
- Abdominal pain

Chapter 22 discusses emergencies that should be sent to the hospital. If the medical assistant has any questions about the patient's concerns and when the patient should be seen, the provider must be consulted.

Sometimes patients arrive at the facility without an appointment scheduled and want to be seen. These patients are called *walk-in patients*. A patient who requires immediate attention will most likely be fit into the schedule. If the patient does not need immediate care, an appointment scheduled for a later time may be the answer. Some facilities require the medical assistant to talk with the provider before having the patient return at a later time. Be sure to follow established office policy.

Scheduling Efficiency. Scheduling patients seems rather easy, but it can be complex. Unfilled time slots in a provider's schedule can reduce the revenue made. Effective and efficient scheduling is important for the business side of the healthcare facility.

- Schedule morning appointments working from noon backward and afternoon appointments working from noon forward.
- Make sure the required time for a patient concern is given. If too much time is given for an appointment that does not require it, the facility misses out on potential revenue. If too little time is given for an appointment, then other patients need to wait, which can affect patient satisfaction.
- Keep missed appointments to a minimum by confirming appointments through email or text messages.
- Create a patient waiting list. In a busy practice, when an appointment becomes open, the medical assistant can contact the next person on the waiting list to see if they are

BOX 23.2 Patient-Centered Care With Scheduling

When scheduling tests and procedures for patients, the medical assistant should consider these patient-centered care tips:

- When a patient needs to fast for a procedure, try to schedule the procedure as early as possible in the morning.
- If a patient is having a procedure in the afternoon and needs to be fasting, find out when the patient must fast. The typically response is "fast from midnight onward," but can this patient start fasting later because the procedure is scheduled later?
- If the patient is having several appointments, such as provider appointments and a procedure, try to schedule the appointments on the same day if possible and without large gaps of wait time between.

available to come in. This works well for annual physical exams if the provider is scheduled out several months.

Scheduling Other Types of Appointments

Scheduling Surgeries, Procedures, and Inpatient Admissions. Medical assistants are involved with scheduling patients for inpatient surgeries, same-day surgeries, and outpatient diagnostic procedures, such as a colonoscopy, magnetic resonance imaging (MRI), and computed tomography (CT) scans (see Procedure 23.4; also Box 23.2). Medical assistants are also involved with scheduling inpatient admissions, especially in areas such as obstetrics.

When a provider orders a surgery, diagnostic procedure, or an inpatient admission for a patient, the medical assistant must provide the hospital, outpatient surgery center, or diagnostic imaging facility with the following information:

- Patient's demographic information (e.g., name, date of birth, address, insurance information)
- Provider's order and any special requests
- Diagnosis (also called *admitting diagnosis*)
- For surgeries:
  - Allergies
  - Type of surgery and anticipated length of surgery
  - Amount of blood to have available for the patient
  - Specific anesthesiologist
  - Assistant surgeon
  - Specific instruments
- For diagnostic procedures:
  - Type of procedure

Many times, the medical assistant must provide the details of the surgery, procedure, or inpatient admission to the patient. It is important to give the patient a written copy of the details. These details include:

- Date, arrival time, and location (address) of the surgery or procedure.
- Required preparations prior to the procedure or surgery:
  - The provider's instructions on how the patient should handle their medications (e.g., take specific medications with a sip of water, stop all medications).
  - When to stop eating food and drinking liquids. If the patient will be given a general or spinal anesthetic,

commonly the person must fast from midnight onward, though this time may vary if the patient has a late afternoon procedure.
  - Any additional preparations, such as an enema or a shower.
- Leaving valuables at home. Sometimes, patients will be requested to bring in certain medications, such as asthma medications.
- The facility may require the patient to bring a photo ID and insurance card.
- For same-day procedures or surgeries, the patient will need someone to drive them home.

After providing the patient with the details, the medical assistant must document the procedure date, time, and location in the patient's health record. The documentation should also include the instructions the patient received.

Home Visits and Extended Care Facility Visits. Some providers make home visits or extended care facility visits to see patients who are not able to come to the facility for an appointment. In many cases the clinical medical assistant will accompany the provider and assist during the visit.

When scheduling these visits, the medical assistant usually confirms the visit with the patient or patient's caregiver. The provider's schedule must be updated to include the visit and travel time to and from the patient's home or the extended care facility.

Telemedicine Visits. With telemedicine visits, the provider uses a webcam, microphone, and internet video chat software to see patients who are at a distance from the healthcare facility. Some facilities use their patient portal for telemedicine visits.

When a telemedicine visit is scheduled, the medical assistant must ensure the patient has the necessary equipment, such as a webcam, computer device, and internet access or a smart phone. The medical assistant may need to coach the patient on how to log on and access the software. Sometimes a practice session helps identify issues and gives the patient confidence in the process.

When medical assistants are working with the virtual video software, they must select a location where the patient cannot be overheard and where the patient cannot overhear others. The background the patient sees should be professional. No other patient materials should be visible.

Pharmaceutical, Equipment, and Supply Representatives. Representatives from pharmaceutical, equipment, and supply companies are frequent visitors to healthcare facilities. They are well trained and bring the provider valuable information on new drugs, equipment, and supplies. The medical assistant is often expected to screen these visitors. As medical assistants learn the provider's preferences, they will identify the representatives the provider wants to see. If in doubt, the medical assistant should ask the provider. If the provider does not want to see the representative, the medical assistant must firmly but tactfully send the person away. Suggest that they leave their literature and cards for the provider to study and say that the provider will contact them if further information is desired.

If the provider wants to see the representative, the medical assistant can provide the person with the provider's available and the potential wait time. The representative can decide whether to wait or return later. Representatives are usually quite understanding and cooperative. Many are willing to wait patiently for a long time for just a brief visit with the provider. In turn, the medical assistant should treat the representative with courtesy, showing as much cooperation as possible.

Many healthcare facilities are limiting and even eliminating visits from pharmaceutical representatives due to the Physician Payments Sunshine Act (part of the Affordable Care Act). Pharmaceutical representatives will often bring samples of the medications that they are going to talk to the provider about. It is important for the medical assistant to understand the policies and procedures for the handling and dispensing of the samples. Most healthcare facilities require that these samples be logged and stored in a locked cabinet. The drug samples are given to patients only with provider approval.

Scheduling Meetings. Often the medical assistant must schedule meetings for the healthcare team and providers. The time may be decided by the providers, or the medical assistant may need to review the providers' schedules and identify a common open time for the meeting. Meetings are commonly held at the beginning or end of the day or before or after lunch.

When scheduling a meeting, the medical assistant must:
- Block the time on the providers' schedules and indicate the meeting name and location.
- Reserve a location for the meeting, if appropriate.
- Create an agenda from the information provided by the providers, office manager, and/or staff (see Procedure 23.5)

Special Circumstances

Late Patients. Every medical practice has a few patients who are habitually late for appointments, which can put a strain on the practice. Such patients can be booked as the last appointment of the day. Then, if closing time arrives before the patient does, the staff has no obligation to wait and other patients have not been inconvenienced. Some medical assistants tell the patient to come in 30 minutes before the scheduled appointment time. Try to work with patients who have occasional difficulties arriving on time, but do not allow the schedule to be constantly disrupted by late patients.

CRITICAL THINKING 23.4

Seth Jones is always late for his appointments. How might Catalina approach him about this issue? What can Catalina do to assist Mr. Jones so that he arrives for appointments on time?

Rescheduling Appointments. Changes sometimes must be made to the appointment schedule. Unexpected conflicts might come up that force a patient to change the appointment time. A change in the provider's schedule may require that a patient's appointment is rescheduled. If the reschedule is due to a provider's absence for a period of time, check to see if the patient wants to be seen by another provider.

When rescheduling an appointment, make sure the first appointment is removed from the appointment book and then set the new appointment. Otherwise, the patient will be expected in the office on 2 days, and time will be wasted with calls and follow-up, only to discover that the appointment was rescheduled. Most computerized scheduling systems will allow the medical assistant to open the appointment and change the date and time or to cut and paste the appointment into the new date and time.

No-Show Patients. The patient who does not arrive for a scheduled appointment or who does not reschedule it is called a *no-show*. There can be a variety of reasons a patient does not arrive for a scheduled appointment, such as:
- Forgot the appointment
- Mixed up the date or time of the appointment
- Owes the facility money and stays away because of an inability to pay for medical services
- May deny they have a condition and feel they do not need to be seen

It is important to determine the reason for failed appointments and to do whatever is possible to remedy the situation. Telephone the patient to make sure no misunderstanding has occurred. If the patient's health requires ongoing care, the provider may write a letter explaining this to the patient. Send the letter by certified mail with return receipt requested. A copy of the letter needs to be added to the patient's medical record for legal protection.

The no-show must be documented in the schedule and in the patient's health record. For computerized scheduling, typically the appointment status can be changed to "no-show." With paper scheduling, "No-show" should be written next to the patient's name. Some facilities use red ink for this notation. The no-show must also be documented in the patient's health record. The documentation protects the facility from legal consequences regarding the patient's care. A patient may try to claim patient abandonment when they have actually been the one to miss the appointments.

Some facilities have a no-show policy. The first time a patient no-shows, it is indicated in the health records. The second time it occurs, the patient may receive a written warning. The third time may cause the provider to take steps to legally terminate the patient-provider relationship (see Chapter 18 for more details). Other facilities will charge patients for no-show visits. Regardless of the no-show policy, it should be explained in the new patient brochure.

VOCABULARY

patient abandonment A form of medical malpractice, also called *negligent termination;* the provider ends the provider-patient relationship without reasonable or adequate notification.

Increasing Appointment Show Rates

Everyone benefits from a full schedule of kept appointments. Appointment show rates can be increased in several ways.

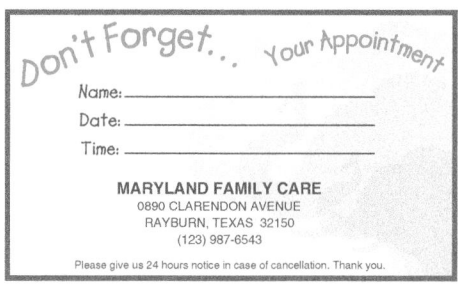

Fig. 23.3 An Example of an Appointment Reminder Card. (From Proctor D, et al: *Kinn's the medical assistant,* ed 13, St. Louis, 2017, Elsevier.)

- *Automated call, email, or text reminders:* Patients can be sent an automated call, email, or text reminder 1 or 2 days before the appointment. They are asked to respond either confirming or canceling the appointment.
- *Appointment cards:* When a patient makes an appointment in person, most healthcare facilities give the patient a reminder card, indicating the date and time (Fig. 23.3). The medical assistant should double-check the information written on the card before giving it to the patient.
- *Confirmation calls:* Some healthcare facilities will make manual calls to patients confirming their appointment. It is important to use the phone number the patient prefers the office to use. Healthcare facilities have policies on what can be left on patient voice mails. Some will want a simple message, such as, "This is Pam at Robert Welch's office confirming your appointment tomorrow at 2 p.m. Please call us if you cannot make the appointment. Our number is 555-212-0909. Thank you!" It is important to ensure that the message does not breach the patient's confidentiality.
- *Emailed reminders:* Most scheduling software can be set up to automatically send email reminders to patients on the day prior to their appointment.
- *Mailed reminders:* Some healthcare facilities send mailed reminders of appointments. These reminders usually accompany questionnaires or other forms the patient needs to complete. They may also include patient instructions if a procedure is going to be performed during the appointment.

Handling Cancellations and Delays

Patient Cancellations. Cancellations occur in every healthcare facility. To minimize the impact of cancellations, keep a list of patients with future appointments who would like to come in sooner. The medical assistant can begin calling those patients to try to get one of them in to fill the available opening. Each cancellation should be noted in the medical record, along with a reason for the cancellation. If the patient simply reschedules an appointment, a notation does not need to be made in the health record unless a pattern develops that might be significant to the patient's medical treatment.

When the Provider Is Delayed. Some days, the provider will be delayed in reaching the office. If you are notified before patients arrive, start calling patients with early appointments and suggest that they come later. If some patients arrive before the office learns of the delay, explain that an emergency has detained the provider. Offer them the option of rescheduling, seeing another provider, or waiting for their provider.

Show concern for the patient, but do not be overly apologetic, which might imply some degree of guilt. Most patients realize that a provider has certain priorities. The patient in the office may be inconvenienced, but it is not a "life or death" matter. If this kind of situation occurs frequently, however, consider devising a different scheduling system.

When the Provider Is Called to an Emergency. Providers are conscious of their responsibilities for responding to medical emergencies, and most patients understand if the medical assistant takes time to explain what has happened. The medical assistant may say, "Dr. Wright has been called away due to an emergency. She asked me to tell you she is very sorry to keep you waiting. There will be at least a 1-hour delay." The medical assistant should then ask the patient, "Would you like to wait? If that is inconvenient, I will be glad to give you the first available appointment on another day. Or perhaps you'd like to have some coffee or do some shopping and return in an hour." It is also possible that another provider may be able to see the patient.

As quickly as possible, call the patients scheduled for later. In many offices, especially those of obstetricians, surgeons, and general practitioners, a whole day's appointments must be canceled. For this reason, it is particularly important to have the daytime telephone number of each patient available so that the appointment can be rescheduled. If at all possible, cancel appointments before the patient arrives in the office to find that the provider is not available. The expediency (ik SPEE dee uh n see) of the office staff in contacting patients who will be affected by an emergency is appreciated.

> **VOCABULARY**
> **expediency** A means of achieving a particular end, as in a situation requiring urgency or caution.

When the Provider Is Ill or Out of Town. Providers get sick, too, and patients scheduled to be seen during the course of the provider's recovery must be informed of this and their appointments rescheduled. They do not need to be told the nature of the illness.

When the provider is called out of town for personal or professional reasons, appointments must be canceled or rescheduled. Usually, the patient is given the name of another provider, or possibly a choice of a few, who will provide care during such absences. For security reasons, only state that the doctor is unavailable. Stating over the telephone that the provider is out of town could lead to attempted burglary or other unauthorized entry on the premises.

PATIENT PROCESSING TASKS

When working at the reception desk, the medical assistant needs to screen the individuals arriving:

- *People with emergent conditions:* Individuals may be bleeding, having chest pain, or feeling very ill. It is important that

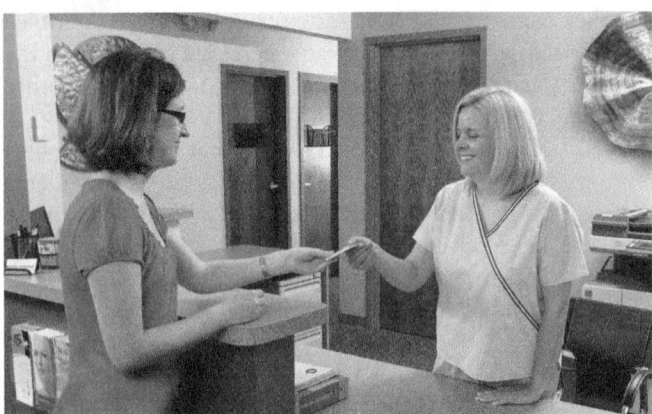

Fig. 23.4 Greet all patients with a warm smile and assist them with forms they need to complete for the health record. (From Proctor D, et al: *Kinn's the medical assistant,* ed 13, St. Louis, 2017, Elsevier.)

the medical assistant immediately contact the triage nurse to see the patient. If the nurse is not available, then the medical assistant should bring the patient back to an exam room and notify the provider right away. Facilities may have procedures in place to indicate when 911 needs to be called immediately.

- *Pharmaceutical and equipment representatives*: The medical assistant should follow the facility's policies and procedures regarding when these representatives are permitted to see the providers.
- *Salespeople and visitors*: The medical assistant needs to find out the reason for the visit and then follow the facility's procedures.

The most common visitors to the facility will be patients and family members who have appointments. We will examine the tasks the medical assistant must perform when patients arrive.

Patient's Arrival

When patients arrive, two important things need to occur. First, they need to know where to go and what to do. Second, they need to be greeted as quickly as possible. Signage is helpful to indicate what patients need to do upon arrival.

Every patient has the right to expect courteous treatment in a provider's office. Regardless of the patient's economic or social status, each person who arrives should receive a cordial, friendly greeting (Fig. 23.4). A personal touch, such as greeting the patient by name, is an easy way to develop patient rapport (Box 23.3). The medical assistant must ensure that their greeting is not inappropriate and does not violate the patient's confidentiality. For instance, the following greetings would violate HIPAA:

"How is your leg ulcer today, Mr. Bowden?"

"Mr. Biller, Dr. Walden will see you now for your shingles."

The following are appropriate greetings for the medical assistant to use as recommended by HIPAA:

"How are you today, Mr. Bowden?"

"Mr. Biller, the doctor will see you now."

The person sitting at the front reception desk should greet each patient as quickly as possible. Some experts say that a person should be greeted within 30 seconds of arriving. If this is not possible, a simple smile and eye contact will acknowledge the person. Make sure to greet the person verbally as soon as possible. If too much time elapses from the person's entrance to

---

BOX 23.3   Patients' Names

- Use the patient's last name and title (e.g., Mrs. Crawford) unless the patient insists on the use of their first name or prefers a nickname.
- Greet any individual you do not know and then ask for their name.
- Learn how to pronounce each patient's name correctly. Incorrect pronunciations may offend or irritate some people.
- Make a note of the phonetic spelling in the health record for reference. Note if the patient prefers a nickname.
- Avoid calling patients "Honey" or "Sweetie."

---

the greeting, the person may feel ignored or unimportant. This can affect a person's perception of the facility and, ultimately, the care provided. If the medical assistant must step away from the reception desk, it is important that they check the reception area for new arrivals as soon as they return.

In facilities where the receptionist is behind sliding glass windows, the environment can appear impersonal to patients. Although the closed glass windows increase patient privacy, they can also give the impression that the staff and provider are off limits to the patients. The glass window should be open as much as possible to give the appearance of openness to others. The policies and procedures manual should indicate when the glass window should be closed.

Sign-in Register. Some facilities will have the patient sign a register. A sign-in register that promotes patients' privacy should be used (Fig. 23.5). Remember, other patients can read the prior patients' information. This is one type of incidental disclosure under HIPAA. This is not considered a violation of HIPAA policy if the information disclosed is appropriately limited, such as:

- Date
- Name
- Arrival time and appointment time
- Appointment with
- Check boxes to indicate changes (but no information can be given)

Features that would cause a HIPAA violation include:

- Insurance information (e.g., name, number)
- Reason for visit
- Demographic information (e.g., address, employer, date of birth)

Infection Control in the Reception Area. It is vital for the medical assistant to take steps to protect the other patients in the reception area. The medical assistant may need to ask a few screening questions to identify patients who are ill with specific symptoms or at risk for specific diseases. These questions are set by the healthcare facility and usually recommended by the Centers for Disease Control and Prevention (CDC). Questions may include the following:

- "Have you traveled outside of the United States in the past 21 days?" Travel to specific countries may be included in the question. Patients who answer yes should be taken to an exam room immediately.
- "Are you coughing?" If patients are coughing, they should be encouraged to use masks. This is especially important during flu season or when other respiratory infections are prevalent.

Patient Sign-In

Date: _____

Please sign-in and notify us if:

• **New patient** • **Phone/address change** • **Insurance change**

No.	Patient Name print	Appt. Time	Arrival Time	Appt. with	New patient (.)	Phone/address change (.)	Insurance change (.)
1	PLEASE						
2	2						
3	3						
4	4						
5	5						
6	6						
7	7						
8	8						
9	9						
10	10						

Fig. 23.5 Sign-in sheets contain basic information about the patient and provide information for the medical assistant about changes that need to be made on the patient's record. (From Proctor D, et al: *Kinn's the medical assistant,* ed 13, St. Louis, 2017, Elsevier.)

BOX 23.4 Facts Listed on Patient Information or Registration Forms

Most patient information or registration forms contain:

- Patient's first, middle, and last name
- Date of birth
- Responsible person's name and relationship to the patient
- Address, telephone number (home and cell phone), and email address
- Name, address, and telephone number of a contact person
- Occupation
- Place of employment
- Social Security number
- Driver's license number
- Nearest relative not living with the patient and their relationship
- Source of referral if any

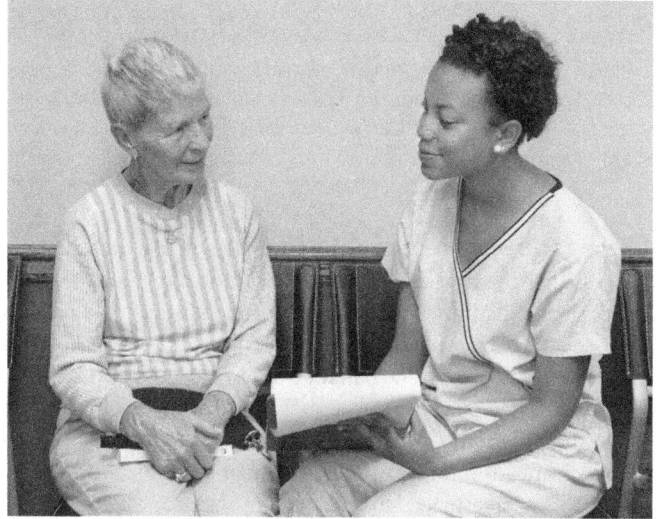

Fig. 23.6 The medical assistant should take time to explain forms the patient does not understand and should always be willing to answer questions. (From Proctor D, et al: *Kinn's the medical assistant,* ed 13, St. Louis, 2017, Elsevier.)

Tissues, along with waste containers and hand sanitizer, should be available for patients in the reception area.

Questions asked at the reception desk can vary as illnesses become predominant in certain areas. For instance, with COVID-19, questions related to key symptoms (i.e., fever, cough, loss of taste or smell) may be asked, and the patient's temperature may be checked. Sometimes patients are given a sticker to indicate they were screened.

Registration for New Patients. When someone visits the provider's office for the first time, the staff must gather information from the new patient, such as demographic and the health history information. The demographic information is usually gathered using the patient information or registration form. The patient's name should appear prominently at the top of the form, followed by other pertinent facts (Box 23.4). The patient's personal history, medical history, and family history may be obtained by using a questionnaire.

There are many ways the healthcare facility can obtain this information. Patients may be mailed the documents a few weeks prior to the appointment or directed to complete the information using the online patient portal. In some facilities, patients complete this information as they wait, prior to the appointment. They may complete paper forms or provide the information using an electronic device. In some cases, the medical assistant may take the patient to a private room where they can ask the questions and enter the information into the electronic health record (EHR).

The medical assistant must be willing to answer any questions either in person or over the phone (Fig. 23.6). The medical assistant must then review the completed form and verify that the required information has been provided. The provider also reviews the health history information and can then add information during the patient visit.

In addition to collecting information from the patient, the provider must give the patient the facility's NPP document. The healthcare provider is legally obligated to give each patient a notice that explains how the health information may be used and shared. HIPAA requires that patients state in writing that they received the NPP document. The healthcare facility may ask the patient to sign a paper or an electronic document. This form is then kept in the patient's health record. If the patient refuses to sign, the provider can still use and disclose the health information as permitted by HIPAA. The refusal needs to be documented in the patient's health record.

Many times, new patients are given a brochure on the facility's policies and procedures (Box 23.5). New patient brochures should be designed in a professional manner. The wording should be at a level that patients understand. When coaching a patient regarding the facility's policies, the medical assistant should summarize the content of the brochure. Do not read the brochure to the patient. Use active listening skills. Make sure to address any questions the patient may have. Procedure 23.6 describes how to create the brochure and coach patients regarding the policies.

CRITICAL THINKING 23.5

Often some time is needed to complete forms when a new patient arrives in the healthcare facility. How might Catalina keep the healthcare facility on schedule when new patients arrive who require health record construction and form completion? What are some ways to trim time from these activities?

Check-in Procedures for All Patients. During the check-in process, the medical assistant must scan or copy both sides of the patient's insurance card. The medical assistant may have to perform verification of eligibility. (This will be described in depth in Chapter 27.) The patient's phone number and address, along with the insurance subscriber's date of birth, should also be verified. Patients must show their insurance cards and picture identification for insurance and identity verification. These verifications take place at every patient visit for eligibility and safety reasons.

Many healthcare facilities are also scanning or copying the patient's legal photo identification. Facilities with EHRs may require a photo of the patient to be taken. The photo is uploaded to the EHR. Between the photo identification and the EHR photo, facilities are trying to reduce the amount of healthcare identify fraud. This fraud occurs when a person obtains healthcare using another person's name and insurance.

Some healthcare facilities insist that copays be collected before the office visit. Signage in the reception area often includes a statement indicating "Copayments are due at the time of the appointment." Ask the patient for payment, using phrases such as, "Your copay today is $15, Mrs. Crawford. Will you be writing a check, or would you like to charge this visit to your Visa?" If the facility is flexible with copayment collection, the medical assistant can give the patient an option. "Mr. Thomas, would you like to pay your copay now?"

BOX 23.5   New Patient Brochure Content

The following topics should be addressed in the new patient brochure:
- Description of the healthcare facility (e.g., type of practice, mission statement)
- Location of the facility or a map with directions
- Contact information (i.e., telephone numbers, emails, and website addresses)
- Providers' names and credentials
- Services offered
- Hours of operation
- How appointments can be scheduled
- Healthcare facility's policies and procedures (e.g., payment policies, appointment cancellations, medication refills, assistance after hours)
- Type of medical insurance accepted

VOCABULARY

verification of eligibility The process of confirming health insurance coverage for the patient.

Patients With Special Needs. After a patient is checked in, the receptionist may have additional duties if the patient has special needs. Some patients arrive in wheelchairs unattended by family or friends. They may need assistance to get to the reception area. Remember to always ask patients if they need assistance before you try to assist them.

If there is a language barrier, the medical assistant may need to get translation assistance for the visit. Typical options for assistance include having a qualified translator present or using translation technology. There are many online programs that can assist with translation in many different languages. It is important for the administrative medical assistant to communicate special needs of patients to the clinical medical assistant. In all special needs cases, it is important to remain professional and treat everyone with respect.

Showing Consideration for Patients' Time

Patients expect to see the provider at the appointed time. There should be signage in the reception area stating that patients should let the receptionist know if they have been waiting for longer than 15 to 20 minutes. If the provider is delayed, the medical assistant should let the patients know (Fig. 23.7). The medical assistant can also offer to reschedule the appointment. Some facilities will offer patients gift cards (e.g., coffee, gas) if an error occurred in scheduling or if the patient needs to reschedule due to a long wait time. These gestures show the patients that the staff recognizes their inconvenience. It is a great customer service practice.

CRITICAL THINKING 23.6

Catalina offers to reschedule patient appointments if the schedule ever falls more than 15 minutes behind. If a patient becomes belligerent about the delays, how can Catalina handle the situation in a professional manner?

Escorting Patients to the Exam Room

In some facilities, the administrative medical assistant may escort the patient to the exam room. In other facilities the clinical

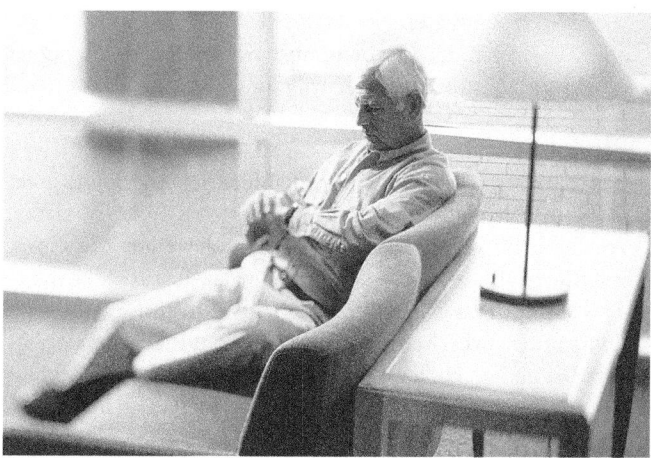

Fig. 23.7 One of the most common patient complaints is the time spent in the reception area. (From Proctor D, et al: *Kinn's the medical assistant*, ed 13, St. Louis, 2017, Elsevier.)

BOX 23.6 Interacting With Friends and Relatives of Patients

Patients are sometimes accompanied by a relative or friend. Be cautious if these individuals want to discuss the patient's illness. Avoid a "too casual" attitude, such as "I'm sure there's nothing to worry about." A show of moderate concern and reassurance that "the patient is in good hands" usually takes care of the situation. Remember that health information cannot be released to anyone, including concerned friends and relatives, without the patient's written consent on the release form.

---

medical assistant comes to the reception area and calls the name of the patient. For confidentiality, it is important to call the patient by the first and last name only. Make sure to clearly pronounce the name. If you are unsure, attempt the pronunciation and then ask the patient. Apologize for pronouncing it incorrectly. Make sure to add the pronunciation to the record for the next visit. Remember, no other information should be given in the public waiting area. When you and the patient are alone or away from the reception area, verify that the patient's date of birth matches your records. If it does not, you have the wrong patient!

Some patients may bring a family member or friend with them to an appointment. On occasion, several people may want to accompany the patient to the exam room. Based on the facility's policy, respectfully explain that the exam room has only two chairs. If the patient still insists, make every attempt to satisfy the patient's needs (Box 23.6). Please be aware that in some cultures, it is expected that multiple people will accompany the patient to see the provider. In those situations, attempt to use a larger room if available.

It is understood that the medical assistant escorts the patient to the exam room. Ask if patients need any assistance, if it appears they might. Do not assume they need assistance – ask first and ask how you can assist them. To show respect for the patient, open doors and walk at the patient's speed.

If a urine specimen is needed, direct the patient to the restroom. Always explain how to collect the specimen and where the specimen should be placed. When you get to the exam room with

the patient, instruct the patient based on the provider's wishes. If the patient needs to undress, explain what clothing items need to be removed and how to put on the gown. Make sure to indicate where the patient needs to sit. If the patient has a risk of falling, have the person sit on the chair instead of the exam table.

If you use the EHR, make sure to log out of the software before leaving the room, and then close the door. If you need to reenter the room, always knock first out of respect for the patient. Pause before opening the door. The pause allows the patient time to prepare and time for them to tell you to enter.

In facilities that use paper health records, often file holders are located on the door or near the door. Place the health record in the holder in such a way that the patient's name is not visible. HIPAA considers names on health records to be incidental disclosures. It is a good practice to protect patient privacy. Many facilities have flags on the door to indicate the status of the patient. Adjust the flagging system so the provider knows the patient is in the room and ready to be seen.

Challenging Situations

Talkative Patients. Any professional office has problem patients. Talkative patients, for example, take up far more of the provider's time than is justified. Many times, the provider and medical assistant will devise a method to help keep everything on schedule. For instance, the medical assistant may have to page the provider after a certain time period. This alerts the provider to the time already spent with the patient. The provider can then complete the visit and move to the next patient.

CRITICAL THINKING 23.7

Catalina has one patient who insists on sitting close to her desk and attempting to chat the entire time she is waiting to see the provider. Even worse, she comes to her appointments at least an hour early. How might Catalina subtly deal with this patient?

Children. Children frequently present special management challenges. The child may be the patient, or they may be accompanying the patient. Parents or guardians are responsible for their children's behavior while at the healthcare facility. If children are doing something that could be harmful, quietly speak to the parents and allow them to handle the situation. The medical assistant should not discipline the child. Strategies to use with bad behavior with children include:

- Move down to the child's level and offer a book or toy.
- Lead the child away from any objects that could be broken or from other patients.
- Say to the child, "Let's come over here and play next to your mom!"

If the child continues to behave badly, call the parent to the exam room early. They may not be seen early but can wait in the exam room instead of the reception area.

In most cases (other than those that involve teens and suspected abuse situations), parents or guardians accompany the child to the exam room. Sometimes parents of older teens want to be present for the visit. Some providers find teens are more honest with their answers if parents are not present. In these situations, allowing the parent to be in the room for the interview may be helpful, but the parent can then wait in the reception area during the physical exam. This will allow the provider to ask follow-up questions if needed without the parent overhearing the answers. In all cases (unless indicated by state law), parental permission is required for minors to be seen.

Angry Patients in the Reception Area. Every medical assistant eventually is confronted with an angry patient. The anger may simply reflect the patient's pain or fear of what the provider may discover during the exam. If possible, invite the patient into a room out of the reception area. Usually the best course is to let the patient talk out the anger. Present a calm attitude and speak in a low tone of voice. Under no circumstances should the medical assistant return the anger or become argumentative. Medical assistants must use good listening skills with angry people and must be empathetic. Notify the facility's administrator of all difficult patients or ask for help from co-workers.

There should be a policy in place for dealing with potentially dangerous individuals. Policies can include:
- Making sure that you can reach the exit if you take the patient to another room
- Having another employee close by
- Knowing under what circumstances you should contact the police or building security for assistance

Patient Checkout

When patients return to the front office for checkout, greet them with a friendly smile and call the individual by name. Form the habit of asking patients if they have any questions. Check the health record to determine when the provider wants the patient to return. Most providers note this information on the encounter form. Make the return appointment. Remember to give the patient choices on the time and day. Give the patient an appointment reminder card. If the patient has no insurance, some facilities have patients pay at checkout.

The medical assistant can convey a sense of caring by terminating the visit cordially. Thank the patient for coming. If the patient will return for another visit, the assistant can say something like, "We'll see you next week." If the patient will not be returning soon, a pleasant "I hope you'll be feeling better soon" is appropriate. In addition, tell patients to call the facility if they have any questions or if they need additional care. Whatever words of goodbye are chosen, all patients should leave the facility feeling that they have received top-quality care and were treated with friendliness, respect, and courtesy.

CLOSING COMMENTS

Going to a healthcare facility can be intimidating and uncomfortable for many patients. It is important that the medical assistant try to put everyone at ease. Cultivate the habit of greeting each patient immediately in a friendly, self-assured manner. Establish eye contact and smile while introducing yourself to the patient. Small talk can help put a patient at ease. Talking about the weather or an uncontroversial topic may make the patient more comfortable.

Asking personalized questions can also help. Providers and staff members sometimes make brief notes in the health record about the current events in the patient's life. On the next visit, the staff or provider can use this information to start a conversation with the patient. For instance, the patient may state she is going to Florida for a vacation. During the next visit, the provider may start the visit off by asking how her Florida trip was. Asking personalized questions will solidify the personal connection with patients. They may feel important, less intimated, and more comfortable. It is a great way to provide excellent customer service.

VOCABULARY

small talk Polite, light conversation about uncontroversial matters.

PATIENT-CENTERED CARE

Working with patients to find an appointment time that works with their schedule may be a time-consuming task. It is important for the medical assistant to remember to be respectful and sensitive to the patient. Professional behaviors that show sensitivity and respect to patients include:
- Being courteous, polite, and welcoming
- Taking time with the patient; not rushing patients
- Maintaining the person's dignity and rights
- Using positive nonverbal behaviors
- Demonstrating a nonjudgmental and accepting attitude
- Focusing your full attention on the patient
- Using summarizing or paraphrasing to clarify what the patient verbalizes. Acknowledge what the patient communicates to you.

BEING PROFESSIONAL

When scheduling and helping patients move through the healthcare facility, the medical assistant has many opportunities to demonstrate professionalism. It is important to remember that we often see patients when they are not at their best, so we must learn not to take all of the responses personally. When an angry patient approaches the reception desk, you should smile politely, ask how you can help the person, and respond in a soothing tone of voice. When a patient calls for an appointment and demands a day and time when the provider is not available, remain calm and explain why that day and time are not an option. As a medical assistant in the front office, you have the opportunity to make an amazing first impression on patients. Remember to always behave professionally.

Role-play this scenario with a peer, who will play the patient: You are answering phones at the front desk, and Sam calls. He wants an appointment today. You review the schedule, and everything is filled for today except for a 5 p.m. appointment slot. You offer him that slot, but it is too late for Sam. He wants one sooner and insists that he needs to come in today. You have spots available tomorrow.

CHAPTER REVIEW

There are two types of scheduling systems, paper-based and computerized. Self-scheduling is gaining in popularity with patients. When establishing the appointment schedule, the staff needs to consider the patient's needs and the provider's preferences and habits. The appointment matrix is used by blocking times the providers are not available and identifying when the facility will be opened. Different types of appointments require varied amounts of time. The medical assistant must identify which type of appointment to use when a patient indicates their reason for the visit.

When adding a patient's appointment to the appointment book, the medical assistant must add the patient's full name, telephone number, and the purpose of the visit. This is typically done in black ink, because the appointment book is a legal document. If it is done in pencil, the medical assistant must go over the pencil with ink at the end of the day to make the permanent document. All no-show and canceled appointments must be indicated on the schedule. The medical assistant must also document the no-show or cancelation in the patient's health record.

There are several types of scheduling, and sometimes more than one can be used in the facility. These types include time-specified, wave, modified wave, open booking, and group or cluster. Advance scheduling and double-booking can be used with other scheduling types. When scheduling patient appointments, the medical assistant needs to give the patient two different appointment time options. Some facilities require the administrative medical assistants to update patient billing information (e.g., address and insurance) during the scheduling process. Additional information is shared with new patients, including directions, parking, and payment options. Besides appointments with providers, the medical assistant is involved with scheduling surgeries, procedures, and inpatient admissions; home, extended care facility, telemedicine, and representative visits.

When a patient arrives for a visit, the medical assistant must ensure the greeting and sign-in register are HIPAA appropriate. Often the medical assistant must ask infection control screening questions when patients arrive. New patients must sign that they received the NPP document. The medical assistant must scan or copy patients' insurance cards and perform verification of eligibility.

In some facilities, the administrative medical assistant may escort the patient to the exam room. In other facilities the clinical medical assistant comes to the reception area and calls the name of the patient. For confidentiality, it is important to call the patient by the first and last name only.

SCENARIO WRAP-UP

Catalina is quickly becoming a part of the team at WMFM Clinic and is developing into a well-liked asset to the staff. When it comes to scheduling, Catalina is flexible and can change the order of the patients seen, if needed, to maximize the use of time and facilities in the office. Because she is so cheerful and friendly, patients do not seem to mind when she asks for their cooperation. She keeps current phone numbers and cell phone information so that she can notify a patient quickly if the providers are running behind schedule. Catalina's proficiency on the computer is also an asset, and she makes frequent use of email to take care of patient problems or rescheduling requests.

Catalina contributes to the efficiency of the healthcare facility by constantly refining her knowledge about her job. She pays attention to the times during the day that do not run as smoothly as others, evaluates the problems at those times, and then corrects them. She also keeps the schedule moving by communicating with the clinical medical assistants, keeping them informed about arriving patients and those who have come early or are running late. She can quickly adjust and substitute a patient who already has arrived. Catalina has learned how to manipulate the schedule to accommodate an emergency. She knows that by making minor adjustments and keeping the waiting patients informed, the staff can handle any emergency.

All medical assistants need to develop skills in flexibility. Establishing a system that works and using it correctly makes patients and staff members more content with their experience in the healthcare facility.

PROCEDURE 23.1   Establish the Appointment Matrix

Task

Establish the matrix of the appointment schedule.

Equipment and Supplies

- Computer with scheduling software or appointment book and black pen
- Office procedures manual (optional)
- Calendar

Scenario

You have been asked to set up the schedule matrix for 1 month for Dr. Julie Walden, Dr. James Martin, and Dr. Angela Perez. The office is open from 8 a.m. to 5 p.m. Monday, Tuesday, Thursday, and Friday. On Wednesday, the office is open from 8 a.m. to 4 p.m. Block off the following times in the appointment schedule:

Dr. Julie Walden

- Lunch: daily 11:30 a.m. to 12:30 p.m.
- Hospital rounds: Mondays and Wednesdays 8 a.m. to 9 a.m.
- Conference: Next Wednesday 1–5 p.m.
- Off Thursdays after 3 p.m.

Dr. James Martin

- Lunch: daily noon to 1 p.m.; no lunch on Wednesdays
- Hospital rounds: Tuesdays and Thursdays 8 a.m. to 9 a.m.
- Nursing home visits: Fridays 8 a.m. to noon
- Meetings: Mondays 4–5 p.m.
- Off Wednesdays after 12 p.m.

Dr. Angela Perez

- Lunch: daily 12:30 p.m. to 1:30 p.m.; no lunch on Mondays
- Hospital rounds: Fridays 8 a.m. to 9 a.m.
- Meetings: Tuesdays 10–noon and Thursdays 3–5 p.m.
- Off Mondays after 12 p.m.

Procedural Steps

1. Using the calendar, determine when the office is not open (e.g., holidays, weekends, evenings).
   - *Paper-based scheduling system*: Using a black pen and the appointment book pages, draw an *X* through each time slot the office is not open. If using the scheduling software, block the times the office is not open. Add the dates to each column.
   - *Computerized scheduling system*: Block the times the office is not open.

   Purpose: Blocking the office's closed times prevents patients from being scheduled when the office is closed.

2. Identify the times each provider has lunch, hospital rounds and nursing home visits.
   - *Paper-based scheduling system*: Using a black pen, write a provider's name on each appointment book page. Draw an *X* through each unavailable time slot. Indicate the reason on the top line of the crossed-out section.
   - *Computerized scheduling system*: Select each provider and block the times the provider is unavailable. Make sure to block the appropriate weeks indicated.

   Purpose: Many providers do rounds in the hospital and cannot see patients in the clinic during those times.

3. Identify the times each provider has meetings and conferences or is off.
   - *Paper-based scheduling system*: Using a black pen, draw an *X* through each unavailable time slot. Indicate the reason on the top line of the crossed-out section.
   - *Computerized scheduling system*: Select each provider and block the time the provider is unavailable. Make sure to block the appropriate weeks indicated.

   Purpose: Providers may have weekly meetings or special times when conferences or meetings are scheduled.

PROCEDURE 23.2   Schedule an Established Patient

Tasks

Manage the provider's schedule by scheduling appointments for an established patient and handling rescheduling and a no-show appointment.

Equipment and Supplies

- Computer with scheduling software or appointment book, black pen, and red pen
- Scheduling guidelines
- Reminder card
- Patient's health record

Scenario

Celia Tapia has just completed her visit today and is checking out at your desk. On the encounter form, you see she needs to schedule a follow-up appointment next week with Dr. Martin. The scheduling guidelines indicate a follow-up appointment is 15 to 20 minutes long.

Procedural Steps

1. Obtain the patient's name. Verify her address and insurance information. Refer to the paperwork for the provider's name and the purpose of the appointment. Obtain any scheduling preferences from the patient.
   - *Computerized scheduling system*: Enter the patient's name and DOB. Verify the correct patient is selected.

   Purpose: To schedule an appointment, the patient's information is required, along with the provider to be seen and the type of appointment required. The patient's address and insurance information are important for billing. Knowing any scheduling preferences or limitations will help you efficiently find an acceptable appointment time for the patient.

2. Identify the length of the appointment by using the scheduling guidelines.

   Purpose: Depending on the appointment type, each provider may require a different length of time for that appointment. Ensuring you schedule the appropriate amount of time will facilitate the flow of patients on that day.

3. Search the appointment book or computerized scheduling system for the first suitable appointment time and an alternate time. Offer the patient a choice of these dates and times. Be respectful and sensitive to the patient if they cannot make the initial options you gave. Provide additional appointment options as needed.

   Purpose: Providing the patient with a choice of dates and times and additional options as needed helps to demonstrate sensitivity when managing appointments. It is an important customer service technique (see the figure).

PROCEDURE 23.2 Schedule an Established Patient—cont'd

SimChart® for the medical office

		Front Office	Clinical Care	Coding & Billing				TruCode

Calendar 📅 Calendar ✉ Correspondence 👥 Patient Demographics 🔍 Find Patient 📋 Form Repository

▼ Calendar View

Add Appointment

	April 2020					
Su	Mo	Tu	We	Th	Fr	Sa
			1	2	3	4
5	6	7	8	9	10	11
12	13	14	15	16	17	18
19	20	21	22	23	24	25
26	27	28	29	30		

Search

Search by patient 🔍

Filter By

Provider:
-Select-

Appointment Type
All
Patient Visit
Block
Other

Exam Room:
-Select-

► Exam Room View
► Provider View

◄ ► **April 19 — 25, 2020**   Day Week Month

	Sun 4/19	Mon 4/20	Tue 4/21	Wed 4/22	Thu 4/23	Fri 4/24	Sat 4/25
8am		Washington, James A. Mar Complete exam			Burgel, Isab James A. Mar Check-up	Yan, Tai I Jean Burke, NP Glucose moni	Miller, Dani James A. Mar
9am			Parker, John Jean Burke, NP Well child c	Patel, Amma A Julie Walden	Parker, John James A. Mar Well child c		
10am		Rainwater, E James A. Mar		Staff Meeting All Staff	Johnson, Cha James A. Mar	Richardson, James A. Mar Prenatal	
11am			Hernandez, C Jean Burke, NP Well child c				Caudill, Rob Jean Burke, NP Hearing test
12pm	Lunch James A. Mar	Lunch James A. Mar	Lunch James A. Mar	Lunch James A. Mar	Lunch James A. Mar	Lunch James A. Mar	Lunch James A. Mar
1pm		Biller, Walt Julie Walden			Tapia, Celia B James A. Mar Annual Exam		
2pm							

Copyright © 2016 Elsevier Inc. All Rights Reserved.

4. Schedule the appointment.
   - *Paper-based scheduling system*: Using a black pen, write the patient's name, phone number, and reason for the visit (per the facility's procedure) in the time slot. Add any other relevant information per the facility's procedures. Make sure to block out the correct amount of time.
   - *Computerized scheduling system*: Create the appointment per the facility's guidelines.

   Purpose: Adding the patient's phone number to the appointment book will help save time if the patient needs to be contacted.

5. Complete the appointment reminder card and ensure the date and time on the card match the appointment time. Give the card to the patient.

   Purpose: Appointment reminder cards help patients remember when their appointments are and reduces the number of no-show appointments.

   Scenario update: Later that day, Celica Tapia calls and says she needs to reschedule her appointment. She is available the day after the scheduled appointment and would like to be seen at the same time she initially had.

6. Follow steps 1 through 4 to reschedule the appointment.
   - *Paper-based scheduling system*: When the new appointment is made, make sure to draw one line through the old appointment on the appointment log and indicate the reason for the change.

   - *Computerized scheduling system*: With the scheduling software, ensure the old appointment time is removed from the schedule. Repeat the appointment date and time to the patient.

   Scenario update: Celia Tapia no-shows for her follow-up appointment.

7. Using the patient's health record, document that the patient failed to show for the follow-up visit with the provider. Indicate in the scheduling system that the patient no-showed.
   - *Paper-based scheduling system*: In the appointment book, using red pen and indicate the patient no-showed.
   - *Computerized scheduling system*: Change the appointment status to no-show.

   Purpose: For legal purposes, the healthcare facility must keep a record of patients who no-show for appointments. By indicating it in the appointment book and in the health record, the practice is covered if any issues should arise. Some medical practices have procedures that include contacting the patient regarding the no-show appointment and finding out the reason. This is then also charted in the health record.

PROCEDURE 23.3 Schedule a New Patient

Tasks

Schedule a new patient for a first office visit and identify the urgency of the visit using established priorities.

Equipment and Supplies

- Computer with scheduling software or appointment book, paper, and black pen
- Scheduling and screening guidelines

Scenario

Patricia Black (DOB 11/25/19XX) calls. She just moved to the area and is a new patient to the practice. Her asthma has flared up over the past 24 hours. Her albuterol inhaler is empty, and she needs a new prescription for it. She states that she is doing okay, but without the albuterol she knows it will get worse within the next few days. According to your screening guidelines, she needs to be seen today. The scheduling guidelines indicate she needs a 40 to 45 minute appointment.

Directions

Role-play this scenario. You are the medical assistant. Your peer will be the patient and can make up any information needed.

Procedural Steps

1. Obtain the patient's demographic information (e.g., full name, birth date, address, and telephone number). Write this information down or enter it into the scheduling software. Verify the information.

   Purpose: It is important to verify the information. If you have difficulty hearing the patient, use a system to verify the spelling (e.g., "A" as in "Alpha").

2. Determine whether the patient was referred by another provider.

   Purpose: You may need to request additional information from the referring provider, and your provider will want to send a consultation report.

3. Determine the patient's chief complaint and when the first symptoms occurred. Use the scheduling and screening guidelines as needed.

   Purpose: You must know the amount of time that will be required for the visit and how quickly the patient needs to be seen based on the chief complaint.

4. Search the appointment book or scheduling software for the first suitable appointment time and an alternate time. Offer the patient a choice of these dates and times. Be respectful and sensitive to the patient if they cannot make the initial options you gave. Provide additional appointment options as needed.

   Purpose: Providing the patient with a choice of dates and times and additional options as needed demonstrates sensitivity when managing appointments. It is an important customer service technique (see the figure).

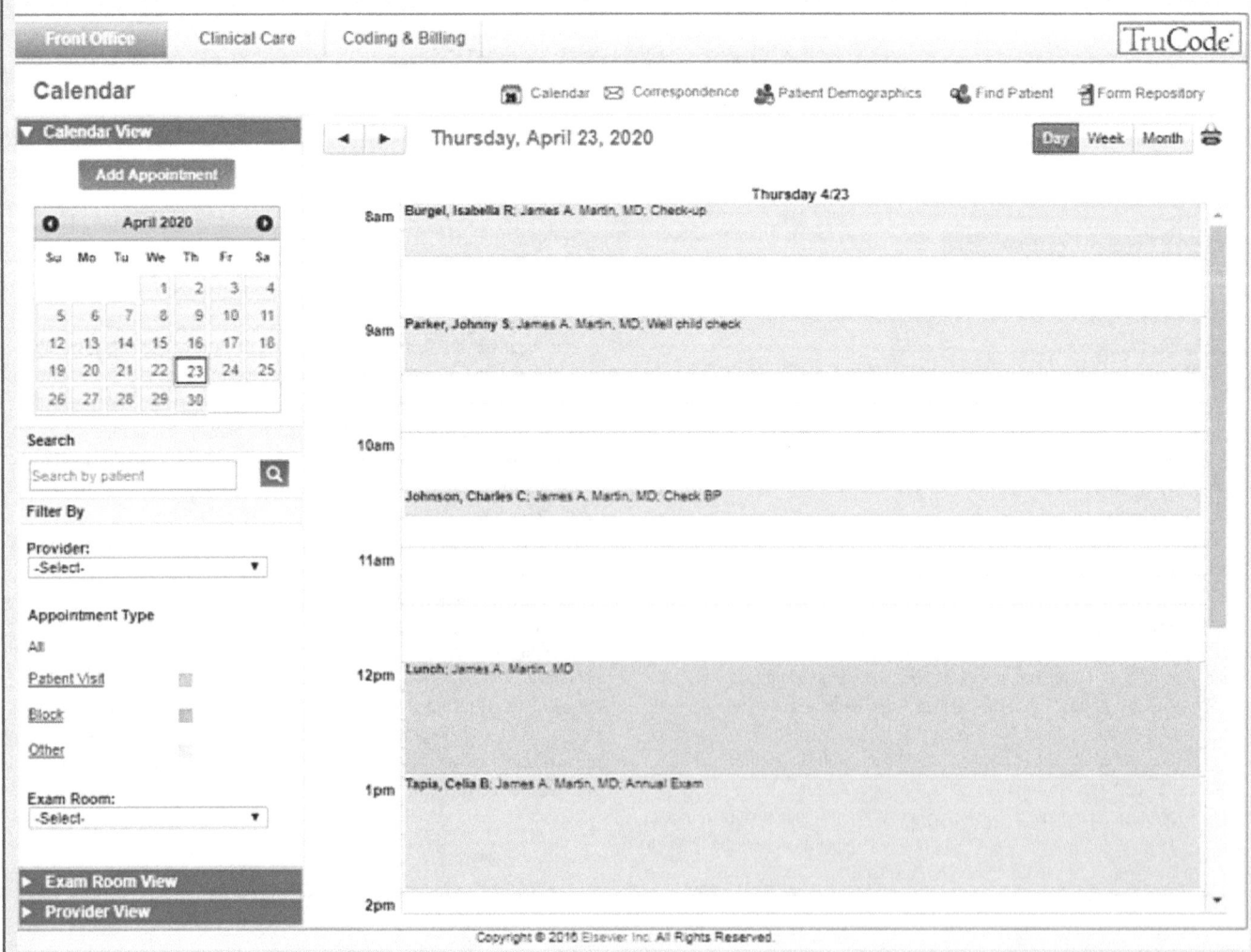

PROCEDURE 23.3 Schedule a New Patient—cont'd

5. Schedule the appointment.
   - *Paper-based scheduling system:* Using a black pen, write the patient's name, phone number, and reason for the visit (per the facility's procedure) in the time slot. Add *NP* for new patient. Add any other relevant information per the facility's procedures. Make sure to block out the correct amount of time.
   - *Computerized scheduling system:* Create the appointment per the facility's guidelines.

   Purpose: The *NP* in the appointment book indicates that this is a new patient. Having the phone number available increases your efficiency if you need to contact the patient.

6. Obtain the patient's insurance information (e.g., insurance company, policy number, and group number). If new patients are expected to pay at the time of the visit, explain this financial arrangement when making the appointment.

   Purpose: Obtaining the patient's insurance information now ensures that the patient is seeing a provider covered by their insurance carrier. Explaining the payment policy before the appointment helps the patient come to the appointment prepared to pay.

7. Provide the patient with directions to the healthcare facility and parking instructions if needed.

   Note: Many facilities will email or mail new-patient paperwork to the patient, who is instructed to complete the forms ahead of time and bring them to the appointment.

8. Before ending the call, ask if the patient has any questions. Reinforce the date and time of the appointment. Politely and professionally end the call, making sure to thank the patient for calling.

   Purpose: It is important to restate the appointment time and date to ensure the patient knows the correct information before ending the call.

   Note: For legal and safety reasons, many healthcare practices encourage patients with urgent same-day appointments to seek emergency care immediately if the condition worsens before the appointment time.

PROCEDURE 23.4 Schedule a Patient Procedure

Tasks

Schedule a patient for a procedure within the time frame needed by the provider, confirm with the patient, and issue all required instructions.

Equipment and Supplies

- Provider's order detailing the procedure required
- Name, address, and telephone number of the facility where the procedure will take place
- Patient's demographic and insurance information
- Patient's health record
- Procedure preparation instructions (optional)
- Telephone
- Consent form (if required for procedure)

Scenario

Monique Jones (DOB 06/23/19XX) has just seen Dr. Martin and is checking out at your desk. She tells you she needs a magnetic resonance imaging (MRI) scan of her left ankle. The provider's order states: "MRI left ankle within one week to rule out stress fracture." The radiology department in your facility performs MRIs.

Directions

Role-play this scenario with a peer. You will be the medical assistant. Your peer with be the patient for steps 1 – 3 and 6 and the radiology department scheduler for steps 4 – 5. Use the following information. Your peer can make up any additional information needed.

Patient's Information:
Address: 1876 Wellington Springs Court, Anytown, AL 12345-1234
Phone: 123-588-9994
Insurance: Blue Cross Blue Shield
Policy/ID: MJ4468871
Group: 78451J

Radiology Department
Walden-Martin Family Medical Clinic
1234 Anystreet
Anytown, Anystate 12345
Phone: 123-123-1248

Preparation for an ankle MRI:

- Arrive 15 minutes early. A consent form is not required.
- You will need to remove all metal and electronic objects from your body. No post-procedure instructions.

Procedural Steps

1. Obtain an oral or a written order from the provider for the exact procedure to be performed. Obtain the patient's name and date of birth.

   Purpose: For you to schedule the procedure, you will need an order from the provider for the procedure to be performed.

2. Gather the patient's demographic and insurance information. Write down the information.

   Note: For some procedures and diagnostic tests, precertification or preauthorization must be completed before the patient is scheduled.

3. Determine the patient's availability within the time frame specified by the provider for the procedure. Determine if the procedure requires a consent form and if needed, identify if it was completed.

   Note: The facility where the procedure is to be performed will need a copy of the consent form. The original form must be added to the patient's health record.

   Purpose: Make sure the patient will be able to comply with the arrangements for the test. The consent form is used to make sure the patient understands the risks, benefits, and alternatives to the procedure.

   Scenario update: Your peer will be the radiology department scheduler.

4. Contact the radiology department and give the scheduler with the following information:
   - Provide the provider's exact order, including the procedure, body location involved (e.g., left ankle), diagnosis, and time frame. Include any urgency for test results.
   - Provide the patient's demographic information (name, DOB, address, telephone number, and insurance information).
   - Establish the date and time for the procedure.

   Purpose: To schedule the procedure, the facility needs the patient's information and the provider's exact order.

5. From the scheduler, obtain information on any patient preparations required prior to the procedure and any post procedure requirements (e.g., driver needed). Write the instructions out for the patient.

   Purpose: The patient needs to be instructed on any preparations and also any post procedure requirements.

   Note: The radiology department may require the provider's order for the procedure. If your facility does not have computerized provider order entry (CPOE), you will need to make arranges to get the order to the radiology department.

   Scenario update: Your peer will be the patient for the following step.

PROCEDURE 23.4   Schedule a Patient Procedure—cont'd

6. Notify the patient of the arrangements and provide the information in a written format.
   - Give the name, address, and telephone number of the diagnostic facility.
   - Specify the date and time to report for the procedure.
   - Give instructions on preparation for the test (e.g., eating restrictions, fluids, medications, enemas).
   - If another facility will be used, the patient will need to bring a form of picture identification and the insurance card.
   - Ask if the patient has any questions and answer the questions.

   Purpose: Make sure the patient understands the necessary preparations and the importance of keeping the appointment. Providing the patient with written instructions reinforces what was discussed and gives the patient a reference for the information.

7. Document the details of the scheduled procedure in the patient's health record. If applicable, create a reminder to check on the procedure results after the appointment date.

   Purpose: Document that the procedure was scheduled. It is legally important to show that what was ordered was scheduled. Creating a reminder for you to check up on the results of the procedure is also important in assisting the provider.

   2/27/20XX 11:05 a.m. Dr. Martin ordered an MRI left ankle within one week to rule out stress fracture. Patient scheduled for an MRI of left ankle on 3/3/20XX 8 a.m. at WMFM Clinic Radiology department. Patient preparation instructions given, and patient verbalized understanding. _____

   _____ Catalina McDowell CMA (AAMA)

PROCEDURE 23.5 Schedule a Meeting and Create an Agenda

Tasks
Schedule a meeting and create an agenda.

Equipment and Supplies
- Computer with internet or a printer
- Email address of the supervisor (the instructor) (optional)

Scenario
You are asked to find a common meeting time between Tuesday through Thursday of next week for a 1-hour meeting with the staff and providers. The office manager wants you to create an agenda for the meeting and include the following topics: continuing education session on infection control, changes in the inventory process, ideas for patient-centered care from scheduling through checkout, and follow-up on last month's meeting. Monthly items always addressed at the beginning of the meeting include monthly birthdays, patient feedback, and updates from the last meeting.

Conference room #3 is always available for a meeting. The office is open 8 a.m. to 5 p.m. Monday, Tuesday, Thursday, and Friday. On Wednesday, the office is open from 8 a.m. to 4 p.m. The following table shows the providers' schedules.

	Dr. Julie Walden	Dr. James Martin	Dr. Angela Perez
Lunch (daily)	11:30 a.m. to 12:30 p.m.	12 p.m. to 1 p.m. (none on Wednesdays)	12:30 p.m. to 1:30 p.m.; none on Mondays.
Hospital rounds	Mondays and Wednesdays 8 a.m. to 9 a.m.	Tuesdays and Thursdays 8 a.m. to 9 a.m.	Fridays 8 a.m. to 9 a.m.
Days off	Thursdays after 3 p.m.	Wednesdays after 12 p.m.	Mondays after 12 p.m.

	Dr. Julie Walden	Dr. James Martin	Dr. Angela Perez
Others	Conference next Wednesday 1–5 p.m.	Nursing home visits Fridays 8 a.m. to noon; Meeting Mondays 4–5 p.m.	Meeting Tuesdays 10 a.m.–noon and Thursdays 3–5 p.m.

Procedural Steps
1. Identify a 1-hour block of time for the meeting. Review the office schedule and the providers' schedules. Schedule the meeting either at the beginning or the end of the day or before or after lunch.
   Purpose: The providers need to be available for the meeting.
   Note: When a time is selected, the medical assistant should block the time in all of the providers' schedules.
2. Using a word processing software, open a new document and type the facility's name at the top. Use Walden-Martin Family Medical Clinic as the facility.
3. Add a few blank lines and then center the following: meeting name, date and time of the meeting, and the location. Use "WMFM Clinic Staff and Provider Meeting" as the meeting name. Use the time selected in step 1.
   Purpose: Agendas need to include the meeting name, date, time, and location.
4. Create a bulleted or numbered list of the items that need to be discussed. Include the items in the order they are to be presented at the meeting.
   Purpose: To help create an organized meeting, the topics should be listed in the order they will be discussed.
5. Proofread the agenda and make any revisions. Email the agenda to the supervisor or print the agenda.
   Purpose: It is important to review the agenda for any mistakes before making it public.

PROCEDURE 23.6 Coach Patients Regarding Office Policies

Tasks
Create a new patient brochure, and then role-play ways to coach patients regarding office policies.

Scenario
You work at Walden-Martin Family Medical (WMFM) Clinic. Your supervisor asks you to create a new patient brochure for the clinic. She wants to make sure patients are informed of the clinic's policies:
- Copayments must be paid at the time of the appointment.
- Bills must be paid within 15 days once billed to the patient.
- Appointments must be canceled 24 hours in advance or the patient will be billed $25.
- Medication refills are done through the patient portal (WMFM Clinic Portal) or when the medical assistant rooms the patient during the visit.
The healthcare facility's information is:
- *Address:* Walden-Martin Family Medical Clinic, 1234 Anystreet, Anytown, Anystate 12345
- *Phone:* 123-123-1234 Fax: 123-123-5678
- *After-hours phone number:* 123-555-1212
- *Type of agency:* Family practice clinic
- *Mission statement:* To provide excellent holistic care to our community members.
- *Providers:* Julie Walden, M.D., James Martin, M.D., Angela Perez, M.D., David Kahn, M.D., and Jean Burke, N.P.

After you complete the brochure, you coach the following patients regarding office procedures:
- Mr. Charles Johnson (he has a question regarding the payment policy)
- Ms. Monique Jones (she has a question regarding the medication refill procedure)

Directions
Use the information provided to create the brochure. Make up any additional information you need. After completing the brochure, role-play the scenarios with a peer. You are the medical assistant and the peer is the patient.

Equipment and Supplies
- Computer with word processing software and printer
- Office procedures manual (optional)

Procedural Steps
1. Using word processing software, design an informational brochure for patients that provides information about the healthcare facility and describes practice procedures. At a minimum, the following information should be included:
   - Description of the healthcare facility (e.g., type of practice, mission statement)
   - Location of the facility or a map with directions
   - Contact information (i.e., telephone numbers, emails, and website addresses)

Continued

PROCEDURE 23.6   Coach Patients Regarding Office Policies—cont'd

- Providers' names and credentials
- Services offered
- Hours of operation
- How appointments can be scheduled
- Healthcare facility's policies and procedures (e.g., payment policies, appointment cancellations, medication refills, assistance after hours)
- Insurance plans accepted

Purpose: Providing patients with a written brochure listing the facility's information, policies, and procedures enables them to use it as a reference.

2. Proofread the brochure. Revise as needed. Print the brochure.

Purpose: It is important to proofread and revise documents as needed before they are made available to patients.

3. Role-play the first scenario with a peer. Give a brief summary of the different parts of the brochure. Use words the patient will understand.

Purpose: By discussing each part of the brochure with the potential patient, you can explain what is printed. Summarize the information without reading the sections to the patient.

4. Ask if the patient has any questions. Actively listen to the patient's concerns. Address those concerns.

Purpose: By actively listening, you will be able to identify issues or confusion the patient is experiencing. It is important that the messages during the conversation are clear for both parties.

5. Role-play the second scenario with a peer. Give a brief summary of the different parts of the brochure. Use words that the patient understands.

Purpose: By reviewing the brochure, you can summarize the policies. If the patient has an immediate question, you can answer it.

6. Ask if the patient has any questions. Actively listen to the patient's concerns. Address those concerns.

Purpose: By actively listening, you will be able to identify issues or confusion the patient is experiencing. It is important that the messages during the conversation are clear for both parties.

24

Technology

LEARNING OBJECTIVES

1. Describe types of personal computers used in ambulatory care facilities.
2. Discuss the difference between input and output hardware, list examples of each type of hardware, and describe computer storage devices and cloud storage.
3. Describe how to maintain computer hardware and explain infection control procedures with computer hardware.
4. Identify principles of ergonomics that apply to a computer workstation.
5. Identify questions to ask when purchasing hardware.
6. Differentiate between system software and application software and provide examples of each.
7. Differentiate between practice management software, electronic health records, electronic medical records, patient portal software, and telemedicine software.
8. Discuss the Health Insurance Portability and Accountability Act's Security Rule safeguards and list examples of each type of safeguard.
9. Discuss technologic advances in healthcare.
10. Describe how to identify reliable health websites.

OUTLINE

▷▷ OPENING SCENARIO

Christiana worked at Walden-Martin Family Medical (WMFM) Clinic as a clinical medical assistant for 5 years. She helped with diagnostic tests and treatment procedures. Christiana enjoyed providing patient care, but she was interested in a change and wanted to use more of her administrative skills. When a front office position opened up, Christiana moved into the administrative role. She is now the lead administrative medical assistant. Besides performing her administrative duties, Christiana is now responsible for the clinic's computer system. She is excited to continue to learn the administrative role and the computer system.

YOU WILL LEARN

1. To describe common hardware and software used in the ambulatory care facility.
2. To explain the medical assistant's role regarding maintaining computer hardware.
3. To describe how to apply infection control principles to a workstation.

4. To discuss how to have an ergonomically correct workstation.
5. To describe computer network security procedures.

INTRODUCTION

When technology was first used in healthcare, it was used in the business departments. Computer software was used for billing and accounting procedures, registration processes, and scheduling.

With the advent of computer technology, what used to take hours to do now takes minutes. Data is collected once, entered, and used for many purposes. Computer software increases accuracy and efficiency and saves money.

When electronic health records (EHRs) were introduced, agencies implemented software to increase the accuracy and efficiency of patient care. The federal government provided financial incentives to use EHRs instead of paper medical records. Currently healthcare workers use "smart" devices for quicker access to information to provide better patient care.

Communication has also changed over the years. Patients use emails and text messages to contact their providers. To help ensure confidentiality, administrators have created tighter network security procedures. Today, medical assistants must be more computer savvy than ever before to meet technologic demands. They must follow procedures to safeguard the privacy and security of patients' records.

CRITICAL THINKING 24.1

When Christiana transitioned into the administrative role, Dr. Kahn hired Michaela as the new clinical medical assistant. Recently the healthcare facility switched from using desktop computers to tablet computers when working with patients in the exam rooms. How might Christiana's experience using the desktop computer in the exam rooms be different from Michaela's use of the tablet computer? Think of the patient's perception; which technology might a patient prefer the medical assistant to use? Why?

VOCABULARY

electronic health record (EHR) An electronic record that conforms to nationally recognized standards and contains health-related information about a specific patient. It can be created, managed, and consulted by authorized clinicians and staff from more than one healthcare organization.

software A set of electronic instructions to operate and perform different computer tasks.

COMPUTERS IN AMBULATORY CARE

Many clinics are using electronic technology in both administrative and patient care areas. Paper medical charts are being replaced with EHRs or used along with the EHR. Technology has increased the efficiency of the office environment. It has made patient information and resources quickly accessible to healthcare staff. Therefore medical assistants need to learn and use computers and technology.

When you think of a computer, thoughts of mobile devices or your personal computer may come to mind. Computers vary greatly on their size, function, and speed. Types of computers including:

- *Supercomputers*: Expensive, very large computers that have incredibly fast processing speeds.
- *Mainframe computers*: Large towering computers that are more common and less expensive than supercomputers. Used by large organizations to store large quantities of information.
- *Minicomputers*: Large multiprocessing machines that support about 200 users at a time. Less powerful than a mainframe computer. A **server** can be a minicomputer.
- *Microcomputer*: Personal computers that have their own central processing unit (CPU).
- *Mobile computers*: Are computers that can be carried, such as laptops, netbooks, tablets, and smartphones.

This chapter will focus on personal computers and mobile computers used in the healthcare setting.

Personal and Mobile Computers

A *personal computer* (PC) is a single-user electronic data processing device. Personal computers can also be mobile computers. Types of personal computers include:

- *Desktop computer*: A larger unit designed for use on a desk. It is used by employees who primarily perform word processing, data entry, and business tasks (e.g., scheduling, bookkeeping, and billing).
- *Laptop computer*: A thin, lightweight, wireless, portable PC with a keyboard; it may include a touchscreen. There is currently a trend toward reducing the size and weight of laptops; those smaller, lighter laptops are often called *notebooks*. Laptops are used by providers and medical assistants in patient exam rooms and at workstations.
- *Tablet PC*: A thin, lightweight, wireless, portable PC that functions with a touchscreen. The most popular operating systems include Android and iOS. Tablets are used by providers and medical assistants in patient exam rooms and at workstations. There are several types of tablet PCs, such as:
  - *Slate-style tablet*: A thin, portable computer with no keyboard. External keyboards are available for many slate-style tablets.
  - *Convertible tablet*: Usually allows the user to use the touchscreen or the physical keyboard. The display can rotate and cover the keyboard, making it appear like a tablet; or, the keyboard makes it look like a small laptop (e.g., notebook).
  - *Hybrid tablet*: May also be called a *hybrid* or *convertible notebook*; it has a removable display, making it look more like a slate tablet.

The PC accepts, stores, and processes data. After processing the information, it generates the data output in a specific form, such as a letter or a patient statement.

The personal computer is a *system unit*, or the primary computer equipment. All other forms of physical equipment used with the PC are called *peripheral devices*. The PC and peripheral devices are hardware. Computer hardware can be divided into input devices, output devices, internal components, secondary storage devices, and network and internet access devices. The following sections describe these categories.

CRITICAL THINKING 24.2

Christiana's keyboard looks different from Dr. Kahn's keyboard in his office. She uses her keyboard during the majority of the day. Why might Christiana have a different keyboard? What type of keyboard might Christiana have?

VOCABULARY

hardware Physical equipment of the computer system required for communication and data processing functions.

operating system System software; it acts as the computer's software administrator by managing, integrating, and controlling application software and hardware. Windows is an example.

output device Computer hardware that displays the processed data from the computer (e.g., monitors and printers).

secondary storage devices Media (e.g., jump drive, flash drive, hard drive) capable of permanently storing data until it is replaced or deleted by the user.

server Computer hardware and software that perform data analysis, storage, and archiving; accepts and responses to requests from devices (clients) made over a network. Also called a *database server* or *data server.*

stylus A pen-shaped device with a variety of tips that is used on touchscreens to write, draw, or input commands.

Input Devices. An *input device* is any peripheral hardware that allows the user to provide data to the computer. Many types of input devices are available on the market. This discussion focuses on those typically used in the ambulatory care setting. Common input devices include keyboards, mice and other pointing devices, touchscreens, webcams, cameras, microphones, scanners, and signature pads.

Keyboard. Keyboards are the most common input devices. The QWERTY keyboard is the standard keyboard for computers. (Q-W-E-R-T-Y are the first six letters, from left to right, just below the number keys on the keyboard.) A wide variety of keyboards are available, including standard, internet, wireless, and ergonomic. Keyboards may have special keys that perform the same functionality as the buttons on Web pages. Numeric keypads are also a feature on many keyboards. Ergonomic keyboards reduce repetitive strain injuries by minimizing muscle strain. These keyboards allow the user's hands to be in a natural position when typing. The two most common ergonomic keyboards are the split-key models and the waved or curved key layout (Fig. 24.1).

Keyboards typically have the following categories of keys:
- *Typing*: Include the numeric and alphabetic keys used for typing.
- *Numeric*: Numeric keypads are in the same position as calculators.
- *Function*: The 12 keys at the top of the keyboard. Each key has a specific purpose. Some software programs allow the function keys to be programmed to complete a specific function.
- *Control*: Allow movement of the cursor and the screen; include Home, End, Insert, Delete, Page Up, Page Down, Control, Escape, Alternate, and four arrow keys.
- *Special purpose*: Include Enter, Shift, Caps Lock, Num Lock, Space Bar, Print Screen, and Tab keys.

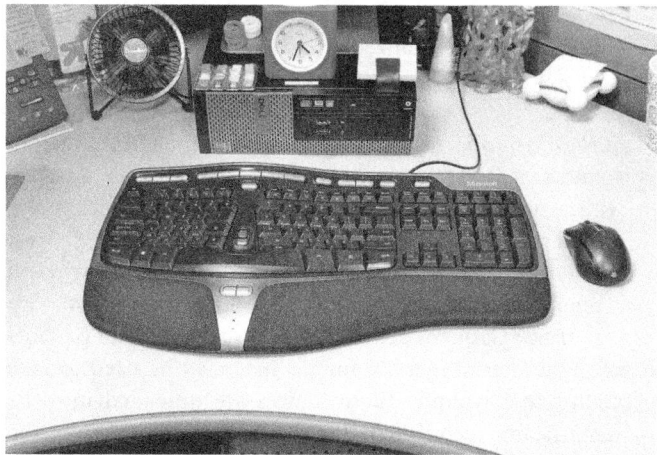

Fig. 24.1 Ergonomic keyboards have different appearances, yet they all reduce repetitive strain injuries. (From Niedzwiecki B, et al: *Kinn's the medical assistant,* ed 14, St. Louis, 2020, Elsevier.)

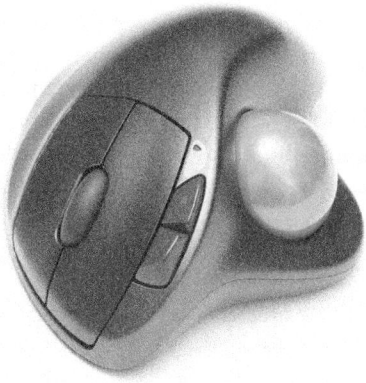

Fig. 24.2 A trackball mouse uses a large ball to control the movement of the cursor/pointer. (From Niedzwiecki B, et al: *Kinn's the medical assistant,* ed 14, St. Louis, 2020, Elsevier.)

Mouse and Touchpad. The mouse and the touchpad are the most common input devices. They make screen navigation much simpler than using the keyboard. A mouse is a palm-sized box with a laser sensor that tracks the movement of the user's hand. The touchpad, found on laptops, is touch sensitive. Both devices send messages back to the computer and move the pointer (cursor) on the screen based on the movement from the mouse or touchpad. The mouse may have left and right buttons and a touchpad may have similar functionality. With a trackball mouse, the user moves the enlarged ball on the top of the mouse to control the pointer (Fig. 24.2).

Touchscreen. A touchscreen is different from a touchpad. A touchscreen allows a person to interact with the computer by touching the display screen with a finger or stylus (STI luhs). Touchscreens can vary, which means the compatible stylus also can vary.
- *Resistive*: Responds to the touch of almost anything that can generate pressure (e.g., finger, plastic stylus, rubber-tip stylus). Found on many handheld electronic devices.

- *Capacitive*: Responds to the electrical characteristics of a finger. Requires a specialized stylus that has more surface area at the point. Found on smart phones and other electrical devices.
- *Surface acoustic wave*: Responds to an inaudible wave of sound that is created on the screen from a finger. A stylus with a rubber or soft tip the size of a pencil eraser is required. Found on kiosks and ordering screens.

Camera, Webcam, and Microphone. Cameras, wireless webcams, and microphones are commonly seen in ambulatory care settings. Cameras are used to capture images of patients before and after surgery. Cameras may also be used to take a picture of a wound. These images are uploaded into the patient's health record. Regardless if a picture is taken in the medical facility or sent by the patient to the provider using the patient portal, the images must remain confidential. Patients must sign a release form before the image can be given to others.

Providers can use webcams, microphones, and internet video chat software to see patients who are at a distance from the healthcare facility. The remote diagnosis and treatment of patients using technology is called *telemedicine*, a form of telehealth. Many times this is done using the patient portal.

Webcams and microphones are also used for meetings and continuing education opportunities. Microphones can be used for dictating notes into a patient's health record. Voice recognition software provides instant transcription into the patient's record.

CRITICAL THINKING 24.3

Dr. Kahn works with a home health agency. Patients and nurses can communicate with him using the internet, microphones, and webcams. How does this technology benefit the patient?

VOCABULARY

patient portal A secure online website that gives patients 24-hour access to personal health information using a username and password.

practice management software A type of software that allows the user to enter demographic information, schedule appointments, maintain lists of insurance payers, perform billing tasks, and generate reports.

telehealth Refers to remote clinical services and nonclinical services, such as provider training, meetings, and continuing education.

Scanner. Scanners in the healthcare setting have become more popular since the use of EHRs has increased. Old medical records are scanned, and the images are uploaded into the patient's EHR. Scanners convert images to digital text through a process called *optical character recognition* (OCR). Types of scanners available include:

- *Handheld scanner*: Used in healthcare to scan identification (ID) bands prior to medication administration and procedures; may also be used for managing the inventory of supplies with the use of bar codes.

- *ID card scanner*: May have other names, including *insurance card scanner*. Used at the reception desk to scan insurance cards, driver's licenses, and so on. Usually information is then saved in the practice management software for billing purposes.
- *Sheet-fed scanner*: Also called an *automatic document feeder (ADF) scanner*. Used to scan loose sheets of paper. May be used to scan test result documents to import into the patient's EHR.
- *Flatbed scanner*: Has a glass panel on which the documents are placed for scanning. May also be used to scan test result documents for importing into the EHR.

Signature Pad. In many ambulatory care settings, signature pads are used in the reception area and in the exam rooms (Fig. 24.3). Patients need to sign several documents, including disclosure authorization forms, consent forms, and the Notice of Privacy Practices (NPP). Patients sign the signature pad. The signature is then imported into the EHR as part of the patient's permanent health record.

Output Devices. The data entered into the computer is then processed by it. The processed data is displayed using *output devices*. Common output devices in the healthcare setting include monitors, printers, and speakers.

Monitor. Monitors display the output as images. Images are created by tiny dots called *pixels*. The higher the number of pixels, the sharper the image. The most common monitor is the liquid crystal display (LCD) monitor. These monitors are easier on the eyes. They also use less electricity. LCD monitors are smaller and lighter than older monitors. Some clinics use LCD monitors in the reception area. Patients can read documents on the monitor before signing the signature pad.

Printer. Printers produce the output on paper. Inkjet and laser printers are the two most common types. Inkjet printers create the images by spraying small drops of ink on the paper. Advantages of inkjet printers include their high-quality printing and that they are inexpensive to purchase. Disadvantages when compared to laser printers include the increased frequency of changing the ink cartridges, which gets expensive, and the slower rate of printing.

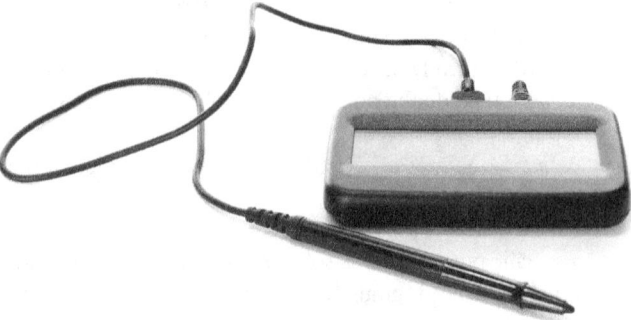

Fig. 24.3 Signature pads allow patients' signatures to be imported into the electronic health record or practice management software. (From Niedzwiecki B, et al: *Kinn's the medical assistant*, ed 14, St. Louis, 2020, Elsevier.)

A laser printer uses a laser, electrical charges, and toner to produce images on paper. Advantages of laser printers over inkjet printers include their high-speed printing, high-quality output, and quality graphics. Laser printers can also support many fonts and font sizes. Toner cartridges are changed less often than inkjet printers. However, the initial cost of laser printers is higher than that of inkjet printers, which is a disadvantage.

Speaker. Speakers for electronic devices come in all shapes and sizes. Typically, speakers are built into the devices used (e.g., monitor, laptop, and tablet). Speakers and sound cards (which will be discussed in a later section) are needed to get sound from the computer.

Internal Components. In desktop personal computers, the internal components are found in the tower or case. Medical assistants would not need to open up the tower or case to problem-solve a computer issue. This may void warranties on the computer equipment. The need to learn about internal components relates more to purchasing hardware and software. The following are internal components that may be of interest when purchasing new hardware or software.

- *Central processing unit* (CPU): Processor or "brains" of the computer; sits on the motherboard. It interprets and executes commands from the software (program).
- *Motherboard*: A platform that is an attachment point for all internal computer parts.
- Primary memory:
  - *Read-only memory* (ROM): Contains hardwire instructions. Used when the computer boots up or starts the system diagnostic checks.
  - *Cache memory*: Provides temporary use of information; contains data and instructions for opened programs. Allows programs to operate more quickly and efficiently
  - *Random access memory* (RAM): Main memory of the computer; used to load and run programs. Required for the computer to operate. If the power is turned off, the memory is lost.
- *Hard drive*: The C drive (C:) of the computer contains the operating system and the related system fields. The C drive includes the hard disk drive (HDD) and the hard drive as one unit. Reads and writes on the hard disk; provides the largest amount of permanent storage for the computer.
- *Optical drive*: Reads and writes (saves) data on removable storage devices, such as compact disks (CDs), digital versatile/video disks (DVDs), and Blu-ray disks (BDs).
- *Sound card*: Also called an *audio card* or *audio adapter*; allows audio information to be sent to speakers or headphones.
- *Video card*: Also called a *graphic card* or *video adapter*; allows the computer to send graphic information to output devices (monitor or projectors).
- *Universal serial bus* (USB) *port*: A connector device that allows hardware to be plugged into the computer. There are multiple types of USB ports, including mini-USB and macro-USB.

CRITICAL THINKING 24.4

Christiana frequently prints documents, including billing statements, appointment reminders, and receipts for payment. What type of printer might be the most economical to use in the front office? Why?

VOCABULARY

boot The process of starting or restarting a computer when the operating system is loaded.

drive A computer device that reads data from and may write data to a storage medium.

media Types of communication (e.g., social media sites); with computers, the term refers to data storage devices.

Secondary Storage Devices. *Secondary storage devices*, or media (ME de ah), are capable of permanently storing data. With many types, the user can write over the existing data or delete the data. These devices can be considered removable, internal (e.g., the hard drive previously discussed), or external. The computer needs a secondary storage device to allow the user to save data. Without a storage device, the computer would be considered a *dumb terminal*. Dumb terminals provide the user access to software, the network, or the internet. They do not allow the user to save data to the hard drive of the computer.

CRITICAL THINKING 24.5

Christiana would like to have a small patient education space in the reception area. She would like to have a computer there with internet access for patients so they can access health information. Christiana knows that cost is an important factor in a small healthcare facility. The computer would also have to be reasonable and reliable. What technology options might she propose to Dr. Kahn?

Types of Storage Devices. The computer storage devices are categorized as follows.

- *Magnetic storage device*: One of the oldest types of storage; uses magnetic technology to read and write data to the device. Examples of magnetic storage devices include the internal hard drive and portable hard drive.
- *Optical storage device (optical disk or disc)*: Uses lasers and lights to read and write data onto optical storage devices. Examples of optical storage devices include the Blu-ray disk (BD), compact disk (CD), and digital versatile/video disk (DVD).
  - *Recordable only* means that data can only be saved once to the disk (e.g., CD-R disk).
  - *Read/write* (RW) allows data to be saved, rewritten (resaved), and deleted many times (e.g., CD-RW).
- *Flash memory device* or *flash drive*: Portable device that has become cheaper and has gained larger storage capacity over the years; connects to the USB port in the computer. Examples of flash memory devices include the jump drive (also called the *USB flash, data stick, pen drive, keychain drive,*

TABLE 24.1	Terms for Data Storage Capacity
Size	**Byte Equivalent**
1 kilobyte (KB)	1024 bytes
1 megabyte (MB)	1024 KB (about 1 million bytes)
1 gigabyte (GB)	1024 MB (about 1 billion bytes)
1 terabyte (TB)	1024 GB (about 1 trillion bytes)

travel drive, or *thumb drive*), memory card, memory stick, and solid-state disk or drive [SSD]). To prevent flash drive data loss or malfunction, make sure to safely remove the drive after it is finished writing or reading data. Operating systems have different steps to do this. For instance, with Windows a person would use the "Safely remove USB Mass Storage Device" icon.

The capacity of storage devices is also a consideration. The storage capacity is measured in bytes. A byte is usually considered a character, such as a number, letter, or symbol. To simplify communication, the storage size is often estimated (Table 24.1). Over the years the capacity of storage devices has increased, and the cost of storage has decreased. Flash drives range in size. Some now can hold more than 2 terabyte (TB), or 2 trillion bytes.

Cloud Storage. The use of cloud storage is becoming more popular. *Cloud storage* is also called file *sharing* or *online storage*. It allows computer files to be stored using the internet and a third-party service. To get started, a person signs up with a cloud storage service. Many companies allow free minimal storage. Others charge monthly fees or fees based on storage size. After signing up, individuals use the internet to send computer files to the service company's servers. The files are copied onto many servers in various locations. This is called *redundancy*. It allows the information to be accessible even if one server goes down and needs repairs.

Cloud systems are gaining in popularity. An authorized user (e.g., an employee with a password) can access the healthcare facility's computer environment from any location with web access and through a wired or wireless connection. The access can occur at any time. For instance, a patient calls the healthcare facility's after-hours number and leaves a message with the answering service. No matter the location, the provider on call can use the cloud to access the EHR when talking with the patient.

Network and Internet Access Devices. Most healthcare facilities have their own private network, or intranet (IN trah net). The intranet allows the employees to communicate with each other and access shared files. Local intranets are generally secure because only authorized personnel can access the network.

The computers and output devices are usually all connected to the facility's private network. An intranet may be limited to the *local area network* (LAN). The local area network can span one building or multiple buildings. Some healthcare agencies have multiple locations over a large area. They may use *wide area network* (WAN) technology, which consists of two or more

LANs. LAN and WAN technology can use telephone lines or fiberoptic cables that increase the speed of transmission.

A *router* must be used to allow multiple devices to be on the same network. Most routers used today have wireless connectivity. A router is peripheral hardware that looks like a small box. Many routers have antennas and use the Ethernet (EE thuhr net). The router allows multiple computers and other devices (e.g., smart devices) to use the same network to send and receive information.

For the computer network to have internet access, the ambulatory care facility must:

- Subscribe to an internet service provider (ISP)
- Have its router connected to a modem (MOE duhm)

Most routers have a specific port that is designed to connect to the Ethernet port of a cable or *digital subscriber line* (DSL) modem. DSL is a high-speed internet service. It uses a modem to translate the computer's digital signals into voltage that is then sent over telephone lines.

Usually, healthcare facilities have a separate network for guests that provides free internet. This protects the facility's main network, which stores confidential patient information. Nonemployees should never have access to the facility's main network.

VOCABULARY

computer network A system that links personal computers and peripheral devices to share information and resources.

Ethernet A communication system for connecting several computers so information can be shared.

file A collection of data or program records stored as a unit with a specific name.

intranet A private computer network that can only be accessed by authorized people (e.g., employees of the facility that owns the network).

modem Peripheral computer hardware that connects to the router to provide internet access to the network or computer.

MAINTAINING COMPUTER HARDWARE

Larger facilities usually have their own information technology (IT) department. The IT staff provides technology assistance and helps maintain the equipment. Other facilities will use external IT support companies or train an employee to handle IT issues.

The medical assistant's role involves preventing computer problems and keeping the hardware clean. To prevent computer problems, the hardware should be located on a stable, even surface, away from heat sources. The ventilation slots should be clear, allowing air to flow into the device to cool the components. The medical assistant should ensure the cables and electric cords are securely plugged in. To prevent accidental spills, liquids and food should be kept away from the hardware.

Routine Cleaning of Hardware

Before cleaning the computer or peripheral components, turn off and unplug the device. Refer to the operator's manual for cleaning instructions.

- If liquids spill on the keyboard, unplug the keyboard. Tip the keyboard upside down to drain out the liquid. Let the keyboard dry overnight. Sticky liquids are more apt to damage the keyboard.
- Use a damp, lint-free cloth to wipe the hardware's casing to remove the grime and dirt.
- Wipe clean all vents and air holes.
- Spray a household glass cleaner on a lint-free cloth, and then wipe the glass monitor screen. Do not spray liquid directly on a component, as the liquid may drip into the device.
- Use a lint-free cloth dampened with water to clean nonglare or antiglare screens.
- Spray a disinfectant on a lint-free cloth or use a disinfectant cloth to disinfect the keyboard.
- Use compressed air dusters (i.e., pressurized air in a can) to blow the dirt out of the keyboard (Fig. 24.4).

CRITICAL THINKING 24.6

Christiana works with an information technology (IT) company that provides hardware, software, and services to the healthcare facility. How might her role with her agency's computer network differ if the healthcare facility had its own IT department?

Working with Disks

When working with a disk, handle it with care and use these guidelines:
- Hold it by the outer edge or center hole.
- Keep disks clean and dust free. Use a clean, lint-free cloth to clean a disk. Wipe in a straight line from the center of the disk toward the outer edge.
- Store disks in cases.
- Keep disks and flash drives out of sunlight and extreme heat or high-humidity environments.

Infection Control Procedures for Computer Hardware.

Many electronic devices are routinely touched by healthcare professionals and patients during the day. One study reported finding several types of harmful bacteria on keyboards. Some types could live for days or months on the keyboard surface. Another study found that keyboards in patient exam rooms were only disinfected 2% of the time, whereas the recommendation was on a daily basis.

Kiosks are being used more often in the reception area for checking in (Fig. 24.5). To help with infection control, some manufacturers are using antimicrobial coatings on kiosks and touchscreens. Some of these coatings kill 99% of all microbes. Clean Touch technology streams a UV-C light across the kiosk's touch surface for 30 seconds after the user steps away. This kills 99.9% of the bacteria and viruses on the kiosk's touch surface. Not all kiosks have infection control features.

It is important for ambulatory care facilities to have procedures for disinfecting technologic devices, including kiosks, keyboards, mice, signature pads, and styluses. Procedures should follow the recommendations from the manufacturers. Usually nonabrasive disinfectant (hospital-grade) wipes or specially made wipes (e.g., antibacterial kiosk wipes) are recommended. Some of the infection control practices for technological devices are:
- Disinfect keyboards daily. Keyboards should also be disinfected when they are contaminated with blood or visibly soiled. Using a disinfectant wipe, clean the surface using friction for 5 seconds in each area.
- Healthcare professionals should wash hands or use hand sanitizer before and after using the keyboard.
- Gloves should not be worn during computer use, unless indicated by the facility's policy.

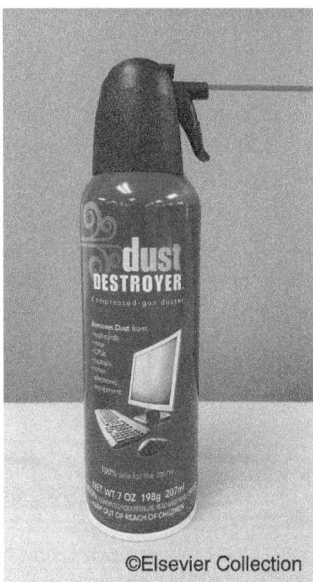

Fig. 24.4 Compressed air dusters provide an efficient means of removing the dust and dirt from keyboards.

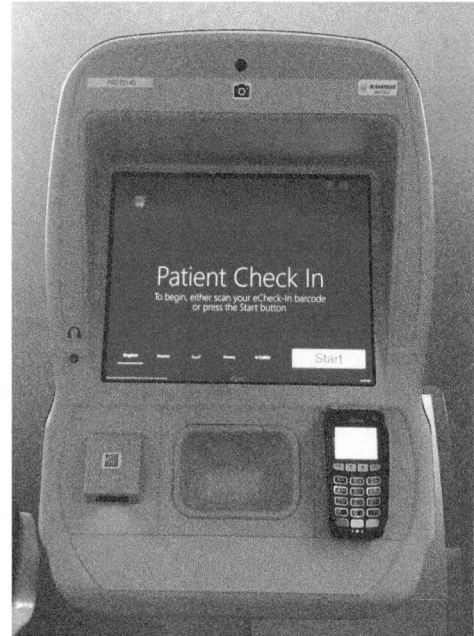

Fig. 24.5 Many healthcare facilities use kiosks in the reception area. (From Niedzwiecki B, et al: *Kinn's the medical assistant*, ed 14, St. Louis, 2020, Elsevier.)

- Touchscreen computer monitors and signature pads should be cleaned and disinfected daily per the manufacturer's guidelines. Avoid applying excessive force to screens.
- Plastic covers can be used to enclose keyboards and other devices. These covers should be disinfected daily.

COMPUTER WORKSTATION ERGONOMICS

It is important to arrange the computer workstation correctly to avoid the risk of repetitive stress injuries. Poor posture and straining can cause physical stress and injury to the body. This results in workers' compensation claims for treatment and services. Ergonomics is the field of study that involves reducing strain and injuries by improving the workstation design.

For an ergonomically friendly workstation, the following factors are important.

- The torso and neck should be vertical and in line.
- The feet need to be flat on the floor or on a footrest (Fig. 24.6A).
- The backrest should help support the upper body; the backrest lumbar support area should be fitted to the small of the back (Fig. 24.6B; see Procedure 24.1).
- The seat should be the appropriate size and height to accommodate the person's body build so that there is no added pressure on the back of the knees or thighs.
- The armrest should support the forearms with the shoulders in a relaxed position (Fig. 24.6C).
- For standing workstations, the legs, torso, head, and neck should be vertical and in line. One foot can be elevated on a step.
- The monitor should be directly in front of the person with the top of the monitor at or just below eye level.
- Use a document holder so that documents are placed at the same distance and height as the monitor (Fig. 24.6D).

- Use an ergonomic split-key or waved keyboard. Place the keyboard at a height and an angle that allow the wrists to be in a neutral position.
- The work surface and mouse should be at elbow level for typing. Your wrist should be supported by a foam wrist rest (Fig. 24.6E).
- Headsets should be used by those answering frequent phone calls to prevent muscle strain.
- Laptop computers and tablets are not ergonomically designed for prolonged use.

Whether you are standing or sitting at a workstation, it is important to change positions every 30 minutes. If you are sitting, adjustments can be made to chairs or backrests. Stretching your fingers, arms, and torso is important. Frequently look away from the computer to a distant object to prevent eyestrain. Stand up and walk around for a few minutes. Preventing repetitive stress injuries is important for all computer users.

VOCABULARY

claim An itemized statement of services and costs from a healthcare facility submitted to the health (insurance) plan for payment.

PURCHASING COMPUTER HARDWARE

In small ambulatory care facilities, the medical assistant may help the provider with computer hardware purchases. In larger facilities, the IT department purchases and installs computer hardware. If the medical assistant is helping with the purchase, identifying the equipment needed is important. Possible questions to ask when buying computers include:

- Who will use it? What will be done on the computer? What operating system and other types of application software will be required? Usually, a software indicates the amount of

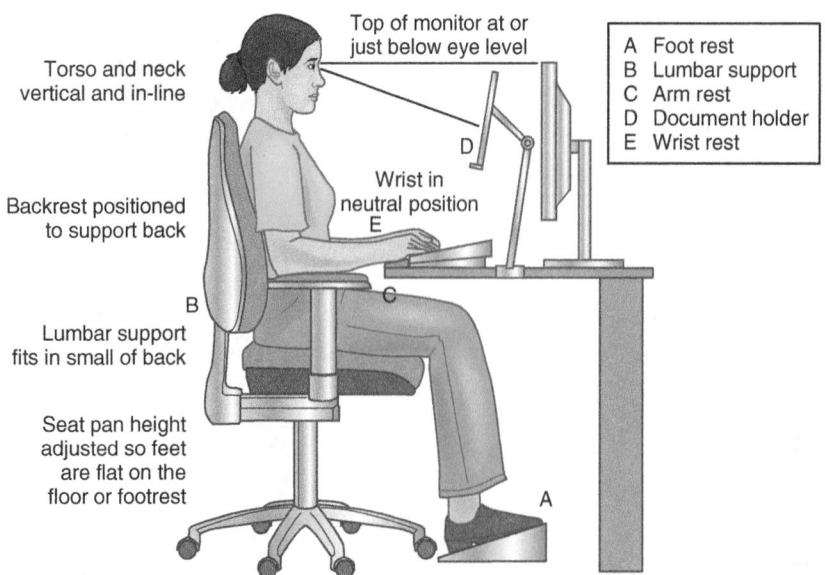

Fig. 24.6 Medical assistants should use an ergonomically correct workstation to prevent repetitive stress injuries. Equipment that helps create this type of workstation includes a footrest (A), lumbar support (B), armrest (C), document holder (D), and wrist rest (E). (From Niedzwiecki B, et al: *Kinn's the medical assistant,* ed 14, St. Louis, 2020, Elsevier.)

memory required to run it. This needs to be taken into consideration when purchasing a new computer.

- Does the computer need to be portable or will a desktop work? If a laptop is selected, will a docking station be needed?
- What size processor is needed? The larger the processer, the quicker the processor will run. What type and size of hard drive is needed? HDD (hard disk drives) are cheaper and larger, but slower compared to an SSD (solid-state drive).
- What amount of RAM is needed? RAM keeps the computer working at fast speeds.

When purchasing a printer, it is important to consider the use of it and how often it will be used. For keyboards, considerations include:

- Will an ergonomic version be needed?
- Will the numeric keyboard be needed?
- Does it need to be wireless?

> **VOCABULARY**
>
> **docking station** Also known as a *universal port replicator;* this hardware device allows laptops to connect with other devices, making it into a desktop computer.
> **interface** An interconnection between systems.

Installing Hardware

If the medical assistant is installing the computer hardware, it is important to read the directions. If you are connecting cables, make sure they are properly placed and securely plugged in. Many computers will automatically detect the connected hardware and start the installation process. Other times you may be required to load the hardware software using the installation directions.

SOFTWARE USED IN AMBULATORY CARE

For hardware to work, the computer must have software. The terms *software* and *program* are mostly synonymous. Programs existed before software. A *program* is a sequence of instructions. It is written in a language understood by the computer. It directs the computer to perform a specific task. *Software* contains several programs that together perform a function. Web browsers, email, games, spreadsheets, and word processors are all types of software.

The two main categories of software are system software and application software.

- *System software*: A collection of programs that operate and control the computer. The system software loads on the computer. It operates in the background while application software is used. Two types of system software are:
  - *Operating systems*: Act as the computer's software administrator by managing, integrating, and controlling application software and hardware. Windows is an example.
  - *Utility software*: Helps the computer function. Examples include file managers, screensavers, backup software, and clipboard managers.
- *Application software*: Also called an *application, app,* or *application program;* it allows the user or other applications to

TABLE 24.2 Types of Application Software Used in the Ambulatory Care Setting

Type of Software	Description
Antimalware software	Used to protect computers against viruses (malware), which damage the computer. An example is AVG AntiVirus Free.
Database software	Allows the user to work with large amounts of data stored in the program. Examples include Microsoft Access, practice management software systems, and electronic health record (EHR) software.
Desktop publishing software	Used to create flyers and newsletters. An example is Microsoft Publisher.
Presentation software	Used to create slides and handouts for presentations. Microsoft PowerPoint and Google Slides are examples.
Spreadsheet software	Used to manage numbers, data, and expenses. Microsoft Excel and Google Sheets are examples.
Telecommunication software	Used to email patients and vendors. An example is Microsoft Outlook, which is also a personal information manager software. Besides email, it includes a calendar, contact manager, task manager, and so on.
Word processing software	Used to compose letters and documents. Examples include Microsoft Word, Google Docs, and Corel WordPerfect.

perform specific tasks. Application software may consist of a single program or a collection of programs. A collection can be called a *software package* or *system.* In the ambulatory care facility, several types of application software are used, including practice management software and electronic health records (Table 24.2).

Practice Management Software

Practice management software (PMS), sometimes called *medical practice management* (MPM) *software,* is used to run the day-to-day business side of the ambulatory care facility. This software interfaces with the EHR software, and each must work with the other *(interoperability).* Information is passed between the practice management software and the EHR software. For instance, a new patient calls for an appointment. During the scheduling process, the person's information is entered into the practice management software. Certain elements of the person's information then move into the EHR software, creating a new health record without requiring any additional time or action on the part of a medical assistant.

Practice management software is used for scheduling appointments, new patient registration, billing, coding, and managing finances. Some of the more useful features of many practice management software programs include:

- *Claim denial management and electronic claim submission*: Insurance claims from patient visits and procedures are submitted electronically using the claim submission feature. The claim denial management feature detects errors on the claim before the submission, thus preventing rejections and a loss of revenue (REV eh noo).

- *Financial and management reporting*: This feature allows for customized reports to be made based on the business activities of the facility. Some of these reports may include the number of patients who no-show for appointments or the amount of revenue each provider brought into the business.
- *Scheduler*: This allows for customization of schedules, adding in providers' out of office times and other events. This feature is used to schedule patient appointments and procedures.
- *Medical coding or encoder*: All visits, procedures, and diagnoses need to be coded. Many practice management software programs include coding features that allow the user to easily select diagnostic and procedural codes when processing billing charges.
- *Insurance eligibility verification*: This allows the staff to verify patients' insurance benefits quickly.

Electronic Health Record and Electronic Medical Record

Many people use the terms electronic medical record (EMR) and electronic health record (EHR) interchangeably. However, there is a significant difference between these two types of software. When patients' records became electronic (or computerized), they were called electronic medical records. The EMR software contains limited information, usually related to medical treatment for one healthcare facility. The EMR was a digital version of the paper medical record.

The electronic health record has advantages over the EMR. The EHR allows sharing of information with other providers outside the facility, including medical laboratories, nursing homes, hospitals, and specialists. The information from all types of healthcare providers can be stored in the EHR, enhancing functionality and patient care.

> **VOCABULARY**
> **electronic medical record (EMR)** An electronic record of health-related information about an individual that can be created, gathered, managed, and accessed by authorized clinicians and staff members within a single healthcare organization. An EMR is an electronic version of a paper record.
> **no-show** To fail to keep an appointment without giving advance notice.
> **revenue** Money collected for providing a product or service.

Patient Portal

A patient portal is a secure online website that allows a patient 24-hour access to his or her health information. The patient needs to enter a secure username and password prior accessing the information. The patient portal may be separate software that interfaces with the electronic health record software and the practice management software. It can also be part of the electronic health record. Patient portal features vary and may allow patients to:

- View health information, such as recent visit information, medications, immunizations, allergies, laboratory results, and diagnostic imaging reports.
- Securely message the provider and receive messages from the provider and staff

- Request prescription refills
- Schedule non-urgent appointments
- Make payments and check insurance benefits and coverages
- Update personal information
- Download forms and complete online forms
- View educational materials
- Attend virtual provider visits.

Web-Based Video Software for Virtual Visits

Telemedicine has been done for years, but during 2020 the use of web-based video products grew quickly as patients and providers need additional options for visits. A variety of products are available for telemedicine, including:

- *Online video applications*, such as FaceTime and Zoom. Security is an important aspect to consider with these online video products. Health Insurance Portability and Accountability Act (HIPAA)-compliant versions are available.
- *Telemedicine specific software*, such as Doxy.me. Features vary with the products and may include:
  - No download requirements for patients. A link can be emailed or texted to a patient. The patient clicks on the link and enters his or her name, before being admitted to the waiting room.
  - Virtual waiting rooms that require the provider to let the patient in for the visit.
  - Document and screen sharing, such as lab results and consent forms.
  - Payment features.
- *Video embedded patient portal*: The patient logs into the patient portal and can access the video software for the virtual visit.

A medical assistant plays an important role in helping to make virtual visits a success. This starts with scheduling the visit. The patient needs to be given directions on how to access the software used for the visit. In most cases, the patient just needs an electronic device (e.g., tablet, PC, or phone) with internet access. The medical assistant should explain the process and what will occur. At the visit, the medical assistant will initiate the visit, much like an in-person visit. The medical assistant obtains the patient's reason for the visit (called the chief complaint), update the medical history, obtain the allergies, review the current medications, and ask if any prescriptions need to be refilled. Once this section of the visit is completed, then the provider sees the patient.

When medical assistants are working with the virtual video software, they must select a location where the patient cannot be overheard and where the patient cannot overhear others. The background the patient sees should be professional or neutral, such as a blank wall. No other patient materials should be visible. Additional etiquette tips include:

- Be punctual to the visit.
- Start by introducing yourself and acknowledge the patient and those with the patient.
- Ask the patient if he or she can hear you and see you.
- Provide the patient with a summary of what will occur during the visit.
- If working in a nonhealthcare setting (e.g., working from home), be dressed appropriately.

- Mute your microphone when you are not talking.
- Keep lag time in mind. Allow the patient to finish talking before you start talking. Usually wait about 2 seconds after the patient's last words before you begin to speak.
- No food should be visible.
- Stay in the patient's view and be mentally and physically present during the conversation.
- Keep your camera on and at eye level. This will help to ensure eye contact with the patient.
- Be professional, just like you would be for an in-person visit.
- Be clear when giving instructions to patients.
- Ask for feedback on the visit, either at the end of the visit or through a survey. This will help you improve your effectiveness and provide better patient satisfaction.

COMPUTER NETWORK PRIVACY AND SECURITY

Vast quantities of confidential information are stored in computer files. Electronic security is becoming more important today. Many healthcare facilities have had their network computer systems compromised by a hacker and malware (MAL wair). Unsecured patient and employee confidential information can lead to identity theft and other criminal actions.

The Health Insurance Portability and Accountability Act (HIPAA) and the Health Information Technology for Economic and Clinical Health Act (HITECH) require privacy, security, and confidentiality of patient records. These acts mandate training and procedures to be used in healthcare facilities to keep electronic records safe. Administrators and employees must work together to keep the computer network safe.

Security Rule

With the anticipated changes in healthcare technology (e.g., the EHR), Congress passed the Health Insurance Portability and Accountability Act of 1996. (HIPAA is discussed at length in Chapter 19.) Given the increase in electronic transactions, HIPAA included provisions for the privacy and security of patients' information. Primary provisions for privacy and security were stated in two standards:

- Standard 2 related to the Privacy Rule: Healthcare facilities, insurance companies, and others need to protect written, electronic, and oral protected health information (PHI).
- Standard 3 related to the Security Rule: Healthcare facilities, insurance companies, and others need to protect the patient information that is electronically stored and transmitted.

Of these two standards, the Security Rule will be discussed in more depth in the following sections.

HIPAA's Security Rule addresses the national standards used to protect electronic protected health information (ePHI). This rule covers the records that are created, used, received, and maintained by the covered entity (EN ti tee). Administrative, technical, and physical safeguards are required by HIPAA and are important to ensure the security of the ePHI.

VOCABULARY

business associate A person or business that provides a service to a covered entity that involves access to PHI. Examples include legal, billing, and management services; accreditation agencies; consulting firms; and claims processing organizations.

covered entity A healthcare facility, healthcare provider, pharmacy, health (insurance) plan, or claims clearinghouse that transmits protected health information electronically.

electronic transaction The electronic exchange of information between two agencies to accomplish financial or administrative healthcare activities.

hacker An unauthorized user who attempts to break into computer networks.

malware Malicious software designed to damage or disrupt a system (e.g., a virus).

protected health information (PHI) Individually identifiable health information stored or transmitted by covered entities or business associates. Includes verbal, paper, or electronic information.

Administrative Safeguards. The administrative safeguards include administrative policies, procedures, and actions to manage the security measures to protect ePHI. The facility must identify a security officer, or an employee who takes on the role to develop and implement policies and procedures that address the Security Rule requirements. The security officer has the responsibility of ensuring the facility's compliance with the HIPAA Security Rule. Besides having a security officer, the facility must have additional administrative safeguards, including:

- *Policies and procedures for assessing and managing risk to ePHI*: The facility must develop, document, and implement policies and procedures and also have a process for periodically reviewing them. Policies and procedures must address all electronic devices and programs that contain ePHI and all users who have access to ePHI. They must also address the review of information system activity (e.g., who is looking at what information).
- *Security risk analysis*: Potential computer network breach threats are identified, the likelihood of occurrence of those threats is determined, and additional safeguards are implemented. The facility should have a plan of action in place in case a threat occurs.
- *Risk management program to prevent the impermissible use and disclosure of ePHI*: The facility must protect against unauthorized or inappropriate access to ePHI. Unauthorized access may include employees and nonemployees. Policies and procedures must include disciplinary measures for unauthorized employee access. These policies and procedures are usually given to employees during orientation, and they may be required to sign a document indicating that they were notified of them.
- *Implementation of employee training*: Employers must provide privacy and security training to new employees. Periodic refresher courses are important for current staff.
- *Execution of business associate agreements*: The healthcare facility (or covered entity) must have a signed agreement from a business associate regarding security of confidential information before any ePHI can be given.

Physical Safeguards. The physical safeguards include the physical measures, policies, and procedures used to protect the computer network and related buildings and equipment from hazards and unauthorized access. These safeguards include:

- *Security policies and procedures*: The healthcare facility must implement policies and procedures that protect the agency and the equipment from unauthorized physical access, tampering, or theft. The facility should use surveillance cameras and alarms. Computers should have identification numbers and security cables for added protection.
- *Inventory of equipment*: The facility needs to have an inventory of all workstation equipment, portable devices, and medical devices that use, collect, or store ePHI.
- *Access restrictions*: The facility must limit what staff members can see on the computer based on job description. Not all staff members have the same access in software programs, such as EHRs and practice management software.
- *Workstation security*: These safeguards protect the workstation computer from unauthorized access (Table 24.3). Software such as the EHR allows each user to have an electronic signature, thus indicating what the person entered. When an unauthorized user gets access to a logged-in workstation, information can be looked at or added to the software (e.g., patient health record). Such activity will appear to be done by the logged-in employee, not the unauthorized user.

Technical Safeguards. Only authorized employees should have access to ePHI. Technical safeguards include technology and policies and procedures that protect the ePHI and access to it. These safeguards include:

- *Encryption*: Software used to encode or change the information into nonreadable or encrypted data (also called *cipher text*), thus preventing unauthorized users from reading the information. An authorized user must enter a password for decryption (dee KRIP shun) to occur and make the text readable again.
- *Data backup*: Depending on the size of the facility, the network may be backed up once to several times a day. Backing up is a process in which the network files are copied using an external hard drive, a server, or an online backup system. To protect the data from a disaster in the medical facility, it is important to store the backup files offsite. When computer data is compromised, either by errors, natural causes (e.g., floods, storm damage), or human causes (e.g., fires, hackers, and malware), the data can be restored using the offsite backup copy.
- *Cloud backup services*: Many healthcare facilities contract with cloud backup services, which copy the network data on a routine basis to protect against data loss. Cloud backup services are like cloud storage services in regard to the ability to access the data anytime and anywhere. Backup companies do not typically provide file sharing services. When computer data is compromised, the data can be restored using the backup copy. Additional technical safeguards are listed in Table 24.4.

CRITICAL THINKING 24.7

As is the case in many small healthcare facilities without an IT department, Christiana must assume a leadership role with the EHRs. She has administrator rights, which means she can assign different levels of access for the various staff members. In such a small healthcare facility, what other security measures should she consider using to ensure the privacy of EHRs? What resources might she use to implement the security measures identified?

TABLE 24.3   Workstation Security

Physical Safeguard	Description
Passwords	Each user should have a strong password, which has more than eight characters and uses a random combination of uppercase and lowercase letters, numbers, and symbols. Frequently change the password and use different passwords for different software. Do not share passwords.
Privacy filters	Devices attached to the monitor that allow visualization of the screen contents only if the user is directly in front of the screen; also called *monitor filters* or *privacy screens*.
Log-out procedures	Users need to log out of the network when leaving a workstation. A logged-in unsupervised workstation allows others to view confidential information. It can also allow individuals to document in an electronic health record (EHR) using your electronic signature.

TABLE 24.4   Additional Technical Safeguards

Technical Safeguards	Description
Audit trail	Record of computer activity used to monitor users' actions within software, including additions, deletions, and viewing of electronic records.
Authentication	Each employee with network access must log in using a unique password. The security officer should be able to see the employee's activity in the network and individual software.
Automatic log-off	After a period of inactivity, the workstation logs off.
Firewall	A program or hardware device that acts as a barrier or filter between the network and the internet. Data coming from the internet must pass through the firewall. Data that do not meet the firewall criteria are not allowed into the network.
Monitoring of log-in activity	Multiple incorrect log-in attempts are flagged, and often the account is then locked. Prevents hackers from cracking passwords.
Unique user identification	Each employee is assigned a unique name or number for identifying and tracking user identity. This allows the security officer to see the individual's activity on the system.
Virus protection software	Also called *antivirus* or *antimalware software*; used to detect and remove malware. Examples include Norton and AVG AntiVirus.

All facilities that are using EHRs and/or practice management software need to have downtime policies and procedures with related supplies available. When the network or a specific software is not available for use, the facility still needs to function. When the network or software becomes usable again, all the patient information collected during the downtime period must be entered into the system.

CRITICAL THINKING 24.8

Some healthcare facilities store network backup copies in fireproof safes onsite. Why is it important to store the backup copy offsite? What would be the advantage of using a data backup internet service that has several data storage locations around the country?

VOCABULARY

decryption The computer process of changing encrypted text to readable or plain text after a user enters a secret key or password.

downtime The interval of time during which something, such as hardware or software, is not functioning.

point-of-care Something designed to be used at or near where the patient is seen; point-of-care tools and apps are resources for the provider to use when working directly with the patient.

CONTINUAL TECHNOLOGIC ADVANCES IN HEALTHCARE

Reception and Waiting Areas

Patients are seeing more technology in healthcare settings today. Receptionists are wearing Bluetooth headsets. These headsets allow them to be more mobile when answering phone calls (Fig. 24.7). Bluetooth is a short-range wireless communication technology. It uses short-wave radio frequencies to interconnect wireless electronic devices such as phones and headsets.

For HIPAA compliance, sign-in sheets are being replaced by sign-in kiosks. Some facilities have patients enter health information using the kiosk or a tablet computer. Some clinics use a camera to take the patient's picture for identification. The health information and the photo are then added to the EHR. Receptionists have card readers to use for collecting payment from patients using credit or debit cards. The card reader machines can be mounted on the computer monitor or are stand-alone units. Many have a printer feature that allows the receptionist to present the patient with a paper receipt.

Many healthcare facilities provide patients with wristbands that have bar code technology. This practice started in the hospital and is now moving into the ambulatory care setting. The wristband is scanned before diagnostic tests are done or medications are administered. This scanning process creates an automatic entry in the patient's EHR. This process is another step in ensuring the patient's safety and accuracy in billing.

Ambulatory surgery centers and walk-in clinics use patient tracking systems in both the reception area and the patient care area. Patients sign in or are signed into the system. Their names go into the queue. For confidentiality purposes, patients may be given a unique number. As patients move from one area of the facility to another, their progress shows on monitors in the reception area. This keeps family members informed of their progress. Patients awaiting appointments or laboratory services can see their number move up in the queue or can observe current wait times. These tracking systems provide cost-effective ways to promote patient satisfaction while improving flow and efficiency.

Patient Care Areas

Many healthcare facilities are using biometrics to log into the network. There are many types of biometrics used, including facial or voice recognition, a palm vein, or a fingerprint. Biometric data is unique and is used to provide additional security to the network.

In the exam room, healthcare workers are using more technology to provide better patient care. Some clinics use wireless mobile workstations, called *computers on wheels* (COWs) or *workstations on wheels* (WOWs). Providers and medical assistants use tablets, smart devices, and wearable computing devices to access EHRs and online resources. Point-of-care tools and apps are available for providers to use in the exam room with the patients. This technology gives providers the latest clinical information. Apps are available to provide patients with visuals of surgical procedures, disease processes, and anatomic structures.

Wearable computing devices allow healthcare employees to access medical records and information while moving around and providing patient care. Mobile devices and apps help providers to make quicker decisions with a lower rate of error and improved patient care outcomes. With advances in Bluetooth smart technology, more medical equipment can work with apps on smart devices.

Because it uses diagnostic imaging to provide detailed information on internal structures, three-dimensional (3D) printing has become popular in healthcare. Implants, medical devices, and prosthetics can be customized for a patient

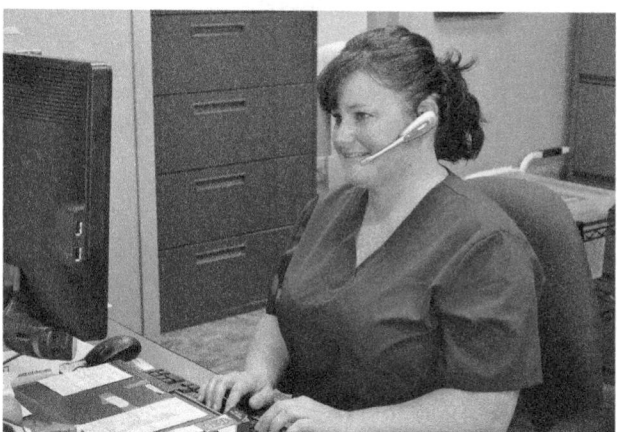

Fig. 24.7 Bluetooth headsets are helpful for receptionists and other healthcare employees who frequently answer or make phone calls. (From Niedzwiecki B, et al: *Kinn's the medical assistant*, ed 14, St. Louis, 2020, Elsevier.)

instead of using a generic model. Surgeons use 3D printing to help with virtual surgical planning. Magnetic resonance imaging (MRI) and computed tomography (CT) create detailed pictures of internal structures. An exact replica of the person's internal structures is created using 3D printing. The replica is used as the surgeons rehearse complicated surgical procedures prior to surgery.

With advancements in EHR software and practice management software, new features and programs are being used. E-prescribing allows providers to send prescriptions to the pharmacy electronically (Fig. 24.8). With voice-recognition software, providers can dictate notes directly into the patient's EHR. Computerized provider/physician order entry (CPOE) software allows orders for medical laboratory tests, diagnostic tests, and medications to be entered into the computer. With laboratory order integration, providers can order laboratory tests and the results are visible in the EHR. In many healthcare facilities, licensed healthcare providers and credentialed medical assistants use CPOE. This improves the efficiency of ordering tests and medications. Some healthcare agencies hire medical scribes. A medical scribe enters patient data into the EHR while the provider examines and treats the patient.

VOCABULARY

e-prescribing The use of electronic software to communicate with pharmacies and send prescribing information. It takes the place of writing a prescription by hand and giving it to a patient; most new or refill prescriptions can be submitted electronically, cutting down on fraud and errors.

Remote Patient Monitoring

Remote patient monitoring (RPM) or *remote patient management* is a method used to gather patient data outside of the traditional healthcare environment. Technologic devices such as smart phones, smart watches, and tablets capture patient data in one location and electronically transmit it to the healthcare provider in another location. This allows healthcare professionals to monitor patients at a distance. RPM has been shown to reduce hospitalizations and readmissions. It can provide an improved quality of life for the patient and reduce costs.

Monitoring programs involve a wide range of data from point-of-care tests. These include vital signs (e.g., blood pressure and pulse), weight, blood oxygen level, blood glucose levels, and electrocardiograms.

CRITICAL THINKING 24.9

Christiana had considered applying for a medical scribe position at a local healthcare facility before she was promoted to lead administrative medical assistant. Why would a strong background in EHR be important for a medical scribe position?

ONLINE WEBSITES FOR PATIENTS

Often, medical assistants need to research health-related topics for patients. The internet has many sites that offer information. The medical assistant must only use websites that are reliable and respected (Table 24.5). The following points should be considered in identifying reliable health websites:

- Government websites (.gov) and educational institution websites (.edu) can be trusted.

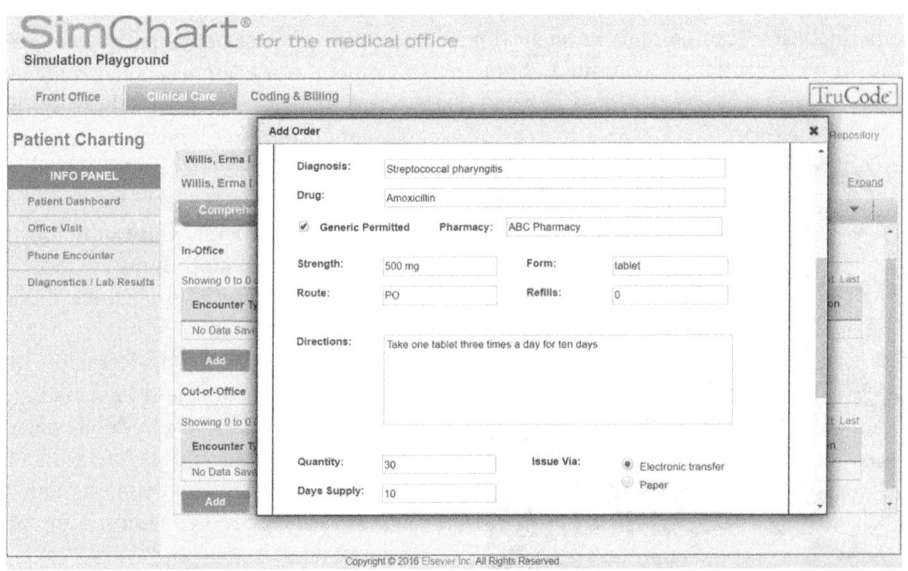

Fig. 24.8 With e-prescribing, providers can enter the prescription information into the electronic health record and send it to the pharmacy. The pharmacist can easily read the information, which reduces the chance of errors.

TABLE 24.5   **Patient Education Websites**

Organization	Website	Description
National Institutes of Health (NIH)	https://www.nih.gov/health-information	Provides information on diseases, including causes, symptoms, and treatments. Also contains Spanish-language materials.
American Diabetes Association	https://www.diabetes.org/	Provides information on diabetes, living with diabetes, food, and fitness.
	https://www.diabetesfoodhub.org/	Provides recipes, a meal planner, and other resources.
Mayo Clinic	https://www.mayoclinic.org/	Provides easy-to-read information on diseases, symptoms, diagnostic tests, and treatments.
Centers for Disease Control and Prevention (CDC)	https://www.cdc.gov/	Provides information on diseases and conditions. It is a great resource for people who are traveling to other countries.
Johns Hopkins Medicine	https://www.hopkinsmedicine.org/patient-education/index.html	Provides information on diseases, treatments, and prevention. Includes additional tools for patients to learn about managing chronic conditions.
Cleveland Clinic	http://my.clevelandclinic.org/health	Provides information on diseases, treatments, procedures, drugs, supplements, diagnostic tests, videos, and tools for patients.
Drugs.com (information comes from many healthcare sources)	https://www.drugs.com/	Provides information about medications and tools (e.g., pill identifier, symptom checker, and medication record).
MedlinePlus (hosted by NIH and US National Library of Medicine)	https://medlineplus.gov/	Provides information on health topics, medications, and supplements. Also includes health and surgery videos, health check tools, and interactive games. Offers information in more than 40 languages.
Familydoctor.org (hosted by the American Academy of Family Physicians)	https://familydoctor.org/	Contains information on diseases and conditions, drugs, procedures, and devices, along with prevention and wellness.
American Heart Association	https://www.heart.org/	Includes heart disease information, management, and prevention. Includes a tracking tool for blood pressure, weight, and exercise.
American Cancer Society	https://www.cancer.org/	Provides information on different cancers, treatment, and support.

- Large, respected healthcare and educational agencies (e.g., Mayo Clinic, Cleveland Clinic, Johns Hopkins) usually have many reliable health-related resources.
- Wikipedia is not reliable.
- If you are reviewing .com or .org websites, evaluate for bias and accuracy (see Procedure 24.2). Research the site by identifying these factors:
  - What is the mission or purpose of the website? Who supports or runs the website? Is advertising present on the website pages?
  - Is the information current or less than 3 years old?
- What is the source of the information? Who is the author of the content? Does a panel of healthcare experts (e.g., doctors, nurses) review the content?
- Do you need to provide your personal information to view the pages? If so, what will the site do with your personal information?

When the medical assistant finds information, it is important to verify the content with the provider before using the materials to coach patients. The medical assistant may also be asked by patients for reputable sites for health education literature. Having a list of reputable websites for commonly seen conditions may be a timesaver for the medical assistant.

CLOSING COMMENTS

With the electronic health record, it is easy to view one's own health record and that of family and friends. Most healthcare facilities do not allow employees to view their own health records. Viewing family and friends' health records without a job-related reason is a breach of confidentiality. *Audit trails* can be done to identify what records a person views and who views a specific patient's record. Many examples can be found in which high-profile individuals were victims of confidentiality breaches. Regardless of their position, employees have been suspended for viewing records without job-related reasons. It is important for medical assistants to remember that others can view their activities in the EHR, and the consequences of breaches can include jail time, fines, and loss of a job.

PATIENT-CENTERED CARE

One of the features of patient-centered care is coordination and integration of care. It is essential for healthcare facilities to have downtime procedures and policies when the EHR is not functioning. Most of the time, EHR system upgrades and maintenance occur outside of the normal ambulatory care hours. Unexpected downtimes during times patients are seen can create chaos if policies, procedures, and supplies are unavailable. With the EHR and PMS being used for accessing lab results, prior patient information, scheduling appointments, billing, and prescriptions, everyday tasks cannot be done.

With EHR unavailability, errors can occur, including duplicate or missed testing, duplicated or missed medications, and so on. Because patient safety is critical, the Safety Assurance Factors for EHR Resilience (SAFER) guides (https://www.healthit.gov) recommend the following practices for facilities:

- Hardware that runs the EHR should be duplicated, and an electric generator with sufficient fuel should be available to back up the EHR during power outages.
- Paper forms need to be available during downtime to replace key EHR functions.
- Backup must be done.
- Downtime policies and procedures need to include accurate patient identification and continuity of operations with regard to patient safety and critical business operations.
- Training and testing of scenarios of downtime and recovery procedures should be done.

Once the EHR system is available, all the downtime documentation and activities need to be added to the EHR. Policies and procedures must address how this should be done in a timely and accurate fashion to prevent any future issues.

BEING PROFESSIONAL

When a medical assistant is using computers while interacting with others, it is important to focus on the customer. Often, the customer feels forgotten when the employee's attention seems to be on the computer. Being attentive to our customers is important. Remember that your customers in healthcare can be co-workers, providers, patients and their family members, and vendors. It is critical that you use eye contact and body language that show your customers you are really listening. Body language that indicates listening includes:

- Turning your head and upper body toward the speaker
- Leaning forward
- Tilting your head and nodding
- Smiling (if appropriate in the situation)

Role-play this scenario with a peer: You are a medical assistant. You are working with a new medical assistant practicum student. Before the student rooms a patient, you talk with the student about the importance of interacting with the patient while working with the computer.

CHAPTER REVIEW

Types of personal computers include desktop computers, laptops, and tablet PCs. An input device is any peripheral hardware that allows the user to provide data to the computer. Common input devices include keyboards, mice and other pointing devices, touchscreens, webcams, cameras, microphones, scanners, and signature pads. The processed data is displayed using output devices. Common output devices in the healthcare setting include monitors, printers, and speakers.

The computer storage devices are categorized as magnetic storage, optical storage, and flash memory devices. Cloud storage is also called *file sharing* or *online storage*. It allows computer files to be stored using the internet and a third-party service.

The IT staff, whether internal or external, will provide technology assistance and help maintain the equipment. The medical assistant should help to prevent computer problems and keep the hardware clean. It is important for ambulatory care facilities to have procedures for disinfecting technologic devices, including kiosks, keyboards, mice, and signature pad styluses. Procedures should follow the recommendations from the manufacturers. It is important to have an ergonomically friendly workstation. The steps to make an ergonomically friendly workstation were discussed in this chapter.

There are a variety of questions to ask when purchasing hardware. For example, for computers, it is necessary to know who will be using the computer, what will be done on it, and what operating system will be used. For printers, it's important to know what it will be used for and how often it will be used. For

keyboards, you need to know if a numeric keyboard is needed, if it needs to be ergonomic, and if it needs to be wireless.

The two main categories of software are system software and application software. The system software loads on the computer. It operates in the background while application software is used. Application software allows the user or other applications to perform specific tasks. Practice management software is used to run the day-to-day business side of the ambulatory care facility. PMS is used for scheduling appointments, new patient registration, billing, coding, and managing finances. The EMR software contains limited information, usually related to medical treatment for one healthcare facility. The EMR is a digital version of the paper medical record. The electronic health record has advantages over the EMR. The EHR allows sharing of information with other providers outside the facility, including medical laboratories, nursing homes, hospitals, and specialists. The information from all types of healthcare providers can be stored in the EHR, enhancing functionality and patient care.

HIPAA's Security Rule addresses the national standards used to protect electronic protected health information. This rule covers the records that are created, used, received, and maintained by the covered entities. Administrative, technical, and physical safeguards are important to ensure the security of the ePHI.

This chapter addressed the use of technology in the ambulatory care facility, including in the reception and patient care areas and for remote patient monitoring. Technologic advances affect administrative and clinical medical assistants, along with providers.

The following points should be considered when identifying reliable health websites:

- Government websites (.gov) and educational institution websites (.edu) can be trusted.
- Large respected healthcare and educational agencies (e.g., Mayo Clinic, Cleveland Clinic, Johns Hopkins) usually have many reliable, health-related resources.

- Wikipedia is not reliable.

A list of reliable health websites was provided in the chapter. When medical assistants review .com or .org websites, they should evaluate for bias and accuracy. Research the site by identifying these factors: the mission or purpose; age of material, source of information, and the need to provide personal information.

SCENARIO WRAP-UP

Christiana has learned a great deal about the healthcare facility's computer network. She is implementing more security measures, such as training staff members to log out of their workstations before leaving the computer. She is also working with a local IT company to increase the network's protection against unauthorized users. She has contracted with an online backup service to protect the network files.

Christiana enjoys her new position and knows that she will need to stay up-to-date on technologic advances and privacy mandates. She plans to do this by reading online articles and attending continuing education events. She understands that learning is an ongoing process that will help her to become the professional she strives to be.

PROCEDURE 24.1 Prepare a Workstation

Tasks

Perform infection control procedures and create an ergonomically friendly workstation.

Equipment and Supplies

- Nonabrasive disinfectant (hospital grade) wipes, or specially made wipes for computer hardware, or wipes as indicated by the keyboard manufacturer
- Gloves (if required for using wipes)
- User guide for keyboard or facility's infection control procedure for computer hardware
- Desktop computer with adjustable monitor
- Office chair with an adjustable seat, armrest, and backrest
- Footrest (if needed)
- Foam wrist rest
- Document holder (optional)
- Hand sanitizer (optional)

Procedural Steps

1. While sitting in the chair, adjust the backrest so it supports the upper body and the lumbar support area fits to the small of the back. Adjust the seat pan height so the feet are flat on the floor or footrest. Adjust the armrest to support the forearms with the shoulders in a relaxed position.
   Purpose: The backrest should support the back. The chair height should not add pressure on the back of the knees or thighs, while allowing the feet to be flat on the floor or footrest.

2. Adjust the monitor so it is directly in front of you and the top of the monitor is at or just below eye level. If you are using a document holder, position it so it is at the same distance and height as the monitor.
   Purpose: Correct positioning of the monitor helps to reduce neck muscle discomfort.

3. Place the keyboard at a height and an angle to allow the wrists to be in a neutral position. Position the mouse so it is at elbow level when using it. Support the wrists with a foam wrist rest.
   Purpose: Supporting the wrists prevents repetitive stress injuries.

4. While sitting with your torso and neck vertical and in line, identify if everything is positioned correctly and comfortably. Make any adjustments as needed.
   Purpose: For ergonomics, the torso and neck need to be vertical and in line. Slouching is not considered ergonomically friendly and can lead to discomfort and potential injuries.

5. Using the keyboard user guide or the facilities infection control procedure for computer hardware, determine the product to use to disinfect the keyboard. Put on disposable gloves if needed. Using a disinfectant wipe, clean the surface using friction for 5 seconds in each area. Discard gloves if worn.
   Purpose: Use only the cleaning products recommended by the manufacturer or the facility when cleaning computer hardware.

6. Wash hands or use hand sanitizer before using the keyboard.
   Purpose: Hand sanitization is an important step for infection control.

PROCEDURE 24.2   Develop a Plan if Computer Access is Unavailable

Tasks

Develop a plan in the event of loss of access for more than 24 hours to the electronic health record (EHR) and practice management software (PMS) to ensure patient care and information integrity.

Equipment and Supplies

- Computer with internet access
- Word processing software
- Printer

Procedural Steps

1. Using reliable internet resources, research the Safety Assurance Factors for EHR Resilience (SAFER) guides. Focus on practices and policies to use during EHR downtime.
2. Create a plan addressing the following points:
   - Downtime: When is it called? Who is in charge? How are people notified?
   - Documentation process during downtime: Who is responsible for collecting data during downtime at the reception desk? During the patient interview (e.g., obtaining the medical history and vital signs)? When the provider examines the patient? What forms should be used? Where are the forms kept?
   - How are orders for medication, procedures, medical imaging, and medical laboratory procedures ordered during the downtime period?
   - How often are ambulatory care employees trained on downtime procedures?
   - Who is responsible for updating the EHR and the PMS with the data captured during the downtime?
3. Compose a one-page paper on your findings. Use double line spacing and a 12-point font size. Include the website you used. Proofread and spell-check your document.

   Purpose: Professional documents need to be spell-checked and proofread.

25

Written Communication

1. Recognize elements of fundamental writing skills, including guidelines for using capitalization, numbers, and punctuation in professional communication.
2. Describe each component of a professional business letter.
3. Differentiate between the formats for business letters.
4. Describe the purpose of templates in professional communication.
5. Discuss memorandums and describe the etiquette for professional emails.
6. Describe how to complete a Health Insurance Portability and Accountability Act compliant fax cover sheet.
7. Describe how to address envelopes and fold business documents for mailing.
8. Describe commonly used postal services in the ambulatory care facility.
9. Explain the medical assistant's role with incoming mail.

OUTLINE

▶ OPENING SCENARIO

Christiana Zwellen is a certified medical assistant (CMA) at Walden-Martin Family Medical (WMFM) Clinic. She had been working as a clinical medical assistant for 5 years. She helped with diagnostic tests and treatment procedures. Christiana enjoyed providing patient care, but she wanted to use more of the administrative skills she had learned. She is organized and enjoys challenges and technology. When a front office position opened up, Christiana moved into the administrative role. She is now the lead administrative medical assistant. Her role involves answering phones, scheduling appointments, greeting patients,

and processing correspondence to patients. She is also responsible for reviewing the clinic's emails. Patients are encouraged to use email to communicate with providers using the patient portal. Christiana has seen an increase in the number of daily emails. She answers those that pertain to appointments. Other emails are forwarded to the providers or their clinical medical assistants. Christiana is excited to continue to learn the administrative role.

YOU WILL LEARN

1. To recognize parts of speech.
2. To compose professional letters.

3. To compose an email.
4. To describe common postal services used in the ambulatory care facility.

INTRODUCTION

Communication has changed over the years. Many people have moved from writing letters to sending emails and text messages. Social media sites have gained popularity. Many of these changes have affected the ambulatory care environment. Patients use emails and text messages to contact their providers. To help ensure confidentiality, administrators have created tighter network security procedures. Restrictions on employee social media postings have also been added.

Today, medical assistants must be more computer savvy than ever before to meet technological demands. As discussed in Chapter 24, they must follow procedures to safeguard the privacy and security of patients' records. The need for proper grammar, punctuation, and word use is greater than ever as medical assistants communicate using letters and electronic technology.

FUNDAMENTALS OF WRITTEN COMMUNICATION

Written communication from an ambulatory care facility is a reflection on the provider and the facility. Medical assistants often compose emails and letters to patients and vendors. A poorly worded message or incorrect punctuation in a letter or an email gives the reader a negative impression of the sender, and thus the clinic. A medical assistant needs to know how to properly write a letter or message to others. It is important that the sentence structure, grammar, spelling, and tone of the message are professional.

Parts of Speech

A *noun* is a word or phrase for a person, place, thing, or idea. A *common noun* names a general group of people, places, things, and ideas (e.g., desk, office). A *proper noun* names a specific person, place, or thing (e.g., Zachary, Boston). A proper noun should start with a capital letter. A *pronoun* is a word that takes the place of a noun (e.g., I, he, she, it, and they) and is not capitalized unless it is at the beginning of a sentence (however, "I" is always capitalized).

A *verb* is a word or a phrase that shows action or a state of being (e.g., talks, walks, is, and are). The *subject* in a sentence is a noun, pronoun, or set of words that performs the verb action. A sentence requires at least one main clause, which contains an independent subject and verb and expresses a complete thought. A *fragment* (or incomplete sentence) is a phrase without a main clause and is a major error in writing. For example:

- Fragment: "Greeted patients before she updated their information."
- Complete sentence: "The receptionist always greeted patients before she updated their information."

It is important to make sure the subject and verb agree. A singular subject (e.g., provider, patient) must be matched with a singular verb (e.g., is, reads, goes). A plural subject (e.g., providers, patients) must be paired with a plural verb (e.g., are, read, go).

- Nonagreement of subject and verb examples:
  - The medical assistant talk to the patient.
  - The patients is waiting for the doctor.
- Agreement of subject and verb examples:
  - The medical assistant talks to the patient.
  - The patients are waiting for the doctor.

Many sentences also contain the following elements:

- *Dependent clauses*: Often begin with words such as although, since, when, because, and if. A dependent clause needs an independent clause (e.g., subject and verb) to be a complete sentence. (Example: The receptionist immediately notified the clinical medical assistant *because the patient felt sick.*)
- *Phrase*: A group of words without a subject or verb. (Example: A warm exam room helps keep the patient comfortable *during a physical exam.*)
- *Adjective*: A word or group of words that describes a noun or pronoun; may come before or after the noun or pronoun it describes. (Example: The *warm* room was full of patients.)
- *Adverb*: A word or group of words that answers how, where, when, or to what extent, thus further describing a verb, adjective, or other adverbs. (Example: The patient spoke *softly.*)
- *Preposition*: A word that indicates a relationship or a location between a noun or pronoun and the rest of the sentence. Commonly used prepositions include near, beside, about, to, with, by, after, and in. (Example: The student sat *beside* the receptionist.)

CRITICAL THINKING 25.1

Christiana needs to compose a letter. How can she be sure she does not have any incomplete sentences in her letter? What parts of speech are required for a complete sentence?

Appropriate Use of Words

When medical assistants compose professional communications, it is important to use language the reader will understand. Refrain from slang, generational terms, and abbreviations used with electronic communication. These can cause miscommunication with the reader. The medical assistant should know the proper use of commonly confused words and misused phrases (Table 25.1). *Homonyms* (i.e., words that sound alike) may not be identified by the software's spell-checker, which can lead to mistakes (Table 25.2). Commonly misused words and phrases include:

- Anyway (not anyways)
- Supposed to (not suppose to)
- Toward (not towards)
- Used to (not use to)

A common mistake is a mismatch between the noun and pronoun number. When referring to plural nouns, use plural pronouns (e.g., we, us, you, they, and them). For example, "When receptionists answer the phone, they need to be polite." When referring to singular nouns, use singular pronouns (I, me, you, she, her, he, him, and it). "They" has also become a singular pronoun, referring

TABLE 25.1 Commonly Confused Words

Words	Examples
As: used in comparisons *Has*: to possess, own, or experience	She is *as* fast as he is on the keyboard. The medical assistant *has* increased his keyboarding speed by using the computer every day.
Lie: to recline or rest on a surface *Lay*: to put or place	I *lie* down to sleep. I *lay* down the book.
Set: to put or place *Sit*: to be seated	She *set* the gown on the table for the patient. *Sit* on the table when you have changed into a gown.
Who: refers to people; he or she did an action *Whom*: refers to him or her	*Who* placed the order for supplies? Mike saw *whom* yesterday?
That: refers to people, things, and groups of people *Which*: refers to things or groups	The letters *that* are on the printer need to be signed. The letters, *which* are on the printer, need to be signed.
Like: means "similar to" *As*: means "in the same manner" and requires a verb	The child is *like* her mother. He works *as* a phlebotomist.
Farther: refers to a measurable distance *Further*: refers to an abstract length	The healthcare facility is *farther* away than I thought. *Further* research is needed before we purchase a new computer.

TABLE 25.2 Meanings of Common Homonyms

Homonyms	Examples
Affect (verb): to influence or transform *Effect* (noun): a result, outcome, consequence, or appearance	The outbreak of influenza will *affect* our patients. The *effect* of influenza was devastating to the city.
Accept (verb): to receive *Except* (preposition): excluding	Will you *accept* this certified letter? She mailed all the envelopes, *except* the certified letter.
Than (conjunction): used to compare *Then* (adverb): tells when	The receptionist was busier *than* the clinical medical assistant. The receptionist finished registering the patient and *then* scheduled the appointment.
There (adverb): indicates place *Their* (pronoun): indicates possession *They're* (contraction): they are	*There* were 25 chairs in the reception area. *Their* children remained in the reception area. *They're* the only patients in the reception area.
Your (pronoun): indicates possession *You're* (contraction): you are	*Your* new job is in pediatrics. *You're* working in pediatrics today.
To (preposition): indicates direction, action, or condition *Too* (adverb): means "also" *Two* (noun): number	She went *to* answer the phone. The medical assistant's phone was ringing, *too*. Her phone has *two* lines.
Where (adverb, noun, pronoun, conjunction): to, at, or in what place *Were* (verb): past tense plural of "be" *Wear* (verb): to have something on your body	*Where* did the patient go? *Were* you finished? *Wear* the gown, please.

to all people, regardless of gender and is used when the gender is unknown. When "they" is used as a subject, the verb should always be a plural, even if "they" represents a single person. The pronoun "their" has replaced the use of "his or her."

To ensure that the message is clear to the reader, make adjustments if necessary:

- Refrain from using two negatives in the same sentence.
- Refrain from using vague expressions or overusing the same words within a paragraph.
- Avoid using run-on sentences, which contain several independent clauses together without the required punctuation.

Proper spelling, use of words, and sentence structure are important because they reflect on the writer and the healthcare facility.

Capitalization

Part of composing written communication is using correct capitalization and punctuation. As mentioned earlier, errors can reflect poorly on the writer and the facility. Professional documents should contain correct capitalization, appropriate punctuation, and the right number format.

The first letter of the first word in a sentence or question should be capitalized. The pronoun "I" is always capitalized. The first letter of proper nouns, including names of people, months, institutions, organizations, countries, and national nouns and adjectives (e.g., French, British), should be capitalized. Common nouns (e.g., girls, women, boys, men) should not be capitalized unless the word is the first word of a sentence.

Punctuation

A sentence can end with one of three types of punctuation: a period (.), a question mark (?), or an exclamation point (!). Use a period for a sentence that makes a statement. Use a question mark after a direct question. Use an exclamation point for sentences that express strong emotion. An exclamation point is rarely used in professional written communication. When quotation marks are used, all punctuation goes inside the closing quotation mark (e.g., "Thank you for coming in today.").

Commas are frequently used in written communication. The rules regarding comma use include:

- Use before a coordinating conjunction (and, but, or, nor, yet, so, and for) when joining two complete sentences. (Example: The last patient left, and the receptionist locked the door.) Do not use a comma if joining a complete sentence with an incomplete sentence.
- Use to separate items in a list of three or more things. (Example: The medical assistant escorted *the mother, the father*, and *the child* to the exam room.)
- Use to separate two interchangeable adjectives. (Example: The patient was a *strong, healthy* child.)
- Use after certain words at the start of a sentence (i.e., yes, no, hello). (Example: *Yes*, the bill was correct.)
- Use to set off a name or title or an expression that interrupts the flow of the sentence. (Examples: Will you, *Michaela*, want an appointment in two weeks? I am, *by the way*, very excited about the job opportunity.)
- Use after a dependent clause that starts a sentence. (Example: *If you have any questions*, let me know.)
- Use to separate the day from the year. (Example: May *24*, 20XX)
- Use to separate the city from its state. (This rule does not apply when addressing envelopes.) (Example: *Madison*, Wisconsin)
- Can be used to separate Sr. or Jr. from the person's name, but this is not mandatory. (Example: Bob Smith, *Sr.*, has arrived for his appointment.)
- Use after a degree or title and to enclose the degree or title if it appears in a sentence. (Example: John Williams, *MD*, will be the speaker for the event.)
- Use to set off nonessential words or phrases. (Examples: Christiana, *the newest secretary*, has arrived. My brother, *Keith*, has an appointment to see Dr. Smith.)
- Use with direct quotations. (Example: She stated, "*I have waited too long.*")

A semicolon (;) is a common punctuation mark used in professional letters and documentation. The semicolon is used before certain words (however, therefore, for example). It is also used when separating phrases in a series or linking two complete sentences (e.g., "The provider is running late; however, our first two patients canceled this morning."). A colon (:) is used to introduce a series of items either in the sentence or bulleted list. A colon is also used after the greeting or salutation in a professional letter.

Quotation marks (" ") are used to set off direct quotes. They are used frequently when documenting a patient's chief complaint, the main reason for the patient's visit. An apostrophe (') is used to show ownership. To show plural possession, the apostrophe is placed after the "s" (e.g., patients').

These are the most common punctuation marks used in professional correspondence and in charting in a patient's health record. Using the correct words and punctuation marks is important when you are composing written correspondence. To reduce the risk of errors, the medical assistant should:

- Perform a spelling and grammar check.
- Proofread the document.
- Double-check the recipient's address.

Many times, the reader develops an impression of the writer, the employer, and the healthcare facility based solely on written correspondence.

Writing Numbers

A few rules apply to writing numbers. Spell out all numbers at the beginning of a sentence. Hyphenate all compound numbers from 21 to 99 (e.g., twenty-three) and all written-out fractions (e.g., two-thirds). For numbers with four or more digits, use commas (e.g., 1,234). It is not advised to include a decimal point or a dollar sign when writing out sums less than a dollar (e.g., 23 cents). Use noon and midnight instead of 12 p.m. and 12 a.m. The format for a.m. and p.m. can vary.

WRITTEN CORRESPONDENCE

Medical assistants are responsible for communicating with vendors or supply companies. They are also required to send written communication to patients and other providers, as directed by their provider-employers. Knowing how to compose a professional letter is an important skill for medical assistants. To compose a letter, you must know the correct content and location for the parts of the letter. Creating an email requires that the writer follow business etiquette guidelines.

Parts of a Professional Letter

A professional letter uses 8.5 × 11-inch paper or letterhead paper. Letterhead paper is 20- to 24-lb. bond paper (e.g., the thicker the paper, the larger the lb. bond number). The letter typically has 1-inch margins on all four sides, though shorter letters may use larger margins. The entire letter should be written using single line spacing. Consistency in line spacing is important for a professional appearance. The font should be simple and easy to read, such as Times New Roman or Calibri, in a 10- or 12-point size. Limit the use of boldface and italics in the letter.

Sender's Address. The sender's address is usually located in the letterhead (Fig. 25.1). Most facilities use preprinted letterhead paper. Letterhead can also be created at the top of the document using the word processing software's header tool. The letterhead may or may not include the provider's name. It should have the clinic's name, street address or post office box, city, state, and ZIP code. Some letterheads have additional contact information, such as phone numbers, a website address, and an email address.

If letterhead is not used for a professional letter, the sender's address is placed at the left margin, 1 inch from the top of the

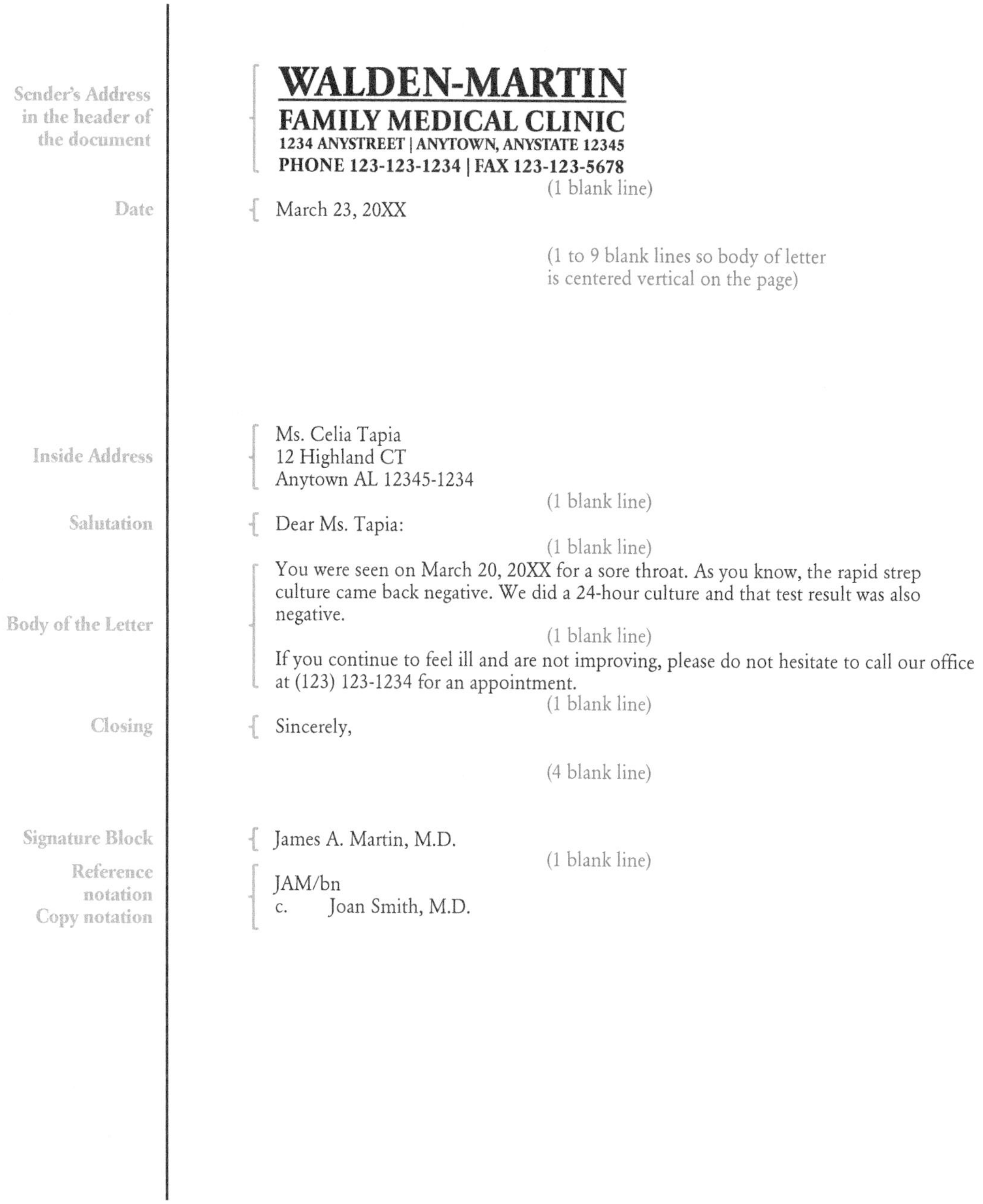

Sender's Address
in the header of
the document

WALDEN-MARTIN

FAMILY MEDICAL CLINIC
1234 ANYSTREET | ANYTOWN, ANYSTATE 12345
PHONE 123-123-1234 | FAX 123-123-5678

(1 blank line)

Date

March 23, 20XX

(1 to 9 blank lines so body of letter
is centered vertical on the page)

Inside Address

Ms. Celia Tapia
12 Highland CT
Anytown AL 12345-1234

(1 blank line)

Salutation

Dear Ms. Tapia:

(1 blank line)

Body of the Letter

You were seen on March 20, 20XX for a sore throat. As you know, the rapid strep culture came back negative. We did a 24-hour culture and that test result was also negative.

(1 blank line)

If you continue to feel ill and are not improving, please do not hesitate to call our office at (123) 123-1234 for an appointment.

(1 blank line)

Closing

Sincerely,

(4 blank line)

Signature Block

James A. Martin, M.D.

(1 blank line)

Reference
notation
Copy notation

JAM/bn
c.   Joan Smith, M.D.

Fig. 25.1 Business Letter Format. When a medical assistant types a letter for a provider, that provider must sign the letter after it has been printed. (From Niedzwiecki B, et al: *Kinn's the medical assistant*, ed. 14, St. Louis, 2020, Elsevier.)

document. Use single spacing and include the facility's address. Do not include the sender's name because that is in the closing section of the letter.

Date. All professional letters must include a date. The date is located either at the left or right margin or starts at the center point of the line (see Fig. 25.1). The location depends on the type of letter format used. When using letterhead, the date line starts on the second line after the letterhead. If letterhead is not used, the date line starts on the second line below the sender's address. In either situation, there should be one blank line between the date and the last line of the letterhead or sender's address.

When keying (typing) the date, write out the name of the month, then the number of the day, followed by a comma and the four-digit year. Make sure to have a blank space between the month and the day and after the comma (e.g., May 14, 20XX). Do not use "th" or "st" after the day (e.g., May 14th, 20XX).

Inside Address. The inside address starts between the second to the tenth line, below the date line. The placement depends on the length of the letter (see Fig. 25.1). If the body of the letter is long, leave one blank line between the date and the inside address. If the body is short, add up to nine blank lines between

TABLE 25.3 US Postal Service Standard Street and Directional Abbreviations

Word	Abbreviation	Word	Abbreviation
Alley	ALY	Road	RD
Avenue	AVE	Route	RTE
Boulevard	BLVD	Street	ST
Bridge	BRG	Terrace	TER
Bypass	BYP	Way	WAY
Center	CTR	North	N
Circle	CIR	South	S
Court	CT	East	E
Crossing	XING	West	W
Drive	DR	Northeast	NE
Estate	EST	Northwest	NW
Highway	HWY	Southeast	SE
Parkway	PKWY	Southwest	SW

the date line and the first line of the inside address. The goal is to have the body of the letter centered vertically on the page.

The inside address is always left justified. It includes the recipient's name and title on the first line. The next lines include the department and healthcare facility name. The last lines include the street address, followed by the city, state, and ZIP code. Always address the letter to a specific person. If the letter relates to a minor, address the letter to the patient's guardian. When writing out the person's name, include the person's personal title (e.g., Miss, Ms., Mrs., Mr., or Dr.). If you are unsure of a woman's title preference, use Ms.

If the inside address will be shown through a window envelope, make sure to use the US Postal Service format and abbreviations for the address (Table 25.3). The format is explained later in the chapter.

Reference Line. The reference line may be used occasionally. It starts on the second line below the inside address at the left margin. The salutation then is placed on the second line below the reference line. The purpose of the reference line is to refer to a specific item, such as a file, case number, or product number. It provides easy reference for the reader and sender (e.g., Reference: Invoice #44549).

Salutation. The salutation is the greeting. It starts on the second line below the inside address. It is always left justified (see Fig. 25.1). For business letters, the salutation should be formal. "Dear" is followed by the person's title and name and then ends with a colon (e.g., Dear Mr. Smith:). Sometime the person's first name may be added (e.g., Dear Mr. Ted Smith:). If the person's gender is not known, use the first and last name without the title (e.g., Dear Sam Smith:). The phrase "To Whom It May Concern" can be used if a person's name is not known.

Subject Line. The subject line is not used very often. The purpose of the subject line is to state the main subject of the letter. It is left justified and placed on the second line below the

salutation. The body of the letter starts on the second line below the subject line. The subject line should be composed using boldface, underlining, or all capital letters to draw the reader's attention (SUBJECT: ORDER NO. 45677-93).

Body of the Letter. The body of the letter starts on the second line below the salutation (see Fig. 25.1). The body is single spaced and either left justified or left justified with the first word of each paragraph indented based on the letter format used. There should be one blank line between paragraphs.

The body of the letter contains the content of the letter. The first paragraph is a friendly opening and states the purpose of the letter. The remaining paragraphs support the purpose of the letter and should be concise. The final paragraph may request a specific action.

Closing. The closing is positioned vertically in the same position as the date (see Fig. 25.1). There should be one blank line between the last line of the body of the letter and the closing. The first word should include a capital letter. Remaining words in the closing should be in lowercase. Typically, "Sincerely" is used; more formal closings include "Yours truly" or "Very truly yours." The word or phrase is followed by a comma.

Signature Block. The signature block includes the signature, typed name, and title of the sender. There should be four blank lines between the closing and the typed name and credentials of the sender. This space allows the person to sign the letter. The person's title is capitalized and is located on the line directly below the typed name (e.g., Director of Walden-Martin Family Medical Clinic). If the medical assistant types the letter for a provider, the provider must sign the letter after it has been printed (see Fig. 25.1).

CRITICAL THINKING 25.2

Christiana is composing several letters. Who would sign each of the following letters?
- A letter to a patient indicating her test results
- A letter to a vendor asking for specific pricing for a new computer
- A letter to a referring physician, thanking him for the patient referral

---

End Notations. Several items may be noted on the letter after the signature block. This may vary among healthcare facilities.
- *Reference notation*: Notes the initials of the person who composed the letter in uppercase followed by the initials of the person who keyed (typed) the letter in lowercase (see Fig. 25.1). A colon (:) or a forward slash (/) divides the two sets of initials (e.g., MR:bn, MR/bn). This notation should be left justified on the second line below the last line of the signature block.
- *Enclosure/attachment notation*: Indicates the number of documents or attachments that accompany the letter. The enclosure notation is left justified. It starts on the second line below the reference notation. If the reference notation is not present, the enclosure notation is placed on the second line below the last line of the signature block. The enclosure notation can be typed in several ways. It can be indicated with either "Enclosure" or "Enc." If more than one enclosure is

BOX 25.1 Suggested Styles for an Enclosure Notation

Any of the following three formats can be used to indicate that an enclosure is included with the letter:

Enclosures: 2

Enclosures (2)

Enclosures:
1. Draft of the policy statement
2. Invoice #45433

TABLE 25.4 Business Letter Formats

Letter Type	Format with Variations
Full block format	• Left justify all elements
Modified block format	• Center point *(most common)* or right justify *(rarely used)* date, closing, and signature block • Left justify all other elements
Semi-block format (or modified block with indented paragraphs)	• Center point *(most common)* or right justify *(rarely used)* date, closing, and signature block • Left justify all other elements • Indent all paragraphs 5 spaces
Simplified letter format	• No salutation or closing • Signature comes right after the body, followed by the sender's name in all capital letters • Left justify all elements

sent, the number of enclosures or the names of the enclosures should be indicated (Box 25.1).

- *Copy notation* (c.): Used to notify the letter's recipient who else received a copy of the letter. The "c" is left justified and goes on the line immediately following the last notation. It is then followed by a period. Use the tab tool to move a half-inch before typing the person's name (e.g., c. John Smith). Additional names should be aligned vertically on the document.
- *Blind copy* (bc.): Used if the sender does not want the recipient to know a copy was sent to another person. The format is the same as it is for "c.," but the "bc." is added only to the office copy of the letter. It is not listed on the letter going to the recipient.

CRITICAL THINKING 25.3

For the letters that Christiana will sign, should she include a reference notation at the bottom of the letter? Why or why not? For the letters prepared by Christiana and signed by Dr. Walden, should she add the reference notation? Why or why not?

Continuation Pages. Letterhead is not used for subsequent pages of a letter. The subsequent pages should be on paper that matches in weight and color. Each sheet after the letterhead must have a heading that includes these elements on separate lines: the recipient's name, the page number, and the date. The name should be on the first line below the top margin, and all three elements should be left justified.

Ms. Celia Tapia

Page 2

March 23, 20XX

Business Letter Formats

Four main formats are used to compose a business letter. The formats vary slightly in the position of certain elements of the letter (Table 25.4). The line spacing between the elements remains the same. It is important for a medical assistant to be able to compose a professional letter.

Full Block Letter Format. The full block format is the most common type of business letter (Fig. 25.2A; see Procedure 25.1). All elements are left justified. This means the elements start at the left margin of the document. Typically, for business letters, "closed" punctuation is used. *Closed punctuation* means the document is typed using the punctuation marks described earlier in this chapter. Closed punctuation gives the letter a professional appearance.

Informal full block–formatted letters can use open punctuation. *Open punctuation* means that minimal punctuation is used in the letter. The body is the only part of the letter that contains the normal grammatical punctuation. No punctuation appears in the sender's or inside addresses, date, salutation, and closing. This is a current trend with electronic technology and letters produced by word processing. Open punctuation should not be used with professional letters.

Modified Block Letter Format. The body and the inside address are left justified with the modified block format. If letterhead is not used, the sender's address is also left justified. The date, closing, and signature block start either at the center point of the line (most common) or are right justified (rarely used) (see Procedure 25.2). If the center point is used, all three elements must start at that point (see Fig. 25.2B). The text flows toward the right margin. The three elements vertically line up in the document. When you use the right justified technique, the text for these three elements finishes in a vertical line at the right margin.

Semi-Block Letter Format. The semi-block letter format can also be called the modified block with indented paragraphs (see Fig. 25.2C). The semi-block format resembles the modified block format with the three elements (i.e., date, closing, and signature block) starting at the center point of the line (most common) or right justified (rarely used). The difference with the semi-block format is the indented paragraph, or paragraphs, in the body of the letter. The paragraphs should be indented five spaces (see Procedure 25.3).

Simplified Letter Format. The simplified letter format is not used as often in healthcare. This format does not use a salutation and closing (see Fig. 25.2D). The signature comes immediately after the body of the letter. The sender's name is keyed in capital letters. With this letter format, the elements are left justified except for the sender's information in the header. The line spacing is the same as in the other formats.

WALDEN-MARTIN
FAMILY MEDICAL CLINIC
1234 ANYSTREET | ANYTOWN, ANYSTATE 12345
PHONE 123-123-1234 | FAX 123-123-5678

May 23, 20XX

Ms. Celia Tapia
12 Highland CT
Anytown AL 12345-1234

Dear Ms. Tapia:

You were seen on May 22, 20XX and had a hepatitis B titer done. Your titer showed that you are immune to hepatitis B.

If you have any questions, please do not hesitate to call our office at (123) 123-1234.

Sincerely,

James A. Martin, M.D.

JAM/cz
c.   Joan Smith, M.D.

A

WALDEN-MARTIN
FAMILY MEDICAL CLINIC
1234 ANYSTREET | ANYTOWN, ANYSTATE 12345
PHONE 123-123-1234 | FAX 123-123-5678

May 23, 20XX

Ms. Celia Tapia
12 Highland CT
Anytown AL 12345-1234

Dear Ms. Tapia:

You were seen on May 22, 20XX and had a hepatitis B titer done. Your titer showed that you are immune to hepatitis B.

If you have any questions, please do not hesitate to call our office at (123) 123-1234.

Sincerely,

James A. Martin, M.D.

JAM/cz
c.   Joan Smith, M.D.

B

WALDEN-MARTIN
FAMILY MEDICAL CLINIC
1234 ANYSTREET | ANYTOWN, ANYSTATE 12345
PHONE 123-123-1234 | FAX 123-123-5678

May 23, 20XX

Ms. Celia Tapia
12 Highland CT
Anytown AL 12345-1234

Dear Ms. Tapia:

You were seen on May 22, 20XX and had a hepatitis B titer done. Your titer showed that you are immune to hepatitis B.

If you have any questions, please do not hesitate to call our office at (123) 123-1234.

Sincerely,

James A. Martin, M.D.

JAM/cz
c.   Joan Smith, M.D.

C

WALDEN-MARTIN
FAMILY MEDICAL CLINIC
1234 ANYSTREET | ANYTOWN, ANYSTATE 12345
PHONE 123-123-1234 | FAX 123-123-5678

May 23, 20XX

ABC Medical Suppliers
545 Supply Ave
Anytown AL 12345-1234

Reference: PO #45938

The packing slip for this order indicated that 2 cases of non-sterile gauze sponges 4"x4", 10 packs (item #1583) were included in the box but were not. The box did contain 2 cases of sterile gauze sponges, though they were not ordered.

Please let me know how you would like to handle this situation. I can be reached at (123) 123-1234.

Thank you.

CHRISTIANA ZWELLEN CMA

D

Fig. 25.2 A, Full block letter format. B, Modified block letter format with the three elements starting at the center point of the line. C, Semi-block letter format with the three elements starting at the center point of the line. D, Simplified letter with a reference line.

TO:	Staff
FROM:	James Martin, M.D.
DATE:	December 15, 20XX
SUBJECT:	Holiday Office Hours

The office will be closed at noon on December 24, 20XX through December 26th. We will reopen at our normal time on December 27, 20XX. We will then close at 3 p.m. on December 31st for the holiday and will reopen at our normal time on January 2, 20XX.

Fig. 25.3 Format for a Memorandum. (From Niedzwiecki B, et al: *Kinn's the medical assistant*, ed. 14, St. Louis, 2020, Elsevier.)

Templates

A template is a sample letter or email that can be personalized for each patient. Many word processing and practice management software programs have prebuilt letter templates. These templates can be used, or a medical assistant can design a template. For routine communication with patients (e.g., normal laboratory results or appointment reminders), a template can be used to save time composing the entire letter or email each and every time.

Some templates allow the user to merge patient data to customize such things as the address, date of the visit, provider's name, and so on. Practice management software, the electronic health record (EHR), or word processing software can be used to merge the patient's data into the letter template. This creates an individualized letter and is an efficient method of providing a customer-friendly document for a patient.

VOCABULARY

electronic health record (EHR) An electronic record that conforms to nationally recognized standards and contains health-related information about a specific patient. It can be created, managed, and consulted by authorized clinicians and staff from more than one healthcare organization.

practice management software A type of software that allows the user to enter demographic information, schedule appointments, maintain lists of insurance payers, perform billing tasks, and generate reports.

template A document or file that has a preset format; this is used as a starting point for composing something and eliminates the need to recreate it each time it is used.

Memorandums

Memorandums, or memos, are communication documents shared within a healthcare facility. They address one topic and provide a message to the reader. Use the portrait orientation for the document, single line spacing, and 1-inch margins. Memorandums typically have four headings:

- **TO:** Include the name of the recipient or recipients and omit the titles (e.g., Mr., Mrs.). With many recipients, each name can be followed by a comma, or each name can be on its own line.
- **FROM:** Include the name of the sender of the memo. It is optional if the sender initials the memo before it is sent.
- **DATE:** Spell out the month and follow it with the day and year (e.g., May 23, 20XX).
- **SUBJECT:** Include the topic of the memo.

The headings are left justified with a blank line between each header (Fig. 25.3). Boldface and capital letters are used for the headings, and a colon (:) follows the heading. The information should be in regular font, with a mix of capital and lowercase letters (see Procedure 25.4). The information should be aligned vertically down the page, using the tab tool in the word processing software. The date should be written out as indicated for professional letters.

The headings may be separated from the body of the memo by a centered black line. The line should extend from 2 inches to the entire width of the page. Whether or not the line is used, there should be two or three blank lines separating the headers from the body of the memo. The body of the memo should be single spaced and left justified. If it consists of multiple paragraphs, skip a single line between paragraphs. The content in the body of the letter should be clear, concise, and informative. The writer does not need to add a closing or signature. Special notations, including reference, copy, and enclosures, can be added to the bottom of the memo. They should be formatted as indicated in the End Notations section.

VOCABULARY

portrait orientation The most common layout for a printed page; the height of the paper is greater than its width.

Professional Emails

The use of electronic communication among ambulatory care center staff and with patients is increasing. Medical assistants need to know how to compose a professional email (see Procedure 25.5). Following email etiquette is important for maintaining a customer-friendly environment. Tips on writing customer-friendly emails include:

- When sending the email to several people, separate each email address by a semicolon (;).
- Add an email address to the cc line if another person needs to receive a courtesy copy of the email.
- If a copy of the email needs to be sent to another person, without the recipient knowing, add the address to the bc line. Blind copying is used on a selected and limited basis.
- Make sure to include a subject on the subject line. Delete any messy FWD: or RE: RE: strings.
- Start with a greeting (salutation). It should include a formal greeting followed by the person's title and name (e.g., "Good morning, Mr. Jones," "Dear Mr. Jones,").

- Be courteous, polite, and respectful in your words and tone. Maintain the appropriate level of formality in the email. Be gracious, using expressions such as "please" and "thank you."
- Refrain from using all capital letters. Many people consider all capital letters to be "shouting" in emails.
- Write out the entire word, and refrain from using abbreviations and emoticons (emojis).
- Use proper capitalization, grammar, sentence structure, and punctuation. Check the spelling in the email before sending it. Most email software has a spell-checker.
- Be concise, accurate, and clear in your message.
- Always end your email with "Thank you" or "Sincerely" and your complete name. For business emails, include contact information after your name. The contact information should include the healthcare facility's address, phone number, and fax number.
- Leave white space (i.e., one blank line) between the salutation, paragraphs, and your complete name.
- Zip large attachments before sending the files. Zip is a computer program that compresses a file or folder, making it smaller and easier to send. The receiver uses an unzip program to extract the contents.
- Many email programs have features such as (!) urgent or a response box that sends an email back to the sender when the email is opened by the recipient. Use the urgent feature only for crucial emails.
- Forward messages with caution. When forwarding messages, always read the content and ensure no confidentiality will be breached.

Some healthcare facilities may also include language in emails related to confidentiality and whom to contact if the email was sent to the wrong address. Medical assistants must adhere to the facility's confidentiality rules when communicating with or about patients. Copies of email communications should be uploaded to the patient's EHR for a permanent record of the electronic communication.

EHR software frequently contains clinical messaging or clinical email features. This feature allows for making email within the EHR. The clinical messaging feature provides secure communication for healthcare employees to converse about the patient. For instance, the message may be sent from the receptionist to the medical assistant regarding a patient who called requesting a refill. The medical assistant can then follow up with the provider regarding the refill.

CRITICAL THINKING 25.4

Christiana answers emails from patients. How might her responses differ from her personal emails to her family and friends?

CRITICAL THINKING 25.5

Christiana receives an email from a patient that is in all capital letters. How might she perceive the situation with the patient? How could she verify her perceptions? How should she handle this situation?

Faxed Communication

Fax (short for facsimile) machines send and receive documents using phone lines. In the healthcare facility, the fax machine may be part of a copy machine, or the computers may have software that allows faxes to be sent and received. As communications technology has advanced, the use of fax machines has decreased, but they are still an important piece of equipment in the ambulatory care center.

When sending a fax, the medical assistant must adhere to rules established by the Health Insurance Portability and Accountability Act (HIPAA) and the Health Information Technology for Economic and Clinical Health Act (HITECH). Healthcare facilities usually have a required face sheet (the first sheet) that includes confidentiality language, which instructs the recipient, if they are not the intended party, to contact the sender (Fig. 25.4). The sender usually discusses how to destroy the records to maintain confidentiality. Besides the confidentiality statement, the face sheet should include the contact information for the sender and recipient, the date, and the total number of pages (see Procedure 25.6).

MAIL

Envelopes

Business letters should be enclosed in standard #10 business-sized envelopes. Standard #10 envelopes measure 4.125 × 9.5 inches. Business envelopes are available with a few variations, including the type of flap, preprinted return address, and presence or absence of a window. The window envelope and the #6¾ envelope, which measures 3⅝ × 6½ inches, may be used for billing statements to patients. The envelopes can be white, manila, or made of recycled paper.

Addressing Envelopes. When the automated mail processing machine at the post office reads the envelope, it reads the bottom line of the recipient's address (i.e., city, state, and ZIP code) before moving up and reading the next line. To ensure timely delivery, use tips when addressing mail:

- Key (type) the envelope using a simple black font of at least 10 points in size. Use all uppercase (capital) letters and no punctuation marks (Fig. 25.5).
- The address should be left justified.
- If you cannot fit the suite or apartment number on the same line as the delivery address, put it on the line above the delivery address, not below it.
- Do not write out directional and street words; instead, use the approved abbreviations (see Table 25.3).
- If using # sign, have a space between # and the number (e.g., #23).
- Put one space between the city and state and two spaces between the state and ZIP code.
- Use the 4 code along with the ZIP code (e.g., 55555-1111) as often as possible. This allows the piece of mail to be directed to a more precise location than when just using the ZIP code.
- Do not put anything (e.g., logo, slogan, attention line) below the last line of the delivery address. The machine will read it, and your letter may be misrouted or delayed. If an attention line is used, it should be at the top of the address.

WALDEN-MARTIN
FAMILY MEDICAL CLINIC
1234 ANYSTREET | ANYTOWN, ANYSTATE 12345
PHONE 123-123-1234 | FAX 123-123-5678

Fax

To: _____   From: _____

Company: _____   Phone: _____

Fax: _____   Date: _____

Phone: _____

Pages: _____

Re: _____

CONFIDENTIAL NOTICE

The material enclosed with this facsimile transmission is confidential and private. The material is the property of the sender and some or all of the information may be protected by the Health Insurance Portability & Accountability Act (HIPAA). This information is intended exclusively for the addressed person or agency indicated above. If you are not the intended individual or entity of this information, you are hereby notified that any use, duplication, circulation, or transmission of the information is strictly prohibited under state and federal law. Please notify the sender immediate using the telephone number indicated above.

Fig. 25.4 A HIPAA-Compliant Fax Cover Sheet. (From Niedzwiecki B, et al: *Kinn's the medical assistant,* ed. 14, St. Louis, 2020, Elsevier.)

Return Address
Use same format as the delivery address

WALDEN-MARTIN FAMILY MEDICAL CLINIC
1234 ANYSTREET
ANYTOWN AL 12345-1235

Postage

CELIA TAPIA
12 HIGHLAND CT
ANYTOWN AL 12345-1234

Delivery Address
1st line: Recipient's Name
2nd line: Company name
3rd line: Post Office box or street address, including Apartment or Suite number
4th line: City, State (2 letter abbreviation), zip code

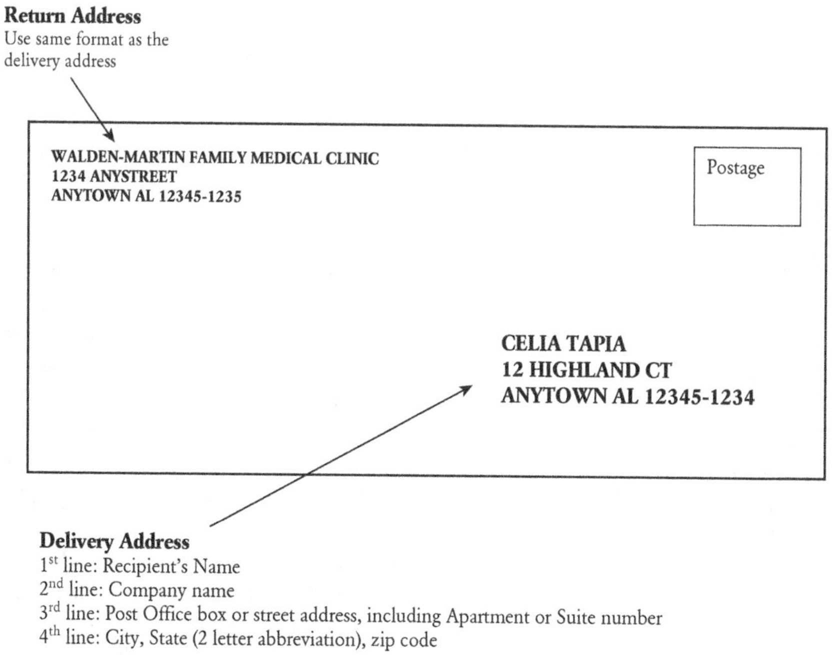

Fig. 25.5 Address Format for an Envelope. (From Niedzwiecki B, et al: *Kinn's the medical assistant,* ed. 14, St. Louis, 2020, Elsevier.)

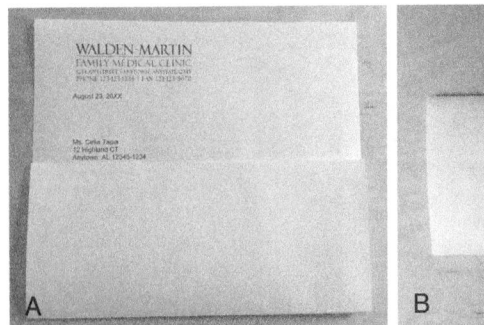

Fig. 25.6 A, For a #10 envelope, fold the bottom to just below the inside address and crease at the fold. B, Fold the top edge down to meet the bottom edge and crease at the fold. (From Niedzwiecki B, et al: *Kinn's the medical assistant*, ed. 14, St. Louis, 2020, Elsevier.)

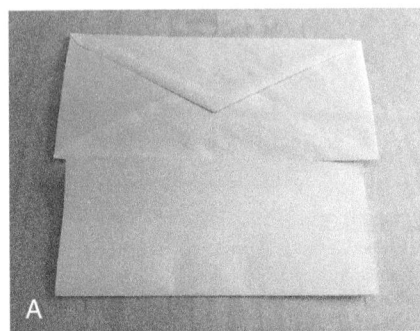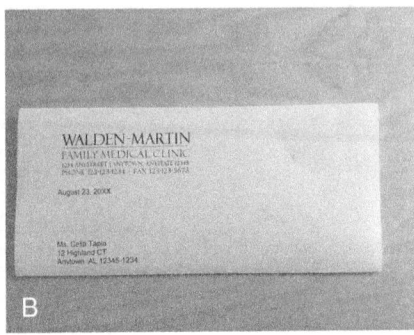

Fig. 25.7 A, For a window envelope, with the print side facing up, place the envelope over or under the top third of the letter. Fold the bottom edge up to meet the bottom edge of the envelope. Crease at the fold. B, With the letter print facing down, fold the top down to the first crease line. Crease at the fold. When the letter is folded, the inside address is visible. (From Niedzwiecki B, et al: *Kinn's the medical assistant*, ed. 14, St. Louis, 2020, Elsevier.)

- For international addresses, key (type) the name of the country in capital letters on the last line.
- Use only approved US Postal Service abbreviations.
- If using a window envelope, the address should start and end at least ⅛" from the edge of the window.

Folding Documents. Depending on the envelope size, the folding process may be different. It is important to fold the document neatly, as this is seen by the reader.

When using a #10 envelope, fold the letter by pulling up the bottom end until it reaches just below the inside address or two-thirds of the way up the letter (Fig. 25.6). Crease at the fold. Then, fold the top of the letter down so that it is flush with the bottom fold and crease the paper. For window business envelopes, fold the letter in a Z pattern. With the letter's print side facing up, place the envelope over or under the top third of the letter (Fig. 25.7). Fold the bottom edge of the paper up to the bottom edge of the envelope and crease at the fold. Then, remove the envelope and flip the letter over so the backside of the document is facing up. Fold the top of the letter down to the prior crease line and crease at the fold. The letterhead and recipient's addresses should then be visible. Place the letter in the envelope so that the recipient's address shows through the window.

For a #6½ envelope, fold the letter by pulling up the bottom end until it is ½ inch from the top edge of the document (Fig. 25.8). Crease at the fold. Then, fold the document vertically starting at the right edge. Bring the right edge two-thirds of the way across the width of the document and crease the paper. Then bring the left edge to the right edge and crease at the fold. Flip the document so the left edge is on the bottom and insert into the envelope.

> **VOCABULARY**
> **zone** A region or geographic area used for shipping.

Postage

After addressing the envelope, you must add postage prior to mailing the letter. The postage depends on the weight, size, urgency for arrival, delivery zone, and services required (Table 25.5). For the ambulatory care facility, there are several postage options for mailings:

- Print postage labels on the US Postal Service (USPS) website (https://www.USPS.com/): Priority Mail Express and Priority Mail shipping labels can be printed on the facility's printer.
- Permit imprints: Used for bulk mailing (200 or more envelopes); requires a fee and permit. Print postage information on the envelope and pay for postage when mailing is sent.
- Precanceled stamps: Complete permit, place precanceled stamps on envelopes, and mail. Cannot return unused stamps.

 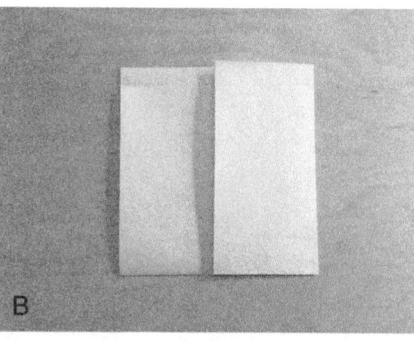 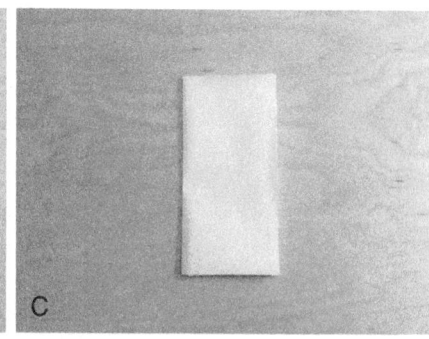

Fig. 25.8 A, For a #6¾ envelope, bring the bottom edge of the document to ½ inch from the top edge. Crease at the fold. B, Fold the document vertically. Bring the right edge two-thirds of the way across the width of the document and crease the paper. C, Bring the left edge to the right edge and crease at the fold. (From Niedzwiecki B, et al: *Kinn's the medical assistant,* ed. 14, St. Louis, 2020, Elsevier.)

TABLE 25.5 US Postal Service Domestic Shipping Sizes

Domestic Shipping	Height (Inches)	Length (Inches)	Maximum Thickness (Inches)
Postcard	3.5–4.25	5–6	0.016
Letter	3.5–6.125 (61/8)	5–11.5	0.25
Large envelopes	6.125–12	11.5–15	0.75
Packages	Maximum length plus girth: 108 inches (130 inches for standard post).		

TABLE 25.6 Summary of the US Postal Service's Domestic Services

Postage Options	Description
Priority mail express	Very expensive; 7-days-a-week delivery service with guaranteed overnight scheduled delivery. Insurance is included. For letters and packages up to 70 lb. Cost based on weight and delivery zone. Flat rate envelopes available.
Priority mail	Expensive; delivery within 3 days. Insurance is included. For letters and packages up to 70 lb. Cost based on weight and delivery zone. Flat rate boxes available.
First-class mail	Most commonly used service. Provides delivery in 3 days or less. For envelopes and packages weighing up to 13 oz. Cost based on size, shape, and weight. Add-on services are available for an extra fee.
USPS retail ground	Delivery in 2–8 days. Used for oversized packages weighing up to 70 lb and measuring up to 130 inches in combined girth and length. Cost based on weight, shape, and delivery zone.
Media mail	Use for sending books, electronic media, and educational material, with delivery in 2–8 days. Cost based on weight.

- Postage meter printing: Lease a postage meter, pay the fee, and print postage directly on the mail or on a meter tape.

The USPS website (http://www.usps.com/) provides valuable resources for addressing and shipping mail. It allows you to buy stamps, schedule a pickup, calculate the shipping costs, look up ZIP codes, and track sent mail.

The medical assistant will use different types of mail services for the healthcare facility's business. It is crucial to understand the different services. For routine mail, the healthcare facility will use First-Class Mail. Table 25.6 summarizes the USPS domestic services available.

The USPS also has a host of optional services that can be added to the standard services for an additional fee. Table 25.7 summarizes additional services available. It is important to note that healthcare facilities use certified mail and return receipt. When using certified mail combined with return receipt, the facility gets a mailing receipt showing the date when the item was mailed. It also gets additional information on when the delivery occurred and the recipient's signature. Many state laws mandate that termination letters be sent by certified mail with return receipt (Fig. 25.9A). The mailing receipt, the return receipt, and a copy of the letter are uploaded into the EHR or filed in the paper medical record (Fig. 25.9B). These items provide proof the law was followed if there is ever a question. For a complete list of services, refer to the USPS website.

VOCABULARY

authorized agent A person who has written documentation that they can accept a shipment for another individual.

bonded A term describing employees for whom an employer has obtained a fidelity bond from an insurance company, which will cover losses from any dishonest acts (e.g., embezzlement, theft) committed by those employees.

girth The measurement around something; when referring to mail, it is the measurement around the middle of the package that is being shipped.

media Types of communication (e.g., social media sites); with computers, the term refers to data storage devices.

termination letters Documents sent to patients explaining that the provider is ending the physician-patient relationship and the patient needs to see other providers.

TABLE 25.7   Optional Services Provided by the US Postal Service

Optional Service	Description
Standard insurance	Protects against loss or damage. Cost is based on the item's declared value.
Registered mail	Used to protect expensive items. Mailed item can be insured up to the maximum amount. A mailing receipt is given; upon request, an electronic verification of delivery or delivery attempt can be sent.
Certified mail	Mailing receipt provides evidence the letter was mailed and, combined with the return receipt, shows delivery information and the recipient's signature.
Signature confirmation	Provides date and time of delivery or when delivery attempt was made, along with the recipient's signature. Copy of delivery record is available upon request.
Return receipt	Provides an automatic electronic or mailed delivery record showing the recipient's signature.
Adult signature restricted delivery	Addressee or authorized agent must verify identity and age (i.e., must be over 21); must sign for delivery.
Restricted delivery	Addressee or authorized agent must verify identity and must sign for delivery.
Certificate of mailing	Provides evidence (i.e., date and time) when an item was mailed. (Limited service because it does not provide evidence of the delivery.)
US Postal Service tracking	Provides updates as an item is being shipped. Will include date and time of delivery or attempted delivery.
Special handling	Used to get preferential handling when shipping very unusual items or items that need extra care.
Collect on delivery (COD)	Recipient pays for merchandise and shipping when the package is received.
Hold for pickup	Option to pick up item from a specified post office within 15 days, depending on service selected.

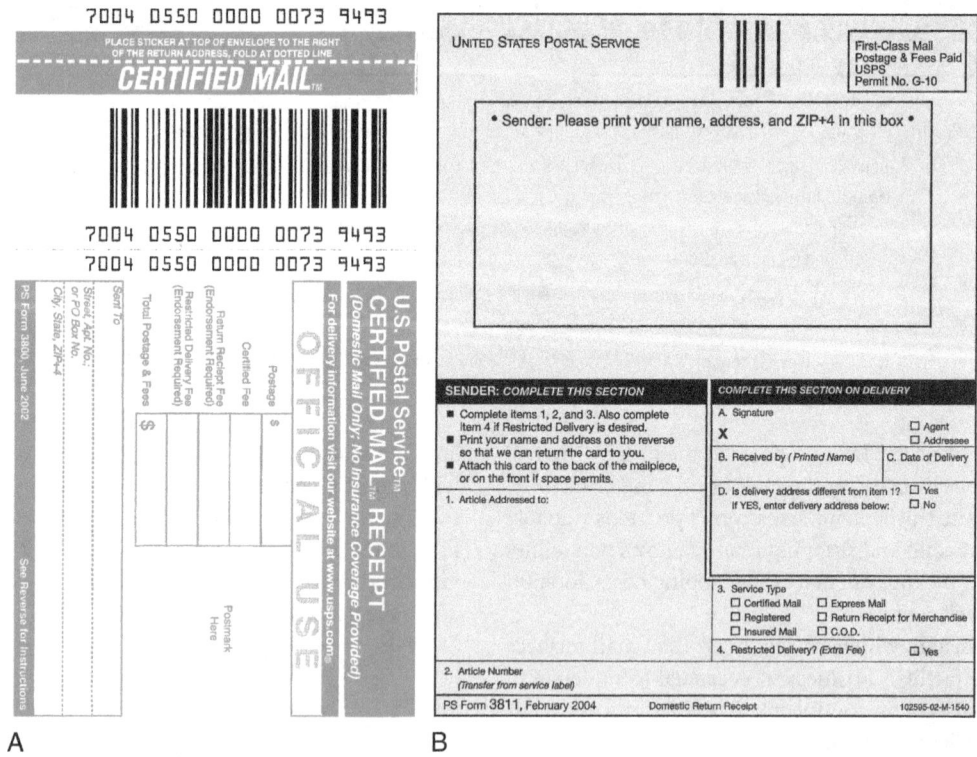

Fig. 25.9 A, Receipt for certified mail. Attach the bottom portion of the receipt to the top of the package or envelope, just to the right of the return address. B, Return receipt used to provide an automatic electronic or hardcopy record showing the recipient's signature. (From Niedzwiecki B, et al: *Kinn's the medical assistant*, ed. 14, St. Louis, 2020, Elsevier.)

Private Delivery Services

The USPS only handles a portion of the mail delivered in the United States. Private companies have grown by offering competitive rates and additional services compared with USPS. Some companies provide national and international services, but others are more locally based. FedEx, UPS, and DHL are very popular national options for shipping letters and packages. Some offer onsite pickup.

Larger cities have courier services that have become popular options for local deliveries. Some companies have drivers who are bonded and trained to handle all aspects of delivery from medical to hazardous deliveries. Some of the services provided include:

- Pickup and delivery of medical specimens (e.g., they take patient laboratory samples to a medical laboratory for testing)
- Transportation of health records and documents from one location to another, complying with HIPAA requirements
- Pickup and delivery of deposits to the bank, with return of cash if requested

The goal for the healthcare facility is to use a mail/courier company that provides the most efficient service at the best price. The medical assistant may have to research the delivery services available in the area to identify the best fit for the facility.

CRITICAL THINKING 25.6

The providers would like to use an offsite laboratory to process specimens. Christiana would like to have a local courier service pick up specimens and deliver them to the offsite laboratory. When researching potential delivery couriers for this activity, what factors should Christiana consider?

Incoming Mail

The medical assistant's responsibility with incoming mail will vary. In large facilities, designated mailroom employees handle incoming mail, and the mail is delivered to each department. The administrative medical assistant sorts the department mail. In smaller facilities, the medical assistant handles all aspects of the incoming mail.

Mail can be collected at the post office or be delivered to the healthcare facility. The medical assistant must sort the mail following the facility's procedure for incoming mail. Providers may request the incoming mail be placed on their desks. In larger departments, mailboxes are used for each person in the department. The medical assistant can easily sort the mail and place it in the individual mailboxes. The mailboxes need to be safe and secure. They should not be in a patient care area.

If there is a question as to who should get a piece of mail, it is important to ask. If there is a question about opening something, it is better to not open it and ask the provider or office manager. If mail is accidentally opened that should not have been, the medical assistant should tape the envelope shut. A note should be included with the envelope to indicate that it was accidentally opened. The note should include the name of the person who opened it and the date. The facility will have a procedure for handling the mail while the provider is on vacation.

CRITICAL THINKING 25.7

Christiana sorts the mail for the healthcare facility. Because the facility is small, the staff does not use the mailbox system. Mail has gotten lost after she placed it on the providers' desks. What other options can Christiana implement to prevent mail from getting lost or misplaced on the providers' desks?

CLOSING COMMENTS

When sending letters and emails to patients, the medical assistant must ensure that a copy is added to the patient's health record. If a copy is not added to the record, then it appears that the patient was never sent a letter or an email. Legally this can be a major issue for the healthcare facility. Having a "paper trail" of communication to the patient helps to provide evidence that the staff notified the patient about test results and updates in the patient care plan.

PATIENT-CENTERED CARE

When patients are having a diagnostic test, it is important to let the patient know prior to the test when they will be given the results. It is also helpful to patients to let them know if the communication will be via a phone call, an email, or a letter. When a patient may receive a potentially life-changing diagnosis, waiting for the news is stressful. The medical assistant should help to ensure that test results are given to the patient as soon as possible and in the manner the patient was told they would be (e.g., via an email or a call).

BEING PROFESSIONAL

When a medical assistant is communicating by email, it is important to watch their tone. Sharp phrases or capitalizing complete words can give the reader a sense that the sender is yelling. The medical assistant should:

- Always maintain a professional tone throughout the letter or email, even if the patient did not originally.
- Have another staff member read an email if the medical assistant is concerned that the message may be perceived in a manner other than what is intended.
- Never send an email response when not in the office or when angry. Wait until strong emotions have calmed down before sending an email. Often it is hard to be professional when one is emotional.

Role-play this scenario with a peer: You and Zach are medical assistants. Zach received an email from a patient with many words in all capital letters. By the tone of the email, Zach states he believes the patient is frustrated at not receiving lab work results, but the lab work results are still not available. Zach wants advice from you on how he should reply to the patient.

CHAPTER REVIEW

This chapter reviewed the parts of speech, including nouns, verbs, subjects, adjectives, adverbs, and so on. It is important to write using complete sentences and not fragments. The medical assistant should know the proper use of commonly confused words and misused phrases.

Part of composing written communication is using correct capitalization and punctuation. Proper nouns, "I," and the first letter of the first word of a sentence or question need to be capitalized. The chapter content also discussed the correct uses for punctuation. Lastly, the medical assistant should remember the rules of writing numbers, including hyphenating all compound numbers from 21 to 99 and spelling out all numbers at the beginning of a sentence.

Components of the professional business letter include:
- Sender's address: Usually in the letterhead of the document.
- Date: Needs to be written out using the month, day, and year format.
- Inside address: Includes the recipient's name, title, and address.
- Reference line: Used occasionally to refer to a specific item (e.g., case number).
- Salutation: The greeting needs to be formal for business letters.
- Subject line: Used occasionally to state the main subject of the letter.
- Body of the letter: Contains the message.
- Closing: Usually "sincerely" is used.
- Signature block: Provides information on the sender, including the signature, typed name, and title.
- End notations, which include:
  - Reference notation: The initials of the sender are followed by the initials of the person who keyed the letter. A colon or forward slash separates the initials.
  - Enclosure/attachment notation: Indicates the number of documents or attachments that accompany the letter.
  - Copy notation: Indicates who received a copy of the letter.
  - Blind copy: Indicates who received a blind copy of the letter; only shown on the office copy of the letter.

Four types of business letter formats include full block, modified block, semi-block, and simplified.

Memorandums, or memos, are communication documents shared within a healthcare facility. They address one topic and provide a message to the reader. They typically have four headings: to, from, date, and subject.

When sending a fax, the medical assistant must adhere to HIPAA and HITECH rules. Healthcare facilities usually have a required face sheet (the first sheet) that includes confidentiality language, which instructs the recipient, if they are not the intended party, to contact the sender. See Procedure 25.6 for details on completing a HIPAA-compliant fax cover sheet.

When addressing an envelope, type the address using a simple black font of at least 10 points in size. Always put one space between the city and state and two spaces between the state and ZIP code. Use only US Postal Service abbreviations.

Procedures 25.1 through 25.3 discuss how to fold a document when using a #10 envelope. Procedure 25.2 discusses how to fold a letter when using a window envelope. Procedure 25.3 discusses how to fold a letter when using a #10 or #6¾ envelope.

The medical assistant will use different types of mail services for the healthcare facility's business. For routine mail, the healthcare facility will use First-Class Mail. Table 25.6 summarizes USPS domestic services available. It is important to note that healthcare facilities use certified mail and return receipt. When using certified mail combined with return receipt, the facility gets a mailing receipt showing the date when the item was mailed. Many state laws mandate that termination letters be sent by certified mail with return receipt.

The medical assistant's responsibility with incoming mail will vary. In large facilities, designated mailroom employees handle incoming mail, and the mail is delivered to each department. The administrative medical assistant sorts the department mail. In smaller facilities, the medical assistant handles all aspects of the incoming mail.

SCENARIO WRAP-UP

Since her promotion, Christiana has learned many helpful administrative procedures. She has also been implementing changes in the administrative area. Her first change was to e-mail, rather than mail, appointment reminders. She uses the appointment reminder feature of the practice management software when e-mailing the notifications to patients. Not only does this save time, but it also saves postage costs. Christiana has also learned how to create letter and memo templates. She uses templates to notify patients about laboratory and diagnostic test results. She continues to create custom letters for patients, yet she saves time by using predesigned templates. Christiana enjoys her new position, and she understands that learning is an ongoing process that will help her to become the professional she strives to be.

PROCEDURE 25.1 Compose a Professional Business Letter Using the Full Block Letter Format

Tasks

Compose a professional letter using technology. Use the full block letter format and closed punctuation. Address the envelope and fold the letter.

Scenario

Jean Burke, NP (nurse practitioner), has requested that you compose a letter to the parent (Lisa Parker) of Johnny Parker (date of birth [DOB]: 06/15/20XX) to let her know that Johnny's throat culture from last Wednesday was negative. If he is not improving or if she has any questions, she should call the office. Lisa Parker's address is 91 Poplar Street, Anytown, AL 12345-1234. You are working at Walden-Martin Family Medical Clinic. The healthcare facility's address is 1234 Anystreet, Anytown, AL 12345. The phone number is 123-123-1234, and the fax number is 123-123-5678.

Equipment and Supplies

- Patient's health record
- Computer with word processing software and printer
- Paper
- #10 envelope

Procedural Steps

1. Obtain the intended recipient's contact information and determine the message you want to convey. Using the computer and word processing software, compose the letter using the full block letter format. Use 1-inch margins on all four sides, portrait orientation, and single line spacing throughout the letter. Use an easy-to-read font (e.g., Times New Roman or Calibri) in a 10- or 12-point size.
   Purpose: Determining the message gives you a focus when composing the letter. You will need the recipient's information to create the letter.
2. Create a letterhead in the header of the document. Include the clinic's name, street address or post office box, city, state, and ZIP code.
   Purpose: The information in the letterhead provides the reader contact information for the clinic.
3. Key (type) the date starting at the left margin. Have one blank line between the date line and the last line of the letterhead.
   Purpose: All letters require a date for legal purposes.
4. Key the inside address starting at the left margin and use the correct spelling and punctuation. Leave one to nine blank lines between the date and the inside address, in order to center the body of the letter on the page.
   Purpose: The body of the letter must be centered vertically from the top to the bottom of the document. More blank lines can be added to move the body to the correct location.

5. Key the salutation starting at the left margin and use the correct spelling and punctuation. Leave one blank line between the inside address and the salutation.
   Purpose: A proper greeting sets the tone of the letter.
6. Use your critical thinking skills to compose a concise, accurate message. Type the message in the body of the letter starting at the left margin. Leave one blank line between the salutation and the first line of the body and then between each paragraph of the body. The message should be clear, concise, and professional. Use proper grammar, punctuation, capitalization, and sentence structure.
   Purpose: Proper grammar helps to convey the message accurately and professionally.
7. Key a proper closing starting at the left margin and use correct spelling and punctuation. Leave one blank line between the last line of the body and the closing.
   Purpose: The closing helps end the message with a professional tone.
8. Key the signature block starting at the left margin and use the correct spelling and punctuation. Leave four blank lines between the closing and the signature block. If you are preparing the letter for a provider, you must include a reference notation.
   Purpose: The signature block provides the reader with the name of the sender of the letter. The reference notation identifies who typed the letter.
9. Spell-check and proofread the document. Check for the proper tone, grammar, punctuation, capitalization, and sentence structure. Check for proper spacing between the parts of the letter. Make any final corrections. Print the document.
   Purpose: The spell-checker identifies only certain errors; proofreading helps you find incorrect word use, improper tone, and errors in formatting.
10. Address the envelope, using either the computer and word processing software or a pen and following the correct format.
    Purpose: Following the Postal Service guidelines on format helps prevent a delay in delivery of the letter.
11. When using a #10 envelope, fold the letter by pulling up the bottom end until it reaches just below the inside address or two-thirds of the way up the letter. Crease at the fold. Then, fold the top of the letter down so that it is flush with the bottom fold and crease the paper.
    Note: If the provider needs to sign the letter, the letter is folded afterward.
    Purpose: The letter must be neatly folded.
12. File a copy of the letter in the paper medical record or upload an electronic copy of the letter to the electronic health record (EHR).
    Purpose: A copy of all correspondence should be kept in the patient's health record.

PROCEDURE 25.2 Compose a Professional Business Letter Using the Modified Block Letter Format

Tasks

Compose a professional letter using technology. Use the modified block letter format (with the center point option). Address the envelope (if needed) and fold the letter.

Scenario

Julie Walden, MD, has requested that you compose a letter to Carl C. Bowden (DOB: 04/05/19XX) to let him know that his hepatitis C laboratory test was negative. If he has any questions, he should call the office. His address is 19 Beale Street, Anytown, AL 12345-1234. You are working at Walden-Martin

Family Medical Clinic. The healthcare facility's address is 1234 Anystreet, Anytown, AL 12345. The phone number is 123-123-1234, and the fax number is 123-123-5678.

Equipment and Supplies

- Patient's health record
- Computer with word processing software and printer
- Paper
- #10 envelope or window business envelope

Continued

PROCEDURE 25.2 Compose a Professional Business Letter Using the Modified Block Letter Format—cont'd

Procedural Steps

1. Obtain the intended recipient's contact information and determine the message you want to convey. Using the computer and word processing software, compose the letter using the modified block letter format. Use 1-inch margins on all four sides, portrait orientation, and single line spacing throughout the letter. Use an easy-to-read font (e.g., Times New Roman or Calibri) in a 10- or 12-point size.

   Purpose: Determining the message gives you a focus when composing the letter. You will need the recipient's information to create the letter.

2. Create a letterhead in the header of the document. Include the clinic's name, street address or post office box, city, state, and ZIP code.

   Purpose: The information in the letterhead provides the reader contact information for the clinic.

3. Key (type) the date starting at the center point of the line, which is usually about 3.25 inches from the margin. Have one blank line between the date line and the last line of the letterhead.

   Note: Starting the text at the center point is not the same as the text being centered on the line. When starting the text at the center point, the text flows towards the right margin.

   Purpose: All letters require a date for legal purposes.

4. Key the inside address starting at the left margin and use the correct spelling and punctuation. Leave one to nine blank lines between the date and the inside address in order to center the body of the letter on the page. If using a window business envelope, adjust the address position to fit the window.

   Purpose: The body of the letter must be centered vertically from the top to the bottom of the document. More blank lines can be added to move the body to the correct location.

5. Key the salutation starting at the left margin and use the correct spelling and punctuation. Leave one blank line between the inside address and the salutation.

   Purpose: A proper greeting sets the tone of the letter.

6. Use your critical thinking skills to compose a concise, accurate message. Type the message in the body of the letter starting at the left margin. Leave one blank line between the salutation and the first line of the body and then between each paragraph of the body. The message should be clear, concise, and professional. Use proper grammar, punctuation, capitalization, and sentence structure.

   Purpose: Proper grammar helps to convey the message accurately and professionally.

7. Key a proper closing. Start the closing at the center point of the line. (The first letter of the closing should align vertically with the first letter of the date.) Use correct spelling and punctuation. Leave one blank line between the last line of the body and the closing.

   Purpose: The closing helps end the message with a professional tone.

8. Key the signature block. Start the signature block at the center point of the line. (The first letter of the signature block should align vertically with the first letter of the date and closing.) Use the correct spelling and punctuation. Leave four blank lines between the closing and the signature block. If you are preparing the letter for a provider, you must include a reference notation.

   Purpose: The signature block provides the reader with the name of the sender of the letter. The reference notation identifies who typed the letter.

9. Spell-check and proofread the document. Check for the proper tone, grammar, punctuation, capitalization, and sentence structure. Check for proper spacing between the parts of the letter. Make any final corrections. Print the document. If needed, address the envelope, using either the computer and word processing software or a pen and following the correct format.

   Purpose: The spell-checker identifies only certain errors; proofreading helps you find incorrect word use, improper tone, and errors in formatting.

10. When using a #10 envelope, fold the letter by pulling up the bottom end until it reaches just below the inside address or two-thirds of the way up the letter. Crease at the fold. Then, fold the top of the letter down so that it is flush with the bottom fold and crease the paper. For window business envelopes, have the letter's print side facing up and place the envelope over the top third of the letter. Fold the bottom edge of the paper up to the bottom edge of the envelope and crease at the fold. Then, remove the envelope and flip the letter over and fold the top of the letter down to the prior crease line and crease at the fold. Place the letter in the envelope so that the recipient's address shows through the window.

    Note: If the provider needs to sign the letter, the letter is folded afterwards.

    Purpose: The letter must be neatly folded.

11. File a copy of the letter in the paper medical record or upload an electronic copy of the letter to the electronic health record (EHR).

    Purpose: A copy of all correspondence should be kept in the patient's health record.

PROCEDURE 25.3 Compose a Professional Business Letter Using the Semi-Block Letter Format

Tasks

Compose a professional letter using technology. Use the semi-block letter format (with the center point option). Address the envelope and fold the letter.

Scenario

Julie Walden, MD, has requested that you compose a letter to Amma Patel (DOB 01/14/19XX) to let her know that her thyroid test was normal, but her vitamin D level was low. Dr. Walden would like Amma to take 15 mcg of vitamin D each morning. She can purchase this over the counter. She needs to have her vitamin D rechecked in 6 months. She can call to schedule a blood test closer to that time. If she has any questions, she should call the office. Her address is 1346 Charity Lane, Anytown, AL 12345-1234. You are working at Walden-Martin Family Medical Clinic. The healthcare facility's address is 1234 Anystreet, Anytown, AL 12345. The phone number is 123-123-1234, and the fax number is 123-123-5678.

Equipment and Supplies

- Patient's health record
- Computer with word processing software and printer
- Paper
- #10 envelope or #6¾ envelope

Procedural Steps

1. Obtain the intended recipient's contact information and determine the message you want to convey. Using the computer and word processing software, compose the letter using the semi-block letter format. Use 1-inch margins on all four sides, portrait orientation, and single line spacing throughout the letter. Use an easy-to-read font (e.g., Times New Roman or Calibri) in a 10- or 12-point size.

   Purpose: Determining the message gives you a focus when composing the letter. You will need the recipient's information to create the letter.

2. Create a letterhead in the header of the document. Include the clinic's name, street address or post office box, city, state, and ZIP code.
   Purpose: The information in the letterhead provides the reader contact information for the clinic.

3. Key (type) the date starting at the center point of the line, which is usually about 3.25 inches from the margin. Have one blank line between the date line and the last line of the letterhead.
   Note: Starting the text at the center point is not the same as the text being centered on the line. When starting the text at the center point, the text flows towards the right margin.
   Purpose: All letters require a date for legal purposes.

4. Key the inside address starting at the left margin and use the correct spelling and punctuation. Leave one to nine blank lines between the date and the inside address in order to center the body of the letter on the page.
   Purpose: The body of the letter must be centered vertically from the top to the bottom of the document. More blank lines can be added to move the body to the correct location.

5. Key the salutation starting at the left margin and use the correct spelling and punctuation. Leave one blank line between the inside address and the salutation.
   Purpose: A proper greeting sets the tone of the letter.

6. Use your critical thinking skills to compose a concise, accurate message. Type the message in the body of the letter starting at the left margin. Leave one blank line between the salutation and the first line of the body and then between each paragraph of the body. Each paragraph should be indented five spaces. The message should be clear, concise, and professional. Use proper grammar, punctuation, capitalization, and sentence structure.
   Purpose: Proper grammar helps to convey the message accurately and professionally.

7. Key a proper closing. Start the closing at the center point of the line. (The first letter of the closing should align vertically with the first letter of the date.) Use correct spelling and punctuation. Leave one blank line between the last line of the body and the closing.
   Purpose: The closing helps end the message with a professional tone.

8. Key the signature block. Start the signature block at the center point of the line. (The first letter of the signature block should align vertically with the first letter of the date and closing.) Use the correct spelling and punctuation. Leave four blank lines between the closing and the signature block. If you are preparing the letter for a provider, you must include a reference notation.
   Purpose: The signature block provides the reader with the name of the sender of the letter. The reference notation identifies who typed the letter.

9. Spell-check and proofread the document. Check for the proper tone, grammar, punctuation, capitalization, and sentence structure. Check for proper spacing between the parts of the letter. Make any final corrections. Print the document.
   Purpose: The spell-checker identifies only certain errors; proofreading helps you find incorrect word use, improper tone, and errors in formatting.

10. Address the envelope, using either the computer and word processing software or a pen and following the correct format.
    Purpose: Following the Postal Service guidelines on format helps prevent a delay in delivery of the letter.

11. When using a #10 envelope, fold the letter by pulling up the bottom end until it reaches just below the inside address or two-thirds of the way up the letter. Crease at the fold. Then, fold the top of the letter down so that it is flush with the bottom fold and crease the paper. When using a #6¾ envelope, pull the bottom edge of the letter up until it is ½ inch from the top edge of the document and crease at the fold. Bring the right edge two-thirds of the way across the width of the document and crease the paper. Then bring the left edge to the right edge and crease at the fold. Flip the document so the left edge is on the bottom and insert the letter into the envelope.
    Note: If the provider needs to sign the letter, the letter is folded afterwards.
    Purpose: The letter must be neatly folded.

12. File a copy of the letter in the paper medical record or upload an electronic copy of the letter to the electronic health record (EHR).
    Purpose: A copy of all correspondence should be kept in the patient's health record.

PROCEDURE 25.4   Compose a Memorandum

Task

Compose a professional memorandum.

Scenario

You are asked by the supervisor to compose a memo that can be posted in the department. You are to remind the staff about the department meeting next Tuesday, at noon in the conference room. Staff can bring their lunches, and beverages will be provided.

Equipment and Supplies

- Computer with word processing software and printer
- Paper

Procedural Steps

1. Determine the message you want to convey. Using the computer and word processing software, compose the memo. Use 1-inch margins on all four sides, portrait orientation, and single line spacing throughout the memo. Use an easy to read font (e.g., Times New Roman or Calibri) in a 10- or 12-point size.
   Purpose: Determining the message gives you a focus when composing the memo.

2. Left justify the headers and use boldface and capital letters, followed by a colon. Headers include TO, FROM, DATE, and SUBJECT. Leave one blank line between each header.
   Purpose: Boldface and capital letters allow the headers to stand out to the reader, making it easier to read the information.

3. Key (type) the information following the headers in regular font, using a mix of capital and lowercase letters. Using the tab tool, align the information vertically down the page. Key the date as indicated for professional letters.
   Purpose: Aligning the information helps the memo look professional.

4. Add a centered black line between the headers and the body (optional). Leave two to three blank lines between the headers and the body of the memo.
   Purpose: The line and extra blank lines help to separate the message in the body from the headers.

5. Key the message in the body of the memo. Left justify the content in the body and use single line spacing. Use proper grammar and correct spelling and punctuation. With multiple paragraphs, skip a single line between paragraphs.
   Purpose: For professional communication, it is important to use proper grammar and correct spelling and punctuation.

6. Write the content of the message in the body of the memo clearly, concisely, and accurately. Add special notations as needed.
   Purpose: Special notations may be used if the memo contains enclosures and so on.

7. Spell-check and proofread the document. Check for the proper tone, grammar, punctuation, capitalization, and sentence structure. Check for proper spacing between the parts of the memo. Make any final corrections. Print the document.
   Purpose: The spell-checker identifies only certain errors; proofreading helps you find incorrect word use, improper tone, and errors in formatting.

PROCEDURE 25.5 Compose a Professional Email

Task

Compose a professional email that conveys the message to the reader clearly, concisely, and accurately.

Scenario

Aaron Jackson (DOB: 10/17/20XX) has an appointment at 11 a.m. next Thursday. Send his guardian an appointment reminder via email. Aaron will be seeing David Kahn, MD. The guardian should bring in any medications Aaron is currently taking. You are working at Walden-Martin Family Medical Clinic. The healthcare facility's address is: 1234 Anystreet, Anytown, AL 12345. The phone number is 123-123-1234, and the fax number is 123-123-5678. Your instructor will supply you with the guardian's name and email address.

Equipment and Supplies

- Patient's health record
- Computer with email software

Procedural Steps

1. Obtain the intended recipient's contact information and determine the message you want to convey.
   Purpose: Determining the message gives you a focus when composing the email. You will need the recipient's information to create the email.
2. Using the computer and email software, key (type) the recipient's email address. If the email has two recipients, use a semicolon (;) after the name of the first recipient. Double-check the email addresses for accuracy.
   Purpose: If the email address is incorrect, the email will not get to the recipient.
3. Key a subject, keeping it simple but focused on the contents of the email.
   Purpose: In many email software packages, the user can search for emails using the subject field. Keeping the subject simple and focused makes it easier for the user to find the message.

4. Key a formal greeting, using correct punctuation.
   Purpose: A proper greeting sets the tone of the letter.
5. Key the message in the body of the email using proper grammar, spelling, punctuation, capitalization, and sentence structure. Avoid abbreviations. The message should be clear, concise, and professional.
   Purpose: Using proper grammar and avoiding abbreviations will convey the message accurately and professionally.
6. Finish the email with closing remarks.
   Purpose: In the closing, you can thank the recipient or encourage them to follow up with concerns or questions. This gives the email a professional tone.
7. Key a closing, followed by your name and title on the next line. Include the clinic's name and contact information below your name.
   Purpose: The email needs to clearly state who is sending it.
8. Spell-check and proofread the email. Check for proper tone, grammar, punctuation, capitalization, and sentence structure. Check for proper spacing between the parts of the email.
   Purpose: White space or spacing between the elements of an email helps separate the parts of the email, making it easier to read.
9. Make any final revisions, select any features to apply to the email, and then send it.
   Purpose: If the email is urgent (!), that feature should be selected before you send the email. If you require a confirmation email when the email is opened, this feature can also be selected.
10. Print a copy of the email to be filed in the paper medical record or upload an electronic copy of the email to the patient's electronic health record (EHR).
    Purpose: A copy of all correspondence should be kept in the patient's health record.

PROCEDURE 25.6 Complete a Fax Cover Sheet

Task

Complete a fax cover sheet clearly and accurately.

Scenario

Lisa Parker, mother of Johnny Parker (DOB: 06/15/20XX), requested his immunization history to be sent to Anytown School, attention: Susie Payne. The school's phone number is 123-123-5784, and the fax number will be supplied by your instructor. The release of medical records has been completed and signed by Lisa, Johnny's guardian/mother. Your phone number is the main clinic number listed on the header of the fax cover sheet.

Equipment and Supplies

- Document to be faxed (optional)
- Fax machine and fax number (optional)
- Pen
- Fax cover sheet (see Fig. 25.4)

Procedural Steps

1. Using a pen and the fax cover sheet, clearly and accurately write your name, phone number, and the date.
   Purpose: The information must be clearly written so the reader can identify who sent the fax.

2. Clearly and accurately write the name of the person receiving the fax. Also include the company, fax number, and phone number.
   Purpose: Being accurate with the information is important so it gets to the correct person.
3. Write the number of pages. The cover sheet must be counted in the total.
   Purpose: It is important to have an accurate count of the total number of sheets faxed.
4. Complete Re: by indicating the subject of the fax. Be general with the subject and refrain from including anything confidential.
   Purpose: It is important to be general when writing the subject. No confidential information should appear in the Re: line.
5. Proofread the fax cover sheet. Verify the name, agency, and contact information of the recipient. Verify the document(s) being sent are correct. Organize the documents so the coversheet is on top and fax to the recipient (optional).
   Purpose: Verifying the information and what is being sent is important for the confidentiality of the records.
   Note: Depending on the type of documents faxed and the facility's policies and procedures, the medical assistant may need to document the activity in the patient's health record.

26

Daily Operations and Safety

LEARNING OBJECTIVES

1. Explain opening and closing tasks that are done by the medical assistant.
2. List the steps involved in completing an inventory and perform an equipment inventory with documentation.
3. Explain the purpose of routine maintenance of administrative and clinical equipment and perform routine maintenance of equipment.
4. Discuss service calls, warranties, and purchasing equipment.
5. Discuss inventory management, inventory management control systems, and ordering supplies.
6. Identify the principles of body mechanics and perform a supply inventory with documentation while using proper body mechanics.
7. Evaluate the work environment to identify unsafe working conditions.
8. Identify critical elements of an emergency response plan to use in the event of a natural disaster or other emergency, and participate in a mock exposure event.
9. Demonstrate the proper use of a fire extinguisher.
10. Recognize the physical and emotional effects on persons involved in an emergency situation.

OUTLINE

▶▶ OPENING SCENARIO

Marie Van Bakel, a certified medical assistant (CMA), is a new medical assistant at Walden-Martin Family Medical (WMFM) Clinic. She was hired to work with the family medicine providers. This is Marie's first job as a new graduate from a medical assisting program. She is excited to work in family medicine. This was the same specialty she worked in during her medical assisting practicum. Because this is a small healthcare facility, Marie's responsibilities are different from what they would be in a larger facility. She and the administrative medical assistant,

Catherine, are the only staff members in the office at the start of the day. The providers make hospital rounds at that time. The providers and the rest of the medical assistants come in later.

Marie and Catherine need to open the office and prepare for the patients. Marie is also responsible for the inventory of clinical supplies and administrative and clinical equipment. During Marie's interview, Dr. Walden expressed her concern about the lack of procedures for ordering and maintaining inventory. She would like Marie to develop those procedures. Having little exposure to supplies and ordering during her practicum, Marie realizes she needs to learn about these procedures.

YOU WILL LEARN

1. To perform duties necessary to open and close the healthcare facility.
2. To perform inventory on equipment and supplies.
3. To order supplies and to perform the procedures done when supplies are received.
4. To follow safety procedures, including using correct body mechanics, evaluating the work environment, and responding to emergencies.

INTRODUCTION

In the ambulatory healthcare facility, the medical assistant has opening tasks to accomplish to prepare the department for patients. At the end of the day, after the last patient leaves, the medical assistant has duties to close the department for the night. Besides performing these daily duties, the medical assistant manages the equipment and supply inventories. Having adequate supplies available to use for patients is critical to the functioning of the department. These topics are addressed in this chapter.

In addition, the medical assistant must be knowledgeable about environmental safety and security. This chapter discusses workplace violence, evaluating the environment, emergency response plans, and the effects of stress. Keeping the work environment safe is an important role for every employee.

OPENING AND CLOSING THE HEALTHCARE FACILITY

Employees who are responsible for opening the ambulatory healthcare facility must arrive before the patients in the morning. These employees must prepare for the day. Preparation time will vary based on the size of the practice and the number of patients on the schedule.

In smaller facilities, a few reliable employees are given keys to unlock the doors and deactivate the alarm system. In larger facilities, employees must use the locked employee entrances. Employees can unlock the doors by entering unique codes into a keypad or by using unique keycards. Both systems are developed to monitor who enters the building. Usually security, custodial, or supervisory personnel are responsible for deactivating the alarm system in larger facilities. Staff members then open the main patient doors at a set time.

Opening Tasks for the Medical Assistant

The clinical medical assistant assists the provider with patient treatments and procedures (e.g., injections, wound care, and diagnostic tests). The administrative medical assistant works in the reception area. In larger facilities, both types of medical assistants have opening duties. If the healthcare facility is small, then the medical assistant may be required to perform both administrative and clinical tasks. Often this is called performing "front office" and "back office" activities.

Clinical Medical Assistant. It is important for the clinical medical assistant to prepare the clinical equipment and exam rooms for

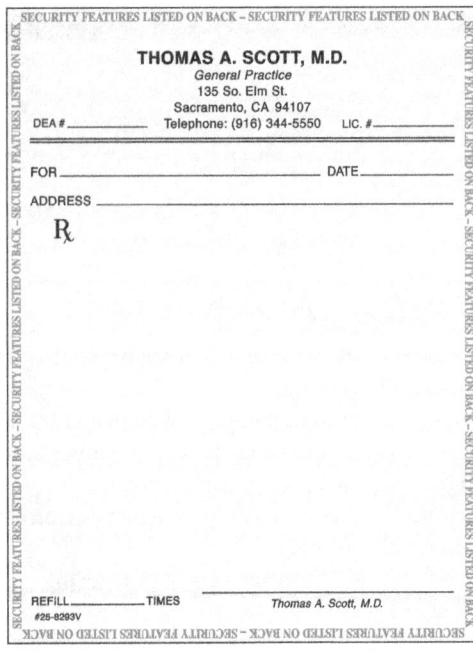

Fig. 26.1 The provider should keep one prescription pad, and extra pads should be locked up. (From Niedzwiecki B, et al: *Kinn's the medical assistant,* ed 14, St. Louis, 2020, Elsevier.)

patient visits. An unprepared area can cause delays in patient care. Facility opening tasks for the clinical medical assistant include:

- Preparing the exam rooms by turning on the lights, ensuring supplies are stocked, and making sure the rooms have been cleaned appropriately and are safe for patients.
- Ensuring prescription pads (if used) are stored outside of the exam rooms, in a locked cabinet (Fig. 26.1). Prescription pads should never be accessible to patients. Some patients or staff might take the pads and try to forge a prescription, which is illegal.
- Unlocking supply cabinets (with the exception of the narcotics cabinet, which remains locked).
- Ensuring restrooms have adequate supplies for patients (e.g., urine specimen containers, cleansing towelettes).
- Performing quality control tests on laboratory equipment and completing refrigerator and freezer temperature logs.

In addition to these tasks, the clinical medical assistant must follow up on outstanding patient issues from the prior day. The medical assistant also needs to handle new diagnostic test reports (e.g., x-ray reports). For agencies using paper health records, this would require:

- Obtaining the patient's paper health record
- Attaching the diagnostic report to the record
- Giving the health record and report to the provider to review

> **VOCABULARY**
>
> **quality control** A process to ensure the reliability of test results, often using manufactured samples with known values.

For facilities with electronic health records (EHRs), this process is completed using the electronic messaging system in the software (Fig. 26.2).

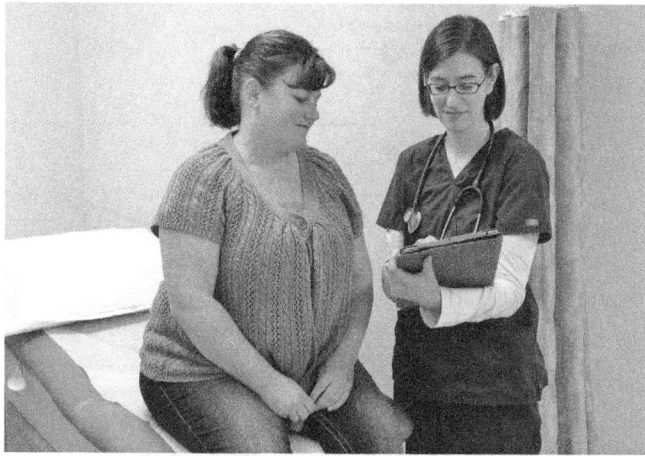

Fig. 26.2 Most providers and their staff members use electronic health records to reduce paperwork and provide better, more efficient patient care. (From Niedzwiecki B, et al: *Kinn's the medical assistant,* ed 14, St. Louis, 2020, Elsevier.)

Often medical assistants notify patients of normal test results and document the notification in the health record. No test result can be given to the patient unless the provider has authorized its release or the facility's procedures allow it. The medical assistant must follow the facility's procedures when notifying the patient of the results.

Administrative Medical Assistant. Opening tasks for the administrative medical assistant include:

- Checking the voice mail or answering service messages. The answering service may email or fax messages to the facility. All messages need to be addressed and documented in the patient's health record.
- Updating the voice mail message.
- Switching on the phone, so patients can reach the facility instead of the answering service.
- Turning on computers, copy machines, and other office equipment.
- Preparing the reception area for patients.
- Printing schedules of the day's appointments. A schedule is kept for the paper health record preparation. Other copies are given to the clinical medical assistants, providers, and the medical laboratory. In some facilities, the EHR allows staff to reference the schedule using the software, thus eliminating the printed schedule.

In addition to these duties, the administrative medical assistant must compile any remaining required paperwork for the day's visits. Usually this is done the prior afternoon. A few patient visits that need to be completed may be added to the schedule. For healthcare facilities with EHRs, required patient education literature (e.g., well-child visit documents) and preprinted paper screening forms may be prepared.

For facilities with paper health records, the medical assistant must do the following:

- Pull the paper health records, using a copy of the appointment schedule.
- Verify that the correct record was pulled for each patient.

- Check off the patient's name on the copy of the appointment schedule.
- Review each record.
  - Have all recently received documents (e.g., laboratory reports, radiograph readings) been placed correctly and permanently attached to the record?
  - Are documents (e.g., laboratory reports) missing that are needed for the visit?
  - Is there enough space available in the progress notes for the provider to write in the record? If not, place additional progress notes pages in the record.
- Arrange the health records in the order in which the patients will be arriving. The record for the first visit of the day should be on top. Larger facilities may alphabetize the health records.

> **VOCABULARY**
>
> **answering service** A commercial service that answers telephone calls for its clients.
> **disinfect** The process of cleaning in order to destroy or prevent the growth of disease-causing microorganisms.
> **progress notes** Documentation in the medical record that can be used to track the patient's condition and progress.
> **restock** The process of replacing the supplies that were used.
> **sanitize** The process of cleaning equipment and instruments with detergent and water in order to remove debris and reduce the number of microorganisms.
> **sterilize** The process of removing all microorganisms.

> **CRITICAL THINKING 26.1**
>
> When Marie, the clinical medical assistant, opens the family medicine office, what jobs does she need to do? What jobs does Catherine, the administrative medical assistant, need to do to prepare for the day?

Closing Tasks for the Medical Assistant

Clinical Medical Assistant. At the end of the day, the medical assistant needs to help with the closing duties. The clinical medical assistant must ensure that all the patients have left by checking the exam and treatment rooms. The clinical medical assistant must:

- Restock the rooms and organize any reading materials.
- Disinfect the exam table, writing table, counters, computer keyboards, and chairs (i.e., those made of plastic, metal, or wood).
- Secure (put away) confidential documents.
- Turn off computers and other devices.
- Sanitize, disinfect, or sterilize equipment and instruments.
- Lock supply and medication cabinets.
- Verify and count the narcotic medication stock, following the facility's procedure.

Administrative Medical Assistant. The administrative medical assistant will complete the following closing duties:

- Preparing the patient records and documents for the next day.

- Turning off the computers, copy machine, and other office equipment.
- Switching phones to voice mail or the answering service.
- Following office procedures for handling money at the end of the day.
- Securing (putting away) any confidential documents.
- Cleaning up the reception area (neatly arranging the magazines, disinfecting toys, and removing garbage and unsolicited advertisements) and turning off the lights, television, stereo, and other devices.

With time being short in the morning, it is important to take care of as much as possible the evening before you leave.

Depending on the facility, the medical assistant may be responsible for turning off the lights, activating the alarms, and locking the doors. In larger facilities, the custodial or security staff handles these responsibilities.

Daily and Monthly Duties

Medical facilities either employ custodial staff or hire cleaning services. This cleaning takes place after the facility closes each day. Larger facilities that employ custodial staff will have the staff clean high-traffic areas several times a day. These areas include the restrooms and the entrances. During wet weather, it is critical that the floors are kept dry to prevent people from slipping and falling.

The medical assistant also is responsible for cleaning and organizing the reception area and exam rooms. During slow times, medical assistants are expected to do extra duties, including restocking medical and office supplies, forms, and patient literature. The cabinets and drawers need to be straightened and reorganized. Medications and supplies that have expiration dates need to be checked monthly. The crash cart and other emergency supplies need to be inventoried at least monthly and after each use (Fig. 26.3). Many facilities use a master list of crash cart supplies with expiration dates. This helps ensure that all supplies are in the crash cart and expiring supplies and medications can be easily identified.

It is important that the healthcare facility be clean and organized. By taking the initiative (i NISH eh tiv) to perform those tasks during quiet times, you will be considered a more valuable employee. Supervisors and providers value employees who look for additional activities that can be done during quiet times.

CRITICAL THINKING 26.2

The office uses a local cleaning service to clean the facility's rooms. The staff members arrive after hours and are gone by the time Catherine and Marie open the office in the morning. Over the past month, Marie has noticed that the rooms do not look as clean as they should. Should she address this concern? If so, with whom should she discuss it?

VOCABULARY

crash cart Medications and equipment (e.g., oxygen, intravenous [IV] and airway supplies) stored in a cart and ready for an emergency.
initiative The ability to determine what needs to be done and take action on your own.

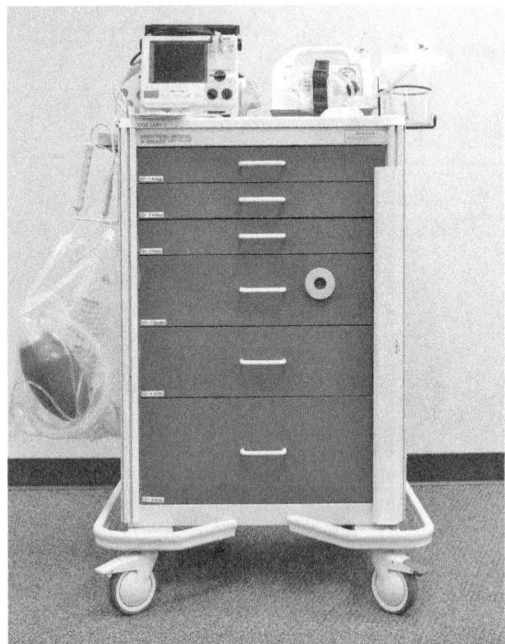

Fig. 26.3 Crash carts must be inventoried monthly or after each use to ensure that medication and supplies have not expired and that all the required supplies are available for an emergency.

EQUIPMENT AND SUPPLIES

Another medical assistant duty is to manage the equipment and supplies in the medical office. In smaller facilities, this may involve ordering and maintaining an inventory control system. In larger facilities, purchasing department employees are hired for such roles.

Equipment

In a healthcare facility, administrative and clinical types of equipment are used. The medical assistant needs to know how to operate, maintain, and handle issues with the equipment. For financial and tax purposes, the purchase cost and age of each item need to be recorded. The process of gathering and creating a list of the equipment in the facility is called managing inventory.

Equipment Inventory. For all clinical and administrative equipment, records need to be maintained. These records are used to replace equipment lost in a disaster or theft. The healthcare facility's accountant also uses the information when preparing tax paperwork. For instance, records should be maintained for the following items:

- Small equipment (e.g., thermometers, glucose monitors), which is deducted as an expense for the year in which it was purchased.
- Large office equipment (e.g., computer hardware, calculators, and copiers), which depreciates (di PREE shee ates) over 5 years.
- Office furniture items (e.g., desks, files, safes, exam tables), which depreciate over 7 years.

The equipment inventory also is used by supervisors to identify equipment that needs to be replaced. Preplanning equipment

Equipment Name	Manufacturer / Serial Number	Location / Facility Number	Purchase Date / Supplier	Cost	Warranty Information
Laser Printer	HP / HP3598XA	Medical Assistant Desk / LP59483	08/01/20XX / Best Office Supplies	$325	Parts and labor expires 07/31/20XX
AT2 Plus ECG / Spirometry	Schiller / WA4893X	Treatment Room / ES00012	05/02/20XX / Medical Equipment Supplies	$2987	Parts and Labor expires 05/01/20XX

Fig. 26.4 An equipment inventory list can be created in a spreadsheet and provides useful information about the administrative and clinical equipment in the facility. (From Niedzwiecki B, et al: *Kinn's the medical assistant,* ed 14, St. Louis, 2020, Elsevier.)

purchases is a financial strategy for the practice. It allows the practice to be prepared and to plan for future investments.

When you are creating an equipment inventory list, it is helpful to use spreadsheet software (Fig. 26.4). In some situations, you may have inventory forms that you can complete (see Procedure 26.1). For all equipment, document the following information:

- Equipment name, manufacturer, and serial number
- Purchase date, cost, and supplier
- Warranty information (e.g., start and end date, warranty coverage)
- Location of the equipment (optional)
- Unique facility number given to that piece of equipment (optional)

The owner's manuals or users' guides and warranty information should be kept at a central location and available to users. Many users' guides are available online. They are used to problem-solve performance issues. They can be used to identify service schedules and routine maintenance. Many users' guides provide a list of parts or supplies needed for the operation of the machine.

VOCABULARY

depreciate To diminish in value (e.g., the value of an item) over a period of time; a concept used for tax purposes.

inventory A detailed list of equipment and supplies owned and stored; the process of counting the supplies in stock.

CRITICAL THINKING 26.3

Marie needs to learn more about managing inventory. She reviews her medical assistant textbook and reads articles online. She decides to start by creating an inventory list of the equipment in the medical office. What are some advantages of having an updated list of administrative and clinical equipment?

Routine Maintenance and Safety. The medical assistant is responsible for monitoring equipment safety and proper functioning. Routine maintenance helps to ensure the best performance of the equipment. Potential issues should not be overlooked. Actions should be taken to prevent injury to staff or patients and costly damage to the equipment. The medical assistant should do the following:

- Check electrical cords on equipment for damage.
- Address any suspected overheating issues.
- Investigate any unusual noise or change in performance.
- Clean and maintain equipment routinely in accordance with the users' guide.

Routine maintenance varies with the equipment. Copiers and printers may require changing of the toner or cartridges. For clinical equipment, maintenance may include changing filters or batteries.

It is important to keep track of routine maintenance. Making a schedule as a reminder for routine maintenance can be helpful. Many facilities use logs to track routine maintenance and service calls (Fig. 26.5). Information commonly found in the routine maintenance log includes:

- Equipment name, serial number, location of machine, and facility's unique equipment number (if applicable)
- Manufacturer's name
- Date of purchase
- Warranty information (e.g., start and end date, warranty coverage)
- Service provider contact information, such as telephone number
- Date and time and description of maintenance activities performed
- Signature of person performing maintenance

Procedure 26.2 explains the steps involved in creating a maintenance log, performing the maintenance, and then documenting the maintenance.

CRITICAL THINKING 26.4

Marie realizes that the facility does not have maintenance logs for the various pieces of equipment. She decides to start making logs, but she realizes she will have to make a lot of logs. How could she create logs in a time-efficient manner? For a small office, describe options that she could use to organize the logs so they are easy to locate and use.

Maintenance Log

Equipment Name: **Laser Printer** Serial #: **HP3598XA** Location: **Medical Assistant Desk**

Facility #: **LP59483** Manufacturer: **HP** Purchased: **08/01/20XX**

Warranty Information: **Parts and labor expires 07/31/20XX**

Frequency of Inspections: **Every 6 months**

Service Provider: **Best Office Supplies**

Date	Time	Maintenance Activities	Signature
12/15/20XX	0956	Replaced toner cartridge	Marie Van Bakel, CMA (AAMA)
02/11/20XX	1235	Service call: Office Repair Company – to fix stray ink marks on copies	Catherine Black, RMA

Maintenance Log

Equipment Name: **AT2 Plus ECG/Spirometry** Serial #: **WA4893X** Location: **Treatment Room**

Facility #: **ES00012** Manufacturer: **Schiller** Purchased: **05/02/20XX**

Frequency of Inspections: **Every 12 months**

Warranty information: **Parts and Labor expires 05/01/20XX**

Service Provider: **Medical Equipment Suppliers**

Date	Time	Maintenance Activities	Signature
10/23/20XX	1123	Replaced battery	Marie Van Bakel, CMA (AAMA)
05/02/20XX	1445	No tracing, cleaned stylus with alcohol	Marie Van Bakel, CMA (AAMA)

Fig. 26.5 Equipment maintenance logs are used by the staff and outside repair agencies to track maintenance activities. (From Niedzwiecki B, et al: *Kinn's the medical assistant,* ed 14, St. Louis, 2020, Elsevier.)

Service Calls and Warranties. When equipment is purchased, a warranty is given for a period of time. The warranty is the manufacturer's guarantee. If the piece of equipment needs to be repaired or has a defective part, the manufacturer will pay for the cost of the repair. In some cases, the item may be replaced. Warranty language includes details on what is covered. Some warranties are not honored if someone other than a "recognized" serviceperson attempts to fix the machine. Extended warranties lengthen the protection time and can be purchased for some equipment.

For complex or expensive equipment, the healthcare facility may contract with a service provider for repairs and routine service checks. This assistance is necessary for some equipment. It also helps to extend the lifetime of those machines. For repairs on other equipment, it might be necessary to ship or bring the machine to the repair service. Usually the cost for onsite repairs is more than if the machine is taken or shipped to the service provider for repairs. One of the main concerns when a piece of equipment breaks down is the effect on the healthcare facility. Some service providers will loan equipment to facilities while the repairs take place. This service greatly lessens the burden on the practice.

Purchasing Equipment. The process of purchasing equipment can vary depending on the size of the organization. Large agencies have purchasing departments. The purchasing staff researches the need and identifies the best equipment to purchase. The medical assistant may be involved with the process in smaller practices.

Many factors are considered when equipment is being replaced:

- Age of the equipment and availability of parts
- Frequency and cost of repairs
- Use of the machine and whether new features will lead to extra billable services

Leasing medical equipment is becoming a popular option for smaller facilities. The healthcare facility pays a fee to lease an item, such as monitoring equipment, diagnostic testing equipment, computer systems, and exam tables. The fee is less than what it would cost to purchase the item. The lease fees are tax deductible and allow the healthcare facility to provide extra billable services.

The medical assistant may help identify potential new equipment models to purchase or lease. Using the internet and contacting the company's salespeople are two ways to get additional information. Some salespeople will meet with the staff and demonstrate the product. In addition to research, the medical assistant may need to explain the usage of the machine and the frequency of repair checks. Usually the supervisor or provider has the final say as to whether the purchase should occur.

> **VOCABULARY**
>
> **billable service** Assistance (i.e., service) that is provided by a healthcare provider and can be billed to the insurance company or patient.

> **CRITICAL THINKING 26.5**
>
> Currently, the providers are using an offsite radiology service. They are contemplating creating a small radiology room where they could take x-rays. How could Marie assist the providers with their plans for a potential purchase of x-ray equipment?

Item Name	Size	Quantity	Item Number	Supplier's Name	Reorder Point	Quantity to Reorder	Cost	Stock Available	Order (✓)
Nonsterile gauze sponges, 8 ply	2"x 2"	100/pkg	NG0022	Midwest Medical	5	25	$2.31/pkg		
Sterile gauze sponges, 12 ply, 2/pkg	2"x 2"	25 pkg/box	NG0042	Midwest Medical	4	20	$3.99/box		

Fig. 26.6 A supply inventory list shows details of items in inventory. For efficiency, use two extra columns ("Stock Available" and "Order") as shown. This list can be duplicated and used for performing inventory. (From Niedzwiecki B, et al: *Kinn's the medical assistant,* ed 14, St. Louis, 2020, Elsevier.)

Supplies

Many supplies are required to run the medical office and treat patients. Supplies include administrative items (e.g., pens, paper, envelopes, and paperclips) and clinical items (e.g., bandages, vaccines, medications, slings, and splints). The medical assistant must make sure there are enough supplies to treat patients. A lack of supplies can greatly affect the services provided to patients. It can be expensive for the healthcare facility to order last-minute because of higher prices to do so. On the other hand, overstocking supplies can be a financial waste to the facility. Many supplies have expiration dates and cannot be used beyond that date. Having adequate amounts of supplies in inventory is crucial.

Inventory Management. Inventory management involves ordering, tracking inventory, and identifying the quantity of product to purchase. The goal of inventory management is to have adequate supplies on hand. It is important not to have too much stock that will expire or take a long time to use.

The medical assistant in charge of ordering and managing supplies must keep a record on each item in inventory. The record can be a manual entry written in a notebook or on index cards. It can also be computerized in a spreadsheet or inventory control system software. For each inventory item, the medical assistant must record:

- Item details: Item name, size, quantity, item number, supplier's name, and cost (Fig. 26.6).
- *Quantity to reorder*: Amount of supplies that need to be ordered. This amount reflects the product used during the buying cycle. For instance, the healthcare facility's buying cycle for 2 × 2 nonsterile gauze (100 per pack) is 1 month. The facility typically goes through 25 packs in 1 month. This would be the quantity used during the buying cycle. It would also be the quantity to reorder each time (see Fig. 26.6).
- *Reorder point*: Point at which low inventory requires the product to be ordered. For instance, when the inventory of 2 × 2 nonsterile gauze packs gets depleted to 5 packs, the medical assistant must reorder (see Fig. 26.6). Five is the reorder point, or the quantity that triggers an order to be placed to replenish the inventory (Box 26.1). The reorder point for medical and administrative supplies can be different for each item because of the usage rate and the time it takes to receive the item after it is ordered.

BOX 26.1   How to Calculate the Reorder Point

The reorder point can be calculated based on the number used per day and the number of days it takes to order and receive the product.

For instance, the practice uses 0.5 pack of 2 × 2 nonsterile gauze per day. It takes 4 days to receive the order from the medical supply company. The medical practice may also want 6 extra days' worth of supplies on hand to prevent issues related to running out of the item. Here is how you would figure out the reorder point:

Stock to cover order time: 0.5 pack per day × 4 days to receive order = 2 packs

Extra stock: 6 days × 0.5 pack per day = 3 packs

Reorder point: 2 packs (stock to cover order time) + 3 packs (6-day supply) = 5 packs

VOCABULARY

buying cycle Refers to how often an item is purchased and depends on how frequently the item is used and the storage space available for it.

Inventory Control Systems. An inventory control system helps to make inventory management work well. Large medical facilities use computerized inventory control systems. These systems monitor usage and inventory in stock. They also identify items that need to be ordered. Smaller facilities may use simple computerized or manual systems.

To help create an efficient computerized system, many medical facilities use bar codes to track inventory, for insurance, and for patient billing for supplies (Fig. 26.7). With this system, each item has a unique bar code. The bar code is scanned with a bar code reader when items are added to or taken from inventory. Software monitors the inventory quantity. For bar codes to work successfully, the staff must be diligent in scanning the bar codes when taking a product from stock. Bar code inventory control systems work successfully in both large and small healthcare facilities.

Several manual systems can also be used to identify supplies that need to be ordered. The following are some of the more common methods used in medical facilities.

- When staff identify a product that needs to be ordered, the item is written in a log. This process is like making a list of what you need at the grocery store. The person responsible

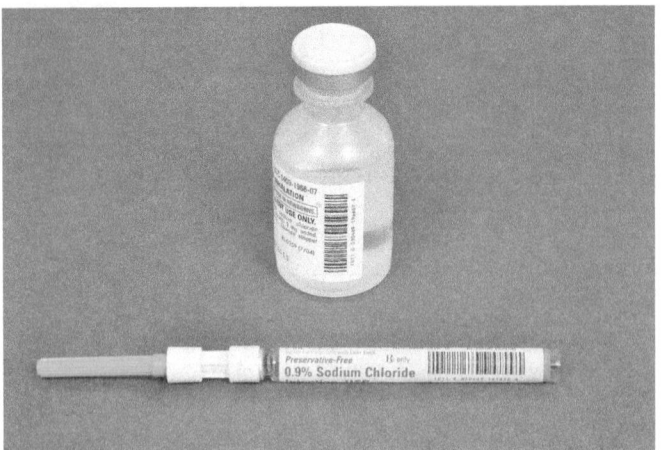

Fig. 26.7 Using bar codes makes inventory control more efficient. (From Niedzwiecki B, et al: *Kinn's the medical assistant,* ed 14, St. Louis, 2020, Elsevier.)

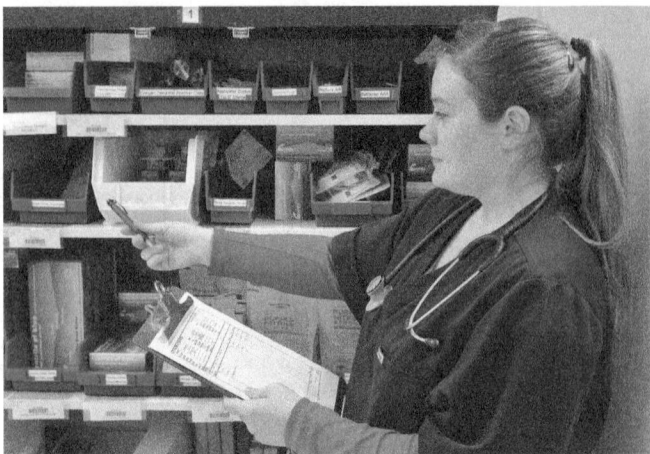

Fig. 26.8 A Medical Assistant Performing an Inventory. (From Niedzwiecki B, et al: *Kinn's the medical assistant,* ed 14, St. Louis, 2020, Elsevier.)

for ordering supplies then prepares the order based on the information in the log.

- Another system includes using product identification slips, which contain the name of the product. The slips or cards are attached to the product or a box/package of items. When the product is used, the slip is put in a special location, such as a box or plastic pocket. The medical assistant uses the slips in the box or pocket to prepare the supply order.
- The two-bin system consists of having a main bin for each item in inventory and then a backup bin for each item. When the main bin is emptied, the backup bin is used, and the product is reordered.
- The medical assistant responsible for ordering performs a hand count of the items in stock to identify what needs to be ordered. This system is explained in the next section.

CRITICAL THINKING 26.6

Marie decides to implement a manual system for inventory. Of the manual systems discussed, which method might work best in the small facility? Discuss your answer.

Taking Inventory. Inventory (counting supplies) must be taken at specific times. Many businesses that use automated inventory control systems hand count their inventory at least once a year. Usually this is done around the close of the business year. These companies compare their hand counts to the computer counts and identify discrepancies. The discrepancies are followed up on. The manual inventory procedure provides the company with information on the actual number of items in stock. With this information, the financial value of the inventory can be calculated and used for financial reports and taxes at the close of the business year.

Some ambulatory care facilities do not use inventory control systems. These facilities must perform inventory or count the items in stock before each buying cycle. This identifies what products need to be ordered.

One of the most frequent errors when performing inventory is to report a different quantity than what is on the supply inventory list. For instance, a medical assistant counts nonsterile sponges. Each package should be counted as 1 and not as 100 each. For example, in Fig. 26.6, if there were 6 packages of nonsterile gauze sponges left in the supply cabinet, it should be noted that the stock available was 6 packages. It should not be indicated as 600 sponges, or 600 each. Counting each item in a box or package when the product is inventoried by box or package creates conflict and confusion when looking at the reorder point.

The medical assistant should use a supply inventory list to be most efficient when counting supplies (Fig. 26.8). The supply inventory list shows all the items in stock. The medical assistant can mark down the inventory counts for each item on the document (see Procedure 26.3). If the supply inventory list is not available, then the medical assistant needs to write down the item number, size, quantity (e.g., 100/box), manufacturer, and any other identifying information. This process takes a lot more time. Using abbreviations can be helpful, such as:

- BTL: Bottle
- BX: Box
- CS: Case
- EA: Each
- PKG: Package
- QTY: Quantity

When you perform an inventory, work in a systematic manner. Start with one supply cabinet, working from top to bottom, before moving on to another cabinet. All stock areas should be inventoried before the supply order is prepared.

VOCABULARY

discrepancy A lack of similarity between what is stated and what is found; for instance, the computer inventory count is different from the physical count.

Price Consideration When Ordering Supplies. When you order supplies, price comparison shopping is important. The healthcare facility must balance the time it takes to get the needed supplies against the money saved when buying from various companies. Some medical offices compare prices only on more expensive items or items that are used in vast quantities. They may compare prices every 6 to 12 months. When you compare prices, consider:

- Shipping and handling charges
- Quantity and amount (e.g., 10 per box), as these must be the same among products
- Quantity discounts or price breaks for buying a certain amount. Quantity discounts or price breaks save money. The more of an item purchased when you order, the cheaper the product becomes, as this example shows:
  - Quantity 1 to 5, $1.50 per each item
  - Quantity 6 to 15, $1.25 per each item

If the medical assistant purchased a quantity of 6, the price per each would be cheaper than if 4 were purchased. Before ordering extra product, consider the storage space available, how quickly the item will be used, and the shelf life or expiration date of the item. Buying too much just to get a price break may not be in the best interest of the healthcare facility.

Some medical facilities join group purchasing organizations (GPOs). These organizations combine orders from many different medical facilities. Combining orders results in volume discounts from specific vendors. GPOs typically purchase both supplies and medications. Physician buying groups (PBGs) offer providers potential cost-saving pricing for vaccines. The drawback is that the provider must exclusively use the vaccines from the contracted manufacturers.

CRITICAL THINKING 26.7

Currently the facility orders its clinical supplies from two vendors. Marie would like to do some cost comparisons to get the best deals on supplies. She does not have a lot of time to spend on the research. How might she approach this situation? Where should she start first? What might be a long-term goal for her?

Ordering Supplies. If the facility is not part of a buying group, the medical assistant might need to order supplies. It is important to select just a few vendors if possible. The medical assistant can use:

- The supplier's printed catalog, though it may only be printed a few times a year and may not provide accurate item availability and pricing.
- The supplier's website store, which would have the most accurate prices, sale prices, and available stock.

Many vendors require the creation of an account before ordering. When creating an account for purchasing supplies, you should use the facility's information (address, fax number, and phone number). Be prepared to give the provider's license number when ordering medications and needles. The medical assistant may need to fax the provider's license number, if required, before ordering. If narcotics are ordered, the company will need a copy of the provider's Drug Enforcement Administration (DEA) registration. Narcotics require special tracking documentation and thus a high level of authorization when they are purchased.

Some medical facilities use purchase order (PO) numbers, giving each order a unique reference number. This PO number should be included on the order sheets, added to the online

information, or provided during the phone order. Vendors add the PO number to the order's documentation (i.e., packing slip and statement). This way both parties can use it as a reference if questions come up. The healthcare facility uses the purchase order number to track the order.

Payment (PYMT) terms may vary among vendors. Payment methods may include credit card, check, money order, or a line of credit. Typically, the *line of credit* (preset borrowing limit) is good for 30 to 60 days. Invoices or billing statements are sent to the facility and should be paid after the purchases have been received. Orders can typically be placed via fax, mail, phone, or online. If the medical assistant is faxing or mailing the order, the vendor usually requires the order to be placed on the vendor's order sheet. The medical assistant should keep a copy of the phoned-in, mailed, or faxed order or a printout of the online order to verify that the order was filled correctly.

VOCABULARY

backordered An order placed for an item that is temporarily out of stock and will be sent later.

invoices Billing statements that list the amount owed for goods or services purchased.

packing slip A document that accompanies purchased merchandise and shows what is in the box or package.

purchase order number A unique number assigned by the ordering facility that allows the facility to track or reference the order.

vendors Companies that sell supplies, equipment, or services to other companies or individuals.

Receiving Orders. Orders can arrive via the mail, a national delivery service (e.g., FedEx, United Parcel Service [UPS]), or a local delivery service. The delivery person may require a signature from an employee. This signature is used to track who received the delivery.

The medical assistant must check the delivery as soon as possible. Some medications, such as vaccines, are shipped in a cold environment and must remain at a cold temperature. These medications need to be placed in the refrigerator or freezer immediately upon arrival. Storage information for medications can be found in the package insert or on the manufacturer's website. If the medication warms up too much, it may be adversely affected. For instance, vaccines that get too warm can have reduced potency. This means they may not protect patients against disease.

When an order arrives, remove the packing slip from the box. Compare the items in the package to the packing slip (Fig. 26.9). Check off all items received. Some vendors may indicate items that are backordered and will be arriving later. Note any discrepancies or differences on the packing slip. Any items that are damaged should be noted on the packing slip. The copy of the original order should be compared against the packing slip, and any differences should be noted. Any discrepancies or damaged items should be addressed with the supply company as soon as possible.

The packing slip should be attached to the copy of the order once the supplies have been reviewed. When the

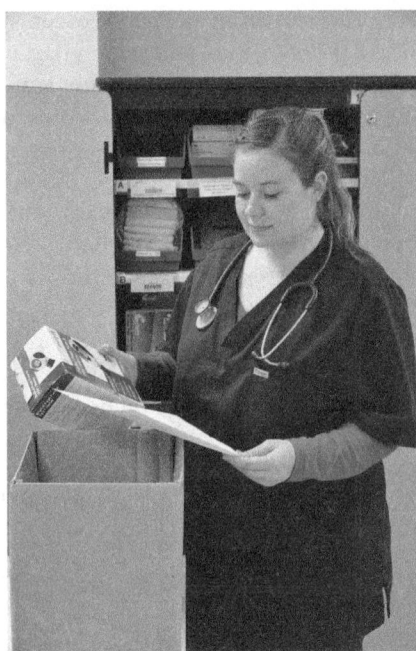

Fig. 26.9 Comparing the packing slip with the contents in the box is an important step in receiving supplies. (From Niedzwiecki B, et al: *Kinn's the medical assistant,* ed 14, St. Louis, 2020, Elsevier.)

complete order has been received, the copy of the order with the packing slips attached should be filed if the order was prepaid. If a line of credit was used, the copy of the order with the attached packing slips is placed in the accounts payable folder to wait for the invoice's arrival. The person responsible for paying the healthcare facility's bills will match the invoice with the copy of the order, ensuring everything was received before paying the bill.

The items received should be put away as soon as possible, and the boxes should be discarded. When you are putting supplies away, it is important to rotate stock. This means the new stock should go in the back and the older stock needs to be moved forward so it can be used first. Any items with expiration dates should be placed with the items expiring first in front, so they are used first. For stock without expiration dates, consider the saying "first in, first out" (FIFO), which means when new stock comes in, it is placed behind the older stock. The older stock needs to be used first. If you are removing expired stock, remember to subtract the quantity from the inventory system.

Vaccine Ordering. For ambulatory care departments that administer vaccines, the Centers for Disease Control and Prevention (CDC) recommends having one person be the vaccine coordinator. The vaccine coordinator must ensure that all vaccines are stored and handled correctly. Some of the vaccine coordinator's duties are:

- Maintaining vaccine inventory information and ordering vaccines
- Overseeing proper storage of the vaccine deliveries
- Managing and monitoring vaccine supplies, including checking expiration dates and rotating stock

- Ensuring the temperature of the refrigerator and freezer are within the normal range

Storing Vaccines. When vaccine deliveries arrive, they need to be unpacked immediately. Per the CDC:

- Each type of vaccine should be placed in its own tray; allow space between the vials promote air circulation. Place newer vaccines behind older vaccines.
- Keep vaccine vials in their original boxes to prevent light exposure. If possible, store diluents with the corresponding vaccines. Never store diluents in the freezer.
- Store vaccines with similar packaging or names on different shelves to prevent mix-ups.
- For frozen and refrigerated vaccines:
  - The refrigerators should maintain temperatures between 36°F to 46°F. The freezer should maintain temperatures between −58°F to 5°F.
  - Position vaccines and diluents 2 to 3 inches from the walls, ceiling, and floor. When using household-grade refrigerators, do not store vaccines directly under cooling vents, in drawers, or on the door shelves.
  - Do not put food or beverages in the vaccine storage refrigerator and freezer.
  - When using a household-grade refrigerator, place bottles of water on the top shelf, the floor, and the door shelves to maintain the temperature.
  - Make sure the door is closed.
  - Post a "DO NOT UNPLUG" warning sign on the unit and near the outlet. If possible, the unit should be connected to electrical outlets that can also be powered by backup generators.

The CDC recommends temperature monitoring equipment (Digital Data Loggers [DDL]) for all vaccine storage units. All vaccine storage units (e.g., refrigerators, freezers, transport containers) must have a temperature monitoring device (TMD). The TMD should be placed in the center of the unit, with vaccines surrounding it. Simple thermometers can show the minimum and maximum temperatures since the last reset. A DDL records a temperature at least every 30 minutes and provides the most accurate storage temperatures. The CDC recommends keeping the digital data from the DDLs for 3 years. This information may need to show compliance when the facility is involved with vaccination programs.

> **VOCABULARY**
> **accounts payable** Money owed by a company to other companies for services and goods; pertains to paying the facility's bills.
> **diluent** A liquid substance that dilutes or lessens the strength of a solution or mixture; it is added to vials of powdered medications to create a solution of the drug for injection.

Temperature Monitoring Logs. The temperature of the refrigerator and freezer should be checked at the start of each workday. If a TMD is used that does not record the minimum and maximum temperature, then the CDC recommends checking the temperature also at the end of the workday. Reset the thermometer if required. The temperature monitoring log sheet needs to be completed with each temperature check (Fig. 26.10). This information should be recorded:

Date	Time	Refrigerator Temperature Range: 36° F to 46° F			Freezer Temperature Range: −58° F to 5° F			Initials	Within Range
		Current	Minimum	Maximum	Current	Minimum	Maximum		
10/11/XXX	0755	40° F	37° F	39° F	3° F	−13° F	−12° F	MVB	Yes
10/11/XXX	1723	38° F	35° F	38° F	−8° F	−28° F	−19° F	BMN	No
10/12/XXX	0752	42° F	36° F	39° F	−13° F	−23° F	18° F	MVB	No
10/13/XXX	0748	47° F	38° F	38° F	−8° F	−27° F	−22° F	MVB	No

Fig. 26.10 An Example of a Temperature Monitoring Log for Vaccines.

- Date and time
- Current temperature or the maximum and minimum temperature record on the device
- Any action taken if the temperature is out of range (too high or too long)
- Name or initials of person who checked and recorded the temperature

If a temperature check was missed, leave a blank entry in the log. If the temperature is out of range, the medical assistant should notify the vaccine coordinator and the supervisor. The vaccines should be labeled "DO NOT USE" and placed in a separate container. The vaccine coordinator or supervisor will need to contact the immunization program or vaccine manufacturer for guidance.

CRITICAL THINKING 26.8

Using Fig. 26.10, the temperature monitoring log, answer the following questions:
- Did all the refrigerator temperatures fall within the required range? Explain.
- Did all the freezer temperatures fall within the required range? Explain.
- If a temperature was outside the required range, what should be done?
- Why was a blank entry left on the log?

SAFETY AND SECURITY

Body Mechanics

The provisions of the Occupational Safety and Health Act (OSH Act) of 1970 are enforced by the Occupational Safety and Health Administration (OSHA). The act requires that employers provide a workplace that is free from serious recognized hazards. Employers must comply with OSH Act standards. In the healthcare environment, most injuries are sprains, strains, and tears. Back injuries are one of the most common injuries. They can result from microtrauma related to repetitive activity over time or from one traumatic experience. Reasons for back injuries include:
- Improper lifting or lifting items too heavy for the back to support
- Reaching, twisting, or bending when lifting
- Bad body mechanics when lifting, pushing, pulling, or carrying items
- Poor footing or constrained posture

Proper body mechanics entails using the appropriate muscles and body movements to maintain correct posture and body alignment. Proper body mechanics will increase coordination and endurance. The risk of strain and injury to the body decreases. Medical assistants need to protect themselves from bodily harm while lifting, reaching, and carrying heavy objects. These are principles of body mechanics:
- To lift an object, maintain a wide, stable base with your feet. Your feet should be shoulder-width apart, and you should have good footing.
- Bend at the knees, keeping your back straight. Lift smoothly, using the major muscles in your arms and legs (Fig. 26.11). Use the same technique when putting the item down. Bending over to lift or to set down a heavy object increases your risk of injury.
- When lifting and carrying heavy items, keep the item directly in front of you to avoid rotating your spine. Carry the item close to your body (Fig. 26.12).
- Keep your movements smooth. Jerky or uncoordinated movements increase the risk for injury.
- When you reach for an object, your feet should face the object. Twisting or turning with a heavy load can cause injury.
- Avoid reaching and straining to get an object. Clear away barriers and use a firm and level surface (e.g., a step stool) to get close to the object. Avoid standing on tiptoes.
- Get help if the item is too heavy to lift by yourself.
- Store heavy objects at waist level or below.

Using proper body mechanics is important to prevent injuries. (See Procedure 26.3, which explains how to use correct body mechanics when performing a supply inventory.)

Providing a Safe Environment

Security and safety are important to the well-being of the ambulatory care staff, patients, and visitors. The healthcare facility can draw unwanted attention from those seeking drugs and money. Having plans in place that can be implemented when security is in question is critical for all.

Medical facilities can be a target for those wanting to steal money, narcotic medications, and prescription pads. The staff should implement measures to limit the amount of money available in the building. Cash and checks from patients should be deposited daily to limit the quantities of money in the facility. Cash drawers should be stored out of the sight of patients and visitors. As mentioned earlier, prescription pads should remain out of the view and reach of patients. Narcotic medications, if present in the healthcare facility, should always be in a double-locked cabinet with the keys

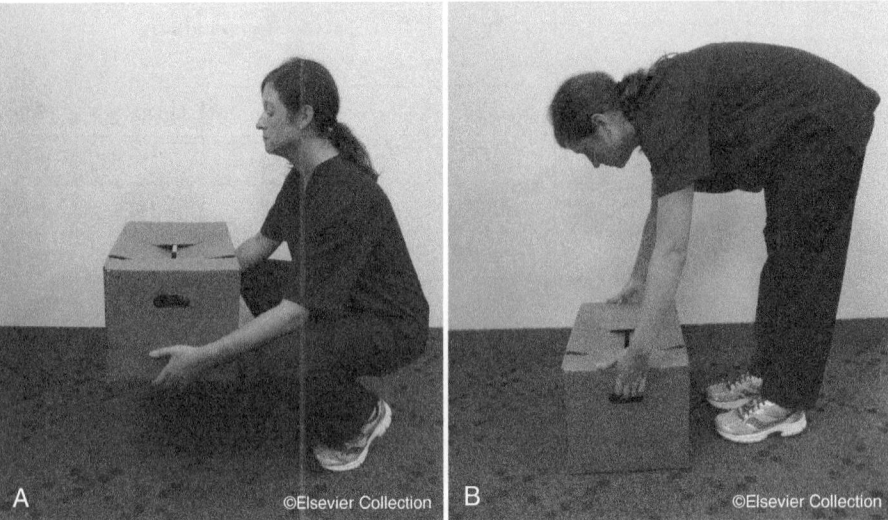

Fig. 26.11 A, Bend the knees for proper lifting technique. B, Improper lifting technique.

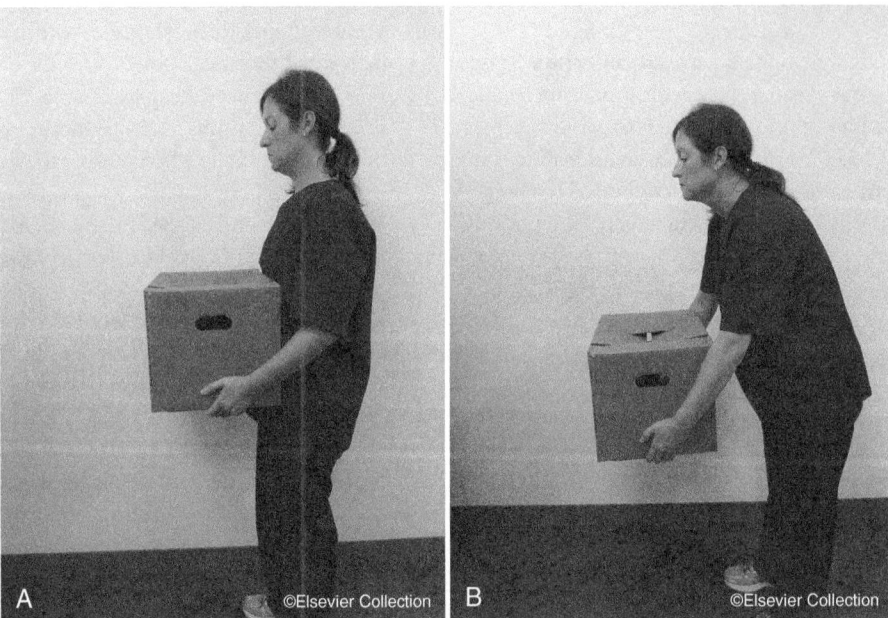

Fig. 26.12 A, Carrying an item close to the body. B, Improper carrying technique.

hidden. Depending on the type of clinic, some will post signs stating there are no narcotic medications on site.

Many facilities have chosen to keep the employee entrance doors locked during business hours. The doors require either a key card or a unique code to enter the building. In high-crime areas, low-staffed clinics, or rural clinics, the doors to the patient care areas are also locked. This prevents the unauthorized entry of people to the patient care areas in the back, thereby increasing security. Tips for ways to stay safe include:

- Stay alert for suspicious people.
- Listen to your instincts if a situation or person makes you feel strange or on edge.
- Try to alert another employee if a situation occurs. Many agencies have code words for emergency situations.
- Use emergency alarms when needed. Many will notify the local police department.

- Keep yourself at a distance from the person (e.g., try to separate yourself from the person by a desk or another piece of furniture).
- Position yourself so you are the closest to the door.
- Discuss the situation with the provider or supervisor if you are uncomfortable rooming a patient.
- Follow the facility's safety procedures.

CRITICAL THINKING 26.9

Over the past 6 months, crime and break-ins have increased in the local area around the clinic. Many people believe the healthcare facility has a supply of narcotic medication in stock, which is not true. What strategies can the staff implement to increase the security of the healthcare facility?

Workplace Violence. Stories of workplace violence are becoming more common. Healthcare employees face an increased risk of work-related assaults, primarily from patients and visitors. In the Guidelines for Preventing Workplace Violence for Healthcare and Social Service Workers, published by OSHA (available at https://www.osha.gov/Publications/osha3148.pdf), increased risk factors for violence in healthcare include:

- Working with patients or family members who have a history of violence, abuse alcohol or other substances, are gang members, or carry firearms or other weapons
- Poorly designed work environments, including inadequately lit hallways, rooms, parking lots, and other areas, which can limit vision of potential situations and interfere with escape plans
- Lack of emergency communication (e.g., alarms, healthcare facility's emergency procedures) and training of employees
- Working in neighborhoods with high crime rates
- High employee turnover
- Long waits for patients in overcrowded, uncomfortable reception areas
- Unrestricted areas, allowing public access to the major areas of the building
- A perception that violence is tolerated, and the police will not be called

OSHA encourages healthcare employees to take "universal precautions for violence." This means that ambulatory care facilities should be prepared for violent situations. Violence can be avoided or lessened by respecting others, protecting the dignity of others, and using teamwork to prevent violence. Medical assistants should report patient incidents or at-risk patient behaviors and situations to the manager.

Healthcare facilities should have violence prevention programs in place. Management and employees should work together to identify hazards and plan preventive strategies. According to OSHA, strategies to secure the workplace environment include:

- Physical barriers (e.g., locked doors, enclosures, bullet-proof windows, security guards)
- Bright, effective lighting and accessible exits
- Closed-circuit video (inside and outside of the building)
- De-escalating (dee es kah LATE ing) areas for patients and visitors
- Secure work areas for those working alone; panic buttons
- Name badges to identify employees

All employees should be trained to handle workplace violence and facility lockdown procedures. Lockdown is used when it is safer to stay where you are. This procedure is used when there is a dangerous person in the building or in the area:

- Lock or barricade the doors. If the person is in the area, lock windows and pull shades.
- Keep away from the windows and doors.
- If the person is in the building, silence cell phones. Contact 911 immediately and hide in a locked room.

Evaluating the Work Environment

It is important to safeguard both the patients and the employees from injuries in the healthcare facility. The medical assistant should continually evaluate the environment for safety. From a flipped-over rug to a burned-out light in the stairway, safety risks can lead to falls and injuries. This section explains how to evaluate the work environment for unsafe working conditions. When problems are fixed or corrected, the environment becomes safer for all. Remember that for all injuries that occur to patients, visitors, and employees, an incident report form must be completed. Incident report forms are discussed in Chapter 19.

Preventing Falls and Injuries. Accidents can be expensive for the healthcare facility because costs can range from loss of employee workdays to lawsuits. Preventing accidents is therefore critical. In the healthcare facility, there are many areas that can be prone to causing slips, trips, and falls. In the winter months, depending on the facility's geographic location, slips and falls can be common because of snow and ice. The healthcare facility should have employees who oversee the sidewalks for patients and visitors. Inside the facility, a number of high-risk situations can result in accidents:

- Water or trash on floors: Standing water on floors should be cleaned up. Signage should be used to indicate wet floors. Paper wrappings, covers, and other items should not be tossed on the floor during procedures, due to an increased risk of injury.
- Dim lighting: Burned-out lightbulbs should be replaced. All stairwells should have adequate lighting.
- Flooring and rugs: Rugs and mats need to be smooth and flat. Flooring that is old and pulling up needs to be replaced. Carpeting with holes can catch a shoe heel, causing the person to trip and fall.
- Cords, cables, and other objects in walkways: Electrical cords, computer cables, boxes, and other potential tripping hazards should never be in the walkway. Hallways and fire doors need to be clear of debris. Unused wheelchairs and walkers should be collapsed if possible and moved out of the way.
- Heavy objects placed on high shelves: These items can fall and injure someone. Reaching for a heavy object can also cause injury. Store heavier items on lower shelves so they do not have to be lifted any higher than necessary.
- Using unsafe objects to stand on: A chair or box could collapse or move when a person stands on it. Use a stable step-stool to reach for things.

> **VOCABULARY**
> **fire doors** Doors made of fire-resistant materials; close manually or automatically during a fire to prevent it from spreading.
> **de-escalating** To reduce the level or intensity; bringing down a person's anger or elevated emotions.

Preventing Electrical Issues and Fires. Malfunctioning equipment can also cause accidents. Any equipment that is not functioning or does not sound normal should not be used until it can be serviced and checked out. The medical assistant should follow the facility's procedure in this situation. Usually, the supervisor is notified if equipment is malfunctioning.

The medical assistant can help prevent injuries and fires in many ways, such as:

- Checking electrical cords and plugs for cracks, fraying, or other damage
- Ensuring power strips are not overloaded
- Not using electricity near water
- Turning off equipment that appears to be overheating or malfunctioning
- Storing potentially flammable chemicals and supplies according to the manufacturers' guidelines
- Keeping combustibles (e.g., paper, cardboard, cloth, flammable chemicals) away from heat sources

Many fires are started by smoking materials. It is important to have adequate No Smoking signs at the facility's doors. Deep, nontip ashtrays should be outside the doors so visitors have an adequate place to dispose of smoking materials.

Cautery equipment and lasers are commonly used in healthcare. Cautery equipment, by design, gets hot. Inappropriate use can cause fires. Lasers can cause health issues (e.g., burns and blindness) and fires. All staff members using or assisting with lasers should take a safety class. Signage should be on the door where the laser is being used. Water should be available if needed. Oxygen, other gases, and combustible chemicals should not be in the room when laser equipment is used.

Procedure 26.4 describes how to evaluate the environment for unsafe working conditions. Remember that when issues are found, it is important to fix them. If you cannot fix the unsafe condition, let your supervisor know immediately. Delays can increase the risk of others being injured.

Emergency Response Plan

A variety of emergency situations can occur and affect the healthcare facility. Each facility should have a plan to respond to these types of situations. An emergency response plan addresses possible workplace emergencies. This document guides the staff on handling emergencies and may protect the business. The occurrence of natural disasters may vary around the country. The emergency response plan should cover only potential emergencies seen at the facility and in the community (Table 26.1). Table 26.2 provides the critical elements that at the minimum must be included in the emergency response plan.

Having a plan is the first step. The employer also needs to train new staff on the procedures. Yearly refresher courses and mock drills help employees remain current on these procedures. The employer should document employee participation at the training sessions.

> **VOCABULARY**
> **workplace emergencies** Unforeseen situations that threaten the employees and visitors; can disrupt services provided.

Evacuation Procedures. Evacuation procedures involve identifying exit routes and implementing procedures for moving employees, patients, and visitors to safe locations. Floor maps with evacuation exit routes and emergency equipment locations should be posted throughout the facility (Fig. 26.13). It is recommended that at least two routes should be identified, which

TABLE 26.1 Potential Emergencies

Event	Type	Examples
Natural	Geologic hazards	Tsunami, volcano, landslide, and earthquake
	Meteorologic hazards	Flood, tornado, hurricane, and ice
	Biological hazards	Foodborne illnesses and communicable disease
Human caused	Accidental events	Hazardous spill, fire, and transportation incident (aircraft, vehicle)
	Intentional events	Robbery, lost person, bomb threat, terrorism, and weapons
	Technology-caused events	Telecommunication, electrical power, water, and cyber security issues

TABLE 26.2 Critical Elements That Must Be in an Emergency Response Plan

Critical Elements	Includes
Methods to report a fire and other emergencies	• How to alert employees of the emergency (e.g., alarms, overhead paging system). • How to alert law enforcement and the fire department.
Evacuation policy and procedure	• Evacuation conditions. • Clear chain of command and designated person to order the evacuation and to account for employees (may be called an *evacuation warden*). • Patient sign-in sheets or schedules that are used to account for patients. • Evacuation procedures, including routes and meeting locations; maps should be posted.
Critical shutdown procedures	• Names of specific employees who must perform certain procedures before leaving. • Critical shutdown procedures (describe what needs to be done); examples include turning off the water, gas, electricity, and oxygen (if piped into the exam rooms).
Emergency escape/exit routes and procedures	• Floor plan, workplace map, safe areas, and procedures.
Rescue and medical duties	• Names of workers who need to perform rescue and medical duties.
Who to contact for additional information	• Names, titles, and contact information of internal and external people who can provide additional information on emergency response plans (internal people would be management and other employees; external people might be community leaders and specialists).

From How to Plan for Workplace Emergencies and Evacuations. https://www.osha.gov/Publications/osha3088.html.

provides a backup route in case the primary route is blocked. Exit routes must follow these conventions:

- Be clearly marked and well lit
- Be wide enough to accommodate several people

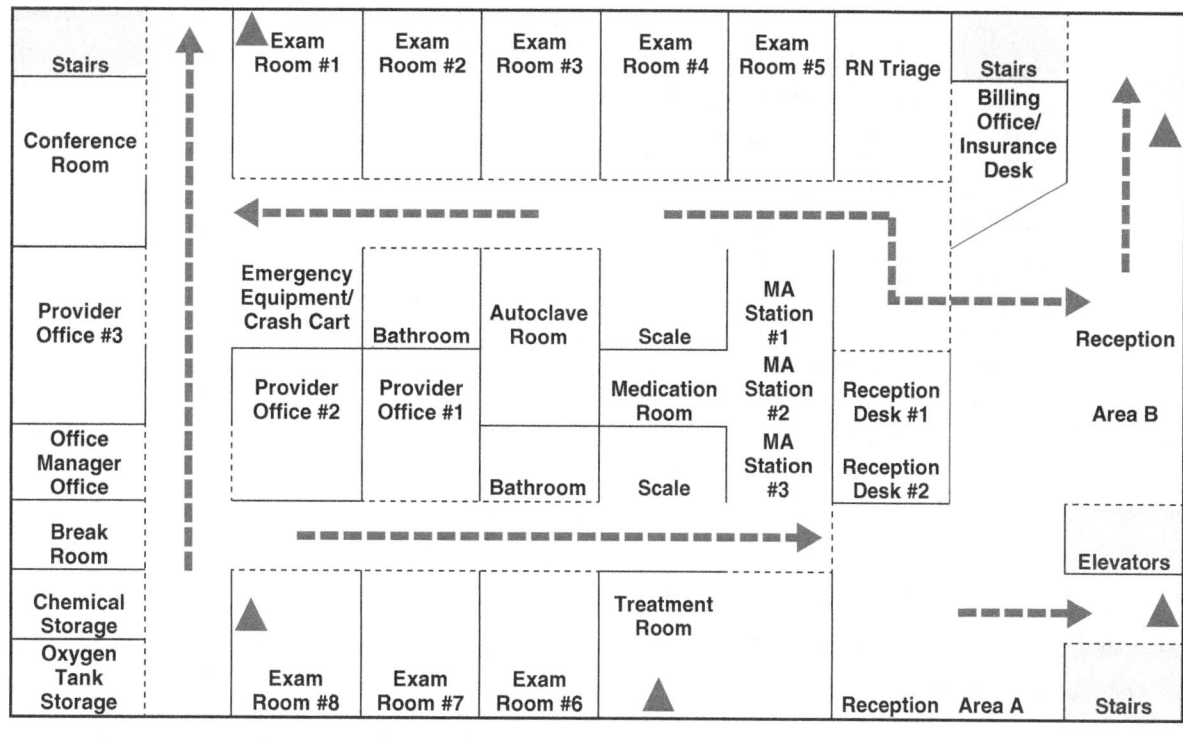

Fig. 26.13 A Floor Map With Exit Routes and Emergency Equipment Indicated.

- Not pass areas where flammable products (e.g., oxygen tanks, chemicals) are stored
- Be clear of debris and obstructions at all times

Some employees must assist those who need help evacuating. According to the Americans with Disabilities Act (ADA), safety requirements are needed for people in multistory buildings who need access to wheelchairs. Areas of rescue assistance are safe places where people in wheelchairs or those who cannot do stairs can await help in emergency situations. Typically, these areas are stairwells that have alarms that communicate with emergency personnel. Evacuation chairs can be used to move people down the stairs.

Evacuation is done by priority, either by location or by people. The evacuation priority by location is:

1. People in immediate danger
2. People located on the floor where the emergency is occurring
3. People on the floors immediately above and below the floor with the situation
4. People on the rest of the floors

Evacuation priority by people means the people nearest the emergency leave first, followed by the ambulatory people, and last the nonambulatory people. As people evacuate by priority, it is important that appointed staff remain behind to verify that everyone is out. All rooms, including restrooms, need to be checked.

Evacuation procedures vary based on the emergency (see Procedure 26.5). There are five types of evacuations:

- *Shelter-in-place evacuation*: Evacuation to an interior room with no windows. In cases of tornados and other severe storms, employees, patients, and visitors should evacuate to shelter-in-place locations. Typically, these locations should

be on the lowest level possible. Shelter-in-place locations are also used when a contaminant (e.g., chemical) is released into the environment.
- *Local evacuation*: Involves moving one or more people out of immediate danger (e.g., evacuating a patient from an exam room where a chemical spill occurred).
- *Horizontal evacuation*: Involves evacuating people off the same floor as the emergency situation.
- *Vertical evacuation*: Involves evacuating people who are located on the floors above and below the situation.
- *Building evacuation*: Involves evacuating everyone from the building to a safe location outside the building.

Fire Response. A medical assistant should be aware of the healthcare facility's fire response procedures. It is important to know how to activate the alarms, evacuate people, and use a fire extinguisher for small fires. The following are fire response actions.

- A wall-mounted fire extinguisher, manual pull station (alarm), warning alarms, smoke alarms, and automatic sprinkler systems should be located throughout the facility per state code. An employee should be assigned to routinely check this equipment and replace it as needed (Box 26.2).
- If you smell smoke or suspect a fire, think of the acronym RACE:
  Rescue individuals threatened by the fire.
  Activate the alarm if you discover the fire or respond if you hear the alarm.
  Confine the fire by closing doors and fire doors to slow the spread of the fire.

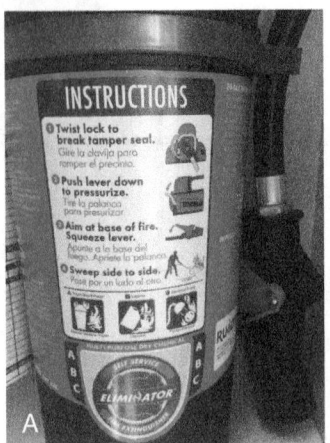 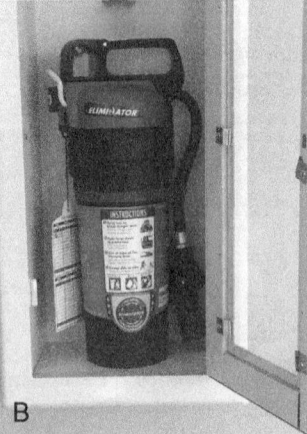

Fig. 26.14 A, The Eliminator is a new type of fire extinguisher. B, Users must follow "TPASS" when using the Eliminator.

TABLE 26.3	**Uses of Fire Extinguishers**
Labeled Class	**Used for**
A	Water extinguisher: Used on *ordinary combustibles* (e.g., paper, wood, rubber, cloth, and many plastics)
B	Carbon dioxide (CO_2) extinguisher: Used on flammable liquids; fires in oils and grease
C	Dry chemical extinguisher: Used on electrical equipment; fires in wiring, fuse boxes, computers, and other electrical sources
ABC	Multipurpose dry chemical extinguisher. Used on ordinary combustibles, flammable liquids, or electrical equipment
D	Fires involving combustible metals: May be found in the medical laboratory
K	Fires involving combustible cooking oils and fats: Found in the kitchen

---

BOX 26.2   New Fire Extinguisher Technology

A new type of fire extinguisher, the Eliminator, has changed the way fire extinguishers are used (Fig. 26.14A). This new fire extinguisher has an ergonomically designed handle and spray hose. Most fire extinguishers need to be serviced and maintained to keep them operable. This extinguisher allows facilities to maintain it more easily and cheaply than other extinguishers. When using the Eliminator, a person must follow "TPASS" (Fig. 26.14B):

T: Twist the lock to break the seal.
P: Push the level down. This will pressurize the extinguisher.
A: Aim the valve nozzle at the base of the fire.
S: Squeeze the valve level.
S: Sweep the valve nozzle from side to side to put out the fire.

Extinguish only small fires; otherwise evacuate individuals from the area.
- Do not use elevators if a fire is suspected. This will reduce the risk of entrapment.
- If a fire is suspected, immediately disconnect oxygen supplies or turn off oxygen tanks to prevent an explosion.
- Use the correct type of extinguisher for the fire (Table 26.3).
- For small fires, use the PASS procedure as you operate a fire extinguisher (see Procedure 26.6).
  Pull the pin.
  Aim the nozzle or hose at the base of the fire.
  Squeeze the handle to release the extinguishing agent.
  Sweep the nozzle or hose from side to side at the base of the fire until the fire is out. Evacuate if you are not successful or doubt your ability to put out the fire.

CRITICAL THINKING 26.10

One morning when the weather is stormy, Marie and Catherine are discussing the facility's emergency policy and procedures. How would you respond to a tornado warning and the need to evacuate to a shelter-in-place? How would you respond if you found a wastebasket on fire in the facility?

Effects of Stress

When a person is involved in an emergency, this can cause physical and emotional signs and symptoms, including:
- Shock, disbelief, irritability, crying, sadness, and anger
- Fear, anxiety, a feeling of numbness, a feeling of powerlessness, and difficulty making decisions
- High blood pressure, high blood glucose levels, back pain, and stomach problems
- Loss of interest in normal activities, trouble concentrating
- Nightmares, sleep problems, and tension

The term general adaptation syndrome (GAS) is used to describe the long- and short-term effects of stress on the body. GAS was originally described by Hans Selye. He felt the syndrome affected the nervous and the endocrine systems. These are the stages:
- *Stage 1 – Alarm reaction*: This is the immediate reaction to the stressor. The "fight-or-flight" response occurs. The body releases the hormones cortisol, adrenaline, and noradrenaline. This provides energy, preparing the body for physical activities. This stage can affect the immune system, causing the person to be more susceptible to illness.
- *Stage 2 – Adaptation stage*: If the stressor continues, the individual's body adapts to the stressor. During this stage, the body begins to repair itself and the hormone levels gradually return to normal.
- *Stage 3 – Exhaustion stage*: At this point, the body's resistance has been diminished by the continued stress. The body is more susceptible to disease.

CLOSING COMMENTS

The medical assistant has many important duties to help the healthcare facility operate. From opening and closing the facility to managing inventory, these duties are important to the success of the facility. Paying attention to detail while performing these duties is important. Keeping the right amount of supplies in stock so providers can treat patients also requires paying attention to details.

The medical assistant also needs to be knowledgeable about the emergency policies and procedures of the healthcare facility. When an emergency occurs is not the time to read the procedure on what to do! It is important for the medical assistant to be calm, cool, and composed during these times. This will help others around you to remain calm.

CHAPTER REVIEW

The medical assistant has many tasks to perform when opening the healthcare facility. Many times, these duties are split between the administrative and the clinical medical assistants. Time must be taken to be prepared. This will make the day run more smoothly.

Just as with opening the facility, the medical assistant has closing duties. It is important not to put tasks off until the next morning. Completing the facility closing tasks will ease the burden in the morning. Besides daily duties, the medical assistant also has monthly duties to keep the facility clean and organized.

for the medical assistant to check them immediately for any items that need to be transferred to the refrigerator or freezer.

There is a lot the medical assistant can do to ensure the safety and security of those in the facility. Using proper body mechanics is an important way for medical assistants to protect themselves from injury. It is also critical for the medical assistant to continually evaluate the work environment for unsafe conditions. Items such as trash on the floor or flipped-over rugs

PATIENT-CENTERED CARE

Safety is a concern for both patients and healthcare professionals. The medical assistant should be alert for potential situations that could turn violent. Treating patients and family members with respect, listening to their concerns, and following through with promises are especially important when working in healthcare. A person who feels respected and listened to is less likely to get angry to the point of violence.

BEING PROFESSIONAL

Being honest, dependable, and reliable are important characteristics for the professional medical assistant. When a mistake or an oversight occurs, it is important for the medical assistant to admit it to the provider or supervisor.

Role-play this scenario: You and Cara are medical assistants. You are responsible for checking the vaccine refrigerator and freezer every morning. Today, you realize that you forgot to do the check yesterday. You tell Cara, and she encourages you to make up information for yesterday. Respond to Cara regarding this situation.

The medical assistant also has a role in managing equipment and supplies. Managing the inventory and ordering supplies are major responsibilities. When the supplies arrive, it is important

are real safety hazards that can take just seconds to correct. All healthcare professionals have an obligation to be current on the facility's emergency policies and procedures. This knowledge will pay off when an emergency occurs.

SCENARIO WRAP-UP

Marie has started to implement an inventory management process that is helping her identify when to reorder and how much to reorder. Initially she hand-counted the inventory, and then she identified how much was used each buying cycle. It took a few months for her to identify trends. She found certain times of the year affected the quantity of products used. For instance, providers tended to use more casting products in the winter and

summer months, which means Marie will need to increase her stock of those items during these times of the year. Marie knows that the more she learns, the more efficient she can become when managing inventory. She has already helped the facility save money by identifying cheaper vendors for commonly used expensive items. Marie loves her new job and the variety of responsibilities she has. She looks forward to continual learning.

PROCEDURE 26.1   Perform an Equipment Inventory With Documentation

Tasks

Perform an equipment inventory. Document the inventory on the equipment inventory form.

Equipment and Supplies

- Equipment inventory form
- Pens
- Administrative or clinical equipment
- Purchase information (e.g., date, cost, and supplier) and warranty information (e.g., start and end date, warranty coverage)

Procedural Steps

1. For the equipment to be inventoried, gather the following information for each piece of equipment:

- Name of equipment, manufacturer, and serial number
- Location and facility number (if applicable)
- Purchase date, cost, supplier, and warranty information

Purpose: It is important to have the essential information required when creating the spreadsheet.

2. Complete an equipment inventory form by adding the gathered information for each item inventoried (see Fig. 26.4).

Purpose: Creating an equipment inventory list on the computer will help you organize the information. It will also help you maintain the information easily.

3. Review the document created. Make any necessary revisions.

Purpose: It is important to proofread your work to ensure it is accurate.

PROCEDURE 26.2   Perform Routine Maintenance of Equipment

Tasks

Perform routine maintenance of administrative or clinical equipment. Document the maintenance on the log.

Equipment and Supplies

- Maintenance log(s)
- Pens
- Information regarding the equipment (i.e., name, serial number, location, facility number, manufacturer, purchase date, warranty information, frequency of inspections, and service provider)
- Administrative or clinical equipment (e.g., oral thermometers)
- Supplies for routine maintenance (e.g., battery)
- Users' guide or owner's manual, if needed

Procedural Steps

1. Gather information on the piece of equipment identified for routine maintenance, including name, serial number, location, facility number, manufacturer, purchase date, warranty information, frequency of inspections, and service provider.

Purpose: It is important to have the essential information required when completing the log.

2. Fill in the equipment details on the log (see Fig. 26.5).

Purpose: Adding the equipment details helps identify the machine. It provides a quick reference to useful information that the service provider might request. The form serves as a log for documenting the maintenance activities performed.

3. To perform the maintenance activities, gather the required supplies. If you are not familiar with the procedure or the required supplies, refer to the users' guide.

Purpose: You need to be familiar with the supplies and the procedure before you start the maintenance.

4. Perform the maintenance activities as directed in the users' guide. Take any required safety precautions necessary to protect yourself and others.

Purpose: Following the outlined procedure in the users' guide will help you successfully complete the maintenance without injuring yourself or others or damaging the machine.

5. Clean up the work area.

Purpose: It is important to clean up after yourself.

6. Using a pen, document the date, time, and maintenance activity performed, and include your signature on the log.

Purpose: The log, indicating the activities performed, will serve as a communication tool for future reference and services needed on that piece of equipment.

PROCEDURE 26.3   Perform a Supply Inventory With Documentation While Using Proper Body Mechanics

Tasks

Perform a supply inventory using correct body mechanics. Document the inventory on the supply inventory form.

Equipment and Supplies

- Supply inventory form
- Pens
- Administrative or clinical supplies to be inventoried
- Purchase information (e.g., item number, cost, and supplier) for supplies in inventory
- Reorder point and quantity to reorder for each item in inventory

Procedural Steps

1. For the supplies in inventory, gather the following information for each item:
   - Name, size, quantity (e.g., purchased individually, 100 per box)

- Item number, supplier's name, cost
- Reorder point and quantity to reorder

Purpose: This information is required as you create the inventory form.

2. For each supply item, enter information on the inventory form. Make sure the appropriate entry is in the right location (see Fig. 26.6). *Note:* The "Stock Available" column will be empty for now.

Purpose: Creating a supply inventory list will help you organize the information and maintain the information easily.

3. Review the document. Make any necessary revisions.

Purpose: Make sure the document is correct so errors do not affect the inventory process.

4. Using the supply inventory list, inventory the supplies in the department. Identify how the supply should be counted (e.g., individually, by the box), and count the number of items in stock.

PROCEDURE 26.3 Perform a Supply Inventory With Documentation While Using Proper Body Mechanics—cont'd

Purpose: By identifying the correct quantity by which the item is inventoried, you will increase the accuracy of the inventory. Counting an item by "each" when it comes as a package can cause confusion when identifying what needs to be ordered.

5. Add the number in the appropriate row under the "Stock Available" header.
   Purpose: Making sure you add the number to the correct column and row will keep your inventory form accurate.
6. Compare the reorder point number to the stock available number. If the stock available number is at or below the reorder point, indicate that the item needs to be reordered by checking the appropriate column.
   Purpose: Identify the supplies that need to be ordered.
7. Make sure the supplies are neatly arranged. The older stock should be in front of the newer stock.
   Purpose: It is important to clean up your workspace. The oldest stock must be moved to the front to ensure it is used first.

8. Repeat steps 5 through 7 until all supplies are inventoried.
9. Use proper body mechanics when lifting and moving supplies by maintaining a wide, stable base with your feet. Your feet should be shoulder-width apart, and you should have good footing. Bend at the knees, keeping your back straight. Lift smoothly with the major muscles in your arms and legs. Use the same technique when putting the item down.
   Purpose: Correct body mechanics will reduce your risk for injury when carrying or lifting heavy objects. See Figs. 26.11 and 26.12 for proper body mechanics when lifting boxes.
10. Use proper body mechanics when reaching for an object. Clear away barriers and use a step stool if needed. Your feet should face the object. Avoid twisting or turning with a heavy load.
    Purpose: Straining when reaching or standing on tiptoes can increase your risk for injury.

PROCEDURE 26.4 Evaluate the Work Environment

Tasks
Evaluate the work environment and identify unsafe working conditions.

Equipment and Supplies
- Work environment evaluation form
- Pen

Procedural Steps
1. Observe the environment for slipping, tripping, or fall risks. Document your findings for the following questions:
   - Is the lighting appropriate? Are any lights burned out? Are any areas dim?
   - Are the flooring and carpeting ripped or pulled up? If rugs/mats are present, are they folded?
   - Is water on the floor? Is signage present warning of the water?
   - Are items cluttering the hallway, making walking difficult?
   - Are cords, cables, and other items in the walkway?
   - Is trash on the floor?
   - Are heavy items on high shelves? Is a sturdy step stool available?
   Purpose: When the floor is cluttered, or the flooring is damaged, the risk of falls increases.
2. Observe the environment for safety and security issues. Document your findings for the following questions:
   - Are rooms available that can be locked and used during workplace violence? Is there limited visibility from the hallway into the room?
   - Are there areas in the building with limited visibility?
   - If the building is accessible to the public, are there any safe zones or areas for staff?
   - Are the emergency call lights in the exam rooms and bathrooms functioning?
   - Are the oxygen tanks (if available) checked per the facility's policy?
   Purpose: Having a safe area in a building is important during a workplace violence situation.
3. Observe the environment for fire risks and electrical issues. Document your findings for the following questions:

- Are electrical cords and plugs free from cracks, fraying, or other damage?
- Are power strips overloaded?
- Is electricity being used near a water source?
- Are flammable chemicals and supplies stored according to manufacturers' guidelines?
- Are combustibles (e.g., paper, cardboard, cloth, flammable chemicals) stored and kept away from heat sources?
Purpose: The risk of fires increases when cords are damaged or power strips are overloaded. Safe storage of chemicals is important to reduce the fire risk.
4. Observe the environment for fire containment and evacuation strategies. Document your findings for the following questions:
   - Are building diagrams posted on walls? Are exit routes indicated? Are two or more exit routes indicated on the map? Are fire alarms and fire extinguishers indicated?
   - Are exit routes uncluttered?
   - Are exit signs visible and lit?
   - Are fire doors unlocked and able to be closed in an emergency?
   - Are interior rooms available for severe storms?
   - Are smoke detectors located throughout the building? Are fire alarms available?
   - Are fire extinguishers available and checked routinely (per the facility's policy)?
   - Are flammable products (e.g., oxygen tanks, chemicals) stored along the exit routes?
   Purpose: Two or more exit routes should be available. Flammable products should not be stored in the location of the exit routes. Closed fire doors will help contain the fire.
5. Based on your observations, summarize your findings. If risks are present, create a list of issues that need to be addressed. Describe what needs to be done for each risk.
   Purpose: Creating a list of issues that need to be addressed is important in a professional setting.

PROCEDURE 26.5 Participate in a Mock Exposure Event

Tasks

Demonstrate self-awareness in an emergency situation. Participate in a mock exposure event and document specific steps taken. Recognize the physical and emotional effects on individuals involved in an emergency situation.

Scenario

You and Beth are in the autoclave room and two chemicals spill, creating toxic fumes. Beth is having trouble breathing. The following staff, patients, and visitors are present.

Rooms	Staff and Reception Areas
1 – Teen and his mother	Reception Area A – Four people waiting
2 – Older woman in a wheelchair	Reception Area B – Five people waiting
3 – Mother with three little children	**Staff**
4 – Adult female	Tim – In MA station 3
5 – Empty	Rose – At the insurance desk
6 – An older couple	Dave and Patty – At the receptionist
7 – Adult male	desk
8 – Empty	Julie Walden, MD – In provider office 1
Procedure room – Empty	Angela Perez, MD – In room 3
	Jean Burke, NP – In room 7

Directions

Create a paper and address the procedure steps. Use reliable Internet resources to research physical and emotional effects of stress on the body. Include your findings in the paper as indicated in the procedure steps. Use 1-inch margins, double spacing, and 12-point font. Length should be at least two pages.

Equipment and Supplies

- Paper
- Pen
- Floor map (see Fig. 26.13)
- Computer with internet access

Procedural Steps

1. Using the scenario, describe how you would handle the emergency exposure situation with Beth.
   - Identify four steps a medical assistant could take to demonstrate self-awareness while responding to this emergency situation.
   - Describe exposure control mechanisms or how you might limit the exposure to other people once you remove Beth from the room.

Purpose: It is important to be self-aware as to how you would respond in emergency situations. Exposure control mechanisms are ways to limit the exposure to other people. How might you contain the situation? How might you prevent others from being affected by the exposure?

Scenario update: Dr. Walden instructs the staff to evacuate from the building. The outdoor safe meeting location is at the back of the parking lot.

2. Document the steps to handle the exposure event and evacuation from the building.
   - Describe what each staff member and provider should do to help with the evacuation procedure and notify 911.
   - Describe the steps (evacuations) in the order that they should occur.
   - Describe how the staff may ensure all individuals are out of the building.

Purpose: It is important to know which individuals need to be evacuated first, second, and so on. Employees should work with individuals in their area unless they have an appointed duty. Making sure all individuals are out of the building is important before the staff leaves the area.

3. Dr. Walden is in charge during the emergency. Describe what her responsibilities include.

Purpose: The evacuation warden's name is listed in the emergency response plan. This person is in charge of the evacuation.

4. Dave took the patient registry. Describe why the patient registry is important.

Purpose: The patient registry lists the patients who have checked in for appointments.

Scenario update: Two weeks after the event, Beth confides to you that she is not doing well. She has recovered from the exposure, but since the event she has had difficulty sleeping. She is anxious when she goes into the autoclave room. She is having trouble concentrating on her job. She mentions she has had two nightmares of emergencies occurring in the department and she gets injured.

5. Do the following:
   - Describe what might be occurring with Beth and the symptoms that relate to it.
   - Discuss what you might encourage her to do about the situation.

Purpose: It is not uncommon after an emergency that individuals involved experience issues related to the emergency.

6. Research the physical and emotional effects of stress on the body. Identify four physical effects and four emotional effects of stress on persons involved in an emergency situation. Cite your resources.

7. Describe how the physical and emotional effects of stress would be different for Beth, you, the providers, and the other employees present.

8. Describe how a medical assistant could limit the physical and emotional effects of stress on each person/group: Beth, the providers, the other employees present in the facility, and yourself.

PROCEDURE 26.6 Use a Fire Extinguisher

Tasks

Select the correct fire extinguisher and demonstrate its correct use.

Scenarios

a. You are working in the medical laboratory, and an electrical fire starts.

b. You are working in the clinic, and a fire starts in a wastebasket.

c. You are working in the medical laboratory, and a chemical fire starts (combustible metal fire).

Equipment and Supplies

- Fire extinguisher

Procedural Steps

1. Using the scenario, identify the type of fire extinguisher required to put out the fire.

Purpose: The correct fire extinguisher must be used to put out the fire. Using the wrong extinguisher can make the fire worse.

2. Hold the extinguisher by the handle with the hose or nozzle pointing away from you. Pull out the pin that is located below the trigger.

Purpose: Pulling the pin allows the extinguisher to be used.

3. Stand about 10 feet from the fire. Aim the extinguisher hose or nozzle at the base of the fire. Keep the extinguisher in an upright position as you work.

Purpose: The most efficient method of putting out fires is to work at the base of the fire.

4. Squeeze the trigger slowly and evenly.

Purpose: Squeezing slowly allows the discharge to come out in a steady flow.

5. Sweep from side to side until the fire is out.

Purpose: As the fire nearest to you is put out, you can move closer to the rest of the fire.

27

Health Insurance Basics

LEARNING OBJECTIVES

1. Define insurance related terminology.
2. List the 10 categories of essential health benefits according to the Affordable Care Act (ACA).
3. Describe various types of government-sponsored insurance plans.
4. Describe different types of private health insurance plans.
5. Discuss traditional health insurance and differentiate among the different types of managed care models.
6. Explain the health insurance contract between the healthcare provider and the health insurance company.

7. Summarize the medical assistant's role in health insurance, including reading a health insurance identification card, verifying eligibility for services, and completing precertifications, preauthorizations, and referrals.
8. Discuss disability insurance, life insurance, long-term care insurance, and liability insurance.
9. Describe the impact that the ACA has had on health insurance in the United States.

OUTLINE

⯈ OPENING SCENARIO

John Bimmell, a registered medical assistant (RMA), has worked for Walden-Martin Family Medical (WMFM) Clinic for 3 years. John started with WMFM Clinic as a receptionist. Donna Potter, the office manager, recognized that John was very detail oriented, so, 2 years ago, she asked him to take charge of the health insurance policies and procedures manual for the practice.

John also trains all new medical assistants on how to verify patient health insurance coverage and eligibility. Because John has learned quite a bit about health insurance, he can answer most of the patients' questions about their coverage, benefits, and/or the exclusions of their policies. He knows where to direct patients who have more complicated questions and how to follow up – one of the most important duties of a professional medical assistant. He has a great attitude about assisting patients with insurance questions and does not hesitate to contact the insurance company on the patient's behalf.

He provides patients with exceptional customer service. When patients call him for assistance, he responds within 24 hours (often within 1 hour) with answers to their questions or a resource to help them. John is willing to help any staff member with other duties when necessary and prides himself on being a patient advocate. He is an enthusiastic team player who puts patients first.

YOU WILL LEARN

1. To identify the various government health insurance plans.
2. To identify private health insurance plans.
3. To recognize the different managed care organizations.
4. To understand what it means to be a participating provider.
5. To understand the medical assistant's role with insurance related activities in the ambulatory care facility.

INTRODUCTION

Insurance is something that is purchased to help protect against loss or harm from specified circumstances. Using automobile insurance as an example, the specified circumstances are those related to a car accident. The insurance could pay for damage done to your vehicle or other vehicles. It could also pay for medical expenses for anyone injured in an accident. With health insurance, the specified circumstances are those related to the policyholder's health. This insurance would pay for hospital expenses, provider expenses, and certain supplies and equipment.

A policy is purchased with a premium. The premium can be paid by:

- An individual
- An employer
- A combination of employer contribution and individual (employee) contribution

The policy is considered a legal contract and will stay in force as long as the premium is being paid. The policy will specify exactly what services are covered. The more services that are covered, the higher the premium cost. The person responsible for the payment of the premium is referred to as a *subscriber*.

Most policies require the patient to pay a portion of the healthcare expenses. This is referred to as *cost-sharing*, which includes the features:

- *Deductible*: A set dollar amount that the policyholder must pay before the insurance company starts to pay for services. Usually the deductible is met on a yearly basis. It can be as low as $100 and as high as $5,000. Generally, plans with higher monthly premiums usually have lower deductibles and plans with lower monthly premiums have higher deductibles.
- *Coinsurance*: The percentage of costs of a covered healthcare service the policyholder pays after the deductible has been paid. The insurance company pays its portion, and the policyholder pays the remaining amount. A typical split is 80/20 – the insurance company pays 80%, and the policyholder pays 20%.
- *Copayment*: Also called copay. A set dollar amount that the policyholder must pay for each office visit. It is possible that copayments differ for different types of office visits. For example, there can be one copayment amount for a primary care provider and a different copayment amount (usually higher) to see a specialist or to be seen in the emergency department.

The policy will specify the dollar amounts for the deductible, coinsurance, and copayment. The premium is not usually considered part of cost-sharing.

In order for the insurance carrier to pay for services, a claim must be submitted. The claim is reviewed by the insurance company to determine if the services provided are covered under the policy. It is important for a medical assistant to be familiar with the different types of insurance so that claims can be submitted accurately. This will result in faster payment for the healthcare facility.

> ### VOCABULARY
> **claim** A formal request for payment from an insurance company for services provided.
> **policy** A written agreement between two parties, in which one party (the insurance company) agrees to pay another party (the patient) if certain specified circumstances occur.
> **premium** The periodic (monthly, quarterly, or annual) payment of a specific sum of money to an insurance company, for which the insurer in return agrees to provide certain benefits.

BENEFITS

The Affordable Care Act (ACA) requires all health plans to cover essential health benefits. There are 10 categories of essential health benefits:

- Ambulatory patient services
- Hospitalization
- Mental health and substance use disorder services
- Prescription drugs
- Preventive and wellness services and chronic disease management
- Emergency services
- Maternity and newborn care
- Rehabilitative and habilitative services and devices
- Laboratory services
- Pediatric services, including oral and vision care

In addition to the essential health benefits, an insurance policy may cover other services. For a group policy, an employer can pick and choose the benefits it wants for employees, such as vision or dental coverage. Medical assistants should contact an insurance company to determine if certain services are covered under a patient's policy.

HEALTH INSURANCE PLANS

There are two types of health insurance plans in the United States:

- Government health insurance plans
- Private health insurance plans

Health insurance plans typically cover health services and procedures that are deemed medically necessary. *Medically necessary* services are those that are necessary to improve the patient's current health. Most insurance policies do not cover elective procedures. *Elective procedures* are medical procedures that are not deemed medically necessary, such as a facelift or another cosmetic procedure. The ACA states that health insurance plans must cover preventive care. *Preventive care* includes services provided to help prevent certain illnesses or that lead to an early diagnosis. Insurance companies must cover preventive care services and cannot impose cost-sharing for those services. Preventive care services include:

- Alcohol misuse screening
- Blood pressure screening
- Cholesterol screening
- Colorectal cancer screening
- Depression screening
- Diabetes (type 2) screening
- Diet counseling
- Hepatitis B and C screening
- Human immunodeficiency virus (HIV) screening
- Immunization vaccines
- Lung cancer screening
- Obesity screening and counseling
- Tobacco use screening
- Sexually transmitted infection (STI) prevention counseling

Government Health Insurance Plans

Government health insurance plans provide coverage with reduced or no monthly premiums for the indigent (IN di juh nt), the elderly, the military, and government employees. There are a number of different plans, but patients need to qualify by:

- Age
- Income
- Government occupation
- Health condition

A patient who is age 65 or older can qualify for *Medicare*. A low-income patient may be eligible for *Medicaid*. Dependents of military personnel are covered by *TRICARE*. Surviving spouses and dependent children of veterans who died in the line of duty are covered by the *Civilian Health and Medical Program of the Veterans Administration* (CHAMPVA). Employees who are injured or become ill due to work-related issues are covered under *workers' compensation insurance*.

VOCABULARY

indigent Poor, needy, impoverished.

resource-based relative value scale (RBRVS) A system used to determine how much providers should be paid for services rendered. It is used by Medicare and many other health insurance companies.

Medicare. Medicare is a federal health insurance program that provides healthcare coverage for individuals who are age 65 or older; people who are disabled; and patients who have been diagnosed with end-stage renal disease (ESRD). Medicare refers to those covered by Medicare as *beneficiaries*. Medicare currently is the world's largest insurance program. In 2020 there were more than 67.7 million beneficiaries, of which almost 93% were age 65 or older.

The Medicare program is administered by the Centers for Medicare and Medicaid Services (CMS), a division of the Department of Health and Human Services (HHS). Laws enacted by Congress regulate the Medicare program. The Medicare plan is divided into four parts (Table 27.1):

- Part A covers inpatient hospital charges. It is financed with special contributions deducted from employed individuals' salaries, with matching contributions from their employers. Due to these contributions and regular Social Security contributions, there is no monthly premium for Part A.
- Part B covers ambulatory care, including primary care and specialists. Beneficiaries are required to pay a monthly premium. As of 2021, the standard monthly premium was $148.50. In addition, beneficiaries are required to meet a yearly deductible of $203 before Medicare covers any services (Box 27.1). Beneficiaries can visit any specialist without a referral.
- Part C is an option for Medicare-qualified patients to turn their Part A and Part B benefits into a private plan that can offer some additional benefits, such as over-the-counter medications, transportation to and from doctor appointments, and adult day care services. The private plan must cover everything that would be covered under Part A and Part B (Box 27.2).
- Part D is a prescription drug program offered to Medicare-qualified individuals that requires an additional monthly premium. To enroll in Part D, you must have either Parts A and B or Part C. When you enroll in a Part D plan, you are responsible for paying your deductible, premium, copayment, and coinsurance amounts. The maximum Medicare Part D deductible for 2021 was $445. Some drug plans charge a $0 yearly deductible, but this amount can vary depending on the provider, your location, and other factors.

Basic medical coverage for Medicare Part B is 80% of the allowed amount after the deductible. This means that patients are responsible for the remaining 20%. The allowed amount is determined using a resource-based relative value scale (RBRVS). The RBRVS is one of the outcomes of the Medicare Physician Payment Reform that was enacted in the Omnibus

TABLE 27.1 Comparing Medicare Plans

	Covered Services	Monthly Premium	Deductible
Part A	Inpatient hospital care, skilled nursing facilities, home healthcare, and hospice services	$0	$1,484 deductible for each benefit period (2021); Days 1–60: $0 coinsurance for each benefit period; Days 61–90: $371 coinsurance per day of each benefit period; Day 91 and beyond: $742 coinsurance per each "lifetime reserve day" after day 90 for each benefit period (up to 60 days over a lifetime)
Part B	Outpatient hospital care, durable medical equipment, provider's services, and other medical services	$148.50	$203 (2021), plus 20% coinsurance for all medical services
Part C	Expanded inpatient hospital and outpatient hospital care benefits	Varies by plan	Varies by plan
Part D	Prescription drugs	Varies by income	Varies by plan

Medicare: Medicare Costs at a Glance. https://www.medicare.gov/your-medicare-costs/costs-at-a-glance/costs-at-glance.html.

BOX 27.1   Medigap

If people have Medicare Part A and Part B, they may choose to purchase a Medigap policy from private health insurance companies. Medigap is Medicare Supplement Insurance that covers the payment "gaps" in Medicare for an individual person. After Medicare pays its share, the Medigap policy pays it share. A Medigap policy can help pay the remaining healthcare costs, such as copayments, deductibles, coinsurance, and services not covered by Medicare. Some policies can also cover medical care costs when a person travels outside of the US.

BOX 27.2   Medicare Advantage Plans

Medicare Advantage Plans (also called Part C or MA Plans) are offered by Medicare-approved private insurance companies. The most common types of Medicare Advantage plans include health maintenance organization (HMO) plans, preferred provider organization (PPO) plans, private fee-for-service (PFFS) plans, and special needs plans (SNPs) plans. The Medicare Advantage Plans provide Medicare Part A and Part B coverage. Most plans provide drug coverage (Part D). Patients need to use healthcare providers who participate in the network. The plans set limits on what the person has to pay out-of-pocket each year for covered services, thus protecting against unexpected costs. An out-of-network coverage option might be available with some plans at a higher cost. The patient must use the Medicare Advantage Plan card to get the Medicare-covered services. A person with a Medicare Advantage Plan does not need a Medigap policy.

Budget Reconciliation Act of 1989 (OBRA '89). Since 1992 the fee schedule for Medicare Part B is determined using the RBRVS. This system consists of three parts:

- Provider work
- Charge-based professional liability expenses
- Charge-based overhead

The provider work component includes the degree of effort invested by a provider in a particular service or procedure and the time it consumed. The professional liability and overhead components are computed by the CMS.

The RBRVS fee schedule is designed to provide nationally uniform payments after adjustment to reflect the differences in practice costs across geographic areas. The fee schedule includes a conversion factor, which is a single national number applied to all services paid under the fee schedule. Conversion factors are changed by Congress, usually annually, at the request of the CMS.

Depending on the contract between the provider and the insurance carrier (especially Medicare, Medicaid, and other government programs), the provider writes off the difference between the RBRVS schedule and their fee. Contracts between the provider of service and the insurance company vary greatly, depending on the insurance. It is important for the medical assistant to know the contract terms for each insurance company. As insurance payments are received, the medical assistant should examine the explanation of benefits (EOB) closely to ensure that all benefits have been reimbursed correctly.

CRITICAL THINKING 27.1

Jana Green is a Medicare patient who has Part A and Part B coverage. Will Medicare cover her office visit with the cardiologist? If so, would the coverage be Part A or Part B? What percent of the bill will she be responsible for?

VOCABULARY

explanation of benefits (EOB) A document sent by the insurance company to the provider and the patient explaining the allowed charge amount, the amount reimbursed for services, and the patient's financial responsibilities.
fee schedule A list of fixed fees for services.

Medicaid. Medicaid is a healthcare program that assists low-income families or individuals in paying for doctor visits, hospital stays, long-term medical and custodial care costs, and more. Because Medicaid programs are state administered, each state's program has a different name, such as Medi-Cal (CA), Buckeye Health Plan (OH), or Mountain Health Trust (PA).

Both state and federal governments split funding responsibilities for Medicaid. To receive federal funding, each state is required to cover certain services, but can decide to cover additional services. The required services include:

- Inpatient hospital services
- Outpatient hospital services
- Nursing facility services
- Early and periodic screening, diagnostic, and treatment (EPSDT) services
- Home health services
- Physician services
- Rural health clinic service
- Federally qualified health center services
- Laboratory and x-ray services
- Family planning services
- Nurse midwife services
- Certified pediatric and family nurse practitioner services
- Freestanding birth center services
- Transportation to medical care
- Tobacco cessation counseling for pregnant women

Eligibility for benefits is determined by the respective states, but most Medicaid recipients also are some or all of:

- Low-income families
- Qualified pregnant women and children
- Recipients of Temporary Assistance for Needy Families (TANF)
- Individuals who receive Supplemental Security Income (SSI)
- Individuals who receive certain types of federal and state aid
- Individuals who are qualified Medicare beneficiaries (QMBs) – Medicaid pays for Medicare Part B premiums, deductibles, and coinsurance for qualified low-income elderly individuals
- Individuals in institutions or receiving long-term care in nursing facilities and intermediate-care facilities

A person eligible for Medicaid in one state may not be eligible in another state and covered medical services may differ.

An ambulatory care facility has the right to limit the number of Medicaid patients it accepts into the practice. The medical office cannot pick and choose which Medicaid patients they are willing to see. There can be no discrimination based on age, sex, gender identity, race, religious preference, or national origin. A physician may choose to participate in the Medicaid program or not to accept Medicaid patients. Participating in the Medicaid program means agreeing to accept Medicaid reimbursement for covered services as payment in full. The physician must write off the difference, if any, between fees charged for services and the amount reimbursed. The physician may not bill the patient for the difference. The Medicaid fee schedule is the lowest of all insurance companies. A provider who accepts Medicaid patients automatically agrees to accept Medicaid's allowed amount as payment in full for covered services. Some patients who are eligible for Medicaid are required to pay a copayment. The provider can only collect the copayment from the patient.

VOCABULARY

eligibility Meeting the stipulated requirements to participate in the healthcare plan.

qualified Medicare beneficiaries (QMBs) Low-income Medicare patients who qualify for Medicaid for their secondary insurance.

Government Managed Care Plans. In an effort to reduce costs and increase the delivery of efficient care, Medicare and many Medicaid programs offer their members the option to join a managed care plan. These managed care plans must cover all services that would be covered under Medicare or Medicaid. The identification cards will look just like the ones issued to people not on Medicare or Medicaid. The government managed care plan may have a copayment that the patient would be responsible for.

Children's Health Insurance Program. The Children's Health Insurance Program (CHIP) is a program for children whose family income is above the Medicaid qualifying income limits, but too low to afford private coverage. CHIP is funded by states and the federal government. CHIP is designed and administered by states, according to federal requirements. The benefits may vary by the state. State CHIP programs must cover:

- Well-child care
- Immunizations
- Provider visits
- Surgical services
- Prescriptions
- Dental care and vision care
- Inpatient and outpatient hospital care
- Laboratory and x-ray services
- Behavioral healthcare
- Emergency services

CHIP programs are similar to managed care plans in that care is covered only through the designated network of providers. The premiums for CHIP are typically 5% of the family monthly income. There are smaller copayments for medical services for CHIP patients.

TRICARE. TRICARE is a program for active duty and retired members of the Uniformed Services, their families, and survivors. Medal of Honor recipients and National Guard/Reserve members and their families are also be covered under this program.

TRICARE is part of the US Military Health System, meaning it provides healthcare at military hospitals, clinics, and some civilian ambulatory care facilities and hospitals. TRICARE is set up to cover many healthcare needs at hospitals around the globe. It is designed to expand access to healthcare, ensure high-quality care, and promote medical readiness.

The Defense Enrollment Eligibility Reporting System (DEERS) registration is required for TRICARE eligibility and enrollment. Those in active duty, retired, or a member of the National Guard/Reserves are automatically registered in the DEERS database and are considered "sponsors." Sponsors must register eligible family members into the DEERS database. Incorrect information in the DEERS database can cause problems with TRICARE claims and with other healthcare benefits. So it is critical that sponsors maintain their DEERS information.

TRICARE offers two types of plans, TRICARE Prime and TRICARE Select (Table 27.2). TRICARE offers a variety of plan options to fit specific health situation or family health needs. Plans differ based on the military branch, the person's healthcare needs, and their military activity status (active duty or retired). In general, TRICARE provides coverage for preventive care, vision and dental care, mental health, pharmacy services, and special programs for individuals with disabilities in need of specialty treatments or in different stages of duty. The healthcare services TRICARE covers vary among enrollees, so it is important to check which specific benefits the plan may cover.

TRICARE can be used with other health insurance plans. By law TRICARE pays after other health insurance, including Medicare. There are a few exceptions to this, including Medicaid and TRICARE supplements. TRICARE is billed first for these exceptions. For those on active duty, TRICARE is their only coverage. They cannot use other health insurance.

Civilian Health and Medical Program of the Veterans Administration. The Civilian Health and Medical Program of the Department of Veterans Affairs (VA) (CHAMPVA) provides coverage for the spouse and the children of a veteran who was permanently disabled or killed in the line of duty or who died of a service-connected disability. To be eligible for CHAMPVA, the person cannot be eligible for TRICARE.

CHAMPVA is a comprehensive healthcare benefits program in which the VA shares the cost of covered healthcare services and supplies with eligible beneficiaries. The program is administered by the Chief Business Office Purchased Care located in Denver, Colorado. Covered services under CHAMPVA include:

- Ambulance service
- Ambulatory surgery
- Durable medical equipment (DME)
- Family planning and maternity
- Hospice and skilled nursing care
- Inpatient, outpatient, and mental health services
- Pharmacy (prescription medicines)
- Transplants

CHAMPVA will pay after Medicare and other insurances, such as Medicare HMOs and Medicare supplement plans for healthcare services and supplies. CHAMPVA will cover many of the costs not covered by Medicare. CHAMPVA does not pay Medicare Part B premiums.

VA Health Care. The Veterans Health Administration (VHA) is the largest healthcare system in the US, with over 1250 healthcare facilities. A veteran with VA health care benefits can seek care at the nearest VA medical center or VA community-based outpatient clinic. Veterans may also be able to seek care from providers in the local community.

TABLE 27.2   Comparing TRICARE Plans

Active Duty Family Members

	TRICARE Prime	TRICARE Select
Annual deductible	None	$150/individual or $300/family for E-5 and above; $50/$100 for E-4 and below
Annual enrollment fee	None	None currently; 1/1/2020 $150/individual or $300/family
Civilian outpatient visit	No cost	Primary care–$21 Specialty–$31
Civilian inpatient admission	No cost	$18.60 a day ($25 minimum)
Civilian inpatient mental health	No cost	$18.60 a day ($25 minimum)
Civilian inpatient skilled nursing facility care	$0 per diem charge per admission; no separate copayment/cost-share for separately billed professional charges	$18.60 a day ($25 minimum)

Retirees (Under 65), Their Family Members, and Others

	TRICARE Prime	TRICARE Select
Annual deductible	None	$150/individual or $300/family
Annual enrollment fee	$289.08/individual or $578.16/family	None
Civilian copays	None	20% of negotiated fee
Outpatient emergency care mental health visit	$12 per visit	$20 Primary $30 Specialty
Civilian inpatient cost-share	$11 a day ($25 minimum) charge per admission	Lesser of $250 a day or 25% of negotiated charges plus 20% of negotiated professional fees
Civilian inpatient skilled nursing facility care	$11 a day ($25 minimum) charge per admission	$250 per diem copayment or 20% cost-share of total charges for institutional care, whichever is less, plus 20% cost-share of separately billed professional charges

TRICARE: Costs. https://tricare.mil/Costs/HealthPlanCosts.

CRITICAL THINKING 27.2

Describe the differences between CHAMPVA and TRICARE. Who sponsors the program? Who is eligible for coverage under the program?

VA health care benefits can be used with other types of healthcare coverage, such as a private insurance plan, Medicare, Medicaid, or TRICARE. Veterans who served in active military, naval, or air service and were not dishonorable discharge may be eligible for VA health care benefits. Eligibility requires veterans to have served 24 continuous months or the full period for which they were called to active duty. A current or former member of the Reserves or National Guard who was called to active duty by a federal order and completed the full active-duty period may also be eligible for VA health care benefits.

When veterans apply for VA health care, they are assigned to 1 of 8 priority groups. The priority groups help ensure veterans who need care immediately get signed up quickly. Enhanced eligibility status, which places the veteran in a higher priority group, can be granted to those that were discharged for a disability resulting from something that occurred in the line of duty, a former prisoner of war, a recipient of a Purple Heart or a Medal of Honor, and a veteran who served in specific locations during specific time periods, such during the Gulf War. Veterans enrolled in the VA health care coverage will receive a Veteran Health Identification Card, which includes their picture.

VA health care coverage can vary by the veteran. All veterans will receive coverage for most healthcare services, but only some will qualify for benefits, such as dental care. Basic healthcare services cover:

- Preventive care services, such as health exams and immunizations
- Inpatient hospital services including surgeries, medical treatments, kidney dialysis, and specialized care, such as organ transplants
- Urgent and emergency care services
- Mental health services to treat behavioral health conditions such as posttraumatic stress disorder (PTSD), military sexual trauma (MST), depression, and substance use

The cost of the VA health care depends on the veteran's income level, disability rating, and military service history. The enrollment process includes a complete financial assessment to help determine if the veteran can qualify for free VA health care.

CRITICAL THINKING 27.3

How does VA Health Care differ from TRICARE and CHAMPVA?

Workers' Compensation. Workers' compensation is a publicly sponsored system that pays monetary benefits to workers who become injured or disabled in the course of their employment.

Workers' compensation is a type of insurance that offers employees compensation for injuries or disabilities sustained as a result of their job.

By agreeing to receive workers' compensation, workers also agree to give up their right to sue their employer for negligence. This is intended to protect both workers and employers. Workers typically give up further recourse in exchange for guaranteed compensation, and employers agree to a certain amount of liability while avoiding potentially greater damage of a negligence lawsuit. All parties (including taxpayers) benefit from avoiding the legal fees involved in a trial.

Most compensation plans offer coverage of medical fees related to injuries that happen as a result of employment. For example, a construction worker could claim compensation if scaffolding fell on their head, but not if they were in a traffic accident while driving to the job site. In other situations, workers can receive the equivalent of sick pay while they are on medical leave. If workers die as a result of their employment, workers' compensation also makes payments to their family members or other dependents. The insurance plan covers:

- Medical care and rehabilitation benefits
- Weekly income replacement benefits
- Death benefits to dependents

The provider accepts the workers' compensation reimbursements as payment in full and does not bill the patient. Time limitations are set for the prompt reporting of workers' compensation cases. The employee is obligated to promptly notify the employer of injury or job-related illness. The employer must then notify the insurance company and refer the employee to a healthcare provider.

All 50 states have passed workers' compensation laws to protect workers against the loss of wages and the cost of medical care resulting from an occupational accident or disease, as long as the employee was not proven negligent. Federal and state legislatures require employers to maintain workers' compensation coverage to meet minimum standards, covering most employees, for work-related illnesses and injuries. The purpose of workers' compensation laws is to provide prompt medical care to an injured or ill worker so that the person may be restored to health and return to full earning capacity in as short a time as possible.

Private Health Insurance Plans

Health insurance plans that are available from commercial insurance companies are considered private plans. The majority of people are part of an employer group plan. Those who are not eligible for an employer plan can purchase insurance on their own. This is referred to as an *individual health insurance plan*. Most private plans use managed care to reduce the costs of delivering quality healthcare.

Employer Group Plans. Many businesses offer a *group policy*, a private health insurance plan purchased by an employer for a group of employees. These plans can cover the employee, their spouse (i.e., domestic partner), and their children. Typically, an employer pays a certain percentage of the premium for full-time employees. This makes the cost of the insurance plan more affordable for the employee. Part-time

---

BOX 27.3 Self-Funded Group Health Plans

Many large companies or organizations have enough employees that they can fund their own insurance program. This is called a *self-funded plan*. Technically, a self-funded plan does not fit the true definition of insurance. The employer pays employee healthcare costs from the funds collected from employee monthly premiums. Usually, the costs of benefits and premiums for self-funded plans are similar to those for group plans. Self-funded plans tend to work best for companies that are large enough to offer good benefit coverage and reasonable premium rates and are able to pay large claims for expensive medical services. Often a third-party administrator (TPA) handles paperwork and claim payments for a self-insured group.

Self-funded healthcare is an arrangement in which an employer provides health or disability benefits to employees with its own funds. This is different from fully insured plans, in which the employer contracts with an insurance company to cover the employees and dependents. In self-funded healthcare, the employer assumes the direct risk for payment of the claims for benefits. The terms of eligibility and coverage are stated in the insurance plan document, which includes provisions similar to those found in a typical group health insurance policy.

---

employees can be part of the group policy, but most employers do not pay a part of the premium for part-time employees. Employers also determine the health insurance benefits under the group policy. Health insurance monthly premiums and benefits can vary from employer to employer. For example, the health insurance plan for Employer A covers chiropractic care, but the health insurance plan for Employer B does not. The premium for a group policy is usually lower than that for an individual plan because of the large pool of employees. The insurance company will receive premiums from a larger number of people, and just a few of them will need a lot of services. The employees' share of the premium is often paid through payroll deductions (Box 27.3).

Individual Health Insurance Plans. An individual health insurance plan is one that is not offered by an employer or another group. An individual policy can cover just one person or a family. These policies can be purchased through a health insurance exchange or directly from an insurance company. Premiums for an individual plan are generally higher than for a group plan.

HEALTH INSURANCE MODELS

There are basically two different models of health insurance today:

- Traditional health insurance
- Managed care organizations

You can find these options in both employer group plans and individual plans.

Traditional Health Insurance

Traditional health insurance plans pay for all or a share of the cost of covered services, regardless of which provider, hospital, or other licensed healthcare provider is used. Because providers are paid for each office visit, test, procedure, or other service they deliver, traditional insurance plans are often called *fee-for-service plans*. This was the first type of health insurance plan offered. Tradition health insurance plans provide the most flexibility for the patient but are also the costliest option.

Policyholders of fee-for-service plans and their dependents choose when and where to get healthcare services. When the policy is purchased, the subscriber is often given a fee schedule, which explains the benefit payment amounts. Benefits are usually paid to the insured, unless the insured has authorized payment to be made directly to the provider. This is referred to as *assignment of benefits*.

The fee schedule amounts can be determined by a process called *usual, customary, and reasonable* (UCR). UCR is the amount paid for a medical service in a geographic area based on what providers in the area usually charge for the same or similar service.

Managed Care Organizations

Managed care organizations (MCOs) are health insurance companies whose goal is to provide quality, cost-effective care to its members. MCOs negotiate reduced rates with contracted providers and hospitals. In return, the managed care plan increases the provider's patient load. Many MCOs require the patient to choose a *primary care provider (PCP)*, who coordinates the patient's care. Managed care plans can also require referrals for their patients to be treated by a specialist, thus limiting patient access to more expensive care. To help further control costs, MCOs require preauthorization for surgical and medical procedures, testing, and medication therapy. It is important that medical assistants be familiar with the various models of managed care to fully understand their effects on healthcare costs.

Models of Managed Care Organizations. Patient care is coordinated through a network of providers and hospitals. There are different types of managed care plans, such as health maintenance organizations (HMOs), preferred provider organizations (PPOs), and exclusive provider organizations (EPOs). They provide healthcare in return for scheduled payments and coordinate healthcare through a defined network of PCPs, hospitals, and other providers.

Health Maintenance Organization. Health maintenance organizations (HMOs) are health plans that are regulated by HMO laws, which require them to include preventive care as part of their benefits package. The goal of the HMO health insurance plan is to reduce the cost of healthcare while still providing quality healthcare. HMO plans typically have the lowest monthly premiums among other health insurance plans, though it is the least flexible for patients. The patient's out-of-pocket expenses are also very low. Patients may not be required to pay a deductible or coinsurance.

Patients are required to select a PCP, who acts as the gatekeeper to more specialized care. The insurance plan will not pay for services that are not included in its provider network; patients are 100% financially responsible for medical expenses incurred outside the HMO network of providers. For example, patients wanting to visit the dermatologist for eczema must visit their PCP first to obtain a referral. If this process is not done, the patient would be fully responsible financially if they made an appointment with a dermatologist directly. The PCP can either treat the patient or refer them to the specialist.

PCPs receive financial incentives when they reduce the cost of patient care. In the earlier example, prescribing medicine to the patient is more cost-effective than referring the patient to the specialist. HMOs always require:

- Referrals from the PCP to specialists
- Precertification and preauthorization for hospital admissions, surgical procedures, outpatient procedures, and treatments

HMOs can be set up using several different models. The payment structure can be different for each of those models (Table 27.3).

CRITICAL THINKING 27.4

Noemi Rodriguez is a patient who called to make an appointment with the endocrinologist because she is having trouble managing her diabetes. She told John over the phone when she was making the appointment that she has Aetna HMO. Will John be able to schedule Ms. Rodriguez's appointment with the endocrinologist? Why or why not? What would she need to make an appointment?

VOCABULARY

gatekeeper The primary care provider, who is in charge of a patient's treatment. Additional treatment, such as referrals to a specialist, must be approved by the gatekeeper.

health insurance exchange An online marketplace where you can compare and buy individual health insurance plans. State health insurance exchanges were established as part of the Affordable Care Act.

preauthorization A process that requires the provider to submit documentation to the payer to show the service or treatment is medically needed, and the payer determines if the service or treatment is medically necessary and covered under the insurance plan. Also called *prior authorization*.

provider network An approved list of physicians, hospitals, and other providers.

referral An order from a primary care provider for the patient to see a specialist or to get certain medical services.

third-party administrator (TPA) An organization that processes claims and provides administrative services for another organization. Often used by self-funded plans.

Preferred Provider Organization. A preferred provider organization (PPO) is a managed care network that contracts with a group of providers. The providers agree on a predetermined list of charges for all services, including those for both normal and complex procedures. The PPO model of managed healthcare uses the fee-for-service concept that many providers prefer. Typically, the patient's financial responsibilities represent, on average, 20% to 25% of the allowed charge, but this depends on the patient's health insurance policy. A provider who joins a PPO does not need to change the manner of providing care and continues to treat and bill patients on a fee-for-service basis. When a patient covered under a PPO plan comes for treatment, the provider treats the patient and bills the PPO. Patients do not need to visit their PCP to obtain a referral to a specialist for more specialized care. And, they typically have more control over healthcare choices.

TABLE 27.3 Health Maintenance Organization (HMO) Models

Model	Structure	Payment Structure
Independent practice association (IPA)	General or family practice provider or provider group that practices independently and may contract with several HMOs. Can see patients outside of the HMO.	Capitation or fee-for-service
Staff	One or more providers hired by an HMO. Providers see only HMO patients.	Salaried
Group	Multispecialty group with or without a primary care provider (PCP; i.e., gatekeeper); may contract with several HMOs.	Capitation or fee-for-service
Network	HMOs contract with multiple provider groups. Those providers can see patients outside of the HMO. Provides wider geographic coverage for members.	Capitation or fee-for-service

PPOs provide their subscribers with a list of participating providers and healthcare facilities from which they can access in-network healthcare at PPO reduced rates. Rates are quite often lower than those charged to non-PPO patients. This gives the patient more choices for providers. If the patient chooses to see a provider who is not in the PPO network, the deductible, coinsurance, and copayments will be higher.

Although patients have the option to visit a specialist when they feel the need, they are still required to obtain preauthorization for more expensive services, such as diagnostic imaging.

CRITICAL THINKING 27.5

Diego Lupez called John; he was upset because he had received a patient statement with a balance owing. He told John that he has full-coverage insurance through his employer and did not know why he had a balance. What information can John share with Mr. Lupez to explain his financial responsibility?

Exclusive Provider Organization. An exclusive provider organization (EPO) combines features of an HMO (e.g., an enrolled group or population, PCPs, and an authorization system) and a PPO (e.g., flexible benefit design and fee-for-service payments). Patients with EPO coverage will not be covered for services outside the designated network of providers (unless there is an emergency), but they may not need to obtain a referral for specialized care. Unlike HMO members, EPO plan members are not required to choose a PCP (Table 27.4). Different plans may require precertification and preauthorization for certain services.

Utilization Management/Utilization Review. Utilization management is a form of patient care review by healthcare professionals who do not provide the care but are employed by health insurance companies. Those doing patient care review are generally nurses. It is a necessary component of managed care to control costs. A *utilization review committee* reviews individual cases to ensure that medical care services are medically necessary. This review is called a *utilization review*. For this committee to function properly, use of the correct diagnosis code is critical. This committee also reviews all provider referrals and cases of emergency department visits and urgent care. For referrals, the committee reviews the referral and either approves or denies it, so it is important to submit accurate documentation. The medical assistant should contact the utilization review department directly; it should never be left to the patient to contact this department.

VOCABULARY

capitation A payment arrangement for healthcare providers. The provider is paid a set amount for each enrolled person assigned to them, per period of time, whether or not that person has received services.

utilization management A decision-making process used by managed care organizations to manage healthcare costs. It involves case-by-case assessments of the appropriateness of care.

PARTICIPATING PROVIDER CONTRACTS

A *participating provider* (PAR) (also called a network provider) is a healthcare provider who signed a contract with an insurance company, managed care plan, or a government health plan to provide services to policyholders. Healthcare providers can apply to become PARs through a process called *credentialing*. Credentialing is the process of confirming the healthcare provider's qualifications, including the healthcare provider's license to practice medicine, affiliated organizations, and their education and professional background.

Once the healthcare provider is credentialed, the health insurance plan issues them a contract to become an in-network PAR. The contract includes a fee schedule that the health insurance company will use to reimburse the provider for health services rendered. By signing the contract, the provider agrees to bill the insurance company directly. The provider also agrees to accept the health insurance plan's fee schedule, even if it is lower than the provider's fee schedule. Specific procedures may be covered in full, such as wellness visits, whereas others may require copayments and coinsurance. When a policyholder seeks care from a participating provider, the fees are discounted compared to seeking care from a nonparticipating provider. Not all participating providers contract with health insurance plans at the same level. "*Preferred providers*" contract with insurers at a higher level and thus services are discounted at a higher rate than those provided by a participating provider.

Contracted Fee Schedules

Payment for services is typically made after the health services are provided. Once the service has been provided to the patient, the healthcare provider must submit a health insurance claim, which includes the diagnosis and procedure codes, in addition to the total charges and any copayments made. Although

TABLE 27.4	**Managed Care Plans**		
Plan	**Providers**	**Access to Specialized Care**	**Deductible, Coinsurance, Copayment**
Health maintenance organization (HMO)	Must see only HMO providers and choose a primary care provider (PCP).	Referral required for specialized care.	Usually no deductible or coinsurance. Copayments required for office visits and prescriptions.
Preferred provider organization (PPO)	No PCP required. There is a network of providers, but out-of-network providers can be seen.	No referral required. Preauthorization needed for expensive services.	Lower deductible and coinsurance if an in-network provider is used. Copayments required for office visits and prescriptions.
Exclusive provider organization (EPO)	Must see network providers. No PCP required.	No referral needed.	Usually no deductible or coinsurance. Copayments required for office visits and prescriptions.

the healthcare provider establishes their own fee schedule, health insurance plans maintain their own rates at which they reimburse.

When setting up a fee schedule a healthcare provider considers time, expertise, and services. In every case, healthcare providers must place an estimate on the value of these services. Fees for medical procedures and services differ from office to office based on the type of practice. An office visit with a family practice provider may cost less than an office visit with a specialist. In the past, most providers worked on a fee-for-service basis; that is, patients were charged for the provider's service based on each individual service performed.

In recent years, health insurance plans, particularly government plans and managed healthcare organizations, have greatly influenced what healthcare providers can be reimbursed by establishing the allowable charge. The *allowable charge* is the maximum that the insurance plan will pay for a procedure or service. The patient cannot be charged for the amount above the allowable charge if the provider and/or the healthcare facility are a PAR provider. For example, if the office visit is $100 but the allowable amount from the insurance company is $80, $80 is the maximum amount for which the patient is responsible. The remaining $20 is a write-off and cannot be billed to the patient or the insurance company.

MEDICAL ASSISTANT'S ROLE

A medical assistant can be involved in many different tasks related to health insurance. Being familiar with the technology and forms that are used will make you more efficient at your job.

Health Insurance Identification Card

When a patient is enrolled in a health insurance plan, they will be issued a health insurance ID card that supplies:

- Health insurance company
- Health plan type
- Subscriber identification number
- Copay amounts
- Health plan name
- Subscriber's name and covered dependents
- Policy group number
- Health plan contact information (e.g., phone numbers and website)

Review Fig. 27.1 for a sampling of different insurance ID cards for common insurance companies. The insurance card contains

information that is used during the billing process. The medical assistant must accurately enter the information from the insurance ID card into the computer software. Most healthcare facilities also require the card to be scanned and the image to be uploaded into the patient's electronic health record. Many facilities also require that a photo ID be scanned and the image uploaded.

Verifying Eligibility

Verification of eligibility is the process of confirming health insurance coverage for the patient. When the medical assistant schedules an appointment, health insurance information should be collected (unless it is an emergency situation). If the healthcare facility is not part of the patient's network of providers, the individual should be informed of this. The patient can then decide if they still want to schedule an appointment. The medical assistant should also verify the *effective date,* or date the insurance coverage began, and confirm that the patient will be covered on the date the medical services are provided (Procedure 27.1). The medical assistant should make it a practice to review each insurer's online insurance web portal, which can verify insurance eligibility, benefits, and exclusions, prior to the patient's appointment. If the online insurance web portal is not available, the medical assistant should contact the provider services department. This phone number should be listed on the patient's health insurance ID card, either on the front or back of the card.

VOCABULARY

online insurance web portal An online service provided by various insurance companies for providers to look up a patient's insurance benefits, eligibility, claims status, and explanation of benefits.

CRITICAL THINKING 27.6

Robert Caudill, an elderly patient, called to make an appointment, but he was unsure what his benefits were. How can John find out what benefits he qualifies for? Is it appropriate for John to educate Mr. Caudill on his health insurance benefits? Why or why not?

In the recent past, the medical assistant would have to call the health insurance company to verify eligibility for each and every patient. Each call to the health insurance company automated

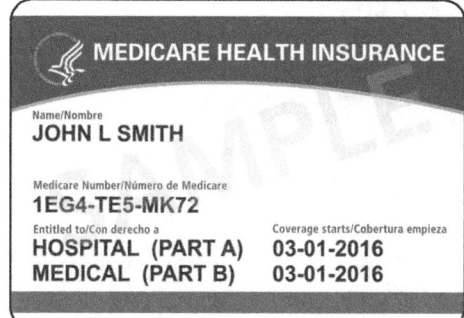

Medicare: The Medicare card uses the patient's social security number as the ID number. The card also details the plan coverages, in this case Part A and Part B.

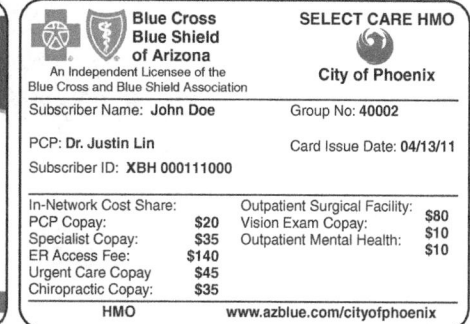

HMO ID Card: Notice the Health Insurance Plan and the HMO Plan are both listed. Common copayments are also listed.
HMO members are required to choose PCP which is designated on their health ID card.

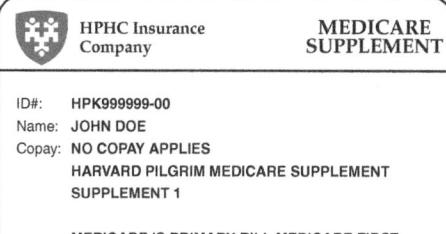

Medicare Secondary Insurance: The ID card states that it is a supplement to Medicare, thus Medicare should be billed as the primary. The ID number does not match the Medicare card.

EPO Plan ID Card: Members are not required to choose a PCP, but can only use their benefits for in-network providers and facilities. Notice the ID number stays the same for the insured and all family members listed.

PPO plan ID card: PPO patients have the most flexibility to visit whichever provider, primary care or specialist they choose. Notice the medical copays are slightly higher than HMO copayments.

Fig. 27.1 A Variety of Different Health Insurance Identification Cards. (From Niedzwiecki B et al: *Kinn's the medical assistant,* ed 14, St. Louis, 2020, Elsevier.)

system would take at least 5 minutes, and the medical assistant would not have access to all of the patient's benefit information unless they spoke to a member services agent, which would take even more time. Today, most privately sponsored health insurance plans have offered online insurance provider portals, which allow for quick and easy verification of eligibility (Fig. 27.2). The healthcare facility will have to apply for access to the online web portal. Once it has been approved, patient benefits can be looked up in their entirety in seconds instead of minutes. Information on a patient's benefit plan can be uploaded to the electronic health record (EHR) very quickly; this process reduces the use of paper in the healthcare facility.

Precertification and Preauthorization

In an effort to control costs, the precertification and preauthorization process is used for certain procedures, treatments, services, and prescription medications. Precertification and preauthorization might be used interchangeably by some, but there is a difference:

- *Precertification*: The process of determining if a procedure or service is covered by the insurance plan and what the reimbursement is for that procedure or service. A notification is sent to the payer (e.g., insurance provider) regarding the service or treatment. The payer then responses indicating if the service is covered under the plan.
- *Preauthorization*: Also called prior authorization. A process that requires the provider to submit documentation to the payer to show the service or treatment is medically needed and the payer determines if the service or treatment is medically necessary and covered under the insurance plan.

Each insurance company has its own precertification and/or preauthorization requirements. Most insurance companies use

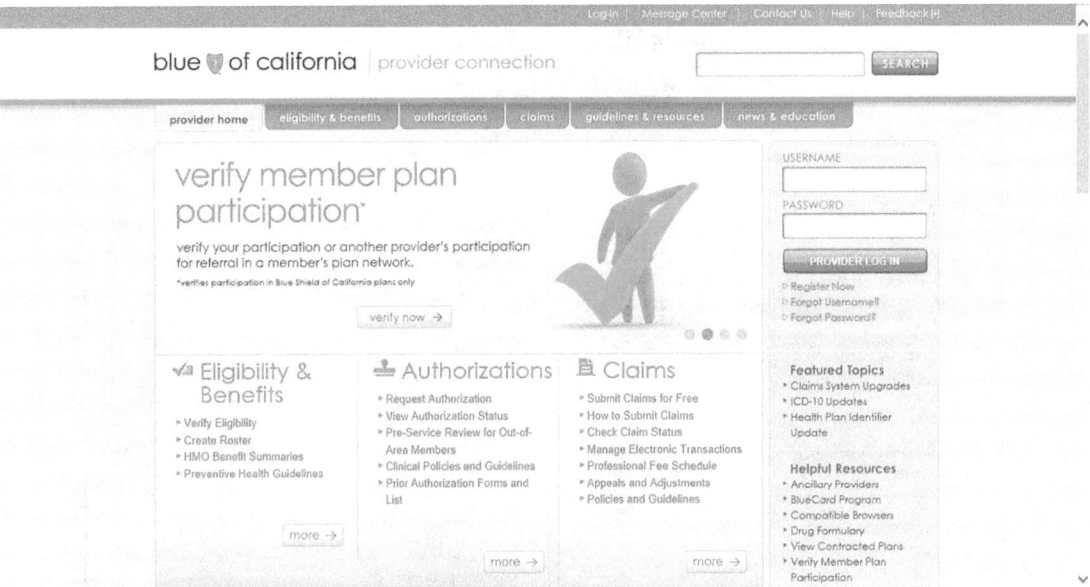

Fig. 27.2 A Provider's Web Portal for Online Health Insurance. (From Fordney MT: *Insurance handbook for the medical office,* ed 14, St. Louis, 2017, Elsevier.)

online Web portals for precertifications and preauthorizations. If the portal is not used, the process is much slower if the paperwork needs to be faxed or mailed to the insurance company. The medical assistant should become familiar with the process completing precertifications and preauthorizations (Procedure 27.2). Both of these processes are similar, though insurance companies may have some differences:

- The medical assistant starts the process by contacting the insurance company's provider services. The contact information is usually on the back of the patient's health insurance ID card.
- The medical assistant will need to provide the insurance company with the diagnostic and procedure codes for the procedure and/or services and the diagnosis. (The diagnostic and procedural codes will be discussed in the following chapters.)
- If medical documentation is required, the medical assistant will need to submit the required information.
- The medical assistant needs to document the contact with the insurance company in the patient's health record, including any information (e.g., numbers) from the insurance company.

A precertification or preauthorization is not a guarantee payment of services. Some insurance companies will have a *predetermination* process that provides the maximum amount the payer will pay for the service or treatment.

Insurance companies can deny coverage for medications, services, or treatments. When this occurs, the patient is then responsible for the cost. Patients have a right to appeal the denial decision. A patient can appeal the denial by following the appeal process, which is usually explained on the insurance company's website.

Referrals

Patients seeking specialized care must first visit their assigned PCP to obtain a referral to a specialist or for more specialized

therapy or care. Patients with HMO plans can only obtain a referral to the specialist by visiting their assigned PCP. If the PCP agrees that the referral is medically necessary for continuing care, the PCP's medical assistant will start the referral process. HMOs will measure how many patients are referred to specialists by individual PCPs. Approval or denial of a referral can take anywhere from a few minutes to a few days. The three types of referrals are as follows:

- A *regular referral* usually takes 3 to 10 working days for review and approval. This type of referral is used when the provider believes that the patient must see a specialist to continue treatment.
- An *urgent referral* usually takes about 24 hours for approval. This type of referral is used when an urgent but not life-threatening situation occurs.
- A *STAT referral* can be approved online when it is submitted to the utilization review department through the provider's Web portal. A STAT referral is used in an emergency situation as indicated by the provider.

A regular referral is the most common type and can be inconvenient for the patient. With most managed care plans, preauthorization needs to be obtained for a referral. Remember this cardinal rule: never tell the patient the referral has been approved unless you have a hard copy of the authorization. A referral is authorized after the approval has been received. When a referral is approved, the PCP's office and the patient should receive a copy of the authorization. Always review the authorization thoroughly and confirm details, such as approved diagnosis and procedure codes and the exact period of time the authorization lasts. The patient will receive a letter with an authorization number and details regarding the approved services. The patient must bring the authorization to the specialist's office on the date of the appointment.

OTHER TYPES OF INSURANCE

When you work in a healthcare facility, the most common type of insurance you will see is health insurance. However, there are other types of insurance that can require the involvement of a healthcare provider. These other types of insurance are discussed next.

Disability Insurance

Disability insurance is a form of insurance that provides income replacement if the patient has a disability that is not work related. The disability means that the employee is unable to perform their work functions or duties. It could involve either short-term disability or long-term disability benefits. Both provide 40% to 70% of the individual's predisability income. Many employers offer a disability policy to their employees. Generally, the employee pays the monthly premium. These policies can also be purchased by an individual.

Short-term disability means that a person is unable to work for 9 to 52 weeks. Long-term disability policies pick up when short-term benefits are exhausted. Long-term disability coverage will pay out until the patient returns to work or for the number of years specified in the policy. Some policies will pay out until the patient reaches the age of 65 and then is eligible for Social Security benefits. There may be a waiting period before benefits can be paid. Sick time can be used for the waiting period days.

Weekly or monthly cash benefits are provided to employed policyholders who become unable to work as a result of an accident or illness. The accident or illness must not be related to work, because that would be covered under workers' compensation. Payments are made directly to the insured and are intended to replace lost income resulting from an illness or other disability. Disability payments are not intended for payment of specific medical bills, and a disability insurance policy should not be confused with a regular health insurance plan.

The medical office may be involved in the examination of the patient to determine the level of disability and when the disability ends. There are forms that must be completed by a healthcare provider and then submitted to the insurance carrier.

Life Insurance

Life insurance provides payment of a specified amount, upon the insured's death, either to their estate or to a designated beneficiary. Annuity life insurance policies provide monthly cash benefits if the policyholder becomes permanently and totally disabled. Sometimes the proceeds from life insurance are used to meet the expenses of the insured person's last illness.

The healthcare facility may be required to complete physical examination forms when a patient is applying for life insurance. If there is an annuity policy, the healthcare provider may have to determine if there is a permanent disability and submit documentation.

VOCABULARY

beneficiary A designated person who receives funds from an insurance policy.

waiting period The length of time a patient waits for disability insurance to pay after the date of injury.

Long-Term Care Insurance

Long-term care insurance is a relatively new type of insurance that covers a broad range of maintenance and health services for chronically ill, disabled, or developmentally delayed individuals. Medical services may be provided on an inpatient basis (e.g., at a rehabilitation facility, nursing home, or mental hospital), on an outpatient basis, or at home.

Liability Insurance

Liability insurance covers losses to a third party caused by the insured. There are many types of liability insurance, including automobile, business, and homeowners' policies. Liability policies often include benefits for:

- Medical expenses resulting from traumatic injuries
- Lost wages
- Sometimes pain and suffering

All liability insurance policies are payable to victims injured by the insured person's home or car, without regard to the insured person's actual legal liability for the accident.

AFFORDABLE CARE ACT

In the early 2000s it became clear that a large number of Americans lacked basic health insurance. *Preexisting conditions*, or health problems that existed prior to the start of a new health coverage, made it difficult for Americans who did not work full time or were self-employed to obtain health insurance. In addition, the health insurance market was discriminating against young adults 18 years or older, who may not have been qualified to receive health benefits because they could not find full-time employment.

In 2010 the Patient Protection and Affordable Care Act (PPACA), also known as the *Affordable Care Act* (ACA), was enacted. It increased the quality, availability, and affordability of private and public health insurance for more than 44 million uninsured Americans. The legislation included new qualifying regulations, taxes, mandates, and subsidies. The federal mandate not only opens opportunities for more Americans to obtain affordable health insurance, but also works to reduce overall healthcare spending in the long run. Other patient protections and provisions under the Affordable Care Act include:

- Insurance companies are prohibited from dropping patient health coverage if the individual gets sick or makes an unintentional mistake on the health insurance application.
- The act eliminated preexisting conditions and gender discrimination, so patients cannot be charged more based on their health status, sexual orientation, or gender identity.
- Young adults can remain on their parent's or guardian's insurance policy until age 26.
- The act created *health insurance marketplaces,* where low- to middle-income Americans can compare plans and lower their costs on healthcare coverage.
- States will expand Medicaid coverage to 15.9 million Americans to include those who qualify for cost assistance through the marketplace.

- Individuals seeking health insurance can apply only during the open enrollment period, which is established by each state.

With more Americans having health insurance, the number of office visits to providers across the country is expected to increase. Thus efficient health insurance management policies should be instituted to meet the new demand for services.

CLOSING COMMENTS

Health insurance and benefits coverage can be confusing to the patient. Medical assistants should educate themselves on the specific details of all plans accepted at the healthcare facility. Managed care has often been criticized in the media for its cost-saving practices. Extra efforts made by medical assistants to overcome these challenges and educate their patients on how to use their health insurance plans will improve the quality of care delivered to their patients. Providers and healthcare facilities need to evaluate their ability to accept the fee schedule of insurance plans they are contracted with, especially since Medicaid's fee schedule is the lowest in the industry.

PATIENT-CENTERED CARE

It is important for patients to understand how their insurance plan works. Many people, especially the elderly, believe that if they have health insurance, all charges for their healthcare will be paid for. To provide excellent customer service, a medical assistant should have a basic understanding of the insurance policies seen most often in the healthcare facility. That way, you can answer questions from patients about their benefits and exclusions. Often healthcare facilities provide their patients with a brochure that explains how health insurance and reimbursement work. The brochures also provide patients with definitions of some of the more common terms used in the insurance claims process. If patients are well advised and comfortable with insurance facts before treatment begins, the medical experience will go more smoothly, and the collection of the amount owed will be easier. The medical assistant must practice good communication skills, patience, and tact when discussing reimbursement and financial responsibilities with patients.

BEING PROFESSIONAL

Patients can be confused or angered when insurance companies deny authorization of services or referrals. Although these decisions are made by insurance companies, many times the blame is put on the medical front office assistants. In situations such as these, it is important for medical assistants to stay calm and listen to the patient's concerns. In most cases, the patient will come to realize that there is nothing the medical assistant can do, but the patient may need to express frustration. Once the patient has calmed down, the medical assistant can then recommend options, such as paying cash or making payment arrangements; the medical assistant can also bring the patient's attention to their insurance member services hotline. Compassionately assure patients that their health is most important and that you will do what you can, so they can receive the appropriate medical treatment.

If the patient continues to escalate the situation and/or becomes belligerent, excuse yourself from the discussion and ask either an office manager or another medical assistant to step in. A medical assistant should never return anger and/or frustration to the patient. Remember, the patient may be mentally compromised and frustrated from extensive healthcare problems, so do not exacerbate the situation by releasing your own anger. If the patient's health is made the primary concern, the healthcare facility can work with the insurance company, so the patient can receive appropriate medical care.

Role-play this scenario with a peer: The peer is a patient who received a prior authorization denial. The patient is upset and really needs the service. Respond to the peer in a respectful and professional manner.

CHAPTER REVIEW

Most patients who visit a provider are covered by some type of insurance plan. The insurance coverage could be from a government plan, such as Medicare, Medicaid, CHIP, TRICARE, CHAMPVA, VA health care, or workers' compensation. It could also be from a private health insurance plan from either an employer group plan or a privately purchased plan. Wherever the coverage is from, it is important for a medical assistant to be familiar with the plans commonly seen in the healthcare facility.

There are basically two different health insurance models, traditional and managed care. Within managed care there are several types, including HMOs, PPOs, and EPOs. Managed care organizations use utilization management/utilization review to help contain the cost of providing healthcare coverage.

Providers who have a contract with a health insurance plan are considered PAR providers and must honor the contracted fee schedule. This means that they will write off the difference between their billed amount and the contracted allowed amount. This reduces the out-of-pocket expenses for the patient.

Medical assistants are responsible for verifying whether or not patients are eligible for services through insurance coverage. This can be done by using online resources, such as a provider's web portal, or by calling the insurance carrier. Medical assistants should also be able to interpret the information found on a patient's insurance identification card.

SCENARIO WRAP-UP

Although he was initially nervous about explaining fees to patients and asking for payment, John has become more comfortable in doing this aspect of his job, because he now understands the business aspect of the practice. Patients understand that providers must charge for their services and have become accustomed to copayments and coinsurance amounts. Many times these fees are collected in advance before the patient sees the provider. This practice saves time on checkout, and most patients believe that the copay is a small cost compared with the entire fee that providers charge to manage their care in one office visit.

John has noticed that the usual, customary, and reasonable fees that Dr. Crawford, a member of the practice, charges his patients directly affect the reimbursements that are paid by various insurance and managed care companies. John has attended several health insurance billing seminars sponsored by Medicare and Blue Cross/Blue Shield, and he believes that this extra training has resulted in a drop in health insurance claim rejections at WMFM Clinic.

PROCEDURE 27.1 Interpret Information on an Insurance Card and Verify Eligibility for Services

Task
To identify essential information on the health insurance identification (ID) card and verify eligibility for services.

Scenario
Ken Thomas (DOB 10/25/19XX) is a new patient of Jean Burke, NP. He wants an appointment today if his insurance covers the visit. You will need to obtain information from his insurance card for billing purposes and then contact the insurance company to verify his eligibility. Jean Burke's national provider identifier (NPI) is 1234567809. (Use the insurance card information in the table. Fill in the current year for 20XX.)

Blue Cross Blue Shield   1234 Insurance Place
                                          Anytown, AL 12345-1234

Insured: Ken H Thomas
Policy/ID #: KT4496785
Group #: 55124T
Effective Date: 01/01/20XX
Copayment information
PCP visits: $25
Emergency visits: $100
Specialist visits: $35
Generic drugs: $10
Brand drugs: $50
Provider Information/Claims/inquiries: 1-800-123-1111 or www.bluecbs.evolve

Directions
Role-play the scenarios with a peer. The peer will be the patient and the insurance representative. You are the medical assistant working at the reception desk.

Equipment and Supplies
- Patient's health insurance ID card, both sides (See above)
- Photo ID (optional)

Procedural Steps
1. Ask the patient for his health insurance ID card. Ask for the patient's photo ID, if required.
2. Review the patient's health insurance ID card and identify the insured on the health insurance ID card. If the patient is someone other than the insured, obtain the relationship with the insured and the insured's date of birth and sex.

Purpose: To submit an accurate health insurance claim, the insured's date of birth and sex are required.
3. Write down the billing information, which includes the patient's name, name of the insurance plan and the contact information, and person's identification number and group number. Check and write down the effective date.
Purpose: To accurately submit the health insurance claim under the correct insurance policy number and group number.
4. Write down the copayment for the visit.
Purpose: The patient will need to pay the copayment prior to the visit.
Scenario update: You try to verify the patient's eligibility using the portal, but the portal is down for maintenance. You need to call the insurance company. With your peer, role play the call. Your peer will be the insurance representative.
5. Contact the insurance company and clearly state the patient's information (policy and group numbers and name).
Purpose: The representative will need to policy and group numbers to find the patient in the company's database.
6. Once the insurance company finds the patient's information, verify the patient's eligibility for services with the provider. Verify the copayment and that the patient can see the provider. Give the insurance representative the provider's NPI.
Purpose: Each provider has a unique NPI, which is used as an identifier with insurance companies.
7. Demonstrate professionalism through verbal communication skills, by stating a respectful, assertive, clear, organized message.
Scenario update: Now your peer will play the patient. You finish the call with the insurance company and notify the patient that he can be seen in 15 minutes. You register the patient and then need to collect his copayment.
8. Ask the patient for the exact amount of the copayment for the visit. Demonstrate sensitivity and professionalism when discussing the copayment and the situation.
Purpose: The patient needs to pay the copayment before his visit.
9. Document the eligibility details in the patient's health record. Include the name of the insurance company, effective date, eligibility to see the provider, and if needed, the name of the insurance representative who assisted you.

08/23/20XX 10:20 am Blue Cross and Blue Shield contacted to verify patient's eligibility. Per Shannon Brown, patient can see Jean Burke, N.P. Effective date 01/01/20XX. Copayment of $25 collected.
_____ John Bimmell RMA

PROCEDURE 27.2   Perform Precertification With Documentation

Task

To obtain precertification from a patient's insurance carrier for requested services or procedures.

Scenario

You are working with Dr. Julie Walden at Walden-Martin Family Medical Clinic. Erma Willis (DOB 12/09/19XX) is seen for excessive snoring, and Dr. Walden orders a sleep study. You need to complete a prior authorization/certification form for the sleep study, which will be conducted by Dr. Jim Sandman. You checked, and there is a signed release of information form.

Insurance Information

Aetna
1234 Insurance Way
Anytown, AL 112345-1234
Member ID Number: EW8884910
Group Number: 66574W

Clinic and Provider Information

Walden-Martin Family Medicine Clinic
1234 Anystreet
Anytown, AL 12345
Provider: Julie Walden, MD
Fax: 123-123-5678
Phone: 123-123-1234
Provider Contact Name: (your name)

Service Information

Place: Walden-Martin Family Medicine Clinic
Service Requested: Sleep study
Starting Service Date: 1 week from today
Ending Service Date: 1 week from today
Service Frequency: once
ICD-10-CM Code: R06.83
CPT Code: 95807
Not related to an injury or workers' compensation

Equipment and Supplies

* *Paper method:* Patient's health record, prior authorization (precertification) request form, copy of patient's health insurance ID card, and pen

* *Electronic method:* Electronic health record system, such as SimChart for the Medical Office (SCMO)

Procedural Steps

1. Gather the information needed.
   * *Paper method:* Gather the health record, precertification/prior authorization request form, copy of the health insurance ID card, and a pen.
   * *SCMO:* Access the Simulation Playground in SCMO.
2. Using the health record, determine the service or procedure that requires precertification/preauthorization.
3. Complete the precertification/prior authorization form.
   * *Paper method:* Using a pen, complete the precertification/prior authorization request form.
   * *SCMO:* Click on the Form Repository icon in SCMO. Select Prior Authorization Request from the left **INFO PANEL**. Use the Patient Search button at the bottom to find the patient. Complete the remaining fields of the form.

   Purpose: This provides information on the ordered procedure or service to the insurance company, which will notify the provider's representative if the procedure or service will be covered under the plan.
4. Proofread the completed form and make any revisions needed.

   Purpose: To ensure the accuracy of the information.

   Scenario update: You sent the completed form to the insurance company.
5. File or save the form.
   * *Paper method:* File the document in the health record after it has been faxed to the insurance carrier.
   * *SCMO:* After printing and faxing or electronically sending the form to the insurance company, save the form to the patient's record.

   Purpose: Copies of all forms completed for the patient need to be maintained in the health record.

28

Diagnostic Coding Basics

LEARNING OBJECTIVES

1. Discuss diagnostic coding, explain where diagnostic statements are found, and define medical necessity as it applies to diagnostic and procedural coding.
2. Identify the structure and format of the ICD-10-CM.
3. Describe how to use the Alphabetic Index to select main terms, essential modifiers, nonessential modifiers, and the appropriate code (or codes) and code ranges.
4. Do the following related to the Tabular List:
   - Explain how to use the Tabular List to select main terms, essential modifiers, nonessential modifiers, and the appropriate code (or codes) and code ranges.
   - List and discuss the conventions used in the Tabular List.

- Summarize coding conventions as defined in the ICD-10-CM coding manual.
5. Explain how to abstract diagnostic statements from the patient's health record.
6. List the eight basic steps required for accurate ICD-10-CM coding, and perform coding using the current ICD-10-CM manual or an encoder.
7. Explain the importance of coding guidelines for accuracy and discuss special rules and considerations that apply to the code selection process.
8. Discuss the importance of maximizing third-party reimbursement, and use tactful communication skills with medical providers to ensure accurate code selection.

OUTLINE

▶ OPENING SCENARIO

Mike Simeone, a recent medical assistant graduate, excelled in his diagnostic coding course. Recently, he found an entry-level coding position at the Walden-Martin Family Medical (WMFM) Clinic. Mike is a little nervous but also excited about using ICD-10-CM coding in his new position. Mike has used

encoder software in some of his classes, which helped him determine the most specific and accurate code to assign. Mike noticed that the new software update in the medical office has the most recent ICD-10-CM codes.

Mike has had some previous experience working in health records, which gives him a strong understanding of the importance of accurate and complete documentation. He knows where to look to find diagnostic statements in providers' orders, treatment plans, progress notes, surgical reports, and other medical reports.

YOU WILL LEARN

1. How the format, layout, and conventions of the ICD-10-CM coding manual will help the medical assistant locate the most accurate and specific diagnostic code.
2. To identify the diagnostic statement from various sources.
3. To apply coding guidelines to coding situations that are seen in the healthcare facility.

INTRODUCTION

A diagnosis (dahy uh g NOH sis) has many purposes in healthcare. Patient treatment plans are based on the diagnosis. Reimbursement (ree im BURS ment) from insurance companies is based, in part, on the correct diagnosis and procedures. Researchers use diagnoses for their studies and other healthcare organizations. Diagnostic coding has been used to standardize diagnoses. It was initially developed to study causes of mortality. Over time, diagnostic coding has been expanded to include all diseases and conditions. The World Health Organization (WHO) has established the International Classification of Diseases. This classification system is in its tenth revision and is known as the *International Classification of Diseases, Tenth Revision, Clinical Modification* (ICD-10-CM). These codes are used for:

- Mortality data
- Epidemiologic (ep i dee mee o LOJ ic) data
- Billing purposes

The ICD-10-CM allows providers to be much more specific in diagnostic coding than was possible with previous revisions. This will, in turn, result in more accurate data collection and billing practices. Every year the Centers for Medicare and Medicaid Services (CMS) reviews the ICD-10-CM coding manual. The update is published on October 1. Additions, revisions, and deletions are made to many of the diagnostic codes, code descriptions, and coding guidelines. *You must always use the current year's coding manual to ensure accurate coding and to comply with regulatory guidelines.*

The Health Insurance Portability and Accountability Act (HIPAA) has mandated that specific code sets be used to help standardize the process of claims submission. The ICD-10-CM is the mandated diagnostic code set.

In this chapter we will look at the structure of the ICD-10-CM codes and how to accurately determine the correct diagnosis code.

WHAT IS DIAGNOSTIC CODING?

Diagnostic coding changes are descriptions of diseases, illnesses, or injuries written in the form of alphanumeric codes. The ICD-10-CM code set uses up to seven characters to identify the disease, condition, or injury. Using the ICD-10-CM can help ensure both accurate health record documentation and efficient claims processing.

The ICD-10-CM code set is available through online resources, within the electronic health record (EHR) as an encoder, or as a print coding manual. The printed coding manual is produced by several publishers and may use different layouts, symbols, color coding, and some other features. For the coding manual, however, the format, conventions, tables, appendices, content, and basic structure are the same.

When you use the ICD-10-CM coding manual, you will be choosing a standardized alphanumeric code for the diagnostic statement assigned by the provider. Diagnostic statements are found in:

- Operative reports
- Discharge summaries
- History and physical exam (H&P) reports
- Reports on *ancillary diagnostic services* (e.g., radiology, pathology, and laboratory reports)

All of these should be used to provide the patient's diagnosis or diagnoses. These reports are used by healthcare providers to code and report clinical information. Diagnostic coding is required for participation in Medicare and Medicaid programs and by most insurance companies. The diagnostic codes are used on insurance claims. The ICD-10-CM codes tell the insurance company why the procedures were done. These codes are linked to the procedures that are performed, using procedural coding. This code linking is used to determine if a procedure or service will be reimbursed. The diagnostic code can show that a procedure or service was medically necessary or a *medical necessity*. If it was not medically necessary, the insurance company will not reimburse for the encounter. The ICD-10-CM codes are also used to keep track of various healthcare statistics related to disease and injury. Practice management software, clearinghouses, and insurance companies recognize these codes, which are used to simplify the coding process; this, in turn, speeds up reimbursement to healthcare providers.

VOCABULARY

diagnosis Determination of the disease or condition that is causing a patient's signs and symptoms.

diagnostic statement Information about a patient's diagnosis or diagnoses that has been taken from the medical documentation.

encoder Software that will apply diagnostic or procedure codes to medical conditions or procedures.

epidemiologic Referring to epidemiology, the branch of medicine dealing with the incidence, distribution, and control of disease in a population. It also involves the prevalence of disease in large populations, in addition to detection of the source and cause of epidemics of infectious disease.

etiology The underlying cause or origin of a disease.

medically necessary Accepted healthcare services that are appropriate for the evaluation and treatment of a disease, condition, illness, or injury, and are consistent with the applicable standard of care. The service can also be called a medical necessity.

mortality The relative frequency of deaths in a specific population.

reimbursement To make repayment for an expense or a loss incurred.

GETTING TO KNOW THE ICD-10-CM

Structure and Format of the ICD-10-CM

The ICD-10-CM has two sections:

- The Alphabetic Index (the ICD-10-CM Index to Diseases and Injuries)
- The Tabular List (officially, the ICD-10-CM Tabular List of Diseases and Injuries)

Determining an ICD-10-CM code starts in the Alphabetic Index and is confirmed in the Tabular List. These codes have three to seven characters (Fig. 28.1). Every ICD-10-CM code begins with an alphabetic letter that indicates the chapter in the Tabular List from

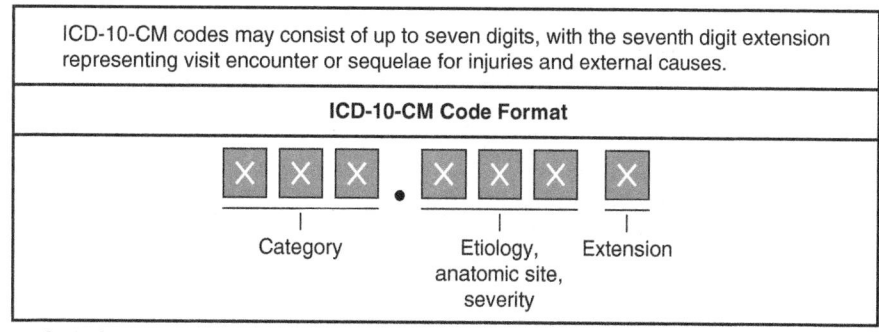

ICD-10-CM codes may consist of up to seven digits, with the seventh digit extension representing visit encounter or sequelae for injuries and external causes.

ICD-10-CM Code Format

| X | X | X | . | X | X | X | | X |

Category — Etiology, anatomic site, severity — Extension

Fig. 28.1 Code Structure and Format of ICD-10-CM Codes. (From Niedzwiecki B: *Kinn's the medical assistant,* ed 14, St. Louis, 2020, Elsevier.)

TABLE 28.1 ICD-10-CM Tabular List of Diseases and Injuries

Chapter	Title	Code Range	Possible Diagnosis[a]	ICD-10-CM Code
1	Certain Infectious and Parasitic Diseases	A00–B99	Measles	B05.9
2	Neoplasms	C00–D49	Colon cancer	C18.9
3	Diseases of the Blood and Blood-Forming Organs, and Certain Disorders Involving the Immune Mechanism	D50–D89	Iron-deficiency anemia	D50.9
4	Endocrine, Nutritional, and Metabolic Diseases	E00–E89	Type I diabetes	E10.9
5	Mental, Behavioral, and Neurodevelopmental Disorders	F01–F99	Dementia	F03.90H65.02
6	Diseases of the Nervous System	G00–G99	Parkinson's disease	G20
7	Diseases of the Eye and Adnexa	H00–H59	Glaucoma	H40.9
8	Diseases of the Ear and Mastoid Process	H60–H95	Otitis media, left ear	H65.02
9	Diseases of the Circulatory System	I00–I99	Hypertensive heart disease	I11.9
10	Diseases of the Respiratory System	J00–J99	Acute sinusitis	J01.90
11	Diseases of the Digestive System	K00–K95	Inguinal hernia	K40.90
12	Diseases of the Skin and Subcutaneous Tissue	L00–L99	Pressure ulcer of right heel	L89.619
13	Diseases of the Musculoskeletal System and Connective Tissue	M00–M99	Rheumatoid arthritis	M06.9
14	Diseases of the Genitourinary System	N00–N99	Endometriosis	N80.9
15	Pregnancy, Childbirth, and the Puerperium	O00–O9A	Ectopic pregnancy	O00.9
16	Certain Conditions Originating in the Perinatal Period	P00–P96	Neonatal jaundice	P59.9
17	Congenital Malformations, Deformations, and Chromosomal Abnormalities	Q00–Q99	Cleft lip	Q36.9
18	Symptoms, Signs, and Abnormal Clinical and Laboratory Findings, Not Elsewhere Classified	R00–R99	Abdominal pain	R10.9
19	Injury, Poisoning, and Certain Other Consequences of External Causes	S00–T88	Left ankle fracture, initial encounter	S82.892A
20	External Causes of Morbidity	V00–Y99	Snowboard accident	V00.318A
			Fall from cliff	W15.XXXA
			Exposure to excessive natural cold, Initial encounter	X31.XXXA
21	Factors Influencing Health Status and Contact With Health Services	Z00–Z99	Pregnancy state	Z33.1
22	Codes for special purposes	U00–U85	Vaping-related disorder	U07.0

[a]All diagnoses presented are not otherwise specified (NOS).

which the code originates (Table 28.1). All the letters of the English alphabet are used except U, which the World Health Organization (WHO) has reserved to assign to new diseases of uncertain etiology (ee tee OL uh jee). Some conditions use more than one alphabetic letter in their code ranges. For example, the codes in Chapter 1, Certain Infectious and Parasitic Diseases (A00–B99), begin with the letter A or B. The second character is always numeric.

The remaining characters can be a combination of letters and numbers. A decimal point is required after the third character.

There are only certain codes that require the seventh character. The following list shows the chapters that require a seventh character, and what the character identifies.

- Chapter 13: Diseases of the Musculoskeletal System – Encounter
- Chapter 15: Pregnancy, Childbirth and the Puerperium – Fetus Identification
- Chapter 18: Symptoms, Signs, and Abnormal Clinical and Laboratory Findings, Not Elsewhere Classified – Coma Scale

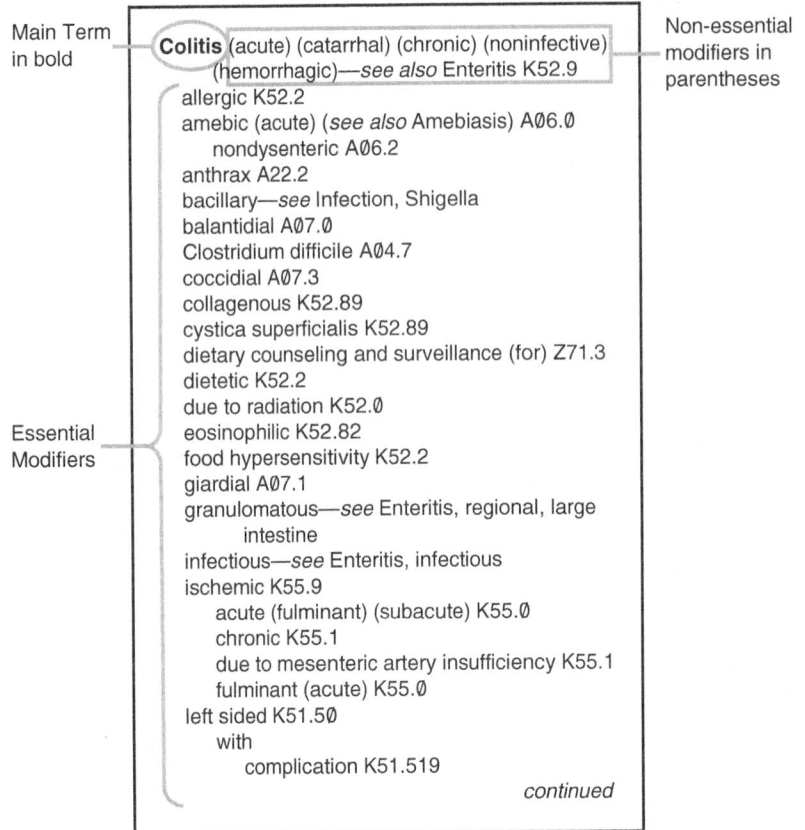

Main Term in bold

Non-essential modifiers in parentheses

Essential Modifiers

Colitis (acute) (catarrhal) (chronic) (noninfective) (hemorrhagic)—*see also* Enteritis K52.9
  allergic K52.2
  amebic (acute) (*see also* Amebiasis) A06.0
    nondysenteric A06.2
  anthrax A22.2
  bacillary—*see* Infection, Shigella
  balantidial A07.0
  Clostridium difficile A04.7
  coccidial A07.3
  collagenous K52.89
  cystica superficialis K52.89
  dietary counseling and surveillance (for) Z71.3
  dietetic K52.2
  due to radiation K52.0
  eosinophilic K52.82
  food hypersensitivity K52.2
  giardial A07.1
  granulomatous—*see* Enteritis, regional, large intestine
  infectious—*see* Enteritis, infectious
  ischemic K55.9
    acute (fulminant) (subacute) K55.0
    chronic K55.1
    due to mesenteric artery insufficiency K55.1
    fulminant (acute) K55.0
  left sided K51.50
    with
      complication K51.519
            continued

Fig. 28.2 ICD-10-CM Alphabetic Index With Main Term, Nonessential Modifiers, and Essential Modifiers.

- Chapter 19: Injury, Poisoning, and Certain Other Consequences of External Causes – Encounter
- Chapter 20: External Causes of Morbidity – Encounter
- Chapter 21: Factors Influencing Health Status and Contact with Health Services – Encounter

As you can see, this character most often indicates the encounter type. The most letters used for an encounter type are A, D, and S:

A: Initial encounter

D: Subsequent encounter

S: Sequela, a complication or condition that occurs as a direct result of a condition

CMS prepares the Official Guidelines for Coding and Reporting to be used with the ICD-10-CM codes, in addition to instructions on how to report the codes on insurance claim forms. The guidelines are a set of rules that have been developed to accompany and complement the official conventions and instructions provided in the ICD-10-CM proper.

The Alphabetic Index

The Alphabetic Index consists of an alphabetic list of diagnostic terms and related codes. This index includes main terms, nonessential modifiers, essential modifiers, and subterms:

- *Main terms:* These terms appear in bold type (Fig. 28.2).
- *Nonessential modifiers:* These terms follow the main term and are enclosed in parentheses. They are supplementary words or explanatory information. They do not need to be in the actual diagnostic statement.
- *Essential modifiers:* These terms are indented under the main term. They can modify the main term by describing different sites or etiology. They must be included in the diagnostic statement.

Let's use the example of *chronic ischemic* (ih SKEE mick) *colitis* (koh LYE tis). You would start with the main term: *Colitis* (see Fig. 28.2). You can see that the main term is followed by the nonessential modifiers (acute, catarrhal, **chronic**, noninfective, hemorrhagic) that do not affect the code assignment. Follow the list to the modifying term: Ischemic. Indented under ischemic, you will find "chronic" with the code K55.1. You will look up K55.1 in the Tabular List.

> **VOCABULARY**
>
> **chronic** Developing slowly and lasting for a long time, generally 3 or more months.

CRITICAL THINKING 28.1

Mike is working with the ICD-10-CM coding manual and is trying to refresh his memory about nonessential and essential modifiers. In your own words, define an essential modifier and a nonessential modifier. Compare your definitions with those of a classmate.

Supplementary Sections of the Alphabetic Index. The Alphabetic Index section includes two important tables.

- *Table of Neoplasms:* This table lists neoplasms by anatomic location and will be described later in the chapter.
- *Table of Drugs and Chemicals:* This table presents a classification of drugs and other chemical substances; it is used to identify poisonings and external causes of adverse effects. The six coding classifications are:
  - Poisoning, Accidental (Unintentional)
  - Poisoning, Intentional Self-Harm

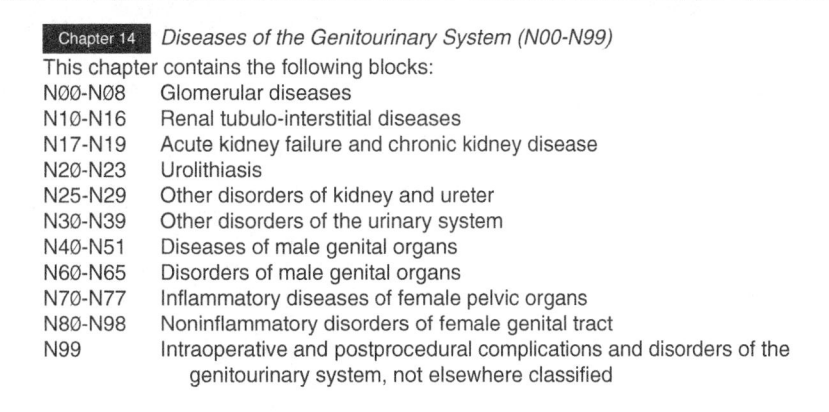

Chapter 14 *Diseases of the Genitourinary System (N00-N99)*
This chapter contains the following blocks:
N00-N08 Glomerular diseases
N10-N16 Renal tubulo-interstitial diseases
N17-N19 Acute kidney failure and chronic kidney disease
N20-N23 Urolithiasis
N25-N29 Other disorders of kidney and ureter
N30-N39 Other disorders of the urinary system
N40-N51 Diseases of male genital organs
N60-N65 Disorders of male genital organs
N70-N77 Inflammatory diseases of female pelvic organs
N80-N98 Noninflammatory disorders of female genital tract
N99 Intraoperative and postprocedural complications and disorders of the genitourinary system, not elsewhere classified

Fig. 28.3 Chapter Blocks in the Tabular List. (From Niedzwiecki B: *Kinn's the medical assistant,* ed 14, St. Louis, 2020, Elsevier.)

- Poisoning, Assault
- Poisoning, Undetermined
- Adverse Effect
- Underdosing

The Tabular List

The Tabular List is divided into 22 chapters. Most chapter titles specify a particular group of diseases and injuries, and all titles are followed by a code range in parentheses; for example, Chapter 1, Certain Infectious and Parasitic Diseases (A00–B99) (see Table 28.1). Some chapters use a body part or an organ system to group the codes; for example:

- Chapter 7, Diseases of the Eye and Adnexa (H00–H59)
- Chapter 9, Diseases of the Circulatory System (I00–I99)

Other chapters group conditions by etiology or the nature of the disease process; for example:

- Chapter 2, Neoplasms (C00–D49)
- Chapter 15, Pregnancy, Childbirth, and the Puerperium (O00–O9A) – groups codes related to the prenatal and postnatal periods
- Chapter 20, External Causes of Morbidity (V00–Y99) – also groups codes related to external causes of injury and poisoning
- Chapter 21, Factors Influencing Health Status and Contact With Health Services (Z00–Z99)

Each chapter is divided into subchapters, or *blocks,* and each subchapter has a designated 3-character code. These subchapter codes and code ranges form the foundation of the ICD-10-CM code set.

In each chapter, all the 3-character block codes begin with the alphabetic letter assigned to that chapter. For example, in Chapter 6, Diseases of the Nervous System (G00–G99), all the block codes (and their versions) begin with G. If a chapter's code range includes two letters [e.g., Chapter 1, Certain Infectious and Parasitic Diseases (A00–B99)], each 3-character block code begins with one of those two letters. The letter is followed by a 2-character number. A summary of the blocks (Fig. 28.3) at the beginning of each chapter provides an overview of the chapter.

As mentioned, the ICD-10-CM coding manual is produced by a variety of publishers, but many of the optional features are similar (remember, the important elements are always the same,

regardless of the publisher). For instance, to enable the coder to better maneuver through the Alphabetic Index, each page has *guide words,* which are the first and last words on that page (this is the same arrangement used for the pages of a dictionary). Each chapter of the Tabular List has a different-colored border strip; in some manuals, this strip shows the chapter title and the range of codes found on that specific page. In the chapters in the Tabular List, the codes for each category/block are arranged alphabetically (by the initial alpha character) and then numerically. Familiarizing yourself with these tools can help you improve your proficiency as you work through the manual to find the most accurate code.

It is important to note that some codes do not need to be extended beyond the 3-character code, and these are considered valid codes; for example, code **I10 {Essential (primary) hypertension}**. If a code has only three characters, do not add a decimal after the 3rd character. If a code has more than three characters, add a decimal point after the 3rd character; for example, **K11.7 {Disturbances of salivary secretion}**. Most ICD-10-CM codes have 4 to 7 characters (Box 28.1).

> **VOCABULARY**
> **specificity** The quality or state of being specific.

> **CRITICAL THINKING 28.2**
>
> Mike is reviewing the Tabular List of the ICD-10-CM coding manual. He notices that each chapter begins with a list of diagnostic categories with a corresponding range of codes. What is this called? How can this feature be used as a tool for accurate ICD-10-CM code assignment?

Conventions Used in the Tabular List. *Conventions* are abbreviations, punctuation, symbols, instructional notations, and related entities that help the coder select an accurate or a specific code. Conventions are found in the Tabular List but not in the Alphabetic Index. Understanding their meaning and using them as guides are crucial to accurate coding. The following table presents the most common conventions.

BOX 28.1 Reporting NEC and NOS Codes

In some cases, because of limited documentation in the patient's health record, the medical assistant can find it difficult to assign an ICD-10-CM code with a higher specificity (spes uh FIS i tee). The ICD-10-CM code set accommodates these coding circumstances by establishing "not elsewhere classified" (NEC) and "not otherwise specified" (NOS) guidelines.

- *NEC* means that the diagnostic statement contains specific wording, but no specific classification exists to match the wording. For example, an NEC code would be assigned if a patient seeks medical attention for chronic postoperative pain. The ICD-10-CM code would be **G89.28 {Other chronic postprocedural pain}**. For all NEC codes, the last character is always 8.

- *NOS* means that the diagnostic statement does not contain any more specific wording. For example, **sinusitis** (sye nuh SYE tis) with no documentation of the specific sinus site is assigned the NOS code **J32.9 {Chronic sinusitis, unspecified}**. The coder should keep in mind that the lack of documentation does not mean that all the patient's sinuses are inflamed. There must be no documentation of the exact site of the sinusitis for a non-NOS code to be assigned. As providers recognize that ICD-10-CM codes are more specific than ICD-9-CM codes, their documentation also is becoming more specific. For all NOS codes, the last character is always 9.

Convention	Explanation	Example
Placeholder Character	ICD-10-CM uses the dummy placeholder X in two different ways. The dummy placeholder can be used as the 5th character in certain six-character codes; this allows for future expansion of the code set without interruption of the six-character structure.	T43.4X1A Poisoning by butyrophenone and thiothixene neuroleptics, accidental, initial encounter (unintentional)
	Specific categories have a 7th character, but may not use the 4th, 5th, or 6th characters. In these cases, the dummy placeholder X is used to fill the empty character spaces. Note that a dummy placeholder would not be needed for codes with fewer than 7 characters.	S50.01XA Contusion of right elbow, initial encounter
Punctuation	Four basic forms of punctuation are used in the Tabular List: brackets, parentheses, colons, and braces. Each form serves a different purpose to help you read and understand the code descriptions.	[ ] Brackets enclose synonyms, alternative wording, or explanatory phrases. ( ) Parentheses are used to enclose supplementary words, which may be present or absent in the statement of a disease or procedure. : Colons are used in the Tabular Index after an incomplete term that needs one or more of the modifiers or adjectives that follow to make it assignable. { } Braces enclose a series of terms, each of which is modified by the statement appearing to the right of the brace.
Instructional Notations	Instructional notations, which are found in both the Alphabetic Index and the Tabular List, are critical to correct coding practices. They are located directly under the main term.	**Includes**: further defines or gives examples of the content of the category **Excludes**: The ICD-10-CM uses two types of exclusion notes: Excludes1: This is a clear "NOT CODED HERE!" message. It means that the excluded code should never be used with the code above the Excludes1 note. For example, code **G14 {Postpolio syndrome}** has this Excludes1 note: sequelae (si KWEL uh) of poliomyelitis (B91). Excludes2: This means "not included here." The excluded condition is not part of the condition represented by the code; however, a patient may have both conditions. When an Excludes2 note is present, the coder may code both conditions if the patient presents with both. For example, code F02 {Dementia (dih MEN shah) in other diseases classified elsewhere} has the following Excludes2 note: **vascular** (VAS kyoo lur) **dementia** (F01.5). This means that vascular dementia is not part of the condition coded as F02; therefore you can code both dementia (F02) and vascular dementia (F01.5) if the patient has both. **Code first/Use additional code**: *Code first* notes appear under *manifestation* codes. Manifestation codes specify the way in which an underlying condition appears, or manifests, as a result of an underlying etiology; the main terms of most manifestation codes include the words "in diseases classified elsewhere." A *Code first* note indicates that the underlying condition must be coded first. For example, Code F02 {Dementia in other diseases classified elsewhere} states, Code first the underlying physiologic condition, such as Alzheimer's (G30.-)

Relational Terms	These terms are used in both the Alphabetic Index and the Tabular List to clarify the context of the disease or injury.

- *And:* In the Tabular List code titles including *and* should be interpreted as meaning "and/or."
- *With:* The term *with* should be interpreted as meaning "associated with" or "due to" when it appears in the Alphabetic Index, or in an instructional note or code title in the Tabular List. In the Alphabetic Index, the word *with* follows immediately after the main term, not in alphabetical order.
- *Due to:* In both the Tabular List and the Alphabetic Index, the term *due to* signifies a relationship between two conditions. This assumption can be made when both conditions are present or when the diagnostic statement indicates this relationship.

MEDICAL TERMINOLOGY

col/o	colon
isch/o	to hold back
sinus/o	sinus
vascul/o	vessel
-ar	pertaining to
-emic	pertaining to blood condition
-it is	inflammation

CRITICAL THINKING 28.3

Mike is looking for the ICD-10-CM code for morbid obesity. From the Alphabetic Index, Mike finds the code E66. When he goes to verify the code in the Tabular List, he finds that the main term, Overweight and obesity, has a symbol indicating that a 4th character is needed. What is Mike's next step to assign the most accurate code? Can Mike just use E66? Why or why not?

PREPARING FOR DIAGNOSTIC CODING

Now that you have a basic understanding of the ICD-10-CM system, let's take a look at how you find the information you need to determine diagnostic codes.

Abstracting Diagnostic Statements

To prepare for diagnostic coding, you must analyze the patient's health record and abstract the diagnostic statement documented in the various reports. Sources of diagnostic statements include the encounter form, treatment notes, discharge summary, operative report, and radiology, pathology, and laboratory reports. Let's take a look at those documents.

Encounter Form. The encounter form (also known as a *superbill*) can be viewed in the EHR or as a paper document. The most commonly used diagnostic and procedure codes are listed on the encounter form. The provider then indicates what services and/or procedures were done and the diagnosis code for the visit. It is important to update the encounter form with the new diagnostic and procedure codes annually. If outdated codes are used, it can delay or reduce the amount paid by the insurance company.

VOCABULARY

abstract To collect important information from the health record.

dementia Loss of cognitive abilities, including memory, concentration, communication, planning, and abstract thinking. May also cause emotional disturbance and personality changes. Results from brain injury, Alzheimer's disease, Parkinson's disease, and other conditions.

encounter form A document used to capture the services/procedures and diagnoses for a patient visit. The fees for the services/procedures are usually included on the encounter form.

sequela An abnormal condition resulting from a previous disease.

History and Physical Exam. The history and physical (H&P) exam are the starting point of the patient's medical evaluation. The H&P includes:

- *Chief complaint (CC) and history of present illness (HPI):* The CC is a statement in the patient's own words that describes the reason for the visit. The HPI provides information on the current illness.
- *Past medical, family, and social histories:* These sections include information on previous illnesses, hospitalizations, surgeries, family members ages and medical conditions, and the patient's social history. The social history includes drug, alcohol, and tobacco use.
- *Allergies and current medications*: A list of the patients allergies and current over the counter and prescription medications are indicated.
- *Review of systems:* The provider includes objective and subjective information from the examination, which is organized by body systems.
- *Diagnostic tests:* Results from laboratory and diagnostic tests are indicated.
- *Problem list:* A list of the patients problems are listed. Usually, the most important problems are listed first.
- *Assessment and plan:* The assessment includes a diagnostic statement. The plan includes the treatments indicated by the provider. The patient may have a number of diagnostic statements in this section.

Progress Notes. Progress notes are the second most common medical document from which diagnostic statements can be abstracted. The format healthcare providers most commonly used for their notes are *SOAP notes*, a system of charting in which information is divided into subjective findings, objective findings, assessment, and plan for treatment. Just as in the H&P, the diagnostic statement can most often be found in the assessment section of the SOAP notes.

Discharge Summary. The discharge summary is used primarily for abstracting diagnostic information for patients who were hospitalized, rather than those seen in a provider's office. The main elements of a discharge summary are:

- Admission date and date of discharge
- H&P findings
- Clinical course during hospitalization
- Health condition on discharge and discharge diagnosis
- Aftercare plan

Diagnostic statements are abstracted from the discharge diagnosis section. This diagnosis would be used to bill for the provider's visits to the patient while the person was in the hospital. The medical office can use a discharge summary as an overview of the patient's condition, especially if the discharge was recent.

Operative Report. For patients who have surgery as an outpatient or inpatient, the operative report also is used to abstract diagnostic statements. An operative report includes:

- Preliminary diagnosis
- Final diagnosis
- Detailed description of the operative procedure from start to finish

The medical assistant uses the final diagnosis when searching for and selecting a diagnostic code.

Radiology, Laboratory, and Pathology Reports. Radiology, laboratory, and pathology reports are used to support and/or establish the diagnostic statement. Any findings from these reports must be documented in the progress notes in the health record so that they can be used for diagnostic coding, charge entry, or insurance billing purposes.

CRITICAL THINKING 28.4

While reviewing an encounter form, Mike notices that the diagnostic statement indicated that the patient needed to be treated for a left inguinal (IN gwin null) hernia (HER nee ah). However, Mike also notes that the surgical report indicates that the left inguinal hernia was obstructed. What should Mike use as the final diagnostic statement? Should he ask the provider which diagnostic statement to use?

VOCABULARY
hernia Protrusion of a loop of intestine through a weakness in the abdominal wall.

STEPS IN ICD-10-CM CODING

Accurate ICD-10-CM coding requires eight basic steps (Table 28.2). The first step involves abstracting the diagnostic statement from the health record and figuring out the main and modifying terms. Use the Alphabetic Index to search for the code or code ranges that best fit the diagnostic statement. The remaining steps are performed using the Tabular List to verify and confirm that the code or codes located in the Alphabetic Index fully match the diagnostic statement and that they are the most specific and accurate diagnostic codes. Procedure 28.1 details the basic coding steps using the ICD-10-CM manual and also encoder software (i.e., TruCode).

Using the Alphabetic Index

After you have abstracted the diagnostic statement from the health record, identify the main term and start searching for the best code, or code range, in the Alphabetic Index. It is important to note that the Alphabetic Index should be used only as a tool to locate the appropriate code or code range. The Tabular List, with its conventions, punctuation, notes, and guidelines, must always be used to confirm that the code or codes selected are accurate and specific and that there are no contraindications to the use of the code found in the Alphabetic Index. For this reason, never assign a code directly from the Alphabetic Index.

Even if only one code is found in the Alphabetic Index, it may be used only if a thorough review of the conventions and instructional notations in the Tabular List does not contraindicate (kon truh IN di keyt) it.

Fig. 28.4 shows an excerpt from the Alphabetic Index for the main term **Cyst**. The first essential modifier is "eyelid." Note the nonessential modifier – sebaceous – in parentheses after eyelid. (Remember, nonessential modifiers add detail, but they do not have to be present in the diagnostic statement for the code to be acceptable for use.) Directly below the essential modifier eyelid are the subterms. Note that there are separate subterms for the left eye and for the right eye. In addition, the diagnostic codes for each eye are further modified by the location of the cyst (upper or lower).

VOCABULARY
contraindicate Suggest that something should not be used.
cyst A small, capsulelike sac that is filled with a semisolid material, such as a keratinous or sebaceous cyst.

Using the Tabular List

Once you have identified the first three characters of the code in the Alphabetic Index, turn to the Tabular List. The chapters in the Tabular List are arranged alphabetically according to the initial letter of the 3-character code or codes assigned to each chapter. For example, Chapter 1 has code range A00–B99; Chapter 2 has code range C00–D49; Chapter 3 has code range D50–D89; and so on.

From the cyst example, you have determined that the code needed is in the H02 code range. Turn to the chapter that includes that range (Chapter 7). Fig. 28.5, an excerpt from the Tabular List, shows **Cysts of eyelid** as a main term, with the code H02.82. (Note that the nonessential modifier, sebaceous, is not shown in parentheses; rather, it appears under the main term in the nonbold phrase "Sebaceous cyst of eyelid.")

In the coding manual you would see the "additional character" symbol, which indicates that code H02.82 requires one more character. All possible diagnoses with 6-character codes are indented below the main term. A closer look at the disorders and their codes shows that the 6th character specifies the right or left eye and the location of the cyst on the eyelid (upper or lower). For the not-specified code, 9 would be the sixth character position.

Encoder Software

Encoder software (e.g., TruCode) is a tool commonly used by coders to assist in medical coding. This software performs computer-aided coding to assign the most accurate code possible. (TruCode is especially helpful to students because it allows them to search the ICD-10-CM coding manual using a few key terms.) The coder types a few key words into a Search box, and the software finds the most likely matches in the Alphabetic Index. The coder then clicks on a specific code, and the software searches the Tabular List. From the Tabular List, the coder can scroll up and down to determine the most accurate code. Encoder software can increase the speed and efficiency of coding for a wide variety of medical cases.

TABLE 28.2 Diagnostic Coding Step-by-Step: Parkinson Disease

Step 1	• Determine the correct diagnosis from the diagnostic statement. Parkinson's disease
Step 2	• Use the main term to look up the diagnosis in the Alphabetic Index. Parkinson disease, syndrome or tremor—see Parkinsonism
Step 3	• Look up the "see" term in the Alphabetic Index. **Parkinsonism** (idiopathic) (primary) G20
Step 4	• Review the essential modifiers under the main term. Parkinsonism (idiopathic) (primary) G20 with neurogenic orthostatic hypotension (symptomatic) G90.3 arteriosclerotic G21.4 dementia G31.83 *[F02.80]* with behavioral disturbance G31.83 *[F02.81]* due to drugs NEC G21.19 neuroleptic G21.11 neuroleptic induced G21.11 postencephalitic G21.3 secondary G21.9 due to arteriosclerosis G21.4 drugs NEC G21.19 neuroleptic G21.11 encephalitis G21.3 external agents NEC G21.2 syphilis A52.19 specified NEC G21.8 syphilitic A52.19 treatment-induced NEC G21.19 vascular G21.4
Step 5	• Choose the correct essential modifier based on the diagnostic statement. Because the diagnostic statement only indicates Parkinson's Disease, code G20 should be chosen.
Step 6	• Look up code G20 in the Tabular List. **G20 Parkinson's disease**
Step 7	• Check for any coding guidelines, conventions, inclusion or exclusion notes, or an additional character symbol. *Includes* — Hemiparkinson *Excludes1* — Idiopathic Parkinsonism or Parkinson disease Paralysis agitans Parkinsonism or Parkinson disease NOS Primary Parkinsonism or Parkinson disease dementia with Parkinsonism (G31.83)
Step 8	• Assign the final ICD-10-CM code. **G20 Parkinson's disease**

CRITICAL THINKING 28.5

Mike has determined a diagnostic statement to be "Perforation of the tympanic (tim PAN ick) membrane in the left ear." What keyword should be used for the TruCode software Search box? What main term will the encoder go to in the Alphabetic Index? What should Mike click to get to the Tabular List? At what point can Mike be sure that he has assigned the most accurate and specific code?

MEDICAL TERMINOLOGY

inguin/o	groin
pharyng/o	throat (pharynx)
tympan/o	eardrum
-al	pertaining to
-ic	pertaining to
sequela (singular)	**sequelae** (plural)

Cyst—*continued*
eyelid (sebaceous) H02.829
infected—*see* Hordeolum
left H02.826
lower H02.825
upper H02.824
right H02.823
lower H02.822
upper H02.821

Fig. 28.4 Excerpt from the Alphabetic Index: Cyst (Main Term), Eyelid (Essential Modifier), Sebaceous (Nonessential Modifier). (From Niedzwiecki B: *Kinn's the medical assistant*, ed 14, St. Louis, 2020, Elsevier.)

UNDERSTANDING CODING GUIDELINES

All ICD-10-CM coding manuals, regardless of the publisher, have comprehensive instructional notations and conventions to

H02.82	Cysts of eyelid
	Sebaceous cyst of eyelid
H02.821	Cysts of right upper eyelid
H02.822	Cysts of right lower eyelid
H02.823	Cysts of right eye, unspecified eyelid
H02.824	Cysts of left upper eyelid
H02.825	Cysts of left lower eyelid
H02.826	Cysts of left eye, unspecified eyelid
H02.829	Cysts of unspecified eye, unspecified eyelid

Fig. 28.5 Excerpt from the Tabular List: Cysts of eyelid. (From Niedzwiecki B: *Kinn's the medical assistant*, ed 14, St. Louis, 2020, Elsevier.)

help the coder select the most accurate diagnostic code or codes. When there is a difference between reference sources (including this text), the current year's ICD-10-CM coding manual is the final authority – this fact cannot be emphasized enough. When coding, you must always refer to and thoroughly review the conventions, instructional notations, code definitions, and other guidelines in the Alphabetic Index and Tabular List in the current year's version of the ICD-10-CM.

The following instructions are designed to provide some additional guidance in selecting diagnostic codes from various chapters in the ICD-10-CM. But they are not to be considered a replacement for the ICD-10-CM coding manual, nor do they provide all the coding information, definitions, or explanations found in the manual. The steps for diagnostic coding (see Procedure 28.1) are the same for all chapters of the ICD-10-CM; however, special rules and considerations apply to some chapters that affect the code selection process.

Coding of Signs and Symptoms

Signs and symptoms are coded only if the provider has not yet determined the final diagnosis. For example, if the provider's notes state "suspected," "probable," "questionable", "rule out" (R/O), or "working diagnosis," the coder should use the patient's documented signs and symptoms, including subjective and objective findings. Subjective findings include the patient's chief complaint or statements about why the patient is seeking medical care. Objective findings are any measurable indicators found during the physical examination, such as a blood pressure reading. If a patient comes in to see the provider because he has had a sore throat and fever for the past 3 days and the provider states "suspected strep throat" as the diagnosis, you would code sore throat and fever.

In the Tabular List, ill-defined conditions, signs, and symptoms are found in Chapter 18, Symptoms, Signs, and Abnormal Clinical and Laboratory Findings, Not Elsewhere Classified (R00–R99).

Conditions, signs, and symptoms in Chapter 18 include:
- Not elsewhere classified (NEC) cases, even after all the facts of the medical case have been examined
- Signs or symptoms that existed on the first encounter but were temporary and for which causes could not be determined
- Conditional diagnosis for a patient who failed to return for further care and the cause of whose condition had not yet been determined

- Medical cases referred elsewhere for treatment before a diagnosis could be made
- Not otherwise specified (NOS) cases in which a more precise diagnosis was not available for any reason
- Certain symptoms, for which supplementary information is provided, that represent important problems in the medical care provided

Coding the Etiology and Manifestation

Etiology refers to the underlying cause or origin of a disease. *Manifestation* describes the signs and symptoms of the disease. In the Alphabetic Index, the etiology and manifestation codes are listed together. The etiology code is always listed first, and the manifestation code is listed beside it in italics and enclosed within brackets. If the diagnosis in the health record indicated cataract (KAT ur ackt) due to myxedema (mick suh DEE mah), you would find the following listed in the Alphabetic Index:
- **cataract** (cortical) (immature) (incipient) H26.9
- the essential modifier would be myxedema E03.9 *[H28]*

E03.9 takes you to the Other hypothyroidism section, which is the etiology for this cataract. H28 takes you to the cataract, which is the manifestation. You would need to verify both codes in the Tabular List and list both codes in the documentation.

> **VOCABULARY**
> **cataract** Progressive loss of transparency of the lens of the eye.
> **myxedema** Advanced hypothyroidism in adulthood.

Coding Organism-Caused Diseases

The two-step process of coding organism-caused diseases begins with the affected anatomic site. In the case of a throat infection caused by enterovirus, you should first assign the diagnostic code for throat infection, or *pharyngitis* (fair in JYE tis). In the Tabular List, code J02.8 {Acute pharyngitis due to other specified organism} is accompanied by the following *Use additional code* note: "Use additional code (B95–B97) to identify infectious agent" (Fig. 28.6). In the Tabular List, the B95–B97 category/block (found in Chapter 1) is titled Bacterial and Viral Infectious Agents. Starting with code B95, search for the code that specifies enterovirus; this happens to be code B97.1 {Enterovirus as the cause of diseases classified elsewhere}. Note that code B97.1 requires a 5th character; however, no other information is provided by the medical record. Therefore you

• J02.8 Acute pharyngitis due to other specified organisms

Use additional code (B95-B97) it identify infectious agent
Excludes1   pharyngitis due to coxsackie virus (B08.5)
                   pharyngitis due to gonococcus (A54.5)
                   acute pharyngitis due to herpes [simplex] virus (B00.2)
                   acute pharyngitis due to infectious mononucleosis (B27.-)
                   enteroviral vesicular pharyngitis (B08.5)

Fig. 28.6 Excerpt from the Tabular List: Acute pharyngitis due to other specified organism.

	Malignant Primary	Malignant Secondary	Ca in situ	Benign	Uncertain Behavior	Unspecified Nature		Malignant Primary
bladder (urinary)	C67.9	C79.11	D090	D30.3	D41.4	D49.4	marrow NEC	C96.9
dome	C67.1	C79.11	D090	D30.3	D41.4	D49.4	unspecified side	C40.10
neck	C67.5	C79.11	D090	D30.3	D41.4	D49.4	marrow NEC	C96.9
orifice	C67.9	C79.11	D090	D30.3	D41.4	D49.4	cartilage NEC	C41.9
ureteric	C67.6	C79.11	D090	D30.3	D41.4	D49.4	clavicle	C41.3
urethral	C67.5	C79.11	D090	D30.3	D41.4	D49.4	marrow NEC	C96.9
overlapping lesion	C67.8	—	—	—	—	—	clivus	C41.0
sphincter	C67.8	C79.11	D090	D30.3	D41.4	D49.4	marrow NEC	C96.9
trigone	C67.0	C79.11	D090	D30.3	D41.4	D49.4	coccygeal vertebra	C41.4
urachus	C67.7	—	D090	D30.3	D41.4	D49.4	marrow NEC	C96.9
wall	C67.9	C79.11	D090	D30.3	D41.4	D49.4	coccyx	C41.4
anterior	C67.3	C79.11	D090	D30.3	D41.4	D49.4	marrow NEC	C96.9
lateral	C67.2	C79.11	D090	D30.3	D41.4	D49.4	costal cartilage	C41.3
posterior	C67.4	C79.11	D090	D30.3	D41.4	D49.4	costovertebral joint	C41.3
blood vessel—*see* Neoplasm,							marrow NEC	C96.9
connective tissue							cranial	C41.0

Fig. 28.7 Excerpt from the Table of Neoplasms. (From Niedzwiecki B: *Kinn's the medical assistant*, ed 14, St. Louis, 2020, Elsevier.)

can assign code B97.19 {Other enterovirus as the cause of diseases classified elsewhere} as the final organism code.

Coding Human Immunodeficiency Virus (HIV) Infection and Acquired Immunodeficiency Syndrome (AIDS)

To correctly code HIV infection and AIDS, it is essential to first understand the descriptions of the codes available. The key is whether the patient has symptoms.

• HIV: This indicates only that the virus is present.
• AIDS: AIDS is a syndrome; a syndrome is defined as a "group of symptoms occurring together." AIDS is the manifestation of signs and/or symptoms that can occur as a result of HIV infection.

Never code a patient as having HIV infection unless it is clearly documented as confirmed. Probable and suspected cases are never coded; instead, the signs and symptoms present should be coded. If a patient is seen for an HIV-related condition, the principal diagnosis should be B20 {Human immunodeficiency virus [HIV] disease}, followed by additional diagnostic codes for all reported HIV-related conditions.

Remember that strict restrictions are placed on the disclosure of medical information about patients with HIV infection and/or AIDS. Make sure the patient has signed the appropriate release of medical information form before any disclosures are made to third parties.

Coding Neoplasms

A neoplasm (NEE uh plaz uh m), or new growth, is coded by the site or location of the neoplasm and its behavior. The Table of Neoplasms (Fig. 28.7) is located just after the Alphabetic Index in the coding manual. This table lists the ICD-10-CM codes for neoplasms by anatomic site in alphabetic order. For coding purposes, neoplasms are further classified into six categories:

• *Malignant Primary:* Identifies the originating anatomic site of the neoplasm. A primary malignancy is defined as the original site or sites of the cancer.
• *Malignant Secondary:* Identifies sites to which the primary neoplasm has metastasized (muh TAS tuh sahyzd) (spread).
• *Ca in situ:* Carcinoma in situ (kahr suh NOH muh in SAHY too) is defined as situated in the original place or position. Tumor cells are undergoing malignant changes but are still confined to the point of origin, without invasion of surrounding normal tissue. The *Ca in situ* column is used only if the provider documents that precise terminology.
• *Benign:* The growth is noncancerous, nonmalignant, and has not invaded adjacent structures or spread to distant sites.
• *Uncertain behavior:* The pathologist is unable to determine whether the neoplasm is benign or malignant.
• *Unspecified nature:* Neither the behavior nor the histologic (hi STOL ah jic) type of neoplasm is specified in the diagnostic statement.

Most coding decisions on malignant neoplasms are between the primary and secondary classifications. Other terms are used:

- *In situ* is used only when the diagnostic statement contains that exact phrase.
- *Unspecified* is used only when no pathologic study has been done, and the neoplasm is still described with a term such as "tumor" or "growth."
- *Uncertain* is used by the provider when it has not been determined whether the neoplasm is malignant or benign.

VOCABULARY

histologic Referring to the study of body tissues.

Six Steps for Coding Neoplasms. The following steps can help determine the most specific and accurate diagnostic code for a neoplasm. These steps can be used in addition to the basic diagnostic steps.

1. In the Table of Neoplasms, find the site (anatomic location) of the neoplasm.
2. Determine, from the documentation, whether the neoplasm is malignant or benign.
3. If the neoplasm is benign, select the correct column in the table by reviewing the diagnostic statement.
4. If the neoplasm is malignant, select the column in the table that best fits its behavior: Malignant Primary, Malignant Secondary, or Ca in situ.
5. Link the appropriate column to the appropriate row.
6. Check the code shown in the table with the code in the Tabular List, to make sure the former complies with the guidelines, conventions, and instructional notations of the latter.

The ICD-10-CM coding manual always provides additional information, definitions, and guidelines for coding neoplasms in the Tabular List, just as it does for all other diseases, illnesses, and injuries.

Coding for Diabetes Mellitus

Diabetes mellitus (DM) (dahy uh BEE tis MEL ih tus) is classified as type 1 or type 2. Patients with DM type 1 develop the disease because the pancreas is unable to produce insulin. In individuals with DM type 2, the pancreas has become unable to maintain the level of insulin the body needs to function, or the person has developed target cell resistance to insulin.

The diabetes mellitus codes are combination codes. This means that they include the type of diabetes mellitus, the body system affected, and the complications affecting that body system. Use as many codes within a particular category/block as necessary to describe all the complications of the disease. These codes should be sequenced according to the reason for a particular encounter. Assign as many codes from category/block E08 to E13 (Diabetes Mellitus) as needed to identify all the patient's associated conditions.

Coding for Complications of Pregnancy, Childbirth, and the Puerperium

Coding for the obstetric patient is like using a specialty code-book within the ICD-10-CM coding manual. This is challenging

for coders who do not code obstetrics often. Some important clinical terms regarding pregnancy are:

- *antepartum* (AN tee PAHR tuh m): pregnancy (applies as soon as a pregnancy test result is positive)
- childbirth: delivery
- *postpartum*: the *puerperium* (pyoo ur Per ee um), or first 6 weeks after delivery
- *peripartum*: the period from the last month of pregnancy to 5 months postpartum

Obstetrics cases use codes from Chapter 15, Pregnancy, Childbirth, and the Puerperium (O00–O9A). Additional codes from other chapters may be used in conjunction with Chapter 15 codes to further specify conditions. If the provider documents that the pregnancy is incidental to the encounter, **Z33.1 {Pregnant state, incidental}** should be used instead of any Chapter 15 codes. This would be the case if the patient were being seen for a sprained ankle. The sprained ankle is not related to the pregnancy but is an incidental diagnosis. It is the provider's responsibility to state that the condition being treated is not affecting the pregnancy. Codes from Chapter 15 are documented only in the maternal health record; they are never used in the health record of the newborn.

Most of the codes in Chapter 15 have a 6th character, which indicates the trimester of pregnancy. Assignment of the final character for trimester should be based on the provider's documentation of the trimester (or number of weeks) for the encounter. This applies to the assignment of trimester for preexisting conditions, in addition to those that develop during or are due to the pregnancy. The provider's documentation of the number of weeks may be used to assign the appropriate code identifying the trimester. The seventh character in this chapter is used to identify the fetus when there is more than one and character options are:

0   not applicable or unspecified
1   fetus 1
2   fetus 2
3   fetus 3
4   fetus 4
5   fetus 5
9   other fetus

MEDICAL TERMINOLOGY

hist/o	tissue
log/o	study of
ante-	before, forward
neo-	new
post-	after, behind
peri-	around, surrounding
-partum	delivery
-plasm	formation

Coding for Burns and Corrosions

The same principles for multiple coding apply to burns. Code each burn separately unless specific combination codes are given in the Tabular List. There are many combination codes. Most burn codes are found in Chapter 19 (Injury, Poisoning, and Certain Other Consequences of External Causes); the applicable code ranges are T20–T32. Because burns are coded by site and degree and by the extent of body surface involvement, all burn cases should have at least two codes, and a third if the wound is infected. Other types of wounds, lacerations, punctures, and so on use a different 5th character to show that they are infected and, therefore, complicated. However, burn codes use the 5th character for other information. Therefore these diagnoses require an additional code to indicate infection.

The ICD-10-CM makes a distinction between burns and corrosions. The burn codes are used for thermal burns (except sunburns) caused by a heat source, such as a fire or hot appliance; burns resulting from electricity; and burns resulting from radiation. Corrosions, on the other hand, are burns caused by chemicals. The guidelines are the same for burns and corrosions.

Current burn codes (T20–T25) are classified by depth, extent, and burn agent (X code). Depth is categorized as first degree (redness), second degree (blistering), and third degree (full-thickness involvement). Burns of the eye and internal organs (T26–T28) are classified by site but not by degree.

Coding for External Causes of Morbidity

External cause codes are intended to provide data for research on injuries and injury prevention strategies. These codes capture:
- How the injury or health condition happened (cause)
- The intent (unintentional or accidental; or intentional, such as suicide or assault)
- The place where the event occurred
- The activity of the patient at the time of the event, and the person's status (e.g., civilian, military)

These codes are often used for workers' compensation claims.

Place of Occurrence Guideline

Codes from category Y92 {Place of occurrence of the external cause} are secondary codes. They are used after other external cause codes to identify the location of the patient at the time of the injury or other condition.

A place of occurrence code is used only once, at the initial encounter for treatment.

No 7th character is used in Y92 codes. Only one code from category Y92 should be recorded on the patient's health record. Do not use place of occurrence code Y92.9 {Unspecified place or not applicable} if the place is not stated or if it is not applicable.

Activity Codes

Category Y93 codes {Activity codes} are used to define the activity the patient was involved in at the time of injury or when the health condition developed. Only one code from category Y93 should be recorded in the patient's health record. An activity code should be used in conjunction with a place of occurrence code (Y92). The activity codes are not applicable to poisonings, adverse effects, misadventures, or sequelae.

Do not assign code Y93.9 {Unspecified activity} if the activity is not stated.

A code from category Y93 can be used with external cause (Y99) and occurrence (Y92) codes if identifying the activity provides additional information about the event.

For example, you are coding a closed right ankle fracture that occurred while the patient was playing soccer in a public park. First, you must identify what should be coded first. In this case, the right ankle fracture is coded first: S92.111A {Displaced fracture of neck of right talus} (Remember, "A" indicates initial encounter). The second code is the activity code; the patient was playing soccer, so the code for this activity is Y93.66 {Activity, soccer}. Remember, if the report did not state an activity, do not add Y93.9 {Unspecified activity}. Finally, when an activity code is used, a place of occurrence code should also be used. In this scenario, the patient was playing in a public park; therefore the place of occurrence code is Y92.830 {Public park}.

Coding for Health Status and Contact With Health Services

In the ICD-10-CM, Chapter 21, Factors Influencing Health Status and Contact with Health Services (Z00–Z99) are used to describe circumstances or encounters with a healthcare provider when no current illness or injury exists, such as:
- inoculations (ih nok yuh LEY shuh n) and vaccinations
- health status
- personal and/or family history of particular diseases
- screening
- observation
- follow-up
- donor counseling
- encounters for obstetric and reproductive services
- supervision of newborns and infants
- routine and administrative examinations
- other health encounters that do not fall into any one of the mentioned categories

MAXIMIZING THIRD-PARTY REIMBURSEMENT

The most important thing to remember in using the ICD-10-CM is to code the diagnosis to the highest level of specificity. Obtaining the correct reimbursement is important to the practice's cash flow, and it depends on proper coding and billing techniques. Some other crucial points to remember when submitting diagnostic codes for claims include:
- Use the current year's ICD-10-CM coding manual and stay informed of all changes, revisions, and additions published for that year, including the codes and the official coding guidelines.
- Code accurately from documented information, making sure the appropriate code or codes are assigned for all parts of the diagnostic statement, with no additions or omissions.
- Be sure the diagnosis codes correspond to the symptoms and treatment. Many codes are specific to age and sex.
- Review data entry to make sure no digits have been transposed.
- Know the insurance carrier's rules and requirements for completion and submission of claims.
- Incomplete or inaccurate codes may result in delay or denial of reimbursement. An inaccurate diagnosis may have a lifelong negative effect on the patient.

PROVIDERS AND ACCURATE CODING

Detailed documentation in the patient's health record can help coders to code to the highest level of specificity. Therefore providers should be trained on how to document the patient's condition in the health records appropriately. Respectfully discuss with providers that diagnostic codes cannot be assigned unless clear documentation is found in the patient's health record. Some providers may feel that because they care for the same type of cases, specialized diagnostic statements should be implied. However, the medical assistant should stress to providers the importance of detailed documentation in the health records. Clear and concise documentation practices ensure that the correct diagnoses are assigned in the patient's health record.

Staff meetings to review third-party requirements should be held regularly by the medical billing supervisor. Medical assistants should be respectful to the healthcare provider when discussing third-party requirements for more detailed documentation. An understanding and patient attitude toward the healthcare provider goes a long way in building a trusting relationship.

CLOSING COMMENTS

Diagnostic coding using the ICD-10-CM, with its almost 70,000 codes, can seem overwhelming. Successful medical coders follow specific steps to assign the most accurate ICD-10-CM code. Encoder software (e.g., TruCode) can search ICD-10-CM codes electronically to aid in faster code lookup. Detailed documentation in the patient's health record and accurate coding work hand-in-hand to maximize reimbursement for services provided. When working with providers on issues related to coding and documentation, show respect and patience. Medical assistants are expected to follow ethical standards by assigning and reporting only codes that are clearly supported by the documentation in the patient's record. When in doubt, a medical assistant should consult the provider for clarification. A coding professional is responsible for maintaining and continually enhancing his or her coding skills and for staying current with the changes in the codes, guidelines, and regulations.

PATIENT-CENTERED CARE

Most patients know little about medical coding, so they may not understand how the codes on their encounter forms relate to their diagnosis. If the patient has questions, explain that the codes represent their diagnosis to the most specific and accurate level. Because the coding system is much like a foreign language to patients, be patient when explaining this process and answering questions. This will help the patient to understand the insurance billing process.

BEING PROFESSIONAL

Although providers may be overly concerned about the need to maximize insurance reimbursements, coders should never feel coerced into fraudulent coding practices. Successful coders rely solely on medical documentation as the source of diagnostic statements. Coders should never assume that additional complications or conditions exist if they are not documented. In these cases, strong communication between the coder and the provider is necessary to clarify the appropriate diagnoses.

Role-play the following scenario with a peer: You are a medical assistant who is doing a provider's coding, and the peer is the provider. The provider is encouraging you to code to the maximum reimbursement, yet you do not see the documentation supporting the reimbursement they are pushing for. Respond to the provider in a respectful and professional manner.

CHAPTER REVIEW

When assigning diagnostic codes, the medical assistant needs to be familiar with the format of the ICD-10-CM coding manual and the various documents in which the diagnostic statement can be found. The ICD-10-CM coding manual is made up of two sections: the Alphabetic Index and the Tabular List. Coding begins in the Alphabetic Index, and the actual diagnostic code is determined in the Tabular List. You should always review the instructional notes to ensure that you have the most specific code.

Diagnostic statements can be found in different health documents. In a clinic setting, the diagnosis is commonly found on the encounter form or in the progress notes. When billing for services provided in the hospital, you may need to review the discharge summary or operative report.

Once the diagnostic statement has been identified, you must follow the coding guidelines and conventions. If the diagnostic statement includes words such as "rule out" or "possible," then you must code the signs and symptoms. When indicated, you should include both the etiology and manifestation codes.

Diagnostic coding can affect reimbursement from the insurance carrier. The diagnostic codes tell the insurance carrier why the services were provided. If the diagnostic code does not match the service provided, the insurance company will not pay for the services provided to the patient. An example would be if the diagnostic code was for pharyngitis, yet the service it was linked to was for a blood glucose test. In this scenario, the insurance company would say that a blood glucose test is not medically necessary for pharyngitis.

Being proficient at diagnostic coding makes you a valuable member of the healthcare team.

SCENARIO WRAP-UP

Mike's experience using the ICD-10-CM coding manual and encoder software on actual medical office cases has made him even more enthusiastic about his new responsibilities, and he enjoys the coding process more. He knows that as he gains experience in ICD-10-CM coding, he will be able to set a positive example for the staff. As Mike progresses with diagnostic coding, he will also be able to help the providers and medical assistant staff be attentive to details when documenting in a health record.

Although the electronic encounter form for entering billing codes is an easy tool, Mike has learned that knowing how to use the ICD-10-CM Alphabetic Index and Tabular List is a necessary skill to ensure accurate coding. He also knows that it is important when coding a diagnosis to make sure the medical documentation matches the encounter form and that all elements of the diagnostic statement are included. Furthermore, he must ensure that the diagnosis listed on the encounter form is fully documented in the patient's health record. Mike is feeling more comfortable about referring to coding guidelines to ensure the most accurate code and to make certain that every character for the ICD-10-CM code is present. Every feature of the manual provides guidance in choosing and confirming a diagnostic code that matches the diagnostic statement on the encounter form and in the health record. Searching for codes in the encoder also has helped Mike develop his coding skills more quickly.

PROCEDURE 28.1 Perform Coding Using the Current ICD-10-CM Manual or Encoder

Task
To perform accurate diagnosis coding using the ICD-10-CM coding manual or an encoder.

Equipment and Supplies
- ICD-10-CM coding manual (current year) *or*
- Encoder software, such as TruCode

Scenario
The encounter form and progress notes both show that the diagnosis for this patient encounter is acute colitis. Locate the most accurate ICD-10-CM code for this diagnostic statement.

Procedural Steps
Alphabetic Index

1. Determine and locate the main terms from the diagnostic statement in the Alphabetic Index.
   Purpose: To provide a starting point for searching the Alphabetic Index.
2. Locate the essential modifiers listed under the main term in the Alphabetic Index.
   Purpose: To ensure further specificity of the codes found in the Alphabetic Index.
3. Review the coding conventions, punctuation, and notes in the Alphabetic Index.
   Purpose: To ensure that no additional searches, exclusions, or similar terms are needed to complete the search in the Alphabetic Index.
4. Choose a tentative code, codes, or code range from the Alphabetic Index that matches the diagnostic statement as closely as possible.
   Purpose: To prevent backtracking and repeated searches in the Alphabetic Index.

Tabular List

5. Look up the codes chosen from the Alphabetic Index in the Tabular List.

Purpose: To begin the process of determining whether the codes selected from the Alphabetic Index are appropriate and accurate.

6. Review notes, conventions, and the Official Coding Guidelines associated with the code and code description in the Tabular List.
   a. Review conventions and punctuation.
   b. Review instructional notations:
      - Includes and excludes notes
      - Code first, code also, and code additional notes
      - *and, or,* and *with* statements

   Purpose: To ensure that the code or codes selected are appropriate for use and to determine whether they require additional codes or further specificity, or are excluded from use.

7. Verify the accuracy of the tentative code in the Tabular List.
   a. Make sure all elements of the diagnostic statement are included in the codes selected.
   b. Make sure the code description does not include anything not documented in the diagnostic statement.

   Purpose: To ensure that the most accurate and specific code is selected and that no contraindication exists to use the code or codes selected.

8. Extend the codes to their highest level of specificity (up to the 7th character, if required). If a 7th character is required and no codes are present for the 4th, 5th, or 6th characters, it is appropriate to use the dummy placeholder X for these positions.

9. Assign the code (or codes) selected from the Tabular List as the appropriate code for the patient's condition as documented in the patient's health record.

   Purpose: To ensure that the health record and/or electronic encounter form contain documentation of the diagnosis code or codes assigned.

Using the TruCode Encoder Software
1. Type in the main term from the diagnostic statement in the Search box, as shown in Fig. 1.

Continued

PROCEDURE 28.1   Perform Coding Using the Current ICD-10-CM Manual or Encoder—cont'd

SimChart® for the medical office   TruCode

| Search for | colitis | in | Diagnosis, ICD-10-CM ▾ | Search | ☐ Find All |

Search Results for `colitis` in ICD-10-CM Diagnosis

Colitis (acute) (catarrhal) (chronic) (noninfective) (hemorrhagic) (see also Enteritis) K52.9

Book: ICD-10-CM Diagnosis

◄ ► Colitis

renal N23
saturnine NEC - see Poisoning, lead
ureter N23
urethral N36.8
    due to calculus N21.1
uterus NEC N94.89
    menstrual - see Dysmenorrhea
worm NOS B83.9
Colicystitis - see Cystitis
Colitis (acute) (catarrhal) (chronic) (noninfective) (hemorrhagic) (see also Enteritis) K52.9
  allergic K52.2
  amebic (acute) (see also Amebiasis) A06.0
    nondysenteric A06.2
  anthrax A22.2
  bacillary - see Infection, Shigella
  balantidial A07.0
  Clostridium difficile A04.7
  coccidial A07.3

1

2. The software will provide a list of main terms that could be related to the diagnosis typed in the Search box. The coder chooses the main term that best represents the diagnostic statement.
3. Based on the main term chosen, a list of essential modifiers is presented (see Fig. 2). The coder must review the diagnostic statement to ensure that all documented modifying terms are identified. If the provider does not document a modifying term, the coder should not assume that a modifying term was implied.

PROCEDURE 28.1   Perform Coding Using the Current ICD-10-CM Manual or Encoder—cont'd

SimChart® for the medical office   TruCode®

Search for   colitis   in   Diagnosis, ICD-10-CM   ▾   Search   ■ Find All

Search Results for `colitis` in ICD-10-CM Diagnosis

Colitis (acute) (catarrhal) (chronic) (noninfective) (hemorrhagic) (see also Enteritis) K52.9

Book: ICD-10-CM Diagnosis Tabular

◀ ▶

	K52.82	**Eosinophilic colitis**
	K52.89	**Other specified noninfective gastroenteritis and colitis**
		Collagenous colitis
		Lymphocytic colitis
		Microscopic colitis (collagenous or lymphocytic)
Ⅰ	**K52.9**	**Noninfective gastroenteritis and colitis, unspecified**
		Colitis NOS
		Enteritis NOS
		Gastroenteritis NOS
		Ileitis NOS
		Jejunitis NOS
		Sigmoiditis NOS

Excludes1:   diarrhea NOS (R19.7)
functional diarrhea (K59.1)
infectious gastroenteritis and colitis NOS (A09)
neonatal diarrhea (noninfective) (P78.3)
psychogenic diarrhea (F45.8)

Copyright © 2015 TruCode LLC. All rights reserved.
CPT copyright 2015 American Medical Association. All rights reserved.

2

4. In the preceding figure, note the yellow area on the left of the chosen diagnosis. In the TruCode program, click on the yellow area, and an instructional notes textbox opens, which includes coding guidelines, which will appear, as shown in Fig. 3. To determine the most accurate code, follow these coding steps.

Noninfective enteritis and colitis (K50-K52)

K50—K52
Includes: noninfective inflammatory bowel disease
K50—K52
Excludes1: irritable bowel syndrome (K58.-) megacolon (K59. 3)

Chapter 11: Disease of the digestive system (K00-K95)

K00—K95
Excludes2: certain conditions originating in the perinatal period (P04-P96)
certain infectious and parasitic diseases (A00-B99)

3

---

5. Once all the menus of essential modifiers have been presented, choose the most accurate and specific code based on the diagnostic statement.

29

Procedural Coding Basics

LEARNING OBJECTIVES

1. Describe the organization of the *Current Procedural Terminology* (CPT) manual.
2. Distinguish between the Alphabetic Index and the Tabular List in the CPT code set.
3. Discuss coding guidelines and explain the importance of modifiers in assigning CPT codes.
4. Identify the required medical documentation for accurate procedural coding.
5. Discuss how to use the Alphabetic Index and Tabular List.
6. Identify common CPT coding guidelines for Evaluation and Management (E/M) procedures, and perform procedural coding of an office visit.
7. Discuss E/M Introductory Guidelines related to Office or Other Outpatient Codes 99202–99215.
8. Review the revised Office or Other Outpatient E/M codes 99202–99215.
9. Discuss time-based coding guidelines.
10. Identify common CPT coding guidelines for surgical procedures. Also discuss coding factors for the Integumentary system, Musculoskeletal system, and Maternity Care and Delivery.

OUTLINE

⟫ OPENING SCENARIO

Kaitlyn Vogt, a medical assisting student, works at Walden-Martin Family Medical (WMFM) Clinic. Kaitlyn really enjoyed learning about diagnostic coding in the *International Classification of Diseases, Tenth Revision, Clinical Modification* (ICD-10-CM), and now she looks forward to learning about procedural coding. Kaitlyn recognizes that a strong understanding of anatomy and physiology are vital to correct diagnostic coding. She also believes the knowledge she has gained will

TABLE 29.1 Comparison of Procedural Code Sets

Code Set	Used For	Code Features	Example	Description	Developer	Updated
ICD-10-PCS	Inpatient hospital procedures	7-digit alphanumeric code	0TTJ0ZZ	Appendectomy	National Center for Health Statistics	Annually, October 1
CPT	Outpatient procedures; professional and technical services	5-digit numeric code; a 2-digit modifier can be added	44970	Laparoscopic, surgical, appendectomy	American Medical Association (AMA)	Annually, January 1
HCPCS	Auxiliary medical treatment, including vaccines, medical transport, drugs, durable medical equipment	5-digit alphanumeric code; a 2-digit modifier can be added	A0428	Ambulance service, basic life support, nonemergency transport	Centers for Medicare and Medicaid Services (CMS)	Annually, October 1

CPT, Current Procedural Terminology; *HCPCS*, Healthcare Common Procedure Coding System; *ICD-10-PCS*, International Classification of Diseases, 10th Revision, Procedure Coding System.

help her in procedural coding. Kaitlyn will be using the *Current Procedural Terminology* (CPT) coding system for most procedures and services provided in the medical office. In addition, she will use the *Healthcare Common Procedure Coding System* (HCPCS; pronounced "hic-pix") for medical products and services not found in the CPT.

As she did with the ICD-10-CM, Kaitlyn is learning that accurate coding begins with the proper analysis of documentation found in the health record. With that information, she will abstract the correct data to assign an accurate procedure code. As does the ICD-10-CM, the CPT has coding guidelines, symbols, and formal steps specific to procedural coding. However, unlike in ICD-10-CM diagnostic coding, in CPT and HCPCS coding Kaitlyn must determine how and when to use modifiers. The office manager wants to give Kaitlyn some experience, so he allows her to review some healthcare records so she can practice coding.

YOU WILL LEARN

1. How the format, layout, and conventions of the CPT and HCPCS manuals help the medical assistant locate the most accurate and specific procedural code.
2. To define upcoding and downcoding and the reasons they should not be done.
3. To identify the documents in which the procedures and services can be found.
4. To apply coding guidelines necessary for procedural coding.
5. When to use a modifier for procedure codes.

INTRODUCTION

Procedural coding changes the written descriptions of procedures and services delivered in a healthcare facility into numeric or alphanumeric codes. These codes are used for a variety of different purposes. They can be used to track the services that are being provided to patients and on claims sent for payment from insurance companies. There are three procedure code sets used for these purposes (Table 29.1):
- International Classification of Diseases, Tenth Revision, Procedural Coding System (ICD-10-PCS)
- Healthcare Common Procedure Coding System (HCPCS) Level 1 codes: Current Procedural Terminology (CPT).

(In this chapter, CPT codes will refer to HCPCS Level 1 codes.)
- HCPCS Level 2 codes. (In this chapter, HCPCS codes will refer to HCPCS Level 2 codes.)

This chapter will focus on the CPT and HCPCS code sets, which are used in ambulatory care settings.

INTRODUCTION TO THE CPT MANUAL

The CPT system was developed and is maintained by the American Medical Association (AMA). It is updated each year and released on January 1. The CPT coding manual consists of descriptive terms and identifying codes for reporting professional and technical services. CPT codes convert written descriptions of procedures and services into numeric codes. They establish a standard system that accurately describes medical and surgical services.

CODE CATEGORIES IN THE CPT MANUAL

There are three different categories of codes in the CPT. Category I codes are used most frequently and are required for insurance claim submission. Category II and Category III codes are used for data collection.

Category I Codes

Category I codes are located in the Tabular List of the CPT manual and arranged by the sections:
- Comprehensive instructions for using the manual, including the steps for coding
- Tabular List, which includes the following six sections:
  - Evaluation and Management
  - Anesthesia
  - Surgery
  - Radiology
  - Pathology and Laboratory
  - Medicine
- Coding Guidelines, Conventions, and Notes
- Appendices (16; A–P)
- The Alphabetic Index

For example, codes beginning with 7 (e.g., 70010–79999—radiologic examination of the mandible, partial, with less than four views) are located in the Radiology section of the manual.

Each code has a description of the service or procedure performed. These codes are 5-digit numeric codes.

Category II Codes

Category II codes are a set of supplemental tracking codes that healthcare facilities use for performance measurement. Category II codes are optional. They cannot be used as a substitute for Category I codes, and they are not used as part of the insurance billing process. When these codes are used, it can reduce the need for abstracting information from the health record. These codes describe clinical components that may be typically included in Evaluation and Management services, or clinical services. In a Category II code, the 5th digit is the letter F. For example, if a patient was seen by the provider for asthma, a Category I code of 99213 could be used for the visit. In addition, a Category II code of 2015F Asthma impairment assessed (Asthma) could be used.

Category II codes are described and listed in their own section, which is located after the Medicine section and before the appendices. Category II codes are reviewed by the Performance Measures Advisory Group. This group is composed of members from various medical organizations and government agencies.

Category III Codes

Category III codes are temporary codes used for emerging and new technology, services, and procedures that have not been officially added to the Tabular List. The 5th digit in a Category III code is the letter T. Category III codes may be used in billing and reporting if:

- no code in the Tabular List correctly describes the technology, service, or procedure performed.
- no Category I code matches the documentation.

In most publishers' editions of the CPT manual, Category III codes are also listed in their own section, after the Medicine section and before the appendices.

ORGANIZATION OF THE CPT MANUAL

The CPT coding manual is separated into the Alphabetic Index and the Tabular List.

Alphabetic Index

CPT coding starts with the Alphabetic Index. It is found in the back of the CPT manual and is an alphabetic listing of main terms. These terms represent the type of surgery, the anatomic site, or eponym (EP uh num) (Fig. 29.1). Much like the Alphabetic Index in the ICD-10-CM manual, the Alphabetic Index in the CPT gives a code, codes, or a code range that must be verified in the Tabular List of the CPT manual.

CRITICAL THINKING 29.1

To practice her coding skills, Kaitlyn is reviewing a surgical report for a gallbladder removal. Will she be able to find the main term "gallbladder" in the Alphabetic Index? Why or why not? What other main term could she be looking for? Once she finds the range of codes in the Alphabetic Index, what is her next step?

Fracture

Acetabulum	
Closed Treatment	27220-27222
Open Treatment	27226-27228
with Manipulation	27222
without Manipulation	27220
Alveolar Ridge	
Closed Treatment	21440
Open Treatment	21445
Ankle	
Bimalleolar	27808, 27810, 27814
Lateral	27786, 27788, 27792, 27808, 27810, 27814
Medial	27760, 27762, 27766, 27808, 27810, 27814
Posterior	27767-27769, 27808, 27810, 27814
Trimalleolar	27816, 27818, 27822-27823
Ankle Bone	
Medial	27760-27762
Bennett's	
See Thumb, Fracture	
Blow-Out Fracture	
Orbital Floor	21385-21387, 21390, 21395
Bronchi	
Reduction	31630
Calcaneus	
Closed Treatment	28400-28405
Open Treatment	28415-28420
Percutaneous Fixation	28406
with Manipulation	28405-28406
without Manipulation	28400

Fig. 29.1 Alphabetic Index: Fractures. (From Niedzwiecki B, et al: *Kinn's the medical assistant,* ed 14, St. Louis, 2020, Elsevier.)

Tabular List

The Tabular List is divided into six sections, with codes listed in numeric order in each section. As in the ICD-10-CM, the codes in the Tabular List include definitions, guidelines, and notes. These enable the coder to select the most specific code based on the procedural statement and service descriptions documented in the health record. The six sections of the Tabular List and their CPT code ranges are:

- Evaluation and Management (99202–99499)
- Anesthesia (00100–01999, 99100–99157)
- Surgery (10021–69990)
- Radiology, including nuclear medicine and diagnostic ultrasound (70010–79999)
- Pathology and Laboratory (80047–89398)
- Medicine (90281–99199, 99500–99607)

Sections are subdivided into *subsections*; *subsections* are subdivided into *subheadings*; and *subheadings* can be subdivided into *categories*. Each level of a section provides more specificity (spes hu FIS i tee) about the procedure or service

---

VOCABULARY

CPT Assistant An online CPT coding journal, supported by the AMA, which addresses subjects such as appealing insurance denials, validating coding to auditors, training staff members, and answering day-to-day coding questions.

eponym In medical terms, a medical diagnosis or procedure named for the person who discovered it.

performance measurement The regular collection of data to assess whether the correct processes are being performed and desired results are being achieved.

specificity The quality or state of being specific.

Section: Surgery (10021-69990)

Subsection: Integumentary System

Subheading: Skin Subcutaneous and Accessory Structures

Category: Débridement

Fig. 29.2 Format of Tabular List.

performed and the anatomic site or organ system involved (Fig. 29.2). Each section and subsection provide coding guidelines and, if needed, a reference to the CPT Assistant. In most instances, all four levels are found, although this is not a hard-and-fast rule.

In the CPT manual, the subsection is listed below the section and indented. The subsection usually describes an anatomic site or an organ system; for example:

- Anatomic site: heart, femur, or skull
- Organ system: digestive, integumentary, or cardiovascular

A subheading is listed below the subsection. It generally refers to a specific procedure or service, but it can also indicate a more specific anatomic site:

- Procedures: esophagoscopy, incision and drainage, or cardiac catheterization
- Specific anatomic site: mitral valve, distal femur, or occipital bone

Category is the lowest level of code description. The subcategory is listed below the subheading. It provides even more specificity about an anatomic site or the procedure or service performed.

UNLISTED PROCEDURE OR SERVICE CODE

Occasionally, even with the most detailed documentation, an accurate code to match the procedure or service performed cannot be found in the CPT manual. For this reason, in each section, nonspecific codes have been provided. These codes are known as Unlisted Procedures and Services. For example, code 29999 is found in the Surgery section, Musculoskeletal subsection. It describes an "unlisted procedure, arthroscopy." Unlisted codes can be used only when no other Category I or Category III code exactly matches the documentation. When an unlisted code is used, a special report must be sent with the insurance claim that describes the procedure or service in detail.

> **VOCABULARY**
> **special report** Additional medical documentation required to confirm the need for the use of unlisted, unusual, or newly adopted medical procedures code.
> **medical necessity** Health-care services or supplies needed to diagnose or treat an illness or injury, condition, disease, or its symptoms and that meet accepted standards of medicine.

CPT CODING GUIDELINES

At the beginning of each section and some subsections are coding guidelines. These guidelines add definitions and descriptions needed to interpret and report the procedures and services in that section or subsection. Coding guidelines enhance the

coder's understanding of when and under what circumstances specific codes may be used. It is important to thoroughly read and apply the coding guidelines provided. Because coding guidelines are updated every year on October 1, it is also important to reread the guidelines after every new edition is released. Selecting a code without reading the guidelines usually leads to selection of the wrong code. Not only will this result in possibly delayed or denied reimbursement, but also, continued inappropriate code selection can be considered fraud or abuse and can result in serious civil or criminal penalties.

Upcoding is the use of a higher level procedure code than is supported in the documentation or by medical necessity. An example would be using E/M code 99213 (low complexity medical decision making and 20-29 minutes of total time) when the documentation supports 99212 (straightforward and 10-19 minutes). This would be considered fraud.

Downcoding is the use of a lower level procedure code than is justified. An example would be using 99213 (low complexity medical decision making and 20-29 minutes of total time) when the documentation supports 99214 (moderate complexity and 30-39 minutes). This also can be damaging to the healthcare facility because it would result in lower reimbursement.

In procedural coding, the coder must always choose the code that most accurately describes the services provided.

Modifiers

Category I code *modifiers* are two-digit, numeric codes that report or indicate:

- Specific criteria
- Specific condition
- Special circumstance

Category II code modifiers are alphanumeric. In either situation, they are used with CPT codes to indicate that a service or procedure performed was altered by specific circumstances (Table 29.2). Modifiers are included with the 5-digit CPT code to supply additional information or to describe extenuating circumstances that affected the procedure or service. For instance, modifier −50 adds the detail that a procedure was performed *bilaterally* (bye LAT er uhl ee), or on both sides of the body. When an assistant surgeon is needed for a surgical procedure, modifier −80 is

TABLE 29.2 Commonly Used CPT Code Modifiers

Modifier	Description
−50	Bilateral procedure. If the procedure was performed on both sides of the body (e.g., both knees, both eyes) and the code description does not indicate that the procedure or service was performed bilaterally, modifier −50 is used.
−62	Two surgeons. When two surgeons work together as primary surgeons performing distinct parts of a procedure, each surgeon should report the procedure they performed to the insurance carrier using modifier −62. This prevents the insurance carrier from possibly rejecting a surgical charge as a duplicate.
−26	Professional component. This modifier is used when a technician performs the service to provide their professional opinion.
−RT, −LT	Indicates the side of the body on which the procedure took place. (e.g., 19100−LT − Breast biopsy, left side)

used. This allows assistant surgeons to submit charges for their time. Modifiers can also show which side of the body a medical procedure was performed on. For example, the code 19100-RT indicates that the right breast was biopsied. A list of modifiers can be found in the CPT coding manual in Appendix A.

CPT CONVENTIONS

Conventions, or special symbols (Fig. 29.3), are used to provide additional information about specific codes. Let's look at a skin graft procedure for a wound that is 50 sq cm:

- Code 15271, Application of skin substitute graft to trunk, arms, legs, total wound surface area up to 100 sq cm; first 25 sq cm or less wound surface area
- Code +15272, each additional 25 sq cm wound surface area, or part thereof

To accurately code for this skin graft, two codes would be used: 15271 and +15272.

In the Tabular List in most CPT manuals, the legend explaining the meanings of the convention symbols is found at the bottom of each page.

CRITICAL THINKING 29.2

Kaitlyn is trying to look up the CPT code for a left arm cyst biopsy. She has found the code, but how can she show that the procedure took place on the left side?

Kaitlyn also came across CPT code 32440 (removal of lung, pneumonectomy), but she needs to also code for the repair of a portion of the bronchus. The code has a (+) in front of it; what does this mean?

DOCUMENTATION FOR CPT CODING

Medical records used for procedural coding can include any or all of:

- Encounter form (Fig. 29.4)
- History and physical report (H&P) and progress notes
- Discharge summary
- Operative report and anesthesia report
- Pathology report and radiology report

Symbols

- ▲ Change or modified procedure descriptor.
- ● New code
- ▶◀ Changed or modified text
- ➲ Reference to *CPT Assistant*, *Clinical Examples in Radiology*, and *CPT Changes*
- + Add-on code
- ⊘ Exemptions to modifier 51
- ⅄ Vaccine pending FDA approval
- ○ Reinstated or recycled code
- \# Out-of-numerical sequence code
- ★ Telemedicine Services
- ✖ Multiple proprietary laboratory analysis tests have identical descriptor.

Fig. 29.3 Current Procedural Terminology (CPT) Conventions. (From Niedzwiecki B, et al: *Kinn's the medical assistant*, ed 14, St. Louis, 2020, Elsevier.)

When comparing the documentation to the codes, make sure all the elements of the description match substantially, with nothing added or missing. For example, review CPT codes 21315 and 21320. Both codes describe the closed treatment of a nasal bone fracture. However, 21315 indicates that there is no stabilization, and 21320 indicates that there is stabilization. The coder reviews the procedures and then assigns the CPT codes with the description that most closely resembles the documentation.

Some providers have CPT and ICD-10-CM codes printed on their encounter forms; however, these codes should be treated only as a reference. Medical coders must also review the health record carefully, abstracting all the procedures and services rendered during an encounter. For example, a provider may circle the procedure for a preventive health visit for a 4-year-old on the encounter form but forget to record the injections provided during the encounter. Upon reviewing the patient's electronic health record (EHR), the medical assistant discovers that the provider's notes state routine injections were administered. If the medical assistant had not reviewed the EHR, the clinic would have lost reimbursement because the claim would not have included all the CPT codes for the visit. Encounter forms should be updated annually to ensure that code additions, changes, and revisions are current.

USING THE ALPHABETIC INDEX

Procedural coding starts with identifying the main term and then locating it in the Alphabetic Index. Although the Alphabetic Index is a comprehensive, alphabetic listing of all main terms, there are no code descriptions. It is not effective to assign a CPT code simply by finding it through the Alphabetic Index. The Alphabetic Index is not a substitute for the Tabular List. Even if an individual is only looking for one code, the Tabular List must be used to ensure the code is accurate.

The Alphabetic Index is used as a guide to search for one or more codes or code ranges. The index is similar to that found in the back of any textbook; it is an alphabetic list of main and modifying terms found in the Tabular List of the coding manual. In a typical index, the term or concept listed in the index is followed by the page numbers on which detailed information is presented in the body of the book. The Alphabetic Index in the CPT coding manual is used in the same way, except that it provides codes or code ranges rather than page numbers. As discussed earlier, the Tabular List is divided into sections, and the procedures and services are listed in numeric order by the Category I code.

The Alphabetic Index is organized by main terms and modifying terms that are indented below the main term. Modifying terms further describe and add information needed to narrow the search for an appropriate procedure or service code. A main term can be a procedure, such as an excision. Each modifying term could provide further information such as:

- Anatomic location
- Organ excised
- Type of instrument used

Julie Walden, M.D.   David Kahn, M.D.
James Marin, M.D.   Jean Burke, N.P.
Angela Perez, M.D.

YOUR NAME CLINIC
Walden-Martin Family Medical Clinic,
1234 Anystreet, Anytown AK 12345
Phone: 123-123-1234   Fax: 123-123-5678

TELEPHONE:
FAX:

PATIENT'S NAME			CHART #			DATE		☐ MEDI-MEDI ☐ MEDICAL ☐ MEDICARE ☐ PRIVATE ☐ SELF PAY ☐ HMO _____

CPT/Md	DESCRIPTION	FEE	CPT/Md	DESCRIPTION	FEE	CPT/Md	DESCRIPTION	FEE	CPT/Md	DESCRIPTION	FEE
OFFICE VISIT—NEW PATIENT			**LAB STUDIES**			**PROCEDURES (continued)**			**INJECTIONS**		
99202	Focused Ex.		36415	Venipuncture		93235	Holter, 24 Hour		90724	Influenza	
99203	Detailed Ex.		81000	Urinalysis		10061	I & D Abscess Comp.		90732	Pneumococcal	
99204	Comprehensive Ex.		81003	—w/o Micro		10060	I & D Abscess Simple		J0295	Ampicillin, 1 gr	
99205	Complex Ex.		84703	HCG (Urine, Pregnancy)		94761	Oximetry w/Exercise		J0696	Rocephin	
OFFICE VISIT—ESTABLISHED PATIENT			82948	Glucose		93720	Plethysmography		J1030	Depo-Medrol 40 mg	
99212	Focused Ex.		82270	Hemoccult		94760	Pulse Oximetry		J2000	Lidocaine 50 cc	
99213	Expanded Ex.		85023	CBC-diff.		10003	Rem. Sebaceous Cyst		J2175	Demerol	
99214	Detailed Ex.		85024	CBC w/part diff		11100	Skin Bx		J3360	Valium 5 mg	
99215	Complex Ex.		85018	Hemoglobin		94010	Spirometry		J1885	Toradol 30 mg IV	
PREVENTATIVE MEDICINE—NEW PATIENT			88155	Pap Smear		92801	Visual Acuity		J1885	Toradol 60 mg IM	
99381	< 1 year old		87210	KOH/Saline Wet Mount		17100	Wart Removal		90720	DTP–HIB	
99382	1–4 year old		87430	Strep Antigen		17101	Wart Removal, 2nd		90746	HEP B—HIB	
99383	5–11 year old		87060	Throat Culture		17102	Wart Removal, 3–15		90707	MMR	
99384	12–17 year old		80009	Chem profile		11042	Wound Debrid.		86580	PPD	
99385	18–39 year old		80061	Lipid profile		**X-RAY**			86580	PPD w/control	
99386	40–64 year old		82465	Cholesterol		70210	Sinuses		90732	Pneumovax	
99387	65+ year old		99000	Handling fee		70360	Neck Soft Tissue		90716	Varicella	
PREVENTATIVE MEDICINE—ESTABLISHED PATIENT			**PROCEDURES**			71010	CXR (PA only)		82607	Vitamin B12 Inj.	
99391	< 1 year old		92551	Audiometry		71020	Chest 2V		90712	Polio	
99392	1–4 year old		29705	Cast Removal		72040	C-Spine 2V		90788	TD Adult	
99393	5–11 year old		2900	Casting (by location)		72100	Lumbosacral		95115	Allergy inj., single	
99394	12–17 year old		92567	Ear Check		73030	Shoulder 2V		95117	Allergy inj., multiple	
99395	18–39 year old		69210	Ear Wax Rem. 1 2		73070	Elbow 2V				
99396	40–64 year old		93000	EKG		73120	Hand 2V				
99397	65+ year old		93005	EKG tracing only		73560	Knee 2V				
			93010	EKG. Int. and Rep		73620	Foot 2V				
			11750	Excision Nail		74000	KUB				
			94375	Flow Volume							

DESCRIPTION	ICD-10-CM

____ Abdominal pain/unspec...... R10.9
____ Abscess............................ L02._
____ Allergic reaction................ T78.40_
____ Alzheimer's disease........... G30
____ Anemia/unspec................. D64.9
____ Angina/unspec.................. I20.9
____ Anorexia........................... R63.0
____ Anxiety/unspec.................. F41.9
____ Apnea, sleep..................... G47.30
____ Arrhythmia, cardiac........... I49.9
____ Arthritis, rheumatoid.......... M06.9
____ Asthma/unspec................. J45.909
____ Atrial fibrillation................ I48.0
____ B-12 deficiency................. E53.8
____ Back pain, low.................. M54.5
____ BPH................................. N40
____ Bradycardia/unspec.......... R00.1
____ Broncitis, acute................. J20._
____ Bronchitis, chronic............ J42
____ Bursitis/unspec................. M71.9
____ CA, breast........................ C50._
____ CA, lung........................... C34._
____ CA, prostate..................... C61
____ Cellulitis........................... L03._
____ Chest pain/unspec............ R07.9
____ Cirrhosis, liver/unspec....... K74.60
____ Cold, common.................. J00
____ Colitis/unspec................... K51.90
____ Confusion......................... R41.0
____ CHF.................................. I50.9
____ Constipation..................... K59.00
____ COPD............................... J44.9
____ Cough.............................. R05
____ Crohn's disease/unspec..... K50.90
____ CVA.................................. I63.9
____ Decubitus ulcer................. L89._
____ Dehydration...................... E86.0

____ Dementia/unspec............... F03
____ Depression, major/unsp...... F32.9
____ Diab I, no complications...... E10.0
____ Diab II, no complications..... E11.9
____   w/kidney complic........... E11.2_
____   w/ophthalmic compl...... E11.3_
____   w/neurolog compl.......... E11.4_
____   w/circulatory compl....... E11.5_
____ Insulin use........................ Z79.4
____ Diarrhea/unspec................ R19.7
____ Diverticulitis...................... K57.92
____ Diverticulosis.................... K57.90
____ Dizziness.......................... R42
____ Dysuria............................. R30.0
____ Edema/unspec................... R60.9
____ Endocarditis...................... I38
____ Esophageal reflux.............. K21.0
____ Fatigue (lethargy).............. R53.83
____ FUO.................................. R50.9
____ Gastritis............................ K29.70
____ Gastroenteritis (colitis)....... K52.9
____ G.I. bleed.......................... K92.2
____ Gout/unspec...................... M10.9
____ Headache.......................... R51
____ Health exam...................... 200.__
____ Hematuria/unspec.............. R31.9
____ Herpes simplex.................. B00.9
____ Herpes zoster.................... B02.9
____ Hiatal hernia...................... K44.9
____ HTN (HBP)......................... I10
____ Hyperlipidemia/unspec....... E78.5
____ Hypothyroidism/unspec....... E03.9
____ Impotence......................... N52._
____ Influenza, respiratory.......... J10.1
____ Insomnia........................... G47.0
____ IBS, diarrhea..................... K58.
____ Lupus, systemic erythim...... M32.9

____ MI, acute.......................... I21._
____ MI, old.............................. I25.2
____ Migraine........................... G43.9
____ Myalgia............................ M79.1
____ Neck pain......................... M54.2
____ Neuropathy....................... G62.9
____ Nausea............................. R11.1
____ Nausea/vomiting................ R11.0
____ Obesity/unspec................. E66.9
____ Osteoarthritis (site)............ M19._
____ Otitis media...................... H66.9_
____ Parkinson's disease........... G20
____ Pharyngitis, acute.............. J02.9
____ Pleurisy............................ R09.1
____ Pneumonia........................ J18.9
____ Pneumonia, viral................ J12.9
____ Prostatitis/unspec.............. N41.9
____ PVD.................................. I73.9
____ Radiculopathy................... M54.1_
____ Rectal bleeding................. K62.5
____ Renal failure..................... N19
____ Sciatica............................ M54.3_
____ Shortness of breath........... R03.02
____ Sinusitis, chr./unspec......... J32.9
____ Syncope............................ R55
____ Tachycardia/unspec........... R00.0
____ Tachy., supraventric........... I47.1
____ Tedinitis/unspec................ M77.9
____ TIA................................... G45.9
____ Ulcer, duodenal/unspec...... K26.9
____ Ulcer, gastric/unspec......... K25.9
____ Ulcer, peptic/unspec.......... K27.9
____ URI/unspec........................ J06.9
____ UTI................................... N39.0
____ Vertigo............................. R42
____ Weight gain...................... R63.5
____ Weight loss....................... R63.4

DIAGNOSIS: (IF NOT CHECKED ABOVE)		TODAY'S FEE	

PROCEDURES: (IF NOT CHECKED ABOVE)	RETURN APPOINTMENT INFORMATION:	REC'D BY: ☐ CASH ☐ CR. CARD ☐ CHECK # _____	AMT. REC'D.
	(DAYS)(WKS.)(MOS.)(PRN)		BALANCE

Fig. 29.4 Encounter Form. (From Niedzwiecki B, et al: *Kinn's the medical assistant,* ed 14, St. Louis, 2020, Elsevier.)

- Special technique
- Other procedures performed at the same time (e.g., obtaining biopsy tissue for examination)

Modifying terms affect the selection of appropriate codes; therefore it is important to review the list of modifying terms when selecting a code or code range.

Searching the Alphabetic Index

Begin the search of the Alphabetic Index by using one of the four primary classifications (or types) of main and modifying terms:

- Procedure or service (e.g., examination, excision, scope, revision, repair, drainage)
- Organ or anatomic site (e.g., clavicle, mandible, humerus, liver, colon, uterus)
- Condition, illness, or injury (e.g., ulcer, fracture, pregnancy, fever)
- Eponym, synonym, abbreviation, or acronym (e.g., Naffziger operation, MRI [magnetic resonance imaging], TURP [transurethral resection of the prostate])

When searching the Alphabetic Index, use:

- the name of the performed procedure or service (anastomosis, splint, repair, stress test, therapy, vaccination).
- the organ or other anatomic site of the procedure (tibia, colon, salivary gland, aorta).
- the condition, illness, or injury (abscess, fracture, cholelithiasis, strabismus).
- synonyms, eponyms, or abbreviations (ECG [electrocardiography], Stookey-Scarff procedure, Mohs' micrographic surgery).

Sometimes searching for a main term may not yield any results. When a main term cannot be found, search by another primary classification in the Alphabetic Index. Let us search the following procedural statement: Removal of Skin Tags on Neck. Begin by identifying the Main terms that closely match the four primary classifications in the Alphabetic Index:

1. Procedure or Service: Removal
2. Organ or Anatomic Site: Neck Skin
3. Condition, Illness, or Injury: Skin Tag
4. Eponym: None in this case

Once all possible main terms have been abstracted, the coder can quickly search through the Alphabetic Index for the code or code range that matches the procedural statement.

Using *See* and *See Also* in the Alphabetic Index

The *see* statement in the Alphabetic Index points to another location in the Alphabetic Index to find the code or code range. The *see also* statement points to additional codes or code ranges in the Alphabetic Index that may be useful to the code found in the original search.

Single Codes and Code Ranges

In the Alphabetic Index, a procedure or service may list a single code or a range of possible codes that may match the documentation. Remember that the Alphabetic Index is an index; it is designed as a guide to the most suitable codes that match the documentation. At this point, the search is only for the closest match or matches to the procedural statement.

Some medical procedures and diagnostic tests can be quite complex. There may be a single code or a code range that may include one main term but has several modifying terms for the main term. For example, the code for Acromioplasty has a range of codes: 23415–23420. The same main term, Acromioplasty, with a modifying term, partial, has a single code: 23130. The code range is shown with a hyphen to indicate that all codes within that range could be appropriate.

In some cases, a single code and a range of codes are listed for the same service or procedure. For example, Catheterization, femur, lists both the single code 27360 and the code range 27070–27071. Once a single code or code range has been found in the Alphabetic Index, the next step is to look up each of those in the Tabular List. Select the code or codes that most closely match the documentation (Box 29.1).

USING THE TABULAR LIST

Once the code or code ranges have been selected from the Alphabetic Index, the next stop is the Tabular List. This is where the procedural coding decision takes place. In the Tabular List, the conventions, symbols, guidelines, notes, and even the punctuation all play a part in choosing the most accurate code possible.

In the Tabular List, look up each code or code range found numerically in the Alphabetic Index. Read the description of each code thoroughly to ensure that the main terms abstracted from the procedural statement in the medical documentation are all included in the code description, with nothing substantial omitted or added. Read the section guidelines and notes to determine whether additional codes should be used, add-on codes or modifiers are required, or use of the code is contraindicated.

Use of the Semicolon

A semicolon (;) at the end of a main description indicates that modifying terms and descriptions follow. Every indented description below a stand-alone code is related to that stand-alone code. To get the full description for an indented code, you

BOX 29.2 Steps for Using the CPT Tabular List

Except for the special considerations required for coding from the Evaluation and Management (E/M) and Anesthesia sections, the following steps apply to all sections of the CPT manual.

1. Look up the code or code range from the Alphabetic Index Search in the Tabular List numerically.
2. Compare the description of the code with the procedural statement from the documentation. Verify that all or most of the health record documentation matches the code description and that there is no additional element or information in the code description that is not found in the documentation.
3. Read the guidelines and notes for the section, subsection, and code to ensure that there are no contraindications to the use of the code.
4. Evaluate the conventions, especially add-on codes (+) and exemption from modifier –51.
5. Determine whether any special circumstances require the use of a modifier or whether a special report is required.
6. Record the CPT code selected in the health record documentation next to the procedure or service performed and in the appropriate block of the insurance claim form.

TABLE 29.3 Commonly Used Place of Service (POS) Codes

Code	Name
01	Pharmacy
02	Telehealth
09	Prison/Correctional Facility
11	Office
12	Home
13	Assisted Living Facility
14	Group Home
15	Mobile Unit
17	Walk-In Retail Health Clinic
18	Place of Employment–Worksite
20	Urgent Care Facility
21	Inpatient Hospital
22	On Campus–Outpatient Hospital
23	Emergency Room–Hospital
24	Ambulatory Surgery Center
31	Skilled Nursing Facility
32	Nursing Facility
34	Hospice
51	Inpatient Psychiatric Facility
60	Mass Immunization Center
65	End-Stage Renal Disease Treatment Facility
71	Public Health Clinic
72	Rural Health Clinic
81	Independent Laboratory

use the description of the stand-alone code up to the semicolon and then include the description of the indented code. Let's look at excision of the spleen as an example. In the CPT manual you will see the following entry:

Hemic and Lymphatic Systems
Spleen
Excision
38100 Splenectomy; total (separate procedure)
38101 partial (separate procedure)
+38102 total, en bloc for extensive disease, in conjunction with other procedure (List in additional to code for primary procedure)

The description for code 38100 is a splenectomy, total. The description for code 38101 is splenectomy, partial. The description for code +38102 is splenectomy, total, en bloc for extensive disease, in conjunction with other procedure. If you were to use +38102, you would also have to have the code for the other procedure. You could not use just +38102 (Box 29.2).

For practice on CPT surgery coding, refer to Procedure 29.1.

COMMON CPT CODING GUIDELINES: EVALUATION AND MANAGEMENT SECTION

Evaluation and Management codes are commonly referred to as E/M codes. These codes are used to reflect what the provider does during the time spent with the patient. To properly code for that, the medical assistant must apply different techniques from the basic steps outlined earlier. Assigning the correct E/M code includes:

- Identifying the section, subsection, category, and subcategory for the procedure or service:
- Reviewing the reporting instructions and guidelines for the code chosen
- Reviewing the level of E/M service
  - Determining the extent of the history obtained and the examination performed
  - Determining the complexity of medical decision making

The E/M section is divided into broad subsections, such as office visit, emergency department visit, hospital visit, and consultation. These subsections are further divided into subcategories, which include the place where the services were rendered, such as:

- Provider's office
- Hospital emergency department
- Skilled nursing facility
- Patient's home
- Patient status
  - New
  - Established

Procedure 29.2, Part A, explains how to perform CPT coding for an office visit. The first two steps in choosing an E/M code are:

1. Identify the place of service (POS)
2. Identify the patient status (new or established)

Identifying the Place of Service

The POS is the healthcare facility where the provider delivered care to the patient. The two most common places of service are "office" and "hospital." Table 29.3 presents a list of common POS locations and their 2-digit identifying numbers, or POS codes.

Identifying the Patient Status

The patient status choices are "new" or "established" patient. A new patient (NP) is one who has not received any professional services from the provider, or from another provider of the exact same specialty and subspecialty who belongs to the same group practice, within the past 3 years.

An established patient (EP) is one who has received professional services from the provider, or from another provider of the exact same specialty and subspecialty who belongs to the same group practice, within the past 3 years.

An advanced practice nurse (APN) and physician assistant (PA) are considered the exact same specialty and subspecialty as the physician.

Once the POS and patient status have been established, the next step in selection of an E/M code is to determine the level of service provided.

Determining the Level of Service Provided for Office/Outpatient E/M Codes

The E/M level of service for office or other outpatient services is based on:
- Medical decision making
- Total time spent by provider

Although the history and physical examination have been eliminated as elements to determine the level of service, providers should perform and document a medically appropriate history and exam. The nature and extent of the history and/or examination are determined by the provider. The extent of the history and examination is no longer an element in selecting an E/M code. The medical decision making and time components are considered for deciding the level of service.

History and/or Examination. Office or other outpatient services include a medically appropriate history and/or physical examination, when performed. The nature and extent of the history and/or provider examination is determined by the provider. The care team may collect information, and the patient or caregiver may supply information directly (e.g., by portal or questionnaire) that is reviewed by the reporting provider or other qualified healthcare professional.

Medical Decision Making. When a provider makes medical decisions, the decisions are based on many years of education and experience. Three elements comprise the medical decision-making process:
1. The number and complexity of problems addressed
2. The amount and/or complexity of data obtained, reviewed, and analyzed
3. The risk of complications and/or morbidity and/or mortality of patient management

Number and Complexity of Problems Addressed. One element in the selection of the code level is the number and complexity of problems addressed at a visit. Multiple new and established problems may be addressed at the same time and may affect medical decision making. The provider's notes during the medically appropriate history and examination should help identify whether the patient's problem is minor, acute, stable, chronic with mild exacerbation, an undiagnosed new problem, or worsening. The level of the problems for medical decision making are:
- *Straightforward*: Self-limited or minor problem
- *Low complexity*: Stable, uncomplicated, single problem, acute uncomplicated illness/injury

- *Moderate complexity*: Multiple problems or significantly ill, undiagnosed problem with uncertain outcome
- *High complexity*: Acute or chronic illness or injury that is life- threatening or decision for hospitalization

Amount and/or Complexity of Data Reviewed and Analyzed. This data includes medical records, tests, and/or other information that must be obtained, ordered, reviewed, and analyzed for the encounter. This includes information obtained from multiple sources or interprofessional communications that are not separately reported. It includes interpretation of tests that are not separately reported. Ordering a test is included in the category of test result(s), and the review of the test result is part of the encounter and not a subsequent encounter. Data is divided into three categories:
1. Tests, documents, orders, or information from independent historian(s) (e.g., parent, guardian, caregiver)
2. Independent interpretation of tests
3. Discussion of management or test interpretation with outside physician or other qualified healthcare professional or appropriate source

Risk of Complications and/or Morbidity or Mortality of Patient Management. The risk of complications, morbidity, and/or mortality of patient management decisions made at the visit is associated with the patient's problem(s), the diagnostic procedure(s), and treatment(s). This includes the possible management options selected and those considered, after shared medical decision making with the patient and/or family. For example, a decision about hospitalization includes consideration of alternative levels of care. Examples may include a psychiatric patient with a sufficient degree of support in the outpatient setting or the decision to not hospitalize a patient with advanced dementia with an acute condition that would generally warrant inpatient care, but for whom the goal is palliative treatment.

Complexity Levels in Medical Decision Making. The complexity of medical decision making is categorized into four levels:
1. Straightforward
2. Low complexity
3. Moderate complexity
4. High complexity

Table 29.4 presents descriptions of the different levels of complexity of medical decision making.

Time. Time is included in the E/M code descriptions only to assist providers in selecting the most appropriate level of E/M service. Beginning with CPT 2021, and except for 99211, time alone may be used to select the appropriate code level for the office or other outpatient E/M services codes. Different categories of services use time differently. It is important to review the instructions for each category to assign the appropriate level. Total time includes face-to-face and non–face-to-face time personally spent by the provider on the day of the visit.

Activities that count for total time include:
- preparing to see the patient (e.g., review of tests).
- obtaining and/or reviewing separately obtained history.
- performing a medically appropriate examination and/or evaluation.

TABLE 29.4 Complexity of Medical Decision Making

Number of Diagnoses or Management Options	Amount and/or Complexity of Data to Be Reviewed	Risk of Complications and/or Morbidity or Mortality	Type of Medical Decision Making
Minimal	Minimal or none	Minimal	Straightforward
Low	Limited	Low	Low complexity
Moderate	Moderate	Moderate	Moderate complexity
High	Extensive	High	High complexity

- counseling and educating the patient/family/caregiver.
- ordering medications, tests, or procedures.
- referring and communicating with other healthcare professionals (when not separately reported).
- documenting clinical information in the electronic or other health record.
- independently interpreting results (not separately reported) and communicating results to the patient/family/caregiver.
- care coordination (not separately reported).

Providers will need to keep track of the total time in all of these activities on the day of the visit. In addition, the total time elements per code are:

New Patient
99202 – 15–29 minutes
99203 – 30–44 minutes
99204 – 45–59 minutes
99205 – 60–74 minutes

Established Patient
99212 – 10–19 minutes
99213 – 20–29 minutes
99214 – 30–39 minutes
99215 – 40–54 minutes

At first, E/M coding can be difficult to understand and put into practice. The E/M coding process provided here can serve as a guide to help medical assistants in determining:

- Place of service
- Patient status
- Level of care provided

You can then select the most accurate E/M code. Using the clinical examples in Appendix C of the CPT manual and comparing them to the medical documentation also can help medical assistants acquire a better understanding of E/M coding.

COMMON CPT CODING GUIDELINES: SURGICAL SECTION

Specific guidelines and notes related to surgery coding must be considered when assigning a CPT code. Always review the current year's guidelines for the Surgery section for the most up-to-date information. The following sections discuss a few of the more common guidelines. When you code procedures and services, be sure to read the guidelines and notes thoroughly for accurate coding assignment.

Surgical Package Definition

A *global period* is the time period from the start of the surgical procedure to a period of time after the procedure. During this time, patient prep, surgical care, and postsurgical care services are provided. A single CPT code is used for these global services. This is an example of *bundling codes* or combining two or more services together under one code. To prevent billing errors and fraud,

documentation in the patient's record must indicate all of the services in the bundle were performed. *Unbundling codes* means to use multiple CPT codes for parts of a procedure, instead of using a single, comprehensive CPT code. Unbundling codes is one of the most common coding errors and can lead to billing fraud.

The CPT code descriptions of global surgical services typically include:
- Local infiltration, digital block, and/or topical anesthesia
- After the decision for surgery, one related E/M encounter on the day of, or the day before, the date of the procedure
- Immediate postoperative care, including documentation in the patient's health record and talking with family and/or other physicians
- Writing orders for postsurgical care
- Evaluating the patient in the post anesthesia recovery area
- Typical postoperative follow-up care (includes care for approximately 6 to 8 weeks after surgery and is usually done at the provider's office)

Integumentary System – Excision of Lesions—Benign or Malignant

Excision of benign lesions includes a simple closure and anesthesia. If a wound (incision, excision, or traumatic lesion) requires intermediate or complex closure, the repair by intermediate or complex closure is coded and reported separately from the incision or excision. For example, if the provider excised a benign lesion measuring 1 cm from the patient's arm that required intermediate repair (closure), two codes would be used:
- 11401 – Excision, benign lesion including margins; excised diameter 0.6 to 1 cm
- 12031 – Repair, intermediate, wounds of scalp, axillae, trunk and/or extremities (excluding hands and feet); 2.5 cm or less

Levels of Closure (Repair).
- *Simple repair:* Performed when the wound is superficial (epidermis, dermis, or subcutaneous) without significant involvement of deeper structures. This includes local anesthesia and chemical or electrocauterization of wounds not closed.
- *Intermediate repair:* Includes simple repair with a need for a layered closure of one or more of the deeper layers of subcutaneous tissue and superficial fascia in addition to the skin closure. Single-layer closure of heavily contaminated wounds that required extensive cleaning or removal of particulate matter also constitutes an intermediate repair.
- *Complex repair:* Includes wounds that require more than layered closure (e.g., scar revision, extensive undermining, or stents or retention sutures). Necessary preparation includes creation of a limited defect for repairs or debridement of

complicated lacerations. Complex repair does not include excision of benign or malignant lesions, excisional preparation of a wound bed, or debridement, or the removal of damaged tissue or foreign objects from a wound, an open fracture, or an open dislocation.

VOCABULARY

debridement The surgical removal of dead, damaged, or infected tissue to improve the function of healthy tissue.

global services For purposes of CPT coding, medical services and procedures performed for the patient before, during, and after a surgical procedure that are included with the assigned CPT code.

Listing Services for Wound Repair.

- The repaired wound or wounds should be measured and recorded in centimeters; it also should be indicated whether the wound was curved, angular, or in a starlike pattern.
- When multiple wounds are repaired, add together the lengths of those in the same classification (simple, intermediate, or complex) and from all anatomic sites that are grouped together into the same code descriptor.
- When wounds of more than one classification are repaired, list the more complicated repair as the primary procedure and the less complicated repair as the secondary procedure, using modifier −59.
- Debridement is considered a separate procedure only when gross contamination requires prolonged cleansing; when a large amount of dead or contaminated tissue must be removed; or when debridement is carried out separately without immediate primary closure.
- Wound repair that involves nerves, blood vessels, and/or tendons should be reported under the appropriate system for repair of those structures. The repair of these associated wounds is included in the primary procedure unless it qualifies as a complex repair, in which case modifier −59 applies.

Musculoskeletal System

Fractures.

- *Closed fracture:* The fractured bone does not protrude through the dermis or epidermis.
- *Open fracture:* The fractured bone cuts through the skin layers and can be directly visualized.
- *Closed treatment:* The fracture site is not surgically opened. The three methods of closed treatment of fractures are:
  - Without manipulation
  - With manipulation
  - With or without traction
- *Manipulation:* Attempted reduction or restoration of a fracture or dislocated joint into its normal anatomic alignment by manually applied forces.
- *Open treatment:* Used when (1) the fractured bone is surgically opened or (2) an opening is made remote from the fracture site to insert an intramedullary nail across the fracture site.
- *Percutaneous skeletal fixation:* Fracture treatment that is neither open nor closed. The fracture fragments are not visualized, but a fixation device (e.g., pins) is placed across the fracture site, usually under x-ray imaging.

Maternity Care and Delivery

The services normally provided in uncomplicated maternity cases include antepartum care, delivery, and postpartum care.

- *Antepartum* care includes:
  - Initial and subsequent history
  - Physical examinations
  - Recording of weight, blood pressure, and fetal heart tones
  - Routine chemical urinalysis
  - Monthly visits up to 28 weeks' gestation
  - Biweekly visits to 36 weeks' gestation
  - Weekly visits until delivery

Any other visits or services provided within this period should be coded separately, including any routine tests (e.g., sonography, routine laboratory tests).

- *Delivery* includes:
  - Admission to the hospital, the admission history, and the physical examination
  - Management of uncomplicated labor
  - Vaginal delivery (with or without forceps or episiotomy), or cesarean delivery

Medical problems complicating labor and delivery should be identified by using the codes in the Medicine and E/M sections in addition to codes for maternity care.

- *Postpartum* care includes:
  - Hospital and office visits after vaginal or cesarean section delivery

COMMON CPT CODING GUIDELINES: PATHOLOGY AND LABORATORY SECTION

Assigning CPT codes for the Pathology section is the same procedure as for the Surgery section. For purposes of coding from the Laboratory section, organ or disease panels are groupings of numerous tests performed to diagnose the health or disease status of specific organ systems. A panel code can be used only if all the tests listed under the code selected were performed. These are considered *bundled codes* and must be billed under the single CPT code (Box 29.3). If they are not all present, the individual tests should be billed using a separate code for each. There are two types of drug testing, qualitative and quantitative. The codes for drug testing are *qualitative;* that is, they are based on the type of drug found. *Quantitative* assays, on the other hand, are performed to determine the amount of drug present.

HCPCS CODE SET AND MANUAL

Healthcare Common Procedure Coding System is a collection of codes and descriptions for procedures, supplies, products, and services not covered by or included in the CPT coding system. As are CPT codes, HCPCS codes are updated annually by

---

CRITICAL THINKING 29.4

Kaitlyn reviewed a coded medical record for a Basic Metabolic Panel with total Calcium that had listed specific CPT codes for each panel test. Is this the correct way to code for the organ panel? According to Box 29.3, how should this organ panel be coded?

the Centers for Medicare and Medicaid Services (CMS). These codes are designed to promote standardized reporting and collection of statistical data on medical supplies, products, services, and procedures.

HCPCS codes have 5 alphanumeric characters, beginning with one letter followed by 4 numbers. HCPCS uses coding conventions for special instructions relating to specific codes (Fig. 29.5). The modifiers for HCPCS are codes composed of 2 alphanumeric characters. The HCPCS modifiers do not change the description of the code, but rather provide additional information or describe extenuating circumstances. Like the CPT manual, the HCPCS manual is divided into an Alphabetic Index and a Tabular List. As with the CPT, procedures and services are looked up in the Alphabetic Index, and the code (or codes) is then confirmed as the most accurate and appropriate using the Tabular List. The HCPCS manual has no subsections, categories, or subcategories; it has only sections. An appendix contains all the HCPCS modifiers and their descriptions.

The coding steps for HCPCS are almost identical to those for CPT codes. Clinical documentation is the starting point for HCPCS coding. The final code selected should add nothing to or omit anything from the description in the medical documentation. The final step is determining whether the code selected can stand alone or requires a modifier to further define or add needed information.

Sometimes HCPCS codes are used along with CPT codes, especially in the medical office setting (Fig. 29.6). For example, a well-baby visit would include the E/M code for the patient visit and HCPCS codes for the administration of immunizations.

BOX 29.3 CPT Tabular List: Basic Metabolic Panel

80047 Basic Metabolic Panel (Calcium, Ionized)
This panel must include the following:
Calcium, ionized (82330)
Carbon dioxide (bicarbonate) (82374)
Chloride (82435)
Creatinine (82565)
Glucose (82947)
Potassium (84132)

The codes in parentheses after the individual tests are CPT codes. Those CPT codes would be used if not all of these tests were ordered at the same time.

Other Basic Metabolic Panel Components
Sodium (84295)
Urea Nitrogen (BUN) (84520)

Humidifiers/Compressors/Nebulizers for Use with Oxygen IPPB Equipment

E0550	Humidifier, durable for extensive supplemental humidification during IPPB treatments or oxygen delivery
E0555	Humidifier, durable, glass or autoclavable plastic bottle type, for use with regulator or flowmeter
E0560	Humidifier, durable for supplemental humidification during IPPB treatment or oxygen delivery
E0561	Humidifier, nonheated, used with positive airway pressure device
E0562	Humidifier, heated, used with positive airway pressure device
E0565	Compressor, air power source for equipment which is not self-contained or cylinder driven
E0570	Nebulizer, with compressor
E0571	Aerosol compressor, battery powered, for use with small volume nebulizer
E0572	Aerosol compressor, adjustable pressure, light duty for intermittent use
E0574	Ultrasonic/electronic aerosol generator with small volume nebulizer
E0575	Nebulizer, ultrasonic, large volume
E0580	Nebulizer, durable, glass or autoclavable plastic, bottle type, for use with regulator or flowmeter
E0585	Nebulizer, with compressor and heater

Fig. 29.6 Healthcare Common Procedure Coding System (HCPCS) Tabular List. (From Niedzwiecki B, et al: *Kinn's the medical assistant,* ed 14, St. Louis, 2020, Elsevier.)

▶ New. Additions to the previous edition.

⮌ Revised. Revisions with the line or code from the previous edition.

✓ Reinstated. A code that was previously deleted and has now been reactivated.

✪ Special coverage instructions. Indicates that there are instructions provided regarding circumstances in which the code might be included for reimbursement.

⦸ Not covered by or valid by Medicare. These codes might result in reimbursement by private health insurance payers but not by Medicare.

✳ Carrier discretion. The individual third-party payer must be contacted to find out if coverage is available.

X ~~Deleted~~ phrases that are removed this year

🅐 Code for a specific age

♀ Code for females

♂ Code for males

Fig. 29.5 Healthcare Common Procedure Coding System (HCPCS) Coding Conventions (from American Medical Association manual). (From Niedzwiecki B, et al: *Kinn's the medical assistant,* ed 14, St. Louis, 2020, Elsevier.)

Procedure 29.2, Part B, explains how to code an office visit involving immunizations.

COMMON HCPCS CODING GUIDELINES

Medical and Surgical Supplies

HCPCS codes for medical and surgical supplies, along with transportation, are A-codes. The HCPCS manual provides some figures that offer guidance as to what the medical and surgical supplies look like, so that they can be billed properly. Medical assistants can code only for surgical supplies purchased by the medical office. For example, pharmaceutical and medical equipment representatives can provide the medical office with some supplies that can be used for patient care. However, it is unethical to bill the patient's insurance company for supplies that were given to the provider for free. All medical and surgical supplies used during patient care should be documented on the encounter form in the patient's health record.

Durable Medical Equipment

HCPCS codes for durable medical equipment are E-codes. Examples of durable medical equipment include crutches, wheelchairs, walkers, and other products that assist patients with mobility. Some equipment is kept in the medical office inventory. If the practice purchases the medical equipment wholesale, it can bill patients and/or their insurance company for the retail value of the equipment. Just as with medical and surgical supplies, it is important for the provider to document the dispensing of durable medical equipment on the encounter form or health record (Procedure 29.3).

CLOSING COMMENTS

The CPT and HCPCS coding manuals are updated and published every year. The updated manuals should be ordered in the early fall so that they arrive in time for the medical assistant to review them. Always use the current year's manuals so that the codes are accurate. The Introduction in each manual discusses and highlights changes and/or new coding guidelines. Annual updates should be uploaded to reflect any coding changes in the encoder to ensure that all codes are up-to-date for the current year.

PATIENT-CENTERED CARE

It is important for anyone who does coding to be able to explain to patients what those codes mean. When statements are sent to patients, many call the healthcare facility and ask for an explanation of the charges. A common question is, "Why is the charge for my office visit so high?" By looking at the CPT E/M code, you can help patients understand that it is not just the face-to-face time that determines the level of an office visit. Most patients understand once all the criteria have been explained to them. Doing this with a pleasant attitude also will help with patient satisfaction.

BEING PROFESSIONAL

Two rules should be followed when you code any procedure or service:
1. Be as specific as possible in code selection and use all pertinent words in the description given in your documentation.
2. Never add or delete any words, modifying terms, or descriptors to the procedure or service code description that change the definition of the procedure or service or that are not documented.

Role-play this scenario with a peer: You are both medical assistants and perform coding. Your peer encourages you to modify descriptions, so the level of service is higher. Respond to your peer in a respectful, professional manner.

CHAPTER REVIEW

In this chapter, you have learned how to determine CPT and HCPCS codes. For both types of codes, the coding process starts with the Alphabetic Index. CPT Category I codes are made up of five numerals. Category II and Category III codes have a letter at the end of the code. You must first determine the main term for the procedure or service and then locate it in the Alphabetic Index. From there you will see a single code, multiple codes, or a code range. All codes must be verified in the Tabular List. Once in the Tabular List, you must look at all the coding conventions to make sure you have the most accurate code.

The Evaluation and Management codes in the CPT require some extra steps because you will need to determine the place of service and the patient status. Once those have been determined, you then need to look at all the codes available in that section, referring to the documentation in the health record if needed. To select the appropriate level of Office or Other Outpatient E/M Service, two components must be considered: medical decision making and the total time for E/M services performed on the date of the encounter.

Medical decision making includes establishing diagnoses, assessing the status of a condition, and/or selecting a management option. Medical decision making may be affected by the provider's role and management responsibility.

Excluding code 99211, time alone may also be used to select the appropriate code level for the office or other outpatient E/M services codes. Time may be used to select a code level in office or other outpatient services whether or not counseling and/or coordination of care dominates the service.

HCPCS codes are used for services and supplies that are not found in the CPT. These codes always start with a letter and are followed by four numerals. In a medical office, HCPCS codes are most often used for medical and surgical supplies and durable medical equipment.

Modifiers are used with both CPT and HCPCS codes to further explain the services provided, such as right or left side. These modifiers can be numeric or alphabetic.

SCENARIO WRAP-UP

Kaitlyn has learned that procedural coding using the CPT is similar in many ways to ICD-10-CM diagnostic coding. The two coding manuals have unique but also similar steps, conventions, and guidelines. She has learned that proper abstraction of procedural data from the health record is equally important for ICD-10-CM and CPT coding. Kaitlyn also has learned that HCPCS codes are used to describe procedures and services not found in the CPT, such as vaccinations, ambulance services, and durable medical equipment.

Kaitlyn uses documentation by the provider in the encounter form to identify the procedures performed. However, she realizes that she also must know how to use the CPT manual because some procedures or services must be coded from the documentation. As with diagnostic coding, Kaitlyn reviews the patient's health record documentation if any questions come up about a claim. She knows that coding to the highest level of specificity helps to ensure accuracy and enables the practice to obtain the maximum reimbursement allowed. She realizes the importance of keeping up-to-date with the CPT and HCPCS codes, so she plans to order the updated manuals every year. As Kaitlyn continues to learn procedural coding, she envisions herself becoming well rounded in her knowledge of the practice's administrative operations.

PROCEDURE 29.1 Perform Procedural Coding: Surgery

Task

To use the steps for CPT procedural coding to find the most accurate and specific CPT surgery code.

Equipment and Supplies

- CPT coding manual (current year) or TruCode encoder software
- Operative report (see Fig. 1)

Operative Report

PATIENT NAME: Sonia Sample
ROOM NUMBER: 222 West
MR NUMBER: 12-34-56

DATE OF PROCEDURE: 04/22/00
PREOPERATIVE DIAGNOSIS: Acute cholecystitis
POSTOPERATIVE DIAGNOSIS: Acute cholecystitis
NAME OF PROCEDURE: 1. Laparoscopic cholecystectomy
                         2. Intraoperative cystic duct cholangiogram
SURGEON: Claude St. John, M.D.
ASSISTANT: Mark Weiss, D.O.
ANESTHESIOLOGIST: Angela Adams, M.D.
ANESTHESIA: General

DESCRIPTION OF THE OPERATION:

The patient was placed in the supine position under general anesthesia. The oral gastric tube was placed. The Foley catheter was placed. The patient received appropriate antibiotics. The abdomen was prepped with iodine and draped in the usual fashion. Using a midline subumbilical incision, we entered the subcutaneous fat to find the aponeurosis of the rectus abdominis. Two stay sutures were placed 0.5 cm from the midline bilaterally, and we left on these sutures, creating an opening in the linea alba.

Under direct vision, the catheter was placed. The Hasson cannula was placed in the abdominal cavity, and all was normal except an acute necrotizing and probably gangrenous gallbladder. There were multiple omental adhesions. Three other trocars were placed in the right subcostal plane in the midline, midclavicular line, and midaxillary line using a #10, #5, and #5 mm trocar, respectively. The gallbladder was punctured and emptied of clear white bile indicating a hydrops of the gallbladder. It was grasped at its fundus and at Hartmann's pouch retracted cephalad and to the right, respectively. We found the cystic duct and the cystic artery after circumferential dissection and isolated the cystic duct completely.

When we were sure that this structure was a deep cystic duct, the clip was placed at the most distal aspect to make an opening immediately proximally, and we placed a Reddick cholangiocatheter into it via #14 gauge percutaneous catheter. The cholangiogram showed normal arborization of the liver radicals. Normal bifurcation of the common hepatic duct. Normal common hepatic duct. Long large cystic duct. The common bile duct had numerous stones within it. They could not be emptied from the common bile duct. There was good flow into the duodenum.

The impression was choledocholithiasis. This was corroborated by the radiologist. The decision was made to prepare the patient most probably for endoscopic retrograde cholangiopancreatography postoperatively, and no further intervention of the common bile duct was done in this setting.

The cholangiocatheter was removed. An attempt was made to milk the bile out, but no stones came out. Three clips were placed on the proximal aspect of the cystic duct and the duct was then cut distally. The artery was isolated and double clipped proximally and single clipped distally and cut in the intervening section. We then peeled the gallbladder off the gallbladder bed with some difficulty because of the intense edema and inflammation. It was then removed from the liver bed completely. Cautery, suctioning, and irrigation were used copiously to create a bloodless field. A last check was made, and there was no bleeding and no bile leaking. A #15 Jackson-Pratt type drain was placed into Morrison's pouch and brought out through the lateral most port. We then removed, with great difficulty, the gallbladder from the umbilicus. Because of its enormous size and a 3 cm stone within it that was very difficult to macerate, the opening of the umbilicus had to be enlarged.

As this was done, we removed the gallbladder completely and sent it for pathologic section. Two separate figure-of-eight 0 PDS were used to close the abdominal fascia. The Jackson-Pratt drain was then sutured in place with 2.0 nylon. The skin was closed throughout with subcuticular 3-0 PDS after copious irrigation of the subcutaneous plane. Mastisol and Steri-Strips were placed on the wound. The patient remained stable although she did have bigeminy during surgery and was on a Lidocaine drip. She will be going to the intensive care unit, but as she left, she was extubated in the recovery room and was fully alert. She is moving all limbs.

I will discuss with the gastroenterologist postoperative endoscopic retrograde cholangiopancreatography.

SPECIMEN: Gallbladder.

Claude St. John, M.D.
CSJ/ld:
D: 04/22/00
T: 04/22/00 9:21 am
CC: Maria Acosta, M.D.

1

Continued

Procedural Steps
Using the CPT Coding Manual

1. Abstract the procedures and/or services from the procedural statement in the surgical report.
2. Select the most appropriate main term to begin the search in the Alphabetic Index.
3. Once the main term has been located in the Alphabetic Index, review and select the modifying term or terms if required.

   Purpose: For additional specificity and to narrow the search for the most accurate CPT code or code range in the Alphabetic Index.
4. If the main term cannot be found in the Alphabetic Index, repeat steps 2 and 3 using a different main term possibly based on the procedural statement.
5. Once the CPT code or code range is identified in the Alphabetic Index, disregard any code or code range containing additional descriptions or modifying terms not found in the health record.
6. Record the code or code ranges that best match the procedural statements in the surgical report.

   Purpose: To prevent repeated reference to the Alphabetic Index by recording all possible matches to the code or code range sought. This saves time and prevents redundant effort.
7. Turn to the Tabular List and find the first code or code range from your search of the Alphabetic Index.

   Purpose: To begin the process of finding the most specific and accurate code.
8. Compare the description of the code with the procedural statement in the surgical report. Verify that all or most of the health record documentation matches the code description and that there is no additional information in the code description that is not found in the documentation.

9. Review the coding guidelines and notes for the section, subsection, and code to ensure that there are no contraindications to use of the code. Review the coding conventions and add-on codes, if any.

   Purpose: To ensure there are no instructions that would prevent the use of the code selected.
10. Determine whether a modifier is needed.

    Purpose: To select any appropriate modifiers that provide additional information for the chosen code to explain certain circumstances or provide additional detail.
11. Determine whether a Special Report is required.

    Purpose: To clarify and add additional detail when an unusual or extenuating circumstance exists or if a Category III or unlisted procedure Category I code is used.
12. Record the CPT code selected in the health record documentation next to the procedure or service performed and in the appropriate block of the insurance claim form.

    Purpose: To complete the documentation and recording requirements.

Using the TruCode Software

1. Abstract the procedures and/or services from the procedural statement in the surgical report.
2. Type the main term into the encoder search box and select the CPT. Then click on Show All Results.
3. If the main term cannot be found through the search, repeat steps 2 and 3 using a different main term based on the procedural statement.
4. Choose the procedure description that is closest to the procedural statement in the surgical report (see Fig. 2).

   Purpose: To prevent upcoding or downcoding errors or other possible fraud and/or abuse circumstances.

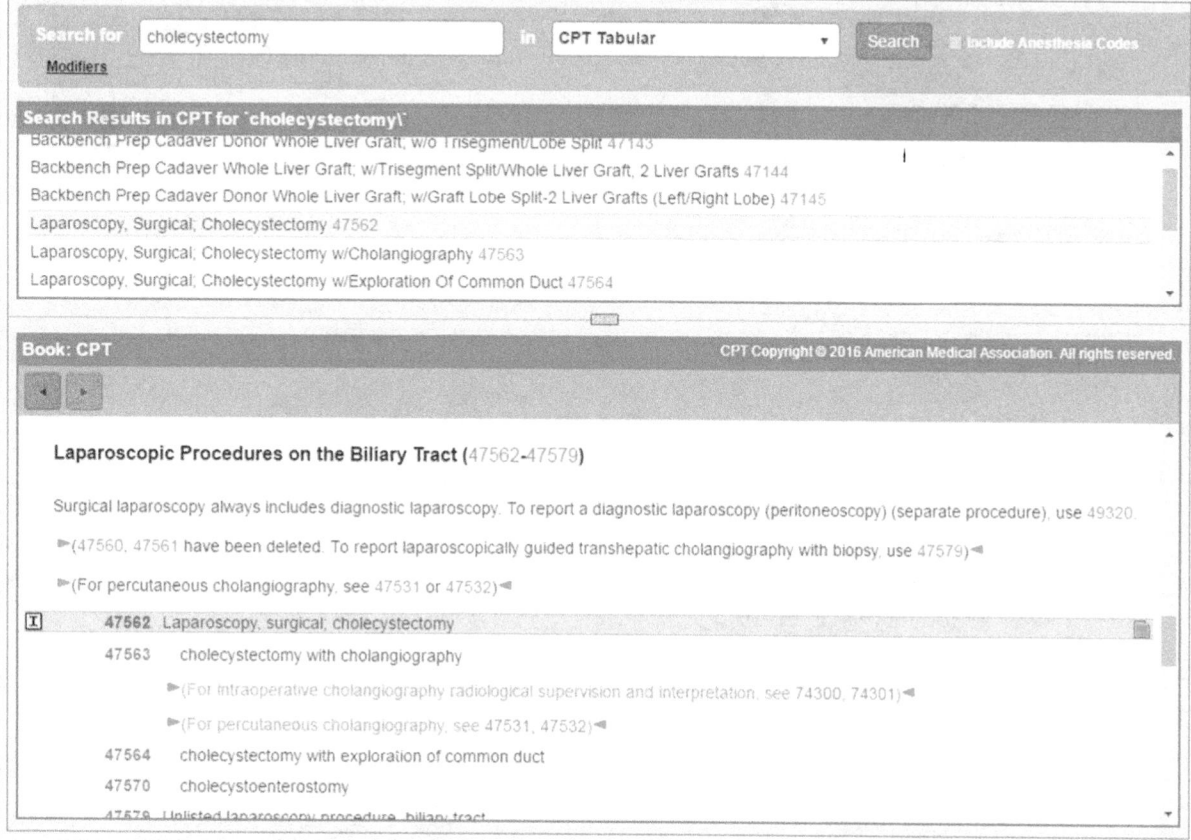

Search for cholecystectomy   in CPT Tabular   ▾   Search   ☑ Include Anesthesia Codes
Modifiers

Search Results in CPT for 'cholecystectomy'

Backbench Prep Cadaver Donor Whole Liver Graft; w/o Trisegment/Lobe Split 47143
Backbench Prep Cadaver Whole Liver Graft; w/Trisegment Split/Whole Liver Graft, 2 Liver Grafts 47144
Backbench Prep Cadaver Donor Whole Liver Graft; w/Graft Lobe Split-2 Liver Grafts (Left/Right Lobe) 47145
Laparoscopy, Surgical; Cholecystectomy 47562
Laparoscopy, Surgical; Cholecystectomy w/Cholangiography 47563
Laparoscopy, Surgical; Cholecystectomy w/Exploration Of Common Duct 47564

Book: CPT   CPT Copyright © 2016 American Medical Association. All rights reserved.

◀ ▶

Laparoscopic Procedures on the Biliary Tract (47562-47579)

Surgical laparoscopy always includes diagnostic laparoscopy. To report a diagnostic laparoscopy (peritoneoscopy) (separate procedure), use 49320.

►(47560, 47561 have been deleted. To report laparoscopically guided transhepatic cholangiography with biopsy, use 47579)◀

►(For percutaneous cholangiography, see 47531 or 47532)◀

[I] 47562 Laparoscopy, surgical; cholecystectomy
     47563   cholecystectomy with cholangiography
          ►(For intraoperative cholangiography radiological supervision and interpretation, see 74300, 74301)◀
          ►(For percutaneous cholangiography, see 47531, 47532)◀
     47564   cholecystectomy with exploration of common duct
     47570   cholecystoenterostomy
     47579 Unlisted laparoscopy procedure, biliary tract

5. Record the CPT code that best matches the procedural statements in the surgical report in the patient's health record.

   Purpose: To prevent repeated reference to the Alphabetic Index by recording all possible matches to the code or code range being sought. This saves time and prevents redundant effort.

PROCEDURE 29.2   Perform Procedural Coding: Office Visit and Immunizations

Task
To use the steps for CPT Evaluation and Management coding and HCPCS coding to find the most accurate and specific CPT E/M and HCPCS codes using the coding manuals or the TruCode encoder.

Equipment and Supplies
- CPT coding manual (current year)
- HCPCS coding manual (current year) or TruCode encoder software
- Progress note

Progress Note for Daniel Miller (DOB 03/12/20XX)
04/08/20XX Daniel was seen today for a follow-up visit for his recent case of otitis media in the left ear. The ear infection has completely cleared, and he is now able to receive his hepatitis B vaccine. The office visit involved a medically appropriate history and examination and straightforward medical decision making. Encounter was 15 minutes in length.

Procedural Steps
Part A: CPT E/M Coding
1. Determine the place of service from the progress note or encounter form.
   Purpose: To determine the most accurate CPT E/M code, the place of service needs to be identified.
2. Determine the patient's status.
   Purpose: To determine the most accurate CPT E/M code, the patient should be identified as new or established.
3. Identify the subsection, category, or subcategory of service in the E/M section.

Purpose: To ensure that the correct place of service and patient status is used and the appropriate level of service is selected.

4. Determine the level of service:
   - Complexity level in medical decision-making based on:
     - The number and complexity of problems addressed
     - The amount and/or complexity of data obtained, reviewed, and analyzed
     - The risk of significant complications and/or morbidity and/or mortality of patient management
   - Total time spent by provider
   Purpose: To ensure that the correct level of service is selected.
5. If necessary, compare the medical documentation against examples in Appendix C, Clinical Examples, of the CPT manual.
   Purpose: To help the coder select the appropriate level of service.
6. Select the appropriate level of E/M service code, and document it in the patient's health record.
   Purpose: To complete the documentation and reporting requirements.

Part B: HCPCS Coding With TruCode Encoder Software
7. Review the provider documentation.
   Purpose: To ensure that all procedures and/or services are listed on the encounter form; that all procedures and services on the encounter form match the health record; and that nothing documented in the health record is missing from the encounter form.
8. Type the main term into the Search box of the encoder and choose the HCPCS Tabular code set for accurate coding (see Fig. 1).

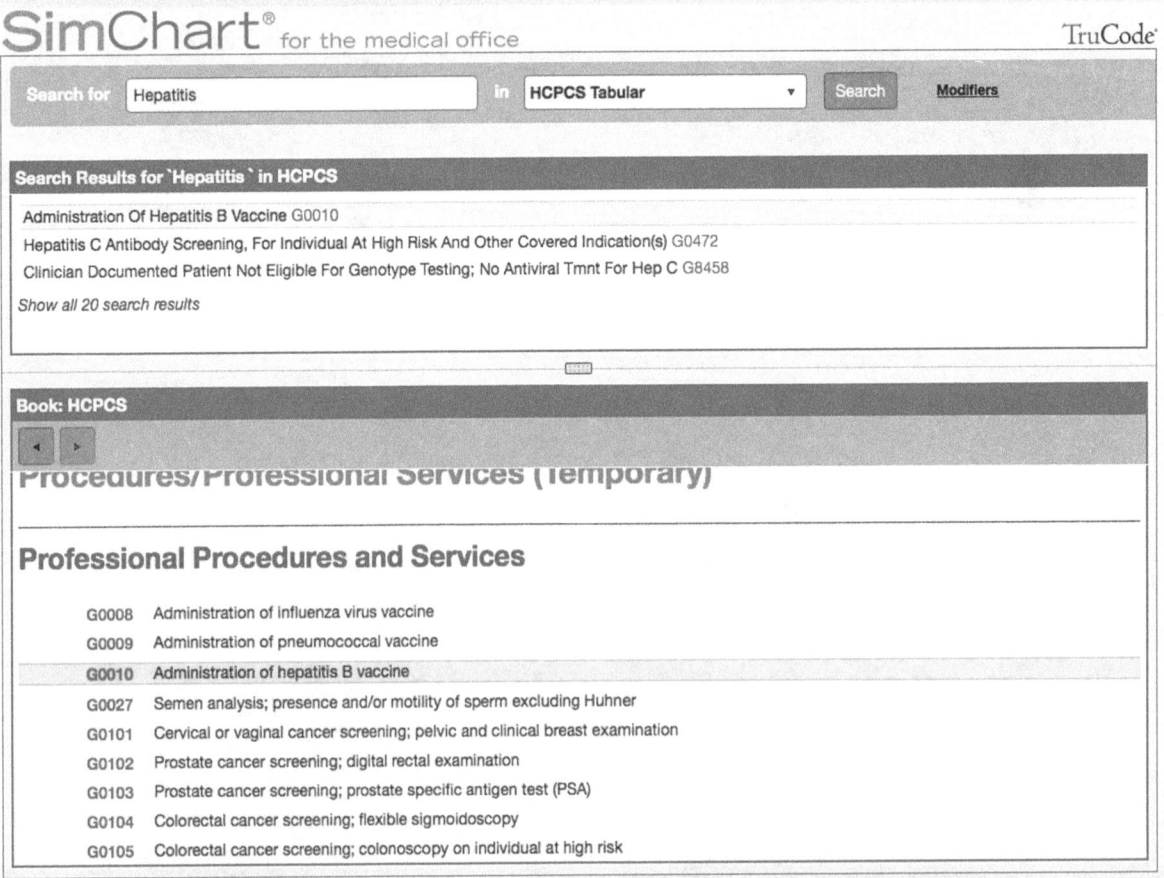

1

9. If no modifying term produces an appropriate code or code range, repeat steps 2 and 3 using a different main term.
   Purpose: To help find the most appropriate code or code range by using alternative methods of searching the Alphabetic Index.
10. Compare the description of the code with the medical documentation.

Purpose: To avoid upcoding and downcoding errors and to ensure there are no contraindications to use of the code selected.

11. Select the appropriate HCPCS immunization code and document it in the patient's health record.
    Purpose: To complete the documentation and reporting requirements.

PROCEDURE 29.3 Working With Providers to Ensure Accurate Code Selection

Task

Communicate respectfully and tactfully with medical providers to ensure accurate code selection.

Background

Using tactful communication skills means using good manners as you provide truthful sensitive information to another person, while considering the person's feelings. Tactful communication skills include verbal and nonverbal communication that shows respect, discretion, compassion, honesty, diplomacy, and courtesy. When you use tactful behaviors, you demonstrate professionalism, and you preserve relationships by avoiding conflicts and finding common ground.

Many times, the medical coder is the expert on the accurate CPT and ICD code selections. The highest level of specificity must be used when coding so that appropriate reimbursement can occur. It is not uncommon for the medical coder to interact with providers and assist them in understanding the coding process. During these interactions, it is crucial that the medical coder provides the information in a professional, organized, and logical manner. Using tactful communication skills is critical to maintaining a healthy working relationship with the providers.

Scenario

You are a new medical coder for the medical practice. You have been on the job for 6 weeks and have been seeing a trend that charges are being downcoded. The required documentation is present in the health records, but the providers have been selecting less specific codes for the appointment types. Your goal today is to explain to the providers accurate code selection for the appointment types.

Directions

Using the scenario, role-play with two peers, who will play the providers. You need to discuss the importance of selecting the correct code for reimbursement. You need to demonstrate respect during the conversation and utilize tactful communication skills.

30

Billing and Reimbursement

LEARNING OBJECTIVES

1. Identify the types of information contained in the patient's billing record.
2. Identify steps for filing a third-party claim.
3. Explain how to submit health insurance claims, including electronic claims, to various third-party payers.
4. Review the guidelines for completing the Centers for Medicare and Medicaid Services claim form, CMS-1500 Health Insurance Claim Form, and complete an insurance claim form.
5. Differentiate between fraud and abuse.
6. Discuss methods of preventing the rejection of claims and display tactful behavior when speaking with medical providers about third-party requirements.
7. Describe ways of checking a claim's status.
8. Review and read an Explanation of Benefits.
9. Discuss reasons for denied claims.
10. Define "medical necessity" as it applies to diagnostic and procedural coding and follow medical necessity guidelines.
11. Explain a patient's financial obligations for services rendered; also, inform a patient of these obligations, and show sensitivity when speaking with patients about third-party requirements.

OUTLINE

OPENING SCENARIO

Ann Snyder, a recent medical assisting graduate, has been hired to work in the billing office for Walden-Martin Family Medical (WMFM) Clinic. During her medical assistant program, her instructor, Grant Wilson, helped her realize that working with health insurance can be quite rewarding. Mr. Wilson worked with Ann and her classmates, answering their questions and helping them to see that medical insurance is not as complicated as it may seem.

Ann is detailed oriented, and she enjoys billing and coding activities. She understands that performing these duties in the provider's office is crucial because tasks related to billing have a significant effect on the healthcare facility. She also understands that income generated is used to pay the clinic's expenses, including payroll, so the facility's staff indirectly counts on accurate and timely billing. Medical assistants who continually develop their coding skills are assets to the practice and can look forward to a long and rewarding career.

Ann gained an understanding of the insurance process while in school. Mr. Wilson showed the students several different explanation of benefits forms (EOBs) from a variety of insurance companies so that the students could learn how the reimbursement process works for a variety of health insurance plans. Ann also learned about the importance of verifying patient billing information, in addition to the steps for obtaining precertification for medical procedures. She also learned how to discuss the patient's billing record professionally. Ann is looking forward to using all the skills she gained in school.

YOU WILL LEARN

1. The importance of collecting accurate billing information.
2. How to complete a CMS-1500 claim form.
3. How to prevent a rejection of the claim.
4. How to use the information found on an explanation of benefits.

INTRODUCTION

Medical billing and reimbursement represent the financial lifeline of the healthcare facility. Collecting accurate patient billing and health insurance information is essential to submitting accurate health insurance claims. Each health insurance company has its own claims submission policies and procedures for timely reimbursement. A successful medical assistant in insurance billing learns the insurance company requirements and submits accurate claims. Many health insurance companies have online provider web portals. This has made the process of checking the status of a claim quick and easy. The medical assistant also needs to be able look at a patient's insurance card and interpret the information found there, including copayment amounts. An explanation of benefits (EOB) from the insurance carrier will indicate the patient's deductible and/or

coinsurance. Clear communication with the patient about their financial responsibilities takes patience and sensitivity.

MEDICAL BILLING PROCESS

The medical billing process starts when a patient makes an appointment and is complete when payment has been received. The following steps are typically taken for medical billing.

1. Collect patient information when the patient calls to schedule an appointment. This includes information about the insured, their employer, demographic information, and health insurance data.
2. When the patient arrives for the appointment, you should:
   - make a copy or scan both sides of the patient's insurance card and government-issued ID card and
   - inform the patient of their copayment responsibility and collect it before services are provided.
3. Verify the patient's eligibility (EL i juh bill i tee), which is explained in Chapter 27.
4. Review patient benefits and exclusions for certain medical procedures and services.
   - If precertification is needed, contact the health insurance company to request it.
5. After services have been provided to the patient, code the diagnosis and procedures, and review the encounter form/superbill for completeness. The charges for the procedure or procedures should be provided automatically by the medical billing software.
6. Complete the CMS-1500 Health Insurance Claim Form (CMS-1500) or an electronic claim form. Submit the form to the insurance company. Electronic claim information may be submitted to a claims clearinghouse.
7. Review the electronic claims submission report to ensure that the claim was submitted accurately. The claims clearinghouse or payer may reject the claim. A *rejected claim* usually contains errors that were identified before the claim was processed by the payer. Discrepancies should be corrected, and the claim should be resubmitted.
8. Meet the timely filing requirements of each of the different health insurance carriers. Health insurance companies do not pay claims submitted after the established filing period, and this balance cannot be billed to the patient.
9. Post payments in the patient's account using the EOB to identify the line items that were paid, reduced, or denied. Patient account statements for the person's financial responsibility should be mailed out. Health insurance claims for patient accounts with secondary insurance should be submitted to the secondary carrier.

CRITICAL THINKING 30.1

The medical billing manager informs Ann that she has noticed an increase in the number of insurance claim rejections that state the patient cannot be identified. Which step of the medical billing process might be addressed to resolve this problem?

TYPES OF INFORMATION FOUND IN THE PATIENT'S BILLING RECORD

The claim submission process begins after the patient receives services from the provider. When a patient makes a first appointment, it is routine to ask the patient for insurance billing information. Much of this information is collected on the patient information form (Fig. 30.1). This form can be sent to the patient ahead of time or completed when the patient comes to the medical office for the first visit. This form should always be completed for every new patient. For established patients, demographic and insurance information should be verified.

Besides collecting accurate billing information, a medical release of information form must also be completed by the patient or guardian. HIPAA does not require the medical release of information form for payment, but the claim form does require a signed and dated medical release of information form to be in the patient's health record.

MANAGED CARE POLICIES AND PROCEDURES

Medical billers should be familiar with procedures commonly used by managed care organizations (MCOs), such as precertification. If the procedures are not followed, the MCO might not pay for the services. For example, pain management services typically require a preauthorization. If a pain management facility were to provide these services to the patient without preauthorization, the MCO could deny all insurance claims. To submit accurate health insurance claims, medical assistants should follow office procedures for applying MCO policies and procedures (Procedure 30.1). Box 30.1 presents more about training offered by MCOs for medical billing purposes.

SUBMITTING CLAIMS TO THIRD-PARTY PAYERS

All health insurance companies accept:
- CMS-1500 as the standard claim form
- ICD-10-CM for diagnostic codes
- Current Procedural Terminology (CPT) and Healthcare Common Procedure Coding System (HCPCS) codes

However, each health insurance company has its own policies and procedures for the submission of claims.

Guidelines for Medicare and Medicaid claims can be found on the administrator websites for each state. MCO plans associated with capitation agreements have specific guidelines on the types of medical services that are billable. Private health insurance plans have their own policies and procedures for submitting claims. The medical assistant should research the health plans commonly seen in the healthcare facility.

The medical assistant can successfully manage the requirements of the different insurance plans by keeping a medical billing manual. The manual should contain the billing policies and procedures for the most common third-party payers. The person in charge of the manual should make sure that every medical biller has a copy and that the policies and procedures are up to date. For example, Medicare's billing procedures and policies are updated on October 1. Whenever an update is released, the medical billing manual also should be updated.

GENERATING ELECTRONIC CLAIMS

Since 2006 Medicare has required that claims be sent electronically. Most health insurance plans have followed suit. If the majority of claims are submitted electronically, why is it important to learn the different fields of the CMS-1500 paper form? The data used to submit electronic claims is the same data used on the CMS-1500. A medical assistant who is familiar with a paper CMS-1500 will have no problem collecting the proper data for an electronic claim.

Electronic claims are insurance claims that are transmitted over the internet from the provider to the health insurance company through *electronic data interchange*. Electronic data interchange is the electronic transfer of data between two or more entities. When submitting electronic claims, a healthcare facility transmits the data for the claim, and the health insurance company accepts it. Most medical billing software is designed to generate electronic claims.

As with paper claims, when electronic claims are submitted, accurate data is essential. When the medical assistant reviews the claim for accuracy, the claim is prepared for submission.

WALDEN-MARTIN
FAMILY MEDICAL CLINIC
1234 ANYSTREET | ANYTOWN, ANYSTATE 12345
PHONE 123-123-1234 | FAX 123-123-5678

Patient Information

Patient Information (Please use full legal name.)

Last Name: _Tapia_   Address 1: _12 Highland Court_
First Name: _Celia_   Address 2: _Apt 101_
Middle Initial: _B_   City: _Anytown_
Medical Record Number: _11012373_   Country: _United States_   State/Province: _AL_
Date of Birth: _05/18/1970_   Zip: _12345-1234_
Age: _42_   Email: _—_
Sex: _Female_   Home Phone: _123-858-1545_
SSN: _857-62-1594_   Driver's License: _—_
Emergency Contact Name: _Arnold Tapia_   Emergency Contact Phone: _123-200-5006_

Guarantor Information (Please use full legal name.)

Relationship of Guarantor to Patient: _Spouse_
Guarantor/Account #: _Tapia, Arnold / 12088787_
Account Number: _12088787_
Last Name: _Tapia_   Address 1: _12 Highland Court_
First Name: _Arnold_   Address 2: _Apt 101_
Middle Initial: _—_   City: _Anytown_
Date of Birth: _05/18/1970_   Country: _United States_   State/Province: _AL_
Age: _42_   Zip: _12345-1234_
Sex: _Male_   Email: _—_
SSN: _812-93-1341_   Home Phone: _123-858-1545_
Employer Name: _Anytown String Shop_   Cell Phone: _—_
School Name: _—_   Work Phone: _—_

Provider Information

Primary Provider: _James A. Martin, MD_   Provider's Address 1: _1234 Anystreet_
Referring Provider: _—_   Provider's Address 2: _—_
Date of Last Visit: _August 28, 2013_   City: _Anytown_
Phone: _123-123-1234_   Country: _United States_   State/Province: _AL_
                                                Zip: _12345-1234_

Insurance Information (If the patient is not the Insured party, please include date of birth for claims.)

Insurance: _Aetna_   Claims Address 1: _1234 Insurance Way_
Name of Policy Holder: _Arnold Tapia_   Claims Address 2: _—_
SSN: _812-93-1341_   City: _Anytown_
Policy/ID Number: _CT5487854_   Country: _United States_   State/Province: _AL_
Group Number: _41554T_   Zip: _12345-1234_
                                                Claims Phone: _180-012-3222_

Secondary Insurance

Insurance: _—_   Claims Address 1: _—_
Name of Policy Holder: _—_   Claims Address 2: _—_
SSN: _—_   City: _—_
Policy/ID Number: _—_   Country: _—_   State/Province: _—_
Group Number: _—_   Zip: _—_
                                                Claims Phone: _—_

"I hereby authorize direct payment of all insurance benfits otherwise payable to me for services rendered. I understand that I am financially responsible for all charges not covered by insurance for services rendered on my behalf to my dependents. I authorize the above prociders to release any information required to secure payment of benefits. I authorize the use of this signature on all insurace submissions."

Signature: _Celia Japia_   Date: _05/06/20XX_

Fig. 30.1 Completed Patient Information Form.

Electronic Claims Submission

Electronic claims are submitted in the 5010-format established by the Health Insurance Portability and Accountability Act (HIPAA) and can be directly transmitted to the insurance carrier or to a claims clearinghouse.

Direct Billing. Direct billing is the process by which an insurance company allows a provider to electronically submit claims directly to the company. Most major insurance companies, including Medicare and Medicaid, provide software packages that are used to enter the patient's and insured's information, charges, and the provider's details.

Many carrier-direct systems are supplied free of charge to the provider, but the direct system can transmit only to specific carriers. If most claims for the healthcare facility are submitted to just one insurance company, direct billing would be a good way to submit claims.

Clearinghouse Submissions. A claims clearinghouse is an organization that acts as a go-between for the healthcare facility and the insurance company. The clearinghouse:

- accepts electronically submitted claims information from healthcare agencies.
- audits the claims for completeness.
- reformats claims to meet the insurance companies' specifications.

The claims are sorted by insurance plans and sent in batches electronically to the appropriate companies. The insurance companies then send a report through the data clearinghouse to:

- confirm the receipt of claims.
- report the status of previously submitted claims.
- serve as claim payment notification.

A clearinghouse charges the healthcare facility a small fee for:

- sending and receiving claims transmissions.
- checking and preparing the claims for processing.
- consolidating claims so that one transmission can be sent to each carrier.
- submitting claims in correct data format to the appropriate insurance payer.

A typical fee is 25¢ per submitted claim. Other services that clearinghouses typically provide include:

- Reporting the number of claims submitted, and the number of errors and their specifics
- Forwarding claims to insurance carriers that accept electronic claims (e.g., Medicare, Medicaid, Blue Cross/Blue Shield, and others) or to another clearinghouse that may hold the contracts with specific payers
- Keeping provider offices updated as new carriers are added to the database
- Generating informative statistical reports

> **VOCABULARY**
> **audit** A process completed before claims submission in which claims are examined for accuracy and completeness.

COMPLETING THE CMS-1500 HEALTH INSURANCE CLAIM FORM

The CMS-1500 Health Insurance Claim Form is the form required by HIPAA for paper claim submission. The form has 33 blocks. These blocks are divided into three sections:

- *Section 1: Carrier.* The first section indicates the type of insurance plan to which the claim is being submitted; this section includes only Block 1.
- *Section 2: Patient and Insured Information.* The second section contains information about the patient and the insured; it includes Blocks 1a through 13.
- *Section 3: Physician or Supplier Information.* The third section contains information about the provider or supplier; it includes Blocks 14 through 33.

Table 30.1 presents a summary of the information needed to complete the CMS-1500 accurately.

Section 1: Carrier – Block 1

Block 1 (Fig. 30.2) shows the type of insurance the patient has. Indicate the type of health insurance coverage for this claim by putting an X in the appropriate box, marking only one box. This information directs the claim to the correct payer.

Section 2: Patient and Insured Information – Blocks 1a Through 13

The CMS-1500 distinguishes between the patient and the insured. The insured is the individual who is directly contracted with the insurance company. For example, if an insurance claim for Sabrina Rudman is submitted and Blue Cross covers her through her employer, she is both the patient and the insured. However, if the insurance claim is for Chris Rudman, her son, Sabrina Rudman is the insured, and Chris Rudman, her dependent, is the patient. Every CMS-1500 requires the name, sex, and birth date of both the insured and the patient, even if they are different individuals. The blocks in Fig. 30.3 highlighted in yellow are for the patient's information, and the blocks highlighted in blue are for the insured's information.

TABLE 30.1 Information Required for Completion of the CMS-1500 Health Insurance Claim Form

Block	Information Needed	Block	Information Needed
	Completed patient registration/intake form	17b	Ordering or referring provider's NPI
	Photocopy of insurance card or cards (front and back)	18	From–To dates if patient encounter included an inpatient hospital stay
	Encounter form	19	Determine whether insurance carrier in Carrier block and Block 1 requires any information to be entered in this field
	Preauthorization or precertification number (when applicable)		
Section 1: Carrier		20	Determine whether an outside laboratory was used; if so, enter charges billed to provider for outside lab services
1	Type of insurance		
		21	ICD-10-CM code or codes for patient's condition, illness, or injury (maximum of four per claim)
Section 2: Patient and Insured Information			
1a	Insured's identification (ID) number (primary insurance)	22	Is Medicaid claim being resubmitted? If yes, provide reference number from original Medicaid claim submitted
2	Patient's full name		
3	Patient's date of birth and sex	23	If prior authorization and/or referral is required, provide authorization (approval) number from insurance payer (preauthorization or precertification number)
4	Insured's name (primary insurance)		
5	Patient's address and telephone number		
	• Permanent address (including apartment number if appropriate)	24A	From–To dates of service for current encounter
	• City, state, ZIP code	24B	Place of service (POS) code
	• Telephone number	24C	If an emergency, put a Y in this box
6	Patient's relationship to insured	24D	CPT and/or HCPCS code
7	Insured's address and telephone number		CPT and/or HCPCS modifier(s) (maximum of four per charge line)
	• Permanent address (including apartment number if appropriate)	24E	Block 21 field or reference number (1, 2, 3, and/or 4)
	• City, state, ZIP code	24F	Total charge for CPT- or HCPCS-coded services listed in Block 24D
	• Telephone number		• If more than 1 day or unit is indicated in Block 24G, multiply the charge for the service(s) coded in Block 24D by the number of days/units in Block 24G; enter the result in Block 24F
9	Other insured's name (secondary insurance)[a]		
9a	Policy or group number (secondary insurance)[a]		
9b	Secondary insured's date of birth and sex[a]		
9c	Secondary insured's employer or school name[a]	24G	Total number of days or units
9d	Secondary insured's insurance plan or program name[a]	24H	EPSDT or Family Plan code (Medicaid or AFDC)
10 a–c	If patient's condition or illness is related to employment, auto accident, or some other type of accident, make sure information is obtained as outlined in Block 1	24I	Qualifier ID code (if no NPI available)
		24J	Rendering (treating) provider's NPI – unshaded field
			PIN (if no NPI is available) – shaded field
10d	Claim codes as designated by NUCC	25	Rendering provider's federal tax ID number (EIN or SSN)
11	Insured's policy, group, or FECA number (primary insurance)	26	Patient's account number with rendering provider
11a	Primary insured's date of birth and sex	27	Determine whether contract or agreement between provider and insurance carrier allows provider to accept assignment
11b	Other claim ID designated by NUCC		
11c	Primary insured's insurance plan or program name	28	Total charges from Block 24F, lines 1–6
11d	Determine whether the patient also is covered by a secondary health insurance plan	29	Amount paid by patient, insured, or other insurance
		30	Balance due (if any amount paid is shown in Block 29)
12	Confirm that the patient's release of information form has been signed, dated, and is in the patient's record	31	Signature of provider performing service or procedure
		32	Address of facility where services were rendered
13	Confirm that the insured's authorization of benefits form has been signed, dated, and is in the patient's record	32a	NPI number of service facility listed in Block 32
		32b	Qualifier ID number and PIN of facility listed in Block 32 (if no NPI available)
Section 3: Physician or Supplier Information		33	Name, address, and phone number of performing (rendering) provider
14	Date of current illness, injury, or pregnancy (LMP)		
15	Determine whether patient has had the same or similar symptoms	33a	NPI of provider listed in Block 33
16	From–To dates if patient was unable to work at current occupation	33b	Qualifier ID number and PIN of provider listed in Block 33 (if no NPI available)
17	Name of ordering or referring provider		
17a	Not required		

[a]Only required if a secondary insurance exists and is to be submitted to the insurance carrier.

AFDC, Aid to Families with Dependent Children; *CPT*, Current Procedural Terminology coding system; *EIN*, Employer Identification Number; *EPSDT*, Early and Periodic Screening, Diagnosis, and Treatment; *FECA*, Federal Employees Compensation Act; *HCPCS*, Health Care Common Procedural Coding System coding method; *ICD-10-CM*, International Classification of Diseases, Tenth Revision, Clinical Modification coding method; *NPI*, National Provider Identifier; *NUCC*, National Uniform Claim Committee; *PIN*, personal identification number; *POS*, place of service; *SSN*, Social Security number; *TANF*, Temporary Assistance for Needy Families.

HEALTH INSURANCE CLAIM FORM

APPROVED BY NATIONAL UNIFORM CLAIM COMMITTEE (NUCC) 02/12

	PICA								PICA	

1. MEDICARE	MEDICAID	TRICARE CHAMPUS	CHAMPVA	GROUP HEALTH PLAN	FECA BLK LUNG	OTHER
☐ (Medicare #)	☐ (Medicaid #)	☐ (Sponsor's SSN)	☐ (Member ID#)	☐ (SSN or ID)	☐ (SSN)	☐ (ID)

Fig. 30.2 Section 1 Carrier (Block 1).

Fig. 30.3 Section 2: Patient and Insured Information (Blocks 1A To 13).

Blocks 1a, 4, 7, and 11 a–d. Information required for the insured includes:

- Patient's health plan ID number
- Name
- Address
- Policy and group numbers
- Birth date (MM/DD/YYYY) and sex
- Employer's name (if applicable)
- Name of the insurance plan
- Whether the insured has another health benefit plan

Blocks 2, 3, 5, 6, and 10 a–c. Required information for the patient includes:

- Patient's name
- Birth date (MM/DD/YYYY) and sex
- Address
- Relationship to the insured
- Patient's status
- Whether the patient's condition is related to their job, an automobile accident, or some other accident

Block 9. Block 9 is for recording information about any secondary insurance plan that may be applicable. The data required includes:

- Other insured person's name
- Policy or group number
- Name of the other insurance plan

When a patient is covered by more than one insurance policy, it is important to determine which policy is considered primary. The primary insurance pays the claim first, and if there is anything left over, it is submitted to the secondary insurance company. One of the most common situations is a patient with coverage under two policies, such as a dependent whose parents each have family coverage through employer group insurance.

In the case of a child whose mother and father both carry the child as a dependent on their employer health insurance plans, primary and secondary insurance status is determined by the *birthday rule*. Whichever parent's birth date falls first in a calendar year is considered to have the primary insurance. The year of the parent's birth is not used. If the mother's birth date is February 20 and the father's birth date is May 1, the mother's insurance is the primary insurance and the father's insurance is the secondary insurance. This means the claim will be submitted to the mother's insurance first, and if there is any balance left, it will be submitted to the father's insurance.

Medicare is usually the primary insurance, and there is a secondary policy to cover the patient's responsibility. In some cases, however, Medicare can be the patient's secondary insurance. This typically happens when a Medicare patient is still covered under an employer-sponsored group policy because the patient works full time.

Medicaid is always the payer of last resort. That means if there is any other type of insurance coverage for the patient, that insurance is responsible for the claim. If there is any balance left over, it will be submitted to Medicaid.

Blocks 12 and 13. Block 12 requires the signature of the *patient* or an authorized person, and Block 13 requires the signature of the *insured* or an authorized person. In Block 12, the signature authorizes the release of any medical or other information necessary to process or adjudicate (uh JOO di keyt) the claim. In Block 13, the signature affirms that the insured has a signature on file authorizing payment of medical benefits directly to the provider (whose name appears in Block 31). The phrase "Signature on File" or "SOF" may be entered in these fields (Box 30.2).

> **VOCABULARY**
> **adjudicate** To settle or determine judicially.

Section 3: Physician or Supplier Information – Blocks 14 Through 33 (Fig. 30.4)

Block 14 – Date of Current Illness, Injury, or Pregnancy (LMP). Block 14 requires the date of the current illness, injury, or pregnancy (LMP). The date should be the date on which the current illness or condition began; the date an injury occurred;

or, in the case of pregnancy, the date of the last menstrual period (LMP), all in MM/DD/YYYY format.

Block 15 – Other Date. This block is used for another date related to the patient's condition or treatment. Enter the applicable qualifier to identify which date is being reported. Qualifiers include:

- 454 Initial Treatment
- 304 Latest Visit or Consultation
- 455 Last X-ray
- 471 Prescription
- 090 Report Start (Assumed Care Date)
- 091 Report End (Relinquished Care Date)
- 444 First Visit or Consultation
- 439 Accident
- 453 Acute Manifestation of a Chronic Condition

Block 16 – Dates Patient Unable to Work in Current Occupation. These dates are used to help determine an employee's long- or short-term disability payments.

Block 17 and 17b – Name of Referring Provider or Other Source. Block 17 is for the name of the provider who referred or ordered the services or supplies. The following qualifier can be added:

- DN Referring Provider
- DK Ordering Provider
- DQ Supervising Provider

The providers' National Provider Identifier (NPI) is entered in Block 17b. Government insurance claims require that NPIs

> ### BOX 30.2 Assignment of Benefits
>
> In the health insurance contract between the third-party payer and the patient, the patient receives the payment when a claim is submitted. For the healthcare facility to receive the reimbursement directly from the insurance company, the patient must sign an *assignment of benefits*. The assignment of benefits transfers the patient's legal right to collect benefits for medical expenses to the provider of those services, authorizing the payment to be sent directly to the provider. In other words, the assignment of benefits authorizes the provider to not only submit the insurance claim on behalf of the patient, but also to be reimbursed directly by the third-party payer. There is usually a statement about the assignment of benefits on the patient information form. When the patient has signed the assignment of benefits, the medical assistant completes Blocks 12 and 13 on the CMS-1500 form with the statement "Signature on File" or "SOF" and the claim filing date.

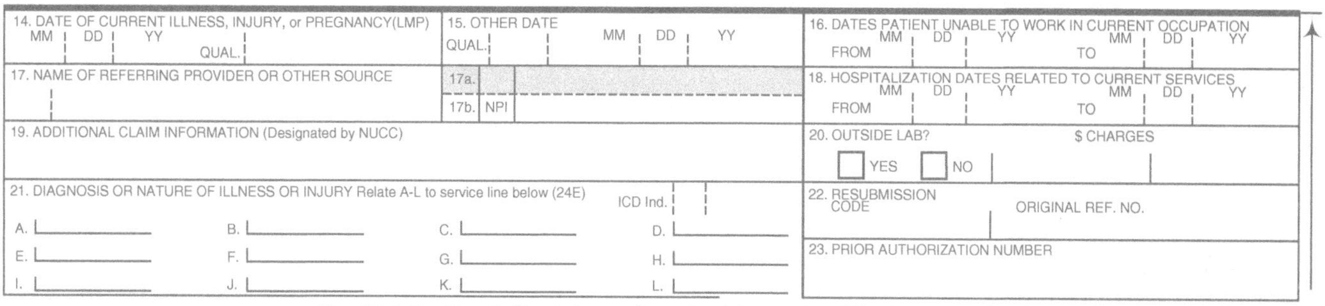

Fig. 30.4 Section 3: Physician or Supplier Information (Blocks 14 to 23).

be used for the referring providers (Block 17b) and rendering providers (Block 24J). Every healthcare entity is required to have an NPI. The NPI is an identifier assigned by the CMS that classifies the healthcare provider by license and medical specialty. The Administrative Simplification provisions of HIPAA required the adoption of standard unique identifiers for healthcare providers and health plans. The purpose is to improve the efficiency of electronic transmission of health information.

Some private insurance companies may require claims to be submitted with the NPI. However, each privately sponsored insurance plan in each state has its own policies and procedures. Medical assistants will find that some third-party payers require NPIs and others do not.

> **VOCABULARY**
> **National Provider Identifier (NPI)** An identifier assigned by the CMS that classifies the healthcare provider by license and medical specialties.

Block 18 – Hospitalization Dates Related to Current Services. If inpatient services are provided, the admission and discharge dates are entered here.

Block 19 – Additional Claim Information. Additional claim information (designated by the National Uniform Claim Committee [NUCC]) is found in Block 19. Some insurance plans ask for specific identifiers in Block 19. The medical assistant should check the instructions from the applicable third-party payer.

Block 20 – Outside Lab Charges. This block applies to diagnostic laboratory services purchased from an independent or a separate provider (who is listed in Block 32). Put an X in the YES box to indicate that the diagnostic test was performed by an entity other than the provider billing for the service (i.e., the provider listed in Block 33), and that the provider in Block 33 paid the laboratory directly. Include the amount the provider was charged by the diagnostic laboratory.

Block 21 – Diagnosis or Nature of Illness or Injury. The ICD-10-CM diagnosis code or codes are entered. Up to 12 diagnostic codes can be entered here. The primary diagnosis should be recorded in the first field. Do not include the decimal point in the diagnosis code. Relate lines A to L to lines of service in Block 24E by the letter of the line. This will link the diagnosis to the service provided.

Block 22 – Resubmission Code and/or Original Reference Number. Both the resubmission code and the original reference number assigned by the insurance payer must be entered in this block. Resubmission codes:
- 7 Replacement of prior claim
- 8 Void/cancel of prior claim

Block 23 – Prior Authorization Number. The preauthorization/precertification number obtained from the insurance company is entered.

Block 24 – Procedures and Charges. Procedure codes, such as the CPT codes and/or HCPCS codes, are listed in Block 24 (Fig. 30.5). Each procedure code is considered a line item; the line numbers are found to the left of Block 24. All data in one line belong to the coordinated CPT/HCPCS code. For claims that require more than six line-items, a second CMS-1500 form should be generated. Check with the insurance company to confirm how to indicate that the claim has multiple pages; some insurance companies require the statement "Continued" or "Page 1 of 2" in Block 28, Total Charges.

Block 24A – Date(s) of Service. Note that there is space for both "From" and "To" dates. If the service was provided on just one

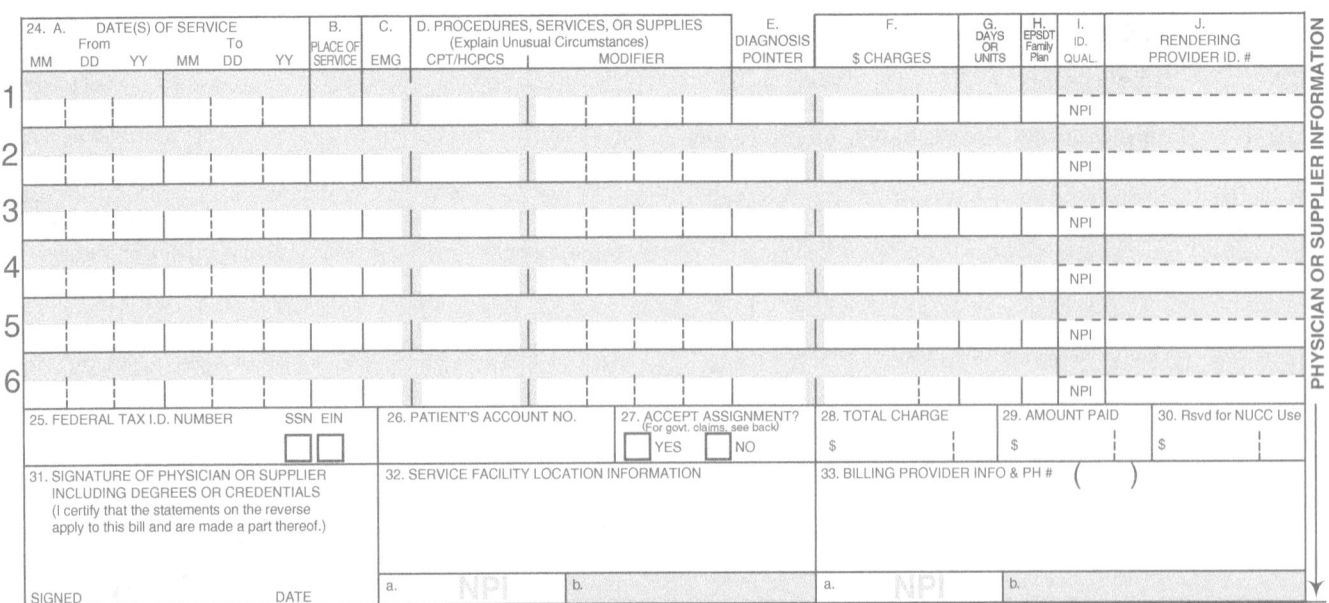

Fig. 30.5 Section 3: Physician or Supplier Information (Blocks 24 to 33).

day, you would only enter a From date, in a MM/DD/YY format. If the service was provided on multiple days, such as an inpatient hospital stay, the first day the service was provided would in the From field and the last day the service was provided would be entered in the To field. The number of times that that service was provided would be indicated in Block 24G.

Block 24B – Place of Service. The Place of Service (POS) codes indicate where the services were provided. The POS for a medical office is 11. (For more information on POS, refer to Chapter 29 and Table 29.3.)

Block 24C – EMG (emergency). A Y in this field indicates that the service was an emergency.

Block 24D – Procedures, Service, or Supplies. There are two sections in this block, CPT/HCPCS and Modifier. There is space for a single 5-digit code and up to four separate 2-digit modifiers. No space is provided for a written description of the code; only the code is required.

Block 24E – Diagnosis Pointer. This block indicates which diagnosis is used for each line item. The letter from diagnosis listed in Block 21 should be used here to link the diagnosis to the service. Do not enter the ICD-10-CM codes in this block.

Block 24F – $ Charges. The dollar amount of the provider's fee for the service is entered here. This fee is calculated in the office based on work, expertise, and time. If a series of services was performed on any one line, multiply the number of days or units (Block 24G) by the charge for one procedure or service and enter the total amount for all days or units. This field is most commonly used for multiple visits, units of supplies, or anesthesia units.

Block 24G – Days or Units. The number of days or units is entered here. Used for multiple visits and units of supplies. If only one service is performed, 1 would be entered.

Block 24H – EPSDT/Family Plan. EPSDT stands for Early and Periodic Screening, Diagnosis, and Treatment, the child health program under Medicaid. This block identifies specific services covered under state health insurance plans. Refer to the appropriate insurance payer's guidelines (typically Medicaid or the Medicaid intermediary) for instructions on completing this block. Leave the block blank for Medicare, TRICARE, and the Civilian Health and Medical Program of the Department of Veterans Affairs (CHAMPVA), group health plans, Federal Employees Compensation Act (FECA)/Black Lung, and most other types of insurance.

Block 24I – ID Qual. Used if the number in Block 24J is not an NPI. The following are the qualifiers:
- 0B State License Number
- 1G Provider UPIN Number
- G2 Provider Commercial Number
- LU Location Number
- ZZ Provider Taxonomy

Block 24J – Rendering Provider ID #. Enter the NPI of the provider who rendered the service, as identification.

Block 25 – Facility Information. The Federal Tax ID Number of the provider filing the claim can be listed as a Social Security number (SSN) or an Employer Identification Number (EIN); mark the appropriate box with an X.

Block 26 – Patient's Account Number. Enter the account number or medical record number assigned to the patient by the provider of the service. This information will be included on the EOB from the insurance company to help with posting the payment.

Block 27 – Accept Assignment?. Put an X in the YES box if the provider will accept assignment; this means that they are a *participating provider (PAR)* and agree to accept the terms of the agreement with the insurance company, and also to accept what the plan states as an allowed amount for the services provided.

Block 28 – Total Charge. This block shows the amount billed on the claim form for all services rendered. To arrive at this amount, add up the charges reported in Block 24F for all the lines of service on the claim form.

Block 29 – Amount Paid. This is the amount received from the patient or other payers.

Block 30 – Reserved for NUCC Use. Some secondary insurance claims use this box for the claim amount due after the primary insurance has paid.

Block 31 – Signature of Physician or Supplier. This is the signature of the authorized or accountable person for the services on the claim, verifying that they provided the services listed, which have been checked for accuracy.

Block 32 – Service Facility Location Information. Enter the name, address, city, state, and ZIP code for the site where the services listed in the claim were provided. Enter the facility's NPI in Block 32a only if it is different from the Billing Provider NPI (Block 24J).

Block 33 – Billing Provider Info & PH #. Enter the address and phone number of the provider asking to be paid on this claim.
    Block 33a. Enter the same NPI number listed in Block 24J.
    Procedure 30.2 shows how to complete a health insurance claim form using the information from an insurance card and an encounter form (Fig. 30.6). With the patient-centered medical home (PCMH) model, completing the claim form can be challenging (Box 30.3).

CRITICAL THINKING 30.3

Ann is reviewing an encounter form that has one CPT code and two HCPCS codes with one diagnosis code for the same office visit. How many lines in Box 24 of the CMS-1500 will she need to use? Will all three CPT/HCPCS codes point to the same diagnosis? Why or why not?

ACCURATE CODING TO PREVENT FRAUD AND ABUSE

In any healthcare environment, accurate coding is essential to prevent fraud and abuse in reimbursement. According to HIPAA:
    Fraud is defined as knowingly and willfully executing or attempting to execute a scheme to defraud any healthcare benefit program or to obtain by means of false or fraudulent

HEALTH INSURANCE CLAIM FORM

APPROVED BY NATIONAL UNIFORM CLAIM COMMITTEE (NUCC) 02/12

PICA	PICA

1. MEDICARE ☑ (Medicare#) MEDICAID ☐ (Medicaid#) TRICARE ☐ (ID#/DoD#) CHAMPVA ☐ (Member ID#) GROUP HEALTH PLAN ☐ (ID#) FECA BLK LUNG ☐ (ID#) OTHER ☐ (ID#) **1a.** INSURED'S I.D. NUMBER (For Program in Item 1): **123-45-6789A**

2. PATIENT'S NAME (Last Name, First Name, Middle Initial): **ROSE DAWSON**

3. PATIENT'S BIRTH DATE: MM **02** DD **17** YY **XX** SEX M ☐ F ☑

4. INSURED'S NAME (Last Name, First Name, Middle Initial): **ROSE DAWSON**

5. PATIENT'S ADDRESS (No., Street): **123 TITANIC PLACE**

6. PATIENT RELATIONSHIP TO INSURED: Self ☑ Spouse ☐ Child ☐ Other ☐

7. INSURED'S ADDRESS (No., Street): **123 TITANIC PLACE**

CITY **NEW YORK** STATE **NY**

8. RESERVED FOR NUCC USE

CITY **NEW YORK** STATE **NY**

ZIP CODE **10001** TELEPHONE (Include Area Code) ( )

ZIP CODE **10001** TELEPHONE (Include Area Code) ( )

9. OTHER INSURED'S NAME (Last Name, First Name, Middle Initial): **ROSE DAWSON**

11. INSURED'S POLICY GROUP OR FECA NUMBER: **123-45-6789A**

a. OTHER INSURED'S POLICY OR GROUP NUMBER: **123-45-6789**

10. IS PATIENT'S CONDITION RELATED TO:

a. EMPLOYMENT? (Current or Previous) YES ☐ NO ☑

a. INSURED'S DATE OF BIRTH: MM **02** DD **17** YY **XX** SEX M ☐ F ☑

b. RESERVED FOR NUCC USE

b. AUTO ACCIDENT? YES ☐ NO ☑ PLACE (State)

b. OTHER CLAIM ID (Designated by NUCC)

c. RESERVED FOR NUCC USE

c. OTHER ACCIDENT? YES ☐ NO ☑

c. INSURANCE PLAN NAME OR PROGRAM NAME: **MEDICARE**

d. INSURANCE PLAN NAME OR PROGRAM NAME: **AARP SECONDARY POLICY**

10d. CLAIM CODES (Designated by NUCC)

d. IS THERE ANOTHER HEALTH BENEFIT PLAN? YES ☑ NO ☐ If yes, complete items 9, 9a, and 9d.

READ BACK OF FORM BEFORE COMPLETING & SIGNING THIS FORM.

12. PATIENT'S OR AUTHORIZED PERSON'S SIGNATURE I authorize the release of any medical or other information necessary to process this claim. I also request payment of government benefits either to myself or to the party who accepts assignment below.

SIGNED **SIGNATURE ON FILE** DATE **01/14/20XX**

13. INSURED'S OR AUTHORIZED PERSON'S SIGNATURE I authorize payment of medical benefits to the undersigned physician or supplier for services described below.

SIGNED **SIGNATURE ON FILE**

14. DATE OF CURRENT ILLNESS, INJURY, or PREGNANCY (LMP): MM DD YY QUAL.

15. OTHER DATE: QUAL. MM DD YY

16. DATES PATIENT UNABLE TO WORK IN CURRENT OCCUPATION: FROM MM DD YY TO MM DD YY

17. NAME OF REFERRING PROVIDER OR OTHER SOURCE: **ROBERT WILSON, MD**

17a. 17b. NPI **11122233344**

18. HOSPITALIZATION DATES RELATED TO CURRENT SERVICES: FROM MM DD YY TO MM DD YY

19. ADDITIONAL CLAIM INFORMATION (Designated by NUCC)

20. OUTSIDE LAB? YES ☐ NO ☐ $ CHARGES

21. DIAGNOSIS OR NATURE OF ILLNESS OR INJURY Relate A-L to service line below (24E) ICD Ind.

A. **E11.22** B. C. D.
E. F. G. H.
I. J. K. L.

22. RESUBMISSION CODE / ORIGINAL REF. NO.

23. PRIOR AUTHORIZATION NUMBER

| 24. A. DATE(S) OF SERVICE | | | | | | B. PLACE OF SERVICE | C. EMG | D. PROCEDURES, SERVICES, OR SUPPLIES (Explain Unusual Circumstances) | | E. DIAGNOSIS POINTER | F. $ CHARGES | | G. DAYS OR UNITS | H. EPSDT Family Plan | I. ID. QUAL. | J. RENDERING PROVIDER ID. # |
From MM	DD	YY	To MM	DD	YY			CPT/HCPCS	MODIFIER							
01	14	XX	01	14	XX	11		99213		1	$125	00	1		NPI	11122233344
															NPI	
															NPI	
															NPI	
															NPI	
															NPI	

25. FEDERAL TAX I.D. NUMBER: **098-76-5432** SSN ☐ EIN ☑

26. PATIENT'S ACCOUNT NO.: **RW125638**

27. ACCEPT ASSIGNMENT? (For govt. claims, see back) YES ☑ NO ☐

28. TOTAL CHARGE $ **125** **00**

29. AMOUNT PAID $ **0**

30. Rsvd for NUCC Use

31. SIGNATURE OF PHYSICIAN OR SUPPLIER INCLUDING DEGREES OR CREDENTIALS (I certify that the statements on the reverse apply to this bill and are made a part thereof.)

SIGNED *Robert Wilson, MD* DATE **01/14/XX**

32. SERVICE FACILITY LOCATION INFORMATION
Feel Better Family Practice
101 Jack Place
New York, NY, 10001
(212) 555-1212
a. **22233344455** b.

33. BILLING PROVIDER INFO & PH # ( )
Robert Wilson, MD
101 Jack Place
New York, NY, 10001
(212) 555-1212
a. **11122233344** b.

NUCC Instruction Manual available at: www.nucc.org PLEASE PRINT OR TYPE APPROVED OMB-0938-1197 FORM 1500 (02-12)

Fig. 30.6 Completed CMS-1500 Health Insurance Claim Form. (From Niedzwiecki B, et al: *Kinn's the medical assistant,* ed 14, St. Louis, 2020, Elsevier.)

BOX 30.3 Patient-Centered Medical Home

The patient-centered medical home (PCMH) is model of patient care. In this model, patient care is looked at from a holistic approach. The healthcare team wants to be able to assist the patient with any issues that come up about their care. This means having multiple team members available. The provider and the medical assistant would provide the primary care. There would also be a nurse who coordinates all of the care for the patient, including issues about home healthcare, financial issues, transportation issues, and so on. Many models include a clinical pharmacist who is available to discuss medication questions and concerns with the patient.

The goal of the PCMH is to improve patient outcomes and reduce costs. There are accreditation processes that must be completed for a healthcare facility to be recognized as a PCMH.

Billing for the services provided can be a challenge for the medical biller. When do you bill for the pharmacist's visit or phone contact? It is important to have billing policies and procedures in place when your healthcare facility is a PCMH so that services are billed consistently and accurately.

---

pretenses, representations, or promises any of the money or property owned by any healthcare benefit program.

Common types of billing fraud include:

- *Double billing*: To submit multiple claims for the same service provided.
- *Phantom billing*: To bill for services not performed and for supplies not given to patients.
- *Unbundling codes*: To use multiple CPT codes for parts of a procedure, instead of using a single, comprehensive CPT code.
- *Upcoding*: To use of a higher-level procedure code than is supported in the documentation or medical necessity.

Abuse in medical billing would be actions that are contrary to ethical standards in the medical office. *Abuse* is an unintended action that directly or indirectly results in an overpayment to the healthcare provider. Abuse is similar to fraud, except that it is unclear if the unethical practice was committed on purpose. The term *intentional* is important when determining whether fraudulent medical billing practices were done on purpose or were an accident.

Common types of billing abuse include:

- Billing for services that are not a medical necessity.
- Misusing codes on claims.
- Increasing the cost excessively for supplies and services.

Violations of the laws governing reimbursement may result in:

- Nonpayment of claims
- Civil monetary penalties (CMPs)
- Exclusion from the payer program
- Criminal and civil liability
- In extreme cases, jail time

These laws may be changed or updated. The person who is responsible for coding must pay close attention to detail and act as a sort of "medical detective" to prevent a case against a provider or clinic.

Guidelines for Reviewing Claims Before Submission

Guidelines can help ensure that clean insurance claims are submitted.

- Proofread the form carefully for accuracy and completeness.
- Make certain any necessary attachments are included with the completed form.

- Follow office policies and guidelines for claim review and signatures.
- Forward the original claim to the proper insurance carrier either by mail or electronically.
- Make sure the patient's and/or insured's name, address, and ID, group, and/or policy number are identical to the information printed on the insurance card.
- Make sure the patient's birth date and sex are the same as in the medical record.
- Enter the word NONE if Medicare is the primary payer for Block 11.
- Make sure the patient has authorized the release of information, and that Block 12 has a handwritten signature, the words "Signature on File," or the acronym SOF.
- Make sure the diagnosis is not missing or incomplete.
- Check that the diagnosis has been coded accurately, according to the ICD-10-CM coding manual and is linked to the treatment.
- List the fees for each charge individually; or, if more than 1 day or unit is entered in Block 24G, the fees must be computed correctly.
- Double-check the provider's federal SSN or EIN and NPI to ensure accuracy.

PREVENTING REJECTION OF A CLAIM

When a claim is submitted to a claims clearinghouse or a *payer* (insurance company), it must first pass specific minimum requirements before it can be processed. If the claim contains invalid or missing data elements required for acceptance into the claim processing system, the claim is considered an *unclean, nonclean,* or *dirty claim*. Unclean claims are rejected, and the provider will receive a letter or report indicating the issues. Discrepancies on the rejected claim should be corrected and the claim should be resubmitted for reimbursement.

Common reasons for rejected claims include incorrect patient information (e.g., name, subscriber number), ineligibility, missing data elements, and a mismatched procedure and ICD code(s). To prevent rejected claims, the medical assistant must understand and comply with the specific guidelines for completing a claim established by the payer. The claim submission guidelines are available from private and government payer websites. Most practice management billing systems have built-in claim scrubbers that help identify errors and create *clean claims* (claims without errors).

VOCABULARY

claim scrubbers Software that finds common billing errors before the claim is sent to the insurance company.

medical necessity Healthcare services or supplies needed to diagnose or treat an illness or injury, condition, disease, or its symptoms and that meet accepted standards of medicine.

Communicating With Providers About Third-Party Requirements

It can be challenging for a provider to keep up with the annual changes made by the government plans, private health insurance companies, and the coding updates. This is why healthcare providers trust their medical office staff to stay up to date on the various changes in the health insurance industry.

Some providers may be so focused on patient care that they feel uncomfortable with change. This may be the case with the encounter form/superbill used in patient care. A provider may feel comfortable using the same form, but over time, some codes may have changed or become obsolete, or new medical services offered may not be listed on the form.

A medical coder should tactfully discuss with the provider the benefits of using an updated encounter form. If the provider is still reluctant to change the form, even though it is outdated, the medical coder may suggest that the form will not be changed, just the codes on it. Adjust the encounter form to include an open text box for the provider to add medical procedures that they perform occasionally.

When communicating with the provider about coding issues, you must always have a respectful attitude. The many changes occurring in medical coding and billing can be overwhelming and confusing for some providers. The approach of coding professionals should be to guide them patiently through these changes.

CHECKING THE STATUS OF A CLAIM

The medical biller should keep track of every submitted claim to ensure timely reimbursement. Clearinghouses send a confirmation report after submission of a claim. The medical biller should always confirm that the claims submitted to the clearinghouse match the claims listed on the confirmation report. If direct billing is used, the medical biller must set up a system to track the claims that were submitted. Medical assistants should maintain this practice to ensure that every claim is submitted correctly.

The claim submission confirmation report also indicates claims that were rejected because they were incomplete. These claims should be corrected and resubmitted electronically immediately. Often these claims are rejected for data entry errors. The medical biller should compare the patient's information in the practice management software to the information on the patient's registration form and scanned insurance card, to ensure accuracy.

It typically takes 10 to 14 business days for insurance companies to process insurance claims electronically. If no response has been received from the insurance company after 30 days, the medical biller should inquire about the status of the claim. This can be done through the company's provider web portal or by a call to the provider services number on the back of the patient's insurance ID card. To verify the claim status, you must provide:

- the insured subscriber's member number and birth date.
- the patient's name and birth date.
- the date of service.

With this information, the insurance company should be able to tell if the claim has been paid, is still in process, was denied, or was never received. The medical biller will use this information for the proper follow-up. This could be:

- Investigating the records at the clinic to see if the payment came in but was applied to the incorrect patient account
- Researching the denial and resubmitting the claim
- Determining why the claim was not received and resubmitting it

The state insurance commission has standards that insurance companies must abide by, including claim processing times and payment guidelines. Medical assistants should keep the commission's contact information in the office medical billing manual as a reference in case a claim should be reported.

EXPLANATION OF BENEFITS

The insurance company sends the patient an explanation of benefits (EOB). The purpose of an EOB is to inform the patient what costs for medical care or products will be covered. An insurance company also send an EOB to the provider, but many times it looks slightly different than the patient's EOB. The provider's version may be called an *explanation of payment* (EOP) or *remittance advice* (RA). An *electronic remittance advice* (ERA) is a digital version of the provider EOB or EOP and provides claim payment explanation to the provider. If the insurance company sends providers payments by checks, an EOP will accompany the check. Most payers, including Medicare, are using ERAs and including information on the electronic fund transfer. (Medicare may send Standard Paper Remit [SPR] in some cases.)

Most EOBs, EOPs, RA, and ERAs contain the following components:

- Patient information and provider information
- Dates of service and a description of the service or product the patient received from the provider
- Amount billed by the provider
- *Provider fee adjustment* (the difference between the amount billed by the provider and the amount the provider agreed to accept as full payment)
- *Copayment* or *copay* (the fixed amount the patient pays for a covered service after the deductible is met)
- *Deductible* (the amount the policyholder pays for covered healthcare services before the insurance plan starts to pay) and amounts not covered by the plan
- *Coinsurance* (the percentage of costs of covered healthcare services the patient pays after the deductible is met)
- Total amount eligible for benefits and the percentage level of benefit coverage
- Amount paid by the health plan and the patient's responsibility
- Remark codes (EOB codes with descriptions are listed to indicate the reason for denial or adjustment.)

Reading an Explanation of Benefits

The EOB contains essential information about the submitted health insurance claim. To properly apply payments to a patient's account, it is vital that the medical assistant understand all the elements of an EOB. When interpreting the EOB, review the steps:

1. Verify that the EOB applies to the correct patient by comparing the account number and date of service on the EOB with the submitted claim.
2. Confirm that the EOB shows the same charged amount as the submitted claim. In other words, the line items and charges should match. Sometimes the EOB summarizes the entire claim in one charged amount. In this case, confirm that the total charged is the same as in the submitted claim.

3. Post the payment and adjusted amount per line item. In the practice management billing software, these are posted on the same line. The patient's responsibility, as determined by the primary insurance EOB, is calculated using the equation:

Charged amount − Payment amount −
Adjustment amount = Patient's responsibility

4. Once the patient's responsibility has been determined, check for a secondary insurance. If one is listed, submit a health insurance claim with the balance due determined by the primary insurance EOB. If no secondary insurance is listed, the patient is billed for the balance due.

5. Review the *remark codes* on the EOB for any additional messages or information about the claim. The remark codes area is where the insurance company indicates the conditions under which the claim was paid. For example, code 01 states that the claim amount allowed was established by the contract between the health insurance plan and the provider. Other remarks codes give the reasons a claim was denied. Some remarks codes indicate that the claim is pending, awaiting specific information.

6. All remarks codes on pending or denied claims should be followed up immediately upon receipt of the EOB, to prevent further delay in payment for other claims.

DENIED CLAIMS

A *denied claim* is a claim that was received and processed by the payer and found to be unpayable. Denied claims usually come back with an EOB, EOP, or ERA. An explanation for why the claim was denied is included in the document and is usually found in the remarks code. A claim may be denied if the following occur:

- The service, equipment, or medication is not a covered benefit under the plan.
- The medical problem began before the person joined the plan.
- The services were provided by a facility or provider outside of the approved network of providers.
- The service, treatment, equipment, or medication is not a medical necessity or is considered experimental.
- Preauthorization for the service was not obtained.

If the issue can be corrected, the medical assistant should and resubmit the claim. Resubmitting the claim after a denial can result in a duplicate claim rejection. To prevent the duplicate claim rejection, the denied claim should be resubmitted with an appeal or a reconsideration request.

The appeals process consists of an internal and external process. When a claim is denied, an internal appeal can be filed. The payer's procedure must be followed, which may include completion of forms and the submission of additional documentation. The internal review must be done within 180 days of receiving the denial. The appeal process may take up to 60 days if the service was already received. The payer will provide the patient with a written decision. If the internal appeal results in a denial, a person can ask for an external review.

Medical Necessity

Insurance companies determine medical necessity based on the diagnostic and procedural codes submitted on the claim. The diagnostic code is the reason that the procedure was necessary. For example, if a claim submitted to the insurance company indicated that a bunionectomy was performed for tonsillitis, the insurer will deny the claim based on medical necessity. Procedure codes are linked to diagnostic codes in the claim. The health record must support the reason for each service provided.

If an insurance claim is denied for medical necessity, the medical assistant should review the claim information and the health record. If there is an error on the claim, such as the wrong diagnostic coded on the encounter form, then a new claim should be submitted with an appeal or a reconsideration request to prevent the duplicate claim rejection.

If an insurance claim is denied for medical necessity and the medical assistant believes that it was coded correctly, an appeal letter should be sent to the insurance company. The appeal letter should identify the denied claim and include a statement from the provider detailing the medical reasoning for performing the procedure. Additional medical reports (e.g., laboratory reports, operative reports, and history and physical examination findings [H&P]) should be sent if they support the provider's treatment decision (Procedure 30.3).

PATIENT'S FINANCIAL RESPONSIBILITY

To help patients understand their health insurance benefits, the medical assistant must be able to explain deductibles, copayments, and coinsurance. The deductible amount is indicated on the EOB. The medical office can contact the insurance company on the patient's behalf to determine the amount of the deductible the patient has already paid in the calendar year.

Once the deductible is paid for the year, the patient may need to pay a copay at the time of service. Copayments can vary by insurance companies and services. A primary care visit may be $15 to $25, and a specialist visit may be around $30 to $50. A visit to the emergency department may be as much as $300. Copays can also be applied to prescription drugs. The medical assistant must make sure that the proper copayments are received and credited to patients' accounts.

After the deductible is met, coinsurance begins. The insurance company and the patient split the cost of the services. An 80/20 split is very common, especially for traditional insurance. This means the insurance company pays 80% of the fee and the insured pays 20%.

Calculating the Coinsurance and Deductible

Consider this example: Mrs. Anita Jones' health insurance plan has a $500 annual deductible, after which the insurance company pays 95% of all charges. Mrs. Jones, therefore, has a 5% coinsurance expense, in addition to the deductible. Mrs. Jones has incurred a $10,000 charge for cardiac surgery performed by her provider.

In Fig. 30.7, Column A shows that Mrs. Jones paid the $500 deductible, and 5% of $9,500. (To calculate this, multiply 9500 by 0.05.) The insurance company then paid the remaining balance of $9,025.

Also, in Fig. 30.7, Column B shows that Mrs. Jones' cardiac surgery cost $20,000. She would pay the $500 deductible and 5% of remaining $19,500 for her coinsurance. (To calculate, multiply 19500 by 0.05.) Her coinsurance is $975. So her total

	Column A	Column B
Total Charge	$10,000	$20,000
Deductible (paid by Mrs. Jones)	$500	$500
Coinsurance (5% paid by Mrs. Jones)	5% of $9500 (Total charge minus the deductible) = $475	5% of 19,500 (Total charge minus the deductible) = $975
Total amount paid by Mrs. Jones	$975	$1475
Total amount paid by insurance	95% of $9500 (Total charge minus the deductible) - $9025	95% of $19,500 (Total charge minus the deductible) - $18,525

Fig. 30.7 Deductible and Coinsurance.

	PAR	NonPAR
Total Charge	$10,000	$10,000
Allowed amount	$8,500	$8,500
$1500 difference between charged amount and allowed amount	Written off as an adjustment	Billed to the patient
Deductible (paid by Mrs. Jones)	$500	$500
Coinsurance (paid by Mrs. Jones)	$8500 – $500 (deductible) X 5% = $400	$8500 – $500 (deductible) X 5% = $400
Total amount paid by Mrs. Jones	$900	$2400
Total amount paid by insurance	$7,600	$7,600

Fig. 30.8 PAR vs. NonPAR.

out-of-pocket expense is $1,475. The insurance company is responsible for payof the balance of $18,525.

Allowed Amount

Another factor to be considered when determining the patient's financial responsibility is whether the provider is a PAR provider or not. To become a participating provider in an insurance network, the provider must agree to accept the insurance plan's fee schedule as payment in full for services rendered. This means that if the provider's fee is higher than the plan's allowed amount, the difference should be adjusted. The *allowed amount* is the maximum amount a plan will pay for a covered healthcare service. For example, a provider may charge $80 for a Level I office visit; however, the insurance plan's allowable amount may be only $60. If the provider is a participating provider, they are obligated to adjust the difference between these two amounts – $20. The patient is not responsible for that $20. However, if the provider is not a participating provider, they can bill the patient for the $20 balance. Because contracts between insurance companies and providers vary greatly, it is important for the medical assistant to closely examine the EOB to ensure that the proper adjustments are done.

Let us look at how this would affect the example in Fig. 30.7. If the allowable amount for Mrs. Jones' $10,000 cardiac surgery is $8,500, the $1,500 difference between the provider's charge and the allowed amount would be either written off or passed on to the patient. Fig. 30.8 demonstrates the differences in the patient's responsibility and provider reimbursement.

CRITICAL THINKING 30.4

The providers in the practice where Ann works are not in network for a preferred provider organization (PPO) that is often used in their geographic area. Many patients are confused when they have to pay a larger out-of-pocket fee for their medical services. How can Ann explain the reason for these higher fees to patients?

BOX 30.4   Advance Beneficiary Notice

The Advance Beneficiary Notice (ABN) is issued by healthcare providers and facilities in situations where Medicare payment is expected to be denied. The ABN notifies patients of the expected noncoverage If patients still want the services from the provider, they need to complete the information on the form and they take financial responsibility of the uncovered fees (see Fig. 30.9).

Discussing the Patient's Financial Responsibility

The *guarantor* is the person legally responsible for the entire bill. It is important that the patient and the guarantor understand what the financial responsibilities are for services provided. Some patients expect insurance to pay all costs simply because they are paying a premium. Often patients do not even read their insurance policies and have no idea what is and is not covered.

The medical assistant may need to educate patients about their policies and help patients work with their insurance company to get answers to questions and make sure they are receiving all the benefits to which they are entitled. If problems come up with the insurance company, it is in the practice's best interest to actively assist the patient. The medical billing staff is usually more knowledgeable than the patient about health insurance. Helping patients with issues can help ensure that providers are compensated for their services.

Medical assistants gain knowledge about the insurance industry when they actively assist patients with their concerns. The more experience a medical assistant has in working with insurance, the more helpful they can be to patients. As mentioned previously, medical assistants should keep a manual of medical billing policies and procedures for most of the insurance plans they handle; this can serve as an excellent source of guidance and suggestions for working with a particular payer.

Always be sure to obtain the guarantor's signature on an agreement to pay for services. Most patient information sheets have a section referring to the guarantor. A statement may be included that serves as an agreement to pay the costs of medical care. States have statutes that deal with guarantors, so be sure the office's policies comply with those laws. It is especially important to secure a written agreement to pay for services when the care will be long term or involves costly treatment or surgical procedures. Procedure 30.4 explains how to inform patients of their financial obligations for services rendered (Box 30.4 and Fig. 30.9).

Showing Sensitivity When Discussing the Patient's Finances

Most patients use health insurance, but they do not always recognize that they will have financial obligations after the insurance plan pays its share. This is common among Medicare patients, who often feel that they should have all their medical expenses paid because they have government insurance. It

A. Notifier: John Doe, MD, College Clinic, 4567 Broad Avenue, Woodland Hills, XY 12345 555-486-9002

B. Patient Name: Mary Judd   **C. Identification Number:** 0920XX7291

Advance Beneficiary Notice of Noncoverage (ABN)

NOTE: If Medicare doesn't pay for **D.** _B12 injections_ below, you may have to pay.
Medicare does not pay for everything, even some care that you or your health care provider have
good reason to think you need. We expect Medicare may not pay for the **D.** _B12 injections_ below.

D.	E. Reason Medicare May Not Pay:	F. Estimated Cost
B12 injections	Medicare does not usually pay for this injection or this many injections	$35.00

WHAT YOU NEED TO DO NOW:
- Read this notice, so you can make an informed decision about your care.
- Ask us any questions that you may have after you finish reading.
- Choose an option below about whether to receive the **D.** _B12 injections_ listed above.
  Note: If you choose Option 1 or 2, we may help you to use any other insurance
     that you might have, but Medicare cannot require us to do this.

G. OPTIONS: Check only one box. We cannot choose a box for you.

☑ **OPTION 1.** I want the **D.** _B12 injections_ listed above. You may ask to be paid now, but I
also want Medicare billed for an official decision on payment, which is sent to me on a Medicare
Summary Notice (MSN). I understand that if Medicare doesn't pay, I am responsible for
payment, but **I can appeal to Medicare** by following the directions on the MSN. If Medicare
does pay, you will refund any payments I made to you, less co-pays or deductibles.

☐ **OPTION 2.** I want the **D.** _____ listed above, but do not bill Medicare. You may
ask to be paid now as I am responsible for payment. **I cannot appeal if Medicare is not billed.**

☐ **OPTION 3.** I don't want the **D.** _____ listed above. I understand with this choice I
am **not** responsible for payment, and **I cannot appeal to see if Medicare would pay.**
H. Additional Information:

This notice gives our opinion, not an official Medicare decision. If you have other questions on
this notice or Medicare billing, call **1-800-MEDICARE** (1-800-633-4227/**TTY:** 1-877-486-2048).
Signing below means that you have received and understand this notice. You also receive a copy.

I. Signature: *Mary Judd*	J. Date: *March 20, 20XX*

According to the Paperwork Reduction Act of 1995, no persons are required to respond to a collection of information unless it displays a valid OMB control number. The valid OMB control number for this information collection is 0938-0566. The time required to complete this information collection is estimated to average 7 minutes per response, including the time to review instructions, search existing data resources, gather the data needed, and complete and review the information collection. If you have comments concerning the accuracy of the time estimate or suggestions for improving this form, please write to: CMS, 7500 Security Boulevard, Attn: PRA Reports Clearance Officer, Baltimore, Maryland 21244-1850.

Form CMS-R-131 (03/11)   Form Approved OMB No. 0938-0566

Fig. 30.9 Advance Beneficiary Notice for Medicare Patients. (From Fordney MT: *Insurance handbook for the medical office,* ed 14, St. Louis, 2017, Elsevier.)

usually falls to the medical assistant to inform patients of their financial responsibilities.

Patients seeking medical care are not usually feeling like themselves because they may be suffering through pain and discomfort. As a result, their behavior may not be typical when the medical assistant suggests discussing their financial responsibilities.

Medical assistants should show patience and sensitivity when discussing a patient's financial obligations (Fig. 30.10). Patients should never be harassed to make a payment or forced into payment arrangements. Medical assistants should always be courteous when discussing payments with patients. In addition, the medical practice should offer a variety of payment options to meet patients' needs, including credit card and online payment options.

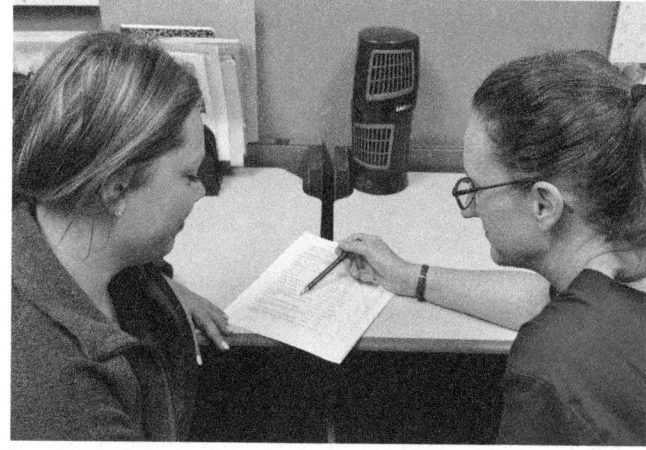

Fig. 30.10 Medical assistants must show respect and sensitivity when discussing financial issues with patients (From Niedzwiecki B, et al: *Kinn's the medical assistant,* ed 14, St. Louis, 2020, Elsevier.)

CLOSING COMMENTS

Accurate insurance billing practices are essential for the financial success of every healthcare facility. Medical assistants are strong assets to the healthcare facility when they can submit claims electronically, manage denied and rejected claims, and discuss financial responsibilities with patients professionally. Medical assistants should always maintain a positive attitude toward patients and keep in mind that those who are ill or facing challenges are not always at their best and may not respond in a positive way when discussing their financial responsibilities.

PATIENT-CENTERED CARE

Most patients are unaware of their benefits and coverage through their insurance policies. The medical assistant should encourage patients to read the entire policy to become familiar with its limitations and exclusions. Inform patients that when they call the insurance company with questions, they should always write down the date, the time, and the name of the person with whom they spoke. Using email is helpful because a record of the correspondence can easily be saved or printed. Making sure that patients have a general understanding of their health insurance coverage is well worth the effort.

Often patients do not dispute the decision or question the insurance company when a claim is denied or *adjusted* (less money was paid). Encourage them to call the company and question denied claims if they do not understand why the claim was denied.

BEING PROFESSIONAL

Being tactful means using good manners as you provide truthful, sensitive information or honest critical feedback to another person. Tactful behaviors include showing respect, discretion, compassion, honesty, diplomacy, and courtesy while you deliver a message. Tactful behaviors encompass both nonverbal and verbal communication, including what you say, how you say it, and your body language during the communication. A critical element of being tactful is considering the other person's feelings and reactions as you deliver the information. When you use tactful behaviors, you demonstrate professionalism, and you preserve relationships by avoiding conflicts and finding common ground.

Many times, the medical biller is the expert on the third-party requirements, and providers rely on the biller to help them understand the requirements. Being tactful with providers as you communicate third-party requirements is critical to your working relationship with the provider and also important in the overall financial scope of the agency. It is crucial to assist the provider in a tactful manner, understanding their role in meeting third-party requirements.

Using the following case study, role-play with two peers how you would display tactful behaviors when communicating with medical providers about third-party requirements: You are the medical biller for your clinic. The two providers have not been communicating with you about procedures that need prior authorization from the insurance companies. As a result, multiple claims are being denied, and the clinic has had to write off much of the cost. Today you are talking with the providers, regarding how to decrease the number of denied claims.

CHAPTER REVIEW

It is important for medical assistants to be familiar with the information needed to submit insurance claims. Not all insurance cards are in the same format. A medical assistant should be able to look at any patient's insurance card and determine the copay amount, identification and group numbers, where claims should be submitted, and where to call to get preauthorization for services.

Most MCOs require precertification/preauthorization. The medical billing specialist should be familiar with how to accomplish this. It can be done with a paper form, or it can be done electronically. If precertification is not done, the services may not be paid for by the insurance company.

Submitting claims can be done either with a paper claim form or electronically. All of the information needed to complete a paper form is also required for an electronic form. If a medical assistant understands the information needed for the paper form, they will know what information needs to be in the computer system for an electronic claim.

Whenever medical assistants work with billing, they need to be sure that they are completing the tasks in a legal and ethical manner. Fraud and abuse should be avoided at all costs. By keeping up-to-date on all regulations for health insurance billing, the medical assistant can avoid fraud and abuse.

After submitting a claim, the medical biller must continue to track the progress of that claim to ensure that payment is received. Once payment has been received, the medical biller must ensure that the payment was correct. Looking for rejections and denials is part of the reimbursement process. Those rejections and denials must be researched and then claims should be resubmitted.

Helping patients understand their financial obligations is one of the responsibilities of a medical assistant. Many patients do not understand what deductibles, copayments, or coinsurance are. Using a sensitive manner in helping them to understand is one way of providing excellent customer service.

SCENARIO WRAP-UP

Ann realizes that the best way to keep track of all the carriers is to keep an up-to-date manual that contains the addresses, phone numbers, and medical billing policies and procedures for each insurance plan that the healthcare facility accepts. This manual can help prevent the rejection and denial of many claims because the claims will be submitted accurately the first time.

The medical assistant's understanding of how to calculate deductibles, coinsurance, and allowed amounts for procedures and services benefits both the provider and the patient. The provider's productivity, income, and losses can be easily tracked, and the patient can be educated as to the exact amounts they are responsible for paying.

Ann also has learned the importance of being courteous to patients when discussing their financial obligations. She has learned how to use the Assignment of Financial Responsibility form to communicate what the patient owes in a clear, straightforward manner.

PROCEDURE 30.1 Show Sensitivity When Communicating With Patients Regarding Third-Party Requirements

Tasks

Communicate in an assertive, professional manner with a third-party representative. Demonstrate sensitivity through verbal and nonverbal communication when discussing third-party requirements with a patient. Display tactful behavior when communicating with a provider regarding third-party requirements.

Scenario

Ken Thomas (DOB 10/25/19XX) saw Jean Burke, NP, for his asthma today. He was prescribed a fluticasone inhaler, 220 mcg, and a refill on his Albuterol inhaler. When Ken stops at the checkout desk to make a follow-up appointment, he looks concerned. You inquire how you can help him, and he states that he is wondering if his new insurance will pick up the fluticasone inhaler. He further explains that he has used the inhaler in the past, with great results, but he recently switched insurance plans, and he is finding it doesn't have the same coverage as his old plan.

Front

AETNA

INSURED: Tapia, Arnold

IDENTIFICATION #: CH1197845   DEPENDENTS: Tapia, Celia B
GROUP #: 33347H   EFFECTIVE DATE: 06/26/2012

CO-PAY: $25   DRUG CO-PAY
SPECIALIST CO-PAY: $35   GENERIC: $10
EMERGENCY DEPT: $35   NAME BRAND: $50

Back

Submit claims to:

Aetna
1234 Insurance Way
Anytown, AK 12345

Member Services: 1-800-123-222

Insured: If a life threatening emergency exists, seek immediate attention.

Role-Play 1

You call the insurance company and discuss the coverage with the insurance carrier's representative. The representative tells you that the fluticasone inhaler is not covered for his condition. The representative gives you names of two other inhalers that would be covered.

When you ask if the drug would be covered through the exceptions process, the representative indicates that the provider must send a letter. The letter must indicate the drug is appropriate for the patient's condition because all other drugs covered by the plan have not been effective or those drugs have side effects that may be harmful to the patient or the patient is allergic to the other drugs.

Role-Play 2

You must explain to Ken, who is upset over his insurance coverage, that he would have to cover the cost of the $250 inhaler.

Role-Play 3

Ken explains he does not have $250 for the inhaler. He asks what else he should do. You mention the exception process, and Ken requests the provider to send a letter. You need to role-play notifying the provider of the third-party requirements.

Directions

Role-play the scenarios with a peer. The peer will play the part of the insurance representative, the patient, and the provider. You need to be professional and assertive with the insurance representative. When working with the patient, you need to show sensitivity. When communicating with the provider, you need to be professional and tactful.

Equipment and Supplies

- Copy of patient's health insurance ID card
- Prescription for new medication

Procedural Steps

1. Obtain a copy of the patient's health insurance ID card and the prescription for the new medication.
   Purpose: Having the required documents will help you to be more efficient as you perform the task.
2. Review the insurance card for coverage information and the phone number for providers.
   Purpose: You will need the phone number from the ID card to call the insurance company. You will also need to provide the insurance representative with the patient's information.
   Scenario: Role-play #1 with a peer. The peer will be the insurance representative.
3. Contact the insurance company and clearly state the patient's information, the patient's question, and the name of the new medication. Write down information provided by the representative.
   Purpose: The insurance representative will need the patient's information and the question to assist you. Speaking clearly as you provide the information will help the listener understand what you are asking.
4. Demonstrate professionalism through verbal communication skills, by stating a respectful, assertive, clear, and organized message, while pronouncing medical terminology and medication names correctly.
   Scenario update: Role-play #2 with a peer. The peer will be the patient.

Continued

PROCEDURE 30.1   Show Sensitivity When Communicating With Patients Regarding Third-Party Requirements—cont'd

5. Explain to the patient the message from the insurance representative using language that can be understood by the patient.

   Purpose: For the patient to understand your message, you need to use language that they can understand.

6. Demonstrate sensitivity to the patient by paying attention to and responding appropriately to the patient's nonverbal body language and verbal message.

   Purpose: Demonstrating sensitivity can be done through verbal messages and body language. Paying attention to the patient and responding appropriately to their message and nonverbal communication are important.

7. Demonstrate sensitivity to the patient by showing empathy and clarifying that you understand what the patient is stating. Give the patient your full attention during the conversation and reserve judgment.

8. Demonstrate sensitivity to the patient by using a pleasant, courteous tone of voice. Use body language to communicate respect (e.g., eye contact if culturally appropriate, keeping arms uncrossed and relaxed).

   Purpose: As the patient's frustration and anger increase, it is important to use a pleasant, courteous, and normal tone of voice. Keeping your body appearance relaxed (e.g., arms uncrossed, hands relaxed) will help to show the patient you are calm.

   Scenario update: Role-play #3 with a peer. The peer will be the provider.

9. Demonstrate tactful behavior when explaining the third-party requirements to the provider.

   Purpose: Providing the patient with choices also shows the patient that you care.

PROCEDURE 30.2   Complete an Insurance Claim Form

Task
To accurately complete a CMS-1500 Health Insurance Claim Form (see Fig. 30.6).

Scenario
Mr. Walter Biller had an appointment with Dr. Walden on November 16, 20XX. He came in for an influenza vaccination, and while he was there, he wanted Dr. Walden to look at his ear because he was having problems hearing. His right ear canal was impacted with cerumen. His ear canal was irrigated, and the cerumen was removed during the visit.

Patient Demographics
Walter B. Biller (patient and insured)
87 Willoughby Lane
Anytown, AL 12345-1234
Phone: 123-237-3748
DOB: 01/04/19XX
SSN: 285-77-7796
HIPAA form on file: Yes – March 19, 20XX
Signature on file: Yes – March 19, 20XX

Clinic and Provider Information
Walden-Martin Family Medical Clinic
1234 Anystreet
Anytown, AL 12345
123-123-1234
POS – 11 Office
Established patient of Julie Walden, MD
Federal Tax ID# 651249831
NPI# 1467253823

Insurance Information
Account Number: 16611
Aetna
Policy/ID Number: CH8327753
Group Number: 33347H

Diagnosis | **ICD-10-CM Code**
Impacted cerumen, right ear | H61.21

Service	**CPT Code**	**Fee**
Est. minimal OV	99211	$24.00
Cerumen removal	69210	$46.00
Vaccine – Flu, 3 Y+	90658	$24.00
Preventive – Flu Administration	G0008	$7.00

Equipment and Supplies
- Patient's health record
- Copy of patient's insurance ID card or cards
- Patient registration/intake form
- Encounter form
- Insurance claims processing guidelines
- Blank CMS-1500 Health Insurance Claim Form

Procedural Steps
Almost all medical billing is done electronically through a practice management billing software. The paper CMS-1500 Health Insurance Claim Form is provided only to help students practice and develop their medical billing skills.

Complete each block (as appropriate) of the CMS-1500 (see Table 30.1 for block descriptions).

1. Gather the documents required to complete the claim form.
2. Complete the claim form using a pen. Use capital letters. Do not use punctuation (commas or dollar signs) unless indicated in the insurance manual or guidelines. Use a hyphen to hyphenate last names.
3. Using a copy of the patient's health insurance ID card, determine the type of insurance, and the insurance ID number. Enter this information into Blocks 1 and 1a.

   Purpose: After selecting the appropriate type of health insurance, the medical assistant can refer to the claims processing guidelines for that plan.
4. Using the ID card, the encounter form, and the registration/intake form, determine the patient's information and the insured individual's information. Accurately complete Blocks 2, 3, 5, 6, 9, and 10 a–c by entering the patient's information. Complete Blocks 4, 7, and 11 a–d with the insured's information.

   Purpose: By distinguishing between the patient and the insured, the medical biller can determine whether the insurer requires additional information for submission of an accurate claim.
5. Complete Blocks 12 and 13 by entering "signature on file" and the date.

   Note: The Assignment of Benefit form should have been signed by the patient and/or the insured at registration. Enter the dates in either the six (6)-digit format (MM/DD/YY) or the eight (8)-digit format (MM/DD/YYYY).

   Purpose: To submit an insurance claim, the medical practice must be authorized to release the service information on behalf of the patient or the insured.
6. Accurately enter the physician or supplier information by completing Blocks 14 through 23. Use the eight (8)-digit format (MM/DD/YYYY) when needed.
7. Using the encounter form, complete Blocks from 24A through 24H. Note the following:
   - *Block 24A:* Enter the dates of service, both From and To. For ambulatory services, enter the same date in the FROM and TO fields. Enter a date for each procedure, service, or supply using an eight (8)-digit format (MM/DD/YYYY).
   - *Block 24F:* Enter the charge for the listed procedure, service, or supply. *Do not use commas when reporting dollar amounts.* The cents column is the small column to the right.

PROCEDURE 30.2   Complete an Insurance Claim Form—cont'd

- *Block 24G:* Enter the number of days or units. This block is usually used for multiple visits, units of supplies, anesthesia units or minutes, or oxygen volume. If only one service was performed, enter 1.
8. Complete Blocks 24I through 27 by entering information on the provider, or on the healthcare facility where the service was provided, and the patient's account number. Check the correct box to indicate acceptance of assignment of benefits.
9. Complete Blocks 28 and 29 by entering the total charges, total amount paid, and the total amount due. Complete Blocks 31 through 33a by entering the provider's and facility's information.

10. Review the claim for accuracy and completeness before submitting. Correct any errors and provide any missing information.
   Note: Before sending the claim, make a copy of the form and file the copy in the patient's insurance claim file.

   Purpose: It is important to double-check the form for accuracy and for required information that has not been provided.

PROCEDURE 30.3   Utilize Medical Necessity Guidelines: Respond to a "Medical Necessity Denied" Claim

Task
To resolve the insurance company's denial of a claim for medical necessity by generating an accurate claim.

Scenario
You are working at the Walden-Martin Family Medicine Clinic, 1234 Anystreet, Anytown, AL 12345 (phone: 123-123-1234). You receive an electronic remittance advice (ERA) indicating that Medicare has denied the following claim for not being medically necessary.

Patient: Norma B. Washington	DOB: 08/07/19XX	Policy/ID Number: 847744144A
Date of Service: 06/13/20XX	ICD: G43.101 (Migraine)	CPT: J3420 (B-12 injection)
Provider: Julie Walden MD		

You do some research and find that the preceding information was the only information sent to Medicare for that encounter. The following information was the correct information for the encounter.

Patient: Norma B. Washington	DOB: 08/01/19XX	Date of Service: 06/15/20XX
ICD: G43.101 (Migraine)	CPT: J1885 (Toradol 15 mg – $15.50) and 90772 (Injection, Ther/Proph/Diag – $25.00)	
ICD: D51.0 (Vitamin B$_{12}$ deficiency anemia)	CPT: J3420 (B$_{12}$ injection – $24.00) and 90772 (Injection, Ther/Proph/Diag – $25.00)	

Billed to: Medicare, 1234 Insurance Road, Anytown, AL 12345-1234

Provider: Julie Walden MD

Equipment and Supplies
- SimChart for the Medical Office or practice management software (PMS) with claim submission tool
- Electronic remittance advice or scenario (see above)

Procedural Steps
1. Review the ERA (scenario) carefully. Compare the submitted information to the health record, claim, and encounter form. Look for errors in the patient's name and date of birth.
2. Compare the ERA (scenario) to the health record, claim, and encounter form. Look for errors in the date of service, the diagnosis, and the procedure codes. The procedure must be medically necessary for the diagnosis indicated.
   Purpose: The procedure codes must indicate an acceptable standard of treatment for the diagnosis listed. Review the patient's health record to determine whether the procedure was medically necessary.
3. Complete the electronic claim using SimChart or PMS. Open the software and navigate to the claim submission tool.
4. Enter the information required on the claim. Make sure to include all the information from the encounter.
5. Proofread the claim form for accuracy before submitting the claim.

PROCEDURE 30.4   Inform a Patient of Financial Obligations for Services Rendered

Tasks
To inform the patient of their financial obligation and to demonstrate professionalism and sensitivity when discussing the patient's billing record. Assist a parent/patient in understanding an Explanation of Benefits (EOB).

Scenario 1
Mr. Walter Biller arrives for his appointment. You need to collect his $20 copay prior to his appointment.

Scenario 2
Lisa Parker and her son are seen at the clinic. Lisa is meeting with you regarding her bill. She received an explanation of benefits form and has questions about it.

She is meeting with you to learn how to read the explanation of benefits and to understand how much she owes.

Directions
Role-play the scenarios with a peer. The peer will be the patient for scenario 1 and the parent for scenario 2. You will be the medical assistant. You need to be professional and sensitive when working with patients regarding payments. You also need to follow the WMFM clinics policy for obtaining payments:
- For patients with copayments, all copayments must be collected before the patient leaves the clinic.
- For patients with balances overdue:
  - Patients must pay 20% of the balance before an appointment can be scheduled.

PROCEDURE 30.4　Inform a Patient of Financial Obligations for Services Rendered—cont'd

- Or patients can establish a 6- or 12-month interest-free payment plan, making the first payment before the next visit can be scheduled.
- Payments can be made using VISA, Mastercard, personal check (no starter checks accepted), or cash. Payments can also be made online.

Equipment and Supplies
- Facility's payment policy
- Copy of patient's insurance card (or see information in the scenario)
- An explanation of benefits form

Procedural Steps
Scenario 1: You need to provide the patient with the information that he owes a copayment for today's visit.
1. Inform the patient of his financial obligation of the copayment.
   Scenario update: He states he does not have the cash with him.
2. Inform the patient of the clinic policy regarding copayments and how the payment can be made.

3. Demonstrate sensitivity and professionalism when discussing the payment.
   Scenario 2: Role-play with a peer who will be the patient.
4. Using the explanation of benefits form, show the parent how to read the information.
   - Show her how to read the services provided, provider charges, allowed amount, and the deductible amount.
   - Show her where to find what the insurance paid and what she is responsible for.
   - Inform the patient of the amount owed for services rendered.
   Scenario update: Patient stated she does not have the money to pay the entire bill today.
5. Inform the patient of the clinic policy regarding overdue accounts and scheduling appointments. Provide the patient with options for the overdue amount based on the clinic policy.
6. Demonstrate sensitivity and professionalism when discussing the payment and the situation.

31

Accounts, Collections, and Banking

LEARNING OBJECTIVES

1. Discuss bookkeeping systems and accounting methods.
2. Perform accounts receivable procedures for patient accounts, including posting charges, payments, and adjustments.
3. Discuss payment from patients and third-party payers.
4. Describe the impact of the Truth in Lending Act on collections policies for patient accounts.
5. Discuss monthly patient account statements.
6. Describe successful collection procedures for patient accounts.
7. Describe types of adjustments made to patient accounts, including a nonsufficient funds (NSF) check and collection agency transactions.
8. Describe procedures to take when accepting cash, checks, debit card, and credit cards for payment.
9. Describe common types of bank accounts and checks, the importance of signature cards, and online banking.
10. Describe banking procedures in the ambulatory care setting, including check writing, preparing bank deposits, and check endorsements
11. Explain the purpose of bank account reconciliation for auditing purposes.
12. Describe the process of paying bills including using petty cash.
13. Discuss the process of employee payroll.

OUTLINE

▶▶ OPENING SCENARIO

Sam Smith has been working in the business office at Walden-Martin Family Medical (WMFM) Clinic for the past 3 years. Her primary job has been working with patient accounts. She has recently been asked to also take on some of the accounts payable responsibilities. This will involve banking procedures and bill paying.

While working with patient accounts, Sam has become familiar with the billing cycle and collection procedures. After the addition of the banking responsibilities to her work duties, Sam met with a bank representative. They discussed some time-efficient ways to bank with mobile depositing and online banking. Sam realizes that she still has much to learn about the daily financial duties in a healthcare facility, including working with the patient account management software, making daily deposits, reconciling bank statements, and many other banking responsibilities.

Sam wants to increase the value of the healthcare facility's bank accounts by looking for bank accounts that pay a higher interest rate and by reducing the office's operational expenses. Sam also wants to encourage patients at the healthcare facility to use debit or credit cards, instead of checks, to pay for services, because she knows that returned patient checks have created problems in the past.

YOU WILL LEARN

1. To define the bookkeeping transactions that occur in a healthcare facility.
2. How to perform accounts receivable procedures, including posting charges, payments, and adjustments.
3. To describe special bookkeeping procedures, including credit balances, NSF checks, and bankruptcy.
4. To understand the need for sensitivity when discussing payment options with patients.
5. How the Truth in Lending Act affects collection policies.
6. To describe successful collection techniques for patient accounts.
7. To explain the purpose of the Federal Reserve Bank.
8. To identify common types of bank accounts.
9. To explain how online banking has made banking processes more efficient.
10. To describe the different methods for patient payments and the precautions needed with each.
11. To manage a petty cash fund.
12. To describe payroll procedures in a healthcare facility.

INTRODUCTION

Managing the finances in a healthcare facility is an important task. Every patient encounter creates a financial transaction for the facility. Transactions generated by the patient encounter include a variety of charges, payments, and adjustments that need to be accounted for on a daily basis. Financial management is essential if the healthcare facility is to pay the business operating expenses. This includes maintaining patient accounts

and performing collection activities and banking duties. If the expenses of operating the healthcare facility exceed the fees collected for services rendered, the business will be forced to close.

A medical assistant who works in the business office is responsible for:

- posting charges and accepting and posting a variety of payments and adjustments.
- endorsing and depositing checks and writing checks for office expenses.
- regularly reconciling bank and credit card statements.

Mobile deposit allows healthcare facilities to deposit checks on the date payments are received, because it is conveniently done in the office. The medical assistant will have to master basic math skills (e.g., addition and subtraction) for all banking functions.

VOCABULARY

adjustment A credit or debit modification on an account.
charge The cost for goods or services that is owed.
patient account A running balance of all financial transactions for a specific patient.
payment The amount paid for goods, services, or a loan.

BOOKKEEPING IN THE HEALTHCARE FACILITY

Bookkeeping is the practice of recording the transactions of a business each day. In the healthcare facility, the medical assistant, manager, or bookkeeper must record the services provided to the patient and financial transactions that occur. All patient charges and all receipts are either entered into the daily journal or the accounting software. In most facilities, when patients pay, they receive a receipt and another receipt is kept by the facility.

Bookkeeping Systems

Single-Entry Bookkeeping. *Single-entry bookkeeping* entails entering one entry in a cash book or journal for each transaction. Commonly, entries track revenue and expenses, much like a checkbook. The healthcare facilities also use an accounts receivable ledger. This contains patient ledger cards showing what each patient owes the facility. Single-entry bookkeeping works if the business is very simple and small. Single-entry bookkeeping is limited because it does not track specific accounts, assets, and liabilities. Errors with entries can go unnoticed.

Double-Entry Bookkeeping. *Double-entry bookkeeping* is more common in ambulatory care settings. For each transaction, two entries are made for the same amount, a debit in one account and a credit in another (Table 31.1). For example, the healthcare facility purchases a car. The debit would be added to the assets account. These means the car increased the total value of resources or increased the asset account. The same cost would be a credit in the liability (debts owed) account. This means the amount of money the facility now owes increased. The double-entry bookkeeping debit and credit concepts are different than the financial definition of *debit* (money owed or paid) and *credit* (you receive money back).

TABLE 31.1 Typical Accounts in a Double-Entry Bookkeeping System

Account	Definition	Account Increased By	Account Decreased By
Assets	Cash and valuable resources (e.g., equipment, land, stocks, supplies) owned by the healthcare facility that could be liquidated or converted to cash	Debit	Credit
Expenses	Costs that the facility incurs (e.g., payroll and supplies)	Debit	Credit
Liabilities	Debts or money owed (accounts payable) to a person or business	Credit	Debit
Equity	The value of the healthcare facility if all of the assets were liquidated and all of the debts were paid off. Equity can be written as: Assets − liability (debts) = Equity	Credit	Debit
Revenue	Money earned from providing services to patients	Credit	Debit

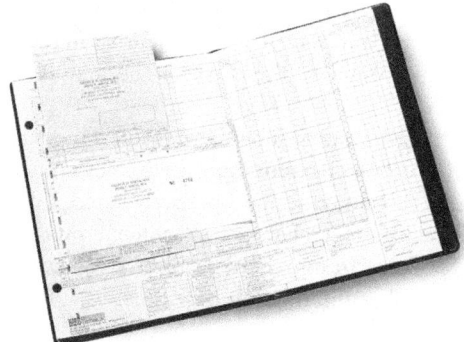

Fig. 31.1 Pegboard Billing System. (Courtesy Bibbero Systems. www.bibbero.com)

With double-entry bookkeeping, debits and credits are equal but opposite entries in the general ledger. The *general ledger* is the healthcare facility's book of financial records. The general ledger contains two columns; the left is for debits and the right is for credits. All of these entries are totaled in a trial balance. If done accurately, the trail balance should have the same number for the credit total and the debit total. Both debits and credits will balance. The information from the general ledger is used to prepare a balance statement. The *balance statement* provides information on the company's assets, liabilities, and equity at a specific time during the year (e.g., end of the year or quarter).

BOOKKEEPING AND ACCOUNTING METHODS

Accounting is a practice of maintaining the financial records of a business. It includes bookkeeping and preparing statements related to the assets, liabilities, and operating results of the business. An accountant uses the data entered during bookkeeping to provide an interpretation and analysis of the financial side of the business. The accountant can prepare the following reports:

- *Balance sheet*: Gives an overview of the financial status. It shows the assets, which are made up of the equity and liabilities: Assets = Equity + Liabilities.
- *Income statement*: Shows the revenue earned minus the expenses. Will show a profit or a loss for the healthcare facility.
- *Statement of cash flow*: Shows the cash flow into and out of the healthcare facility and addresses operations, financing, and investments.

The accountant can prepare monthly, semiannual, and annual summaries. These summaries allow the provider and office manager to improve business practices by eliminating unprofitable services and better budgeting of expenses. At the end of the fiscal year, the accountant prepares annual summaries and business tax returns are filed with the Internal Revenue Service (IRS).

Accounting and bookkeeping methods can be manual, computerized, or virtual. The following sections describe these methods.

> **VOCABULARY**
>
> **cash flow** Movement of cash into and out of the healthcare facility.
> **fiscal year** An accounting period of 12 months during which a company determines earnings and profit; the business determines the beginning of its fiscal year.
> **incurs** Acquires or sustains.
> **pegboard system** A manual bookkeeping system that uses a day sheet to record all financial transactions for the date of service and maintains patient account balances by using physical ledger cards.

Manual Bookkeeping and Accounting

Manual accounting uses physical registers and account books to keep the financial records. Manual accounting is a slow process, and all calculations are performed manually. Financial statements are prepared at the end of a quarter or period and give an overall picture of the finances. The pegboard system is a commonly used manual accounting method.

Pegboard System. The pegboard system is considered a "one-write system" of manual bookkeeping (Fig. 31.1). The system was so named because the forms are held in place by a row of pegs on the side of the board. With the pegboard system, the forms overlay each other. All the forms used in any system must be compatible so that they can be aligned perfectly on the board. When a person writes the information on the top form, the information is transferred to the other forms.

The pegboard system can be used for many different financial activities, including:

- *Patient accounts*: The medical assistant writes the information once, which enters information on the encounter form, receipt, patient account ledger card, and the daily journal or day sheet. The day sheet includes all information about the services rendered, charges, and receipts from the day.

- *Writing checks*: When the medical assistant writes a check, the figures are transferred onto the journal in the proper columns. This eliminates the need for check stubs and double posting.

The pegboard system allows the medical assistant to keep control over cash, collections, and receivables and ensures that every cent is accounted for and properly entered. It provides a record of every patient, charge, and payment, plus a daily recap of earnings – a running record of receivables and an audited summary of cash – and requires little time.

Computerized Bookkeeping and Accounting

With computerized bookkeeping and accounting, all financial transactions are entered into the software. The software can be part of the practice management software, or the healthcare facility can purchase software, such as QuickBooks or Sage. An advantage of computerized bookkeeping and accounting is that all calculations are done by the computer. Trial balance and financial reports or statements can be done quickly and easily. The equity of the business can be determined. Use of the bookkeeping/accounting software requires training. The hardware and software can be more expensive than manual bookkeeping and accounting.

Virtual Bookkeeping and Accounting

Virtual bookkeeping and accounting are becoming more popular in ambulatory care facilities. The virtual bookkeeper uses software to post financial transactions, review and update statements, and reconcile accounts. The virtual bookkeeper usually has remote access to the healthcare facility's server, accounting software, and financial documents.

A healthcare facility may decide to have a medical assistant, the office manager, or a bookkeeper enter the financial transactions into accounting/bookkeeping software. The facility may hire a virtual accountant or a virtual accounting firm to perform the accounting tasks needed, such as preparing reports, balancing the accounts, and preparing tax paperwork. If the healthcare facility uses a virtual accountant, the medical assistant, manager, or bookkeeper enters the financial transactions using the software indicated by the virtual accountant.

ACCOUNTS RECEIVABLE

Business transactions are usually divided into accounts receivable and accounts payable activities.
- *Accounts receivable (A/R)*: The money owed to the business that has not yet been received. In ambulatory care facilities, the providers provide services to patients. The patient and/or a third party, such as an insurance company, pays the facility for the services provided. A record of what is owed to the facility and by whom is found in the accounts receivable. When a payment is made on the patient account, the received payment becomes cash on hand.
- *Accounts payable (A/P)*: The money a business owes to its vendors and for payroll. The ambulatory care expenses include rent, utilities (e.g., electricity), supplies, equipment, and so on. All invoices, statements, and operating expenses are included in accounts payable. When expenses

have been paid, they are no longer categorized as accounts payable.

This chapter will discuss the accounts receivable activities followed by the accounts payable activities in the ambulatory care facility.

Posting to the Patient Ledger

When a patient is seen by a healthcare provider, services are provided, such as an examination and immunizations. With a manual bookkeeping system, these services are added to the encounter form and charges are calculated based on the fee schedule (Fig. 31.2 and Box 31.1). A summary of the encounter form activities and the charges are added to the *daily journal* (also called a *day sheet*) and the patient's *ledger* (also called a *ledger card*). The daily journal is also used to record charges and receipts from payments received that day.

All transactions, such as charges and payments, are posted to the patient's ledger daily (Procedures 31.1 and 31.2). In this way, the ledger becomes the source for answering questions from patients about their financial obligations. The patient ledger should include all information related to collecting the balance due, such as:
- Name and address of the guarantor
- Insurance identification information
- Home, work, and cell phone numbers
- Any special instructions for billing
- Emergency or alternative contact information

The patient ledger (Fig. 31.3) provides a running balance, the result of all of the different financial transactions performed in the account, including charges, payments, and adjustments.

When the healthcare facility uses a computerized system, the process for capturing charges to the posting in the ledger can vary. Some facilities use paper encounter forms, and information is keyed into the software. The assigning of the fees based on the fee schedule can be done manually or may be automated. Other facilities have automated the encounter form, and providers complete the encounter form online. The entire billing process is then done through the software.

VOCABULARY

cash on hand The amount of money the healthcare facility has in the bank that can be withdrawn as cash.

fee schedule A list of fixed fees for services.

guarantor The person legally responsible for the entire bill. This is usually the patient, but in the case of a minor it would be a parent or legal guardian.

Posting Payments From Patients

When patients pay in person, a receipt should be given to the patient showing the amount paid. If handwritten, the original receipt is given to the patient and the copy is used to post the payment to the ledger. If the facility uses software, an electronic receipt can be given to the patient.

Other payments may be received from patients by mail or electronically. All payments need to be logged in the daily journal if manual systems are used. With a computerized system, the payments are posted to the patient's account and daily reports can be created to show the daily payments.

At the end of the day, the medical assistant must reconcile payments received during the day. If the facility uses a manual

STATE LIC.# C1503X
SOC. SEC. # 000-11-0000
PIN # _____

Walden-Martin Family Medical Clinic
1234 Anystreet, Anytown, AK 12345-1234

Phone: 555-486-9002

☐ Private ☒ Bluecross ☐ Ind. ☐ Medicare ☐ Medi-cal ☐ Hmo ☐ Ppo

Patient's last name	First		Account #:	Birthdate	Sex ☒ Male	Today's date
Thomas	Ken		11594111	10 / 25 / 1961	☐ Female	09 / 17 / 20XX
Insurance company	Subscriber			Plan #	Sub. #	Group
Blue Cross Blue Shield	Ken Thomas				KT4496785	55124T

ASSIGNMENT: I hereby assign my insurance benefits to be paid directly to the undersigned physician, I am financially responsible for non-covered services.
SIGNED: Patient, or parent, if minor **Ken Thomas** Today's date 09 /17 / 20XX

RELEASE: I hereby authorize the physician to release to my insurance carriers any information require to process this claim.
SIGNED: Patient, or parent, if minor **Ken Thomas** Today's date 09 /17 /20XX

✓	DESCRIPTION	CODE	FEE	✓	DESCRIPTION	CODE	FEE	✓	DESCRIPTION	CODE	FEE
	OFFICE VISITS	NEW	EST.		Venipuncture	36415			OFFICE PROCEDURES		
	Blood pressure check		99211		TB skin test	86580			Anoscopy	46600	
	Level II	99202	99212		Hematocrit	85013			Ear lavage	69210	
	Level III	99203	99213		Glucose finger stick	82948			Spirometry	94010	
X	Level IV	99204	99214	$175	IMMUNIZATIONS				Nebulizer Rx	94664	
	Level V	99205	99215		Allergy inj. X1	95115			EKG	93000	
	PREVENTIVE EXAMS	NEW	EST.		Allergy inj. X2	95117			SURGERY		
	Age 65 and older	99387	99397		Trigger pt. inj.	20552			Mole removal (1st)	17110	
	Age 40 - 64	99386	99396		Therapeutic inj.	96372			(2nd to 14th)	17003	
	Age 18 - 39	99385	99395		VACCINATION PRODUCTS				Flat warts (1st - 14th)	07110	
	Age 12 - 17	99384	99394		DPT	90701			15 or more	17111	
	Age 5 - 11	99383	99393		DT	90702			Biopsy, 1 lesion	11100	
	Age 1 - 4	99382	99392		Tetanus	90703			Addt'l. lesions	11101	
	Infant	99381	99391		MMR	90707			Endometrial Bx	58100	
	Newborn ofc		99432		OPV	90712			Skin tags to 15	11200	
	OB/NEWBORN CARE				Polio inj.	90713			Each addt'l. 10	11201	
	OB package		59400		Flu	90662			I & D abscess	10060	
	Post-partum visit N/C				Hemophilus B	90645			SUPPLIES/MISCELLANEOUS		
	LAB PROCEDURES				Hepatitis B vac.	90746			Surgical tray	99070	
X	Urine dip		81000		Pneumovax	90670			Handling charge	99000	
	UA qualitative		81005		VACCINE ADMINISTRATION				Special report	99080	
	Pregnancy urine		81025		Age: Through 18 yrs. (1st inj.)	90460			DOCTOR'S NOTES:		
	Wet mount		87210		Age: Through 18 yrs. (ea. addt'l. inj.)	90461					
	kOH prip		87220		Adult (1st inj.)	90471					
	Occult blood		82270		Adult (ea. addt'l. inj.)	90472					

DIAGNOSES ICD-10-CM

_____ Abdominal pain/unspec.. R10.9
_____ Absess................L02._
_____ Allergic reaction.......T78.40_
_____ Alzheimer's disease.....G30
_____ Anemia/unspec........D64.9
_____ Angina/unspec........I20.9
_____ Anorexia.............R63.0
_____ Anxiety/unspec........F41.9
_____ Apnea, sleep.........G47.30
_____ Arrhythmia, cardiac....I49.9
_____ Arthritis, rheumatoid...M06.9
_____ Asthma/unspec......J45.909
_____ Atrial fibrillation......I48.0
_____ B-12 deficiency........E53.8
_____ Back pain, low.......M54.5
_____ BPH.................N40
_____ Bradycardia/unspec....R00.1
_____ Broncitis, acute.......J20._
_____ Bronchitis, chronic.....J42
_____ Bursitis/unspec.......M71.9
_____ CA, breast...........C50._
_____ CA, lung............C34._
_____ CA, prostate.........C61
_____ Cellulitis.............L03._
_____ Chest pain/unspec....R07.9
_____ Cirrhosis, liver/unspec...K74.60
_____ Cold, common........J00

_____ Colitis/unspec.........K51.90
_____ Confusion............R41.0
_____ CHF.................I50.9
_____ Constipation.........K59.00
_____ COPD...............J44.9
_____ Cough..............R05
_____ Crohn's disease/unspec..K50.90
_____ CVA.................I63.9
_____ Decubitus ulcer.......L89._
_____ Dehydration..........E86.0
_____ Dementia/unspec......F03
_____ Depression, major/unsp...F32.9
_____ Diab I, no complications...E10.0
_____ Diab II, no complications...E11.9
_____   w/kidney complic......E11.2_
_____   w/ophthalmic compl...E11.3_
_____   w/neurolog.compl.....E11.4_
_____   w/circulatory cmpl.....E11.5_
_____ Insulin use............Z79.4
_____ Diarrhea/unspec.......R19.7
_____ Diverticulitis..........K57.92
_____ Diverticulosis.........K57.90
_____ Dizziness.............R42
_____ Dysuria..............R30.0
_____ Edema/unspec........R60.9
_____ Endocarditis..........I38
_____ Esophageal reflux.....K21.0
_____ Fatigue (lethargy).....R53.83

_____ FUO................R50.9
_____ Gastritis.............K29.70
_____ Gastroenteritis (colitis)...K52.9
_____ G.I. bleed............K92.2
_____ Gout/unspec.........M10.9
_____ Headache............R51
_____ Health exam........200._
_____ Hematuria/unspec....R31.9
_____ Herpes simplex......B00.9
_____ Herpes zoster.......B02.9
_____ Hiatal hernia........K44.9
_____ HTN (HBP).........I10
_____ Hyperlipidemia/unspec...E78.5
_____ Hypothyroidism/unspec..E03.9
_____ Impotentce..........N52._
_____ Influenza, respiratory...J10.1
_____ Insomnia............G47.0
_____ IBS, diarrhea........K58.
_____ Lupus, systemic erythim..M32.9
_____ MI, acute...........I21._
_____ MI, old..............I25.2
_____ Migraine............G43.9
_____ Myalgia.............M79.1
_____ Neck pain..........M54.2
_____ Neuropathy.........G62.9
_____ Nausea............R11.1
X Nausea/vomiting......R11.0
_____ Obesity/unspec......E66.9

_____ Osteoarthritis (site)......M19._
_____ Otitis media..........H66.9_
_____ Parkinson's disease.....G20
_____ Pharyngitis, acute.......J02.9
_____ Pleurisy.............R09.1
_____ Pneumonia..........J18.9
_____ Pneumonia, viral......J12.9
_____ Prostatitis/unspec......N41.9
_____ PVD................I73.9
_____ Radiculopathy.......M54.1_
_____ Rectal bleeding......K62.5
_____ Renal failure.........N19
_____ Sciatica.............M54.3_
_____ Shortness of breath....R03.02
_____ Sinusitis, chr./unspec....J32.9
_____ Syncope............R55
_____ Tachycardia/unspec....R00.0
_____ Tachy., supraventric....I47.1
_____ Tendinitis/unspec.....M77.9
_____ TIA................G45.9
_____ Ulcer, duodenal/unspec..K26.9
_____ Ulcer, gastric/unspec....K25.9
_____ Ulcer, peptic/unspec....K27.9
_____ URI/unspec..........J06.9
X UTI.................N39.0
_____ Vertigo.............R42
_____ Weight gain.........R63.5
_____ Weight loss.........R63.4

Diagnosis/additional description:	Doctor's signature/date	
Headache	*Dr. Martin*	09-17-20XX

Return appointment information:	-with whom	Rec'd by:	Total today's fee	$175
Days Wks. (Mos.) 1 month	(Self) other	☐ Cash	Co-payment	$50
PLEASE RMEMBER THAT PAYMENT IS YOUR OBLIGATION, REGARDLESS OF INSURANCE OR OTHER THIRD PARTY INVOLVEMENT.		☐ Check ☐ Credit # _____	Amount rec'd today	

Fig. 31.2 Encounter Form With Charges. (Courtesy Bibbero Systems. www.bibbero.com)

BOX 31.1 Encounter Form and Superbills

Encounter forms are also called *superbills*, *charge slips*, or *fee tickets*. They are preprinted forms that are used to capture the charges for services provided during a patient visit. The forms include the most common services provided, along with procedural and diagnostic codes, which are required for billing insurance companies. The components of an encounter form include:

- *Provider's information*: Name, National Provider Identifier (NPI), facility address, phone number, email, provider's signature, and if applicable, a referring provider and their NPI.

- *Patient's information*: Name, address, phone number, date of birth (DOB), and insurance information.
- *Visit information*: Diagnosis and procedure codes (International Classification of Diseases [ICD] and Current Procedural Terminology [CPT]) with descriptions and related information, such as modifiers and fees charged.

---

daily journal or day sheet to record payments received, the daily activity must be calculated. As payments are received, the medical assistant completes a row on the day sheet by indicating the patient account and adding the amount received in the payment column. If the facility accepts credit cards, cash, checks, and electronic payments, they may have a column for each type of payment. At the end of the day, each column is totaled and then a final total of all payments received is calculated. If the facility uses a computerized system, the type of payment received is indicated as the payment is entered into

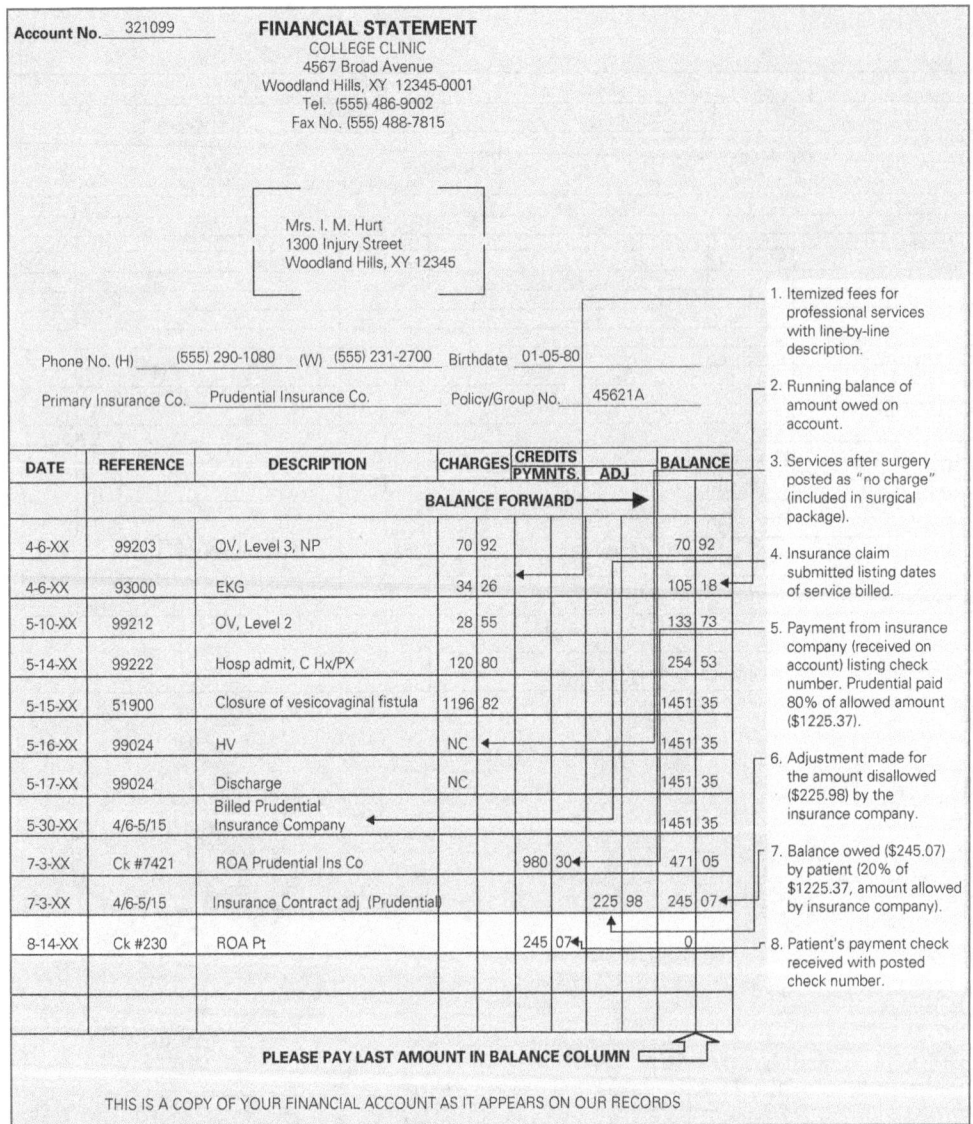

Account No. 321099

FINANCIAL STATEMENT
COLLEGE CLINIC
4567 Broad Avenue
Woodland Hills, XY 12345-0001
Tel. (555) 486-9002
Fax No. (555) 488-7815

Mrs. I. M. Hurt
1300 Injury Street
Woodland Hills, XY 12345

Phone No. (H) (555) 290-1080 (W) (555) 231-2700 Birthdate 01-05-80

Primary Insurance Co. Prudential Insurance Co. Policy/Group No. 45621A

DATE	REFERENCE	DESCRIPTION	CHARGES	CREDITS PYMNTS.	ADJ	BALANCE
		BALANCE FORWARD				
4-6-XX	99203	OV, Level 3, NP	70 92			70 92
4-6-XX	93000	EKG	34 26			105 18
5-10-XX	99212	OV, Level 2	28 55			133 73
5-14-XX	99222	Hosp admit, C Hx/PX	120 80			254 53
5-15-XX	51900	Closure of vesicovaginal fistula	1196 82			1451 35
5-16-XX	99024	HV	NC			1451 35
5-17-XX	99024	Discharge	NC			1451 35
5-30-XX	4/6-5/15	Billed Prudential Insurance Company				1451 35
7-3-XX	Ck #7421	ROA Prudential Ins Co		980 30		471 05
7-3-XX	4/6-5/15	Insurance Contract adj (Prudential)			225 98	245 07
8-14-XX	Ck #230	ROA Pt		245 07		0

PLEASE PAY LAST AMOUNT IN BALANCE COLUMN

THIS IS A COPY OF YOUR FINANCIAL ACCOUNT AS IT APPEARS ON OUR RECORDS

1. Itemized fees for professional services with line-by-line description.
2. Running balance of amount owed on account.
3. Services after surgery posted as "no charge" (included in surgical package).
4. Insurance claim submitted listing dates of service billed.
5. Payment from insurance company (received on account) listing check number. Prudential paid 80% of allowed amount ($1225.37).
6. Adjustment made for the amount disallowed ($225.98) by the insurance company.
7. Balance owed ($245.07) by patient (20% of $1225.37, amount allowed by insurance company).
8. Patient's payment check received with posted check number.

Fig. 31.3 **Patient Ledger.** (From Fordney WT: *Insurance handbook for the medical office*, ed 14, St. Louis, 2017, Elsevier.)

the software. At the end of the day, reports can be printed to show the day's activity.

If the facility accepts cash payment, the money in the cash drawer must be counted nightly. Cash drawers always contain money (a *starting balance*) at the beginning of the day so change can be made if needed. The starting balance must be subtracted from the nightly balance. The remaining amount should match the amount of cash received from payments. The totals from the checks received during the day are added up and the final total must match the total on the daily report or the day sheet.

Payment at the Time of Service. For the most part, patients are expected to pay their copayment at the time of service unless previous arrangements have been made (Fig. 31.4). Patients without health insurance should pay after the visit has been completed. When an appointment is made, patients should be informed that payment is expected at the time of service. That way they are not surprised when asked for payment at

the healthcare facility. The medical assistant may say, "Your charge for today is $25. Will that be cash, check, or credit or debit card?" If a patient asks to be billed, the medical assistant may say, "Our normal procedure is to pay at the time of service unless other arrangements are made in advance." Box 31.2 describes how to display sensitivity when requesting payment from patients.

Posting Payments From Third-Party Payers

Payments for services for patients can come from a third-party payer. A *third-party reimbursement* is payment from a party other than the patient or the patient's family. The most common third-party payers in ambulatory care are government programs and private insurance companies.

When third-party payments are posted in manual or computerized ledgers, each payment is posted on a separate line along with the corresponding health insurance claim information (Procedure 31.3). All payment amounts posted should match

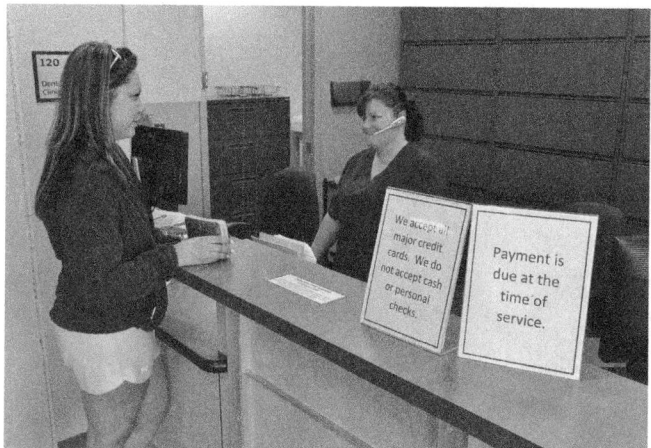

Fig. 31.4 Most healthcare facilities display a sign informing patients that payments are due at the time of service. (From Niedzwiecki B, et al: *Kinn's the medical assistant*, ed 14, St. Louis, 2020, Elsevier.)

BOX 31.2   Displaying Sensitivity When Requesting Payment

Informing patients of the amount they will be required to pay before they arrive for the appointment can help with the payment process. Use tact and good judgment when collecting payments. Understand that it can be uncomfortable for the patient to talk about money. Requests for payment should be made in a private setting. Do not be embarrassed to ask for payment for the valuable services that have been provided. Give each patient individual attention and personal consideration; also, be courteous and show a sincere desire to help the patient with financial problems.

CRITICAL THINKING 31.1

Adam Page comes to the front desk to pay his copay with a credit card. His card is declined. How can Sam handle the situation? What options could be offered to Mr. Page to make a payment at the time of service?

the total amount shown on the explanation of benefits (EOB) (Fig. 31.5). Adjustments must also be posted to the ledger and are discussed in the following section. Once the third party pays the insurance claim and adjustments have been made, if needed, the remaining balance is owed to the provider by the patient. This can be written as a formula:

Insurance payment amount + Adjustment amount
+ Patient responsibility = Total charged

VOCABULARY

explanation of benefits (EOB) A document sent by the insurance company to the provider and the patient explaining the allowed charge amount, the amount reimbursed for services, and the patient's financial responsibilities.

Posting Adjustments

Adjustments are used to either credit or debit a patient's account. A *credit adjustment* is posted to the patient's ledger when an amount needs to be subtracted from a patient's balance. An example would be when the provider's fee exceeds the amount allowed stated on the EOB. The difference between the billed amount and the allowed amount would need to be adjusted (written off). Credit adjustments should always be posted to the patient account

record at the same time as the payment. The patient ledger should have a column for the adjustments. *Remember: payments and credit adjustments are both credits.* Payments are money that is received in the healthcare facility, and credit adjustments simply reduce the balance that the patient owes on the account. When the payments and credit adjustments are subtracted from the charged amount, the balance is either the patient's responsibility or the amount billed to the secondary insurance.

Before continuing to post to the next EOB line item, confirm that the payment amount, the adjusted amount, and the patient responsibility/secondary insurance balance exactly match the amounts calculated on the EOB.

A *debit adjustment* is posted to the patient ledger when an amount needs to be added to the patient's balance but is not a charge for services. An example would be if a check the patient had written to the healthcare facility was returned for nonsufficient funds. The amount had initially been credited to the account, but the healthcare facility never actually got the funds. A debit adjustment must be made to add the amount of the check back to the patient's balance (Box 31.3 and Fig. 31.6).

CRITICAL THINKING 31.2

The bank calls Sam to inform her that three of the patient checks deposited last week were NSF. What steps should Sam take to collect the NSF check amounts from the patients? Are there additional charges she can add to the patients' balances to cover the inconvenience?

Credit Balances

A *credit balance* occurs when a patient has paid in advance, or an overpayment or duplicate payment is made. For example, an overpayment occurs if the patient makes a partial payment, and later the insurance payment is more than the remaining balance. When this happens, the patient account will show a credit balance, or the amount that the provider owes. The medical assistant should investigate to whom the credit balance is owed (i.e., the patient or the insurance company). The first place to look is

BOX 31.3   Nonsufficient Funds (NSF) Checks

Nonsufficient funds (NSF) checks occur when a patient pays with a check without having sufficient funds in the bank to cover the payment. The bank will return the check to the healthcare practice marked NSF and will charge the practice's bank account a returned check fee. The payment posted to the patient account must be reversed. It is important to note that the original payment is not deleted; instead, a charge line item is added to the patient account record with the amount of the NSF check. Many medical offices add additional line items for NSF fee charges, but this is up to the discretion of the provider.

If the healthcare facility receives NSF checks, call the signers of the checks immediately and ask them to stop by the office to pay the amount needed to cover the check and the additional fee. Most offices require that such payment be made by another form of payment, preferably credit card. Legal remedies are available for the provider if the check remains unpaid.

Many NSF problems can be cleared up quickly and easily with courtesy and tact, assuming the situation was simply a mistake or an oversight. Bad checks may be reported to several organizations, and once the writer is in their databases, the person will have difficulty writing a check to any business. Turn the account over to a qualified collection agency if you are unable to collect on the account within a short time.

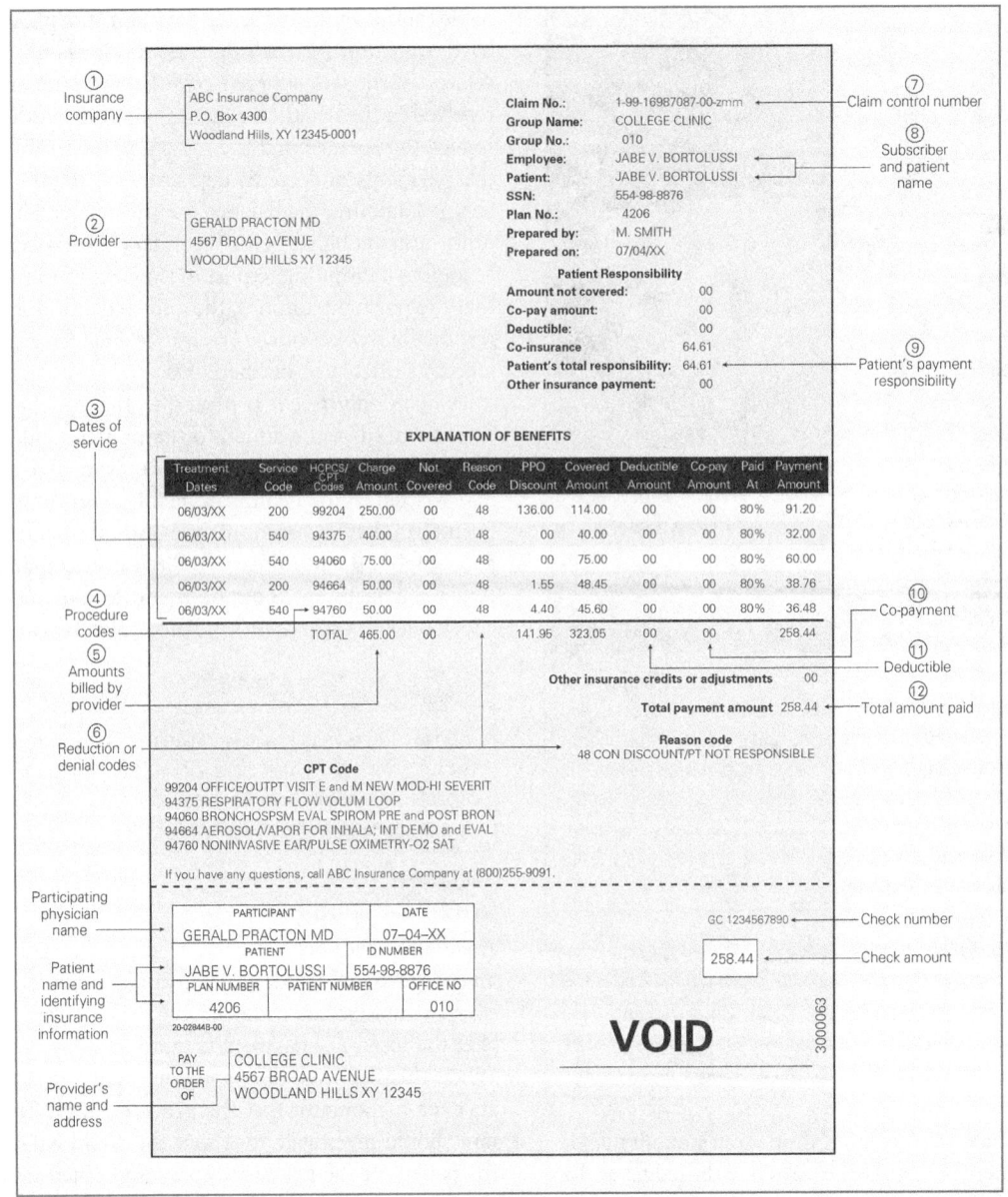

Fig. 31.5 **Explanation of Benefits (EOB).** (From Fordney WT: *Insurance handbook for the medical office,* ed 14, St. Louis, 2017, Elsevier.)

The healthcare facility receives two checks for a patient, Kelly Washington, from Blue Cross for the same date of service. One check is for $438, and the other is for $534. Can Sam post the larger payment and just refund the smaller payment to Blue Cross? What must Sam do before she posts either payment?

Sam received a claim denial for a patient, Clara Martin, for date of service 1/11/20XX. The denial stated that Ms. Martin was not covered on this date of service. Sam reviewed her notes in the patient's account and found the verification of eligibility that was done on 1/11/20XX for Clara Martin. What should Sam do to prepare to call the insurance company?

the EOB from the insurance company. This document shows the exact amount of the patient's financial responsibility. The medical assistant should confirm that all the line items match the corresponding amounts on the EOB because many credit balances are created when an error is made in payment posting. If the patient's payment exceeded the amount indicated on the EOB, the provider must send a check for the balance to the patient. A credit balance creates a *debit* in the patient account, or an amount that is due by the provider to the patient or the insurance company, depending on which party made the overpayment. A debit adjustment is done showing that the patient or insurance company was refunded. This debit adjustment should bring the account balance to zero.

Most patient account management software can enter charges, payments, and adjustments. As discussed previously, charges increase what is owed to the provider. Third-party and patient payments reduce what is owed to the provider. Adjustments can either increase or decrease what is owed to the provider.

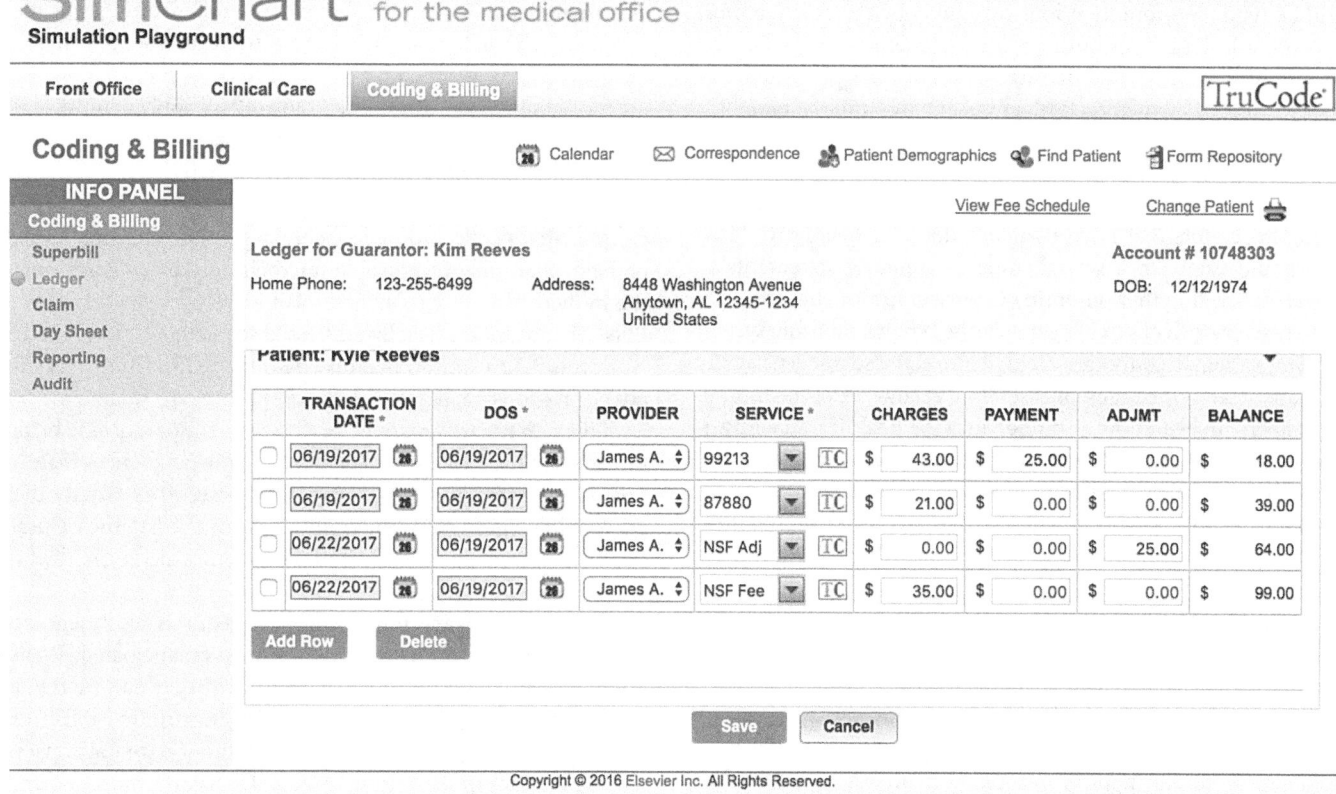

Fig. 31.6 Nonsufficient Funds Adjustments in SimChart for the Medical Office.

If a medical assistant has questions required a claim or payment from a third-party, a third-party representative can be contacted. Box 31.4 and Procedure 31.1 present tips for interacting with third-party representatives.

Payment Agreements

With the increase in high-deductible insurance plans, there has been an increase in the need for payment agreements. If the patient is having an elective procedure, payment can be made before or at the time of service. If the procedure or therapy is expensive, the patient may need to spread the payments out over time. Therefore the medical assistant must explain to the patient the fees and the office credit policies. In most healthcare practices, the appropriate staff member sits down with the patient for a financial consultation before a payment arrangement contract is offered. The payment arrangement contract states the monthly payment; how many months it must be paid; the payment due date; whether interest will be charged; and the penalties of nonpayment. If the patient is going to be making more than four payments, the Truth in Lending Act comes into play.

> **VOCABULARY**
> **interest** Money that is paid in exchange for borrowing or using another person's or organization's money.

Truth in Lending Act. It is considered an offer of credit when the healthcare facility allows the patient to make more than four payments on their balance. When offering credit options for patients, the healthcare facility should be in compliance

> **BOX 31.4 Interacting With Third-Party Representatives**
>
> Most health insurance companies offer an online provider web portal for verification of eligibility and claim status. However, in some circumstances medical assistants must speak with third-party representatives. This can be a time-consuming process involving waiting on hold for long periods. Nevertheless, medical assistants must interact professionally. Here are some tips for interacting with third-party representatives:
> - Before calling provider services, have all documents readily accessible to discuss the patient account.
> - When the representative answers, refrain from telling them how long the wait was; the person usually does not have much control over wait times.
> - Document the details of the phone conversation with the health insurance representative in the patient account record, including the representative's name and the date and time of the call.
> - If the conversation is a follow-up call, share the details collected from the previous call from notes documented in the patient account record.

with Regulation Z of the Truth in Lending Act (TILA). TILA is enforced by the Federal Trade Commission (FTC) and is part of the Consumer Credit Protection Act. TILA requires that individuals be provided certain information when credit is extended, including:

- the annual percentage rate (APR).
- the monthly interest rate.
- the total costs to the borrower.
- when payments are due.
- the amount of any late payment charges and when they will be applied.

If the healthcare facility and patient agree that payment will be made in more than four installments, the practice must provide a Federal Truth in Lending Statement (Fig. 31.7). This should be in place even if no finance fees are charged. The statement is signed by the practice's representative and the patient.

Monthly Patient Account Statements

Healthcare facilities should send monthly statements for all patient accounts that have a balance due. The healthcare facility should establish a set schedule for sending statements to patients. Sending them monthly is most common, but they can be sent every 2 weeks or even quarterly. When a monthly system is used, patient accounts are divided into equal segments, usually alphabetically. One segment is sent out each week of the month. This keeps an even flow of money into the healthcare facility. It can also spread out patients' calls about their statements.

Statements should be printed on clean, good-quality paper. Payment options, such as check, e-check, online payments, and/ or debit or credit card, should be presented clearly. The statement should provide itemized details on:

- Date(s) of service
- Services provided
- Insurance payments and adjustments
- Patient payments, including copayments

Envelopes should be printed with "Address Service Requested" in the appropriate place to maintain up-to-date mailing lists. A self-addressed return envelope included with the statement is convenient for the patient and encourages prompt payment. The statement should also indicate how old the balance is, such as 30, 60, 90, 120, or >120 days. For accounts that are more than 60 days past due, some offices apply neon-colored stickers to emphasize the need to pay the balance as soon as possible, thus avoiding further collection activity.

Billing Minors. According to federal regulations, minors cannot be held financially responsible for their account balance unless the individual is an emancipated (ih MAN suh pay tid) minor. Bills for minors are usually addressed to the **guarantor.** If a bill is addressed to a minor, parents could take the attitude that they are not responsible because they never received a statement.

If the parents are separated or divorced, the parent who brings the child in for treatment is responsible for payment. Whatever financial agreement exists between the parents is strictly their personal business and should not concern the healthcare practice. The responsible parent should be so informed from the first appointment.

If a minor appears in the office and requests treatment, you should determine if the person is legally emancipated. If they are, they will be financially responsible. Minors can be treated for certain conditions, such as sexually transmitted infections (STIs), pregnancy, and birth control, without parental consent. State laws differ in these cases. Medical assistants must be familiar with their state laws and office polices to determine where the statement should be sent.

> **VOCABULARY**
> **emancipated minor** A minor who has been granted emancipation by the court; the minor can assume the rights and responsibilities of adulthood.
> **indigent** Poor, needy, impoverished.

Medical Care for Those Who Cannot Pay. The medical profession traditionally has accepted the responsibility of providing medical care occasionally for individuals who are unable to pay for these services. There are government programs to help care for the medically indigent (IN di juh nt), but there are still patients who are not covered. In many instances, medical care for the indigent is available through social service agencies. Medical assistants should learn about local organizations and agencies that can aid patients in obtaining the necessary assistance. The provider can provide only medical services. Other agencies can:

- help pay for hospitalization.
- arrange for and help pay for special therapy, rehabilitation, or medications.

Unfortunately, another segment of the population consists of uninsured or underinsured employees who are not eligible for public assistance, are not covered under a group policy, and cannot afford the high premiums for private medical insurance. Give special attention to helping these people arrange payment of their medical bills. If a provider knows in advance that a patient cannot pay for services and decides to still provide care, complete records must still be kept on the patient. The only

---

Walden-Martin Family Medical Clinic
1234 Anystreet, Anytown AL 12345-1234

Telephone 123-123-1234

FEDERAL TRUTH IN LENDING STATEMENT
For professional services rendered

Patient ___Quinton Brown___
Address ___4554 Browning Street Anytown,___
___AL 12345-1234___
Parent _____

1. Cash Price (fee for service)	$	1200.00
2. Cash Down Payment	$	200.00
3. Unpaid Balance of Cash Price	$	1000.00
4. Amount Financed	$	1000.00
5. FINANCE CHARGE	$	–0–
6. Finance Charge Expressed As Annual Percentage Rate		–0–
7. Total of Payments (4 plus 5)	$	1000.00
8. Deferred Payment Price (1 plus 5)	$	1000.00

"Total payment due" (7 above) is payable to _James A. Martin MD Taylor_ at above office address in __five__ monthly installments of $ _200.00_. The first installment is payable on __May 1__ 20 _xx_, and each subsequent payment is due on the same day of each consecutive month until paid in full.

___4-15-20xx___   ___Quinton Brown___
Date   Signature of Patient; Parent if Patient is a Minor

FORM 9402 COLWELL SYSTEMS, INC., CHAMPAIGN, ILLINOIS

Fig. 31.7 Truth in Lending Statement. (Courtesy Colwell Systems, Champaign, IL.)

difference in procedure is that an adjustment would be made to the account so that the balance would be zero.

Fees in hardship cases. Sometimes a healthcare practice is faced with the problem of deciding whether to reduce or cancel a fee in a hardship case. Before adjusting or canceling a fee, the provider or medical assistant should have a frank discussion with the patient about their financial situation. Find out whether the patient is entitled to or qualifies for medical assistance. If the patient's injuries are the result of a car accident, there may be medical insurance through the automobile policy. The patient may qualify for local or state public assistance, such as crime victim assistance. Maintain information about such agencies in the area and direct the patient to the appropriate one.

If the provider is aware of the hardship before services are provided, the fee can be discussed, and payment arrangements made. The healthcare facility may suggest that a medically indigent patient seek care at a clinic that provides public assistance. Providers should be free to choose their form of charity and should not feel obligated to substantially reduce or cancel a fee when the circumstances are known in advance.

The provider and the patient may agree on a fee, but special circumstances may come up that create a hardship. If the provider agrees to reduce the fee, the patient should be told that the reduction will occur only after the adjusted amount is paid in full. For instance, if a fee of $500 is reduced to $350, the full amount of the $500 charge should appear on the ledger, and when $350 has been received, the remainder can be written off as an adjustment.

Make fee reductions the exception rather than the norm. Problems can come up when a provider begins to reduce the fees. Patients may begin to expect fees to be reduced in all circumstances. Take great care in reducing the fee for care of a patient who dies. This could be misinterpreted and result in a suit for malpractice. The family may suspect that the fee was reduced because the provider knew they made an error.

Collection Procedures

Collection is the process of using all legal resources available to collect payment for past due patient account balances. Sometimes patients may have difficulty meeting all of their financial obligations. The patient may have lost a job or insurance coverage. An emergency could arise that depletes finances. When patients must choose between paying their medical bills and having electricity, the provider is often forced to wait for payment. Although a few patients absolutely refuse to pay for their medical care, most are honest and willing to pay but may need help with a payment plan. As discussed earlier, terms can be arranged for collecting payment in full when the office and the patient cooperate with each other. The medical assistant should attempt to work out a plan that the patient can abide by, and the patient should be expected to make promised payments. For those patients who do not pay their bill, further action is necessary.

Fair Debt Collection Practice Act. The Fair Debt Collection Practices Act (FDCPA) is designed to eliminate abusive, deceptive, and unfair debt collection practices. If the medical assistant is responsible for collection practices, it is important that the FDCPA is followed. Fair debt collection practices under the FDCPA include:

- Collection calls cannot be made before 8 a.m. and after 9 p.m. in most states, unless the person as agreed to it.
- Calls cannot be made to place of employment if the people indicated they are not allowed to get calls there.
- The person can send a letter by mail to ask for contact to stop. The healthcare facility can confirm it received the letter and what action it will be taking; all other contact must stop.
- If the debtor is represented by an attorney, the healthcare facility cannot communicate to the debtor regarding the debt.
- Within 5 days from first contact with the debtor, the healthcare facility must send a written validation notice indicating the amount of money owed, the name of the creditor, and what to do if the person does not think the debt is theirs.
- Collectors cannot threaten violence or harm, use obscene or profane language, or repeatedly use the phone to annoy the person.

The statute of limitations (SOL) of the FDCPA determines the length of time a debt collector can collect an unpaid balance. The SOL varies by state and is usually between 3 and 6 years. If the SOL expires, the debt collector cannot pursue the person owing the money.

Preparing Patient Accounts for Collection Activity. Before you begin collection action, it is essential to determine which accounts have a balance due and how old the account balance is. Some accounts are grouped together, or "aged," according to the dates of the last payment activity, whereas others are grouped according to the original date of service (Fig. 31.8). Common account aging categories are:

- Current
- 31–60 days
- 61–90 days
- 91–120 days
- >120 days

Most bills with balances less than 30 days old are probably waiting for the health insurance to pay, so no collection action is needed. Patient account balances more than 90 or 120 days old require a final demand letter before the account is turned over to a collection agency. Always allow the provider to review and approve the list of patient accounts being sent to a collection agency.

The medical assistant can use a variety of techniques to collect patient accounts, such as collection phone calls, collection letters, emails, and text messages. Often more than one technique must be used to obtain payment. Always be courteous and kind when using all collection techniques.

Collection Telephone Calls. Whenever attempts are made to collect a debt, the Fair Debt Collection Practices Act must be kept in mind. A telephone call at the right time, with the right presentation, is more successful than notes, patient account statements, or collection letters. The personal contact call often prompts patients to mail in their payment or to make payments over the phone with a credit card. If the staff does not have enough time to make calls, the collection letter is the next best approach. If collections are a serious problem, it may be worth an extra salary to hire a person to make the phone calls.

Patient Account Aging Report: Walden-Martin Family Medical Clinic
Starting Date: 9/1/2017   Ending Date: 9/30/2017   Report Date 9/30/2017

Jacob Abraham (3406) — Guarantor: Self — Last Payment: 7/12/2017 15.00 — Home: 954-233-9033 Work: NA

Date	Code	Billed	Current	31–60	61–90	91–120	>120	Total
7/12/2017	99201	45.00			45.00			45.00
7/12/2017	Cash	(15.00)			(15.00)			(15.00)
Patient Total		30.00	0.00	0.00	30.00	0.00	0.00	30.00

Frank Bullock (3412) — Guarantor: Wife — Last Payment: 8/20/2017 45.00 — Home 954-388-0196 Work: 954-233-5803

Date	Code	Billed	Current	31–60	61–90	91–120	>120	Total
8/20/2017	99205	195.00		195.00				195.00
8/20/2017	Check	(45.00)		(45.00)				(45.00)
Patient Total		150.00	0.00	150.00	0.00	0.00	0.00	150.00

Cynthia Dearing (3433) — Guarantor: Self — Last Payment: 7/25/2017 10.00 — Home: 953-518-2100 Work: 954-333-9003

Date	Code	Billed	Current	31–60	61–90	91–120	>120	Total
6/12/2017	99386	185.00				185.00		185.00
7/15/2017	BCBS	(160.00)				(160.00)		(160.00)
7/25/2017	Check	(10.00)				(10.00)		(10.00)
Patient Total		15.00	0.00	0.00	0.00	15.00	0.00	15.00

Kirsha Macken (3462) — Guarantor: Parent — Last Payment: 7/10/2017 50.00 — Home: 954-736-7227 Work: FT Student

Date	Code	Billed	Current	31–60	61–90	91–120	>120	Total
4/23/2017	58900	230.00					230.00	230.00
4/23/2017	Cash	(50.00)					(50.00)	(50.00)
7/10/2017	99214	90.00			90.00			90.00
7/10/2017	90658	30.00			30.00			30.00
7/10/2017	Cash	(50.00)			(50.00)			(50.00)
Patient Total		250.00	0.00	0.00	70.00	0.00	180.00	250.00

Larry Nerod (3501) — Guarantor: Self — Last Payment: 6/22/2017 15.00 — Home: 953-736-7227 Work: 954-332-001

Date	Code	Billed	Current	31–60	61–90	91–120	>120	Total
6/22/2017	99204	140.00				140.00		140.00
6/22/2017	CCard	(15.00)				(15.00)		(15.00)
Patient Total		125.00	0.00	0.00	0.00	125.00	0.00	125.00

Emanuel Perez (3513) — Guarantor: Self — Last Payment: 7/12/2017 46.00 — Home: 956-303-2070 Work: 953-322-5500

Date	Code	Billed	Current	31–60	61–90	91–120	>120	Total
7/12/2017	68500	403.00			403.00			403.00
7/12/2017	Check	(46.00)			(46.00)			(46.00)
Patient Total		357.00	0.00	0.00	357.00	0.00	0.00	357.00

			Current	31–60	61–90	91–120	>120	Total
Report Totals			0.00	150.00	457.00	140.00	180.00	927.00
Percent of Total			0.00%	16.18%	49.3%	15.10%	19.41%	100.00%

Fig. 31.8 Sample Aging Report.

Make the call in private and have the patient's financial record and insurance information available. Call only between 8 a.m. and 9 p.m. Determine the identity of the person with whom you are speaking. Use the person's full name. Include suffixes, such as "Thomas Melborn, III." This may sound too formal, but it helps to ensure that the correct person is on the phone. Be respectful. One can be friendly and professional at the same time. After a brief greeting, state the purpose of the call. Make no apology for calling, but state the reason in a friendly, businesslike way. Ask the patient whether it is a convenient time to talk. Open the call with a phrase such as, "This is Alice, Dr. Walden's medical assistant. I'm calling about your account." A well-placed pause at this point in the call sometimes gets an immediate response from the debtor with regard to the nonpayment. Keep the conversation brief and to the point; do not make threats of any kind. The medical assistant can offer payment plans but must follow the facility's policies. Try to get a definite commitment – payment of a certain amount by a certain date. Document the call in the patient's record. Follow up on promises made by the patient. Before a final demand for payment is made, a letter must be sent indicating that legal or collection proceedings will be started.

> **VOCABULARY**
>
> **salary** A fixed compensation periodically paid to a person for regular work.

Collection Letters. Some experts believe that a printed collection letter or reminder enclosed with a statement is more effective than a personal letter. Letters that are friendly requests for an explanation of why payment has not been made are effective in most cases. These letters should indicate that the provider is sincerely interested in the patient's health and well-being and wants to help resolve the financial obligation. Invite the patient to the office to explain the reasons for nonpayment so that payment arrangements can be made. To lessen the patient's embarrassment, these letters can suggest that previous statements may have been overlooked.

When receiving these letters, most patients make some effort to explain their failure to make payment. If a patient really is having financial difficulties, they may be able to get some type of assistance. If it is a temporary financial problem, the provider and the patient may work together to come up with a satisfactory installment plan for payment.

The medical assistant is often given a free hand in designing collection patterns and composing collection letters. Many medical assistants compose a series of collection letters using example letters they have found effective. Such a series usually includes at least five letters in varying degrees of forcefulness. The medical assistant should sign the letter. Do not put "collections" in a reference or subject line, because it can be confused with a collection agency.

Sometimes even people with poor paying habits will pay, as long as they are treated with respect and consideration. The medical assistant should never go beyond the authority granted by the provider in pursuing collections. If questions come up about special collection problems, always check with the provider or office manager before proceeding. The provider and the medical assistant should agree on general collection policies. In all cases when an account is to be assigned to a collection agency, make sure the provider is aware and approves.

Personal Finance Interviews. Personal finance interviews with patients can sometimes be more effective than a whole series of collection letters. Often speaking with a patient face-to-face can result in a better understanding of the problem, and an agreement about future payment plans can be reached. When it is known in advance that the patient requires extensive treatment, the matter of payment should be discussed early in the course of treatment. The credit policy should be explained, and some agreement should be reached on a payment plan.

Because medical services are far more intangible (in TAN juh buhl) than any commercial service, collection efforts must not be delayed too long. Most responsible, sincere patients will call the provider's office after receiving a second statement and explain the delay in payment or ask for a payment plan. This is best accomplished in a private, personal interview.

If the account ultimately must be referred to a collection agency, find a good agency with a high recovery rate. All collection activity is costly. Know when to stop and call on the services of a professional collection agency.

Special Collection Situations

Tracing skips. When a patient account statement is returned marked "Moved—no forwarding address," you may consider this account a *skip*. This could be an innocent error on the part of the patient, who may have forgotten to provide a forwarding address to the post office. The patient could also be attempting to avoid liability for debts. Whichever is the case, immediate action should be taken. Do not wait until the next billing cycle to attempt to trace the debtor.

The medical assistant can:
- Use the online white pages or social networking sites, such as Facebook, to search for the patient's name.
- Review the patient's original office registration card.
- Call the telephone number listed in the patient account record. Occasionally a patient may move without leaving a forwarding address but will transfer the old telephone number.
- Check the guarantor's place of employment for information.

Investigate the search results carefully so that collection efforts are directed at the right person. If all attempts fail, turn the account over to a collection agency without delay. Do not keep a skip account too long because as time passes, the trail may become so cold that even collection experts would not be able to follow it.

Claims against estates. The patient account for a deceased patient may be handled a little differently from regular accounts. Courtesy dictates that a bill should not be sent immediately, but do not delay longer than 30 days. The executor will expect to receive the statements from all healthcare providers. Use the following format to address the statement:
- Estate of (name of patient)
- c/o (spouse, next of kin, or executor if known)
- Patient's last known address

A will generally is filed within 30 days of a death. The name of the executor usually can be obtained by sending a request to the Probate Department of the Superior Court, County Recorder's Office, in the county where the person lived. The time limits for filing an estate claim are determined by the state where the person resided.

An itemized statement should be sent to the executor of the estate by certified mail, return receipt requested. If no response is received in 10 days, contact the executor or the county clerk where the estate is being settled and obtain forms for filing a claim against the estate. This claim against the estate must be made within a certain time. This time frame varies from 2 to 36 months, depending on the state where it is filed.

The executor of the estate either accepts or rejects the claim. If it is accepted, the executor will send an acknowledgment of the debt. Payment can be delayed because of the legal complications involved in settling an estate. If the claim has been accepted, the provider eventually receives the payment. If the executor rejects the claim, file a claim against the executor according to state laws. The time limit in such cases starts with the date on the letter of rejection.

States have different time limits and statutes with regard to these issues. The medical assistant should contact the provider's attorney or the local court for the exact procedure to follow. The provider may prefer to turn such matters over to their legal counsel immediately.

Bankruptcy. *Bankruptcy* is a federally authorized procedure in which people are legally declared unable to meet their debts. Bankruptcy laws were passed to ensure equal distribution of the assets of an individual among the individual's creditors. These are federal laws that apply in all the states. When notified that a patient has declared bankruptcy, do not send statements or make any attempt to collect on the account from the patient.

Chapter 7 bankruptcy is usually a "no asset" situation. Because the provider's charges are considered an unsecured debt, there is little purpose in pursuing collection. Chapter 13 is known as wage-earner bankruptcy, which means that the patient-debtor pays to a trustee a fixed amount agreed upon by the court. This money is passed on to the creditors. During this period, none of the creditors can attach the debtor's wages or otherwise attempt to collect the debt. However, the debts are paid in order, secured debts first. Consequently, the provider may never receive payment from a debtor who has filed for bankruptcy.

VOCABULARY

executor An individual assigned to make financial decisions about the estate of a deceased patient.
intangible Something of value that cannot be touched physically.
trustee The coordinator of financial resources assigned by the court during a bankruptcy case.
unsecured debt Debt that is not guaranteed by something of value; credit card debt is the most common type of unsecured debt.

Using a Collection Agency. The medical assistant should try every means possible to collect on accounts before they become delinquent. An account should be sent to a collection agency as soon all collection activities have been exhausted. If the patient has failed to respond to the final letter or has twice failed to send a promised payment, the account should be considered uncollectable. Skips should be sent immediately.

Even though the collection agency will keep 40% to 60% of the amount owed, waiting only reduces the chances of recovery by the professional collector. If the healthcare facility finds that the case deserves special consideration, it will ask the provider's advice before proceeding further.

The collection agency represents the healthcare facility. Therefore the healthcare facility should ensure that its patients are treated with as much respect and dignity as possible throughout the collection process. There are many different collection agencies. If one does not work out, prepare to switch to another that can better represent the healthcare practice.

A collection agency needs certain data to begin collection procedures on overdue accounts:

- Guarantor's full name
- Spouse's full name
- Last known address
- Full amount of the debt
- Date of the last entry (charge, payment, or adjustment) on the account
- Occupation of the debtor
- Employer's address and phone number

When an account goes to collections, many healthcare agencies will zero out the patient's ledger and indicate the amount was turned over to collections. The zero balance can be achieved by posting a negative adjustment, which would be subtracted from the balance, and indicating it was a collection write-off. This prevents the debt from appearing on the A/R report and statements from being sent to the patient. The account should be flagged, which can be done in billing software.

The healthcare facility can make no further collection attempts. Refer the patient to the collection agency if they contact the office about the account. Promptly report any payments made directly to your office to the collection agency and pay the collection agency's fee.

Posting collection agency transactions. The healthcare facility pays the collection agency a percentage, usually between 25% to 50% of the amount collected. The healthcare facility may also pay a fee for each account managed by the collection agency along with a communication fee (e.g. a charge for each call or letter sent to the debtor). The older the account, the higher the collection agency's fee may be. Some debts can also be purchased by collection agencies for cents on the dollar.

The collection agency deducts its fees from the total money collected and pays the remaining amount (netback) back to the healthcare facility. When posting the collected amount to the patient's ledger, the medical assistant must first post an adjustment for the amount send to the collection agency, if the account was zeroed out. Next the medical assistant must post the payment from the collection agency and a credit adjustment for the collection agency's fees. For instance, a collection agency charges 50% of the balance collected. The collection agency collects a $62.80 payment and sends the healthcare facility a $31.40 payment. The collection agency keeps $31.40 to cover its fees. The medical assistant posts the $31.40 payment to the patient's ledger and adds a $31.40 credit adjustment. If the initial balance due was $62.80, the balance would now be zero (Fig. 31.9; see Procedure 31.3).

Small Claims Court. Many healthcare facilities find small claims court a satisfactory, inexpensive means of collecting delinquent accounts. State law places a limit on the amount of debt for which relief may be sought in small claims court. This limit should be determined before the small claims court process is started.

Parties to small claims actions are not represented by an attorney at the hearing but may send another person to court on their behalf to produce records supporting the claim. Providers often send their medical assistant with records of unpaid accounts to show the judge.

If the court awards a judgment for the amount owed, the plaintiff in small claims court may also recover the costs of the suit. For a very small investment in time and money, the provider who uses this method saves the time of a civil court action and eliminates attorneys' fees.

After being awarded a judgment, the healthcare facility must still collect the money. The only person in a small claims action who has the right of appeal is the defendant. An appeal by the defendant may have the judgment set aside. The plaintiff cannot file an appeal in a small claims action; the decision of the court is final.

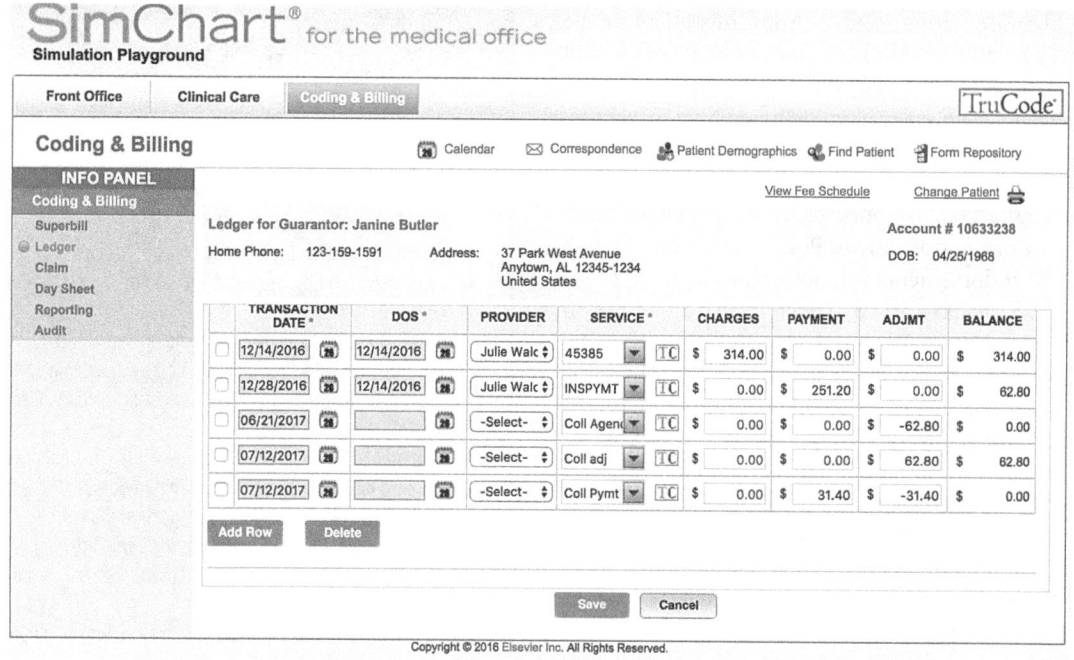

Fig. 31.9 Posting A Collection Agency Payment in SimChart for the Medical Office.

The necessary papers for filing action and full instructions on the course to follow may be obtained from the clerk of the local small claims court. It would be wise for a medical assistant who has never appeared in court to attend once as a spectator to preview the procedure; this should allow them to feel more at ease when appearing for the provider.

Patient Payment Management

Cash Payments. Some patients may prefer to pay in cash instead of by check or debit or credit card. Cash transactions can occur with little or no paperwork; therefore an audit trail is harder to establish.

To prevent the mismanagement of cash, many healthcare facilities do not allow patients to pay cash for services. Healthcare facilities that have a no-cash payment policy should post a sign in the lobby to inform patients of this in advance. If a patient does not have a bank account, the medical staff can kindly refer the patient to a local money order dealer. Patients may see this as an inconvenience, but the medical assistant should explain that the policy is intended to protect the patient's account.

If your healthcare facility chooses to accept cash payments, keep in mind the following precautions:
- Make sure the cash is not counterfeit (KOWN ter fit). Use a marker or tool designed for this purpose to confirm its authenticity. If you suspect that the cash may be counterfeit,

do not accept the payment, and contact the local law enforcement office.
- Establish a checks-and-balance system in which the employee accepting cash must document cash payments on a register and in the patient's account to establish an audit trail.
- Inform patients that change cannot be made for larger bills.

Checks. Most payments sent through the mail are in the form of a personal check. Patients may also write a check when they are making a payment at the time of service. If it is the healthcare facility's policy to accept checks, then certain precautions need to be taken:
- Inspect the check carefully for the correct date, amount, and signature.
- Do not accept a check with corrections on it.
- Ask for a state-issued picture ID and compare the signature on the ID to the check signature.
- Do not accept a government check, payroll check, unnumbered check, or a non-personalized check, such as a starter check. When a person opens a new checking account, starter checks will be used until the regular checks are printed. Starter checks have low check numbers and do not include the person's personal information. Starter checks may not have the name and address of the financial institution.
- Do not accept a third-party check. For example, Mrs. Richards, a patient, receives a check written to her by her neighbor for $30. Mrs. Richards brings the check to her visit with the provider and presents it to the clinic to pay her copayment. If the check is accepted and subsequently returned by

the bank, obtaining reimbursement from the patient or the neighbor may be difficult. A check from the patient's health insurance carrier is the only exception.

- The facility may have special guidelines about accepting out-of-town checks. They may accept checks from nearby locations.
- When accepting a postal money order for payment, make sure it has only one endorsement. Postal money orders with more than two endorsements will not be honored.
- Do not accept a check marked "Payment in Full" unless it does pay the account in full, up to and including the date on which it is received. If a check so marked is less than the amount due, you will be unable to collect the balance on the account once you have accepted and deposited such a check. It is illegal to cross out the words "Payment in Full."
- Do not accept a check written for more than the amount due; returning cash for the difference between the amount of the check and the amount owed is poor policy. If the check is not honored by the bank, your office suffers the loss not only of the amount of the check, but also of the amount returned in cash.

CRITICAL THINKING 31.6

A new patient wants to pay for his services at the end of the office visit. The charge is $75. The patient writes a check for $100 and asks Sam for $25 in currency in return. How should Sam handle the situation?

Debit Cards and Credit Cards. Most debit cards are connected to a checking account. When the debit card is used, the amount of the transaction is immediately withdrawn from the available balance in the account. A personal identification number (PIN) is assigned to the card for cash withdrawal and point-of-sale (POS) purchases. The cards usually have a MasterCard or Visa logo and can be used wherever they are accepted. In most situations, when there are not enough funds in the account to make a purchase, the card is declined unless the account has some type of overdraft protection. Substantial fees may be charged if the bank elects to pay the debit when the account has insufficient funds. The medical assistant may see various types of debit cards in the provider's office (Box 31.5). Many states issue a debit card to individuals receiving child support payments or some types of state financial assistance.

Credit cards are a common method of payment from patients. Drawbacks of credit card payments include the small processing fee that is deducted from the amount deposited into the healthcare facility's bank account. There is also an increased risk of fraud with credit cards.

To help reduce fraud, magnetic strip cards are being replaced with cards imbedded with EMV chip technology. These chip cards offer advanced security for in-person payments, but the EMV chip cards require a special terminal to read the chips. If a healthcare facility accepts credit or debit cards, it is important to have a terminal that processes the EMV chip cards. Businesses that cannot process the chip cards may be liable for fraud losses to their customers.

Many credit card processing terminals can accept both credit cards and debit cards, and some can also process check

BOX 31.5   Precautions for Accepting Credit and Debit Cards

Just as the medical assistant must take precautions when accepting checks, care must be taken when accepting a credit or debit card as payment for medical services. These guidelines help prevent credit card and debit card fraud:

- Check the person's photo ID with every credit or debit card transaction. The person's name on the ID must match the name on the card. Follow the healthcare facility's policy on verifying identity if the name on the state-issued ID does not match the name on the credit card.
- Accept EMV chip cards.
- Swipe credit or debit cards, insert chip cards into the reader, or tap chip cards to the reader. Do not accept cards that cannot be tapped, inserted, or swiped. Just typing in a credit or debit card number can increase the risk for fraud.
- Use Address Verification Service (AVS). The financial facility issuing the card confirms the person's billing address. If the address does not match, the medical assistant can decline the card.
- Review the receipt to ensure that the cardholder's name, last four digits of the account number, and the signature on the card matches the credit or debit card information.

Some patients may use a prepaid credit card, which is purchased with cash and does not have the patient's name printed on it, to make payments on their accounts. These cards, if allowed by office policy, work a lot like a debit card.

If you suspect fraud is occurring, follow the healthcare facility's policy. The card issuer's authorization center should be called. State "code 10 authorization request" to the operator. If the patient presenting the card is nearby, "code 10" will alert the operator to ask "yes" or "no" questions. Keep calm and avoid alarming the patient. If a patient becomes belligerent (buh LIG er ent) about the card transaction, refer the person to the office manager.

payments electronically. Debit card transactions use a PIN but do not need a patient's signature. Credit card transactions do not need a PIN, but patients may need to sign.

Near field communication (NFC) is wireless technology that enables short-range communication between compatible devices. The NFC technology is used with contactless payment systems. Payments can be made when a phone, watch, or other device, linked to a credit or debit card, is placed near the processing terminal (Fig. 31.10). If office policy allows this type of payment to be made, special equipment will be purchased to accommodate it.

Although using the credit card processing terminal incurs per-transaction charges, valuable time is saved because an office employee does not need to visit the bank branch to make the daily deposit. Debit and credit card transactions also can reduce the chances of money mismanagement in the office, such as embezzlement (Box 31.6).

VOCABULARY

belligerent Hostile and aggressive.

embezzlement The misuse of funds for personal gain.

EMV chip technology Global technology that includes embedded microchips that store and protect cardholder data; also called *chip and PIN* and *chip and signature*.

fidelity bond An insurance policy that protects an employer for loss resulting from a fraudulent or dishonest act by an employee.

surety bond A surety agency guarantees payment of a sum of money to a third party in the event the client fails to fulfill certain obligations.

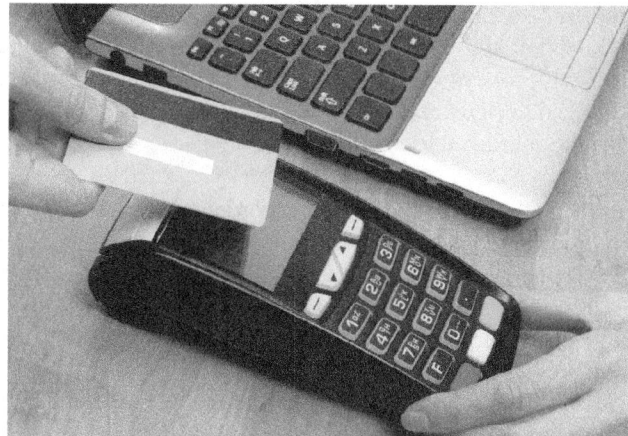

Fig. 31.10 Paying With A Contactless Credit Card With Near Field Communication (NFC) Technology. (ratmaner/iStock.com.)

BOX 31.6 Bonding

When an employee is responsible for handling money in the ambulatory care facility, the facility should carry a special business insurance called a **fidelity bond**. A fidelity bond provides the facility protection against the losses incurred from an employee's fraudulent or wrongful acts. A fidelity bond can protect against physical and monetary losses. It is part of the facility's risk management strategy plan.

When an employee commits a wrongful act, the ambulatory care facility may be exposed to legal or financial penalties. The fidelity bond covers such damages. Other actions that are covered by fidelity bonds include:

- Acts of forgery
- Robbery and burglary of the safe
- Destruction of company property
- Illicit transfer of funds
- Theft from the business or from patients

Some ambulatory care facilities may require employees who handle financial transactions to purchase and carry a surety bond. *Surety* is a person or an organization that agrees to take legal responsibility for another person's debt. A **surety bond** provides security against losses incurred when an employee steals from the facility.

Online Payment Options. Many offices choose to accept payment online. Patients can use their patient portal to make payments by debit or credit card, electronic check, or direct transfer. If your office uses this for payments, it should be noted in patients' bills, so they know they have this option for payments.

ACCOUNTS PAYABLE

Managing accounts payable may be the responsibility of the medical assistant. There are many aspects of accounts payable, which will be discussed in the next section.

Banking in Today's Business World

Banks can be used to centralize all financial transactions for a healthcare facility. The bank account tracks all deposits, withdrawals, and transfers. Monthly bank account balances can help healthcare facilities establish and maintain a monthly operational budget. Banks also provide opportunities to earn interest and to invest for future financial gain. Overall, banks organize funds for the financial management of the healthcare facility.

Fees for banking services depend on the bank and services used (Table 31.2). The type of bank the medical practice will use is a decision made by the provider and the office manager, depending on the needs of the medical practice.

Congress created the Federal Reserve Banking System, which monitors the movement of money, in the form of checks, from one bank account to another. A *routing transit number* (RTN) is a nine-digit code printed on the bottom left side of checks. An RTN is assigned to every banking institution under the Federal Reserve Banking System. It identifies the bank upon which the check was drawn. RTNs are also used for direct deposits and the transfer of funds between banks. The first two digits indicate the Federal Reserve district where the bank is located. The third digit indicates the specific district office. And the rest of the digits represent the individual accounts that belong to the bank. Bank account numbers are assigned to each individual account. No two account numbers in the same financial institution can be the same. Although the Federal Reserve Bank (Fig. 31.11) manages all banks in the United States, healthcare facilities can choose from a number of different types of banks with which to do business.

- *Retail banks*: Offer basic banking services to the public; these banks have hundreds of branches to provide easy consumer access.
- *Commercial banks*: Offer business banking services to businesses of all sizes; they are equipped to handle large volumes of check deposits and credit card transactions.
- *Credit unions*: Nonprofit banking institutions owned by members; credit unions use the funds deposited to make loans to their members, which enables them to offer loans at lower than market rates.
- *Online banks*: Offer basic banking services at competitive rates because all banking transactions are done online; there are no branch locations to visit.

The medical assistant will most likely manage only the bank accounts set up for the income and operational expenses of the healthcare facility.

Common Types of Bank Accounts

Checking accounts. By placing an amount of money in a bank, a depositor can set up a checking account. Simply stated, a checking account is a bank account against which checks can be written, or debit cards used, and funds can be transferred to the payable party. Banks typically charge a monthly account maintenance fee. In addition, there may be fees associated with banking services, such as transferring funds to other banks or using the checking overdraft (see Table 31.2).

Savings account. Money that is not needed for current expenses can be deposited into a savings account. In most cases, savings accounts earn a higher interest rate than checking accounts. Interest rates fluctuate with the financial market.

A standard savings account earns interest at the lowest prevailing rate and has no minimum balance requirement and no check-writing privileges. However, penalties apply for withdrawing funds from a savings account more than six times per month. The provider may deposit a certain percentage of discretionary income into a savings account each month to earn interest. The money in a savings account can be transferred to a checking account when needed.

Money market savings account. An insured money market savings account combines features of checking and savings accounts. A minimum balance is required (anywhere from $500 to $5,000). It earns interest at money market rates (usually a higher percentage rate than for a regular savings account), and it allows only a specified number of checks (frequently three) to be written per month. Such checks are usually written to transfer funds to a checking account. Some businesses transfer excess funds from the business checking account to a money market account over the weekend or over an extended holiday period to earn higher interest on the funds.

Signature Cards. When an account is opened at a bank branch, any account signers are required to provide their handwritten signatures on a physical or electronic card, which is kept on file with the bank. If a check comes through and some suspicion arises that the depositor's signature has been forged, bank personnel compare the signature on the check with the original on the signature card.

The task of paying bills is often delegated to a responsible medical assistant. In this case, any staff member who has been authorized to sign the healthcare facility's checks must go to the bank and add their handwritten signature to the signature card. Only those whose names appear on the signature card are authorized to sign checks, and the bank is responsible for verifying any questionable signatures.

Checks. A *check* is a bank draft, or an order to pay a certain sum of money, on demand to a specified person or entity. When a check is presented for payment, the *drawee* (the bank on which the check is drawn or written) pays the specified sum of money written on the face of the check to the *holder* (the person presenting the check for payment).

A check is considered a negotiable (ni GOH shee uh buhl) instrument. For a check to be negotiable, it must:

- be written and signed by the drawer (the person who writes the check).
- contain a promise or order to pay a sum of money.
- be payable on demand or at a fixed future date.

The check should have the amount written as a number and as text to confirm the amount. Finally, the check must be signed and dated by the drawer of the account.

VOCABULARY

discretionary income Money in a bank account that is not assigned to pay for any office expenses.

negotiable instrument A document guaranteeing payment of a specific amount of money to the payer named on the document.

TABLE 31.2   Common Banking Fees

Fee	Description	Average Fee	Waivable?
Monthly maintenance fee	Fee for using the bank account	$0 to $35 per month	Some bank accounts waive monthly account maintenance fees if a specific balance is maintained in the account or if direct deposit is used.
Overdraft fee	Fee for the bank paying a check or debit when the balance is not in the account	$25 to $40 per occurrence	Not usually. To avoid the fee in the future, tie the checking account with an overdraft account just in case the balance is low.
Returned deposit fee	Fee charged when a deposited check is returned from the drawer's account	$5 to $10 per occurrence	Not usually. However, the practice can require the check drawer to cover this expense because the check did not clear their account.
Hard copy statement fee	Fee for the bank to send paper copies of bank statements	$5 to $10 per statement	This fee can be avoided by downloading all electronic bank statements when they are released.
Nonsufficient funds (NSF) fee	Fee charged when a check is written against an account with not enough funds and the check is returned unpaid	$25 to $40 per occurrence	Not usually. To avoid the fee in the future, tie the checking account with an overdraft account just in case the balance is low.
Transaction fee	Fee charged when too many transactions are made on a bank account	$.50 to $1 per transaction	Online banking is usually free, but nowadays banks are charging fees to visit bank branches and to complete transactions with customer service over the phone.

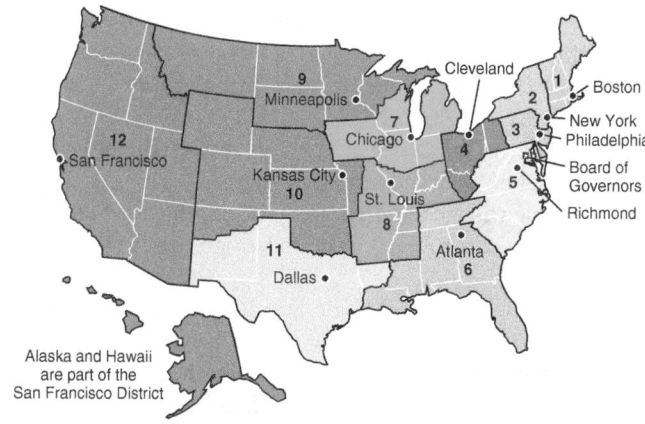

Fig. 31.11 The 12 Federal Reserve Districts. (From Niedzwiecki B, et al: *Kinn's the medical assistant,* ed 14, St. Louis, 2020, Elsevier.)

Types of negotiable instruments. There are several types of negotiable instruments.

- *Personal check*: Drawn by a bank against funds deposited to a personal account in another bank. May be used by patients for copayments and other financial responsibilities.
- *Cashier's check*: A bank's own check, drawn on itself and signed by the bank cashier or other authorized official. Obtained by paying the bank the amount of the check plus the fee, in cash. Usually used by a customer who does not have a checking account.
- *Money order*: Purchased at banks, some retail stores, and the US Postal Service. Often used to pay bills by mail when a person does not have a checking account. The maximum face value varies, depending on the source. Cashier checks are preferable to money orders when larger amounts need to be paid.
- *Business check*: The professional office usually uses a ledger-type book with three checks per page and a perforated stub at the left side of the check. The stubs serve as the checking account register, where the balance of the account is tracked. The checks and matching stubs are numbered in sequence and preprinted with the depositor's name and account number. Accounting software can also print checks, or business checks can be prepared through online banking.
- *Voucher check*: This may be a detachable voucher form, or it could be attached to an EOB. The voucher portion is used to itemize or specify the purpose for which the check was drawn. The voucher portion of the check is removed before the check is presented for deposit. The voucher is then used to post the payment in the patient account ledger (Fig. 31.12).

How checks are processed from one bank to another. Checks received by the drawee's bank are turned over daily to a regional banking clearinghouse, which clears each one. The identifying code numbers, printed on the face of the check with magnetic ink, enable this "clearing" process to be accomplished quickly and efficiently. Checks due from and to all banks outside a specific region are settled by electronic entries. The bank keeps the canceled checks, and an electronic copy of the check is returned to the drawer, or the writer of the check. When the drawer needs proof of payment, a copy of the check can be requested from the bank, or the drawer can review monthly bank statements for printed copies of cleared checks. Check copies can also be obtained online through the banking portal.

Online Banking. Internet banking has changed the way financial institutions manage money. People once had to fight traffic and wait in line at crowded banks; now, they can bank from their offices any time of day. A healthcare facility's banking transactions, such as paying bills and transferring funds between accounts, can be done online. In addition, staff members have access to supply companies online and can easily review costs from the office instead of driving to numerous companies to compare prices.

Online banking is a means of performing banking services electronically via the internet. All banks and credit unions have this capability, and most of them offer both basic and advanced services. With basic services, a customer usually can:

- Check account balances
- Transfer funds between accounts in the same bank
- Pay bills electronically and create checks
- Determine whether a check has cleared the bank
- Download account information
- View images of transactions

More advanced services include being able to deposit checks online.

A major concern with online banking is fraud. Concern that unauthorized users may gain access to the healthcare facility's account balances is valid. Some experts believe that online banking involves a slightly greater risk of fraud than does conventional banking. Despite the disadvantages, studies show that internet banking is now mainstream.

Electronic fund transfer. Electronic fund transfer (EFT) is the online transfer of money from one bank account directly to another account. Some types of EFT include:

- *Direct deposit*: An EFT directly from the account of the payer to that of the party being paid. Used to electronically pay employees.
- *Wire transfer*: A fast way to send money; usually used for large, infrequent payments.
- *Automated teller machines (ATMs)*: A way to withdraw cash, make deposits, and transfer funds between accounts without going to a bank.
- *Electronic checks* or *e-checks*: An online process in which the medical assistant provides the healthcare facility's bank account number and routing number and approves the payment.

Paper checks can be converted into EFTs. A patient writes a check for services provided. The medical assistant scans the routing and account numbers on the bottom of the check. The check is then stamped "void" and handed back to the patient. The scanning process sends the payment information to the bank electronically. When this is done in the healthcare facility, a sign should be present to notify patients that payments by check will be processed in that way.

Banking Procedures in the Ambulatory Care Setting. Healthcare facilities use bank accounts to deposit funds (as cash, checks, debit card, or credit card transactions) and to pay their operational expenses by electronic fund transfer, check, or credit card. Accounting software is compatible with many online banking portals. That means that daily transactions can be downloaded directly into the accounting program. Attentive medical assistants who download daily can manage all account balances on a regular basis. Office expenses and invoices can be entered into the accounting software as accounts payable, and payments can be scheduled for entered invoices. Checks to vendors can be printed at any time from the accounting software, documenting the transaction – and documented transactions make bank reconciliation (rek uh n sill ee AY shun) a snap!

> **VOCABULARY**
> **reconciliation** To bring into agreement.

How to write a check. Checks are written in ink or produced using software. Write or key the check by the following steps:
1. Date the check using one of these formats: May 23, 20XX; 05/23/20XX; or 5/23/20XX.
2. On the "Pay to the Order of" line, correctly write or key the person's name or the company's name.
3. On the line with the dollar sign, write out the exact amount of the check starting next to the dollar sign (e.g., $135.00, not $135).
4. On the line below the recipient's name, write out the amount, making sure to start at the left edge. The cents are written in a fraction. Draw a single line through the rest of the line to prevent any additions (e.g., One hundred thirty-five and 50/100—————).
5. On the Memo line, indicate the purpose of the payment (optional).

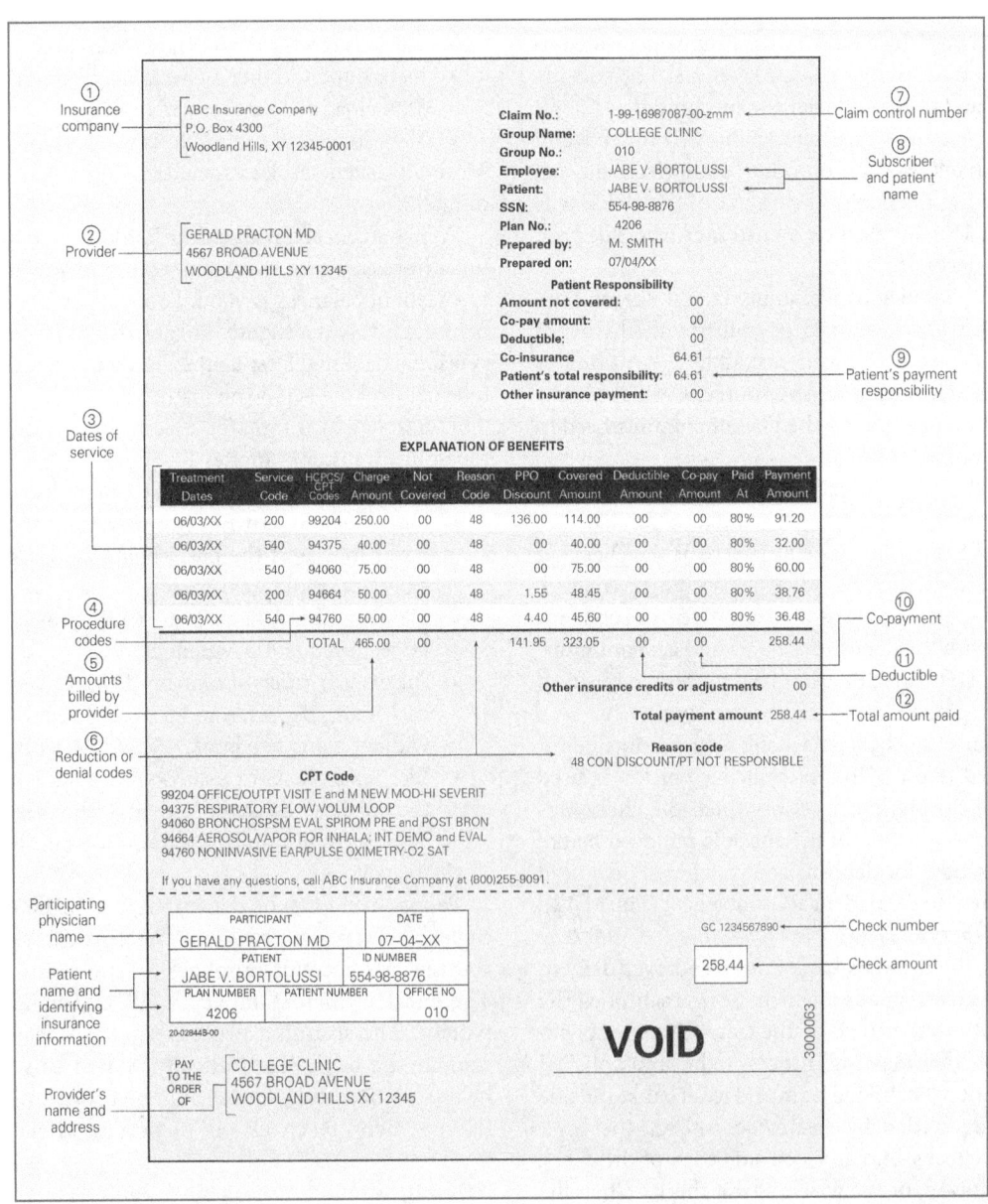

Fig. 31.12 Sample Voucher Check. (From Fordney WT: *Insurance handbook for the medical office,* ed 14, St. Louis, 2017, Elsevier.)

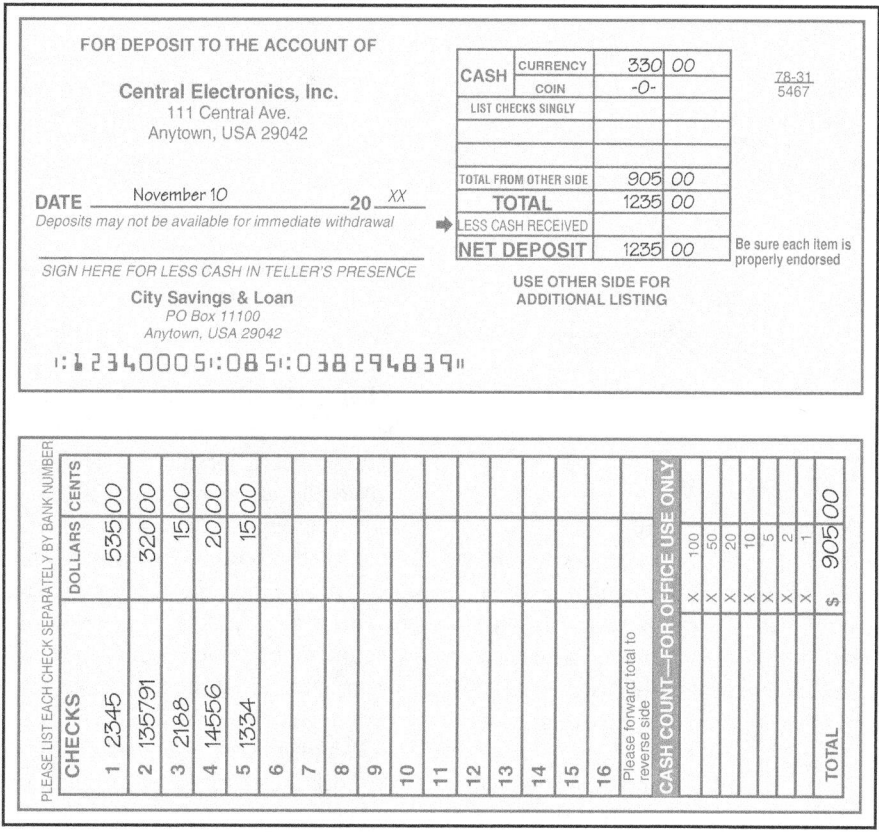

Fig. 31.13 Front and Back of A Deposit Slip. (From Niedzwiecki B, et al: *Kinn's the medical assistant,* ed 14, St. Louis, 2020, Elsevier.)

6. The check needs to be signed to be valid. If the provider is signing the check, clip the invoice to the check and place it on the provider's desk for a signature. If you are responsible for signing checks, your name must be on the signature card on file at the bank. For checks over a certain amount, two signatures will be needed.

If you make a mistake when writing the check, it cannot be altered by crossing out or changing anything that was written. You will need to void the check and rewrite another check. Write "VOID" on the stub and on the check. File the voided check with other accounting documents for auditing purposes. If you are using accounting software, indicate the check number has been voided in the software.

Preparing the bank deposit. If the facility does not use EFT, the medical assistant should make daily bank deposits. This minimizes the risks of keeping large sums of money on hand and also makes the money available for paying expenses. Depositing checks daily is important for these reasons:

- Checks may have a restricted time payment or may be lost, misplaced, or stolen over time.
- A stop-payment order may be placed on a check, or it may be returned for insufficient funds.
- Prompt processing is a courtesy to the payer.

Prompt check processing ensures that the money is available for the healthcare facility to use or to be used to build interest.

The medical assistant must prepare a deposit slip (ticket) that accompanies the funds being deposited. The deposit slip, which can be paper or electronic, itemizes the cash or checks being deposited. It provides the information for the bank account into which the funds need to be deposited (Fig. 31.13). All details of the daily deposit should be recorded in the accounting software program; each check should be entered separately (Procedure 31.4). The check number, payer, and check amount should also be recorded in the accounting software so that the deposit amount from the software matches the bank deposit record. Many banks will not credit deposits made after 3 p.m. until the following business day.

Another option is using remote deposit or mobile deposit. A deposit can be made without visiting the bank. Depending on the volume of checks to deposit, a healthcare facility can use a check scanner, flatbed scanner, or a mobile device to capture check images (Fig. 31.14). Checks are scanned individually and documented as a bank transaction on the monthly statement. Mobile deposits can save staff time and do not require a deposit slip because the software (app) is linked to the bank account being used. When mobile deposits are used, the daily deposit amount must match the exact daily deposit amount in the accounting software.

Check endorsements. An *endorsement* is a signature plus any other writing on the back of a check by which the endorser transfers all rights in the check to another party. Endorsements are made with either a pen or rubber ink stamp. The medical assistant needs to endorse the back of the check in the box indicated. Regardless of how checks are deposited, they all need to be endorsed.

Four principal kinds of endorsements can be used.

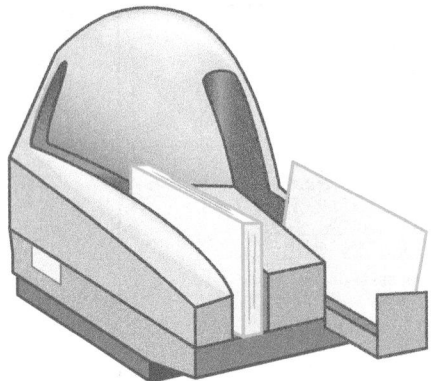

Fig. 31.14 Mobile Check Scanner. (From Niedzwiecki B, et al: *Kinn's the medical assistant,* ed 14, St. Louis, 2020, Elsevier.)

Pay to the Order of
Midwest National Bank
Main Branch
For Deposit Only
ROBERT SPALDING
301-012697

Fig. 31.15 Example of A Restrictive Endorsement. (From Niedzwiecki B, et al: *Kinn's the medical assistant,* ed 14, St. Louis, 2020, Elsevier.)

- *Blank endorsement*: The payee signs only their name, making the check payable to the bearer. This is the simplest and most commonly used type of endorsement. It should be used only when the check is to be cashed or deposited immediately.
- *Restrictive endorsement*: This type is commonly used. It specifies the purpose of the endorsement and is used when preparing checks for deposit to the provider's checking account (Fig. 31.15).
- *Special endorsement*: This includes words specifying the person to whom the endorser makes the check payable. For instance, a check written to Helen Barker as the payee may be endorsed to the provider by writing on the back of the check as follows:
  Pay to the order of
  Theodore F. Wilson, MD
  Helen Barker
  The check is still negotiable but requires Dr. Wilson's signature or endorsement.
- *Qualified endorsement*: The effect of the endorsement is qualified by disclaiming or destroying any future liability of the endorser. Usually the words "without recourse" are written above by an attorney who accepts a check on behalf of a client but who has no personal claim in the transaction.

Any endorsement should exactly match the name on the Pay To line of the check. If the name of the payee is misspelled, the payee usually must endorse the check the way the name is spelled on the face, followed by the correctly spelled signature.

A stamp can be used to endorse checks from patients and other sources. As they arrive, these checks should be recorded in the ledger and immediately stamped with the restrictive endorsement "For Deposit Only." This is a safeguard that prevents the cashing of lost or stolen checks. Most banks accept routine stamp endorsements that are restricted to For Deposit Only if the customer is well known and maintains an established account.

A signature can also be used as an endorsement. Some insurance checks or drafts require a personal signature endorsement; a stamped endorsement is not acceptable. This is stated on the back of the check. In such cases ask the payee to endorse the check, then stamp immediately below the signature the restrictive endorsement For Deposit Only.

Overdraft. When a depositor writes a check for more than the amount available in the account, the account is *overdrawn.* Issuing a check for more than the amount on deposit in the bank is illegal. Such a check is said to "bounce." Should this happen through error or oversight and a check is written by an established depositor, the bank may honor the check and notify the depositor that the account is overdrawn. If the bank pays or covers the check, it issues an overdraft on the depositor's account. Considerable fees ($25 to $40) normally are charged for an overdraft. If the bank does not cover the amount of the check, it will be returned as NSF.

Stop-payments. A depositor or check writer who wants to take back the check has the right to request that the bank stop payment on it. Stop-payment orders should be used only when absolutely necessary, because most banks charge a fee for this service. A stop-payment request may be made for a lost check or a disagreement about a purchase or payment.

Bank Statements and Reconciliation. The bank creates a statement at the end of each month. The medical assistant can download the bank statement directly into the accounting software, which has a reconciliation feature. The process of reconciliation starts with the beginning balance. Add all deposits and subtract all checks and other debit transactions. This will then leave the ending statement balance. The ending balance should match the ending balance on the bank statement. If it does, the account has been reconciled.

Bank statement reconciliation is used as an audit or to ensure that the bank is managing the funds in the account accurately and no fraud has occurred (Box 31.7). It can also help to locate any errors made in the checking account register. Any errors on the bank statement should be immediately reported to the bank. Bank statements typically contain (Figs. 31.16 and 31.17):

- Beginning balance and ending balance
- Deposits made
- Checks paid and online payment transactions
- Transfer transactions
- Bank charges
- Ending balance

What to do when the balances do not match. When there is a large number of transactions from check deposits and bill payment activities, it can be challenging to match the closing balance of the bank statement with the closing balance indicated in the accounting management software. Keeping accurate records of deposits and bill payment activities makes the bank reconciliation much smoother. All deposit copies should be maintained with a copy of the calculator tape totaling the day's deposit. Every online bill pay transaction should be recorded accurately in the accounting management system.

If you have carefully recorded every transaction and the balances still do not match, ask yourself these questions:

BOX 31.7 Preventing Check Fraud in the Healthcare Facility

The National Check Fraud Center suggests the following steps to minimize the chance of check fraud in the healthcare facility:

- Check bank statements immediately after receiving them. If check fraud is not reported within 30 days of receipt of a monthly statement, the bank usually does not have to reimburse the loss.
- Make sure all extra checks, deposit slips, bank statements, and records are stored securely (e.g., locked in a file cabinet or a secure electronic folder).
- Bank statements and records should be maintained for up to 7 years and then shredded before disposal.

For more information on how to prevent check fraud or what to do if fraud occurs, consult the National Check Fraud Center's website: http://ckfraud.org/.

- Is your math correct? Could a deposit, check, or online bill pay amount be transposed?
- Did you forget to include one of the outstanding checks?
- Did you fail to record a deposit, or did you record one twice?

Most banks ask to be notified within a reasonable time (e.g., 10 days) of any error found in the statement. The bank statement should be reconciled as soon as it is received. Most banks provide a form for reconciliation (bank statement reconciliation formula) on the last page of the bank statement:

Bank statement balance	$ ________
Minus outstanding checks	$ ________
Plus deposits not shown	$ ________
Corrected bank statement balance	$ ________
Checkbook balance	$ ________
Minus any bank charges	$ ________
Corrected checkbook balance	$ ________

If the two corrected balances agree, stop there. If they do not agree, subtract the lesser figure from the greater figure; the difference usually provides a clue to the error. For instance, if

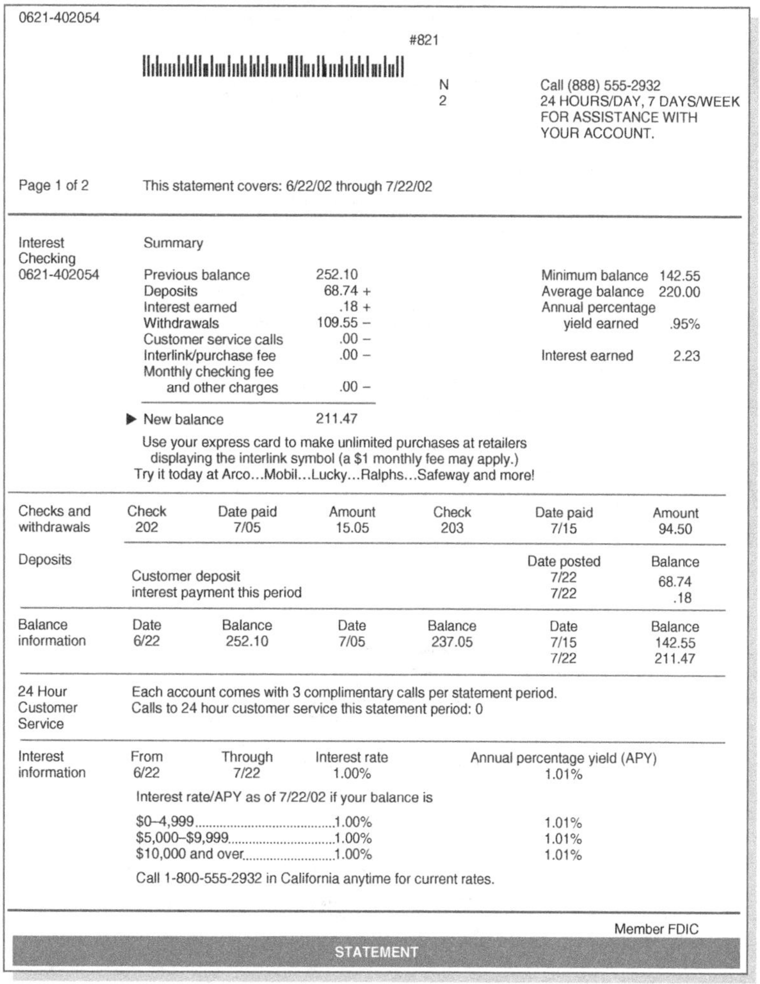

0621-402054

#821

N
2

Call (888) 555-2932
24 HOURS/DAY, 7 DAYS/WEEK
FOR ASSISTANCE WITH
YOUR ACCOUNT.

Page 1 of 2 — This statement covers: 6/22/02 through 7/22/02

Interest Checking 0621-402054 — Summary

Previous balance	252.10	Minimum balance	142.55
Deposits	68.74 +	Average balance	220.00
Interest earned	.18 +	Annual percentage yield earned	.95%
Withdrawals	109.55 –		
Customer service calls	.00 –		
Interlink/purchase fee	.00 –	Interest earned	2.23
Monthly checking fee and other charges	.00 –		
▶ New balance	211.47		

Use your express card to make unlimited purchases at retailers displaying the interlink symbol (a $1 monthly fee may apply.)
Try it today at Arco...Mobil...Lucky...Ralphs...Safeway and more!

Checks and withdrawals	Check	Date paid	Amount	Check	Date paid	Amount
	202	7/05	15.05	203	7/15	94.50

Deposits		Date posted	Balance
	Customer deposit	7/22	68.74
	interest payment this period	7/22	.18

Balance information	Date	Balance	Date	Balance	Date	Balance
	6/22	252.10	7/05	237.05	7/15	142.55
					7/22	211.47

24 Hour Customer Service — Each account comes with 3 complimentary calls per statement period. Calls to 24 hour customer service this statement period: 0

Interest information	From	Through	Interest rate	Annual percentage yield (APY)
	6/22	7/22	1.00%	1.01%

Interest rate/APY as of 7/22/02 if your balance is

$0–4,999	1.00%	1.01%
$5,000–$9,999	1.00%	1.01%
$10,000 and over	1.00%	1.01%

Call 1-800-555-2932 in California anytime for current rates.

Member FDIC

STATEMENT

Fig. 31.16 Example of A Regular Checking Account Statement. (From Niedzwiecki B, et al: *Kinn's the medical assistant,* ed 14, St. Louis, 2020, Elsevier.)

the shortage is $35, examine all the transactions for $35 on the statement and checkbook register and determine whether one of them has a posting error. Check the math and make sure all figures were added and subtracted correctly. Look at each figure and make sure none has been transposed. These tips usually catch the mistake.

Paying Bills to Maximize Cash Flow

It is important to establish a systematic plan for paying bills. Some offices use an online bill paying system and pay bills as soon as they are received. Some pay bills monthly. In establishing the procedure for accounts payable, a medical assistant should keep in mind that most vendors allow 30 days to pay. When each invoice is received, check the "terms," which are usually located at the top of the document. Sometimes a bill will be discounted if it is paid within a specified time, such as 10 days. Such discounts usually are indicated at the bottom of invoices or billing statements. If the terms say, "Net 30," this means the total amount of the bill is due within 30 days.

Remember to allow a certain number of days for mailing (2 to 5, depending on where the payment is sent). If the business checking account is an interest-bearing one, do not pay bills before their due date. This way, the funds in the account continue to earn interest until the check is cashed. Also, if the practice has a weekly service (e.g., a laundry or cleaning service) that bills several times a month, accumulate the invoices and issue only one check per month.

Invoices and Statements. The vendor usually includes an invoice for payment with delivery of the merchandise. An invoice describes the products delivered and shows the amount due. Always verify that the items listed on the packing slip and invoice are included in the delivery.

Invoices should be placed in a designated accounts payable folder until paid. The healthcare facility may make more than one purchase from the same vendor during the month and send only a single payment at the end of the month for all deliveries.

> ### CRITICAL THINKING 31.7
>
> Sam does not recall ordering a certain item from the office supply company. However, it was included in her last shipment and was shown on the packing list. How can she determine whether the item was ordered?

This worksheet is provided to help you balance your account

1. Go through your register and mark each check, withdrawal, Express ATM transaction, payment, deposit or other credit listed on this statement. Be sure that your register shows any interest paid into your account, and any service charges, automatic payments, or Express Transfers withdrawn from your account during this statement period.

2. Using the chart below, list any outstanding checks, Express ATM withdrawals, payments or any other withdrawals (including any from previous months) that are listed in your register but are not shown on this statement.

3. Balance your account by filling in the spaces below.

ITEMS OUTSTANDING	
NUMBER	AMOUNT

Enter
The new balance shown on this statement .... $_____

Add
Any deposits listed in your register $_____
or transfers into your account which $_____
are not shown on this statement. $_____
+$_____

Total..............+ $_____
Calculate the subtotal.................................... $_____

Subtract
The total outstanding checks and withdrawals from the chart at left..................− $_____

Calculate the ending balance
This amount should be the same as the current balance shown in your check register.................... $_____

TOTAL $

If you suspect errors or have questions about electronic transfers

If you believe there is an error on your statement or Express ATM receipt, or if you need more information about a transaction listed on this statement or an Express ATM receipt, please contact us immediately. We are available 24 hours a day, seven days a week to assist you. Please call the telephone number printed on the front of this statement. Or, you may write to us at United Trust Company, P.O. Box 327, Anytown, USA.

1. Tell us your name and account number or Express card number.

2. As clearly as you can, describe the error or the transfer you are unsure about, and explain why you believe there is an error or why you need more information.

3. Tell us the dollar amount of the suspected error.

You must report the suspected error to us no later than 60 days after we sent you the first statement on which the problem appeared. We will investigate your question and will correct any error promptly. If our investigation takes longer than 10 business days (or 20 days in the case of electronic purchases), we will temporarily credit your account for the amount you believe is in error, so that you may have use of the money until the investigation is completed.

Fig. 31.17 Reverse Side of A Bank Statement, Which is Used for Reconciling A Checking Account.
(From Niedzwiecki B, et al: *Kinn's the medical assistant,* ed 14, St. Louis, 2020, Elsevier.)

TABLE 31.3 **Payroll Forms**		
Form Number	**Name**	**Description**
SS-4	Application for Employer Identification Number (EIN)	All employers that withhold taxes from employees' paychecks must have a 9-digit EIN number.
SS-5	Application for a Social Security Card	All employees need a Social Security number.
W-2	Wage and Tax Statement	Used to report the total amount of federal, state, and other taxes withheld from the employee's paycheck. Used by the employee to file personal income taxes. Sections: • Copy A: Submit to Social Security Administration (SSA) by January 31 of the following year. • Copy 1: Submit to state tax department. • Copy B: Used by the employee to file federal tax return. • Copy C: Kept by the employee. • Copy 2: Used by the employee to file state tax return. • Copy D: Retained by the employer for 4 years. Copies B, C, and 2 must be given to the employee by January 31 of the following year.
W-3	Transmittal of Wage and Tax Statement	Used to report total income and Federal Insurance Contribution Act (FICA) taxes withheld from the employee's paychecks. Employer sends form to the SSA.
W-4	Employee's Withholding Certificate	New hires must provide their tax status (e.g., single) and how many allowances they are claiming. This information is used when the employer withholds money from their paycheck for income taxes.
	State Tax Withholding Form	Used by the employer to determine the amount of income tax to be withheld from the employee's paycheck.
940	Employer's Annual Federal Unemployment Tax Return	Used to report the employer's annual Federal Unemployment Tax Act (FUTA) tax.
941	Employer's Quarterly Federal Tax Return	Reports federal income and FICA taxes. Must be filed each quarter.
8109	Federal Tax Deposit Coupon Book	Used to deposit federal payroll taxes taken out of employee's paychecks.
1099	Miscellaneous Income	Reports all types of income except for wages; filed with the Internal Revenue Service (IRS).
I-9	Employment Eligibility Verification	Used to verify a person's identity and employment authorization. All US employers must ensure the form is completed by both the new hire and the employer. The form requires the new hire to provide the employer with documents that prove identity and employment authorization.

Petty Cash. *Petty cash* is a small amount of money kept on hand for small, miscellaneous expenses, such as postage due, deliveries, and minor office supplies. Although it is a small amount of money, records still need to be kept and expenses tracked.

To start a petty cash fund, a check is written for "cash" and cashed. An assortment of bills and coins is obtained. Usually a petty cash fund start with $25 to $50. The money is kept in a cash box out of sight. Printable petty cash logs are available online, or a customized log can be made. It is important to include such columns as date, number, paid to/received from, purpose, approved by, cash out, cash in, and balance (Procedure 31.5).

When a payment must be made from petty cash, the person should present a receipt, or a voucher should be filled out. The voucher should indicate the date, time, transaction number, purpose, amount paid, and the signature of the person receiving the money. The log should be completed with the information from the receipt or voucher. All receipts and vouchers must be kept with the log until the petty cash log is reconciled. To reconcile petty cash, the total payments from the receipts and vouchers are calculated. The total payments are subtracted from the starting balance. The total should match the total cash in the box. When adding money to the petty cash fund, write a check for cash and cash it as indicated earlier. Complete the log to indicate cash was added to the fund.

Employee Payroll

In an ambulatory healthcare facility, the payroll may be a manual or computerized process. Payroll services are also available. A medical assistant maybe responsible for processing employee payroll for the healthcare facility. Employees can be paid either on an hourly basis or with a salary. If employees are salaried, their gross pay will always be the same dollar amount. If the employee is paid hourly, the gross pay will depend on how many hours the person worked during the pay period. The hourly rate is multiplied by the number of hours worked to determine these individuals' gross pay. In either situation, the gross amount earned is used to determine how much is withheld for taxes.

Table 31.3 describes payroll-related forms the employer needs to file. Mandatory and voluntary deductions are calculated and subtracted from the gross amount earned. Mandatory payroll deductions include:

- Federal Insurance Contributions Act (FICA) tax: Made up of Medicare and Social Security taxes. The employee and employer contribute to the FICA tax equally.
- Federal income tax
- State and local taxes
- Wage garnishments: Court order or order from a government agency to withhold money from an employee's paycheck due to that person's unpaid debt.

Voluntary payroll deductions include:

- Health insurance premiums
- Retirement plans, such as an Individual Retirement Account (IRA)
- Life insurance premiums
- Job-related expenses, such as union dues and uniforms

After the deductions are taken the from the gross amount, the net pay remains. The medical assistant will either write a check or process the direct deposit so the funds are transferred to the employees' accounts.

It is important for the healthcare facility to keep exact records regarding payroll, withholding, and deductions. The employer is responsible for submitting the withheld tax amounts to the federal and state governments in a timely fashion. These are usually submitted on a quarterly basis (i.e., every 3 months).

> **VOCABULARY**
> **gross** The amount earned before any tax deductions or adjustments.

CLOSING COMMENTS

Patient accounts management and collections are critical responsibilities in the healthcare facility, and a responsible medical assistant is a great asset in this important area. Always maintain a positive attitude with patients when discussing financial matters. Remember that people who are ill or facing challenges are not always cordial, so they may not respond positively to discussion of their patient account balances. Make every attempt to work with each patient to develop a financial plan for settling the account balance. The healthcare facility works hard to collect every dollar, so effective financial management is essential for practice success.

An equally important financial aspect for the healthcare facility is accounts payable. This must also be handled in an efficient manner. Being aware of the different banking options can help with depositing funds and paying bills. Making sure that there are policies in place for patient payment methods is crucial. Patients should also be made aware of those policies.

> **PATIENT-CENTERED CARE**
>
> It should be emphasized that patients are financially responsible for balances on their accounts. Patients should be informed of the healthcare facility's payment policy at the very first appointment. If a patient submits an NSF check, the medical assistant should call the patient and explain the problem, requesting that they correct the matter as soon as possible. It is important to remember that most overdrafts are simply the result of mathematical errors or a delay in deposited funds being available for withdrawal. Therefore the medical assistant should be patient and courteous when discussing NSF issues with patients. However, patients need to know that overdrafts are costly not only to them but also to the healthcare facility.

> **BEING PROFESSIONAL**
>
> Role-play this scenario with a peer: You, the medical assistant, have asked the patient to pay the copayment prior to the appointment. The patient (your peer) just attempted to use a credit/debit card, and it was rejected. Ask the patient for another form of payment in a respectful and professional manner.

CHAPTER REVIEW

Bookkeeping is the practice of recording the transactions of a business each day. Two types of bookkeeping are single-entry and double-entry systems. Single-entry bookkeeping entails entering one entry in a cash book or journal for each transaction. Double-entry bookkeeping requires two entries for each transaction, a debit in one account and the same amount as a credit in an opposite account. Accounting is a practice of maintaining the financial records of a business. Three types of bookkeeping and accounting are:

- Manual, which includes the pegboard system
- Computerized, which requires all financial transactions to be entered into the software
- Virtual, which is becoming more popular

Business transactions are usually divided into accounts receivable and accounts payable activities. A/R is the money owed to the business, and A/P is the money a business owes. All patient financial transactions are posted to the patient's ledger, including:

- Payments from the patient.
- Payments from third-party payers, such as insurance companies.
- Adjustments, which can credit or debit the patient's account. Credit adjustments are posted to the patient ledger when an amount needs to be subtracted from

a patient's balance. Debit adjustments are posted to the patient ledger when an amount needs to be added to the patient's balance but is not a charge for services.

- Credit balance, which occurs when a patient has paid in advance or an overpayment or a duplicate payment is made.

Monthly statements should include dates of service, services provided, insurance payments and adjustments, and payments, including copayments. Special guidelines must be considered when billing minors and hardship cases.

Collection is the process of using all legal resources available to collect payment for past due patient account balances. Fair debt collection practices under the FDCPA must be followed. The SOL of the FDCPA determines the length of time a debt collector can collect an unpaid balance. Collection calls can be made, and collection letters can be sent, but FDCPA rules must be followed. Tracing skips, billing an estate, and using a collection agency are all collection activities that a medical assistant may be involved with.

When a patient pays their bill, the medical assistant must follow the facility's policy regarding accepting cash, checks, and credit card and debit card payments. Debit and credit card transactions can reduce the chances of money mismanagement in the office, such as embezzlement. Online payments have also become more popular.

The medical assistant might be involved with the banking procedures in the healthcare facility. Common types of bank accounts include checking, savings, and money market savings. When an account is opened at a bank branch, the account signer is required to provide their handwritten signature on a physical or electronic card, which is kept on file with the bank. If a check comes through and some suspicion arises that the depositor's signature has been forged, bank personnel compare the signature on the check with the original on the signature card.

Online banking, including EFTs, and checks are typical ways the medical assistant will pay the bills owed by the healthcare facility. Using a computerized accounting system for check writing will help with documentation of transactions. Besides paying bills, the medical assistant may need to prepare the bank deposit, which includes endorsing checks, and reconcile bank statements.

Petty cash is a small amount of money kept on hand for small, miscellaneous expenses, such as postage due, deliveries, and minor office supplies. Although it is a small amount of money, records still need to be kept and expenses tracked. The person receiving the payment must present a receipt, or a voucher needs to be completed to help track the payment.

The medical assistant may also be involved with preparing the employee payroll. If the employee is salaried, their net pay will always be the same dollar amount. If the employee is paid hourly, the net pay will depend on how many hours the person worked during the pay period. The hourly rate is multiplied by the number of hours worked to determine these individuals' gross pay. Mandatory and voluntary deductions must be deducted from the gross amount. The remaining amount is the net.

SCENARIO WRAP-UP

Sam has learned a lot about the different types of bookkeeping transactions performed daily in the healthcare facility. As she has gained more experience, she has come to appreciate the important role of patient accounts collection in the practice's cash flow and ability to cover its operating expenses.

After the visit with the bank representative, Sam implemented a few changes in bank account management, which have increased productivity in the office. For one, Sam requested that the bank send a mobile deposit machine so this could be done in-house, which has saved Sam a lot of time.

Sam has also set up an online bill pay system and manages all invoice payments through the banking portal online. She sits down once a month and sets up all payments for the month. In this way, she can budget the office expenses for the month and can transfer unused funds to a money market account that pays a higher interest rate.

Sam is working closely with the providers at WMFM Clinic to make some financial policy changes in the office to streamline banking processes. As of January 1 of the new year, the sign at the healthcare facility's lobby window will explain that cash will no longer be accepted for services and that a $35 fee will be charged for NSF checks.

PROCEDURE 31.1   Post Charges and Payments to a Patient's Account

Tasks

Create a new patient account ledger card. Post charges and payment manually to the patient's account.

Scenario

Ken Thomas (DOB 10/25/19XX) is a new patient of Dr. Martin. He makes his $50 copayment at the time of the office visit. He provides you with two phone numbers: cell phone (123) 784-1118 and his wife's cell phone (123) 125-4725. His address is 398 Larkin Avenue, Anytown, AL 12345-1234. The effective date of his insurance was January 1 of this year.

Equipment and Supplies

- Patient account ledger card
- Encounter form/superbill (use Fig. 31.2)
- Black Pen

Procedural Steps

1. Create the patient account by entering the following information on a patient account ledger card. Use the information found in Fig. 31.2.

- Patient's full name, address, and at least two contact phone numbers
- Date of birth (DOB)
- Health insurance information, including the subscriber number, group number, and effective date
- Subscriber's name and date of birth (if the subscriber is not the patient)

Purpose: To keep all insurance and collection information available with the patient account record balance for reference.

2. Using the completed encounter form in Fig. 31.2, enter the charges manually on the ledger card for the patient's account record. Use today's date. Enter the CPT Code as the service description.

3. Total all the charges on the encounter form for the services rendered. Then subtract the copayment made from the total charges. The previous balance, if any, is added to this new total.

Use the following worksheet to calculate the new balance.

Total Charges	$_____
Amount paid (copayment)	$_____
+ Previous balance (if any)	$_____
= New Balance Due	$_____

PROCEDURE 31.2   Post Charges and Payments to a Patient's Account Using SimChart for the Medical Office Software

Task

To enter charges and payments to the patient's account record using software.

Scenario

Ken Thomas (DOB 10/25/19XX) is a new patient of Dr. Martin. He makes his $50 copayment by check at the time of the office visit.

Equipment and Supplies

- SimChart for the Medical Office
- Encounter form/superbill (use Fig. 31.2)

Procedural Steps

1. After logging into SimChart, go to the Simulation Playground. Locate the established patient by clicking on Find Patient; enter the patient's name and click Go. When the name appears, verify the date of birth (DOB), click on the radio button, and click Select. The patient's health record will open in the Clinical Care tab. If there is no encounter shown, create an encounter by clicking on Office Visit under Info Panel on the left, click Add New, select a visit type and provider, and click on Save. Once an encounter has been created, either return to the Patient Dashboard and click on the Superbill link on the right (found under the weight) or click on the Coding and Billing tab and select Superbill on the left Info Panel.

Purpose: Verifying the DOB ensures you have the correct patient.

2. Click on the encounter (in blue) found in the Encounters Not Coded section located on the Superbill screen. Using the information from Fig. 31.2, enter the diagnosis code in the Diagnosis field in the Rank 1 row. Scroll down to the office visit section and document "1" in the Rank column for a comprehensive new patient. Enter the charge and the code as indicated in Fig. 31.2. Click Save. Go to page 4 of the superbill. Enter the copay amount. Scroll down and select the "I am ready to submit the Superbill" checkbox at the bottom of the screen. For the signature on file, click the checkbox for Yes. Select the date. Click Submit Superbill.

3. Click on Ledger on the left. If needed, search for your patient. Type in your patient's name and click Go. When the name appears, verify the DOB, click on the radio button, and click Select.

4. Click the arrow to the right of the patient's name in the ledger. (The arrow is above the Total Ledger Balance box.)

5. Enter the date, DOS (date of service), provider, and PTPYMTCK (for patient payment by check) in the Service column; enter the charge and payment (copay amount) and the copay amount in the payment column. Click Save, and the balance will be autocalculated for you.

Purpose: In the ledger, it is important to indicate how the patient paid.

PROCEDURE 31.3   Post Payments and Adjustments to a Patient's Account

Task

To post payments and adjustments to a patient account ledger.

Scenario

Blue Cross Blue Shield paid $84 (check #326421) for the wellness visit for Monique Jones (06/23/19XX). The provider's fee is $23 more than allowed by the insurance company. Document a credit adjustment for the $23. Monique paid the remaining $28 by check (#2364).

Equipment and Supplies

- Patient account ledger card and a black pen, or SimChart for the Medical Office (SCMO) software

Procedural Steps

1. Find the patient's ledger.

- *Ledger card*: Find the patient's ledger card and confirm you have the correct patient. If her ledger is blank, add the following information: date of service was 1 month ago, service description is Z00.00, and the charge is $135.

- *SCMO*: Using the Simulation Playground, click the Coding & Billing tab. Select Ledger from the left Info Panel. Search for Monique Jones using the Patient Search fields and click Go. Verify her DOB and select the radio button for Monique Jones. Click Select. Click the arrow to the right of the patient's name in the ledger. Charges submitted on claims will auto-populate the ledger. If her ledger is blank, add the following information: Enter the date and DOS

PROCEDURE 31.3 Post Payments and Adjustments to a Patient's Account—cont'd

(date of service; make it 1 month ago), Z00.00 in the Service column, and $135 in the charge column.

Purpose: All transactions need to be posted to the correct account.

2. Enter the payment made by the insurance company and the adjustment.
   - *Ledger card:* Enter the insurance payment, check number, and adjustment. Complete the row of information, including the balance.
   - *SCMO:* Click Add Row. Enter the date, DOS (date of service), INSPYMT (for insurance payment) in the Service column, payment, and the adjustment (−$23).

Purpose: In the ledger, it is important to indicate how much the insurance paid and the adjustment.

3. Enter the patient's payment.
   - *Ledger card:* Enter the patient's payment, check number, and complete the row of information, including the balance.
   - *SCMO:* Click Add Row. Enter the date, DOS, PTPYMTCK (for patient payment by check) in the Service column, and the payment. Click Save, and the balance will be autocalculated for you.

Purpose: In the ledger, it is important to indicate how the patient paid.

PROCEDURE 31.4 Perform End-of-Day Reconciliation and Prepare a Bank Deposit

Task

Calculate the total payments received, reconcile the cash drawer, and prepare a bank deposit for currency and checks.

Scenario

You are a medical assistant at Walden-Martin Family Medicine Clinic and are responsible for closing activities, which involves end of day reconciliation and preparing a bank deposit. The healthcare facility's account number 123-456-78910, and the bank is Clear Water Bank, Anytown, Anystate

Equipment and Supplies

- Cash drawer (with currency and checks)
- Day sheet showing cash and check payments
- Calculator and black pen
- Bank deposit slip or SimChart for the Medical Office (SCMO)

Procedural Steps

1. Using the day sheet, calculate the total cash received for the day. Write down the total.

   Purpose: A total is needed when checking the amount of cash in the cash drawer.

2. Count the bills and coins in the cash drawer and write down the totals.
3. Calculate the total cash received for the day, by subtracting the starting amount from the amount in the cash drawer at the end of the day. Write down the total. Verify the total matches the cash total on the day sheet. If the totals do not match, recalculate the totals and recount the currency.

Note: The supervisor should be notified if the totals do not match. The cash received for the day is removed from the cash drawer and placed in a zippered bank deposit bag.

4. Compare the checks listed on the day sheet with the checks in the cash drawer. Verify the check number and the amount. Correct any errors on the day sheet and make sure all information is correct. Calculate the total amount from the checks. Write the total down.

   Scenario update: Prepare the deposit slip for the cash and checks received today.

5. Prepare the paper or electronic deposit slip.
   - *Paper method:* Using a black pen, write the date on the deposit slip.
   - *SCMO:* Enter the Simulation Playground in SCMO. Click on the Form Reposicon. On the INFO PANEL, click on Office Forms and then select Bank Deposit Slip. Add the date in the date field.
6. For the cash received today, count the currency (bills) to be deposited. Enter the amount in the CURRENCY line, completing the dollar and cent boxes on the deposit slip. Do the same steps for the coins to be deposited. Enter the total amount of currency and coins in the TOTAL CASH line.
7. Enter the total amount from the checks in the CHECK line, completing the dollar and cent boxes on the deposit slip. For each check to be deposited, enter the check number, the dollars, and cents. List each check on a separate line. Calculate the total to deposit and add the number in the bottom box. Indicate the number of items deposited in the TOTAL ITEMS box. Verify the information.

   Purpose: The bank requires that each check be listed separately; this also helps when verifying the checks before the deposit.

   Note: Ensure each check is endorsed before finalizing the deposit.

PROCEDURE 31.5 Complete and Reconcile a Petty Cash Log

Tasks

Add entries to a petty cash log and calculate the amount of money left in the petty cash fund.

Scenario

You need to start a petty cash fund, enter the following cash disbursements, and calculate the amount of money left in the box.

- 3/4/20XX Started with $50
- 3/8/20XX $12.50 for postage (number 001)
- 3/16/20XX $1.50 parking fee (number 002)
- 3/22/20XX $10.63 lunch for the provider (number 003)
- 3/23/20XX $15.23 donuts for the staff (number 004)
- 3/25/20XX $3.25 parking fee (number 005)
- 3/28/20XX $4.20 postage (number 006)

Directions

For this project, you can make up any additional information you need to complete the log.

Equipment and Supplies

- Petty cash log and black pen or a computer with an electronic petty cash log
- Calculator

Procedural Steps

1. Complete the petty cash log either using a pen or electronically. For all 20XX in the scenario, replace with the current year.

   Purpose: The log should contain enough information to show that the cash disbursement is well documented.

2. Add in the petty cash activity listed in the previous scenario. Add any extra information as indicated by the directions.
3. Calculate the balance for each row, after the money has been added or removed.

   Purpose: The balance is a running balance for the fund and gives a quick update on what should be in the cashbox.

   Scenario update: The petty cash fund needs to be brought back up to $50.

4. For the last entry in the log, complete the information using 3/28/20XX and indicate the amount of cash added to the fund. Calculate the new balance

32

Infection Control

LEARNING OBJECTIVES

1. Describe the characteristics of pathogenic microorganisms.
2. Explain the differences among acute, chronic, latent, and opportunistic infections.
3. Apply the chain of infection process to the ambulatory care environment.
4. Describe Standard Precautions, Bloodborne Pathogen Standard, and Transmission-Based Precautions.
5. List potentially infectious body fluids.
6. Describe when and how to perform hand hygiene.
7. Discuss the use of personal protective equipment and how to remove it while following Standard Precautions.
8. Describe how to minimize the risk of injury in the workplace.
9. Describe housekeeping controls and protocols for disposal of biologic chemical materials.
10. Summarize the management of postexposure evaluation.
11. Apply the concepts of medical and surgical asepsis to the healthcare setting.
12. Differentiate among sanitization, disinfection, and sterilization procedures.

OUTLINE

OPENING SCENARIO

Rosa Lucia is a certified medical assistant working for Walden-Martin Family Medical (WMFM) Clinic. She is quite concerned about contracting an infectious disease while caring for her patients. Rosa learned about Standard Precautions while enrolled in her medical assisting program and now must implement that knowledge in the workplace. She remembers that two important factors in preventing the spread of infection are (1) understanding how to break the chain of infection and (2) recognizing the importance of correct and frequent hand washing.

YOU WILL LEARN

1. To identify the various infectious agents.
2. To recognize the components of the chain of infection.
3. To describe how Standard Precautions, Bloodborne Pathogen Standard, and Transmission-Based Precautions impact healthcare.
4. To use standard precautions, follow safe work practices, and use personal protective equipment.
5. To differentiate among sanitization, disinfection, and sterilization.

INTRODUCTION

To gain an understanding of the importance of infection control, you must first understand how disease is transmitted. Disease-causing microorganisms can be spread from person to person by a number of different pathways. Healthcare professionals need to be aware of these and how they can be interrupted. One of the easiest ways to prevent the spread of disease is to wash your hands or use alcohol-based hand sanitizers. This is commonly referred to as *hand hygiene*. Every procedure must begin and end with effective hand hygiene practices. Another important way to stop the spread of disease is to use specific techniques appropriate for the situation, such as medical aseptic technique and sterile technique. In this chapter we will discuss the fundamental concepts that should be used whenever you are faced with an infection control issue, most of which were established by the Occupational Safety and Health Administration (OSHA). The guidelines presented in this chapter are basic to all clinical skills, and following them can reduce the transmission of disease organisms and lessen the severity of disease. They also may save a patient's or co-worker's life, or even your own.

DISEASE

Disease is defined as a specific illness with a recognizable group of signs and symptoms and a clear cause. Diseases can be infectious or noninfectious. *Noninfectious disease* cannot be spread from person to person. Instead these types of diseases are caused by something unique to a particular individual. Some common examples of noninfectious diseases are hereditary disease, autoimmune disease, drug-induced disease, and degenerative disease. *Infectious diseases* are caused by microscopic organisms *(microbes)* that invade the body and cause harmful changes to body cells, structures, or chemistry. When people have signs and symptoms of an infectious disease, they are said to have an *infection*.

Microbes are almost everywhere. We carry them on our skin, in our bodies, and on our clothing. They can be on your desk, in ice, the soil, the air, and even in boiling water. The only places free of microbes are sterilized medical equipment and supplies and internal body tissues and organs. Any healthy body organs and tissues that are not connected to the outside are generally free of all microorganisms. Pathogens enter the body by being ingested, injected, or inhaled or in some cases can move through mucous membranes. There are five types of infectious agents: bacteria, viruses, *fungi* (FUHN jahy), *protozoa* (proh tuh ZOH uh), and *helminths* (HEL minths).

Not all microbes that enter the body cause disease; in fact, some are helpful. Some microbes live on or even in the body. They compete with pathogens, which makes it difficult for the disease-causing microbes to actually cause disease. These competing microbes are known as *normal flora* and are essential for healthy living. Microbes that do not live permanently on or in the body but are present are called *transient flora*. Transient flora is a bit like hitchhikers. They are picked up when a person touches an object and use that person as a free ride. They are often picked up on the hands and carried onto doorknobs, desktops, or other items that are touched. These are often disease-causing microbes. If they "hitch" a ride into the mouth, nose, eyes, or other body orifice, they enter the body and cause disease.

Even when a microbe is known to cause disease, it will not do so in every case. The immune system (see Chapter 9) works to control pathogens to prevent disease. In some cases, individuals may have acquired a pathogen but do not develop a disease. This could be because their immune system kills the pathogen, or it may be because that person is not susceptible to that specific disease process. Even if particular people do not develop disease, as long as they carry that pathogen, they risk spreading it to others. In this case we refer to that person as a *carrier*.

VOCABULARY

autoimmune disease Illness caused by the immune system mistakenly attacking structures or systems within the body.

degenerative disease Illness caused by cells or tissues that have deteriorated over time.

hereditary disease A condition passed from parents to offspring through the genes.

ingested Swallowed, as food, into the body.

medical aseptic technique Strategies used to maintain medical asepsis (or to destroy disease-causing organisms); also called the clean technique.

microbes Microscopic organisms including bacteria, viruses, fungi, and parasites.

pathogen A disease-causing organism or agent.

sterile technique A set of specific procedures performed to keep a sterile field, a surgical incision, and any other invasive procedure (e.g., injections) free of microorganisms; also called surgical aseptic technique.

susceptible Likely to be harmed by a particular thing.

Bacteria

Bacteria are small single-celled organisms. Bacteria are classified according to their shape, or morphology (Box 32.1). Some bacteria can produce resistant external structures, called **spores**, that make treatment difficult.

Bacteria is present in our environment. We have bacteria in and on our bodies, of which most is harmless. Some types of bacteria in

BOX 32.1 Bacteria Morphology

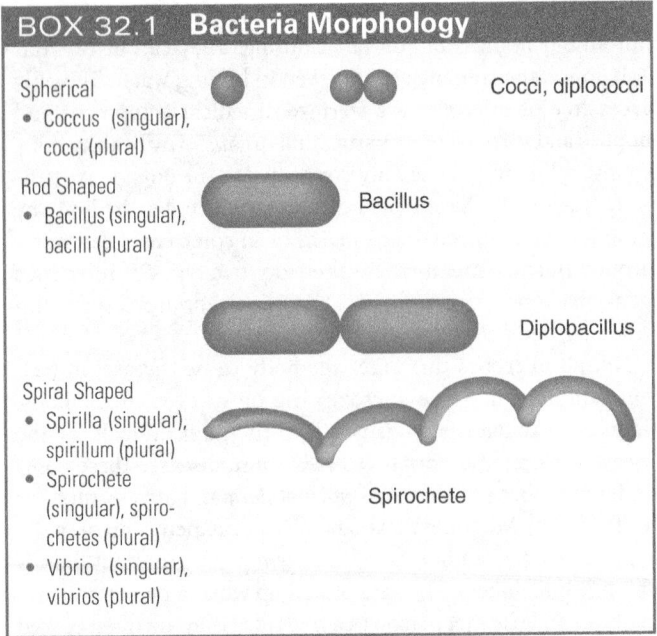

Spherical
- Coccus (singular), cocci (plural)

Cocci, diplococci

Rod Shaped
- Bacillus (singular), bacilli (plural)

Bacillus

Diplobacillus

Spiral Shaped
- Spirilla (singular), spirillum (plural)
- Spirochete (singular), spirochetes (plural)
- Vibrio (singular), vibrios (plural)

Spirochete

BOX 32.2 Microbiome

Did you know that the normal flora in the typical human is made of bacteria, fungi, and protozoa? It is also made up of so many cellular organisms that it accounts for up to 5 pounds of an individual's weight! Just like fingerprints, no two people's microbiomes are exactly alike, and they also change over time. The microbiome is made up of multiple different microbes that an individual comes into contact with throughout their life. The microbiome is extremely important because it has many jobs that help the body. For example, the microbiome:
- assists the immune system by fighting off disease-causing microbes.
- assists the body in breaking down food components, such as complex carbohydrates and fibers.
- creates vitamins the body needs to survive (including vitamin B_{12} and vitamin K)

our bodies help with digestion and make vitamins, such as vitamin K and some B vitamins. Other bacteria destroy pathogens. Our normal flora is made up of a large portion of bacteria (Box 32.2).

Less than one percent of bacteria can cause disease. Bacteria, commonly found in our normal flora, can cause disease if moves into an area of the body where it is not commonly found. For example, *Escherichia coli* (*E. coli*) are common bacteria found in the intestinal tract. If *E. coli* gets into the urethra and travels to the bladder, a person can get a urinary tract infection (UTI). The leading cause of UTIs in females is caused from *E. coli*.

Some types of bacteria can multiply rapidly and overwhelm the body's natural defenses, causing disease. Other types of bacteria produce and secrete toxins in their environment. Some bacteria create toxins, which are released when they die. Toxins damage cells and neutralize antibodies. Examples of diseases

VOCABULARY

interferon A protein formed when a cell is exposed to a virus; the protein blocks viral action on the cell and protects against viral invasion.

spores A thick-walled, dormant form of bacteria that is very resistant to disinfection measures.

toxins Substances created by microorganisms, plants, or animals that are poisonous to humans; can cause disease.

caused by toxins include diphtheria, tetanus, botulism (a type of food poisoning), and pertussis (whooping cough).

When people have bacterial infections, they are typically treated with antibiotics. *Antibiotics* kill bacteria or inhibit their growth. The disease-causing bacteria can be destroyed by the antibiotic, thus curing the disease. Antibiotics can also destroy good bacteria, which may lead to a secondary infection. A *secondary infection* is an infection that occurs during or after the treatment for another infection, either due to the treatment or changes in the immune system. An example of a secondary infection is a vaginal yeast infection after taking an antibiotic for another infection.

Antibiotic Resistance Bacteria. Infectious bacteria that once were easily treated with antibiotics are growing increasingly resistant to the actions of these drugs. Bacteria can fight against antibiotics and find new ways to survive. These defense strategies are called *resistance mechanisms*. Bacteria not killed by antibiotics can multiply, and some can give their resistance directly to other pathogens.

The antibiotic resistant bacteria can spread within and between healthcare facilities. These infections are called *healthcare-associated infections* (HAIs). The antibiotic resistant bacteria can quickly spread in the community and between countries. Each year in the U.S., at least 2.8 million people have antibiotic resistant infections, which are difficult to impossible to treat. More than 35,000 people die yearly as a result. Antibiotic resistance is one of the world's most significant public health problems. To limit bacteria resistant infections, it is important to:
- Wash hands and keep wounds clean.
- Only use antibiotics when they are prescribed for you. Remember antibiotics do not kill viruses and thus should not be taken for viral infections, such as influenza and the common cold.
- Complete the entire course of antibiotics. Never share antibiotics with another person.

Viruses

Viruses are the smallest of all pathogenic microbes. They are unable to reproduce on their own. Viruses inject their own genetic material (either deoxyribonucleic acid [DNA] or ribonucleic acid [RNA]) into cells. This genetic material takes over the cell's nucleus and forces it to reproduce more viruses. This will eventually kill the cell. Once the cell dies, the newly formed viruses are released into the body to find new cells. Because viruses grow inside otherwise normal body cells, viruses can be very difficult for immune cells to recognize. When a cell is invaded by a virus, it will often release a substance called interferon to help protect the body from a viral infection. Interferon leaves the infected cell and acts somewhat like Paul Revere, warning neighboring cells that "a virus is coming!" The neighboring cells then produce antiviral proteins inside the cells. These proteins are like security guards for the cell. They protect the cell by staying inside the cell and killing any foreign genetic material that enters. This works to slow the infection from spreading because it takes longer for the virus to find a cell it can use to reproduce. This causes it to remain outside of the cell, allowing the immune cells longer to fight it.

Common viral diseases include influenza, herpes, hepatitis B and C, and acquired immunodeficiency syndrome (AIDS), which is caused by the human immunodeficiency virus (HIV).

Antiviral medications can be used to treat viral infections. Antiviral medications work by stopping the infection process in different ways. They work best if taken soon after the illness begins. Antiviral medications can lessen the severity of the illness and shorten the time a person is ill. With severe illness, interferon and antiviral medications may be prescribed. Treatment for mild to moderate viral infections is commonly *palliative,* or focused on relieving symptoms, to help patients feel better as their immune system fights off the pathogen.

Fungi

Fungi are single celled or very complex multicellular organisms that reproduce by releasing spores. Just like bacteria, fungi are found in the environment and on and in our bodies. Many types of fungi do not cause disease. Common types of fungi include yeast, molds, and mushrooms. Fungi must have food, water, and oxygen to survive. They generally like to grow in warm, moist environments. Fungal infections are most often seen on the skin but can occur in the body. Examples of fungal disease are:
- *Candidiasis* (kan di DAHY us sis), a yeast infection that causes such infections as vaginal candidiasis and thrush (oral candidiasis).
- *Tinea* (TIN ee uh), which includes such infections as ringworm, athlete's foot, and jock itch.

Fungal infections are typically treated with antifungal medications.

MEDICAL TERMINOLOGY

immun/o	immune, immunity
myc/o	fungus
inter-	between
-al, -ic	pertaining to

Parasites

A *parasite* is an organism that lives on or in a host, taking nutrients and getting protection from the host. Parasites are different from normal flora because they generally harm the host instead of helping it.

Protozoa are unicellular parasites that can replicate and multiply rapidly once inside the host. Protozoa are commonly transmitted by vectors, most commonly insects. They are most commonly seen in tropical climates, which have large insect populations. Examples of diseases caused by protozoa include:
- Giardiasis, which is typically caused by the ingestion of water contaminated by feces.
- Malaria, in which mosquitoes serve as vectors; the parasite enters the body through the mosquito's bite.

Helminths are multicellular organisms and include tapeworms, roundworms, and flatworms (flukes [flooks]). Tapeworms live in the intestines of some animals and can be transferred to humans who eat undercooked meat from infected animals. Most parasitic roundworm eggs are found in the soil and enter the human body when a person picks them up on the hands and then transfers them to the mouth. Roundworms eventually end up or live in human intestines and cause infection and disease. Flatworms with an external sucker are referred to as *flukes.* Flukes are found in raw or improperly cooked fish.

VOCABULARY

host The living organism that the pathogen resides within.
vector Animals or insects that that transmit a pathogen (e.g., ticks).

TYPES OF INFECTION

Acute Infection

An *acute infection* has a rapid onset of symptoms that can be quite severe but lasts a relatively short time. An acute infection goes through several stages, and the patient moves through them relatively quickly, generally over a few days to weeks.

Stages of an Infection. Many infectious diseases take time to fight off the initial immune response and infect enough of the body to develop signs and symptoms. An acute infection will go through the following stages:
- *Incubation*: It starts at the time of exposure and ends when the signs and symptoms appear. It is important to know that even though there may be no signs of disease in patients, they are still infectious. The incubation stage or period can last anywhere from minutes to weeks. Incubation times change disease to disease, as well as person to person (Table 32.1). Depending on how quickly the pathogen spreads through the body, it may take longer for an individual to develop symptoms.
- *Prodromal*: The short period of time when the first symptoms appear.
- *Acute*: The disease is at its peak, and symptoms are fully developed.
- *Declining*: The symptoms of the disease start to subside. If patients have been prescribed antibiotics, this when they may decide to stop taking them. It is important to stress to patients that they must take all of the medication. For some diseases, such as mononucleosis, the declining stage can take several weeks or even months.
- *Convalescent*: In this stage, patients will regain their strength and return to a state of good health.

TABLE 32.1	Common Disease Incubation Times
Disease	**Incubation Time**
Botulism	18–36 hours
Influenza	1–4 days
Gonorrhea	1–14 days
Strep throat	2–5 days
Impetigo	10 days
Infectious mononucleosis (mono)	28–42 days

Chronic Infection

A *chronic infection* is one that persists for a long period of time, sometimes for life. In some cases, patients are *asymptomatic*, or without symptoms, for part or all of the duration of the disease. Even though there may be no noticeable symptoms, the infection is still considered a disease because it will cause damage to the body. In these cases, in which there are no symptoms, the patient can still be contagious to others. The most common chronic infections are bloodborne pathogen infections and some sexually transmitted infections (STIs).

Latent Infection

A *latent infection* is a persistent infection in which the symptoms cycle through periods of relapse and remission. Cold sores and genital herpes are latent viral infections caused by the herpes simplex virus (HSV) types 1 and 2, respectively. The virus enters the body and causes the original lesion. It then lies dormant in nerve cells away from the surface until a certain trigger (illness with fever, sunburn, or stress) causes it to leave the nerve cell and seek the surface again. Once the virus reaches the superficial tissues, it becomes detectable for a short time and causes a new outbreak at the site. Another herpes virus, varicella-zoster, causes chickenpox (varicella). This virus may lie dormant along a nerve pathway for years and later erupt as the painful disease shingles (herpes zoster).

VOCABULARY

fomites Objects that are likely to carry infectious organisms.
relapse The recurrence of the symptoms of a disease after apparent recovery.
remission The partial or complete disappearance of the clinical and subjective characteristics of a chronic or malignant disease.
transmission To pass or spread disease.

Opportunistic Infections

Opportunistic (AH per too NIS tik) *infections* are caused by organisms that are not typically pathogenic but that cause disease under certain circumstances. A host with an impaired immune system response is more likely to get opportunistic infections. The person's immune system may not be able to fight off the pathogen before it causes disease.

CHAIN OF INFECTION

Regardless of the type of infectious disease, certain factors are required in order for it to spread from person to person. These factors make up what we know as the links in the chain of infection. Break the chain, and you break the infection process (Fig. 32.1). The steps or *links* in the chain of infection are:

1. *Infectious agent*: A pathogen must be present in order to create the disease process.
2. *Reservoir host*: A place for the pathogen to grow. Animate reservoirs can be a person, animal, insect, and birds. Inanimate reservoirs include water, soil, food, feces, and equipment. Different pathogens use different reservoirs.
3. *Portal of exit*: The pathogen must exit the reservoir. For a person, the portal of exit can include blood, respiratory tract and secretions, urine, feces, wounds, and other body fluids.

4. *Mode of transmission*: The pathogen must be transmitted to a new host. Transmission can occur by direct contact or indirect contact.
5. *Portal of entry*: The pathogen must enter a potential host. Portal of entries can include the mucous membranes, nonintact skin, and the respiratory, genitourinary, and digestive tracts.
6. *Susceptible host*: The potential host must be capable of supporting the growth of the infecting organism. For example, when individuals are vaccinated against a disease, they greatly reduce their risk of getting the disease. There are many different factors that can be used to determine if someone is susceptible to a disease. Some of these include:
   - Genetic factors
   - Quantity of organisms
   - State of the individual's health or poor health
   - Stress
   - Poor nutrition and poor hygiene

Direct and Indirect Transmission

After exiting the reservoir host, the organism needs a mode of transmission. Transmission can be either direct or indirect.

- *Direct transmission* occurs from direct contact with a pathogen or droplet spread. Direct contact can be from an infected person through skin-to-skin contact, sexual intercourse, or contact from infectious feces and body fluids (e.g., blood, urine, and saliva) or with infected food, soil, or water.
- *Indirect transmission* occurs when a pathogen leaves the reservoir and is transferred to the susceptible host through inanimate objects, air particles, or vectors.

Types of Transmission. *Droplet transmission* is very common for viral or bacterial diseases. It can be either direct or indirect transmission. Pathogens travel on respiratory droplets that exit the reservoir host through coughing, sneezing, or talking. These can be propelled through the air and land on a susceptible host. They may also land on inanimate objects, such as doorknobs, tables, or other surfaces that act as fomites (FOH mahyts), holding pathogens until they are picked up by a susceptible host. The common cold, influenza, and whooping cough (pertussis) can be spread by droplet transmission.

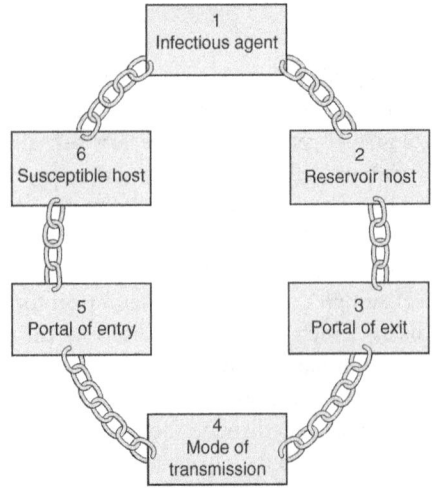

Fig. 32.1 The Chain of Infection. (From Niedzwiecki B, et al: *Kinn's the medical assistant,* ed 14, St. Louis, 2020, Elsevier.)

Airborne transmission occurs when pathogens are very light and can stay suspended in the air, often attached to dust particles. They infect a susceptible host through inhalation. Airborne transmission is especially concerning because pathogens can travel through ventilation systems and air ducts, potentially infecting a person who was never in the same area as the reservoir host. Airborne transmission can occur with diseases such as tuberculosis, measles, and varicella.

Vector transmission occurs when the pathogen is carried to a susceptible host through an outside agent. This typically occurs when insects or other animals that harbor pathogens transmit them to humans. West Nile virus, malaria, and the Zika virus are examples of vector-transmitted diseases.

Food-borne transmission occurs when pathogens are spread to susceptible hosts that eat contaminated food or drink contaminated beverages. Food-borne diseases include hepatitis A, cholera, and giardiasis.

Bloodborne transmission occurs when pathogens are transferred through contact with blood or other contaminated body fluids. Often the pathogens that are transferred with bloodborne transmission cannot live long outside a human host and cannot survive indirect transmission. Bloodborne transmission is seen most commonly in individuals who come into close contact with body fluids. At-risk individuals include:

- Those using injectable drugs who share needles
- People having unprotected sexual intercourse with multiple partners
- Healthcare workers who clean up spills and have accidental exposure through needlesticks or cuts from contaminated items

Hepatitis B, hepatitis C, and AIDS are examples of diseases spread by bloodborne transmission and will be discuss later in the chapter. At least 20 other pathogens can be spread by bloodborne transmission.

Sexual transmission occurs when a pathogen is spread through intimate contact, specifically intercourse or other sexual acts. Although bloodborne pathogens can also be spread through sexual intercourse, there are many other STIs that are transmitted specifically through sexual intercourse. Examples of STIs include gonorrhea and chlamydia.

Nosocomial infection occurs when pathogenic microbes are spread within the healthcare facility. These are also called *healthcare-associated infections.*

Breaking the Chain

In order to prevent infectious disease from spreading, the chain of infection must be broken. The first line of defense is to stop the transmission process through the use of *Standard Precautions.* This would include wearing gloves and surgical masks, performing proper wound care, correct disposal of contaminated

products, and hand washing. Using Standard Precautions helps control the ability of infectious material to spread from one host to another. The use of sanitization, disinfection, and sterilization procedures will do a lot to prevent the transmission of pathogens. Antiseptics (an tuh SEP tiks) and germicides (JUR muh sahyds) (e.g., Wavicide and Cidex) should be used to keep patients safe and patient areas clean.

VOCABULARY

antiseptics Substances that inhibit the growth of microorganisms on living tissue (e.g., alcohol and povidone-iodine solution [Betadine]); they are used to cleanse the skin, wounds, and so on.

disinfection The process of eliminating most to all pathogenic microorganisms except for spores.

germicides Agents that destroy pathogenic organisms.

inhalation The act of breathing in.

sanitization Reducing the number of pathogens to a level at which they cannot be harmful.

sterilization The process that kills all microorganisms and any spores on surfaces.

The Body's Natural Protective Mechanisms. Once a pathogen has come in contact with a susceptible host, it is up to the host's first line of defense to keep the pathogen out of the body. The first line of defense includes barrier mechanisms and chemical substances. The barrier mechanisms act to keep antigens out of the body and include:

- *Physical mechanisms*: Intact skin and the mucous membranes that line all organs that exit the body.
- *Movements*: Cilia sweep or move particles out of the airway and intestinal peristalsis move pathogens out of the body (e.g., diarrhea). Sweat, urine, and tears also move pathogens out of the body or off the body surface.
- *Reflexes*: Coughing and sneezing helps move particles and pathogens out of the airway.

Chemical substances such as hydrochloric acid in the stomach, enzymes (EN zahym) (such as lysozymes in tears and saliva), and mucus prevent antigens from entering into the body tissues.

If the pathogen enters the body, there is a second line of defense, which uses chemical and cellular responses to fight off disease. This triggers the body's inflammatory response, which in turn brings extra blood flow to the area where the pathogen is present. This allows white blood cells and antibodies to fight the pathogen. The inflammatory response produces swelling, redness, and heat due to the increased blood flow to the area. It can also cause pain if the swelling pushes against nerves. When a disease process is more systemic, the inflammatory response will still cause swelling, redness, and heat, but it looks slightly different. We often see fever, swollen lymph glands, and fatigue. For more information on how the immune system responds to disease, see Chapter 9.

CRITICAL THINKING 32.2

Tommy Anderson, a 5-year-old patient, is in the office because of an outbreak of impetigo. Rosa must apply the concepts of the chain of infection and infection control methods to teach Tommy and his mother how to prevent the spread of the infection to other members of the family. What procedures should she follow after Tommy's visit to prevent the spread of the infection to other patients, other staff members, and herself?

CRITICAL THINKING 32.3

Rosa's next patient appears to have a localized inflammatory response to a splinter. What signs and symptoms should she expect the patient to show?

Rosa answers a telephone call from a patient who had surgery 3 days ago. The patient is concerned that the incision site is red, swollen, and hot. Is this a normal postoperative response? How might Rosa know whether the response is abnormal?

REGULATORY STANDARDS FOR THE HEALTHCARE SETTING

Standard Precautions and Transmission-Based Precautions

By 1985 significant concern had arisen about the increasing number of people infected with HIV and hepatitis B virus (HBV). In order to help slow the spread of these diseases and to standardize infection control efforts across the U.S., the Centers for Disease Control and Prevention (CDC) created the *Universal Precautions*. With Universal Precautions, healthcare workers had to treat all blood and certain body fluids from all patients as if they contained infectious bloodborne pathogens. Personal protective equipment (PPE) was used to prevent exposures, and hand washing was recommended immediately after glove removal.

In 1996, Standard Precautions and Transmission-Based Precautions were introduced, replacing Universal Precautions. *Standard Precautions* are the minimum infection prevention practices that all healthcare workers must use for all patients. Healthcare workers must take precautions when there is a risk of potential exposure to blood, body fluids (except sweat), nonintact skin, and mucous membranes. Healthcare workers need to perform hand hygiene and use PPE. Standard Precaution also address:

- Respiratory hygiene/cough etiquette: Use tissue to cover the mouth and nose when coughing and sneezing. Discard tissue and perform hand hygiene.
- Sharps safety and safe injection practices
- Sterile instruments and devices
- Clean and disinfected environmental surfaces

Besides developing Standard Precautions, the CDC created Transmission-Based Precautions, which serve as an additional level of basic infection control. These precautions are used in addition to Standard Precautions when working with patients who have infections and include strategies to use to prevent contact, droplet, and airborne transmission. Failure to follow Standard Precautions and Transmission-Based Precautions can lead to infection transmission between patients and staff. Standard Precautions and Transmission-Based Precautions are discussed later in the chapter.

VOCABULARY

bloodborne pathogen A pathogen present in blood that can be transmitted to an individual who is exposed to the blood or body fluids of an infected individual. Can include HIV, hepatitis B virus (HBV), and hepatitis C virus (HCV).

personal protective equipment (PPE) Clothing, eye protection, gloves, or other garments or equipment designed to protect the wearer's body from injury or infection.

CRITICAL THINKING 32.4

Rosa is caring for an injured 3-year-old child with an open wound on his right knee. She puts on disposable gloves to clean the wound, and the mother demands to know why. How can she explain her actions?

Bloodborne Pathogen Standard

In 1991 OSHA published the Bloodborne Pathogen Standard in response to the significant health risk associated with workplace exposure to blood and other potentially infectious materials. The Bloodborne Pathogen Standard addressed ways to minimize or eliminate the risk of bloodborne pathogen exposures.

As technology advanced, companies developed safer products, which decreased the risk of exposures. In response to the advancements, Congress passed the Needlestick Safety and Prevention Act in 2000. The Needlestick Safety and Prevention Act directed OSHA to revise the Bloodborne Pathogen Standard, requiring employers to identify and make use of safer medical devices. As a result of the revisions, the Bloodborne Pathogen Standard requires employers to protect workers from occupational exposures to blood or other potentially infectious materials (OPIM) (Box 32.3). The standard requires the employer to:

- *Have a written exposure control plan*: Each facility must identify potential exposure risks. The plan needs to be reviewed and updated annually.
- *Hepatitis B Vaccination:* Offered free to all employees with occupational exposure to blood and OPIM.
- *Training*: Employees need annual training on the bloodborne pathogen standard, the facility's Exposure Control Plan, bloodborne pathogens, hepatitis B vaccination, how to reduce exposures, and postexposure activities.
- *Maintain a sharps injury log*: This log must include a description any parenteral (pa REN ter uhl) employee exposure, the device involved in the incident, and the details of how and where the incident occurred. An employer who fails to comply with OSHA's Bloodborne Pathogens Standard could face a maximum penalty of $7,000 for the first violation and up to $70,000 for repeated violations.
- *Personal protective equipment*: PPE must be provided by the employer and used by the employees when there is a risk of exposure to blood or OPIM.
- *Identify and use engineering controls:* This includes equipment that minimizes the exposure risk, such as sharps disposal containers and safety needles. All needles must have a safety device to cover the needle after use. It also requires that whenever possible needles be avoided, such

---

BOX 32.3 Other Potentially Infectious Materials

Items contaminated with any of the following potentially infectious materials require special handling.

- Body fluids
  - Semen
  - Vaginal secretions
  - Cerebrospinal fluid (CSF)
  - Synovial fluid
  - Pleural fluid
  - Pericardial fluid
  - Peritoneal fluid
  - Amniotic fluid
- Any unfixed tissue
- Any pathogenic microorganism
  - Saliva in dental procedures
  - Any body fluid that is visibly contaminated with blood
- All body fluids in situations in which it is difficult or impossible to differentiate between body fluids

as by implementing the use of needleless intravenous (IV) systems.

- *Identify and use work practice controls*: These practices reduce the risk of exposure by changing the way a task is performed. Work practice controls include handling and disposing contaminated sharps, handling specimens, and cleaning contaminated surfaces and equipment.
- *Signs and labels need to be used to communicate hazards*: Signs must be posted on containers and in the location of where blood or OPIM are stored. Facilities can use red bags or red containers to communicate hazards.

VOCABULARY

parenteral To take into the body by any route other than the digestive tract.

CRITICAL THINKING 32.5

Your office manager asks you to prepare a fact sheet for your co-workers that summarizes the details of OSHA's Bloodborne Pathogens Standard. What should you include?

PREVENTING DISEASE TRANSMISSION

A medical assistant must follow the Standard Precautions, Transmission-Based Precautions, and the Bloodborne Pathogen Standard in the ambulatory care facility. The following sections will discuss strategies to prevent disease transmission by applying these precautions.

Hand Hygiene

Hand hygiene is one of the most important steps to control the spread of infectious disease. Proper hand washing is the best approach to hand hygiene. Although proper hand washing is considered the best approach to hand hygiene, studies have shown that correct use of alcohol-based hand sanitizers significantly reduces the number of microorganisms on the skin. It also takes less time than traditional hand washing and causes less irritation to the skin (Fig. 32.2).

Hand Washing. Proper medical aseptic hand washing involves using soap, running water, and friction (Procedure 32.1). The temperature of the water does not appear to affect the microbe removal according to the CDC. Warm water is suggested since hot water can cause drying of the skin. Using soap is more effective than not using soap. The surfactants in the soap help lift the dirt and microbes from the skin surface. The lathering of soap and scrubbing the hands creates friction that also helps to lift the dirt and microbes from the skin. Remember that your fingers have four sides, and fingernails have two sides. Using running water helps rinse off the microbes and dirt. With the fingertips pointing downward, start by rinsing the wrists and move towards the fingertips.

A water-soluble lotion may be rubbed into the hands after they have been washed and dried to prevent cracking. Dry, cracked, chapped skin is no longer intact and can provide a means of entry for microorganisms. It can also create a place on

the hands that will harbor pathogenic bacteria, which can then be passed onto patients.

There are certain times hand washing must be done and hand sanitizer is not appropriate:

- When first arriving for a shift. Hand washing should be done for at least 1 minute at the beginning of the shift. For subsequent hand washing, the CDC recommends 20 seconds.
- If the hands are visibly soiled.
- After using the restroom.

Alcohol-Based Hand Sanitizer. When using an alcohol-based hand sanitizer, apply the label-recommended amount to the palm of one hand (Procedure 32.2). Rub the hands together, covering all surfaces. It should take 20 to 30 seconds to rub it into the skin. Continue rubbing it in until your hands are dry. Antimicrobial-impregnated wipes (e.g., towelettes) are not a substitute for an alcohol-based hand sanitizer.

Hand Hygiene Recommendations. Medical aseptic hand washing or alcohol-based hand sanitizer should be used in the following situations:

- Before and after contact with the patient or their immediate care environment
- After removing gloves.
- After handling one specimen and before handling another specimen
- Before performing an invasive procedures, such as administering an injection
- After contact with blood, OPIM, or contaminated surfaces
- When hands move from a contaminated body site to a clean body site during patient care

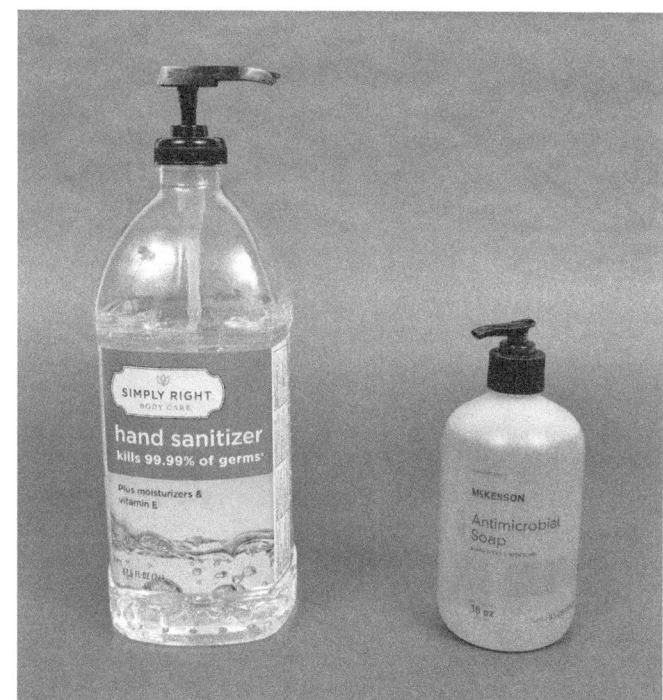

Fig. 32.2 Alcohol-Based Hand Sanitizer and Soap. (From Niedzwiecki B, et al: *Kinn's the medical assistant,* ed 14, St. Louis, 2020, Elsevier.)

- Before you leave the facility
- Before and after eating

The CDC recommends that artificial nails should not be worn. Studies show that even after careful hand hygiene, healthcare workers with artificial nails have more pathogenic microbes under their nails and on their fingertips than workers with natural nails. Artificial nails also cause nail changes that contribute to the transmission of microbes. The CDC also recommends that natural nail tips should be no longer than ¼ of an inch to prevent microbial growth under the nail.

It is important to remember that microbes can be present on jewelry. Because of this, jewelry should be removed. If the medical assistant chooses to wear minimal jewelry, such as a wedding band or wristwatch, these must be able to be washed or easily removed and sanitized.

Personal Protective Equipment

Personal protective equipment, or barrier protection, are specialized clothing or equipment that is worn for protection against blood and OPIM, according to OSHA. PPE should be used when there is a chance of exposure to blood or OPIM. This prevents or minimizes the entry of infectious material into the body (Fig 32.3). Examples of personal protective equipment include:

- *Gloves*, which protect the hands.
- *Shoe covers, impermeable gown/aprons, and laboratory coats*, which protect the clothing and skin.
- *Surgical masks and respirators*, which protect the nose and mouth. Respirators (e.g., N95) protect the respiratory system from airborne infectious agents. Respirators must be fit tested.
- *Protective eyewear* (e.g., goggles), which protect the eyes.
- *Face shields*, which protect the face, nose, mouth, and eyes.

Protective equipment contaminated with blood or OPIM must be removed and placed in a designated area or biohazardous waste container. The hands or any other exposed areas must be washed or flushed as soon as possible.

Utility gloves, such as household cleaning type rubber or plastic gloves, may be reused if they are intact (i.e., have no cracks, tears, or punctures). All personal protective equipment (PPE) must be removed before the medical assistant leaves the medical facility.

Gloves. Gloves are the most commonly used PPE in a healthcare facility. According to the Bloodborne Pathogen Standard, gloves must be worn if the medical assistant might be:

- Touching a patient's blood, body fluids, mucous membranes, or skin that is not intact.
- Handling items and surfaces contaminated with blood and OPIM.
- Performing venipuncture, finger sticks, injections, and other vascular procedures.
- Assisting with any surgical procedure. If a glove is torn during the procedure, the glove should be removed, the hands washed carefully, and new gloves put on as soon as possible.
- Handling, processing, and disposing of all blood and body fluid specimens.
- Cleaning and decontaminating spills of blood or OPIM.

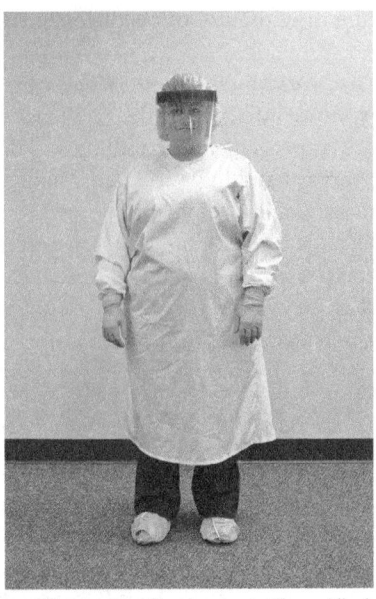

Fig. 32.3 Personal Protective Equipment. (From Niedzwiecki B, et al: *Kinn's the medical assistant*, ed 14, St. Louis, 2020, Elsevier.)

When using gloves it is important to remember to work from clean to dirty to prevent any spread of pathogens. Do not touch your face or hair or adjust your PPE with contaminated gloves. Limit touching other surfaces except as necessary with contaminated gloves. Change gloves after each patient; never use the same gloves for more than one patient. Change torn or heavily soiled gloves. When you remove your gloves, it is important to do so carefully so that no material or pathogens on the gloves become dislodged or move onto the skin (Procedure 32.3). It is also important to remember to use hand hygiene after removing gloves.

Environmental Protection

Environmental protection refers to minimizing the risk of injury by isolating or removing any physical or mechanical health hazard in the workplace. This includes a number of precautions:

- Read warning labels on biohazardous waste containers and equipment.
- Minimize splashing or spraying of OPIM. Blood that splatters onto exposed areas of the skin or mucous membranes is a proven mode of HBV transmission.
- Contaminated needles and other sharps should never be recapped, bent, broken, or resheathed. Needle units must have protective safety devices to cover the contaminated needle after injection.
- Contaminated sharp instruments, such as operating scissors, should not be processed in a way that requires employees to reach into containers to grasp them.
- Immediately after use, dispose of syringes and needles, scalpel blades, and other disposable sharp items in a labeled, leakproof, puncture-resistant biohazard container. The container must be located as close as possible to the area where the item is used.
- All specimens must be placed in a container that prevents leakage during collection, handling, processing, storage,

transport, and shipping. Avoid contaminating the outside of the container or the label with the specimen substance. The container must have a biohazard label to alert others that it holds potentially infectious material. Gloves should be worn when handling containers with specimens.

- Equipment requiring repair that has been contaminated with blood or body fluids should be decontaminated before being repaired in the office or transported for repair.
- Smoking, eating, drinking, applying cosmetics or lip balm, and handling contact lenses are prohibited in work areas where there is a reasonable likelihood of contamination by pathogens.
- Food and beverages cannot be kept in refrigerators, freezers, or cabinets or on countertops where infectious materials could be present.
- Bandage any breaks or lesions on your hands before gloving.

Housekeeping Controls

The Bloodborne Pathogens Standard requires certain housekeeping measures to ensure a sanitary work area. A schedule must be posted for the cleaning and decontamination of each work area where exposures could occur. Documentation of these procedures must include information about the surface cleaned, the type of waste encountered, and procedures performed in the designated area (Box 32.4).

- After accidental spills of blood or OPIM, at the end of each procedure, and at the end of each shift, work surfaces must be immediately cleaned and then disinfected with a disinfectant (dis in FEK tuh nt) registered with the Environmental Protection Agency (EPA).

BOX 32.4 Protocols for Disposal of Biologic Chemical Materials

The Medical Waste Tracking Act set the standards for governmental regulation of medical waste; however, that law expired in 1991. The states were then given responsibility for regulating the disposal of medical waste. Each state varies in its degree of regulation, ranging from no regulation to strict rules. The following are some examples of regulations covering the disposal of hazardous materials.

- Biomedical waste should be collected in containers that are leakproof and strong enough to prevent breakage during handling; the containers must be labeled with the biohazard symbol.
- Workers who handle biomedical waste should observe Standard Precautions.
- Biologic waste containers and boxes should not be held in the healthcare facility for longer than 30 days.
- Boxes for disposal of chemicals should be labeled with the chemicals' names and any other pertinent data. They must be adequately sealed to prevent breakage or leakage.
- Each healthcare facility must hire a biomedical waste disposal service whose employees are trained to collect and haul away biomedical waste in special containers (usually cardboard boxes or reusable plastic bins) for treatment at a facility designed to handle biomedical waste.

The cost to the healthcare facility for biomedical waste disposal is typically based on the weight of the contaminated items collected (i.e., the weight of filled sharps containers, biohazard boxes, and bags).

- All reusable containers must be disinfected and decontaminated on a routine basis.
- Sharps are instruments intended to cut or penetrate the skin. They include lancets, scalpel blades, needles, and syringe/needle combinations. Sharps must be placed in red, hard plastic sharps container after use. When placing items into the sharps container, always place the sharp end in first. Never attempt to reach inside a sharps container. Sharps containers must be kept as close as possible to the work area. Sharps containers should be replaced when they are about 75% filled; never overfill them. Close the lid securely before removing and replacing the sharps container.
- Never pick up spilled material or broken glassware with your hands. Brooms, brushes, dustpans, and pickup tongs or forceps should be used. The material should be placed immediately into an impervious (im PUR vee uhs) biohazardous waste container at the spill site (Fig. 32.4). Use an absorbent, professional biohazardous spill preparation as directed to decontaminate the site.
- Handle soiled linen as little as possible and always wear gloves or other protective equipment during disposal. Linens soiled with blood or body fluids should be double-bagged and transported in labeled, leakproof biohazard bags.
- Contaminated materials and/or infectious waste must be handled with extreme caution to prevent exposure. Biohazardous waste must be collected in impermeable, red polyethylene or polypropylene biohazard-labeled bags or containers and sealed (Fig. 32.5). This waste must be disposed of in accordance with all federal, state, and local regulations. Disposal methods include treatment by heat, incineration, steam sterilization, chemical treatment, or other equivalent methods that will render the waste inactive before it is placed in a landfill.

The CDC has developed a checklist that ambulatory care facilities can use to systematically assess employee adherence to infection prevention. It helps to ensure that the facility has policies and procedures in place and has adequate supplies available to prevent infections at the site. If the answer to any of the questions is no, the facility must do all it can to correct the problems with either staff or supplies (Table 32.2).

VOCABULARY

disinfectant Any chemical agent used on nonliving objects to destroy or inhibit the growth of harmful organisms; disinfectants are not effective against bacterial spores.

impervious Not permitting penetration.

Transmission-Based Precautions

Transmission-based precautions help provide an additional level of protection and are used in addition to Standard Precautions. Transmission-based precautions include airborne, droplet, and contact precaution. In ambulatory care facilities, the placement of the patient, PPE used, and the transport of the patient are key issues with transmission-based precautions. Facilities should have policies and procedures regarding early

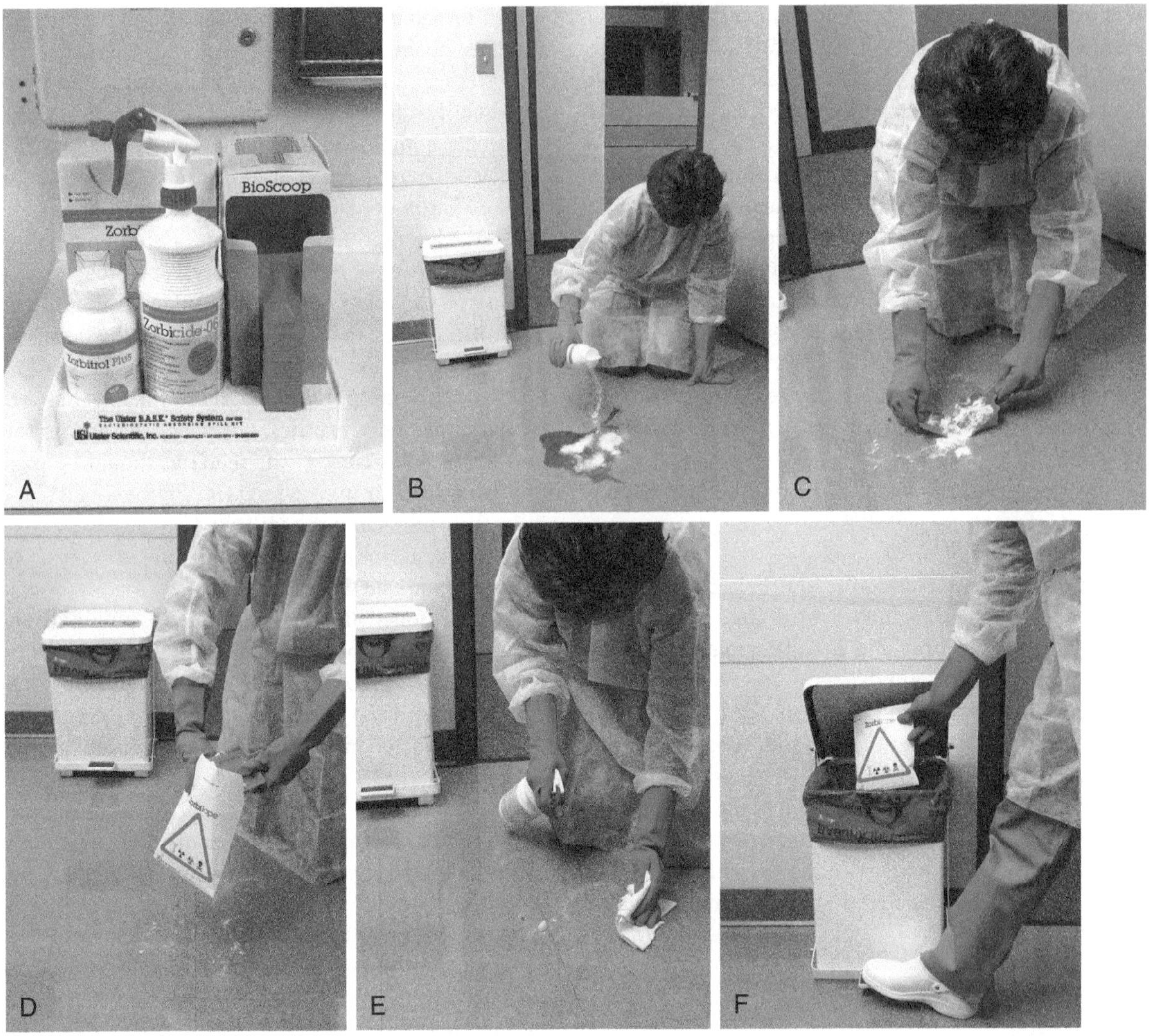

Fig. 32.4 Cleaning Up Spilled Material. A, Cleanup kit with printed instructions. B, Sprinkle congealing powder over the spill. C, Scoop up the spill. D, Place the contents in a biohazard bag. E, Wipe the area thoroughly with a germicide. F, Place all contaminated material in a biohazard bag or container. (From Niedzwiecki B, et al: *Kinn's the medical assistant,* ed 14, St. Louis, 2020, Elsevier.)

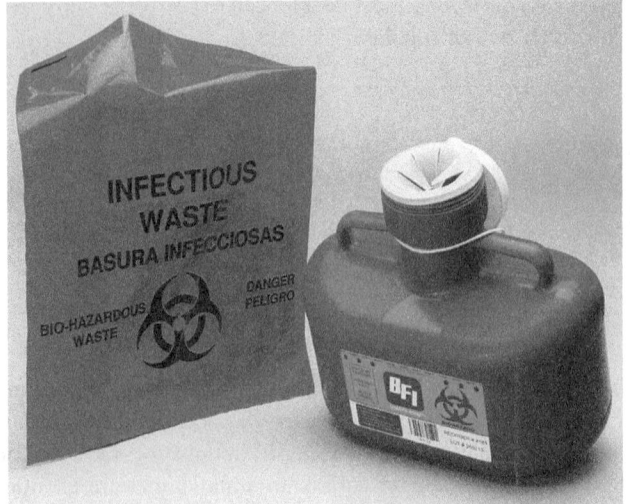

Fig. 32.5 Biohazard Bag and Biohazard Sharps Container. (From Niedzwiecki B, et al: *Kinn's the medical assistant,* ed 14, St. Louis, 2020, Elsevier.)

		If Answer Is No,
	Practice	Document Plan
Facility Policies	Performed	for Remediation

TABLE 32.2   Modified CDC Infection Prevention Checklist

1. Administrative Policies and Facility Practices

Facility Policies	Practice Performed	If Answer Is No, Document Plan for Remediation
a. Written infection prevention policies and procedures are available, current, and based on evidence-based guideline, regulations, or standards.	Yes No	
b. Infection prevention policies and procedures are reassessed at least annually or according to state or federal requirements and updated if appropriate.	Yes No	
c. At least one individual trained in infection prevention is employed by or regularly available to the facility.	Yes No	
d. Supplies necessary for adherence to Standard Precautions are readily available.	Yes No	

TABLE 32.2 Modified CDC Infection Prevention Checklist—cont'd

Facility Policies	Practice Performed		If Answer Is No, Document Plan for Remediation
e. Healthcare personnel for whom contact with blood or other potentially infectious material is anticipated are trained on the OSHA Bloodborne Pathogens Standard upon hire and at least annually.	Yes	No	
f. The facility maintains a log of needlesticks, sharps injuries, and other employee exposure events.	Yes	No	
g. Following an exposure event, post-exposure evaluation and follow-up, including prophylaxis as appropriate, are available at no cost to employee.	Yes	No	
h. Hepatitis B vaccination is available at no cost to all employees at risk of occupational exposure.	Yes	No	
i. Postvaccination screening for hepatitis B surface antibodies is conducted.	Yes	No	
j. All personnel are offered annual influenza vaccination at no cost.	Yes	No	
k. All personnel with potential exposure to tuberculosis (TB) are screened for TB upon hire and annually (if negative).	Yes	No	

2. Surveillance and Disease Reporting

a. Updated list of reportable diseases is readily available to all personnel.	Yes	No	

3. Hand Hygiene

a. Facility provides training and supplies necessary for adherence to hand hygiene.	Yes	No	

4. Personal Protective Equipment (PPE)

a. Facility provides training and supplies for appropriate PPE.	Yes	No	
b. Impermeable gowns are worn during procedures in which contact with blood or body fluids is anticipated.	Yes	No	
c. PPE is removed and discarded prior to leaving the exam room.	Yes	No	
d. Hand hygiene is performed immediately after removal of PPE.	Yes	No	

5. Environmental Cleaning

a. Policies and procedures exist for routine cleaning and disinfection of environmental surfaces.	Yes	No	
b. Cleaning procedures are periodically monitored and assessed to ensure that they are consistently and correctly performed.	Yes	No	
c. The facility has a policy/procedure for decontamination of spills of blood or other body fluids.	Yes	No	

aThe complete checklist is available at the CDC website for Infection Prevention in Outpatient Settings Modified from the Occupational Safety and Health Administration. www.cdc.gov/HAI/settings/outpatient/checklist/outpatient-care-checklist.html.

detection and management of potentially infectious patients. The administrative medical assistant at the reception desk has an important role in identifying patients with potentially infectious conditions.

Airborne Precautions

Airborne precautions provided additional protection and are used when the patient have a known or suspected infection that is spread by airborne transmission. Such conditions can include tuberculosis, measles, and chickenpox. Airborne precautions include:

- Placing a potentially infectious patient in a negative pressure examination room or an examination room instead of waiting in the reception area. (Not all ambulatory care facilities have negative pressure examination rooms.) The door should remain closed at all times.
- Using a respirator, gloves, face shield, and an impermeable gown when working with the patient.
- Having the patient wear a surgical mask outside of a negative pressure examination room.

> **VOCABULARY**
> **negative pressure** A ventilation system designed so the air flows from the hallways into an isolation room. This prevents the contaminated air from passing from the isolation room to other parts of the building.

Droplet Precautions

Droplet precautions are used to prevent or limit contact with secretions from the nose and lungs. Conditions that require droplet precautions include influenza, pertussis (whooping cough), mumps, and coronavirus (Covid-19). Many facilities have signs at the entrance regarding respiratory hygiene/cough etiquette for patients with signs and symptoms of a respiratory infection. Tissue, hand sanitizer, and a waste container may be available. Additional droplet precautions include:

- Having the patient wear a surgical mask. Typically, adult and child size masks are available at or near the reception desk.
- Using a surgical mask, gloves, face shield, and an impermeable gown when working with the patient (Procedure 32.4).

For patients with signs and symptoms of coronavirus, facilities may require staff to use a respirator instead of a surgical mask. Patients should be immediately placed in an examination room. After the patient leaves, the examination room should be disinfected, and some agencies may limit the immediate use of the room.

Contact Precautions

Contact precautions are used to prevent the spread pathogens by direct contact or indirect contact, such as touching an item the patient touched. Contact precautions are used with *C. difficile*, norovirus, and Methicillin-resistant *Staphylococcus aureus* (MRSA), a staph infection resistant to antibiotics. Contact precautions include wearing an impermeable gown and gloves when coming in contact with the patient or something the patient touched.

Hepatitis B Vaccination

Healthcare professionals are considered at increased risk for contracting HBV. Because of this OSHA requires that all healthcare employers provide vaccination free of charge to all employees at risk for occupational exposure to bloodborne pathogens. The hepatitis B vaccine series should be started within 10 days of employment. Depending on the brand, the single antigen vaccine schedules vary:

- Heplisav-B requires two intramuscular injection doses 1 month apart.
- Engerix-B and Recombivax HB require three intramuscular injection doses. The second dose is given at least 4 weeks after the first. The third dose is usually given 6 months after the first.

If the employee does not complete the series, the current recommendation by the CDC is to continue with the series from the point where it was interrupted. The series does not need to be restarted. After the original series is completed, additional boosters are not currently recommended. However, if this changes in the future, boosters must be made available to eligible employees without cost.

After the hepatitis B series, most healthy individuals develop adequate antibody responses to confer immunity. In fact, about 90% of healthy adults show appropriate antibody levels after immunization. Despite this, healthcare workers with a high risk of exposure should have a titer drawn 1 to 2 months after completing the series. The antibody testing will show if the person is immune (has enough antibodies to protect against HBV). If the antibody testing shows the person is nonimmune, one more dose of hepatitis B vaccine and repeated antibody testing is recommended. If the person is still nonimmune, the person should receive the rest of the hepatitis B series and be retested. If the final test result is nonimmune, the healthcare worker should be counseled on HBV precautions and the need to obtain hepatitis B immune globulin (HBIG) prophylaxis for any exposures.

Employees have the right to decline hepatitis B immunization, but they are required to sign a declination form (Fig. 32.6). The hepatitis B declination form must be kept on file as a record of their refusal. The statement can be signed only after the employee has received training on HBV and the hepatitis B vaccine (e.g., the efficacy, safety, method, and benefits of vaccination). In addition, the employee must be informed that the vaccine will be administered free of charge. Employees who change their mind may receive the vaccine at a future date with the charge covered by the employer.

> **VOCABULARY**
>
> **titer** A test that measures the amount of antibodies found in a person's blood

Exposure Events

When a sharps injury occurs, the healthcare worker has the following estimated risk:

- HBV: Healthcare workers who have received the hepatitis B vaccine and have developed immunity to the virus are at virtually no risk for infection. For an unvaccinated person, the risk from a single needlestick or a cut exposure to HBV-infected blood ranges from 6% to 30%.
- HCV: The estimated risk for infection after a needlestick or sharps injury is 0.2%.
- HIV: The estimated risk of HIV infection from a sharps injury is about 0.3% or 1 in 300. Approximately 1 in 7 people have HIV, but most do not know they have it.

Exposure events include incidents in which an employee is exposed to potentially contaminated body fluids. This typically happens if the employee has an accidental needlestick, is exposed to patient fluids through a cut or other broken skin, has body fluids splashed or spattered onto their mucus membranes or into their eyes, or suffers a human bite. If this type of event happens, certain steps must be followed to reduce the risk of infection.

Steps to Take After an Exposure

If a blood or OPIM exposure occurs, a medical assistant must know the immediate steps to take. If you have an exposure to blood or OPIM, do the following:

- With a needlestick or an exposure to a cut or a body surface, wash the area with soap and warm, running water for 10 to 15 minutes as soon as possible after the exposure. Chlorine-based antiseptics and 10% iodine solution can also be used to clean the area.
- Flush splashes to the nose or mouth with water.
- Irrigate the eyes. Continuously flush them with water as soon as possible for a minimum of 15 minutes using an eye wash unit. A stationary unit connected to warm, running water is the best method for properly flushing potentially infectious material out of the eyes. (This will be discussed in detail in Chapter 52.)
- Report the incident to the supervisor and immediately seek medical treatment.

Hepatitis B Vaccine Declination

I understand that due to my occupational exposure to blood or other potentially infectious materials I may be at risk of acquiring hepatitis B virus (HBV) infection. I have been given the opportunity to be vaccinated with hepatitis B vaccine, at no charge to myself. However, I decline hepatitis B vaccination at this time. I understand that by declining this vaccine, I continue to be at risk of acquiring hepatitis B, a serious disease. If in the future I continue to have occupational exposure to blood or other potentially infectious materials and I want to be vaccinated with hepatitis B vaccine, I can receive the vaccination series at no charge to me.

Name: _____   Date: _____

Fig. 32.6 Sample Hepatitis B Declination Form. (From the Occupational Safety and Health Administration. https://www.osha.gov/SLTC/etools/hospital/hazards/bbp/declination.html.)

> **CRITICAL THINKING 32.6**
>
> Rosa's office has been especially busy today. While administering an injection to a frightened 6-year-old child, a co-worker accidentally sticks herself with the needle. She tells Rosa about the incident, but she does not know what to do next. What steps should be taken to manage the situation?

Postexposure Follow-up

The employee must immediately receive a confidential medical evaluation.

- The provider caring for the exposed employee must receive written details of the exposure incident, including the route and circumstances surrounding the incident. All documentation related to the exposure must meet the following requirements:
  - All information regarding the incident must remain confidential.
  - An incident report must be filed that documents the details surrounding the exposure incident, the route or type of exposure, and the identity, if known, of the source individual. The source individual is the person, living or dead, whose blood or OPIM was the source of the occupational exposure.
  - The documentation must be kept for at least the duration of the worker's employment plus 30 years.
- The source individual is screened for HBV, HCV, and HIV, unless the disease status is known. Depending on state regulations, consent may or may not be required from the source individual to perform the screening. If consent is required but not given, the employer must document that consent was not received from the source individual. If screening is done, OSHA requires that the employee be informed of the results of the source individual's tests.
- Depending on the situation, the exposed employee may be tested for HBV, HCV, and HIV if consent is given. Factors such as the exposed employee's HBV immunity status and the source patient's known disease status can affect the situation. If the employee refuses the tests but blood is drawn, the sample must be stored 90 days for the worker to decide whether screening is wanted.
- If the employee has not been vaccinated against HBV, vaccination is offered.
- The injured employee must receive a copy of the healthcare provider's written opinion within 15 days of completion of the evaluation.
- The exposed employee must receive health counseling about the risk of illness or other adverse outcomes of exposure and the potential for and consequences of transmission of the disease to family, patients, and others.

Postexposure Management

Postexposure management for specific bloodborne pathogens include:

- *Hepatitis B virus (HBV):* Postexposure prophylaxis (PEP) includes the hepatitis B vaccine series for unvaccinated people and may also include the hepatitis B immune globulin.
- *Hepatitis C virus (HCV):* Immune globulin and antiviral agents (e.g., interferon with or without ribavirin) are not recommended for PEP of hepatitis C; determine the HCV status of the source and the exposed person; provide follow-up HCV testing for the employee if the source is HCV positive.
- *Human immunodeficiency virus (HIV):* Four-week PEP regimen of two drugs (zidovudine [Retrovir] and lamivudine [Epivir], Epivir and stavudine [Zerit], or didanosine [Videx]

and Zerit) for most HIV exposures, and a third drug for HIV exposures that pose an increased risk of transmission; employees should receive follow-up counseling, postexposure testing, and medical evaluation, regardless of whether they receive PEP. After baseline testing at the time of exposure, follow-up testing could be performed at 6 weeks, 12 weeks, and 6 months after exposure.

ROLE OF THE MEDICAL ASSISTANT IN ASEPSIS

Breaking the chain of infection is one of the most important things a medical assistant can do to stop disease from spreading within the ambulatory care setting. Asepsis is one of the few procedures that will directly affect the health of the patient, the provider, and the staff.

The spread of pathogens in the ambulatory care setting can be controlled only through the effective, consistent application of the Bloodborne Pathogens Standard and by proper sanitization, disinfection, and sterilization of supplies, equipment, and work surfaces.

Asepsis (ey SEP sis) is the state of being free of infection or infectious material. *Medical asepsis* is defined as the use of practices to reduce disease-causing organisms; also considered the clean technique. By using principles of medical asepsis, we can prevent the spread of disease. The goal is to eliminate or minimize pathogens by following OSHA's Bloodborne Pathogens Standard and disinfecting objects as soon as possible after contamination. This creates a healthcare environment as free of pathogens as possible.

The most effective barrier against infection is intact skin. If the skin and mucous membranes are intact, medical asepsis can be used for most noninvasive procedures, such as pelvic and proctologic examinations. Instruments and objects used in medical aseptic procedures must be sanitized and disinfected or sterilized before being used on another patient. Medical aseptic procedures may include the use of impermeable gowns and surgical masks, but these are not sterile and are worn to protect the healthcare worker more than the patient.

> **VOCABULARY**
> **noninvasive procedures** Procedures that do not penetrate human tissue.

Another practical application of medical aseptic technique is to set up work areas in the medical office's laboratory. One side of the laboratory is the "clean" side, where only noninfectious procedures are performed. The other side is the "dirty" side, where potentially infectious materials are processed or cleaned.

Surgical asepsis is the use of practices to eliminate all microorganisms. This technique is used for any procedure that enters the body's skin or tissues, such as surgery or injections. Anytime the skin or a mucous membrane is punctured, pierced, or incised, surgical aseptic techniques are practiced. This means that everything that comes in contact with the patient should be sterile, including gloves, drapes, and instruments. Minor surgery, urinary catheterization, injections, and some specimen collections, such as blood collection and biopsies, are performed using surgical aseptic technique.

The medical assistant must develop the skills needed for performing aseptic procedures properly. It is important that these techniques be done on such a routine basis that they become an unbreakable habit. The use of disposable items is highly recommended for infection control purposes. The use of disposable instruments minimizes the need for sanitization, disinfection, and sterilization. However, when disposable equipment is used, the assistant must follow recommended disposal guidelines to ensure infection control.

Sanitization

Instruments and other items used in the healthcare facility must be carefully cleaned before proceeding with disinfection or sterilization. *Sanitization* (SAN i tah zaa shun) is the cleaning process that reduces the number of microorganisms to a safe level. This cleansing process removes debris such as blood and other body fluids from instruments or equipment. This debris can protect the microorganisms from disinfection or sterilization (Procedure 32.5).

The medical assistant should always wear gloves while performing sanitization. Thick utility gloves will help protect your hands when working with instruments that have sharp or pointed edges. Gloves prevent possible personal contamination with potentially infections material that may be present on the articles being cleaned. The procedure should be completed immediately after use of the instruments. Instruments left out or left to "soak" present an infection risk to others who may come into contact with them. A separate workroom or the decontamination side of the utility room is used to prevent cross-contamination of clean instruments and equipment. If sanitization cannot be done immediately, rinse the used items under cold water immediately after the procedure, place them in a detergent solution, and clean them as soon as possible. Never allow blood or other substances to dry on an instrument.

When you are ready to sanitize instruments, rinse each instrument in cold running water. Sharp instruments should be kept separate from the other instruments. Metal instruments may damage the cutting edges, and sharp instruments may damage other instruments or injure you. When cleaning sharp instruments, it is important that you have time set aside that can be uninterrupted so you can focus on preventing injury. Open all hinges and scrub serrations and ratchets with a small scrub brush or toothbrush. Rinse the instruments in hot water and then check carefully that they are in proper working order before they are disinfected or sterilized. The items should be lightly hand dried with a towel to prevent spotting and allowed to air dry before further processing. Sanitization is a very important step, and it cannot be overlooked or done carelessly.

Sound waves can also be used to sanitize instruments. When *ultrasonic sanitization* is used, the instruments are placed in an ultrasonic bath of cleaner and water. Sound waves cause the solution to vibrate, which loosens the materials attached to the instruments. Ultrasonic cleaners are beneficial because they do not damage even the most delicate instruments, and workers do not run the risk of an accidental sharps injury.

Disinfection

Disinfection is the process of killing pathogenic organisms or of rendering them inactive. It is not always effective against spores, tuberculosis bacilli, and certain viruses. For hard surfaces, such as exam tables and countertop surfaces, several different types of disinfectants are available, depending on the level of disinfection needed (Box 32.5). It is important to follow the facility's policies on which disinfectant to use and the manufacturer's guidelines to ensure that the disinfectant is used properly. Some common errors that can cause chemicals to lose their effectiveness are:

- Instruments are not thoroughly sanitized. Attached organic matter inhibits or prevents the action of the disinfectant. No chemical can kill unless it reaches all instrument surfaces; therefore complete sanitization is absolutely necessary.
- The disinfectant solution is left in an open container, and evaporation changes its concentration.
- Solutions are not changed after the recommended period for use has expired.
- Solutions are not prepared properly or are not mixed properly before use.
- The manufacturer's recommended temperature for use and storage is not maintained.

Chemical disinfectants cannot be used on skin or tissues because they can damage them. Therefore antiseptics, such as alcohol, are used on the skin to reduce the number of pathogens. Alcohol is the most widely used antiseptic, but studies indicate that it is not as effective as other products in inhibiting the growth and reproduction of microorganisms on the skin's surface. Other antiseptic chemicals, such as povidone-iodine solution (Betadine), are effective antimicrobial agents that are safe to use on a patient's skin. Always check with a patient for allergies or sensitivities before placing anything on their skin.

CRITICAL THINKING 32.7

Rosa is responsible for orienting the new medical assistant in the office's sanitization and disinfection procedures. Outline the important concepts and methods of each procedure.

BOX 32.5 Levels of Disinfectants

The Centers for Disease Control and Prevention (CDC) defines three levels of disinfectants:

- *Low-level disinfectants* can kill most vegetative bacteria, some fungi, and some viruses. These are used for exam tables and countertops. Example: hydrogen peroxide.
- *Intermediate-level disinfectants* can kill mycobacteria, vegetative bacteria, most viruses, and most fungi, but they do not kill spores. They are used for noncritical items, such as stethoscopes and percussion hammers. Example: isopropyl alcohol.
- *High-level disinfectants* will kill all microorganisms except large numbers of bacterial spores. They are used for semicritical items, such as a flexible fiberoptic sigmoidoscope. Example: Cidex OPA.

Sterilization

Sterilization is essential for surgical asepsis. Sterilization can be achieved with moist heat, dry heat, ultraviolet light, ionizing radiation, gas, or chemicals. Some chemicals, such as Cidex, are effective enough to kill all organisms and achieve sterilization, but the usual immersion time for these chemicals is 10 hours or longer. Medical facilities typically use the autoclave method, which uses moist heat. Steam under pressure in the autoclave offers an excellent method of sterilization because it kills all pathogens and spores. You will learn more about surgical asepsis and the sterilization process in Chapter 39.

CLOSING COMMENTS

One of the medical assistant's main responsibilities is to perform sanitization, disinfection, and sterilization procedures with precision and total effectiveness. There is no room for compromise. These procedures have a huge impact on infection control. Patients should have absolute confidence that they are being treated in an aseptic atmosphere and under aseptic conditions. This assurance is just as important for the protection of the provider and staff as it is for the patient. Allowing the provider to assume that the correct aseptic techniques were used when preparing a procedure and allowing them to use contaminated equipment on a patient may result in a malpractice lawsuit. Honesty on the part of the medical assistant builds self-respect and contributes to professional achievement.

PATIENT-CENTERED CARE

The medical assistant should take every opportunity to educate patients about the infection process and ways to prevent the transmission of disease. The best time to instruct a patient in aseptic techniques that can be used at home is while performing the aseptic procedure. Consider these examples:
- While washing your hands, explain to the patient that this routine is particularly important for patients who are very young or old or who seem to get sick frequently. Instruct the patient that the hands should be washed before and after meals; after sneezing, coughing, or blowing the nose; after using the restroom; before and after changing a dressing; and after changing an infant's diaper.
- Advise the patient to carry an alcohol-based hand sanitizer and to use it as indicated throughout the day.
- Explain to the patient that coughing or sneezing into a bent elbow is an effective method for preventing the spread of disease.
- Instruct the patient in the differences between sterile and clean dressings and bandages. Demonstrate each step in changing a dressing properly and explain how to dispose of contaminated items.

BEING PROFESSIONAL

Part of working in healthcare is to do everything possible to help patients live healthier lives. Even when you are not face-to-face with a patient, there are things that can be done to help provide information on how to improve health. Medical assistants can work with providers and their manager to provide information to patients. Here are some examples of what can be done:
- Set up an information table in the waiting room with take-home pamphlets and literature.
- Mail, email, or post on the healthcare facility's website a periodic newsletter to patients about infection control, especially during flu season.
- Demonstrate and explain aseptic procedures to patients and family members, inviting them to participate.
Role-play with a peer the following scenario. You and Jo (your peer) are medical assistants. Dr. Martin has asked the WMFM Clinic staff to come up with ideas to help patients understand the importance of living healthy lives and what they can do to help them keep healthy. Jo states she sees no value in this activity. How do you respond to Jo in a professional manner?

CHAPTER REVIEW

To understand infection control, you must first know what can cause disease. The different pathogenic microorganisms include viruses, bacteria, fungi, protozoa, and helminths. The chain of infection starts with those infectious agents. In order for it to grow, the pathogen must have a reservoir host that provides all of the proper conditions. The next link in the chain is the means or portal of exit, mode of transmission, and means or portal of entry. It ends with a susceptible host. Breaking any one of those links will stop the spread of infection. If someone does become infected with a pathogen, the inflammatory response and the immune response will try to take care of the pathogen.

OSHA standards have been developed to reduce the risk of infection for both patients and healthcare professionals. Following the Bloodborne Pathogens Standard is crucial for infection control.

Sanitization is washing with soap and water to remove blood and other debris so that disinfection and sterilization can occur. Disinfection removes most pathogens but is not effective against spores. Sterilization is destruction of all microbial life.

SCENARIO WRAP-UP

Implementing Standard Precautions throughout daily practice is crucial to the welfare and protection of both the patient and the healthcare worker. Rosa must be sure to wash her hands routinely or to use an alcohol-based hand sanitizer. She also must familiarize herself with the office's exposure control plan, follow OSHA's Bloodborne Pathogens Standard, use PPE when needed, follow environmental protection guidelines, use appropriate procedures for cleaning up contaminated spills and other housekeeping controls, and understand postexposure follow-up if an accidental exposure occurs. In addition, Rosa must follow guidelines for sanitization, disinfection, and sterilization of appropriate instruments and equipment.

PROCEDURE 32.1 **Perform Hand Hygiene: Medical Aseptic Hand Washing**

Task

Minimize the number of pathogens on the hands, thus reducing the risk of transmission of pathogens.

Equipment and Supplies

- Sink with warm running water
- Liquid soap in a dispenser (bar soap is not acceptable)
- Disposable nailbrush or orange stick
- Paper towels in a dispenser
- Water-based lotion
- Covered waste container with foot pedal

Procedural Steps

1. Remove all jewelry except your wristwatch, if it can be pulled up above your wrist, and a plain wedding ring.
   Purpose: Jewelry can harbor microorganisms.
2. Turn on the faucet and regulate the water temperature to lukewarm.
   Purpose: Water that is too hot can cause skin to become dry and chapped.
3. Wet your hands, apply soap, and lather using a circular motion with friction while holding your fingertips downward (Fig. 1). Rub well between your fingers. If this is the first hand wash of the day, use a nailbrush or an orange stick and clean under every fingernail. Inspect your nails thoroughly.
   Purpose: Friction removes soil and contaminants from the hands and wrists.

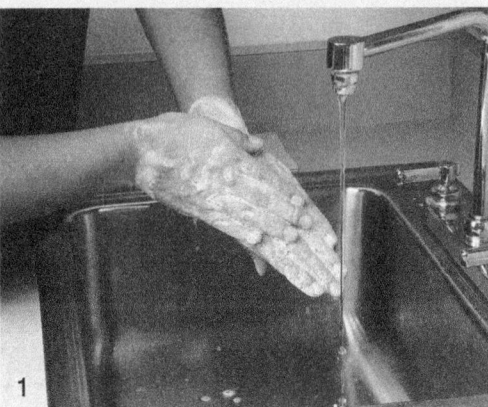

4. Rinse well, holding your hands so that the water flows from your wrists downward to your fingertips (Fig. 2).
   Purpose: Soil and contaminants will wash off the skin and down the drain.

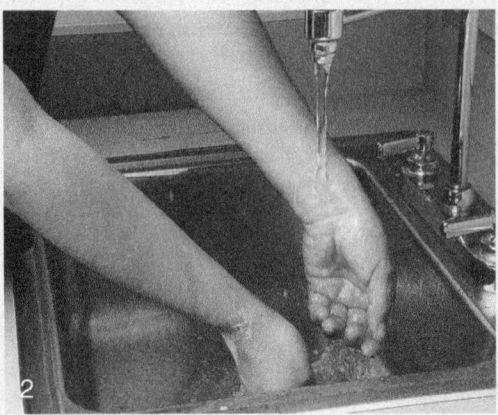

5. If this is the first hand wash of the day or if your hands are obviously contaminated, wet your hands again and repeat the scrubbing procedure using a vigorous, circular motion over the wrists and hands for at least 1 to 2 minutes.
   Purpose: Time is required for friction and motion to eliminate all possible soil and contaminants.
6. Rinse your hands a second time, keeping the fingers lower than your wrists.
   Purpose: To ensure removal of all transient flora.
7. Dry your hands with paper towels. Do not touch the paper towel dispenser as you are obtaining towels (Fig. 3).
   Purpose: Touching the dispenser contaminates your hands, and you will need to start over.

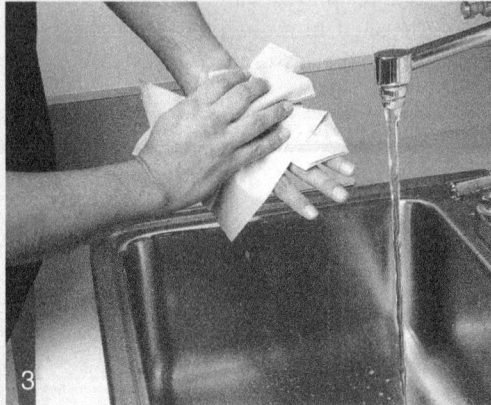

8. If the faucets are not foot operated, turn them off with a dry paper towel (Fig. 4).
   Purpose: The faucet is dirty and will contaminate your clean hands.

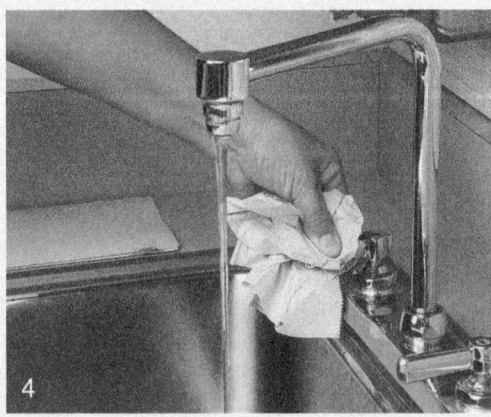

9. After you finish drying your hands and turning off the faucets, place used towels into a covered waste container.
   Purpose: Always discard contaminated waste in a covered waste container immediately to eliminate the source of infection.
10. If needed, apply a water-based antibacterial hand lotion to prevent chapped or dry skin.
    Purpose: Chapped skin eliminates the first line of defense against infectious organisms.
11. Repeat the procedure as indicated throughout the day.
    Purpose: To eliminate contaminants and prevent the transmission of pathogens to yourself and others.

PROCEDURE 32.2 Perform Hand Hygiene: Applying an Alcohol-Based Hand Sanitizer

Task

Minimize the number of pathogens on the hands, thus reducing the risk of transmission of pathogens.

Equipment and Supplies

- Alcohol-based hand sanitizer

Procedural Steps

1. Inspect hands to ensure they are not visibly soiled.

   Purpose: If hands are visibly soiled, then the medical aseptic hand wash should be performed.

2. Remove watch or push it up on your arm and remove rings.

   Purpose: Watches and rings can harbor microorganisms.

3. Apply alcohol-based hand sanitizer to the palm of one hand; gel or lotion should be dime sized, and foam should be walnut sized.

   Purpose: Using too much alcohol-based hand sanitizer can be drying to the skin. Dry skin cracks and chaps, creating portals of entry for microorganisms.

4. Thoroughly spread sanitizer over all surfaces of both hands, including around and under fingernails.

   Purpose: All surfaces need to be exposed to the alcohol-based hand sanitizer to effectively kill all microorganisms.

5. Rub hands until dry (20 to 30 seconds).

PROCEDURE 32.3 Remove Contaminated Gloves and Discard Biohazardous Material

Task

Minimize exposure to pathogens by medical aseptically removing and discarding contaminated gloves.

Equipment and Supplies

- Disposable gloves
- Biohazardous waste container with labeled red biohazard bag

Procedural Steps

1. With the dominant hand, grasp the glove of the opposite hand near the palm and begin removing the first glove (Fig. 1). The arms should be held away from the body with the hands pointed down.

   Purpose: Holding the hands down and away from the body helps prevent possible contamination.

2. Pull the glove inside out (Fig. 2). After removal, ball it into the palm of the remaining gloved hand.

   Purpose: Taking off the glove inside out prevents transmission of pathogens to another surface.

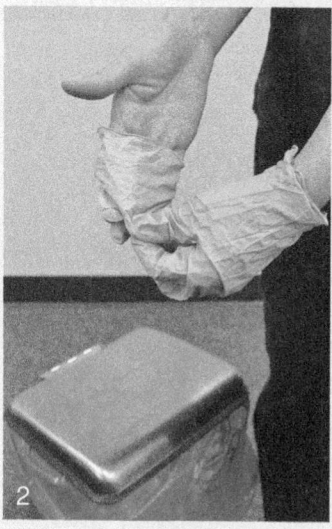

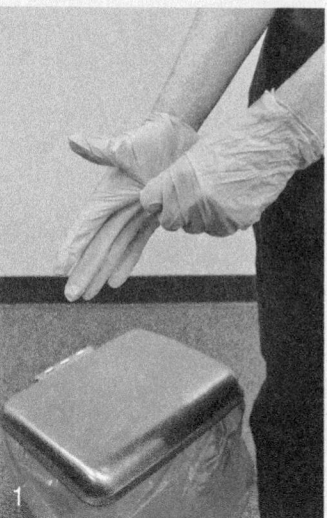

Continued

PROCEDURE 32.3   Remove Contaminated Gloves and Discard Biohazardous Material—cont'd

3. Insert two fingers of the ungloved hand between the edge of the cuff of the other contaminated glove and the hand (Fig. 3).

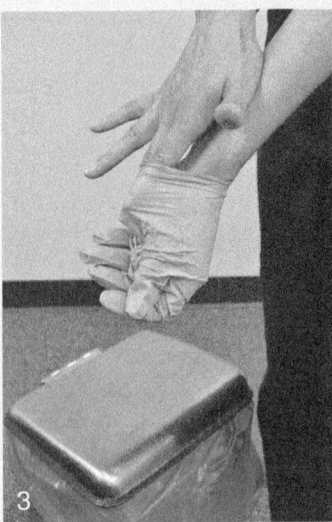

4. Push the glove down the hand, inside out, over the contaminated glove being held, leaving the contaminated side of both gloves on the inside.

   Purpose: This technique protects the wearer from the contaminated surfaces of both gloves.

5. Properly dispose of the inside-out, contaminated gloves in a biohazardous waste container (Fig. 4).

   Purpose: To prevent the spread of infection.

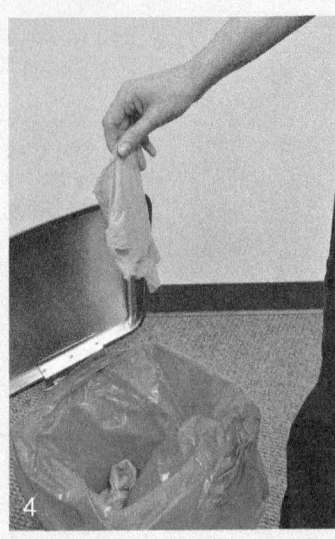

6. Perform a medical aseptic hand wash as described in Procedure 32.1 or sanitize the hands with an alcohol-based sanitizer (Procedure 32.2)

   Purpose: To minimize the number of pathogens on the hands, thereby reducing the number of transient flora and the risk of transmission of pathogens.

PROCEDURE 32.4   Remove Full-Body Personal Protective Equipment

Task

Minimize exposure to pathogens by aseptically removing and discarding a contaminated gown.

Equipment and Supplies

- Gloves
- Disposable impermeable gown
- Surgical mask or face shield
- Hand sanitizer
- Biohazardous waste container with labeled red biohazard bag

Procedural Steps

1. Leave patient care area and check surroundings carefully before removing personal protective equipment (PPE). Be sure there is a biohazardous waste container present and that there are no other individuals near. Assess your body for contaminated areas (Fig. A).

   Purpose: It is important to carefully remove PPE and immediately discard it appropriately to prevent it from contaminating clean areas or surfaces. Being aware of areas of high contamination will allow for special caution to be taken around these areas.

2. Carefully remove gloves by following the process in Procedure 32.3. Drop them into the biohazardous waste container (Fig. B).

   Purpose: Removing the gloves first prevents contamination to the body as ties are released.

3. Carefully reach behind and untie to top knot on the gown, then the waist tie. Be careful not to allow the hands to touch the gown other than the ties (Fig. C).

   Purpose: This allows the gown to be loosened to be removed. Avoiding touching the gown will prevent the hands from becoming contaminated.

4. Reach inside the cuff of one arm and pull the hand in. Then hold the outside of the other cuff through the gown and pull the second hand in.

   Purpose: This keeps the hands free from contamination on the outside of the gown.

5. Peel the gown away from the neck and shoulders, turning it carefully inside out toward the inside. Be careful to touch only the inside of the gown with the ungloved hands. Drop the gown into the biohazardous waste container (Fig. D).

   Purpose: Touching only the inside prevents the hands from becoming contaminated from materials on the outside of the gown.

6. Use hand sanitizer to remove any potential contaminant on your hands.

   Purpose: This will remove any unseen pathogenic material on the hands and prevent it from spreading as the other PPE is removed.

7. Using one hand, grasp eye protection from the side away from the eyes. Carefully remove from the face. If disposable, drop in the biohazard bin. If reusable, set aside to be cleaned and disinfected.

   Purpose: Grasping the eye protection on the side away from the eyes is important to avoid getting potential contaminants from the hands into the eyes.

Continued

PROCEDURE 32.4 Remove Full-Body Personal Protective Equipment—cont'd

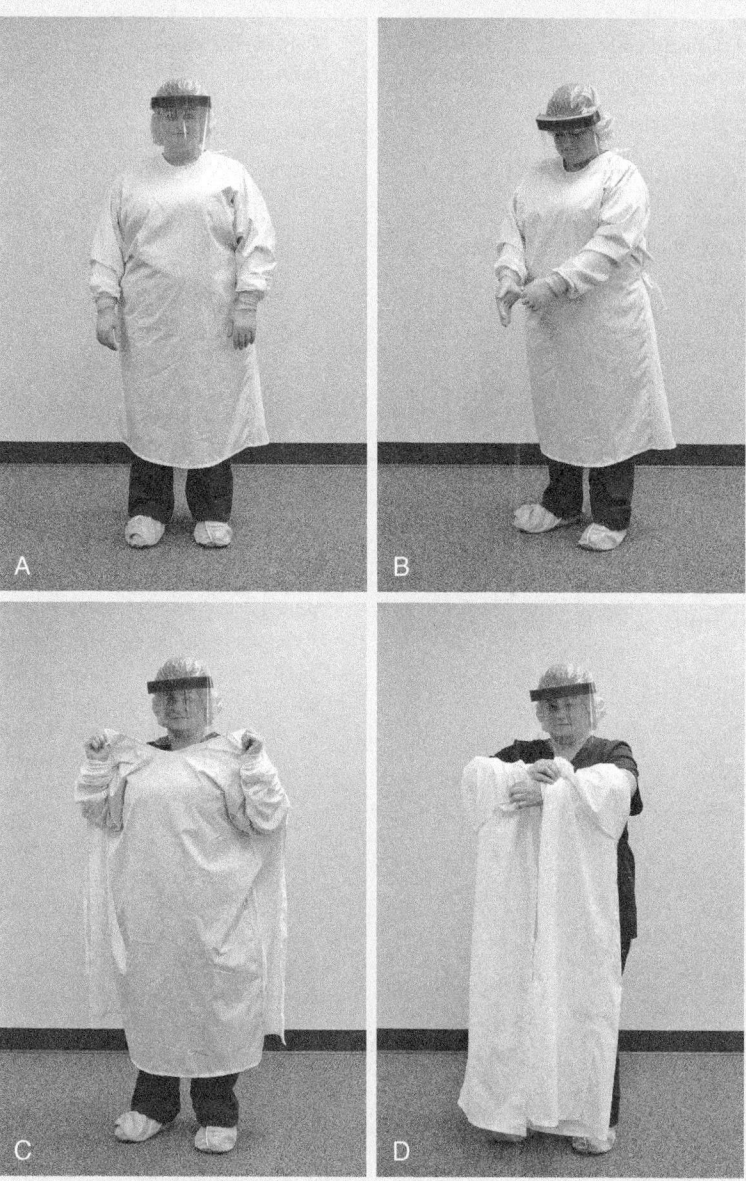

8. Remove the surgical mask carefully by untying the bottom tie, then the top tie or by removing the ear loops. Lift away from the face while holding the ties or loops and place in the biohazardous waste container.
   Purpose: Loosening the bottom of the mask prevents it from falling while still partially fastened, which can spread contamination.

9. Perform a 1- to 2-minute hand wash.
   Purpose: Procedures that require full-body PPE are considered high risk for contamination. A full aseptic hand wash is required when these procedures are performed.

PROCEDURE 32.5   Sanitize Soiled Instruments

Task

Remove all contaminated matter from instruments in preparation for disinfection or sterilization while following Standard Precautions and wearing appropriate personal protective equipment (PPE).

Equipment and Supplies

- Sink with cold and hot running water
- Sanitizing agent or low-sudsing soap with enzymatic action
- Decontaminated utility gloves (e.g., household cleaning type rubber or plastic gloves) that show no signs of deterioration
- Chin-length face shield or goggles and surgical mask if contamination with bloodborne pathogens is possible
- Impermeable gown
- Disposable brush
- Disposable paper towels
- Gloves
- Disinfectant cleaner prepared according to the manufacturer's directions
- Covered waste container with foot pedal
- Biohazardous waste container with labeled red biohazard bag

Procedural Steps

1. Put on an impermeable gown, surgical mask, and face shield or goggles if the potential for splashing of infectious material exists (Fig. 1).
   Purpose: To provide personal protection against potentially infectious matter.

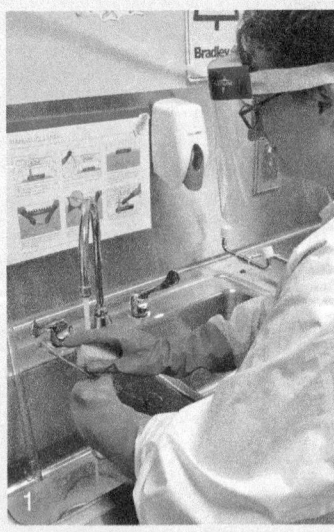

2. Put on utility gloves.
   Purpose: To provide personal protection against potentially infectious matter and sharp instruments.
3. Separate the sharp instruments from other instruments to be sanitized.
   Purpose: To prevent possible self-injury and exposure to infectious matter.

4. Rinse the instruments under cold running water.
   Purpose: To help remove debris and body fluids.
5. Open hinged instruments and scrub all grooves, crevices, and serrations with a disposable brush (Fig. 2).
   Purpose: Microorganisms can hide under contaminants and may not be destroyed by the disinfection process.

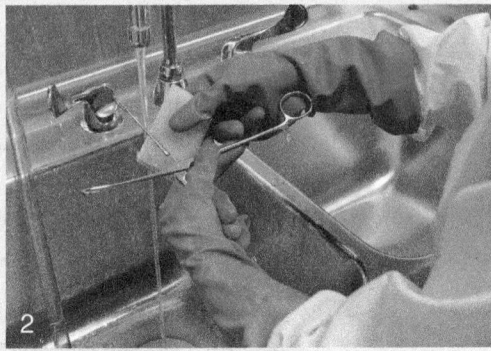

6. Rinse well with hot water.
   Purpose: Hot water removes all soap and contaminant residue.
7. Towel-dry all instruments thoroughly and dispose of contaminated towels and disposable brush in a biohazardous waste container. Do not touch the paper towel dispenser as you are obtaining towels.
   Purpose: All contaminated material must be discarded in a labeled biohazard container or a labeled red biohazard bag. Touching the dispenser with the utility gloves contaminates the dispenser. Wet instruments can rust or become dull.
8. Remove the utility gloves and wash your hands according to the steps in Procedure 32.1.
   Purpose: To remove any possible contaminants.
9. Towel-dry your hands and put on gloves. Decontaminate the utility gloves and work surfaces using disinfectant.
   Purpose: To prevent personal exposure to contaminants. All equipment and working surfaces should be cleaned and decontaminated with a disinfectant to prevent transmission of infectious organisms.
10. Dispose of the contaminated towels in a covered waste container.
    Purpose: All contaminated material must be disposed of in a labeled biohazard container or a labeled red biohazard bag.
11. Place sanitized instruments in a designated area for disinfection or sterilization.
    Purpose: Sanitized instruments must be removed from the cleaning area to prevent possible cross-contamination.
12. Remove the gloves according to Procedure 32.3. Dispose of the gloves in a biohazardous waste container. Sanitize the hands.
    Purpose: To prevent the spread of infectious organisms and to remove any possible contaminants.

33

Vital Signs

LEARNING OBJECTIVES

1. Do the following related to temperature:
   - Convert temperature readings between the Fahrenheit and Celsius scales.
   - Describe factors that affect the body temperature.
   - Describe abnormal temperatures, including different fever patterns.
   - Discuss common types of thermometers used in ambulatory care.
   - Obtain and record an accurate patient temperature using different types of thermometers.
2. Do the following related to pulse:
   - Describe factors that affect the pulse rate.
   - Identify common pulse sites.
   - Describe pulse rate, volume, and rhythm.
   - Cite the average pulse rate for various age groups.
   - Obtain and record radial and apical pulse rates.
3. Do the following related to respiration:
   - Describe factors that affect the respiration rate.

- Describe the rate, rhythm, and depth of respirations.
- Cite the average respiratory rate for various age groups.
- Obtain and record a respiration rate.
4. Do the following related to blood pressure:
   - Describe factors that affect the blood pressure.
   - Differentiate between the different types of hypertension.
   - Differentiate between hypotension and orthostatic hypotension.
   - Describe blood pressure equipment and how to select the appropriate cuff size.
   - Describe factors that affect the accuracy of blood pressure measurements.
   - Obtain and document a blood pressure.
   - Cite the average blood pressure ranges for various age groups.
5. Discuss and perform pulse oximetry.
6. Measure and document height and weight.
7. Describe how to calculate the body mass index (BMI).

OUTLINE

OPENING SCENARIO

Carlos Ricci, CMA (AAMA), works at Walden-Martin Family Medical (WMFM) Clinic. Carlos graduated from a medical assistant program 3 years ago and enjoys working with patients at the WMFM Clinic. One of Carlos' primary responsibilities is to accurately measure and record each patient's vital signs before the patient is seen. Over the past 3 years, he has come to understand the importance of accurately obtaining and recording vital sign measurements.

YOU WILL LEARN

1. To recognize why vital signs are an important part of the patient examination.
2. To identify the factors that can affect vital signs and how to minimize them.
3. To list the most common types of thermometers and describe how they should be used.
4. To locate the pulse sites.
5. To identify the characteristics of a pulse and describe what must be assessed.
6. To identify the characteristics of respirations and describe what must be assessed.
7. To obtain a blood pressure.
8. To define pulse oximetry.
9. To accurately determine a patient's height and weight.

INTRODUCTION

Vital signs are measurements of a patient's essential body functions. Almost every patient who visits the healthcare facility will have at least some vital signs measured. These signs are the body's indicators of internal homeostasis (hoh mee oh STAY sis) and the patient's general state of health. A good understanding of the physiology and theory behind each vital sign will help to ensure accurate readings.

Medical assistants are often responsible for obtaining vital sign measurements. Accurate measurement and documentation of vital signs are essential. A change in one or more of the patient's vital signs may indicate a change in general health. This in turn influences diagnostic and treatment decisions by the healthcare provider. Because it is so important that vital sign measurements are accurate, they should never be measured in an indifferent or casual manner.

The *vital signs* (also called *cardinal signs*) include the patient's temperature (T), pulse rate (P), respiration rate (R), and blood pressure (BP). Additional measurements that provide information to the provider about the patient's general health include pulse oximetry, height (ht), and weight (wt). These measurements are taken at the same time as the vital signs and are often reported with them.

Understanding vital signs and factors that affect them are important when recognizing abnormalities and potential medical emergencies. Any abnormal vital sign measurements should always be brought to the provider's attention as soon as possible. If it is suspected that the patient's vital signs may be temporarily influenced, the medical assistant may be asked to take the vital signs later in the visit. This gives the patient time to be calm and comfortable, allowing for a more accurate measurement.

VOCABULARY

homeostasis The internal environment of the body that is compatible with life. A steady state that is created by all the body systems working together to provide a consistent and unvarying internal environment.

metabolism The chemical process that occurs within a living organism to maintain life; the process the body uses to obtain or make energy from the food eaten.

vital signs Measurements of a patient's essential body functions including temperature, pulse rate, respiratory rate, and blood pressure. Also referred to as cardinal signs.

MEDICAL TERMINOLOGY

home/o	constant
-ism	condition, process
-stasis	to stand, place, stop, control

TEMPERATURE

Body temperature is defined as the balance between heat lost and heat produced by the body. It is measured in degrees Fahrenheit (F) or degrees Celsius (C) (Box 33.1). The process of chemical and physical change in the body that produces heat is called metabolism. Body temperature is a result of this process. The

---

BOX 33.1 Temperature Conversions

There are many options for converting temperatures between the Fahrenheit and Celsius scales. Most electronic health records (EHRs) will do the conversion when the temperature is entered. Online options also are available. If you need to do the conversion manually, the following formulas will help you out.

Fahrenheit to Celsius	Celsius to Fahrenheit
$°C = (°F − 32) ÷ 1.8$	$°F = (°C × 1.8) + 32$
Example: 101°F	*Example:* 39°C
$°C = (101 − 32) ÷ 1.8$	$°F = (39 × 1.8) + 32$
$°C = 69 ÷ 1.8$	$°F = 70.2 + 32$
$°C = 38.3$	$°F = 102.2$

CRITICAL THINKING 33.1

Using the correct formula, convert the following temperatures from one system to the other:

1. 99°F = _____ °C
2. 102°F = _____ °C
3. 38°C = _____ °F
4. 39.5°C = _____ °F

core body temperature is maintained within a normal range by the hypothalamus. The average body temperature varies from person to person.

Factors Affecting the Body Temperature

Many factors affect a person's metabolism, which then changes the body temperature. When the metabolism increases so does the temperature; when it decreases, so does the temperature.

Factors that may affect body temperature include:

- *Age:* The body temperature of infants and young children fluctuates (FLUHK choo eyts) more rapidly in response to external environmental temperatures, causing younger people to have a higher average temperature. Aging adults lose the insulation of subcutaneous fat and thermoregulatory control, causing older adults to have a lower average temperature.
- *Stress, strong emotions, and physical activity:* These can increase the metabolic rate, causing an elevation in temperature.
- *Sex:* Hormone secretions result in fluctuations of the core body temperature in women throughout the menstrual cycle. During the second part of the cycle, the temperature may go up by 1 degree or more.
- *Time of day:* Vital signs such as systolic blood pressure, pulse and respiration rates, and body temperature are lower in the morning upon waking and increase slightly over the day. This daily change is due to the *diurnal* (dahy UR nl) *variation* or *circadian rhythm*, the daily cycle of biological activities that are influenced by the sleep-wake cycle. Throughout the day, the body temperature changes between 0.9 to 1.8 °F (0.5 to 1°C). In a healthy adult, this diurnal variation ranges from 97.7° to 99.5°F (36.5° to 37.5°C); the average daily temperature is 98.6°F (37°C).
- *External factors:* Cold exterior temperatures tend to cause the body temperature to decrease slightly. Warm temperatures and high humidity can cause the body temperature to increase.
- *Illness:* A disease process can increase an individual's metabolic activity, thus increasing the internal heat production and the body temperature. The increase in body temperature inhibits the growth of some bacteria and viruses.
- *Diseases:* Certain endocrinology diseases, such as hypothyroidism and Graves disease, can lower the metabolism, thus decreasing the body temperature. Hyperthyroidism can increase the metabolism, causing the body temperature to increase.

When the core body temperature elevates, the blood vessels near the surface of the body dilate causing the skin to look redder. With the increase in blood flow near the surface of the

body, heat is lost from the body, thus lowering the temperature. The sweat production is increased by the hypothalamus. When the sweat evaporates from the skin, it helps to lower the body temperature.

When the core body temperature is lower than average, the blood vessels near the surface of the body constrict. This limits the blood flow near the surface of the skin and less heat is lost. When the hypothalamus senses the lowered temperature, it triggers shivering, which produces heat, thus increasing the body temperature.

VOCABULARY

febrile Pertaining to an elevated body temperature.
fluctuate To shift back and forth.
malaise A condition of general bodily weakness or discomfort, often marking the onset of a disease.
pyrexia A febrile condition or fever.

Abnormal Temperatures

Hypothermia, an abnormally low body temperature, occurs when the body temperature is below 95°F (35°C) rectally. A *fever* or pyrexia (pahy REK see uh) occurs when the oral temperature is at or above 99.5°F (37.5°C), according to MedlinePlus (https://medlineplus.gov/). *Hyperthermia* or *hyperpyrexia* is an abnormally high body temperature, with a temperature of 106°F (41°C) or higher. Hypothermia and hyperthermia are medical emergencies.

Higher than average body temperature is often the first warning of an illness or other change in the patient's current condition. Infection is the most common cause of fever in both children and adults. Infants do not usually develop febrile (FEB ruh l) illnesses during the first 3 months of life; if one is present, it usually is very serious. However, a fever is very common in young children and accounts for an estimated 30% of ambulatory care visits. When the body encounters disease, it will make efforts to increase the body temperature in an attempt to make the body less hospitable to the pathogen causing the disease. An *antipyretic medication*, such as acetaminophen, can be taken to bring down a fever.

As a fever goes up the patient will often feel cold and experience goose bumps, chills, and even shivering. The superficial blood vessels (those near the surface of the skin) constrict. The small papillary muscles at the base of hair follicles also constrict, creating "goose bumps." Chills and shivering may follow, producing internal heat. As this process repeats itself, more heat is produced, and the body temperature rises above the normal range.

Patients also often complain of headaches, increased thirst, and general malaise. Patients will appear flushed, and the skin will feel hot to the touch. When the body begins to return to homeostasis, the fever "breaks" and the temperature begins to return to normal. When this happens, the patient will usually complain of feeling hot and will often sweat as the body works to lower the temperature.

Fevers are classified according to the 24-hour pattern they follow. The three most common patterns (Fig. 33.1) are:

- *Continuous fever:* The temperature remains above normal and rises and falls only slightly in a 24-hour period, with less

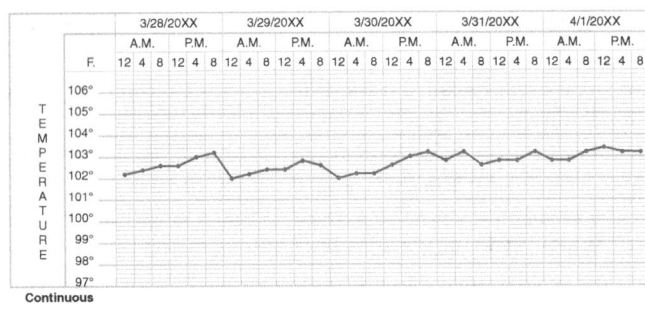

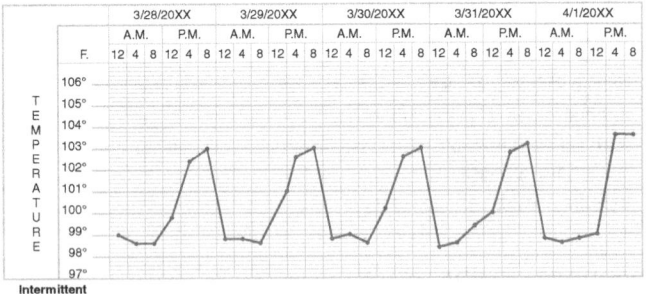

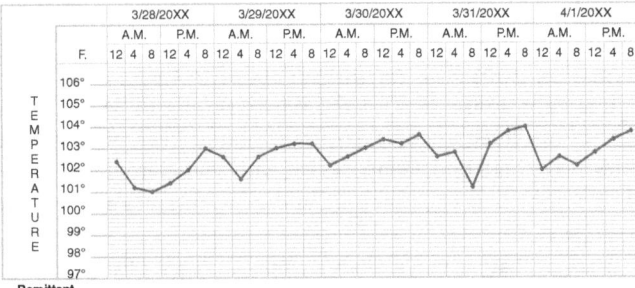

Fig. 33.1 Fever Patterns.

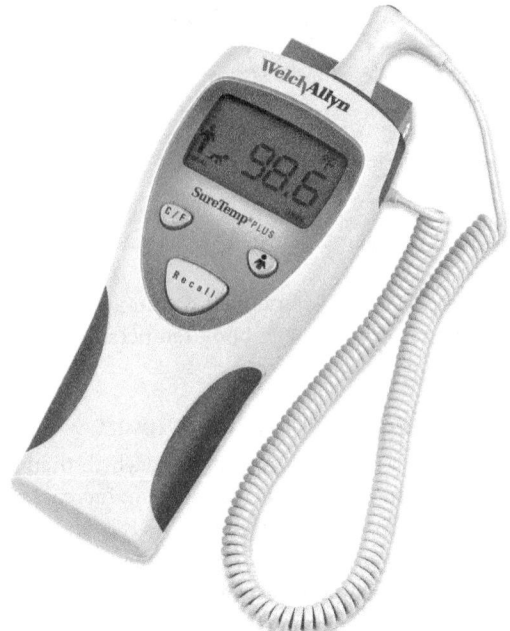

Fig. 33.2 Digital Thermometer. (Courtesy Welch Allyn.)

BOX 33.2 Temperatures

The average normal oral temperature is 98.6°F (37°C). Rectal, tympanic, and temporal artery temperatures are considered 1°F (0.6°C) higher than an oral temperature. Axillary temperatures are about 1°F (0.6°C) lower than an oral temperature. Usually, infrared temperatures are also 1°F lower than an oral temperature. With these variations, it is important to include the site used when documenting the temperature.

---

than 3 degrees difference between the highest point and the lowest point.

- *Intermittent fever*: The fever comes and goes, alternating between elevated and normal levels.
- *Remittent fever*: The fever fluctuates considerably (i.e., by more than 3 degrees) but remains elevated and does not return to the normal range.

It is important to remember that there is quite a bit of variation in temperatures.

Thermometers

The most common type of thermometer used in the ambulatory care facility is a digital thermometer. These are battery operated. The digital thermometer reads a temperature quickly (usually between 10 and 60 seconds) and displays the reading on a screen. Disposable covers fit snugly over the probe and are easy to remove quickly. Since the covered probe is the only part of the thermometer to come into contact with the patient, the risk of cross-contamination is very small.

Thermometers also vary in style based on the site where they will be used to take a temperature. Taking a temperature under the tongue, in the armpit, or in the rectum requires a digital thermometer with a long, narrow probe (Fig. 33.2). These thermometers are typically referred to as "digital thermometers." A tympanic thermometer is a digital thermometer that has a small cone shaped probe. A temporal artery thermometer has a

small, round probe that is moved across the forehead and reads the temperature off the temporal artery. A noncontact infrared thermometer uses a small infrared laser to detect the temperature of the skin surface where it is aimed (Box 33.2).

Although all of these sites are generally considered appropriate for taking accurate temperatures, there are some things that must be considered when determining which is best for a specific patient.

Age	Birth–3 months: Infrared, temporal artery, or rectal
	3–6 months: Infrared, axillary, temporal artery, or rectal
	6 months–5 years: Infrared, axillary, temporal artery, or tympanic
	5 years or older: Infrared, oral, axillary, temporal artery, or tympanic
Condition	Mouth breathing: oral not an option
	Ear infection or occlusion: tympanic not an option
	Diarrhea: rectal not an option
	Open wound or rash on forehead: temporal artery not an option
	If the environmental temperature is below 60.8°F (16°C) or above 104°F (40°C): an infrared thermometer should not be used.

PROCEDURE 32.4 Remove Full-Body Personal Protective Equipment—cont'd

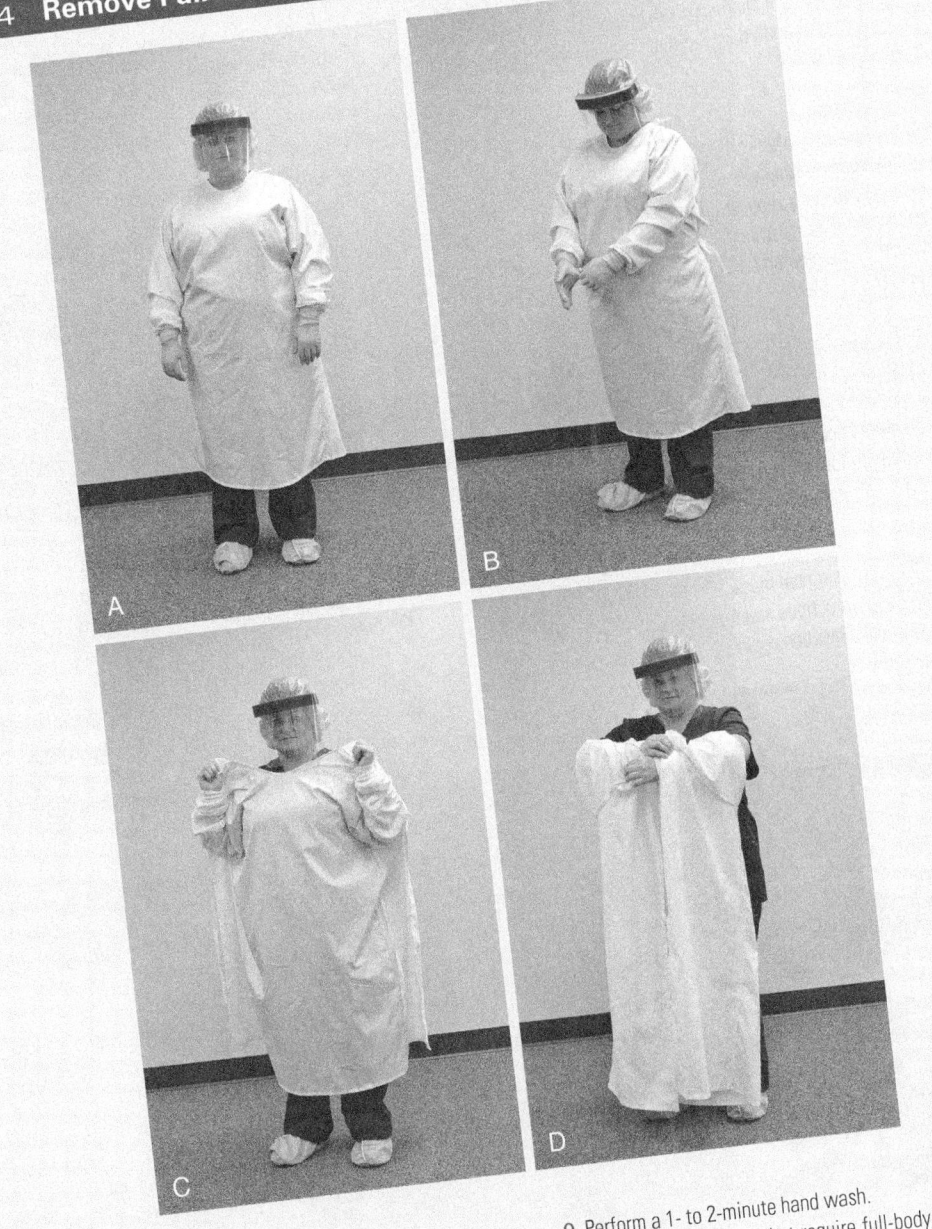

8. Remove the surgical mask carefully by untying the bottom tie, then the top tie or by removing the ear loops. Lift away from the face while holding the ties or loops and place in the biohazardous waste container.
Purpose: Loosening the bottom of the mask prevents it from falling while still partially fastened, which can spread contamination.

9. Perform a 1- to 2-minute hand wash.
Purpose: Procedures that require full-body PPE are considered high risk for contamination. A full aseptic hand wash is required when these procedures are performed.

---

ious: oral not an option

ties may have only one or two types meters available.

care providers may have specific s. Check with your provider on eferences.

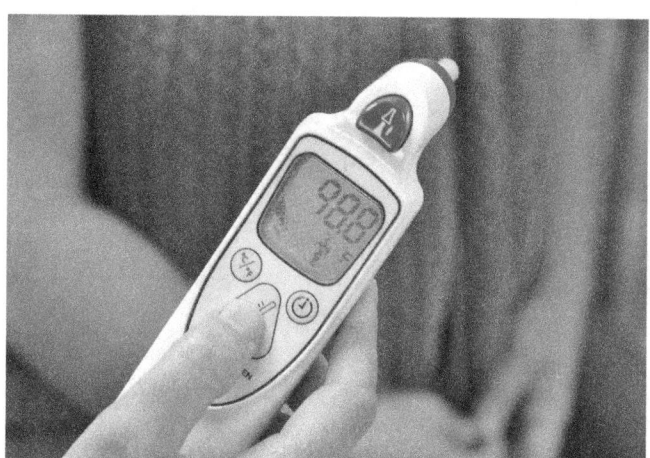

Fig. 33.3 Tympanic Thermometer. (From Niedzwiecki B, et al: *Kinn's the medical assistant,* ed 14, St. Louis, 2020, Elsevier.)

ures are taken by placing the ongue on either side of the GWEE), the vertical fold of). This area has a rich blood mouths and use their lips place. For children under annot do this, the medical ethod as the oral tempera-

e, ask patients if they have rink (including chewing activities may artificially If the patient answers yes hould choose a different wait 10 to 15 minutes ow the oral temperature

e-taking techniques in the

meter in his mouth swimmer's ear) rmometer is available

nen tte

e of the safest sites more comfortable the least accurate longest to regis- re facilities may its.
e medical assis- the probe. This creating a seal 3.2).

ild had an axil- le is full today, y today or first ? What is the

Rectal Temperature. A digital thermometer with a red probe is used for rectal temperatures (Procedure 33.3). It is typically only used for babies in ambulatory care. Some facilities limit the use of rectal thermometers and encourage the use of other thermometers that are less invasive and just as accurate.

If a rectal temperature is to be taken, it is important to lubricate the probe tip with a water-soluble lubricant (e.g., KY jelly). Hold the baby securely with the legs elevated and insert the probe approximately ½ inch or just past the anal sphincter muscle. For older children, insert the probe ⅝ inch and 1 inch for adults. It is important not to insert the probe too far to avoid damage to the colon. Hold the probe carefully and continue to secure the legs throughout the procedure to prevent rectal damage. When you eject the probe cover, take extra care not to contaminate the base unit. If there is any chance that the patient's body fluids touched the unit, wipe it with disinfectant before returning it to the storage area.

Tympanic Temperature. The tympanic membrane of the ear shares a blood supply with the hypothalamus, which regulates body temperature. This makes the tympanic (*aural*) temperature one of the more accurate temperature sites if done correctly. It is also less invasive, so it is considered to be very safe. The tympanic temperature is one of the fastest methods of temperature reading, with results measured in about 2 seconds.

The tympanic thermometer consists of a handheld unit equipped with a small cone-shaped probe, which is covered with a disposable probe cover (Fig. 33.3). The probe is placed in the ear canal and gently seals the external opening of the canal. The sensor uses infrared energy to read the temperature off the tympanic membrane. In order to get an accurate reading, the tip of the tympanic thermometer probe must be in line with the tympanic membrane. To do this the ear canal should be pulled straight. In children younger than age 3 years, the pinna of the ear should be gently pulled down and back. For patients older than 3 years, the pinna of the ear should be gently pulled up and back (Procedure 33.4).

If a person is experiencing ear pain, such as with otitis media or otitis externa (swimmer's ear), the ear should not be used

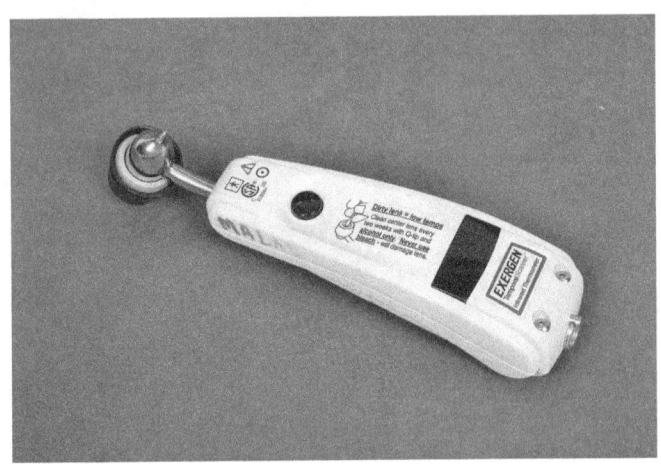

Fig. 33.4 Temporal Artery Thermometer. (From Niedzwiecki B, et al: *Kinn's the medical assistant,* ed 14, St. Louis, 2020, Elsevier.)

for a temperature. If there is pain in both ears, another method should be chosen. In addition, if the patient has or has a history of impacted cerumen (si ROO muh n), do not use a tympanic thermometer because the reading may be inaccurate.

VOCABULARY

cerumen A waxy secretion in the ear canal; commonly called earwax.

Temporal Artery Temperature. In recent years, the temporal artery temperature has become the preferred method of temperature taking in many ambulatory care facilities. When taken correctly, it is as accurate as the tympanic temperature. It is appropriate for all age groups and has fewer physical issues that can cause an incorrect reading. Like the tympanic thermometer, the temporal artery thermometer uses an infrared beam to read the temperature.

When using the temporal artery thermometer, the probe is scanned across the forehead and behind the ear (Fig. 33.4). The infrared beam reads the temperature off the temporal artery, which lies about 1 mm below the skin. Because the artery is so close to the skin, it provides good surface heat conduction, allowing the thermometer to obtain a fast, accurate, and noninvasive measurement of body temperature.

To prepare for the procedure, anything obscuring the forehead or the side of the face must be removed. Bangs should be pushed back off the forehead. If there is perspiration on the forehead, gently dry the area with a clean cloth or paper towel. To perform the procedure, place the probe in the center of the forehead, halfway between the eyebrows and the hairline. Depress the button on the scanner and gently stroke the probe across the forehead toward the hairline (at the temple), keeping the probe flat on the patient's skin. Keeping the button depressed, lift the scanner from the temporal area and lightly place the probe behind the earlobe. Release the button and remove the probe (Procedure 33.5).

As the scanner moves across the forehead, repeated temperature measurements are taken and the highest measurement is recorded. This takes about 3 seconds. Depending on the facility's infection control procedures, disposable covers can be used

on the scanner, or it can be cleaned between patients with an alcohol wipe.

Noncontact Infrared Temperature. In recent years concern about cross-contamination between patients has increased, and efforts to reduce patient contact where possible have been made. In response to this, the use of noncontact infrared thermometers has increased in popularity. These thermometers also use an infrared light, but with noncontact thermometers the unit does not touch the patient – only the light does. The infrared beam is aimed at the area of the temporal artery, and the temperature is taken (Fig. 33.5). These thermometers are very easy to use, easy to clean and disinfect, and measure the temperature very quickly (under 5 seconds). However, they are not as accurate as the temporal artery thermometer (Procedure 33.6).

PULSE

A patient's pulse rate reflects the palpable beat of the arteries as they expand and relax in response to contraction of the heart. With every beat, the heart pumps an amount of blood, known as the stroke volume, into the aorta. The blood moves into the arteries that branch off the aorta. This causes an increase in arterial pressure, and the arteries dilate. When the heart relaxes, less blood moves through the arteries, and arterial pressure decreases. Each contraction and relaxation of the heart muscle is a heartbeat. The resulting expansion and relaxation of the arteries create a pulsation. This pulsation can be felt through an artery that is close to the body surface and can be pushed against a bone. Palpating a peripheral (puh RIF er uh l) pulse gives the rate, rhythm, and volume of the heartbeat and local information about the condition of the artery used.

VOCABULARY

peripheral Refers to an area outside of or away from an organ or structure.
stroke volume The amount of blood that moves through the arteries when the heart beats.

Factors Affecting the Pulse Rate

Factors that can affect the pulse rate include:
- *Age*: Children tend to have more rapid pulse rates than adults.
- *Body position*: The pulse rate tends to be faster in the sitting position compared to the supine position. It tends to increase when an individual stands.
- *Diseases*: Hyperthyroidism, anemia, a fever, and an electrolyte imbalance can cause an increase pulse. Hypothyroidism, myocarditis, obstructive sleep apnea, and inflammatory disease, such as rheumatic fever and lupus, can cause a decrease pulse rate.
- *Sex*: Women tend to have slightly faster pulse rates (70 to 80 bpm) than men (60 to 70 bpm).
- *Health status*: Well-conditioned athletes tend to have pulse rates of 50 to 60 beats per minute. Consistent aerobic exercise strengthens the heart muscle (the myocardium) so that

---

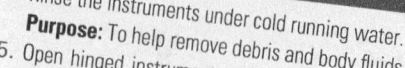
anitize Soiled Instruments

ruments in preparation for disinfection
Precautions and wearing appropriate

h enzymatic action
ehold cleaning type rubber or plastic
n

rgical mask if contamination with

he manufacturer's directions

ed biohazard bag

, and face shield or goggles if
rial exists (Fig. 1).
st potentially infectious matter.

tially infectious mat-

to be sanitized.
o infectious matter.

4. Rinse the instruments under cold running water.
   Purpose: To help remove debris and body fluids.
5. Open hinged instruments and scrub all grooves, crevices, and serrations with a disposable brush (Fig. 2).
   Purpose: Microorganisms can hide under contaminants and may not be destroyed by the disinfection process.

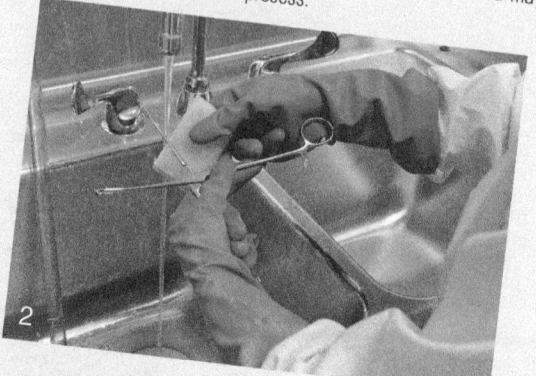

6. Rinse well with hot water.
   Purpose: Hot water removes all soap and contaminant residue.
7. Towel-dry all instruments thoroughly and dispose of contaminated towels and disposable brush in a biohazardous waste container. Do not touch the paper towel dispenser as you are obtaining towels.
   Purpose: All contaminated material must be discarded in a labeled biohazard container or a labeled red biohazard bag. Touching the dispenser with the utility gloves contaminates the dispenser. Wet instruments can rust or become dull.
8. Remove the utility gloves and wash your hands according to the steps in Procedure 32.1.
   Purpose: To remove any possible contaminants.
9. Towel-dry your hands and put on gloves. Decontaminate the utility gloves and work surfaces using disinfectant.
   Purpose: To prevent personal exposure to contaminants. All equipment and working surfaces should be cleaned and decontaminated with a disinfectant to prevent transmission of infectious organisms.
10. Dispose of the contaminated towels in a covered waste container.
    Purpose: All contaminated material must be disposed of in a labeled biohazard container or a labeled red biohazard bag.
11. Place sanitized instruments in a designated area for disinfection or sterilization.
    Purpose: Sanitized instruments must be removed from the cleaning area to prevent possible cross-contamination.
12. Remove the gloves according to Procedure 32.3. Dispose of the gloves in a biohazardous waste container. Sanitize the hands.
    Purpose: To prevent the spread of infectious organisms and to remove any possible contaminants.

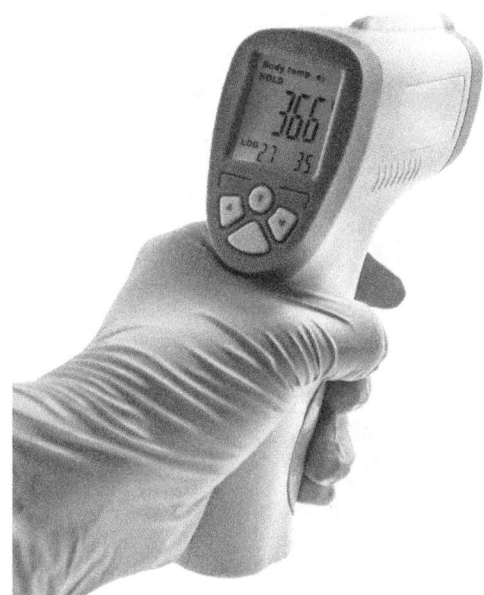

Fig. 33.5 Noncontact Infrared Thermometer. (Vladyslav Danilin/iStock.com)

each heart contraction ejects an increased volume of blood into the arterial system.

- *Physical activity*: The pulse rate will increase with physical exertion. The pulse will decrease when the patient is at rest, dropping to as low as 45 to 50 bpm when the patient is asleep.
- *Psychological state*: Stress, nervousness, and anxiety can cause the pulse rate to increase.
- *Certain drugs and nicotine*: Medications can work to increase or decrease the pulse rate. Nicotine, stimulants, such as cocaine or methamphetamine, and drinking too much caffeine and alcohol can also increase the pulse.

Pulse Sites

The most common pulse sites are the temporal, carotid, brachial, radial, femoral, popliteal, and dorsalis pedis arteries (Fig. 33.6). Although the apical pulse may be felt in some people, it is generally taken by listening with a stethoscope. Typically, the radial and apical pulses are used in the ambulatory care setting.

Temporal (TEM per uhl) pulse	Located in the temple area of the skull, parallel and lateral to the eyes (Fig.33.7). It is seldom used as a pulse site but may be used as a pressure point to help control bleeding from a head injury.
Carotid (kuh ROT id) pulse	Located between the larynx (voice box) and the sternocleidomastoid muscle in the front and to the side of the neck (Fig. 33.8). It most frequently is used in emergencies and to check the pulse during cardiopulmonary resuscitation (CPR). It can be felt by pushing the muscle to the side and pressing against the larynx.

Brachial (BREY kee uh l) pulse	Felt at the inner (*antecubital* [an tuh KYOO bit uhl]) aspect of the elbow. It also can be felt in the groove between the biceps and triceps muscles on the inner surface of the middle upper arm. This is the artery that is felt and listened to when blood pressure is measured (Fig. 33.9). This is the best choice of palpated pulse sites in young children and the one that is checked on infants and young children receiving CPR.
Radial (REY dee uh l) pulse	The most commonly used site for counting the pulse rate. It is found on the thumb side of the wrist, 1 inch below the base of the thumb (Fig. 33.10).
Femoral (FEM er uh l) pulse	Located at the site where the femoral artery passes through the groin (see Fig. 33.6). The examiner must press deeply below the inguinal (ING gwuh ml) ligament to palpate this pulse.
Popliteal (pop LIT ee hu l) pulse	Found at the back of the leg behind the knee (see Fig. 33.6). Palpation of this pulse requires the patient to be in a recumbent position with the knee slightly flexed. The popliteal artery is deep and difficult to feel. It is palpated and also monitored with a stethoscope when a leg blood pressure measurement is necessary. The provider checks blood flow through the popliteal artery if a circulatory system problem, such as a blood clot, is suspected in the lower leg.
Dorsalis pedis (dawr SAL is PEE diss), or pedal pulse	Felt across the arch of the foot, just slightly lateral to the midline, beside the extensor tendon of the great toe. This pulse may be congenitally absent in some patients. Because a good pulse rate at this site is an indicator of normal lower limb circulation and arterial *sufficiency* (suh FISH uh n see), the provider checks the pedal pulses in patients with *peripheral* (phy RIF er uh l) *vascular* (VAS kyuh ler) problems, such as diabetes mellitus. Because this pulse is very difficult to feel, it is often checked with an ultrasound unit (Fig. 33.11).
Apical (Ey pi kih l) pulse, or apical heart rate	The heartbeat at the apex of the heart. This is generally heard with a stethoscope. It is used for infants and young children because the radial pulse is difficult to palpate in young patients. Apical rates are also recorded on adult patients who have irregular or difficult-to-feel radial pulses to ensure an accurate heart rate reading (Procedure 33.7).

Characteristics of a Pulse

When taking a pulse, you must be aware of three specific factors: rate, rhythm, and volume. When counting the rate, you must also be aware of rhythm and volume. Each of these characteristics relays valuable information about the heart contractions. Variations from normal should be noted.

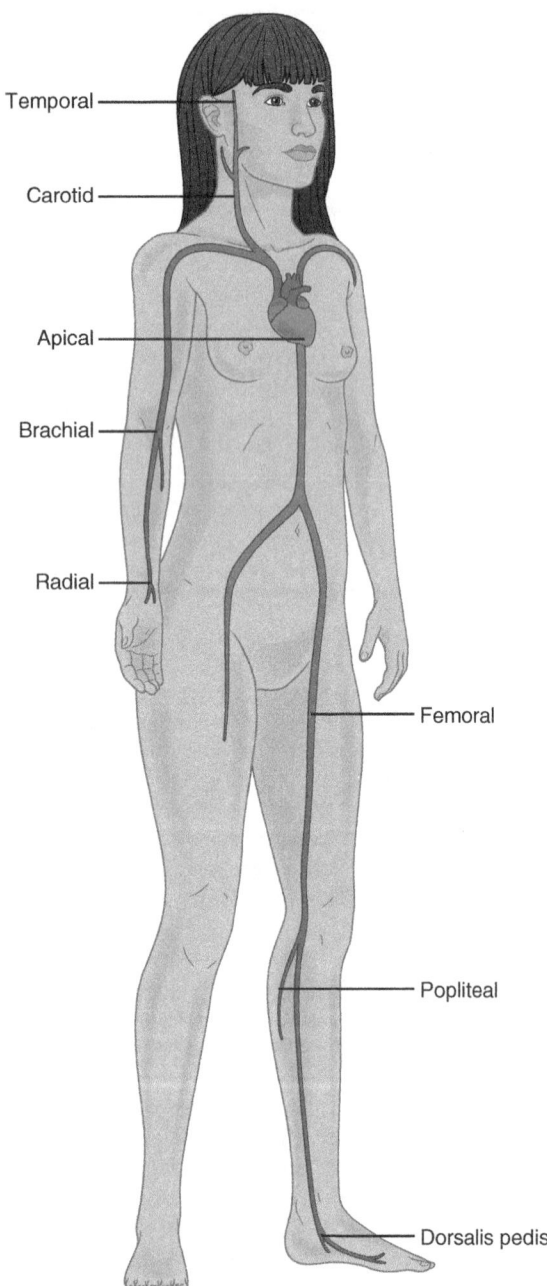

Fig. 33.6 Pulse Sites. (From Niedzwiecki B, et al: *Kinn's the medical assistant*, ed 14, St. Louis, 2020, Elsevier.)

Rate. The rate of the pulse is the number of beats (pulsations) that occur in 1 minute, which should be recorded as beats per minute (bpm). Taking the pulse for a full 60 seconds allows for the most accurate recording (Table 33.1). If the pulse rate is counted at any site other than the radial artery, the site used needs to be documented with the rate.

Rhythm. The pulse rhythm is the time between pulse beats. The pulse rhythm is documented as "regular" or "irregular." A "*regular*" or normal rhythm pattern has an even tempo, which indicates that the *intervals* (or spacing) between beats are of equal duration. An "irregular" or abnormal rhythm pattern does not have an even tempo. The intervals between beats are different.

Common abnormalities include:

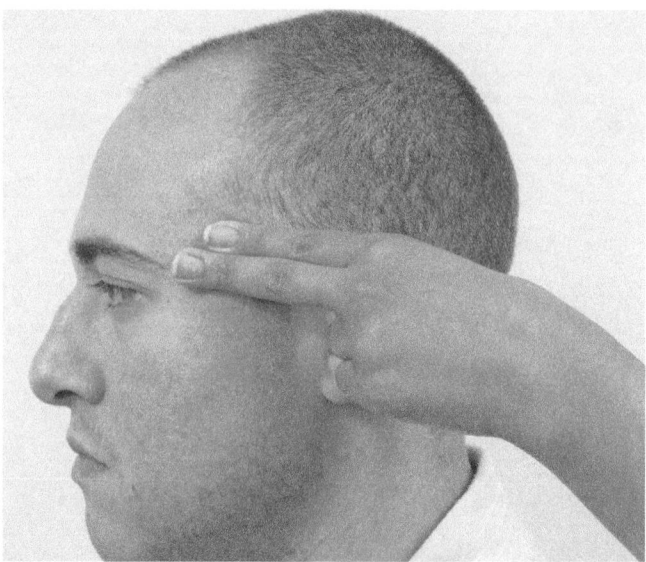

Fig. 33.7 Temporal Pulse. (From Niedzwiecki B, et al: *Kinn's the medical assistant*, ed 14, St. Louis, 2020, Elsevier.)

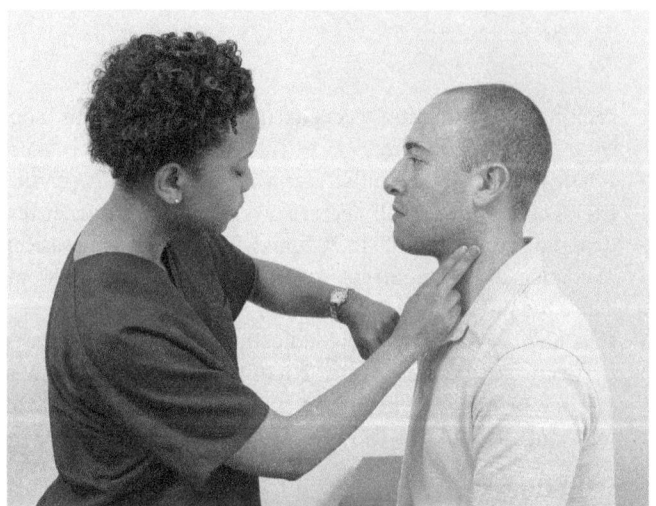

Fig. 33.8 Carotid Pulse. (From Niedzwiecki B, et al: *Kinn's the medical assistant*, ed 14, St. Louis, 2020, Elsevier.)

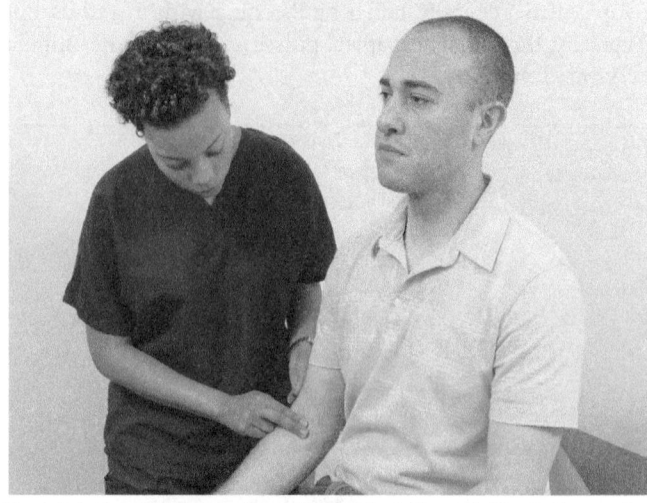

Fig. 33.9 Brachial Pulse. (From Niedzwiecki B, et al: *Kinn's the medical assistant*, ed 14, St. Louis, 2020, Elsevier.)

- *Intermittent pulse*: A pulse in which beats occasionally are skipped. This occurs in healthy individuals during exercise or after drinking a caffeinated beverage.
- *Sinus arrhythmia*: An irregular heartbeat that originates in the sinoatrial node.
- *Respiratory sinus arrhythmia*: A common irregularity in children and young, healthy adults. The heart rate increases when the person inhales and decreases with exhaling.

An irregular pulse should be indicated for the provider, because this may indicate heart disease. If an irregular rhythm is detected, the pulse should be counted for a full minute to ensure accuracy.

Volume. The volume (*pulse amplitude* [AM pli tood]) can be assessed by feeling the strength of the pulse. The force of the heart contraction and the condition of the arterial wall (whether hard or soft) influence the volume of the pulse. With heart disease, the pulse may be regular and only vary by the volume. The pulse volume is described and recorded using the following three-point scale:

3+	Full, **bounding** pulse	Pulsation is very strong and does not disappear with moderate pressure.
2+	Normal pulse	Pulsation is easily felt but disappears with moderate pressure.
1+	Weak, **thready** pulse	Pulsation is not easily felt and disappears with slight pressure.

Counting a Radial Pulse Rate

The radial pulse is the most common pulse site used in ambulatory care. To record an accurate radial pulse, the patient should be in a comfortable position, with the artery to be used at the same level as or lower than the heart (Procedure 33.8). The extremity should be well supported and relaxed. The patient may be lying down or sitting.

As with all palpated pulse readings, the pads of the first two or three fingers are placed over the artery. Never use your thumb to determine the pulse rate. The thumb has its own pulse, and you may confuse your pulse rate with the patient's rate. Push the radial artery against the bone until the strongest pulsation is felt. Too much pressure occludes the artery, and too little pressure prevents detection of irregularities or of all the beats.

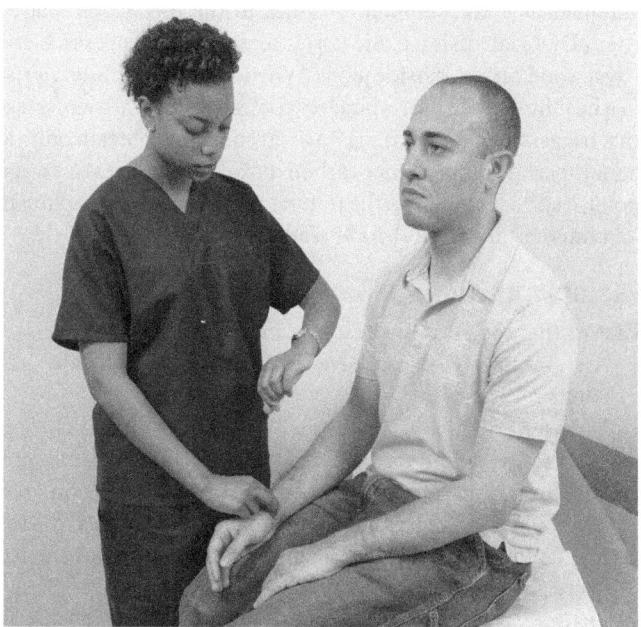

Fig. 33.10 Radial Pulse. (From Niedzwiecki B, et al: *Kinn's the medical assistant,* ed 14, St. Louis, 2020, Elsevier.)

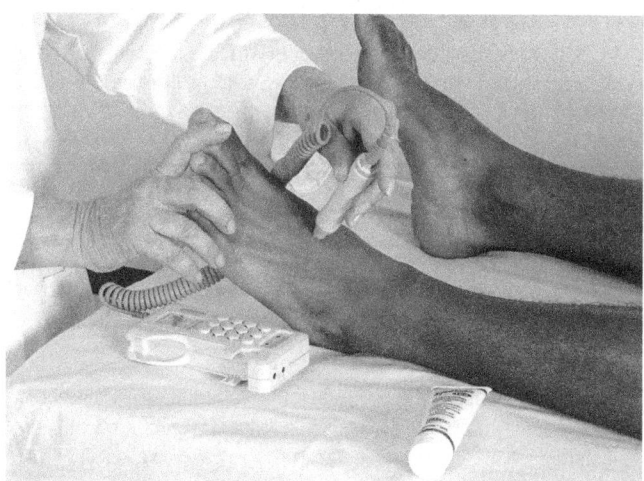

Fig. 33.11 Doppler Ultrasound Unit Measuring the Pedal Pulse. (From Jarvis C: *Physical examination and health assessment,* ed 7, St. Louis, 2016, Saunders.)

TABLE 33.1	Normal Vital Signs by Age					
	PULSE RATES		**RESPIRATION RATES**		**BLOOD PRESSURE RANGES**	
Age	Range (beats/min)	Average	Range (breaths/min)	Average	Systolic	Diastolic
Newborn	120–160	140	30–50	40	60–96	30–62
1–2 years	80–140	120	20–30	25	78–112	48–78
3–6 years	80–120	100	18–26	22	78–112	50–79
7–11 years	75–110	95	16–22	19	85–114	52–79
Adolescence	60–100	80	12–20	16	94–119	58–79
Adulthood	60–100	80	12–20	16	100–119	60–79

Commonly, the radial pulse is counted for a 30-second interval, with the result multiplied by 2 to come to a beat-per-minute reading. If the pulse is irregular or if the medical assistant is new at taking a pulse, the rate should be counted for 1 full minute.

Counting an Apical Pulse Rate

For an apical pulse (AP), the patient can be sitting or lying down. Place the stethoscope at the junction of the fifth intercostal space at the left midclavicular line for older children and adults. For infants and young children, the apical pulse can be heard at the fourth intercostal space at the left mid-clavicular line.

You will hear a *lub dub* sound. Each *lub dub* sound is one heartbeat. The apical pulse should always be auscultated (AW skuh l teyt ed) for 1 full minute to detect any irregularities in rate and rhythm. The pulse should be documented with the notation (AP) beside the recorded count.

A radial pulse and an apical count may be requested if the patient is taking cardiac drugs or has bradycardia (bradi KAHR dee uh) or tachycardia (tak i KAHR dee uh). Normally, the heartbeat rate and the pulse rate are the same. To determine the presence of a pulse deficit, the provider may listen to the apical beat while the medical assistant counts the pulse at another site (usually the radial pulse).

CRITICAL THINKING 33.4

Mrs. Arnez has a documented thready pulse. What site should Carlos use to measure the pulse? Why should he take the pulse for a full minute?

VOCABULARY

auscultate To listen to with a stethoscope.
bounding Describes a pulse that feels full because of the increased power of cardiac contraction or as a result of increased blood volume.
bradycardia A slow heartbeat; a pulse below 60 beats per minute.
exhalation The act of breathing out. The diaphragm relaxes, allowing air to be expelled from the lungs.
external respiration The exchange of oxygen and carbon dioxide between the body and atmosphere that occurs within the lungs.
inhalation The act of breathing in. The diaphragm contracts and drops down drawing air into the lungs.
internal respiration Exchange of oxygen and carbon dioxide between the bloodstream and body cells.
pulse deficit A condition in which the radial pulse is less than the apical pulse; it may indicate a peripheral vascular abnormality.
tachycardia A rapid but regular heart rate; one that exceeds 100 beats per minute.
thready Describes a pulse that is thin and feeble.
occlude To close, shut, or stop up.

MEDICAL TERMINOLOGY

cleid/o	clavicle (collarbone)
mastoid/o	mastoid process
stern/o	sternum

RESPIRATION

The body cells require oxygen, and when this is used, they create carbon dioxide as a waste product. Respiration works to remove the carbon dioxide and provide a steady flow of oxygen to the cells. One complete inhalation (in hull LAY shun) and exhalation (ex hull LAY shun) cycle is called a *respiration*. During the inhalation phase, the diaphragm contracts and drops down. The *intercostal* muscles pull the ribs up and outward. This causes the lungs to expand and fill with air. During the exhalation phase, the diaphragm returns to its normal elevated position, and the intercostal muscles relax. This causes the lungs to expel the waste air from the body.

Internal respiration occurs at the cellular level. This term is used when this exchange occurs within the body, between the blood and the body cells. External respiration relates to the flow of air into and out of the lungs, and the transfer of oxygen and carbon dioxide that occurs within the lungs. This is what is referred to when counting the respiration rate.

Respiration can be controlled to a certain extent, and because of this, it is considered a voluntary function. However, when people are not consciously altering their breathing, they will breathe automatically. The respiratory center in the medulla oblongata (muh DOO lah ob lon GAH tah) is sensitive to changes in blood oxygen and carbon dioxide levels. When carbon dioxide levels rise in a healthy person, the respiratory control center sends a message that triggers breathing. This is why we can hold our breath only for a short period of time. Once carbon dioxide levels rise to a certain point, a stimulus is sent to the respiratory muscles (the diaphragm and intercostal muscles) and breathing begins involuntarily.

Factors Affecting the Respiration Rate

Factors that can affect the respiration rate include:

- *Age*: Younger children have a higher respiration rate than adults.
- *Diseases*: Metabolic acidosis, anemia, asthma, chronic obstructive pulmonary disease (COPD), head trauma, and pain from rib fractures can increase the respiration rate. Metabolic alkalosis, diabetic ketoacidosis, liver and kidney failure, electrolyte imbalance, and hypothyroidism can decrease the rate.
- *Environmental*: Being in a higher altitude and exposure to cold temperatures will increase the respiration rate.
- *Physical activity*: Physical exertion will increase the respiration rate.
- *Psychological state*: Anxiety and panic can increase the respiration rate.
- *Certain drugs and nicotine*: CNS depressant substances, such as opioids and alcohol, can decrease the respiration rate.
- *Chemicals*: Certain industrial chemicals and dangerous levels of carbon monoxide can slow the respiration rate.

Characteristics of Respirations

Normally a person's breathing is relaxed, automatic, and relatively silent. Respiratory disease and other chronic conditions can influence the characteristics of an individual's respirations and cause changes in the normal breathing sounds and pattern.

When a provider listens to a patient's breath sounds, unusual sounds and patterns can be valuable tools in patient diagnosis.

When assessing a patient's respirations, you must note three important characteristics:

- *Rate*: The rate of respiration is the number of respirations per minute. Fig. 33.12 shows sample breathing rate patterns recorded with a spirometer. Table 33.1 lists normal respiratory ranges for patients in various age groups.
- *Rhythm*: Rhythm refers to the breathing pattern, the space between each breath. A steady breathing pattern with similar spaces between breaths is normal in adults and most children; however, the breathing pattern for infants varies. Automatic interruptions, such as sighing, are also considered normal. The terms "regular" or "irregular" are used to document rhythm.
- *Depth*: The depth of respiration is the amount of air inhaled and exhaled. When a patient is at rest, normal respirations have a consistent depth, which can be noted as you watch the rise and fall of the chest. *Shallow breathing* occurs when a person inhales and exhales abnormally small volumes of air. *Gasping breathing* occurs when a person is breathing sharply or with effort. The terms "normal," "deep," "shallow," and "gasping" should be used to document depth.

Abnormal Respirations. Because normal breathing causes very little sound, distinctly noticeable breath sounds that occur during the breathing process are a sign of respiratory problems. Though many of these abnormal breathing characteristics can be noticed without assistance, the provider will often listen closely to the lungs with a stethoscope to determine the specific characteristics of the breath sounds (Table 33.2).

When an individual cannot breathe in enough oxygen to supply all body cells with oxygenated blood, normal skin coloring, particularly around the mouth and the nail beds, changes to a bluish, dusky color. This coloration, which indicates an increased level of carbon dioxide in the blood, is called cyanosis. The patient also may have other signs and symptoms, such as vertigo (VUR tih goh), chest pain (angina), and numbness in the fingers and toes.

VOCABULARY

cyanosis Abnormal blue coloration to tissues caused by an excess of carbon dioxide.

vertigo A false sensation that you or your environment is spinning or moving.

MEDICAL TERMINOLOGY

cost/o	rib
hal/o	to breathe
a-	without, no, not
brady-	slow
dys-	difficult, painful, abnormal, bad
ex-	out
hyper-	excessive, too much, above
in-	in, into
inter-	between
tachy-	fast
-al	pertaining to
-ation	process, condition
-pnea	breathing

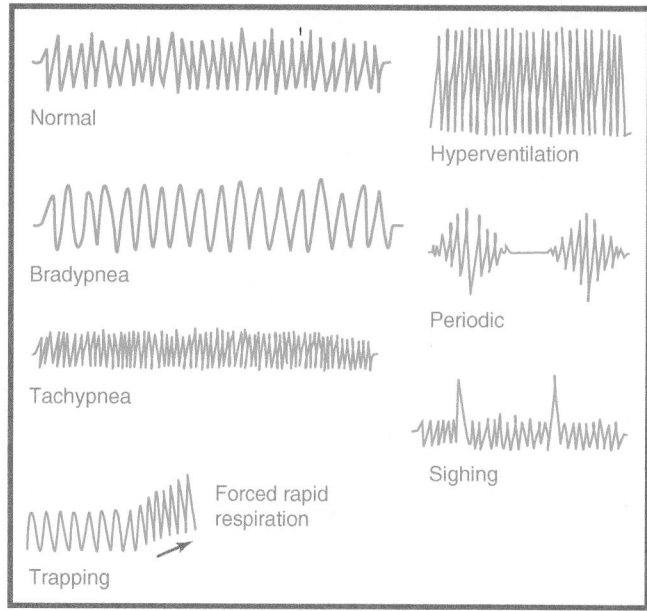

Fig. 33.12 Respiratory rate patterns, called *spirograms*, are recorded using a spirometer. (From Niedzwiecki B, et al: *Kinn's the medical assistant*, ed 14, St. Louis, 2020, Elsevier.)

Counting Respirations

Because most people can control their breathing to a certain extent, do not mention that you will be counting the person's respirations (see Procedure 33.8). Patients may self-consciously alter their breathing rate when they know they are being watched. Count the respirations while appearing to count the radial pulse. Keep your eyes alternately on the patient's chest and your watch while you count the pulse rate; then, without removing your fingers from the pulse site, determine the respiratory rate (Fig. 33.13). If the patient is lying down, the arm on which you are taking the radial pulse may be crossed over the chest so that respirations can be felt with the rise and fall of the chest. Another way of observing respirations is to watch the movement of the patient's shoulders with each inspiration. Count the respirations for 30 seconds and multiply the number by 2. Do not use the 15-second interval because this count can vary by a factor of ±4, which is significant when dealing with such a small number. Record the respiration rate, rhythm, and depth in the health record.

BLOOD PRESSURE

A BP reading reflects the arterial blood pressure, or the pressure of the blood on the arterial walls. Blood pressure is read in millimeters of mercury (mm Hg) and record as fraction. There are actually three BP readings:

- *Systolic* (SIS tol ic) *pressure*: The greatest pressure in the arteries, which occurs when the heart is contracting. It is the first sound heard and is documented as the numerator (top) in the BP fraction.
- *Diastolic* (dye AS tol ic) *pressure*: The lowest pressure in the arteries, which occurs when the heart is relaxed. It is the last sound heard and is the denominator (bottom) in the BP fraction. Systole and diastole make up the cardiac cycle.

TABLE 33.2 Abnormal Respirations

Respiratory Characteristic	Description	Common Illness
Apnea (AP nee ah)	Abnormal, periodic cessation of breathing; often with a large gasp as the patient starts breathing again.	• Sleep apnea
Bradypnea (brad IP nee ah)	Abnormally slow breathing rate.	• Excessive use of sedatives (including alcohol and narcotics) • Spinal cord or head injuries
Dyspnea (DISP nee uh)	Difficulty breathing, breathlessness, or air hunger. Also known as shortness of breath.	• Asthma • Broken ribs • Cardiac issues • Pulmonary embolism • Low blood volume • Chronic obstructive pulmonary disease (COPD)
Hyperpnea (hye PURP nee ah)	Excessively deep breathing exchanging high volume of air.	• Physical activity most common cause; breathing returns to normal within a few minutes • Panic disorder
Hyperventilation (hye pur ven tih LAY shun)	Abnormally fast or deep breathing.	• Excessive use of stimulants • Drug overdoses (with the exception of drugs with a sedative effect). For example, an aspirin overdose will cause hyperventilation. • Severe pain • Panic disorder • Infection in the lungs
Orthopnea (or THOP nee ah)	Difficulty with breathing when lying down; breathing is easier when sitting or standing.	• Heart failure • Pulmonary edema • Pneumonia • Severe obesity
Rales (rayls)	Inspiratory auscultatory sounds resembling crackles or popping sounds; caused by fluid in the airway or alveoli. Can be described as moist, dry, fine, or coarse.	• Pneumonia • Croup • Heart failure
Rhonchi (RON kye)	Auscultatory sounds resembling snoring. Occurs when air flow is partially blocked through the large airways.	• COPD • Pneumonia • Cystic fibrosis
Stertorous (STER tore us)	Very labored and creates a raspy snoring sound.	• Snoring (structural blockage when the respiratory passages relax) • Sleep apnea
Stridor (str I DOR)	High-pitched, wheezing sound noted on inspiration, caused by disrupted airflow.	• Partial airway blockage; often noted with choking • Inflammation in larynx or trachea
Tachypnea (tak IP nee ah)	Rapid, shallow breathing.	• Sepsis • Diabetic ketoacidosis • Carbon monoxide poisoning • Asthma
Wheezing (WHEE zeeng)	Hoarse whistling sound, caused by narrowing in the large airways.	• Asthma • COPD

• **Pulse pressure:** The difference between the systolic and diastolic blood pressures (30 to 50 mm Hg is considered normal). This can be affected by medications and some disease processes.

Factors Affecting the Blood Pressure

There are many factors that can affect the blood pressure, including:

• *Blood volume:* Total amount of blood in the body. Dehydration, hemorrhage, and diuretic (DIE ah ret ik) medications lower the blood volume, thus decreasing the blood pressure. An increase in blood volume will increase the blood pressure.

• *Strength of ventricular contractions:* The greater the force of the contraction, the more blood is pumped into the arteries, thus increasing the blood pressure.

• **Peripheral resistance** *to blood flow:* Any factor that increases the resistance to blood flow through the arteries will increase the blood pressure. Factors that increase resistance include a narrowed lumen, lack of elasticity of the arterial walls, and an increase in the viscosity of the blood. Fatty cholesterol deposits called *atherosclerotic plaque* (ath uh roh skluh ROH tic plak) can narrow the arterial lumen. The vessel elasticity can decrease with advancing age, certain lifestyle factors, and the presence of arteriosclerosis (ar teer ee oh sklah ROH sis). Polycythemia (pol ee sie THEE mee ah) and blood

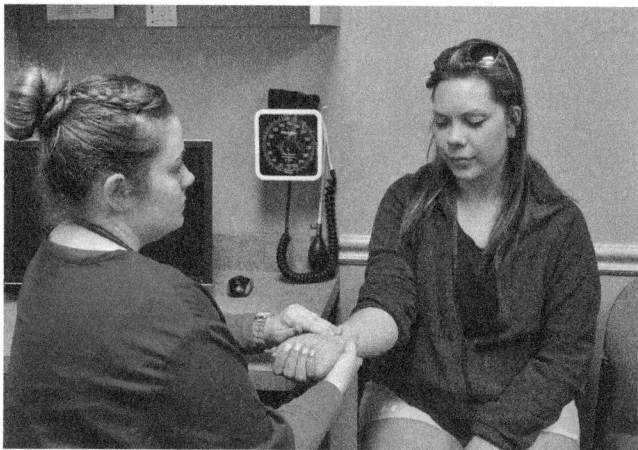

Fig. 33.13 Hand Position When Counting Respirations. The hands should be left in place as if still counting the patient's pulse. (From Niedzwiecki B, et al: *Kinn's the medical assistant,* ed 14, St. Louis, 2020, Elsevier.)

transfusions can increase the blood viscosity. (For more information, see Chapter 10.)

- *Physical activity, stress, and stimulants* (e.g., caffeine) can cause a temporary increase in blood pressure.

CRITICAL THINKING 33.5

Tina Anderson, a 36-year-old patient who is obese, is wearing a heavy knit sweater, and Carlos needs to obtain a respiratory count. What could he do to obtain an accurate measurement of Tina's respiratory rate?

VOCABULARY

arteriosclerosis Thickening, decreased elasticity, and calcification of arterial walls.

hypertension Chronically high blood pressure, generally readings of more than 129/80 for an extended period of time.

peripheral resistance The resistance of the arteries to blood flow.

pulse pressure The difference between the systolic and diastolic blood pressures (30 to 50 mm Hg is considered normal).

Hypertension

One reading of high blood pressure is not necessarily a concern because of the likelihood of temporary factors increasing the blood pressure. Chronic high blood pressure is dangerous because this leads to stress and eventual damage to the blood vessels. This is known as hypertension (HTN) (Table 33.3). Hypertension is often referred to as the "silent killer" because symptoms of chronic high blood pressure tend to be mild and go unnoticed. Individuals may go long periods of time without knowing that they have a problem. Signs and symptoms of hypertension include blurred vision, vertigo, fatigue, flushing, angina, dyspnea, headache, and nosebleeds (*epistaxis* [ep uh STAK sis]). About 47% of the adults in the U.S. have hypertension according to Million Hearts (https://millionhearts.hhs.gov). Hypertension increases the risk for stroke and heart disease, two leading causes of death.

Hypertension can occur in people of all ages (including young children) and in people of all ethnic origins. Those at highest risk for developing hypertension and hypertension-related illnesses are:

- Middle-aged and older adults
- Individuals of African American descent
- Patients with diabetes mellitus
- Patients with kidney disease

Because few people notice symptoms of high blood pressure, it is especially important that every patient be screened at every appointment. Hypertension is most often diagnosed during a patient visit for another problem.

Temporary Hypertension. As with other vital signs, the blood pressure will change throughout the day. Some patients experience an elevated blood pressure at the start of their visit, although it is normal in other settings. This is called *white coat hypertension,* or white coat syndrome. Usually, the blood pressure is repeated either after the patient has relaxed for 5 minutes or at the end of the visit.

If patients have a high blood pressure measurement during a healthcare visit, they are often asked to track their blood pressure. Home monitoring is discussed later in the chapter. Only when abnormal readings show consistently over time is hypertension diagnosed.

Essential Hypertension. Essential hypertension (or *primary hypertension*) is the most common type of hypertension. Essential hypertension is considered idiopathic (id ee uh PATH ik), but it is associated with obesity, elevated cholesterol levels, a family history, and metabolic syndrome. It also is more common in older adults.

Treatment of essential hypertension depends on the severity of the hypertension. Treatment can include:

- *Lifestyle changes:* Low salt, fat, and cholesterol diet, exercise, smoking cessation, and weight loss.
- *Medications:* Antihypertensive medications and diuretics to reduce the blood pressure. Some antihypertensive medications cause vasodilation, while others decrease the stroke volume. Diuretics decrease the blood volume. It is common for patients to start on one medication and then additional medications are added as needed to lower the blood pressure.

A patient-centered treatment approach should be implemented to motivate patients to maintain compliance with hypertension management. The medical assistant can play an active role by providing ongoing education and support to ensure compliance with provider-recommended treatment.

CRITICAL THINKING 33.6

Mr. Samuel Long, a 43-year-old patient, recently was diagnosed with essential hypertension. What should Carlos discuss with Mr. Long to emphasize the dangers of his disease and to teach him about possible lifestyle modifications that he must make to improve his health? Are any community resources available that might help Mr. Long and his family effectively manage his disease?

Secondary Hypertension. *Secondary hypertension* occurs when the reason for the high blood pressure is clearly known and directly related to an underlying pathologic condition. Once the condition

TABLE 33.3   Stages and Treatment of Hypertension

Blood Pressure	Treatment
Normal <120 systolic AND <80 diastolic	If readings fall into this category, follow a balanced diet and get regular exercise. Continue to monitor blood pressure in case of future increase in readings.
Elevated 120–129 systolic AND <80 diastolic	Lifestyle modification: reduced sodium; low saturated- and trans-fat diet; regular aerobic activity; moderate alcohol intake; smoking cessation; weight loss; stress reduction.
Hypertension – Stage 1 130–139 systolic OR 80–89 diastolic	Continue with lifestyle modifications. Drug therapy for patients with cardiovascular risk, diabetes mellitus, or chronic kidney disease.
Hypertension – Stage 2 ≥140 systolic OR ≥90 diastolic	Continue with lifestyle modifications. Common for providers to use combination blood pressure medications, specifically for patients with comorbidities such as diabetes mellitus or chronic kidney disease.
Hypertensive Crisis >180 systolic >120 diastolic	Requires emergency medical attention.

Information from the American Heart Association. https://www.heart.org/en/health-topics/high-blood-pressure/understanding-blood-pressure-readings.

is corrected, the blood pressure will return to normal ranges. Commonly, renal disease, complications of pregnancy, endocrine imbalance, and brain injuries can cause secondary hypertension.

Hypotension

Hypotension occurs when the blood pressure drops below normal and there is not enough pressure to push the blood through vital organs. Common symptoms of hypotension are dizziness or lightheadedness, fatigue, nausea, blurred or fading vision, syncope, and loss of concentration.

In some cases, patients may experience a sharp decrease in blood pressure and an increase in the pulse rate when they change position, specifically when they stand quickly. This is known as orthostatic (postural) hypotension. It can be related to dehydration, heart failure, or blood pressure medications. If patients symptoms of hypotension, it is important to notify the provider, since it can lead to falls.

VOCABULARY

calibrated Determined by or checked against a standard (as in readings).

essential hypertension Elevated blood pressure of unknown cause that develops for no apparent reason; sometimes called primary hypertension.

hypotension Blood pressure that is below normal (systolic pressure below 90 mm Hg and diastolic pressure below 50 mm Hg).

idiopathic Of unknown cause.

orthostatic (postural) hypotension A temporary fall in blood pressure when a person rapidly changes from a recumbent position to a standing position.

syncope Fainting; a brief lapse in consciousness.

Blood Pressure Equipment

The blood pressure is taken with a stethoscope and a *sphygmomanometer* (sfig moh man NAW meh ter), or blood pressure cuff. The sphygmomanometer consists of an inflatable cuff, an inflation bulb with a control valve, and a pressure gauge (Fig. 33.14A). The device may be handheld, wall mounted, or a floor model (Fig. 33.14B). Some systems have a trigger-style air release valve. These can be pumped up and then the air slowly released simply by pushing the trigger (Fig. 33.15). With the more traditional sphygmomanometers, the valve must be unscrewed.

Sphygmomanometers are delicately calibrated (KAL uh breyt d) instruments that must be handled carefully. They should be recalibrated regularly and checked for accuracy. The needle on the aneroid dial sphygmomanometer should rest within the small square or circle at the bottom of the dial. If

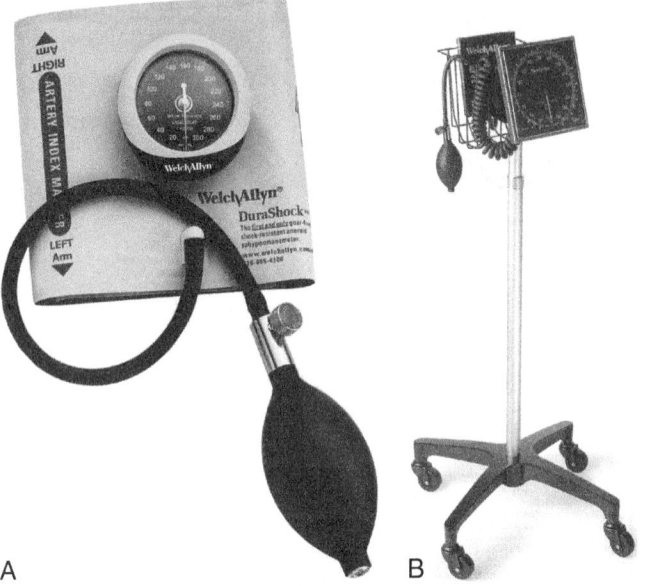

Fig. 33.14 A, Aneroid dial system with an inflatable cuff. B, Aneroid floor model with a large slanted face. (From Niedzwiecki B, et al: *Kinn's the medical assistant,* ed 14, St. Louis, 2020, Elsevier.)

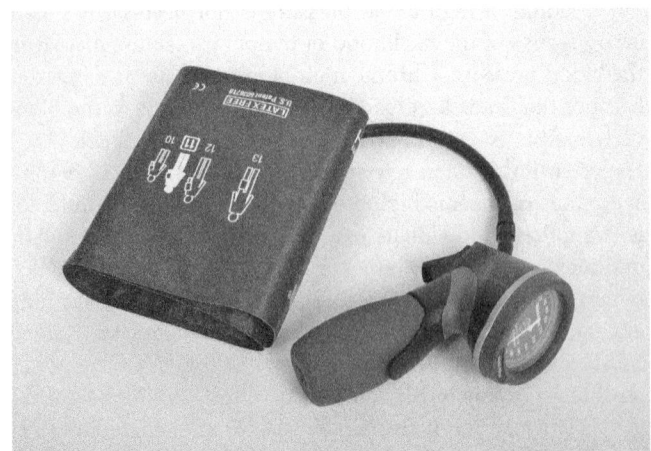

Fig. 33.15 Trigger-Release Aneroid Blood Pressure Valve. (From Niedzwiecki B, et al: *Kinn's the medical assistant,* ed 14, St. Louis, 2020, Elsevier.)

the sphygmomanometer is not correctly calibrated, the patient's blood pressure measurement will be inaccurate.

Automatic blood pressure machines are also used in ambulatory care. Machines range in size and usually a variety of cuff sizes are available. Typically, the machine is used for one reading. Some machines have automatic settings that allow the medical assistant to set how often a reading is needed. These machines are useful during procedures or situations where constant blood pressure monitoring is required. If the automatic BP reading seems inaccurate, the medical assistant should do a manual BP.

MEDICAL TERMINOLOGY	
cardi/o	heart
man/o	scanty or pressure
my/o	muscle
sphygm/o	pulse
hypo-	deficit, too little, below
-meter	instrument to measure

Appropriate Cuff Size. To obtain a correct blood pressure measurement, the cuff used must be the proper size. The inflatable part (the bladder) of a cuff should cover about 80% of the circumference of the upper arm. The bladder width should equal at least 40% of the upper arm's circumference.

To help with this, most blood pressure cuffs have predetermined markings on the internal side (the side placed on the patient's arm). As long as the cuff is secured within these lines, it should be the accurate size (Fig. 33.16). Table 33.4 presents the various sizes of blood pressure cuffs available.

Obtaining an Accurate Blood Pressure

To obtain an accurate blood pressure measurement, the patient should relax and be quiet for 5 minutes. Avoiding caffeine, exercise, and smoking for 30 minutes prior to the reading is recommended. The arm must rest 1-2 minutes between readings if repeated measurements are taken. Seven additional factors that must be considered when obtaining an accurate blood pressure include:

1. *Empty a full bladder*: If the patient has a full bladder and needs to use the restroom, this should be done prior to taking the blood pressure. Dealing with a full bladder can add 10 mm Hg to the BP reading.
2. *Use the correct cuff size*: Using a too small a cuff can add 2-10 mm Hg and a too large a cuff can decrease the reading by 5 mm Hg.
3. *Support the back and feet*: The person should be sitting in a chair with the back supported. The feet should be flat on the floor or on a footstool. An unsupported back, slouching, or dangling feet can increase the BP reading by 6 mm Hg.
4. *Keep legs uncrossed*: Large veins in the legs can be squeezed when legs are crossed. This can increase the BP reading by 2-8 mm Hg.
5. *Support the arm at heart level*: The arm should be supported on a table or counter, so the BP cuff is at the level of the heart. The arm should be relaxed. The hand should not be

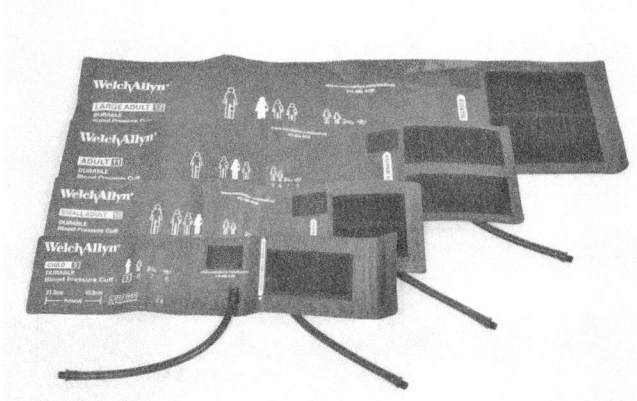

Fig. 33.16 Variety of Blood Pressure Cuff Sizes. (From Niedzwiecki B, et al: *Kinn's the medical assistant*, ed 14, St. Louis, 2020, Elsevier.)

TABLE 33.4	Blood Pressure Cuff Sizes	
	ARM CIRCUMFERENCE	
Cuff	**Centimeters**	**Inches**
Small adult	22–26	8.7–10.2
Adult	27–34	10.6–13.4
Large adult	35–44	13.8–17.3
Adult thigh	45–52	17.7–20.5

From Target:BP at https://targetbp.org/patient-measured-bp/implementing/smbp-selecting-the-right-cuff-size/. Accessed 4/24/2021.

clenched. An unsupported arm can increase the BP reading by 10 mm Hg.
6. *Place the cuff on a bare arm*: Have the patient roll up the sleeve, remove the arm from the sleeve, or change into a gown. Ensure the clothing above the cuff is not tight since it can restrict the blood flow and alter the BP reading. Placing the cuff over clothing can elevate the BP reading by 5-50 mm Hg.
7. *Refrain from engaging in a conversation*: The medical assistant should encourage the patient not to talk during the procedure. Talking and active listening during the reading can increase the BP reading by 10 mm Hg.

Measuring the Blood Pressure

The goal of the procedure is to use the inflatable cuff to stop the circulation through an artery. The stethoscope is placed over the artery just below the cuff. As the cuff is slowly deflated to allow the blood to flow again, cardiac cycle sounds are heard through the stethoscope. Readings are taken when the first (systolic) and last (diastolic) sounds are heard (Procedure 33.9).

On the first visit, the ambulatory care facility's policy might require the medical assistant to take the blood pressure in both arms. The blood pressure can be different between the arms.

Cuff Placement. The medical assistant must select an appropriately sized blood pressure cuff. The bladder of the cuff should be completely deflated before using it. The cuff should be wrapped smoothly around the upper arm. The bladder of the cuff should be centered over the brachial artery. Most cuffs

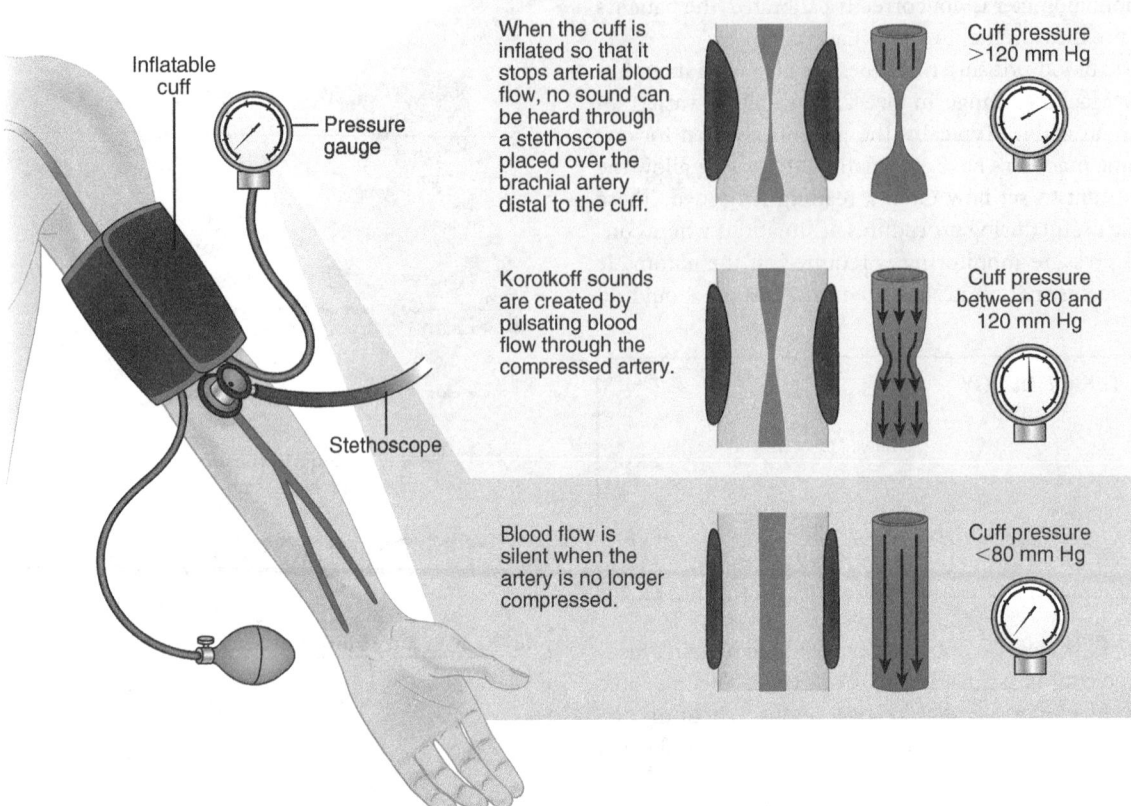

Fig. 33.17 The Science of Taking a Patient's Blood Pressure. (From Niedzwiecki B, et al: *Kinn's the medical assistant,* ed 14, St. Louis, 2020, Elsevier.)

have a marking that must be placed over the brachial artery. The lower edge of the cuff should be 1 inch (2.5cm or about 2 finger widths) above the elbow or antecubital space. This allow plenty of room to place the stethoscope without touching the cuff.

Obtain an Estimated Systolic Pressure. The medical assistant must know how far to inflate the cuff. An over inflated or under inflated cuff could lead to an inaccurate blood pressure measurement. The medical assistant should first estimate the systolic pressure by using the *palpatory method.*

- Apply the cuff to the upper arm as previously described.
- Find and continue to palpate the radial pulse.
- Inflate the cuff to the point where the radial pulse can no longer be felt. Inflate the cuff an additional 30 mm Hg.
- Slowing deflate the cuff. Note the reading on the gauge when the pulse reappears. This is the estimated systolic pressure.

If you need to document the reading, use a "P" to indicate the systolic reading was palpated. For example, if you first felt the radial pulse return at 122 mm Hg, the palpated blood pressure is recorded as 122/P.

The medical assistant should let the arm rest for 1-2 minutes before taking the blood pressure. The blood pressure cuff can remain in place. The medical assistant should add 30 mm Hg to the estimated systolic pressure. This is the how much the cuff needs to be inflated when taking the blood pressure. The

medical assistant should smoothly and evenly deflate the cuff at about 2 mg Hg (one mark) per second.

When documenting the blood pressure, the medical assistant must indicate the blood pressure reading, the position of the patient, the location (e.g., right arm), and the cuff size. Table 33.1 lists normal BP ranges for patients of various age groups.

Korotkoff Sounds. Korotkoff sounds are heard during auscultation of the blood pressure. Vibrations of the arterial wall produce these sounds when the blood surges back into the vessel after it has been compressed by the blood pressure cuff. The sounds are classified into five distinct phases, which include (Fig. 33.17):

I. *Appearance of clear tapping sound.* This is the systolic blood pressure.

II. *Sounds become softer and longer.* Occasionally blood pressure sounds completely disappear during this phase, only to reappear later. This is called an auscultatory (AW skuh l tah tohr ee) gap. The silence may continue as the needle falls another 30 mm Hg. Auscultatory gaps can occur with hypertension and certain types of heart disease. It is important to report the gap to the provider.

III. *Sounds become clearer, crisper, louder and continue rhythmically.*

IV. *Sounds become softer and muffled.* Controversy surrounds whether the diastolic blood pressure in children and adolescents should be the start of phase IV or V.

V. *Sounds disappear.* Record this as the diastolic pressure. Continue to deflate the cuff for 10 mm Hg past the last sound to ensure the accuracy of the diastolic pressure.

VOCABULARY

auscultatory gap A period during which Korotkoff sounds fade away and reappear later at a lower pressure point as the cuff deflates.

CRITICAL THINKING 33.7

Vital signs are documented in a paper record in this order: temperature (T), pulse (P), and respirations (R). Blood pressure is recorded after TPR. Depending on the electronic health record (EHR) system, they may be ordered differently. Correctly document the following vital signs:

1. Oral temperature 101.2°; apical pulse 90 regular rhythm; respirations 22 regular rhythm, shallow volume; and orthostatic blood pressure in the right arm is 138/88 supine in the right arm and 110/70 standing in the right arm
2. Tympanic temperature 36.8°; radial pulse 66, irregular rhythm, normal volume; respirations 18, regular rhythm, normal volume; and bilateral blood pressure 128/76 in the left arm, sitting, and 132/80 in the right arm, sitting
3. Temporal artery temperature 102.4°; apical pulse 102, irregular rhythm; and respirations 27, regular rhythm, normal volume
4. Axillary temperature 97.7°; carotid pulse 58, irregular rhythm; respirations 24, regular rhythm, deep volume; and palpated systolic blood pressure 62

Taking a Blood Pressure Using the Thigh. If the patient's arms cannot be used for a blood pressure, a thigh blood pressure can be obtained. If using the thigh to take a blood pressure, the patient should be in the prone position if possible. The leg should be level with the heart. Locate the popliteal artery. Wrap a thigh-sized cuff around the thigh, placing the cuff edge 1 inch above the bend of the knee. The bladder should be centered over the popliteal artery. Place the stethoscope over the popliteal artery and proceed to take the blood pressure. Typically, the systolic pressure in the popliteal artery is 20-30 mmHg higher than when taking the BP using the arm.

Taking Orthostatic Vital Signs. Orthostatic vital signs may be done to evaluate patients who are at risk for hypovolemia due to loss of fluid (e.g., vomiting, diarrhea), syncope, or are at risk for falls. As a person moves positions, a significant change in vital signs can increase the person's risk of falling. Procedure 33.10 describes the process of obtaining orthostatic vital signs. The following are considered abnormal when performing orthostatic vital signs:

- A drop in the blood pressure of ≥20 mm Hg
- A drop in the diastolic BP of ≥10 mm Hg
- Lightheadedness or dizziness during position changes.

Automated Ambulatory Blood Pressure Monitoring

Ambulatory blood pressure monitors can be used to check patients' blood pressures throughout the day. Typically, patients wear the monitor for up to 2 days. The blood pressure is automatically taken and recorded. The provider reviews the patient's blood pressure readings to check for elevated readings over the course of the day.

Home Blood Pressure Monitoring

A variety of manual cuffs and automatic blood pressure monitors are available in stores for patients to purchase for home BP monitoring (Fig. 33.18). Patients should check to see if their insurance covers the cost of the machine.

American Heart Association (https://www.heart.org) recommends patients purchase validated automatic home monitors. The blood pressure monitors should be for the upper arm since they are more reliable than the wrist blood pressure monitors. Blood pressure monitors that transmit readings to providers or store blood pressure readings in the memory are recommended. Providers can review these readings to check the effectiveness of the blood pressure management strategies.

When the medical assistant instructs patients how to take their blood pressure reading at home, it can be helpful to have patients bring in their monitors. The medical assistant can check the patient's technique and verify the accuracy of the blood pressure measurement. The patient should be encouraged to bring the machine into the facility every 6 to 12 months check the accuracy of the reading.

Patients should be coached on the importance of relaxing for at least 5 minutes before taking the reading. Avoiding caffeine, exercise, and smoking for 30 minutes prior to the reading is recommended. They should use the same arm for the reading. They should check their BP at various times throughout the day. The medical assistant should also review the patient's position and other factors that impact the accuracy of the reading.

PULSE OXIMETRY

Pulse oximetry (ok SIM i tree) is a method of evaluating the oxygen saturation of the blood. It is also referred to as saturation of peripheral oxygen (SpO_2). Many ambulatory care settings use pulse oximeters to assess a patient's oxygenation status with disorders such as pneumonia, bronchitis, emphysema, or asthma. In many cases the SpO_2 will be checked routinely with the vital signs.

To perform the procedure, the medical assistant clips a probe on the patient's earlobe or finger (Fig. 33.19, Procedure 33.11). Fingernail polish must be removed before the clip is applied. If the patient has artificial nails, the earlobe should be used. A beam of infrared light passes through the tissue. The light is blocked by oxygenated hemoglobin within the blood. A sensor placed on the other side of the finger registers how much light was blocked to estimate the oxygenation of the blood. The reading is displayed as a percentage on the digital screen.

The infrared light also measures the patient's pulse rate, which also is shown on the screen. The pulse should not be recorded off the pulse oximeter for the initial vital sign reading. Instead this should be used to make sure the pulse oximeter is reading correctly. If the pulse on the device closely matches the manual pulse, the oxygenation reading also is considered accurate.

A normal pulse oximetry reading is 95% or higher. Treatments, such as oxygen and bronchodilator therapies, usually are started when readings are 90% to 92% or lower. Pulse oximeters will not read oxygenation correctly in patients who

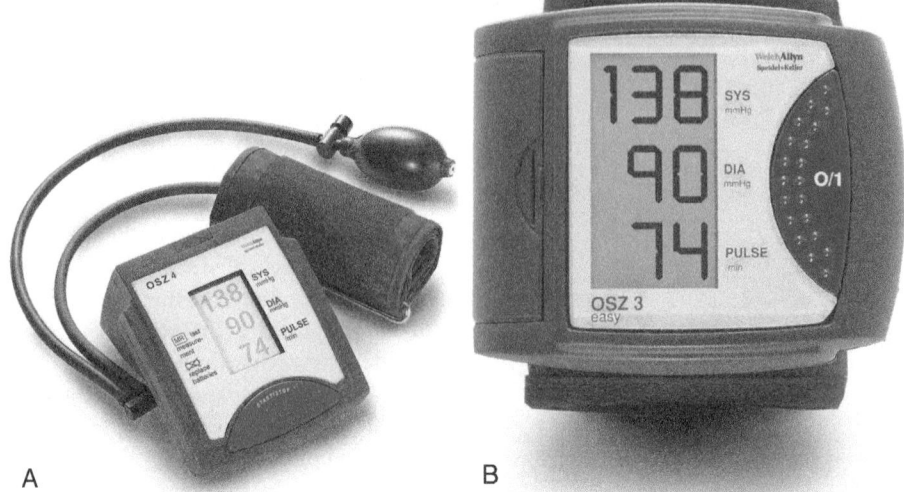

Fig. 33.18 **Personal Blood Pressure Systems.** A, Digital arm cuff. B, Digital wrist cuff. (From Niedzwiecki B, et al: *Kinn's the medical assistant,* ed 14, St. Louis, 2020, Elsevier.)

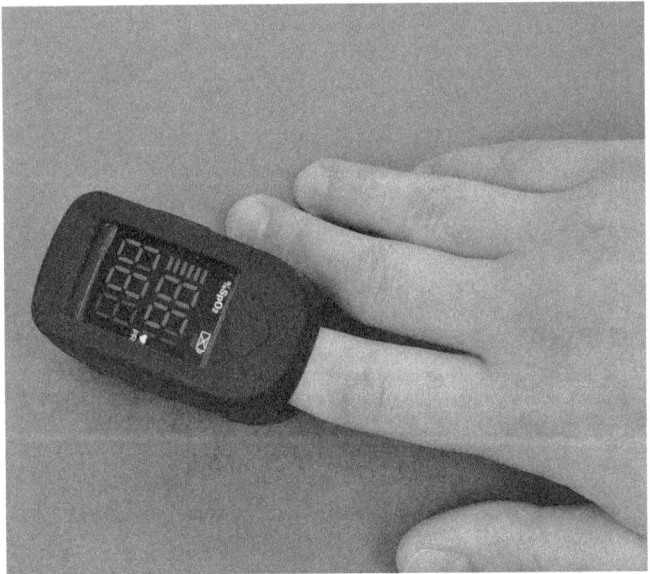

Fig. 33.19 **Pulse Oximeter.** (From Niedzwiecki B, et al: *Kinn's the medical assistant,* ed 14, St. Louis, 2020, Elsevier.)

have been exposed to carbon monoxide, since carbon monoxide binds to oxygen receptor sites on the hemoglobin, blocking oxygen.

ANTHROPOMETRIC MEASUREMENTS

Anthropometry (an thruh POM i tree) is the science that deals with measurement of the size, weight, and proportions of the human body. These measurements often are included in the initial recording of vital signs. Because they are indicators of the patient's state of health and well-being, height and weight measurements and the associated BMI are discussed as aspects of the vital signs.

A patient's weight and height can be helpful in diagnosis, and the medical assistant must obtain these readings with accuracy and empathy (Procedure 33.12). In ambulatory care,

weight and height are measured routinely as the patient is taken to the examination room. To safeguard patient confidentiality, the scale should be located in a private area where other people cannot see the patient's weight. Safeguard the patient's confidentiality by not repeating the measurement out loud. Others nearby might hear this private patient information. If this is the patient's first visit, anthropometric measurements are recorded in the history database and are used as reference information during future visits as needed.

Height

Height can be measured in inches or centimeters (Box 33.3). Measurement is accomplished by using a wall ruler or a scale with a height bar attachment. Patients should stand with their feet to the wall, or when the scale is used, with the feet toward the back of the weighing platform. They should stand straight, and the parallel bar should be gently lowered to touch the top of the head. Before you take height measurements, it is important to ask the patient to remove their shoes, which can add to the height reading.

For adult patients, the height should be checked at the first visit and is generally documented in feet and inches. Because adult height generally does not change significantly over time, follow facility policies regarding height checks after the initial visit for adult patients. Some providers require height measurements on older adults yearly. For children, the height should be checked at every visit to clearly document growth in the child.

Weight

Weight can be a sensitive issue for many patients. Maintain a professional attitude when obtaining a patient's weight. Weigh the patient in a private area. Make sure heavy items are removed from pockets and that the patient is not holding a purse. Shoes and coats should also be removed.

The medical assistant should select the most appropriate scale for the patient. Infant scales are used to weigh newborns and babies. Some scales can weigh heavier patients. When

BOX 33.3 Height Conversions

Convert Feet and Inches to Inches
Height equivalent: 1 feet (ft) = 12 inch (in)
  Multiply the number of feet by 12 and add the inches.

Example
  A patient's height is 6 ft 3 in. Convert the height to inches.
  Step 1: (Convert the feet to inches.) 6 x 12 = 72 in
  Step 2: (Add the remaining inches.) 72 + 3 = 75 in
  Answer: The patient is 75 inches.

Convert Inches to Feet and Inches
Height equivalent: 12 inch (in) = 1 feet (ft)
  Divide the number of inches by 12. Calculate the remaining inches, multiply the feet by inches, and subtract the inches from the total inches.

Example
  A patient's height is 52 in. Convert the height to feet and inches.
  Step 1: (Convert the inches to feet.) 52 ÷ 12 = 4 ft
  Step 2: (Calculate the remaining inches.) 4 x 12 = 48 inches
  Step 3: (Calculate the remaining inches.) 52 − 48 = 4 inches
  Answer: The patient is 4 feet 4 inches.

Convert Inches to Centimeters
Height equivalent: 1 inch (in) = 2.54 centimeter (cm)
  (If the height is in feet and inches, convert the height to inches, following the above steps.) Multiply the number of inches by 2.54. Round the answer to the nearest tenth.

Example
  A patient's height is 67 in. Convert the height to centimeters.
  Step 1: (Calculate the number of centimeters.) 67 x 2.54 = 170.18 cm
  Step 2: (Round to the nearest tenth.) 170.18 = 170.2 cm
  Answer: The patient is 170.2 cm.

Convert Centimeters to Inches
Height equivalent: 1 inch (in) = 2.54 centimeter (cm)
  Divide the number of centimeters by 2.54. Round the answer to the nearest tenth.

Example
  A patient's height is 100 cm. Convert the height to inches.
  Step 1: (Calculate the number of inches.) 100 ÷ 2.54 = 39.37 in
  Step 2: (Round to the nearest tenth.) 39.37 in = 39.4 in
  Answer: The patient is 39.4 in.

BOX 33.4 Weight Conversions

To Convert Kilograms to Pounds
Weight equivalent: 1 kg = 2.2 lb
  Multiply the number of kilograms by 2.2. Round the number to the nearest tenth.

Example
  A patient weighs 68 kg.
  68 × 2.2 = 149.6 lb

To Convert Pounds to Kilograms
1 kg = 2.2 lb
  Divide the number of pounds by 2.2 kg. Round the answer to the nearest tenth.

Example
  A patient weighs 120 lb.
  120 ÷ 2.2 = 54.5 kg

BOX 33.5 Body Mass Index (BMI)

The provider may ask the medical assistant to calculate the patient's BMI. The BMI is the relationship of weight to height that mathematically correlates the patient's measurements with health risks. It is a more accurate predictor of weight-related diseases than traditional height-weight charts because it provides a good estimate of the degree of body fat. The table below shows the correlation between a patient's BMI and the risks for disease.

To calculate the BMI, use this formula: $(lb) ÷ (inches)^2 × 703 = BMI$. (*Tip:* If your calculator does not have the square function, divide the weight by height twice and then multiple the answer by 703. For example, if the weight is 40 lbs and the height was 36 inches, you would punch the following into your calculator: 40 ÷ 36 ÷ 36 × 703 = 21.7 [BMI].

Body Mass Index	Classification	Disease Risk
≤18.5	Underweight	Low
18.5–24.9	Normal weight	Low
25–29.9	Overweight	Increased
30–34.9	Obese	High
35–39.9	Obese	Very high
≥40	Extremely obese	Extremely high

CRITICAL THINKING 33.9

Calculate these weights and round your answers to the nearest tenth.
  1. A patient weighs 87 kg. Convert the weight to lb.
  2. A patient weighs 148 lb. Convert the weight to kg.
  3. A patient is 84 lb. Convert the weight to kg.
  4. A patient is 26 kg. Convert the weight to lb.

CRITICAL THINKING 33.8

Convert these heights and round your answers to the nearest tenth.
  1. A patient is 6 feet 1 inch tall. Convert the height to cm.
  2. A patient is 162.5 cm tall. Convert the height to inches.
  3. A patient is 64 inches tall. Convert the height to feet and inches.
  4. A patient is 63 cm tall. Convert the height to inches.

- *Flat scales or scales built into the floor*: Patients with mobility limitations do not need to step up onto the scale. The scale is flat with the floor.
- *Wheelchair scale*: Patients can be weighed while in their wheelchair. The wheelchair weight will need to be deducted from the total to find the patient's weight.

Certain medical specialties and specific medical problems may require continuous monitoring of weight. Hormone disorders (e.g., diabetes), growth patterns (seen in children), and eating disorders (e.g., obesity, bulimia) require accurate weight

patients have mobility limitations, safety is important. Having the patient hold onto another person or an assistive device (e.g., walker) while on the scale can impact the accuracy of the weight. Scales that can be used for mobility limitations include:
- *Handrail scale*: Patients can use the side handrails to stabilize themselves while getting an accurate weight.

checks as part of every medical visit. In addition, pregnant patients must have their weight monitored to make sure they are gaining weight appropriately while watching for too much weight gain, which may indicate fluid retention. Patients with cardiovascular disorders who tend to retain fluid should have their weight checked each time they are seen in the office. Many healthcare facilities document weight in kilograms, but most Americans understand the pound measurements better (Box 33.4).

If the provider prescribes weight measurement at home, make sure the patient understands the importance of getting weighed at the same time each day in clothing of similar weight. Body weight may vary considerably from early morning to late afternoon, so it is usually best if the patient is weighed in the morning. If it is important that the patient be weighed each day, make sure you remind the patient to document each weight and notify the clinic as directed if there are major shifts.

Body Mass Index

Many providers use the BMI (Box 33.5) to determine the risk for certain diseases, so the medical assistant may have to use the accurately measured height and weight to determine and record the patient's BMI. This is typically done using a BMI chart that converts the patient's height and weight ratio into a BMI number, or with a wheeled device that calibrates the BMI when the height and weight intersect. BMI numbers also can be determined using an online conversion calculator. Electronic health record (EHR) systems automatically calculate and document the patient's BMI after the height and weight measurements are entered.

CRITICAL THINKING 33.10

Mrs. Johnson is being seen at WMFM Clinic for the first time. In what order should Carlos take her vital signs and her anthropometric measurements? Should blood pressure be measured in both arms, with the patient both sitting and standing? If so, what is the rationale?

CLOSING COMMENTS

Taking accurate vital signs and anthropometric measurements is an important aspect of a medical assistant's responsibilities. These measurements give the provider a strong indication of the patient's overall health. Being confident in the process of obtaining these measurements is crucial. Taking vital signs will become second nature over time, but a medical assistant must always take care to be as accurate as possible. It is also important to remember that our patients may be concerned about those measurements. Practicing empathy and using good listening skills are also part of being a good medical assistant.

PATIENT-CENTERED CARE

Measuring and documenting vital signs and anthropometric measurements are crucial parts of the medical assistant's responsibilities. We must keep in mind that the results can cause patients anxiety and concern. For example, if you have patients who are struggling to maintain a healthy blood pressure, it is important that you are sensitive to their concerns. If you have patients who are having difficulty maintaining or losing weight, they can be quite apprehensive, embarrassed, or even depressed about weight results. Being aware of patients' concerns about vital signs and anthropometric measurements and showing sensitivity to their needs are part of being a medical assistant.

BEING PROFESSIONAL

Vital signs and anthropometric measurements are used by the healthcare provider to make determinations about the patient's health and treatment decisions. It is essential that these measurements are taken carefully, accurately, and completely. If you are ever uncertain of a specific measurement, it should be repeated. If there is still a question about the measurement, ask another medical assistant to also check the vital sign in question to verify your readings. Always remember to pass along abnormal and concerning readings to the provider as soon as possible.

Role-play this scenario with a peer. You are the student, and your peer plays Carlos. You are working as a medical assistant student at WMFM Clinic, and your mentor is Carlos. Truong Tran is a young adult male who is being seen in the office today. When you take Truong's vitals, you are surprised to find his blood pressure and pulse are quite high. Carlos asks you to have the patient sit for a few minutes and then recheck the BP and pulse. You do as Carlos indicates and find that they are still high. However, as a student you are not yet confident in your ability to be accurate in all of your readings. You are nervous because this reading is so unexpected. Explain the situation and ask your peer to recheck Truong's vital signs.

CHAPTER REVIEW

A medical assistant should be familiar with the different sites for taking a temperature and the different thermometers used. Using the correct site and thermometer will ensure that a proper temperature is obtained.

Pulse and respiration are often measured at the same time. This way patients are unaware that you are watching them breathe. Until you are proficient at taking a radial pulse, it should be counted for a full minute. An apical pulse is done using a stethoscope. You will hear two sounds, lub dub. Each lub dub is one heartbeat.

When you take a blood pressure, it is important to use the correct-size cuff and have it positioned correctly over the brachial artery. By taking a palpated systolic blood pressure first, you can be certain that you do not miss the first Korotkoff sounds.

Pulse oximetry is often done when there is question about the blood's ability to transport enough oxygen. A finger or earlobe can be used for this procedure. If a finger is used, it should be free of fingernail polish.

Weight and height are anthropometric measurements that are typically taken at a healthcare facility. Weight is usually taken at every visit. Height is usually measured annually for adults, unless the patient has a specific medical condition. These measurements should be taken in a private location for the comfort of the patient. Accurate weight and height measurements are crucial for an accurate BMI calculation. Many providers use the BMI to counsel patients about lifestyle changes.

SCENARIO WRAP-UP

Carlos recognizes the significance of measuring and documenting each patient's vital signs and anthropometric measurements. The providers at WMFM Clinic rely on Carlos to provide this information accurately. Carlos has never let these procedures become routine. He is always focused on the task because vital signs are an important reflection of a person's health status.

Carlos knows that a number of factors can alter a patient's vital signs, including the external environment, smoking, drinking hot beverages, exercise, anxiety, and pain. Carlos evaluates patient factors such as age, sex, level of compliance, and the presence of disease to determine the best method of accurately measuring vital signs. In addition, Carlos is sensitive to the need for safeguarding the patient's privacy. When he was first hired by WMFM, he was concerned about privacy and confidentiality when he discovered that the patient scale was in the hall next to the waiting room. After he discussed this with the office manager, the scale was moved to an examination room so that patients could be weighed in privacy.

Carlos attended a workshop last year on the AHA guidelines for the diagnosis and treatment of hypertension, and he is prepared to explain those recommendations to patients. He recognizes his role in motivating patients diagnosed with prehypertension to stick with recommended lifestyle changes and follow the provider's treatment protocol.

PROCEDURE 33.1 Obtain an Oral Temperature Using a Digital Thermometer

Tasks
Accurately obtain a patient's oral temperature using a digital thermometer and document the reading in the patient's health record.

Equipment and Supplies
- Patient's health record
- Digital thermometer and a probe cover
- Biohazardous waste container

Procedural Steps
1. Wash hands or use hand sanitizer.
   Purpose: To ensure infection control.
2. Assemble the needed equipment and supplies.
3. Greet the patient. Identify yourself. Verify the patient's identity with full name and date of birth. Explain the procedure to be performed in a manner that the patient understands. Answer any questions the patient may have about the procedure.
   Purpose: Identification of the patient prevents errors, and explanations are a means of gaining implied consent and patient cooperation.
4. Make sure the patient has not eaten, consumed any hot or cold fluids, smoked (including vaping), or exercised during the 15 minutes before the temperature is measured.
   Purpose: The temperature will be inaccurate if hot or cold food or fluids have been consumed. Chewing also increases the temperature in the mouth, which can cause a false high recording. Smoking or vaping also is known to increase oral temperature. Exercise can temporarily increase all temperatures, and the medical assistant should wait 15 minutes after strenuous physical exercise before taking any temperature.
5. Apply the probe cover to the probe (Fig. 1).
   Purpose: To ensure infection control.

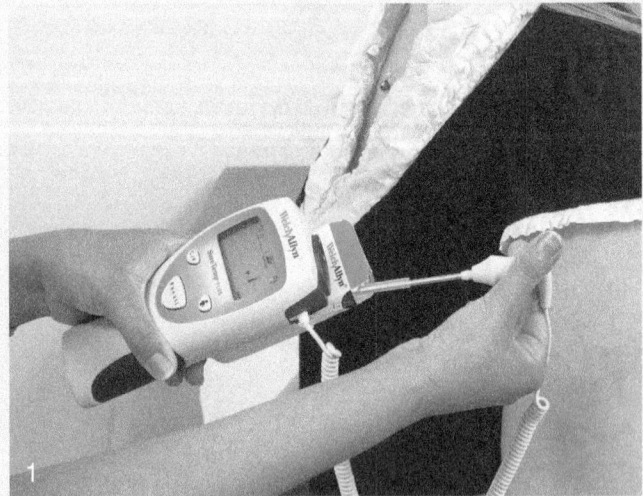

6. Place the probe under the patient's tongue (Fig. 2) and instruct the patient to close the mouth tightly without biting down on the thermometer. Help the patient by holding the probe end, or the patient can hold the probe end if that is more comfortable.
   Purpose: Air seeping into the mouth interferes with an accurate body temperature reading.

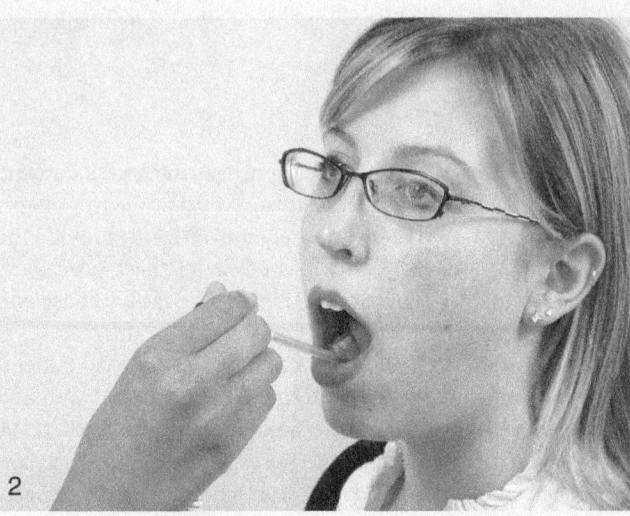

7. When a beep is heard, remove the probe from the patient's mouth and immediately eject the probe cover into an appropriate biohazardous waste container.
   Purpose: The probe cover is contaminated and must be discarded in a biohazardous waste container. This should be done immediately to reduce any chance of cross-contamination.
8. Accurately note the reading on the display screen of the thermometer.
9. Wash hands or use hand sanitizer. Disinfect the equipment as indicated.
   Purpose: To observe infection control measures and Standard Precautions.
10. Accurately document the reading in the patient's health record.
    Purpose: Procedures that are not documented are considered not done.
    6/28/20XX 10:05 a.m. T: 98.6°F _____ C. Ricci, CMA (AAMA)

PROCEDURE 33.2 Obtain an Axillary Temperature Using a Digital Thermometer

Tasks

Accurately obtain a patient's axillary temperature using a digital thermometer and document the reading in the patient's health record.

Equipment and Supplies

- Patient's health record
- Digital thermometer and a probe cover
- Supply of tissues
- Patient gown (optional)
- Waste container

Procedural Steps

1. Wash hands or use hand sanitizer.
   Purpose: To ensure infection control.
2. Gather the needed equipment and supplies.
3. Greet the patient. Identify yourself. Verify the patient's identity with full name and date of birth. Explain the procedure to be performed in a manner that the patient understands. Answer any questions the patient may have about the procedure.
   Purpose: Identification of the patient prevents errors, and explanations are a means of gaining implied consent and patient cooperation.
4. Apply a probe cover to the probe.
5. Expose the axillary region. If necessary, provide the patient with a gown for privacy.
6. Pat the patient's axillary area dry with tissues if needed.
   Purpose: To ensure an accurate reading. Do not rub the area because this may cause an elevated reading.
7. Place the probe tip into the center of the armpit, making sure the thermometer is touching only skin, not clothing.
   Purpose: To obtain the most accurate axillary reading; contact with clothing alters the reading.

8. Instruct the patient to hold the arm snugly across the chest or abdomen until the thermometer beeps (Fig. 1).
   Purpose: To prevent air from leaking in and interfering with the temperature reading.

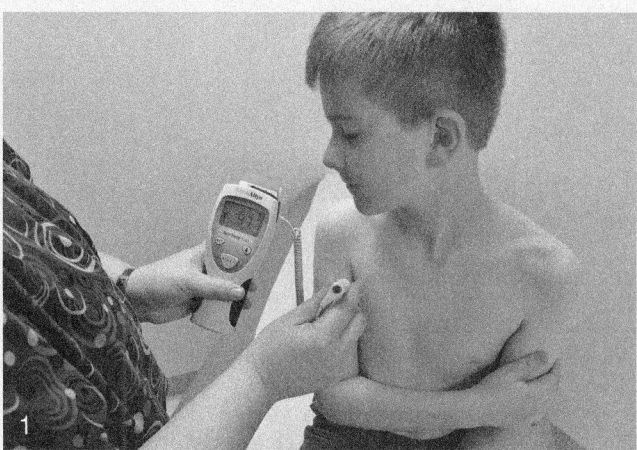

9. Remove the thermometer probe from the axillary area and accurately note the digital reading.
10. Dispose of the probe cover in the waste container. Disinfect the thermometer if indicated.
    Purpose: To ensure infection control.
11. Wash hands or use hand sanitizer.
12. Accurately document the reading in the patient's health record.
    Purpose: Procedures that are not recorded are considered not done.
    Note: When documenting axillary temperatures, most facilities either document "axillary" or write a circled "A" behind the temperature.
    6/29/20XX 10:05 a.m. T: 98.2°F (Axillary)————C. Ricci, CMA (AAMA)

PROCEDURE 33.3 Obtain a Rectal Temperature in an Infant Using a Digital Thermometer

Tasks

To obtain an infant's rectal temperature using a digital thermometer and document the reading in the patient's health record.

Equipment and Supplies

- Patient's health record
- Digital thermometer with red probe and a probe cover
- Water soluble lubricant (KY jelly)
- 2 x 2 gauze (optional)
- Gloves
- Biohazardous waste container
- Waste container
- Tissue

Procedural Steps

1. Wash hands or use hand sanitizer.
   Purpose: To ensure infection control.
2. Assemble the needed equipment and supplies. Make sure that the red probe is used.
3. Greet the patient's parent or caregiver. Identify yourself. Verify the patient's identity with full name and date of birth. Explain the procedure to be performed in a manner that the patient's parent or caregiver understands. Answer any questions about the procedure.
   Purpose: Identification of the patient prevents errors, and explanations are a means of gaining implied consent and cooperation.

4. Instruct the parent or caregiver undress the infant.
5. Put on gloves.
   Purpose: To ensure infection control.
6. Apply the probe cover to the probe. If using a tube of water-soluble lubricant, apply a small amount to the gauze. Lubricate the first two inches of probe with water-soluble lubricant.
   Purpose: To ensure infection control.
7. Gently insert the thermometer probe ½ inch for infants. Hold the child's legs still while holding the thermometer in place until a beep is heard.
8. Remove the probe. Note the reading on the display screen of the thermometer.
9. Eject the probe cover into a biohazardous waste container. Using the tissue, wipe any lubricant from the rectal area. Discard tissue in the biohazard waste container.
   Purpose: The probe cover is contaminated and must be discarded in a biohazardous waste container.
10. Remove the gloves and discard them into an appropriate waste container.
11. Wash hands or use hand sanitizer and disinfect the equipment as indicated.
    Purpose: To observe infection control measures and Standard Precautions.
12. Document the reading in the patient's health record.
    Purpose: Procedures that are not documented are considered not done.
    Note: When documenting rectal temperatures, most facilities either document "rectal" or write a circled "R" behind the temperature.
    6/29/20XX 2:10 p.m. T: 100.7°F (Rectal)_____C. Ricci, CMA (AAMA)

PROCEDURE 33.4 Obtain a Temperature Using a Tympanic Thermometer

Tasks

Accurately obtain a patient's temperature using a tympanic thermometer and document the reading in the patient's health record.

Equipment and Supplies

- Patient's health record
- Tympanic thermometer and a probe cover
- Alcohol wipes (optional)
- Waste container

Procedural Steps

1. Wash hands or use hand sanitizer.
   Purpose: To ensure infection control.
2. Gather the necessary equipment and supplies.
3. Greet the patient. Identify yourself. Verify the patient's identity with full name and date of birth. Explain the procedure to be performed in a manner that the patient understands. Answer any questions the patient may have about the procedure.
   Purpose: Identification of the patient prevents errors, and explanations are a means of gaining implied consent and patient cooperation.
4. Clean the probe lens with an alcohol wipe if indicated. Place a disposable cover on the probe (Fig. 1).
   Purpose: To ensure a clean surface and prevent cross-contamination.

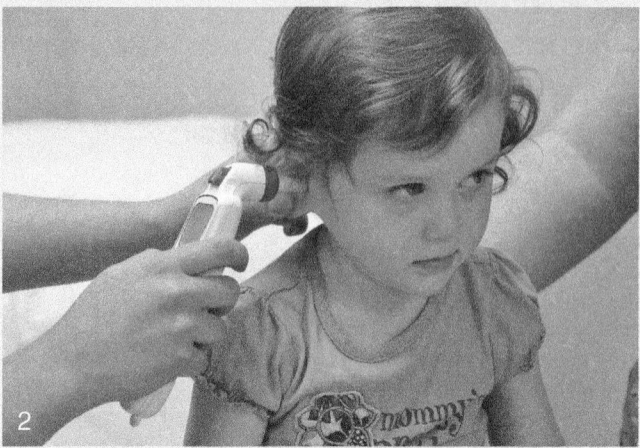

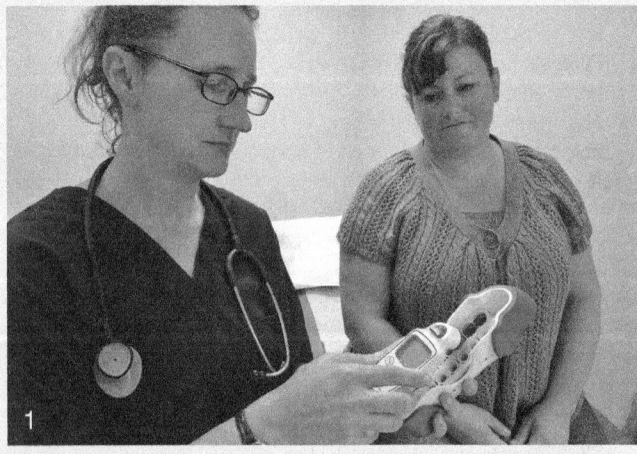

5. Insert the probe into the ear canal far enough to seal the opening. Do not apply pressure. For children younger than age 3, gently pull the earlobe down and back (Fig. 2); for patients older than age 3, gently pull the top of the ear (pinna) up and back (Fig. 3).
   Purpose: The external ear must be pulled gently to open the external auditory canal and expose the tympanic membrane for an accurate reading.

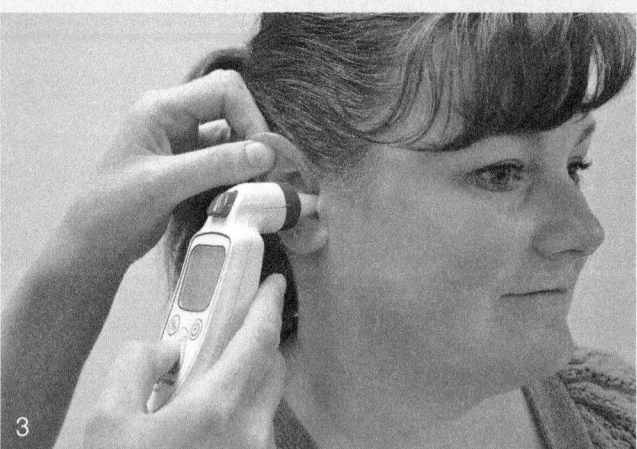

6. Press the button on the probe as directed. The temperature will appear on the display screen in 1 to 2 seconds.
7. Remove the probe, accurately note the reading, and discard the probe cover into a waste container without touching it.
   Purpose: The probe cover is contaminated and must be discarded in a waste container.
8. Wash hands or use hand sanitizer. Disinfect the equipment and clean the probe lens if indicated.
   Purpose: To ensure infection control. See the manufacturer's manual for cleaning the probe tip. Many recommend cleaning the probe lens with alcohol wipes.
9. Accurately document the reading in the patient's health record
   Purpose: Procedures that are not recorded are considered not done.
   Note: When documenting tympanic temperatures, most facilities either document "tympanic" or indicate the ear used, such as "left ear," after the temperature.
   7/11/20xx 2:20 p.m. T: 101.2°F (Tympanic) ————C. Ricci, CMA (AAMA)

PROCEDURE 33.5   Obtain a Temperature Using a Temporal Artery Thermometer

Tasks

Accurately obtain a patient's temperature using a temporal artery thermometer and document the reading in the patient's health record.

Equipment and Supplies

- Patient's health record
- Professional temporal artery thermometer
- Probe cover (if indicated by facility's policy)
- Alcohol wipes (optional)
- Waste container

Procedural Steps

1. Wash hands or use hand sanitizer.
   Purpose: To ensure infection control.
2. Gather the necessary equipment and supplies.
3. Greet the patient. Identify yourself. Verify the patient's identity with full name and date of birth. Explain the procedure to be performed in a manner that the patient understands. Answer any questions the patient may have about the procedure.
   Purpose: Identification of the patient prevents errors, and explanations are a means of gaining implied consent and patient cooperation.
4. Remove the protective cap on the probe. Depending on the facility's infection control procedures, disposable covers can be used on the scanner, or it can be cleaned by lightly wiping the surface with an alcohol wipe.
   Purpose: To ensure infection control.
5. Push the patient's hair up off the forehead to expose the site. Gently place the probe on the patient's forehead, halfway between the edge of the eyebrows and the hairline, at the center of the face (just above the nose).
   Purpose: This places the probe directly over the temporal artery.
6. Depress and hold the SCAN button, and lightly glide the probe sideways across the patient's forehead to the hairline just above the ear (Fig. 1). As you move the sensor across the forehead, you will hear a beep and a red light will flash
   Purpose: This verifies that the scanner is recording temperatures as it moves across the surface of the temporal artery.

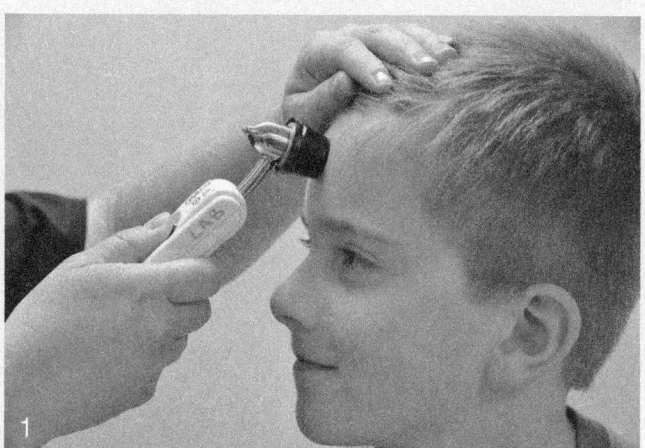

7. Keeping the button depressed, lift the thermometer, and place the probe behind the earlobe (Fig. 2). The thermometer may continue to beep, indicating that the temperature is rising.
   Purpose: To continue scanning of the temporal artery until the highest temperature is recorded on the thermometer.

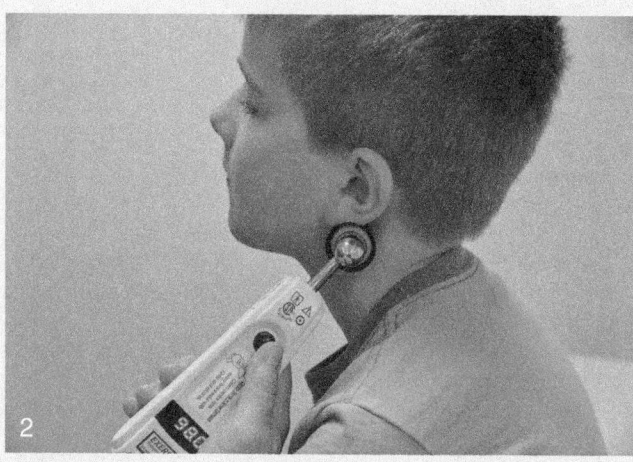

8. When scanning is complete, release the button and lift the probe. Accurately note the temperature recorded on the digital display.
   Note: The scanner automatically turns off 15 to 30 seconds after release of the button.
9. If a probe cover was used, eject it directly into a waste container. Disinfect the thermometer if indicated and replace the protective cap.
   Purpose: To ensure infection control. Depending on the facility's infection control procedures, disposable covers can be used on the scanner, or it can be cleaned between patients with a disinfectant wipe.
10. Wash hands or use hand sanitizer.
11. Accurately document the reading in the patient's health record.
    Purpose: Procedures that are not recorded are considered not done.
    Note: When documenting temporal artery temperatures, most facilities use (TA) after the temperature.
    8/1/20XX 11:20 a.m. T: 101.6°F (TA) ————————C. Ricci, CMA (AAMA)

PROCEDURE 33.6   Obtain a Temperature Using a Noncontact Infrared Thermometer

Tasks
Accurately obtain a patient's temperature using a non-contact infrared thermometer and document the reading in the patient's health record.

Equipment and Supplies
- Patient's health record
- Healthcare professional noncontact infrared thermometer
- Alcohol wipes

Procedural Steps
1. Wash hands or use hand sanitizer.
   Purpose: To ensure infection control.
2. Gather the necessary equipment and supplies.
3. Greet the patient. Identify yourself. Verify the patient's identity with full name and date of birth. Explain the procedure to be performed in a manner that the patient understands. Answer any questions the patient may have about the procedure.
   Purpose: Identification of the patient prevents errors, and explanations are a means of gaining implied consent and patient cooperation.
4. Push the patient's hair up off the forehead to expose the site. Hold the probe close to the forehead without touching (generally about 6 to 12 inches away; follow the guidelines for the specific model of thermometer being used). Aim the probe halfway between the edge of the eyebrows and the hairline, at the center of the face (just above the nose).
   Purpose: This places the probe directly over the temporal artery.
5. Depress and hold the SCAN button and hold until the unit beeps and displays the temperature.
   Purpose: Holding the thermometer in place until the read is complete will ensure a more accurate reading.
6. When scanning is complete, release the button and lift the probe. Accurately note the temperature recorded on the digital display. The scanner automatically turns off 15 to 30 seconds after release of the button. Following the facility's policies, use alcohol or other disinfectant to clean the unit
   Purpose: To ensure infection control. Even though the unit does not touch the patient, it can be exposed to droplet transmitted pathogens. It is important to ensure that the unit is cleaned between each use.
7. Wash hands or use hand sanitizer.
8. Accurately document the reading in the patient's health record.
   Purpose: Procedures that are not recorded are considered not done.
   Note: When documenting infrared temperatures, most facilities use "(infrared)" after the temperature.
   8/1/20XX 11:20 a.m. T: 101.6°F (Infrared)————————C. Ricci, CMA (AAMA)

PROCEDURE 33.7   Obtain an Apical Pulse

Tasks
Accurately determine and record the patient's apical heart rate.

Equipment and Supplies
- Patient's health record
- Watch with a second hand
- Patient gown (optional)
- Stethoscope
- Alcohol wipes

Procedural Steps
1. Wash hands or use hand sanitizer. Clean the stethoscope earpieces and diaphragm with alcohol wipes.
   Purpose: To ensure infection control and to follow Standard Precautions.
2. Greet the patient. Identify yourself. Verify the patient's identity with full name and date of birth. Explain the procedure to be performed in a manner that the patient understands. Answer any questions the patient may have about the procedure.
   Purpose: Identification of the patient prevents errors, and explanations are a means of gaining implied consent and patient cooperation.
3. If necessary, assist the patient in disrobing from the waist up and provide the patient with a gown that opens in the front. Assist the patient into the sitting or supine position.
   Purpose: To expose the chest and provide privacy and warmth. Position allows for easier access to the apical site at the apex of the heart.
4. Hold the stethoscope's diaphragm against the palm of your hand for a few seconds.
   Purpose: To warm the diaphragm, promoting patient comfort.
5. Place the stethoscope at the left midclavicular line at the fifth intercostal space over the apex of the heart (Figs. 1 and 2). Do not touch the bell end of the stethoscope.
   Purpose: This is the point of maximum contractile strength, where the heartbeat can be heard best. Touching the bell end of the stethoscope may interfere with the sound.

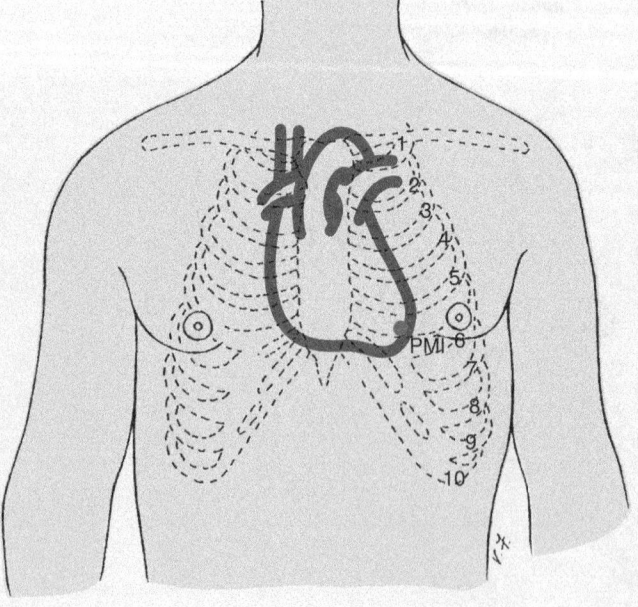

1

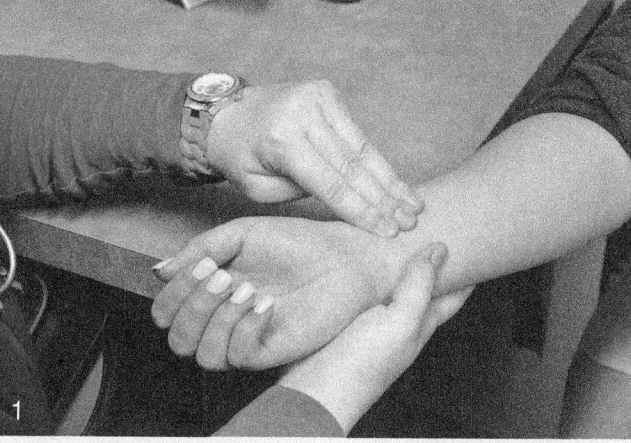

6. Listen carefully for the heartbeat. Accurately count the pulse for 1 full minute. Note any irregularities in rhythm and volume.
   Purpose: The apical pulse is always measured for 1 full minute to obtain the most accurate reading.
7. Help the patient to sit up and dress.
8. Disinfect the stethoscope with an alcohol wipe.
   Purpose: To ensure infection control.
9. Wash hands or use hand sanitizer.
10. Accurately document the reading in the patient's heart record.
    Purpose: Procedures that are not recorded are considered not done.
    Note: When documenting the apical pulse, most facilities will indicate "AP" followed by the rate and rhythm.
    3/3/20XX 4:10 p.m. AP: 93 irregular————————C. Ricci, CMA (AAMA)

PROCEDURE 33.8   **Assess the Patient's Radial Pulse and Respiratory Rate**

Tasks

Accurately determine and document a patient's radial pulse rate, rhythm, and volume and respiratory rate, rhythm, and depth.

Note: Respirations should be assessed immediately after the radial pulse while the medical assistant is appearing to take the pulse, so the patient does not artificially alter breathing patterns.

Equipment and Supplies

- Patient's health record
- Watch with a second hand

Procedural Steps

1. Wash hands or use hand sanitizer.
   Purpose: To ensure infection control.
2. Greet the patient. Identify yourself. Verify the patient's identity with full name and date of birth. Explain the procedure to be performed in a manner that the patient understands. Answer any questions the patient may have about the procedure.
   Purpose: Identification of the patient prevents errors, and explanations are a means of gaining implied consent and patient cooperation.
3. Place the patient's arm in a relaxed position, palm at or below the level of the heart.
   Purpose: The patient's radial artery is more easily palpated when the patient is relaxed and in this position.
4. Gently grasp the palm side of the patient's wrist with your first two or three fingertips approximately 1 inch below the base of the thumb (Fig. 1).
   Purpose: This position puts your fingertips directly over the radial artery. Press firmly (but do not press too hard, or you will occlude the artery and feel nothing).

5. Accurately count the beats for 1 full minute using a watch with a second hand or if indicated by the instructor, count for 30 seconds and multiply by 2.
   Purpose: Counting for 1 full minute allows you to obtain an accurate count, including any irregularities in rhythm and volume. Once you become more adept at taking a pulse, you can reduce this to 30 seconds and multiply that number by 2 to record the patient's heart rate.
6. While counting the beats, also assess the rhythm and volume of the patient's pulse.
7. While continuing to hold the patient's arm in the same position used to count the radial pulse, observe the rise and fall of the patient's chest (see Fig. 33.13). If you have difficulty noticing the patient's breathing, place the arm across the chest to detect movement.
   Purpose: The respiratory count may be altered if the patient is aware that you are counting their breaths; placing the arm across the chest allows you to feel or see the rise and fall of the chest wall.
8. Inhalation and exhalation make up one complete breathing cycle or respiration. Accurately count the respirations for 30 seconds and multiply by 2.
   Purpose: Counting for 30 seconds allows you to obtain an accurate count and determine any irregularities in rhythm or depth or unusual breathing patterns. If respirations are abnormal in any way, count for 1 full minute.
9. While counting, also assess the rhythm and depth of the patient's respirations.
10. Release the patient's wrist.
11. Wash hands or use hand sanitizer.
    Purpose: To ensure infection control.
12. Accurately document the readings in the patient's health record.
    Purpose: Procedures that are not recorded are considered not done.
    5/6/20XX 8:35 a.m. P: 72 regular, 1+ ; R: 18, regular, normal ———————————————————————C. Ricci, CMA (AAMA)

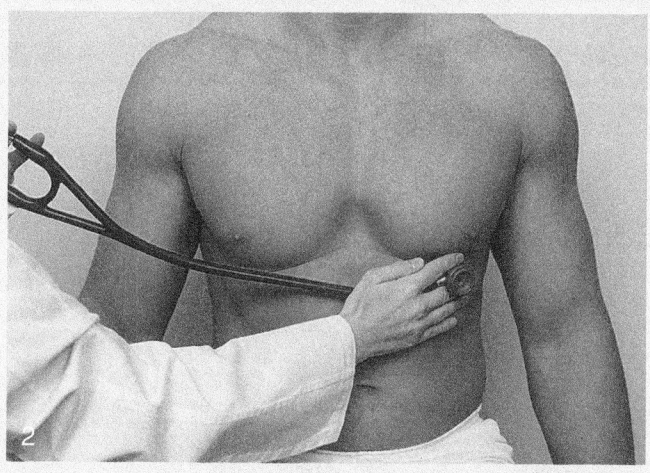

PROCEDURE 33.9   Determine a Patient's Blood Pressure

Tasks

Accurately perform and record a blood pressure measurement that is correct in technique, accurate, and comfortable for the patient.

Equipment and Supplies

- Patient's health record
- Sphygmomanometer
- Stethoscope
- Alcohol wipes

Procedural Steps

1. Wash hands or use hand sanitizer.
   Purpose: To ensure infection control.
2. Assemble the equipment and supplies needed. Clean the earpieces and diaphragm of the stethoscope with alcohol wipes.
   Purpose: For infection control and to follow Standard Precautions.
3. Greet the patient. Identify yourself. Verify the patient's identity with full name and date of birth. Explain the procedure to be performed in a manner that the patient understands. Answer any questions the patient may have about the procedure.
   Purpose: Identification of the patient prevents errors, and explanations are a means of gaining implied consent and patient cooperation.
4. Select the appropriate arm for application of the cuff (no mastectomy on that side, no injury or disease).
   Purpose: The pressure of the cuff temporarily interferes with circulation to the limb. *Caution:* If a female patient has had a mastectomy, the blood pressure should never be taken on the affected side. Compressing the arm may cause complications. If she has had a bilateral mastectomy, another site, such as the popliteal artery, must be used, which requires use of a thigh cuff.
5. Seat the patient in a comfortable position with the back and legs supported. Legs should be uncrossed. The arm should be supported by a table, so the cuff will be at heart level. The palm should be facing up.
   Purpose: To expose the brachial artery; also, to promote patient relaxation and ensure a true reading. Crossed legs may increase the blood pressure, and positioning of the arm above heart level may cause an inaccurate reading.
6. Roll the sleeve to about 5 inches above the elbow, or have the patient remove the arm from the sleeve.
   Purpose: Tight clothing prevents an accurate reading.
7. Select the correct cuff size.
   Purpose: An incorrect cuff size prevents accurate measurement of blood pressure. The cuff should fit comfortably around the patient's arm, and the bladder should be located over the brachial artery between the lines designated on the cuff. Pediatric, normal adult, and large adult cuff sizes should be available. Thigh cuffs may be needed for obese patients.
8. Palpate the brachial artery at the antecubital space in both arms. If one arm has a stronger pulse, use that arm. If the pulses are equal, select the right arm.
   Purpose: A stronger pulse is easier to measure; the right arm is the universal arm of choice.
9. Center the cuff bladder over the brachial artery with the connecting tube away from the patient's body and the tube to the bulb close to the body (Fig. 1).
   Purpose: Pressure must be applied directly over the artery for an accurate reading. The cuff and its tubing should not touch the stethoscope. Noise from the tubing can interfere with a correct reading.

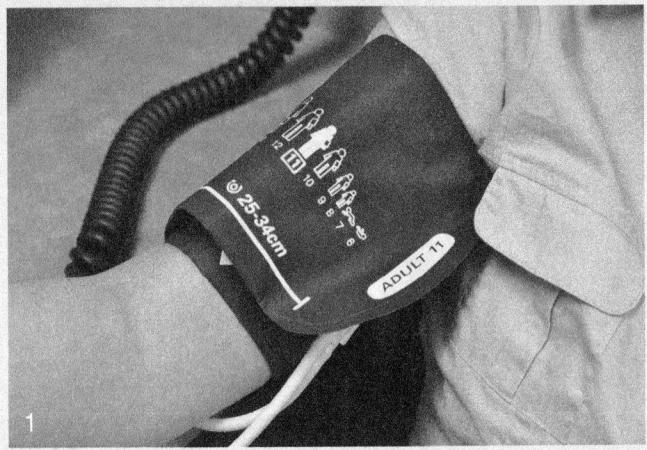

10. Place the lower edge of the cuff about 1 inch above the palpable brachial pulse, normally located in the natural crease of the inner elbow and wrap it snugly and smoothly.
    Purpose: To help ensure an accurate reading. The cuff should be high enough on the arm that the stethoscope does not touch it and so that cuff sounds do not interfere with listening to the blood pressure sounds. A loose cuff results in an inaccurate reading.
11. Position the gauge of the sphygmomanometer so that it is easily seen.
    Purpose: An aneroid gauge should show the needle within the zero mark.
12. Palpate the radial pulse, tighten the screw valve on the air pump, and inflate the cuff until the pulse can no longer be felt. Inflate an additional 30 mm Hg and then deflate the cuff. Note the reading when the pulse can be felt. Deflate the cuff. Wait 1 to 2 minutes before taking the BP.
    Purpose: The point where the radial pulse is no longer felt provides an estimate of the systolic pressure. Pumping the cuff above that level ensures that phase I of the Korotkoff sounds will be heard.
13. Insert the earpieces of the stethoscope turned forward into the ear canals.
    Purpose: With the earpieces in this position, the openings follow the anatomic line of the ear canal and the blood pressure will be accurately heard.
14. Place the stethoscope's diaphragm over the palpated brachial artery for an adult patient or the bell for a pediatric patient. Press firmly enough to obtain a seal but not so tightly that the artery is constricted. Only touch the edges of the stethoscope head.
    Purpose: Forming a seal around the head of the stethoscope aids listening for blood pressure sounds. Placing your fingers directly over the stethoscope head will cause interference with the sound.
15. Close the valve and squeeze the bulb to inflate the cuff, rapidly but smoothly, to 30 mm above the palpated systolic level, which was previously determined (Fig. 2).

Continued

PROCEDURE 33.9 Determine a Patient's Blood Pressure—cont'd

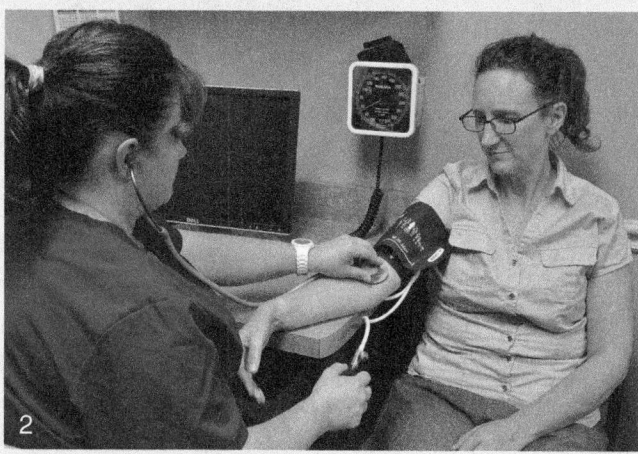

2

16. Open the valve slightly and deflate the cuff at a constant rate of 2 mm Hg per second.
Purpose: Careful, slow release allows you to listen to all sounds.

17. Listen throughout the entire deflation; accurately note the point on the gauge at which you hear the first sound (systolic), the last sound (diastolic), and until the sounds have stopped for at least 10 mm Hg.

18. Do not reinflate the cuff once the air has been released. Wait 1-2 minutes to repeat the procedure if needed.
Purpose: Not allowing the blood to refill in the brachial artery results in inaccurate readings.

19. Remove the cuff from the patient's arm.

20. Remove the stethoscope from your ears. If needed, write down the reading and arm to reference when documenting.

21. Clean the earpieces and the head of the stethoscope with an alcohol wipe and return both the cuff and the stethoscope to storage.

22. Wash hands or use hand sanitizer.
Purpose: To ensure infection control.

23. Accurately document the readings in the patient's health record. Include the reading, the arm, the person's position, and the cuff size used.
Purpose: Procedures that are not recorded are considered not done.
3/7/20XX 4:25 p.m. BP 126/66 left arm, sitting (adult cuff)————————————————————————————————C. Ricci, CMA (AAMA)

PROCEDURE 33.10 Determine a Patient's Orthostatic Vital Signs

Tasks
Perform orthostatic vital signs and document in the patient's health record.

Equipment and Supplies
- Patient's health record
- Sphygmomanometer
- Stethoscope
- Watch with a second hand
- Alcohol wipes
- Exam table

Procedural Steps
1. Wash hands or use hand sanitizer.
Purpose: To ensure infection control.

2. Assemble the equipment and supplies needed. Clean the earpieces and diaphragm of the stethoscope with alcohol wipes.
Purpose: For infection control and to follow Standard Precautions.

3. Greet the patient. Identify yourself. Verify the patient's identity with full name and date of birth. Explain the procedure to be performed in a manner that the patient understands. Answer any questions the patient may have about the procedure.
Purpose: Identification of the patient prevents errors, and explanations are a means of gaining implied consent and patient cooperation.

4. Help the patient lie comfortably in a supine position on the examination table. Pull out the table extender, if necessary, for them to rest their feet. Allow the patient to rest in this position for 5 minutes.
Purpose: Allowing the patient to rest before beginning will allow their blood pressure to come to baseline for this position.

5. Take the patient's pulse and blood pressure (as indicated in Procedures 33.8 and 33.9) with the patient lying down. Do not remove the cuff from the arm.
Purpose: Allowing the cuff to stay on the arm will allow the same arm to be used in additional measurements without having to put it on and take it off the arm.

6. Help the patient into a sitting position and ask the patient if they are experiencing any dizziness, weakness, or visual changes with the position change. Watch for any change in skin coloring or in the patient's behavior.

Purpose: This identifies any symptoms of hypotension the patient may be experiencing.

7. Once the patient has been sitting for 1 minute, repeat the pulse and blood pressure.
Purpose: This will provide blood pressure readings in the new position.
Note: If the patient has symptoms associated with the position change or if the sitting blood pressure is less than 90 systolic and/or 60 diastolic, have the patient lay back down and immediately notify the provider.

8. Assist the patient to stand. Ask the patient about dizziness, weakness, or visual changes associated with the position change. Note any change in the patient's appearance or behavior.

9. Immediately repeat the blood pressure and pulse readings after the patient has stood up.
Purpose: A quick change in positioning with an immediate read of BP and pulse will indicate if the patient is experiencing orthostatic hypotension.

10. Ask the patient to continue standing and repeat the pulse and blood pressure measurements after 3 minutes.
Purpose: BP and pulse readings that return to normal after the patient has stood for a few minutes indicate a different problem than if the readings stay low (or high).

11. Clean the earpieces and the head of the stethoscope with an alcohol wipe and return both the cuff and the stethoscope to storage.

12. Wash hands or use hand sanitizer.
Purpose: To ensure infection control.

13. Clearly document each blood pressure and pulse reading along with the position and any symptoms the patient experienced in the patient's health record.
Purpose: Documenting the reading along with the position and symptoms experienced will allow the provider to make connections in positional BP/P and make diagnostic and treatment decisions.
3/9/20XX 2:20 p.m. (Lying) BP 120/72 right arm, (adult cuff); P: 68 regular, 1+. (Sitting 1 min) BP 116/ 64; P: 84 regular, 1+. (Standing, initial VS) BP 110/58; P: 96 regular, 1+. (Standing 3 min) BP 112/66; P: 88 regular, 1+. Had dizziness initially after standing that resolved within 1 min. Pt resting on the exam table. Dr. Walden notified.————————————C. Ricci, CMA (AAMA)

PROCEDURE 33.11   Perform Pulse Oximetry

Tasks

Accurately assess the oxygen saturation in the blood using a pulse oximeter.

Equipment and Supplies

- Patient's health record
- Pulse oximeter and probe of the appropriate size

Procedural Steps

1. Wash hands or use hand sanitizer. Assemble the equipment.
   Purpose: Standard Precautions must be followed to prevent the spread of disease.
2. Greet the patient. Identify yourself. Verify the patient's identity with full name and date of birth. Explain the procedure to be performed in a manner that the patient understands. Answer any questions the patient may have about the procedure.
   Purpose: An informed patient is more cooperative.
3. Turn on the monitor and attach the probe to the finger (preferred). Fingernail should be free of artificial nail and polish. If the finger cannot be used, use the ear lobe, and apply sensor so it is flush with the skin.

4. The light-emitting diode (LED) should be placed on top of the nail. If the patient is wearing nail polish or has artificial nails, these may have to be removed to get a strong pulse signal. Accurately note the reading.
   Purpose: To measure the pulse and oxygen saturation level.
5. Sanitize the patient probe and the external portion of the monitor with an aseptic cleaner.
   Purpose: To follow Standard Precautions.
6. Wash hands or use hand sanitizer.
   Purpose: To ensure infection control.
7. Accurately document the oxygen saturation (SpO_2) percentage and pulse in the patient's health record. Include the date and time; if the patient is receiving supplemental oxygen, record the amount in liters.
   Purpose: Procedures that are not documented are considered not done.
   4/7/20XX 1:25 p.m. SpO_2 96% on room air. P: 76_____C. Ricci, CMA (AAMA)

PROCEDURE 33.12   Measuring a Patient's Weight and Height

Tasks

Accurately weigh and measure a patient's height. Document the measurements in the patient's health record.
Note: Make sure the scale is located in an area away from traffic to maintain the patient's privacy.

Equipment and Supplies

- Patient's health record
- Balance beam scale with a measuring bar
- Paper towel

Procedural Steps

1. Wash hands or use hand sanitizer.
   Purpose: To ensure infection control.
2. Greet the patient. Identify yourself. Verify the patient's identity with full name and date of birth. Explain the procedure to be performed in a manner that the patient understands. Answer any questions the patient may have about the procedure.
   Purpose: Identification of the patient prevents errors, and explanations are a means of gaining implied consent and patient cooperation.
3. Have the patient remove shoes. Place a paper towel on the scale platform. Check to see that the balance bar pointer floats in the middle of the balance frame when all weights are at zero.
   Purpose: A floating pointer indicates that the scale is properly adjusted and in balance.
4. Make sure the patient has removed any heavy objects from pockets and removed a jacket if wearing one. Make sure the patient is not holding anything, such as a jacket or purse. Help the patient onto the scale as needed.
5. Move the large weight into the groove closest to the patient's estimated weight. The grooves are calibrated in 50-lb increments. If you choose a groove that is more than the patient's weight, the pointer will immediately tilt to the bottom of the balance frame. You then must move it back one groove (Fig. 1).

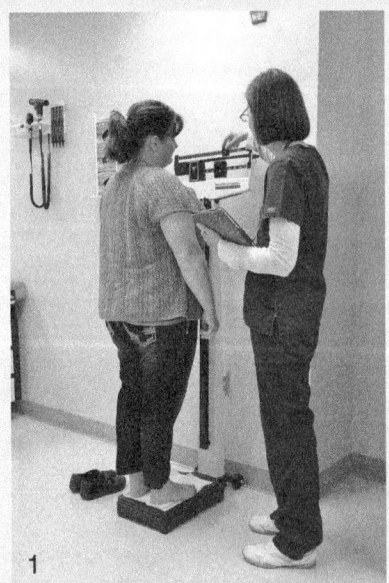

1

6. While the patient is standing still, slide the small upper weight to the right along the pound markers until the pointer balances in the middle of the balance frame.
   Purpose: The pointer floats between the bottom and the top of the frame when both lower and upper weights together balance the scale with the patient's weight.
7. Leave the weights in place.
8. Ask the patient to step off the scale and move the height bar to a point above the patient's height. Extend the bar and ask the patient step back on the scale. On some scales, the patient may need to turn with their back to the scale.
9. Adjust the height bar so that it just touches the top of the patient's head (Fig. 2).

Continued

PROCEDURE 33.12 **Measuring a Patient's Weight and Height—cont'd**

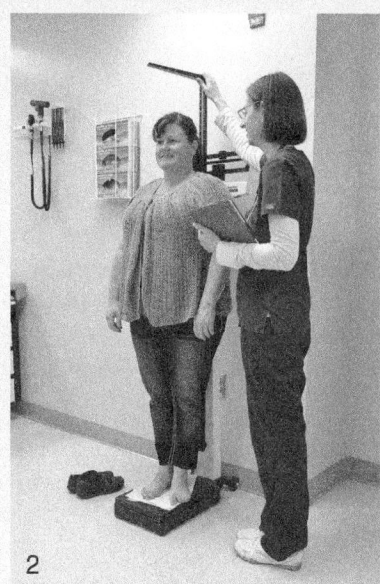

13. Accurately read the height. Read the marker at the movable point of the ruler and document the measurement to the nearest quarter of an inch on the patient's health record (e.g., Ht: 5' 6.5") (Fig. 3).

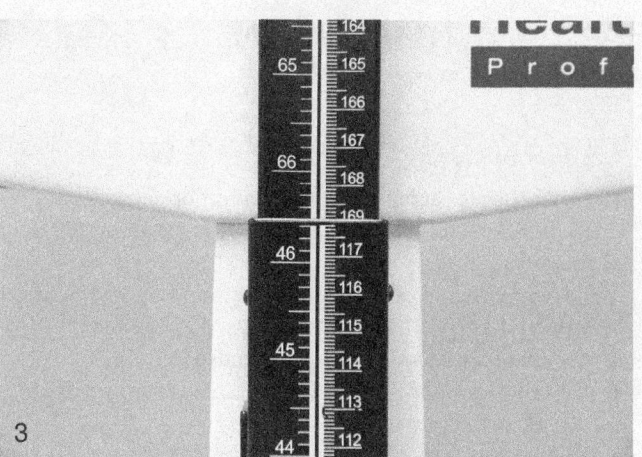

10. Leave the elevation bar set.
    Purpose: To maintain the height recording while protecting the patient from possible injury.
11. Assist the patient off the scale. Make sure all items that were removed for weighing are given back to the patient.
12. Accurately read the weight scale. Add the numbers at the markers of the large and small weights and document the total to the nearest quarter of a pound in the patient's health record (e.g., Wt: 136.5 lb).

14. Use the patient's weight and height to determine the body mass index (BMI).
15. Return the weights and the measuring bar to zero.
16. Remove the paper towel and dispose of in the waste container. Wash hands or use hand sanitizer.
17. Accurately document the results in the patient's health record. Use the patient's weight and height to determine the BMI if the EHR program does not do it automatically.

5/26/20XX 11:07 a.m. Wt: 136.5 lb, Ht: 5'6.5"; BMI 21.7————————
————————————————————————C. Ricci, CMA (AAMA)

34

Patient Interview

LEARNING OBJECTIVES

1. Demonstrate therapeutic communication feedback techniques to obtain information when gathering a patient history.
2. Respond to nonverbal communication when interacting with patients.
3. Compare open-ended and close-ended questions.
4. Describe how a medical assistant can show sensitivity to diverse patient groups.
5. Discuss how a medical assistant should prepare for a patient interview.
6. Identify barriers to communication and their impact on the patient interaction.
7. Detect a patient's use of defense mechanisms and the resultant barriers to therapeutic communication.
8. Describe information found in each components of the medical history.
9. List questions that can be asked to obtain a concise description of the patient's symptoms.
10. Differentiate between a sign and a symptom and list examples of each.
11. Explain documentation guidelines.
12. Define common abbreviations used in healthcare.

OUTLINE

▶▶ OPENING SCENARIO

Chris Isaacson, CMA (AAMA), works for Walden-Martin Family Medical (WMFM) Clinic. He is responsible for initial patient interviews, taking medical histories, and documentation. Chris struggles with gathering the information needed from some patients. They do not always respond openly and honestly. Chris wonders what he can do to help his patients feel more comfortable and willing to open up and share the necessary information.

YOU WILL LEARN

1. To use therapeutic communication techniques when obtaining a patient's medical history.
2. To recognize nonverbal communication.
3. To recognize communication barriers.
4. Questions to ask to obtain information for all components of the medical history.
5. To document a patient's medical history following established guidelines.

INTRODUCTION

Medical assistants are directly involved in gathering information from patients about their health. Good healthcare needs to focus on the total patient, not only on a disease process. This holistic (hoh LIS tik) perspective includes finding out about all areas of patients' lives that can affect their health, which includes not only physical health, but also mental, emotional, environmental, and spiritual health. Because of this the assessment process should reflect the entire patient, not just a report about signs and symptoms. Individual lifestyles and environmental factors can be complicating factors or may even be the cause of disease. All aspects of a patient's health should be considered when information is gathered about the patient's chief complaint. For example, if a patient smokes or works in a stressful occupation, they may be more prone to hypertension. Health professionals should consider all patient factors when gathering information about the patient's health status. Holistic patient care recognizes that illness is the result of many factors, not just physical ones.

VOCABULARY

chief complaint A statement in the patient's own words that describes the reason for the visit.

clarification Gathering additional information to make a concept or idea easier to understand.

holistic Considering the patient as a whole; includes the physical, emotional, social, economic, and spiritual needs of the person.

Patient care begins when the patient first contacts the office. The medical assistant has the opportunity to interact with patients to ensure that they feel comfortable during the process and that all of the necessary information is obtained.

Interviewing patients and preparing documentation are important responsibilities for a medical assistant. You must know the components of a medical history and the techniques for interviewing patients. These will gather important information to help the provider diagnose and treat the patient. The more complete the medical history, the better able the provider will be to treat the patient.

THERAPEUTIC COMMUNICATION

To provide high-quality patient care, we must communicate effectively with the patient and provide a warm, caring environment. Positive interactions with the patient are vital. A medical assistant must always remember that each patient is an individual with certain anxieties. These anxieties often cause people to act and react in different ways; therefore effective verbal and nonverbal communication with each patient is essential.

It is the responsibility of the healthcare professionals to lead in developing a healthy relationship with their patients. The interpersonal nature of the patient–medical assistant relationship means that the focus should be on the patient's needs. Medical assistants can bring out either a positive or a negative response simply by the way they treat and interact with patients.

The medical assistant is usually the first person with whom the patient communicates, and because of this, you play a vital role in therapeutic patient interactions (Procedure 34.1).

A key component to building a trusting relationship with patients is good communication. Communication is an interactive process involving the sender of the message, the receiver, and feedback. At any given time, the roles of the sender and receiver change or overlap. Feedback lets us know that the receiver got the message and how they interpreted it. This completes the communication cycle by providing a means for us to know exactly what message the patient received and whether it requires clarification (KLAR uh fa kay shuh n).

For example, as a medical assistant, one of your responsibilities will be to provide patient education on how to prepare for diagnostic studies. Let's say you have to explain to an older adult patient how to prepare for a colonoscopy. You provide a detailed explanation of the preparation procedure and a handout explaining the step-by-step process. How do you really know whether the patient understands? You ask the patient to provide feedback by explaining the process back to you. As a member of the healthcare team, you must become an effective communicator. You will play a vital role in collecting and documenting patient information. If your methods of communication are faulty, the quality of patient care may be seriously impaired.

Active Listening

Hearing is a physical act. Someone speaks, and we hear what the person has said. Listening is much more than this. It includes making sure that we understand what is being communicated. Active listening is when we take an active role in the communication even when we are not acting as the communicator. This includes making efforts to concentrate on what is being said and striving to understand what is being communicated.

Listening is not a passive role in the communication process; it is active and demanding. For the duration of the patient interview, no one is more important than this particular patient. Helpful listening guidelines include:

- Listen to the main points in the discussion.
- Listen to the way things are said and the tone of the patient's voice.
- Respond to both verbal and nonverbal messages.
- Be patient and nonjudgmental.
- Do not interrupt.
- Never intimidate your patient.
- Do not be preoccupied with other things.

Therapeutic Communication Techniques

Active listening involves using therapeutic communication techniques. These techniques encourage patients to expand on and clarify the content and meaning of their messages. Therapeutic communication techniques are very useful tools when a patient is agitated or upset. They can also be used to help clarify the important details of the chief complaint. Table 34.1 describes common therapeutic communication techniques

TABLE 34.1	**Active Listening Techniques**	
Process	**Description**	**Value**
Restatement	Paraphrasing or repeating the patient's statements with phrases such as, "My understanding of what you are saying is..." or "You are telling me the problem is..."	Checks your interpretation of the patient's message for validation. Helps the patient know that you understand the meaning of what is being said. Allows the opportunity for additional information to be shared.
Reflection	Repeating the main idea of the conversation while also identifying the sender's feelings. For example, if the mother of a young patient is expressing frustration about her child's behavior, a reflective statement identifies that feeling with the response, "It sounds like you are frustrated about..."	Shows the patient your acknowledgment of their feelings
Clarification	Clarification seeks to summarize or simplify the sender's thoughts and feelings and to resolve any confusion in the message. Questions or statements that begin with "Give me an example of..." or "Explain to me about..." or "So what you're saying is..." are good examples of clarification.	Clarification statements help patients focus on the message and give the medical assistant the opportunity to clear up any misconceptions.
Silence	Allows time to gather thoughts and answer questions	Nonverbally communicates your acceptance of the patient and a willingness to wait until the patient is ready to answer
Acknowledgment	Recognizes the patient's importance in the patient-medical assistant relationship	Shows the importance of the patient's role and respect for autonomy
Summarizing	Provides an opportunity for the listener to recap and review what was said	Helps the patient separate relevant from irrelevant material; provides clarity to the interview
Establishing guidelines	Shares the goals of what will occur	Informs the patient of what to expect during the interview

that are used during the patient interview process. (See Chapter 17 for additional information on therapeutic communication.)

Nonverbal Communication

When people think of communication, they normally think of speaking with each other. However, there is so much more to communication than what we express verbally. Experts say that more than 90% of communication is nonverbal. Much of what we communicate to our patients is conveyed through the use of body language. Our nonverbal actions, such as gestures, facial expressions, and mannerisms, are learned behaviors that are greatly influenced by our family and cultural backgrounds. It is important to remember while conducing patient interviews that nonverbal communication can seriously affect the therapeutic process.

Commonly nonverbal communication is unintentional and instinctive. Even small changes in our gestures and stance can make a big impression on those we are communicating with. Just as with verbal communication, nonverbal communication can relay both positive and negative messages. Most of the negative messages communicated through body language are unintentional.

The body language naturally expresses our feelings. Carefully observing nonverbal communication can help the medical assistant be aware of the patient's feelings. This enables you to adapt your behavior to these feelings. You can deliberately select your response, either verbal or nonverbal, to have a favorable effect on others. By being aware of nonverbal communication from our patients, we can be more aware of their individual needs. We can provide emotional support, defuse fear or anger, and better convey we care. By being aware of patients' nonverbal communication, we can provide an

opportunity for patients to release pent-up feelings and create an open environment to discuss their feelings. Table 34.2 lists some nonverbal behaviors by patients that may indicate anxiety, frustration, or fear.

> **CRITICAL THINKING 34.1**
>
> List nonverbal behaviors that you have when you are bored, angry, happy, and frustrated. List nonverbal behaviors you have observed in others for these four feelings.

The Medical Assistant's Nonverbal Behaviors. Your tone of voice can put a patient at ease. Your facial expression and the ease and confidence of your movements demonstrate a sincere interest to the patient. Therapeutic use of space and touch are also important ways of sending nonverbal messages to your patients. You should establish eye contact if culturally appropriate, sit in a relaxed but attentive position, and avoid using furniture as a barrier between you and the patient. Give the patient your undivided attention and let your body language inform each patient that you are interested in their medical problems (Fig. 34.1 and Procedure 34.2).

The key to successful patient interaction is congruence (kuh n GROO uh ns) between verbal and nonverbal messages. In order to be seen as honest and sensitive to the needs of your patients, you must be aware of your nonverbal behavior patterns. The nonverbal message the patient receives from the medical assistant's listening behavior should be "You are a person of worth, and I am interested in you as a unique individual."

Nonverbal behavior – your body language – can have either a positive or a negative effect on patient interactions. Positive nonverbal behaviors enhance the patient's experience in the

TABLE 34.2 Observations of Nonverbal Communication in Patients

Area	Observation	Indication
Breathing patterns	Rapid respirations, sighing, shallow thoracic breathing	Anxiety, boredom, pain
Eye patterns	No eye contact, side-to-side movement, looking down at the hands	Anxiety, distrust, embarrassment
Hands	Tapping fingers, cracking knuckles, continuous movement, sweaty palms	Anxiety, worry, fear
Arm placement	Folded across chest, wrapped around abdomen	Anxiety, worry, fear, pain
Leg placement	Tension, crossed or tucked under, tapping foot, continuous movement	Frustration, anger

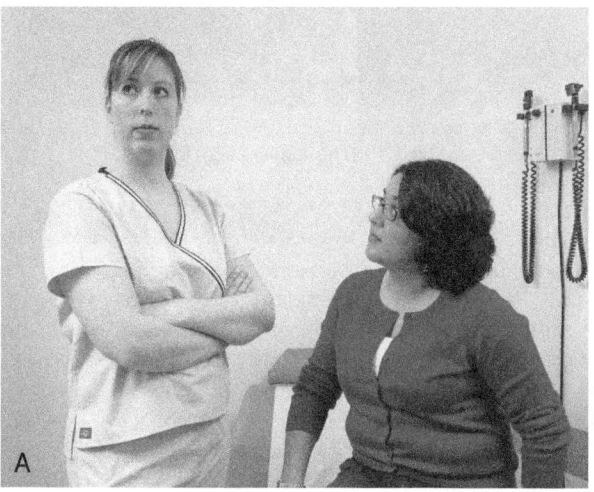 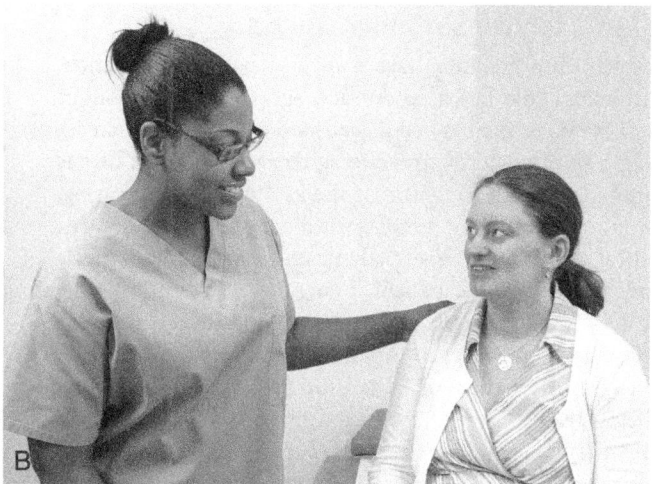

Fig. 34.1 A, Ineffective nonverbal language. B, Therapeutic nonverbal language. (From Niedzwiecki B, et al: *Kinn's the medical assistant,* ed 14, St. Louis, 2020, Elsevier.)

healthcare setting. Communication experts recommend these measures:

- When gathering a health history, lean toward the patient to show interest.
- Face the patient squarely and at eye level to make the process more comfortable and to demonstrate sensitivity and empathy.
- Eye contact, if culturally appropriate, is essential for therapeutic communication unless the patient is from a culture that discourages this.
- Do not use a closed posture, such as crossing your arms or legs, since that indicates disinterest.
- Be sensitive to the patient's personal space when possible. Maintain a comfortable distance from the patient, at least an arm's length, when conducting the interview.
- Be careful with body gestures, such as hand and arm movements. Gestures such as nodding your head when the patient talks can display interest, but too much body movement can be distracting.
- Your tone of voice should reflect your interest in the patient. Speaking too quietly or too loudly can detract from therapeutic communication.
- Continually observe the patient's body language during the interview; watch for signs of confusion, boredom, worry, and so on so that you can respond appropriately.
- Documenting in an electronic health record (EHR) can be distracting to both the medical assistant and the patient.

Remind yourself to look at the patient frequently and use encouraging body language to maintain a personal interaction.

> **VOCABULARY**
> **congruence** Agreement; the state that occurs when the verbal expression of the message matches the sender's nonverbal body language.

Closed and Open-Ended Questions

Sometimes, when interviewing patients, we are looking for very specific information. Other times we need the patient to feel free to share whatever they feel they need to share. Depending on the information we are looking for, we will use either closed or open-ended questions.

Closed questions, also called *direct questions,* are used to gather specific information. This type of question limits the response to one or two words. Often the response is yes or no. Use this form of question when you need confirmation of specific facts. Here are some examples:

- "Do you have a headache?"
- "What is your birth date?"
- "Have you ever broken a bone?"

Open-ended questions or statements are used to gather more general information. They can be used when trying to understand something from the patient's perspective. An open-ended question requires more than a simple one- or two-word answer.

This type of question or statement encourages patients to respond in a manner they find comfortable. It allows patients to express themselves fully and provide comprehensive information. Open-ended questioning is an effective method of gathering more details about the chief complaint or health history. Consider these examples:

- "What brings you to the doctor?"
- "How have you been getting along?"
- "You mentioned having dizzy spells. Tell me more about that."

Sensitivity to Diverse Patient Groups

Most healthcare facilities have a diverse patient population. The diversity could be based on race, age, culture, religion, or physical qualities, such as being deaf/hard of hearing. Whatever the origin of the diversity, practicing respectful patient care is extremely important. Empathy is the key to creating a caring, therapeutic environment. Empathy is different from sympathy. A medical assistant who is empathetic understands and respects the individuality of the patient. Being empathetic means the medical assistant attempts to see the patient's health problem through that person's eyes. An empathetic medical assistant can recognize the effect of all holistic factors on the patient's well-being.

Empathetic sensitivity to diversity requires you to examine your own values, beliefs, and actions. You cannot treat all patients with care and respect until you first recognize and evaluate personal biases. We think and act a certain way for many reasons. The first step in understanding the process is to evaluate your individual value system. Why do you have certain attitudes or beliefs about the worth of individuals or things?

Many factors influence the development of a value system. Value systems begin as learned beliefs and behaviors. Families and cultural influences shape the way we respond to a diverse society. Other factors that influence reactions include socioeconomic and educational backgrounds. To develop therapeutic relationships, you must recognize your own value system to determine whether it could affect how you interact with patients. Preconceived ideas about people because of their age, race, religion, income level, ethnic origin, sexual orientation, or gender can act as barriers to the development of a therapeutic relationship. You cannot treat your patients empathetically unless you can connect with them in some way. Personal biases or prejudices are huge barriers to the development of therapeutic relationships (Fig. 34.2).

Box 34.1 presents strategies for working with diverse patient populations.

> **VOCABULARY**
> **empathy** The ability to understand another's perspective, experiences, or motivations.
> **rapport** A relationship of harmony and accord between the patient and the healthcare professional.
> **sympathy** Feeling sorrow or concern for what the other person has gone through.

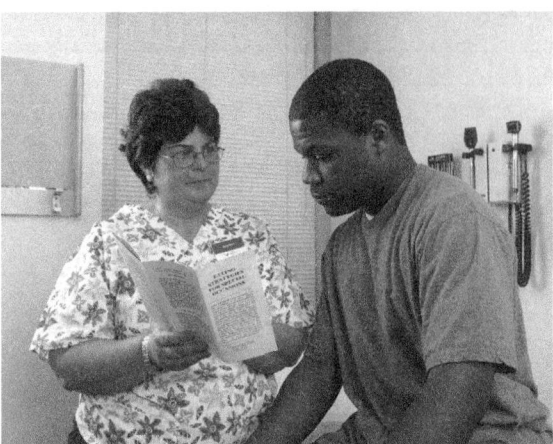

Fig. 34.2 Respectful Patient Care. (From Niedzwiecki B, et al: *Kinn's the medical assistant,* ed 14, St. Louis, 2020, Elsevier.)

> **CRITICAL THINKING 34.2**
>
> Honestly evaluate your personal biases. What do you find unacceptable in people? Do you prejudge an individual based on their affiliation with a particular group or because of a certain lifestyle decision? Do these biases create barriers to the development of therapeutic relationships? If so, how can you get beyond these barriers?
>
> Consider the following scenarios, and discuss them with your classmates:
> - While you are conducting a patient interview, the patient informs you that he has tested positive for the human immunodeficiency virus (HIV). Do you think this will affect your therapeutic relationship?
> - You are responsible for recording an in-depth interview on a homeless person with very poor hygiene. Will this cause a problem with your professional manner?
> - Your office manager tells you that an inmate of the county prison is being brought in this afternoon for an examination. Do you think his status will affect your interaction with the patient?
> - You are attempting to interview a 20-year-old patient who brought her two young children with her to the office today. She is a single mother who is pregnant with her third child and receives public assistance. What do you think? Will you have difficulty being empathetic?

INTERVIEWING THE PATIENT

When the patient appointment begins, there is a time that is known as the *initial patient interview.* This interview is where the medical assistant gathers the patient's medical history and information regarding the reason for their visit. This is the first and most important part of the data collection that will take place during the visit. The medical history identifies the patient's health strengths and problems and is a bridge to the next step in data collection, the physical examination performed by the provider. At this point, patients know everything about their own health status and you know nothing. Your interview skills help collect the necessary information and build rapport (ra POHR) for a successful working relationship.

Consider the interview a type of contract between you and your patient. The contract consists of spoken and unspoken language and addresses what the patient needs and expects from the healthcare visit. The patient interview consists of three

BOX 34.1 Sensitivity to Diverse Patient Populations

Regardless of the type of healthcare facility you work in, you will care for a wide variety of patients. The medical assistant should take the initiative to learn about the cultures represented in the healthcare practice. Some points to consider about diverse groups include:

- Patients of Asian backgrounds may have been raised in a culture that considers it extremely rude to establish eye contact. Americans view an unwillingness to establish eye contact as a sign of distrust or embarrassment; however, for people from Japan or China, lack of eye contact may be a way of demonstrating respect.
- Personal space may be an issue for patients from diverse backgrounds. If a patient appears very uncomfortable with touch or lack of personal space, attempt to accommodate them as much as possible during the office visit.
- Research has shown that older people face unique communications problems in the healthcare environment. The healthcare facility should have tools available to help patients with hearing or vision issues. When caring for an aging individual, it is important to focus patient teaching and information on the patient, rather than the family member who may be present.
- Patients may use their religious beliefs and values to understand and cope with their health problems. Sometimes the beliefs may conflict with the provider's recommendations. Healthcare workers must remember to respect patients' religious beliefs and their rights to make their own decisions.

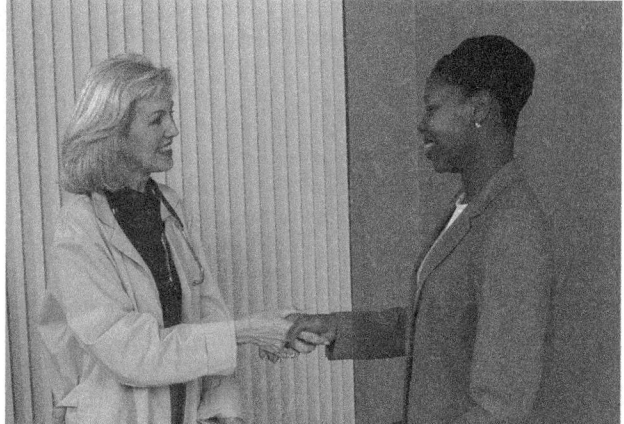

Fig. 34.3 Greeting the Patient. (From Niedzwiecki B, et al: *Kinn's the medical assistant,* ed 14, St. Louis, 2020, Elsevier.)

- The reason the patient is seeking healthcare (e.g., chief complaint)
- The patient's perception of the problem
- The characteristics of the problem
- The patient's medical history
  - During this time, use active listening skills and a combination of open-ended and closed statements and questions to gather the details of the patient's history and current health problem. During the interview, the medical assistant should:
  - *Take careful notes while focusing on the patient*: It is important to document the information from the patient, but your focus must remain on the patient. Focusing too much on documentation (e.g., on the computer screen) can diminish the patient's sense of importance and hinder therapeutic communication. The medical assistant should be familiar with the electronic health record (EHR) medical history templates used. This will help with efficiency and documentation, while yet allowing the medical assistant to focus on the patient.
  - *Share the documented information with the patient*: Patients can find it disturbing not knowing what is being documented in the health record. Newer exam room configurations are making it easier for patients to view computer screens or paper health records. Many facilities are encouraging healthcare professionals to share their documented information with patients. The sharing of information helps build trust between the patient and the healthcare team.

Conclude the interview by summarizing the results of your interaction. The closing of the interview should clarify the patient's chief complaint, the purpose of the visit, and the patient's expectations of care. This is the patient's opportunity to add any details or to explain further the characteristics of the health problem.

stages: the preparation and introduction, obtaining the information, and the closing.

Preparation and Introduction

When preparing for and completing a patient interview, the medical assistant should:

- *Ensure privacy and prevent interruptions*: Make sure the conversation is private. The door should be closed. The patient needs to feel sure that no one can overhear the conversation or interrupt. An interruption can destroy in seconds what you have spent many minutes building up.
- *Prepare comfortable surroundings*: Conducting the interview in comfortable surroundings reduces the patient's anxiety. Keep the distance between you and the patient at arm's length. Arrange chairs so that you and the patient are comfortably seated at eye level and the desk or table does not act as a barrier between you.
- *Greet, introduce yourself, verify the patient, and explain the purpose*: At the beginning of the interview, introduce yourself (Fig. 34.3). Verify the patient's identity to ensure you have the correct patient. Ask the patient's complete name and date of birth. Explain what you will be doing. For example: "Mr. Coleman, my name is Stacey, and I am a certified medical assistant who works with Dr. Perez. What is your full name and date of birth? I have some questions to ask you about your health history."

Obtaining the Information and the Closing

After the brief introduction, move on to the body of the interview, where the information is obtained. This is when you use various therapeutic communication techniques to determine:

Communication Barriers

Communication is rarely a straightforward process. Not only is it important to take into consideration verbal and nonverbal communication and cultural differences, but there are also many barriers that can come up that stop effective communication. The medical assistant must work to avoid or correct situations that can cause a breakdown in communication with the patient.

Providing Unwarranted Assurance. Mrs. Miller says to you, "I know this lump is going to turn out to be cancer." The typical reply is almost automatic: "Don't worry, I'm sure everything will be fine." This type of answer indicates that her anxiety is insignificant and denies her the opportunity to further discuss her fears. A reflective response, such as "You sound really worried about…" acknowledges her feelings and demonstrates empathy and a willingness to listen to her concerns.

Giving Advice. Mrs. Thompson has just finished talking to the doctor. She looks at you and says, "Dr. Rowe says I need surgery to get rid of these gallstones. I just don't know. What would you do?" If you tell her how you would handle the situation, you may have shifted the accountability for decision making from her to you. She has not worked out her own solution. Does this woman really want to know what you would do? Probably not. You could respond to her question by saying, "Based on what the doctor told you, what do you think you should do?" or "Do you need further information to make your decision?" If the patient continues to question the provider's recommendations, the medical assistant should encourage further discussion with the provider.

Using Medical Terminology. You must adjust your vocabulary to fit the patient. The more the patient understands about what is happening and how to manage the problem, the better the outcome. Misinterpreted communication is the most common error in patient care. One of the biggest problems for the patient is understanding medical terminology. Closely observe the patient's body language as they receive instructions or patient education. If the patient shows signs of not understanding the procedure, ask the patient to repeat back to you the information or instructions. This demonstration–return demonstration form of providing feedback ensures that the patient completely understands what is happening. It also gives the medical assistant the opportunity to clarify any misconceptions.

Leading Questions. During the interview, you ask the patient, "You don't smoke, do you?" By asking questions in this manner, you indicate the preferred answer. Telling you that they do smoke would surely meet with your disapproval. Keep your questions positive. A better way of asking would be, "Have you ever smoked?" or "Do you use tobacco?"

Talking Too Much. Some medical assistants associate helpfulness with verbal overload. The patient may let the interviewer talk at the expense of their own need to explain what is wrong. Always remember that when interviewing a patient, you should listen more than you talk. Pay close attention to the patient's body language to make sure you are giving the patient ample opportunity to discuss the health problem.

Defense Mechanisms. Many individuals respond to anxiety-provoking situations by automatically relying on defense mechanisms. Defense mechanisms are used consciously or unconsciously to block an emotionally painful experience. It is understandable that patients facing a traumatic diagnosis or a difficult treatment feel the need to protect themselves from the reality of the situation. Ensuring compliance with treatment becomes an issue if the patient is in denial, projecting feelings onto the healthcare worker, or repressing the need for treatment or diagnostic follow-up.

The medical assistant must be sensitive to patients' use of defense mechanisms. (See Chapter 17 for additional information on defense mechanisms.) Consistently applying therapeutic communication techniques to interactions with patients will help to overcome the defense mechanisms. For example, Mrs. Alicia Simone, a 48-year-old patient, has just been told she has breast cancer. The following are defense mechanisms she might display to protect herself from the psychological reality of her disease.

- *Denial*: The patient completely rejects the information. Example: "I couldn't possibly have breast cancer. You must be mistaken."
- *Suppression*: The patient is consciously aware of the information or feeling but refuses to admit it. Example: "I don't think the test is accurate. My mammograms are always normal."
- *Reaction formation*: The patient expresses her feelings as the opposite of what she really feels. Example: If she is angry at the medical assistant for insisting that a biopsy be scheduled, she may express the opposite emotion: "I appreciate your trying to help me, but I just can't come to the hospital that day."
- *Projection*: The patient accuses someone else of having the feelings that she has. Example: If the patient is angry about the diagnosis, she may say to the medical assistant, "You don't have to lose your temper about this," even though the medical assistant's demeanor is completely professional.

- *Rationalization*: The patient comes up with various explanations to justify her response. Example: "I think the results are wrong. I didn't follow the directions for the tests like I should have, and besides, there's no history of breast cancer in my family."
- *Undoing*: The patient tries to reverse a negative feeling by doing something that indicates the opposite feeling. Example: If the patient feels angry and violated about the diagnosis but she finds those feelings unacceptable, she may say, "Don't worry, dear, I'm not upset with you for telling me about this."
- *Regression*: The patient reverts to an old, usually immature behavior to vent her feelings. Example: Perhaps instead of discussing the diagnosis and the need for treatment, she just storms out of the office. Or she may say, "I can't possibly schedule a procedure without discussing this with my mother."
- *Sublimation*: The patient redirects her negative feelings into a socially productive activity. Example: Mrs. Simone eventually becomes an active member of a local support group for women recovering from breast cancer.

CRITICAL THINKING 34.4

Mr. Gonzales, a 48-year-old patient recently diagnosed with hypertension, did not show up today for his follow-up appointment. Chris calls to find out why he failed to keep the appointment, and the patient tells Chris he forgot to come, even though an appointment reminder call was made yesterday. He also tells Chris he has not been taking his medicine and does not understand why it is so important for him and his wife to meet with the dietitian. Is this patient using defense mechanisms? How should Chris respond? What communications skills might promote a therapeutic relationship?

MEDICAL HISTORY

Collecting the History Information

A new patient is asked to complete a health history form. This form is useful for diagnosing and treating the patient. This self-history also allows the patient to be more involved in the process. The form may be mailed to the patient's home before the appointment or may be completed in the office during the first visit. Some healthcare facilities use electronic forms. These can be emailed to the patient before the first appointment and incorporated into the patient's electronic health record (EHR) when the completed form is emailed back. The patient may also be able to complete the form online through a patient portal. If a paper form is used, it can be scanned into the patient's EHR after it is completed.

In some cases, the medical assistant may be asked to sit with a patient and complete the medical history form or a portion of the medical history. The medical assistant must:

- Conduct the interview in a private area, free of distractions and where others cannot overhear anything.
- Listen to the patient in a nonjudgmental manner.
- Document the information in an organized manner, exactly as given by the patient, without opinion or interpretation.

The provider will take the information gathered from the medical history and correlate (KAWR uh leyt) it with the physical findings from the examination. The complete medical history and the physical exam are the starting point for the provider to determine what the patient needs. These form the foundation for all patient-physician contacts. EHR systems help by incorporating the information gathered from the medical history and the physical examination directly into the health record (Fig. 34.4).

Components of the Medical History

The medical history is the foundation of a patient's health record. When interviewing a patient during the visit to the facility, a more complex medical history form is typically used. For subsequent visits, a simpler form is used. The following sections discuss the components of the medical history. Additional information about the components is also found in Chapter 21.

Demographics. The patient's demographics (dem uh GRAF iks) includes the patient's full name, address, contact information, occupation, and so on. The patient demographics are obtained on the patient's first visit. Usually, the administrative medical assistant will check with the patient for any changes to the demographics on subsequent visits.

VOCABULARY

correlate To establish an orderly relationship or connection.
demographics Statistical data of a population. In healthcare this includes the patient's name, address, date of birth, employment, and other details.

Past Medical History. A patient's past medical history (PMH) or past history (PH) is a summary of the patient's previous health prior to the visit. During a patient's initial visit to the facility, a comprehensive history is obtained. Subsequent visits will obtain any new information from the last visit. The past medical history includes the dates and details about:

- Previous illnesses/injuries, including usual childhood diseases [UCD], dental conditions (and last dental exam), and behavior health conditions
- Previous hospitalizations and surgeries.
- Medications and immunizations
- Allergies
- Gynecologic and obstetric history (for women)

CRITICAL THINKING 34.5

List two closed and open-ended questions or statements to obtain information about a patient's past medical history.

Immunization History. Some patients may bring an immunization record to the initial visit, but many do not. Many states have an immunization database that healthcare professionals can access to obtain a patient's past immunization history. When a vaccine is administered either by public health departments or by healthcare facilities, the immunization information is added to the state's immunization database. It is important to realize that the state's

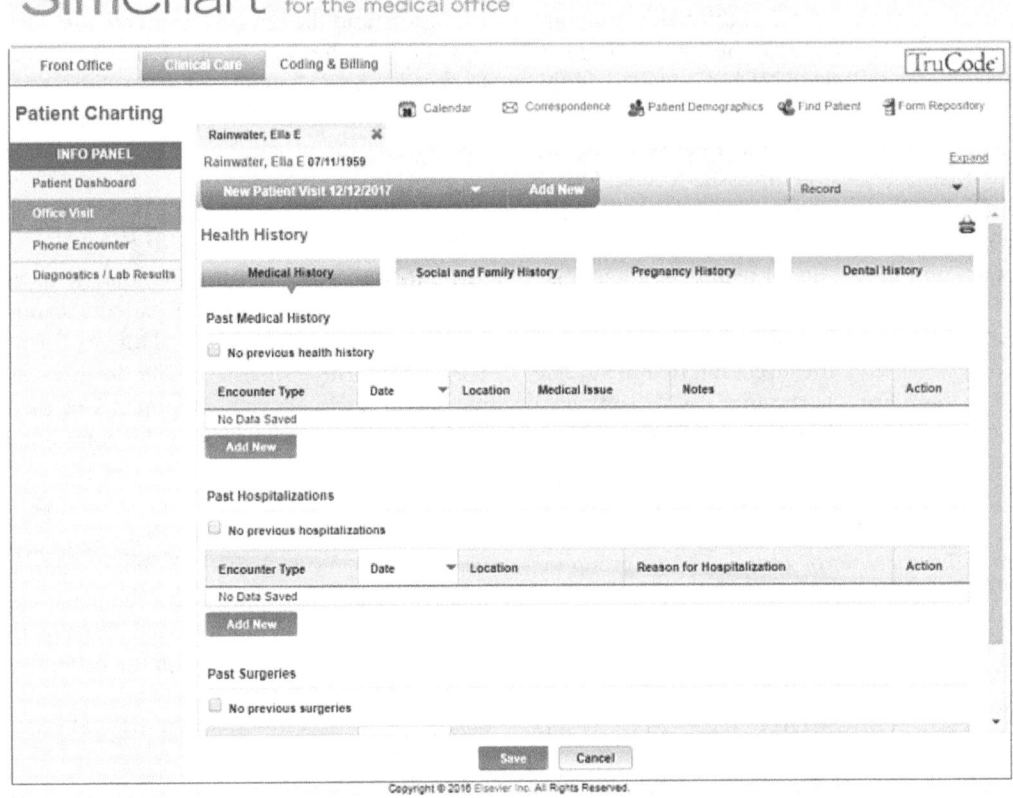

Fig. 34.4 Example of an Electronic Health Record (EHR) System.

database may not contain the patient's complete immunization history. Depending on the patient's age, if the patient lived in other states, and if facilities did not access the database, there can be gaps in the immunization history.

During an initial visit, the medical assistant may need to use the information in the state's database to update the facility's immunization record on the patient. During subsequent visits, the medical assistant might be required to review the immunization history and flag for the provider any vaccines that are due.

Allergy history. An allergy history contains a list of the patient's medication, food, and environmental allergies. The allergy list is frequently used when a provider is prescribing medications and vaccines or when a procedure will be done. Examples of food allergens that are found in medications and medical products include the following:

- *Egg*: Probiotics, some vaccines
- *Gelatin*: Several types of tablets, capsules, and suppositories in gelatin capsules; vaccines; gelfoam surgical sponges used to stop bleeding
- *Peanut oil*: Valproic acid, dimercaprol, and progesterone capsules
- *Milk proteins* (e.g., lactose, casein): Many tablets, capsules, granules, and powder forms; vaccines, probiotics, dry powder inhalers such as Diskus, Flexhaler, HandiHaler, and Turbuhaler
- *Soy*: Some metered-dose inhalers (MDIs), such as Combivent.
- *Food dyes*: Give color to tablets and liquids

When procedures are done that use products containing latex, the patient's allergy list is checked for such an allergy.

The allergy history is obtained during the initial visit. During each subsequent patient interaction, the allergy history must be reviewed and revised as needed. The electronic health record software will a field or checkbox that the medical assistant must complete after reviewing the allergy history during each visit.

Social and Occupational Histories. The social history (SH) includes information about the patient's personal habits and lifestyle. The SH includes living situation, marital status, diet, and sleep patterns. It also includes tobacco (e.g., cigarettes, chew, vaping), alcohol, and drug use. (See Chapter 21 for additional information.) Occupational history (OH) contains information on the person's employment. All these factors can have an impact on a patient's overall health and also help to highlight risk factors.

During the initial visit, the social and occupational histories are obtained. During each subsequent visit healthcare facilities may require the medical assistant to ask specific screening questions. These screening questions are used to collected required information and focus on prevention and quality patient care. Common screenings include the following:

- *Alcohol misuse screening:* An alcoholic drink is classified as a 12-oz bottle of beer, a 5-oz glass of wine, or a 1.5-oz shot of liquor. The recommendations are no more than one drink per day for a female and two drinks per day for a male adult.

- *Nicotine or tobacco screening*: The questions focus on whether or not tobacco products are used, product used, how much is used per day, the history of use, and quitting behaviors (e.g., strategies used in the past or thoughts of quitting).
- *Drug abuse screening*: The questions focus on prescription drug use for nonmedical reasons and illegal drug use.

CRITICAL THINKING 34.6

List two closed and open-ended questions or statements to obtain information about a patient's social and occupational histories.

Family History. The family history (FH) includes familial diseases (e.g., diabetes mellitus) and hereditary diseases that grandparents, parents, and siblings have. For deceased family members, information on the cause of death and the age at death is usually obtained. Age of living family members are also obtained.

CRITICAL THINKING 34.7

List two closed and open-ended questions or statements to obtain information about a patient's family history.

Review of Systems. Review of systems (ROS) or systems review (SR) is obtained through a logical sequence of questions about the state of health of body systems, beginning with the head and proceeding downward (Fig. 34.5). The questions gather information from patients about their general health and help detect other conditions or concerns. Usually, prior to the initial visit, the patient received the questionnaire in either a paper or digital form. The review of system questions may be intermixed with the past medical history questions for some healthcare facilities. During the initial visit, the medical assistant checks the questionnaire for completeness. The provider will use the form to ask the patient additional questions about his or her concerns. The ROS form provides a baseline for the provider. The ROS is usually done for the initial visits and may be done during annual wellness visits.

For female patients, their *last menstrual period* (LMP), pregnancy history, and method of birth control if sexually active can be part of the ROS. The LMP is documented as the date of the first day of the woman's last period.

CRITICAL THINKING 34.8

Select a body system. List two closed and open-ended questions or statements to obtain information about the patient's state of health regarding that body system.

Chief Complaint and History of Present Illness. *Chief complaint* (CC) is the purpose of the patient's visit. Generally, this is documented in the patient's own words. When documenting the patient's own words, it is important to use quotation marks ("").

The history of present illness (HPI) provides additional information about the current health problem. The history of current problem should be a concise chronologic description of the patient's symptoms from when it initially started to the present time. The HPI elaborates on the chief complaint, and both need to be obtained at each patient's visit.

When the medical assistant is obtaining the HPI, the acronym, "OLDCARTS," should be used. Asking these questions will help the medical assistant gather a concise description of the patient's symptoms:

- *Onset*: When did it begin?
- *Location*: Where is it located?
- *Duration*: How long has it been going on?
- *Characterization*: How would you describe it? For instance, with pain is it crushing, sharp, burning, or dull? Is it constant or intermittent?
- *Alleviating and aggravating factors*: What makes it better? What makes it worse? If medication was taken for it, what was taken? How often is it taken? Is it effective? When was the last dose?
- *Radiation*: Does it stay in one location or move?
- *Temporal factor*: Is it better or worse at different times of the day?
- *Severity*: Using a scale of 0 to 10, with 0 being none and 10 being the worst, how does it rate? (This scale is typically used for pain, 0 being no pain and 10 being the worst pain ever.) (Fig. 34.6)

When the medical assistant is obtaining the HPI, asking about signs and symptoms that commonly come together are important. For instance, if a patient a cough, the medical assistant should find out if it is productive or nonproductive. Does the person have chest congestion? A fever? A sore throat? Asking about related signs and symptoms help provide a concise HPI. Learning to take a concise HPI is a skill that needs to be practiced and refined.

VOCABULARY

baseline An observation or value that represents the normal or beginning level of a measurable quality; used for comparison.

chronologic Arranged in the order of time.

familial Occurring in or affecting members of a family more than would be expected by chance.

hereditary Passed from parents to offspring through the genes.

history of present illness (HPI) Describes the signs and symptoms from the time of onset.

productive Producing mucus or sputum.

sign Something that is measured or observed by others; also called objective data. Examples of signs include redness, swelling or edema, blood pressure, and pulse.

symptom Something that is only perceived by the patient; also called subjective data. Examples include pain, headache, dizziness, and nausea.

CRITICAL THINKING 34.9

A patient's chief complaint is right-sided abdominal pain. List three closed and open-ended questions or statements to obtain more information about the patient's present illness for the HPI.

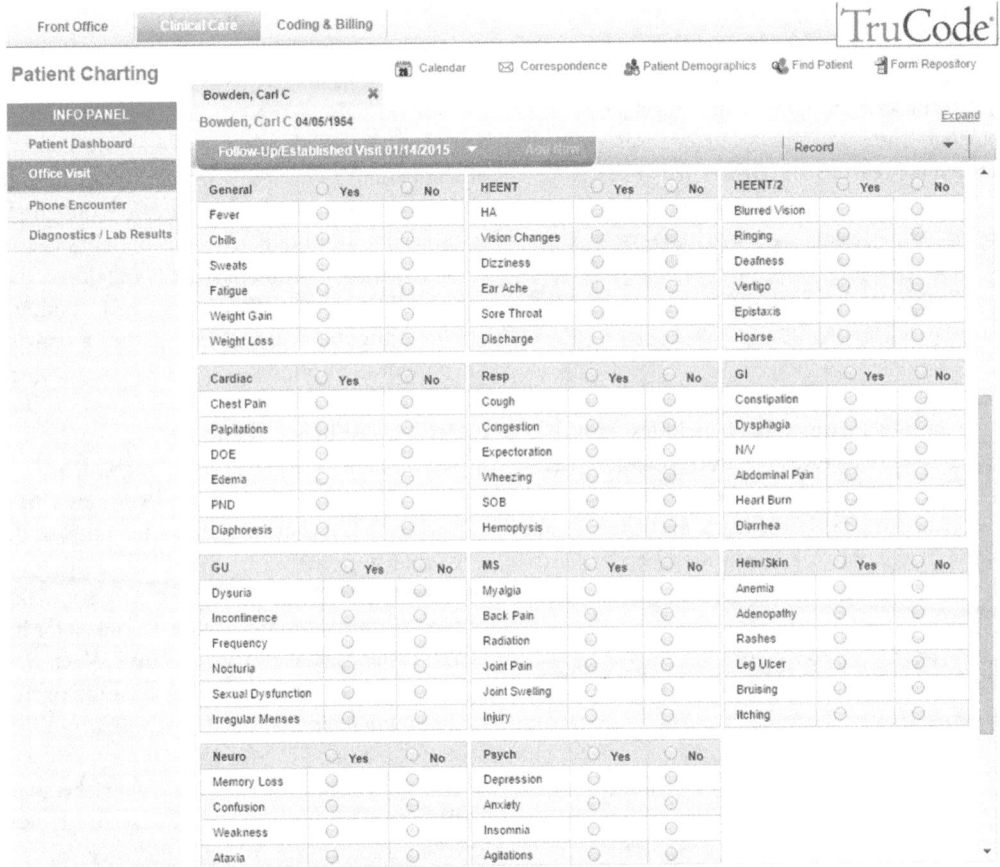

Fig. 34.5 Example of review of systems (ROS) questions in an electronic health record (EHR).

Symptoms and signs. A *symptom* of a disease is subjective and perceived only by the patient. A symptom can include pain, discomfort, nausea, dizziness, and so on. It cannot be measured or observed by another person. The medical assistant may have the patient rate symptoms, such as pain, to help gauge the severity. Symptoms of the greatest significance in identifying a disease are called *cardinal symptoms*. For example, crushing chest pain and difficulty breathing are cardinal symptoms of a possible heart attack.

A *sign* of a disease is objective and perceived by the provider. A sign can be measured or observed. A fever, vomiting, swelling, and redness are signs since they are observable or measurable. During the HPI, patients commonly provide signs and symptoms they have experienced. The signs may also be perceived by the provider. For instance, patients may state they had a fever. During the visit, the patient's temperature is measured. Patients may indicate swelling in a certain location. The provider can observe the swelling (*edema*).

DOCUMENTATION

Various methods can be used for documentation, depending on the healthcare provider's preference or the facility's EHR system. However, certain documentation procedures have been standardized to meet the legal requirements for maintaining medical records accurately and concisely. Complete, accurate documentation is one of the primary responsibilities of a medical assistant.

Documentation Guidelines

Medical assistants should follow these documentation guidelines:

- Check that the name on the record matches the patient. Confirm the patient's identity by asking for the full name and date of birth.
- All unusual complaints, symptoms, or reactions must be noted in detail. Include complete information about the *onset* (when the problem started), *duration* (how long episodes last), and *frequency* (how often episodes occur) of each reported sign and symptom. *Example:* Pt reports night cough, which started 2 days ago, lasts approximately 10 minutes, and occurs 3–4 times per night.
- Describe objective data, such as the presence of a wound, using correct anatomic medical terminology. *Example:* Observed wound on left distal anterior leg approximately 2 cm long and 1 cm wide.
- If the patient reports pain, record the quality and intensity of the pain using a pain scale of 0 to 10. *Example:* Pt c/o dull pain at wound site, a 4 on a scale of 0–10.

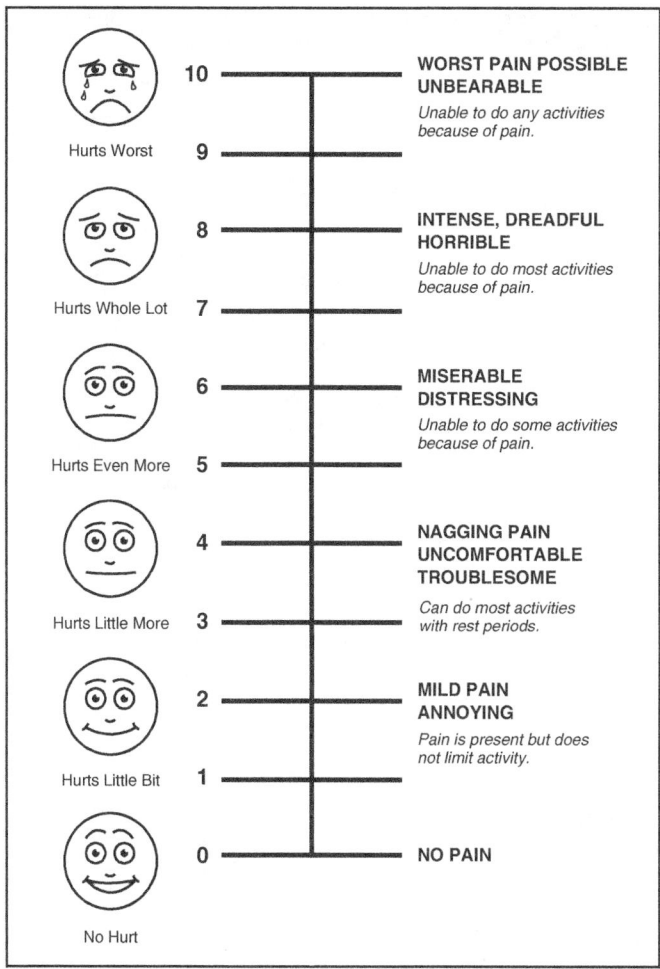

10 — WORST PAIN POSSIBLE
UNBEARABLE
Unable to do any activities because of pain.

Hurts Worst 9

8 — INTENSE, DREADFUL
HORRIBLE
Unable to do most activities because of pain.

Hurts Whole Lot 7

6 — MISERABLE
DISTRESSING
Unable to do some activities because of pain.

Hurts Even More 5

4 — NAGGING PAIN
UNCOMFORTABLE
TROUBLESOME
Can do most activities with rest periods.

Hurts Little More 3

2 — MILD PAIN
ANNOYING
Pain is present but does not limit activity.

Hurts Little Bit 1

0 — NO PAIN

No Hurt

Fig. 34.6 Wong-Baker Faces Pain Rating Scale.

- If the patient's comments are entered in the patient's own words, enclose them in quotation marks. *Example:* Pt states, "I fell against a stone foundation while cutting the grass and slashed my leg."

- Document the complete medication history, including both prescription and OTC medications, along with vitamins, minerals, and herbal supplies. Include the name, dose (amount taken), number of times taken during the day, why it is taken, and any other pertinent details. *Example:* Pt reports taking ibuprofen 400 mg orally for pain every 6 hours. Last dose taken 45 minutes ago.
- Record details about the previous history of the current CC. *Example:* Pt reports having a similar cough 3 weeks ago.
- Learn to be observant and to note anything that seems pertinent.
- Use accurate abbreviations, symbols, and terminology that is approved by the facility (Table 34.3).
- Review your documentation immediately after completion so that you can detect errors while the information is fresh in your mind.
- If details are omitted, add an addendum. Include the current date and time. Refer to the original entry. Include the reason for the addition and the new information.

When the medical assistant is documenting in a paper health record, these guidelines should be followed:

- Do all charting in black ink except for noting allergies in red ink; never use pencil.
- Write in a clear, legible manner.
- Do not leave any blank spaces on the paper record, and do not skip lines between documentation entries.
- Start the entry with the complete date (month, day, and year) and time.
- Sign the entry and add the appropriate initials after your name (e.g., CMA). (The EHR entry will automatically include your name and title on the entry.)
- Never scribble, erase, or use whiteout on an error. For legal purposes, it is crucial that the corrected error be readable.
- Correct the error by drawing one line through it. Write "error" above the corrected word or words and date and initial the correction. Then write in the correction.

TABLE 34.3 Medical Abbreviations

Abbreviation	Definition	Abbreviation	Definition
abd	abdomen	FUO	fever of unknown origin
ABG	arterial blood gases	fx	fracture
ac	before meals	GC	gonorrhea
ACLS	advanced cardiac life support	GI	gastrointestinal
ad lib	as desired	GTT	glucose tolerance test
AFP	alpha-fetoprotein	GU	genitourinary
AKA	above the knee amputation	HCT	hematocrit
ASAP	as soon as possible	Hgb	hemoglobin
ASHD	atherosclerotic heart disease	HIV	human immunodeficiency virus
BE	barium enema	h/o	history of
bid	twice a day	HPI	history of present illness
BM	bowel movement	hs	at bedtime or hour of sleep
BMR	basal metabolic rate	HTN	hypertension
BOM	bilateral otitis media	Hx	history
BP	blood pressure	I&D	incision and drainage
BUN	blood urea nitrogen	I&O	intake and output
bx	biopsy	IG	immunoglobulin
$\overline{c}$	with	lytes	electrolytes
C&S	culture and sensitivity	MI	myocardial infarction
CA	cancer	NG	nasogastric
CABG	coronary artery bypass graft	NKA	no known allergies
CAD	coronary artery disease	NPO	nothing by mouth
CBC	complete blood count	N/V	nausea and vomiting
CC	chief complaint	$\overline{P}$	after
CHF	congestive heart failure	PE	pulmonary embolism
CHO	carbohydrate	prn	as needed
CNS	central nervous system	pt	patient
c/o	complains of	PE	physical examination
COPD	chronic obstructive pulmonary disease	PT	physical therapy
CPK	creatinine phosphokinase	q	every
CPR	cardiopulmonary resuscitation	RBC	red blood cells
CSF	cerebrospinal fluid	R/O	rule out
CT	computed tomography	ROM	range of motion
CVA	cerebrovascular accident	R/T	related to
CXR	chest x-ray	Rx	prescription
DAT	diet as tolerated	$\overline{s}$	without
dc	discontinue	SOB	shortness of breath
D&C	dilation and curettage	s/s	signs and symptoms
DDx	differential diagnosis	STI	sexually transmitted infection
DM	diabetes mellitus	STAT	immediately
DNR	do not resuscitate	Sx	symptoms, surgery
DVT	deep vein thrombosis	Tx	treatment
Dx	diagnosis	UA	urinalysis
ECG	Electrocardiogram	URI	upper respiratory infection
EENT	eyes, ears, nose, throat	UTI	urinary tract infection
FBS	fasting blood sugar	VS	vital signs
f/u	follow up	WNL	within normal limits

Modified from Proctor D, et al: *Kinn's The Medical Assistant*, ed 13, St. Louis, 2017, Elsevier.

CLOSING COMMENTS

Having good communication skills is an important trait of a good medical assistant. This is not only essential as you deal with the provider and co-workers, but also as you work with patients. Helping the patient feel comfortable will help them feel that they can open up and more easily speak with the healthcare staff. This is important, to ensure that all the necessary information is available for the provider. Being aware of communication barriers and defense mechanisms is the first step to overcoming them and to keeping an open line of communication with the patient.

PATIENT-CENTERED CARE

When medical assistants perform patient interview using virtual video software for telehealth, they must:

- Make sure patients know how to use the software prior to the visit. This may result in coaching the patient prior to the visit on how to access the software and the technology requirements.
- Select a location for the visit that will provide privacy and confidentiality. The background should be professional or neutral, such as a blank wall.
- Keep the camera at eye level, to help ensure eye contact with the patient. The camera must be on during the visit. The microphone should be muted when the medical assistant is not talking.
- Be punctual to the visit and make sure the patient can hear and see you.
- Greet the patient, introduce themselves, verify who the patient is, and explain what will occur.
- Allow the patient time to finish talking. Be professional, just like the patient is in the facility for an in-person visit.

BEING PROFESSIONAL

While working to build a trusting relationship with patients, it is also important to remember to maintain professional boundaries. Although we want patients to feel comfortable, it is important that we keep our focus on the patient. When working with patients who are seen frequently, it is easy to start to think of them as friends. With a friend you are likely to share personal information that is not appropriate to share with a patient. Patients may feel that they cannot share important health-related information because you are their friend and it would be embarrassing to share that information with a friend.

Self-boundaries can also be thought of as professional boundaries. You need to treat patients with respect and keep the relationship professional. Be friendly to patients and always keep the focus on the patient.

During your practicum it is likely that you will get to know many of the patients at your site. Assume that you are a student at WMFM Clinic, and you have seen one of the regular patients, Kyle Reeves, several times. At one of his visits Kyle mentions to you that he is having a party at his house over the weekend and would really like you to come. As he describes the party, it sounds like a lot of fun, and you would like to attend. Keep in mind that even as a student you are held to the same professional standards as a full-time employee. Role-play this situation with a peer. You are the student medical assistant, and your peer is Kyle. Respond to Kyle's invitation.

CHAPTER REVIEW

In this chapter we discussed therapeutic communication techniques and how they should be used in the patient interview process. To be an effective medical assistant, you need to be able to communicate effectively and compassionately. This includes using both verbal and nonverbal communication and actively listening to both verbal and nonverbal communication from the patient.

Active listening techniques, such as using open-ended questions, restatement, reflection, clarification, and being sensitive to cultural differences, are essential to ensuring good communication with patients. By building a good rapport with the patients, a medical assistant can better gather the necessary information, which will assist the provider in their diagnosis and treatment decisions.

The medical history is an important part of the patient interview and an important part of holistic healthcare. To obtain an accurate medical history, you must be familiar with the information needed and use therapeutic techniques to obtain it.

The barriers to a good interview include defense mechanisms. By recognizing defense mechanisms and how they influence communication, we can overcome this barrier and ensure the correct information is carried forward.

SCENARIO WRAP-UP

Chris has met with the office supervisor and reviewed essential techniques for gathering patient information. Therapeutic communication includes demonstrating respectful patient care, using active listening skills, observing nonverbal behaviors, and using a combination of both open-ended and closed-ended questions to gather the best possible detail about the patient's chief complaint. The supervisor gave Chris a variety of information on meeting the needs of a diverse patient population and also gave him suggestions on how to develop empathetic, helping relationships with patients. Chris feels much better prepared to meet the communication needs of each patient he sees.

PROCEDURE 34.1 Obtain and Document Patient Information

Tasks
Use restatement, reflection, and clarification to obtain patient information and document patient care accurately.

Equipment and Supplies
- Medical history form or EHR system with the patient history window opened
- If using a paper form, a red pen for recording the patient's allergies and a black pen to meet legal documentation guidelines
- Quiet, private area

Directions
Complete this procedure with another student playing the role of the patient. To make the experience more realistic, choose a student about whom you know very little. To maintain the students' privacy, students do not have to share any confidential information.

Procedural Steps
1. Greet the patient. Identify yourself. Verify the patient's identity with full name and date of birth. Explain what you need to do with the patient and answer any questions the patient may have.
   Purpose: To make the patient feel comfortable and at ease.
2. Take the patient to a quiet, private area for the interview and explain why the information is needed.
   Purpose: A quiet, private area is necessary to protect confidentiality and prevent interruptions. An informed patient is more cooperative and therefore more likely to provide useful information.
3. Complete the medical history form by using therapeutic communication techniques, including restatement, reflection, and clarification. Use active listening skills. Make sure all medical terminology is adequately explained.

Purpose: Therapeutic communication techniques help the medical assistant gather complete information; the self-history is designed to save time and to involve the patient in the process.

4. Use appropriate nonverbal communication. Speak in a pleasant, distinct manner, remembering to maintain eye contact with your patient, if culturally appropriate.
   Purpose: Positive nonverbal behaviors create a friendly, caring atmosphere.
5. Demonstrate empathy and remain sensitive to the diverse needs of your patient throughout the interview process.
   Purpose: Incorporate awareness of your personal biases into treating all patients with respect despite their diverse backgrounds.
6. Ask the patient for his or her demographic information, which is required on the form or in the EHR. Report patient information concisely and accurately.
7. Ask the patient for the chief complaint and the history of present illness information. Use quotation marks around the patient's words if used in the documentation. Report patient information concisely and accurately.
   Purpose: The provider needs this information to make an accurate assessment and diagnosis.
8. Ask the patient for his or her past medical history. For the paper form, write the allergies in red ink. Report patient information concisely and accurately.
   Purpose: The presence of an allergy may alter medication and treatment procedures.
9. Ask the patient for his or her social, occupational, and family histories. Report patient information concisely and accurately.
10. If using a paper form, record all information legibly and neatly. Review information for correct spelling. Ensure the form is complete. If using the EHR, log out. Thank the patient for his or her time.
    Purpose: To maintain a medical record that is understandable and defensible in a court of law.

PROCEDURE 34.2 Perform a Telehealth Patient Interview

Tasks
Perform a telehealth patient interview and input the patient data into the electronic health record or electronic medical record. Observe the patient and respond appropriately to nonverbal communication. To use restatement, reflection, and clarification to obtain patient's information and document patient information accurately.

Equipment and Supplies
- Medical history form for established patient or EHR system with the patient's history window opened
- If using a paper form, a red pen for recording the patient's allergies and a black pen to meet legal documentation guidelines
- Virtual video software and internet access

Scenario
You need to complete a telehealth patient interview before the patient is seen by the provider. Yesterday, you coached the patient on how to use the software.

Directions
Role-play the scenario with a peer, who will be the patient, and you are the medical assistant.

Procedural Steps
1. Greet the patient. Identify yourself. Verify the patient's identity with full name and date of birth. Explain what you need to do with the patient and answer any questions the patient may have.
2. Using the form or the EHR, ask the patient's chief complaint and history of present illness. Accurately and concisely document the information obtained. Pay close attention to the patient's body language on the screen to determine whether what the patient is telling you is congruent with their body language.

Purpose: Nonverbal language naturally expresses the patient's true feelings. Closely observing body language will help you reach more accurate conclusions about the patient's information.

3. Ask the patient about their current medications and allergies, social history, and any updates on medical history since last visit. Accurately and concisely document the information obtained.
4. Obtain the patient's information using therapeutic communication techniques, including restatement, reflection, and clarification. Use active listening skills.
   Purpose: Therapeutic communication techniques help the medical assistant gather complete information; using feedback techniques and making sure the patient understands medical terms can help to relieve anxiety.
5. Correctly use and pronounce medical terminology during the interaction. Make sure all medical terminology is adequately explained.
6. Use appropriate nonverbal communication. Speak in a pleasant, distinct manner, remembering to maintain eye contact with your patient, if culturally appropriate. Select the appropriate verbal response to demonstrate your sensitivity to their discomfort, frustration, and anxiety.
   Purpose: Positive nonverbal behaviors create a friendly, caring atmosphere.
7. Demonstrate empathy and remain sensitive to the diverse needs of your patient throughout the interview process.
   Purpose: Displaying sensitivity to and awareness of the patient's nonverbody language demonstrates your concern for the patient and can help defuse the patient's concerns.
8. If using a paper form, record all information legibly and neatly. Review information for correct spelling. Ensure the form is complete. If using the EHR, log out. Thank the patient for his or her time.

35

Physical Examination

LEARNING OBJECTIVES

1. Describe the medical assistant's role in preparing for the physical examination.
2. Summarize the instruments and equipment the provider typically uses during a physical examination.
3. Describe the principles of body mechanics that should be used while transferring a patient.
4. Describe positioning and draping a patient for various examinations.
5. Describe the methods of examination.
6. Discuss the typical sequence for a routine physical examination.
7. Describe how to perform and document vision screening tests, including the distance visual acuity, near visual acuity, and the Ishihara test.
8. Describe hearing screening testing, including tuning fork testing and audiometric testing.
9. Describe the role of a medical scribe.

OUTLINE

▶▶ OPENING SCENARIO

Chris Isaacson, CMA (AAMA), works for Walden-Martin Family Medical (WMFM) Clinic. Chris is responsible for assisting with physical examinations. His duties include preparing and maintaining the examination room and equipment; getting the patient ready for specific physical examinations; and gowning, draping, and positioning the patient as needed. Because Chris assists with examinations, he must be familiar with the physical examination procedure and the order in which the provider needs various pieces of medical equipment. Throughout the physical examination process, Chris needs to be aware of proper body mechanics.

YOU WILL LEARN

1. To prepare the equipment for a physical examination.
2. To position patients properly for all aspects of the physical examination.
3. To use proper body mechanics when working in a healthcare facility.
4. To perform vision and hearing screening tests.
5. To accurately scribe for a physical exam.

INTRODUCTION

The physical examination is a vital step in providing healthcare. During the physical examination, the provider is present with the patient and uses a variety of methods to determine a diagnosis (Dx). The diagnosis is based on information gathered from the patient about symptoms; contributing family, personal, and social histories; and a complete physical examination. This diagnosis is then used to determine the appropriate treatment for the patient. The most common types of diagnosis we see in the ambulatory care center are:

- *Differential diagnosis* (DDx): This type of diagnosis focuses on finding multiple options for what is causing the symptoms and follows a process of elimination until only one possible disease remains. This is often considered a diagnosis by ruling out.
- *Working diagnosis (clinical diagnosis)*: This is a diagnosis obtained from the clinical findings of the provider without validation from imaging or laboratory findings. It is considered a verification diagnosis, with the provider ordering tests to validate the diagnosis.
- *Final diagnosis*: This is the diagnosis that is verified by testing. It is the final diagnosis after all the ruling out has been done and imaging and laboratory testing have verified the working diagnosis.

Introduction to the Physical Examination

After the interview is complete, the patient is prepared for the physical examination. During the examination, the healthcare provider methodically checks all the body's systems. For each system, the provider mentally compares the system with established norms. Normal and abnormal findings are documented in the patient's health record. (Some facilities just charting by exception.) The physical examination typically starts with the head and progresses downward to the feet. However, the order may vary, depending on the provider's specialty.

A sign can be observed or measured by the provider or medical assistant. They are the indicators of health or disease that a provider detects when examining a patient. The provider feels, sees, hears, or measures the signs that often are associated with a certain disease or abnormal condition. For example, a mass that a provider *palpates*, or feels, in the patient's abdomen is an objective finding and a sign of an abnormal condition. In addition, objective data can be measured and recorded, and repeat measurements can be taken to confirm the presence of or changes in the sign. The patient's temperature, pulse, respirations, and blood pressure are objective signs the medical assistant measures and regularly records. Signs and symptoms work together to help the provider determine how to best treat the patient.

A medical assistant must also know how to best assist the provider during the physical examination. Understanding what supplies and instruments are needed will make the visit go more smoothly for both the patient and the provider. During a complete physical exam, the patient is placed in various positions to facilitate examination. It is often the medical assistant's responsibility to assist the patient into the correct position and drape them for modesty.

VOCABULARY

charting by exception (CBE) A method of documentation based on established standards of practice. Only abnormal findings or exceptions to the predefined normal findings are documented.

diagnosis Determination of the disease or condition that is causing a patient's signs and symptoms.

sign Something that is measured or observed by others; also called objective data. Examples of signs include redness, swelling or edema, blood pressure, and pulse.

symptom Something that is only perceived by the patient; also called subjective data. Examples include pain, headache, dizziness, and nausea.

PHYSICAL EXAMINATION

The purpose of a physical examination is to determine the patient's overall state of well-being. All major organs and body systems are checked during a physical examination. As providers examine the entire body, they interpret the findings. By the time the examination has been completed, the provider has formed a working diagnosis of the patient's condition. Often laboratory and other diagnostic tests are ordered to supplement and finalize this diagnosis.

The physical exam is not only used to refine the patient's diagnosis, but also to help the provider plan or revise treatment for the patient, evaluate drug therapy, and determine the patient's progress.

Before the examination, the medical assistant has the opportunity to make sure that the patient feels comfortable during the examination process and that all the necessary medical information has been obtained. The medical assistant's duties include:

- preparing and maintaining the examination room and equipment.
- preparing the patient.
- assisting the provider during the physical examination.

Preparing the Examination Room

The medical assistant is responsible for making sure the examination room is ready for any procedure that might be performed during the physical examination. The area should be as comfortable as possible for the patient and free of any potential dangers, such as contaminated equipment. You should prepare the examination room as follows:

- Check the area at the beginning of each day and between patients to make sure it is completely stocked with equipment and supplies.
- Make sure all equipment is functioning properly. You must understand how to take care of and operate all equipment and instruments. You should refer to user guides supplied by manufacturers as needed.
- Regularly check expiration dates on all packages and supplies. Discard expired materials and replace with new materials.
- Make sure the room is private, well lit, and at a comfortable temperature for the patient during the physical examination.
- Clean and disinfect the area daily and between patients to prevent the spread of infection and to ensure patients' comfort. When the patient leaves the room, discard the used exam table paper. Using disinfectant wipes, clean the table and any other potentially contaminated surface. When the table dries, replace the exam table paper.
- Arrange drapes, gowns, and all other patient supplies before the patient enters the room so that they are ready for use.
- To save time during the exam, prepare the instruments and equipment needed. Arrange them for easy access, before the provider enters the room.
- Make sure the examination room has all materials required for observing Standard Precautions, including gloves, soap, paper towels, biohazardous waste containers, sharps containers, impervious gowns, and face guards. Sharps containers are replaced when they are about 75% filled.

CRITICAL THINKING 35.1

List five tasks the medical assistant needs to do to prepare an examination room.

Assisting the Patient

The medical assistant assists the patient prior to, during, and after the examination. Getting the patient ready for the examination includes taking care of paperwork before the provider enters the examination room:

- Introduce yourself. Verify the patient's identity by asking for the full name and date of birth. Verify the information with the health record. Address the patient by his or her preferred name, making sure to show respect at all times. Pay close attention to the patient's nonverbal language to make sure he or she understands what to expect.
- Measure and record the patient's vital signs, height, and weight. Calculate the body mass index (BMI), if needed.
- Ask the patient for the reason for the visit and explain the examination procedure to the patient. Be prepared to answer the patient's questions and ease any fears. If needed, refer the patient's questions to the provider.
- Make sure the health record is complete. Document current medications and allergies. Identify any medications that need refills.
- Ask whether patients need to empty their bladder before the examination, because a full bladder may interfere with the examination and may be uncomfortable for the patient.

Some procedures (most commonly pelvic ultrasounds) require a patient to have a full bladder.

- Obtain specimens (e.g., urine, blood) if the provider has ordered them or if there is a standing order for the tests.
- Help the patient physically prepare for the examination. Explain to the patient what clothing should be removed and in what direction to put on the gown (open to the front or to the back, depending on the type of examination). Provide a drape to ensure the patient's privacy and help as needed.
- Assist the patient into and out of various examination positions as needed. As the provider proceeds with the examination, make sure the patient remains unexposed by adjusting the drape and gown.
- Throughout this sequence of events, explain what is happening and consistently maintain the patient's privacy and confidentiality.
- Help the patient with dressing as needed after the examination.

CRITICAL THINKING 35.2

Why is it important that the medical assistant introduce himself or herself before starting a procedure?

VOCABULARY
standing order An order applies to all patients who meet specific criteria.

Assisting the Provider

Prior to the provider entering the examination room, the medical assistant should conduct any diagnostic tests, such as hearing and visual screenings, that are either preordered or part of the provider's standing orders. During the physical examination, the medical assistant should be prepared to help the provider to make the process as efficient as possible. During the examination, the provider may expect the medical assistant to:

- Hand instruments and equipment as requested and provide supplies as needed.
- Alter the position of the light source to better illuminate the area being examined and turn lights on and off during specific phases of the examination.
- Position and drape the patient during different phases of the examination.
- Assist in collecting and properly labeling specimens such as urine, Pap test specimens, and throat cultures.
- Conduct follow-up diagnostic procedures as ordered, including an *electrocardiogram* (ECG), urinalysis, and phlebotomy.
- Document patient data in the health record, completing all forms required.
- Schedule post-examination diagnostic procedures, such as mammography, an x-ray examination, or a colonoscopy.

MEDICAL TERMINOLOGY

cardi/o	heart
electro-	using electricity
-gram	a record or recording

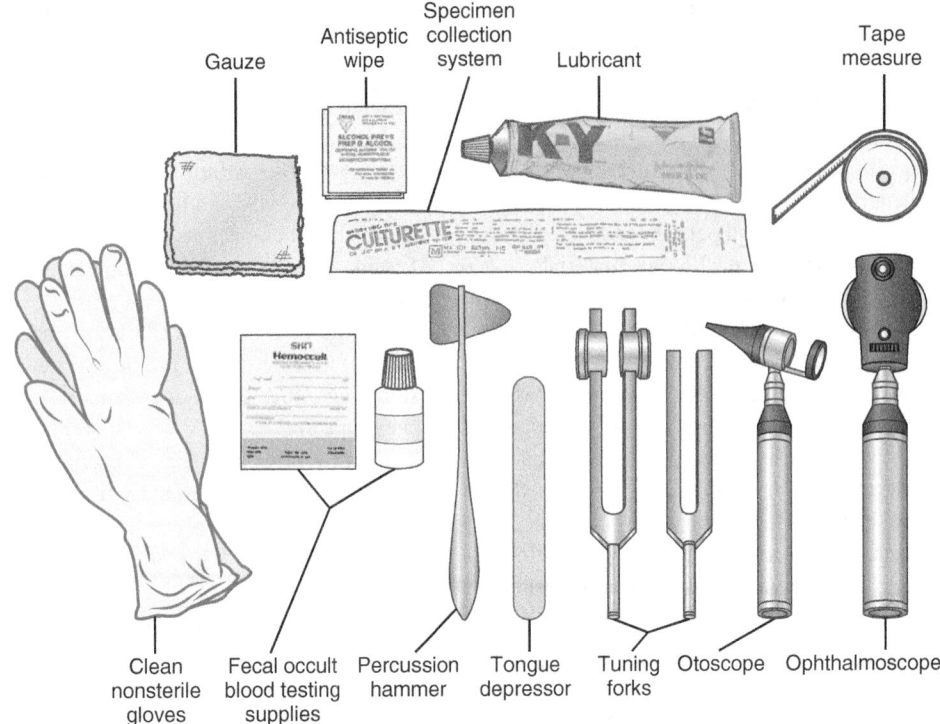

Fig. 35.1 Instruments for the Physical Examination. (From Niedzwiecki B, et al: *Kinn's the medical assistant*, ed 14, St. Louis, 2020, Elsevier.)

Supplies and Instruments Needed for the Physical Examination

The instruments typically used during the physical examination are shown in Fig. 35.1. These are used to assist the physician in the exam. All equipment must be in good working order, properly disinfected, and readily available for the provider's use during the examination. The instruments most frequently used for a physical examination are described in Table 35.1. Physical examinations are typically performed from the head to the feet. The instruments are listed in the order in which the provider typically would request them.

> **VOCABULARY**
>
> **auscultate** To listen with a stethoscope.
>
> **peripheral neuropathy** Occurs as a result of damage to the peripheral nervous system. The patient can experience multiple symptoms including tingling, numbness, weakness, burning pain, muscle wasting, and organ dysfunction.

PRINCIPLES OF BODY MECHANICS

Medical assistants should use proper body mechanics consistently throughout the work environment when sitting or standing, lifting or carrying objects, pushing or pulling, or transferring patients. Without consistent application of correct anatomic alignment, injuries, especially lower back injuries, easily occur.

Proper body alignment begins with good posture. Maintaining posture requires a combination of muscle efforts. Good posture keeps the spine balanced and aligned while a person is sitting or standing. A person in good body alignment can maintain balance without undue strain on the musculoskeletal system.

When you reach for an object, avoid twisting or turning; instead, move the feet to face the object needed. This prevents undue strain on the lumbar region. Do not cross the legs while sitting, because this interferes with circulation to the legs and feet. When sitting, keep the popliteal area (behind the knees) free of the edge of the chair. Pressure in this area interferes with circulation and may damage nerves behind the knees. Do a mental check of your posture regularly. Hold the head erect, the face forward and the chin slightly up, the abdominal muscles contracted up and in, the shoulders relaxed and back, the feet pointed forward and slightly apart, and the weight evenly distributed to both legs, with the knees slightly bent. Always be on the alert for poor body mechanics that may cause injury.

Transferring a Patient

Patients may need assistance in moving from a chair to the exam table or back again. Patients can be transferred in multiple ways, but all should focus on correct body mechanics. If the patient is in a wheelchair, move the chair at a 45-degree angle toward the footrest that extends from the bottom of the exam table (Fig. 35.4). Make sure the patient's strong side is beside the exam table so the transfer moves toward the patient's strong side. Lock the wheels of the wheelchair and lift the footrests of the wheelchair out of the way. Explain the procedure to the patient and ask the individual for assistance.

If one side of the patient is stronger than the other, always provide support on the strong side. Support the patient close to your body on the strong side, with one hand under the axillary region

TABLE 35.1 Instruments Needed for the Physical Examination

Instrument	Use
Ophthalmoscope	To inspect the inner structures of the eye. It consists of a stainless steel handle containing batteries and an attached head, which has a light-magnifying lens and an opening through which the eye is viewed.
Tongue depressor	A flat, wooden blade used to hold down the tongue when the throat is examined.
Otoscope	To examine the external auditory canal and tympanic membrane. It has a stainless steel handle containing batteries or is part of a wall-mounted electrical unit. The head of the otoscope has a light that is focused through a magnifying lens; it should be covered with a disposable ear speculum. The light also may be used to illuminate the nasal passages and throat.
Tuning fork	An aluminum, fork-shaped instrument that consists of a handle and two prongs (Fig. 35.2). The prongs produce a humming sound when the provider strikes them against their hand. Tuning forks are available in different sizes, and each size produces a different pitch level. A tuning fork is used to check the patient's auditory acuity and to test bone vibration. A tuning fork can also be used to test for diabetic peripheral neuropathy, by testing the patient's vibration sense.
Tape measure	A flexible ribbon ruler that is usually printed with inches and feet on one side and centimeters and meters on the reverse side. Measurements may be used to assess length and head circumference in infants, wound size, and so on.
Stethoscope	A listening device used when certain areas of the body are auscultated (AW skuh l teyt d), particularly the heart and lungs. This instrument is available in many shapes and sizes. All have two earpieces that are connected to flexible rubber or vinyl tubing (Fig. 35.3). At the distal end of the tubing is a diaphragm or bell (many have both); when it is placed securely on the patient's skin, it enables the provider to hear internal body sounds.
Reflex hammer	Sometimes called a *percussion hammer.* This stainless steel instrument has a hard rubber head that is used to strike the tendons of the knee and elbow to test the neurologic reflexes.
Gloves	Gloves protect the healthcare worker and the patient from microorganisms. According to Standard Precautions, gloves must be worn whenever the potential exists for contact with body fluid, broken skin or wounds, or contaminated items.
Additional supplies	Gauze, cotton balls, cotton-tipped applicators, disposable tissues, specimen containers, fecal occult blood test cards, Pap test supplies for female patients, lubricating jelly for vaginal and rectal examinations, and laboratory request forms should be easily accessible during the examination.

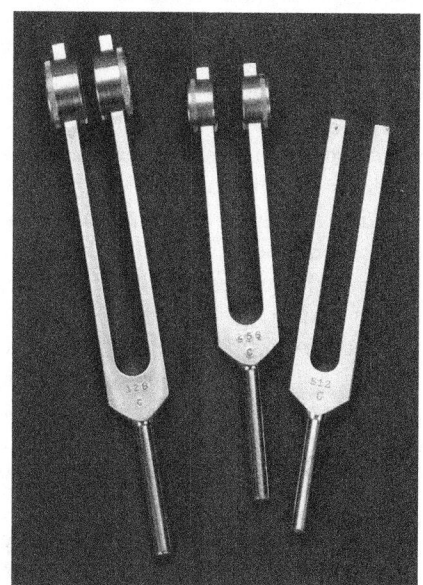

Fig. 35.2 Tuning Forks. (From Niedzwiecki B, et al: *Kinn's the medical assistant,* ed 14, St. Louis, 2020, Elsevier.)

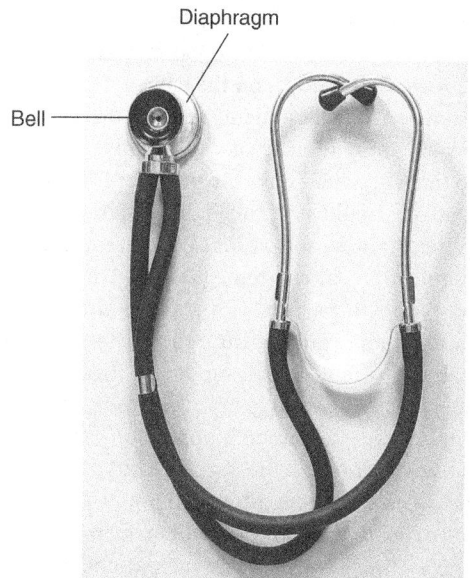

Fig. 35.3 Stethoscope. (Modified from Ball JW, et al: *Seidel's guide to physical examination,* ed 8, St. Louis, 2015, Mosby.)

and the other either grasping the patient's hand or holding the forearm. When bending, always bend at the knees and maintain the back's three natural curves, allowing the leg muscles to help in lifting. Give the patient a signal and lift as the patient assists. Help the patient step up onto the footrest with the strong leg first, then pivot. Ease the patient down onto the table, bending your knees while keeping your back aligned. Make sure the patient is comfortable and safely positioned on the table.

A *gait belt* is a safety device that is used to help when transferring or walking with the patient. The gait belt helps you support the patient while keeping your body in proper alignment to prevent back injuries. A gait belt should be used if the patient is weak and at risk of falling. Follow these steps to use a gait belt:

• Place the belt around the individual's waist over clothing with the buckle in front.

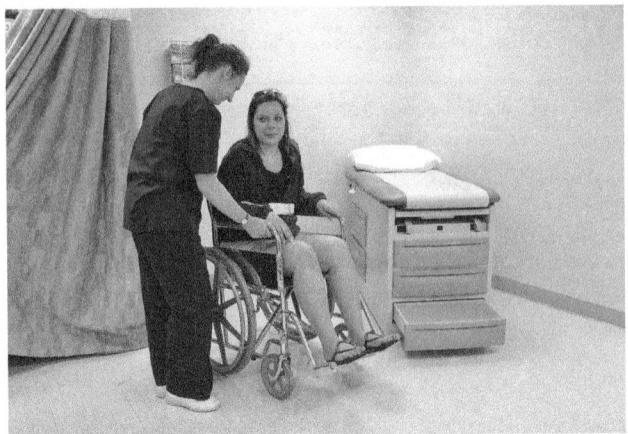

Fig. 35.4 Wheelchair at a 45-Degree Angle at the End of the Exam Table. (From Niedzwiecki B, et al: *Kinn's the medical assistant,* ed 14, St. Louis, 2020, Elsevier.)

- Insert the belt through the teeth of the buckle and pull it tight to lock it. The belt should be tight, with just enough room to place your fingers under it.
- Grip the belt tightly, bend your knees, and keep your back straight.
- Ask the patient to assist you; then lift, using your arm and leg muscles.
- Avoid twisting or turning as you help the patient stand.
- Keep your body close to the patient with your knees in front of theirs at all times to stabilize the patient and prevent falls.
- Complete the transfer without bending or twisting your body; encourage the patient to bear as much weight as possible and to gently sit down on the table.
- After transferring the patient, remove the gait belt for the provider's examination; replace it to help transfer the patient back to the wheelchair after the provider is finished.
- If the patient should start to fall during a transfer, do not try to stop the fall because you may be injured. Use the gait belt to help guide the patient to the floor as gently as possible.

You may need to remain with patients until the examination has been completed to ensure their safety. If the provider prefers that the patient be in a supine position, place one arm across the patient's shoulders and the other under the knees and smoothly lower the patient's upper body to the table while raising the legs. Support the legs as you pull out the table extension. Use the same pivoting techniques with proper body mechanics to help transfer the patient from the exam table back to the locked wheelchair. If the patient must hold onto you, have the person hold your waist or shoulders, not your neck (Procedure 35.1).

Before a transfer is attempted, the medical assistant must make sure that the people involved can be safe while transferring. Be sure to ask for help whenever necessary, specifically for large patients or patients who are completely immobilized and cannot assist with the transfer. If the patient begins to slip during the transfer, use the gait belt to shift the individual's weight so the patient returns to the table or chair without falling. The goal is to never have a patient fall or any injury to occur with any transfer. If there is ever any concern or doubt about the ability to move safely, ask for help.

CRITICAL THINKING 35.3

Mr. Brown had a stroke and has weakness on the left side of his body. You need to transfer him from the wheelchair to the exam table. Describe how you would position the wheelchair next to the exam table.

POSITIONING AND DRAPING THE PATIENT FOR THE PHYSICAL EXAMINATION

Various patient positions are used to facilitate a physical examination. The medical assistant instructs the patient and assists the patient into these positions, ensuring as much ease and modesty as possible. The medical assistant may also help the patient maintain the position during the examination with as little discomfort as possible. Never leave patients' side if they are in a position that could result in a fall.

Draping the patient with a sheet protects the individual from embarrassment and keeps the patient warm. However, the sheet must be positioned so that it allows complete visibility for the examiner and does not interfere with the examination. During the general examination, each part of the body is exposed one portion at a time. The following sections describe a number of the positions used during medical examinations.

Sitting, Full Fowler, and Semi-Fowler Positions

The sitting position is one of the most common positions for a physical examination for children and adults. This position is useful for examinations and treatments of the head, neck, chest, and upper back. In the sitting position, the patient sits at the end of the exam table with his or her legs dangling over the side of the table (Procedure 35.2).

The full Fowler position is useful for examinations and treatments of the head, neck, and chest, and for patients who have difficulty breathing while lying down. In the full Fowler position, the patient sits on the exam table with the head of the table elevated 90 degrees; the footrest may be extended for patient support and comfort.

The semi-Fowler position is useful for postoperative examination, for patients with breathing disorders, and for patients suffering from head trauma or pain. The semi-Fowler position is a modification of the full Fowler position. The head of the exam table is positioned at a 45-degree angle. The footrest may be extended for patient support and comfort.

Drape placement for these three positions varies depending on how the gown is opened and the type of physical examination done. To maintain the patient's modesty, the drape is adjusted to cover any exposed area that is not being examined from the upper chest to the legs.

VOCABULARY
trauma A physical injury or wound caused by external force or violence.

Supine (Horizontal Recumbent) and Dorsal Recumbent Positions

The supine position or horizontal recumbent position is used for the examination of the front of the body, including the head, chest (e.g., heart and breast exam), abdomen, and extremities. In this position, the patient lies flat with the face upward and the lower legs supported by the table extension (Procedure 35.3). The patient's gown should open down the front. The drape is placed lengthwise from the top of the chest to the legs.

The dorsal recumbent position relieves muscle tension in the abdomen. This position may be used for examination of the rectal, vaginal, and perineal (pair ih NEE uhl) areas. It can also be used as a substitute position for the supine position if the patient is experiencing back discomfort. In the dorsal recumbent position, the patient lies face upward with the knees flexed so the feet are flat on the table. The drape is placed in a diamond shape, with one corner on the patient's chest and the opposite corner over and between the legs (see Procedure 35.3). The perineal area should be covered along with any other exposed area from the top of the chest to the legs.

Lithotomy Position

The lithotomy (li THOT uh mee) position is similar to the dorsal recumbent position, with the exception that the patient's feet are placed in the stirrups. The lithotomy position is used primarily for vaginal examinations that require the use of a speculum and for Pap tests. The patient should not be placed in the lithotomy position until the provider is present and ready for the vaginal exam. This position can be uncomfortable for the patient and may make the patient feel more vulnerable or exposed.

To place the patient in the lithotomy position, pull out the stirrups on the exam table. With the patient in the dorsal recumbent position, have the patient slide the buttocks down to the bottom edge of the table. Assist the patient in placing the feet in stirrups. Adjust the stirrups as needed and lock in place. If the heels are too close to the buttocks, the possibility of leg cramps increases, and it is more difficult for the patient to relax the abdominal muscles. The drape placement is the same as the dorsal recumbent position. The provider lifts the drape away from the pubic area when the examination begins (Procedure 35.4).

Left Lateral Position

The left lateral position is used for rectal examinations, for instillation of rectal medication, and for some perineal and pelvic examinations. The patient is placed on the left side. The left arm and shoulder are drawn back behind the body so that the body's weight is predominantly on the chest. The right arm is flexed upward for support. The left leg is slightly flexed, and the buttocks are pulled to the edge of the table. The right leg is sharply flexed upward. The drape extends diagonally from under the arms to below the knees. The provider can raise a small portion of the sheet from the back of the patient to expose the rectum sufficiently. The remaining portion of the drape covers the patient's chest area and thighs (Procedure 35.5).

Prone Position

The prone position is used for examination of the back and for certain surgical procedures. This position is opposite of the supine position and is another of the recumbent positions. Patients lie face down on the table on their stomach or the ventral surface of their body. The drape should cover from the middle of the back to below the knees, with the gown opening in the back (Procedure 35.6).

Knee-Chest Position

The knee-chest position is used for rectal and proctologic (prok TOL loj ick) examinations. The patient starts in the prone position and then moves to the knee-chest position. The patient will need assistance to assume the knee-chest position correctly. The patient rests on the knees and the chest with the head turned to one side. The arms can be placed under the head for support and comfort, or they can be bent and placed at the sides of the table near the head. The thighs are perpendicular to the table and slightly separated. The buttocks extend up into the air, and the back should be straight. The patient's gown should open in the back. Depending on the exam, a fenestrated drape or a drape sheet will be used. The drape should be placed diagonally over the buttock with a corner falling toward the knees and a corner resting on the back (Procedure 35.7).

Most patients have difficulty maintaining this position, so they should not be placed into it until it is required. The medical assistant must remain next to the patient for assistance and support the entire time the knee-chest position is needed. If the correct knee-chest position cannot be obtained, the patient may have to be placed in a knee-elbow position. This position puts less strain on the patient and is easier to maintain.

VOCABULARY

fenestrated drape A disposable sheet with a hole or window that exposes only the area the provider needs to see.

perineal Pertaining to the area between the vaginal opening and the rectum (perineum).

CRITICAL THINKING 35.4

Determine the correct patient position and method of gowning and draping for:
- Insertion of a rectal suppository
- Annual Papanicolaou (Pap) test
- Examination of the back
- Patient with dyspnea
- Breast examination

METHODS OF EXAMINATION

Examinations are performed as both a routine confirmation of wellness and a means of diagnosing disease. Healthcare providers use six specific methods to examine the human body. All six are part of a complete physical examination.

Inspection

During the inspection, the provider uses observation to detect significant physical features or objective data. This method of examination ranges from focusing on the patient's general appearance (general state of health, including posture, mannerisms, and grooming) to more detailed observations, including body contour, gait, symmetry, visible injuries and deformities, tremors, rashes, and color changes. Inspection will be done before palpation or percussion so that there will be no changes made to the appearance of the skin.

Palpation

With *palpation* (PAL pey taa shuh n), the provider uses the sense of touch (Fig. 35.5A). A part of the body is felt with the hand to determine its condition or the condition of an underlying organ. Palpation may involve touching the skin or performing a firmer exploration of the abdomen for underlying masses. With this technique, the provider is assessing these factors:

- *Temperature*: Does the body seem to be the correct temperature (not too hot or too cold)?
- *Vibration*: Is there any area of the body that seems to be shaking or moving very quickly (e.g., shivering)?
- *Consistency*: Are there distinct differences between body areas that should be similar?
- *Form*: Is the shape and size of any specific area correct for the patient's age and build?
- *Rigidity*: Does the area seem to be appropriately firm (or soft)?
- *Elasticity*: Can the area be stretched or compressed and return to normal?
- *Moisture*: Is there any wetness present?
- *Texture*: How does the surface feel; is it appropriately textured or smooth?
- *Position*: Is everything where it should be?

Palpation is performed with one hand, both hands (bimanual), one finger (digital), the fingertips, or the palmar aspect of the hand. Some exams are done *bimanually*, with both hands palpating in different ways and different positions.

Percussion

Percussion (per KUSH un) involves tapping or striking the body, usually with the fingers or a small hammer. This will cause sounds, vibratory sensations, or involuntary reactions. Percussion can help to determine the position, size, and density of an underlying organ or cavity. The examiner both hears and feels the effect of percussion. It is helpful in determining the amount of air or solid matter in an underlying organ or cavity. The two basic methods of percussion are direct percussion and indirect percussion. *Direct percussion* is performed by striking the body with a finger or a reflex hammer. With *indirect percussion*, which is used more frequently, the provider places their hand on the area and then strikes the placed hand with a finger of the other hand (see Fig. 35.5B). Both a sound and a sense of vibration are evident. The examiner assesses the sound in terms of pitch, quality, duration, and resonance.

Auscultation

For *auscultation* (aw skul TAY shun), the provider uses a stethoscope to listen to sounds from the body. Auscultation is a complex method of examination because the provider must distinguish between a normal sound and an abnormal sound (see Fig. 35.5C). It is particularly useful for evaluating sounds originating in the lungs, heart, and abdomen, such as a murmur, a bruit (broot), and bowel sounds.

VOCABULARY

bruit An abnormal sound or murmur heard on auscultation of an organ, vessel (e.g., carotid artery), or gland.

extension The process of stretching out; increasing the angle of a joint.

flexion The process of reducing the angle of a joint.

gait The manner or style of walking.

manipulation Movement or exercise of a body part by means of an externally applied force.

murmur An abnormal sound heard during auscultation of the heart that may or may not have a pathologic origin; it is associated with valve disease or a congenital heart defect.

palpation The use of touch during the physical examination to assess the size, consistency, and location of certain body parts.

percussion Tapping or striking the body to create sounds, vibratory sensations, or involuntary reactions.

symmetry Similarity in size, form, and arrangement of parts on opposite sides of the body.

Mensuration

Mensuration (men sue RAY shun) is the process of measuring. Measurements that are recorded include:

- Height and weight
- Size and depth of a wound
- Size of the uterus during pregnancy
- Pressure of a grip
- Length and diameter of an extremity

Measurements are taken with a flexible tape measure, a circular wound measurement device (Fig. 35.6), or a specialized piece of equipment (e.g., a goniometer [go nee OHM eh ter]).

Manipulation

Manipulation (mah nip you LAY shun) is the passive movement of a joint to determine the range of extension or flexion of a part of the body. Insurance and industrial reports often request this information in detail. For example, a patient involved in a work-related accident that caused joint damage may have to perform assisted range-of-motion (ROM) exercises to the joint, with subsequent measurements of joint flexion and extension to demonstrate improvement or lack of it.

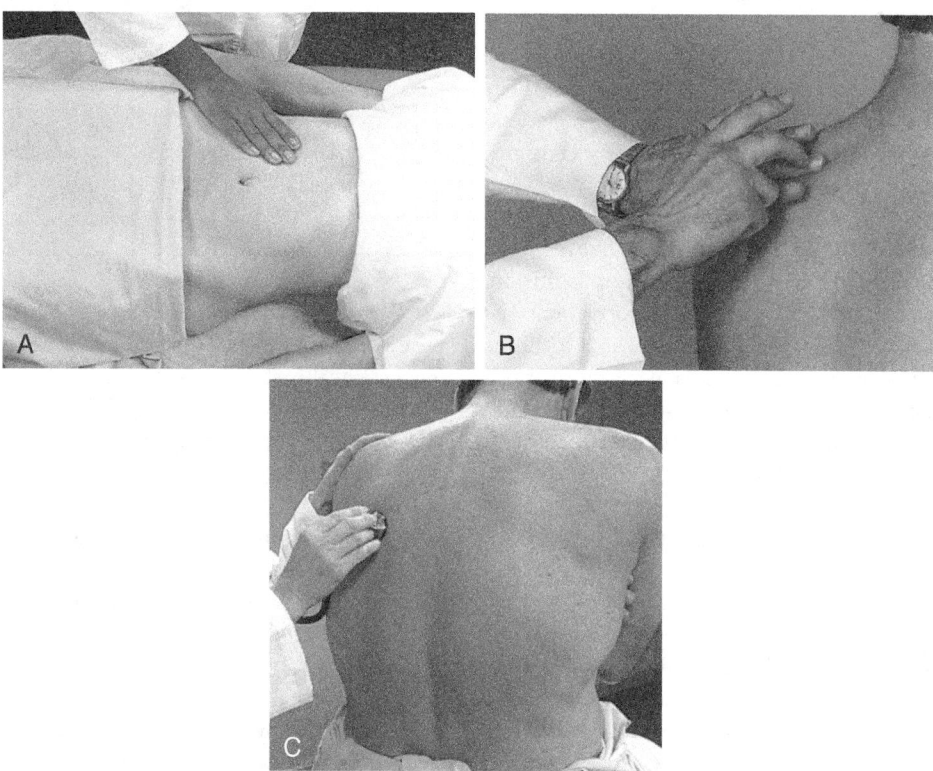

Fig. 35.5 A, Demonstration of palpation. B, Demonstration of percussion. C, Demonstration of auscultation. From Ball JW, et al: *Seidel's guide to physical examination,* ed 8, St. Louis, 2015, Mosby.

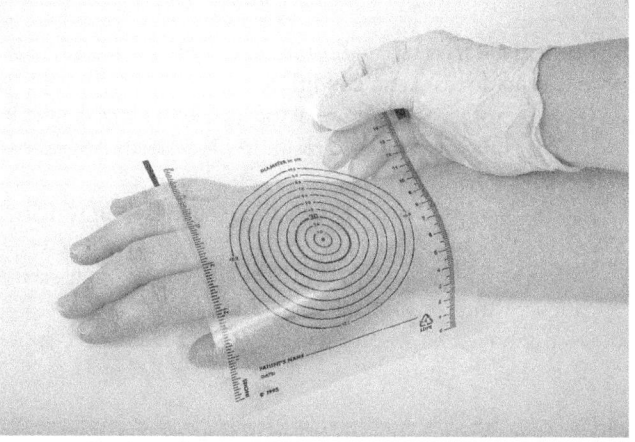

Fig. 35.6 Circular Wound Measurement Device.

EXAMINATION SEQUENCE

The physical examination sequence is fairly standard. Variations may occur, depending on the provider's specialty, the reason for the examination, and the provider's preference. Patients are more cooperative and less anxious if they understand what is expected of them. Start by giving the patient a brief explanation of the examination process.

Many healthcare facilities provide the option for patients to have a chaperone present during physical examinations. For more information about chaperones, see Box 35.1. When the provider begins the examination, the medical assistant should keep conversation to a minimum and remain inconspicuous (in kuhn SPIK yoo uhs).

> ### BOX 35.1 Chaperones During Physical Examinations
>
> It is becoming common for chaperones to be present during physical examinations. Having a third person in the exam room provides protection for both the patient and the provider. A medical assistant may be asked to be a chaperone.
>
> A chaperone can reassure the patient about the professional character of the healthcare facility. The patient has the right to refuse having a chaperone present in the room, but most are accepting. When the chaperone is another health professional, such as a medical assistant, they can serve two purposes: as a chaperone and as an assistant to the provider.
>
> If a healthcare facility is going to have chaperones present, there should be a written policy that describes the role of the chaperone. This policy should allow for a private conversation between the patient and the provider.

The examination usually starts with the patient seated at the end of the exam table. If patients need support while they are sitting, they can be placed in the full Fowler position. Standard overhead lights are generally sufficient most of the time. For examinations that need additional lighting, it is very common for special instruments to be used that light up to provide optimal visualization. In some cases, additional lighting may need to be used. When placing these lights, take care not to shine a light directly into the patient's eyes. This can be done by turning on lights while they are directed away from the patient and carefully moving the light toward the area. Procedure 35.8 presents the steps for assisting with the physical examination.

> **VOCABULARY**
> **inconspicuous** Not noticeable or prominent.

General Appearance

The provider starts the physical examination by observing the patient's appearance using an inspection technique. The medical assistant will also make judgment calls about the general appearance while taking the patient's history and vital signs. Anything unusual should be reported to the provider. When you evaluate the general appearance, it is important to note whether the patient appears disoriented or in distress, well-nourished or undernourished, and answers questions with ease or confusion.

The patient's gait often provides important information. The patient may limp, walk with the feet wide apart, have a shuffle step, or have difficulty maintaining their balance. Posture also is checked for indications of pain, stiffness, or difficulty with limb movement. Because it is common for the provider to come in after the patient has sat down in the room and to leave before the patient leaves, the medical assistant is often the one to relay concerns about a patient's gait. It is important for the medical assistant to pay attention to the patient's gait as they come back to the examination room and report any concerns to the provider.

Also, while assessing the general appearance, the provider notes body build and proportions. Any *gross* (immediately obvious) deformities are recorded. Sometimes abnormalities in height or body proportion may be caused by hormonal imbalances.

Speech

Speech is evaluated throughout the examination process as the provider and patient interact. It is important to take note of speech patterns and any abnormalities because speech may reveal a pathologic condition. The following are some basic speech defects.

- *Aphonia* (ey FOH nee uh): The inability to speak because of loss of the voice, which is commonly seen with vocal cord injuries, severe *laryngitis* (lar uh n JAHY tis), or overuse of the voice
- *Aphasia* (ah FAY zhah): Partial or complete loss of the ability to articulate ideas or understand written or spoken language. This is usually caused by a stroke (cerebrovascular accident [CVA]), brain tumor, infections, injuries, or dementia. Four main types include:
  - *Motor aphasia, or Broca aphasia*: Patients know what they want to say but have an inability to speak or to organize the muscular movements required to speak. The person may only be able to say three to four words at once.
  - *Sensory aphasia, or Wernicke aphasia*: A person hears the voice or sees the print but cannot make sense of the words. The person can speak, but the words or sentences may not be coherent.
  - *Anomic aphasia*: A person understands speech and words when reading, but has a hard time finding the correct word for places, events, and objects.
  - *Global aphasia*: The severest form of aphasia. A person cannot speak, understand speech, read, or write.

Speech assessment is important in well-child checkups. A delay in speech development can indicate an issue such as a neurologic deficit or possibly autism spectrum disorder. Often the delay in normal milestones related to speech is the first sign of these issues.

Skin

The condition of the skin can be an indicator of the patient's general health status. Abnormalities in the skin's color and/or texture can be a clue to many different disease processes. This can be more difficult to evaluate, because there is such a wide range of normal skin colors and even textures. Because of this, changes in skin color and texture are often more telling than a one-time assessment. Specific things to look for in the skin are extreme dryness, scaling, extended time for wound healing, and frequent breaks in the skin. Specific problems of the skin will often be referred for evaluation by a dermatologist.

The skin can also provide a strong indication of a patient's hydration level. If dehydration is suspected, skin turgor (TUR ger) is checked by pinching the skin on the posterior surface of the hands. The tissue is observed to see how quickly it returns to the normal location. A delay indicates a decrease in tissue fluid, confirming the diagnosis of dehydration.

Fingernails and toenails often give some indication of a person's health.

- Brittle nails are a normal result of aging but can also be due to certain diseases and conditions.
- Clubbing of the fingertips is associated with some congenital heart or lung diseases that result in *hypoxia* (decreased oxygen in the tissues).
- *Koilonychia* (koy low NIK EE ah) is a condition in which the nails are abnormally thin and concave from side to side and the edges are turned up, like a spoon. This is often seen in patients with iron-deficiency anemia.
- Deep grooved horizontal lines, known as *Beau lines,* appear after an acute illness but will grow out and disappear.

Head, Eyes, Ears, Nose (Sinuses), and Throat (Mouth)

The head and related structures are generally evaluated together and recorded as HEENT (head, eyes, ears, nose, and throat). Once the provider makes the overall observations of the patient's general condition, the physical examination typically begins with the head and face and moves downward to the feet. The face reflects the patient's state and tells the provider a great deal about how the patient handles stress and illness. The skull, scalp, and face are palpated for size, shape, and symmetry. The distribution or lack of hair and hair texture may indicate hormonal changes. Excessive hair, especially facial hair in females, indicates a hormonal imbalance. As the head is palpated, the provider assesses possible nodules, masses, or signs of trauma.

A complete examination of the eyes is technical and requires expensive equipment and the expertise of an ophthalmologist or optometrist. However, a primary care provider performs some basic examinations and treatments of the eye. The ophthalmoscope is used to examine the interior of the eye. It projects a bright, narrow beam of light through the lens and illuminates the interior parts of the eye and retina. It is helpful for detecting disorders of the eyes and certain systemic disorders, such as capillary changes that occur with diabetes mellitus.

Eyes. The eyelids are examined for edema, which may be the result of nephrosis, heart failure, allergy, or thyroid deficiency. *Blepharoptosis* (bleff ah rop TOH sis), also called *ptosis*, is drooping of the upper eyelid. It can be caused by normal aging, damage to the third cranial nerve, muscular weakness, and also diseases such as *myasthenia gravis* (mye ah STHEE nee ah GRAV us) and a CVA.

The pupils of the eyes are normally round and equal. Normal pupils constrict rapidly in response to light. This is demonstrated by shining a bright, pinpoint light into one eye from the side of the patient's head. The pupil of an illuminated eye constricts, and the pupil of the other eye constricts equally. This test is called *light and accommodation*. An older patient's eyes do not accommodate as well as those of a younger person. Each eye is checked this way. The patient then is asked to look at the provider's finger as it is moved directly toward the patient's nose to check for eye coordination. To document normal findings, the provider will use the acronym PERRLA, which means "pupils equal, round, and reactive to light and accommodation."

Ears. The ears are examined with an otoscope covered with a disposable speculum. The external ear is checked first for inflammation of the external auditory canal or for earwax *(cerumen)*. The *tympanic membrane* (eardrum) is examined and should appear pearly gray. Scars on the eardrum are frequently the result of earlier, chronic ear infections or perforations. The color of the eardrum is important to the diagnosis because it may indicate fluids such as blood or pus behind the eardrum in the middle ear. The patient may be asked to swallow several times to allow observation of movement of the tympanic membrane, which occurs because of pressure changes in the eustachian (you STAY shahn) tube. The eustachian tube equalizes air pressure between the middle ear and the throat. The ability of the tympanic membrane to move is crucial to the hearing process.

The otoscope is also often used to view the internal mucosa of the nasal cavity. This is assessed for color and texture. The sinuses cannot be seen, but the frontal and maxillary (MAK suh ler ee) sinuses may be examined by firm palpation over the area and by transillumination (trans i LOO muh ney shun).

> **VOCABULARY**
>
> **emphysema** Thinning and eventual destruction of the alveoli; a type of chronic obstructive pulmonary disease (COPD).
> **nodules** Small lumps, lesions, or swellings that are felt when the skin is palpated.
> **symmetric** Similar in size, form, and arrangement of parts on opposite sides of the body.
> **transillumination** Inspection of a cavity or organ by passing light through its walls.

Mouth and Sinuses. The mouth, or oral cavity, is usually thought of in terms of oral hygiene and dental care. This is important, but the health of the mouth and related structures can also affect the overall health of the entire body. Dental hygiene includes the condition of the teeth, how the patient cares for the teeth and gums, and whether the teeth of the upper and lower jaws meet properly (occlude) for chewing. Healthy gums are pale pink, glossy, and smooth and do not bleed when pressure from a tongue depressor is applied. Poor dental hygiene is known to lead to things such as pneumonia and heart disease. The palatine tonsils are usually visible. The provider may use a tongue depressor and a piece of gauze to grasp the tongue to examine it carefully. The floor of the mouth is examined by both inspection and palpation for enlarged lymph nodes, salivary gland function, and ulcerations. The insides of the cheeks and the gum line are also examined for any abnormal marks or color. The provider may use the otoscope light to help with the examination.

When disorders of the eyes, ears, nose, and throat are observed and the provider believes that the condition warrants the attention of a specialist, the patient is referred to an *ophthalmologist* (OF thahl mol uh jist) or an *otorhinolaryngologist* (oh toh rahy noh lar ing GOL uh jist) (ear, nose, and throat specialist).

Neck

The neck is examined for ROM by having the patient move the head in various directions. The thyroid gland is given special attention for symmetry, size, and texture. The provider manually palpates the thyroid area while the patient swallows several times because this action elevates the thyroid lobes. The carotid artery is palpated and auscultated for possible bruits. The lymph nodes are palpated. *Lymphadenopathy* (lim fad uh NOP ah thee) (enlargement of the lymph nodes) can occur if the patient has an infection of the face, head, or neck.

Chest

While the patient is still in the sitting position, the chest, heart, and lungs are examined. The chest is examined for symmetric expansion. A tape measure may be used, especially if variation exists between the upper and lower chest. For example, a patient with a history of emphysema (em fi SEE mah) may have a barrel-shaped chest. The provider may also use percussion to determine the density of lung tissues.

Placing a stethoscope on the patient's back, the examiner auscultates lung sounds. The patient is asked to take deep, regular breaths. This may produce slight dizziness, but the patient should be assured that it is only the result of the deep respirations and will rapidly pass. The provider notes the types of respirations and the presence of lung sounds in all lobes.

Because considerable concentration is required to interpret heart sounds, the provider must have complete silence when listening to the patient's heart. In patients with heart disease, the provider may spend an extended time listening to heart sounds. If lung or heart abnormalities are found, the provider typically orders further diagnostic tests, including blood analysis, x-ray evaluation, and an electrocardiogram (ECG). Once the results of these studies have been analyzed, the provider may refer the patient to a *cardiologist* (kar DEE ol oh jist) for treatment of a heart condition, or a *pulmonologist* (PULL mun ahl oh jist) or a respiratory care specialist for treatment of a breathing disorder.

MEDICAL TERMINOLOGY	
aden/o	gland
blephar/o	eyelid
lymph/o	lymph, lymphatic tissue
ophthalm/o	eye
ot/o	ear
pulmon/o	lung
rhin/o	nose
-logist	one who specializes in the study of
-pathy	disease condition
-ptosis	drooping
-scope	instrument to view

Abdomen

For the abdominal part of the examination, the patient is lowered into the dorsal recumbent or supine position and the drape is lowered to the pubic hairline. The gown is raised to just under the breasts. The patient's arms may be placed at the side, or the hands may be crossed over the chest or under the head. Relaxation of the abdominal muscles is needed for the abdominal examination. To assist in this goal and to promote patient comfort, a small pillow can be placed under the head and knees. The provider auscultates the abdomen in all quadrants to confirm the presence of complete bowel sounds and palpates the abdomen for any abnormalities. The provider also may use percussion to determine the density, position, and size of underlying abdominal organs.

Reflexes

The patient's reflexes are checked with the patient sitting in the Fowler position or supine. While the patient is sitting, the biceps are checked with the patient's arm flexed and supported by the examiner. The knee jerk (*patellar reflex*) and the ankle jerk (*Achilles reflex*) are checked using a reflex hammer.

The plantar reflexes are tested with the patient in an upright or a supine position. The *Babinski reflex* is a normal reflex in infants. When the sole of the foot has been firmly stroked, the big toe then moves toward the top surface of the foot and the other toes fan out.

Breast and Testicles

Careful breast examination is part of the physical examination for every female, even if she is asymptomatic. The breasts are examined both by inspection, with the patient in the Fowler position, and by inspection and palpation with the patient in the supine position. The arm on the side that is being examined is bent and tucked under the head. Breast cancer is the most common malignancy in women, and early detection is the key to successful treatment.

In the past patients were encouraged to complete a monthly breast self-examination (BSE) at home. However, current research has shown that this may lead to unnecessary stress and overuse of diagnostic testing. This is due to patients not being clearly trained and becoming very concerned over normal changes in breast tissue. Some providers still encourage females to do monthly BSE, and others do not. It is most important for females to be aware of changes in their breasts and to report these to the provider. Concerns to report to the provider include:

- Visual changes (e.g., puckering, dimpling, or changes in size or shape)
- A hard lump within the breast or under the armpit
- An abnormal discharge from the nipple

It is also important to note that men have breast tissue to over their pectoral muscles and can also suffer from breast cancer. Men who have concerning lumps or visual changes to the chest area should consult their healthcare provider.

For male patients who have reached puberty or are 14 years of age or older, the provider performs a testicular examination. The provider looks for lumps, swelling, shrinking, or any other signs of a problem. As with the BSE there has been a strong push historically to have all male patients perform testicular self-examinations (TSE); however, there are no set guidelines in recommending this to patients. Currently this recommendation is based on provider preference and facility policies. Medical assistants should know and understand their providers' preferences and the facility policies and use these as guidelines for patient education. Regardless of whether a TSE is recommended, men should be advised to consult with their healthcare provider if they notice any abnormalities in this area.

CRITICAL THINKING 35.5

Alice Greenbaum, a 68-year-old patient of Dr. Walden, is scheduled for an annual physical examination, including a breast check and Pap test. Mrs. Greenbaum appears anxious and asks Chris whether the gynecologic examination is necessary. How should Chris answer this patient? What might help to ease the patient's fears and prepare her for the examination?

Rectum

The rectal examination usually follows the abdominal examination or may be part of the examination of the genitalia. It can be done on both males and females to evaluate for problems such as internal hemorrhoids and gastrointestinal bleeding. A rectal exam should be performed in all men over age 50 as this is the least intrusive way for a provider to evaluate the prostate. Preserving the patient's comfort and dignity is vital during these types of examinations. For this part of the examination, the provider needs gloves and water-soluble lubricating jelly (e.g., KY jelly). The examination light should be directed at the perineal area during the examination.

Fecal occult blood test specimens are often collected at the time of the digital rectal examination. If this is a procedure the provider performs, be sure to include the necessary collection folder with the examination equipment. Patients diagnosed with gastrointestinal (GI) disorders may be referred to a *gastroenterologist* (gas troh en tuh ROL uh jist).

MEDICAL TERMINOLOGY

enter/o	small intestine
gastr/o	stomach

VISION AND HEARING SCREENINGS

There are some basic screening procedures that medical assistants perform during a physical examination. Some of the more common ones are screenings related to the eye and ear. Eye procedures would include distance visual acuity (ah KYOO ih tee), near visual acuity, and color vision screening. Ear procedures would include hearing screening using tuning forks or audiometers. In order to measure visual and auditory acuity most accurately, it is necessary to understand the disorders that can cause issues here.

VOCABULARY

acuity Test of the clearness or sharpness of vision.

CRITICAL THINKING 35.6

Chris is performing visual acuity examinations. Dr. Martin asks him whether he understands the causes of refractive errors. Chris has difficulty explaining why refractive errors occur. So he tells Dr. Martin that he will research the topic and get back to him. What have you learned about the different refractive disorders and why they occur?

Distance Visual Acuity

Determining distance visual acuity (DVA) is frequently part of a complete physical examination, especially for children. Often the DVA is completed by the medical assistant before the provider enters the room (Procedure 35.9). The DVA chart can consist of letters, numbers, or pictures printed in lines of decreasing size. This test uses one of three charts:

- Snellen chart: The most commonly used chart; it displays various letters of the alphabet (Fig. 35.7A).
- Tumbling E chart: This chart is used for individuals with limited knowledge of the English alphabet. It displays the letter E, which faces in different directions. To avoid confusion, the medical assistant should review what is meant by "facing" before the patient starts the test (Fig. 35.7B). The patient can use their fingers to show the direction the E is facing.

- Symbol chart. This is used for young children who do not yet know their alphabet. It uses symbols that indicate common items, such as a cup or a boat. Children are asked what picture they see. As with the E chart, it is important to review the possible symbols with patients before starting. Also be aware that what we may consider a cup, a child could call by a different name, such as a mug or a glass.

All of these charts are based on the same principle. People with normal vision can read the symbol on the top line of the chart at 200 feet. In each of the succeeding rows, from the top down, the size of the symbols is reduced so that a person with normal vision can see them at distances of 100, 70, 50, 40, 30, 20, 15, and 10 feet, consecutively.

The patient must not be allowed to study the chart before taking the test. The room or hall should be long enough that the 20-foot distance can be marked off accurately, and it must be free of interruptions from patient and staff traffic. The chart should be hung at the patient's eye level and illuminated with maximum light, without glare on the chart. To complete the test the patient should be asked to read the chart from the top down with each eye individually, and then with them both together. The patient should be advised to cover the eye not in use but not to press in on the eye. This could make the vision blurry and invalidate the test when that eye is being used. Also, it is possible for patients to memorize the order of the letters, specifically from one eye to the next. Because of this it is good practice to ask the patient to read the letters in reverse order or randomize the order that they read the letters as they move through the test.

During a normal physical exam, the provider generally needs to know if the patient's vision is adequate for a healthy lifestyle. If the patient normally wears corrective lenses as part of their normal daily routine, they should wear the corrective lenses when being tested for distance vision. The medical assistant should indicate in the medical record that the test was done with corrective lenses. You cannot always see corrective lenses, so it is a good practice to always ask patients without glasses if they are wearing contact lenses.

When documenting the DVA test results, record the findings for each eye separately and as fractions. The numerator (top number) is the distance of the patient from the chart (usually 20 feet), and the denominator (bottom number) is the lowest line read satisfactorily by the patient. For example, if the patient was able to successfully read the 40 line with the left eye, this should be documented as left eye 20/40. "Satisfactory" means the patient did not squint or strain when reading the line. The patient also was able to correctly identify a majority of the characters on that line. The number of mistakes allowed to be considered a pass will depend on the expectations of the provider and what exactly they are looking for. (The standard of two or fewer errors is commonly used for lines with five or more characters.) Be sure to understand your facility's policies with regard to how many figures per line can be missed in determining whether the reading of that line is successful. If a facility allows a line to be considered "passed" with errors, make sure this is also clearly documented. For example, if a patient successfully reads the 20/15 line with two errors using both eyes, the finding would be documented: both eyes 20/15 −2. The medical assistant should

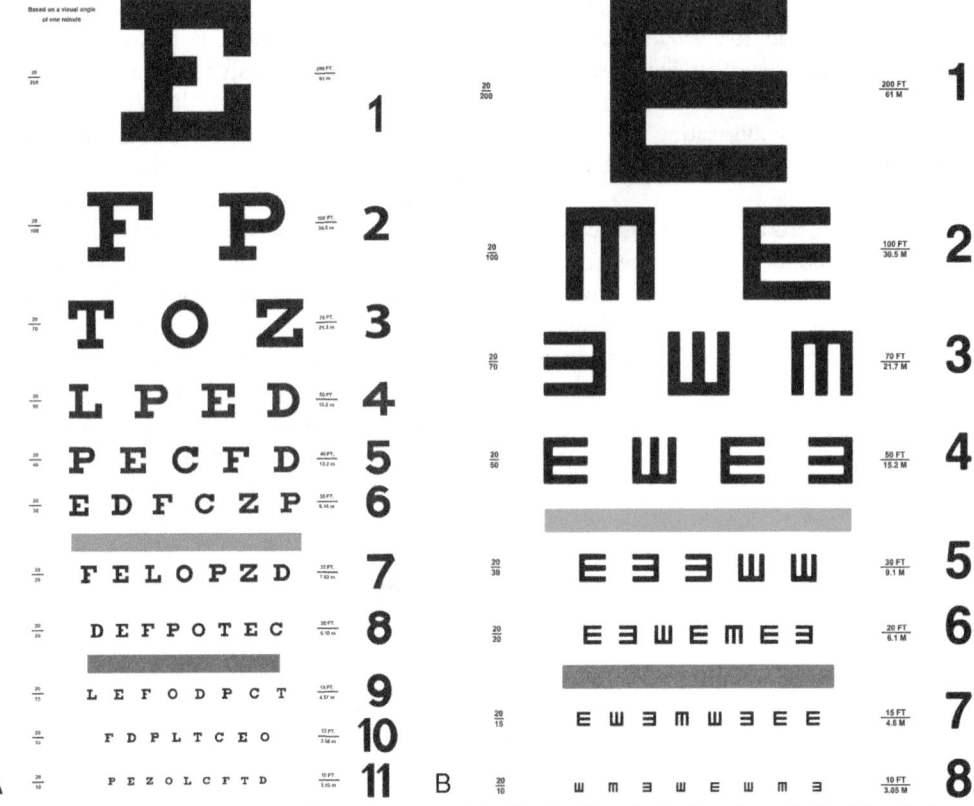

Fig. 35.7 Distance Visual Acuity Charts Developed by Dr. Snellen. A, Snellen chart. B, Tumbling E chart. (A courtesy joebelanger/iStock.com; B courtesy grebeshkov/iStock.com.)

BOX 35.2   Interpreting Snellen Results

- The patient stands 20 feet from the chart.
- Each result is a record of how well the patient can see compared with normal vision.
  - *Example*: A patient with a 20/40 reading can see that line correctly standing at 20 feet, but an individual with normal vision can see the same line correctly at 40 feet, so the patient's vision is not as acute as someone with normal vision.
  - *Example*: A patient with a 20/15 reading can see that line accurately standing at 20 feet, but a person with normal vision must stand at 15 feet to have the same vision, meaning the patient's vision is better than someone with normal vision.

---

document the outcomes of the test, specifying the results for each eye and for both eyes. Box 35.2 provides more information about interpreting Snellen results.

The Joint Commission no longer recommends the use of medical abbreviations for the eyes and ears because they are frequently confused or misinterpreted. The medical assistant must now document right eye, left eye, and both eyes.

Near Visual Acuity

Near visual acuity (NVA) can be tested with the near vision acuity chart (Fig. 35.8). The test should be given in a well-lit room, with the patient holding the card approximately 14 to 16 inches away. As with the Snellen examination, the near visual acuity test is given for each eye, starting with the right eye. The eye

not being tested should be covered with an occluder but remain open. The patient should be monitored for indications of difficulty, such as squinting or tearing. The patient reads the card, starting at the top, until reaching the smallest print that can be read. The medical assistant should document the number at which the patient had no more than two errors for each eye and also the two eyes together, whether corrective lenses were worn, and any signs of eyestrain.

CRITICAL THINKING 35.7

Susie Anthony, a 19-year-old patient, was seen for a general eye examination. The provider orders a routine Snellen test, and Chris administers it. Susie wears contact lenses. With her right eye, she reads without errors to the 20/25 line; however, she squints and makes three errors at the 20/20 line. With her left eye, Susie makes two mistakes at the 20/20 line; with both eyes she reads the 20/25 without errors. How should Chris document this procedure?

Ishihara Test

The most common test for color vision is the Ishihara test. The Ishihara test is a simple, convenient, and accurate procedure. It detects total color blindness, in addition to the red-green blindness prevalent in congenital blindness (Procedure 35.10). The test assesses the perception of primary colors and shades of colors.

The test booklet contains plates made up of colored dots in numeric patterns. The numbers are one color, and the background dots are a different color. Patients with average visual acuity can read the number within the dot matrix without difficulty. Patients

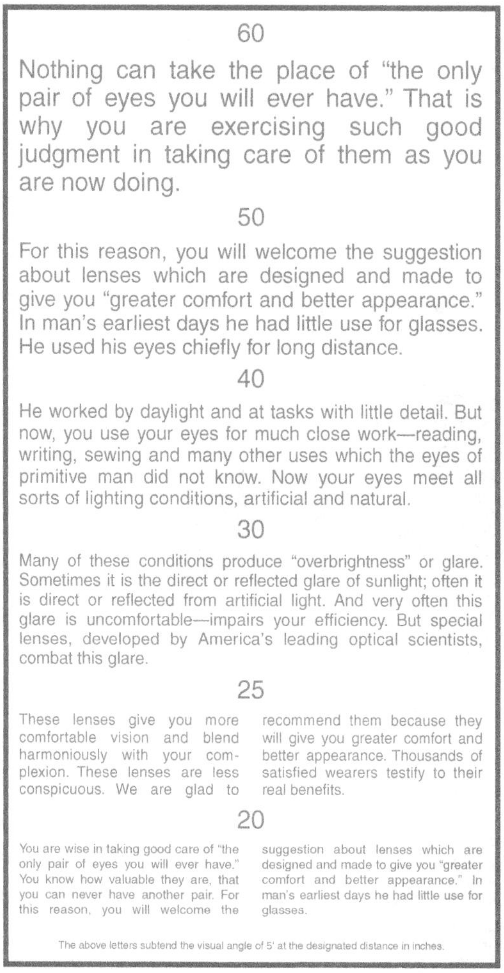

60

Nothing can take the place of "the only pair of eyes you will ever have." That is why you are exercising such good judgment in taking care of them as you are now doing.

50

For this reason, you will welcome the suggestion about lenses which are designed and made to give you "greater comfort and better appearance." In man's earliest days he had little use for glasses. He used his eyes chiefly for long distance.

40

He worked by daylight and at tasks with little detail. But now, you use your eyes for much close work—reading, writing, sewing and many other uses which the eyes of primitive man did not know. Now your eyes meet all sorts of lighting conditions, artificial and natural.

30

Many of these conditions produce "overbrightness" or glare. Sometimes it is the direct or reflected glare of sunlight; often it is direct or reflected from artificial light. And very often this glare is uncomfortable—impairs your efficiency. But special lenses, developed by America's leading optical scientists, combat this glare.

25

These lenses give you more comfortable vision and blend harmoniously with your complexion. These lenses are less conspicuous. We are glad to recommend them because they will give you greater comfort and better appearance. Thousands of satisfied wearers testify to their real benefits.

20

You are wise in taking good care of "the only pair of eyes you will ever have." You know how valuable they are, that you can never have another pair. For this reason, you will welcome the suggestion about lenses which are designed and made to give you "greater comfort and better appearance." In man's earliest days he had little use for glasses.

The above letters subtend the visual angle of 5' at the designated distance in inches.

Fig. 35.8 Near Vision Acuity Chart.

with color vision defects are unable to read the number, or they see a totally different number. A section of plates is included that contains colored line trails through a background of dots. These plates are designed to be used with children and adults who are unable to read numbers. In this situation, the patient uses a finger to follow the dotted trail through the picture.

The test should be administered in a quiet room that is well illuminated by sunlight, not by artificial lighting. If this is not doable, create the best situation possible by adjusting lights to resemble the effect of natural daylight. The test uses 14 color plates. The basic test consists of plates 1 through 11. Plates 12 through 14 are used if the patient appears to be having difficulty with red-green differentiations. The medical assistant records the number of plates read correctly. If the score is 10 or higher, the patient is within the average range (normal finding). If the score is 7 or lower, the patient is suspected of having a color deficiency, and the ophthalmologist performs additional assessment tests using more precise color vision testing equipment.

Tuning Fork Testing

Tuning fork tests measure hearing by:

- Air conduction: Sound waves moving through the air. Hearing loss related to air conduction is called *sensorineural hearing loss.*

- Bone conduction: Sound vibrations through cranial bones to the inner ear. Hearing loss related to bone conduction is called *conductive hearing loss.*

If there are hearing losses noted in both, the condition is called a *mixed hearing loss.*

Tuning forks are available in different sizes, each with a different frequency. The most commonly used tuning fork is the 512 hertz (hurts) (Hz), which means that it vibrates 512 cycles per second, the level of normal speech patterns (Fig. 35.9A). To activate the fork, the provider holds it by the stem and strikes the tines softly on the palm of the hand. Striking the tines too forcefully creates a tone that is too loud for diagnostic use. The two tests used to evaluate hearing are the Weber and Rinne tests. Both of these procedures are commonly used to evaluate conductive and sensory losses.

The *Rinne test* is designed to test for sensorineural hearing loss. In this test, the stem of the vibrating fork is placed on the patient's mastoid process, and the patient is instructed to raise a hand when the sound disappears. The fork is quickly inverted so that the vibrating tines are approximately 1 inch in front of the external ear canal. If hearing is normal, the patient should still hear a sound. In normal hearing, the sound is heard twice as long by air conduction as by bone conduction (Fig. 35.9B).

The *Weber test* is used to find issues with conductive hearing loss. In the Weber test the vibrating tuning fork is placed in the center of the top of the head, and the patient is asked in which ear the tone is louder or if the tone is the same in both ears. Because the patient is hearing the tone by bone conduction through the head, a normal result is hearing the sound equally in both ears (Fig. 35.9C).

VOCABULARY

hertz The unit of measurement used in hearing examinations; a wave frequency equal to 1 cycle per second.

Audiometric Testing

An audiometric test may be done in an otology, a pediatrics, or a family practice and is performed by medical assistants. Audiometry measures the lowest intensity of sound an individual can hear (Fig. 35.10). Audiometers can vary greatly. Some machines require headphones to be placed over the ears. Other machines are handheld. The medical assistant inserts ear tip into the ear and within one minute the hearing can be screened. The medical assistant must receive training on the audiometer before screening patients with the machine.

Regardless of how the specifics of the individual machine work, each ear is tested by delivering a single frequency at a specific intensity. The test starts with low-frequency tones and works to very high frequencies. This is because hearing loss typically starts with high frequencies. Starting with low frequencies makes it more likely that the patient will hear the first tones and be more comfortable with the test as the tones get higher.

Patients are asked to signal when they hear the sound. The results are printed on a graph, called an *audiogram,* or the medical assistant charts the results on a graph sheet (Procedure 35.11). An adult with normal hearing can hear tone frequencies below 25 decibels, and children with normal hearing can hear

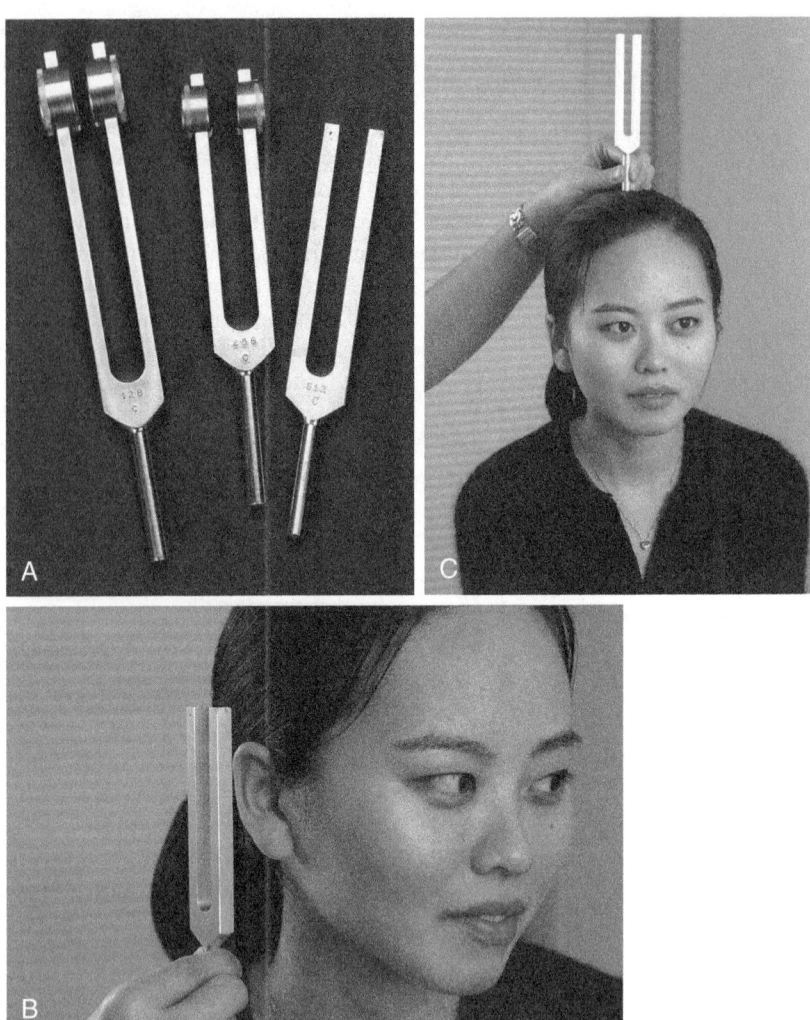

Fig. 35.9 A, Turning forks. B, Weber test. C, Rinne test. (From Niedzwiecki B, et al: *Kinn's the medical assistant,* ed 14, St. Louis, 2020, Elsevier.)

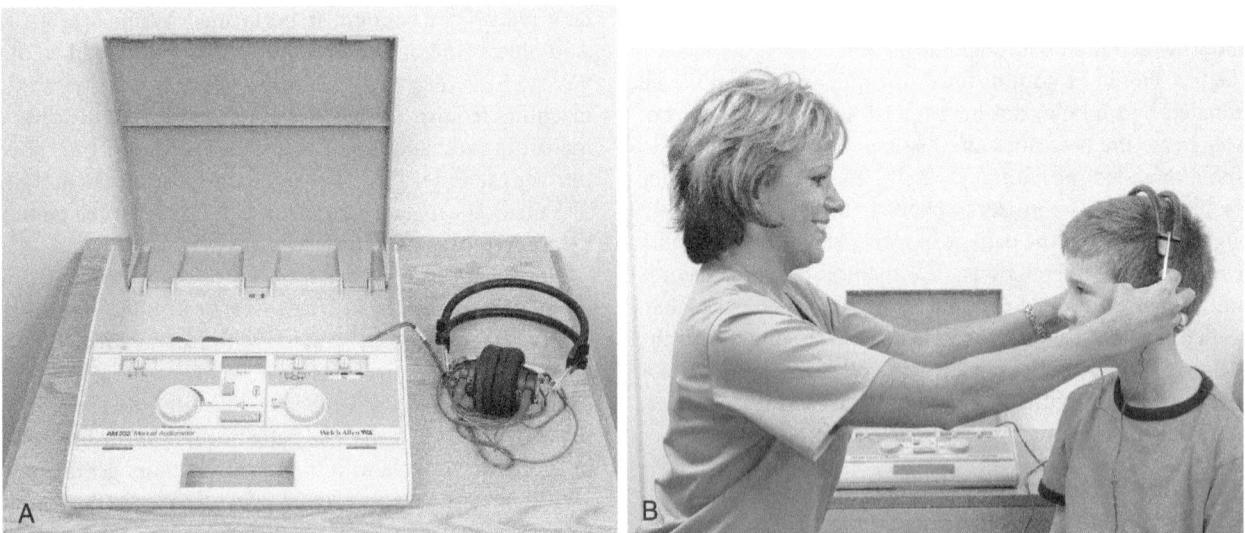

Fig. 35.10 Audiometer With Headset. (From Niedzwiecki B, et al: *Kinn's the medical assistant,* ed 14, St. Louis, 2020, Elsevier.)

those below 15 decibels. If initial screening indicates a hearing deficit, the provider may recommend an appointment with an audiologist (aw dee OL uh jist) for audiometric evaluation.

> **VOCABULARY**
> **audiologist** An allied healthcare professional who specializes in the evaluation of hearing function, detection of hearing impairment, and determination of the anatomic site of impairment.

MEDICAL SCRIBE

The role of medical scribe is relatively new to healthcare. A medical scribe is in the exam room with the provider during the visit. The provider examines the patient and verbalizes the findings. The medical scribe documents the findings in the electronic health record (EHR). This allows the provider to focus on the patient without needing to use the computer. The provider is more efficient with this medical model and can see more patients without reducing the quality of care. This also ensures that documentation is done in a timely manner.

After the visit, the provider will review the notes entered by the medical assistant and sign them. It is important that the notes show the scribe's signature and the provider's signature. EHR systems are set up to do this automatically. If you are asked to scribe in an EHR system, make sure that you do so under your individual login. You can never document using the provider's login.

When a provider orders a medication, the medical assistants may be asked to prepare patient's prescriptions for the provider to sign. The medical assistant may also print off patient education information and send referral requests if the patient is to be referred. It is essential that the medical assistant be very familiar with the documentation system before taking on this role.

A person can obtain a degree in medical scribing, but it is also a job that a medical assistant can do. With training in medical terminology, anatomy, disease processes, treatment protocols, and the physical exam process, a medical assistant has the knowledge required to scribe. To excel at scribing, the medical assistant must be discreet, organized, attentive, and show attention to detail.

CLOSING COMMENTS

Medical assistants play a vital role in the physical examination process. Being familiar with the supplies needed and making sure that they are available in the examination room make the process more efficient. Using good body mechanics helps to protect you and your patient. Whether the medical assistant is directly assisting with the examination or performing screening tests, their role in the physical examination is essential. Using what you have learned in this chapter will help to make you a valued medical assistant.

PATIENT-CENTERED CARE

Being kind and showing respect are two traits that are essential for every medical assistant. This is very much the case as the medical assistant assists with the physical examination. People do not tend to enjoy having a physical examination. It can be very intrusive and often requires patients to expose their body in ways that could make them feel quite uncomfortable. Working to safeguard the patient's privacy as much as possible with adequate gowning and draping helps prevent unnecessary exposure and embarrassment for patients. Knowing the exam sequence and having the equipment ready can reduce the time the patient is in uncomfortable positions. Supporting the provider in equipment handling, completing testing, and assisting with documentation can allow the patient to have more time in conversation with the provider and help them feel as if they are being heard.

BEING PROFESSIONAL

Understanding the physical examination process and documentation of that exam will show that the medical assistant is competent and can do a lot to help the patient feel comfortable. You are working at WMFM Clinic and are asked to set up an exam room for a physical exam to be done by a new provider.

Role-play the scenario with a peer. Make a list of things that a new provider may have preferences for regarding examinations. Your peer will play the provider. Using the list, ask about the provider's preferences and gather information on what the provider would like set out for the examination.

CHAPTER REVIEW

This chapter focused on how to prepare for the physical examination. It is important to have the room well supplied so that the exam can proceed efficiently. Knowing the instruments needed for the exam will help you to assist the provider. Knowing the positions needed will help you to assist the patient. Using good body mechanics will help to keep you and your patient safe.

The methods of examination were presented. Understanding each of the methods and when it is used will allow you to better help the provider. Knowing the positions and methods of examination needed for each part of the examination sequence will make the examination go more smoothly.

We discussed vision and hearing screening tests. These tests are often part of a complete physical examination. A Snellen chart is used to assess distance visual acuity. Near visual acuity can be assessed with a chart showing type in different sizes. Ishihara plates are used to assess color vision. For hearing screening, a set of tuning forks can be used, in addition to an audiometer.

In the last section of this chapter we discussed medical documentation and scribing. Because medical assistants are often present in the examination room to assist and to chaperone, they can also work to help the provider be more productive by assisting in the documentation of the visit. Close attention to detail and a clear understanding of what is going on is essential for good scribing.

SCENARIO WRAP-UP

Chris has taken on the responsibility of making sure all the exam rooms are fully supplied and the equipment is in working order. This requires going through each exam room at least once per day, and it has helped him feel more comfortable working in the exam room assisting the provider with examinations. Chris knows what is needed and where it can be found at any time.

He is also able to place patients in all the appropriate positions during the examination. In addition, he can provide complete vision and hearing screenings when needed. Chris has realized the importance of proper body mechanics and how to use these to safeguard himself while also keeping his patient's safe and secure.

PROCEDURE 35.1 Use Proper Body Mechanics

Task
Safely transfer a patient from a wheelchair to an exam table using proper body mechanics.

Equipment and Supplies
- Patient's health record
- Wheelchair
- Exam table with pull-out footrest
- Gait belt

Procedural Steps
1. Wash hands or use hand sanitizer.
   Purpose: Hand sanitization is an important step for infection control.
2. Greet the patient. Identify yourself. Verify the patient's identity with full name and date of birth. Explain the procedure to be performed in a manner that the patient understands. Determine how much assistance the patient will need to transfer from the wheelchair to the exam table. Do not proceed if you think you will need additional help.
   Purpose: To promote the patient's cooperation during the transfer and prevent personal injury.
3. Place the wheelchair at a 45-degree angle toward the footrest at the base of the exam table.
4. Lock the brakes on the wheelchair and move the footrests of the wheelchair out of the way (Fig. 1).
   Purpose: Never transfer a patient into or out of a wheelchair until the brakes are locked on both sides of the chair.

5. Place the gait belt around the patient's waist over clothing with the buckle in front. Insert the belt through the teeth of the buckle and pull it tight to lock it. The belt should be tight with just enough room to place your fingers under it.
6. Request that the patient place both feet flat on the floor with the hands on the armrests.
   Purpose: This position helps you grasp the gait belt; the patient can use the wheelchair armrests to help push up into an upright position, and feet flat on the floor help with patient stability.
7. Stand directly in front of the patient with your feet apart, back straight, and knees bent (see Fig. 2).
   Purpose: This position helps you maintain good body mechanics during the transfer.

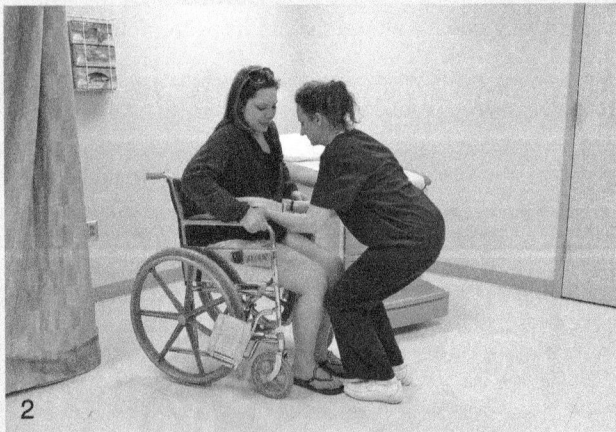

8. Slide your fingers under the gait belt on opposite sides of the patient's waist.
9. Instruct the patient at the count of 3 to push off from the armrests while you at the same time grasp the gait belt and, using your leg muscles, straighten your knees so that the patient is in a standing position.
   Purpose: This position allows the patient to assist as much as possible while you are using the large muscles of your legs to help lift the patient.
10. Ask the patient to step up onto the footrest at the bottom of the exam table and assist the person in pivoting and sitting down on the exam table. Remove the gait belt until the provider has completed the examination (see Fig. 3).

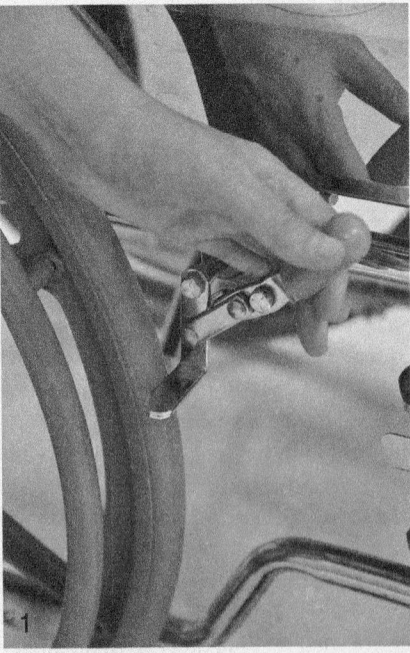

PROCEDURE 35.1 Use Proper Body Mechanics–cont'd

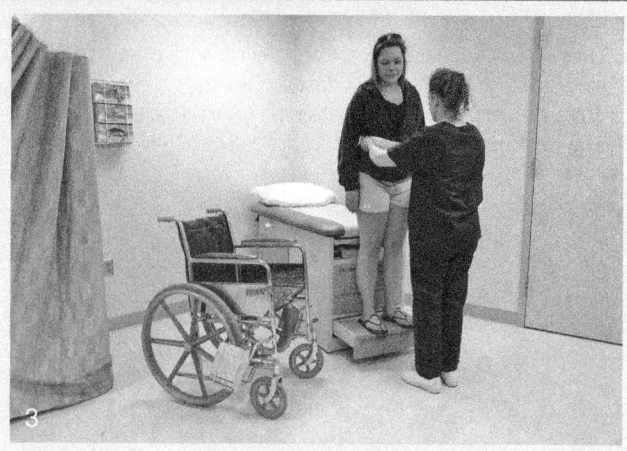

11. After the examination is complete, place the wheelchair at an angle next to the exam table and lock the wheels. Replace the gait belt. Make sure the patient is positioned at the edge of the table.
    Purpose: To prepare for transfer back to the wheelchair.
12. Place yourself directly in front of the patient with your back straight and your knees bent. Slide your fingers under the gait belt on opposite sides of the patient's waist.
13. Grasp the gait belt on both sides at the waist. Instruct the patient at the count of 3 to push off from the exam table and, using your leg muscles, straighten your knees so that the patient is in a standing position on the footrest.
14. Maintaining your hold on the gait belt, ask the patient to step down. Pivot the person so that they can slowly sit in the wheelchair; at the same time, bend your knees but keep your back straight.
15. Remove the gait belt. Replace the wheelchair footrests and unlock the brakes on the wheelchair.

PROCEDURE 35.2 Sitting, Full Fowler, and Semi-Fowler Positions

Tasks

Position and drape the patient for examinations of the head, neck, and chest, or position and drape patients who have difficulty breathing when lying flat.

Equipment and Supplies

- Patient's health record
- Exam table, pillow, and table paper
- Patient gown and drape
- Disinfectant wipes
- Gloves
- Waste container

Procedural Steps

1. Wash hands or use hand sanitizer.
   Purpose: Hand sanitization is an important step for infection control.
2. Greet the patient. Identify yourself. Verify the patient's identity with full name and date of birth. Explain the procedure to be performed in a manner that the patient understands. Answer any questions the patient may have about the procedure.
   Purpose: To promote the patient's understanding and cooperation during the examination.
3. Give the patient a gown. Explain what clothing must be removed for the examination being done and whether the gown should open in the front or the back. Provide assistance as needed. Give the patient privacy while changing. Knock on the examination room door before reentering to make sure the patient has completed undressing and gowning.
4. For the sitting position: Instruct the patient to sit at the end of the exam table. The person's legs can dangle over the edge of the table (Fig. 1). Ensure the patient is not dizzy and is safe to sit at the edge of the table. Cover the patient with a drape, ensuring all exposed areas from the patient's upper chest to legs are covered.
   Purpose: Draping the patient provides warmth and privacy while giving the provider access to the examination site.

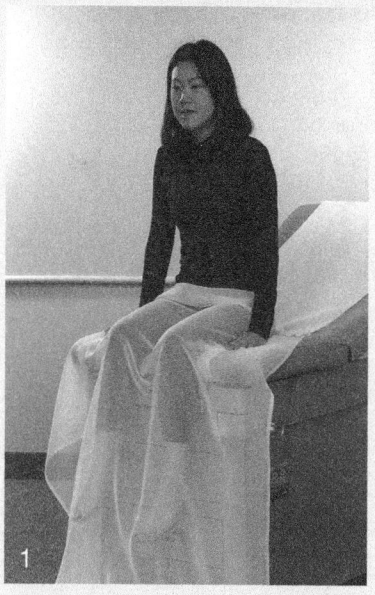

5. For the full Fowler position: Position the head of the exam table to a 90-degree angle. Assist the patient into the full Fowler position. Extend the footrest as needed for patient comfort. Cover the patient with a drape, ensuring all exposed areas from the patient's upper chest to legs are covered.
6. For the semi-Fowler position: Position the head of the exam table to a 45-degree angle. Assist the patient into the semi-Fowler position (Fig. 2). Position the pillow so the patient is comfortable. Extend the footrest as needed for patient comfort. Cover the patient with a drape, ensuring all exposed areas from the patient's upper chest to legs are covered.
7. After the examination has been completed, assist the patient as needed to get off the table and get dressed.

Continued

PROCEDURE 35.2   Sitting, Full Fowler, and Semi-Fowler Positions–cont'd

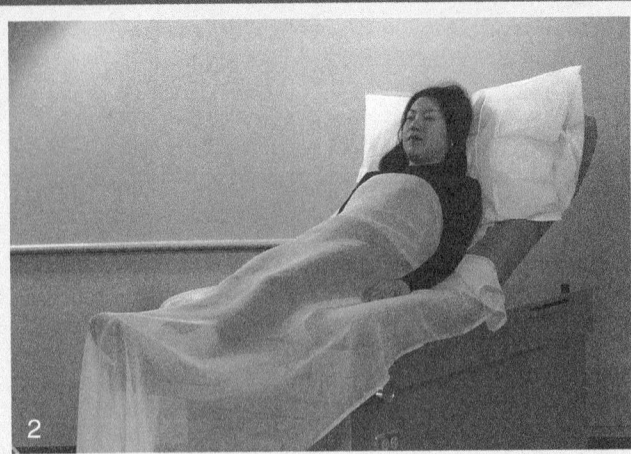

8. Put on gloves and use disinfectant wipes to clean the exam table and all potentially contaminated surfaces. Dispose of the used gloves and exam table paper in the waste container. Wash hands or use hand sanitizer.
   Purpose: To ensure infection control and to prevent the transmission of pathogens from one patient to another.
9. Allow the exam table to dry before pulling clean paper over the table.

PROCEDURE 35.3   Supine (Horizontal Recumbent) and Dorsal Recumbent Positions

Tasks

Position and drape the patient for examinations of the abdomen, heart, and breasts in the horizontal recumbent (supine) position and exams of the rectal, vaginal, and perineal areas in the dorsal recumbent position.

Equipment and Supplies

- Patient's health record
- Exam table, pillow, and table paper
- Patient gown and drape
- Disinfectant wipes
- Gloves
- Waste container

Procedural Steps

1. Wash hands or use hand sanitizer.
   Purpose: Hand sanitization is an important step for infection control.
2. Greet the patient. Identify yourself. Verify the patient's identity with full name and date of birth. Explain the procedure to be performed in a manner that the patient understands. Answer any questions the patient may have about the procedure.
   Purpose: To promote the patient's understanding and cooperation during the examination.
3. Give the patient a gown. Explain the clothing that must be removed for the examination being done and whether the gown should open in the front or in the back. Provide assistance as needed. For the supine position, the gown should be open in the front. Give the patient privacy while changing. Knock on the examination room door before reentering to make sure the patient has completed undressing and gowning.
4. Do not place the patient in the necessary positions until the provider is ready for that part of the examination.
   Purpose: To ensure the patient's privacy, comfort, and modesty.
5. For the supine (horizontal recumbent) position: Pull out the table extension that supports the patient's legs. Help the patient lie flat on the table with the face upward (Fig. 1). Place the drape so it is lengthwise from the top of the chest to the legs.
   Purpose: Draping the patient provides warmth and privacy while giving the provider access to the examination site.
6. For the dorsal recumbent position: Have the patient lie flat on the back and flex the knees so the feet are flat on the table (Fig. 2). Place the drape so it is in a diamond shape, with one corner on the patient's chest and the opposite corner over and between the legs.

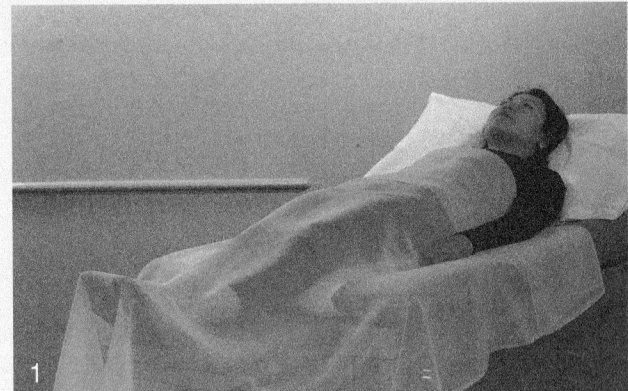

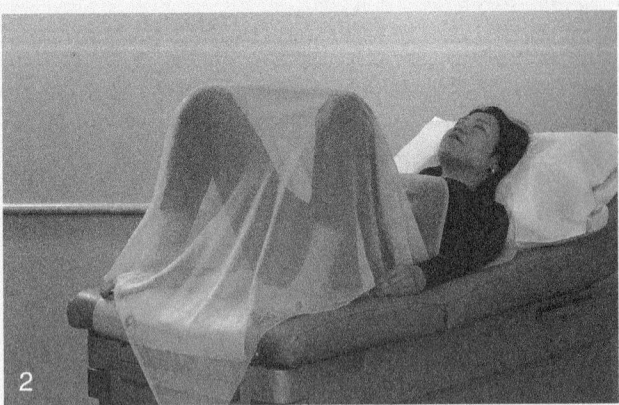

7. After the examination has been completed, assist the patient as needed to get off the table and get dressed.
8. Put on gloves and use disinfectant wipes to clean the exam table and all potentially contaminated surfaces. Dispose of the used gloves and exam table paper in the waste container. Wash hands or use hand sanitizer.
   Purpose: To ensure infection control and to prevent the transmission of pathogens from one patient to another.
9. Allow the exam table to dry before pulling clean paper over the table.

PROCEDURE 35.4 Lithotomy Position

Tasks

Position and drape the patient primarily for vaginal and pelvic examinations and Pap tests.

Equipment and Supplies
- Patient's health record
- Exam table, pillow, and table paper
- Patient gown and drape
- Disinfectant wipes
- Gloves
- Waste container

Procedural Steps

1. Wash hands or use hand sanitizer.
   Purpose: Hand sanitization is an important step for infection control.
2. Greet the patient. Identify yourself. Verify the patient's identity with full name and date of birth. Explain the procedure to be performed in a manner that the patient understands. Answer any questions the patient may have about the procedure.
   Purpose: To promote the patient's understanding and cooperation during the examination.
3. Give the patient a gown. Instruct the patient to undress from the waist down with the gown open in the back. If the provider also will be doing a breast examination, the patient should undress completely and put on the gown so that it opens in the front. Provide assistance as needed. Give the patient privacy while changing. Knock on the examination room door before reentering to make sure the patient has completed undressing and gowning.
4. Have the patient sit on the exam table. Do not place the patient in the lithotomy position until the provider is ready for that part of the examination.
   Purpose: To promote the patient's privacy, comfort, and safety.
5. Pull out the table extension that supports the patient's legs and help the patient lie face upward on the table. Pull out the stirrups, adjust their extension length for the patient's comfort, and lock them in place.
6. Reinsert the table extension and have the patient move toward the foot of the table with her buttocks on the bottom table edge. Gently place the

patient's legs in the stirrups, checking for comfort. The patient's arms can be placed alongside the body or across the chest (Fig. 1).

Note: Some offices may stock cloth or paper stirrup covers to protect the patient and make the position more comfortable.

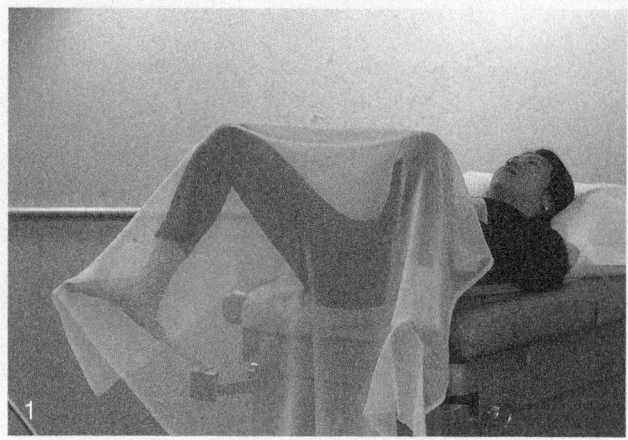

7. Place the drop in a diamond shape, with one corner on the patient's chest and the opposite corner over and between the legs. The perineal area should be covered along with any other exposed area from the top of the chest to the legs.
   Purpose: To provide warmth and privacy for the patient while giving the provider access to the examination site.
8. After the examination has been completed, assist the patient as needed to get off the table and get dressed.
9. Put on gloves and use disinfectant wipes to clean the exam table and all potentially contaminated surfaces. Dispose of the used gloves and exam table paper in the waste container. Wash hands or use hand sanitizer.
   Purpose: To ensure infection control and to prevent the transmission of pathogens from one patient to another.
10. Allow the exam table to dry before pulling clean paper over the table.

PROCEDURE 35.5 Left Lateral Position

Tasks

Position and drape the patient for examination of the rectum, instillation of rectal medication, perineal examination, and some pelvic examinations.

Equipment and Supplies
- Patient's health record
- Exam table, pillow, and table paper
- Patient gown and drape
- Disinfectant wipes
- Gloves
- Waste container

Procedural Steps

1. Wash hands or use hand sanitizer.
   Purpose: Hand sanitization is an important step for infection control.
2. Greet the patient. Identify yourself. Verify the patient's identity with full name and date of birth. Explain the procedure to be performed in a manner that the

patient understands. Answer any questions the patient may have about the procedure.
   Purpose: To promote the patient's understanding and cooperation during the examination.
3. Give the patient a gown and explain what clothing must be removed for the examination being done. Tell the patient that the gown should open in the back. Provide assistance as needed. Give the patient privacy while changing. Knock on the examination room door before reentering to make sure the patient has completed undressing and gowning.
4. Do not place the patient in the left lateral position until the provider is ready for that part of the examination.
   Purpose: To promote the patient's privacy, comfort, and safety.
5. Help the patient turn onto the left side; the left arm and shoulder should be drawn back behind the body so that the patient is tilted onto the chest. Flex the right arm upward for support, slightly flex the left leg, and sharply flex the right leg upward. Help the patient move the buttocks to the side edge of the table (Fig. 1).

Continued

PROCEDURE 35.5   Left Lateral Position–cont'd

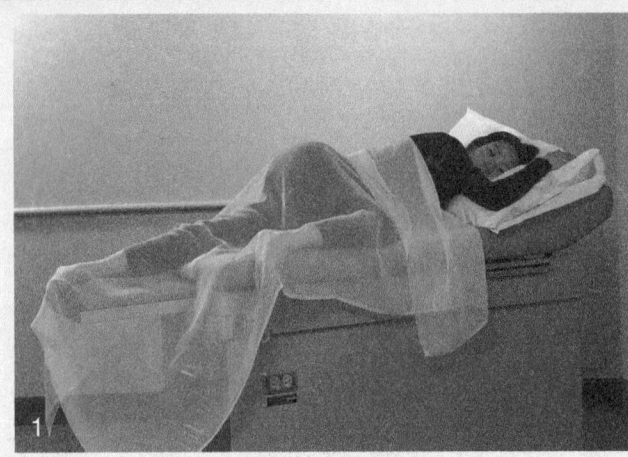

6. Place the drape on the patient diagonally from under the arms to below the knees.
   Purpose: Draping the patient provides warmth and privacy while giving the provider access to the examination site.
7. After the examination has been completed, assist the patient as needed to get off the table and get dressed.
8. Put on gloves and use disinfectant wipes to clean the exam table and all potentially contaminated surfaces. Dispose of the used gloves and exam table paper in the waste container. Wash hands or use hand sanitizer.
   Purpose: To ensure infection control and prevent the transmission of pathogens from one patient to another.
9. Allow the exam table to dry before pulling clean paper over the table.

PROCEDURE 35.6   Prone Position

Tasks
Position and drape the patient for examination of the back and certain surgical procedures.

Equipment and Supplies
- Patient's health record
- Exam table, pillow, and table paper
- Patient gown and drape
- Disinfectant wipes
- Gloves
- Waste container

Procedural Steps
1. Wash hands or use hand sanitizer.
   Purpose: Hand sanitization is an important step for infection control.
2. Greet the patient. Identify yourself. Verify the patient's identity with full name and date of birth. Explain the procedure to be performed in a manner that the patient understands. Answer any questions the patient may have about the procedure.
   Purpose: To promote the patient's understanding and cooperation during the examination.
3. Give the patient a gown and explain what clothing must be removed for the examination being done. Tell the patient that the gown should open in the back. Provide assistance as needed. Give the patient privacy while changing. Knock on the examination room door before reentering to make sure the patient has completed undressing and gowning.
4. Do not place the patient in the prone position until the provider is ready for that part of the examination.
   Purpose: To promote the patient's privacy, comfort, and safety.
5. Pull out the table extension and help patients lie down on their stomach (Fig. 1).

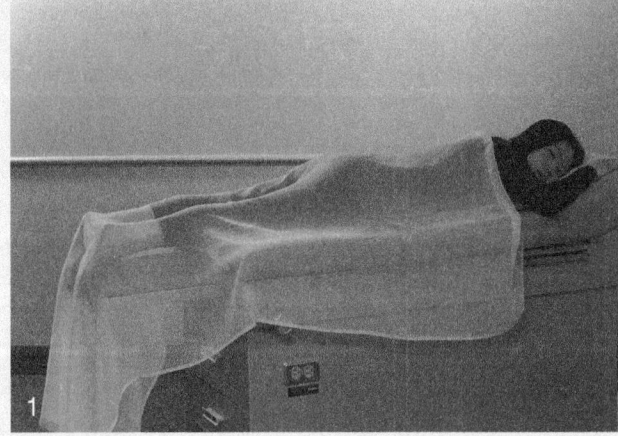

6. Place the drape over the patient so it covers the middle of the back to below the knees.
   Note: For female patients, the drape should be large enough to cover from the breasts to below the that the patient is not exposed accidentally if she is asked to roll over.
   Purpose: Draping the patient provides warmth and privacy while giving the provider access to the examination site.
7. After the examination has been completed, assist the patient as needed to get off the table and get dressed.
8. Put on gloves and use disinfectant wipes to clean the exam table and all potentially contaminated surfaces. Dispose of the used gloves and exam table paper in the waste container. Wash hands or use hand sanitizer.
   Purpose: To ensure infection control and to prevent the transmission of pathogens from one patient to another.
9. Allow the exam table to dry before pulling clean paper over the table.

PROCEDURE 35.7 Knee-Chest Position

Tasks

Position and drape the patient for examinations of the back and rectum and for certain surgical procedures.

Equipment and Supplies

- Patient's health record
- Exam table, pillow, and table paper
- Patient gown and drape
- Disinfectant wipes
- Gloves
- Waste container

Procedural Steps

1. Wash hands or use hand sanitizer.
   Purpose: Hand sanitization is an important step for infection control.
2. Greet the patient. Identify yourself. Verify the patient's identity with full name and date of birth. Explain the procedure to be performed in a manner that the patient understands. Answer any questions the patient may have about the procedure.
   Purpose: To promote the patient's understanding and cooperation during the examination.
3. Give the patient a gown and explain what clothing must be removed for the examination being done. Tell the patient that the gown should open in the back. Provide assistance as needed. Give the patient privacy while changing. Knock on the examination room door before reentering to make sure the patient has completed undressing and gowning.
4. Do not place the patient in the knee-chest position until the provider is ready for that part of the examination.
   Purpose: To promote the patient's privacy, comfort, and safety.
5. Pull out the table extension if necessary. Help the patient lie down on their back and then turn over into the prone position. Ask the patient to move up onto the knees, spread the knees apart, and lean forward onto the head so that the buttocks are raised. A pillow can be placed under the chest to help provide support.

Tell the patient to keep the back straight and turn the face to either side. The patient should rest their weight on the chest and shoulders (Fig. 1).

Note: If the patient has difficulty maintaining this position, an alternative is to place weight on bent elbows with the head off the table.

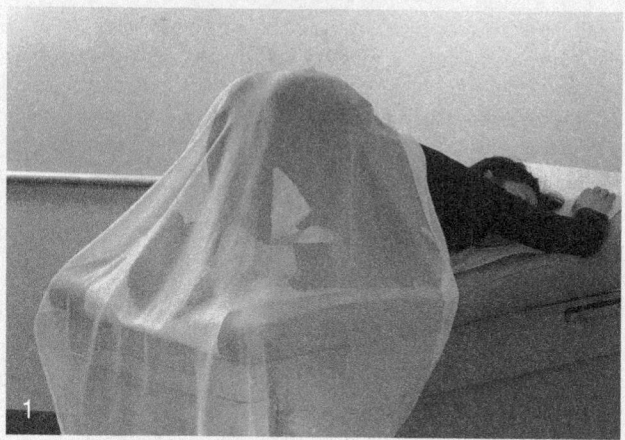

6. Place the drape diagonally over the buttock with a corner falling toward the knees and a corner resting on the back.
   Purpose: Draping the patient provides warmth and privacy while giving the provider access to the examination site.
7. After the examination has been completed, assist the patient as needed to get off the table and get dressed.
8. Put on gloves and use disinfectant wipes to clean the exam table and all potentially contaminated surfaces. Dispose of the used gloves and exam table paper in the waste container. Wash hands or use hand sanitizer.
   Purpose: To ensure infection control and to prevent the transmission of pathogens from one patient to another.
9. Allow the exam table to dry before pulling clean paper over the table.

PROCEDURE 35.8 Assist the Provider With a Patient Exam

Tasks

Aid the provider in the examination of a patient by preparing the patient and the necessary equipment and ensuring the patient's safety and comfort during the examination.

Equipment and Supplies

- Patient's health record
- Scale with height measurement bar
- Stethoscope and sphygmomanometer
- Thermometer and probe cover (if needed)
- Exam table, table paper, and pillow
- Examination light
- Mayo stand or table with paper procedure towels
- Otoscope with disposable speculum
- Ophthalmoscope
- Gauze
- Penlight
- Tuning fork
- Tongue depressor
- Cotton balls
- Percussion hammer
- Specimen bottles and laboratory requisition form
- Lubricating gel
- Cotton-tipped applicators
- Tape measure
- Fecal occult blood test supplies
- Gloves
- Patient gown and drape
- Disinfectant wipes
- Biohazardous waste container
- Waste container

Procedural Steps

1. Wash hands or use hand sanitizer. Ensure room is clean and has been disinfected for the next patient.
   Purpose: Hand sanitization is an important step for infection control.
2. Obtain and organize supplies and instruments for the physical exam. Check any expiration dates on items. Cover the mayo stand, table, or counter with a paper procedure towel and then place items on the paper in the order the provider will use them. Cover supplies with an additional paper towel or drape if per facility policy.
   Purpose: Old items with expired expiration dates cannot be used. To promote time management and ensure that all needed equipment and supplies are ready.
3. Greet and identify the patient, introduce yourself, and determine whether the patient understands the procedure. If the patient does not, explain what to expect. Refer any unanswered questions to the provider.

Continued

PROCEDURE 35.8 Assist the Provider With a Patient Exam–cont'd

Purpose: To promote the patient's understanding and cooperation during the examination.

4. Review the medical history with the patient and ask the purpose of the visit. Review current medications and document any changes or prescription refills needed. Document the interview results.
   Purpose: To verify that all information is current and complete.

5. Obtain and record the patient's vital signs, height, weight, and body mass index (BMI). Instruct the patient on how to collect a urine specimen, if ordered, and hand the patient a properly labeled specimen container.
   Purpose: To gather data needed before the examination begins.

6. Hand the patient a gown and drape. Explain what clothes should be removed for the examination and whether the gown should open in the front or the back. Help the patient with undressing as needed (most patients prefer to undress in privacy). Knock on the door before reentering the room to protect the patient's privacy.
   Purpose: To assist the patient in preparing for the examination and to safeguard the patient's privacy, comfort, and safety.

7. Assist the patient as needed in sitting at the foot of the exam table; place the drape over the patient's lap and legs. If the patient is an older adult, confused, or feeling faint or dizzy, do not leave them alone.
   Purpose: To provide for the patient's warmth and privacy and to prevent a fall or injury.

8. Place the patient's paper health record in the designated area or make sure the computer is ready for the provider to log in and access the patient's electronic health record (EHR). Be careful to safeguard patient confidentiality during this step of the procedure.

9. Assist during the examination by handing the provider instruments as needed and by positioning and draping the patient.

10. When the provider has completed the examination, allow the patient to rest for a moment, then help the patient from the table. Assist with dressing, if necessary. Use proper body mechanics if assistance in transfer is needed.
    Purpose: To ensure the patient's stability and safety and to protect yourself from injury.

11. Return to the patient and ask whether they have any questions. Give the patient any final instructions, and schedule tests as ordered by the provider or the next appointment.
    Purpose: To clarify instructions, eliminate any misunderstandings, and allow the patient to discuss any concerns. If the patient's misunderstandings or concerns are beyond your scope of experience or skill, arrange for the provider to speak with the patient again.

12. Put on gloves. Dispose of any biohazard waste in designated biohazardous waste containers. Dispose of exam table paper and other waste in the waste container. Use disinfectant wipes to clean the exam table and any other potentially contaminated surface. Disinfect all equipment.
    Purpose: To prevent cross-contamination with any potentially infectious materials.

13. Remove the gloves, discard them in the waste container, and wash your hands or use hand sanitizer.
    Purpose: To ensure infection control.

14. Allow the exam table to dry before pulling clean paper over the table. Replace used supplies and prepare the room for the next patient.

PROCEDURE 35.9 Measuring Distance Visual Acuity

Task
Determine the patient's degree of visual clarity at a measured distance of 20 feet using the Snellen chart and established protocols.

Equipment and Supplies
- Patient's health record
- Provider's order or standing order
- Snellen eye chart
- Occluder and disinfectant or disposable eye occluder
- Pen or pencil and paper

Procedural Steps
1. Wash hands or use hand sanitizer.
   Purpose: Hand sanitization is an important step for infection control.
2. Prepare the area. Make sure the room is well lit and that a distance marker is 20 feet from the chart.
3. Greet the patient. Identify yourself. Verify the patient's identity with full name and date of birth. Explain the procedure to be performed in a manner that the patient understands. Answer any questions the patient may have about the procedure.
4. Instruct the patient not to squint during the test. The patient should not have an opportunity to study the chart before the test is given. If the patient wears corrective lenses, they should be worn during the test.
   Purpose: Explanations help gain the patient's cooperation and alleviate apprehension. Squinting can temporarily improve vision.
5. Position the patient in a standing or sitting position at the 20-foot marker. Check that the Snellen chart is positioned at the patient's eye level.
   Purpose: Twenty feet is the standard testing distance.

6. If the occluder is not disposable, disinfect it before the procedure starts. Then instruct the patient to cover the left eye with the occluder and to keep both eyes open throughout the test to prevent squinting (Fig. 1).
   Purpose: Traditionally, the right eye is tested first.

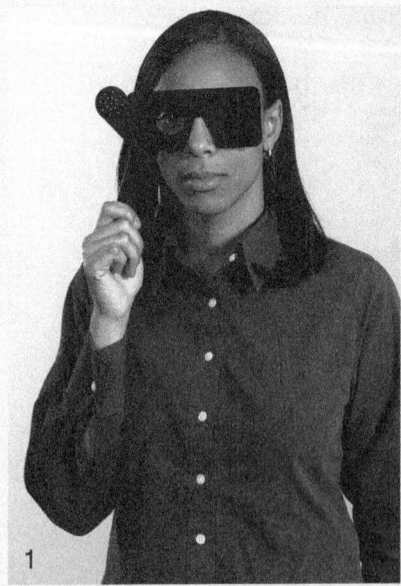

7. Stand beside the chart and point to each row as the patient reads it aloud, starting with the 20/70 row (Fig. 2).

PROCEDURE 35.9 Measuring Distance Visual Acuity–cont'd

Purpose: Starting with larger letters gives the patient confidence and allows for accommodation of vision.

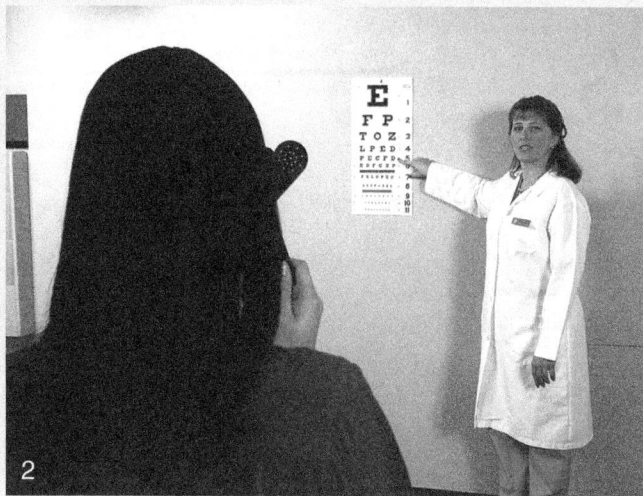

8. Proceed down the rows of the chart until the smallest row the patient can read with a maximum of two errors is reached. If one or two letters are missed, the outcome is recorded with a minus sign and the number of errors (e.g., 20/40 –2). If more than two errors are made, the previous line should be documented. Record any of the patient's reactions while reading the chart.

Purpose: Reactions such as squinting, leaning, tearing, or blinking may indicate that the patient is having difficulty with the test.

9. Repeat the procedure with the left eye, covering the right eye. Have the patient read the line backwards. Record any of the patient's reactions while reading the chart.

Purpose: Patients can quickly memorize the chart. By having the patient read the line backwards, the medical assistant can help ensure the accuracy of the results.

10. Repeat the procedure with both eyes uncovered. Record any of the patient's reactions while reading the chart.

11. Disinfect the occluder, if it is not disposable, and wash hands or use hand sanitizer.

Purpose: To follow infection control procedures.

12. Document the procedure in the patient's record, including the date and time, visual acuity results, and any reactions by the patient. Also record whether corrective lenses were worn.

Purpose: Procedures that are not recorded are considered not done.

Documentation Exercise

The medical assistant conducts a Snellen exam on Carlene Anderson, who wears contacts. The results are as follows: right eye 20/60; left eye 20/30, but she missed one letter at the 20/30 line; both eyes 20/40. Carlene does not squint or strain during the exam.

Correct Documentation

8/01/20XX 2:20 p.m. DVA completed using the Snellen chart. Right eye 20/60, left eye 20/30 –1, both eyes 20/40 corrective lenses. No squinting noted.
———————————————————— Kim Tau, CMA (AAMA)

PROCEDURE 35.10 Assess Color Acuity Using the Ishihara Test

Task
Assess a patient's color acuity correctly using established protocols and record the results.

Equipment and Supplies
- Patient's health record
- Provider's order or standing order
- Room with natural light, if possible
- Ishihara color plate book
- Pen, pencil, and paper
- Watch with a second hand

Procedural Steps
1. Assemble the equipment and prepare the room for testing. The room should be quiet and illuminated with natural light.
   Purpose: Natural light is needed to test colors correctly.
2. Greet the patient. Identify yourself. Verify the patient's identity with full name and date of birth. Explain the procedure to be performed in a manner that the patient understands. Answer any questions the patient may have about the procedure. Use a practice card during the explanation and make sure the patient understands that they have 3 seconds to identify each plate.
   Purpose: To make sure you have the right patient. Also, an informed patient is a cooperative patient. The first plate is a practice plate and is designed to be read correctly.
3. Hold up the first plate at a right angle to the patient's line of vision and 30 inches from the patient. Be sure both of the patient's eyes are kept open during the test (Fig. 1).

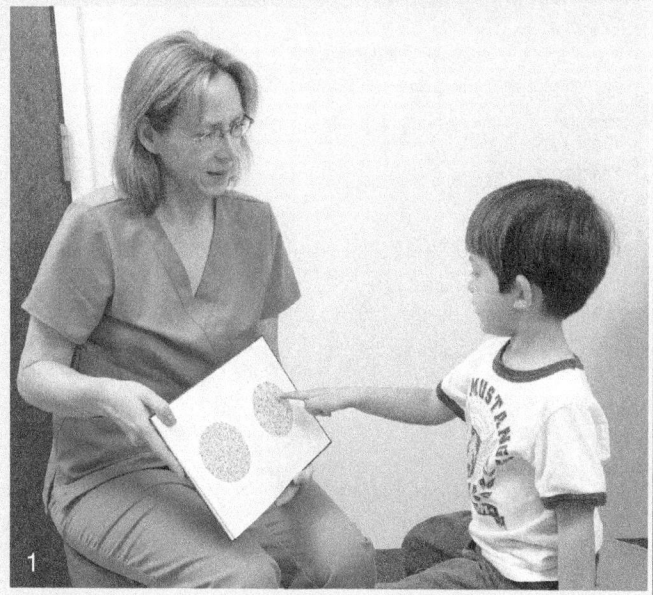

4. Ask the patient to tell you the number on the plate. Record the plate number and the patient's answer (Fig. 2).

Continued

PROCEDURE 35.10   Assess Color Acuity Using the Ishihara Test—cont'd

2

5. Continue this sequence until all 11 plates have been read. If the patient cannot identify the number on the plate, place an X in the record for that plate number. Your record should look like this:
   Plate 1 = pass, Plate 2 = pass, Plate 3 = X, Plate 4 = pass, and so on
6. Include any unusual symptoms in your record, such as eye rubbing, squinting, or excessive blinking.
7. Place the book back into its cardboard sleeve and return it to its storage space.
   Purpose: The Ishihara color plates must be stored in a closed position away from external light to protect the colors.
8. Document the procedure in the patient's health record, including the date and time, the testing results, and any patient symptoms shown during the test.
   Purpose: Procedures that are not recorded are considered not done.

PROCEDURE 35.11   Measuring Hearing Acuity With an Audiometer

Task
Perform audiometric testing of hearing acuity using established protocols.

Equipment and Supplies
- Patient's health record
- Provider's order or standing order
- Audiometer with adjustable headphones or handheld audiometer with probe cover
- Graph paper (optional)
- Quiet area

Procedural Steps
1. Wash hands or use hand sanitizer, assemble the equipment, and bring the patient into a quiet area.
   Purpose: The testing room should be free of distractions and noise so the patient can concentrate completely on the hearing evaluation.
2. Greet the patient. Identify yourself. Verify the patient's identity with full name and date of birth. Explain the procedure to be performed in a manner that the patient understands. Answer any questions the patient may have about the procedure.
   Purpose: To make sure you have the right patient. Also, explanations help gain the patient's cooperation and ease apprehension.

3. Explain that the audiometer measures whether the patient can hear various sound wave frequencies through the headphones. Each ear is tested separately. When the patient hears a frequency, they should raise a hand or push the button to signal the medical assistant.
   Purpose: Patient education is needed for compliance with the examination.
4. If using headphones, place over the patient's ears, making sure they are adjusted for comfort. If using a handheld audiometer, apply the probe cover.
5. Test the first ear and make a note of the results. Stagger the timing of the tones if audiometer is not automatic.
   Purpose: If the tones are rhythmic, the patient may indicate hearing a tone when the tone was not heard.
6. Test the second ear and make a note of the results. Stagger the timing of the tones if audiometer is not automatic.
7. Document the results in the patient's health record. If a graph is used, document the results on the graph.
   Note: The audiometer tests each ear separately, starting at a low frequency. If the machine does not automatically record the results, the medical assistant documents the patient's response to the frequencies on a graph or audiogram. Results for the left ear are marked with an X, and those for the right ear are marked with an O (Fig. 1).

PROCEDURE 35.11 Measuring Hearing Acuity With an Audiometer–cont'd

8. Disinfect the audiometer according to the manufacturer's guidelines.
9. Wash hands or use hand sanitizer.

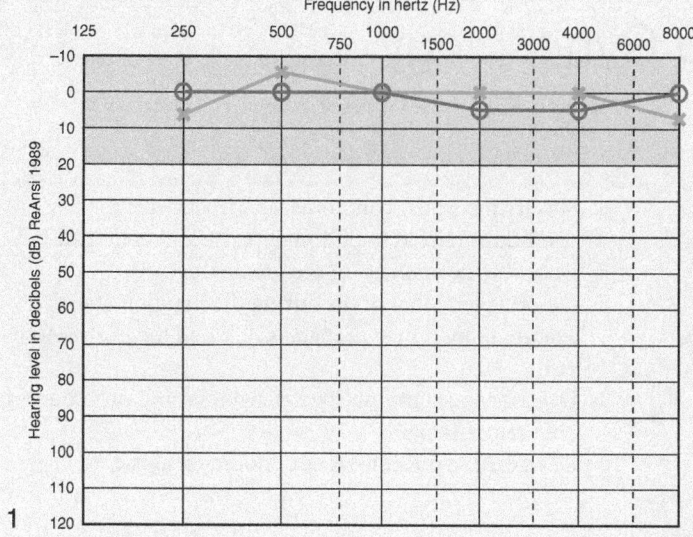

1

36

Assisting in Obstetrics and Gynecology

LEARNING OBJECTIVES

1. Describe the medical assistant's role with preparing for, setting up, and assisting with gynecologic examinations.
2. Describe the medical assistant's role with specimen collection for a Pap test and vaginal infections.
3. Discuss post-examination duties for the medical assistant.
4. Describe cryotherapy, a colposcopy, and a loop electrosurgical excision procedure, including patient preparation and postprocedure instructions.
5. Differentiate between contraception types, including barrier methods, hormonal contraceptives, intrauterine devices, and permanent methods.
6. Specify the signs, symptoms, and treatments for conditions related to perimenopause and menopause.
7. Describe the contents of the prenatal record.
8. Describe tests that occur during the first prenatal examination, return prenatal visits, and the postpartum visit.
9. Describe the common specialized tests and procedures for obstetric patients.
10. Describe the possible signs of domestic abuse.

OUTLINE

 OPENING SCENARIO

Beth St. John, RMA has been working in the obstetrics and gynecology (OB/GYN) department for about 5 years. She loves what she

does and feels grateful that she can be there for her patients as they go through the pregnancy process. She also gets a lot of satisfaction from working with patients who come in with gynecologic issues. She especially likes the patient education that she can do with all of her patients. Her supervisor recognizes that Beth enjoys teaching and has asked her to mentor a medical assistant student, Jill Snow, who is just starting her practicum. Beth is excited to share how she works with patients in the OB/GYN department.

YOU WILL LEARN

1. To recognize the components of a gynecologic examination.
2. To recognize the components of prenatal and postpartum examinations.
3. To assist providers with specialty examinations.
4. To assist providers with gynecologic procedures.
5. To assist with special testing done during pregnancy.

INTRODUCTION

Most examinations are similar between men and women. However, there are significant differences in the exams that deal with sex-related issues. The branch of medicine that deals with diseases of the reproductive system in women is called *gynecology* (gy neh KAW loh jee). Gynecologic issues affect reproductive organs, hormones that directly affect the reproductive system in women, and breast tissue. *Obstetrics* (awb STE triks) is a branch of gynecology that specifically deals with pregnancy, labor, and the postpartum period. Frequently a provider practices both specialties and is known as an *OB/GYN provider*. Assessment of the female reproductive system is an important part of healthcare.

It is very important that medical assistants be familiar with signs and symptoms of diseases and conditions related to this specialty. This is because it is common for patients to be uncomfortable talking about sexual matters. They may hesitate to bring up issues they are having in this area. If medical assistants are familiar with potential issues, they can identify areas of concern even if patients are not upfront. Gynecologic and obstetric issues are very emotionally charged. The medical assistant needs to be sensitive, aware of the patient's emotional state, and give support when needed. The medical assistant is responsible not only for assisting the provider, but also for providing support and comfort to the patient. This would include assisting her in being as comfortable as possible during the visit. Providing this care to the patient will help build a trusting relationship between medical assistant and patient. When a trusting relationship is established, the patient is more likely to share the information. This information is needed by the provider to give her the best possible care.

CRITICAL THINKING 36.1

Because of the sensitive nature of reproductive issues, it is common for patients coming into an OB/GYN practice to be very shy and not want to talk about problems they may be having. What are some things you can do to help a patient feel more at ease and comfortable while in the office?

GYNECOLOGIC EXAMINATIONS

The medical assistant will often be responsible for:
- Preparing the patient for a gynecologic examination
- Setting up for a gynecologic examination

- Assisting the provider during the examination
- Performing post-examination duties

All of these should be done with close attention to detail and mindfulness as to the patient and her needs.

Preparing for a Gynecologic Examination

When a patient makes an appointment for a gynecologic examination, she should be advised not to douche, use any vaginal medications or spermicidal products, or have sexual intercourse for 2 days before the examination. All these activities can affect the vaginal discharge, which can alter the results of some gynecologic examinations. If possible, it is also important not to schedule gynecologic examinations during the patient's menstrual period.

VOCABULARY

douche Irrigating the vagina for hygienic reasons. Usually water is used, and occasionally other substances for cleaning or odor control are also used.

Setting Up for a Gynecologic Examination

If the medical assistant knows a gynecologic examination will occur, the room is set up prior to rooming the patient. A medical assistant is responsible for setting up the examination room and making sure that all the supplies are available for a gynecologic examination. All items should be placed within easy reach for the provider and organized in a logical manner. There is not a specific requirement for item placement; rather, follow the provider's preference. The following is a list of supplies needed for a routine gynecologic examination.

- Patient's health record
- Patient gown and drape
- Lubricant
- Examination light
- Vaginal speculum
- Gynecologic swabs
- Fecal occult blood test cards with developer
- Biohazardous waste container
- Supplies needed for specimen collection and transport:
  - For liquid-based Pap test: cervical spatula, plastic-fronded broom, and vial containing liquid preservative
  - Direct smear Pap test: cervical spatula, microscope slide, fixative, and lead pencil (or other recommended method for labeling slide)
  - Other tests: sterile swabs, specialized swabs, dropper bottle with saline and/or 10% solution of potassium hydroxide (KOH), microscope slide, and lead pencil for labeling slide
  - Transport bags or cases, as required by the receiving lab
  - Patient information labels for each specimen container and laboratory requisition slips

---

CRITICAL THINKING 36.2

Preparing for a general physical examination was discussed in Chapter 35. What are some of the major differences between preparation and set up for a general physical and a gynecologic examination?

Assisting With a Gynecologic Examination

The medical assistant is responsible for obtaining the patient's vital signs and gynecologic history prior to the start of the gynecologic examination.

Gynecologic History. Before the provider enters the room, the medical assistant should obtain a full gynecologic history.

- Age at *menarche* (first menstrual period)
- Details about the menstrual (MEN stroo al) cycle, including:
  - Date of the first day of the last menstrual period (LMP)
  - Regularity of menstrual periods
  - The amount and duration of menstrual flow
  - A history of menstrual disturbances and their treatment
- Any current indicators of infection, including vaginal discharge, pelvic pain, and/or unusual itching, and urinary difficulties
- Description of any breast abnormalities and the date of the patient's last mammogram
- Date and results of the last Pap test
- Sexual history, including:
  - Number of partners currently
  - Number of partners over the patient's life
  - Any sexually transmitted infection (STI) history
- Number of times pregnant and the number of pregnancies carried to more than 20 weeks
- Lifestyle factors, including diet, exercise, smoking, and alcohol use

After documenting the patient's history and chief complaint, the medical assistant should prepare the patient for the examination (Procedure 36.1).

Preparing the Patient. Gynecologic examinations may be uncomfortable for some patients. To prevent unnecessary embarrassment and discomfort, the procedure should be fully explained to the patient before starting. This should be done using terms that are easy for the patient to understand. The medical assistant should also remain in the examination room to provide reassurance to the patient and legal protection for the provider.

Before the examination starts, the patient should be instructed to empty her bladder, completely disrobe, and put on an examination gown. Although it is typical to have the gown open in the front, some providers may prefer the gown open in the back. Be sure to check for provider preferences before instructing the patient. It is also common to provide a sheet for the woman to place over her lap. It can be used by the medical assistant to drape the patient appropriately throughout the procedure.

Breast Examination. Traditionally the first part of the gynecologic examination is the clinical breast examination (CBE). The CBE is done to screen for abnormalities in the breasts that could indicate breast cancer. The current recommendation regarding the CBE is that it may not be necessary with every well-woman exam. The decision of whether a CBE needs to be done is up to the individual provider. Some providers may determine that it is not necessary, and others may continue to do the CBE with

every examination. The medical assistant needs to be prepared to assist with this portion of the exam if necessary.

The CBE begins with the patient in the sitting position for a visual check of the breasts. The gown should be adjusted so that the breast tissue can be easily exposed. After the visual inspection, the patient will be placed in the supine position. The medical assistant should be prepared to help the patient to lie down on the examination table. The footrest should be extended, and a small pillow may be placed under the patient's head for comfort. If needed, the gown and drape should be adjusted to protect the patient's modesty. The provider will use palpation over the entire breast and into the armpit area to look for any abnormalities, such as:

- Abnormal thickening of breast tissue
- Unusual texture to the skin or the underlying tissue
- Lumps in the breast or under the arms
- Unusual nipple discharge

When the examination is complete, the gown is readjusted to cover the breasts.

Abdominal and Pelvic Examination. While the patient is in the supine position, the provider will palpate the abdomen. This is done to confirm normal symmetry (SIM i tree) of the pelvic organs and to detect any masses. The provider also watches for any signs of discomfort or pain that could indicate a problem.

The need for an annual pelvic examination is currently somewhat debated. The American College of Obstetricians and Gynecologists (ACOG) recommends that pelvic examinations be done at the discretion of the healthcare provider when indicated by medical history or symptoms. Some providers still choose to do these as part of the annual well-woman examination. Other providers may do it every 3 years or when a complaint or concern justifies the exam. Remember that this is the call of the healthcare provider. The medical assistant needs to be prepared to assist in this exam if necessary.

For the pelvic examination, the patient is placed in the lithotomy (li THOT uh mee) position. The medical assistant should help the patient into this position and keep her totally covered. It is important that the patient never be placed in this position until the provider is ready to begin the examination. The provider will uncover the patient's pelvic area when the examination begins. During the examination, the medical assistant should stand nearby to observe the patient and quickly assist the provider as necessary.

> **VOCABULARY**
> **perineal** Pertaining to the area between the vaginal opening and the rectum (perineum).
> **symmetry** Similarity in size, form, and arrangement of parts on opposite sides of the body.

Examination of the External Genitalia. First, the provider inspects the external genitalia (jen ih TAY lee ah) and palpates the perineal (pair ih NEE al) area. The patient may be asked to bear down to show any abnormalities or muscular weaknesses. This can be common in women who have had previous vaginal deliveries that caused a laceration to this area. Discoloration, sores, or other visible abnormalities can be a sign of a larger problem and will need to be further evaluated.

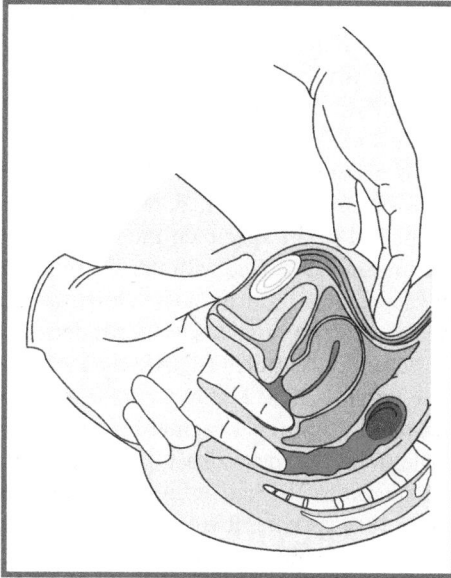

Fig. 36.1 Bimanual Examination. (From Niedzwiecki B, et al: *Kinn's the medical assistant*, ed 14, St. Louis, 2020, Elsevier.)

Internal Examination. Next, the vaginal speculum (SPEK yuh luh m) is inserted for examination of the cervix and the vaginal canal. The provider will inspect the tissues and obtain vaginal specimens if needed. Before the provider inserts the speculum, it should be warmed, either in a warming drawer or run under warm tap water. Have the patient take some deep breaths to help relax the abdominal muscles. This allows the speculum to move in easily without any pain or injury to the patient.

The normal cervix points posteriorly (toward the back) and has a smooth, pink appearance. Abnormalities most frequently seen are ulcerations (erosions or sores), Bartholin (BAR thoh lin) cysts, and cervical polyps. Healed lacerations from childbirth are common and are considered a normal finding. The vaginal wall is reddish pink and has a corrugated appearance from the overlapping tissue lining. The vaginal discharge should be clear. Vaginal infections can cause the vaginal discharge to appear frothy (bubbly), milky white, green, or blood-tinged.

After inspecting the vaginal wall, the provider may collect specimens. The medical assistant is responsible for labeling each specimen and preparing it for transport to the cytology laboratory. Be sure to follow all laboratory instructions during the preparation to avoid having to repeat the collection process.

Bimanual Examination. After removal of the vaginal speculum, the provider will do a bimanual examination. For a bimanual examination, two gloved fingers are lubricated with a water-soluble jelly (lubricant) and inserted into the vaginal canal. The provider's other hand deeply palpates the abdomen over the pelvic organs (Fig. 36.1). The uterus is examined for shape, size, and consistency, and its position is noted. A normal uterus is freely movable with limited discomfort. A *laterally displaced uterus* is usually the result of pelvic adhesions or displacement caused by a pelvic tumor. The fallopian tubes and ovaries are also evaluated. Normal tubes and ovaries are difficult to palpate. The provider examines the cervix and may have to press firmly in the pelvic area, causing minor discomfort for the patient.

BOX 36.1   Pap Test Results

The Bethesda System is often used to report the results of a Pap test. This system looks at the squamous cells and the glandular cells separately. The squamous cell grading goes from negative to severe.

Squamous Cells
- *Negative for intraepithelial lesion of malignancy.* Normal epithelial cells, no precancerous findings.
- *Atypical squamous cells (ASC).* Most common abnormal finding and is divided into two groups:
  - *Atypical squamous cells of undetermined significance (ASC-US).* Squamous cells do not appear completely normal. The cause is unclear but could be related to an HPV infection.
  - *Atypical squamous cells, cannot exclude a high-grade squamous intraepithelial lesion (ASC-H).* Lesions might be at higher risk of being precancerous than ASC-US lesions.
- *Low-grade squamous intraepithelial lesions (LSILs).* Mild abnormalities caused by HPV infection. Often return to normal in younger women.
- *High-grade squamous intraepithelial lesions (HSILs).* Severe abnormalities that have a higher likelihood of progressing to cancer if left untreated.
- *Carcinoma in situ (CIS).* Severely abnormal cells that resemble cancer cells. Remain on the surface of the cervix and have not spread.
- *Squamous cell carcinoma:* Cervical cancer

Glandular Cells
- *Atypical glandular cells (ACG).* Glandular cells do not appear normal and the cause is unclear.
- *Endocervical adenocarcinoma in situ (AIS).* Severely abnormal cells are found, but they have not spread beyond the glandular tissue of the cervix.
- *Adenocarcinoma:* Cancer of the endocervical canal and possibly endometrial, extrauterine, and other cancers.

A digital rectal exam may be done at this time. This involves the insertion of a gloved finger into the rectum. A small amount of stool is left on the glove and can be used for a fecal occult blood test. The medical assistant should have the fecal occult blood test card open and ready. The provider will place the sample on the card before removing the gloves.

VOCABULARY

Bartholin cyst Caused from a blockage of the Bartholin's gland resulting in fluid backing up into the gland, causing a painless swollen area on the side of the vaginal opening.
corrugated Shaped with alternating ridges and grooves.

Specimen Collection. During a pelvic examination, there are several types of specimens that may be collected.

Cervical Cancer Screening. In the past, Pap testing was the only method to screen for cervical cancer. Today, cervical cancer screening includes 3 approaches:
- *Human papillomavirus (HPV) testing:* Looks for the presence of high-risk HPV types in cervical cells. A cervical specimen is obtained and analyzed. The results are reported as either negative or positive, with positive being high risk for an HPV infection.
- *Pap testing:* Looks for cervical cell changes. The results of the Pap test are often reported to the provider using the Bethesda System (Box 36.1).

- *HPV/Pap cotesting*: Checks the same cell sample for both high-risk HPV types and cervical cell changes.

The United States Preventive Service Task Force recommends women ages 21 to 29 to have a Pap test every 3 years. Women 30 to 65 should have either a high-risk HPV or cotesting every 5 years or a Pap test alone every 3 years. Cervical cancer screening is not recommended for women under 21 years of age. For women over 65 years of age, screening requirements are based on their medical history.

For the HPV/Pap cotesting, the same specimen is used for both tests. There are two methods for collecting specimens for a Pap test or cotesting, the liquid-based method and the direct smear method.

- *Liquid-based method*: The most common and considered the most accurate. The specimen is collected with a plastic-fronded broom or a cervical spatula (or both). The provider will insert the collection device through the speculum and collect the cells from the cervix. The broom or spatula is rinsed in a vial containing liquid preservative. This suspends the cells within the preservative.
- *Direct smear method*: A cervical spatula is used to obtain the specimen. Cells are placed (smeared) directly on a microscope slide. A fixative must be applied immediately to the slide to preserve the cells and ensure they are securely fixated on the slide for transport.

Regardless of which method is used, the specimen is sent to a lab for evaluation.

A *maturation index* may be done with a Pap test. A maturation index is used to evaluate the estrogen (ES truh juh n) and progesterone balance. This test can assist in the diagnosis and treatment of infertility issues, amenorrhea (ah men uh REE ah), menopause, or postmenopausal bleeding. If the provider orders a maturation index, it must be clearly indicated on the cytology request form.

VOCABULARY
amenorrhea Lack of menstrual flow.

Vaginal infections. Common vaginal infections were discussed in Chapter 14. Tests for these infections are often done during a pelvic examination. The collection device and transfer container used may be different, depending on the test being done. It is important that the medical assistant know what tests the provider may want to run and have the appropriate testing supplies available.

- *Bacterial infections*: Generally a sterile swab is used to collect mucus from the cervix. The swab is transported to the lab in a sterile container. Bacteria from the cervical mucus are grown out on a petri plate. It will take about 24 to 48 hours to get results.
- *Fungal infections*: Used for yeast infections. Commonly cervical mucus is collected on a sterile swab. The mucus is then placed on a slide. A drop of 10% solution of potassium hydroxide (KOH) is added to the slide. The KOH dissolves other cellular debris so the yeast buds can be seen under a microscope.
- *STI testing*: The specimen collection method depends on the type of test done, for example:

- *Trichomoniasis*: A small sample of cervical mucus is taken with a sterile swab and placed on a slide. A small drop of sterile saline is placed over the sample, and the slide is viewed under the microscope.
- *Chlamydia and gonorrhea*: The preferred collection method is using a swab to collect the vaginal specimen. Once the specimen is obtained, the lower portion of the swab is placed in the specimen tube. The tube is sealed, and the specimen is mixed with the transport media.

Recent advancements in technology allow specimens to be evaluated for cellular components, specifically deoxyribonucleic acid (DNA) and ribonucleic acid (RNA). The DNA probe analysis of vaginal fluid is seen as highly accurate and is often used to test for bacterial and fungal vaginal infections. With DNA testing, a sterile swab is used to collect the specimen and placed in a transport medium. The size of the swab and the transport medium can be very specific. It is important that the medical assistant be aware of laboratory requirements for all DNA probe analysis tests. Having the correct swabs for the provider and using the correct transfer tube are critical.

MEDICAL TERMINOLOGY

cephal/o	head
men/o	menses, menstruation
perine/o	perineum
a-	without, no, not
micro-	small
-al	pertaining to
-rrhea	discharge, flow
-y	condition; process of

CRITICAL THINKING 36.3

Beth has a patient coming due to unusual vaginal discharge. She anticipates that the provider will need to do a vaginal examination and gather some specimens for testing. What supplies should she have prepared for the examination?

Post-Examination Duties

When the examination is finished, the medical assistant should help the patient into a sitting position. If the patient needs help dressing, the medical assistant should aid her as needed. If not, the medical assistant should leave the room to give the patient privacy to dress. Before leaving the room, the medical assistant may need to remove examination equipment, supplies, or specimens using Standard Precautions. Once the patient has left, the room should be sanitized, disinfected, and restocked as necessary.

Special Procedures

There are several gynecologic special procedures that a patient may undergo after having received abnormal findings from the pelvic exam, HPV test, or Pap test. These are often done in the office, and the medical assistant may be asked to assist with them.

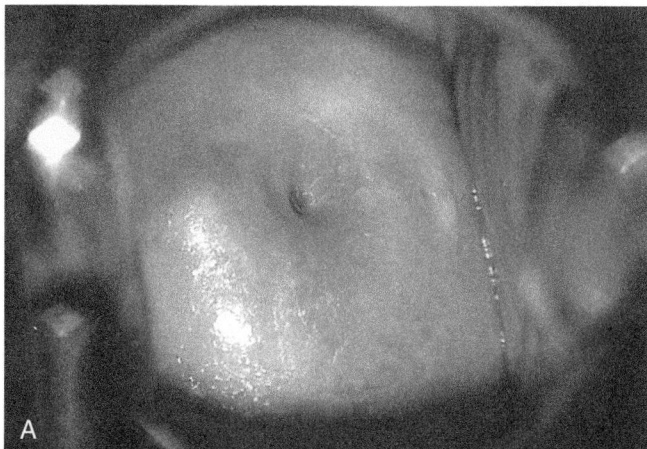
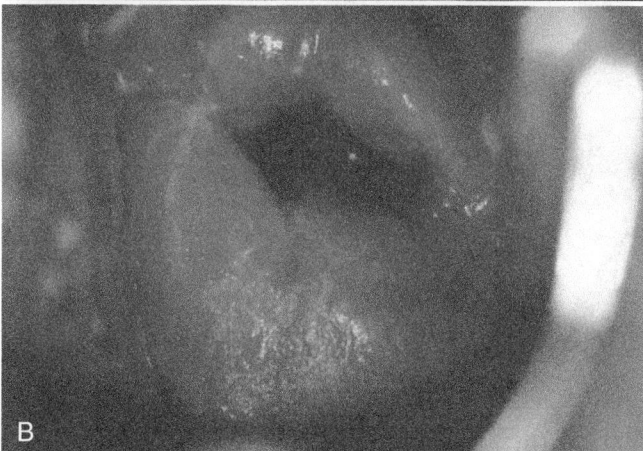

Fig. 36.2 Colposcopic appearance of a normal cervix (A) and an abnormal cervix (B). (A from Swartz MH: Textbook *of physical diagnosis*, ed 7, Philadelphia, 2014, Saunders; B from Pfenninger JL, Fowler GC: *Pfenninger and Fowler's procedures for primary care*, ed 3, Philadelphia, 2011, Saunders.)

cells will turn brown, whereas cancerous areas will not. Cervical biopsies can also be done if suspicious areas are seen. When the medical assistant receives the tissue sample from the provider, the provider will indicate the location. The provider uses the face of a clock for determining the location of the biopsy. It is very important to accurately label each specimen container with the location of the biopsy (e.g., 2:00). Should the biopsy result indicate further treatment, the provider will know the area of concern.

A colposcopy is a relatively safe procedure performed in an ambulatory care facility. Discomfort may occur during the examination. If a biopsy is taken, medication is applied to the area to control the bleeding. Monsel solution, a commonly used medication, is a yellow liquid frequently applied with a swab.

After the procedure, the patient should use a sanitary pad due to bleeding. Within 1 to 2 days, the patient may have a coffee ground–like vaginal discharge. This is caused by the combination of blood and the Monsel solution. Depending on the provider, patients may be instructed not to use tampons, douche, or have intercourse for 7 to 10 days after the procedure.

> **VOCABULARY**
>
> **necrosis** Death of cells in an organ or a tissue; generally due to damage or lack of blood supply.

MEDICAL TERMINOLOGY	
colp/o	vagina
cry/o	extreme cold
necr/o	death, dead
-itis	inflammation
-osis	abnormal condition
-scope	instrument used to view
-scopy	process of viewing
-therapy	treatment

Cryotherapy. *Cryotherapy*, also called *cryoablation*, is used to freeze and destroy abnormal cervical tissue. A cryoprobe is placed on the abnormal tissue. Compressed nitrogen gas flows through the cryoprobe causing the metal to freeze. The tissue is frozen, allowed to thaw, and refrozen. This process causes cellular necrosis, and in approximately 1 month, the dead cells are replaced with healthy cells. The patient may experience some pain and cramping during the procedure and a slight watery discharge for up to a week. The patient should be advised to call the provider's office if any signs of infection, foul-smelling discharge, or pain develop. Advise the patient not to engage in sexual intercourse for 1 month and to expect a heavier than usual menstrual flow for the first cycle after the procedure.

Colposcopy With or Without a Biopsy. *Colposcopy* is the visual examination of the vagina and cervical surfaces with a *colposcope* (Fig. 36.2). The colposcope is a microscope with a light source and a magnifying lens. It is used during a vaginal examination to examine tissue and evaluate abnormal cells.

After the provider examines the tissue with the colposcopy, additional procedures can be done. An acetic acid wash can be done, which turns the abnormal tissue white. A diluted iodine solution wash (e.g., Lugol's or Schiller's solution) can be done and normal

Loop Electrosurgical Excision Procedure. A loop electrosurgical excision procedure (LEEP) is used to collect biopsies or to treat abnormal tissue (Fig. 36.3). With this procedure, a local anesthetic is injected into the cervix and a fine wire loop is inserted into the vagina. A high-frequency electrical current running through the wire is used to remove thin layers of abnormal tissue from both the cervix and the endocervical canal. Some patients feel faint during the procedure. Allow the patient time to rest after the procedure if needed.

After the procedure, the patient should use a sanitary pad due to bleeding. Mild cramping, spotting, and a dark-colored discharge is normal for several days. Depending on the provider, patients may be instructed not to use tampons, douche, or have intercourse for up to 4 weeks after the procedure.

CONTRACEPTION

At the time of a gynecologic examination, a provider may discuss *contraception* (con trah SEP shun) (also called *birth control*) with the patient. There are many different methods of contraception, and ultimately it's the patient's choice. To make an informed choice, a patient should know the risks, benefits, side

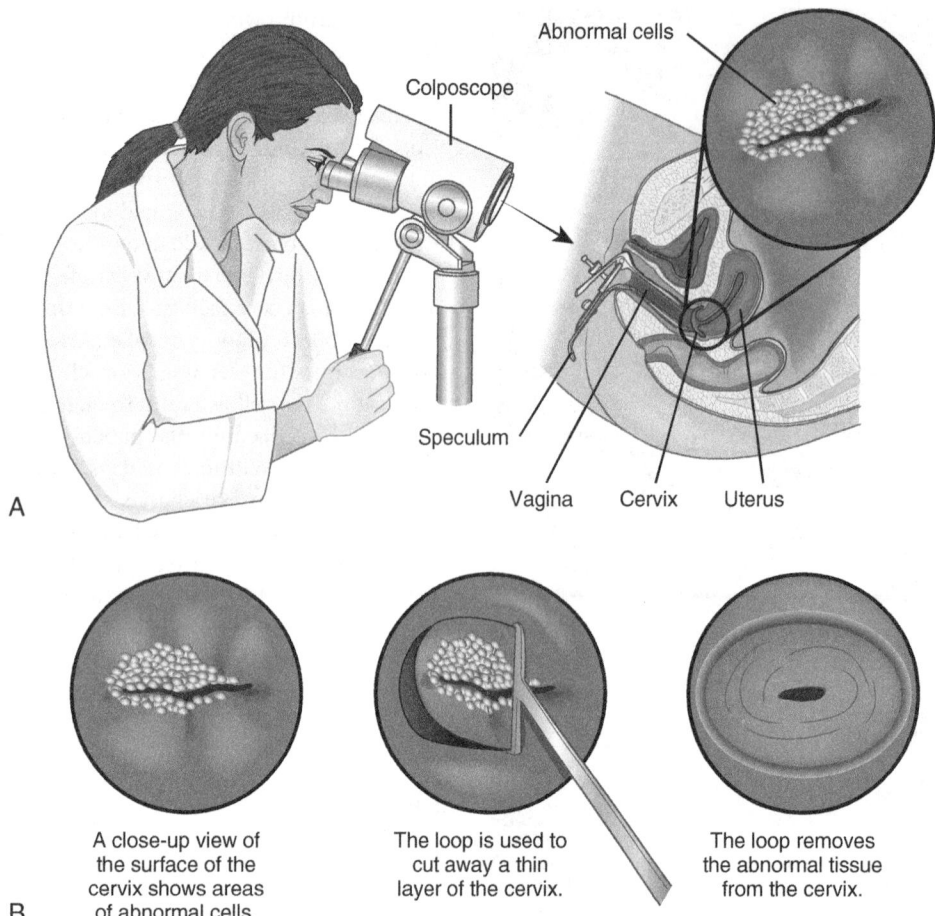

Fig. 36.3 Colposcopic view of the cervix (A) and loop electrosurgical excision procedure biopsy of abnormal cells (B). (From Niedzwiecki B, et al: *Kinn's the medical assistant,* ed 14, St. Louis, 2020, Elsevier.)

effects, costs, failure rates, and convenience of each method. It is common for the medical assistant to help provide patient education on contraceptive methods. The medical assistant must be familiar with the different methods, including risks, benefits, side effects, and so on. Fig. 36.4 summarizes various contraceptive methods and their effectiveness.

The patient's history may also affect the type of contraception selected.

- *Allergies*: A patient with a latex allergy would want to avoid latex condoms. A patient with a copper allergy would need to avoid an intrauterine device (IUD) that uses copper as a spermicide.
- *Health conditions*: A patient with a history of blood clots needs to avoid hormone-based birth control.
- *Smoking*: A patient who smokes may be advised by the provider to avoid oral contraceptives. The combination of smoking and oral contraceptives can increase the risk for blood clots, which may cause a heart attack, stroke, or pulmonary embolism.

Barrier Methods

Barrier methods of contraception can kill sperm (through the use of a chemical spermicide) and/or prevent them from entering the cervical os. Barrier methods are inexpensive and include condoms, diaphragms (DY ah frams), cervical caps, and sponges. If a person uses the barrier method, it must be used applied or inserted each time the person has intercourse.

Condoms must be put on prior to sexual intercourse and removed immediately after. Condoms are the only contraceptive device that offers some protection against STIs. If a person has multiple partners and uses another type of contraceptive, condoms are still recommended to help protect against STIs.

A *cervical cap* is a thimble-sized, domed barrier device that fits over the end of the cervix. It provides a barrier to keep sperm from entering the cervical os. A cervical cap is commonly used with spermicidal jelly (Fig. 36.5). A cervical cap can be inserted up to 12 hours before intercourse and can stay in place up to 72 hours after without reduction in effectiveness and safety.

A *sponge* is a small, disk-shaped device made of soft plastic foam. The sponge is inserted into the vagina, covering the cervix. It continuously releases a spermicide that kills sperm. A sponge can be inserted up to 24 hours before intercourse and must be kept in place for at least 6 hours after intercourse. The sponge must be removed within 24 to 30 hours after insertion to prevent toxic shock syndrome, a rare life-threatening infection.

A *diaphragm* is a reusable barrier device that is specifically fitted to the patient. Like the cervical cap, it should be used with spermicidal jelly to maximize effectiveness. Because it is a reusable device, the user must follow these guidelines:

- Before repeated intercourse, add spermicide to the outside of the diaphragm with an applicator.
- Wait 6 hours after intercourse to remove the diaphragm.

Effectiveness of family planning methods

Most effective	Reversible		Permanent		How to make your method most effective

Less than 1 pregnancy per 100 women in a year

Implant
0.05 %*

Intrauterine device (IUD)
LNG - 0.2 % copper T - 0.8 %

Male sterilization (vasectomy)
0.15 %

Female sterilization (abdominal, laparoscopic, hysteroscopic)
0.5 %

How to make your method most effective
After procedure, little or nothing to do or remember. **Vasectomy and hysteroscopic sterilization:** Use another method for first 3 months.

6-12 pregnancies per 100 women in a year

Injectable
6 %

Pill
9 %

Patch
9 %

Ring
9 %

Diaphragm
12 %

Injectable: Get repeat injections on time.
Pills: Take a pill each day.
Patch, ring: Keep in place, change on time.
Diaphragm: Use correctly every time you have sex.

18 or more pregnancies per 100 women in a year

Male condom
18 %

Female condom
21 %

Withdrawal
22 %

Sponge
24 % parous women
12 % nulliparous women

Fertility-awareness based methods
JANUARY
24 %

Spermicide
28 %

Condoms, sponge, withdrawal, spermicides: Use correctly every time you have sex.
Fertility awareness-based methods: Abstain or use condoms on fertile days. Newest methods (standard days method and twoday method) may be the easiest to use and consequently more effective.

Least effective

* The percentages indicate the number out of every 100 women who experienced an unintended pregnancy within the first year of typical use of each contraceptive method.

CS 242797

Condoms should always be used to reduce the risk of sexually transmitted infections.

Other methods of contraception

Lactational amenorrhea method: LAM is a highly effective, temporary method of contraception.
Emergency contraception: Emergency contraceptive pills or a copper IUD after unprotected intercourse substantially reduces risk of pregnancy.

Adapted from World Health Organization (WHO) Department of Reproductive Health and Research, Johns Hopkins Bloomberg School of Public Health/Center for Communication Programs (CCP). Knowledge for health project. Family planning: a global handbook for providers (2011 update). Baltimore, MD; Geneva, Switzerland: CCP and WHO; 2011; and Trussell J. Contraceptive failure in the United States. Contraception 2011;83:397–404.

Fig. 36.4 Effectiveness of Family Planning Methods. (Adapted from World Health Organization (WHO) Department of Reproductive Health and Research, Johns Hopkins Bloomberg School of Public Health/Center for Communication Programs (CCP). *Knowledge for health project. Family planning: a global handbook for providers (2011 update).* Baltimore, MD; Geneva, Switzerland CCP and WHO; 2011; and Trussell J: Contraceptive failure in the United States, *Contraception* 83:397–404, 2011.)

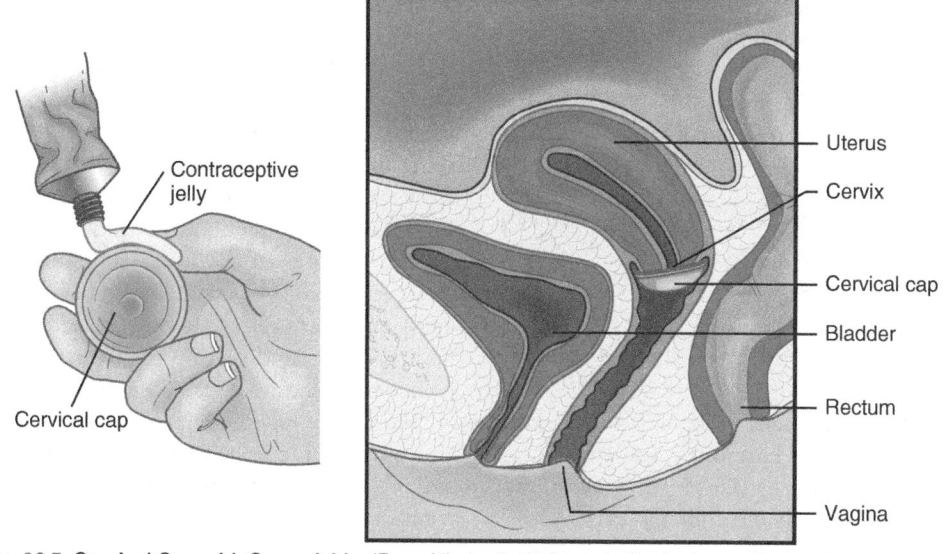

Fig. 36.5 Cervical Cap with Spermicide. (From Niedzwiecki B, et al: *Kinn's the medical assistant,* ed 14, St. Louis, 2020, Elsevier.)

- After removal, wash the diaphragm with soap and water and allow it to air dry. Before storing, and with each use, hold the diaphragm up to a bright light to check for holes or cracks.
- Have the diaphragm refitted if you:
  - Gain or lose more than 10 pounds
  - Have a miscarriage, give birth, or undergo any type of pelvic surgery
  - Have difficulty voiding (urinating) or having a bowel movement with the diaphragm in place
  - Have repeated urinary tract infections
- Replace the diaphragm every 2 years.

Hormonal Contraceptives

Hormonal contraceptives are a highly effective and reversible form of contraception. They work by:

- Preventing ovulation
- Changing the cervical mucosa
- Affecting sperm mobility
- Preventing thickening of the endometrial wall

Hormonal contraceptives include oral birth control, patches, implants, vaginal rings, and Depo-Provera injections.

Besides being used for birth control, hormonal contraceptives can be used to treat a wide range of gynecologic conditions, including menstrual irregularities, premenstrual syndrome (PMS) symptoms, and anovulation. However, to be effective, hormonal contraceptives must be taken exactly as prescribed. Pills must be taken at the same time every day. The patch and ring need to be changed exactly on time. Depo-Provera must be received every 3 months. Waiting even an extra week can increase the risk of pregnancy. Although hormonal contraceptives tend to be considered highly effective, failure rates increase substantially in those who do not use as prescribed.

Hormonal contraceptives, especially, oral contraceptives, can have serious side effects. With oral contraceptives, obesity, age 35 years or older, and being a smoker are risk factors for blood clots that can lead to a heart attack, stroke, and pulmonary embolism. Estrogen and a type of progestin (proh JES tin) called desogestrel have been found to increase the risk of blood clots. Women on hormonal contraceptives should be instructed to look for signs and symptoms of blood clots. Using the mnemonic ACHES can be a helpful memory tool:

- **A**bdominal pain (new and severe)
- **C**hest pain (new and severe)
- **H**eadaches (new or more frequent)
- **E**ye problems (blurred vision or vision loss)
- **S**evere leg pain

MEDICAL TERMINOLOGY	
ovul/o	ovum
an-	no, not, without
-ation	process, condition

Oral Contraceptives. There are many variations in oral contraceptives with different levels of hormones. These can have different effects on the woman's body. Two main types of oral contraceptives include combination pills and mini pills.

Combination birth control pills contain two hormones, estrogen and progestin. These hormones cause cervical mucus to thicken and the lining of the uterus to thin. This prevents fertilization and implantation of the egg. Combination pills may also be used to treat acne and premenstrual dysphoric (dis FOR ik) disorder (PMDD), along with multiple other hormone-related health conditions. It is important to remember that these are often used for health conditions and not only to prevent pregnancy.

With combination pills, one tablet is taken daily. Combined pills are typically packaged as 21 active pills and 7 inactive pills (non–hormone containing). During the 7 days of inactive pills, menses (period) occurs. To reduce the number of periods, some combination pill formulations have increased the number of active pills to 84 with 7 inactive pills. Amethyst is a combination pill that is designed to be taken continuously for 1 year; it has no inactive pills.

Progestin-only pills, or "mini-pills," contain progestin. The hormone causes the thickening of cervical mucus and thinning of the uterine lining. Mini-pills are packaged as 28 active pills.

VOCABULARY
anovulation Failure of the ovaries to release an ovum at the time of ovulation.
osteoporosis Abnormal thinning of the bone structure, causing bones to become brittle and weak.
premenstrual dysphoric disorder (PMDD) A mood disorder that includes depression, irritability, fatigue, changes in appetite or sleep, and difficulty in concentrating; it occurs 1 to 2 weeks before the onset of the menstrual flow.
premenstrual syndrome (PMS) A poorly understood group of symptoms that occur in some women on a cyclical basis; breast pain, irritability, fluid retention, headache, and a lack of coordination are some of the symptoms.

Depo-Provera. Depo-Provera is an injectable contraceptive that contains high doses of progestin. Each dose prevents pregnancy for up to 3 months. The injection must be administered within the first 5 days of the menstrual period and must be repeated every 3 months. If the patient waits longer than 13 weeks to receive a new dose, the effectiveness of the injection has already worn off. The patient should be asked to complete a pregnancy test before receiving another dose. Using Depo-Provera for 2 years or longer may increase the risk of bone loss and the eventual development of osteoporosis. However, the risk of blood clots and cardiovascular disease are less with this type of hormonal birth control than others.

Other Types of Hormonal Contraceptives. A *transdermal contraceptive patch,* also called a birth control patch, is a 1¾-inch square that slowly releases estrogen and progestin through the skin into the blood stream. The patch is worn for 3 consecutive weeks and then is removed. The patient remains without a patch for 1 week, allowing menstruation to occur. The patch can be applied to the buttocks, lower abdomen, and upper body, but the breasts should be avoided. Women should be advised not to apply any creams or oils to the application site. The woman can bathe, shower, and swim while wearing the patch. If the patch comes off, it should be replaced immediately.

The *vaginal ring contraceptive device* is made of flexible plastic and is inserted into the vagina. The ring slowly releases estrogen and progestin in order to prevent pregnancy and provide effective contraceptive action for 1 month after insertion. Like the patch the

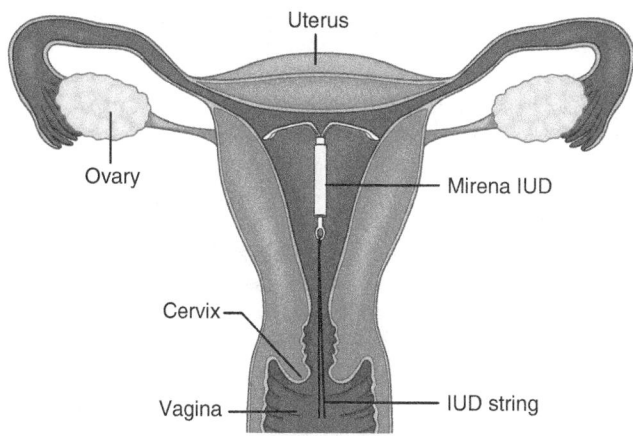

Fig. 36.6 Intrauterine Device (IUD). (From Niedzwiecki B, et al: *Kinn's the medical assistant,* ed 14, St. Louis, 2020, Elsevier.)

ring is normally kept in place for 3 weeks and then removed for 1 week, allowing menstruation. The device is 2 inches in diameter and can be inserted anywhere in the vagina. The deeper it is placed, the less likely it is to be felt after insertion. When the patient first starts using the ring, an additional method of birth control must be used for the first week. If the ring falls out, it should be rinsed with warm water and reinserted within 3 hours. If it is out for longer than 3 hours, contraception is not certain, and the patient should use another birth control method for 1 week.

A *contraceptive implant*, also called a birth control implant, is a flexible rod, about the size of a match, that is inserted under the skin of the upper arm. The birth control implant releases a low, steady dose of progestin. This suppresses ovulation, thickens cervical mucus, and thins the endometrial wall to prevent implantation. It prevents pregnancy for up to 3 years after insertion. Risks are similar to those for other types of hormonal birth control. When a woman decides she wants to get pregnant, she must have her provider remove the implant.

Intrauterine Device

An *intrauterine device* (IUD) is a T-shaped plastic frame with threads attached that is inserted into the uterus by the provider (Fig. 36.6). Two common types of IUDs include:
- *Copper IUD*: Can remain in place as long as 10 years. It may temporarily increase vaginal bleeding and menstrual pain after it is placed. The copper acts to slow the movement of sperm, in addition to blocking the sperm's progress.
- *Hormonal IUD*: Can remain in place for 3 to 5 years. It releases progestin, which reduces sperm mobility and prevents the thickening of the endometrial wall during the menstrual cycle. The hormonal IUD results in both decreased menstrual flow and cramping.

Usually, the IUD can be removed by the provider in the ambulatory care facility. If the IUD perforates the uterine wall and migrates to into the abdomen, laparoscopic surgery is necessary.

Permanent Methods

Both male and female patients can undergo surgical procedures that are considered permanent contraceptive methods. Vasectomies in the male were addressed in Chapter 14.

During a bilateral tubal ligation in a female, a portion of both fallopian tubes is excised or ligated. The procedure can be done after childbirth or during an abdominal surgery, such as a cesarean section. Tubal ligation reversals require major surgery and may not be effective. Most tubal ligations cannot be reversed.

VOCABULARY

excised Surgically removed.
ligated Tied or otherwise closed off.

CRITICAL THINKING 36.4

When directed by the provider, Beth provides patient education regarding contraceptives. Beth has asked Jill to create a reference sheet that covers all birth control options, their characteristics and side effects, and any patient education details that might be appropriate. What should Jill include?

MENOPAUSE

Menopause is the permanent ending of menstruation as a result of the end of ovarian function. It usually occurs between 45 and 55 years of age but can occur as early as the 30s and as late as the 60s. Menses may stop suddenly, flow may decrease over time, or the time between menses may lengthen until menstruation completely stops. Menopause can be diagnosed only retrospectively. Only after 12 months of amenorrhea is a woman said to be in menopause, and the years after this are called *postmenopause*.

Perimenopause begins when hormone-related changes start to appear, and it lasts until the final menses. The total time for this depends greatly on the individual. It can be a relatively short time or last as long as 10 years. During perimenopause, women are still ovulating. The changes with estrogen and progesterone can cause hot flashes, sleep disorders, concentration problems, mood swings, irritability, migraines, vaginal dryness, urinary incontinence, and dry skin.

Medical treatment of menopause focuses on:
- Managing uncomfortable symptoms
- Preventing conditions associated with a drop in blood levels of estrogen, such as osteoporosis and coronary artery disease.

The provider may prescribe low-dose oral contraceptives to balance estrogen and progesterone levels or short-term hormone replacement therapy (HRT) to treat symptoms. HRT is only used less than 5 years. Long-term use of HRT can increase the risk for heart attack, stroke, breast cancer, and blood clotting.

Strategies to treat the symptoms of menopause include medications, vitamins, dietary changes, relaxation, and exercise.
- *Hot flashes*: Gabapentin, clonidine, antidepressants and vitamin E; avoiding caffeine and spicy foods.
- *Osteoporosis*: Alendronate, risedronate, ibandronate, and raloxifene; consuming a low-fat diet high in calcium and vitamin D; regular weight-bearing exercise such as walking.
- *Vaginal dryness*: Estrogen administered locally by vaginal tablet, ring, or cream; KY jelly and vaginal lubricant; soy products or supplements.

- *Mood changes*: Vitamin B$_6$ helps create natural serotonin, a neurotransmitter that affects mood.
- *Sleep disorders*: Relaxation techniques.

MEDICAL TERMINOLOGY	
oste/o	bone
por/o	passage

CRITICAL THINKING 36.5

Beth and Jill room Rose Conrad, a 53-year-old patient. Mrs. Conrad is here to see Dr. Walden regarding her hormone replacement therapy, which she has been on for 3 years. Mrs. Conrad is willing to have Jill in the room during her discussion with Dr. Walden so that Jill can observe and learn. Mrs. Conrad recently read that her therapy may be dangerous. Dr. Walden agrees that if she is concerned, she can stop taking the medication; however, Dr. Walden recommends that Mrs. Conrad try some alternative therapies. What suggestions might Dr. Walden make for nonpharmaceutical treatment of perimenopausal symptoms?

OBSTETRICS

Pregnancy can be the most exciting and most terrifying experience for a patient, especially the first time around. As a medical assistant working in obstetrics, it is important to be able to reassure the patient while remaining professional. Patient education is vital for a woman who is planning to become pregnant or has just discovered that she is pregnant. Box 36.2 presents important tips the medical assistant can provide to these women. The next section will discuss the examinations and procedures related to prenatal and postpartum care.

Prenatal Record

At the first prenatal examination, an extensive health history will be taken. This history can help to identify any risk factors for the patient and the fetus. Frequently, the first prenatal visit is the first comprehensive physical examination that the patient has had in a long time. The health history can point out pregnancy-related risk factors and overall health-related risk factors that can also be addressed. Along with a general health history, the following information should be collected when creating the prenatal record for a patient:

- Demographic information
- Menstrual history
- Obstetric history
- Medical and surgical history
- Family and social history

The prenatal record will continue to be updated throughout the pregnancy. There will be clinical data added at each prenatal visit. You will also be checking with the patient to see if there have been any changes or additions to the initial demographic and history information. This information will supply the provider with the information needed to provide excellent care during the patient's pregnancy.

Menstrual History. The prenatal record should include the first day of the last menstrual period. This is used to help determine the *estimated date of delivery* (EDD) or due date. It is also

BOX 36.2   Patient Education: Obstetrics

A woman who is planning a pregnancy or who has just found out that she is pregnant may benefit from some simple guidelines for healthy living.

- *Nutrition:* Before pregnancy, emphasize the need for folic acid to prevent neural tube defects. The woman can take a supplement or can eat dark green, leafy vegetables. Many women have iron-deficiency anemia, and eating foods high in iron (red meat, spinach, or enriched cereal) is helpful. A pregnant woman needs about 1000 mg of calcium a day. During the first trimester, most women do not need any extra calories. During the second trimester, most women need about 340 extra calories a day. During the third trimester, daily calorie needs increase to 450.
- *Foods to avoid:* Fish high in mercury, such as orange roughy, shark, and swordfish. Foods that may contain bacteria: raw or rare fish, shellfish, meats, poultry, and eggs; unpasteurized juices, milk, or soft cheese; prepared meat salads; raw sprouts, and cold deli meat.
- *Limit caffeine and added sugars.* Encourage water and decaffeinated beverages.
- *Alcohol:* Alcohol passes through the placenta to the fetus and can cause fetal alcohol spectrum disorder (FASD). (See Chapter 6 for more information.) No amount of alcohol is considered safe during pregnancy.
- *Weight gain:* The recommendations are based on the woman's weight prior to pregnancy and if it is a multiple birth pregnancy. For women who are at normal weight prior to pregnancy and are having one baby, a gain of 25-35 pounds during pregnancy is recommended.
- *Smoking and Secondhand Smoke:* Smoking during pregnancy increases the risk of preterm birth, low birth weight, birth defects of the mouth and lip, and nicotine withdrawal at birth. Smoking during and after pregnancy increases the risk for sudden infant death syndrome (SIDS). With exposure to smoke after birth, infants can have weaker lungs and an increased risk in health problems.
- *Recreational drug use:* Recreational drugs are known to pass through the placenta to the fetus and can cause serious problems, including a higher risk of stillbirth. Regular use of certain drugs can cause neonatal abstinence syndrome (NAS). With NAS, the baby has to go through withdrawal upon birth. There is no "safe" drug; even those that are considered mild can have serous effects on the fetus's development and the newborn baby.
- *Medicine:* All chemicals pass through the placenta. A pregnant woman should never take any medicine (even over-the-counter drugs) without the knowledge and approval of her obstetrician. If the medical assistant is managing telephone screening, having a list of provider-approved medications next to the phone helps in answering patients' questions.
- *Sexually transmitted infection (STI) screening:* State law may require screening during pregnancy. Many STIs are asymptomatic in women but treatable. Infants are at risk for serious health problems if exposed to certain STIs in utero or during the birth process.

important to know the normal cycle length for the patient and if this last menstrual period was "normal." The medical assistant should also ask if the patient was using contraception when she became pregnant. If she was, the method being used should be documented.

Obstetric History. The provider will need to have a complete history of previous pregnancies. This will help to determine any risk factors for the current pregnancy. The following information should be included in the obstetric history (Fig. 36.7):

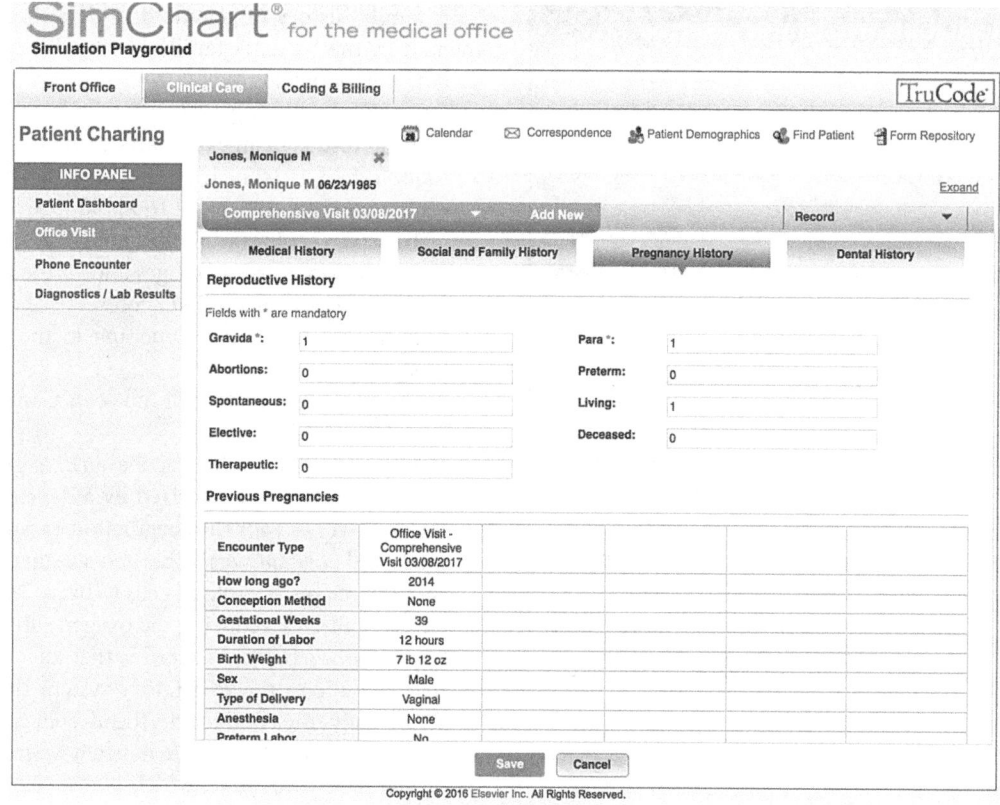

Fig. 36.7 Pregnancy History Form from SimChart for the Medical Office.

- Dates of previous deliveries
- Types of previous deliveries (vaginal or cesarean); if cesarean, the type of incision should be noted
- Birth weight and gestational age of previous infants
- Complications of previous pregnancies

A prenatal record includes documenting the gravida, para, and abortion information (Table 36.1). A medical assistant should be able to determine those numbers after obtaining the obstetric history from a patient. To calculate:

- *Gravida* (G): Number of pregnancies including the current pregnancy. A multiple birth pregnancy, such as twins or triplets, is counted as one.
- *Para* (P): Number of viable births or births >20 weeks (age of viability). A multiple birth pregnancy is counted as one. Stillbirths are also included in the para.
- *Abortion* or *abortus* (A or Ab): Termination of a pregnancy before the fetal age of viability (before 20 weeks' gestation), includes both spontaneous (miscarriage) and induced (elective) abortions.

For example, a 10-week pregnant woman, has 3 living children (a 6-year-old daughter and 3-year-old twin sons). She had a miscarriage at 13 weeks and a stillbirth at week 32. Her history would be G5, P3, Ab1.

The terminology TPAL may also be used in an obstetric history.

- T (Term births): Births after 37 weeks' gestation
- P (Preterm births): Births prior to 37 weeks' gestation
- A (Abortus or abortions): Includes spontaneous (miscarriage) and induced (elective) abortions
- L (Living children)

TPAL may be written as numbers separated by hyphens, such as 2-2-0-4. This means 2 term infants, 2 premature infants, 0 abortions, and 4 living children.

CRITICAL THINKING 36.6

Jill is interviewing a new OB patient. The patient tells Jill that this is her fourth pregnancy, and she has two children. She had two early miscarriages. What would her gravida number be? What would her para number be? What would her abortion number be?

MEDICAL TERMINOLOGY

para-	near, abnormal, beside
multi-	many
nulli-	none
primi-	first
-gravida	pregnancy

Medical and Surgical History. There are medical and surgical conditions that could affect a patient's current pregnancy. Common chronic conditions are:

- *Endocrine diseases*: Diabetes mellitus and thyroid disorders
- *Cardiovascular diseases*: Hypertension, mitral valve prolapse, and bleeding disorders
- *Respiratory disease*: Asthma
- *Autoimmune disorder*: Systemic lupus erythematosus
- *Reproductive diseases*: Pelvic inflammatory disease (PID), which can cause scarring of the fallopian tubes, which in turn

TABLE 36.1   Obstetric History Terms

Term	Definition
primigravida (pree ma GRAV i duh)	A woman who is pregnant for the first time
multigravida (muhl ti GRAV i duh)	A woman who has been pregnant two or more times
nulligravida (nuh li GRAV i duh)	A woman who has never been pregnant
primipara (pree ma PEAR uh)	A woman who has carried one pregnancy to the age of fetal viability
multipara (muhl ti PEAR uh)	A woman who has carried two or more pregnancies to the age of fetal viability
nullipara (nuh li PEAR uh)	A woman who has not carried a pregnancy to the age of fetal viability
spontaneous abortion	Natural death of an embryo or fetus before the fetal age of viability. Also called a *miscarriage*
therapeutic or *elective abortion*	A procedure for the planned termination of a pregnancy
stillbirth	Fetal death after 20 weeks' gestation. Also called *intrauterine fetal death* (IUFD)

increases the risk of an ectopic (eck TAH pick) pregnancy. If there is a history of prior ectopic pregnancy, the patient would be at risk for another one. A history of preeclampsia (pree eh KLAMP see ah) increases the risk of getting it with a future pregnancy.

These conditions can affect both the mother and the fetus. In order to help both, the provider needs to be aware of those conditions and the treatment that is being followed for each. This treatment may need to change or be adjusted during pregnancy.

A history of certain STIs can put the patient at risk for complications. For example, genital herpes and other infections can be transmitted to the newborn during delivery. If the provider is aware of those conditions, plans can be made to protect both the mother and the baby.

If the patient has had any type of abdominal surgical procedure, it could affect the pregnancy and/or delivery. If there is a history of a uterine puncture or any uterine incision, the patient and provider will need to talk about a possible cesarean section.

VOCABULARY

ectopic pregnancy Implantation of the embryo in any location other than the uterus.

preeclampsia A form of toxemia during pregnancy, characterized by high blood pressure, fluid retention, and protein in the urine. May progress to eclampsia.

viability Ability to live.

Family History. There are many conditions that have a genetic component to them. Obtaining an accurate family history can help to determine if the patient and/or the infant is at risk. Additional testing may be included during the prenatal period for a patient with certain factors in the family history. Conditions that could be of concern include diabetes, hypertension, heart disease, autoimmune disease, kidney disease, seizures, depression, thyroid disease, and preeclampsia.

A family history of genetic disorders should also be documented in the patient's family history. These disorders could include the following:

- *Down syndrome*: A genetic disorder in which abnormal cell division results in an extra chromosome 21.
- *Neuro tube defects*, such as:
  - *Spina bifida* (SPY nah BIF id dah): A condition in which the spinal column has an abnormal opening that allows protrusion of the meninges and/or the spinal column.
  - *Meningocele* (meh NING goh seel): The protrusion of the meninges through an opening in the spinal column or skull.
  - *Anencephaly* (an en SEF uh lee): Congenital absence of part or all of the brain.
- *Hemophilia* (hee moh FEE lee ah): A group of inherited blood disorders characterized by a deficiency of one of the factors necessary for the coagulation of blood.
- *Sickle cell anemia*: An inherited anemia characterized by crescent-shaped red blood cells (RBCs). This causes RBCs to block capillaries, reducing the oxygen supply to the cells.
- *Cystic fibrosis* (CF): A disorder that affects all the exocrine cells but affects the respiratory system the most. Mucus is abnormally thick and blocks the alveoli, causing dyspnea.
- *Phenylketonuria* (PKU): A deficiency in the enzyme phenylalanine hydroxylase, which is responsible for converting phenylalanine into tyrosine.

Other family history information that should be noted would include a history of twins in the family, food allergies, and a family history of recurrent miscarriages or stillbirths.

MEDICAL TERMINOLOGY

encephala/o	brain
hem/o	blood
mening/o, meningi/o	meninges
spin/o	spine
bi-	two
-cele	herniation
-fida	split
-philia	attraction, affinity
-y	process of; condition

Social History. The following information is included in the social history.

- *Use of tobacco and alcohol, and recreational drug use.* These substances can cause significant issues with the fetal development. Discussion of the use of these and assistance to quit during pregnancy should be discussed with the provider. It is important to make sure the patient understands that this information will not be reported to law enforcement, even if the patient admits to illegal drug use.
- *Dietary preferences and restrictions.* Finding out if the pregnant patient follows a particular diet, such as vegan or vegetarian, will provide the opportunity for patient education regarding the nutritional needs during pregnancy.
- *Exercise.* A discussion about exercise habits can help the patient minimize unnecessary weight gain in pregnancy, improve undesirable pregnancy-related symptoms, and keep

the mother healthy while pregnant. However, it is important that the provider discuss physical activities that should be avoided when pregnant.

- *Living accommodations* (including if the patient has a stable home, if she lives with others, and so on). Discussing living accommodations can alert the provider if there is a need to get a social worker involved. It is important to make sure there is a safe environment for the mother and baby.
- *Safety practices* (e.g., wearing a seatbelt). This provides a great opportunity to discuss safety habits and their importance during pregnancy.
- *Employment.* A discussion about employment can point out any occupational duties that could be affected by pregnancy, such as working with certain chemicals.

First Prenatal Examination

The physical examination during a first prenatal visit includes a complete physical examination and a pelvic examination. This is done so the provider can have a good overall assessment of the woman's health status. The medical assistant is often responsible for preparing the room and the patient for this examination.

When preparing the room, the medical assistant needs to ensure that the supplies and equipment necessary are available. This includes those needed for a physical exam and a pelvic exam, in addition to the equipment for performing pelvic measurements and anything needed to collect required lab specimens. The medical assistant will also need to collect vital signs, weight, and acquire a urine sample for urinalysis and possible pregnancy test.

A physical exam will be completed with special attention to the heart, lung, and thyroid. This is done to rule out any abnormalities that will need to be monitored during the pregnancy. Next, the provider performs an obstetric examination that includes measurement of the height of the uterus and a pelvic examination. It is common for a Pap test to be done at this time, in addition to basic screening for vaginal infections.

The EDD will be determined at this visit. There are a number of different ways to determine the due date. The most popular method is using a gestational wheel (Fig. 36.8). With this method the arrow is lined up with the first date of the LMP. The EDD is shown at the 40-week mark. The EDD may also be calculated by the electronic health record (EHR) or determined by ultrasound.

Laboratory Tests. Along with the physical exam, a series of lab tests are performed during the initial prenatal visit. Some of these tests may be repeated toward the end of the pregnancy, depending on state laws and the mother's health history.
- Blood test
  - *Blood type and Rh factor with antibody screening* for possible Rh incompatibility to determine if precautions need to be taken to avoid hemolytic disease of the newborn (Fig. 36.9 and Box 36.3).
  - *Hematocrit and/or hemoglobin levels* to check for anemia. Anemia can be problematic in a newly pregnant woman because there will be increased demands for oxygen and nutrients throughout the body.
  - *Rubella titer* to determine whether the mother is immune to German measles. A rubella infection during pregnancy

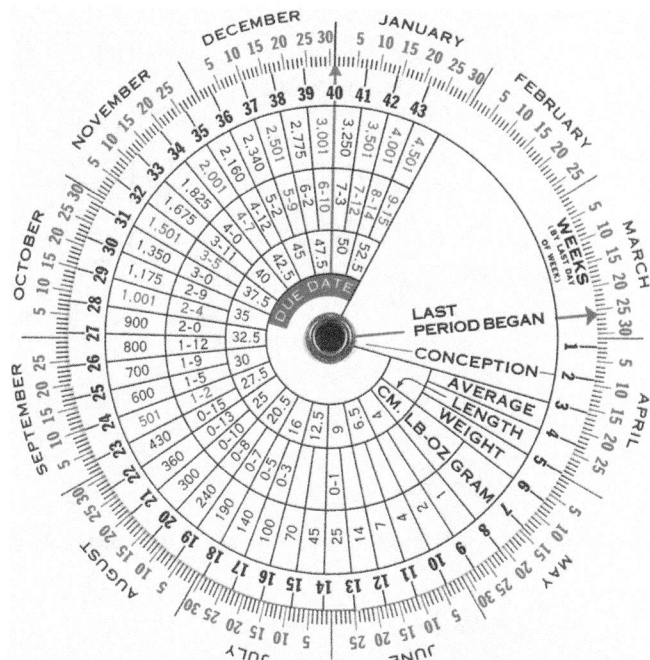

Fig. 36.8 Gestational Wheel. (From Jarvis C: *Physical examination and health assessment,* ed 6, St. Louis, 2012, Saunders.)

can cause multiple birth defects, including deafness, vision disorders, and intellectual disabilities.
  - *Syphilis screening.* If the result is positive, antibiotic treatment is initiated to protect the fetus from congenital syphilis.
  - *Hepatitis B screening,* because the virus can be passed to the fetus in utero.
  - *Human immunodeficiency virus (HIV) screening* is suggested. If the result is positive, treatment of the mother greatly reduces the risk of transmission to the fetus.
- Vaginal swab: Gonorrhea and chlamydia cultures to prevent infection of the baby at birth.
- Urine test
  - Urinalysis to detect protein, white blood cells, or glucose.
  - Pregnancy test to verify the pregnancy. Early prenatal visits often occur before the woman shows physical signs of pregnancy.

Prenatal Resources. Newly pregnant women and their partners often have strong emotions tied to a new pregnancy. Excitement, nervousness, and uncertainty are all normal responses to pregnancy and will often be even stronger in first-time pregnancies. Any specific concerns that the patient has should be reported to the provider. The medical assistant may need to define common obstetric terms when working with patients (Box 36.4). The medical assistant should also be prepared to suggest community resources that can aid new parents, such as:
- Childbirth and parenting classes
- Infant cardiopulmonary resuscitation (CPR) courses
- Nutritional counseling and assistance, such as Special Supplemental Nutrition Program for Women, Infants, and Children (WIC), which helps lower income expectant mothers get nutritious food.

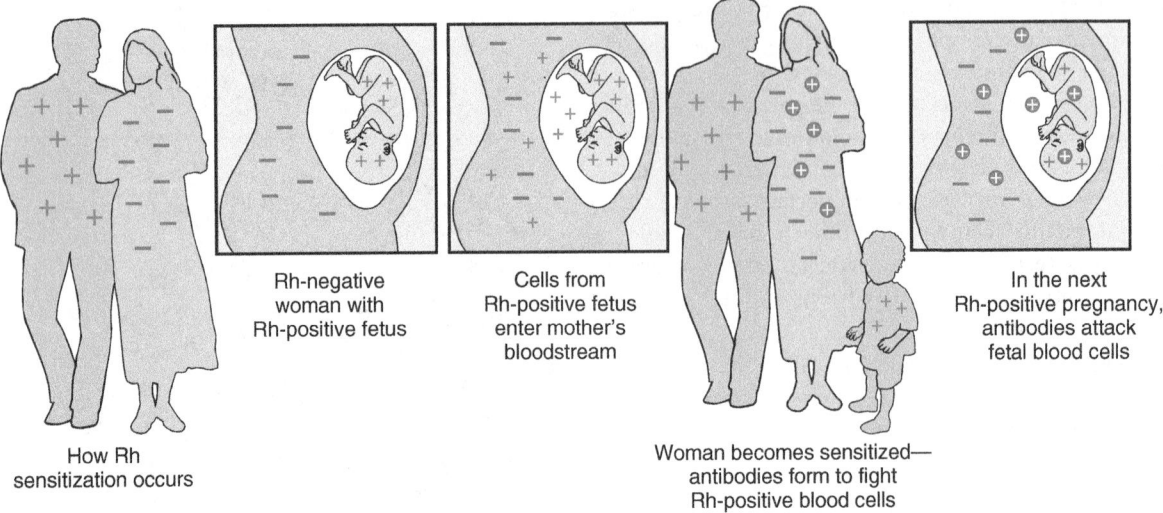

Fig. 36.9 Hemolytic Disease of the Newborn. (From Hagen-Ansert SL: *Textbook of diagnostic sonography,* ed 7, St. Louis, 2012, Mosby.)

BOX 36.3   Hemolytic Disease of the Fetus and Newborn

To determine if someone's blood type is Rh positive or Rh negative, the blood is tested for the presence of D antigens. Rh-positive blood has D antigens present. Rh-negative blood does not. If the blood type with Rh factor shows that the mother has Rh-negative blood, there is a concern that hemolytic disease of the fetus and newborn (HDFN) could develop if the fetus is Rh positive. HDFN is also known as *erythroblastosis fetalis* and *hemolytic disease of the newborn* (HDN). The condition occurs if the mother has Rh negative blood and fetus has Rh positive blood. If the fetal red blood cells move into the mother's circulation, the mother's body forms antibodies to the Rh-positive factor. Future Rh-positive pregnancies will be in jeopardy because the mother's anti-Rh antibodies will cross the placenta and destroy fetal blood cells.

HDN can be prevented by giving the mother Rh immune globulin products. A medication called RhoGAM, or anti-D immune globulin, is given around 28 weeks' gestation to Rh-negative mothers, regardless of the father's Rh type. After delivery, the cord blood is tested, and a dose of RhoGAM is given within 72 hours of delivery only if the baby is Rh positive. MICRhoGAM (a smaller dose of RhoGAM) or RhoGAM is also given for miscarriages or abortions. The immune globulin prevents the infant's Rh-positive cells from stimulating the mother's immune system, thus preventing HDN.

Return Prenatal Visits

Unless there are complications requiring a woman to be seen more often, most return prenatal visits follow a regular schedule:

- Every 4 weeks through 28 weeks' gestation.
- Every 2 weeks through 35 weeks' gestation.
- Every 1 week until delivery.

As with the initial prenatal visit, the medical assistant is often responsible for preparing the room and the patient before the provider enters the room. The medical assistant should take the patient's weight at every appointment and ask questions about the patient's diet and health habits. Typically, women gain 2 to 4 pounds during the first trimester and then 1 pound per week through the rest of the pregnancy. It is not uncommon for women to lose a small amount of weight early in pregnancy

---

BOX 36.4   Common Obstetric Terms

When working in obstetrics, the medical assistant should be familiar with these terms:

- *Braxton Hicks contractions*: Called "false labor," occurs typically during the third trimester when the uterus briefly tightens.
- *Cesarean section* (C-section): Infant is delivered through a surgical incision in the abdomen.
- *Colostrum*: A thick, yellowish fluid secreted from the breasts during pregnancy and during the first few days after childbirth.
- *Contractions*: Tightening of the uterine muscles. Frequency and intensity increase during labor until the child is born.
- *Effacement*: Thinning or shortening of the cervix; occurs before and during early labor. Expressed as a percentage.
- *Engorgement*: The breasts are swollen, hard, and painful because of being overly full of milk.
- *Episiotomy*: An incision made at the vaginal opening to assist with the delivery and prevent tearing and sutured after delivery.
- *Fetal distress*: The fetus shows signs of stress, usually occurs during labor. Fetal heart rate may decrease, and meconium may be seen in the amniotic fluid.
- *Induced labor*: Labor is started using artificial means, such as medication (e.g., Pitocin).
- *Linea nigra*: A dark vertical line that appears on the abdomen during pregnancy.
- *Lochia*: Postpartum vaginal discharge.
- *Premature birth*: Also called preterm birth, occurs when a baby is born before 37 weeks of pregnancy.
- *Presentation*: The way the baby is positioned in the uterus. *Vertex presentation* means the head will be delivered first. *Breech presentation* means the feet, shoulders, or buttocks are down and are delivered first. Some breech presentations require a C-section delivery.
- *Preterm labor*: Labor that occurs before 37 completed weeks of pregnancy.
- *Quickening*: Initial fetal movements felt by the women. May feel like light tapping or fluttery feeling.
- *Rupture of membranes*: Also called "water breaking." The amniotic sac ruptures and flush rushes out. Occurs before the baby is delivered.
- *VBAC*: Vaginal birth after previous cesarean section.

due to changes in appetite and nausea, which are common with early pregnancy. Too little weight gain could indicate a nutritional problem and could cause problems with the fetus's development. Too much weight gain could lead to health effects on the mother and could also affect the fetus.

The medical assistant should also ask the mother to leave a urine sample. At each visit the urine should be checked for protein and sugars. This is an early indicator of *gestational* (ges TA shun all) *diabetes mellitus* (GDM) and preeclampsia (PRE i KLAMP see ah), which can create pregnancy complications (Box 36.5). Vital signs are taken at each prenatal visit, with a specific emphasis on blood pressure. Blood pressure elevations, even if staying within normal range, can be an early indicator of preeclampsia.

Fetal Heart Tones. A Doppler ultrasound monitor needs to be available for each prenatal appointment. This is used to listen to the baby's heart tones starting at 9 to 12 weeks' gestation. It is important to remember that a fetal heart rate is much faster than an adult rate; it should be between 120 and 160 beats per minute. A slow fetal heart rate is a sign of fetal distress and should be followed up on by the provider immediately. If the medical assistant is assessing the fetal heart tones and gets a reading between 60 and 100 beats per minute, it may be because the mother's heart tones are being picked up. If this is the case, adjust the Doppler and try again. If the fetus's heart rate is not easily found, notify the provider.

Fundal Height Measurements. A flexible tape measure needs to be available for the provider to take fundal height measurements. As the uterus grows during pregnancy, it will rise into the abdominal cavity. Between 8 and 13 weeks' gestation the fundus can be palpated above the symphysis pubis. The fundal height is measured from the symphysis pubis to the fundus of the uterus. The height is measured in centimeters (cm). The measurement should match the number of weeks the patient has been pregnant through the first and second trimesters. For example, if the patient is 25 weeks pregnant, the provider would expect to see a fundal height measurement of 25 cm (Fig. 36.10). If the fundal height does not match the number of weeks pregnant, this could signal an issue with the pregnancy. Fundal height measurements that are either larger or smaller than expected could indicate:

- Inaccurate delivery date (inaccurate conception date)
- Slow fetal growth (intrauterine growth restriction)
- A significantly larger than average baby (*fetal macrosomia*)
- Too little amniotic fluid (*oligohydramnios* [oh lih goh hy DRAM nee ohs])
- Too much amniotic fluid (*polyhydramnios* [paw lee hy DRAM nee ohs])

If the provider suspects an issue, an ultrasound would likely be ordered to determine what was causing the unusual measurements.

VOCABULARY
fundus The top of the uterus.

BOX 36.5 Conditions and Diseases During Pregnancy

Pregnancy Related Conditions
During pregnancy, the healthcare provider monitors for pregnancy related conditions, such as:

- *Eclampsia* (eh KLAMP see ah): Extremely serious form of hypertension secondary to pregnancy. Patients are at risk for coma, convulsions, and death.
- *Ectopic pregnancy.* Implantation of the embryo in any location other than the uterus.
- *Hyperemesis gravidarum* (hy per EM eh sis grav ih DAIR um): Excessive vomiting that causes weakness, dehydration, and fluid and electrolyte imbalance.
- *Gestational diabetes.* Develops during pregnancy. The hyperglycemia can affect the health of the pregnancy and the baby. (See Chapter 7 for additional information.)
- *Placenta previa* (plah SEN tah PREE vee ah): Placenta that is positioned in the uterus so that it covers the opening of the cervix.
- *Placental abruption* or *abruptio placentae* (ah BRUP she oh plah SEN tee): Premature separation of the placenta from the uterine wall; may result in a severe hemorrhage that can threaten both infant and maternal lives.
- *Preeclampsia* (pree eh KLAMP see ah): Abnormal condition of pregnancy with unknown cause, marked by hypertension, edema, and proteinuria.

Infectious Diseases During Pregnancy
There are several infectious diseases that can harm the growing fetus during pregnancy. Examples of these diseases include:

- *Congenital Rubella Syndrome* (CRS): If a woman gets rubella during pregnancy, the risk increases for a miscarriage or a stillborn. The developing fetus may be at risk for severe birth defects.
- *Cytomegalovirus* (CMV): If a woman gets CMV, a common virus, during pregnancy, the baby may have spleen, liver, and brain problems. Babies with CMV may have growth problems and hearing loss.
- *Toxoplasmosis:* This parasite is spread from cat litter. If the pregnant woman becomes infected, the baby may be born without serious symptoms. The child can develop blindness and mental disabilities later in life.
- *Zika* (ZEE kuh) virus: A mosquito-borne virus that typically causes a mild fever, rash, and joint pain. Zika is concerning during pregnancy since the virus can be passed to a fetus. It can cause certain birth defects such as *microcephaly* (abnormally small head associated with incomplete brain development).

See Chapter 14 for additional information on conditions and diseases during pregnancy.

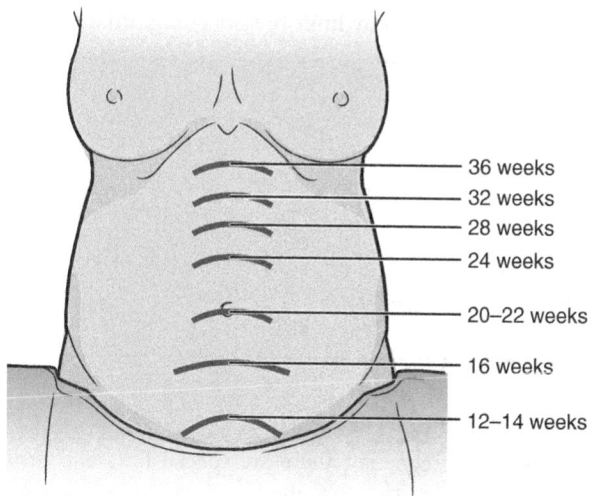

Fig. 36.10 Fundal Height Measurement.

- 36 weeks
- 32 weeks
- 28 weeks
- 24 weeks
- 20–22 weeks
- 16 weeks
- 12–14 weeks

Postpartum Visit

The patient should return about 6 weeks after delivery for a postpartum visit. At this visit, the provider will do a pelvic examination to make sure that everything is healing. If a cesarean section was done, the incision site will also be checked to see how it is healing. When preparing for this visit, set up for a pelvic examination. The provider will examine the cervix, vaginal canal, and perineum for healing. The perineum can tear during a vaginal delivery, which then requires suturing. Along with evaluating how the patient is healing, the postpartum visit is a good time to address any questions or concerns the patient may have. The following are some common topics.

- *Emotional health*: Postpartum depression, also called the *baby blues*, is quite common after delivery. It is generally due to the quick shift in hormones, loss of sleep, and significant disruption of the daily routine. All mothers should be screened for depression at the postpartum visit (Box 36.6).
- *Contraception*: After a new baby is born, the mother may want to use contraception.
  - If the mother is breastfeeding, the provider may recommend the mini-pill over the combination birth control pill.
  - If the patient previously used a diaphragm, the fit would need to be checked.
  - If an IUD is to be used, it is commonly placed during the postpartum visit.
- *Infant feeding*: Women should be checked for breast engorgement, mastitis, nipple irritation, or other issues related to lactation. It is often said that breastfeeding is best, and there is a lot of research to back up this claim. Mothers who are breastfeeding can be given provider-approved material on breastfeeding issues and information on local support groups. Some women are successful with breastfeeding, whereas other women struggle. Those who struggle can feel many negative emotions. Some women have personal reasons for not breastfeeding. Mothers who cannot, or choose not, to breastfeed should never be led to feel inadequate or shamed for this. It is important to remember that there are several medical issues that may limit breastfeeding. Infant formula does a very good job at maintaining appropriate nutrition levels in infants.

MEDICAL TERMINOLOGY	
hydr/o	water
olig/o	scanty, few
poly-	many, much, excessive, frequent
post-	after, behind
-amnios	amnion, inner fetal sac
-partum	parturition (delivery)

Special Tests and Procedures

Throughout the pregnancy, there are special tests and procedures that may done to assess the status of the pregnancy. In the next section we will explore some of the more common tests and procedures.

BOX 36.6   Postpartum Depression

- The incidence of postpartum depression (PPD) is not clear, but an estimated 10% to 20% of women struggle with major depression before, during, and after delivery of a baby. Fewer than half of these are diagnosed in routine office visits.
- Postpartum depression can be diagnosed a month to a year after childbirth. Women with a history of depression during pregnancy should be monitored for signs of postpartum depression for a minimum of 4 months.
- Risk factors include a history of depression, abuse, or mental illness; smoking or alcohol use; anxiety during pregnancy and fears over childcare; lack of financial resources and secure relationships; a fussy or colicky infant; and lack of social support.
- Symptoms of postpartum depression include anorexia and insomnia; irritability and anger; overwhelming fatigue; loss of interest in sex and lack of a feeling of joy in life; feelings of shame, guilt, or inadequacy; severe mood swings; difficulty bonding with the baby; withdrawal from family and friends; and thoughts of harming herself or the baby.
- Postpartum depression must be detected as soon as possible so that treatment can begin; untreated postpartum depression may last for a year or longer. Treatment includes both counseling and antidepressant medication.
- The 10-question Edinburgh Postnatal Depression Scale (EPDS) is a valuable and efficient way of identifying patients at risk for perinatal depression (between the 28th week of pregnancy and the 28th day after birth). Healthcare professionals working with the perinatal population should use the EPDS as a routine part of postnatal care, because the EPDS is a valid and reliable means of detecting PPD. This screening tool is user friendly, easy to administer, and easy to score. A score of 10 to 12 is considered the cutoff for PPD; the mother should be referred for further evaluation or treatment. Users may reproduce the scale without further permission, providing they respect the copyright by quoting the names of the authors and the title and the source of the paper in all reproduced copies. The EPDS can be accessed at the American Academy of Pediatrics website: https://www.aap.org/en-us/advocacy-and-policy/aap-health-initiatives/practicing-safety/Documents/Postnatal%20Depression%20Scale.pdf%23search=postnatal%20depression.

Ultrasound. Ultrasound examinations are typically done once during the first trimester and then again between 18 and 20 weeks' gestation (Fig. 36.11). These are done in order to assess the mother's organs, the implantation site, and fetal growth and development and also to confirm the age of the fetus. The sex of the baby can also be determined during the later ultrasound. Although it is important to get a urine sample with the prenatal visits, this should be avoided during the ultrasound visit. The patient needs a full bladder for the ultrasound.

Ultrasound uses sound waves that travel well through fluid. Having a full bladder during ultrasounds early in the pregnancy provides a great "window" for the sound waves, allowing for the best possible images. The patient should be instructed to drink two or three 8-ounce glasses of water 1 hour before the scheduled ultrasound. It can be very uncomfortable for a patient to have a full bladder, especially when pregnant. Because of this, it is very important that ultrasound appointments be on time and the patient is not left to wait.

Triple/Quad Screen. Between weeks 15 and 18 of pregnancy, the provider may suggest that the patient have a maternal blood screen to detect any risk of fetal and chromosomal disorders. This could be a Triple Screen Test (also known as AFP Plus, multiple marker test, and multiple marker screen) or a Quad

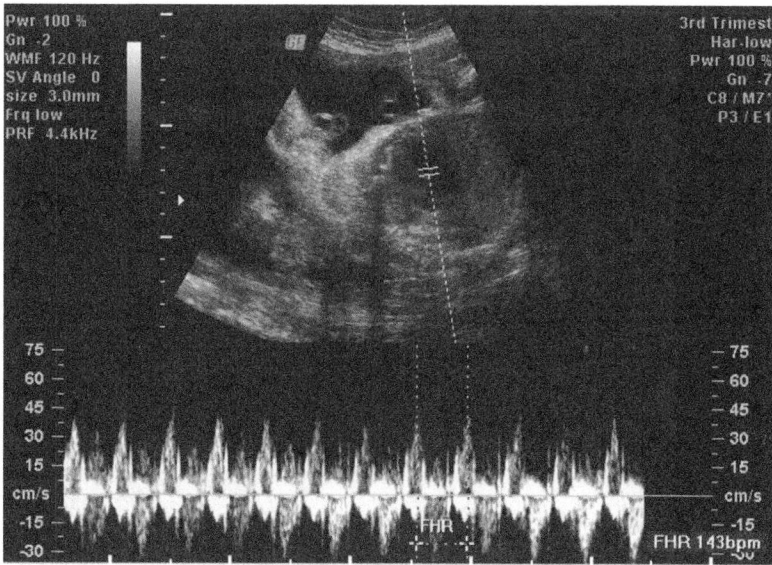

Fig. 36.11 Ultrasound Image of a Fetus.

Screen Test (also known as the quadruple marker test). Both tests screen for:

- Alpha-fetoprotein (AFP): Protein made by the fetus. Elevated levels may indicate a potential defect.
- Human chorionic gonadotropin (hCG): A hormone produced by the placenta. Low levels may indicate potential issues with the pregnancy. Elevated levels may indicate a molar pregnancy or a multiple birth pregnancy.
- Estriol: This type of estrogen is produced by the placenta and the placenta. Low levels may indicate a risk of Down syndrome.

The Quad Screen Test also looks at the level of Inhibin-A, which is a hormone made by the placenta. It may indicate Down syndrome.

The provider will discuss the accuracy of the tests with the patient. They are recommended in women who have a family history of these conditions.

Glucose Challenge Test. Between 24 and 28 weeks of pregnancy, the provider will typically order a glucose challenge test. This is used to determine if the mother is at risk for developing GDM. Some factors can increase the risk of developing GDM:

- A body mass index (BMI) before pregnancy of 30 or higher
- A first-degree relative (mother, father, sibling or child) with type 2 diabetes

For a glucose challenge test the patient will be asked to ingest a relatively high amount of glucose. Typically, a glucose solution drink is used, but glucose chewable tablets can also be used for the test. One hour later, the blood glucose level is checked. A level of 130 to 140 milligrams per deciliter (mg/dL) is considered normal. If the result is higher than that, a glucose tolerance test may be ordered.

The glucose tolerance test involves having the patient fast overnight before coming in for a blood glucose reading. The patient will then drink another glucose solution and have her blood glucose level checked every hour for the next 3 hours. If two out of the three readings are higher than normal, the patient would be diagnosed with gestational diabetes.

Group B Strep Test. Group B streptococcus (GBS) is a common bacterium found in the digestive tract and the genital area of adults. It is so common that it is found in about 1 in 4 pregnant women. GBS does not generally cause problems for adults who carry it, but if it is present in women during delivery, it can cause serious illness for a newborn baby. GBS can be passed to the baby during childbirth, causing meningitis, pneumonia, and life-threatening septicemia. Between 32 and 36 weeks' gestation, the provider usually tests for GBS by taking a swab of vaginal secretions. If the patient tests positive for GBS, she will receive intravenous (IV) antibiotics during labor. This significantly lowers the risk of the baby getting GBS disease.

> **VOCABULARY**
>
> **septicemia** A systemic infection marked by pathologic microbes in the blood as a result of an infection that has spread from elsewhere in the body.

Chorionic Villus Sampling. Chorionic villi are tiny placental projections, the cells of which have the same genetic material found in fetal cells. Chorionic villus sampling (CVS) involves the removal of a small piece of the chorionic villi, either transvaginally or through a small incision in the abdomen (Fig. 36.12). Cellular screening is done between weeks 11 and 14 of pregnancy gestation and provides early detection of genetic or chromosomal disorders. Results are generally available within a few days. Potential complications include miscarriage, Rh sensitization (for Rh-negative mothers), and uterine infection. Due to the serious potential complications, CVS generally is done only if there is a high risk of genetic or chromosomal disorders.

Amniocentesis. *Amniocentesis* is a test that may be done after 14 weeks of pregnancy. It can be done to:

- Test for genetic conditions, such as Down syndrome
- Diagnose a fetal infection
- Check the fetal lung maturity prior to delivery
- Treat polyhydramnios
- Test for paternity

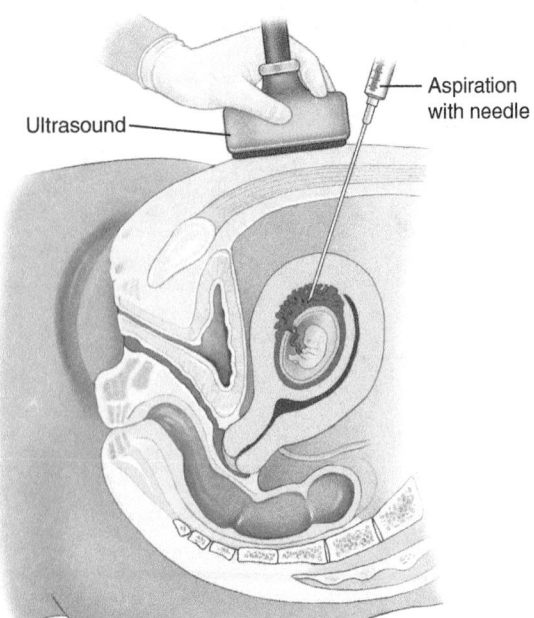

Fig. 36.12 Chorionic Villus Sampling. (From Shiland B: *Medical terminology and anatomy for* ICD-10 *coding*, St. Louis, 2012, Mosby.)

During the procedure, a needle is inserted into the placenta guided by an ultrasound. Less than 1 ounce (30 mL) of amniotic fluid is drawn out and sent to the laboratory for testing (Fig 36.13). Potential complications include leaking of amniotic fluid, miscarriage, fetal injury, Rh sensitization, and infection.

RECOGNIZING DOMESTIC ABUSE

Abuse was discussed in Chapter 19, and all of the recommendations, reporting requirements, and warning signs also are true for pregnant women. It is unfortunately common for domestic abuse to increase during pregnancy. This is often due to a number of factors:

- The partner is upset because of an unplanned pregnancy.

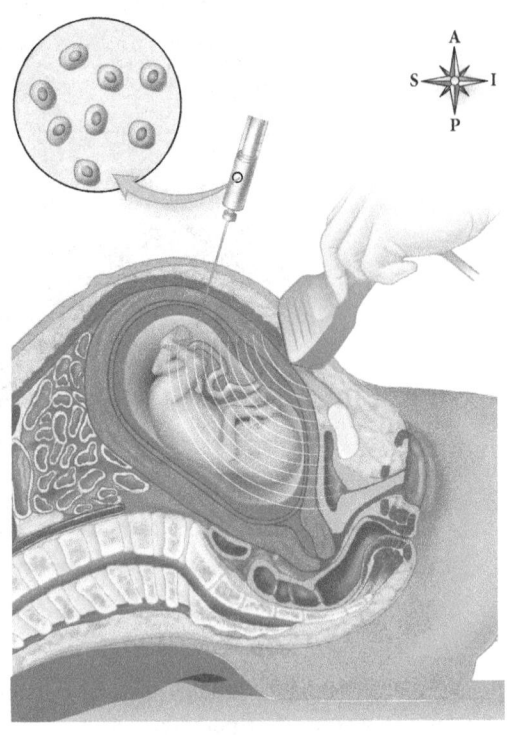

Fig. 36.13 Amniocentesis. In amniocentesis, a syringe is used to collect amniotic fluid. Ultrasound imaging is used to guide the tip of the syringe needle to prevent damage to the placenta and fetus. (From Patton KT, Thibodeau GA: *The human body in health and disease*, ed 7, St. Louis, 2018, Elsevier.)

- There is increased stress in the need to plan for a child, especially with finances.
- The partner resents the shift in attention away from them and to the new baby.

It is always important to watch for signs of abuse in all patients. This responsibility increases when dealing with vulnerable populations, such as pregnant women and their unborn children. Be sure to report any concerns to the provider immediately.

CLOSING COMMENTS

Working in OB/GYN can be a very rewarding experience. Patients being seen for conditions related to OB/GYN are often put in positions that feel compromising and uncomfortable. Being mindful of this and providing support to your patients can make the trying experience more tolerable for them. When working with obstetric patients, you have an opportunity to develop a strong relationship with your patients, because you are seeing them on a regular basis. Using good communication techniques and active listening skills will help to build that relationship. By building that solid patient-provider relationship, you become part of providing the best possible care for your patient.

PATIENT-CENTERED CARE

Given the intimate nature of OB/GYN visits, women visiting the healthcare facility for an OB/GYN issue often experience very strong emotions. This could be the result of anxiety over the examination or potential test results, or perhaps excitement over a new pregnancy. This can make the experience even more memorable for the patient, and it is the duty of the medical assistant to do all that they can to prioritize the patient's experience. There are three specific strategies that can be used to help improve your patient's experience:

- Active listening: Demonstrate to your patient that you respect their opinions and hear their concerns.
- Clear communication: Make sure that the patient is well aware of what to expect and what will be expected of them.
- Personal warmth: A patient will notice if you are distracted or rushed. It is important to do your best to minimize stress and tension.

BEING PROFESSIONAL

To provide excellent customer service while working in obstetrics and gynecology, a medical assistant should:

- Behave in a professional manner at all times because this can be an uncomfortable and embarrassing situation for the patient.
- During patient education sessions, make sure that the patient truly understands the content.

- Stay current with the new topics and technology related to obstetrics and gynecology.
- Treat all patients as you would want to be treated.

Role-play the following scenario with a peer, who will be the patient: Casey is a new patient at your clinic. As you take her vital signs, she tells you that she has never had a well-woman examination before and is very nervous about what is going to happen. Address Casey's nervousness and anxiety.

CHAPTER REVIEW

Obstetrics and gynecology are very closely linked. Gynecology is the study of the female reproductive system. Obstetrics deals with pregnancy, labor, and the postpartum period. In order to sustain a pregnancy, the reproductive system needs to be healthy. The gynecologic examination, which includes a breast and pelvic examination, is done to determine if there are any abnormalities in the female reproductive system. Obstetric examinations are done to evaluate the health of the mother and the infant. For both of these exams the medical assistant is involved in the following ways:

- Setting up for the examination
- Preparing the patient for the examination
- Obtaining vitals and any other preordered measurements or specimens

- Assisting the provider and patient during the examination
- Providing patient education as directed by the provider
- Processing specimens obtained during the examination
- Cleaning and restocking the examination room

Whether the patient is being seen for a gynecologic examination or an obstetric examination, the medical assistant has a duty to look for signs of abuse. If the medical assistant sees those signs, they must be reported to the provider.

As always, medical assistants have a duty to provide excellent customer service to all patients. This can be done by behaving in a professional manner, having resources available for all patients, and treating everyone (patients and co-workers) as you would want to be treated.

SCENARIO WRAP-UP

Jill Snow has enjoyed her time in the OB/GYN department and has learned a lot from Beth. She was able to observe several procedures and saw how Beth prepped the patient and the exam room for those procedures. Beth has been an amazing mentor for Jill. She has taken the time to explain the reasons for each procedure and the way it is done. Beth's knowledge and expertise in OB/GYN, along with her willingness to teach others, has made Jill decide to pursue a position in this field after she graduates. Beth's supervisor recognizes her talents in this area and has asked her to take over the practicum program for their department.

PROCEDURE 36.1 Set Up for and Assist the Provider With a Gynecologic Examination

Tasks

Prepare equipment for a gynecologic examination and assist the provider by placing the patient in the appropriate positions.

Equipment and Supplies

- Patient's health record
- Fecal occult blood test kit
- Water-soluble lubricant
- Vaginal speculum
- Liquid preparation container or slide and fixative
- Cervical spatula or plastic-fronded broom
- Laboratory requisition form and labels for specimen containers
- Cotton-tipped applicator
- Mayo stand or tray with paper procedure towel
- Gloves
- Patient gown and drape

- Disinfectant wipes
- Biohazardous waste container
- Waste container

Procedural Steps

1. Wash hands or use hand sanitizer. Ensure room is clean and has been disinfected for the next patient.
   Purpose: Hand sanitization is an important step for infection control.
2. Obtain and organize supplies and instruments for the gynecologic examination. Place on a tray or Mayo stand in a logical order.
   Purpose: Having the equipment in a logical order allows you to assist the clinician in an efficient manner.
3. Greet the patient. Identify yourself. Verify the patient's identity with full name and date of birth. Explain the procedure to be performed in a manner that is understood by the patient. Answer any questions the patient may have about the procedure.

Continued

PROCEDURE 36.1   Set Up for and Assist the Provider With a Gynecologic Examination—cont'd

Purpose: It is important to identify the patient in two different ways to ensure that you have the correct patient. Explaining the procedure can make the patient feel more comfortable and helps to reduce anxiety.

4. Ask if the patient needs to empty her bladder; collect a urine specimen if needed.
   Purpose: An empty bladder will make the pelvic examination more comfortable for the patient.

5. Instruct the patient to undress and put on the gown with the opening in front or as indicated by the provider. Instruct patient to sit on the exam table and place the drape over her lap. Assist the patient if needed or give the patient privacy to change.
   Purpose: The patient will need to be completely undressed for the examination. The first position used for the gynecologic examination is the sitting position. In this position the provider will visually inspect the breasts.

6. Assist the patient into the supine position, providing a pillow under her head for comfort. Pull out the leg extension on the examination table.
   Purpose: For the rest of the breast examination and the abdominal examination, the patient will need to be in the supine position.

7. With the stirrups in place on the examination table, assist the patient into the lithotomy position. The leg extension should be pushed in.

Purpose: The lithotomy position is used for the pelvic examination.

8. When the examination is complete, assist the patient into the sitting position. Instruct the patient that she can get dressed. Assist patient as needed or give the patient privacy to change.
   Purpose: At the end of the examination the patient can get dressed.

9. After the patient has left the exam room, put on gloves. Prepare specimens for transport to the laboratory. Dispose of any biohazard waste in designated biohazardous waste containers. Dispose of exam table paper and other waste in the waste container. Use disinfectant wipes to clean the exam table and any other potentially contaminated surface. Disinfect all equipment.
   Purpose: To prevent cross-contamination with any potentially infectious materials.

10. Remove the gloves, discard them in the waste container, and wash your hands or use hand sanitizer.
    Purpose: To ensure infection control.

11. Allow the exam table to dry before pulling clean paper over the table. Replace used supplies and prepare the room for the next patient.

37

Assisting in Pediatrics

LEARNING OBJECTIVES

1. Describe childhood growth and developmental patterns.
2. Measure and document a child's height, weight, head circumference, and chest circumference.
3. Calculate a patient's body mass index.
4. Describe Erikson's psychosocial development stages for children.
5. Describe common childhood diseases.
6. Describe common childhood immunizations and the current pediatric immunization schedule.
7. Explain the type of information on the Vaccine Information Statement and how to document vaccinations.
8. Discuss therapeutic approaches for working with infants, toddlers, preschoolers, school-aged children, and adolescents.
9. Describe the Apgar scoring system.
10. List the frequency of well-child visits as recommended by the American Academy of Pediatrics.
11. Discuss sick-child visits and telephone screening questions to obtain information about the patient's symptoms.
12. Describe how to obtain pediatric vital signs.
13. Specify child safety guidelines for injury prevention and management of suspected child abuse.

OUTLINE

▶ OPENING SCENARIO

Allison Kwong, CMA (AAMA), who has 2 years of experience, has accepted a new position with the pediatric department of the Walden-Martin Family Medical (WMFM) Clinic. Allison's primary responsibility will be to assist in the clinical area, but she also will rotate through the message screening center in the office.

Office policy states that telephone screening employees should manage problems using the protocols signed by the providers. All advice given to patients must be from the protocols. Any questions and anything not addressed by the protocols must be addressed with the provider. The policy also indicates that all phone communication and advice given must be documented in the patient's health record.

Although Allison has worked in the healthcare field for 2 years, she does not have much experience with pediatrics. She is glad that she has been assigned a mentor for the first few weeks.

YOU WILL LEARN

1. The normal growth and development patterns of children.
2. To recognize the common childhood diseases.
3. The Centers for Disease Control and Prevention (CDC) schedule of immunizations.
4. Common vaccines and combination vaccines used in pediatrics.
5. The difference between a well-child visit and a sick child visit.
6. How to assist with pediatric examinations, including obtaining vital signs.

INTRODUCTION

Pediatrics (pee dee A triks) is the medical specialty that deals with the development and care of children and with the treatment of childhood diseases. Pediatric patients range in age from newborn to 17 years of age. Some providers may consider pediatric patients to be under 21 years of age. Due to the unique considerations necessary with pediatric patients, medical specialties often have providers who specialize in seeing children within that specialty. For example, specialties such as surgery, cardiology, and psychiatry have pediatric specialists who focus on the care of children in these areas.

Approximately 50% of the patients who visit a pediatric office are not sick. Rather, they come to the healthcare facility for well-baby or well-child visits. These visits are important because they help the provider track the growth and development of the child. They can also be used to identify any developmental issues that may be arising.

Pediatric care actually starts before the child is born, with good prenatal care. This was discussed in Chapter 36. Good healthcare (both before and after birth), along with confidence and enthusiasm by the parents, can have a significant impact on an infant's physical and emotional well-being. Medical assistants can help provide good healthcare and encourage confidence through the use of therapeutic communication. Using sensitivity and empathy in our approach to patients can help the patient and family develop trust in the staff, the facility, and even the provider. This trust forms the basis of good medical care.

NORMAL GROWTH AND DEVELOPMENT

Although the terms *growth* and *development* are often used together, they actually mean very different things. *Growth* refers to measurable changes, such as height and weight. The potential height of any individual is determined by genetic factors. However, environmental factors, nutritional status, and the presence of disease at key times in a child's life can slow growth and limit height. Weight also has a genetic element but is more strongly influenced by nutrition, disease, and environmental factors.

Development refers to specific stages of physical, cognitive (mental), and social growth. A child's development is determined by a combination of prenatal, nutritional, and environmental factors. Disease and disorders (including mental illness) can also influence developmental progress. Development is evaluated by identifying when the child performs key skills or developmental milestones. Example of these milestones include taking a first step, learning to speak, or using the toilet independently.

Children have their own pattern of growth and development. Growth patterns and individual milestones vary by each child. A comprehensive health history and clear documentation from appointment to appointment are important. The provider uses these to evaluate trends in growth and development specific to that child.

Growth Patterns

Physical growth is one of the most visible changes in childhood. Infants grow very quickly during the first year of life. Growth patterns include:

- 5-6 months of age: Birth weight doubles
- 1-year-old: Triples the birth weight, length increases by 50%, and the head circumference equals the chest circumference
- 2-year-old: Gains about 5 pounds in 1 year and reaches about half of his or her adult height.
- 3- to 6-year-olds: Gains 4-5 pounds yearly and grows 2-3 inches each year

By school age, the child usually slims down, taking on characteristics most commonly associated with a preschooler.

Growth tends to slow down from age 6 to 12 years, but as the child nears puberty, growth will speed up again. This is referred to as a *growth spurt*. Between the ages of 12 and 18, girls will typically gain about 20 to 25 pounds and 5 to 6 inches in height. Boys will gain about 15 to 20 pounds and gain 4 to 5 inches in height. During this time the adolescent will reach sexual maturity. The specific timing of this varies greatly from person to person. In girls, sexual maturity is signaled by the onset of the menstrual cycle. In boys, it is determined by the presence of sperm in the semen.

Height is gained through skeletal growth. Skeletal growth is considered complete when the epiphyseal (eh PIFF ih see uhl) plates of the long bones of the extremities have completely fused. This generally occurs in girls between the ages of 15 and 16. It generally occurs in boys between the ages of 17 and 18.

> **VOCABULARY**
> **epiphyseal plate** A thin layer of cartilage located at the ends of a long bone where new bone forms. Also called the *growth plate*.

Measurements. In order to properly evaluate growth patterns, the provider will need regular and accurate measurements. These should be completed at each visit and include:

- Height or length
- Weight (Procedure 37.1)
- Head circumference (measured until age 3) (Procedure 37.2)
- Chest circumference (optional) (see Procedure 37.2)

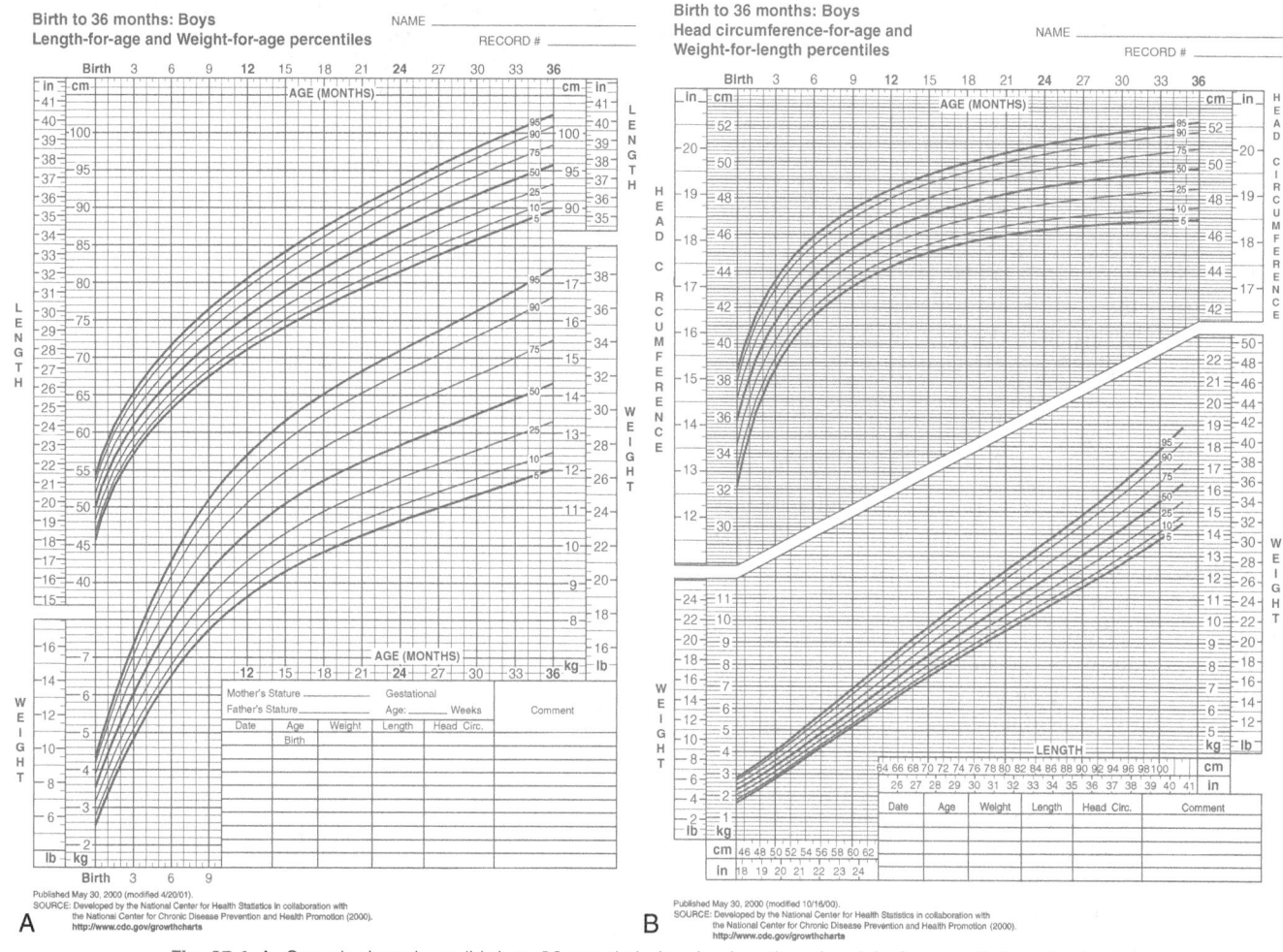

Fig. 37.1 A, Growth chart: boys (birth to 36 months) showing length and weight for age. B, Growth chart: boys (birth to 36 months) showing head circumference for age and length for weight.

- Body mass index (BMI) (for children 2 years and older)

During routine well-child visits, the medical assistant should measure the head circumference for children under 3 years of age. The circumference measurement provides information on the child's growth and development. The size of the child's head reflects the growth of the brain. Brain growth is 50% complete by 1 year of age, 75% by age 3, and 90% by age 6. Routine head measurement is recommended in children until 36 months of age and in older children whose head size is not within norms. If the circumference of the head deviates greatly from normal measurements, hydrocephalus (hi droe SEF ah luhs) or microcephaly (MY krow SEF ah lee) may be suspected.

The provider will determine if the chest circumference needs to be measured. Usually the head circumference of a newborn is about 2 cm larger than the chest circumference. Both measurements are equal between 6 months and 2 years. After 2 years of age, the chest circumference is larger.

Along with the head circumference, the medical assistant should measure the child's length and weight. These measurements are documented on the growth chart, which is used to compare a child's individual growth pattern with national standards. The growth chart also helps the provider track the child's growth over time. Early detection of abnormal growth patterns is important so that treatment can be started early, avoiding long-term complications.

The CDC has published 20 different growth charts, 10 for each sex. Growth charts are birth sex specific and vary by age groups:

- *Birth to 36 months*: Designed to have length and weight by age on one side and head circumference for age and weight for length on the other side (Fig. 37.1).
- *2 to 20 years*: Designed to have stature (height) and weight for age on one side, and BMI for age on the other side.

Many electronic health record (EHR) systems contain a growth chart tool. When the measurements are charted, the tool automatically plots the measurements on the appropriate growth chart and calculates the percentile and the BMI if relevant.

VOCABULARY

hydrocephalus An abnormal accumulation of cerebrospinal fluid that causes enlargement of the skull and compression of the brain.

microcephaly Abnormally small head associated with impaired brain development.

MEDICAL TERMINOLOGY	
cephal/o	head
micro/o	small
auto-	self
hydro-	water
-y	process of, condition

Calculate the Body Mass Index. The BMI is a measurement that compares the relationship between height and weight. If the BMI is not calculated by the EHR, the medical assistant can use the following formula to calculate the BMI:

$$BMI = \frac{Weight(lb)}{Height(in)^2} \times 703$$

For example: A child is 40 pounds (lb) and 36 inches (in). Round the BMI to the nearest tenth. Calculate: $40 \div (36)^2 \times 703 = BMI$. Answer: 21.7 (*Tip*: If your calculator does not have the square function, divide the weight by height twice and then multiple the answer by 703. For this problem you would punch the following into your calculator: $40 \div 36 \div 36 \times 703$.)

Childhood growth patterns will cause variations to BMI, causing normal BMI in children to change depending on the child's age. Because of this, growth charts are used to evaluate BMI in children. The CDC's weight status categories include:

- Underweight: Less than the 5th percentile
- Normal or health weight: 5th percentile to less than the 85th percentile
- Overweight: 85th percentile to less than the 95th percentile
- Obese: Equal to or greater than the 95th percentile

CRITICAL THINKING 37.1

Calculate the following BMIs. Round your answer to the nearest tenth.
1. Weight 60 pounds and length 38 inches
2. Weight 84 pounds and length 53 inches
3. Weight 22 pounds and length 21 inches
4. Weight 46 pounds and length 34 inches
5. Weight 52 pounds and length 36 inches
6. Weight 72 pounds and length 50 inches

Developmental Patterns

Children develop rapidly during the first year of life as the infant progresses from reflex activities (e.g., grasping fingers and sucking) to learning to manipulate simple objects (e.g., pulling open drawers or throwing toys out of the crib). In addition to these motor skills, the child learns verbal patterns, progressing from cooing and crying for attention to speaking their first words. Development continues throughout childhood with clear patterns based on age (Table 37.1).

During the preschool stage, the child becomes increasingly independent and initiates activities. Preschoolers have mastered many gross motor skills and are perfecting their fine motor development. Verbal communication has increased to full simple and even complex sentences but remains quite literal. Nonverbal communication skills are also being mastered. The

TABLE 37.1 Early Developmental Milestones

Age	Developmental Milestones
2-month-old	Begins to smile. Coos and turns head towards sound. Looks at faces. Begins to follow things with eyes. Can hold head up and begins to push up when lying on tummy.
4-month-old	Smiles spontaneously. Babbles. Reaches for toys. Uses hand-eye coordination. Holds head steady, unsupported. Brings hand to mouth.
6-month-old	Knows familiar faces. Likes to look at self in a mirror. Makes "ah" and "oh" sounds. Responds to own name. Passes things between hands. Makes sounds to show joy and displeasure. Rolls over in both directions. Begins to sit without support.
9-month-old	May be afraid of strangers and clingy to familiar adults. Understands "no." Uses fingers to point at things. Plays peek-a-boo. Stands while holding on. Sits without support and pulls self up to stand. Crawls.
1-year-old	Cries when parent(s) leave. Puts out arms or legs to help with dressing. Responds to simple spoken requests. Tries to say words you say. Says "mama" and "dada." Shakes, bangs, and throws objects. Follows simple directions. Walks holding onto furniture. May stand alone.
18-month-old	May have temper tantrums. Says several single words. Says and shakes head "no." Knows ordinary things, such as spoon and telephone. Scribbles. Walks along and may pull toys while walking.
2-year-old	Copies others. Shows defiant behavior by doing things he or she has been told not to do. Says 2-4-word sentences. Knows names of familiar people and body parts. Begins to sort shapes and colors. Can build towers with 4 or more blocks. Kicks ball and begins to run.
3-year-old	Shows increased *autonomy* (aw TON uh mee) or the ability to function independently. Walks and is toilet trained. Sits at the table and eats with the family. Makes simple sentences. Understands "no." Imitates the parents by using verbal gestures. The vocabulary consists of up to 900 words.

vocabulary now includes more than 2000 words. During this period children need to develop social skills, such as sharing and taking part in peer group activities.

School-aged children have perfected fine motor skills and can paint, draw, and play an instrument. They enjoy team activities and are expanding their reading and writing skills. Their intellectual skills are developing, and social skills are going through refinement as a sense of self-achievement and self-worth is developed. During this time, the child learns and tests the rules for socializing outside the immediate family as an independent individual.

During adolescence, the individual attempts to establish an adult identity. The teenager proceeds by trial and error, experimenting with adult roles and behavior patterns. Traditional values learned in childhood may be questioned, and peer relationships take on new importance. During this time teenagers must develop the emotional maturity and motivation to make reasonable decisions. They look to family members for encouragement and guidance in making decisions that will help them develop self-confidence and to become patient, in addition to less impulsive and self-centered.

The CDC has published typical milestones for different age groups, which can be helpful for providers and parents. The milestones cover social, emotional, language/communication, cognitive, and movement/physical development. For each age group the milestones (what a child of that age usually can do) in these areas are listed. This resource is available at the website: https://www.cdc.gov/ncbddd/actearly/milestones/index.html.

CRITICAL THINKING 37.2

Allison receives a call from the mother of a 6-month-old child. The woman is concerned that her child may not be reaching his developmental milestones. What type of information about the child's growth and development should Allison gather? If Allison is unable to answer the mother's questions, what should she do?

Psychosocial Development Stages

One well known psychologist in the area of child development was Erik Erikson. His theory is based on stages of development that the individual must pass through and master. Each stage focuses on a developmental crisis, which an individual must resolve in order to move on to higher levels of development.

When you work in pediatrics, it can be helpful to understand Erikson's stages and how you can help patients as they work to master each stage. (See Chapter 17 for more information.) According to Erikson, the following are the stages that children must master:

- *Trust versus mistrust:* Infants learn to rely on caregivers; mistrust occurs if needs are not met.
- *Autonomy versus shame and doubt:* Toddlers learn language skills and gain independence. They may feel shame and doubt if they cannot meet parental expectations or are overprotected.
- *Initiative versus guilt:* Preschoolers actively seek out new experiences. Children become hesitant if restrictions or reprimands make them feel guilty or afraid to try more challenging skills.
- *Industry versus inferiority:* School-aged children enjoy finishing projects and receiving recognition. They develop feelings of inferiority if not accepted by peers or if they cannot please their parents.
- *Identity versus role confusion:* Adolescents face many physical and hormonal changes in this stage. Teenagers work at figuring out who they are and where they fit. They are looking for a direction for their lives. If they are unable to establish an identity and sense of direction, they become role confused.

PEDIATRIC DISEASES AND DISORDERS

Pathogenic microbes have the potential to make any susceptible host sick, regardless of age. However, it is important to understand that the disease process in pediatric patients comes with a few special considerations. Children are constantly changing both physically and functionally. Immature organ systems,

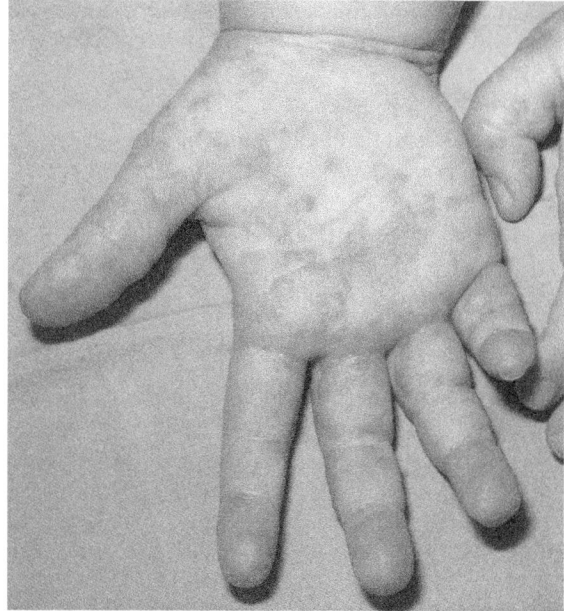

Fig. 37.2 Vesicular Palm Lesion in Hand-Foot-and-Mouth Disease. (From Fitzpatrick JE, Morelli JG: *Dermatology secrets plus,* ed 4, St. Louis, 2011, Mosby.)

immature immune systems, and low overall body size can increase the risk to the child and increases the potential for long-term harm from disease. This section will discuss a few disease processes that are either unique to children or have special considerations in the pediatric patient.

Common Childhood Diseases

The following three diseases are common childhood diseases seen in primary care settings.

- *Conjunctivitis:* Also called *pink eye.* A common, highly contagious eye infection in children. Usually caused by viruses or bacteria but can also be related to allergies. Signs and symptoms include blurred vision, crusts that form on the eyelid while sleeping, eye pain, itching and redness of the eyes, and increased tearing.
- *Fifth disease:* Also called *erythema infectiosum, parvovirus B19,* or *slapped cheek rash.* Caused by the human parvovirus B19. Signs and symptoms included fever, headache, and nasal drainage. An intermittent rash appears on the body and face and may take about 2 weeks to completely disappear.
- *Hand-foot-and-mouth disease:* Also called *coxsackievirus infection* or *HFM disease.* Most commonly caused by the coxsackievirus A16. Children under 10 are most often affected, though it can affect teens and adults. Signs and symptoms include fever, headache, loss of appetite, sore throat, oral ulcers, and rash with small blisters on the feet, hands, and groin area (Fig. 37.2).

Reye Syndrome

Reye syndrome occurs in children who were given aspirin during a viral infection, such as chickenpox (varicella). The signs and symptoms include confusion, mental changes, loss of consciousness, seizures, double vision, hearing loss, speech difficulties, and weakness in the arms and legs. It can be fatal.

To prevent Reye syndrome, never give children aspirin unless ordered by the provider.

Failure to Thrive

Failure to thrive is not a disease but a situation. It is a sign of health problems that is very specific to young children. This term is used to refer to children whose current weight or rate of weight gain is much lower than that of other children of similar age and sex. An infant or a young child whose weight is consistently below the 3rd percentile on standardized growth charts, or who is 20% below the ideal body weight for length, may be diagnosed with failure to thrive. Physical, mental, and social skills also are delayed in these children. This could include failure to roll over, smile, coo, stand, or walk at age-appropriate developmental levels. Children with failure to thrive need more calories than usual –approximately 150% of their normal calorie load – to catch up to their target weight.

Failure to thrive can be caused by either *physiologic* or *psychological* factors. Some examples include:

- *Physiological:* problems with genes (e.g., Down syndrome), organs, or hormones; damage to the central nervous system or brain making feeing difficulty; heart, lung, or blood conditions; metabolism, malabsorption issues, chronic infections, gastroesophageal reflux disease (GERD). (For more information on GERD in pediatrics, see Chapter 12.)
- *Environmental:* lack or loss of bonding between parent and child, poverty, problems with child-caregiver relationship, exposure to parasites or toxins, and poor eating habits.

Because failure to thrive is diagnosed based on the child's physical development, accurate height, weight, and head circumference measurements are essential and must be completed at each visit. A comprehensive family history is also important to rule out genetic growth abnormalities or a history of malabsorption problems, such as cystic fibrosis or celiac disease. Because both medical and environmental factors are evaluated in the treatment of children with this problem, the family must be considered as a whole when trying to determine the cause. In the case of nonorganic (nahn or GAN ik) causes, the family will often have to be involved in order to address the issues effectively. Treatment may include the use of support groups and parental counseling.

> **VOCABULARY**
> **nonorganic** Not having an organic or physiologic cause; a disorder that does not have a cause that can be found in the body.
> **suppurative** Characterized by the formation and/or discharge of pus.

Colic

Colic is the frequent, prolonged, and intense crying or fussiness in a healthy infant. If a child develops colic, it typically starts at about 3 weeks of age, gets worse between 4 to 6 weeks of age, and gets better by 12 to 16 weeks of age. During an episode, the infant draws up the legs, clenches the fists, and cries inconsolably. This generally occurs in the late afternoon and evening hours. Possible causes include gas pains, hunger, overfeeding, issues tolerating milk, sensitivity to stimuli, and emotions. Often the exact cause is unknown.

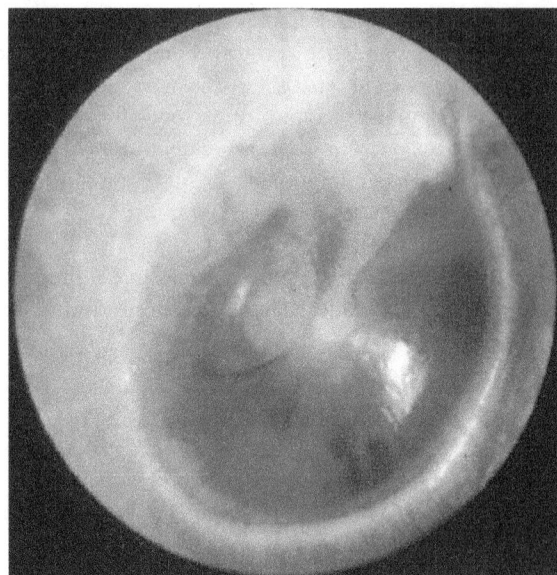

Fig. 37.3 Otitis Media With Effusion (Also Called *Serous Otitis Media*). (From Swartz MH: *Textbook of physical diagnosis,* ed 5, Philadelphia, 2006, Saunders.)

Diet modifications (such as switching formula) will often be advised with mixed results. Parents are encouraged to use soothing strategies, such as a pacifier, rocking the baby, or taking a car ride or walk with the baby in a stroller. It is important for parents to take self-care strategies, such as expressing feelings, taking a break, and do not judge oneself.

Otitis Media

Infection or inflammation of the middle ear, known as *otitis media* (OM), is common in children under 3 years of age. It is most often seen when higher than normal amounts of sinus drainage are present, such as with a respiratory infection (e.g., a cold) or with allergies. In adults the *eustachian* (u stay shee ahn) tubes are angled downward to allow for optimal drainage. However, in young children the eustachian tubes are shorter and more horizontal, making it more difficult for fluid to drain easily. Otitis media with effusion occurs when there is thick fluid behind the *tympanic membrane* (eardrum) (Fig. 37.3). Chronic suppurative otitis media (CSOM) is a chronic ear infection that continues even when treated (Fig. 37.4). Chapter 8 provides additional information on otitis media.

Because OM can be caused by irritation, viruses, or bacteria, it is not always easy to determine the best course of treatment. In 2019 the American Academy of Pediatrics (AAP) and the American Academy of Family Physicians (AAFP) reaffirmed guidelines for the diagnosis of OM. The groups also outlined management of OM in healthy children 6 months to 12 years of age:

- Pain should be assessed, and the provider should recommend treatment to reduce the pain.
- Antibiotic therapy should be given for acute OM with severe signs and symptoms, including moderate to severe earache, ear pain for >48 hours, or a temperature of 102.2°F (39°C) or higher.

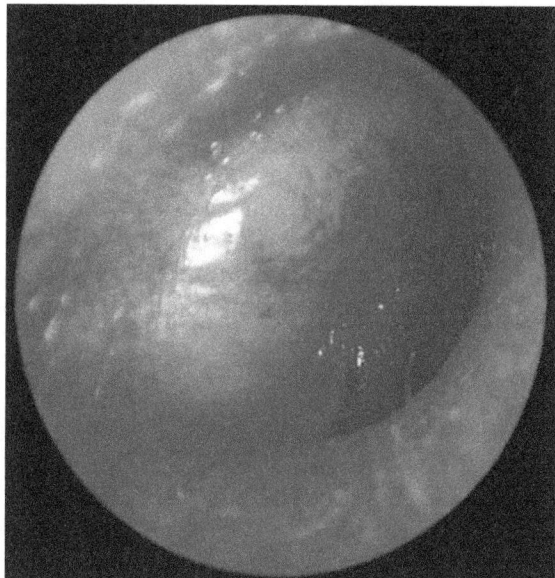

Fig. 37.4 **Chronic Suppurative Otitis Media.** (Courtesy Michael Hawke, MD. From Zitelli BJ, Davis HW: *Atlas of pediatric physical diagnosis*, ed 5, St Louis, 2007, Mosby.)

- For children 6 to 23 months old, antibiotic therapy should be prescribed for bilateral acute OM regardless of the severity of the symptoms.
- For children 6 to 23 months old with unilateral acute OM or children >2 years with nonsevere acute OM, antibiotics may be prescribed, or the provider may have the parent/guardian call if the child gets worse or does not improve within 48 to 72 hours of the onset of symptoms. At that time, the provider would prescribe an antibiotic.
- Prophylactic antibiotics should not be given.
- For recurrent acute OM, tympanostomy tubes can be offered if the child had 3 acute OM in 6 months or 4 in 1 year with 1 infection in the past 6 months. This surgical procedure involves making a small incision in the tympanic membrane and a tube is inserted. The tube drains the fluid and balances the pressure between the outer and middle ear. The tube typically stays in place for 6 to 12 months and falls out as the child grows.

Diarrhea

Diarrhea is caused by bacteria, viruses, and parasites. It can also be caused by certain medications, food intolerances, stress, anxiety, a liquid diet, and diseases, such as inflammatory bowel disease. Diarrhea is diagnosed when there are three or more watery or apparently abnormal stools within 24 hours. *Acute diarrh*ea is diarrhea that occurs for less than 4 weeks. If the diarrhea lasts longer than 4 weeks, it is considered *chronic diarrhea*. Although diarrhea is not unique to children, there are specific considerations when it is present in children.

Children may not have other symptoms with diarrhea. Diarrhea can cause dehydration and electrolyte imbalance because of fluid loss. Since young children are so small, it does not take many watery stools to lead to dehydration.

Medical intervention is needed if diarrhea continues for longer than 1 day or is severe (more than 6 in 24 hours). Medical intervention is also needed if the child is showing signs of dehydration, such as:

- Dry mouth and dry, cracked lips
- No tears when crying
- Little to no urine for 6 to 8 hours
- Sunken eyes or sunken soft spot on the head of infants
- An increase in the pulse and respiration rates.
- Weight loss
- Lethargy (LETH er jee) or less activity than normal

Diarrhea can also cause diaper rash and excoriation (ik skawr ee EY shun n), which can be very painful.

When a child is seen for diarrhea, the provider will often recommend the use of oral rehydration solution (ORS), such as Pedialyte, to avoid dehydration. Usually, it is recommended to give 1 teaspoon (5 mL) of an ORS every 1 to 5 minutes and increase the amount as tolerated. Breastfed babies should continue to breastfeed, and ORS can be given between feedings. According to Mayo Clinic, older children can be given diluted sports drinks (1 part sports drink to 1 part water) (https://www.mayoclinic.org). For mild to severe dehydration, soft drinks, juices, full-strength sports drinks, and tea are not recommended. They lack the correct balance of electrolytes and can lead to more diarrhea.

As the child improves, provide the child with small, nutritious meals. A bland diet is recommended and includes formula, eggs, chicken, pasta, rice, bread, popsicles, potatoes, fruits, and vegetables. Fried and spicy foods or foods that cause gas are not recommended.

Generally diarrhea will resolve on its own, and medical intervention is more to prevent dehydration and treat other related issues. For diarrhea caused by a bacterial infection, the provider will prescribe an antibiotic. Children who are severely dehydrated may be given intravenous (IV) fluids. The child should not be given over-the-counter (OTC) antidiarrheal medications.

VOCABULARY

excoriation Inflammation and irritation of the skin.
lethargy The state of being drowsy and dull, listless, and unenergetic.

CRITICAL THINKING 37.3

Allison receives a call from the grandmother of a 3-year-old child who has had diarrhea since last night. What are some questions Allison should ask to determine the seriousness of the problem? Should the child be seen today, even though appointments are already overbooked?

Obesity

Obesity now affects nearly 20% of all children and adolescents in the United States. The level of body fat changes as the child grows. Higher levels are seen in the first few years and during puberty. Lower levels are seen during the school-age years.

Obesity in children is diagnosed if their BMI is equal to or higher than the 95th percentile.

Factors that can cause obesity include a high calorie diet, lack of exercise, family members with obesity issues, stress and anxiety, limited resources, and certain medications (e.g., prednisone, paroxetine, gabapentin, and amitriptyline). Childhood obesity is known to cause significant health issues such as:

- Asthma, sleep apnea, high blood pressure, and high cholesterol
- Impaired glucose tolerance, insulin resistance, and type 2 diabetes
- Joint problems, musculoskeletal discomfort, fatty liver, gallstones, and GERD
- Anxiety, depression, low self-esteem, and social issues, such as bullying
- Obesity in adulthood with greater disease risk factors

To overcome obesity, the focus includes a healthy diet and increased levels of physical activity. Because there is a significant social component to obesity, often a family approach is needed. Encouragement is important because of the psychological impact obesity can have. It is also good practice to refer these patients to community education and support programs.

CRITICAL THINKING 37.4

Juanita Johnston is a 12-year-old patient who was recently diagnosed as being obese. You are asked to help Juanita and her mother access online information about healthy nutrition options. What websites would be most appropriate for Juanita and her family? What other community resources can you recommend to support the family in making healthier nutrition decisions?

Autism Spectrum Disorder

Autism spectrum disorder (ASD) is a developmental disorder with symptoms that appear by age 2. The child has difficulty interacting and communicating with others. ASD occurs in all ethnic and socioeconomic groups and affects every age group; however, it does tend to be more prevalent in boys than in girls.

The communication issues and behaviors, such as repetitive behaviors and limited interests, affect the person's ability to function at school and at home. Children with autism have impaired social interactions. They will often avoid eye contact and find comfort in repetitive motion and/or sounds. In more severe cases children avoid communicating with others and show limited interest in their surroundings. Many children with autism are extremely sensitive to noise, touch, or other sensory stimulation. There can be a wide range of symptoms and severity; thus it is known as a "spectrum" disorder. Treatment involves coordinated educational and behavioral interventions to help the child develop social and language skills. (See Chapter 15 for more information on autism.)

IMMUNIZATIONS

Over the years immunizations have helped dramatically reduce potentially lethal childhood infections. Two main types of vaccines are inactivated and live virus, which are also called *attenuated* (or weakened). (See Chapter 46 for more information on vaccines.) When a vaccine is administered, it stimulates artificial active immunity. The body creates immunity against the disease. Most vaccines require multiple doses over a specific period of time to produce full immunity. A booster may be needed in future years as the immunity decreases.

Vaccines undergo years of testing to ensure their safety and effectiveness. There are also strict established protocols for manufacturers to ensure that vaccines are created with proper potency and stability. The package inserts describe proper storage for vaccines to maintain their potency. (Vaccine ordering and storage is discussed in Chapter 26.)

Vaccine package inserts include information on the use, *route* (how it is administered), adverse (unexpected or life-threatening) reactions, and common symptoms the patient may experience. Although severe side effects of vaccines are rare, they are possible. The medical assistant must watch patients for common symptoms and adverse reactions to immunizations.

Immunization Schedule

The vaccine schedules are reviewed each year and updated as new vaccines become available and/or research indicates a better method or timing for giving the vaccine. Fig. 37.5 shows the immunization schedule from the CDC for children from birth through 18 years of age. The most current immunization schedules can be found at the CDC's website: https://www.cdc.gov/vaccines/schedules/index.html.

The CDC recommends immunizations for all individuals, except for those for whom a particular vaccine would pose an unacceptable risk. Each state has developed its own immunization program and methods of enforcement. Parents/guardians do have the right to refuse immunizations. However, depending on the state, this could limit the child's ability to participate in public education or use certain daycare services.

Table 37.2 and Box 37.1 discuss common childhood immunizations. *Combination vaccines* contain two or more vaccines in a single injection, which reduces the number of injections given. Table 37.3 describes combination vaccines for childhood immunizations.

Prior to Administering Vaccines

Prior to administration, patients or parents/guardians should complete a screening questionnaire. The questionnaire is designed to identify patients who should not receive the vaccines due to current medical conditions, allergies (such as latex, eggs, yeast, and gelatin), or a recent dose of immunoglobulin. Besides having the questionnaire completed, the medical assistant should:

- Provide the Vaccine Information Statement (VIS) to the patient/parent. The VIS provides information on the reasons to get the vaccine, the schedule, risks (or common side effects), and when to contact the provider regarding adverse reactions. The National Childhood Vaccine Injury Act requires that all patients get the appropriate VIS prior to every dose of vaccine administered. The specific list of vaccines that require the VIS are listed on the CDC's website at https://www.cdc.gov/vaccines/hcp/vis/about/facts-vis.html. For more information on the VIS, refer to Chapter 46.

Table 1 Recommended child and adolescent immunization schedule for ages 18 years or younger, united states, 2020

These recommendations must be read with the notes that follow. For those who fall behind or start late, provide catch-up vaccination at the earliest opportunity as indicated by the green bars. To determine minimum intervals between doses, see the catch-up schedule (Table 2). School entry and adolescent vaccine age groups are shaded in gray.

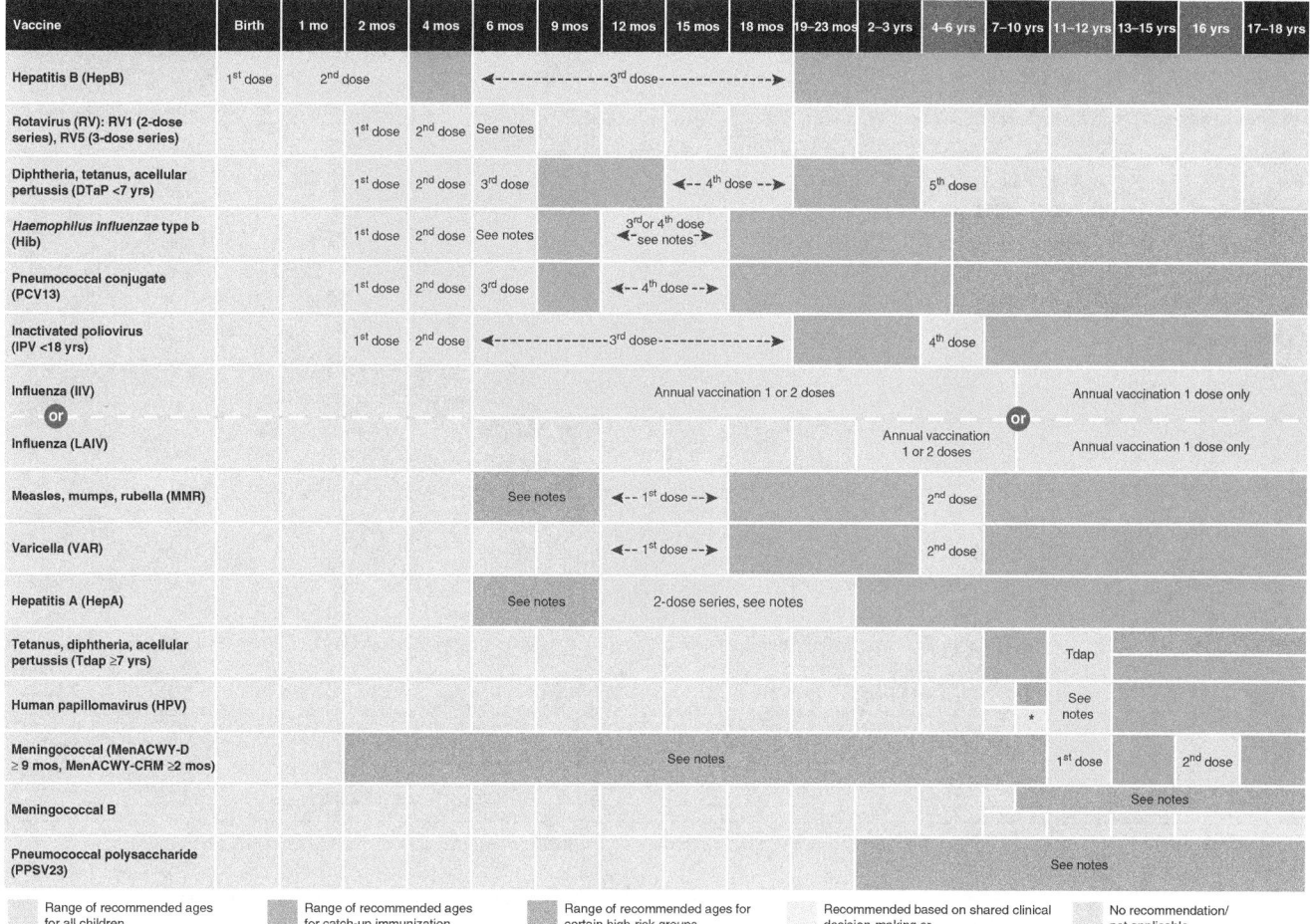

Fig. 37.5 Recommended Immunization Schedule for Children Ages Birth to 18 Years. (From the Centers for Disease Control and Prevention. https://www.cdc.gov/vaccines/schedules/downloads/child/0-18yrs-child-combined-schedule.pdf.)

TABLE 37.2 Childhood Immunizations

Vaccine	Trade Name (number of doses)	Route of Administration	Contraindications[a]	Side Effects
DTaP *Diphtheria, tetanus, pertussis*	Daptacel and Infanrix *(requires 5 doses)*; found in combination vaccines	IM	Moderate or severe acute illness; neurologic problem; complication after previous dose (e.g., fever, convulsions)	Mild fever, anorexia, irritability, drowsiness
Td *Tetanus and diphtheria*	Tenivac *(given every 10 years to people ≥ 7 years)*	IM		
Hep A *Hepatitis A*	Havrix and Vaqta *(require 2 doses)*	IM	Hypersensitivity to product, acute infection, or fever	Localized injection site reaction, fever, headache
Hep B *Hepatitis B*	Engerix-B and Recombivax HB *(require 3 doses)*; HEPLISAV-B *(requires 2 doses)*; found in combination vaccines	IM	Moderate or severe acute illness; hypersensitivity to yeast; severe cardiovascular disease	Fever, pain at site, headache, malaise, vomiting
Hib *Haemophilus influenzae*	PedvaxHIB *(requires 3 doses)*; ActHIB and Hiberix *(requires 4 doses)*; found in combination vaccines	IM	Not routinely given to children older than 5; moderate or severe acute illness	Minimal

Continued

TABLE 37.2   Childhood Immunizations—cont'd

Vaccine	Trade Name (number of doses)	Route of Administration	Contraindications[a]	Side Effects
HPV *Human papillomavirus*	Gardasil-9 *(requires 2 or 3 doses depending on age)*	IM	Hypersensitivity to ingredients, including yeast; pregnancy	Relatively few; mild headache and GI upset
IIV *Influenza (quadrivalent)*	Afluria, Fluarix, FluLaval, Fluzone, Flucelvax (many types) *(a dose is given each fall)*	IM	Allergy to eggs; recent fever	Uncommon; fever, local irritation at injection site, general malaise
IPV *Inactivated poliovirus*	IPOL *(requires 4 doses)*; found in combination vaccines	Subcut or IM	Moderate or severe acute illness	Uncommon
MenACWY *Meningococcal*	Menactra and Menveo *(requires 2 doses)*	IM	Moderate or severe acute illness; history of allergic reaction to MCV4; hypersensitivity to yeast (MenACWY)	Uncommon
MenB *Meningococcal*	Bexsero and Trumenba *(requires 2 doses)*			
MMR *Measles, mumps, rubella*	M-M-R II *(requires 2 doses)*	Subcut *(live virus)*	Moderate or severe acute illness; immunocompromised patients (may be given if HIV positive); pregnancy or possible pregnancy in 3 mo	Fever
PCV *Pneumococcal*	Prevnar 13 (PCV13; *requires 4 doses for children 6 weeks through 5 years; or 1 dose for ages 6–17)*; Pneumovax 23 *(requires 1 dose for high risk children ≥ 2 years)*	IM or subcut	Moderate or severe acute illness; hypersensitivity to yeast	Drowsiness, local irritation at site, mild fever
RV *Rotavirus*	Rotarix (RV1; *requires 2 doses*); RotaTeq (RV5; *requires 3 doses*)	PO	Hypersensitivity; history of intussusception	GI upset and blood disorders
VAR *Varicella*	Varivax *(requires 2 doses)*; found in a combination vaccine	Subcut *(live virus)*	Confirmed history of chickenpox; pregnancy or possible pregnancy in 1 mo; moderate or severe acute illness; immunocompromised patients	No salicylates for 6 wk afterward to prevent risk of Reye syndrome

GI, Gastrointestinal; *HIV*, human immunodeficiency virus; *IM*, intramuscular; *mo*, month; *PO*, oral; *subcut*, subcutaneous; *wk*, week.
[a]Mild illness is not a contraindication.

TABLE 37.3   Combination Vaccines

Combination Vaccine Name	Combination of Vaccines	Notes
Pediarix	Hepatitis B, DTaP, and IPV	Requires 3 doses. For children > 6 weeks to 7 years old.
TWINRIX	Hepatitis A and hepatitis B	Requires 3 doses. Recommended for people > 18 years
Pentacel	Hib, DTaP, and IPV	Requires 4 doses. Given to children ages 2 to 18 months
Kinrix and Quadracel	DTaP and IPV	Use as a fifth shot in the DTaP series, given to children 4 to 6 years old.
Vaxelis	DTaP, polio, hepatitis B, and Hib	Three doses required. Use for infants 6 weeks through less than 1 year old.
ProQuad	MMR and varicella (referred to as MMRV)	Two doses required. Use for children ages 1 through 12 years of age.

DTaP, Diphtheria, tetanus, pertussis; *IPV*, inactivated poliovirus; *Hib*, *Haemophilus influenzae*; *MMR*, measles, mumps, rubella.

BOX 37.1   Types of Diphtheria, Tetanus, and Pertussis Vaccines

There are many types of diphtheria, tetanus, and pertussis (also called *whooping cough*) vaccines. Diphtheria is abbreviated with a D, tetanus with a T, and pertussis with a P. Types of vaccines include:

- **DT**: Generic vaccine available
- **Td**: Tenivac and generic vaccines available
- **DTaP**: Daptacel, Infanrix, Kinrix, Pediarix, Pentacel, Quadracel, and Vaxelis are trade names of the available vaccines
- **Tdap**: Adacel and Boostrix are available vaccines

The upper-case letter indicates that the vaccine contains a full-strength dose of that vaccine. A lower-case letter indicates a smaller dose of that vaccine. For example, Td contains a full-strength dose of the tetanus vaccine and a smaller dose of diphtheria vaccine. It is important how you write or type the name of the medication in the patient's health record.

- Coach the parent/patient on the vaccine, using the most current VIS in the person's primary language. Answer any questions the parent may have. (The most current VIS and VIS in other languages are available at https://www.cdc.gov/vaccines/hcp/vis/index.html and https://www.immunize.org/vis/.)

- Have the parent complete and sign an informed consent if required by the state or healthcare facility.

After Administering Vaccines

After administering the vaccine, the medical assistant must:
- Document the following information in the patient's health record (Procedure 37.3):
  - The date, type of vaccine, amount, site of administration, and any side effects the patient experienced.
  - The edition date of the VIS and the date the VIS was provided to the parent/patient.
  - The office address, name, and title of the person who administered the vaccine.
- Document the immunization in the state's patient immunization record, if applicable. Many states have an electronic immunization record system that can be accessed in any healthcare facility. It can also be used by schools to verify students' immunization records.
- Provide the patient/parent with a record of the immunization, either by updating a paper record or by providing a printed copy of the immunization record.

CRITICAL THINKING 37.5

Allison will be administering pediatric immunizations during the well-baby visits scheduled for today. To prepare for this responsibility, she looked up the primary vaccinations, their routes of administration, contraindications, and possible side effects. The first child arrives for her 4-month checkup. She has been receiving all her previous immunizations on schedule. What immunizations should the child receive, and how should they be administered? The baby's father asks whether she will get sick from the vaccines. What should Allison tell him? What does Allison need to do to meet the requirements of the National Childhood Vaccine Injury Act?

CARING FOR PEDIATRIC PATIENTS

Children do not understand things or process things the same way adults do. Because of this, normal everyday things could seem very exciting or very frightening to them. The key to working with young children is to use an age-specific approach. Getting down on the child's level, establishing eye contact, and using a gentle but firm voice are ways of gaining the child's confidence and cooperation (Fig. 37.6). The best technique can change with the patient's age. Box 37.2 provides techniques for therapeutic communication for various age ranges.

With pediatric patients the parents are responsible for making healthcare decisions and much of the communication is often directly with the parent (Fig. 37.7). However, children should never be ignored, and when possible, the child should be included in the discussion about their health and treatment. Children often fear the unknown, so explaining all procedures in language that the child understands is very important. Although the parent will make all health-related decisions, allowing older children the opportunity to make certain decisions can help them feel more comfortable and be more cooperative with the

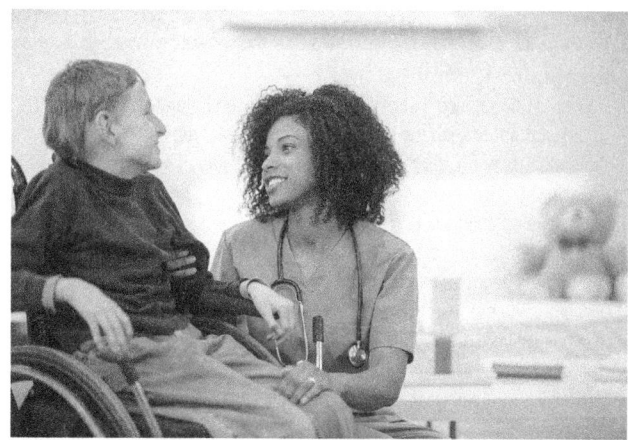

Fig. 37.6 Getting down on the child's level and establishing eye contact helps the child feel important. (FatCamera/iStock.com.)

TABLE 37.4 Apgar Scoring System[a]

Clinical Sign	ASSIGNED SCORE		
	0	**1**	**2**
Heart rate	Absent	<100 beats per minute	>100 beats per minute
Respiratory effort	Absent	Slow and irregular	Good and crying
Muscle tone	Limp	Some flexion of the arms and legs	Active movement
Reflex irritability	No response	Grimace	Coughing, sneezing, or vigorous cry
Color	Blue and pale	Body pink and extremities blue	Pink all over

[a]Readings are taken by the provider at 1 minute and 5 minutes after birth. At *1 minute:* If the score is 7 or lower, some nervous system problems are suspected. If the score is below 4, resuscitation usually is necessary. At *5 minutes:* If the score is at least 8, the child probably is reacting normally.

visit. For example, Heather, a 13-year-old patient with diabetes, is having some changes to her medication dosing and will need an insulin injection during her visit. She could be asked to choose the site of the injection. Or, if she has been administering the medication herself at home, she could be allowed to do the same in the office.

Apgar Score

An infant's first physical assessment comes at the time of delivery, when the provider assesses the newborn's ability to thrive outside the uterus. The Apgar score is a system for evaluating the infant's physical condition at 1 and 5 minutes after birth (Table 37.4). Developed by pediatrician Virginia Apgar, the scoring system evaluates the heart rate, respiratory effort, muscle tone (flexion, movement), reflex irritability (grimace, coughing, crying), and color (appearance). These parameters are each rated 0, 1, or 2. The maximum total score is 10. Infants with low scores require immediate medical attention.

BOX 37.2   Therapeutic Approaches for Pediatric Patients

Newborn to 12 Months
- Crying is normal; use distraction, but do not overstimulate.
- It is important to keep the infant close to the caregiver; either have the parent hold the infant or keep the parent in the child's line of vision.
- Involve the parent as much as possible, depending on the task and the parent's level of comfort.
- Place a familiar object near the infant and keep frightening ones out of view.
- An infant's negative response to strangers usually develops at approximately 8 months; do not take the rejection personally.
- Do not restrain the infant any more than necessary but be ready to use restraint at times (e.g., when giving an injection) to keep the infant safe.
- Encourage the caregiver to cuddle and hug the child after the procedure is complete.
- Unpleasant procedures are associated with other objects, so do not use play areas for treatment, and do not use a favorite toy or object during the procedure; offer it afterward for comfort.

Toddlers and Preschoolers (2 to 6 Years)
- Toddlers and preschoolers often fear visits to the doctor; ignore temper tantrums and negative behavior.
- Praise the child as much as possible.
- Perform unpleasant procedures as quickly as possible; the fear of the procedure is worse than the actual discomfort.
- Allow the child to keep on as much clothing as possible for security and comfort.
- Use words familiar to the child, and do not use words the child could misinterpret. For example, "The test uses dye" (the child may think you mean "die"); "The doctor will put you to sleep so it doesn't hurt" (the family dog may have been put to sleep).
- Explain a procedure as the child would sense it; that is, what it will look like, how it will smell, how it will feel, and so on.

- Allow the child to handle equipment when possible.
- Do not use the child's favorite doll or stuffed animal to demonstrate; the child may believe the toy feels pain.
- Explain procedures to the parents away from the child when possible; the child may misinterpret the information.

School-Aged Children (7 to 11 Years)
- Allow choices when possible, such as which arm to use for an injection.
- A parent or caregiver should always be present during examinations.
- Remove only as much clothing as needed for the examination or procedure.
- Explain procedures in concrete terms; use pictures and diagrams when possible.
- Give the child time to ask questions.
- School-aged children often are curious, and they can be cooperative if they know what is expected of them.
- Address the conversation to the child; involve the child in decision making as much as possible.
- Provide privacy.

Adolescents (12 to 18 Years)
- Adolescents are self-conscious and strongly influenced by peers.
- Privacy is very important to them.
- Address how a procedure might affect the adolescent's appearance.
- Do not be judgmental; listen without condemning.
- Encourage the adolescent to verbalize their concerns and fears.
- The adolescent may regress to more childish behaviors when sick.
- Teenagers want to be treated as adults; they want to know what is being done and why.
- To promote honest discussion about lifestyle issues, encourage the teenager to see the provider without the parent present.

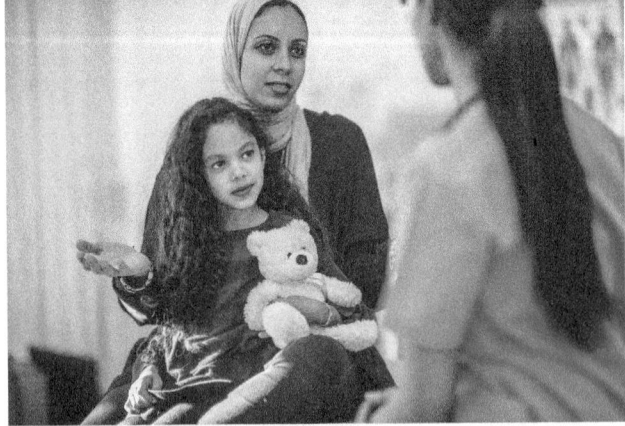

Fig. 37.7 Interacting With a Child and Parent. (FatCamera/iStock.com.)

Well-Child Visits

The frequency of well-child visits varies with the provider and the community. The American Academy of Pediatrics recommends the following pattern:

- 2 to 5 days
- 1 month
- 2 months
- 4 months
- 6 months
- 9 months

CRITICAL THINKING 37.6

Based on what you have learned about therapeutic approaches for the pediatric patient, what would be the best way to deal with the following patient situations?
1. A crying 3-month-old being seen for a well-child visit
2. A 10-month-old with otitis media
3. A 2-year-old who needs the dressing changed on an infected wound
4. A 5-year-old scheduled for vision and hearing screening
5. An 8-year-old who needs a throat culture to rule out a strep infection
6. A 12-year-old who needs a penicillin injection in the ventrogluteal site
7. A 15-year-old girl who complains of abdominal pain and is accompanied by her mother

- 12 months
- 15 months
- 18 months
- 2 years
- Annually

Well-child visits focus on maintaining the child's health and monitoring for any developing conditions. These visits include:
- *A medical history*: The provider reviews any current and past health concerns. A review of body systems is typically done, including the child's sleep patterns and nutritional status. Additional information is obtained about the child's use of electronic/TV and safety devices (e.g., bike helmets,

BOX 37.3 Lead Paint Exposure

Children are especially vulnerable to lead levels in their environment. High blood lead levels can result in serious brain injury, including seizures, coma, and death. Lower levels can cause learning problems, stunted growth, and behavior disorders. The most common causes of lead exposure are lead-based paint in homes and on imported toys, and chronic exposure to lead-contaminated dust and water. The Centers for Disease Control and Prevention (CDC) recommend a screening blood test for lead levels in all children between 1 and 2 years of age. For children who show elevated levels, follow-up should include home and school environmental testing to determine the cause of lead exposure.

TABLE 37.5 Important Questions for Telephone Screening of Pediatric Problems

Complaint	Screening Questions
Pain	• What are the onset, frequency, and duration of the pain? • On a scale of 1 to 10, how severe is the pain? • Where is the exact location? • Was any accident involved (include details)? • Has the pain gotten worse over time? • Has the pain interfered with sleep? • Is there associated fever, vomiting, diarrhea, or rash?
Gastrointestinal	• What are the onset, duration, and frequency of the symptoms? Has the child been vomiting longer than 24 hours without improvement? • Is the child drinking and/or eating? • Is the child dehydrated (e.g., dry mouth, no urination in 8 to 10 hours, listless)? • If the child has diarrhea, have there been more than five or six watery stools in 12 hours? • Does the child have other symptoms (e.g., vomiting, fever of 101°F [38.3°C], rapid breathing)?
Respiratory	• What are the onset, duration, and frequency of the symptoms? • How would you describe the child's breathing? • Has the child been diagnosed with a breathing disorder? • Is a prescribed treatment being used? • Are any other signs or symptoms present (e.g., severe headache, stiff neck, fever, cough)? • If the child is coughing, what does it sound like? • Are there signs of a sore throat or earache?

car seats). The provider will also obtain information on the home environment (e.g., drugs, firearms, cigarettes smoke, and lead paint) (Box 37.3).

- *A physical examination:* The medical assistant assists the provider by obtaining the height/length, weight, and head circumference (if appropriate for the age).
- *A developmental assessment:* Most ambulatory care facilities have parents complete developmental survey tools. These tools are designed for children of different ages and provide information to the provider on the child's developmental milestones, including language, fine motor, and gross motor skills.
- *An immunization review:* The provider will review the past immunizations and recommend current vaccines that are due.

When the child is young and unable to speak, the provider will obtain the information from the parents. As the child gets older, the provider will ask the child questions. Not only does it allow the provider to get information from the child, but it also allows the provider to assess the child's language skills. The parents can clarify the information as needed. Close observation of the child and the parent/child interaction also can give a lot of information.

Sometimes the provider may ask to see a younger child alone, without the parents present. Usually this occurs when the child looks to the parent for approval before answering or performing a skill. The provider may want to assess the child's independent abilities. Commonly providers request to see teenage patients without the parents present. The adolescent's answers to questions regarding alcohol, drugs, seat belts, and sexual activity might be more truthful if the parent is out of the room. The medical assistant should reassure the parents that as soon as the exam is over, they will be asked to return to the examination room.

Sick-Child Visits

Sick-child visits occur whenever needed, usually on short notice. For this reason most pediatric offices keep open appointments in the schedule to accommodate calls for sick-child visits. The length and frequency of this type of visit depends entirely on the child and the illness.

The medical assistant is frequently the first point of contact for a sick child and the child's caregiver. Often this occurs when the parent calls to request an appointment for the sick child. The medical assistant will often be asked to

determine if the child should be seen immediately or if the problem can wait for an opening in the schedule. Offices will have protocols in place to help the medical assistant make this decision. However, if there is ever any doubt about how it should be handled, the medical assistant should ask provider for advice. Usually the provider prefers to see the child rather than delay seeing a patient with a potentially serious condition. When a parent calls in to request an appointment for a child, it is important for the medical assistant ask clear and specific questions to get a good idea of what is going on (Table 37.5). When such a call comes in, it is important to focus on:

- *Onset* (when symptoms first started)
- *Frequency* (are symptoms constant, or do they cycle through recurrences)
- *Duration* (how long the episodes last) of the problem
- *Treatments* that have been attempted and their effectiveness

The telephone conversation should be documented in the patient's health record and include the reason for the call, information obtained, action taken, whether the provider or standing orders were consulted, any advice or provider orders given, and if an appointment was scheduled. The child should be seen right away if they are young (under 2 years old) and the parent reports:

- Frequent cycles of crying, lethargy, or vomiting that last longer than 24 hours
- Diarrhea (more than six stools in the past 24 hours)
- Signs of dehydration such as a decrease in the number of wet diapers or no tears
- Fever of 101°F (38.3°C) or higher

CARING FOR ADOLESCENT PATIENTS

Adolescence begins with the onset of puberty, a time when the child's reproductive system matures. This is a period marked by rapid changes in the endocrine and musculoskeletal systems. The adolescent undergoes rapid growth spurts and the development of secondary sexual characteristics.

Privacy is very important to most adolescent patients. It is important to respect their privacy as much as possible during the examination. For example, if the patient will be required to disrobe, it is important to keep exposure to a minimum. Adolescents often want to know what is going on during the examination, what to expect, and what the findings mean. Keeping them informed in a language they can understand is important. Patients should be encouraged to ask question, which should be answered as completely and clearly as possible. Take every opportunity to teach your patients about their disease and to share information about significant wellness factors.

Medical History and Screenings

Health examinations for patients in this age group should include:

- Screening for height and weight.
- Reviewing vaccination history and administering vaccines as indicated.
- Gathering data about diet and exercise routines. Eating disorders (e.g., *anorexia nervosa* and *bulimia nervosa*) often start in the adolescent years.
- Assessing for high-risk behaviors, such as substance abuse, smoking, alcohol use, and sexual behavior.
  - If the patient is sexually active, the examination should include screenings for sexually transmitted infections (STIs). According to the CDC, half of all STIs each year are among people 15 to 24 years of age (https://www.cdc.gov/healthyyouth/). A Pap test and screening for human papilloma virus (HPV) are no longer recommended for teens. The recommendation is to start at age 21, regardless of when the person started having sex.
  - If the patient uses tobacco, alcohol, or illegal drugs, the provider should screen for drug or alcohol abuse and refer the patient if necessary.
- Gathering information on physical activities and the use of safety equipment, such as seat belts and helmets. (Accidental death is the number one cause of death in this age group in the United States.)
- Assessing mental health, specifically for depression or suicidal tendencies. (Suicide is the second leading cause of death in this age group.)

Depression and Suicide. The diagnoses of depression and anxiety are more common in teens than in younger children. About 20% of teens experience depression before adulthood. A teen's risk of suicide increases about 12% with depression. Three in 10 teens with depression have a substance use disorder.

The sudden shift in hormones that comes with puberty can make it difficult for the developing brain of the adolescent to process strong emotions. The normal changes in behavior and the teenage "moodiness," as it is often described, can be difficult to distinguish from a real problem for many parents. Because of this, it is essential that every teenager be screened for depression during their healthcare visit. Some signs of depression in adolescents are:

- Irritable or angry, extremely sensitive to criticism
- Unexplained aches and pains
- Chronic headaches, abdominal discomfort, anorexia, and chronic fatigue
- Unprovoked or excessive aggressiveness
- Drug or alcohol use; sexual promiscuity
- Obsession with death, talking about dying, writing suicide notes
- Giving away prized objects; withdrawing from social groups
- Sudden change in normal behavior patterns

> **VOCABULARY**
> **anorexia** Loss of appetite for food.

ASSISTING WITH THE PEDIATRIC EXAMINATION

As with other examinations the medical assistant is often responsible for:

- Obtaining vital signs
- Measuring height, weight, and head circumference
- Updating the health history
- Performing ordered screening tests (e.g., vision, hearing, urinalysis, and hemoglobin checks)
- Administering immunizations
- Providing patient and caregiver support

Each step should be explained in a language the child (and parent) can understand. Children can feel nervous, and efforts should be made to help them feel at ease. Children younger than age 2 may feel better if the parent holds them or remains very close (Fig. 37.8). Preschool children enjoy playing, so making a game out of the situation is helpful (Fig. 37.9). Whatever the child's age, the medical assistant should be sensitive to their individual needs and should adapt the examination and procedures as much as possible to meet those needs.

The sequence of the provider's examination varies and frequently is based on the child's cooperation. The provider will probably leave procedures and tests that are likely to cause the most objections until the end of the appointment. The provider is constantly evaluating the child's development by watching the child's alertness and responses to determine if they are age appropriate. With infants and young children of preschool age, the parent is closely questioned about the child's eating, sleeping, and elimination habits. A school-aged child is usually a little more cooperative during an examination and can answer most questions without parental assistance. Adolescent patients should be given the option of not having parents present during an examination. This allows the privacy that many adolescents prefer and may permit teenagers to respond more honestly about lifestyle factors.

Vital Signs

Vital signs were discussed in Chapter 33. When you take vital signs, some adjustments may be necessary, depending on the age and size of the patient (Table 37.6).

Temperature. Depending on the child's age and level of cooperation, the temperature may be obtained by the axillary, oral, rectal, tympanic, or temporal artery method. The rectal and temporal artery methods are considered most accurate in infants; however, the temporal artery method is easiest, quickest, and less invasive. It is important to remember that the younger the child, the more immature the ability to regulate body heat. Therefore the temperature of an infant may fluctuate easily and rapidly.

Routes for temperatures include:
- Birth–3 months: Infrared, temporal artery, or rectal
- 3 months–6 months: Infrared, axillary, temporal artery, or rectal
- 6 months–5 years: Infrared, axillary, temporal artery, or tympanic
- 5 years and older: Infrared, oral, axillary, tympanic, or temporal artery

Pulse and Respiration Rates. The child's pulse rate is affected similarly to that of an adult. It can increase as a result of activity, anxiety, illness, and environmental temperature. If the child is younger than age 3, an apical pulse should be obtained. In infants and young children, the apical pulse can be heard at the fourth intercostal space at the left midclavicular line. For older children, place the stethoscope at the junction of the fifth intercostal space and the midclavicular line on left side of the patient's chest. Always count the beats for 1 full minute for accuracy. After age 3 a radial pulse can be obtained. The pulse rate decreases with age. The pulse rate in a child will be higher than in an adult.

The medical assistant should closely observe the child's chest when counting the respiratory rate. When obtaining the respiration rate in infants, the rate should be counted for a full minute. Infants have *periodic breathing*, which means they can brief pauses causing an irregular breathing pattern. The medical assistant can gently place a hand on the infant's chest/abdomen, which can help when counting the respiration rate. The respiration rate decreases with age.

Blood Pressure. It is recommended that blood pressure (BP) be checked for children aged 3 years or older, unless the child

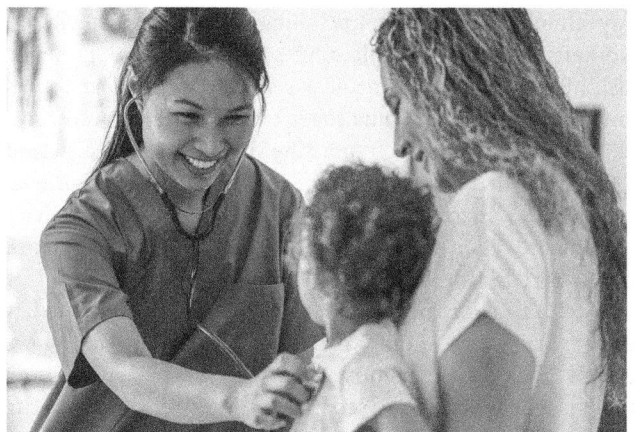

Fig. 37.8 Sometimes a pediatric patient is more comfortable when held by a parent. (FatCamera/iStock.com.)

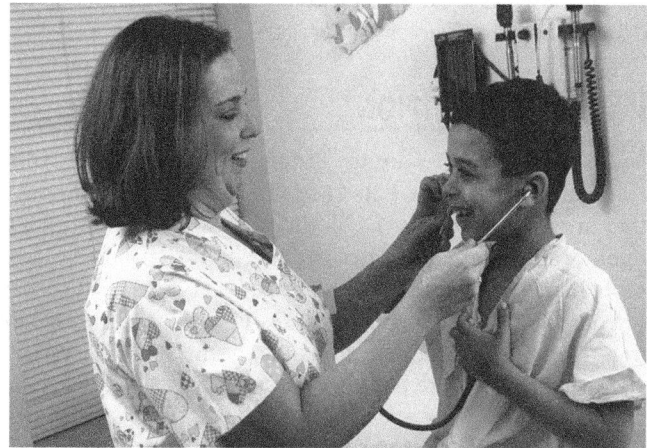

Fig. 37.9 Making a Game Out of a Procedure. (From Niedzwiecki B, et al: *Kinn's the medical assistant*, ed 14, St. Louis, 2020, Elsevier.)

TABLE 37.6	Reference Ranges for Pediatric Vital Signs					
	PULSE RATES		**RESPIRATION RATES**		**BLOOD PRESSURE RANGES**	
Age	Range (beats/min)	Average	Range (breaths/min)	Average	Systolic	Diastolic
Newborn	120–160	140	30–50	40	60–96	30–62
1–2 years	80–140	120	20–30	25	78–112	48–78
3–6 years	80–120	100	18–26	22	78–112	50–79
7–11 years	75–110	95	16–22	19	85–114	52–79
Adolescence	60–100	80	12–20	16	94–119	58–79

BOX 37.4 Signs of Child Abuse

Obvious Signs
- Previously filed reports of physical or sexual abuse of the child
- Documented abuse of other family members
- Different stories from the parents and the child on how an accident happened
- Stories of incidents and injuries that are suspicious
- Injuries blamed on other family members
- Repeated visits to the emergency department for injuries

Examination Findings
- Trauma to the nervous system
- Internal abdominal pain
- Discolorations/bruising on the buttocks, back, and abdomen
- Elbow, wrist, and shoulder dislocations

Changes in Child's Behavior
- Too eager to please the parent
- Overly passive and too compliant
- Aggressive and demanding
- Parenting the parent (role reversal)
- Delays in the normal growth and development patterns
- Erratic school attendance

Physical Indicators
- Poor hygiene
- Malnutrition
- Obvious dental neglect
- Neglected well-baby procedures (e.g., immunizations)

---

has a condition that requires BP checks prior to age 3. The cuff must be the appropriate width to obtain an accurate reading, A pediatric stethoscope with a bell should be used. Blood pressure readings increase with age, so a child's reading will be lower than that of an adult.

Pain

Accurately judging the level of pain a young patient is experiencing can be difficult. Often fussiness and body movements are the only indication of pain in infants too young to verbally communicate. If the child is able to communicate, the Wong-Baker FACES Pain Rating Scale could be used. This scale shows simple drawings of faces that express varying levels of pain on a 0 to 10 scale (see Chapter 34, Fig. 34.6).

INJURY PREVENTION

Unintentional injuries are the leading cause of death and disability in children ages 1 to 14 in the United States. Although they are considered preventable, injuries still cause more childhood deaths than all diseases combined. In the United States, more than 9000 children die each year – about 25 deaths a day – from injuries. The primary causes of childhood deaths are unintentional suffocations, drowning, burns, and motor vehicle accidents. Falls are the leading cause of nonfatal injuries in children.

Young children are totally dependent on caregivers to keep them safe, so constant supervision and a childproof environment are essential for this age group. Older children need to be aware of health hazards and should be encouraged to protect

themselves from injury (e.g., use bike helmets, protective padding when skateboarding, seat belts, and so on).

Healthcare workers play a major role in injury prevention. The medical assistant is responsible for making sure the ambulatory care office is safe and parents are educated about potential hazards. Parental education on accident prevention should be reviewed at each well-child visit.

CHILD ABUSE

The Child Abuse Prevention and Treatment Act states that all threats to a child's physical and/or mental welfare must be reported. Most states mandate specific professionals to report any child maltreatment, including school personnel, social workers, healthcare providers, nurses, mental health professionals, childcare providers, medical examiners or coroners, and law enforcement officers. Some states require anyone who suspects child abuse or neglect to report the situation. In most states the identity of the reporter is considered confidential information and is not given to the child's parent or guardian. The individual making the report is also protected under the law from any liability for reporting suspicions of child abuse.

If child abuse, neglect, or exploitation is suspected, the medical assistant should consult with the provider immediately (Box 37.4). In most states the medical assistant and the provider can make separate reports to the authorities. However, state laws vary, so state and local reporting protocols should be outlined in the office procedures manual. (See Chapter 19 for additional information on child abuse, neglect, and exploitation.)

CLOSING COMMENTS

Working in pediatrics can be one of the most challenging and rewarding jobs a medical assistant can have. The patient population is diverse. You are dealing with all ages. You must also

establish a solid relationship with the patient's parents and/or caregivers. Having solid communication skills will help to develop those relationships.

PATIENT-CENTERED CARE

In a pediatric practice the child usually is joined by one or both parents during visits to the provider. Parents need reinforcement, praise, and understanding in dealing with the health and welfare of their child. Provide parents with information to help them understand their child's behavior and improve their parenting skills. Understanding the normal behavioral characteristics of a particular developmental stage may increase the parents' confidence and reinforce expectations for the child.

The waiting room is an ideal place for parent education. Use the space and resources available to provide up-to-date information on child health issues and on local resources for support and assistance. If the provider has pamphlets available, discuss them with the parents. Answer questions when possible or alert the provider so that questions can be answered during the office visit. Every opportunity should be taken to teach parents about sound healthcare.

BEING PROFESSIONAL

Patients and parents or guardians have a right to refuse treatments and procedures. A medical assistant must respect their rights and not attempt to sway the patient/parent in one direction. A medical assistant should know how to handle the situation if a patient refuses a procedure or treatment. It is important to follow the facility's policy and procedure in such a situation. Most times the following apply when a patient refuses treatment or procedures:
- Show sensitivity to the patient/parent's rights by being respectful and professional. Remember, it is the right of the patient/parent to refuse.
- Ask the patient/parent if they have questions regarding the procedure. If so, let the provider know.
- Notify the provider of the refusal.
- Document the refusal in the health record. Make sure to include which provider was notified.

Role-play this scenario with a peer: Your peer will play the role of a parent. You are the medical assistant. You are reviewing the VIS for HPV, and the parent tells you they are not interested in having the child get the vaccine. Respond to the parent.

CHAPTER REVIEW

In this chapter we have discussed the growth patterns that children go through. Understanding those patterns can help you deal with all of the patients seen in pediatrics. In addition, it will help you recognize when there is a potential problem about which the provider should be informed. Erik Erikson's development theories can also provide insight on how to work with patients of all ages.

Working with a child can be challenging, but if you can establish a positive relationship with the child, things will go more smoothly. Adolescent patients pose their own set of challenges, some of them legal. You should be aware of the laws in your state on the treatment and release of information regarding adolescents.

For well-child visits, the medical assistant will obtain certain vital signs, based on age. It is important to remember the normal range for most changes in vital signs that correspond to the age of the patient.

There are certain diseases and disorders that are more common in children than adults. Colic, diarrhea, and failure to thrive are conditions that can be very upsetting for parents and caregivers. The medical assistant's role is to reinforce the instructions and information given by the provider regarding these conditions.

Immunizations are a big part of well-child visits. Following the CDC's schedule of immunizations can help ensure that the vaccines protect the child. The VIS is a part of the immunization procedure. A VIS must be given to an adult patient or to the parents or caregivers of a child before the immunization is given, and all their questions must be answered. Documentation is the key for immunizations. Be sure to document all needed information.

It is important to be aware of any signs of abuse or neglect in children. Any suspected abuse must be reported immediately to the proper authorities.

SCENARIO WRAP-UP

After working with the telephone screening staff, Allison has come to realize the importance of becoming familiar with childhood diseases and disorders, and the management policy of her provider-employers. Many times Allison has had to refer to the office procedures manual to make sure she is asking the right questions and gathering all the information needed for the provider who will make the daily response calls.

From working in the clinical area, Allison has also realized that a pediatric practice actually has two groups of patients: the child and the caregivers. She must be sensitive to the needs of both groups and develop communication skills that

build trust with the child and their parents. Allison is working on developing a comprehensive education site in the office for interested parents and is creating a community resource guide for interested caregivers. She recognizes the need to stay up-to-date on the CDC's recommendations for childhood immunizations, and she routinely refers to the CDC's website to make sure the office has the most recently published VIS forms. Allison regularly attends her local American Association of Medical Assistants (AAMA) chapter meetings to maintain her certification and to continue to learn about the pediatric practice specialty.

PROCEDURE 37.1   Measure an Infant's Length and Weight

Task

Measure an infant's length and weight accurately so that growth patterns can be monitored and recorded.

Equipment and Supplies

- Patient's health record
- Infant scale with paper cover
- Flexible measuring tape
- Examination table paper
- Pen
- Pediatric length board, if available
- Age and sex-specific infant growth chart
- Gloves
- Disinfectant wipes
- Waste container

Procedural Steps

Measuring an Infant's Length

1. Wash hands or use hand sanitizer; assemble the necessary equipment.
   Purpose: To ensure infection control.
2. Greet the patient and parent or caregiver. Identify yourself. Verify the patient's identity with full name and date of birth. Explain the procedure to be performed in a manner that is understood by the patient and the parent or caregiver. Answer any questions about the procedure.
   Purpose: To alleviate anxiety and gain the child's trust.
3. Undress the infant. The diaper may be left on.
4. Cover the examination table with smooth, flat paper. Ask the caregiver to place the infant on their back on the examination table. If the table is a pediatric table with a headboard, ask the caregiver to hold the infant's head gently against the headboard while you straighten the infant's leg and note the location of the heel on the measurement area. If there is no headboard, ask the caregiver to gently hold the infant's head still while you draw a line on the paper at the top of the baby's head and at the heel after extending the leg (Fig. 1).

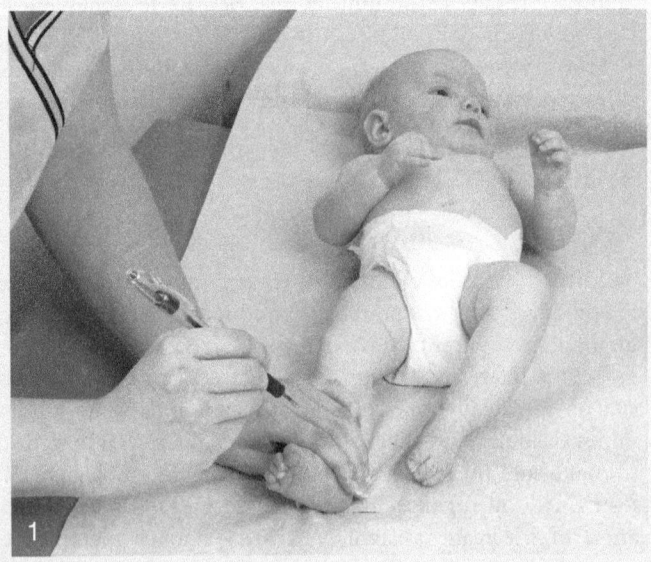

5. Measure the infant's length with the tape measure to the nearest 0.5 cm or ¼ inch and record it. Document the results in either inches or centimeters, depending on office policy, on the infant's growth chart, in the progress notes, and in the caregiver's record if requested.
   Note: Some providers may require the length to be measured to the nearest ⅛ inch.

Weighing an Infant

6. If the scale is not a digital model, prepare the scale by sliding weights to the left; line the scale with disposable paper to reduce the risk of pathogen transmission.
7. If the diaper is clean and dry, it can remain on (depending on the healthcare facility's procedures).
   Purpose: It is important to get the most accurate weight possible, and a wet or soiled diaper will add to the total weight.
8. Place the infant gently on the center of the scale, keeping your hand directly above the infant's trunk for safety (Fig. 2).
   Purpose: To protect the infant from possible injury.

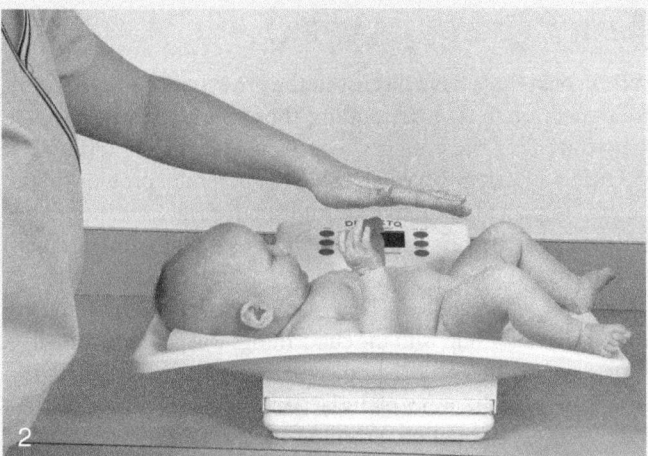

9. The scale is not a digital model, slide the weights across the scale until balance is achieved. Read the infant's weight while they are still. Read the weight in either pounds and ounces or to the nearest tenth of a kilogram, depending on the facility's procedures.
10. If the scale is not a digital model, return the weights to the far left of the scale and remove the baby. Discard the paper lining the scale. If the scale became contaminated during the procedure, follow Occupational Safety and Health Administration (OSHA) guidelines for use of gloves and disposal of contaminated waste. Disinfect the equipment according to the manufacturer's guidelines.
    Purpose: For infection control.
11. Wash hands or use hand sanitizer.
12. Document in the patient's health record and on the growth chart, the length in either inches or centimeters and the weight in pounds and ounces or to the nearest tenth of a kilogram, depending on the facility's policy.
    8/24/20XX 10:20 a.m. Wt 17 lb 4 oz. Length 27.5 in _____
    _____ A. Kwong, CMA (AAMA)

PROCEDURE 37.2   Measure the Head and Chest Circumference of an Infant

Tasks

Obtain an accurate measurement of the circumference of an infant's head and chest and plot the head circumference result on the patient's growth chart.

Equipment and Supplies

- Patient's health record
- Flexible disposable tape measure
- Age- and sex-specific growth chart
- Pen

Procedural Steps

1. Wash hands or use hand sanitizer.
   Purpose: To ensure infection control.
2. Greet the patient and the parents or caregivers. Identify yourself. Verify the patient's identity with full name and date of birth. Explain the procedure to be performed in a manner that is understood by the patient (if old enough) or the parent or caregiver. Answer any questions about the procedure. If the child is old enough, gain his or her cooperation through conversation.
   Purpose: To alleviate anxiety and gain the child's trust.
3. Place an infant in the supine position, or the infant may be held by the parent. An older infant may sit on the examination table.
4. Hold the tape measure with the zero mark against the infant's forehead, slightly above the eyebrows and the top of the ears. Ask the parent for assistance if necessary.
5. Bring the tape measure around the head, just above the ears, until it meets (Fig. 1).

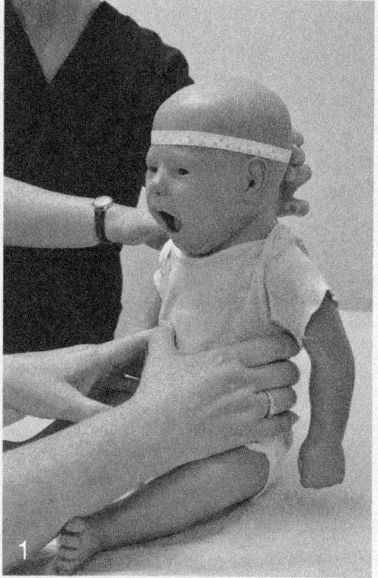

6. Read to the nearest 0.5 cm or ¼ inch. Remember the reading or write it down.
7. Position the infant on his or her back on the exam table. Using the tape measure, wrap it around the infant's chest at the nipple line. The tape measure should be tight without leaving marks on the infant's skin.
   Purpose: Measuring the chest circumference on a child under 2 years of age requires the child to be on his or her back. If the child is older than age 2 and can sit on the exam table, the procedure can be done with the child in the sitting position.
8. Read the measurement to the nearest 0.5 cm or ¼ inch. Remember the reading or write it down.
9. Dispose of the tape measure. Wash hands or use hand sanitizer.
   Purpose: To ensure infection control.
10. Document the measurements in the health record. Record the head circumference measurement on the growth chart.
    Purpose: A procedure is not done until it is recorded.
    8/24/20XX 10:30 a.m. Head circumference 48 cm. Chest circumference 48.5 cm.
    _____ A. Kwong, CMA (AAMA)

PROCEDURE 37.3   Use the Immunization Schedule and Document Immunizations Task

Task

Identify recommended immunizations using an immunization schedule. Document vaccines on the immunization record in the electronic health record.

Equipment and Supplies

- CDC Immunization Schedule (see Fig. 37.5)
- Electronic health record or SimChart for the Medical Office (SCMO)

Scenario

Pedro Gomez (07/01/20XX), a five-year-old child has a wellness check. The mother has completed the vaccine screening questionnaire. She answered the questions, gave her signed consent, and there are no concerns. You administered Kinrix and MMRV per the provider's orders and now need to document the vaccines.

Procedural Steps

1. Using the CDC Immunization Schedule, identify the recommended vaccines for the following patients who were up to date with their vaccines until this visit:
   a. 4-month child
   b. 4-year-old child
   c. 16-year-old teen
2. Log into the EHR or SCMO (into the Simulation Playground) and find the patient's record. Create an office visit encounter for today's wellness visit with Dr. James Martin.
3. Document that the patient has no known allergies to drugs, foods, or environmental items.

Continued

PROCEDURE 37.3   Document Immunizations—cont'd

4. Using the vaccine record screen, document the following immunizations that were given today as ordered by Dr. Martin. In the Reaction field, document the patient's reaction and the VIS edition date (e.g., no reaction; VIS 07/20/XX):

   a. Kinrix (fifth dose of DTaP and fourth dose of IPV), 0.5 mL, IM in the left deltoid, Elsevier #3263, Exp. (one year from today), no reaction. (DTaP VIS edition date 07/20/XX and IPV VIS edition date 06/01/XX)

   b. Second dose of MMRV (MMR and Varicella), 0.5 mL, subcut in the left anterolateral thigh, Elsevier #5569, Exp. (6 months from today), no reaction. (MMR VIS edition date 08/22/XX and Varicella VIS edition date 03/11/XX)

Note: When documenting combination vaccines, each type of vaccine must be documented separately. For example, MMRV would be documented in the MMR section and also in the Varicella section.

Purpose: The documentation should be documented on the correct dose line. For instance if the immunization is the third dose, it needs to be documented on the third dose line.

5. Log out of the EHR or SCMO.

38

Assisting in Geriatrics

LEARNING OBJECTIVES

1. Explain changes in anatomy and physiology caused by aging.
2. Differentiate between common cardiovascular conditions seen in older adults.
3. Discuss symptoms and common complications of type 2 diabetes mellitus
4. Describe the risks and treatments for osteoporosis.
5. Describe the stages of Alzheimer disease.
6. Discuss strategies to use when communicating with a hearing-impaired or visually impaired adult.
7. Describe strategies for healthy eating and sleeping for older adults.
8. Identify strategies to prevent falls.
9. Discuss community resources typically available for older adults.
10. Describe vaccines recommended for adults age 65 and older.
11. Summarize the role of the medical assistant in caring for aging patients.
12. Discuss strategies for effective communication with aging patients.

OUTLINE

▶▶ OPENING SCENARIO

Bill Novelli, CMA (AAMA), works at Walden-Martin Family Medical (WMFM) Clinic. Although patients of all ages are seen in the practice, many patients are age 65 or older. Through his work with Dr. Stephanie Kennedy, Bill has learned to recognize the unique communication needs of aging individuals and the importance of using family and community resources to maintain optimum health in this special population.

YOU WILL LEARN

1. To describe the changes in anatomy and physiology in body systems in geriatric patients.

2. Strategies to use when communicating with older adults.
3. Strategies to help promote wellness in the older population
4. To describe the medical assistant's role with caring for the older patient.

INTRODUCTION

According to the Centers for Disease Control and Prevention (CDC), the life expectancy at 65 years of age is an additional 18.2 years for men and 20.8 years for women. According to US Census Bureau (https://www.census.gov):

• By 2034, there will be 77 million adults age 65 years and older.
• Most people over 65 years of age have been married at some point. By age 85, more than twice as many women have been

widowed compared to men. There are more older women than there are older men.

- Thirty-five percent of women live alone compared to 21% of men. Seventy-two percent of men live with a spouse or partner compared to 49% of women.
- About 75% of the older population is Caucasian. The proportions of the other racial groups were less than their respective representations in the total populations.
- About 11% of people age 85 years and older live in group quarters (e.g., long-term care facilities).

Most older people have at least one chronic medical condition, and many have multiple conditions (comorbidity). Hypertension, arthritis, heart disease, cancer, and diabetes are the most common health problems in the elderly. A significant number of older adults also have asthma, emphysema, and complications from a past cerebrovascular accident (CVA) (stroke). Heart disease, cancer, and chronic lower respiratory disease are the leading causes of death.

VOCABULARY

comorbidity The presence of two or more chronic diseases or conditions in a patient.

Aging

To provide quality care to aging patients, medical assistants must understand the aging process, including the physical and sensory changes that occur with aging. This knowledge enables medical assistants to recognize the special needs of the aged and to develop therapeutic management and communication skills that can help them effectively care for the older patient.

Aging is a complex physiologic, psychological, and social process. Old age is not an illness, but rather a normal life process that people experience in different ways. As people age, changes occur in their physical appearance and abilities. These changes can have a profound effect on the individual's ability to interact with their environment. Personal and environmental factors, such as lack of exercise, poor nutrition, substance abuse, chronic stress, and air pollutants, can cause age-related changes to occur much sooner and be more pronounced. The increase in the number of individuals over 65 and the active role they play in society are doing a lot to help dispel common myths about aging.

According to the National Institute on Aging (https://www.nia.nih.gov), there are misconceptions about aging and the older adult:

- *It is normal for older adults to be depressed and lonely.* Loneliness can lead to feelings of sadness and depression. Studies have shown that older adults are less likely to be depressed than younger adults. Older adults who feel depressed may appear tired, have issues sleeping, or seem irritable. Heart disease, stroke, or cancer can be conditions that cause depressive symptoms.
- *Older adults need less sleep.* Older adults need the same amount of sleep as younger adults. Sleep patterns change with aging, and it is important to get adequate sleep.
- *Older adults cannot learn new things.* Older adults have the ability to learn new things, create new memories, and improve their skills. Trying and learning new skills can help improve cognitive abilities in the older adult.

- *Older adults will get dementia.* Dementia is not a normal part of aging. The risk for dementia may increase with age, but not everyone will get dementia.
- *Older adults should take it easy and avoid exercise so they do not get injured.* Being active will help an older adult manage some chronic conditions. Physical activity and exercise also help keep people more independent as they age.
- *If a parent has Alzheimer disease, then all of the children will get it too.* The risk for Alzheimer disease is higher if there is a family history of it, but it does not necessarily mean that all descendants will get it. Environmental and lifestyle factors, such as exercise, diet, exposure to pollutants, and smoking, can increase the risk for Alzheimer disease.
- *Older people have to give up driving.* About 1 in 5 drivers are age 65 or older.

CRITICAL THINKING 38.1

When Bill first started working with aging patients, he believed many of the myths about people over age 65. Through his work with Dr. Kennedy, he has come to realize that many of these myths have no foundation in actual practice. Based on the myths mentioned in the text, what do you think about these beliefs on aging? Share your thoughts with your classmates.

CHANGES IN ANATOMY AND PHYSIOLOGY

The aging process brings about changes in all of the body's systems. The following sections describe the changes that occur with aging.

Cardiovascular System

Changes occur in the heart with age. The left ventricle may increase in size, causing a smaller stroke volume. The walls of the heart can become stiffer, leading to heart disease. Valves become thicker and stiffer, causing heart murmurs. With the loss of cells in the sinoatrial (SA) node, the heart rate is slower. Electrocardiogram (ECG) changes can be seen. Atrial fibrillation is more common in older adults.

Baroreceptors in the carotid arteries and aorta detect changes in blood pressure and help maintain a fairly constant blood pressure with position changes. With age, the baroreceptors become less sensitive, making older people more at risk for orthostatic hypotension when changing positions.

Changes also occur in the blood and blood vessels. It can take longer for red blood cells to be produced, putting the person at risk for anemia. The number of neutrophils decreases, making it harder to resist infections. The arterial walls thicken and become stiffer, increasing the blood pressure.

The risk of certain cardiovascular diseases increases with age. The following cardiovascular conditions are prevalent in older adults:

- *Anemia*: Caused by malnutrition, bleeding from the gastrointestinal tract, chronic infection, or a side effect of medication.
- *Arteriosclerosis* (ar teer ee oh sklah ROH sis): Over time deposits buildup on the arterial walls and begin to calcify. The calcification decreases the elasticity of the walls, which impacts constriction and dilation of the vessels.

- *Congestive heart disease*: A leading cause of illness, disability, and death among adults age 65 and older. Age-related changes to the cardiovascular system are a major cause of heart disease. Disease and lifestyle habits, such as a lack of exercise, poor diet, and stress also contribute to this.
- *Hypertension*: Heart and blood vessel changes can increase the blood pressure. Hypertension increases the workload of the heart, which can cause hypertrophy (hahy PUR troh fee) and weakening of the myocardial (mahy uh KAHR dee all) wall. Hypertension can lead to congestive heart failure, arrhythmias (ey RITH mee uh), coronary artery disease, CVA, peripheral artery disease, and renal failure.
- *Orthostatic (postural) hypotension*: The blood pressure drops suddenly as a person changes position, such as moving from sitting to standing. Certain cardiac medications can increase the risk for orthostatic hypotension. Orthostatic hypotension can lead to falls in older adults.

Proper management of cardiovascular disease and healthy lifestyle habits can help maintain the health of an aging population and reduce mortality (mawr TAL i tee) rates. Management of heart diseases includes monitoring the blood pressure and cholesterol and blood glucose levels. Regular screening checks for orthostatic hypotension should be done. Healthy lifestyle habits include regular exercise, weight control, and a diet rich in fruits, vegetables, and whole grains.

VOCABULARY

arrhythmia Heart beats with an irregular or abnormal rhythm.

calcify Harden by deposition of or conversion into calcium compounds.

hypertrophy The enlargement of an organ or tissue due to an enlargement of its cells.

mortality The relative frequency of deaths in a specific population.

MEDICAL TERMINOLOGY

arteri/o	artery
cardi/o	heart
my/o	muscle
thromb/o	clotting, clot
hyper-	excessive, too much, above
phleb-	vein
-al	pertaining to
-itis	inflammation
-osis	abnormal condition
-sclerosis	abnormal condition of hardening
-trophy	nourishment, development

Endocrine System

Changes occur in the endocrine system with age. The pituitary gland in the brain decreases in size. The thyroid gland in the neck becomes nodular. Thyroid hormone production and metabolism remains for the most part unchanged. Parathyroid hormone affects phosphate and calcium levels. This hormone rises with age, which can lead to osteoporosis.

The average fasting glucose levels increase 6 to 14 milligrams per deciliter (mg/dL) every decade after age 50. The cells become less sensitive to insulin (increase in insulin resistance), which can lead to type 2 diabetes mellitus.

Changes occur with the adrenal cortex hormones. Aldosterone, which regulates fluid and electrolyte balance, decreases with age. This can cause lightheadedness and orthostatic hypotension. Cortisol is involved with the metabolism of glucose, protein, and fat. Cortisol also has anti-inflammatory and anti-allergy effects. The release of cortisol decreases with age, but the blood level remains about the same.

With aging, men often have a lower level of testosterone. After menopause, women have lower levels of estrogen hormones.

Changes in hormone levels vary with age. Some increase, some decrease, and others remain unchanged. Examples include:

- *Hormones that decrease with age*: Aldosterone, calcitonin, growth hormone, and renin. Estrogen and prolactin levels decrease significantly in women. Testosterone decreases gradually in men with age. Melatonin levels decrease with age, which may affect the normal sleep/wake cycles. Growth hormone levels decrease with age. This causes a decrease in lean body mass and an increase in body fat in the abdominal area.
- *Hormones that remain mostly unchanged*: Cortisol, epinephrine, insulin, and thyroid hormones - Triiodothyronine (T3) and Thyroxin (T4).
- *Hormones that increase with age*: Follicle-stimulating hormone (FSH), luteinizing hormone (LH), norepinephrine, and parathyroid hormone.

Type 2 Diabetes Mellitus. One of the most common endocrine system disorders seen in the aging population is type 2 diabetes mellitus (DM). According to the CDC in 2020, about 11.5 million people age 65 and older have been diagnosed with diabetes, 2.9 million have undiagnosed diabetes, and 24.2 million have prediabetes.

As indicated in the prior section, insulin resistance occurs with age and the body needs more insulin. The pancreas cannot make enough insulin to meet the demands of the body. People with type 2 diabetes may be asymptomatic initially. Early symptoms include polydipsia, polyuria, polyphagia, weight loss, fatigue, blurred vision, frequent infections, and slow-healing wounds.

The complications of diabetes mellitus develop over time. Two factors increase the risk of complications: the longer a person has DM and the more uncontrolled the blood glucose. The following list provides possible complications of diabetes mellitus:

- *Cardiovascular disease*: DM increases the risk for coronary artery disease with *angina* (chest pain), *atherosclerosis* (narrowing of the arteries), myocardial infarction (MI) (heart attack), and CVA.
- *Neurologic disorders*: Type 2 diabetes increases a person's risk of dementia-related disorders (e.g., Alzheimer disease). With hyperglycemia and a decrease in blood flow, over time

---

VOCABULARY

polydipsia Extreme thirst.

polyphagia Excessive hunger.

polyuria High levels of urine output.

BOX 38.1   Factors That Can Affect Diabetes Management in Older People

- Modifying lifestyle risk factors may be more difficult because of poor nutrition, inability to exercise, and long-standing habits, such as smoking and a diet high in saturated fats and calories.
- Previously diagnosed health conditions, such as hypertension and heart disease, in addition to an age-related decline in kidney and liver function, increase the challenge of treating diabetes.
- Older people are more likely to be prescribed multiple medications, which increases the risk of adverse drug interactions.
- Elderly patients with diabetes are more prone to hypoglycemia and may not recognize and respond quickly to the signs of low blood glucose levels.
- Diabetic complications can develop quickly because of a long history of prediabetes before diagnosis.
- Older people may have decreased physical and/or mental abilities that make it difficult for them to understand and adhere to a complicated treatment regimen.
- Older patients may not be able to afford the medications and supplies needed to maintain health.

diabetic neuropathy can occur. A person with diabetic neuropathy can have other types of neuropathies, including peripheral and autonomic neuropathies. *Peripheral neuropathy* causes burning, tingling, pain, and numbness in the extremities. The symptoms start in the fingers and toes and work up the arms and legs. *Autonomic neuropathy* causes changes with the heart rate, blood pressure, digestive system, bladder, sweat glands, eyes, and reproductive organs.

- *Kidney disease*: Hyperglycemia damages the tiny blood vessels (glomeruli) in the kidney. This causes chronic kidney disease (CKD), which can lead to kidney failure if untreated.
- *Poor healing of wounds*: Diabetes can increase the risk of infections. Infections can increase the blood glucose level. With hyperglycemia, nutrients and oxygen can be prevented from getting to the cells. The immune system may not be as efficient. If a wound does not heal, the person may be at risk for an amputation.
- *Depression*: Is common in patients with type 2 DM.
- *Periodontal disease*: Gum infections and tooth loss can occur, which also increases hyperglycemia.
- *Blindness and eye conditions*: Glaucoma, diabetic retinopathy, and cataracts can lead to vision loss.

Treatment for Type 2 DM involves healthy eating, regular exercise, weight loss if obese, medications (e.g., antihyperglycemics, insulin), and glucose monitoring. Box 38.1 lists unique considerations for older adults.

It is recommended that people with diabetes have their eyes checked every 4 to 6 months. Early prevention and screening can prevent blindness with diabetic retinopathy. Dental cleans and exams are recommended twice a year.

VOCABULARY

cataracts Clouding of the lens, leading to decreased vision.
diabetic retinopathy Diabetes mellitus damages the blood vessels in the retina, leading to loss of vision and eventual blindness.
dysphagia Difficulty swallowing.
glaucoma A condition in which the fluid pressure in the eye increases; this can lead to blindness if not treated.

MEDICAL TERMINOLOGY

angi/o	vessel
neur/o	nerve
retin/o	retina
-pathy	disease condition

CRITICAL THINKING 38.2

Quite a few of the elderly patients at WMFM Clinic have type 2 diabetes. Based on what you have learned about the difficulty of managing diabetes in aging people, what factors do you need to consider when conducting patient education for an elderly person with diabetes? Are there any community resources that might be useful for patients and their families?

Digestive System

Age related changes in the digestive or gastrointestinal (GI) system can cause older patients to have malnutrition. Tasting, chewing, and swallowing can change. As people age, they have less taste buds and a diminished sense of smell. Dysphagia (dis FAY jee ah) and dental issues are more common.

With age, the stomach cannot accommodate as much food because of decreased elasticity. The stomach empties slower. The amounts of hydrochloric acid and intrinsic factor decrease. Hydrochloric acid helps with protein digestion and kills pathogens. Intrinsic factor is a protein that is needed to help the body absorb vitamin B_{12}. A lack of intrinsic factor leads to pernicious anemia.

The lactase levels decrease with age, leading to lactose intolerance. Bacterial overgrowth (excessive growth of certain intestinal bacteria) is more common with age. This leads to bloating, weight loss, pain, and reduced absorption of certain nutrients (e.g., iron, calcium, and vitamin B_{12}).

Age-related changes can be seen with the accessory organs. The pancreas decreases in weight as some tissue is replaced with scar tissue, although these changes do not affect the organ's ability to produce digestive enzymes and sodium bicarbonate. The liver gets smaller and blood flow decreases. Liver function test results, however, are unchanged. Metabolism of many substances decreases, which affects drug metabolism. Older adults may experience dose-related side effects. The production and flow of bile decreases with age, leading to more gallstones.

With the aging process, gastroesophageal reflux disease (GERD) is the most common upper digestive disorder. GERD can be caused by the slowed gastric emptying, aging muscles, extra weight gain, and medications, such as antihypertensive and antidepressant medications. Treatment for GERD includes medications to reduce or block acid production. Antacids can neutralize the stomach acid. Continuous high doses of antacids can cause acid rebound, metabolic alkalosis, and problems with pre-existing conditions, such as hypertension and congestive heart failure. Taking antacids with magnesium can cause diarrhea.

Constipation is a common concern with older adults. With the decreased peristalsis, increased water absorption can occur as the fecal content slowly moves through the large intestine,

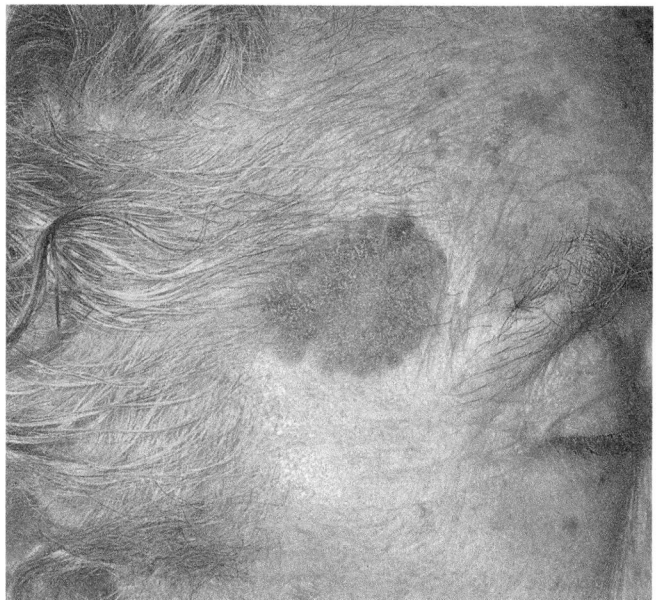

Fig. 38.1 Seborrheic keratosis. (From Habif TP: *Clinical dermatology: a color guide to diagnosis and therapy*, ed 6, St. Louis, 2016, Mosby.)

leading to harder stools. Other contributing factors to constipation include the lack of fluids and exercise, low-fiber diets, and certain medications, such as antidepressants, diuretics, antacids containing aluminum or calcium, and medications for Parkinson's disease.

Integumentary System

With aging, the skin undergoes changes. The epidermis thins. The number of melanocytes decrease, and the remaining melanocytes increase in size. The skin looks paler, thinner, and translucent. Age spots commonly appear in sun-exposed areas, such as the face and back of the hands. Changes in the connective tissue reduce the skin's strength and elasticity. Those that work outdoors tend to have a leathery, weather-beaten appearance to their arms and face. This is called *solar elastosis* (EE las TOE sis). Skin growths, such as skin tags, warts, seborrheic keratosis, and actinic keratosis, are more common in older people (Fig. 38.1). Older adults are more prone to bruising (*senile purpura*) due to fragile blood vessels in the dermis.

Sebaceous glands produce less oil, causing drier skin. Women experience this after menopause, and men may not notice the decrease until after age 80. The number of collagen (KAW lah jen) cells in the dermis declines, causing the skin to sag and wrinkle. Atrophy occurs with the subcutaneous fat layer, increasing the risk for skin injury and an inability to maintain the body temperature. With sweat glands producing less sweat, this also leads to overheating and a higher risk of heat stroke.

Hair growth patterns tend to change. Some individuals may experience *alopecia* (al oh PEE sha), the complete or partial loss of hair from the head or other parts of the body. Hair may also start to grow in areas it did not previously. Woman may notice more facial hair growth. Hair in the nose and ears becomes

coarser and longer. Nails, particularly toenails, thicken. It is not unusual for nails to split, making them more susceptible to fungal infections.

The medical assistant should use caution when working with other adults. Their skin can tear easily. Fragile blood vessels can break easily, leading to bruising. Aging skin is slower to repair itself, and wound healing may be up to 4 times slower.

Skin changes relate to environmental factors, nutrition, genetic makeup, and other factors. Sun exposure is the greatest factor in skin changes. Protecting the skin throughout the life span is important. Wearing a hat, protective clothing, and good quality sunscreen will protect the older adult from sunburn. Strategies to prevent dry skin include:
- Use a room humidifier to moisten the air.
- Bathe less frequently and use warm rather than hot water.
- Use a mild soap or cleansing cream.
- Wear protective clothing in cold weather.
- Moisturize dry skin.

CRITICAL THINKING 38.3

Rose Deluca, a 71-year-old patient of Dr. Martin, is unhappy with her constant dry skin that has occurred in the past several years. Based on what Bill knows about the normal changes that occur in the skin as people age, how can he explain these changes to Mrs. Deluca? What can he suggest to help with dryness?

VOCABULARY

actinic keratosis A wartlike growth that can become malignant. Usually seen in middle to older adults due to excessive exposure to the sun. Also called senile or solar keratosis.

age spots Hyperpigmented flat dark areas on the skin that occur in irregular shapes; also called liver spots, sunspots, and senile lentigo.

atrophy Degeneration of cells, causing a reduction or "wasting away" of tissues.

collagen The most abundant structural protein found in skin and other connective tissues. It provides strength and cushioning to many parts of the body.

seborrheic keratosis A benign epidermal tumor that ranges in color from light tan to black. It appears flat or slightly raised; waxy or scaly; round or oval. Typically appears on the face, shoulders, chest, and back.

Musculoskeletal System

Changes are seen in the musculoskeletal system with aging. The following are common skeletal system changes that occur with age:
- Bones lose calcium and other minerals, which reduces the bone mass or density. Bone density starts to decrease around age 30 to 40 in both males and females. It accelerates in women after menopause. The loss of bone density makes the bones more brittle, leading to osteoporosis and fractures.
- The disks between the vertebrae wear and tear with age. They can dehydrate and the cartilage can stiffen, causing the disk to bulge.
- Loss of height from the compression and curving of the spinal column occurs, which can cause a more stooped posture.

- The long bones in the body become more brittle because of the mineral loss.
- Joints become stiffer and less flexible. Synovial fluid decreases and cartilage may wear away, causing degenerative changes. This can lead to inflammation, stiffness, pain, and deformities.
- Lean body mass decreases, partly due to atrophy of the muscle tissue. Muscle fibers shrink. Lost muscle tissue is replaced slower and replaced with a tough fibrous tissue. This creates the thin, bony appearance in the hands.
- Muscles are less toned and become rigid with age.

Osteoporosis is a common problem, especially for women. The bones break easier. Compression fractures of the vertebrae reduce mobility and cause pain. Fatigue, weakness, and reduced activity tolerances occurs because of the muscle weakness. Stiff joints and debilitation osteoarthritis are common. The risk of falls increases because of gait changes, instability, and loss of balance. *Fasciculations* (fah SIK yeh LAE shuhns) (involuntary muscle tremors and fine movements) are more common with age. People who are unable to move an extremity may get muscle contractures

Osteoporosis. Osteoporosis (OS tee oh pah roe sis) is a condition that causes bones to become brittle and weak. Healthy bone is constantly being broken down and remodeled. When a person has osteoporosis, bones are being broken down quicker than new bone can be created. The bones become very porous. This leads to weak bones that are easily fractured, especially in the wrist, hip, and spine.

Increased risks for osteoporosis include menopause, family history, small body frame, white or Asian descent, hormonal imbalance, dietary deficiencies (low calcium intake), long-term corticosteroid use, celiac disease, kidney or liver disease, cancer, and some autoimmune conditions. A sedentary lifestyle, tobacco use, and excessive alcohol consumption are also risk factors for osteoporosis.

Weight-bearing exercises to maintain bone density as well as calcium and vitamin D supplements are recommended to prevent osteoporosis. Medications that are used to prevent and/or treat osteoporosis include:

- *Bisphosphonates*: Prevents and treats bone loss. Alendronate (a LEN droe nate) (Binosto, Fosamax), ibandronate (i BAN droh nate) (Boniva), risedronate (ris ED roe nate) (Actonel, Atelvia) are oral tablets. Zoledronic (ZOE le dron ik) acid (Reclast, Zometa) is given as an intravenous (IV) medication. Common side effects include heartburn, nausea, and abdominal pain. When taking an oral medication, the patient must:
  - Take the medication on an empty stomach in the morning. Take with 6 to 8 ounces of plain water.
  - Remain sitting or standing for 30 minutes after taking the tablet. Do not eat or drink for 30 to 60 minutes after taking the tablet.
- *Raloxifene* (ral OX i feen) (Evista): Used to prevent and treat osteoporosis. It can reduce the risk of spinal fractures. The medication is administered as a daily oral tablet that can be taken with or without food. Thrombi in the legs (known as

deep vein thrombosis [DVT]) or thrombi in the lungs (pulmonary embolism) are side effects of the medication.

- *Denosumab* (den OH sue mab) (Prolia): Increases bone density. Administered as a subcutaneous injection every 6 months.
- *Teriparatide* (terr ih PAR a tyd) (Bonsity, Forteo): A synthetic form of parathyroid hormone. It causes the body to build new bone and increases bone strength and density, thus decreasing the risk for fractures. Administered as a daily subcutaneous injection. Can cause nausea, heartburn, dizziness, depression, or leg cramps.
- *Romosozumab* (roe moe SOZ ue mab) (Evenity): Increases bone formation and decreases bone breakdown. Administered subcutaneously monthly. Can cause hypocalcemia.

VOCABULARY

dementia Loss of cognitive abilities, including memory, concentration, communication, planning, and abstract thinking. May also cause emotional disturbance and personality changes. Results from brain injury, Alzheimer disease, Parkinson's disease, and other conditions.

hypocalcemia Abnormally low level of calcium in the blood.

osteoporosis Abnormal thinning of the bone structure, causing bones to become brittle and weak.

porous Having many small spaces or holes.

thrombi Blood clots that block the flow of blood (singular, thrombus).

MEDICAL TERMINOLOGY

arthr/o	joint
oste/o	bone
-penia	lack, deficiency

CRITICAL THINKING 38.4

The family of Rita Schaeffer, a 73-year-old patient, is concerned about the risk of falls. Mrs. Schaeffer recently was diagnosed with osteoporosis, and she lives alone. What information should Bill give the family to help them prevent accidents in their mother's home? Also, Mrs. Schaeffer's 45-year-old daughter is concerned about developing osteoporosis. What steps should the daughter take to prevent the disease?

Nervous System

With age, the brain and spinal cord lose nerve cells. With the degeneration of nerve cells, waste products, such as beta amyloid, collect in the brain leading to the formation of plaques and tangles. An older adult can have a loss of reflexes, which can lead to safety and mobility issues. Slowing of thought and memory is a normal part of aging. Severe memory issues, such as dementia, is not normal. Symptoms of dementia include being unable to do normal activities of living (e.g., eating, dressing, grooming). A person has problems solving problems and controlling emotions. To be diagnosed with dementia, a person needs to have at least two or more problems with brain function (e.g., memory, language).

Some conditions can cause serious memory problems that resemble dementia. Once the condition is corrected, the memory problems should go away. These conditions include:

BOX 38.2 Alzheimer's Disease

According to the Alzheimer's Association:

- It is estimated that 1 in 9 people or 6.2 million people age 65 and older have Alzheimer's dementia in 2021 and 72% are age 75 or older.
- Almost 66% of those with Alzheimer's in US are women.
- About 1 in 3 older adults die with Alzheimer's or another dementia.
- On average, adults age 65 and older survive 4 to 8 years after the diagnosis of Alzheimer's disease, yet some live as long as 20 years.
- About 1 in 3 caregivers to someone with Alzheimer's is age 65 or older.
- About 66% of caregivers live with the person with Alzheimer's.

From Alzheimer's Association. https://www.alz.org/alzheimers-dementia/facts-figures. Accessed May 5, 2021.

- Emotional problems, such as depression, stress, and anxiety.
- Side effects of certain illegal and legal drugs, including prescription and over the counter (OTC).
- Alcoholism and malnutrition.
- Blood clots, tumors, or infections in the brain.
- Delirium and head injury, such as a concussion.
- Thyroid, kidney, and liver problems.

The best way to ensure mental functioning later life is to remain mentally and physically stimulated. Ways to maintain mental function are:

- Exercise regularly
- Keep socially active
- Practice stress-reduction activities
- Quit smoking and drink alcohol in moderation
- Use hearing aids and glasses if needed
- Receive treatment for depression, diabetes, hypertension, and high cholesterol levels

Alzheimer Disease. Alzheimer (ALTS high mer) disease (AD), also called senile dementia, is a degenerative disease of the brain. It is characterized by disorientation, memory failure, speech disturbance, and a loss of mental capacity. Alzheimer disease is the most common cause for dementia (Box 38.2). An increased amount of microscopic neurofibrillary tangles and amyloid plaques in the cerebral cortex and the loss of neurons are seen with AD. A definitive diagnosis of Alzheimer disease occurs upon examination during an autopsy.

During the early stage of AD, the person may be able to function independently. People may have problems coming up with the right word or name. They may have difficulty completing tasks and forgetting information just read. They have issues planning and organizing and commonly misplace objects.

The middle-stage of AD is the longest and may last for years. The symptoms become more pronounced. People may:

- Have personality and behavioral changes, such as delusions. They may become confused, moody, suspicious, compulsive, repetitive, and angry.
- Forget their personal history, such as their address or schools they attended
- Become incontinent of urine and stool
- Have sleep pattern changes

People in the late stage of Alzheimer disease have severe dementia symptoms. They lose the ability to respond to others. They have problems swallowing, moving, and walking. They require 24/7 care. They become susceptible to infections, such as pneumonia. Hospice can be helpful during the late stage.

Current treatments may only keep symptoms from getting worse for a limited time; no cure is available. Medications that help treat cognitive symptoms include:

- *Cholinesterase inhibitors*: Boost the acetylcholine in the brain, which is depleted with AD. Common medications include donepezil (doe NEP e zil) (Aricept), rivastigmine (ri va STIG meen) (Exelon), and galantamine (ga LAN ta meen) (Razadyne).
- *Memantine* (MEM an teen) (Namenda) is used for moderate to severe AD.

Supportive care for family members is essential. The medical assistant can be especially helpful in recommending educational workshops, support groups, and stress management skills for caregivers.

VOCABULARY

amyloid plaques Masses or clumps of proteins that form between neurons and disrupt cellular function.

delusions Unshakable belief in something untrue; may be accompanied by hallucinations and/or paranoia.

elastin A highly elastic protein in connective tissue that allows tissues to resume their shape after stretching or contracting; found abundantly in the dermis of the skin.

neurofibrillary tangles Abnormal structures composed of twisted protein fibers within nerve cells.

Pulmonary System

At around age 20 to 25, the lungs reach maturity. By age 35, lung function starts to decline. People who smoke can increase the aging of their lungs. As a person ages, the following respiratory system changes occur:

- Chest wall and thoracic spine deformities cause increased work of breathing.
- The diaphragm grows weaker, leading to a decreased ability to inhale and exhale.
- Weakness in respiratory muscles causes the coughing reflex to be less effective.
- Changes in elastin (ih LAS tin) and collagen cause the lungs to lose their elasticity. This leads to an inability to keep the airway completely open.
- Alveoli lose their shape, which causes air to be trapped in the lungs. This leads to a decrease in gas exchange and lung capacity.

With these changes, an older person has more difficult breathing and coughing effectively to clear mucus from the lungs. These factors put the older adult at greater risk for pneumonia and aspiration.

The larynx also changes with aging. This will cause a change in the pitch and quality of the voice. The voice often sounds quieter and slightly hoarse. Although the voice sounds weaker, it generally does not interfere with the ability to effectively communicate.

Sensory Organs

Vision. Visual changes can occur with age. The eyes may appear to sink in their sockets, as the supporting fat pads become smaller. The cornea becomes less sensitive, so eye injuries may not be as noticeable. Arcus senilis (AHR kuhs suh NAHY lis) is common with aging. The pupil size may decrease about 60%, and the pupils may be slower to react to light changes. The lens becomes yellowed, less flexible, and slightly cloudy. The vitreous liquefies and shrinks. The vitreous separates from the retina, causing vitreous detachment, which does not require treatment. Floaters in the vision increase. Collagen and proteins in the vitreous become "stringing" and float in the vitreous, casting a shadow on the retina. Eye glands produce less tears and oil, thus dry eyes are more common. The eye muscles are less efficient with rotating the eye, reducing the peripheral vision.

By the early to mid-40s age-related presbyopia (prez bee OH pee uh) develops, making it difficult to focus on objects close at hand. This will require the use of corrective lenses in order to see things near to the eye, such as for reading. Age-related macular degeneration (AMD) and cataracts are the most common causes of blindness in older adults.

Older people need more light in order to read, but too much light can cause problems with glare. Glare can be a particularly uncomfortable visual experiences for the aging eye. Exposed light bulbs (e.g., those used in chandeliers) and light from highly reflective surfaces can produce excessive glare. The aging eye also struggles when going from light to dark or dark to light. This can make going from a well-lit room into a dim hallway very difficult to navigate.

Vision changes increase the risk for falls and accidents. Stairs become an increased hazard because the edges of the steps cannot be seen clearly. Box 38.3 provides suggestions on how to assist a visually impaired older adult.

VOCABULARY

age-related macular degeneration A condition in which the cells of the macula lutea degenerate, causing blurred vision and ultimately blindness.

arcus senilis A white or gray opaque ring around the cornea that commonly occurs in people over age 50 years. Can be caused from fat deposits or hyaline degeneration.

Ménière disease Chronic disease of the inner ear causing recurrent episodes of vertigo, progressive sensorineural hearing loss, and tinnitus.

ototoxic A medicine or substance capable of damaging cranial nerve VIII (vestibulocochlear nerve) or the organs of hearing and balance.

presbycusis Age-related hearing loss.

presbyopia Far-sightedness caused by changes to the eye related to aging.

Hearing. The ear structures help with maintaining balance and with hearing. With age, older adults may have problems maintaining their balance with sitting, standing, and walking. Changes in hearing typically begin around age 30 and slowly progress as the individual ages. Age-related hearing loss is generally caused by a loss of cochlear cilia, which results in the inability to hear high-frequency sounds. As individuals age, the hearing progressively worsens until lower frequency sounds are also affected. By age 65, 1 out of 3 people have lost enough

---

BOX 38.3   Suggestions for Helping the Visually Impaired Older Adult

- When escorting an older person, regardless of whether they are visually impaired, allow patients to place their hand above your elbow. It is easier for the person to follow your movements. This method also provides a source of support and security.
- Use high levels of evenly distributed, glare-free light.
- Ask the pharmacist to use large lettering when labeling medicine bottles.
- Use paper that has a nonglare finish and large size font for forms and educational materials.
- Make distinct differences (e.g., size of containers or color coding with bright primary colors) for pills that are similar in size and color.
- Place all objects within the visual field and prevent clutter.

BOX 38.4   Suggestions for Helping the Hearing-Impaired Older Adult

- Stand in the patient's direct line of vision and gently touch the person to get their attention.
- Use gestures, pictures, and large, bold print to communicate.
- Talk in short sentences into the ear with better hearing.
- Do not increase the volume of your speech. This also raises the frequency of the voice, which is the hearing most impaired in aging people. Use expanded speech; lower the tone of your voice and talk in distinct syllables.
- Avoid background noise. Give instructions in a quiet room with the door closed. If the patient has a hearing aid, make sure it is on.

---

cilia to be diagnosed as having presbycusis (prez by cue sees). Hearing impairment can be compounded by otosclerosis (oh toh sklair ROH sis), Ménière (meyn YAIRZ) disease, long-term exposure to intense noise, and certain ototoxic drugs, such as aspirin. Impacted cerumen and otitis media can also increase hearing loss in the short term, but it tends to resolve when the condition is corrected.

Hearing loss can have a profound psychological effect on aging people, causing depression, social withdrawal, and feelings of isolation. Hearing loss can make it difficult for these individuals to take part in a typical conversation. Because hearing loss generally occurs gradually over time, it is often not noticed until it is severe and psychological effects are occurring. Symptoms of presbycusis include:

- Lack of attention when addressed
- Inappropriate responses
- Asking to have statements repeated
- Speaking too loudly
- Increasing the volume of devices, such as the television and radio

Hearing aids are often used to help those with hearing loss. They are small electronic devices that use a microphone to pick up sound and amplify it directly into the ear of the person using it. Hearing aids can be very helpful in improving hearing and correcting the social isolation that comes with hearing loss. It is important to remember that hearing aids may also increase background noises, so areas with a lot of background noise can still be problematic for those with hearing loss.

Along with hearing loss, some individuals may experience tinnitus. Tinnitus causes a continuous sensation of ringing in the ears. This can make it difficult to understand speech and can make sleeping difficult. The medical assistant can provide support to those with hearing loss and their families. Box 38.4 provides suggestions on how to assist a hearing-impaired older adult.

MEDICAL TERMINOLOGY	
ot/o	ear
tox/o	poison
presby-	old age
-cusis	hearing
-ic	pertaining to
-opia	vision condition
-sclerosis	abnormal condition of hardening

Taste and Smell. Taste and smell play an important role in our lives. They help us enjoy food and also allow us to detect dangers, such as gases, smoke, and spoiled foods. As a person ages, changes occur that can affect a person's ability to taste and smell.

With age, taste buds decrease in size and number. After age 60, the sensitivity to the five tastes declines. The sense of taste can also be affected by the decrease in the saliva production due to certain medications. The sense of smell declines by age 70, which can be related to the loss of nerve endings and low amounts of mucus in the nose. Mucus helps odors stay in the nose longer, allowing the nerve endings to detect the odors. Diseases, smoking, and exposure to harmful particles in the air can accelerate the loss of taste and smell.

If people are experiencing a loss of taste and smell, it is important to talk with their provider. If a medication is causing the issue, switching medications may help improve the senses. Using more spices when cooking can increase the interest in food. It is also important to ensure carbon monoxide and smoke detectors are working.

Touch. With the sense of touch, we become aware of pain, pressure, temperature, vibration, and body position. Receptors in the skin, muscles, joints, tendons, and internal organs detect these sensations. With decreased blood flow to the nerves, spinal cord, and brain, these sensations can be reduced or changed. In addition, malnutrition, diabetes, confusion, and nerve damage can also affect the sensations. Older people may become more sensitive to light touches because their skin is thinner.

With the changes in the receptors, a person may have a difficult time determining the temperature of the environment and water. Burns, frostbite, hypothermia, and hyperthermia related conditions can occur. After age 50, many people have less sensitivity to pain. This can lead to injuries, such as pressure ulcers.

To help keep older adults safe:
- Lower the water heater temperature to no higher than 120°F.
- Dress according to the thermometer.
- Inspect feet for injuries daily.

Urinary System

In older adults, the kidney tissue and number of nephrons are reduced up to 20%. The renal arteries can harden. This causes the kidneys to filter blood more slowly. The kidneys become less able to regulate water balance. Older adults are at more risk of dehydration when the weather is hot or if they have diarrhea. The bladder wall becomes stiffer and less stretchy with age. The bladder cannot hold as much urine as before. Bladder muscles weaken. The urethra may be obstructed by an enlarged prostate gland or a prolapse of the bladder or vagina. Older adults are at more risk for chronic kidney disease, urinary tract infections (UTIs), and incontinence.

Urinary incontinence (in KON tn uh nens), the involuntary loss of urine, is a significant problem for aging patients. Urinary incontinence can be caused from UTIs, vaginal infections, constipations, structural changes related to age, confusion, and certain medications. Difficulty with mobility can also cause episodes of incontinence. Incontinence is both an emotional and a physical problem. To avoid the risk of an embarrassing accident, people with this problem may avoid social occasions or activities they enjoy. They may minimize the amount of fluids they drink, which can lead to dehydration. Treatment for incontinence consists of timed voiding. The person urinates on a set schedule. Lifestyles, such as weight loss, limiting caffeine and alcohol, and preventing constipation, can also help limit incontinence.

Reproductive System

Reproductive system changes occur with age. In females, the vagina, uterus, cervix, and ovaries decrease in size. Less vaginal secretions are produced, leading to vaginal dryness and an increased risk for bacterial and fungal infections. Women in this age group who are sexually active should be advised to use a lubricant to avoid damage to the vaginal canal.

With men, the prostate can increase in size, causing difficulty with urination. This is treated with medications to reduce the size of the prostate, making it easier to void. In more severe cases surgery can be used to remove part of the prostate to improve urination. Surgery is avoided if possible because it can lead to impotence. Erectile dysfunction (ED) can also occur with age. Common conditions that lead to ED include heart disease, hypertension, tobacco use, alcoholism, diabetes, metabolic syndrome, Parkinson disease, prior pelvic surgeries and treatments, obesity, depression, and stress. Drugs that can cause ED include antidepressants, antihistamines, antihypertensives, and pain medications. Sperm production declines after age 50, but men can remain virile well into old age.

> **VOCABULARY**
> **virile** Having strength, energy, and a strong sex drive.
> **void** To urinate.

It is important that healthcare professionals dismiss the myth that older patients have lost interest in sexual intercourse, because many older adults maintain interest in sexual activities. Illness and some drugs can interfere with sexual function. Declining health can make sexual activities more of a health risk due to the physical activity and increased heart rate. Patients need to be helped to feel comfortable and should not be embarrassed to discuss their concerns openly with their provider.

PROMOTING WELLNESS

As a person ages, it is important to maintain as much independence as possible. Living a healthy lifestyle and ensuring a safe living environment can help to decrease the risk of disease and accidents.

Nutrition

Older adults may face challenges that affect their nutrition, including:

- *Changes in mobility*: Limitations with mobility may make cooking and shopping harder for an older person.
- *Changes in the home life*: The person may now be living alone and cooking for one.
- *Income*: Little money may be left for food after paying bills and purchasing medications.
- *Physical changes*: The sense of smell and taste decrease. The person may have chewing or swallowing issues.
- *Medication side effects*: Dry mouth and a decreased appetite can be side effects of medications.

As a person ages, good nutrition is important. Besides giving a person energy and nutrients, it can also help to prevent certain diseases, such as hypertension, heart disease, and type 2 diabetes mellitus. Strategies to eat healthy include:

- *Eat nutrient dense food.* Choose different types and colors of fruits and vegetables. Eat whole grain foods, such as oatmeal, brown rice, and whole-wheat bread. Eat fat-free or low-fat dairy products that have added vitamin D and calcium. Incorporate fish, lean meats, poultry, eggs, beans, nuts, and seeds into your diet.
- *Avoid empty calories.* Limit foods that contain a lot of calories and only a few nutrients, such as chips, baked goods, candy, soda, and alcohol.
- *Select foods that are low in fat and cholesterol.* Dietary cholesterol is found in animal-based foods, such as egg yolks, meat, shellfish, and cheese. Healthier options included baked and boiled foods, instead of fried foods.
- *Avoid saturated and trans fats.* Saturated fats are found in butter, whole milk, fatty meats, coconut oil, and palm oil. Trans fats are found in foods made with hydrogenated and partially hydrogenated oils, such as margarine and commercially prepared baked goods.
- *Drink enough noncaffeinated liquids.* Some people lose their sense of thirst as they age. Limitations in mobility may also cause older people to limit their fluid intake. Drinking adequate fluids, such as water, will help prevent dehydration.
- *Be physically active.* Exercise will help a person feel hungry.

Dietary counseling and annual dietary screenings should be a part of routine care for aging patients

Adequate Sleep

As individuals age it is common not to sleep as heavily, which reduces the amount of time spent in the deepest stages of sleep. This often increases complaints of sleeping difficulties. Because the quality of sleep declines, the amount of time spent sleeping may be longer than in a younger person. Physical and emotional distress can also cause disturbed sleep that leaves the person feeling tired. Lack of sleep can result in restlessness, disorientation, increased emotional disturbances, and speech problems (including word pronunciation). Things that may interfere with sleep include:

- Medications, caffeine, and alcohol
- Depression and pain
- Environmental or physical changes
- Parkinson disease (because of difficulty changing positions)
- Congestive heart failure (CHF)
- Chronic obstructive pulmonary disease (COPD)
- Diabetes mellitus (which increases nocturia [nok TOO R ee uh])

The symptoms of sleep problems are often confused with dementia. Patients who have dementia symptoms should be asked to track their sleeping patterns. Medications, diet, exercise routines, and a change of lifestyle can also affect sleeping. If sleeping issues are present, medications can be used, but these should be used only in the short term. There is a high risk of drug dependence, especially in the elderly population. Side effects are also often more pronounced in this population, such as next-day drowsiness and temporary memory loss. Simple modifications of behavioral patterns related to sleeping patterns may improve sleep. Examples of modifications that can be tried are:

- Taking fewer naps
- Completing exercise several hours before bedtime
- Changing eating times
- Reducing the amount of alcohol and caffeine ingested
- Changing medications or the time the medications are taken

VOCABULARY

nocturia Frequent urination at night.

decubitus ulcers Sores or ulcers that develop over a bony prominence as the result of ischemia from prolonged pressure; also called *bed sores* or *pressure sores*.

Preventing Falls

Falls cause the greatest number of injuries in people over age 80. Injuries from falls are most commonly fractures of the bones. Serious fractures, such as those of the hip, require the patient to be immobile for extended periods of time, which can increase musculoskeletal issues and also puts the person at risk for decubitus (deh KYOO bih tus) ulcers and pneumonia.

Although the risk for falls and complications is higher in the elderly population, they are still largely preventable (Box 38.5). The medical assistant can play an active role in helping the patient and family members be aware of risk factors and suggest safety measures. Suggestions that can help patients prevent falls are:

- Have regular vision tests.
- Understand the side effects of medications, especially those that cause vertigo and orthostatic hypotension. With orthostatic hypotension, rise slowly and stand still for a moment, with support, before moving.
- Limit the use of alcohol.
- Use assistive devices, such as a cane or walker, for support if needed. The assistive device should be sized appropriate. The person should be taught how to use the assistive device, including doing stairs and switching positions.

BOX 38.5 Suggestions for Helping the Older Adult With Mobility, Dexterity, and Balance

- Encourage the person to use assistive devices, such as adaptive silverware, a tub seat or shower chair, an electric razor, and reaching devices.
- Assist the person with gripping devices as needed (wait for the patient to place their hand around a cup or help them with it before letting go).
- Provide older adults with enough time to complete tasks independently.
- For a post-stroke patient who is ambulatory but has one weak side, use a gait belt when transferring the patient from a chair to an examination table.
- The provider may recommend physical therapy for range-of-motion exercises.
- Encourage activity approved by the provider; lack of activity results in a decline in the ability to function.

- Wear well-fitting low-heeled, rubber-soled shoes with good support.
- Avoid going outside in icy weather.
- Engage in regular weight-bearing exercise for muscle and bone strength.
- Assess the home for possible danger areas: poorly lit areas, throw rugs, torn carpeting or flooring, cords across the walkway, no grab bars in the bathroom and shower, and no handrails on the stairs. Dangerous areas should be fixed. Local emergency numbers should be available.

Living Arrangements

People generally prefer to "age in place." This means that they want to live in their own home environment as long as possible. Most individuals in this age group live close to their children and are in frequent contact with them. Some older adults may live with family members. Typically, yearly screenings are done to ensure older adults feel safe in their homes and are feel from abuse and neglect.

Many resources are available to ensure the elderly have appropriate living arrangements and care.

- Outreach programs, such as Meals on Wheels, deliver nutritious meals to the homes of older adults.
- Senior centers serve as a focal point for many activities and a source of information.
- Transportation services provide rides to providers' appointments, adult day care centers, shopping centers, and community events.
- Adult day care centers provide socialization, recreation, meals, and in some centers physical therapy, occupational therapy, and transportation. These centers offer supervision for older adults who may be taken care of by family members in the evening but need care during the day.
- Home health agencies provide services, including in-home assistance in activities of daily living (ADLs), medication administration, wound care, and speech and occupational therapy services.
- Assisted living facilities, also called *retirement homes* or *board-and-care homes,* are used by seniors who need some assistance with ADLs but are primarily independent.

- Skilled nursing facilities (SNFs) provide 24-hour medical care and supervision. Residents also receive physical therapy, occupational therapy, speech therapy, close nutritional observation, and transportation when needed.
- Many local resources are typically available to help support caregivers.

Vaccinations

Part of the preventive practices for older adults is making sure they are up to date with their vaccinations. It is important to remember that patients may have reasons for refusing vaccines and that is their right. Some insurance providers do not cover all the recommended vaccines for older adults. Patients may request a quote prior to deciding about the vaccines.

Vaccines recommended for older adults include:

- *Influenza vaccine*: An annual flu vaccine is recommended for most adults. The annual influenza vaccine is typically available in early fall.
- *Pneumococcal vaccine*: Recommended that all people over 65 years of age or older receive 1 dose of Pneumovax 23 (PPSV23) to prevent pneumonia. Those that have been previously vaccinated prior to age 65 may qualify for a one-time repeat vaccination if their last vaccine was 5 or more years ago.
- *Zoster vaccine*: Recommended for anyone 60 and older to prevent shingles. Shingrix (RZV) consists of 2 doses, separated by 2 to 6 months regardless of a previous history of varicella or shingles. If patient was previously vaccinated with Zostavax (ZVL), 2 doses of Shingrix is recommended at least 2 months after ZVL.
- *Tetanus and diphtheria*: Given every 10 years; but can be given sooner for wound management.

Additional vaccine series or boosters may be recommended for older adults, such as Hepatitis A and Covid-19.

MEDICAL ASSISTANT'S ROLE IN CARING FOR THE OLDER PATIENT

Elderly patients in the ambulatory care setting present a specific set of needs that require a certain amount of accommodation by the staff. For example, aging patients typically require more time to perform tasks and have questions answered (Procedure 38.1). It is important to provide the time needed to prepare for examinations, ask questions, receive and understand answers, and have procedures explained. A system that is sensitive to the needs of older patients should:

- Schedule longer periods for appointments
- Have adequate lighting in the waiting room
- Provide forms in large print
- Have examination rooms equipped with furniture, magazines, and treatment folders especially designed for older adults

Depression is common in this age group but too often overlooked. The medical assistant may be able to identify risk factors for depression through conversations with the individual and family members. Depression screenings should be done at each

GERIATRIC DEPRESSION SCALE (SHORT FORM)

Choose the best answer for how you have felt over the past week:

1. Are you basically satisfied with your life? YES / **NO**
2. Have you dropped many of your activities and interests? **YES** / NO
3. Do you feel that your life is empty? **YES** / NO
4. Do you often get bored? **YES** / NO
5. Are you in good spirits most of the time? YES / **NO**
6. Are you afraid that something bad is going to happen to you? **YES** / NO
7. Do you feel happy most of the time? YES / **NO**
8. Do you often feel helpless? **YES** / NO
9. Do you prefer to stay at home, rather than going out and doing new things? **YES** / NO
10. Do you feel you have more problems with memory than most? **YES** / NO
11. Do you think it is wonderful to be alive now? YES / **NO**
12. Do you feel pretty worthless the way you are now? **YES** / NO
13. Do you feel full of energy? YES / **NO**
14. Do you feel that your situation is hopeless? **YES** / NO
15. Do you think that most people are better off than you are? **YES** / NO

Answers in **bold** indicate depression. Although differing sensitivities and specificities have been obtained across studies, for clinical purposes a score >5 points is suggestive of depression and should warrant a follow-up interview. Scores >10 are almost always depression.

Fig. 38.2 Geriatric Depression Scale. (From Niedzwiecki B, et al: *Kinn's the medical assistant,* ed 14, St. Louis, 2020, Elsevier.)

appointment to help identify if depression is present. Fig. 38.2 is an example of a common depression screening tool.

As people age, they frequently experience a loss of control over their lives. Part of the medical assistant's job is to help aging people maintain their dignity and independence while in the ambulatory care setting. Remember, each patient, regardless of their education, socioeconomic status, or age, deserves to be treated with compassion and respect. Ask the patient directly what is wrong. Listen carefully and be specific and sincere when responding. When a patient is talking, take time to allow them to complete the sentence; do not finish it for the person. Give the patient your full attention rather than continuing with other tasks while the individual is speaking. Older people may take a little longer to process information, but they are capable of understanding. Do not hurry through explanations or questions; rather, take time to review a form or give instructions as needed.

Effective Communication

Strategies for effective communication with aging patients include:

- Address the patient as Mr., Mrs., or Ms. unless the patient has given you permission to use their first name.
- Introduce yourself and explain the purpose of a procedure before performing the procedure.
- Face the aging person and softly touch the individual to get their attention before beginning to speak.
- Use expanded speech, gestures, demonstrations, or written instructions in block print.
- If the message must be repeated, paraphrase or find other words to say the same thing.
- Observe patients' nonverbal behavior for cues indicating whether they understand.
- Provide adequate lighting without glare.
- Allow patients time to process information and take care of themselves unless they ask for assistance.
- Conduct communication in a quiet room without distractions. Involve family members as needed for continuity of care.
- When leaving a telephone message, remember to speak slowly and clearly and repeat the message in the same manner. It is difficult to interpret a message, and even more difficult to write it down, if the message was delivered in a hurried manner.
- Use referrals and community resources for support.
  - *Alzheimer's Association*: Provides information and support for people with Alzheimer disease and dementia and their families. (https://www.alz.org/)
  - *American Council of the Blind*: Provides referrals to state and other organizations that provide services and equipment for the blind. (https://acb.org/)
  - *American Speech-Language-Hearing Association*: Offers information on hearing aids, hearing loss, and communication problems in older people and provides a list of certified audiologists and speech pathologists. (https://www.asha.org/)
  - *Arthritis Foundation Information Line*: Makes referrals to local chapters and provides information on various types of arthritis. (https://www.arthritis.org/)
  - *American Diabetes Association*: Provides information and support for those with diabetes. (https://www.diabetes.org/)
  - *National Institute on Aging Information Center*: Provides information on aging health issues for patients, families, and healthcare professionals. (https://www.nia.nih.gov/)
  - *National Meals-on-Wheels Foundation*: Provides information on local Meals on Wheels chapters, which deliver nutritious meals to older adults. (https://www.mealsonwheelsamerica.org/)

- *National Hospice and Palliative Care Organization*: A nonprofit organization committed to improving end-of-life care and expanding access to hospice care. (https://www.nhpco.org/)

CRITICAL THINKING 38.5

New staff members in the practice are complaining of having to repeat information to older patients, who, they say, do not pay attention when procedures are explained. Dr. Kennedy has decided to invite a gerontologist from the local university to present an in-service workshop on healthy aging. She asks Bill to coordinate the in-service workshop and prepare materials requested by the guest speaker. What information about caring for the ambulatory aging patient should be included in the workshop?

CLOSING COMMENTS

Elderly patients typically have multiple health problems that are frequently complicated by physical, psychological, and environmental factors. To provide quality care for these individuals, you must look at their health issues in a holistic way, taking into consideration all the factors that affect their ability to follow treatment plans and improve their health status. Part of the process involves identifying resources that might help aging people be better equipped to take care of themselves. Consistently using community and online resources may mean the difference between being able to stay in the home or having to go to long-term care. The professional medical assistant can play a crucial role in providing assistance to aging patients.

PATIENT-CENTERED CARE

The medical assistant must keep in mind the sensorimotor changes that accompany aging and also the importance of respectful patient communication when conducting patient education with older patients. Remember, the aging process does not affect a person's ability to learn; it just may take longer to process the information, and the material may need to be repeated for understanding. Showing sensitivity to the needs of aging learners ensures successful patient education and improves compliance with prescribed treatment plans. The following are general guidelines for effective patient education with older adults:

- The patient may have short-term memory loss, so you may need to repeat the information using different words.
- The patient may be distracted more easily, so learning in a group may be difficult.
- The patient may take longer to process information, so teach at a pace that matches the patient's needs.
- Provide the patient with handouts that have large print and block letters for reviewing information at home.
- Involve family members as needed for continuity of care; supply provider-approved websites for reference.

BEING PROFESSIONAL

Elderly patients often come with unique challenges to the medical assistant. Impaired hearing, eyesight, movement, and other factors can complicate a normal routine. A few things to keep in mind with elderly patients:

- Do not rush. Elderly patients need more time to get around. Do not hurry them, because they can get stressed and become unstable when they are rushed.
- Offer physical assistance. You may offer them a wheelchair, but do not assume that every older patient needs one.
- Use clear communication. Speak to the patient and listen as the patient speaks to you. Do not ignore the patient and speak only to a caregiver.
- Be polite. It is essential that you keep your feelings aside and focus on the patient.

Role-play the following scenario: You are working at WMFM Clinic, and it has been a very busy day. You are a bit behind in getting patients checked in, and you have a large amount of paperwork and a lot of phone calls to return. You feel very stressed and are hoping to move through the next few patient intakes quickly so you can get to your paperwork and phone calls.

Your next patient is Jana Green, an 85-year-old woman who is here to talk to the doctor about her medications. Mrs. Green is here with her daughter. You know from previous appointments that Mrs. Green is very independent and is proud that she can still get around herself and is not dependent on a wheelchair or walker. As you call Mrs. Green back to her appointment, she seems to struggle to get up and walks slowly to the door. As Mrs. Green approaches you, she apologizes for being slow. How can you respond to Mrs. Green in a respectful way? What are the next steps you can take to help ensure a good patient experience for Mrs. Green?

CHAPTER REVIEW

In this chapter we discussed the impact of a growing aging population on society and what that means to the healthcare system. Most older people have at least one chronic medical condition and may have multiple conditions. As healthcare professionals, we need to be aware of the stereotypes and myths associated with aging. To provide respectful care, medical assistants should be educated about the realities of aging and the elderly population.

The changes in the anatomy and physiology caused by aging were discussed. All body systems are affected by the aging process. There are normal changes that occur, but these changes can be intensified by poor health habits. It is important to stress the importance of regular exercise, a healthy diet, and an annual physical examination with health screenings.

Because aging affects the patient's ability to live on their own, the healthcare facility may need to provide living options for its patients. A knowledge of the assisted living and skilled nursing facilities in your area can help you help your patients and their families.

SCENARIO WRAP-UP

Bill has learned to understand the special needs of aging patients. He used to think that most older people were chronically sick and would ultimately end up in long-term care facilities. Now he understands that most aging people lead healthy, active lives and that the disorders that occur in later life usually are the result of lifestyle factors, such as diet and lack of exercise. Bill also has learned how to communicate effectively with older patients and to conduct patient interviews so as to evaluate the patient's physical, mental, emotional, and nutritional health.

PROCEDURE 38.1   Understand the Sensorimotor Changes of Aging

Task

With a partner, role-play an older adult in order to better understand the needs of aging people.

Directions

Work with a peer as you role-play common concerns of older adults. You will be the older person. You will need to complete the "Prepare" step before your peer completes the "Partner's directions."

Equipment and Supplies

- Yellow-tinted glasses, ski goggles, or laboratory goggles
- Pink, white, yellow "pills" (e.g., various colors of Tic Tacs)
- Petroleum jelly (e.g., Vaseline)
- Cotton balls
- Eye patches
- Tape
- Utility gloves
- Tongue depressors
- Elastic bandages
- Medical forms in small size font
- Pennies
- Button shirts
- Walker

Procedural Steps

1. Role-play vision and hearing loss.
   - *Prepare:* Put two cotton balls in each ear and an eye patch over one eye. Follow your partner's instructions.
   - *Partner's instructions:* Stand out of the line of vision (to prevent lip-reading). Without using gestures or changing your voice volume, tell your partner to cross the room and pick up a book.
2. Role-play yellowing of the lens of the eye.
   - *Prepare:* Line up "pills" of different pastel colors. Put on yellow-tinted glasses or goggles. Follow your partner's instructions.

- *Partner's instructions:* Tell the "older adult" to pick up a certain color of pills.
3. Role-play difficulty with focusing.
   - *Prepare:* Put on goggles smeared with petroleum jelly and follow your partner's directions.
   - *Partner's instructions:* Stand at least 3 feet in front of your partner and motion for them to come to you. Your partner is deaf, so talking will not help.
4. Role-play loss of peripheral vision.
   - *Prepare:* Put on goggles with black paper taped to the sides.
   - *Partner:* Stand to the side, out of the field of vision, and motion for your partner to follow you.
5. Role-play aphasia and partial paralysis.
   - *Prepare:* You are unable to use your right arm or leg. Place tape over your mouth.
   - *Partner's instructions:* Stand at least 3 feet away with your back to your partner and wait for instructions.
   - *Task:* The "older adult: needs to let the partner know he or she needs to go to the bathroom.
6. Role-play problems with dexterity.
   - *Prepare:* Put thick gloves on your hands.
   - *Tasks:* Try to sign your name, button a shirt, tie your shoes, and pick up pennies.
7. Role-play problems with mobility.
   - *Prepare:* Use the walker to cross the room.
   - *Partner's instructions:* After your partner starts to use the walker, hand him or her a book to carry.
8. Role-play changes in sensation.
   - Prepare: Put a rubber utility glove on.
   - Tasks: Turn on very warm water. Test the difference in temperature between the gloved hand and the ungloved hand.
9. Summarize and share with the group your impressions of the effects of age-related sensorimotor changes.

39

Surgical Equipment and Supplies

LEARNING OBJECTIVES

1. Describe common features found on instruments.
2. Describe the purpose of each of the five categories of instruments and give examples for each category.
3. Explain the purpose of surgical drapes.
4. Differentiate between the types of wound closures.
5. Describe care and handling of instruments in ambulatory care.
6. Explain how to sanitize instruments.
7. Differentiate between sanitization, disinfection, and sterilization.
8. Describe how to use pouches and autoclave paper.
9. Differentiate between chemical and biological indicators.
10. Explain how load, use, and unload the autoclave.
11. Describe storage and shelf life for sterile supplies.
12. Describe record keeping and quality control for autoclaving.
13. Describe chemical sterilization.
14. Describe surgical solutions and medications used in ambulatory care.

OUTLINE

▷▷ OPENING SCENARIO

Susie Rana, CMA (AAMA), works for the Walden-Martin Family Medical (WMFM) Clinic. Susie was hired to work as an administrative medical assistant at the front desk, but one of the clinical medical assistants unexpectedly quit, and the office manager has offered Susie the position. Susie is excited about this opportunity, especially the chance to work with Dr. Juanita Perez, but she is also concerned about her skill level in sterile procedures. At least she is familiar with a number of the patients, most of the staff, and the types of outpatient surgeries performed in the facility. Before she can assist with surgeries, Susie must demonstrate her knowledge of surgical instruments and how to maintain them.

YOU WILL LEARN

1. To identify common surgical instruments.
2. To describe surgical drapes and wound closures.
3. To properly sanitize instruments.
4. To properly prepare instruments for the autoclave.
5. To correctly handle autoclaved packages.

INTRODUCTION

Over the years advancements in medicine have allowed many procedures to be moved out of the hospitals and into the ambulatory care center. The medical assistant often takes on the role of managing equipment and supplies for these procedures. It is

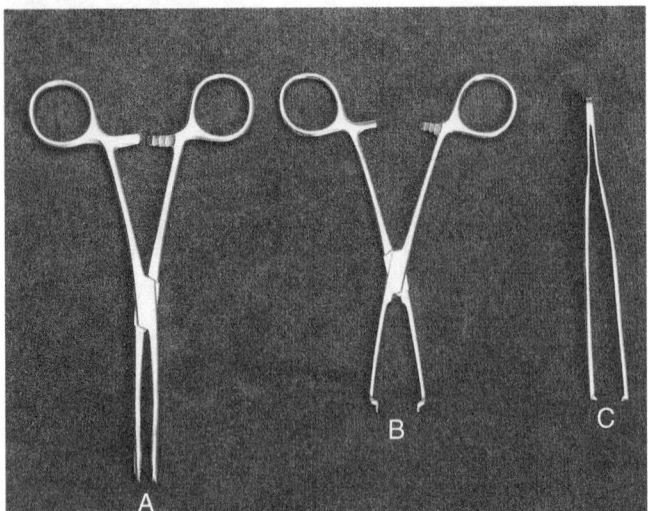

Fig. 39.1 A and B, Ring-handle forceps. C, Spring-handle thumb forceps. (From Niedzwiecki B, et al: *Kinn's the medical assistant,* ed 14, St. Louis, 2020, Elsevier.)

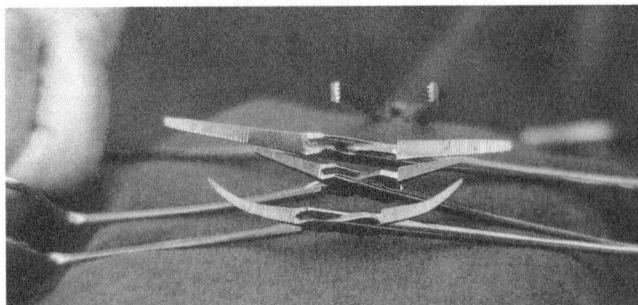

Fig. 39.2 Instruments With Serrations. (From Niedzwiecki B, et al: *Kinn's the medical assistant,* ed 14, St. Louis, 2020, Elsevier.)

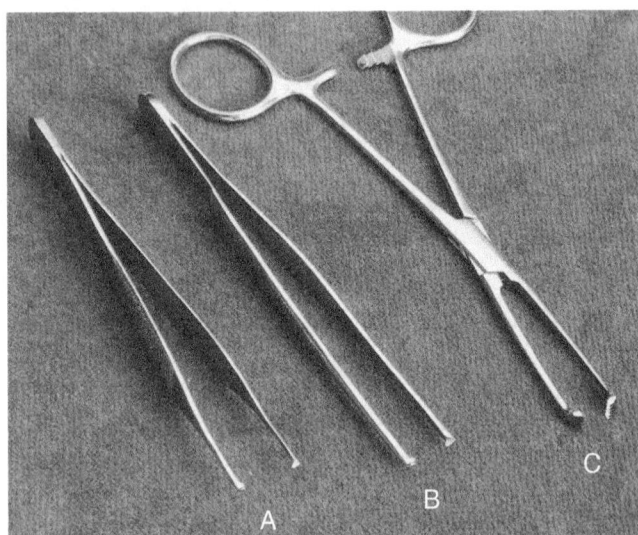

Fig. 39.3 A and B, Toothed jaws. C, Teeth of Allis tissue forceps. (From Niedzwiecki B, et al: *Kinn's the medical assistant,* ed 14, St. Louis, 2020, Elsevier.)

the medical assistant's responsibility to verify that all equipment and supplies are available and properly prepared before the procedure starts. To do this the medical assistant must be familiar with the different types of equipment used, their functions, and how to properly care for them.

Medical equipment used in surgical procedures includes many different instruments. Instrument names can be confusing. An instrument may be named for its use (e.g., splinter forceps for removing splinters); for the person who developed it (e.g., Kelly clamps, named after Howard Kelly); or for the part of the body where it is used (e.g., rectal speculum). It is also common for instruments to have multiple names. Learning the different instruments by identifying characteristics and use can help the medical assistant navigate the confusion associated with instrument names.

SURGICAL INSTRUMENTS

Medical assistants must know which instruments are used for each procedure. They should be able to identify and understand the function of the surgical instruments preferred by the provider. Instruments have clearly identifiable parts and can be visually differentiated from one another. The basic components are the handle, the closing mechanism, and the part that comes in contact with the patient, commonly called the *jaws.*

Instruments have either ring handles (finger rings) (Fig. 39.1 A-B) or spring handles (Fig. 39.1 C); these sometimes are called *thumb-handled* or *thumb grasp* instruments. Scissors are an example of a ring-handled instrument; forceps (tweezers) have spring handles. Some instruments have a hinge-type mechanism called a *box lock.*

Many ring handled instruments have *ratchets* that are located just below or next to the ring handle (see Fig. 39.1 A-B). When one ratchet connects with another ratchet on the instrument, it locks the jaws in place. Thus ratchets are considered a locking mechanism for the jaws of the instrument. Instruments can have different size ratchets, allowing the jaws to remain open in various positions.

The *jaws* (tips) of these instruments may be straight or curved. The type used depends on the procedure and the provider preference. The surface inside the jaws may be smooth, partially serrated,

or fully serrated (Fig. 39.2). *Serrations* are rows of tiny teeth found on the jaws of instruments. The serrations may be crisscross, horizontal, or lengthwise. Serrations on instruments are used to prevent materials or tissues from slipping when they are being held.

The tips of the jaws may be plain or toothed (Fig 39.3 A-C). Tissue forceps usually are toothed instruments and are identified by the number of intermeshing teeth (e.g., 1 × 2, 2 × 3, 3 × 4). Allis forceps (see Fig. 39.3C) are used to grasp delicate, soft tissues, so the teeth are finer, shallower, and more rounded. Other forceps have teeth that are sharper and deeper. Still others have sharp, hooklike, single or double teeth, such as a tenaculum. Toothed instruments commonly have ratchets for locking into towels or human tissues.

Surgical instruments are generally placed into one of five categories according to their use. These categories are:

- Clamping and occluding instruments
- Grasping and holding instruments
- Cutting and dissecting instruments
- Retracting instruments
- Probing and dilating instruments

Clamping and Occluding Instruments

Clamping and occluding instruments are used to apply pressure, occlude vessels, or secure tissue. The jaws may be fully or partly serrated, without teeth. The jaws may be curved or straight. The hemostatic forceps is the most common type of clamping and occluding instruments (Table 39.1).

TABLE 39.1 Clamping and Occluding Instruments

Instrument	Description
Hemostatic forceps A, Kelly hemostatic forceps. B, Mosquito hemostatic forceps. (From Niedzwiecki B, et al: Kinn's *the medical assistant*, ed 14, St. Louis, 2020, Elsevier.)	• Jaws may be fully or partly serrated, without teeth. They may also be curved or straight. • Used to clamp small vessels or hold tissue. • Mosquito forceps (4 inches) are smaller and used for very small vessels. Kelly forceps (6 to 7 inches) are larger. (Needle holder [Fig. C] and smooth-tip needle holder [Fig. D] - see Table 39.2 for more information)

Grasping and Holding Instruments

Grasping and holding instruments are used to grasp tissue and hold it in place. They may also be used to hold materials and other instruments or grasp items during a procedure. Table 39.2 lists common grasping and clamping instruments.

Cutting and Dissecting Instruments

Cutting and dissecting instruments have sharp edges used to **dissect**, incise (cut), scrape, and puncture tissue. The most common cutting instruments are scissors and scalpels. The jaws of scissors can be curved or straight. The tips can be sharp/blunt, blunt/blunt, or sharp/sharp.

Scalpels are unique in that they are generally disposable. The entire instrument may be disposable, or a disposable blade can be attached to a reusable handle. After the procedure, the blade is discarded in a sharps biohazard container, and the handle is sterilized. Handles and blades come in different sizes. The handle and blade used are based on the provider's preference. A number 3 handle is most commonly used in ambulatory care. A number 15 blade is used for short shallow incisions and is most common. Number 10, 11, and 12 blades may be used for specialty incisions. Table 39.3 lists common cutting and dissecting instruments.

VOCABULARY

dissect To cut or separate tissue with a cutting instrument or scissors.

Retracting Instruments

Retracting instruments hold tissue away from the surgical wound (incision). Smaller retractors are more often seen in ambulatory care. The Senn retractor is a popular choice for ambulatory care facilities (Fig. 39.4). The flat end is generally blunt, and the three-pronged end may be sharp or dull. Senn retractors are used to retract small incisions or to secure a skin edge for suturing.

Probing and Dilating Instruments

Probes and dilators are used both for surgery and for examinations. *Probes* are used to explore wounds, search for a foreign body in the wound, and to enter a fistula. *Dilators* are used to stretch a cavity or opening for examination or before insertion of another instrument to obtain a specimen. Table 39.4 lists common probes and dilators found in ambulatory care.

Miscellaneous Instruments

Although most of the instruments used in minor surgeries fit into the previously described categories, there are some common instruments that may not. These instruments include:

- *Biopsy forceps*: Works to both grasp and cut tissue. It is used during minimally invasive endoscopic procedures for collecting the biopsies. The forceps is threaded through the endoscope and is used to collect the tissue.
- *Ear curettes*: Used to remove foreign matter from the ear canal (Table 39.5).

TABLE 39.2   Grasping and Holding Instruments

Instrument	Description	
Needle holder C, Needle holder. D, Smooth-tip needle holder.	• 4 to 7 inches long. • Jaws may be serrated or may have a groove in the center. • Have shorter and stronger than hemostat jaws. • Used to grasp a suture needle firmly.	(See Table 39.1.)
Splinter forceps **Plain thumb (dressing) forceps** Plain thumb (dressing) forceps (Fig. A) Splinter forceps (Fig. B)	• Manufactured in lengths from 4 to 12 inches with serrated jaws (no teeth). • Used to insert packing into or remove objects from deep cavities. • Fine tip for foreign object retrieval.	 A B
Towel forceps A, Small sharp towel forceps. B, Large sharp towel forceps. C, Small atraumatic towel forceps. D, Large atraumatic towel forceps. (From Niedzwiecki B, et al: Kinn's the medical assistant, ed 14, St. Louis, 2020, Elsevier.)	• Various lengths from 3 to 6½ inches. • May have sharp or atraumatic (dull-edged) tips. • Used to hold drapes in place during surgery.	 A B C D
Allis tissue forceps	• Used to grasp tissue, muscle, or skin surrounding a wound.	
Toothed tissue forceps	• Manufactured in 4- to 18-inch lengths with a pincher grip. • Used to grasp tissue, muscle, or skin surrounding a wound.	 A B

TABLE 39.2   Grasping and Holding Instruments—cont'd

Instrument	Description
Foerster sponge forceps	• Straight or curved, with or without serrations. • Used to hold gauze squares to sponge the surgical site and as transfer forceps to arrange items on a sterile tray.
Bozeman sponge forceps	• Designed to hold sponges or dressings. • Used to swab the surgical area or apply medication.
Tenaculum forceps	• Very sharp, pointed tips. • Used to hold tissue (e.g., the cervix) while a tissue specimen is obtained or to lift the cervix so that the fornix can be seen.
Wilde ear forceps (Fig. B)	• Angled, with serrated tips or toothed tips; allows easier access to the ear canal and nasal cavities. • Used for nasal packing, grasping delicate tissue or ear tubes. • Can be used to remove foreign bodies. (Biopsy forceps [Fig. A] and ear curette [Fig. C] - see Table 39.4 for more information)

TABLE 39.3   Cutting and Dissecting Instruments

Instrument	Description
Scalpels Disposable scalpel (see figure) (From Niedzwiecki B, et al: *Kinn's the medical assistant,* ed 14, St. Louis, 2020, Elsevier.)	• May be fully disposable or have a disposable blade with a reusable handle. Available in many sizes and styles. • Safety disposable units, blades, and reusable handles available. • Used to cut and dissect tissue.
Lister bandage scissors (Fig. A)	• Blunt probe tip. • Easily inserted under bandages with relative safety. • Used to remove bandages and dressings.
Operating scissors (Fig. B)	• 5 to 6 inches long. • Curved or straight blade tips. • Used to cut and dissect tissue.
Suture scissors	• Blade has beak or hook to slide under sutures. • Used to remove sutures.
Iris scissor	• Curved or angled blades with sharp/sharp tips. • Used for dissection and precise procedures, such as eye surgery.

TABLE 39.3 Cutting and Dissecting Instruments—cont'd

Instrument	Description	
Uterine curette	• Available in several sizes. • Hollow and spoon shaped; used for scraping. • Used to remove polyps, secretions, and bits of placental tissue.	
Skin Punch or Surgical Punch	• Circular hollow blade attached to a pencil-like handle. • Available as disposable, reusable, and automated instrument. • Used for biopsy procedures.	

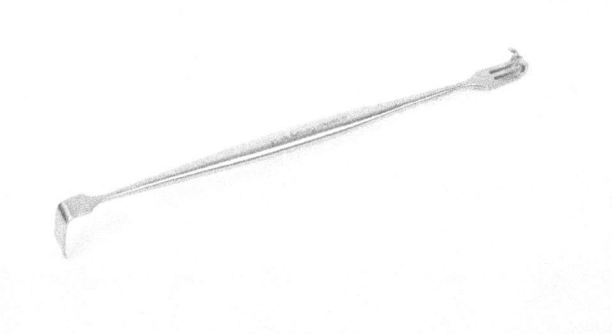

Fig. 39.4 Senn Retractor.

Highly specialized practices may also have additional instrumentation that the medial assistant will need to become familiar with when working in that particular facility.

SURGICAL DRAPES

Surgical drapes are often used in minor surgeries and within a **sterile field**. Surgical drapes come in a large variety of sizes and are generally disposable. They come in two general types:
• *Fenestrated* drapes: Sterile drapes with a hole in the center, which is placed over the operative area. This is used to keep the surgical site clean and provide a sterile field around the area (Fig. 39.5).
• *Nonfenestrated* drapes do not contain a center hole through which to work. These drapes are often used to cover areas not involved in the surgery.

WOUND CLOSURE

After minor surgery or with a laceration repair, the wound is typically closed. The wound edges are well approximated using wound closure materials to hold them in place while the wound heals.

VOCABULARY

laceration A wound caused by the tearing of soft body tissue.
sterile field An area free of microorganisms that is used in a surgical procedure to reduce the risk of infection
well approximated The margins or edges of the wound fit neatly together.

Suture

The word *suture* is used to mean both the surgical material (e.g., thread) used to close a wound and the process of joining two surfaces or edges together along a line by sewing. The primary purpose of a suture is to hold the edges of a wound together until natural healing occurs. Good material for sutures needs to have certain characteristics:
• Easy to handle
• Holds a secure knot
• Nonallergenic, will not cause a localized tissue reaction
• Has adequate strength without cutting through tissue
• Can be sterilized

Sutures come in both natural and synthetic materials. They may break down on their own over time (*absorbable*) or need to be removed (*nonabsorbable*). The provider will request a certain type of suture based on the specific properties of the suture material and the wound needing to be closed.

TABLE 39.4   Probing and Dilating Instruments

Instrument	Description
Probes A, Probe. B, Grooved dilator. C, Lacrimal duct probes.	• Lengths range from 4 to 12 inches; available with or without bulbous tip. • May be smooth or may have a grooved director. • Used to find foreign bodies embedded in dermal tissue or muscle or to trace a wound tract.
Trocars and obturators D, Double-ended cannula. E, Sharp trocar. F, Cannula. G, Blunt-tipped obturator. (From Niedzwiecki B, et al: *Kinn's the medical assistant,* ed 14, St. Louis, 2020, Elsevier.)	• Available in various sizes. • Consist of a sharply pointed stylus (STAHY luh s) (obturator [OB tuh reyt or]) contained in a cannula (KAN yuh luh). • Used to withdraw fluids from cavities or for draining and irrigating with a catheter.
Specula A, Long nasal speculum. B, Short nasal speculum. C, Graves vaginal speculum. D, Anal speculum, self-retaining. (From Niedzwiecki B, et al: *Kinn's the medical assistant,* ed 14, St. Louis, 2020, Elsevier.)	• Most common dilators used. • Valves are spread apart, dilating the opening to open a body orifice or cavity. • Most common of these is the vaginal speculum used during gynecologic examinations. Vaginal specula can be stainless steel (reusable) or plastic (disposable) and can also have a light source for illumination.

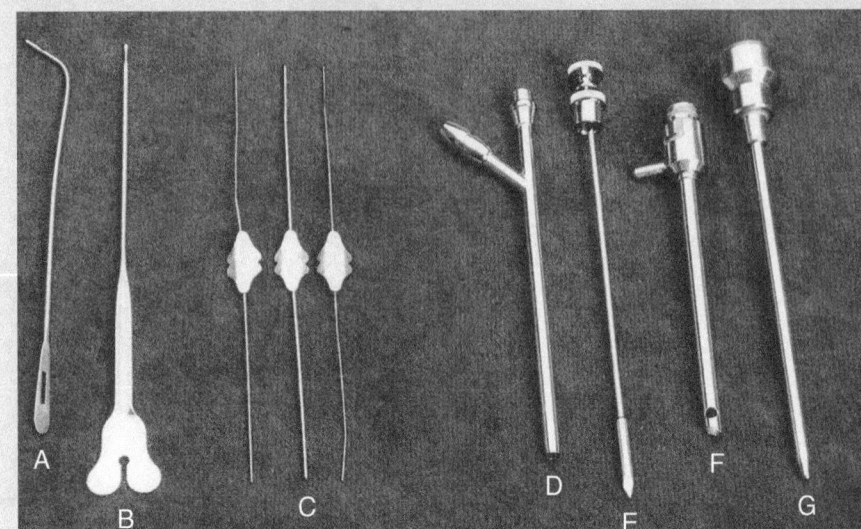

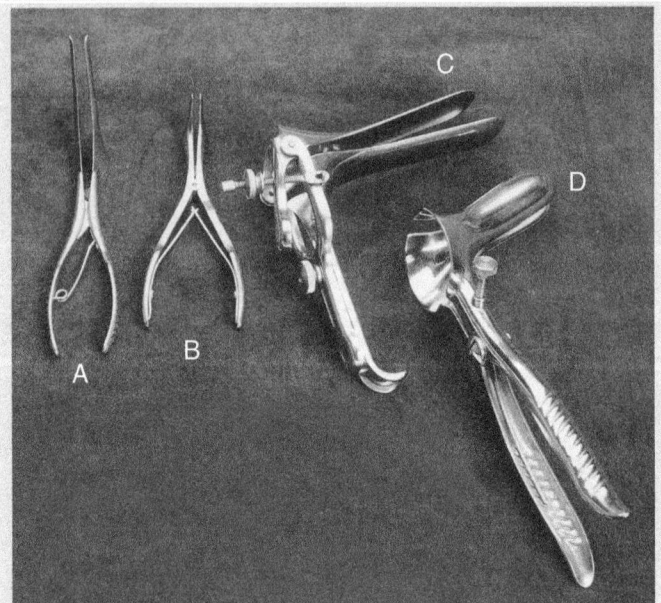

TABLE 39.5   Miscellaneous Instruments

Instrument	Description	
Biopsy forceps	• Available in different lengths and styles. • Inserted with the jaws closed so as not to damage tissue.	(See Table 39.2)
Ear curette	• Manufactured in various sizes, available in standard and disposable models. • Can have a loop or spoon at the end; may be blunt or sharp (to scrape). • Used to remove foreign matter from the ear canals.	(See Table 39.2)

VOCABULARY

cannula A hollow, flexible tube that can be inserted into a vessel, organ, or cavity of the body to withdraw or instill fluid, monitor information, and visualize a vessel or cavity.

obturator A metal rod with a smooth, rounded tip that is placed in hollow instruments to reduce injury to body tissues during insertion.

stylus A metal probe that is inserted into or passed through a catheter, needle, or tube used for clearing purposes or to facilitate passage into a body orifice.

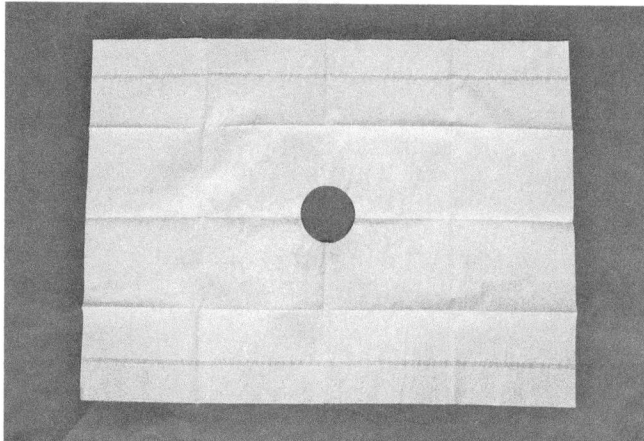

Fig. 39.5 Fenestrated Drape. (From Niedzwiecki B, et al: *Kinn's the medical assistant,* ed 14, St. Louis, 2020, Elsevier.)

Nonabsorbable suture material is used in many minor surgical procedures because wounds tend to be superficial and in places that are not overly difficult to access. Common materials for nonabsorbable sutures include natural suture (silk) and synthetic suture (nylon [Ethilon], polypropylene [Prolene], Novafil, and polyester). Polypropylene suture does not adhere to the tissues, thus pulls out better than other suture. Nonabsorbable sutures are generally left in place until healing has occurred. This can vary based on the location:

- Facial sutures: about 3 to 5 days to minimize scarring
- Scalp and arm sutures: about 7 to 10 days
- Trunk, legs, hands, feet, and joint sutures: about 10 to 14 days
- Palms and soles: about 14 to 21 days

Usually, after 48 hours the sutured area can be cleaned with a mild soap and water.

Absorbable sutures are dissolved by the body's enzymes during the healing process. They are often used when a deep incision or laceration requires multiple layers of sutures to fully close the wound. They are also used if suture removal will be difficult, such as when placing sutures in the mouth. Common absorbable suture materials include natural suture (gut) or synthetic materials such as Vicryl, Monocryl, Dexon, PDS, and Maxon. These materials remain in place (about 2 weeks or more, depending on the material), allowing the wound to heal completely before they are fully absorbed.

Suture material is available in a variety of sizes. The diameter of the suture strand determines its size (Box 39.1). Lengths of the suture material are also listed on the package.

CRITICAL THINKING 39.1

The provider asks for the thinnest suture available. You find the following: 0, 1, 3-0, and 2-0. What do you give the provider? Which would be the thickest suture?

Needles. Suture needles are chosen according the tissue and depth of the wound. Usually surgical needles are made from stainless steel and are either straight or curved. Curved needles are more common and come in a variety of sizes. Curved suture needles allow the provider to penetrate the tissue and come up the other side more easily than do straight needles.

BOX 39.1 Suture Sizes[a]

The size of suture refers to the diameter of the thread. The thicker the diameter, the stronger the suture thread. Suture is typically measured by a USP (U.S. pharmacopoeia) numeric scale. The USP scale runs from 7 (the largest) to 11-0 (the smallest). It is important to remember the more zeros the size has, the finer the thread. The number in front of the hyphen indicates the number of zeros. For instance, 2-0 is 00 and 5-0 is 00000. If these two suture threads were compared, 5-0 would be the thinnest. The following table provides additional information on suture sizes.

Suture Size	Diameter
6-0	0.07 mm
5-0	0.10 mm
4-0	0.15 mm
3-0	0.20 mm
2-0	0.30 mm
0	0.35 mm
1	0.40 mm
2	0.50 mm

[a]Sutures are sized according to the US Pharmacopoeia (USP) scale.

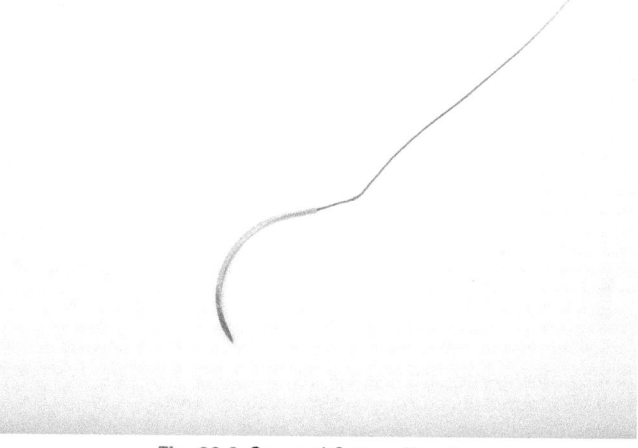

Fig. 39.6 Swaged Suture Needle.

The following are parts of a suture needle.
- *Swaged end*: The section of the suture needle that is fused with the suture thread (Fig. 39.6).
- *Shaft or needle body*: Grasped by the needle holder.
- *Needle point*: Sharpest point that pierces the skin. The most common needle points are:
  - *Cutting needle*: Most common needle body found in ambulatory care. This type has a triangular shape that allows for suturing through the subcutaneous tissue and skin.
  - *Taper-point needle*: Used for easily penetrated, delicate tissues, such as subcutaneous tissue.

The type of suture material, the length of suture material, and the type of needle included are listed on the package (Fig 39.7).

Surgical Staples

Surgical staples are used to close deep incisions or lacerations. This is the quickest way to close a long incision. They are usually made of stainless steel and titanium and are available in different sizes. Absorbable staples are available, but not as common. Staples are straight, curved, or circular. They are used on the legs, arms,

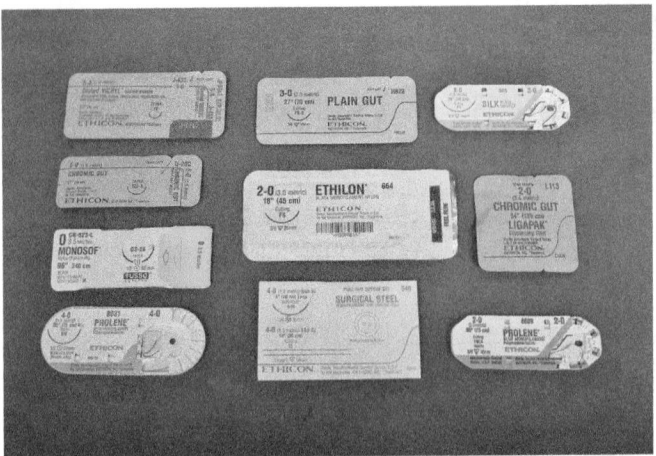

Fig. 39.7 Suture Packets Labeled According to Size, Type, Length, and Type of Needle Point and Shape. (From Niedzwiecki B, et al: *Kinn's the medical assistant,* ed 14, St. Louis, 2020, Elsevier.)

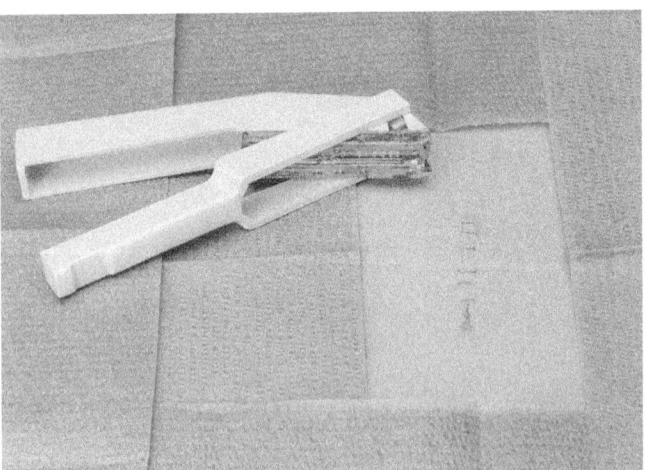

Fig. 39.8 Disposable Skin Stapler. (From Niedzwiecki B, et al: *Kinn's the medical assistant,* ed 14, St. Louis, 2020, Elsevier.)

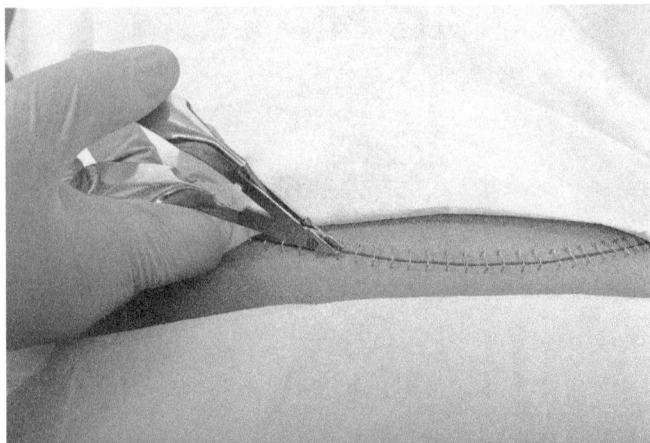

Fig. 39.9 Surgical Staple Remover. (From Niedzwiecki B, et al: *Kinn's the medical assistant,* ed 14, St. Louis, 2020, Elsevier.)

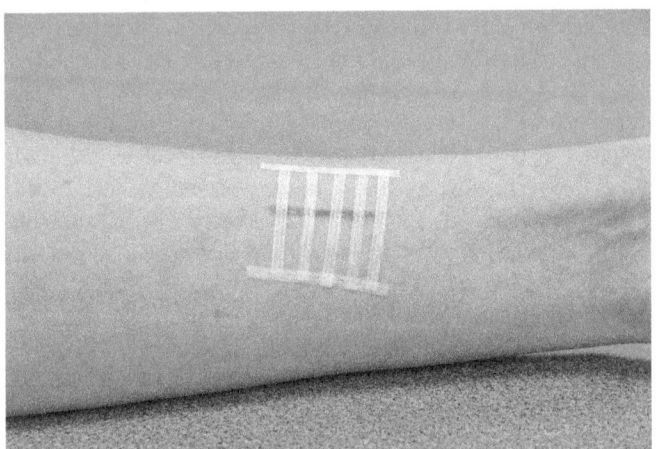

Fig. 39.10 Wound Closed With Steri-Strips. (From Niedzwiecki B, et al: *Kinn's the medical assistant,* ed 14, St. Louis, 2020, Elsevier.)

back, abdomen, and scalp. They are not usually used on the face, feet, or neck. Staples do not allow for precise wound edge alignment; thus they can cause scarring. Surgical staples are applied using a skin stapler and are removed with specific staple instruments, such as a surgical staple remover (Figs. 39.8 and 39.9).

Staples are usually left in for up to 15 days, depending on the location. Usually the stapled area can be cleaned with mild soap and water by 48 hours after the procedure. Often adhesive skin closure strips are applied over the incision when the staples are removed to help with healing.

Adhesive Skin Closure Strips

Adhesive skin closure strips, also called Steri-Strips, are placed over the wound, pulling the edges together (Fig 39.10). Compound benzoin tincture is generally used prior to the application of adhesive skin closure strips to help the strips adhere. It is carefully applied to the edges of the wound. The tincture can cause a burning sensation if it touches the wound. Adhesive skin closure strips are generally used for small, clean lacerations in areas of the body that are protected for significant movement and stress. The patient should be instructed to keep the area clean and dry. The strips will fall off, usually within 2 weeks.

Tissue Adhesive

Tissue adhesive, similar to glue for the skin, can also be used to close superficial wounds. Common examples of tissue adhesives are Histoacryl, Dermabond, and SurgiSeal. Advantages of using a tissue adhesive include:

- No local anesthetic (an uh s THET iks) injections required prior to the wound repair
- Takes less time to place than sutures or Steri-Strips
- Creates a flexible, water-resistant protective bond across the wound edges, allowing normal healing to occur
- Many have antibacterial properties to protect against infection
- Eliminates the need for suture removal and minimizes scarring
- Helpful in patients with a fear of needles

Tissue adhesives are commonly used to close facial lacerations, especially in young children. They are not as strong as sutures and should be avoided in areas that experience a lot of movement and stress.

The patient should keep the adhesive area dry for the first 24 hours. After that the area can be cleaned. The person should not soak the area. Tape should not be placed over the adhesive. Usually adhesives wear off in about 7 to 10 days.

VOCABULARY
anesthetic An agent that causes partial or complete loss of sensation.

Describe patient education for staples, sutures, adhesive skin closure strips, and tissue adhesive.

CARE AND HANDLING OF INSTRUMENTS

Instruments that are not disposable are most commonly made of fine-grade stainless steel. Stainless steel resists rust and keeps fine edges and tips longer. However, even the best stainless steel may develop water spots and stains and become damaged over time. Mistreatment can cause small nicks in the blades and damage to the other parts of the instrument. Care should be taken to avoid dropping instruments, because this can damage them and cause nicks in the blades. It is important that the medical assistant properly care for each instrument to maximize its life and ensure every part is in safe working order. Any damaged or malfunctioning instrument must be discarded to prevent complications during a surgical procedure.

All instruments should be carefully examined when they are purchased and after they are cleaned, before they are sterilized for their next use.

- Scissors should be tested to see whether they cut evenly along the full blade. Do not use the scissor if it does not cut a piece of cloth cleanly.
- Clamps and gripping instruments should be checked to make sure teeth and serrations interlock completely and the jaws are even on the sides and tip.
- Hinges must work freely but should not be too loose.
- Thumb- and spring-handle instruments must have the correct tension and meet evenly at the tips.

Before an instrument or a piece of equipment can be used in a procedure, it must first be sanitized, before it can be disinfected or sterilized. Sanitizing removes the inorganic and organic materials on the instrument or equipment. If these materials were left on the item, it would interfere with the effectiveness of the high-level disinfection or sterilization. It is essential that you understand the concepts of sanitization and disinfection before learning sterilization methods. All three of these procedures are typically done in the utility room, though some facilities may have a special room for sterilization procedures. Written sanitization, disinfection, and sterilization procedures should be in place for each workplace.

> **VOCABULARY**
> **disinfection** The process of killing pathogenic organisms or rendering them inactive.
> **sanitization** The cleansing process that removes organic material and reduces the number of microorganisms to a safe level.
> **sterilization** The process that kills all microorganisms and any spores on surfaces.

Utility Room Setup

To ensure proper sterilization for surgical aseptic procedures, an area or utility room should be set aside for just this purpose. The area should be divided into three sections per the Centers for Disease Control and Prevention (CDC): sanitizing, packaging, and sterilization areas.

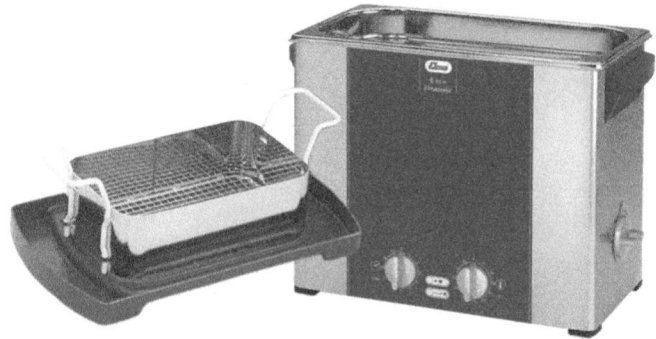

Fig. 39.11 Elmasonic E Ultrasonic Cleaner Unit. (Courtesy Tovatech Elma Ultrasonic, South Orange, NJ.)

In the sanitizing or decontamination area, equipment and instruments are received, sorted, and decontaminated (sanitized). All equipment and instruments must undergo the sanitizing process first before they are either disinfected or sterilized. For the equipment that will be disinfected, a special area is usually reserved for this process. Some solutions require items to soak in the chemical for a period of time to achieve disinfection. Personnel working in the decontamination area should wear household cleaning type rubber or plastic gloves. Face masks, eye protection (goggles or full-length face shields), and appropriate gowns should also be worn. This area should have a sink, receiving basins, proper sanitizing and disinfecting agents, brushes, and the household cleaning gloves.

The packaging area is used for inspecting, assembling, and packaging the clean, dry instruments and equipment. Personnel working in this area should wear disposable gloves, since the equipment has not been disinfected and contains pathogens, such as hepatitis B virus. This area should have autoclave wrapping paper or cloth, tape, sterilizer indicators, autoclave pouches, and gloves.

The sterilization area is used to sterilize instruments and equipment. Personnel working with the hot autoclave should wear heat-resistant autoclave gloves for unloading the autoclave. This area should have clear, clean plastic bags in which to store sterile packs.

Sanitizing Instruments

Chapter 32 discusses sanitizing instruments. The following summarizes the important steps:

- If immediate cleaning is not possible, the instruments should be rinsed well and submersed completely in the solution. Never allow blood or other substances to dry on any instrument because it will be difficult to remove and could damage the instrument.
- To sanitize instruments, rinse first and then place instruments in a basin full of cold water and a mild detergent designed to be used with surgical instruments.
- Heavier instruments should be on the bottom of the basin and lighter, more delicate instruments on the top.
- Always unlock and/or open each instrument before placing it in the solution. This will allow the solution to get to all areas of the instrument.
- After scrubbing instruments, rinse thoroughly, and allow to dry.
- Some delicate instruments, such as microsurgical and lensed instruments, should always be washed by hand. Mechanical washing with an ultrasonic device is best used with sharp instruments to prevent injuries (Fig. 39.11).

STERILIZATION USING AN AUTOCLAVE

In prior chapters, you learned that *asepsis* means free from infection or infectious materials. *Surgical asepsis* is the use of practices to eliminate all microorganisms. These practices or procedures are called sterile technique. *Sterile technique* is a set of specific procedures performed to keep a sterile field, a surgical incision, and any other invasive procedure (e.g., injections) free of microorganisms. (See Chapter 40 for more about sterile technique.) *Sterilization* is a process that kills all microorganisms and any spores on surfaces. All supplies and equipment used in a surgical procedure must be sterilized to maintain surgical asepsis and to prevent wound contamination and infection. Sterilization can be achieved using moist heat, dry heat, ultraviolet or ionizing radiation, gas, or chemicals.

The most common type of sterilization used in the ambulatory care center is steam under pressure in the autoclave (Fig. 39.12). Pressurized steam is fast, convenient, and dependable. The pressure allows for high heat, and when combined with moisture it creates a very effective mechanism for killing all microorganisms. The autoclave holds heat and pressure consistently for long enough to kill all microorganisms and spores on items in the chamber.

Wrapping Instruments

Once an item has completed a sterilization cycle in the autoclave, it is considered **sterile** until it comes into contact with a nonsterile surface. This presents a problem when the item needs to be removed from the autoclave and stored. To maintain the sterility of the equipment, it needs to be carefully wrapped. This way the outside of the wrapper can be handled while the interior is kept sterile.

Autoclave wrapping material must be permeable (PUR mee uh buh l) to allow steam to enter the package and fully sterilize everything in it. It also must be impervious (im PUR vee uh s) to contaminants, preventing pathogens from entering during storage and handling. Because there are such strict requirements for autoclave wrapping, only wrapping specifically designed for use in the autoclave should be used. There are generally two types of autoclave wrapping material used in ambulatory care facilities, peel-apart polypropylene pouches and disposable double-ply autoclave paper.

VOCABULARY

impervious Not permitting penetration.
permeable Allowing penetration.
spore A thick-walled, dormant form of bacteria that is very resistant to disinfection measures.
sterile Free of all microorganisms.

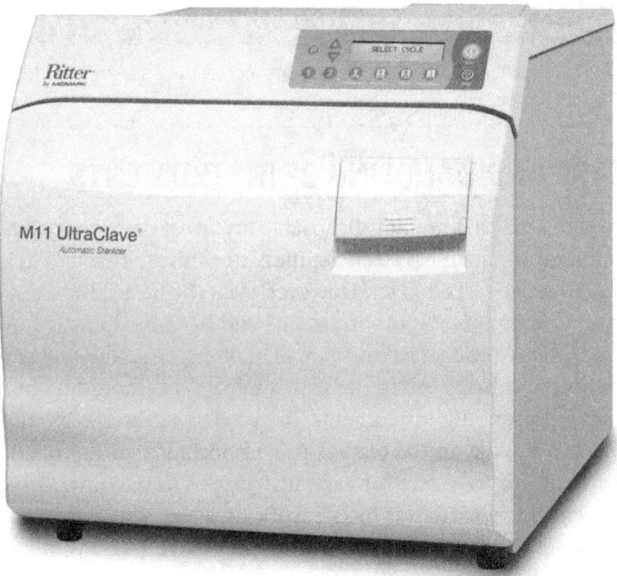

Fig. 39.12 **Steam Autoclave.** (Courtesy Midmark Corp., Dayton, OH.)

Peel-Apart Pouches. The peel-apart polypropylene pouches have a puncture-resistant plastic front sealed to an autoclave paper backing (Fig. 39.13). Hinged instruments should be left open to allow for steam penetration into the hinges and all surfaces (Procedure 39.1). Gauze should be wrapped loosely around any sharp points to prevent them from tearing the paper, which would contaminate the pack. Using a permanent marker, the pouch should be labeled with:

- The contents of the package. Although an instrument can be seen through the puncture-resistant package, details such as size may not be easily visible.
- The date the pouch was sterilized.
- The initials or name of the person who wrapped and sterilized the equipment.

Autoclave Paper. Autoclave paper is often used for large or odd-sized equipment or when several instruments are wrapped together (known as an *autoclave pack*). When you wrap an autoclave pack (Procedure 39.2), it is important to remember these rules:

- Discard autoclave paper that is torn or has holes.
- Be sure the autoclave paper is large enough to cover the items to be sterilized.

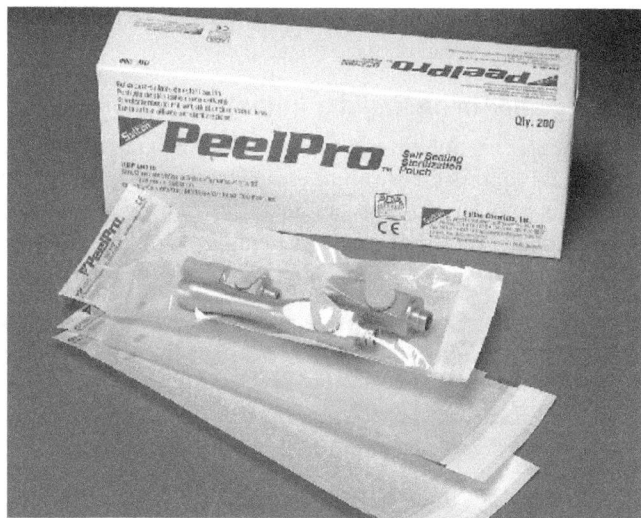

Fig. 39.13 Sterilization Pouches. (Courtesy Practicon, Inc., Greenville, NC.)

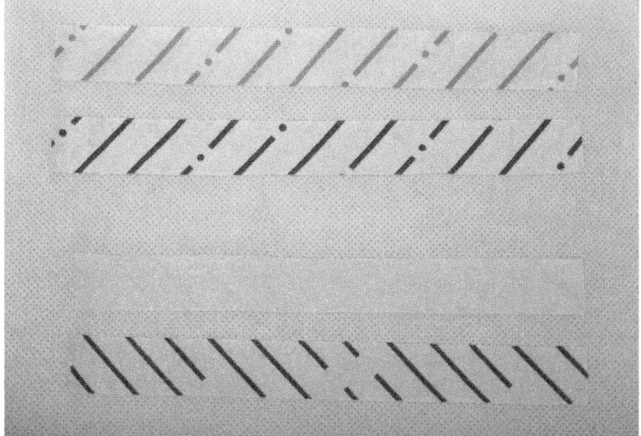

Fig. 39.14 Autoclave Tape.

- Wrap all hinged instruments in the open position to allow full steam penetration of the joint.
- Place a gauze square around the tips of sharp instruments to prevent them from piercing the wrapping material.
- If a stainless steel tray is used to hold instruments in the pack, place a surgical towel double-folded on the tray and then position the instruments. This helps to protect the instruments.
- Seal the pack with autoclave tape (Fig. 39.14).
- Label each pack. Include all instruments in the pack, the sterilization date, and the name or initials of the person who wrapped the pack. Use a permanent marker.

CRITICAL THINKING 39.6

Susie discovers a number of packages of paper-wrapped sterile instruments that appear to have water marks on them, although the packaging is now dry. The indicator tape shows that they have been autoclaved. What should she do with these packs? Why?

Sterilization Indicators. Putting instruments in the autoclave for a cycle does not guarantee sterilization. Sterilization occurs when steam penetrates to the center of the articles with the proper pressure and temperature for the required amount of time. To tell if this occurred and the item is now sterile, an indicator is used. These sterilization indicators must be used routinely to determine if all microorganisms and their spores have been destroyed. There are two basic types of sterilization indicators, chemical and biological. Generally both should be used to be certain sterilization has taken place.

Chemical sterilization indicators contain a special ink that changes colors once critical parameters (e.g., temperature, steam, or exposure time) have been met. Chemical sterilization indicator strips vary. With some, the ink changes colors when a certain temperature, steam quality, and/or exposure time have been reached. Some indicators address all 3 parameters. The medical assistant should know what the indicator looks like when the parameters have been met. Common examples of chemical sterilization indicators include autoclave tape and the printed indicators on autoclave pouches (see Fig. 39.14). Chemical sterilization indicator strips should also be placed in the center of each autoclaved pouch and package. This is to indicate if parameters were met at the center of each pack.

The CDC recommends that *biological sterilization indicators* be used at least once a week to verify the autoclave is working properly and that all requirements are being met for proper sterilization. Some facilities do this more often. Biological indicators may come in strips or in vials. They contain a small sample of bacteria and spores that is generally very resilient, can survive at high temperatures (up to 121°C [250°F]), and grow easily in laboratory conditions. If all the bacteria are killed in the biological indicator, it is determined that sterilization has taken place. The biological indicator should be placed in the center of the largest pack that is routinely sterilized within the autoclave. It is then carefully removed, and the bacteria are cultured to determine if there is growth. It is common for these vials/strips to be sent to the lab to be cultured, but some facilities may do this in house. If these are cultured in house, it is important to note that any growth in 48 hours demonstrates failed sterilization. Results from biological indicator testing must be clearly documented, and any failed tests must be investigated. The causes of the failure must be resolved before the autoclave is used again.

If for any reason the integrity of the sterilization process is in question, the load should be considered contaminated and autoclaved again. Reasons for concern include:
- Any load that fails to convert a chemical sterilization indicator
- Any loads processed after a biological test indicates that the autoclave is not working properly.

The equipment autoclaved with the failed indicator and any subsequent loads before the indicator results are available must be recleaned, repackaged, and reautoclaved.

Loading and Using the Autoclave

When pouches and packs are put in the autoclave, they should be resting on their edges and not be overly crowded (Procedure 39.3). Using stainless steel racks can also help prevent the instruments from being packed too tightly. Some instruments may be autoclaved unwrapped if they do not need to remain sterile for use. For example, although vaginal speculums do not need to be sterilized for use (the vagina is a body cavity that is naturally open to the external environment), they must be sanitized and sterilized to prevent cross-contamination among patients. They can be placed, unwrapped, on a perforated stainless steel tray in the autoclave and then stored in a clean area for future use. It is important not to pack items too tightly in the autoclave chamber. To be effective, the moisture must come in contact with all surfaces being sterilized.

When an autoclave is used, it is important to follow the guidelines and recommendations that come with the particular machine. If the recommendations are not followed, the instruments may not be properly sterilized (Table 39.6). The recommended temperature for sterilization in an autoclave is 121°C to 123°C (250°F to 255°F) with 15 pounds per square inch (psi) pressure. The effective time for sterilization depends on what is being sterilized. In general, unwrapped items are sterilized for 20 minutes; small, wrapped items for 30 minutes; and large items or packages for 40 minutes. To time sterilization it is important to remember that the time does not start until the autoclave reaches full temperature and pressure. Table 39.7 provides tips for improving autoclave effectiveness.

Autoclaves are highly specialized machines and as such require particular care. Every office should have specific protocols to follow for maintenance. Most offices have daily, weekly, monthly, quarterly, and yearly maintenance requirements written into the office policies. Maintenance includes proper cleaning, inspection, quality assurance testing, and regular inspection by a licensed autoclave specialist. When an autoclave is cleaned, only an approved autoclave cleaner should be used. It is also important to use distilled water when cleaning and refilling the

autoclave. Minerals from nondistilled water or chemicals in cleaning solutions can damage the autoclave.

Venting and Unloading the Autoclave

Once the sterilization time has elapsed, the autoclave should be vented. This allows the steam to escape and the instruments to dry. Some autoclaves do this automatically, and some will need to be manually vented. If manually venting is required, wait for

TABLE 39.6 Common Factors Influencing the Effectiveness of Sterilization

Causes	Potential Problem
Improper sanitization of instruments	Protein and salt debris may prevent direct contact with pressurized steam and heat in the autoclave.
Improper packaging	Prevents penetration of the sterilizing agent; packing material may melt.
Wrong packaging material for the method of sterilization Excessive packaging material	Reduces penetration of the steam and heat.
Improper loading of the sterilizer Overloading	Increases heat-up time and reduces penetration of pressurized steam and heat to the center of the sterilizer load.
No separation between packages, even without overloading	May prevent or reduce thorough contact of the sterilizing agent with all the items in the chamber.
Improper timing and temperature Incorrect operation of the sterilizer	Insufficient time at proper temperature to kill organisms.

Adapted from the Centers for Disease Control and Prevention (CDC): Infection Control. https://www.cdc.gov/infectioncontrol/guidelines/disinfection/sterilization/sterilizing-practices.html.

TABLE 39.7 Tips for Improving Autoclave Techniques

Problem	Causes	Correction
Damp autoclave paper	Clogged chamber drain; items removed from chamber too soon after cycle; improper loading	Remove strainer; free openings of lint. Allow items to remain in sterilizer an additional 15 min with door slightly open. Place packs on edge; arrange for least possible resistance to flow of steam and air.
Stained autoclave paper	Dirty chamber	Clean chamber with mild detergent solution; never use strong abrasives, such as steel wool; rinse thoroughly after cleaning.
Corroded instruments	Poor sanitization; residual soil; exposure to hard chemicals (e.g., iodine, salt, and acids); inferior instruments	Improve sanitization process; do not allow soil to dry on instruments – sanitize first. Do not expose instruments to hard chemicals; if exposure occurs, rinse immediately. Use only top-quality instruments.
Spotted or stained instruments	Mineral deposits on instruments; residual detergents from cleaning; mineral deposits from tap water	Wash with soft soap and detergent with good wetting properties. Rinse instruments thoroughly with distilled water.
Instruments with soft hinges or joints	Corrosion or soil in joint; instrument parts out of alignment	Clean with warm, weak acid solutions (e.g., 10% nitric acid solution); rinse thoroughly. Have instrument realigned by qualified instrument repair professional.
Steam leakage	Worn gasket; door closed improperly	Replace gasket; reopen door and shut carefully; have serviced if unable to close door properly.
Chamber door does not open	Vacuum in chamber (check chamber pressure gauge)	Turn on controls to start steam pressure; wait until equalized, then vent and open door.

the pressure gauge to read "0" before attempting to vent the machine. Using heat-resistant gloves, stand back from the door and open the door approximately ¼ inch. A rush of steam may escape; this is considered normal.

The dry time depends on the machine and size of the load – follow the manufacturer's guidelines for dry time. Dry time is usually about 15 to 20 minutes. Do not remove the packs until they are fully dry. Wet packs can act like a sponge, attracting outside moisture and microorganisms. Touching a wet pack allows microorganisms on your hands to penetrate the wrappings, making the contents of the pack nonsterile.

Dry, wrapped packs may be removed with clean, dry hands. However, it is a good idea to wear heat-resistant gloves to reduce the possibility of burns from hot instruments inside the packs. If possible allow the packs to cool in the autoclave with the door open. Do not place the packs on cold surfaces, because hot packs may cause condensation, and moisture will contaminate the contents.

Storage and Shelf Life

All sterile packs and pouches should be handled with care. Avoid crushing, compressing, or puncturing the packs and pouches. Store the sterile packs and pouches in dry, dust-free, covered shelves or in drawers.

The shelf life of sterile packs and pouches can vary by facility. The CDC reports that sterile pouches can keep equipment sterile for up to 9 months. Sterile packs have a shelf life of 30 days. Some facilities have switched from a date shelf life to "event related." With event-related practices, the product should remain sterile until some event causes the item to become contaminated. All sterile packages should be inspected before use to verity the package is not wet, damaged, or torn in any way. Even if a pack has recently been sterilized, it is considered contaminated if the pack becomes torn, wet, dropped on the floor, or damaged in any way. If this happens, the items should be removed from the wrap or pouch, sanitized, disinfected, wrapped in new autoclave paper or placed in new autoclave pouches, and autoclaved again.

Record Keeping and Quality Control

Good record keeping is vital to ensuring that high quality is maintained within a facility. When dealing with sterilization practices, good records show that the equipment is working well and that sterilization is being done properly and consistently. Sterilization documentation should include:

- Records on the purchase date and manufacturer of all sterilization equipment
- Equipment maintenance and cleaning records
- Quality control checks (including results from all biological indicators)
- Sterilization logs

Each time equipment is sterilized, it should documented in a sterilization log. The sterilization log includes the date, temperature, pressure, and time the items in the autoclave were exposed. It should also include the results from visible chemical indicators and be initialed. If any issues occurred, notes should be added to the log indicating what actions were taken to correct the issues. Sterilization logs need to be kept for 3 years unless otherwise indicated by state and federal guidelines or laws.

If there are issues with sterilization, all items must be removed from the packaging and washed, rinsed, dried, and rewrapped. Items cannot be reautoclaved in the same packages. Keeping logs of what is autoclaved each time will help save time identifying equipment when sterilization issues occur.

CHEMICAL STERILIZATION

Some items cannot be exposed to the high temperature and pressure of the autoclave. In these cases a sterilizing chemical solution is commonly used. This is a specialized chemical solution made to destroy all microorganisms and spores. For it to work effectively, it must be used exactly as specified by manufacturer's guidelines. Often these chemicals may need to be mixed, and they have specific requirements for how long they are active before they need to be replaced. When the solution is prepared, it needs to be marked with the date of preparation and the expiration date.

Materials to be sterilized in a chemical solution will need to be submerged in this chemical bath with a closed lid for approximately 8 hours (this may vary, depending on the solution). Items are removed with sterile forceps and must be rinsed with sterile water to remove all traces of the chemical before the items are used on a patient. When you work with sterilization chemicals, it is very important that you wear gloves and make sure all the solution is completely rinsed off the equipment. Sterilization fluid is highly caustic, and it is important that contact with the skin and eyes is avoided. Special airflow and venting may be required. See the chemical's safety data sheet for safety information.

Because it is difficult to keep instruments sterile when removing them from the sterilization liquid and rinsing them, this method is often considered not very practical in the ambulatory care center. In the ambulatory care facility, chemical sterilization fluids are used most commonly with instruments that do not need to be sterile but should be sterilized between patients to avoid cross-contamination. A common example of this is endoscopes.

> **VOCABULARY**
> **caustic** Capable of burning, corroding, or destroying living tissue.

SURGICAL SOLUTIONS AND MEDICATIONS

It is very common for sterile procedures to require the use of medications and other liquid solutions. The medical assistant is often responsible for maintaining up-to-date supplies, preparing the solutions for the sterile field, and using solutions to clean and irrigate as needed.

Sterile water is kept in two forms. Multiple-dose or single-use vials are used as a diluent for medications. Larger containers of sterile water are for rinsing instruments that have been in a chemical disinfectant solution.

Sterile normal saline solution is also stocked in two sizes. The small vial is used for injection (e.g., 0.9% Sodium Chloride Injection USP single-dose vials; Bacteriostatic 0.9% Sodium Chloride Injection USP multiple-dose vials). A larger plastic container of sterile saline (e.g., 0.9% Sodium Chloride Irrigation USP) is used for cleaning, rinsing, and irrigating wounds. Once a sterile solution bottle is opened for a procedure, the remaining solution must be discarded.

Anesthetics

Even minor surgical procedures require the use of anesthetics. *Local anesthetics* produce a temporary numbing at the site by blocking the generation and conduction of nerve impulses. Local anesthetics can be injected locally, sprayed, or applied topically to the site. When injected locally, the provider may give several small injections of the anesthetic around the procedure site. Sometimes, a topical or spray anesthetic will be applied prior to the injections of the local anesthetic. This prevents the patient from feeling the injections. Many different types of local anesthetics are available, but all share the same suffix, -caine. Common anesthetics include lidocaine (Xylocaine), procaine (Novocaine), chloroprocaine (Nesacaine) and bupivacaine (Sensorcaine).

Local injectable anesthetics are commonly purchased in multiple-dose vials of 30 to 50 mL. They are also available in various strengths, such as 0.5%, 1%, and 2%. They begin acting relatively quickly, within 5 to 15 minutes. They last 1 to 3 hours, depending on the type of anesthetic.

When highly vascular areas are involved, local anesthetics containing epinephrine (ep uh NEF rin) may be used. Epinephrine causes vasoconstriction (vey zoh kuh n STRIK shuh n) at the site, which keeps the anesthetic in the tissues longer, prolonging its effect. It also minimizes bleeding. However, epinephrine is not used in areas where decreased circulation may cause problems with healing, including the ears, nose, fingers, toes, and genital areas. In these areas the use of epinephrine can damage the tissues.

Vapocoolant sprays, such as ethyl chloride, lower the tissue temperature in the application area, numbing the pain receptors. In addition, petroleum jelly should be applied to the surrounding areas to protect them from the freezing action of the spray. Because ethyl chloride is highly flammable, it should never be used in the presence of electrical cauterizing equipment.

VOCABULARY

diluent A liquid substance that dilutes or lessens the strength of a solution or mixture; it is added to vials of powdered medications to create a solution of the drug for injection.

vasoconstriction Contraction of the muscles, causing narrowing of the inside tube of the vessel.

Cleaning Solutions

Before surgery, the surgical site must be disinfected with an antiseptic skin cleansing preparation to reduce the number of pathogens. Research indicates that chlorhexidine gluconate products (Hibiclens) and povidone-iodine (Betadine) are safe and effective antiseptics. For some surgical procedures, the patient is instructed to take a Hibiclens shower the morning of the procedure.

The provider's hands and those of the medical assistant should be scrubbed to reduce the chances of wound contamination, even though the hands will be covered by sterile gloves. Surgical scrub preparations should:

- be effective against bacterial spores
- work to reduce transient bacteria
- show evidence of persistent activity on the skin
- work despite the presence of organic matter, such as blood or wound drainage

Other Solutions

When tissue or biopsy specimens are sent to the laboratory for analysis, a 10% formalin solution is typically used to preserve the specimen. When a specimen is obtained, the provider will place it in a container with formalin solution. The medical assistant must label the container with this information:

- Patient's name and date of birth
- Date of collection
- Type of specimen
- Any other information required by the facility or laboratory accepting the specimen

Sometimes the provider may want to use topical silver nitrate ($AgNO_3$) solution or coated applicator sticks. These help to stop localized bleeding. The applicators must be kept in a light-proof container. The applicator sticks are convenient for use in the mouth and nose and are often used for *epistaxis* (ip uh STAK sis) (nosebleed).

CRITICAL THINKING 39.7

Susie is ready to do an inventory of supplies in the minor surgery room. What solutions and medications should she make sure are on hand for the busy surgical schedule planned for next week?

CLOSING COMMENTS

Minor surgeries in the ambulatory care center have become very common in recent years. The medical assistant must be knowledgeable about procedures commonly performed in the facility and the medications and equipment needed. Having a good understanding of the procedures will help the medical assistant know what equipment to have ready before hand.

Preparing equipment means proper maintenance, cleaning, sterilizing, and storage of that equipment. The medial assistant is often responsible for managing equipment and making sure it is available for procedures. Make sure you are aware of sanitization, disinfection, and sterilization processes and machinery. A successful surgery begins with appropriately maintained and sterilized equipment.

PATIENT-CENTERED CARE

A complete understanding of Standard Precautions is important for the medical assistant to maintain a safe patient environment. When you are preparing instruments for minor surgery, pay careful attention to the sterilization of equipment. A few things to keep in mind when using an autoclave to sterilize equipment include:

- Before starting a cycle always check to make sure there is adequate fluid in the machine and there is no visible damage.
- Do not use an autoclave that has failed a biological indicator test. Be sure to always include a chemical indicator strip in every package to be autoclaved.
- Carefully check each item before it is placed in a sterilization pouch or pack. Make sure it is in good working order.
- Wear proper gear when cleaning instruments and when removing them from the autoclave to avoid injury.
- Never remove anything from the autoclave until it is fully dry.

BEING PROFESSIONAL

It is very important to make sure that all sterilization equipment is in good working order. If it is not, every effort should be made to get the problem fixed as quickly as possible. The equipment should not be used until the problem is corrected.

Role-play the following scenario with a peer: You and Sam are responsible for making sure equipment is properly cleaned and sterilized each day and ready for use. After sanitizing, disinfecting, and wrapping instruments for sterilization, Sam finds a small crack in the rubber seal on the autoclave. Sam tells you it should not cause a problem. You believe it could keep the autoclave from properly sealing and getting up to the correct pressure. How would you handle this situation?

CHAPTER REVIEW

In this chapter we began by discussing what is needed to set up for minor surgery. A medical assistant must know the basic instruments that are used for the various procedures that are performed in an ambulatory care facility. You must also know how to handle the instruments after they have been used.

Sanitizing instruments involves washing them with a low-sudsing detergent to remove organic matter and to reduce the number of microorganisms. After the instruments have been sanitized, they must be prepared for the autoclave. They should be wrapped with the appropriate material and then loaded properly into the autoclave. You must be familiar with how the autoclave in your healthcare facility works. It is important to check the sterilization indicators when removing packs from the autoclave. It is also important to perform all quality assurance measures to ensure that the autoclave is functioning properly.

If sterilization of equipment that cannot be autoclaved is needed, chemical sterilization may be used. The chemicals used for sterilization can be very dangerous, and the medical assistant should take special care to prevent them from touching their skin or the patient.

There are many medications and other solutions commonly used in surgery. It is important for the medical assistant to know which of these will be needed and to make sure they are available and have not expired.

SCENARIO WRAP-UP

Susie is enjoying her review of surgical equipment. At first she found that preparing instruments for sterilization – specifically, wrapping those instruments appropriately – was challenging. With some practice she now finds that she enjoys the process and that having a properly assembled, wrapped, and sterilized equipment packet is quite rewarding. She is looking forward to assisting with the procedures and using the equipment she has prepared.

PROCEDURE 39.1 Wrap Instruments Using a Peel-Apart Pouch for Sterilization in an Autoclave

Task
Place dry, inspected, and sanitized instrument(s) inside appropriate peel-apart pouch for sterilization and storage without contamination.

Equipment and Supplies
- Dry, inspected, and sanitized instruments
- Peel-apart autoclave pouch (with internal and external chemical indicators)
- Sterilization strip
- Permanent marker
- Gloves

Procedural Steps
1. Wash or sanitize your hands. Collect supplies and put on gloves. Collect already inspected, sanitized instruments to be placed in the pouch.
   Purpose: Gloves must be worn to prevent the spread of pathogens, since instruments are only sanitized, not disinfected.
   Note: Use an autoclave pouch large enough to accommodate the opened instrument. Make sure to be wearing gloves before touching sanitized instruments.

2. Place the pouch on a clean, flat surface. Using a permanent marker, label the pouch with the date, including the year, contents, and your initials.
   Purpose: Staff members will need to know what is in the pouch, when it was autoclaved, and who performed the task.

3. Open any hinged instruments. If the instrument is sharp, its teeth or tip should be shielded with cotton or gauze.
   Purpose: To prevent puncture of the package or injury to the operator.

4. Open the pouch on the unsealed side, by the adhesive strip. Place the handle of the instrument in the pouch first. If the instrument is hinged, ensure it remains opened.
   Purpose: When the autoclaved pouch is opened, the handle should be the first part of the instrument removed from the pouch.

5. Remove the paper on the adhesive strip. Fold the flap on the perforation line. Seal the adhesive to the plastic by pressing firmly with your fingers.
   Purpose: If a flap is folded at an angle, not using the perforation line, it may not seal. This would allow bacteria to enter the pouch.

6. Inspect the pouch to ensure it is adequately sealed.
   Purpose: Inadequately sealed pouches are considered unsterile.

PROCEDURE 39.2   Wrap Instruments and Supplies for Sterilization in an Autoclave

Task
Place dry, inspected, and sanitized supplies and instruments inside appropriate wrapping materials for sterilization and storage without contamination.

Equipment and Supplies
- Dry, inspected, and sanitized instruments
- Double-ply autoclave paper
- Autoclave tape
- Sterilization strip
- Permanent marker
- Gloves

Procedural Steps
1. Wash or sanitize your hands. Collect supplies and put on gloves. Collect already inspected, sanitized instruments or equipment to be wrapped.
   Purpose: Gloves must be worn to prevent the spread of pathogens, since instruments and equipment are only sanitized, not disinfected.
   Note: Make sure to be wearing gloves before touching sanitized instruments and equipment.
2. Place the double-ply autoclave paper on a clean, flat surface.
3. Place the instruments diagonally at the approximate center of the double-ply autoclave paper. Make sure the size of the square is large enough for the items (see Fig. 1).
   Purpose: Each of the four corners must fold over and completely cover the instruments, with a few extra inches of overlap for folding.

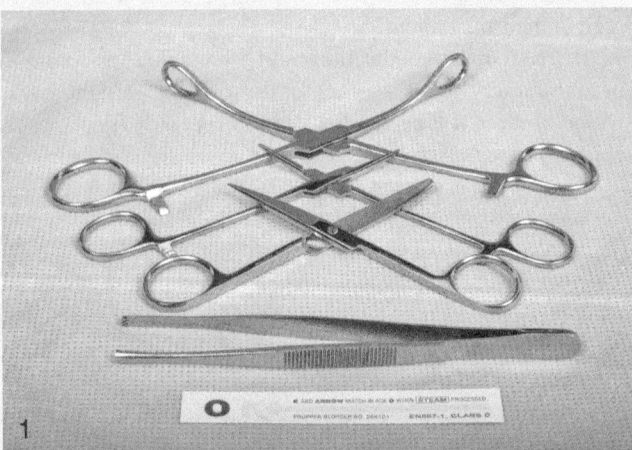

4. Open any hinged instruments. If the instrument is sharp, its teeth or tip should be shielded with cotton or gauze.
   Purpose: To prevent puncture of the package or injury to the operator.
5. Place a sterilization strip in the center of the pack to check for sterilization standards.
   Purpose: To ensure that the autoclave is reaching effective levels of heat and pressure to destroy all microorganisms.
6. Bring up the bottom corner of the wrap and fold back a portion of it.
   Purpose: This folded-back flap is the only part of each wrapper corner that can be touched when a sterile package is opened (see Fig. 2).

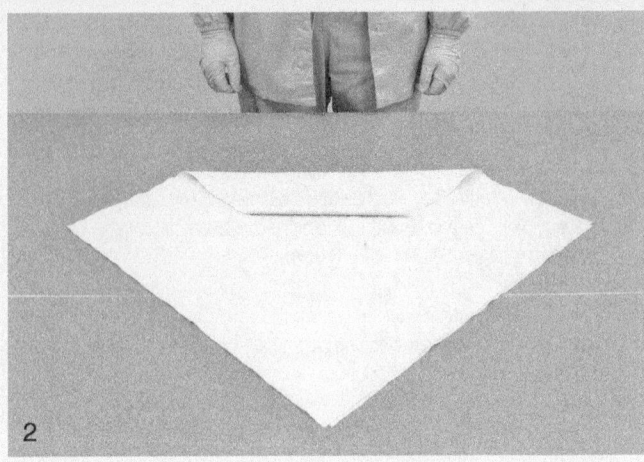

7. Repeat the previous step with each corner, making sure to turn back a portion each time (see Figs. 3 and 4).

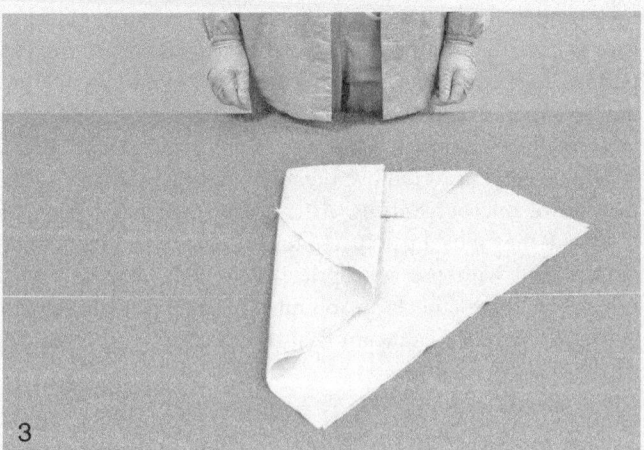

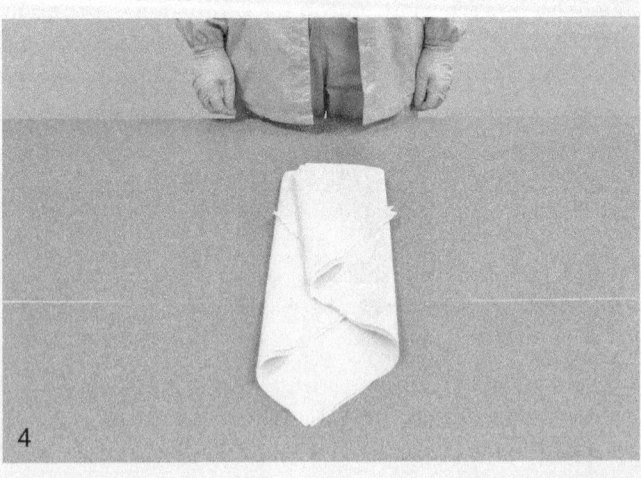

PROCEDURE 39.2 Wrap Instruments and Supplies for Sterilization in an Autoclave—cont'd

8. Fold the last flap over (see Fig. 5).

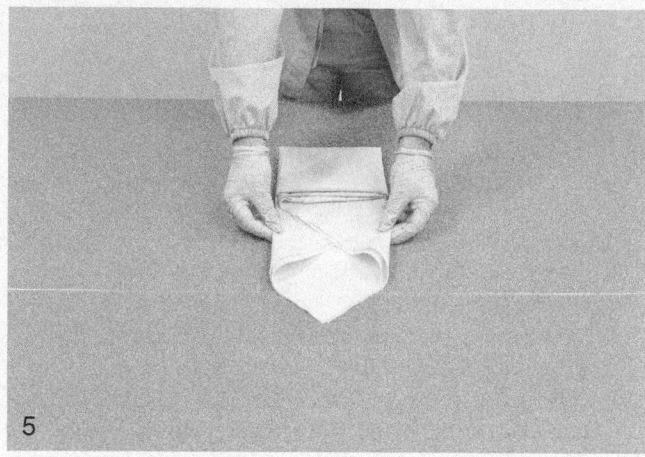

5

Purpose: Staff members will need to know what is in the pack, when it was autoclaved, and who performed the task.

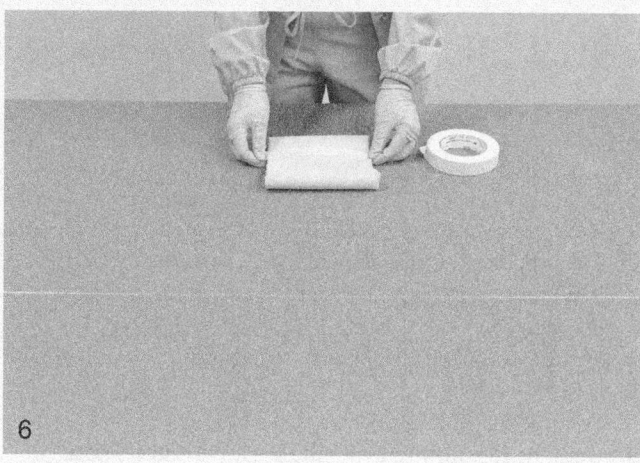

6

9. Secure with autoclave tape (see Fig. 6) and label the package with the date, including the year, contents, and your initials.

PROCEDURE 39.3 Operate the Autoclave

Task
Sterilize properly prepared supplies and instruments using the autoclave.

Equipment and Supplies
- Autoclave
- Wrapped items ready to be sterilized
- Heat-resistant gloves

Procedural Steps
Note: The specific instructions for operating an autoclave may vary based on the model number and manufacturer. Refer to the instructions that accompany the autoclave to be sure the appropriate steps are followed.
1. Check the water level in the reservoir and add distilled water as necessary.
   Purpose: Too much or too little water may alter the effectiveness of the equipment. Tap water leaves lime deposits in the chamber.
2. Turn the control to "Fill" to allow water to flow into the chamber. The water flows until you turn the control to its next position. Do not let the water overflow.
3. Load the chamber with wrapped items, spacing them for maximum circulation and penetration.
   Purpose: To ensure sterilization of all items.
4. Close and seal the door.
   Purpose: The door must be closed, or the heated water in the chamber evaporates.

5. Turn the control setting to "On" or "Autoclave" to start the cycle.
6. Watch the gauges until the temperature gauge reaches at least 121°C (250°F) and the pressure gauge reaches 15 pounds of pressure.
   Purpose: The proper temperature and pressure must be reached before sterilization can begin.
7. Set the timer for the desired time.
8. At the end of the timed cycle, turn the control setting to "Vent."
   Purpose: This releases the steam and pressure. The water at the bottom of the chamber drains back into the reservoir. Newer autoclaves automatically perform this step.
9. Wait for the pressure gauge to reach zero.
10. Standing behind the autoclave door, carefully open the chamber door.
    Purpose: To allow steam to escape faster. Be careful to prevent accidental burns.
11. Leave the autoclave control at "Vent" to continue releasing heat.
    Purpose: To dry the items faster.
12. Allow complete drying of all articles.
13. Using heat-resistant gloves, remove the items from the chamber and place the sterilized packages on dry, covered shelves or open the autoclave door and allow the items to cool completely before removal and storage.
14. Turn the control knob to "Off" and keep the door slightly ajar.
    Purpose: To allow the inside of the autoclave to dry completely.

40

Surgical and Special Procedures

LEARNING OBJECTIVES

1. Differentiate between medical asepsis and surgical asepsis.
2. Describe the medical assistant's role in minor surgery, including preparing the patient, positioning, and skin preparation.
3. Demonstrate a surgical hand scrub and how to prepare the skin for surgery.
4. Discuss the principles of sterile technique.
5. Demonstrate how to apply sterile gloves and set up a sterile field.
6. Describe how to prepare for common surgical procedures, including biopsies, cyst removal, incision and drainage, ingrown toenail removal, and laceration repair.
7. Demonstrate how to assist with minor surgery.
8. Describe the medical assistant's postoperative responsibilities.
9. Demonstrate the application of adhesive skin closure strips and the removal of sutures and staples.
10. Differentiate between types of bandages, dressings, and tape.
11. Demonstrate changing a dressing, obtaining a wound culture, and applying tubular and elastic bandages.
12. Describe special procedures, including electrosurgery, cryosurgery, laser surgery, microsurgery, endoscopic procedures, and therapeutic injections and joint aspirations.
13. Demonstrate inserting and removing straight and indwelling Foley catheters.

OUTLINE

▶ OPENING SCENARIO

Susie Rana, CMA (AAMA), works for Walden-Martin Family Medical (WMFM) Center. Susie was recently asked if she would train to assist with outpatient surgeries in the facility. Susie is able to identify different surgical equipment and knows how to sterilize and handle the equipment. She now must demonstrate that she is able to set up a sterile field without contaminating the field. She also must show she can perform wound care skills, including applying a sterile dressing and changing bandages.

YOU WILL LEARN

1. To describe the medical assistant's role with minor surgery.
2. To describe principles of sterile technique.
3. To apply sterile gloves and set up a sterile field.
4. To list unsterile and sterile equipment and supplies used for common surgical procedures.
5. To assist with minor surgery, including passing instruments to the provider.
6. To perform wound care by obtaining a culture and applying dressings and bandages.

7. To describe the different phases of wound healing.
8. To explain special procedures done in the ambulatory care facility.
9. To insert a straight catheter and an indwelling Foley catheter using sterile technique.

INTRODUCTION

Medical assistants are often asked to assist with minor surgical procedures in the ambulatory care facility. This chapter will focus on preparing for and assisting with minor surgery and special procedures. The role of medical assistants in minor surgery includes:

- Preparing the patient and the sterile field
- Assisting the provider as needed
- Taking care of the patient after the procedure
- Documenting appropriately
- Preparing any specimens for transport to the lab

Careful attention must be paid when you are assisting with or participating in any surgical procedure. Surgical procedures increase the risk of infection to the patient. To minimize this risk, it is important that all individuals involved be clearly aware of their role and avoid any "breaks" in technique. In a sterile field, infection control is essential.

MINOR SURGERY ROOM

The room set aside for minor surgeries in an ambulatory care facility is often called the *procedure room*. This room should be near a workroom with a sink and an autoclave (often referred to as the *utility room*). The procedure room should have a sink and cabinets to hold surgical supplies, wound care equipment, medications, and biopsy containers. Countertops serve as a side or back table during the procedures. It is important that procedure rooms be set up in a way that makes it easy to disinfect the area. Countertops and other areas within the room should remain uncluttered to allow for easy access to the patient and necessary supplies.

The procedure room should have bright lighting, vital signs equipment, and a portable instrument stand (Mayo stand) (Fig. 40.1). Often procedure rooms have special examination tables that are more adjustable than those found in general examination rooms.

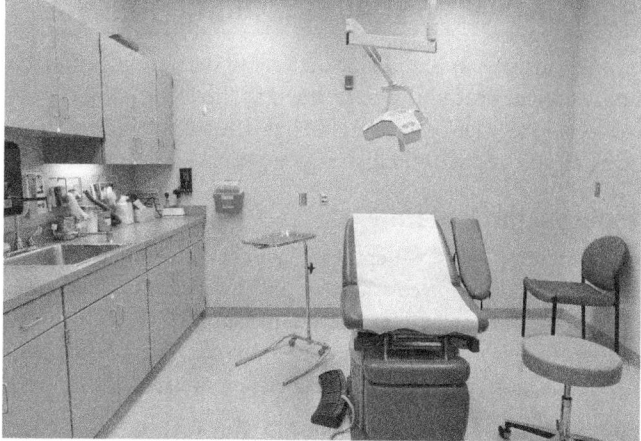

Fig. 40.1 Typical Surgical Procedure Room in an Ambulatory Care Setting. (From Niedzwiecki B, et al: *Kinn's the medical assistant,* ed 14, St. Louis, 2020, Elsevier.)

SURGICAL ASEPSIS

Asepsis (ey SEP sis) was discussed in Chapter 32. It is important to use medical asepsis to ensure that the examination room is free of pathogenic organisms and safe for patients. Medical asepsis will help prevent spreading infection from patients to other patients and staff members.

Surgical asepsis should be used with any procedure that invades the body's tissues. Anytime the skin or a mucous membrane is punctured or pierced, as with minor surgery, surgical aseptic must be practiced. With surgical asepsis everything that comes in contact with the surgical site must be sterile, including surgical gowns, drapes, instruments, and the gloved hands of the provider and assistants. Biopsies, cyst removals, dressing changes to open wounds, and urinary catheterizations are performed using sterile technique.

As with medical asepsis, surgical asepsis begins with a hand wash. A surgical hand wash is different from a medical aseptic hand wash because it is designed to remove transient microbes and reduce resident flora from the forearms, hands, and fingernails (Procedure 40.1). Surgical asepsis directly affects the health and well-being of the patient and the healthcare professionals and must be practiced without fail.

CRITICAL THINKING 40.1

During orientation, Susie notices that many procedure room cabinets are kept locked. When she asks about this, she is told it is to keep patients and their family members out of them. The cabinets contain expensive and dangerous supplies and equipment, such as sharp instruments, needles, and medications. Susie knows that patients are often asked to wait in the procedure room until the provider is available for their surgery. As part of her orientation Susie is shown where extra keys are kept. She is told to take a set when assisting in the procedure room so she can access the supplies in the cupboards. Susie wonders if locking the cabinets may cause a problem if equipment is needed during a procedure. She also does not think that patients are likely to get into the supplies. Do you feel that locking the cabinets is a good practice? Why or why not?

VOCABULARY

asepsis The condition of being free of infection or infectious material.
biopsy Process of viewing living tissue that has been removed for the purpose of diagnosis or treatment.
medical asepsis The use of practices to reduce disease-causing organisms; also considered the clean technique.
sterile Free of all microorganisms.
sterile field An area free of microorganisms that is used in a surgical procedure to reduce the risk of infection.
sterile technique A set of specific procedures performed to keep a sterile field, a surgical incision, and any other invasive procedure (e.g., injections) free of microorganisms.
surgical asepsis The use of practices to eliminate all microorganisms.

ASSISTING WITH SURGICAL PROCEDURES

The medical assistant should have a clear understanding of all the minor surgical procedures performed in the facility. This information is used when preparing the patient, assisting before and during the procedure, and instructing patients on wound care.

Preparing the Patient

Prior to minor surgery, patients can have concerns and fears about the pain, disfigurement, cost, and the possible diagnosis (in the case of a biopsy). The medical assistant must be sensitive to a patient's concerns and fears and address questions asked by the patient. The medical assistants can answer general questions within their scope of practice and the facility's policies. Other questions must be referred to the provider. The medical assistant must reassure the patient that any questions will be answered prior to the surgery.

If the procedure is scheduled in advance, the medical assistant should call the patient the day before the procedure. The medical assistant should answer the patient's questions and review any specific preoperative instructions. These instructions may include information such as shaving, cleansing enemas, food intake restrictions, special bathing, and/or administration of a sedative medication. The patient may be required to have a driver after surgery. The medical assistant should encourage the patient to leave jewelry and other valuables at home.

When the patient arrives for the procedure, typically the process is the same as with other patients. The patient's vital signs and medical history are obtained. The medication and allergy lists are reviewed and updated as needed. In addition, the medical assistant should:.

- Have the patient use the restroom. Collect a urine specimen if required.
- Have any ordered blood tests done.
- Check that the preoperative home preparation and dietary restrictions were completed.
- Ensure the patient has completed the necessary informed consent form(s) (Box 40.1),

CRITICAL THINKING 40.2

Susie is preparing a patient for a biopsy of a suspected cancer of the skin. The consent form has been signed and is in the health record. While Susie is chatting with the patient during completion of the final setup for the procedure, it becomes clear the patient thinks she is having a "skin tag" removed from her back. What action should Susie take, if any? What is the significance of what the patient said in this situation?

Positioning. The medical assistant must instruct the patient to change into a gown, if required for the procedure. The surgical site needs to be completely exposed to avoid accidental contamination during the procedure. Tight clothing may act as a tourniquet. Clothing may be stained during the procedure. Use standard precautions if assisting a patient with an opened wound.

Once the patient is ready for the procedure, the medical assistant should help the patient get comfortable on the exam table. Being uncomfortable can lead to the patient moving during the procedure, which can be problematic. The patient's position will depend on the procedure being done.

BOX 40.1   Informed Consent

The provider must have the patient's written informed consent before beginning any surgical procedure. An informed consent is unique in that it must be obtained by the provider. Although a medical assistant may explain the procedure and answer the patient's questions, the provider must take time to sit with the patient and obtain the informed consent. Without an informed consent signed by both the provider and the patient it is not legal to perform a surgical procedure. (See Chapter 18 for more information on informed consents.)

CRITICAL THINKING 40.3

You are helping prepare a female patient for a cyst removal from her right forearm. She is wearing a long-sleeved shirt that is quite tight. You tell her she will need to remove the shirt for the procedure, but she does not feel it is necessary. She states that she can fold the shirt up above the cyst, and even though it is tight, she is fine with that. What would you say to explain to the patient why it is necessary to remove the clothing?

Skin Preparation. It is not possible to sterilize the skin without damaging skin cells and tissues. The goal of adequate skin preparation for a surgical procedure is to reduce the number of transient flora and limit harmful organisms at the incision site. Skin prep includes cleansing the patient skin before surgery with surgical soap and antiseptic and shaving the area if needed (Procedure 40.2).

Patients may be instructed to cleanse the surgical site at home the morning of the surgical procedure. Chlorhexidine solution or wipes can be used for this type of preparation. In the ambulatory care facility, iodine, alcohol, or chlorhexidine-based solutions are used to prepare the site. Disposable skin prep trays and electric razors should be available.

Preparing the Room

If you assist with a minor surgical procedure, you need to know the provider's preferences for instruments, supplies, and wound care. All procedures require medical asepsis and many also require surgical asepsis. Procedures requiring surgical asepsis will include a sterile field for sterile items and a nonsterile area for other supplies and equipment. The following section discusses the principles of sterile technique and setting up and maintaining a sterile tray.

CRITICAL THINKING 40.4

Why is it necessary to consider individual provider preferences when setting up a room for a surgical procedure?

Sterile Technique With Sterile Fields. Sterile technique must be followed to keep the sterile field sterile. The principles of sterile technique include:

1. A Mayo stand or table covered with a sterile drapes is sterile only at waist level. The drape below the surface of the table or tray is not considered sterile. The edges of the table serve as the line between the sterile and nonsterile

area. Anything that falls below the edge of the table is considered nonsterile.

2. If a sterile field does not cover the entire Mayo stand or table, a 1-inch margin around the field is considered unsterile.

3. Only sterile items can be placed on a sterile field.
   - Before opening supplies, the medical assistant should check the package to ensure the integrity. Do not use supplies if they appeared crushed or the outer wrapper is soiled, ripped, wet, or if sterilization indicators have not changed colors. Check the expiration date. Do not use if expired. Any supplies that fall onto the floor should not be used.
   - If a nonsterile item is placed on the field, the field must be discarded and another one set up.

4. When opening sterile packages, such as peel packs and supply packets, the glued edges are not sterile. The inner edge of the glued area is the line between the sterile and nonsterile area. The sterile field and sterile item should not touch the unsterile edge nor the outer unsterile surface of the sterile package.

5. The inside of a sterile package remains sterile if the package is peeled open properly. It should be opened the entire way, and the contents then tossed onto the field without the person crossing over the sterile area. A two-person transfer can be used. One person opens the sterile supplies. The other person, who is wearing sterile gloves, removes the contents from the package and places them on the sterile tray.

6. Pour only sterile solutions into sterile bowls. The unused portion should be discarded after the procedure. If the solution is kept for a future procedure, the sterility of the liquid cannot be guaranteed and will jeopardize the sterility of the procedure.

7. Consider a sterile field contaminated if it has been wet, cut, or torn.

8. Sterile supplies are opened just before the procedure.

9. Sterile supplies and sterile fields must always be in view. They are considered contaminated if you turn your back to them or they are left unattended.

10. Unsterile items should never cross over the sterile field.

11. Do not touch or reach over a sterile field or sterile item if you are not sterile (wearing sterile gloves or gown).

12. Keep sterile gloved hands above waist level at all times; do not let hands drop below the waist. If the hands fall below the waist, they are considered contaminated, and handwashing/gloving should be repeated.

13. If using a sterile gown, the gown is considered sterile in the front, from the axilla to the waist. The cuffs are considered unsterile and need to be covered with sterile gloves. Then the sleeves are considered sterile from the cuffs to 2 inches above the elbows. All other areas are considered unsterile.

14. Do not cough or talk over or near a sterile field. Air currents carry bacteria and viruses.

Constant attentiveness and absolute honesty are essential for maintaining sterile techniques. Any break in sterile technique could lead to serious wound contamination, which can lead to infection and other serious complications. To maintain sterile technique, it helps to keep in mind: *Everything sterile is white and everything that is not sterile is black – there is no grey!* If you are in doubt about the sterility of anything, consider it contaminated.

Sterile surfaces must *never* come in contact with nonsterile surfaces. If this occurs, the sterile surface is immediately considered contaminated, or nonsterile. This is considered a *break* in sterility. During any procedures needing sterile technique, a *break* in the sterile field will require everything to stop so that the problem can be corrected immediately. This often means that the medical assistant must discard the sterile tray and reset it up.

Hair and contaminated sterile gloves are two of the greatest sources of contamination with a sterile field. Hair that falls freely over the shoulders gives off a cloud of bacteria with every movement. It must always be secured back and up, not touching the shoulders.

Procedure 40.3 describes applying sterile gloves. A medical assistant must be diligent when applying sterile gloves and using sterile gloves. As mentioned in the prior section, gloves must remain above the waist and in view. Remember to only touch sterile items. If gloves become contaminated, they need to be replaced.

CRITICAL THINKING 40.5

After completing a surgical scrub before a minor surgical procedure, Susie remembers that she forgot to lay out the practitioner's sterile glove package. She opens up the storage cabinet and quickly adds this to the collection of sterile supplies. The sterile drape, gauze, and instruments are unopened and on the counter. Can she put on her sterile gloves? Why or why not?

Creating a Sterile Field. A sterile field is any sterile surface on which sterile items are placed. In the ambulatory facility it is common for the sterile field to be set up on a Mayo stand (Fig. 40.2). The sterile field is created by draping sterile towels (either disposable or from autoclaved packs) over a Mayo stand or table (Procedures 40.4 and Procedure 40.5). Sutures, scalpels, and other instruments needed are added to the field. The surgical site on the patient's skin is prepared and then draped with sterile towels or a fenestrated drape, thus creating a sterile field. A sterile field can also be created by opening up a sterile pack. For instance, when opening a sterile glove pack, the paper that surrounds the gloves is a sterile field. For some procedures, the sterile field surrounding a sterile supply or instrument may be used.

VOCABULARY

fenestrated drape A surgical drape with an opening in the center. The size of the opening depends on the size of the surgical field.

Preparing for Specific Surgical Procedures. The procedures seen in the ambulatory care facility will vary by the facility. The specific supplies used for the procedures will also vary and are determined by the provider performing the procedure.

Biopsies. Several types of biopsies are done in the ambulatory care facility, including:

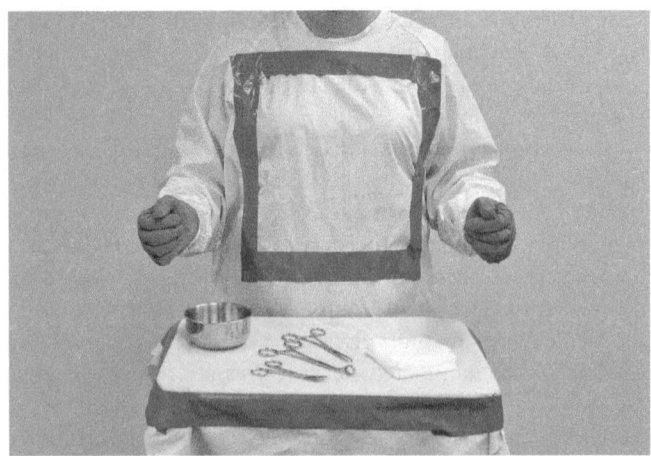

Fig. 40.2 Sterile Field *(red outline)*.

- *Needle biopsy*: A needle is used to remove fluid or tissue. With a *core needle biopsy*, a wide gauge needle is used to remove a tissue specimen. With a *fine-needle aspiration (FNA) biopsy*, a fine gauge needle is used to remove a fluid specimen. Computerized tomography (CT) or an ultrasound may be used during the biopsy to locate the area of concern. Needle biopsies using local anesthesia can be done in the ambulatory care setting, while biopsies requiring sedation or full anesthesia are done in a surgical center.
- *Punch biopsy*: A surgical punch (a circular hollow blade attached to a pencil-like handle) is used to remove a small round piece of tissue. A punch biopsy is used to obtain a specimen for skin, vulvar, and cervical cancers.
- *Shave biopsy*: A small blade is used to remove a skin abnormality and a small layer of surrounding skin.

The medical assistant must prepare a nonsterile area and a sterile area for a biopsy procedure. The following items should be included unless otherwise indicated by the provider:

- *Nonsterile area*: Gauze soaked with povidone-iodine solution (skin prep), sterile gloves for the provider, anesthetic medication vial, alcohol pads, Monsel's solution (optional), dressing material (antibiotic ointment, bandage, nonstick bandage, tape), and gloves. For specimen collection, a labeled specimen container (with preservative [10% formalin solution] or normal saline if required), specimen bag for transport, and a laboratory requisition form is needed.
- *Sterile area*: 10 mL syringe and safety needle, stack of sterile 4 × 4 gauze, sterile cotton-tipped swabs (optional), and fenestrated drape. For needle biopsy: needle and syringe. For punch biopsy: surgical punch, operating scissor, and needle holder and suture (optional). For shave biopsy: disposable scalpel and tissue forceps.

Cyst Removal. A sebaceous (epidermoid) cyst is a noncancerous cyst of the sebaceous gland. When the gland becomes blocked, sebum (oily secretion) builds up, creating the cyst. These cysts can occur anywhere on the body except on the palms of the hand and soles of the feet. The cyst is attached to the skin and moves freely over the underlying tissue. To remove the cyst, the provider dissects around it and usually tries to remove the entire cyst from the wound intact. The contents of the cyst are drained first, and it may spray when the incision is

made. Wearing the appropriate personal protective equipment (e.g., face shield) is important.

The medical assistant must prepare a nonsterile area and a sterile area for a cyst removal procedure. The following items should be included unless otherwise indicated by the provider:

- *Nonsterile area*: Gauze soaked with povidone-iodine solution (skin prep), sterile gloves for the provider, anesthetic medication vial, alcohol pads, dressing material (antibiotic ointment, bandage, nonstick bandage, tape), and gloves. For specimen collection, a labeled specimen container (with preservative [10% formalin solution] or normal saline if required), specimen bag for transport, and a laboratory requisition form is needed.
- *Sterile area*: 10 mL syringe and safety needle, stack of sterile 4 × 4 gauze, fenestrated drape, mosquito forceps, dressing forceps, operating or Iris scissor, disposable scalpel, tissue forceps or tooth forceps. If suturing will be required, suture, a needle holder, and scissor should be included.

Incision and Drainage. Incision and drainage (I&D) is a minor surgical procedure used to treat abscesses. Local anesthesia is used to numb the area and an incision is made in the abscess, which helps to drain the fluid and pus. The contents of the abscess may spray when the incision is made. Wearing the appropriate personal protective equipment (e.g., face shield) is important.

The medical assistant must prepare a nonsterile area and a sterile area for an I & D procedure. The following items should be included unless otherwise indicated by the provider:

- *Nonsterile area*: Gauze soaked with povidone-iodine solution (skin prep), sterile gloves for the provider, anesthetic medication vial, alcohol pads, dressing material (antibiotic ointment, bandage, nonstick bandage, tape), and gloves. For specimen collection, a labeled culture swab, specimen bag for transport, and a laboratory requisition form is needed.
- *Sterile area*: 10 mL syringe and safety needle, stack of sterile 4 × 4 gauze, fenestrated drape, mosquito forceps, dressing forceps, operating scissor, disposable scalpel, tissue forceps or tooth forceps, and irrigation fluid and supplies. If suturing will be required, suture, a needle holder, and scissor should be included.

Some providers may pack the wound, which needs to be changed every day.

Ingrown Toenail Removal. An ingrown toenail occurs when the edge of the nail grows into the skin of the toe. It commonly occurs with the great (large) toe. Ingrown toenails can occur from poorly fitting shoes, foot or toe deformities, untrimmed toenails, and toenails trimmed too short or cut with rounded edges. The skin near the toenail edge becomes red, infected, and painful. In moderate to severe cases, part or all of the nail must be removed (nail avulsion).

The medical assistant must prepare a nonsterile area and a sterile area for a nail avulsion procedure. The following items should be included unless otherwise indicated by the provider:

- *Nonsterile area*: Gauze soaked with povidone-iodine solution (skin prep), sterile gloves for the provider, anesthetic medication vial, alcohol pads, bandage scissors, Monsel's solution (optional), dressing material (antibiotic ointment, bandage, nonstick bandage, tape), and gloves

- *Sterile area*: 10 mL syringe and safety needle, stack of sterile 4 × 4 gauze, fenestrated drape, iris scissor, 2 straight hemostats, sterile rubber band (optional), nail splitter (optional), and sterile cotton-tipped swabs (optional)

Usually, the patient is in a supine position and the knee is flexed so the foot is flat on the table. After the wound is dressed, the patient should receive verbal and written home care instructions, which may include:

- Nail will regrow back in 2 to 4 months.
- Keep the wound dry for 24 hours. Then wound can be cleaned with soap and water. Do not scrub wound.
- Keep wound moist with an antibiotic ointment and cover with a non-stick bandage.

Laceration Repair. Depending on the type of wound, the provider may decide to close the wound up to 18 hours after the injury (Fig. 40.3, Box 40.2). Wound irrigation may be done to help remove debris and bacteria before the wound is closed. Even though lacerations are considered contaminated, surgical asepsis is used during the repair procedure. Depending on the type of injury and the patient's last tetanus booster, an updated booster may be given.

The medical assistant must prepare a nonsterile area and a sterile area for a laceration repair. The following items should be included unless otherwise indicated by the provider:

- *Nonsterile area*: Gauze soaked with povidone-iodine solution (skin prep), sterile gloves for the provider, anesthetic medication vial, alcohol pads, dressing material (antibiotic ointment, bandage, nonstick bandage, tape), and gloves.
- *Sterile area:* 10 mL syringe and safety needle, stack of sterile 4 × 4 gauze, fenestrated drape, needle holder, suture, tissue or toothed forceps, scissor, and irrigation fluid and supplies.

Assisting the Provider During Surgery

The provider ultimately is responsible for the patient. The medical assistant is responsible for ensuring that everything the assistant and the provider will use in caring for the surgical patient is accounted for, ready for use, and prepared in a safe and sterile manner. Every team has preferences about the sequence it follows during routine minor surgery. Once a routine has been established, it should be followed in every case.

Passing Instruments. The medical assistant is often responsible for handing sterile instruments to the provider during the procedure. This requires the medical assistant to be wearing

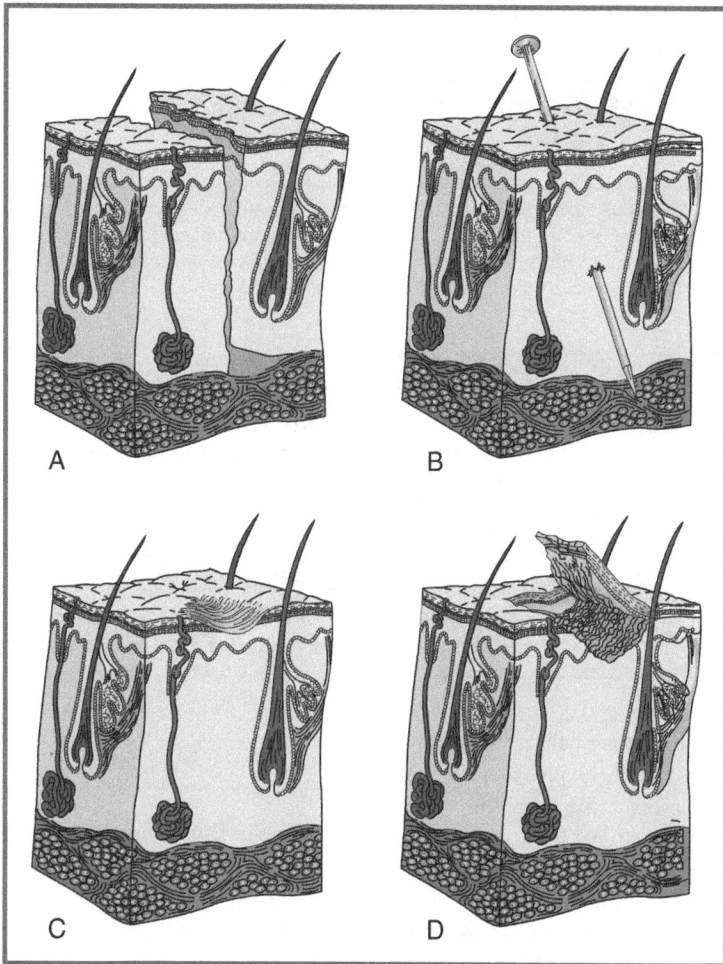

Fig. 40.3 Types of Wounds. A, Laceration – a jagged, irregular breaking or tearing of tissues, usually caused by blunt trauma. B, Puncture – piercing of the skin by a pointed object, such as a pin, nail, splinter, or bullet. C, Abrasion – a superficial wound made by scraping of the skin. D, Avulsion – tissue forcibly torn or separated, caused by accidents.

Continued

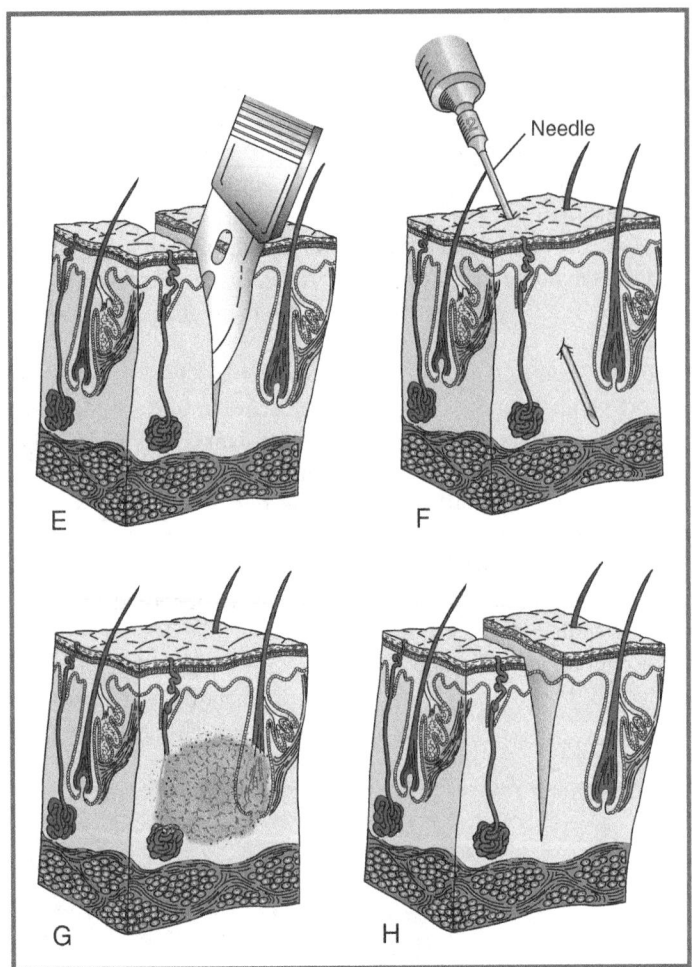

Fig. 40.3, cont'd E, Surgical incision – a neat, clean cut. F, Hypodermic puncture – an injection under the skin. G, Contusion – a closed, nonpenetrating wound in which blood from broken vessels accumulates in tissues. H, Incision – a neat, clean cut from sharp objects, such as glass, knives, or metal. (From Niedzwiecki B, et al: *Kinn's the medical assistant*, ed 14, St. Louis, 2020, Elsevier.)

BOX 40.2 Types of Wounds

A wound can be intentional (such as a surgical incision) or accidental, and it may be open or closed. An *open wound* has an outward opening, and the skin is broken, exposing underlying tissues. Open wounds may be classified according to the appearance of their openings (see Fig. 40.3). A *closed* (or non-penetrating) *wound* does not have an outward opening, but the underlying tissues are damaged, as in a hematoma, contusion, or bruise. Closed wounds usually are the result of some type of blunt trauma to the body. A clean or aseptic wound is not infected with pathogens, but septic wounds are infected.

sterile gloves. As teams work together, they will begin to anticipate needs. Instrumentation is logical; if the provider requests the needle holder and suture, scissors must be readily available because it likely will be needed next. To limit unnecessary speaking, the provider may use hand signals to let the medical assistant know which instrument is needed.

While gaining experience the medical assistant watches, listens, and learns to judge what will be needed or performed next. Pass instruments with a firm, purposeful motion so that the provider does not have to look up. Wait until you feel the

provider grasp the instrument so that it does not drop onto the patient or the floor. Be especially careful with instruments with sharp edges and work to protect the patient, provider, and yourself from injury. Procedure 40.6 describes how to pass instruments to the provider.

CRITICAL THINKING 40.6

While Susie is assisting in a nonsterile procedure, she passes an instrument to the provider. Susie feels the instrument cut through her glove. She quickly and secretly looks at it and notices a "very tiny" nick in her glove. Because this is a nonsterile procedure, she decides to say nothing and continues assisting with the procedure. Is her reasoning sound here? What is the best approach to handling this situation? Why?

Specimen Collection. If a specimen is collected during a procedure, it is placed in a sterile specimen cup or basin. Do not remove the specimen from the sterile field until the procedure is completed or the provider has asked you to do so. The provider may want to examine the specimen again during the procedure. After the procedure is complete, place the specimen in an appropriate container. The specimen container should be

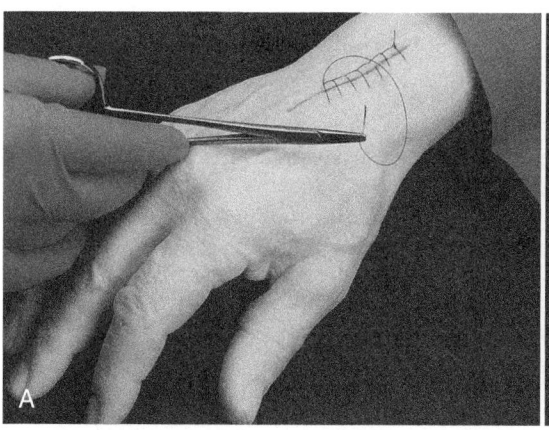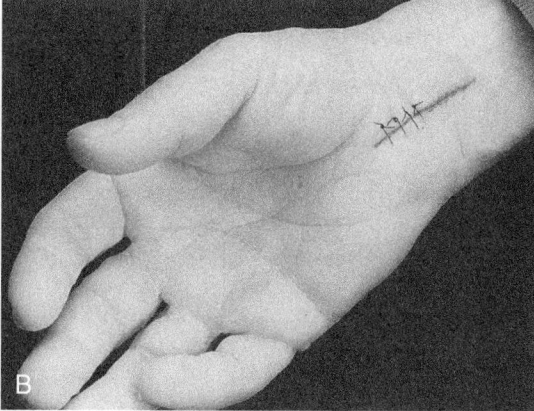

Fig. 40.4 A, Continuous (i.e., running) suture placement. B, Interrupted suture placement. (From Niedzwiecki B, et al: *Kinn's the medical assistant,* ed 14, St. Louis, 2020, Elsevier.)

labeled with the patient name, patient number, date, time, and biopsy location before it is sent to the laboratory for analysis. The specimen container may be placed in a specimen bag for transport to the laboratory. A laboratory requisition form typically accompanies the specimen container.

Wound Closure. As the procedure is completed, it may be necessary to close the wound. Whatever method is chosen, the edges of the wound should be well approximated (uh PROK suh meyt d) but not so tightly closed that blood circulation is cut off to any of the tissue. This is generally done with tissue adhesive, adhesive skin closure strips, staples, or sutures (Procedure 40.7).

The most common wound closure is sutures. Sutures hold the wound better than tissue adhesive or Steri-Strips and scar less than staples. Usually, the provider will use either a running stitch or an interrupted stitch (Fig. 40.4).

VOCABULARY

well approximated The margins or edges of the wound fit neatly together.

CRITICAL THINKING 40.7

A common saying among providers when doing sutures is to "approximate not strangulate." What do you think this means? Why would this be important to remember when closing a wound?

Postoperative Responsibilities. When the wound is closed, the medical assistant may be asked to clean the area and bandage the wound. Sterile normal saline may be poured over the wound area to cleanse it (known as a *wound lavage*), or the area is cleansed with an antiseptic and blotted dry using sterile dry sponges. Care must be taken not to disturb the wound edges or sutures. Next, a sterile dressing is placed over the incision, and a bandage is applied to support the dressing. The medical assistant may also be required to change this dressing during the patient's follow-up visits.

The patient should be given time to rest after surgery. If a sedative was administered, make sure the patient has recovered sufficiently to avoid injury during the trip home. If the patient

was given a topical or local anesthetic, explain that the anesthesia effect will wear off and that some discomfort may be felt at the operative site. Check with the provider about instructions for managing pain. If medication is prescribed or over-the-counter medication is recommended, review the purpose of the medication and the directions for use with patients and their companion.

Remember that postoperative care extends for the total recovery period and not just for the time of the surgery and immediately thereafter. Medical assistants are often responsible for teaching patients to care for themselves after surgery. A postoperative patient may have trouble comprehending or remembering instructions, because of this all instructions should be given both verbally and in writing. They should be simple to understand by the patient. Preprinted instruction forms for specific surgeries or a general form with checked boxes for particular postoperative instructions can be given to inform anyone assisting the patient at home (Fig. 40.5).

Explain to patients the importance of calling the provider if they have any questions or concerns. Tell patients to call immediately if they notice any increasing redness, bleeding from the surgical wound, fever, swelling, or increasing or severe pain, because these may be signs of an infection. Make sure there is a follow-up appointment scheduled before the patient leaves the facility. Never allow the patient to leave the facility without the provider's knowledge and approval. It is important to call patients in about 24 hours to see how they are doing. Often patients ignore problems or feel uncomfortable calling because they do not want to be a nuisance.

After caring for the patient, the medical assistant should clear the sterile field, following Standard Precautions. Wear gloves while cleaning up the contaminated equipment and supplies. All sharps (e.g., needles and blades) should be the first items removed from the sterile field. Place sharps in the biohazardous sharps container. Place contaminated disposable supplies in the biohazardous waste container. Wrappings and other noncontaminated disposable supplies should be placed in the waste container. Move nondisposable supplies to a clean basin to be removed for sanitizing, disinfection, and sterilization for future use. Any blood spills or other contaminated areas need to be cleaned up appropriately. Disinfect all surfaces in the room, including the exam table, Mayo stand, counters, and tables. After everything is cleaned, remove your gloves and wash your hands.

POSTOP INSTRUCTIONS FOR _____

☐ Elevate your arm.
☐ Elevate your leg.
☐ Limit food intake to _____.
☐ Limit activity to _____.
☐ Do not bathe or shower.
☐ Sponge bath only.
☐ Change dressing as instructed.
☐ Call the office for fever, redness, pain, swelling, or bleeding.
☐ Take_____ every 4 hours as needed for pain.
☐ Return to school/work in _____days.
☐ Call the office tomorrow before _____p.m.
☐ Your next appointment is on M T W Th F S_____ at _____ .

Fig. 40.5 An Example of Preprinted Postoperative Patient Instructions. (From Niedzwiecki B, et al: *Kinn's the medical assistant*, ed 14, St. Louis, 2020, Elsevier.)

TABLE 40.1	**Phases of Wound Healing**
Healing Phase	**Description**
Hemostasis (hee muh STEY sis) *phase*	Blood vessels contract to slow bleeding. Blood platelets form a network that acts as a glue to plug the wound. After a cascade of chemical reactions, fibrin is released into the wound and clotting begins. Fibrin continues to collect red blood cells and the clot dries into a scab.
Inflammatory phase	Macrophage clear away bacteria and dead tissue. Within 1 to 4 days the fibrin threads contract and pull the edges of the wound together under the scab. During this phase, edema, *erythema* (redness), heat, and pain can occur.
Proliferation phase	Lasts 5 to 20 days. As new tissue of collagen and extracellular matrix form, the wound contracts and seals. A new network of blood vessels must occur.
Remodeling or Maturation phase	Starts around day 21 and may last for a year or more. The wound fully closes. The collagen fibers lie closer together, creating stronger tissue and reducing the scar thickness.

FOLLOW-UP CARE

Depending on the type of wound or surgical procedure, patients may return to the ambulatory care facility for follow-up care. The patient may need the wound closures to be removed or for a dressing to be changed. If the wound looks infected, the provider may also order for a wound culture.

When providing wound care, the medical assistant must be familiar with the phases of wound healing (Table 40.1). Being young, in good health, and having adequate nutrition can help promote healing. Adequate protection and rest of the injured area also enhance the healing process. Additional reinjury to the area can delay healing and increase scarring. Wounds are susceptible to infection because the normal skin barrier is broken. Any necrotic tissue present in the wound can increase the risk of bacterial growth. If necrotic tissue is present, the provider may perform wound debridement. Should the medical assistant have questions on the appearance of the wound or if the wound looks infected, the be notified.

Some wounds fail to show signs of healing in 30 days. These wounds are called *chronic wounds*. Pressure, trauma, bacterial infection, poor circulation, smoking, poor nutrition, and inappropriate treatments can lead to chronic wounds. Patients should be coached to:

- Wash hands prior to changing dressings.
- Keep the dressing clean and dry; minimize pressure on the wound.
- Focus on eating a healthy diet.

Chronic wounds are treated with antibiotics, compression stockings and bandages, and hyperbaric oxygen therapy.

VOCABULARY

debridement The surgical removal of dead, damaged, or infected tissue to improve the function of healthy tissue.

exudate Fluids with high concentrations of protein and cellular debris that have escaped from the blood vessels and have been deposited in tissues or on tissue surfaces.

hemostasis The stoppage of bleeding.

hyperbaric oxygen therapy Treatment in which a patient is placed in a sealed chamber and breathes oxygen at higher-than-atmospheric pressure. The high-pressure oxygen can stop bacteria growth and increase the blood oxygen concentration, which can help with the healing process.

Wound Closure

Nonabsorbable sutures and staples will be removed at the follow-up appointment. It is often the responsibility of the medical assistant to remove the sutures or staples (Procedures 40.8 and Procedures 40.9). Before removing sutures or staples, the medical assistant should:

- Address any concerns about wound healing with the provider.

TABLE 40.2   Types of Dressings

Dressing Type	Description	Uses
Alginate	Nonadhesive pad made from seaweed. Forms a gel over the wound when in contact with exudate. Can absorb up to 20 times its weight. Helps reduce the risk of bacterial infection.	Used for wounds with moderate to heavy exudate, pressure ulcers, and surgical wounds; not for dry wounds and third-degree burns.
Composite	Multi layered adhering dressing that absorbs drainage and provides a bacterial barrier.	Used for surgical wounds and pressure ulcers. Used for wounds with minimal to heavy exudate.
Foam	Soft and highly absorbent. Allow moisture to enter the wound but keeps bacteria out.	Used for wounds with moderate exudate (e.g., laceration, pressure ulcers); not used for dry wounds.
Gauze Sponge and Gauze Roll	Made from 100% cotton. Absorbs drainage. Economical and all-purpose dressing. Gauze roll can be used as a dressing or a bulky bandage.	Used for all types of wounds. Roll used for extremities and heads.
Hydrocolloid	Consist of an inner colloidal layer and an outer water-impermeable layer. Absorbs wound exudate. Impermeable to bacteria. Provides a moist healing environment.	Used for wounds with light to moderate exudate, pressure sores, superficial burns, and traumatic wounds.
Hydrogel	Controls the moisture level in the wound, which helps with natural debridement and promotes cell growth.	Used for dry or mostly dry wounds; any wound with dead tissue.
Medical Grade Honey	Dressing with medical grade honey. Promote a healing environment. Can assist in the debridement process and inhibits bacterial growth.	Used for acute and chronic wounds; pressure ulcers, leg ulcers, and surgical wounds.
Non-adherent Pad	Does not stick to the wound.	Wounds with light to moderate drainage; skin tears and acute wounds.
Transparent film	A transparent adherent dressing that that is impermeable to liquids, bacteria, and water. Allows oxygen into the wound.	Used for pressure ulcers and second-degree burns. Not used for wounds with heavy exudate.

- Make sure it is the proper time to remove them according to the provider's note in the patient's health record. They should not be removed early.
- Read the patient's health record and identify the number of suture or staples placed.

After the medical assistant removes the sutures or staples, it is important to document the appearance of the wound and the number of sutures or staples removed.

Wound Culture

To perform a wound culture, the medical assistant will need:
- A provider's order
- A culture swab with the patient's label, specimen bag for transport, and the laboratory requisition form
- Supplies to clean the wound (such as betadine)
- Dressing and bandages

The provider may have the medical assistant rinse the wound with normal saline to remove contaminated material (e.g., necrotic tissue and dried exudate [EKS you date]). If the wound is dry, the swab should be moistened with sterile normal saline (NS). This helps with the collection. If the wound is moist, no saline is needed.

To collect the specimen, the medical assistant should gently roll the swab stick from margin to margin using a zig-zag motion, using enough pressure to accumulate fluid on the swab. If pus is seen, it should be swabbed. The swab should only touch the wound. After the collection, the swab should be placed in a labeled tube. If the tube has formalin, squeeze the tube to release the formalin to preserve the specimen before sending it to the laboratory.

Dressing Change

When a provider orders a dressing change, it may be a sterile or clean dressing change. With a *sterile dressing change*, the medical assistant uses clean gloves to remove the old dressing. The

dressing is inspected for drainage (exudate). Types of exudate include:
- *Sanguineous* (sang GWIN ee us): The exudate contains blood. It appears bright red and may be thick in consistency.
- *Serosanguineous* (SEE roe sang GWIN ee us): The exudate contains serum and blood. It appears pink and thinner than the sanguineous drainage.
- *Serous* (SEE rus): The exudate contains serum. It appears thin and watery, may be clear or slightly yellow.
- *Seropurulent* (SEE row PYUE rue lent): The exudate that contains both serum and pus. It appears as a thin watery pus. The color can vary and may include white, green, brown, yellow, pink, and gray. This drainage is usually a sign of infection.
- *Purulent* (PYURE uh lent): The exudate contains pus. It appears as a thick, cloudy liquid that may be brown, green, yellow, or gray. This type of exudate is a sign of infection.

The wound is inspected for signs of infection. Wound closures are checked to ensure they are intact. Sterile gloves and sterile technique are used to apply the new dressing (Procedure 40.10).

When a medical assistant performs a clean dressing change, clean gloves are used to remove the old dressing. Draining is checked as well as the wound. Clean gloves are used to apply the sterile dressing and bandages. The medical assistant should avoid contaminating the sterile dressing as it is placed on the wound. This can be achieved by only touching the edges of the dressing, which will not be placed on the wound.

Dressings. A *dressing* is a sterile covering placed over a wound. Table 40.2 describes common types of dressings found in ambulatory care facilities. Many times the providers will order specific dressings to be applied by the medical assistant. For some procedures, a *pressure dressing* may be applied. This type of dressing applies pressure over the area to prevent bleeding or collection of fluid in the tissues.

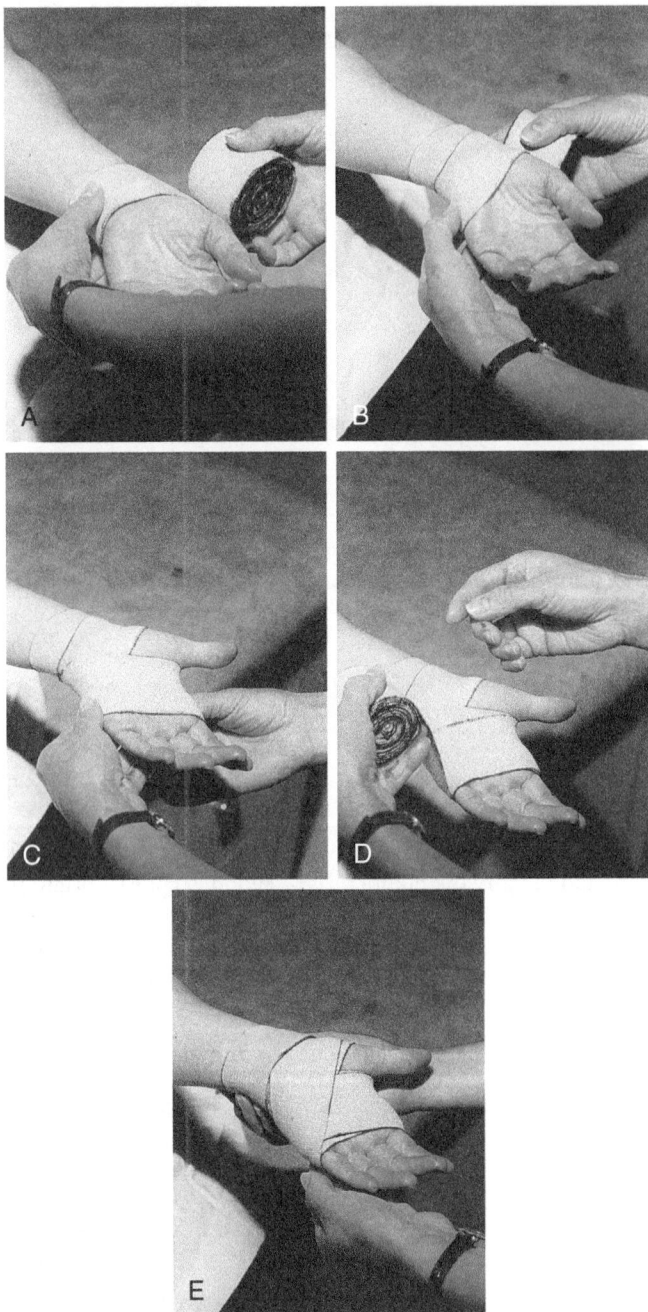

Fig. 40.6 A, A combination of recurrent and figure-eight turns is used for the hand. B, Bandaging starts at the wrist. C, Applying a roller bandage to the hand. D, Roller bandage in place on the hand. E, Consistent tension is maintained while the bandage is applied. (From Proctor D, et al: *Kinn's the medical assistant,* ed 13, St. Louis, 2017, Elsevier.)

For optimal wound healing, a dressing needs to create and maintain a moist environment. It should allow gaseous exchange but be impermeable to bacteria and other contaminates. Dressings should protect the wound from additional trauma and can be removed without causing trauma. In addition, a dressing should be comfortable, inexpensive, and require infrequent changes.

Sometimes the provider may prefer no dressing or bandage on small wounds. This is called *open wound healing*. This is not as common as it causes an increased risk for contamination of the wound. The new cells also dry out, leading to slower healing and more pain.

Bandages. A *bandage* holds dressings in place and protects the wound from injury and contamination. A bandage may also be used to maintain direct pressure over the wound. Bandages can restrict movement and provide support. Not all dressings need to be covered by bandages. Types of bandages include:

- *Roller*: A strip of gauze or material is wrapped over a dressing on an extremity or head. A roller dressing can help immobilize the injured area and provide pressure over the area (Fig. 40.6, Procedure 40.11). Examples include Kerlix, Kling, gauze roll, and elastic bandage (e.g., ACE Wrap).

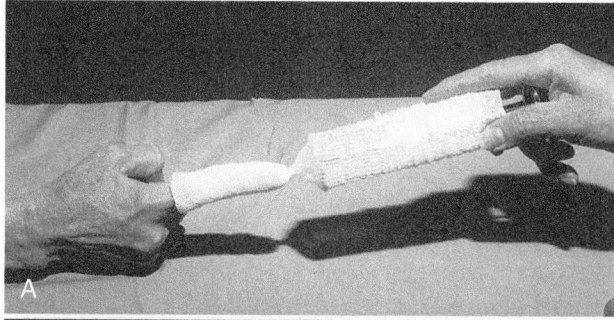

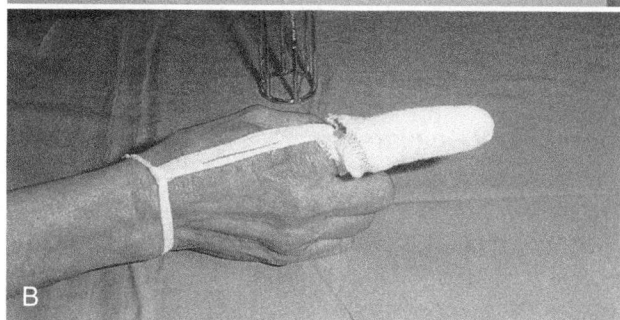

Fig. 40.7 A, Tube gauze is applied with even tension and is twisted at the fingertip before the next layer is applied. B, Tube gauze bandage has been applied and secured by tying at the wrist. (From Niedzwiecki B, et al: *Kinn's the medical assistant,* ed 14, St. Louis, 2020, Elsevier.)

BOX 40.3   Remember: CSMT When Bandaging

When applying bandages, you should assess these factors:

Color: Should be the same as the opposite extremity; report any bluish or white fingers or toes

Sensation: Should be able to feel fingers/toes; report any numbness

Movement: Should be able to move fingers/toes; report if unable to move fingers/toes

Temperature: Should be the same as the opposite extremity; report any cool/cold fingers/toes

---

- *Gauze Pads*: Placed over dressings and used to help absorb drainage. An example includes abdominal (ABD) pad.
- *Tubular* or *Tube*: Used for fingers, toes, arms, and legs. Help to keep the dressing in place and may also provide bulk to protect the wound (Fig. 40.7, Procedure 40.12).

Bandages require special skill to apply properly. Bandages that are too loose fall off, and those that are too tight can compromise circulation and do further harm to the patient. It takes practice and attention to get bandages applied correctly (Box 40.3).

Bandages need to be held in place either by clips, tapes, or ties. Common types of tape found in ambulatory care include:

- *Micropore paper tape*: The adhesive is hypoallergenic and can be used long-term without causing irritation.
- *Transpore polyethylene tape*: Hypoallergenic plastic surgical tape that is translucent and easy to tear.
- *Durable cloth tape*: Is flexible and comfortable tape. It sticks well to skin, but not always the best to secure cloth dressings or bandages.

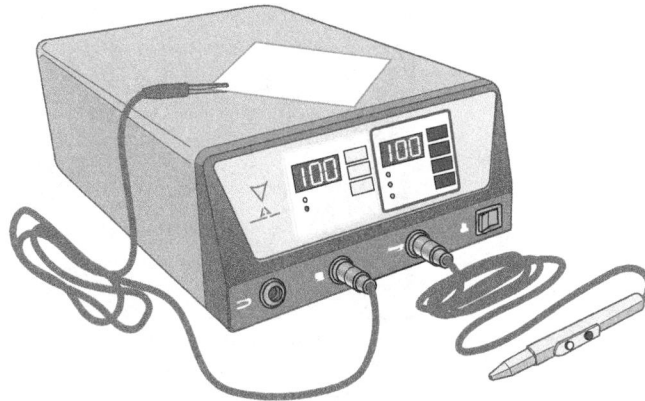

Fig. 40.8 Electrosurgical Unit. (From Niedzwiecki B, et al: *Kinn's the medical assistant,* ed 14, St. Louis, 2020, Elsevier.)

BOX 40.4   Important Tips About the Grounding Pad

- Carefully inspect the pad, cable, and skin before the procedure.
- Place the pad close to the operative site.
- The pad must be tight against the patient's skin and applied to a fleshy area, such as the thigh.
- Do not place the pad over a bony area, body hair, or metal implants or a pacemaker.
- Carefully inspect the pad site on the skin after the procedure for signs of burns.

When removing tape from a bandage, always remove it by pulling toward the wound. If it is adhering to a hairy area of the body, lift the outer tape edge with one hand and slowly and gently separate the underlying hair and skin from the tape with the thumb of your other hand. Peel the skin from the bandage, not the bandage from the skin. An adhesive remover can also be used to loosen the tape from the skin. Never "rip" tape from the body because it may injure the skin.

SPECIAL PROCEDURES

Electrosurgery

Electrosurgery is commonly known as *electrocautery*. In electrosurgery an electrosurgical unit (ESU) uses a small probe with an electric current running through it to cauterize the tissue (Fig. 40.8). This process seals blood vessels, which minimizes bleeding. Electrosurgery is often used to destroy problematic tissue, to obtain a tissue specimen for examination, and to stop bleeding.

An ESU needs a power source, the *active electrode* (a pencil-like instrument with a tip for the electrical current to run through), and a ground cable and pad. The grounding pad is a gel-covered adhesive electrode that is attached to the patient. This provides a safe return path for the electrosurgical current (Box 40.4).

VOCABULARY

cauterize To destroy tissue through burning. Used to remove tissue and/or close off blood vessels.

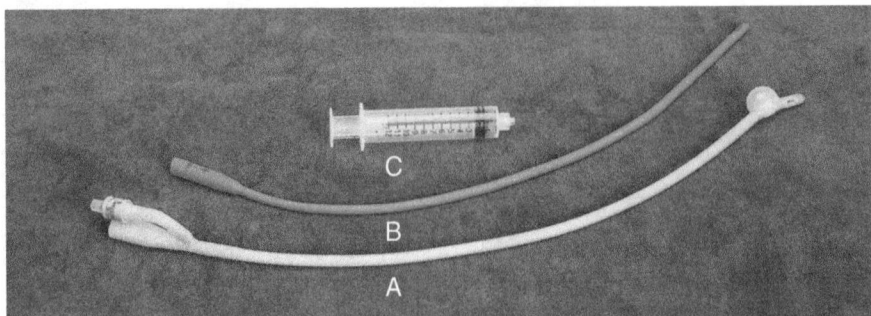

Fig. 40.9 Urinary Catheters. A, Foley catheter with inflated balloon. B, Straight catheter. C, A 12-mL Luer-Lok syringe used to inflate the balloon in the Foley catheter. (From Niedzwiecki B, et al: *Kinn's the medical assistant*, ed 14, St. Louis, 2020, Elsevier.)

Cryosurgery

Cryosurgery (KRY oh sur juh ree) involves the use of a very-low-temperature probe (usually below −20°C [4°F]) to destroy tissue by freezing it on contact. This low temperature is achieved by circulating liquid nitrogen through the tip of the probe. It is commonly used to destroy unwanted tissue on the skin, such as with warts or skin cancers.

Laser Surgery

Laser is an acronym for *l*ight *a*mplification by *s*timulated *e*mission of *r*adiation. Lasers are currently used for many procedures. Some of these include removal of lesions, warts, or moles and cosmetic surgical procedures (e.g., permanent hair removal).

Because a laser beam is so small and precise, it can be used to safely treat specific tissue with minimal damage to surrounding tissues and limited scar formation. Several types of lasers are used, including carbon dioxide, yttrium-aluminum-garnet (YAG), and pulsed dye lasers. Each laser has a specific use.

The medical assistant should complete a full laser safety program before assisting in laser procedures. Laser equipment requires very careful handling, care, and maintenance. Laser light destroys tissue and can harm the patient and staff members if improperly handled.

CRITICAL THINKING 40.8

You are a medical assistant working in a dermatology clinic. The clinic has recently obtained laser equipment for hair removal. As a medical assistant, what do you need to do in order to be qualified to assist with laser hair removal?

Microsurgery

Microsurgery involves the use of an operating microscope to perform delicate surgical procedures. Surgical microscopes are expensive, delicate instruments that require extreme care in handling and cleaning. A medical assistant must acquire a basic knowledge of the operation and care of an operating microscope before assisting in these types of procedures. The basic components of an operating microscope are the light source, eyepieces (also called the *oculars*), lenses, and cord. There may also be accessory pieces, depending on the surgery. Examples of these include cameras, video recorders, and an observer lens.

Endoscopic Procedures

An endoscope is a medical device consisting of a miniature camera mounted on a flexible tube with an optical system and light source. They are used to examine the area inside an organ or a cavity. Direct visualization with an endoscope is used for diagnostic purposes or to perform surgical procedures. Common examples of endoscopic procedures are colonoscopy, sigmoidoscopy, bronchoscopy, colposcopy, and cystoscopy.

There are several different types of endoscopes, including rigid, semirigid, and flexible. The type of endoscope used depends on the specific procedure being performed. Accessories will also depend on the specific procedure and may include things such as light cables and light source, suction, camera, and irrigation ports.

All endoscopes are delicate and expensive. They require extreme care in handling to protect them from damage. All equipment must be checked before and after use. Special care must also be taken in sanitizing, disinfecting, and sterilizing endoscope equipment. Always follow the manufacturer's recommendations for use, care, and maintenance, because the standard sterilization process and common disinfectants will damage the endoscope.

Therapeutic Injections and Joint Aspiration

Some medical issues can be improved with the use of a needle either to introduce medication (injection) or to withdraw fluid. Therapeutic injections and joint aspirations are used to treat localized problems, commonly in the joints. These procedures require that the needle be introduced directly into the joint. This procedure is performed with sterile technique by the provider with the assistance of the medical assistant. It is important that the technique be done in a sterile manner to avoid an infection in the joint.

VOCABULARY

localized Restricted or limited to a particular place.

Urinary Catheterization

A urinary catheter is a hollow, flexible tube that is inserted into the bladder through the urethra. It is used to collect urine. There are two primary types of urinary catheters (Fig. 40.9):

- An *indwelling catheter* is inserted into the bladder, drains the urine, and is removed. A straight catheter, a type of indwelling catheter, can be used to obtain a urine specimen.
- An *indwelling Foley catheter* is used to help patients who are unable to *void* (urinate) on their own. It is placed with the tip in the bladder and left in place to allow urine to be removed from the body and drained in a collection bag. The tip of the catheter contains a balloon, which is filled. This holds the catheter in the bladder (Procedure 40.14).

Some facilities and state statutes allow medical assistants to insert catheters. The medical assistant must use the correct-sized catheter to prevent tissue damage (Table 40.3). It is critical that the medical assistant insert the catheter using sterile technique to minimize the risk of a urinary tract infection (UTI).

Depending on the state statutes and the facility's policy, the medical assistant may also discontinue indwelling catheters. Sometimes after an indwelling catheter is removed, the patient may have *urinary retention* (inability to void) or void small amounts, not emptying the bladder as normal. The patient may experience:

TABLE 40.3	Urinary Catheter Sizes[a]	
Age	Weight	Catheter Size
Newborn	Up to 2500 g	5 Fr
0–2 years	3.4–12 kg	6–8 Fr
3–6 years	12–21 kg	8–10 Fr
7–8 years	21–27 kg	10–12 Fr
9–12 years	27–45 kg	12–14 Fr
>12 years	45 kg+	16 Fr

[a]Larger sizes may be needed for very large patients. Check with the provider when determining the appropriate catheter size.

- Abdominal discomfort and pain
- If voiding, a weak stream, voiding small amounts
- Urinary incontinence

Patients should be instructed to monitor when and how much they void. Usually a person should void 6 hours after the removal of an indwelling Foley catheter. If a patient suspects an issue, they should call the provider immediately.

CLOSING COMMENTS

Assisting with minor surgery can be challenging and rewarding. There are many things to remember, but the key piece is to always maintain sterile technique. Whether it is in handling instruments, setting up trays, or assisting the provider, sterile technique must be followed to protect your patients.

PATIENT-CENTERED CARE

A medical assistant's duties may include calling the patient the day before surgery to confirm the scheduled surgical procedure and appointment time. Explaining the procedure and what to expect during and after surgery prepares the patient and helps calm the person's fears or concerns.

- Lying still during surgery is important and eating a light meal the night before should be encouraged.
- Bathing before coming to the ambulatory care facility helps reduce the number of bacteria on the skin, and comfortable, loose clothing should be worn.
- Patients should be informed that they may need someone to accompany them home.
- Make sure the patient has an appointment for a return visit and examination.

Sometimes in the course of general conversation, the medical assistant can pick up hints of concerns the patient may have and can direct the conversation into a discussion of these concerns. Patients should also be encouraged to call the provider immediately if they suspect an infection or have a sudden increase in pain at the surgical site.

BEING PROFESSIONAL

Often patients need to be instructed on changing dressings at home. The medical assistant should talk with the patient to determine who will perform the dressing change and what supplies will be used. Having the person who will be doing the dressing change present during the instructions is critical. If patients do not have the supplies, the medical assistant can provide the patient with a list of supplies to purchase. Providing the patient with possible locations to purchase the supplies is also beneficial.

Role-play the following scenario with a classmate: Sallie Jones had a cyst removed, and you have been asked to dress the wound. In the future, Sallie will need to have the dressing changes at home. The dressing is located on her back. Role play identifying who will change the dressing and provide the patient with ideas of where to purchase the dressings.

CHAPTER REVIEW

In this chapter we discussed various types of surgical procedures common to the ambulatory care facility. The more you work with your provider, the more comfortable you will be with each of the procedures. When assisting the provider, you must maintain sterile technique. Nonsterile items should never pass over the sterile field. If this does happen, you should admit it so that the items can be made sterile again.

We also discussed the phases of wound healing. It is important for medical assistants and their patients to understand what is happening with the wound and the care that must be taken during each phase.

Dressings and bandages are often applied after a minor surgical procedure. Dressings are considered sterile and are applied directly to the wound. Bandages can be used to hold dressings in place. When you apply bandages, it is important to start at the proximal point and work toward the distal point. After applying the bandage, the medical assistant should assess the site using the CSMT mnemonic.

Lastly, we discussed other examples in which sterile procedure is necessary. In some cases the medical assistant will assist with these procedures; in other cases the medical assistant may perform them. Regardless, it is important that sterile technique be observed in order to reduce the risk of patient complications.

SCENARIO WRAP-UP

Susie is finding her clinical medical assisting position at the WMFM Clinic rewarding, exciting, and challenging. She enjoys coming to work every day and has learned all aspects of her position much more quickly than most of her peers. Susie frequently reads the latest information on new developments in minor surgery practice. Her concern for her patients' well-being makes her stand out, and the providers constantly get positive comments on her level of professionalism.

Susie has made a few errors in sterile technique since starting the clinical assistant position, but she has learned from each

situation and has never covered up a mistake. Whenever she realized that she had not followed procedure, she discussed the issue with her supervisor and with Dr. Perez. In this way errors can be corrected, if possible, and she most likely will not make the same or similar mistakes again.

Susie is a team player who consistently tries to anticipate the needs of the provider and patient both before and during surgery. Her cooperative, supportive manner is appreciated by everyone on the clinical staff.

PROCEDURE 40.1   Perform a Surgical Hand Scrub

Task
Scrub the hands with surgical soap, using friction, running water, and a disposable sterile brush to sanitize the skin before assisting with any procedure that requires surgical asepsis.

Equipment and Supplies
- Sink with foot, knee, or arm control for running water
- Surgical soap in a dispenser
- Towels (sterile towels if indicated by the facility's policy)
- Nail file or orange stick
- Sterile disposable brush

Procedural Steps
1. Remove all jewelry. Roll long sleeves above the elbows. Inspect your fingernails for length and your hands for skin breaks.
   Purpose: Jewelry harbors bacteria and is not permitted in surgical asepsis.
2. Turn on the faucet and regulate the water to a comfortable temperature, being careful to stand away from the sink to prevent contamination of clothing from contact with the sink or countertop.
3. Keep your hands upright and held at or above waist level (Fig. 1).
   Purpose: Water running from the unscrubbed area above the elbow down to the hands can carry bacteria back onto the hands. All areas below the waist are considered contaminated during all surgical procedures.

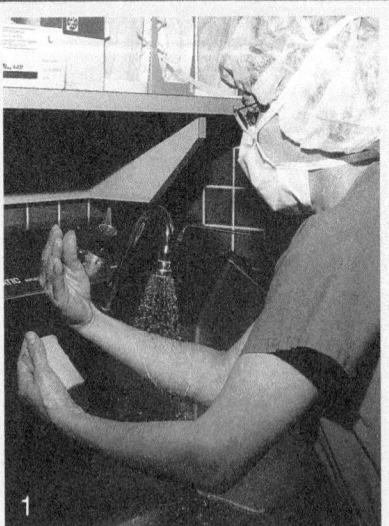

4. Clean your fingernails with a file, discard it (in most situations you will drop the file into the sink and discard it later to prevent contamination by lowering your hands and/or touching a waste container), and rinse your hands under the faucet without touching the faucet or the inside of the sink basin (Fig. 2).

PROCEDURE 40.1 Perform a Surgical Hand Scrub—cont'd

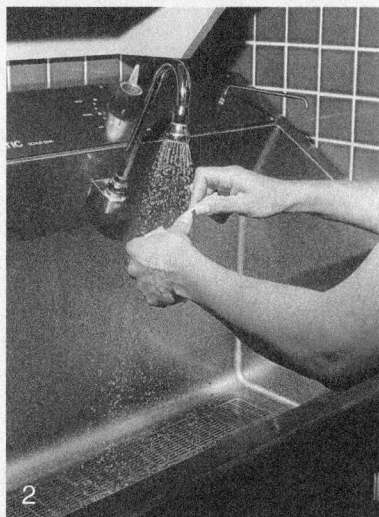

5. Allow the water to run over your hands from the fingertips to the elbows without moving the arm back and forth under the water.

   Purpose: Water running from the elbow down to the hands can carry bacteria back onto the hands.

6. Apply surgical soap from the dispenser to the sterile brush (or use a prepared disposable brush) and start the scrub by scrubbing the palm of the hand in a circular fashion.

7. Continue from the palm to the base of the thumb, then move on to the other fingers, scrubbing from the base, along each side, and across the nail, holding the fingertips upward and remembering to rub between the fingers (Fig. 3). After the fingers have been completely scrubbed, clean the posterior surface of the hand in a circular fashion and then proceed to the wrist. The scrubbing process should take at least 5 minutes for each hand and arm.

   Purpose: The surfaces of the fingers have four sides that all need to be thoroughly cleaned.

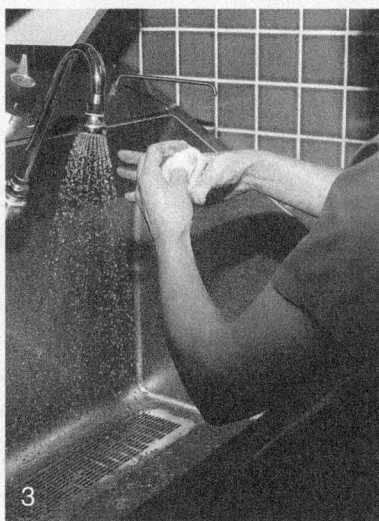

8. Do not return to a clean area after you have moved to the next part of the hand.

Purpose: Once an area has been scrubbed, it is considered surgically clean, and rubbing that area again contaminates it.

9. Wash the wrists and forearms in a circular fashion around the arm while holding your hands above waist level (Fig. 4).

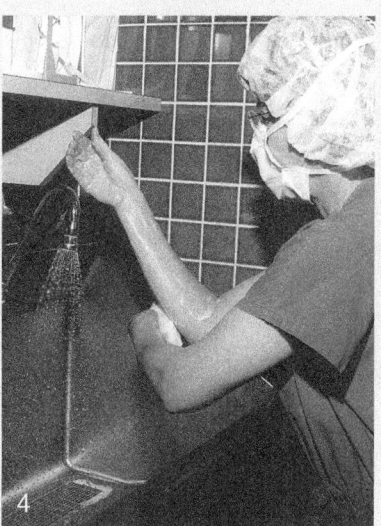

10. Rinse the arms and forearms from the fingertips upward, holding the fingers up, without touching the faucet or the inside of the sink basin (Fig. 5).

    Purpose: Keep the fingers higher than the rest of the arm to prevent contamination from water running downward from the elbow. Touching the dirty faucet and/or basin causes contamination.

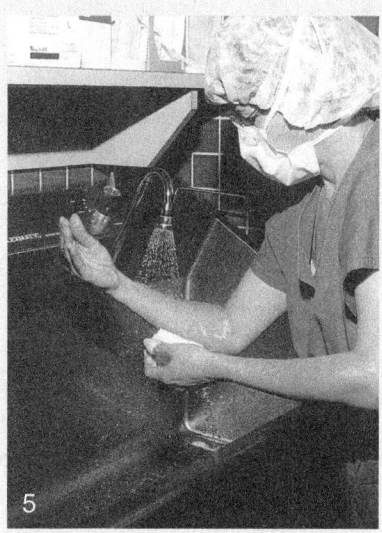

11. Apply more solution without touching any dirty surface and repeat the scrub on the other side, remembering to wash and use friction between each finger with a firm, circular motion.

12. Scrub all surfaces, being careful not to abrade your skin. The second hand and arm should take at least 5 minutes.

13. Rinse thoroughly, keeping your hands up and above waist level. Discard the scrub brush without lowering the arms below the waist (Figs. 6 and 7).

Continued

PROCEDURE 40.1   Perform a Surgical Hand Scrub—cont'd

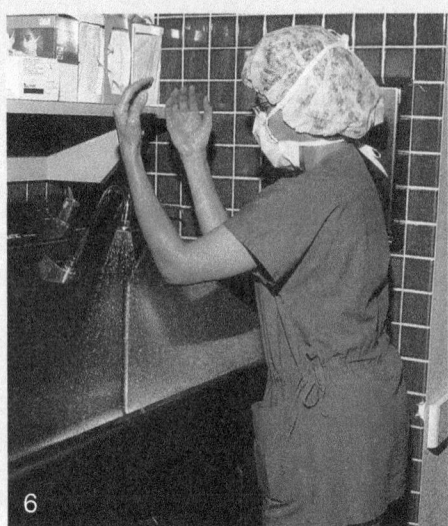

6

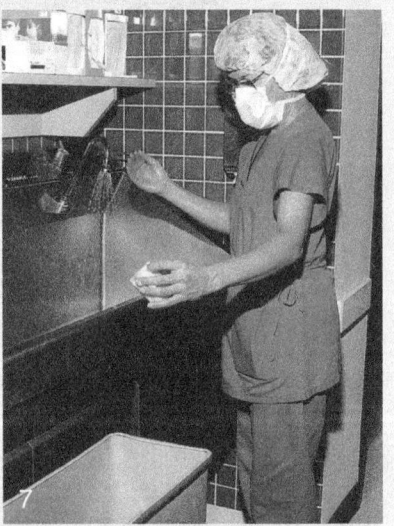

7

14. Turn off the faucet with the foot, knee, or forearm lever, if available.
    Purpose: To prevent clean hands from touching the contaminated faucet handles.
15. Dry your hands with a sterile towel, being careful to keep the fingers pointing upward and your hands above the waist. Do not rub back and forth, dragging contaminants from the dirtier area of the upper arm down toward the hands. Use the opposite end of the towel for the other hand.
    Purpose: To keep your clean hands from touching the part of the towel that comes in contact with your forearms, which are not as clean as your hands. If you are to gown and glove for a procedure, you must use a sterile towel.
16. Using a patting motion, continue to dry the forearms. Discard the towel and keep your hands up and above waist level (Fig. 8).

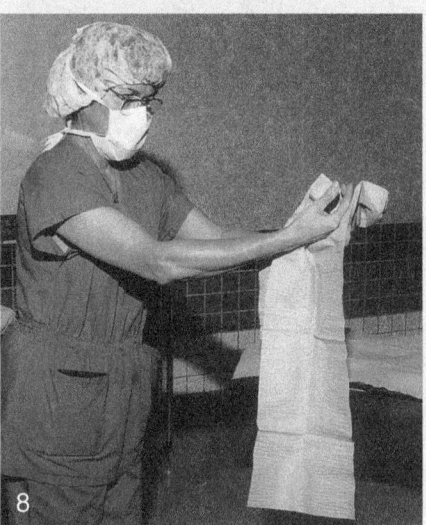

8

PROCEDURE 40.2   Perform Skin Prep for Surgery

Tasks
Prepare the patient's skin and remove hair from the surgical site to reduce the risk of wound contamination.

Equipment and Supplies
- Disposable skin prep kit, or collect the following: waterproof pads, gauze sponges, cotton-tipped applicators, soap, antiseptic or antiseptic swabs (e.g., Betadine swabs), sterile towel, gloves, and optional: cotton balls, nail pick, and scrub brush.
- Electric clippers
- Two small bowls
- Sterile normal saline solution
- Sterile drape
- Biohazardous waste/sharps containers
- Waste container
- Patient's health record

Procedural Steps
1. Wash your hands or use hand sanitizer.
   Purpose: To follow Standard Precautions.
2. Greet the patient. Identify yourself. Verify the patient's identity with full name and date of birth. Explain the procedure to be performed in a manner that is understood by the patient. Answer any questions the patient may have on the procedure. Verify the patient's allergies.
   Purpose: To ensure cooperation and demonstrate awareness of possible patient concerns.
3. Ask the patient to remove any jewelry and clothing that might interfere with exposure of the site. Provide a gown if needed.
4. Assist the patient into the proper position for site exposure. Provide a drape if necessary, to protect the patient's privacy. Expose the site. Use a light if necessary.
5. If hair is present and needs to be removed per the provider: put on gloves. Using an electric clippers, shave in the direction of hair growth using short

PROCEDURE 40.2   Perform Skin Prep for Surgery—cont'd

strokes. Remove any stray clipped hair. Discard disposable clipper had in the sharps container.

Purpose: Shaving will be required if the hair will obstruct the surgical procedure. In the past, shaving was required for all surgeries, but recent studies have shown no increase in surgical site infection (SSI) rates if patients are not shaven.

6. Place a waterproof underpad under the area to be scrubbed. While wearing gloves, open the skin prep pack and add the soap to the two bowls.

7. Start at the incision site and begin washing with the soap on a gauze sponge in a circular motion, moving from the center to the edges of the area to be scrubbed (Fig. 1).

Purpose: A circular motion from inside to outside drags contaminants away from the incision site.

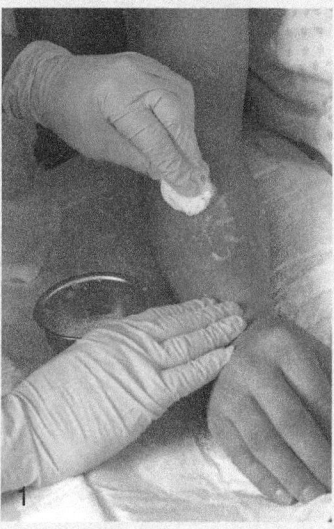

8. After one complete wipe, discard the sponge and begin again with a new sponge soaked in the antiseptic solution.

Purpose: After one circular sweep, the sponge is contaminated with skin bacteria and debris.

9. Repeat the process, using sufficient friction for 5 minutes (or follow facility's policy for the length of time required for a particular prep).

10. Rinse the area with sterile normal saline solution (Fig. 2).

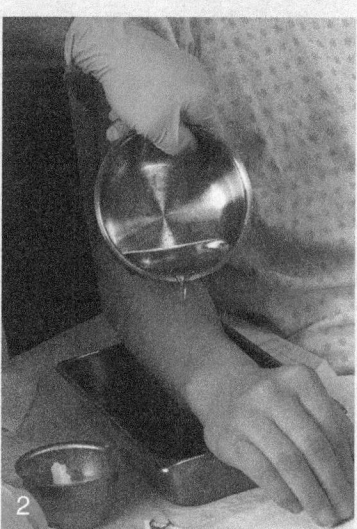

11. Dry the area, using the same circular technique with dry sponges. The area may be dried by blotting with a sterile towel.

12. Paint on the antiseptic with the cotton-tipped applicators or gauze sponges, using the same circular technique and never returning to an area that has already been painted.

13. Place a sterile drape and/or towel over the area.

14. Answer all the patient's questions to relieve anxiety about the upcoming surgical procedure.

15. Discard the waste in the appropriate waste container. Discard disposable clipper had in the sharps container if required or disinfect the clipper per facility's policy. Remove gloves and sanitize hands.

16. Document completion of the skin prep in the patient's health record.

PROCEDURE 40.3   Put on Sterile Gloves

Task
Put on sterile gloves correctly before performing sterile procedures.

Equipment and Supplies
- Pair of packaged sterile gloves in your size

Procedural Steps
1. Perform the surgical hand scrub as explained in Procedure 40.1 before putting on sterile gloves.

2. Open the glove pack, being careful not to cross over the open area in the middle of the pack. Remember, a 1-inch area around the perimeter of the glove wrapper is considered not sterile.

Purpose: The open glove pack is a sterile field.

3. With your nondominant hand, pick up the glove for your dominant hand with your thumb and forefinger, grabbing the edge of the folded cuff closest to you, which is the inside of the glove, being careful not to cross over the other sterile glove (Fig. 1).

Purpose: The inside of the glove will be next to your skin and is considered not sterile. This sets up your dominant hand to do the more difficult step, which is to put on the second glove.

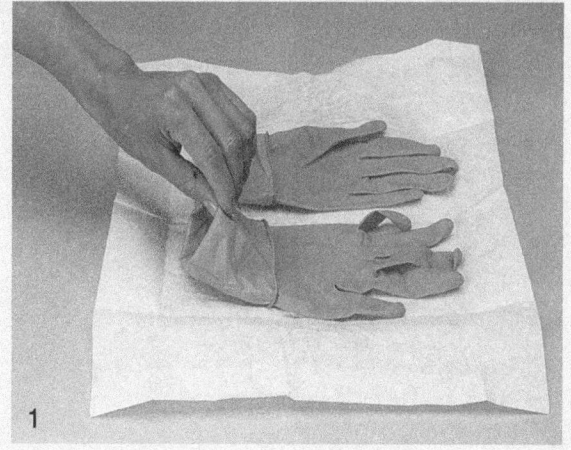

4. Lift the glove up and away from the sterile package.

Purpose: To prevent accidental contamination from touching the glove on the 1-inch area around the perimeter of the glove wrapper.

Continued

PROCEDURE 40.3   **Put on Sterile Gloves—cont'd**

5. Hold your hands up and away from your body and slide the dominant hand into the glove (Fig. 2).

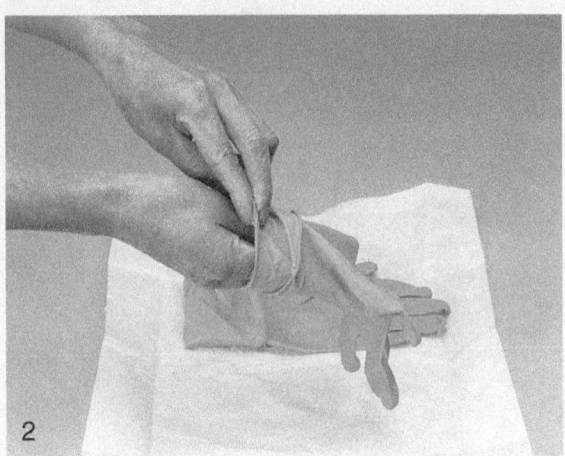

6. Leave the cuff folded (Fig. 3).
   Purpose: You will unfold the cuff later.

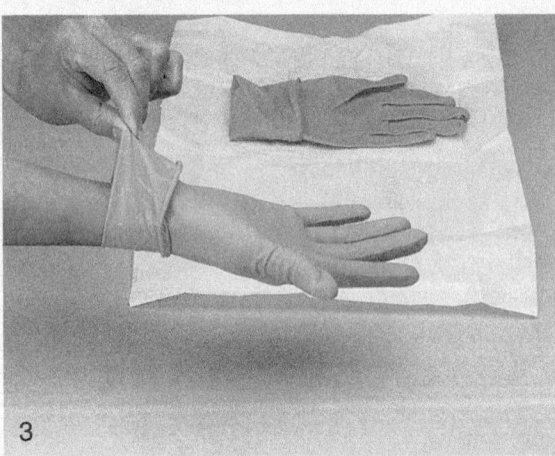

7. With your gloved dominant hand, pick up the second glove by slipping your gloved fingers under the cuff, extending the thumb up and away from the glove (thumbs up position), so that your gloved fingers touch only the outside of the second glove (Fig. 4).
   Purpose: Sterile surfaces must always touch sterile surfaces.

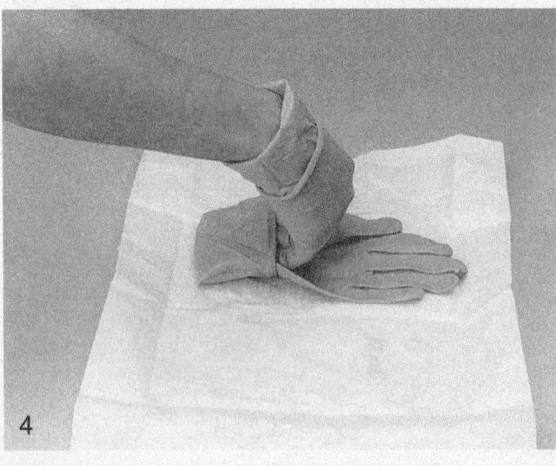

8. Slide your nondominant hand into the glove without touching the exterior of the glove or any part of the gloved hand (Figs. 5 and 6).

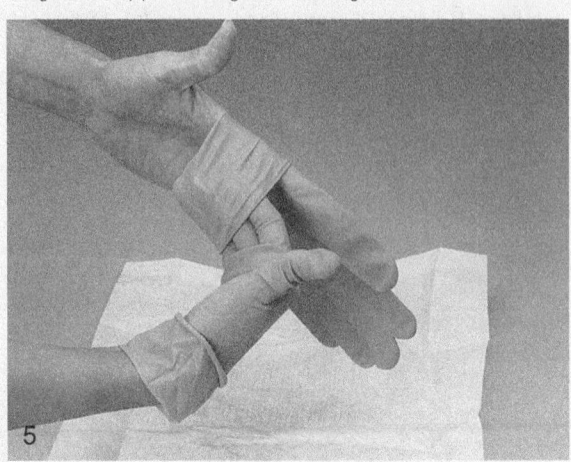

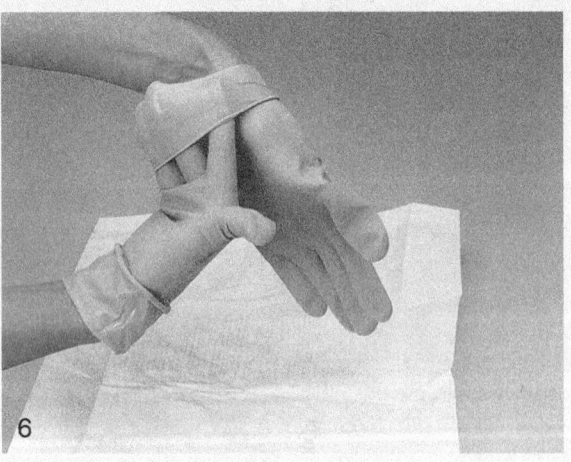

9. Still holding your hands away from you, unroll the cuff by slipping the fingers into the cuff and gently pulling up and out. Do not touch your bare arm or the internal surface of the glove with any part of the sterile glove (Fig. 7).

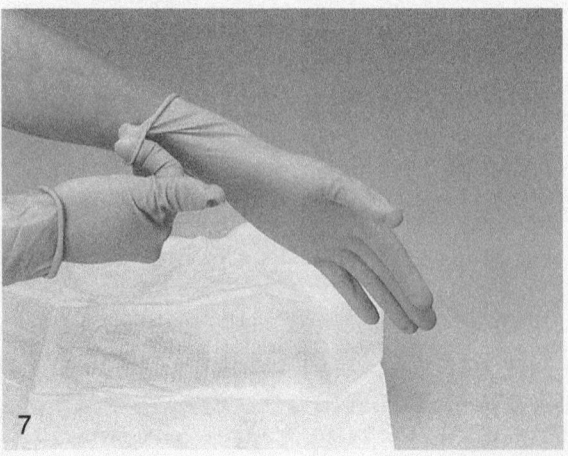

10. Now, slip your gloved fingers up under the first cuff and unroll it, using the same technique (Fig. 8).

PROCEDURE 40.3   Put on Sterile Gloves—cont'd

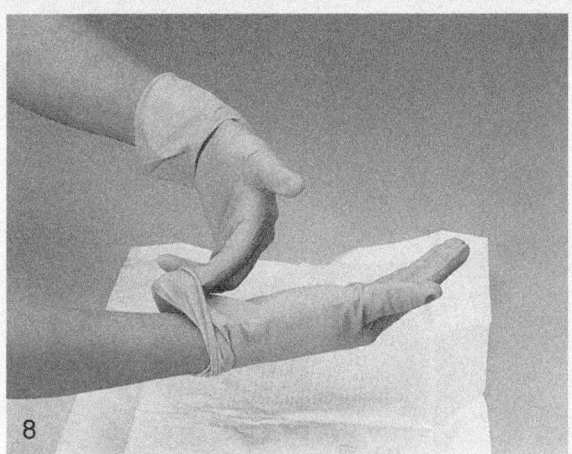

Purpose: To reduce the number of transient flora on your hands and forearms; moisture on your hands contaminates the pack.

PROCEDURE 40.4   Prepare a Sterile Field, Use Transfer Forceps, and Pour a Sterile Solution into a Sterile Field

Tasks

Open a sterile instrument pack using correct aseptic technique and create a sterile field; move sterile items on a sterile field or transfer sterile items to a gloved team member; pour a sterile solution into a sterile stainless-steel bowl or container sitting at the edge of a sterile field.

Equipment and Supplies

- A sterile instrument pack wrapped with autoclave paper that, when opened, will serve as a sterile table drape or field
- Mayo stand or countertop
- Disinfectant and gauze sponges or disinfectant wipes
- Sterile item to move or transfer
- Sterile wrapped transfer forceps
- Unopened bottle of sterile solution
- Sterile bowl or container
- Sink or waste container

Procedural Steps

1. Check that the Mayo stand or countertop is dust free and clean. If it is not, disinfect it and allow it to air dry.
   Purpose: Although some areas cannot be sterile, steps must be taken to keep contamination to a minimum; moisture on a tray contaminates the pack.
2. Wash or sanitize your hands and make sure they are completely dry.
   Purpose: To reduce the number of transient flora on your hands and forearms; moisture on your hands contaminates the pack.
3. Gather supplies. Check the label of the ordered solution. Check the solution name and the expiration date. Do not use the solution if it is expired.
   Purpose: The label needs to be checked three times before the solution is used on the patient.
4. If an autoclaved pack is used, check the indicator tape for a color change.
   Purpose: Autoclave indicator tape changes color after the sterile processing cycle.
5. Open the outside cover (Fig. 1). Position the package so that the outer envelope flap is at the top and with the tab facing you.
   Purpose: This positions the pack for correct opening so that you do not have to cross over the sterile pack to open it.

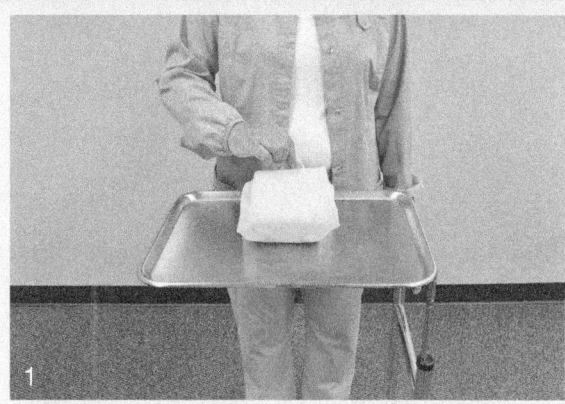

6. Open the outermost flap (Fig. 2). Next, open the first flap away from you. You can cross over the uncovered portion of the Mayo stand because it is not sterile. Do not cross over the pack.

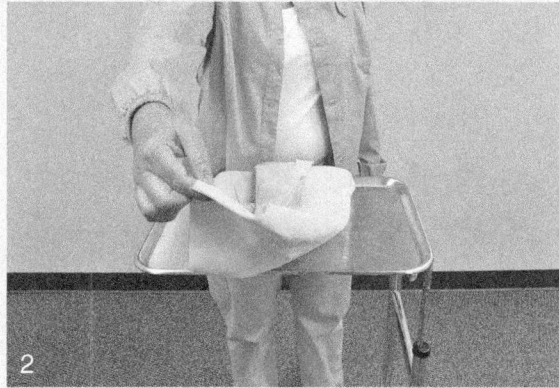

7. Open the second corner, pulling to the side (Fig. 3).
   Purpose: To prevent contamination of the sterile field.

Continued

PROCEDURE 40.4 Prepare a Sterile Field, Use Transfer Forceps, and Pour a Sterile Solution into a Sterile Field—cont'd

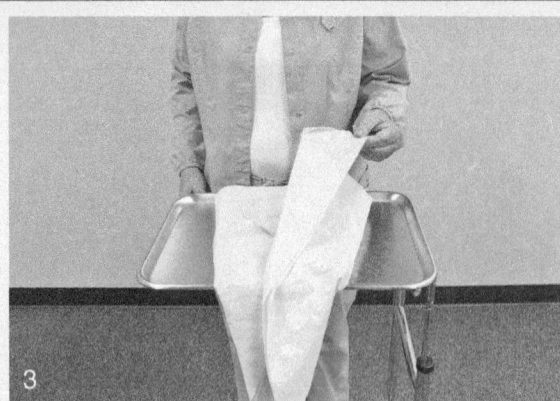

8. Be careful to lift the flaps by touching only the small, folded-back tab and without touching or crossing over the inner surface of the pack or its contents. Open the remaining two corners of the pack (Fig. 4).

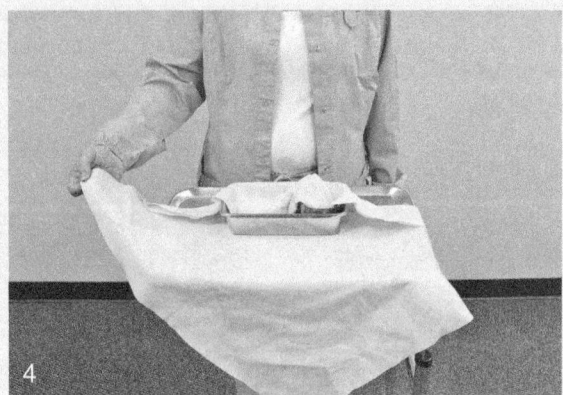

Note: You now have a sterile drape as a sterile field from which to work and for the distribution of additional sterile supplies and instruments (Fig. 5).

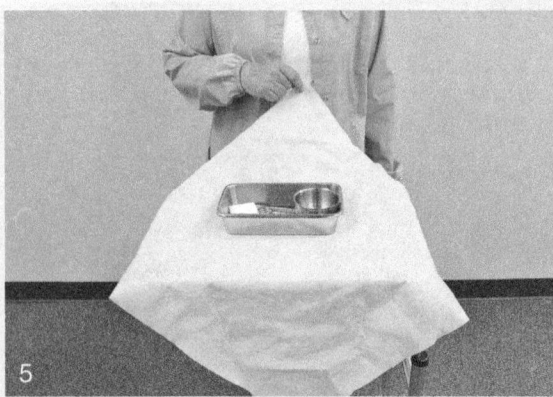

9. Open a package containing sterile transfer forceps (Fig. 6). Using sterile technique, handle the sterile forceps by the ring handle only. Always point the forceps tips down.

Purpose: If the tips are turned upward, any solution encountered will run onto the nonsterile area and then back down over the sterile end when the tips are turned down again, thus contaminating the forceps.

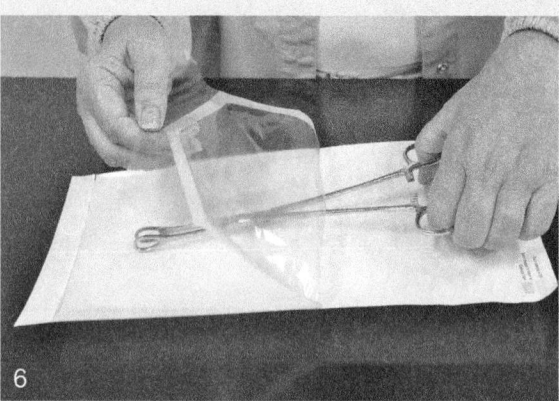

10. Grasp an item on the sterile field with the sterile forceps, points down, and move it to its proper position for the procedure, making sure not to cross the sterile field with the hand or contaminated end of the forceps (Fig. 7).

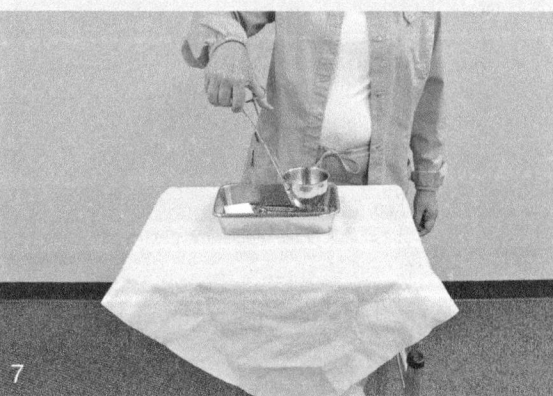

11. Set the forceps aside after one-time use.
    Note: The sterile bowl should be placed, using sterile transfer forceps, near one edge of the field and the perimeter of the 1-inch barrier.
12. Check the label of the solution for the second time.
13. Lift or unscrew the cover of the bottle. Listen for the vacuum release sound. If there is no vacuum, assume the fluid is not sterile and select another bottle. Do not touch the rim or inside of the cover. Hold the cover with the nondominant hand.
    Purpose: The rim of the bottle and inside the cover are considered sterile. Sterile solutions are single patient use. The unused portion must be discarded after the procedure.
14. Place your hand over the label. Pour away from the label without allowing any part of the bottle to touch the bowl and without crossing over the sterile field (Fig. 8).
    Purpose: Spills down the side of the bottle can stain the label or make it unreadable. The bottle exterior is not sterile, so it cannot pass over the sterile field.

PROCEDURE 40.4   Prepare a Sterile Field, Use Transfer Forceps, and Pour a Sterile Solution into a Sterile Field—cont'd

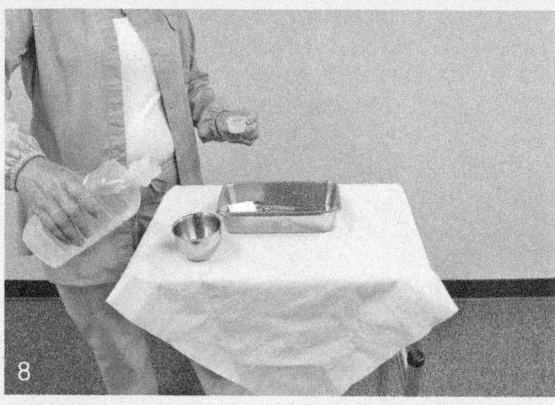

15. Tilt the bottle up to stop the pouring while it is still over the bowl.
Purpose: Solutions spilled on the sterile field may contaminate the field.

16. Check the label of the solution for the third time. Replace the cover on the bottle if the solution will be kept until the end of the procedure (per facility policy).

PROCEDURE 40.5   Two-Person Sterile Tray Setup

Task
Perform a sterile tray setup for a cyst removal.

Directions
This procedure involves two people. One person will act as the nonsterile person, and the other will have on sterile gloves and will place the items on the sterile tray.

Equipment and Supplies
Nonsterile area:
- Gauze soaked with skin prep solution (e.g., povidone-iodine)
- Sterile gloves for the provider
- Anesthetic medication vial and alcohol pads
- Dressing material (antibiotic ointment, bandage, nonstick bandage, tape),
- Gloves
- Labeled specimen container, specimen bag for transport, and a laboratory requisition form
- Patient's health record

Sterile tray:
- Mayo stand
- Sterile drape
- 10 mL syringe and safety needle
- Sterile 4 × 4s gauze
- Fenestrated drape
- Instruments (per provider's preference): Mosquito forceps, dressing forceps, operating or Iris scissor, disposable scalpel, and tissue forceps or tooth forceps
- Suture, a needle holder, and scissor (if suturing will be done)

Procedural Steps
Nonsterile Person
1. Check that the Mayo stand or countertop is dust free and clean. If it is not, disinfect it and allow it to air dry.
Purpose: Although some areas cannot be sterile, steps must be taken to keep contamination to a minimum; moisture on a tray contaminates the pack.
2. Wash or sanitize your hands and make sure they are completely dry.
Purpose: To reduce the number of transient flora on your hands and forearms; moisture on your hands contaminates the pack.
3. Gather all supplies and equipment. Inspect all sterile packs for holes and tears. Check indicators. Discard any packs that are not sterile.
4. Assemble supplies in the nonsterile area.
5. Place the package containing the sterile drape on a flat surface near the Mayo stand/tray. Check the integrity of the outer package. Open the package without touching the barrier field.

6. Pick up the barrier field, by the corner, as you move away from the table and allow it to unfold without touching anything else (Fig. 1). Drape over the Mayo stand.
Purpose: This maintains the sterility of the barrier field, creating the sterile field on the Mayo stand.

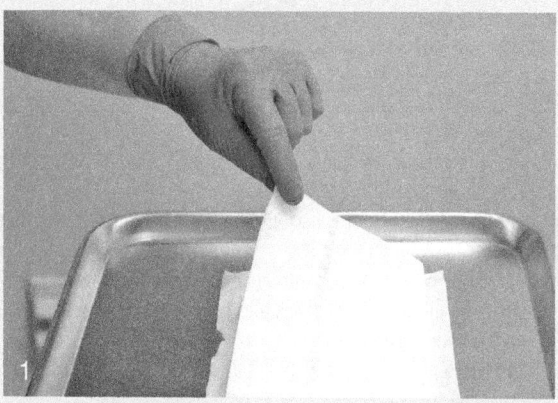

7. Slowly pull the sides of the peel pack of sterile 4 × 4s away from each other. Maintain control of the item inside the package by opening the package only far enough for a sterile person to grab the item. Allow the sterile person to take the 4 × 4s. Recheck the wrapper for holes and check the internal indicator strip (if present) before the sterile person places the item on the sterile field. Discard the wrapper.
Purpose: By inspecting the package after the item has been removed, you can ensure that it is truly sterile.
8. Repeat step 7 with the suture pack, syringe, and safety needle.
9. Repeat step 7 with the scalpel and instrument pack(s).
10. Repeat step 7 with the fenestrated drape.

Sterile Person
1. Perform the surgical hand scrub as explained in Procedure 40.1.
Purpose: To reduce the number of transient flora on your hands and forearms; moisture on your hands contaminates the pack.
2. Apply sterile gloves as explained in Procedure 40.3.
3. Remove an item from a peel pack and maintain sterile technique.
4. After the nonsterile person has indicated that the peel pack has not been compromised, place the item on the sterile tray. Repeat for all items. Arrange items on the sterile tray.
5. Maintain sterility of sterile field and sterile supplies.

PROCEDURE 40.6   Assist With Minor Surgery

Tasks
Perform a sterile tray setup for a cyst removal.

Equipment and Supplies
Nonsterile area:
- Gauze soaked with skin prep solution (e.g., povidone-iodine)
- Sterile gloves for the provider
- Anesthetic medication vial and alcohol pads
- Dressing material (antibiotic ointment, bandage, nonstick bandage, tape)
- Gloves
- Labeled specimen container, specimen bag for transport, and a laboratory requisition form
- Patient's health record

Sterile Tray:
- Mayo stand
- Sterile drape
- 10 mL syringe and safety needle
- Stack of sterile 4 × 4 gauze
- Fenestrated drape
- Instruments (per provider's preference): Mosquito forceps, dressing forceps, operating or Iris scissor, disposable scalpel, and tissue forceps or tooth forceps
- Suture, a needle holder, and scissor (if suturing will be done)

Procedural Steps
1. Wash or sanitize your hands. Gather equipment and supplies. Assemble supplies in the nonsterile area. Check the anesthetic medication label for the right name and route, ensuring it is the medication the provider requested. Verify the medication has not expired.
   Purpose: To follow Standard Precautions. Medications need to be checked 3 times prior to use.
2. Greet the patient. Identify yourself. Verify the patient's identity with full name and date of birth.
3. Explain the procedure to be performed in a manner that is understood by the patient. Answer any questions the patient may have on the procedure. Verify the patient's allergies.
   Purpose: To ensure cooperation and demonstrate awareness of possible patient concerns.
4. Prep the patient's skin with surgical soap and antiseptic solution as explained in Procedure 40.2. Explain the prep procedure to the patient.
   Purpose: To ensure infection control and to demonstrate awareness of possible patient concerns.
5. Complete the second anesthetic medication label check. Perform the surgical hand scrub as explained in Procedure 40.1.
6. Assemble sterile field with supplies and equipment. Ensure all sharp equipment conspicuously placed on the sterile field. Maintain sterile technique. Position the Mayo stand near the patient and the operative site.
   Purpose: To prevent contamination of supplies and provide easy access for the provider.
7. Perform the third anesthetic medication label check. After the provider drapes the site, assist by preparing wiping the local anesthetic vial rubber stopper with an alcohol pad. Hold the vial of local anesthetic so that the provider can read the label. Hold the vial upside down as the provider inserts needle and withdraws the medication (Fig. 1).
   Note: In many facilities, a person wearing sterile gloves places the drape on the surgical site. When applying the drape, the person should wrap both

of their sterile gloved hands around the ends of the drape. This protects the sterile gloves from touching the patient when the drape is placed.
   Purpose: The medical assistant must hold the vial of local anesthetic medication since it is unsterile and the provider is wearing sterile gloves. The medication label must be checked before a medication is administered.

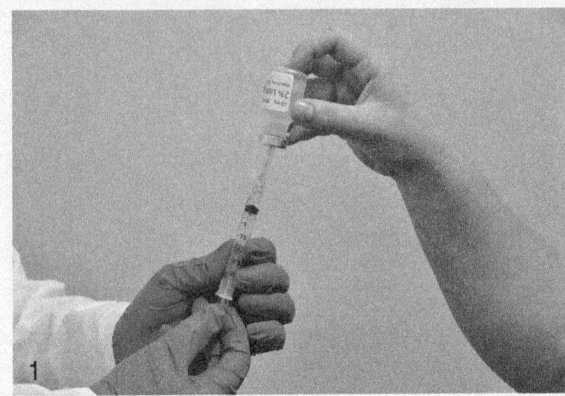

8. While the provider injects the local anesthetic, apply sterile gloves (see Procedure 40.3).
9. Position yourself so you have access to the sterile tray and are within reach to the provider and surgical site.
10. Pass the scalpel, blade down and handle first, to the provider, or the provider will reach for it. If passing the scalpel, place your fingers at the top, near the middle of the scalpel (Fig. 2). Give a verbal cue that you are passing the scalpel. The provider will take the scalpel with the thumb and forefinger in the position ready for use.
    Purpose: Giving a verbal cue when passing a sharps helps prevent injuries.

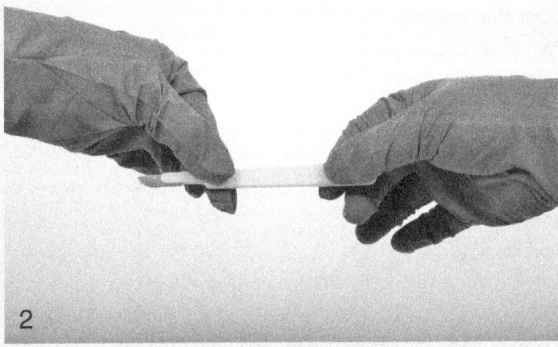

11. Pass the forceps and scissors. Pick up a ring handle instrument, holding near the tip, and pass it to the provider. The ring handles can be placed in the provider's palm. If the instrument has a curved tip, pass the instrument so the curved tip is facing the provider's opposite hand. When passing scissors, the tips should be closed. When passing an instrument with ratchets, have the instrument open (to the smallest opening) using the first ratchet.
    Purpose: When handing the instruments in this way, it becomes more efficient for the provider.
12. Hold sterile gauze sponges in your hand or with a dressing forceps. Use the sponges as needed to pat or sponge the wound in the surgical area. Dispose of soiled sponges in the biohazard waste container.

PROCEDURE 40.6 Assist With Minor Surgery—cont'd

13. Load the needle holder with the suture. Hold the needle holder in the right hand and the suture packet in the left hand. Open the needle holder jaws. Push the tips of the needle holder into the packet as you grasp the needle just below the swagged point. The needle should be about 1-2 mm from the tip of the needle holder. Clamp the jaws shut. Rotate the packet slightly, so the needle tip release as you pull out the suture.

14. Hold the needle holder near the hinge and pass the needle holder to the provider (Fig. 3). Give a verbal cue that you are passing the needle holder. Assist with cutting the suture at the surgical site, if indicated by the provider.

    Purpose: Giving a verbal cue when passing a sharps helps prevent injuries.

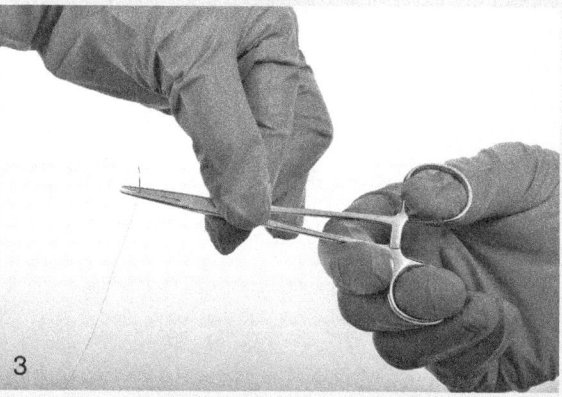

15. When the provider is finished, clean the surgical site using sterile technique. Apply the dressing and bandage indicated by the provider. Monitor the patient and provide verbal and written home care instructions.

16. Collect the specimen using Standard Precautions, place it in a labeled specimen container. Please container in a specimen bag for transport. Remove all sharps from the sterile tray and discard in the sharps biohazard container. Collect all the instruments. Discard waste in the appropriate waste container. Remove your gloves.

17. Wash your hands or use hand sanitizer. Document the patient education provided.

PROCEDURE 40.7 Apply Adhesive Skin Closure Strips

Tasks

Apply adhesive skin closure strips to a wound and document the procedure in the patient's health record.

Equipment and Supplies

- Patient's health record and provider's order
- Sterile gloves or clean gloves (per facility's procedure)
- Adhesive skin closure strips (e.g., Steri-strips)
- Compound benzoin tincture (optional)
- Sterile gauze
- Waste container
- Scissor and forceps
- Dressing/bandages (optional)

Provider's order: Apply adhesive skin closure strips to laceration on right arm.

Procedural Steps

1. Wash your hands or use hand sanitizer. Read the provider's order. Assemble the necessary supplies.

    Purpose: For infection control.

2. Greet the patient. Identify yourself. Verify the patient's identity with full name and date of birth. Explain the procedure to be performed in a manner that is understood by the patient. Answer any questions the patient may have on the procedure. Verify the patient's allergies.

    Purpose: To ensure cooperation during the procedure.

3. Instruct the person to lie or sit still during the procedure. Position the patient comfortably.

4. Put on gloves. Using a sterile gauze, clean and dry the skin at least 2 inches around the wound. Apply a thin layer of compound benzoin tincture on the skin up to the wound edge. Avoid getting the tincture in the wound.

    Purpose: The compound benzoin tincture can cause burning if it gets into the wound. It can also impair wound healing,

5. Remove the adhesive strip card from the package. Trim the size of the strips if needed. Remove the top of the card by the perforation.

    Purpose: Removing the tab makes it easier to grasp the strip.

6. Using a sterile forceps, grasp the end of the adhesive strip and lift straight up.

    Purpose: This prevents the strip from curling.

7. When the tincture becomes tacky on the skin, apply the strips. Apply the first adhesive strip perpendicular to the wound edge starting at the middle of the wound. Attach half of the adhesive strip to the wound margin and press adhesive strip firmly in place with gloved finger.

    Note: Do not stretch the strip across the wound.

Continued

PROCEDURE 40.7   Apply Adhesive Skin Closure Strips–cont'd

8. Using the forceps or a finger, approximate wound edges. Then firmly press the other half of adhesive strip to the other side of the wound.

9. Place the next strip 1/8" from the first strip. Continue to apply strips until the wound edges are well approximated. Space the strips 1/8" from each other.

   Note: If a strip needs to be removed and replaced, gently and slowly lift the edge of the strip moving towards the wound. Use a finger to support the wound. Once one side is removed to the edge of the wound, repeat the process on the other side.

10. Apply an adhesive strip parallel to wound approximately ½ inch from the ends of the other strips, creating a railroad track appearance.

    Purpose: Besides securing the other strips, the parallel adhesive strips can reduce stress and can decrease the risk of blisters.

11. Apply a dressing/bandage per the provider's order. Instruct the patient on wound care. (Patients can shower or wash the area with the adhesive strips with mild soap and water. Gently pat the area dry. Do not pull or rub strips off. They will fall off on their own within 10-14 days.)

    Purpose: Patient education is a required part of patient care. The patient needs to know how to care for the wound at home.

12. Clean up the area. Discard the waste in the appropriate waste container. Remove your gloves and discard them in the appropriate waste container. Wash or sanitize hands.

13. Document the procedure and the instructions on wound care given to the patient.

    Purpose: A procedure that is not documented was not done.

PROCEDURE 40.8   Remove Sutures

Task

Remove sutures from a healed incision using sterile technique and without injuring the closed wound.

Equipment and Supplies

- Sterile gloves or clean gloves (per facility's procedure)
- Adhesive skin closure strips or adhesive bandage strips (e.g., Band-Aids) (optional)
- Skin antiseptic swabs (e.g., Betadine swabs)
- Biohazardous waste/sharps containers
- Waste container
- Patient's health record
- Provider's order
- Sterile suture removal kit: Suture removal scissors, gauze, and thumb dressing forceps

Provider's order: Remove sutures from healed incision on left arm.

Procedural Steps

1. Wash your hands or use hand sanitizer. Read the provider's order. Assemble the necessary supplies. Read the patient's health record to determine the number of sutures inserted.

   Purpose: The medical assistant must know how many sutures were inserted prior to starting the procedure. The count of how many were inserted must match the count of those removed.

2. Greet the patient. Identify yourself. Verify the patient's identity with full name and date of birth. Explain the procedure to be performed in a manner that is understood by the patient. Answer any questions the patient may have on the procedure.

   Purpose: To ensure cooperation during the procedure.

3. Instruct the person to lie or sit still during the procedure. Position the patient comfortably and support the sutured area.

4. Check the incision line to make sure the wound edges are well approximated and there are no signs of infection, such as inflammation, edema, or drainage.

   Purpose: Sutures should not be removed unless the site is completely healed with the wound edges together. Infection at the site will interfere with the healing process. Removing sutures before the site is completely healed may result in the wound edge separating.

5. Put on gloves. Using antiseptic swabs, cleanse the wound to remove exudate. Clean the site from the inside out, starting at the top of the wound

and working your way down. Use a new swab if the step must be repeated. Remove gloves and discard them.

   Purpose: Dried exudate on sutures may make removing them without traumatizing the wound more difficult. Cleansing the wound reduces the possibility of wound infection.

6. Open the suture removal pack while maintaining the sterility of the contents.

7. Place sterile gauze next to the wound site.

   Purpose: To receive the removed sutures.

8. Put on sterile or clean gloves (per the facility's policy).

9. Grasp the knot of the suture with the dressing forceps without pulling. Cut the suture at skin level.

10. Lift, do not pull, the suture toward the incision and out with the dressing forceps.

11. Place the suture on the sterile gauze sponge and check that the entire suture strand has been removed.

    Purpose: Suture fragments left in a wound may cause irritation and/or infection and may prolong the healing process.

12. If any bleeding occurs, blot the area with a sterile gauze sponge before continuing. Continue in the same manner until all sutures have been removed.

13. Remove the gauze holding the sutures. Count the sutures removed. Dispose of sutures in the biohazardous waste container. Place sharps (e.g., scissor) in the sharps biohazardous container.

14. Apply adhesive skin closure strips or an adhesive bandage strip if ordered by the provider. Instruct the patient to keep the wound edges clean and dry and not to place excessive strain on the area.

15. Clean up the area. Discard the waste in the appropriate waste container. Wash or sanitize hands.

14. Document the procedure, wound condition, number of sutures removed, whether adhesive skin closure strips or an adhesive bandage strip were applied, and the instructions on wound care given to the patient.

    Purpose: A procedure that is not documented was not done.

Documentation Example

07/30/20XX 10:20 a.m. Per Dr. Walden's order, sutures removed. Wound edges well approximated with 5 intact sutures. No sign of infection. Site was cleaned with Betadine, and 5 sutures were removed. Pt instructed on home wound care and to notify provider if drainage changes, inflammation increases, or fever occurs. _____ Susie Rana, CMA (AAMA)

PROCEDURE 40.9   Remove Surgical Staples

Task

Remove surgical staples from a healed incision using sterile technique and without injuring the closed wound.

Equipment and Supplies

- Sterile gloves or clean gloves (per facility's procedure)
- Adhesive skin closure strips or adhesive bandage strips (e.g., Band-Aids)
- Skin antiseptic swabs (e.g., Betadine swabs)
- Biohazardous waste/sharps containers
- Waste container
- Patient's health record
- Provider's order
- Surgical staple remover kit: Surgical staple remover and 4 × 4-inch gauze

Provider's order: Remove surgical staples from healed incision on left calf.

Procedural Steps

1. Wash your hands or use hand sanitizer. Read the provider's order. Assemble the necessary supplies. Read the patient's health record to determine the number of staples inserted.

    Purpose: The medical assistant must know how many staples were inserted prior to starting the procedure. The count of how many were inserted must match the count of those removed.

2. Greet the patient. Identify yourself. Verify the patient's identity with full name and date of birth. Explain the procedure to be performed in a manner that is understood by the patient. Answer any questions the patient may have on the procedure.

    Purpose: To ensure cooperation during the procedure.

3. Instruct the person to lie or sit still during the procedure. Position the patient comfortably and support the stapled area.

4. Check the incision line to make sure the wound edges are well approximated and there are no signs of infection, such as inflammation, edema, or drainage.

    Purpose: Staples should not be removed unless the site is completely healed with the wound edges together; infection at the site will interfere with the healing process; removing staples before the site is completely healed may result in the wound edge separating.

5. Put on gloves. Using antiseptic swabs, cleanse the wound to remove exudate and destroy microorganisms around the staples. Clean the site from the inside out, starting at the top of the wound and working your way down. Use a new swab if the step must be repeated. Remove gloves and discard them.

    Purpose: Dried exudate on staples may make removing them without traumatizing the wound more difficult. Cleansing the wound reduces the possibility of wound infection.

6. Open the staple removal pack while maintaining the sterility of the contents. Place sterile gauze next to the wound site.

    Purpose: To receive the removed staples.

7. Put on sterile or clean gloves (per the facility's policy).

8. Gently place the bottom jaw of the staple remover under the first staple (Fig. 1). Tightly squeeze the staple remover handles together.

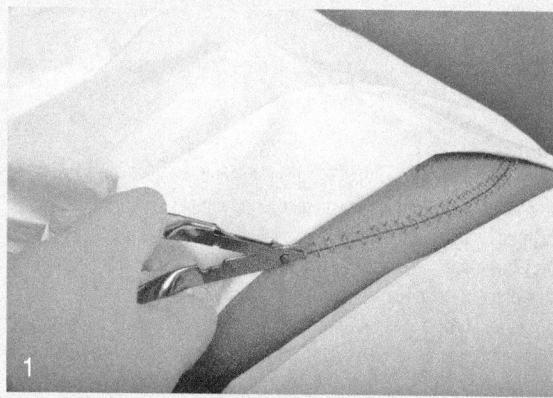

9. Carefully tilt the staple remover upward until the staple lifts out of the wound. Place the removed staple on a 4 × 4-inch gauze square.

10. If any bleeding occurs, blot the area with a sterile gauze sponge before continuing. Continue the process until all staples have been removed.

11. Remove the gauze holding the staples. Count the staples removed. Dispose of staples in the biohazardous sharps container.

12. Apply adhesive skin closure strips or an adhesive bandage strip if ordered by the provider. Instruct the patient to keep the wound edges clean and dry and not to place excessive strain on the area.

13. Clean up the area. Discard the waste in the appropriate waste container. Wash or sanitize hands.

14. Document the procedure, wound condition, number of staples removed, whether adhesive skin closure strips or an adhesive bandage strip were applied, and the instructions on wound care given to the patient.

    Purpose: A procedure that is not documented was not done.

Documentation Example

07/30/20XX 10:35 a.m. Per Dr. Walden's order, staples removed. Wound edges well approximated with 8 intact staples. No sign of infection. Site was cleaned with Betadine, and 8 staples were removed. Pt instructed on home wound care and to notify provider if drainage changes, inflammation increases, or fever occurs. _____ Susie Rana, CMA (AAMA)

PROCEDURE 40.10   Obtain a Wound Culture and Apply a Sterile Dressing

Tasks

Perform a dressing change and obtain a wound culture. Apply a sterile dressing while maintaining aseptic technique. Instruct and prepare the patient for the procedure. Explain the rationale for the procedure. Document the procedure.

Scenario

Dr. Walden orders a dressing change. You are to apply a sterile dressing after you obtain a culture of the wound drainage. As you are beginning the procedure, the patient has questions regarding personal protective equipment (PPE) and the reason for the wound culture. You need to explain the rationale for wearing PPE and why a wound culture is obtained

Directions

Role-play the scenario with a peer. The peer will be the patient, and you are the medical assistant. After the role-play, the rest of the procedure is done on a mannequin. You need to report the wound appearance to the provider (your instructor).

Equipment and Supplies

- Gloves
- Biohazardous waste container
- Sterile water or hydrogen peroxide (optional)
- Disposable ruler

Continued

PROCEDURE 40.10   Obtain a Wound Culture and Apply a Sterile Dressing—cont'd

- Culture swab
- Lab requisition, label, and plastic specimen bag for transport
- Sterile gloves
- Antiseptic swabs
- Sterile dressing and abdominal (ABD) pad
- Tape
- Mannequin with a wound
- Patient's health record

Provider's order: Change dressing and apply a sterile dressing. Culture wound drainage.

Procedural Steps

1. Wash your hands or use hand sanitizer. Assemble supplies on a Mayo stand and place a biohazardous waste container within easy reach.
   Purpose: For infection control.
2. Greet the patient. Identify yourself. Verify the patient's identity with full name and date of birth. Verify the patient's allergies.
3. Instruct and prepare the patient for the procedure. Explain the procedure to be performed in a manner that is understood by the patient. Explain what will occur, what the patient should do during the procedure, how long the procedure will take, and what the patient will sense (e.g., feel, smell). Answer any questions the patient may have on the procedure.
   Purpose: To ensure cooperation and demonstrate awareness of possible patient concerns.
   Scenario update: The patient questions why you need to change gloves so much during the procedure. They also ask why the wound culture needs be done.
4. Based on the patient's comments, explain the reason for changing your gloves during the procedure and also for the wound culture. Demonstrates empathy and appropriate nonverbal communication when addressing the patient's questions and concerns.
   Scenario update: The rest of the steps can be done on a mannequin.
5. Put on gloves. Loosen the tape on the old bandage from the edges to the middle, toward the wound. Remove the bandage and dressing, one at a time. If the dressing is stuck, use a small amount of sterile water or hydrogen peroxide to loosen it (per facility's policy).
6. Check for drainage on the dressing and bandage. Note the color of the drainage. Measure any drainage using a disposable ruler, then discard everything in the biohazardous waste container.
   Purpose: The information on the drainage is needed when documenting the procedure.
7. Assess the wound. If present, count the sutures or staples. Check if they are intact. Check the wound for signs of infection.
   Purpose: This information is needed when documenting the procedure.
   Scenario update: You notice signs of infection at the wound. Report signs of an infected wound to the provider (your instructor).
8. Report relevant information concisely and accurately to the provider.
   Purpose: The provider needs to be informed if the site shows signs of infection.
   Scenario update: The provider orders a wound culture.
9. Culture the wound, by gently rolling the swab stick from margin to margin using a zig-zag motion, using enough pressure to accumulate fluid on the swab. The swab should only touch the wound. After the collection, place the swab in a labeled tube and squeeze the tube to release the formalin if needed. Place the tube in the laboratory transport bag.

10. Remove your gloves and discard them in the biohazardous waste container. Wash your hands or use hand sanitizer.
    Purpose: For infection control.
11. Open and arrange sterile supplies in the order they will be used. Apply the principles of sterile technique.
    Purpose: To prevent contamination of supplies and provide easy access for the provider.
12. Apply sterile gloves (see Procedure 40.3). State that the nondominant hand will be nonsterile and the dominant hand will be sterile.
13. With the nondominant hand, pick up the antiseptic swab container. With the dominant hand, grasp an antiseptic swab without touching the package. Clean from the center of the wound to the edge; use one roll of the swab and discard it in the waste container. Start with a new swab where you left off with the previous swab. Continue until all the exudate is removed.
14. With the dominant hand, remove the sterile dressing without touching the package. Place the sterile dressing material over the wound and cover the wound completely. With the dominant hand, place an ABD pad over the dressing as a bandage.
15. Remove and discard the sterile gloves. Secure the bandage with tape.
    Purpose: The bandage needs to be secure, so it does not fall off.
16. Provide patient education as needed for wound care.
    Purpose: Patient education is a required part of patient care. The patient needs to know how to care for the wound at home.
17. Complete the lab requisition for the culture. Apply gloves and clean up the area. Discard all biohazardous waste in biohazardous waste containers. Discard all other waste in the regular waste containers. Disinfect the tables.
    Purpose: The specimen cannot be processed by the laboratory if it is not labeled or if the requisition is not completed.
18. Remove your gloves and dispose of them appropriately. Wash your hands or use hand sanitizer.
    Purpose: For infection control.
19. Using the patient's health record, document the name of the provider ordering the dressing change, the wound's appearance, the number of intact sutures or staples (if present), the culture obtained, the wound care performed, and the patient education provided.
    Purpose: A procedure that is not documented was not done.
20. In the written response section, discuss the implications for failing to comply with CDC regulations in healthcare settings.

Documentation Example

10/12/20XX 2:15 p.m. Per Dr. Walden's order, dressing change completed to wound on L mid forearm. Area slightly inflamed, moderate amount serosanguineous drainage noted. Site cleansed and sterile dressing applied. Pt instructed on home wound care and to notify provider if drainage changes, inflammation increases, or fever occurs. _____ Susie Rana, CMA (AAMA)

Written Response

You failed to wear gloves when changing a patient's dressing. During the procedure, you got blood on your hands. Discuss the implications for failing to comply with CDC regulations in healthcare settings. Answer the following questions:

1. How might your actions (of not wearing gloves) impact the patient's health and safety?
2. How might your actions (of not wearing gloves) affect your health and safety?

PROCEDURE 40.11 Apply an Elastic Bandage

Tasks

Apply an elastic bandage to the forearm using the spiral wrap technique and to the ankle using a figure-eight wrap technique. Document the procedure.

Equipment and Supplies

- Patient's health record
- Two 3- or 4-inch elastic bandages with clip or Velcro closures
- Provider's order

Provider's order: Apply an elastic bandage to the right arm and right ankle.

Procedural Steps

1. Wash your hands or use hand sanitizer. Read the provider's order. Assemble the necessary supplies.
   Purpose: For infection control.
2. Greet the patient. Identify yourself. Verify the patient's identity with full name and date of birth. Explain the procedure to be performed in a manner that is understood by the patient. Answer any questions the patient may have on the procedure.
   Purpose: It is important to answer the patient's questions before starting a procedure.
3. Hold the roll so the bandage can be rolled away from you (Fig. 1). Using the patient's arm, perform a circular turn at the starting point. Secure a turned down corner of the bandage in the first circle around the arm.

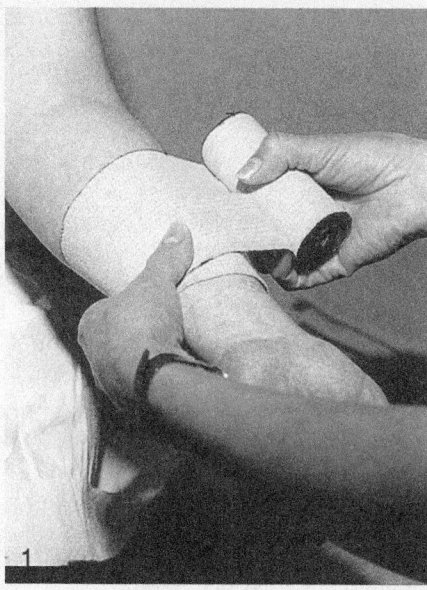

Purpose: Performing a circular turn at the starting point helps to anchor the bandage.

4. Keep the roll close to the patient and keep it facing upward (Fig. 2). With each successive turn, overlap the previous bandage turn by half. Maintain even tension and spacing as you continue to apply the bandage up the forearm.

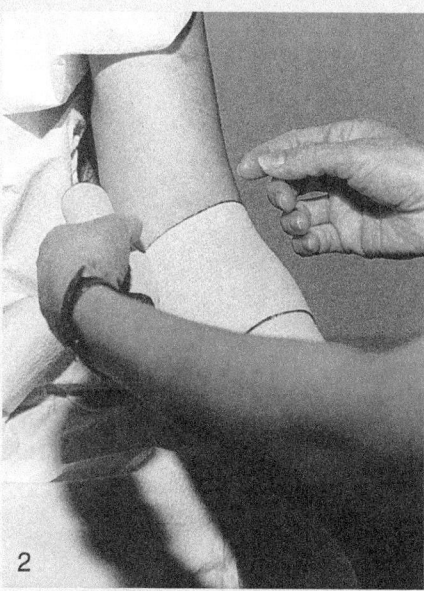

Purpose: To maintain even, light pressure over the entire area.

5. When crossing a joint, slightly flex the joint (Fig. 3).

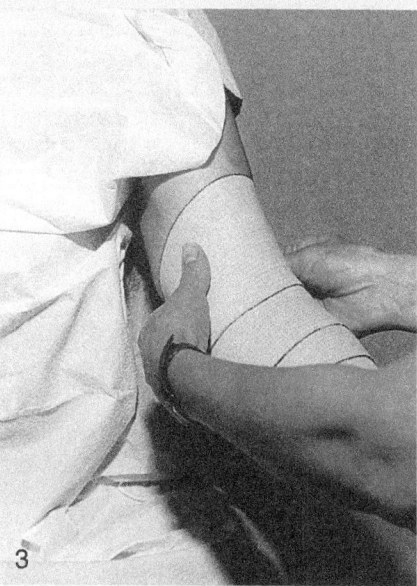

Purpose: To facilitate patient comfort and maintain normal circulation.

6. Ensure the bandage is smooth (Fig. 4). Fasten the end of the bandage with clips, Velcro, or tape.

Continued

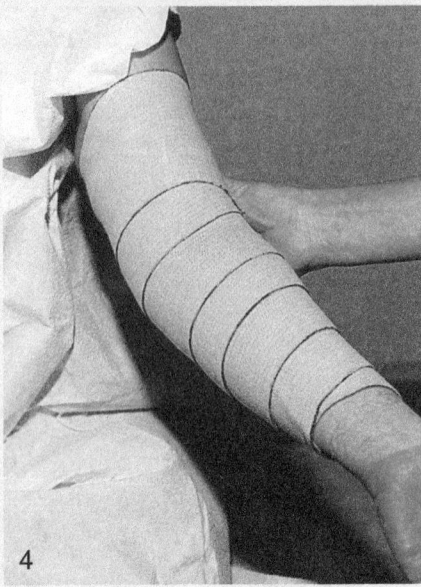

4

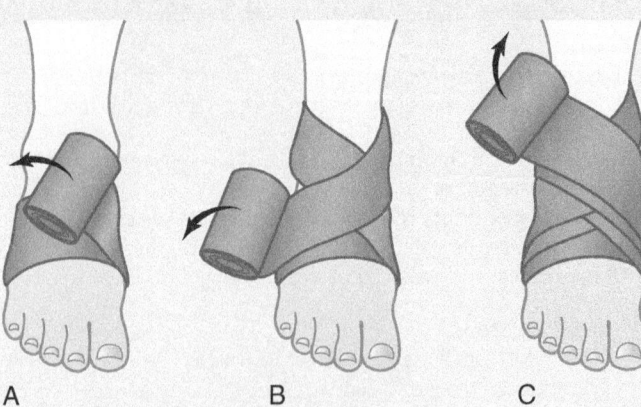

A B C

7. Hold the roll so the bandage can be rolled away from you. Using the patient's ankle, perform a circular turn at the starting point near the most distal part of the foot (near the toes). Secure a turned down corner of the bandage in the first circle around the foot.

Note: The patient's ankle should be at a 90-degree angle. Make sure the end of the bandage is not on the bottom of the foot, which would cause discomfort.

Purpose: Performing a circular turn at the starting point helps to anchor the bandage.

8. Keep the roll close to the patient and keep it facing upward. Slowly circle the bandage around the arch of the foot and then around the ankle (Figs. A and B). With each successive turn, overlap the majority of the previous bandage turn. Maintain even tension and spacing as you continue to apply the bandage on the foot and up the ankle (see Fig. C). The bandage should be smooth.

Purpose: To maintain even, light pressure over the entire area.

9. Fasten the end of the bandage with clips, Velcro, or tape.

10. Check the nail beds for cyanosis; ask the patient whether the bandages are comfortable or feel too tight. Check the pulse on the wrapped extremities. Have the patient move the fingers and toes on the wrapped extremities.

Purpose: To ensure that the bandage is not acting as a tourniquet if applied too tightly.

11. Document the procedure in the patient's health record. Include the name of the provider ordering the bandage, the procedure done, how the patient tolerated the procedure, and instructions given to the patient.

Purpose: The procedure is not completed until it is recorded, dated, and signed.

Documentation Example

10/18/20XX 9:10 a.m. Per Dr. Walden's order, an elastic bandage using a spiral wrap technique was applied to the right forearm, and an elastic bandage using a figure-eight wrap technique was applied to the right foot and ankle. Pt denies bandage too tight. Fingers warm to touch. Explained to patient how to replace bandage if needed and how to check for good circulation in the fingers and toes. Patient verbalized understanding of the information and described signs of poor circulation. _____ Susie Rana, CMA (AAMA)

PROCEDURE 40.12 Apply a Tubular Gauze Bandage

Tasks

To apply a tubular gauze bandage to a patient's finger. Document the procedure.

Equipment and Supplies

- Gloves
- Tubular gauze bandage appropriate size for extremity
- Metal applicator appropriate size for extremity
- Bandage scissor
- Patient's health record
- Provider's order

Provider's order: Apply a tubular gauze bandage to the left hand index finger.

Procedural Steps

1. Wash hands or use hand sanitizer. Read the provider's order. Assemble the necessary supplies.

Purpose: For infection control.

2. Greet the patient. Identify yourself. Verify the patient's identity with full name and date of birth. Explain the procedure to be performed in a manner that is understood by the patient. Answer any questions the patient may have on the procedure

Purpose: To ensure cooperation during the procedure.

3. Instruct the person to lie or sit still during the procedure. Position the patient comfortably.

4. Determine the appropriate applicator and tubular gauze for to use. Apply the tubular gauze to the metal applicator. Add enough gauze for 4 to 6 layers and then extra for tying the gauze if needed. Use the scissor to cut the gauze.

5. Place the applicator over the area to bandage. Hold the edge of the gauze near the base of the finger. Move the applicator toward the tip of the finger as the material slides off the applicator.

6. As the applicator moves beyond the tip of the finger, give the applicator a full half-turn. Place the applicator over the finger and repeat the process until the desired amount of gauze is applied to the finger. Be careful not to create a tourniquet effect when you reverse the applicator.

7. Cut the gauze and tie the gauze to the wrist.

Purpose: This secures the gauze, so it stays on the finger.

8. Check the bandage to ensure it is not too tight and the finger has adequate circulation. Instruct the patient how to check for adequate circulation and what to do if the patient has concerns.

9. Disinfect the applicator. Clean up the work area. Wash or sanitize hands.

Purpose: For infection control.

10. Document the procedure and the patient education in the patient's health record.

Purpose: The procedure is not completed until it is recorded, dated, and signed.

PROCEDURE 40.13 Urinary Catheterization: Insertion of a Straight Catheter to Obtain a Urine Specimen

Task
Place a urinary catheter to collect a urine specimen using sterile technique.

Equipment and Supplies
- Patient's health record
- Gloves
- Waterproof pad (optional)
- Provider's order
- Straight catheterization tray kit, containing:
  - Waterproof pad
  - Fenestrated drape
  - Sterile gloves
  - Presaturated antiseptic swab sticks or antiseptic solution (povidone-iodine or chlorhexidine), sterile cotton balls, and sterile forceps
  - Water-soluble lubrication jelly packet
  - Specimen container with lid
  - Urethral catheter (properly sized)
  - Outer basin tray
- Specimen label
- Mayo stand
- Biohazardous waste container
- Waste container
- Disinfectant wipes for cleaning

Provider's order: UA using a straight catheter for specimen collection.

Procedural Steps
1. Wash your hands or use hand sanitizer. Read the provider's order. Assemble the necessary supplies.
   Purpose: A provider's order is required to gather a urine specimen by a straight catheterization.
2. Greet the patient. Identify yourself. Verify the patient's identity with full name and date of birth. Explain the procedure to be performed in a manner that is understood by the patient. Answer any questions the patient may have on the procedure.
   Purpose: It is important to answer the patient's questions before starting a procedure.
3. Place a waterproof pad on the lower part of the examination table (optional). Provide a drape for the patient. Instruct the person to remove clothing from the waist down and sit on the examination table with the drape over the patient's lap. Give the patient privacy.
   Purpose: To ensure cooperation during the procedure. Having the patient disrobe will allow access to the perineal area.
4. Before entering the room, give a courtesy knock. Ensure adequate lighting.
   Purpose: Adequate lighting is necessary to safely complete the procedure.
5. Position the patient. Place a drape to cover the patient and expose only required anatomic areas.
   Female patient: On the back with the knees flexed and the thighs relaxed so that the hips rotate to expose the perineal area.
   Male patient: Supine with the legs extended and slightly apart.
   Purpose: This provides access to the urethra.
6. Open the kit. Put on sterile gloves using sterile technique (see Procedure 40.3).
7. Using the waterproof pad from the kit, wrap the edges of the pad around your sterile gloved hands. Place the pad between the patient's legs, creating a sterile field.
   Purpose: Wrapping the hands around the edges of the pad protects the sterile gloves from contamination.
8. Working in the sterile field, prepare supplies. Open the antiseptic swab sticks or open the antiseptic solution and pour it over the cotton balls. Open the lubricant packet. Lubricate the tip of the catheter about 1.5 to 2 inches.

Purpose: Lubricant will minimize discomfort and reduce the risk of urethral trauma during the procedure.
9. Clean the perineal area.

Female Patient
- Separate the labia with the fingers of your nondominant hand. This will contaminate the hand, and it can no longer be used in the sterile field. This hand will continue to hold the labia until the catheter is inserted.
- With the dominant hand, pick up a swab stick or use the forceps and pick up a cotton ball. Using the swab stick or cotton ball, wipe down the center over the urinary meatus toward the rectum. If you use the swab stick, rotate the swab as you wipe. Discard the swab stick or cotton ball.
- Repeat the previous step and wipe down both the right and left sides. Discard the swab stick or cotton ball after each wipe (each side).

Male Patient
- Gently grasp the penis shaft and hold it at a right angle to the body with the nondominant hand. If the patient is uncircumcised, use this hand to gently retract the foreskin. (After the catheter is inserted, make sure to push the foreskin back to the original position.) This will contaminate the hand. This hand will continue to hold the penis until the catheter is inserted.
- With the dominant hand, pick up a swab stick or use the forceps and pick up a cotton ball. Using the swab stick or cotton ball, wipe the center of the urinary meatus and work outward in a circular manner. If you use the swab stick, rotate the stick as you wipe. Discard the swab stick or cotton ball after the first circle. Continue, using another new swab stick or cotton ball for each progressively larger circle.
   Purpose: This will reduce the number of microbes in the area of catheter insertion and minimize the transmission of microorganisms.
10. Place the sterile collection cup in the sterile tray. Place the tray between the patient's legs. Place the end of the catheter in the sterile collection cup. Pick up the catheter with the sterile dominant hand approximately 2 to 3 inches from the tip.
    Purpose: The sterile cup will catch urine as it starts to flow. Holding the catheter closer to the tip will help to control it during insertion. Holding the catheter too close to the tip risks contaminating the sterile hand by touching the patient during insertion.
11. Insert the catheter. If you meet resistance while inserting the catheter, do not force the catheter. Discontinue the procedure if continued resistance is met or if the patient is having unusual discomfort or pain. Talk with the provider.

Female
- Ask the patient to bear down gently to help expose the urethral meatus.
- Insert the catheter 2 to 3 inches into the meatus until urine starts to flow.
- Do not force the catheter.
  Note: If urine does not appear, the catheter may be in the patient's vagina. You may leave the catheter in place as a landmark and insert another sterile catheter into the urinary meatus. The catheter in the vagina is no longer sterile. Do not reuse that catheter. Do not allow the new catheter to come into contact with the previous catheter.

Male
- With the nondominant hand (which is holding the penis at a right angle to the body), pull up slightly on the shaft.
- Ask the patient to bear down gently and slowly insert the catheter through the urethral meatus. Advance the catheter 6 to 8 inches until urine flows.
- Do not force the catheter. Ask the patient to take deep breaths and try again.
  Note: If the catheter does not advance in the male patient, do not force it. The patient may have an enlarged prostate or urethral obstruction.

Continued

PROCEDURE 40.13   Urinary Catheterization: Insertion of a Straight Catheter to Obtain a Urine Specimen—cont'd

12. Once the specimen is obtained, secure the cover on the container. Make sure not to touch the inside of the container or cover. Set the specimen container on the Mayo stand.

    Purpose: The inner surface of the specimen container and cover are sterile and needs to remain sterile.

13. Remove the catheter by pulling out slowly and smoothly. Wrap the used catheter in the waterproof pad.

    Purpose: This will prevent accidental spilling of urine from the catheter.

14. Discard all biohazardous waste in the biohazardous waste container. Discard all other waste in the waste container. Remove your gloves and discard them in the biohazardous waste container. Wash or sanitize your hands.

15. After the patient has dressed and left the room, put on gloves and disinfect the examination table and Mayo stand. Label the urine specimen.

16. Remove the gloves and dispose of them appropriately. Wash your hands or use hand sanitizer.

17. Using the patient's health record, document the procedure. Include the ordering provider's name, the size of the catheter inserted, how the patient tolerated the procedure, and the urine output.

Documentation Example

12/11/20XX 10:10 a.m. Per Dr. Walden's order, urine specimen obtained through use of 16 Fr straight catheter. Patient tolerated the procedure well with minimal discomfort. 50 mL of clear, pale yellow urine obtained. Specimen sent to lab.
_____ Susie Rana, CMA(AAMA)

PROCEDURE 40.14   Urinary Catheterization: Insertion of an Indwelling Foley Catheter

Task
Insert an indwelling catheter with a drainage bag using sterile technique.

Equipment and Supplies
- Patient's health record
- Gloves
- Waterproof pad (optional)
- Provider's order
- Straight catheterization tray kit containing:
  - Waterproof pad
  - Fenestrated drape
  - Sterile gloves
  - Presaturated antiseptic swab sticks or antiseptic solution (povidone-iodine or chlorhexidine), sterile cotton balls, and sterile forceps
  - Water-soluble lubrication jelly packet or syringe
  - Indwelling urethral catheter connected to a urine drainage bag
  - Prefilled syringe with fluid
- Mayo stand
- Biohazardous waste container
- Waste container
- Disinfectant wipes for cleaning

Provider's order: Insert Foley catheter.

Procedural Steps

1. Wash your hands or use hand sanitizer. Read the provider's order. Assemble the necessary supplies.

   Purpose: A provider's order is required to insert a Foley catheter.

2. Greet the patient. Identify yourself. Verify the patient's identity with full name and date of birth. Explain the procedure to be performed in a manner that is understood by the patient. Answer any questions the patient may have on the procedure.

   Purpose: It is important to answer the patient's questions before starting a procedure.

3. Place a waterproof pad on the lower part of the examination table. Provide a drape for the patient. Instruct the person to remove clothing from the waist down and sit on the examination table with the drape covering the patient's lap. Give the patient privacy.

   Purpose: To ensure cooperation during the procedure. Having the patient disrobe will allow access to the perineal area.

4. Before entering the room, give a courtesy knock. Ensure adequate lighting.

   Purpose: Adequate lighting is necessary to safely complete the procedure.

5. Position the patient. Place a drape to cover the patient and expose only the required anatomic areas.

   Female patient: On the back with the knees flexed and the thighs relaxed so that the hips rotate to expose the perineal area.

   Male patient: Supine with the legs extended and slightly apart.

   Purpose: This provides access to the urethra.

6. Put on clean gloves. Open the outer kit wrap.

   Purpose: Standard Precautions should be observed while cleaning the area and preparing the patient for the procedure.

7. Cleanse the perineal area with wipes from the kit or a with a washcloth, warm water, and soap or a perineal cleanser, according to facility policy.

   Purpose: Cleaning removes any secretions and reduces the risk of urinary tract infection (UTI).

8. Remove and dispose of gloves. Use hand sanitizer to perform hand hygiene.

9. Carefully open the catheterization kit, avoiding contaminating the sterile interior.

   Purpose: This will serve as your sterile field and keep supplies needed free of microbes.

10. Put on sterile gloves using sterile technique (see Procedure 40.3).

11. Using the waterproof pad from the kit, wrap the edges of the pad around your sterile gloved hands. Place it between the patient's legs, creating a sterile field.

    Purpose: Wrapping hands around edges protects the sterile gloves from contamination.

12. Place the fenestrated drape on the patient, only exposing the perineum or penis.

    Purpose: This will provide a sterile surface around the patient, which works to minimize the risk of contamination of the supplies and minimize the risk of UTI.

13. Working in the sterile field, prepare supplies. Open antiseptic swab sticks or open the antiseptic solution and pour it over the cotton balls. Open the lubricant packet or use the lubricant jelly syringe and place the water-soluble jelly on the tray. Remove the plastic upper tray from the bottom tray and place it nearby.

    Purpose: The upper plastic tray will remain as a sterile field.

14. In the lower tray, place the water-filled syringe to the inflation port on the catheter. If required by the facility's procedures, check the Foley catheter's balloon. Push the plunger of the syringe, filling the balloon. Make sure the balloon fills correctly and there are no leaks or tears. Withdraw the fluid from the balloon. Keep the syringe attached to the catheter. Make sure the tubing to empty the Foley bag is closed.

    Purpose: Checking the integrity of the balloon helps reduce the risk of the catheter malfunctioning and falling out.

15. Lubricate the tip of the catheter about 1.5 to 2 inches. Make sure to keep the catheter sterile.

PROCEDURE 40.14 Urinary Catheterization: Insertion of an Indwelling Foley Catheter—cont'd

Purpose: Lubricant will minimize discomfort and reduce the risk of urethral trauma during the procedure.

16. Clean the perineal area:

Female Patient

- Separate the labia with the fingers of the nondominant hand; this will contaminate the hand, and it can no longer be used in the sterile field. This hand will continue to hold the labia until the catheter is inserted.
- With the dominant hand, pick up a swab stick or use the forceps and pick up a cotton ball. Using the swab stick or cotton ball, wipe down the center over the urinary meatus toward the rectum. If you use the swab stick, rotate the swab as you wipe. Discard the swab stick or cotton ball.
- Repeat the previous step and wipe down both the right and left sides. Discard the swab stick or cotton ball after each wipe (each side).

Male Patient

- Gently grasp the penis shaft and hold it at a right angle to the body with the nondominant hand. If the patient is uncircumcised, use this hand to gently retract the foreskin. (After the catheter is inserted, make sure to push the foreskin back to the original position.) This will contaminate the hand. This hand will continue to hold the penis until the catheter is inserted.
- With the dominant hand, pick up a swab stick or use the forceps and pick up a cotton ball. Using the swab stick or cotton ball, wipe the center of the urinary meatus and work outward in a circular manner. If you use the swab stick, rotate the stick as you wipe. Discard the swab stick or cotton ball after the first circle. Continue, using another new swab stick or cotton ball for each progressively larger circle.

  Purpose: This will reduce the number of microbes in the area of catheter insertion and minimize the transmission of microorganisms.

17. Pick up the catheter and the lower tray with the sterile dominant hand. Place the bottom tray between the patient's legs. Make sure to hold the catheter approximately 2 to 3 inches from the tip.

    Purpose: Holding the catheter closer to the tip will help to control it during insertion. Holding it too close to the tip risks contaminating the sterile hand by touching the patient during insertion.

18. Insert the catheter. If you meet resistance while inserting the catheter, do not force the catheter. Discontinue the procedure if continued resistance is met or if the patient is having unusual discomfort or pain. Talk with the provider.

Female

- Ask the patient to bear down gently to help expose the urethral meatus.
- Insert the catheter 2 to 3 inches into the meatus until urine starts to flow. Then advance the catheter an additional 1 to 2 inches to ensure it is in the bladder.
- Release the labia with the nondominant hand and hold the catheter in place as the dominant hand inflates the balloon. Disconnect the syringe and gently pull on the catheter until you feel resistance.

  Note: If urine does not appear, the catheter may be in the patient's vagina. You may leave the catheter in place as a landmark and insert another sterile catheter into the urinary meatus. The catheter in the vagina is no longer sterile. Do not reuse that catheter. Do not allow the new catheter to come into contact with the previous catheter.

Male

- With the nondominant hand (which is holding the penis at a right angle to the body), pull up slightly on the shaft.
- Ask the patient to bear down gently and slowly insert the catheter through the urethral meatus. Advance the catheter 6 to 8 inches until urine flows. Then advance the catheter an additional 1 to 2 inches to ensure it is in the bladder.

- Hold the catheter in place with the nondominant hand while the dominant hand inflates the balloon. Disconnect the syringe and gently pull on the catheter until you feel resistance.

  Note: If the catheter does not advance in the male patient, do not force it. The patient may have an enlarged prostate or urethral obstruction.

19. Secure the catheter on the thigh with tape or a catheter holder. Allow enough slack to prevent tension. Ensure the catheter is not secured too tightly, affecting movement or blocking urine drainage.

    Purpose: The catheter holder has an elastic band that is placed round the thigh and a Velcro strip that is used to secure the catheter.

20. Discard all biohazardous waste in the biohazardous waste container. Discard all other waste in the waste container. Remove your gloves and discard them in the biohazardous waste container. Wash your hands. After the patient has dressed and left the room, put on gloves and disinfect the examination table and Mayo stand.

21. Remove the gloves and dispose of them appropriately. Wash your hands or use hand sanitizer.

22. Using the patient's health record, document the procedure. Include the ordering provider's name, size of the catheter inserted, how the patient tolerated the procedure, and the urine output.

Documentation Example

12/11/20XX 10:10 a.m. Per Dr. Walden's order, 16 Fr Foley catheter inserted. Patient tolerated the procedure well with minimal discomfort. Within 5 minutes, 100 mL of clear, pale yellow urine drained. Patient instructed on how to drain urine from bag and how to maintain Foley catheter system at home. _____
_____Susie Rana, CMA (AAMA)

Scenario update: The patient returns for removal of the indwelling Foley catheter.

23. Wash your hands or use hand sanitizer. Read the provider's order. Assemble the necessary supplies. Place a waterproof pad on the lower part of the examination table.

    Purpose: A provider's order is required to remove a Foley catheter.

24. Greet the patient. Identify yourself. Verify the patient's identity with full name and date of birth. Explain the procedure to be performed in a manner that is understood by the patient. Answer any questions the patient may have on the procedure. Instruct the person to remove clothing from the waist down and sit on the examination table; provide a drape for them to place over their lap. Put on nonsterile gloves.

25. Measure the contents of the catheter bag. Empty urine from the bag. Remove any securement or anchor device from the patient's thigh.

26. If indicated by the facility's procedures, clean around the meatus and catheter using soap and water or an antiseptic solution. Always wipe away from the urethral meatus and use a new cloth or swab with each wipe.

    Purpose: This will reduce the transfer of microorganisms into the urethra.

27. Attach a syringe to the inflation port on the catheter. Verify the balloon size on the catheter. Withdraw that amount of fluid from the balloon.

    Purpose: A partially deflated balloon will cause trauma to the urethral wall.

28. Remove the catheter by pulling out slowly and smoothly. If resistance is met, it might mean that fluid is still in the balloon. Reattach the syringe and pull back any remaining fluid. Continue to remove the catheter and wrap the used catheter in the waterproof pad

    Purpose: This will prevent accidental spilling of urine from the catheter.

29. Discard waste in the appropriate waste containers. Wash or sanitize your hands. Using the patient's health record, document the procedure

Documentation Example

12/28/20XX 10:10 a.m. Per Dr. Walden's order, indwelling Foley catheter removed. Patient tolerated the procedure well with minimal discomfort. Drained 250 mL of clear, pale yellow urine._____Susie Rana, CMA (AAMA)

41

Patient Coaching With Health Promotion

LEARNING OBJECTIVES

1. Describe the medical assistant's role as a coach.
2. Discuss the stages of grief and how the health belief model helps to explain what factors influence a person's health beliefs and practices.
3. Describe the three domains of learning.
4. Explain how a medical assistant can adapt coaching to the patient.
5. Describe the teaching-learning process.
6. Discuss how a medical assistant can coach on disease prevention.
7. Describe how a medical assistant can coach on health maintenance and wellness, including different types of self-exams and screenings.
8. Perform a monofilament foot exam.
9. Describe how a medical assistant can coach on diagnostic procedures and treatment plans.
9. Describe care coordination and patient navigation, develop a list of community resources, and facilitate referrals.

OUTLINE

 OPENING SCENARIO

Suzanne Peterson, CMA (AAMA), has worked for Walden-Martin Family Medicine (WMFM) Clinic for 5 years. Her favorite part of her job is coaching patients on health topics, diagnostic tests, and treatment plans. Her patients know they can contact Suzanne if they have questions between appointments. Suzanne answers the questions she can and talks with the providers for other questions. She feels that it is very important for patients to understand how to self-manage their conditions and to know when to contact their providers.

Over the years, Suzanne has seen the role of the medical assistant expand. She has learned the importance of screening patients during the initial interview. The information that she enters into the electronic health record is then used to collect data on how well the clinic provides patient care. She has also learned the importance of patient care coordinators. She hopes WMFM Clinic implements a care coordinator program soon.

YOU WILL LEARN

1. To apply the basics of teaching and learning, including the domains of learning and how to adapt coaching to patients.
2. To perform common coaching as required for disease prevention, including cough hygiene, nicotine cessation, and vaccinations.
3. To perform coaching as required for health maintenance, including self-exams and screenings.
4. To perform coaching as required for common diagnostic tests.
5. To perform coaching as required for treatment plans, including medication administration.
6. To coordinate care, navigate patients, and make community resource referrals.

INTRODUCTION

Healthcare is changing, and the role of the medical assistant is changing, too. Some of the current challenges in healthcare include:
- Pressure to reduce costs.
- Shorter primary care provider visits, yet an increased need for data collection to incorporate patient interviews and outcome measurements (e.g., test results).
- Patients leaving the facility not understanding what they were told.
- An unwillingness on the part of patients to adhere to treatment plans (e.g., not taking medication or not taking it correctly, not making lifestyle changes that would improve their health).

Many experts have researched ways to meet these challenges. Several studies have examined patient medication adherence (ad HEER uh ns) or compliance (kuhm PLIE uhns). Medication adherence means patients are taking the right dose at the right times as prescribed by the provider. Research has shown that medication adherence with chronic diseases is low. This leads to the progression of the disease and more medical visits for the patient. Ultimately, nonadherence to medication is increasing the cost of healthcare.

Why is it that patients do not take their medication correctly? This question has been a focus of many studies. Common reasons include:
- Forgetfulness and confusion on how to take it
- Side effects and cost of the medication
- Feeling it is not helping

Research has shown that many patients are confused after seeing their providers. Patients do not always understand the treatment plan designed to manage their conditions. Confusion about medication and home care is prevalent. Many patients are not able to manage their disease adequately between provider visits; thus their condition worsens. To solve this problem,

ambulatory care facilities are moving toward coaching and care coordination. This chapter focuses on the medical assistant's role in coaching and care coordination.

> **VOCABULARY**
> **adherence** The act of sticking to something.
> **compliance** The act of following through on a request or demand. "Patient compliance" sounds negative, thus *patient adherence* is now being used.
> **cessation** A bringing to an end.

COACHING

Coaching provides patients with skills, knowledge, support, and confidence to manage their disease between provider visits. One study found that coaching by medical assistants increased the patients' compliance with medication regimens and lifestyle changes. Coaching is extremely valuable for patients. The medical assistant can coach patients in many areas.

- *Disease prevention*: Provide patients with information on preventing the disease or the spread of disease. Medical assistants can provide information on respiratory hygiene, recommended vaccines, and nicotine cessation (se SAY shuhn).
- *Health maintenance*: Provide patients with information on routine screenings and show patients how to do self-exams (e.g., foot, breast, and oral self-exams).
- *Diagnostic tests*: Instruct patients prior to diagnostic tests. This can include special preparation (e.g., fasting and bowel cleansing preparations).
- *Treatment plans*: Instruct patients on home care and follow-up as ordered by the provider. Research has shown that coaching can help patients understand information from the visit. It can ensure patients understand how they need to proceed and addresses any concerns before patients leave the facility. Coaching educates patients on self-management of diseases, thus increasing compliance with the treatment plans.
- *Specific needs*: Patients have unique concerns. These can include personal, family, social, financial, and culture-related issues. By closely working with the patient, the medical assistant can provide emotional support and create a bond with the patient. This bond helps the patient feel comfortable. With encouragement, the patient may be more willing to call the medical assistant with questions and concerns between visits.
- *Community resources*: By listening to patients and by asking questions, the medical assistant can identify patients' unique needs. Patients have many needs that affect their health. For instance, if a patient has a limited income, does the patient purchase the prescribed medication, or food? Community resources exist to address many needs, including low-cost medications, food banks, transportation, medical supplies, assisted living, and so on.

This chapter provides information on specific aspects of patient education required for these coaching areas. But first, let us examine health beliefs and practices and how to adapt education to patients' needs.

TABLE 41.1   Stages of Grief and Dying

Stage	Description	Adaptive Interactions
Denial	Refuses to accept the fact (i.e., diagnosis or prognosis). May refuse to discuss the diagnosis. May not remember the health coaching. Denial is a defense mechanism that allows the person to ignore what is happening.	Provide handouts that explain the disease and treatment. Encourage family member(s') support with the treatment. Provide online and community resources (i.e., support groups).
Anger	Anger can be directed at oneself or others. Anger can surface at unrelated times and be directed toward unrelated issues.	Use therapeutic communication techniques (e.g., reflection) to acknowledge the patient's feelings about the issue. Recognize the real cause of the anger.
Bargaining	Attempts to bargain with the higher power the person believes in (e.g., God). Sometimes the patient will bargain with the provider to make lifestyle changes at a later time.	Work with the healthcare team regarding the bargaining requests. Help provide opportunities for the patient to make decisions.
Depression	People feel sadness, fear, and uncertainty. They may grieve the loss of their health or independence. They may dread the change that is occurring.	Encourage the use of community and healthcare resources to help ease the change process for the patient and family members.
Acceptance	Has come to terms with the situation.	Provide coaching on aspects of the disease and self-care management.

MAKING CHANGES FOR HEALTH

Often, healthcare professionals see patients who do not comply with the treatment plan. They may not take the prescribed medication, or maybe they do not make the recommended lifestyle changes. If the diagnosis is life-threatening or life-changing, grief and loss can occur. Other times, patients may not perceive the change as necessary. The following sections examine theories that may explain why patients do not comply with the treatment plan.

Stages of Grief

Elisabeth Kübler-Ross studied people's reactions to death and dying. She found that people experienced similar stages. Over the years, these stages have been applied to grief and loss. When a patient and the family get a life-threatening or life-changing diagnosis, they can feel grief and loss. People go through the stages of grief in their own way and at their own pace (Table 41.1). This process can take weeks to months. Patients may not be open to making the recommended changes. Healthcare professionals may view this as the patient not wanting to comply with the treatment plan. Sometimes a patient must accept a diagnosis before compliance occurs. It is important for the medical assistant to be supportive, to use empathy when communicating with patients, and to adapt interactions to help with the stages of grief.

> **CRITICAL THINKING 41.1**
>
> Suzanne has seen many patients dealing with grief. Why might a patient who is grieving not adhere to a treatment plan?

Health Belief Model

The health belief model helps explain what factors influence a person's health beliefs and practices. The first part of this model deals with a person's perception of their chance of developing a disease. For example:

- Jess is in her 20s and has lost her mother, sister, and grandmother to breast cancer. She feels her chance of developing breast cancer is significant.
- Sam has an older brother with heart disease that is being managed by medication, diet, and exercise. Sam blames the

disease on his brother's stressful job. Sam does not have a stressful job, so he feels he will not get heart disease. Even though Sam receives education on a heart-healthy lifestyle, he ignores the information.

The second part of this model deals with a person's perception of the severity of the disease. A person's perception is influenced by:

- Personal factors (e.g., age, gender, race, employment)
- Social factors (e.g., peers, personality, family)
- Perceived threats of the disease
- Cues to action (e.g., mass media campaigns, social media, advice from family, friends, and healthcare providers and professionals)

In the prior examples, Jess has lost three family members to breast cancer. She perceives breast cancer as being a severe disease. Sam, on the other hand, may not perceive the severity of heart disease, because his brother's heart disease is being managed.

The third part of the model focuses on whether the person will take preventive action. A person weighs the benefits of and barriers to taking the preventive actions. For example, Jess may decide to have a double mastectomy as a preventive strategy. For many it may seem severe, but for Jess, she is willing to take such a preventive action. Sam, on the other hand, may not see the benefit of following a heart-healthy lifestyle. He may feel that he must "give up" his current lifestyle and make changes.

It is important to remember this model when coaching patients on preventive actions. Start with identifying if the person perceives they are at risk for a disease. Exploring the patient's beliefs and educating the patient on the facts, in addition to getting rid of the myths, can be helpful. Discussing the severity of the disease or what the disease can lead to is the next important step. Finally, offering the patient help in eliminating or diminishing the barriers and helping the person see the benefits of the preventive action are important.

> **CRITICAL THINKING 41.2**
>
> Suzanne has had patients state they do not want to give up their lifestyle and follow the provider's recommendations for better health. How might a medical assistant address this issue with a patient?

TABLE 41.2 Strategies and Barriers With the Three Domains of Learning

	DOMAIN		
	Cognitive	**Psychomotor**	**Affective**
Involves	Learning new concepts and information	Learning new skill or procedure	A change in attitude or emotions that will influence the person's behavior
Teaching strategies to use	Discussion, written information, online videos, computer instruction	Demonstration and return demonstration	Discussion, role-play, and simulations
Barriers to learning	Memory or cognition issues; language barriers	Tremors and paralysis; sensory limitations (e.g., visual impairment, hearing impairment)	Anxiety, denial, pain, fatigue, or stress; cultural customs; previous experience; poor coping skills
Strategies for adapting to barriers	Keep it simple. Provide easy-to-read handouts. Use an interpreter and provide handouts in the patient's primary language if possible	Use adaptive equipment, such as a magnifying glass and a magnifier for syringes	Provide analgesics as ordered by the provider, help to minimize barriers, provide home instructions, and include additional family member(s) if possible

BASICS OF TEACHING AND LEARNING

Domains of Learning

Learning is the process of gaining new knowledge or skills through instruction, experience, or study. We learn new information in three different ways or domains: cognitive, psychomotor, and affective. These domains are discussed in the coming sections.

Cognitive Domain. The *cognitive domain* of learning involves the mental processes of recall, application, and evaluation. We learn new information by listening to what is said and by reading written words. Many experts believe we have three ways to store memories:

- *Sensory stage*: For a memory to be created, we must pick up something from our senses (e.g., touch, hearing, sight). Our senses are constantly picking up perceptions. Many will be forgotten in a split second. We will pay attention to just a few, and they will move to the short-term memory. The deciding factor between what is forgotten and what moves into the short-term memory is based on its importance to us.
- *Short-term memory*: This is our temporary working memory. If nothing is done with the memory, it will fade within 30 seconds. The short-term memory can only handle about seven units of information at once. By chunking information into meaningful units or attaching it to something we already know, we can increase the amount in our short-term memory.
- *Long-term memory*: The more we use short-term memories, the quicker they enter our long-term memory. We can add endless memories to our long-term memory, but without use (recall), those memories can fade.

Our goal for patient education is to put the information into patients' long-term memory. Not everything we tell the patient will be picked up and remembered. We hope the important information will be. The following tips can be used to help patients remember critical information.

- *Present the information at an appropriate level for the patient.* Most studies show that patient education literature should be at a sixth-grade reading level. According to the US National Library of Medicine's website (https://medlineplus.gov/), patient educational materials should be between a seventh- and eighth-grade reading level. If the patient's primary language is not English, then a lower reading level is needed.
- *Build on the patient's prior knowledge about the topic.* Start by finding out what the patient knows about the topic. Clarify any inaccurate information and then provide new information that builds on the existing knowledge.
- *Present information in small chunks in a clear, well-organized manner.* Do not overwhelm the patient; keep to the facts and keep it simple. For complex topics, meeting with the patient over several days may help the patient to retain the information.
- *Provide the information in two different ways.* For example, discuss the information with the patient and then provide a written handout.
- *Tell the patient, "This is important to remember," and repeat important information several times during the session.* Be aware that if everything is "important to remember," nothing will be remembered. Do not overuse this strategy.
- *Have the patient "teach back" the information you provided.* This allows you to check what the patient recalls and if it is accurate. Teaching back also enhances the patient's ability to remember the information.

Table 41.2 provides strategies to use for the cognitive domain. The *barriers*, or reasons learning does not occur effectively, are also listed. These barriers are important for the medical assistant to limit if possible.

Psychomotor Domain. The *psychomotor domain* is the "doing" domain. We learn new skills and procedures by watching demonstrations and assisting with something. Many people would prefer to attempt a skill versus reading about it or discussing it. They learn best through the psychomotor domain. Table 41.2 provides some barriers to the psychomotor domain.

Some tips to help patients remember critical information include:

- Provide written step-by-step directions for the patient to follow and then take home.
- Give timely feedback on the person's performance.
- Have the patient teach back the skill or do a return demonstration to check for accuracy (Fig. 41.1).

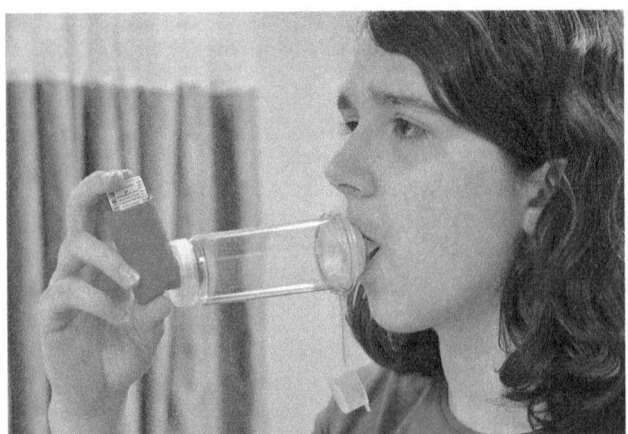

Fig. 41.1 Have Patients Do a Return Demonstration.

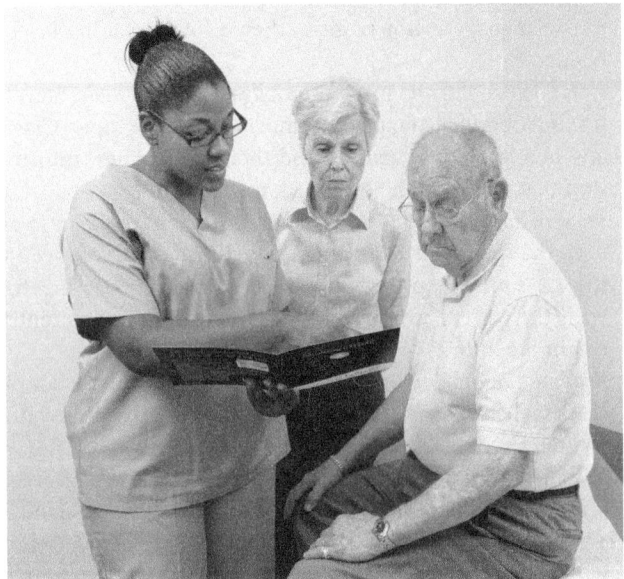

Fig. 41.2 Teaching the family member along with the patient can provide the patient with more support. (From Niedzwiecki B, et al: *Kinn's the medical assistant,* ed 14, St. Louis, 2020, Elsevier.)

- Repeated practice doing the skill helps with recall and retention of the steps.
- Make sure to use the equipment and supplies the patient will be using at home.

Affective Domain. The *affective domain* is the "feeling" domain. It includes our feelings, emotions, values, and attitudes. Our emotions and values are very important. They affect our motivation, confidence, and priorities. When our personal values conflict with the new information presented, a barrier to learning can occur. Pain is another example of an affective barrier. If you are instructing a patient on wound care and they are in pain, they may not remember what you said. Additional barriers to the affective domain are listed in Table 41.2.

Make sure that you address (as much as you can) any affective domain barriers prior to educating a patient. If another family member has accompanied the patient, it can be helpful to instruct both the patient and the family member (Fig. 41.2). Written home instructions should also be given.

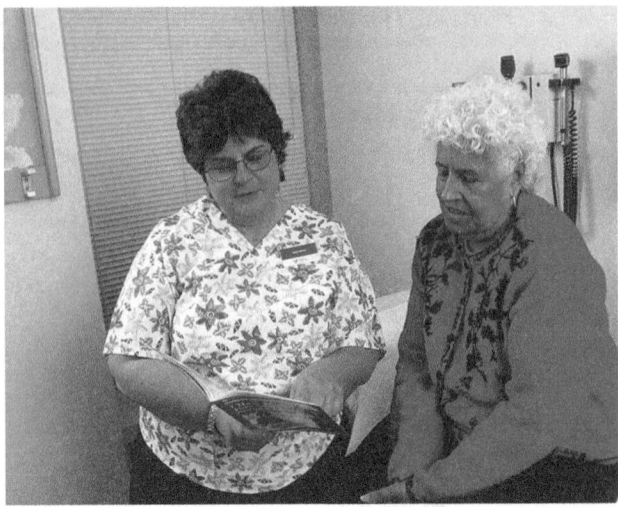

Fig. 41.3 When coaching a patient, make sure to be at the patient's level. Referencing materials as you talk can be helpful to the patient. (From Niedzwiecki B, et al: *Kinn's the medical assistant,* ed 14, St. Louis, 2020, Elsevier.)

Adapting Coaching to the Patient

When you coach patients, it is important to recognize that they are individuals. One way of presenting new information to a patient may not work for another patient. It is important for the medical assistant to consider the barriers to learning and possible ways to help the patient overcome those barriers. It is also important for the medical assistant to remember the patient's developmental level and possible cultural diversity issues that may affect learning.

Developmental Level. As we grow and develop, our thought processes and behaviors change. We learn differently. We can understand more complex concepts than when we were younger. It is important for the medical assistant to consider the person's developmental level when coaching. For instance, young children are concrete thinkers. What you say is what they believe you will do. For example, if you say, "I am going to take your blood pressure," a 2-year-old child would have no idea what you are going to do. If you say, "I am going to give your arm a hug," then the child may have a better understanding of what you are going to do. Coaching techniques you use for teens will be different from those you use with older adults (Fig. 41.3). Also, referencing materials as you talk can be helpful to the patient.

Erikson's psychosocial developmental stages can be useful when considering the developmental level of patients. Understanding the goal of each stage can help a medical assistant to coach patients in that age group. Table 41.3 provides coaching tips based on the developmental stages.

CRITICAL THINKING 41.3

In the family practice environment, Suzanne sees patients of all ages. Explain why the methods she uses with 2-year-old children should differ from those she uses when working with teens. What strategies could she use when coaching both populations?

TABLE 41.3   Erikson's Psychosocial Development Stages With Coaching Tips

Development Stage	Goals of Stage	Coaching Tips
Trust versus mistrust (age range 0–1.5 years [*infancy*])	Must develop trust, with the ability to mistrust should the need arise.	Use a calm, soothing voice, hold child securely. Involve the parent(s) as much as possible. Keep routines consistent as much as possible (if it is time for the infant to eat, allow the child to eat unless eating/drinking is restricted for a medical reason).
Autonomy versus shame and doubt (age range 1.5–3 years [*toddler*])	Must explore and manipulate things in their "world" to develop autonomy and self-esteem.	Use simple, familiar words. Allow child to handle equipment and make choices. Use play to teach the child.
Initiative versus guilt (age range 3–6 years [*preschool*])	Encourage to try new activities. Must assume responsibilities and learn new skills. Will make child feel purposeful and increase self-esteem.	Use familiar words and simple explanations and demonstrations. Allow the child to handle equipment and make choices. Explain a procedure as the child would sense it (e.g., how it feels, looks).
Industry versus inferiority (age range 6–12 years [*school age*])	Must seek to finish tasks. Recognition for accomplishments is important.	Use engaging simple tools to communicate information (videos, gaming software, and pamphlets). Encourage discussion, questions, and making choices. Use concrete terms (with pictures and diagrams) when explaining procedures.
Identity versus role confusion (age range 12–18 years [*adolescence*])	To know who you are as a person and how you fit into the world around you. Creates a meaningful self-image.	Provide privacy and independence. Encourage responsible decision making. Encourage discussion and questions. Address how a procedure might affect the adolescent's appearance. Promote honest discussion about lifestyle issues.
Intimacy versus isolation (age range 18–25 years [*young adult*])	Can vary. Develops friendships; takes on commitments.	Identify motivating factors. Find out what they know about the topic; correct any inaccuracies. Build on prior information. Listen to their concerns and provide resources as needed.
Generativity versus stagnation (age range about 25–60 years [*middle adulthood*])	Achieve a balance between the concern for the next generation (having a family) and being self-absorbed.	
Ego integrity versus despair (age range 60 or older [*late adulthood*])	Reflect on one's life and come to terms with it instead of regretting the past.	Communicate with dignity and respect. Use simpler language. Speak clearly. Allow time to respond. Find out what they know about the topic; correct any inaccuracies. Build on prior information. Listen to their concerns and provide resources as needed.

Cultural Diversity. *Culture* is the set of behaviors, ideas, and customs shared by a specific group of people that distinguishes the members from other people. Some characteristics of a culture group may include its language, religious beliefs, geographic origin, ethnicity, history, sexual orientation, and socioeconomic class. Culture can be learned from prior generations and passed on to future generations. It is dynamic and evolving. Our culture frames and shapes how we feel about our health and the world around us. Factors affected by a person's culture that healthcare professionals should consider include:

- Role of the family and community: Who makes the healthcare decisions? Who pays for the healthcare? Who needs to be present during healthcare discussions?
- Religion: What are the beliefs about illness? Will the person's religious beliefs affect adherence to the treatment?
- Views on health, wellness, death, and dying
- Views on complementary therapies (e.g., chiropractic care, massage) and alternative therapies (other practices used in place of conventional medicine)
- Views on gender roles and relationships
- Beliefs related to food, diet, illness, and health
- Beliefs regarding sexuality, fertility, and childbirth

In the United States, disease conditions are seen as more of a scientific situation. Science plays a major role in medicine. Many other cultures take more of a holistic approach. A *holistic approach* focuses on the interrelationship among the physical, mental, social, and spiritual aspects of the person's life. A holistic approach is broader than a scientific approach to health and illness.

Many cultures have similar practices, such as:
- *Coining and spooning*: Rubbing a silver coin or spoon vigorously on the skin. These practices leave red marks on the skin. Do not confuse the marks with signs of abuse.
- *Cupping*: Applying suction to the skin, which can leave marks. Do not confuse these marks with signs of abuse.
- *Acupressure*: Applying firm pressure on specific points on the body.
- *Acupuncture*: Inserting fine needles into acupuncture points (specific sites on the body).

It is important to remember that not every member of the same culture has the same health beliefs (Fig. 41.4). Differences are typically seen between the generations. The healthcare professional should not assume patients have specific health beliefs. However, being aware of possible cultural beliefs and practices of a group is important (Box 41.1). It can help the medical assistant ask related questions to identify a patient's beliefs and practices.

CRITICAL THINKING 41.4

In the family practice environment, Suzanne sees patients from a variety of cultures. If you worked in a similar place, what would you do if you noticed red circles on a child's back? You are unsure as to what caused the circles.

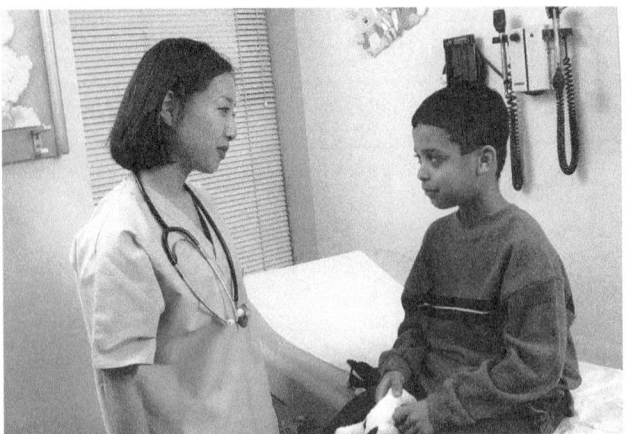

Fig. 41.4 Patients come from a variety of backgrounds and cultures. (From Niedzwiecki B, et al: *Kinn's the medical assistant,* ed 14, St. Louis, 2020, Elsevier.)

Communication Barriers. Coaching patients with communication barriers can be a challenging process. Hearing, vision, and language barriers are common in healthcare. It is estimated that 2% of people in the United States have a visual impairment, 3% have a hearing impairment, and 9% have limited English proficiency. It is important to overcome these barriers when coaching patients.

For healthcare agencies accepting federal funds, the Civil Rights Act requires that all patients have equal access to services. People with vision, hearing, or speech impairments use different ways to communicate. The Americans with Disability Act requires effective communication with patients who have impairments. This may mean offering a qualified medical interpreter or other interpretation services free of charge. Large-print materials and written instructions are also required. Translated written materials are needed for non-English-speaking patients.

BOX 41.1   Cultural Differences

African Americans
- Extended family and church play important roles.
- May have a key family member who must be consulted on healthcare decisions.
- Older members may look at their health as being up to God's will, although younger members seek health screening and treatments as needed.

Cambodians
- Good health means the person is balanced; believe in the balance of hot and cold.
- Illness may be seen as punishment for sins in a past life.
- Typically use traditional healing practices before seeking conventional medicine. May use herbs, cupping and coining, acupuncture, and acupressure.
- They may not be interested in preventive care and screenings.

Chinese
- May use acupuncture, massage, and herbs, seeking care from traditional practitioners for less severe illnesses.
- Respectful of elders, teachers, and healthcare professionals. May affect how a person interacts and discusses health topics with the healthcare professional. The person may not ask questions or discuss concerns.

Hispanics/Latinos
- May have strong family and religious beliefs. Family is respected and plays an important role. May view an illness as God's will.
- May use home remedies or follow folk healer's advice over conventional medicine.
- Sickness is caused by a person having too much heat or cold. Foods and herbs are used to bring back the balance. (Heat and cold are not temperature related.) Cold diseases have more unseen symptoms, such as a chest cold and an earache. Hot diseases have more visible symptoms, such as vomiting, fever, and sore throat.
- Males often answer questions and give consent. Make sure to address the patient also. Friendliness and respectfulness are very important.

Hmong
- Lack words in native language for medical terms and some body organs.
- May seek care from folk medicine doctors and shaman.
- Herbs, massage, coining or spooning, and cupping can be used.
- Accessories may be worn around wrists, necks, or ankles for health or religious reasons.

- Respecting older family members is very important. Often oldest male in the family is the decision maker. Extended family is very important.
- Eye contact is considered rude.
- Touching the head of a child is not accepted. The head is considered sacred.

Native Americans
- May place a lot of value in family and spiritual beliefs.
- State of health occurs when living in total harmony with nature. Illness is the imbalance between the person and nature.
- May use a traditional tribal medicine person.
- Often avoid direct eye contact out of respect and concern for the loss of one's soul.

Russians
- May view healthcare with some mistrust, based on past experience.
- May not be used to asking questions and participating in a discussion with a provider.
- Some practice home remedies and bonki. *Bonki* is practiced by pressing glass cups against the person's shoulders to ease the symptoms. Bruising can occur, which should not be confused with abuse.
- Family likes to receive news about patient's condition and prognosis and may not give bad news to the patient. This lessens the person's anxieties and promotes calmness.

Somalis
- Believe that individuals do not prevent illness, which is only done through prayer and living a life according to their religion.
- Use traditional spiritual healers.
- May not take medication if they feel healthy.
- Healthcare decisions are made by the family, and the father gives consent for procedures.
- Male and female circumcisions are performed; being uncircumcised means the person is unclean.

Vietnamese
- Illness is often explained by mystical beliefs.
- Health is the balance between the hot and cold poles that govern the bodily functions.
- Use alternative therapies, such as acupuncture, coining, spooning, and cupping.

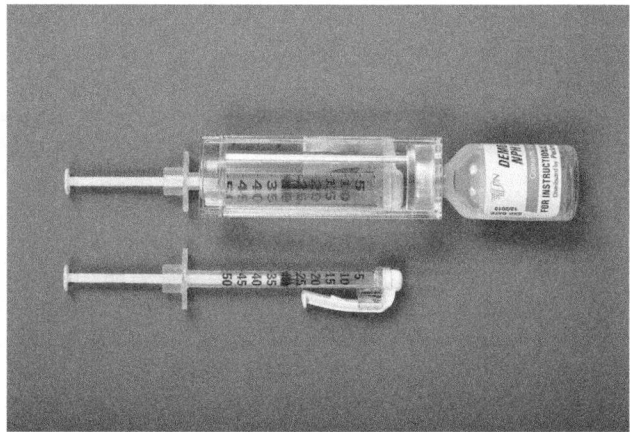

Fig. 41.5 Syringe magnifiers are used by people with visual impairments. The magnifiers increase the size of the calibration markings on the syringes.

The following sections provide tips for communicating with patients. It is important to listen to patients concerning what works best for them.

Patients With impaired vision. When you work with patients who have impaired vision, it is important to ensure the room has adequate light. Position the patient so they do not have to look directly toward the light source. Make sure the patient is wearing glasses or contacts if needed. When teaching a patient with impaired vision, the following points are important:

- Consider the impact of color contrast and glare on the materials used. Use a large black and white font (larger than 14 points) or electronic copy that can be enlarged. Use bold markers for handwritten information.
- Ask the patient how they prefer the information. Provide the patient with large-print directions or brochures.
- Have adaptive equipment available or information on resources for such equipment. For instance, you need to show a patient how to draw up insulin using a syringe. Having a syringe magnifier can help the patient see the calibration markings on the syringe (Fig. 41.5).
- Face the patient directly. Make eye contact, if culturally appropriate. Use a normal tone of voice.
- Gestures and other nonverbal cues are not as helpful with visual impairments.
- Encourage the patient to use their own magnification aids.
  Patients With impaired hearing. When teaching a patient with impaired hearing, the following points are important:
- Face the person when speaking.
- Determine if the person has better hearing in one ear than the other. Position yourself so your voice is close to the better-hearing side.
- If the patient has a hearing aid, encourage the patient to use it.
- Use a low-pitched voice and speak clearly, slowly, and distinctly. Pause between sentences or phrases. Speak naturally; do not shout. Limit medical terms.
- Say the person's name before you begin a conversation.

- Keep your hands away from your face when talking.
- Speak louder if you are wearing a mask.
- If an interpreter is present, look at the patient, not the interpreter.
- Limit extra noises in the environment.
- Attempt to rephrase or find a different way to say something if the patient has difficulty understanding a phrase.
- Provide important information in writing.
- Have the person repeat back important information.
  Patients With language barriers. When teaching a patient who has a language barrier, these points are important:
- Address the patient by their last name (e.g., Mrs. Martinez, Mr. Nguyen).
- Be respectful and courteous.
- Use simple phrases. If medical terminology must be used, make sure to define it for patients.
- Use an interpreter or an interpretation service. Focus on the patient and not on the interpreter.
- Use translated materials.
- Pictures and models can be helpful during the coaching session.

Teaching-Learning Process

Teaching opportunities vary greatly in ambulatory care. Sometimes a patient wants to know what a certain medication is for. Other times, the medical assistant needs to coach a patient on a diagnostic test.

Always take a moment to look over any information you provide to patients. Make sure you know the content before you review it with the patient. Providing information that conflicts with the handout will confuse the patient.

The medical assistant should start the coaching process by finding out what the patient knows about the topic. A simple way to do this is by asking a few questions, such as, "Have you had an ultrasound before? If so, what do you remember about it?" This helps the medical assistant identify what the patient knows. From there the medical assistant can begin teaching.

When coaching patients, it is important to follow these steps to ensure the coaching is relevant to the patient's needs:

1. *Identifying the patient's educational needs*: What does the patient need to learn? What are the patient's motivations and concerns? What is the patient's learning style? It is important to identify the patient's learning goals or the main reason for learning the content.
2. *Identifying barriers to learning*: It is important to identify barriers to learning and using strategies to overcome those barriers. Be sure to consider the patient's individual needs (e.g., primary language, developmental level, barriers to learning). Teaching aids, such as brochures, online resources, models, health-related apps, and drawings can be helpful to overcome certain barriers. For patients with lower reading levels or English as a second language, using more pictures can be helpful (Box 41.2). Using different teaching strategies can also help reduce barriers to learning. For skills, demonstration and role-play with demonstration

---

BOX 41.2 Tips on Patient Education Materials

The following are some guidelines for medical assistants who are responsible for developing or ordering educational supplies.

- The material should be written in lay language at a sixth- to eighth-grade level to promote understanding.
- Good pictures can help patients understand the information.
- Information should be well organized and clearly described.
- All material should be checked for accuracy. (Providers will want to approve the information ahead of time.)
- Handouts should be attractive and professional.
- Copies should be available in languages other than English when possible and in large print for visually impaired clients.
- Disease information literature from medical and pharmaceutical companies that includes advertising of their products should not be used. (This type of information can create confusion if the patient is not using the product advertised.)

---

are effective strategies. Discussion, videos, and internet sites can be helpful for teaching about a disease, diagnostic tests, or treatment.

3. *Coaching the patient on the topic*: It is important to start with the basics and build from there. Keep the information simple, focused, and appropriate for the individual patient. Reinforce important information. If teaching a skill, make sure to have the equipment available that the patient will use at home. This will promote the patient's comfort with the task.

4. *Evaluating the patient's learning*: After teaching important points, have the patient summarize what you stated. Keeping the patient involved will help them retain more information. Throughout the teaching session, make sure to ask the patient for feedback on whether they understand what you are discussing. Instead of just saying, "Do you understand?" ask specific questions to evaluate the patient's learning; for example, "What are four symptoms of low blood sugar?" Summarize the important points at the end of the teaching session. Answer any questions the patient may have. Identify areas in which the patient needs more information. If there will be more than one session, summarize what will occur during the next meeting

5. *Documenting the coaching*: It is important to document the content taught to the patient, how the patient responded, evidence that the patient learned the content, handouts given, and any plans for follow-up. Make sure to include the provider's name and any adaptations you made to individualize the teaching/learning experience. Evidence may include statements such as, "Pt safely and accurately walked 20 feet using the walker." "Pt stated six signs and symptoms of hypoglycemia."

COACHING ON DISEASE PREVENTION

Medical assistants coach patients of all ages on disease prevention. It is important to help patients understand ways to prevent

diseases in their lives. Common disease prevention coaching by age group includes the following:

- School-age children: Teaching about hand washing.
- Teens and adults: Teaching about ways to prevent sexually transmitted infections (STIs) and the risks of using cigarettes, smokeless tobacco, and e-cigarettes.
- All age groups: Teaching about respiratory hygiene/cough etiquette. Coaching patients and parents on the vaccines recommended for that specific age (Procedure 41.1). Childhood immunization schedules can be found on the website for the Centers for Disease Control and Prevention (CDC), https://www.cdc.gov/vaccines/schedules/downloads/child/0-18yrs-child-combined-schedule.pdf. Common adult vaccines usually include:
  - Influenza yearly.
  - Tetanus and diphtheria (Td) every 10 years and substitute tetanus, diphtheria, and acellular pertussis vaccine (Tdap) once.
  - Recombinant zoster vaccine (RZV), Shingrix, two doses for adults age 50 or older.
  - 13-Valent pneumococcal conjugate vaccine (PCV13), one dose usually after age 65 unless given before based on the patient's health.
  - 23-Valent pneumococcal polysaccharide vaccine (PPSV23 or PPSV), one to two doses, depending on patient's health

Additional vaccines can be given based on the situation (e.g., traveling or job related); adulthood immunization schedules can be found on the CDC's website, https://www.cdc.gov/vaccines/schedules/downloads/adult/adult-combined-schedule.pdf.

Cough Etiquette

It is important for everyone to be aware of respiratory hygiene/cough etiquette. The Centers for Disease Control and Prevention (CDC) encourages the use of respiratory hygiene/cough etiquette to prevent the transmission of all respiratory infections:

- Cover your mouth and nose with a tissue when coughing or sneezing.
- Discard the tissue in the nearest waste container.
- Wash your hands or use an alcohol-based hand sanitizer.

Sexually Transmitted Infections

Teaching teens and adults how to prevent STIs is important.

- *Abstinence* (not having any type of sex) is the most reliable way to prevent STIs.
- Long-term mutual monogamy (an agreement to be sexually active with just one person) with an uninfected partner is also a reliable way to prevent STIs.
- Reducing the number of partners reduces the risk. All partners need to be tested.
- Use latex condoms, although they are not 100% effective.
- Avoid sharing underwear and towels.
- Wash after intercourse.
- Avoid anyone with a genital rash, sore, discharge, or other symptoms.
- Get vaccinated for hepatitis B and human papilloma virus (HPV).

Cigarettes, Smokeless Tobacco, and E-Cigarettes

Teaching children, teens, and adults about the health risks associated with cigarettes, smokeless tobacco, and e-cigarettes is important. Often manufacturers of such products market to children and teens, making the products look attractive.

Tobacco smoke contains more than 7000 chemicals, of which 250 are harmful and at least 69 can cause cancer. One in five deaths are related to smoking. According to the CDC, smokers are more likely to develop heart disease, lung cancer, and strokes. Smoking can cause problems in all parts of the body, and quitting has numerous health advantages, which are discussed in length in Chapter 11.

Secondhand smoke causes lung cancer, strokes, low-birthweight babies, and heart disease. Children exposed to secondhand smoke have increased risks of sudden infant death syndrome (SIDS), ear infections, bronchitis, pneumonia, colds, and asthma. *Thirdhand smoke* is the residue or chemicals from the smoke that gets on skin, clothing, furniture, carpeting, and so on. This can be harmful to little children and animals that spend time on the floor. This residue – and its chemicals – can be both breathed in and ingested. They can be transferred from the carpet, clothing, and so on to hands and then into a person's mouth.

The CDC reports that at least 28 cancer-causing chemicals have been found in smokeless tobacco (e.g., chew and dip). Smokeless tobacco can cause cancer of the mouth, pancreas, and esophagus.

According to the US Surgeon General, e-cigarettes heat liquids to form an aerosol that is then inhaled. Many people call this *vaping*. The liquids typically contain nicotine, flavorings, and other additives. E-cigarettes are considered tobacco products because they contain nicotine that comes from tobacco. The nicotine makes e-cigarettes addictive. The additives can pose health risks.

Local resources and prescriptive medications are available if a person wants to quit using these products. Websites (e.g., https://smokefree.gov) and quit lines are also available (e.g., National Cancer Institute Smoking Quitline: 1-877-44U-QUIT).

COACHING ON HEALTH MAINTENANCE AND WELLNESS

Often with health maintenance and wellness, the provider establishes standing orders for specific education to be given based on the patient's history or age. When the medical assistant rooms a patient, a health history is obtained and screening questions are asked. Based on the patient's answers, the medical assistant may need to provide coaching on specific topics per the provider's standing orders. For instance, a patient states they smoke one pack of cigarettes daily. The provider's standing order for smokers requires the medical assistant to provide information on the hazards of tobacco use and resources for quitting. Another example would be a patient who is turning 45. Because colon cancer screenings typically start at age 45, the provider's standing order would be to provide this information to the patient.

The following sections discuss self-exams that can be taught to patients and the screenings that are commonly done. The medical assistant completes some screenings, whereas others require the medical assistant to educate the patient on the tests to be performed.

Self-Exams

The purpose of self-exams is to identify changes in one's body. Sometimes these changes can be the first sign of a disease. Self-exams are typically done monthly. To help maintain a person's health, the early diagnosis of a disease such as cancer is important.

Breast Self-Exam. Breast cancer can affect both females and males, though males are at a lower risk. Breast cancer is the second most common cancer in females after skin cancer. The risk of breast cancer increases with age. About 1 in 8 women will have invasive breast cancer. Typically, the survival rate is higher the earlier the cancer is diagnosed.

It is important for all women to know what is normal with their breasts. Any abnormality should be reported to their provider. Warning signs of breast cancer include:

- Change in the skin (redness, warmth, darkening of the color, dimpling, puckering)
- Lump or hard area inside the breast or in the axilla area
- Change in the size or shape of the breast
- Change in the nipple (inverted or pulling in appearance; rash, sore, or drainage)
- Pain that does not go away

Some providers still recommend a monthly breast self-exam (BSE) to be done after the menses. Procedure 41.2 describes how to perform a BSE. It is helpful for the medical assistant to provide the patient with a brochure showing the technique. It is also recommended to demonstrate the technique on a model (Fig. 41.6). If possible, the patient should demonstrate the technique back to the medical assistant. This practice helps the medical assistant determine if the patient understood the coaching.

Testicular Self-Exam. According to the American Cancer Society, males at any age can develop testicular cancer. Many causes of testicular cancer are unknown. It is more common in men who had abnormal testicle development, an undescended testicle, and a family history of the cancer. Symptoms of testicular cancer include:

- Swelling or a lump in the testicle
- A heavy sensation in the scrotum
- Pain in a testicle or in the scrotum, abdomen, and groin

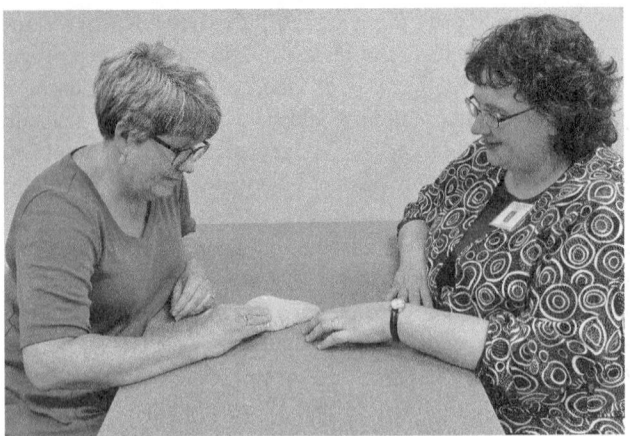

Fig. 41.6 Coaching a Patient on the Breast Self-Exam.

About 50% of those diagnosed are between 20 and 34 years of age. It is estimated that 1 in 263 males will get testicular cancer.

If the cancer is found early (before it has spread), there is a good chance of a cure. The American Cancer Society recommends that providers perform a testicular exam as part of a routine physical exam. Some providers recommend that after puberty (around age 15) males should do a monthly testicular self-exam (TSE) after a shower (Procedure 41.3). Again, it is helpful for the patient to have a brochure and to practice the technique on a model during the coaching session.

Skin Self-Exam. Skin cancer is the most common type of cancer in the United States. The three most common types of skin cancer are basal cell, squamous cell, and melanoma. Basal cell and squamous cell carcinomas are curable. Melanoma is more dangerous and can cause death. These three types of skin cancers are caused by overexposure to ultraviolet (UV) light. UV exposure comes from the sun, tanning beds, and sun lamps. UV rays are an invisible kind of radiation that penetrates and changes skin cells.

Certain people have a greater risk than others for skin cancer. Risk factors for skin cancer include:

- Skin that is lighter than normal skin color; burns, freckles, or reddens easily; becomes painful in the sun
- Family or personal history of skin cancer
- History of sunburns (especially early in life) or indoor tanning
- Exposure to sun through work or play
- Green or blue eyes
- Red or blond hair
- Certain types and a large number of moles

Experts recommend monthly skin self-exams. It is important to watch for changes in moles. To remember how moles may change, use the ABCDE rule:

Asymmetry: One half of the mole does not match the other half.
Border: The edges of the mole are blurred or irregular.
Color: The mole is not the same color throughout and has shades of tan, brown, black, red, white, or blue.
Diameter: The mole is larger than 6 mm, about the size of a pencil eraser or pea; but it could be smaller.

Evolving: The mole changes over time.
Any change in moles, including in the size, shape, color, elevation, or symptom (e.g., bleeding, itching, or crusting), should be reported immediately (Fig. 41.7).

When doing the monthly skin check, start at the scalp and work toward the soles of the feet. Use mirrors to exam the back of the ears and the back. Many people miss mole changes on the back of their ears. When examining hands and feet, make sure to check between the fingers and toes and to check the nail beds. Check all skin surfaces. Document the location of the moles and their appearances. Any changes seen, or any suspicious-looking mole, should be reported to the provider immediately.

Oral Cancer Self-Exam. Oral cancer includes cancer of the lips, tongue, throat, salivary glands, pharynx, larynx, and sinuses. Here are some facts about oral cancer:

- Men get oral cancer twice as often as women.
- Using tobacco, drinking alcohol, or having oral HPV are risk factors for oral cancer.
- About 25% of those with oral cancer had no risks.
- Most oral cancers occur after age 40.

It is estimated that more than 40,000 new cases of oral cancer are diagnosed yearly with almost 9000 related deaths. Early detection is important for oral cancer. Signs and symptoms of oral cancer include:

- White or red patches in the mouth or on the gums, tongue, or lips
- Numbness or pain in the mouth; pain with chewing or talking
- Long-term hoarseness or sore throat
- Swelling in the jaw area or constant earache
- Bleeding in the mouth or a long-term sore
- Feeling of a lump or something stuck in the throat

Oral cancer screening is routinely done by the dentist and should occur every 6 months. It is important for people to do a monthly oral cancer self-exam. Any changes in appearance or sores that do not heal should be reported to the dentist immediately. According to the American Dental Hygienists Association, an oral cancer self-exam consists of looking for lumps and color changes and then feeling for lumps and swelling. To do an oral cancer self-exam, follow these steps:

1. Check the head and neck for lumps, bumps, or swelling. Is one side of the face larger than the other?
2. Check the skin on the face for changes. Is there a color change? Are there sores, moles, or growths?
3. Check for any lumps or tenderness in the neck.
4. Check the upper and lower lip for sores and color changes. After the visual inspection, feel for any changes in texture or lumps.
5. Check the inner cheek for any color changes (red, white, or dark patches). Then palpate the cheeks with a thumb on the outside and a finger inside. Are any lumps found?
6. Check the roof of the mouth for lumps and color changes. Feel for any lumps.
7. Check the floor of the mouth, using your tongue, for any lumps; also check for color changes. Examine all angles. Feel the tongue with a finger for any lumps or tenderness.

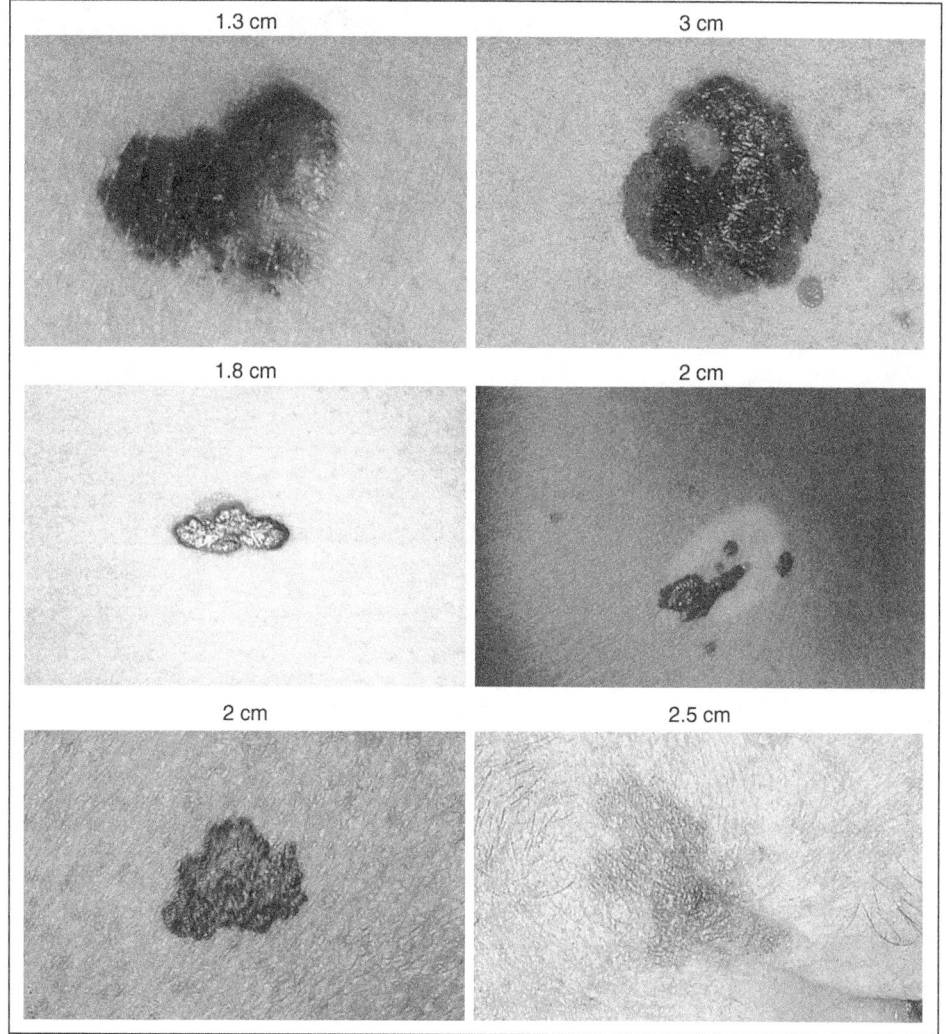

Fig. 41.7 Malignant Melanomas. Note the presence of the ABCDE characteristics. (From Rothrock J: *Alexander's care of the patient in surgery,* ed 14, St. Louis, 2011, Mosby.)

Regular Screenings

Medical assistants in primary care typically need to talk with patients about the recommended regular screenings for different diseases. Suggested times for screenings are based on an adult with an average risk. If a patient has family members with the disease, that person may have a higher than normal risk. This means the patient may need to be screened earlier and more often than other adults. Regular preventive screenings are summarized by age in Table 41.4; they include:

- *Blood pressure*: Patients at higher risk include African Americans, those who are overweight, and those with previously higher than normal blood pressure readings.
- *Bone density*: This screening provides information on the strength of the patient's bones and if the patient has osteoporosis. Women have a higher risk than men, and it increases with age.
- *Cholesterol*: Adults with a family history of high cholesterol levels or who have high cholesterol need more frequent testing.
- *Colorectal cancer screening*: The American Cancer Society recommends that regular screening start at age 45. Other organizations recommend starting regular screenings at age

50. Screening can either be stool based or visual exams (see Table 41.4).
- *Dental exam*: The American Dental Association recommends a dental exam and cleaning yearly. Dental health can affect the overall health of the body.
- *Dilated eye exam*: It is important to have a dilated eye exam if a person has a risk of eye disease (e.g., glaucoma). The CDC recommends dilated eye exams for:
  - Patients with diabetes (recommended annually)
  - African American patients age 40 years or older (recommended every 2 years)
  - Patients older than 60 years of age (recommended every 2 years)
  - Patients with a family history of glaucoma (recommended every 2 years)
- *Fall risk screening*: The CDC and the American Geriatric Society recommend yearly fall risk screening for adults age 65 or older. If the screening shows the person is at risk, it is recommended that the patient have a fall assessment (Box 41.3). Having dizziness, light-headedness, or an irregular or rapid pulse puts the older person at risk for falls.

TABLE 41.4   Preventive Recommendations

	Age 18–39	Age 45–64	Age 65+
Blood pressure	Age 18–39: Every 3–5 years; Age 40–44: Annually	Annually	
Bone density (Females)			Every 2 years
Cholesterol	Every 4–6 years		
Fall risk screening			Annually
Fecal stool tests (gFOBT, FIT)		Age 45–75: Annually Age 75+: Individual decision	
Stool DNA test (Cologuard)		Age 45–75: Every 3 years Age 75+: Individual decision	
Colonoscopy		Age 45–75: Every 10 years Age 75+: Individual decision	
Dental exam	Annually		
Dilated eye exam		Age 60+: Every 2 years	
Lung cancer screening		Age 55–80 who meet the criteria: Annual low-dose computed tomography (LDCT)	
Mammogram (Females)	Age 40–44: Annually (optional)	Age 45–54: Annually Age 55+: Every 1–2 years	
Pap test	Age 21–29: Every 3 years; age 30–65: every 3 years or if having an HPV test then every 5 years.		Individual decision
Prostate cancer (DRE or PSA test)		Age 50–69: Individual decision	
Diabetes mellitus type 2	Every 3 years or more frequent if patient has hypertension or obesity		

DRE, Digital rectal exam; *FIT,* fecal immunochemical test; *gFOBT,* guaiac fecal occult blood test; *HPV,* human papilloma virus; *PSA,* prostate-specific antigen.
From Healthfinder.gov. https://healthfinder.gov/HealthTopics/Category/doctor-visits; and American Cancer Society, https://www.cancer.org/.

BOX 41.3   Fall Risk Screening and Assessment

STEADI (Stopping Elderly Accidents, Deaths & Injuries) is a program established by the CDC to help screen, assess, and intervene when older adults are at risk for falls. According to the CDC, factors that can cause falls include:

- Advanced age, fear of falling, and poor vision
- Previous falls, muscle weakness, and gait and balance problems
- Postural hypotension
- Chronic conditions, such as arthritis, stroke, incontinence, Parkinson disease, dementia, and diabetes mellitus
- Poor stair design and lack of handrails
- Lack of bathroom grab bars
- Dim lighting or glare
- Objects in the walkway, tripping hazards, and slippery or uneven surfaces
- Improper use of assistive devices

The medical assistant can help screen patients by using screening tools available from the CDC or asking the following questions:

- Do you feel unsteady when standing or walking?
- Do you worry about falling?
- Have you fallen in the past year? If so, how many times? Were you injured?

More information on the STEADI program is available on the CDC's website: https://www.cdc.gov/steadi/.

- *Lung cancer screening:* Patients who are 55 to 80 years old, have a history of heavy smoking, and are currently smoking or quit in the previous 15 years should be screened for lung cancer. (Heavy smoking means smoking one pack of cigarettes a day for 30 years or two packs for 15 years.)

- *Mammogram:* This x-ray of the breasts helps to identify breast cancer. See Table 41.4 for the American Cancer Society recommendations. Mammogram screening recommendations vary by organization.
- *Pap test:* This test is used to identify cervical cancer.
- *Prostate cancer:* Risk factors include being 50 years old or older, being African American, exposure to Agent Orange, and having a father, brother, or son who had prostate cancer. No specific test exists for prostate cancer. The digital rectal exam (DRE) and the prostate-specific antigen (PSA) test are used. The provider may offer either test after age 50. Frequency is based on the patient's history.
- *Blood glucose test:* Adults should be screened for type 2 diabetes mellitus every 3 years or more often, depending on their medical history.

One-Time Screenings

The medical assistant may also need to coach patients on one-time screening as indicated by the provider. People are recommended to have the following screenings at least once, unless a person's risk is greater than average:

- *Abdominal aortic aneurysm:* Males between 65 and 75 years of age who have smoked at one time in their lives should receive this screening. This population has the highest risk of having an abdominal aortic aneurysm (AAA).
- *Human immunodeficiency virus (HIV) screen:* People 15 to 65 years old need to get an HIV blood test at least once in their lifetime. All pregnant women need to be tested. People

with a high risk for HIV should have testing annually, if not more often. High-risk factors include multiple sexual partners, sexual partners who have or may have HIV, and those who use injectable illegal drugs.

- *Hepatitis C*: This condition is passed through blood from an infected person. A person with risk factors should be tested. Risk factors for hepatitis C include:
  - Born between 1945 and 1965
  - History of a blood transfusion or organ transplantation before 1992
  - Use of injected illegal drugs
  - Chronic liver disease, HIV, or acquired immunodeficiency syndrome (AIDS)

Additional Screenings

When rooming patients, medical assistants have to perform different screenings. Either the patient's age or the patient's responses will trigger the need for the screening. Screenings have increased throughout the years. This is due to increased data collection requirements and focusing on prevention and quality patient care. The following are common screenings.

- *Alcohol misuse screening*: Drinking in moderation means that females have no more than one drink a day and males have no more than two drinks per day. (An alcoholic drink is classified as a 12-ounce (oz) bottle of beer, a 5-oz glass of wine, or a 1.5-oz shot of liquor.) Drinking more than the recommended daily amount may lead to health issues.
- *Nicotine or tobacco screening*: Various tools are used. Tools typically focus on whether or not tobacco products are used, how much is used per day, the history of use, and quitting behaviors (e.g., strategies used in the past or thoughts of quitting).
- *Drug abuse screening*: Various tools are used. Tools focus on prescription drug use for nonmedical reasons and illegal drug use. Tools usually identify any history of or recent drug abuse. Common signs of drug abuse include:
  - Poor hygiene; changes in eating and sleeping patterns
  - Loss of interest in favorite things
  - Very energetic, talking fast, very sociable
  - Tired, sad, nervous, agitated, and bad moods
  - Missing school, work, or appointments
  - Spending money excessively
  - Slowed reaction time, paranoid thinking
- *Intimate partner violence screening*: This screening covers domestic abuse. It is important to remember that both males and females can be victims of domestic abuse. Many psychological and health problems come from violence, including substance abuse, obesity, depression, brain trauma, pregnancy complications, and chronic pain. Intimate partner violence includes controlling behaviors, physical abuse, sexual abuse, and emotional or verbal abuse.
- *Elderly safety screening*: These screening tools focus on how safe the older person feels at home and screen for abuse and neglect. Box 41.4 provides types and symptoms of elder abuse and neglect.
- *Neurologic Status Exam*: This screening tool is used to test the patient's cognitive functions and provides a baseline of

neurologic information for the provider (Fig. 41.8 and Procedure 41.4). Part of the exam also requires gathering information from the patient's caregiver.

- *Functional status screening*: Several tools are available for primary care providers to use for older patients. By using a functional status screening tool, the provider obtains information on the patient, such as:
  - Physical functions with daily activities (e.g., grooming, bathing, walking, and eating)
  - Psychological health (e.g., mood and anxiety)
  - Role function (e.g., employed or volunteer)
  - Social function (e.g., interacting with others or isolating self)
- *Depression screening*: Several tools are used to screen for depression. The screening tools ask questions related to moods, thoughts, and feelings. The number of questions will vary depending on the tools. For instance, the Patient Health Questionnaire–2 (PHQ-2) asks two questions that focus on the frequency of depressed mood and anhedonia over the previous 2 weeks. If the patient screens positive, then the Patient Health Questionnaire–9 (PHQ-9) is given to see if the patient meets the criteria for a depressive disorder (Fig. 41.9). (The first two questions of the PHQ-9 are the two questions on the PHQ-2 tool.)
- *Peripheral neuropathy screening*: Screening questions focus on loss of feeling or a "pins and needles" sensation in the feet and hands. Besides asking the patient screening questions, the medical assistant may also need to do a monofilament foot test and coach the patient on foot care (Box 41.5 and Procedure 41.5). Proper foot care can help to limit foot sores and identify suspicious areas sooner.

VOCABULARY

anhedonia The inability to feel or experience pleasure during a pleasurable activity.

COACHING ON DIAGNOSTIC TESTS

It is important for the medical assistant to provide the necessary teaching for diagnostic and laboratory tests ordered for patients. For tests to be completed, the patient needs to be prepared. Some tests require fasting, whereas others do not. The medical assistant needs to provide answers to these questions:

- What is the test?
- Where does the patient need to go for the test? When is the test scheduled?
- Does the test require fasting? If so, for how long? If no foods or beverages can be consumed, does this include water?
- Should patients continue or stop taking their medications? This may require a discussion with the provider.

It is important to give patients the correct answers. Tables 41.5 and 41.6 provide information on common procedures and medical laboratory tests. Remember, patient preparation may vary based on the facility.

WALDEN–MARTIN   Instructor: Becky Swisher
FAMILY MEDICAL CLINIC
1234 ANYSTREET | ANYTOWN, ANYSTATE 12345
PHONE 123-123-1234 | FAX 123-123-5678

Neurological Status Exam

The Neurological Status Examination tests the individual's sense of cognitive functions and quickly allows the provider to screen for cognitive impairment and/or loss. In addition to testing language recall and motor skills, the NSE also allows you to test an individual's orientation to time, detail, and attention.

There are five sections. Each section of the test involves relating a series of questions or commands to a patient; the patient should receive one point for each correct answer. Conduct the test without interruptions in a well-lit, private exam room. Instruct the patient to listen carefully and to answer each question as accurately as possible. In the event that there is a caregiver accompanying the patient, ask the Caregiver Questions and record the responses (these are not part of the final score).

Read each question once and document the patient's response. Do not time the patient's answers or duration of the test overall; once completed, score the test immediately. To do so, add only the number of correct responses. The individual can receive a maximum score of 10 points; a score below 4 indicates cognitive impairment.

Patient Name: _____   Date of Birth: _____
Performed By: _____   Date: _____

Caregiver Questions (if available): (Yes, No, Not Aware)

	Yes	No	Not Aware
Name of Caregiver: _____			
• Does the patient have difficulty remembering recent events or conversions?	☐	☐	☐
• Does the patient have difficulty performing activities of daily living (bath, driving, cooking, etc.)?	☐	☐	☐
• Have you noticed changes to speech patterns?	☐	☐	☐

Patient Interview

Sequencing:

Read the following statement to the patient three consecutive times: **"Drive the red car to Washington Street."** Then ask the Patient to restate the sentence; you will ask the patient to recall the statement later in the test.

	Yes	No
The patient was able to repeat the exact statement to you	☐	☐

Total: _____

Time Orientation:

Ask the patient the following questions:

	Correct	Incorrect
• What is today's date?	☐	☐
• What season is it?	☐	☐
• What is the day of the week?	☐	☐

Total: _____

Drawing:

Give the individual a piece of paper and ask him/her to copy a design of the two intersecting shapes. One point is awarded for correctly copying the shapes. All angles on both figures must be present, and the figures must have one overlapping angle.

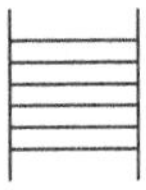

	Correct	Incorrect
	☐	☐

Total: _____

Information:

Ask the patient the following questions:

	Correct	Incorrect
• Who is president of the United States?	☐	☐
• How may stars are on the American flag?	☐	☐

Total: _____

Recall:

Ask the patient to restate the sentence that you asked him/her at the beginning of the procedure. One point is given for repeating each of the following words.

	Correct	Incorrect
• Drive	☐	☐
• Red car	☐	☐
• Washington Street	☐	☐

Total: _____

Total Exam Score: _____

Fig. 41.8 Neurological Status Exam Form. (From Niedzwiecki B, et al: *Kinn's the medical assistant,* ed 14, St. Louis, 2020, Elsevier.)

PATIENT HEALTH QUESTIONNAIRE-9 (PHQ-9)

Over the last 2 weeks, how often have you been bothered by any of the following problems?
(Use "✓" to indicate your answer)

	Not at all	Several days	More than half the days	Nearly every day
1. Little interest or pleasure in doing things	0	1	2	3
2. Feeling down, depressed, or hopeless	0	1	2	3
3. Trouble falling or staying asleep, or sleeping too much	0	1	2	3
4. Feeling tired or having little energy	0	1	2	3
5. Poor appetite or overeating	0	1	2	3
6. Feeling bad about yourself — or that you are a failure or have let yourself or your family down	0	1	2	3
7. Trouble concentrating on things, such as reading the newspaper or watching television	0	1	2	3
8. Moving or speaking so slowly that other people could have noticed? Or the opposite — being so fidgety or restless that you have been moving around a lot more than usual	0	1	2	3
9. Thoughts that you would be better off dead or of hurting yourself in some way	0	1	2	3

FOR OFFICE CODING ___0___ + _____ + _____ + _____

=Total Score: _____

If you checked off any problems, how difficult have these problems made it for you to do your work, take care of things at home, or get along with other people?

Not difficult at all	Somewhat difficult	Very difficult	Extremely difficult
☐	☐	☐	☐

Fig. 41.9 Example of a Depression Screening Tool: Patient Health Questionnaire–9 (PHQ-9).

BOX 41.4   Types and Signs of Elder Abuse and Neglect

- *Physical abuse*: Fractures, rope marks, cuts, bruising, dislocations, broken glasses, giving too little or too much medication, bleeding, and sudden changes in the person's personality or behavior
- *Sexual abuse*: Unexplained sexually transmitted infections, bruising in the genital region, and reports from the older person
- *Emotional abuse*: Not communicating, withdrawn, agitated, and symptoms that mimic dementia
- *Neglect*: Malnutrition, dehydration, lack of proper living conditions, and failing to treat health problems
- *Abandonment*: Leaving the person in a public place
- *Financial abuse*: Stealing from the older person, forging signatures on financial transactions, and any other illegal action that represents a financial loss for the older person

BOX 41.5   Foot Care for Patients With Neuropathy

The medical assistant can coach the patient on proper foot care. It is important for patients to check their feet daily and also to care for their feet daily. The following points should be reinforced with patients who have neuropathy:

- Check your shoes for damaged areas or stones before putting them on. Wear good-fitting shoes at all times to protect your feet.
- Check your feet when taking off your shoes. Look at all sides of your feet and between the toes. Check for redness, blisters, swelling, sores, and so forth.
- Keep your toenails trimmed to a proper length.
- Wash your feet every day with lukewarm water and soap. Dry well with a soft towel. Use lotion, lanolin, or oil on dry skin, but do not put it between the toes because this could cause an infection.
- Seek medical care immediately for foot sores.
- Avoid putting pressure for long periods of time on areas with nerve damage.
- Use an elbow instead of the toes or hands to check the bathwater temperature.

MEDICAL TERMINOLOGY

bi/o	life, living
hem/o	blood
-occult	secret or hidden

CRITICAL THINKING 41.6

Sometimes Suzanne has a patient who refuses to follow the preparation steps for a diagnostic test. How might you handle this situation?

TABLE 41.5   Common Patient Instructions for Common Procedures

Procedures	Description	Common Patient Instructions
X-ray	X-ray particles pass through the body, and an image is recorded. Many different types of x-rays.	Provide overview of test and why it is being done. X-rays are painless, although some body positions may be uncomfortable. • Patients may be asked to hold the breath during the procedure to get a clear x-ray. • Screen for pregnancy.
Computed tomography scan (CT scan, CAT scan)	Uses x-rays to create pictures of cross sections of the body. Several types of CT scans exist; each may have different preparations. Patient will lie on a narrow table that slides into the center of the CT scanner. The x-ray beam will rotate around the patient, creating separate images (slices) of the body.	Provide overview of test and why it is being done. May require an intravenous (IV) or oral contrast medium. If so: • Check allergies (contrast medium and iodine). • Check if patient has kidney disease or is on dialysis. • Nothing by mouth (NPO) for 4–6 hours before test. • Address if medications need to be stopped. • IV contrast medium may cause a slight burning feeling and a metallic taste in the mouth; flushing can occur.
Bone density scan (also called dual-energy x-ray absorptiometry [DEXA] scan)	Uses low-dose x-ray test that measures calcium and other minerals in the bone. The measurement shows the strength and thickness of the bones and is used to diagnose osteoporosis.	Provide overview of test and why it is being done. • Patient must stop taking calcium supplements 24 to 48 hours before the test. • Avoid wearing metal jewelry or clothes with metal buttons or buckles. • Patient must lie still in a supine position on a table. The scanning machine will pass over the lower spine and hip. A photon generator will pass beneath the patient. The two images are combined, and a computer image is created.
Magnetic resonance imaging (MRI)	Uses powerful magnets and radio waves to create images of the body. Does not use radiation. Several types of MRIs exist; may have different preparations. Patient will lie on a table. The machine makes loud noises. No metal is allowed in the room.	Provide overview of test and why it is being done. May require contrast (see CT scan contrast medium information). • May require being NPO for 4–6 hours. • Must identify if patient is claustrophobic (afraid of or anxious about closed spaces). • Due to strong magnets, must screen for artificial heart valves, brain aneurysm clips, heart pacemaker or defibrillator, cochlear (inner ear) implants, recent artificial joint, vascular stents, or history of working with metal. • Must remove all metal from patient, including removable dental work (e.g., plates).
Mammography	An x-ray picture of the breasts used to find tumors. The breast will be compressed on a flat surface for the x-ray.	Provide overview of test and why it is being done. • Do not use any perfume, deodorant, powders, or ointments on the arms or breast on the day of the test; may interfere with the results of the x-ray. • Undress from the waist up and remove all jewelry from the neck and chest area. • Screen for pregnancy, breastfeeding, or if the patient has had a breast biopsy.
Positron emission tomography (PET) scan	Imaging test that uses an IV radioactive substance (tracer) to identify disease in the organs and tissues. Patient will lie on a table that slides into the tunnel-shaped PET scanner.	Provide overview of test and why it is being done. • May require patient to be NPO for 4–6 hours (with exception of water) before the scan. • Medications may be held (check with the provider). • IV tracer will be given, which may cause a sharp sting. Afterward the patient needs to rest for 1 hour. During the test, the patient must lie still to prevent blurry images. • Screen for claustrophobia, pregnancy, and allergies to contrast medium and iodine.
Ultrasound (US)	Uses high-frequency sound waves to create the image of the organs and structures.	Provide overview of test and why it is being done. May require special preparation based on the type of US done. • Patient will need to expose the area. • A clear, water-based gel is applied to the skin, and a transducer (handheld probe) moves over the area.
Electroencephalogram (EEG)	Detects electrical activity in the brain using the electrodes that are placed on the scalp.	• Avoid caffeine. • Wash hair the night before or the day of the test. Do not use conditioner. See Procedure 41.6.
Colonoscopy	An endoscope is inserted through the anus and used to visualize the colon.	Provide overview of test and why it is being done. • Clear liquid diet day before and NPO day of test. • Colon prep as ordered. • Sedation is usually given. Patient may feel cramping or the urge to have a stool when the air is pumped into the colon. See Procedure 41.7.

TABLE 41.6   Patient Instructions for Common Medical Laboratory Tests

Test	Use	Common Patient Preparation
Creatinine	Used to monitor kidney health and disease.	May need to fast overnight. May need to refrain from eating meat for a period of time, because it could increase the creatinine level.
Guaiac fecal occult blood test (gFOBT)	Fecal specimen exam to detect occult or hidden blood, which may indicate gastrointestinal (GI) bleeding. Intestinal bleeding may be an indicator of colon cancer.	Seven days prior to the test: • Stop taking aspirin and nonsteroidal anti-inflammatory medications (e.g., ibuprofen, naproxen, and indomethacin). • Do not take vitamin C supplements. Three days before the test: • Do not eat red meat or raw fruits or vegetables (e.g., horseradish, turnips, broccoli, melons, and radishes). Stool samples are collected over several days, and cards are prepared and sent to the laboratory.
Fecal immunochemical test (FIT)	Fecal specimen exam to detect human hemoglobin protein, which may indicate GI bleeding.	No preparation required. Stool sample is collected by the patient and sent to the laboratory.
Cologuard stool DNA test (FIT-DNA)	Used to detect blood in the stool. Computer analysis looks at the DNA in the stool, checking for cancer and precancerous cells.	No preparation required. Stool sample is collected by the patient and returned to a specific medical laboratory for testing.
Glucose tests	Used to determine the blood glucose level.	For a fasting glucose test, the patient needs to be NPO (except for water) for at least 8 hours. Other glucose tests may require fasting and eating at specific times.
Lipid profile	Used to monitor cholesterol levels and treatment.	May require NPO (except for water) prior to the test.
Pap test	Used to screen for cervical cancers and some uterine or vaginal infections.	Do not schedule the test during the menstrual period. For 2 days prior to test: • Refrain from sexual intercourse. • Do not douche or use vaginal medications or spermicidal products.

CRITICAL THINKING 41.7

Suzanne has seen more providers ordering the fecal immunochemical test (FIT) rather than the guaiac fecal occult blood test. What are the advantages of the FIT?

COACHING ON TREATMENT PLANS

Many facilities have the medical assistants meet with the patients after the providers finish. The medical assistants review the treatment plan with the patients. They answer any questions, explore any issues the patients may have, and provide additional instructions. As mentioned, this type of coaching has been shown to increase patients' adherence to the treatment plans. Additionally, it provides patients with a lifeline should they have questions or concerns at home.

Medical assistants coach patients on treatments to do at home. These could include:

- Taking medications
- Caring for casts and splints, applying hot or cold therapy, and using assistive devices (discussed in Chapter 43)
- Testing blood glucose levels and coagulation using home monitors (discussed in Chapter 55)
- Monitoring the blood pressure (discussed in Chapter 33)

Medication Administration at Home

It is important for patients to know how to take medications at home. Some helpful questions are:

- When should the patient take the medications and how should they take them?
- Do the medications need to be taken on an empty stomach?

- Can they be taken with the other medications?
- Do they need to be taken at bedtime?

Some patients are on a lot of medications. It is important that the medications are taken correctly. When updating the patient's current medications list, the medical assistant commonly finds discrepancies. For example, the patient may be taking the medication differently from how it was ordered. Any discrepancy found needs to be communicated to the provider.

The medical assistant may coach the patient on the proper ways to take medication. Sometimes the medical assistant may need to help patients find ways to remember to take medications. Many patients use medication boxes that they, a family member, or a pharmacy set up. The boxes typically are arranged for 7 days a week with one or more boxes per day (Fig. 41.10). The medications are placed in each box based on the administration time. Some have boxes for morning, noon, and night medications.

If patients are receiving injections at home, they will need to know how to safely dispose of the needles. Patients can dispose of needles in biohazardous sharps containers. These containers are available at local pharmacies and medical supply stores. An internet search can identify local sites that take biohazardous sharps containers from patients. Some drug companies have mail-back programs for specific medications. (For more information, visit https://safeneedledisposal.org.)

Discarding Medications. It is important to encourage patients to discard expired, unwanted, or unused medications. This will help prevent misuse and theft. To get rid of controlled substances, take the medications in their original prescription bottles to a medicine take-back facility. Usually, Drug Enforcement

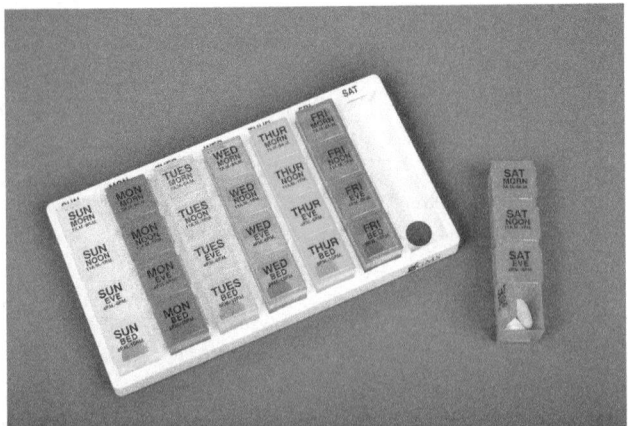

Fig. 41.10 Daily medication boxes can help patients remember to take their medications.

Administration (DEA) representatives are available to take control of the controlled substances. Another option is to contact a DEA-authorized collector. The DEA's website has more information on both programs (https://www.deadiversion.usdoj.gov).

If these programs are not available, some medications are labeled with specific disposal instructions. Many times, the label recommends flushing controlled substances down the sink or toilet. The website for the Food and Drug Administration (FDA) contains a complete list of medications that can be discarded by flushing (https://www.fda.gov/).

If the label does not indicate flushing, then mix the medications in an unpalatable substance (dirt, used coffee grounds, or kitty litter). Place the mixture in a plastic bag. Seal and discard it in the household trash. Make sure all personal information and the prescription number have been scratched out on empty pill bottles.

CARE COORDINATION

Care coordination provides personalized patient- and family-centered care in a team-based environment. Advantages of care coordination include:

- Greater efficiency in providing patient care
- Reduced costs
- Better patient care
- Individualized patient guidance and services
- Encourages patients to focus on goals and self-management
- Reduces hospital emergency department visits and readmissions
- Ensures the patient's needs and preferences for healthcare services are met

The care coordinator communicates between the patient and the healthcare team. Care coordinators ensure patients get timely care and do not fall through the cracks. In the ambulatory care setting, care coordination can be set up in different

ways. It has been shown to be successful in primary and specialty care areas. The overall goals include:

- Help patients understand why and what services are needed
- Schedule and sequence appointments
- Provide instructions and directions to patients
- Ensure that test results are available to the providers during patient appointments
- Communicate the patient's needs and concerns to providers

A patient navigator (also called a *patient advocate*) has been described as a type of care coordinator. The navigator program was established at the Harlem Hospital Center in 1990. The goal was to assist cancer patients in accessing quality healthcare. Based on the success of patient navigators, the Patient Navigator, Outreach and Chronic Disease Prevention Act of 2005 funded additional positions. Today, patient navigators typically guide chronically ill patients through the healthcare system. They identify patients' financial, cultural, physical, and emotional barriers. Then, they work closely with the healthcare team and the patients to ensure barriers are eliminated and patients get timely care.

In the ambulatory care setting, medical assistants can be care coordinators. A person must have strong interpersonal skills to be successful as a care coordinator. The medical assistant must listen to the patient and family to identify their needs and concerns. The care coordinator must be compassionate yet provide firm guidance with patients who are difficult.

The following are possible areas involved with care coordination.

- Interview patients to identify their needs and barriers to wellness and healthcare.
- Provide patients with resources based on their needs and barriers.
- Schedule and sequence appointments.
- Make sure the required information is communicated to and from specialty departments.
- Assist with reducing language barriers by identifying bilingual providers and translators.
- Discuss special needs patients have with their healthcare team.
- Identify community resources, which may include:
  - Transportation and medical equipment
  - Adult day care, assisted living, and long-term care
  - Educational programs and support groups
  - Low-cost medication programs
  - Low-cost preventive screening and immunizations

Procedure 41.8 describes the process of creating a current list of community resources and referring patients or family members.

> **VOCABULARY**
>
> **patient navigator** A person who identifies patients' barriers, works closely with the healthcare team and patients, and guides the patients through the healthcare system; may also be called a *patient advocate*.

CLOSING COMMENTS

It is an exciting time to become a medical assistant. The medical assistant's role is changing to meet healthcare needs. Studies have shown that medical assistants play an important role in coaching and helping patients comply with treatment and lifestyle changes. It is important for the medical assistant to coach the patient in a manner that helps the patient understand and retain the information. Adapting the coaching to the patient's communication barriers, developmental stage, and cultural practices will help the patient complete the treatment plan.

BEING PROFESSIONAL

When coaching patients, the medical assistant must observe the patient's nonverbal and verbal communication. It is important for the medical assistant to listen to the patient and be open to questions from the patient. If the medical assistant does not know the answers to questions or if the questions are outside the medical assistant's scope of practice, the provider should be notified.

Role-play this scenario with a peer: You are a medical assistant who is working with a patient (your peer). The patient asks you a question about a surgical procedure that they will be having soon. The question is beyond the scope of your practice. How would you answer the patient in a respectful and professional manner?

PATIENT-CENTERED CARE

The focus of patient-centered care is to have patients make decisions about their healthcare. To make such decisions, patients need to be given information on such topics as diseases, tests, and treatments. Patient education materials are used to help patients learn more about different topics. With the advances in technology, patient education materials are no longer available just on paper. Apps can help providers explain procedures and diseases to patients. YouTube links and other websites provide videos and information on diseases, procedures, and treatments.

When you use patient education materials from apps and online sites, it is important to use only provider-approved sites. The information must be current and from a reputable source. The following are possible online websites for patient education materials.

- National Institutes of Health (NIH) from the US Department of Health and Human Services (https://www.nih.gov/health-information)
- Centers for Disease Control and Prevention (CDC) (https://www.cdc.gov/)
- MedlinePlus from the US National Library of Medicine (https://medlineplus.gov/)
- American Diabetes Association (ADA) (http://www.diabetes.org/)
- American Heart Association (AHA) (https://www.heart.org/en/health-topics)
- Drugs.com (https://www.drugs.com/)
- Mayo Clinic (https://www.mayoclinic.org/)
- Cleveland Clinic (http://my.clevelandclinic.org/health/)
- Stanford Health Care (http://healthlibrary.stanford.edu/resources/bodysystems/)
- Familydoctor.org from the American Academy of Family Physicians (https://familydoctor.org/)

CHAPTER REVIEW

This chapter focused on coaching patients and coordinating care. It is helpful for the medical assistant to understand why patients may not always comply with the treatment plan. When a patient is diagnosed with a life-changing condition, the person can experience grief. It may take some time before the person complies with the recommended treatments. In other situations, the health belief model helps healthcare professionals understand why a person may or may not make the recommended lifestyle changes. Factors such as the perceived risks and severity of the disease, along with the barriers to and benefits of prevention, affect compliance.

There are three domains of learning: cognitive, psychomotor, and affective. For each domain, specific teaching strategies are used. For instance, the psychomotor domain includes learning new skills. Demonstration and return demonstration are teaching strategies that can be used for this domain. Along with the domains come barriers to learning. These barriers must be overcome, or the medical assistant must adapt to these barriers to help the patient learn the content.

Besides adapting coaching to deal with the barriers to learning, a medical assistant must also consider the patient's developmental level and cultural diversity. Erikson's psychosocial developmental stages help a medical assistant understand the developmental goals for different ages. Specific coaching techniques can be used to teach patients of different developmental stages. Cultural diversity is all around us.

Knowing general cultural practices for the populations typically seen in the ambulatory care setting is important. Adapting coaching to meet a person's cultural practice will increase the compliance with the treatment plan. For this to occur, the medical assistant must be open and respectful with the patient. It is important for the medical assistant to ask questions and then help the patient incorporate the changes into their lifestyle.

Medical assistants can provide coaching to patients in these areas:

- *Coaching on disease prevention*: Examples include discussing good hygiene practices, recommended vaccinations, preventing STIs, and nicotine (tobacco) cessation.
- *Coaching on health maintenance and wellness*: Examples include self-exams and information related to specific screenings.
- *Coaching on diagnostic tests*: Patients need to be aware of what to expect and how to prepare for tests.
- *Coaching on treatment plans*: Patients need to be instructed on home medication administration, therapies, and assistive devices. Proper coaching will help patients adhere to the treatment plan.
- *Coaching on community and healthcare resources*: Through care coordination or healthcare navigation, the medical assistant has the opportunity to provide information about community resources that will help the patient.

SCENARIO WRAP-UP

During Suzanne's yearly review with her supervisor, she mentioned that she was interested in becoming a care coordinator. She and the supervisor discussed how the program might assist the providers and patients. Suzanne agreed to research the role and bring a proposal to her supervisor in the coming weeks.

The supervisor would then take it to the provider meeting and discuss the care model with all of the WMFM Clinic providers. Both are excited to pursue new changes in the practice and continue to provide patients with the best possible care.

PROCEDURE 41.1   Coach a Patient on Disease Prevention

Tasks
Coach a patient on the recommended vaccinations for their age. Adapt the coaching for any communication barrier and the patient's developmental life stage. Document the coaching in the patient's health record.

Scenario
You are working with Dr. David Kahn. You need to room Charles Johnson (date of birth [DOB] 03/03/19XX), and his record indicates he has not been seen in several years. Charles has significant hearing loss, and he communicates by signing. His wife interprets for him. You look in his health record and see that he is due for influenza, Td, and recombinant zoster (shingles) vaccines. Per the provider's standing order, you need to coach adult patients on potential vaccines they are due for during the initial rooming process.

Directions
Role-play this scenario with two peers, who will play Charles and his wife. You are the medical assistant.

Equipment and Supplies
- Vaccine Information Statements (VIS) (available at https://www.immunize.org/vis/)
- Patient's health record

Procedural Steps
1. Wash hands or use hand sanitizer.
   Purpose: Hand sanitization is an important step for infection control.
2. Greet the patient. Identify yourself. Verify the patient's identity with full name and date of birth. Explain what you will be doing.
   Purpose: It is important to identify the patient in two different ways to ensure that you have the correct patient. Explaining the procedure can make the patient feel more comfortable and helps to reduce anxiety.
3. Arrange the chairs so the patient can see both you and the person signing. Speak slowly. Pause as needed to allow person signing to finish with the last statement. Look at the patient when communicating.
   Purpose: The medical assistant must focus on the patient and not the person signing or the interpreter. Speaking slowly and pausing allows the person to sign what you are saying.

4. Use simpler language when talking. Speak clearly. Communicate with dignity and respect. Allow time for the patient to respond. Listen to the patient's concerns.
   Purpose: When working with older patients, it is important to treat them with respect and dignity. Listening is important.
5. Ask the patient if he has received vaccines somewhere else over the past few years.
   Purpose: It is important to verify that the health record is accurate.
   Scenario update: The patient has not seen any healthcare providers over the past few years. The only vaccines he has received were given at this facility.
6. Describe the vaccines that are due. Use the VIS for each vaccine as you coach the patient on the purpose of the vaccine.
   Purpose: The VIS is written for patients and describes the vaccine, disease(s) it prevents, and adverse reactions (side effects).
   Scenario update: The patient knows the shingles vaccine is not covered and costs more than $200. He refuses the shingles vaccine, and he does not believe in getting the influenza vaccine. He is interested in getting the Td vaccine.
7. Ask the patient which vaccines he is interested in getting. If he refuses, be respectful of his choice. Any reason he gives for the refusal should be communicated to the provider.
   Purpose: Patients have the right to refuse. Any treatment refused must be communicated to the provider.
8. Document the coaching in the patient's health record. Include the provider's name, what was taught, how the patient responded, and any vaccines refused.
   Purpose: It is important to document the procedure in the health record to show it was done.
   07/16/20XX 1305 Per Dr. Kahn's order, instructed pt on the RZV, influenza, and Td vaccines. Pt stated he was not interested in the influenza vaccine or the RZV. He also stated his insurance wouldn't cover the RZV, and he didn't have the money to pay for it. He is interested in receiving the Td vaccine. Reviewed the Td VIS (07/15/20XX) with the patient. Pt stated he understood and would call if he had any issues. Due to pt's hearing impairment, pt's wife interpreted for pt during the visit._____ Suzanne Peterson, CMA (AAMA)

PROCEDURE 41.2   Coach a Patient on the Breast Self-Exam

Tasks
Coach a patient to do a breast self-exam (BSE) while considering the patient's cultural beliefs and developmental life stage. Document your teaching in the patient's health record.

Scenario
You are working with Binh, a 17-year-old Vietnamese patient. She has a strong family history of breast cancer. The patient can fluently speak English and understands it well. For this patient, Dr. David Kahn ordered: breast self-exam (BSE) coaching.

Directions
Role-play this scenario with another peer, who will be the patient.

Equipment and Supplies
- Breast self-examination brochure (optional)
- Breast model
- Provider's order
- Patient's health record

PROCEDURE 41.2   Coach a Patient on the Breast Self-Exam—cont'd

Procedural Steps

1. Wash hands or use hand sanitizer.

   Purpose: Hand sanitization is an important step for infection control.

2. Read the provider's order. Assemble the equipment.

   Purpose: It is important to know the provider's order before starting the procedure.

3. Greet the patient. Identify yourself. Verify the patient's identity with full name and date of birth. Explain the procedure to be performed in a manner that the patient understands. Answer any questions the patient may have about the procedure.

   Purpose: It is important to identify the patient in two different ways to ensure that you have the correct patient. Explaining the procedure can make the patient feel more comfortable and helps to reduce anxiety.

4. Provide privacy and independence during the session. Encourage the patient to ask questions and discuss her concerns.

   Purpose: It is important to adapt the coaching to the patient's developmental stage. Privacy and independence are important to someone who is 17. Encouraging questions and discussions is also effective.

5. Ask the patient if she is familiar with breast self-examinations. Ask about her thoughts on illness and if she does alternative therapies. Explain the importance of doing a self-exam.

   Purpose: In the Vietnamese culture, illness is often explained by mystical beliefs. Asking the patient her thoughts might be helpful for the medical assistant during the coaching session.

6. Explain to the patient that she will need to undress and look at her breast in the mirror to identify any changes.
   - Let her know that she will need to check to see if they are the usual size, shape, and color.
   - She should also look for swelling, redness, rash, dimpling, puckering, or bulging of the skin.
   - She should check to see if the nipple position or appearance has changed.
   - Finally, she should check to see if any fluid is coming from the nipple by placing her thumb and index finger on the tissue by the nipple and pulling outward toward the end of the nipple (Fig. 1).

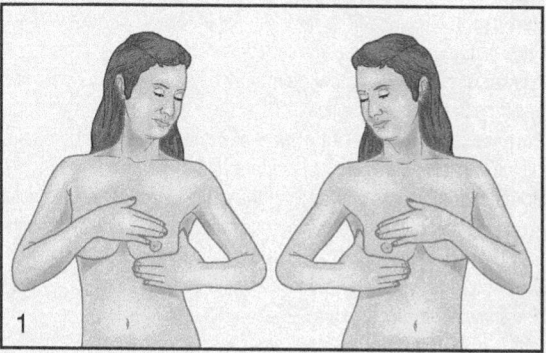

   Purpose: Changes in the appearance may indicate an issue.

7. Instruct the patient that she needs to change positions and continue to check the appearance of the breasts. She needs to place her hands on her hips and press down. This tightens the chest muscle under the breasts. While in this position, she should turn from side to side to see the outer part of the breasts. Instruct her to clasp her hands behind her head or raise her arms and look at the outer part of the breasts again (Fig. 2).

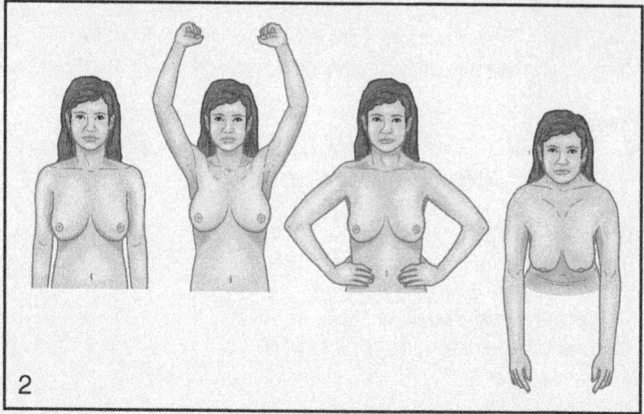

   Purpose: Sometimes changing the arm position may cause an abnormality to appear.

8. Instruct the patient to bend forward and roll her shoulders and elbows forward while tightening her chest muscles. While in this position, she can check for changes in the shape of the breasts

   Purpose: Abnormalities may be seen in this position.

9. Instruct the patient to palpate the breast using one of the following two techniques. Use the model as you explain the technique.
   - *Lying down technique:* Instruct the patient to check the breast while lying down. Have her do the following: Tuck a small pillow under the side being checked. Tuck one arm under the head, and with the other hand check the opposite breast (e.g., right hand checks the left breast). Use the first two or three finger pads. With fingers together, use a circular motion and a firm, smooth touch to check the entire breast. Start at the top outer breast tissue and move around the breast in a circular pattern. When the top of the breast is reached again, move in 1 inch toward the nipple and complete another circle around the breast. Repeat until the entire breast from the armpit to the cleavage is checked. Then place fingers flat on the nipple and feel for any changes beneath the nipple. Repeat these steps on the other breast.
   - *Shower technique:* Place the right hand on the right hip. With a soapy left hand, feel for changes in the right axilla area. Use two or three finger pads to press on the breast. Move in an up-and-down pattern over the breast tissue. Make sure to cover from the bra line to the collarbone. Repeat on the opposite side.

   Purpose: This position allows the patient to check the entire breast. The entire breast, including under the arm and up to the collarbone, needs to be checked for changes.

10. Have the patient select a technique that she will use. Encourage the patient to demonstrate the technique on the breast model. Coach the patient on ways to improve the exam if needed.

    Purpose: It is important to have the patient demonstrate the skill to check the accuracy her technique.

11. Answer any questions the patient may have. Provide the patient with a brochure to take home (optional).

    Purpose: It is important to answer any questions the patient has and if possible provide her with a brochure to take home.

12. Document the patient education in the patient's health record. Include the provider's name, the order, what was taught, how the patient responded, how the patient did the demonstration, and any handouts provided.

    Purpose: It is important to document the patient education in the health record to show it was done.

    07/19/20XX 1505 Per Dr. Kahn's order, instructed pt on the BSE. Instructed the patient on how to check for changes in the breast. Explained the lying down and showering techniques. Pt opted for the showering technique. She demonstrated how to palpate the breast tissue correctly using a breast model. All her questions were answered. Provided her with the "BSE" brochure and encouraged her to perform it monthly. _____ Suzanne Peterson, CMA (AAMA)

PROCEDURE 41.3   Coach a Patient on the Testicular Self-Exam

Tasks

Coach a patient to do a testicular self-exam (TSE) while considering the patient's developmental life stage. Document your teaching in the patient's health record.

Scenario

You are working with Dr. David Kahn. For Truong Tran (DOB 05/30/19XX), he ordered: testicular self-exam (TSE) coaching.

Directions

Role-play this scenario with another peer, who will be the patient.

Equipment and Supplies

- Testicular self-examination brochure (optional)
- Testicular model
- Provider's order
- Patient's health record

Procedural Steps

1. Wash hands or use hand sanitizer.
   Purpose: Hand sanitization is an important step for infection control.
2. Read the provider's order. Assemble the equipment.
   Purpose: It is important to know the provider's order before starting the procedure.
3. Greet the patient. Identify yourself. Verify the patient's identity with full name and date of birth. Explain the procedure to be performed in a manner that the patient understands. Answer any questions the patient may have about the procedure.
   Purpose: It is important to identify the patient in two different ways to ensure that you have the correct patient. Explaining the procedure can make the patient feel more comfortable and helps to reduce anxiety.
4. Ask the patient what he knows about the self-exam. Clarify any inaccuracies. Build on the patient's prior knowledge of the topic during the session. Identify the patient's motivating factor for learning about the self-exam. Listen to the patient's concerns.
   Purpose: It is important to adapt the coaching to the patient's developmental stage. Because of the patient's age, identifying motivating factors is important.
5. Explain to the patient that the best time to do the self-exam is after a warm shower or bath.
   Purpose: The scrotal skin is more relaxed.
6. Demonstrate on the model while discussing the technique. Instruct the patient to examine each testicle gently with both hands.
   - Roll the testicle between the thumb and fingers (Fig. 1).
   - Show the patient the epididymis, the soft, curved structure behind and on top of the testicle (Fig. 2).
   - Then show the patient how to examine the vas deferens, which is the tube that runs up the epididymis (Fig. 3).
   Purpose: This allows the person to do a better self-exam.

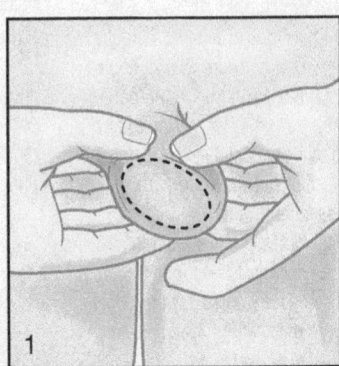

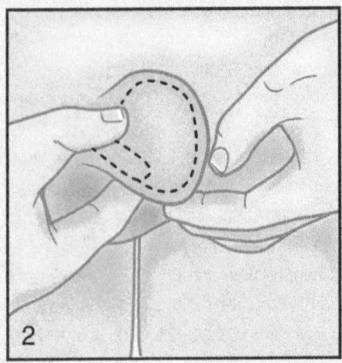

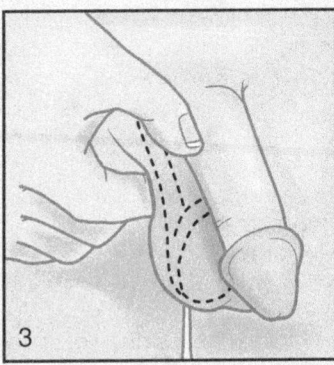

7. Instruct the patient to feel for any abnormalities and lumps. These could be painless or painful. Instruct the person to look for changes in the size, texture, or shape.
   Purpose: Any changes should be reported to the provider for possible follow-up.
8. Have the patient demonstrate the technique on the model. Coach the patient on ways to improve the exam if needed.
   Purpose: It is important to have the patient demonstrate the teaching to check for accuracy of technique and correct understanding.
9. Answer any questions the patient may have. Provide the patient with a brochure to take home (optional).
   Purpose: It is important to answer any questions the patient has and if possible provide him with a brochure to take home.
10. Document the patient education in the patient's health record. Include the provider's name, the order, what was taught, how the patient responded, how the patient did the demonstration, and any handouts provided.
   Purpose: It is important to document the patient education in the health record to show it was done.
   07/19/20XX 1505 Per Dr. Kahn's order, instructed pt on TSE. Instructed the patient on how to check for changes in the testes. Explained the technique and encouraged the patient to do monthly checks after a warm shower/bath. Pt provided an accurate return demonstration. His questions were answered. Gave pt the "TSE" brochure. _____ Suzanne Peterson, CMA (AAMA)

PROCEDURE 41.4 Perform a Neurological Status Exam

Tasks

Administer and score a Neurological Status Exam.

Scenario

Dr. David Kahn has ordered a Neurological Status Exam form to be completed on Robert Caudill (DOB 10/31/19XX). Mr. Caudill is accompanied by his caregiver.

Directions

Role-play this scenario with two other peers. One will play the patient and the other will be the caregiver.

Equipment and Supplies
- Patient's health record
- Order for the neurologic status exam
- Neurologic status exam form (see Fig. 41.8) or SimChart for the Medical Office (SCMO)

Procedural Steps

1. Wash hands or use hand sanitizer.
   Purpose: Hand sanitization is an important step for infection control.
2. *SCMO:* Click on the Form Repository and select the Neurological Status Exam on the INFO PANEL. Read the form.
   Paper form: Read the directions for the test.
   Purpose: To complete the test accurately, the directions need to be followed. Know the directions before completing the exam with the patient.
3. Greet the patient. Identify yourself. Verify the patient's identity with full name and date of birth. Explain the procedure to be performed in a manner that the patient understands. Answer any questions the patient may have about the procedure.
   Purpose: It is important to identify the patient in two different ways to ensure that you have the correct patient. Explaining the procedure can make the patient feel more comfortable and helps to reduce anxiety.
4. *SCMO:* Click on Patient Search. Select the patient and verify the DOB. Click Select and the patient's name and DOB will autofill into the form field. Key in the information for the performed by and the date fields.
   Paper form: Complete the following information on the exam form: patient name, date of birth, performed by, and date.
   Purpose: The patient information needs to be completed on the form. Your name and the date also need to be completed.
5. Ask for the caregiver's name and clearly ask the caregiver related questions from the form. Accurately document the information obtained.
   Purpose: The caregiver's information is important for the completion of the exam.
6. Perform the patient interview, following the directions on the form. Clearly provide the patient with the directions and the questions. Accurately document the information obtained from the patient.
   Purpose: Accurately documenting the information is critical for the accuracy of the exam.
7. Accurately score the test as indicated by the directions.
   SCMO: Key the scores in the total fields. Save the form when completed.
   Paper form: Write the scores on the total line. Give the completed form to the provider.
   Purpose: The score is important for the provider for diagnostic purposes.

PROCEDURE 41.5 Perform a Monofilament Foot Exam

Tasks

Perform a monofilament foot exam to screen for peripheral neuropathy. Provide health maintenance coaching by giving the patient foot care instructions. Document test results in the patient's health record.

Scenario

For patients with diabetes mellitus, Dr. David Kahn's standing orders include a monofilament foot exam and foot care instruction coaching. Your next patient has diabetes mellitus.

Directions

Role-play this scenario with another peer. The peer will be the patient.

Equipment and Supplies
- 10 g monofilament tool
- Gloves
- Paper towel
- Waste container
- Provider's order or standing order
- Patient's health record

Procedural Steps

1. Wash hands or use hand sanitizer.
   Purpose: Hand sanitization is an important step for infection control.
2. Read the provider's order. Assemble the equipment.
   Purpose: It is important to know the provider's order before starting the procedure.
3. Greet the patient. Identify yourself. Verify the patient's identity with full name and date of birth. Explain the procedure to be performed in a manner that the patient understands. Answer any questions the patient may have about the procedure.
   Purpose: It is important to identify the patient in two different ways to ensure that you have the correct patient. Explaining the procedure can make the patient feel more comfortable and helps to reduce anxiety.
4. Ask the patient to remove socks and shoes and rest the feet on the paper towel. The paper towel should be placed under the person's feet either on the floor or on the exam table step.
   Purpose: This prepares the patient for the test.
5. Using your hand, demonstrate that the monofilament is flexible and not sharp. Also demonstrate the monofilament on the patient's hand. Put gloves on.
   Purpose: This alleviates the patient's anxiety. Demonstrating on the patient's hand allows the patient to know how it feels.
6. Instruct patients to close their eyes. Tell patients to say "yes" when they feel the monofilament on the foot.
   Purpose: The patient's eyes must be closed for this test to be accurate.
7. Start with the great toe and place the monofilament perpendicular to the skin. Press the monofilament until it bends, hold for 1 second, and release (Fig. 1). Pause to give the patient an opportunity to confirm it was felt. A confirmation is a positive or normal response. The test result is abnormal if the patient cannot feel in one area.
   Purpose: It is important to hold the monofilament for 1 second for accurate results.

Continued

PROCEDURE 41.5 Perform a Monofilament Foot Exam—cont'd

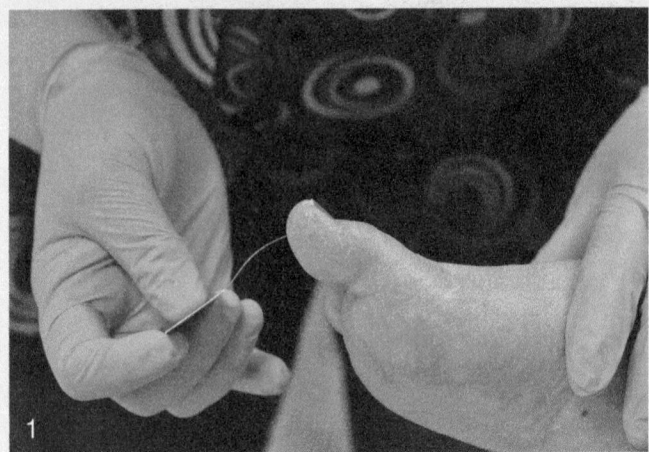

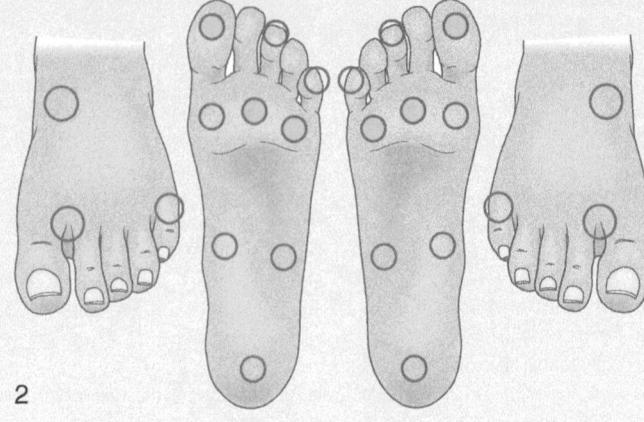

8. Do not cue the patient if no confirmation is given. Just move to the next location. Randomly test 9 to 12 locations on the anterior and posterior side of each foot or as the provider indicates (Fig. 2). If a patient does not feel the site, check it three times randomly. Make sure to space out testing times (e.g., the time between each check).
   Purpose: If the test is done in a rhythmic way, the patient may confirm the feeling without really feeling the test.
9. Discard supplies in the waste container. Remove gloves and wash hands.
   Purpose: Washing hands is important for infection control.
10. Coach the patient on proper foot care to prevent sores. Include when to check the feet, what to look for, and how to care for the feet daily. Suspicious areas need to be watched carefully and reported to the provider if they do not return to normal.
   Purpose: Careful monitoring can help prevent serious foot sores.

11. Document the test results in the patient's health record. Include the provider's name, the order, and the results of the test. For the test, the first number indicates the total number of sites felt, and the last number indicates the total times done. Indicate all sites where the patient did not feel the test. If the provider indicates specific areas to test, documentation should reflect these areas. Include any teaching done.
   Purpose: It is important to document the patient education in the health record to show it was done.
   07/19/20XX 1625 Per Dr. Kahn's order, performed a monofilament exam on both feet. Right foot 9/12 and left foot 12/12. Right posterior great toe 0/3. Pt coached on foot care. Stressed daily foot care and inspections. Pt listed the daily foot care required. Pt indicated what and where on his feet he needs to examine daily. All the pt's questions were answered. The "Feet Guide for Neuropathy" brochure was given to the patient. _____
   _____ Suzanne Peterson, CMA (AAMA)

PROCEDURE 41.6 Coach a Patient for an Electroencephalogram (EEG)

Tasks
Coach a patient on the preparation needed for an electroencephalogram. Document in the patient's health record.

Directions
Role-play the scenario with a peer, who is the patient. Your instructor is the provider. Make up the location, date, and time of the procedure.

Patient Instructions
Purpose of the EEG:
- An EEG is done to check for changes in the brain activity and can be helpful when diagnosing different disorders.
Patient preparation:
- Avoid caffeine on the day of the test.
- Take daily medications unless the provider indicates to hold medications until after the test.
- Wash hair the night before or the morning of the test, but do not use conditioners or any other hair care products.
- If you are to sleep through the EEG test, stay up later the night before the test or avoid sleeping.
During the test:
- Electrodes (patches with wires) will be attached to your head either with adhesive or by using a special cap.
- There will be little or no discomfort during the test.

- The technician may ask you questions during the test.
After the test:
- The technician will remove the electrodes.
- If sedation was used, you cannot drive after the test and for the rest of the day. Plan to have someone bring you home. Rest for the remaining part of the day.

Equipment and Supplies
- Patient instructions
- Patient's health record
Order: Provide EEG instructions.

Procedural Steps
1. Wash hands or use hand sanitizer.
   Purpose: Hand sanitization is an important step for infection control.
2. Greet the patient. Identify yourself. Verify the patient's identity with full name and date of birth. Explain what you will be doing in a manner that the patient understands. Answer any questions the patient may have.
   Purpose: It is important to identify the patient in two different ways to ensure that you have the correct patient. Explaining the procedure can make the patient feel more comfortable and helps to reduce anxiety.
3. Explain the purpose of an EEG.
   Purpose: The patient needs to understand why the EEG is being done.
4. Explain how the patient should prepare for the test.
   Purpose: Appropriate preparations are needed for quality test results.

PROCEDURE 41.6   Coach a Patient for an Electroencephalogram (EEG)—cont'd

5. Explain what the patient should expect during and after the test.

    Purpose: Explaining what to expect during and after the procedure will help reduce the patient's anxiety about the procedure.

6. Ask the patient to teach back the preparation to you. Clarify any misconceptions or inaccuracies. Answer any questions the patient may have. Give the patient a phone number to call if he has questions.

    Purpose: Using the teach-back method to evaluate the patient's understanding will help identify any misunderstandings the patient may have.

7. Let the patient know when to anticipate the results from the EEG. Also, give the patient the appointment information for the EEG, including the location, date, and time.

    Purpose: Letting patients know when to expect test results helps to alleviate confusion and anxiety.

8. Document the teaching in the patient's health record. Include the provider's name, what was taught, how the patient responded, and any written directions (including appointment information) sent home with the patient.

    Purpose: A procedure is not complete until it has been documented accurately in the patient's health record.

    9/12/20XX 1508 Per Dr. Kahn's order, EEG instructions were given to the pt. Pt's questions were answered. Patient taught back the instructions accurately. Patient was given the "Having an EEG" booklet. Pt was notified of appointment on 9/20/20XX at 9 a.m. at AnyTown Neurology Clinic. _____

    _____Suzanne Peterson, CMA (AAMA)

PROCEDURE 41.7   Coach a Patient on Health Maintenance: Colonoscopy

Tasks

Coach a patient on the colonoscopy preparation. Document the coaching in the health record.

Scenario

You work at WMFM Clinic. You are working with Dr. David Kahn, who has asked you to coach Charles Johnson (DOB 03/03/19XX) on the colonoscopy patient instructions. Dr. Kahn wants Charles to take his antihypertensive medication the morning of the procedure, 1 hour after finishing the preparation solution.

The ambulatory surgical center requires that Charles not eat or drink anything starting at midnight on the day of the procedure. He needs to arrive 90 minutes before the procedure, which is scheduled at 11 a.m. He will be receiving IV sedation during the procedure and will need a driver to take him home.

Patient Instructions

Purpose of the colonoscopy:

- To detect abnormal changes in the large intestine and rectum.

Dietary preparations:

- Two days before the procedure: Do not take fiber supplements or eat foods high in fiber (e.g., nuts, seeds, whole grains, and raw or cooked fruits and vegetables).
- One day before the procedure: Do not eat solid foods, just drink clear liquids (e.g., broth, gelatin, coffee, tea, clear juice, popsicles, and sport drinks). Do not drink red liquids or eat red gelatin. Do not drink or eat dairy products or alcohol.
- On the day of the procedure: Do not eat solid foods or drink liquids other than the preparation solution from midnight onward.

Colon cleansing:

- Split the preparation solution (e.g., GoLYTELY, Colyte) and take half the evening before the procedure. Take the rest of the solution in the morning. The solution must be completed at least 2 hours before the procedure.
- Usually within 1 hour of starting the preparation solution, liquid stools can occur and continue until 2 hours after completing the solution. Chills, headache, cramping, weakness, nausea, vomiting, and bloating can occur when taking the solution. Drinking the preparation more slowly can help reduce the severe vomiting and cramping.

During the test:

- Sedation is usually given. You will be lying on your side on the exam table.
- The colonoscope will be inserted into your rectum. Air or carbon dioxide is pumped into the intestine to help the provider see the lining of the colon. This can cause some cramping.

- The procedure takes about 30 to 60 minutes.

After the test:

- You will need to recover about an hour after the test.
- Do not drive. Plan to have someone bring you home.

Directions: Role-play the scenario with a peer, who is the patient. Your instructor is the provider. Make up the location, date, and time of the procedure.

Equipment and Supplies

- Patient instructions
- Patient's health record

Procedural Steps

1. Wash hands or use hand sanitizer.

    Purpose: Hand sanitization is an important step for infection control.

2. Greet the patient. Identify yourself. Verify the patient's identity with full name and date of birth. Explain what you will be doing in a manner that the patient understands. Answer any questions the patient may have.

    Purpose: It is important to identify the patient in two different ways to ensure that you have the correct patient. Explaining the procedure can make the patient feel more comfortable and helps to reduce anxiety.

3. Use simpler language when talking. Speak clearly. Communicate with dignity and respect. Allow time for the patient to respond. Listen to the patient's concerns.

    Purpose: When working with older patients, it is important to treat them with respect and dignity. Listening is important.

4. Ask the patient if he has ever had a colonoscopy. If so, ask him what he remembers about it.

    Purpose: It is important to find out what the patient already knows about the topic.

5. Discuss the purpose of the colonoscopy and the preparation involved. Refer to the written instructions that the patient will be taking home.

    Purpose: Referring to the written directions that will be sent home with the patient helps eliminate confusion.

6. Explain what the patient should expect during and after the procedure.

    Purpose: Explaining what to expect during and after the procedure will help reduce the patient's anxiety about the procedure.

7. Ask the patient to teach back the preparation to you. Clarify any misconceptions or inaccuracies. Answer any questions the patient may have. Give the patient a phone number to call if he has questions.

    Purpose: Using the teach-back method to evaluate the patient's understanding will help identify any misunderstandings the patient may have.

Continued

PROCEDURE 41.7 Coach a Patient on Health Maintenance: Colonoscopy–cont'd

8. Let the patient know when to anticipate the results. Also, give the patient the appointment information for the procedure, including the location, date, and time.

   Purpose: Letting patients know when to expect test results helps to alleviate confusion and anxiety.

9. Document the coaching in the patient's health record. Include the provider's name, what was taught, how the patient responded, and any written directions (including appointment information) sent home with the patient.

Purpose: It is important to document the procedure in the health record to show it was done.

08/14/20XX 1105 Per Dr. Kahn's order, instructed pt on the colonoscopy preparation. Patient taught back the instructions accurately. Gave the patient the "Colonoscopy Patient Directions" booklet. Pt was notified of appointment on 08/25/20XX at 11 a.m. at AnyTown Surgical Center. _____
_____ Suzanne Peterson, CMA (AAMA)

PROCEDURE 41.8 Develop a List of Community Resources and Facilitate Referrals

Tasks
As a patient navigator, develop a current list of community resources that meet the patient's healthcare needs. Discuss the resources with the patient and facilitate referrals to the chosen resources.

Scenario 1
Robert Caudill (DOB 10/31/19XX) was just diagnosed with dementia. He currently lives with his daughter, Ruby, who works full time. Ruby is feeling overwhelmed with being his only caregiver and realizes that she needs to find someone to care for her father while she is working.

Scenario 2
Leslie Green (DOB 08/03/20XX) just tested positive for pregnancy. She does not feel that she has a support system to help her make decisions.

Scenario 3
Ella Rainwater's husband of 30 years died suddenly 1 month ago. Ella (DOB 07/11/19XX) stated that she feels alone and has no one to talk to. Her daughter feels that Ella needs the support of others who have gone through the same thing.

Directions
For steps 1 and 2, research resources for these scenarios. For the remaining steps, role-play a scenario with two peers.

Equipment and Supplies
- Computer (with internet) or a telephone book
- Paper and pen
- Community Resource Referral Form or other referral form
- Patient's health record

Procedural Steps
1. Using the scenarios, identify the possible types of community resources that would assist each patient or family. Identify three different types of resources (e.g., medical equipment, support group) that would meet each patient's needs.

   Purpose: A variety of community resources are available for patients and families who are dealing with chronic illnesses and death. Such resources range from day care, meals, transportation, medical equipment, assisted living, and support groups to reduced costs for medications.

2. Using the internet or the phone book, identify two local resources for each of the three kinds of resources (i.e., find two assisted living resources, two medical equipment suppliers, and so on). Make a list of six resources for the patient and family. Include the following:
   - Organization's name
   - Address and contact information
   - Summary of the services provided
   - Cost and other relevant information

   Purpose: As the patient navigator or care coordinator, it is important for you to provide patients and families with the contact information for various community resources. This information can help the family find the best solution for the situation.

   Scenario update: Role-play the scenario indicated by the instructor.

3. Provide the patient or family member with the list of six resources. Describe the services offered and any costs.

4. Allow the patient or family member time to review the services. Answer any questions.

   Purpose: It is important that the patient and family members understand the services available.

5. Use professional, tactful verbal and nonverbal communication as you work with the patient or family member.

   Purpose: Patients and family members are more apt to respond positively to assistance if the medical assistant's communication is professional, empathetic, and tactful. Talking down to patients or acting superior are unprofessional behaviors that negatively affect the working relationship with patients.

6. Role-play making the community referrals. Have the patient or family member decide on two or more services they are interested in. Complete the referral document. Have the patient provide any additional information required on the form. Call the community resource agency and provide the referral information to the representative (a peer).

   Note: Some community referrals (e.g., support groups) will require the patient to make contact and not the healthcare professional.

   Purpose: The referral document is used by many organizations to capture the patient's preferences and to help process the referral.

7. Document the patient education and the referrals in the health record.

   Purpose: It is important to document all patient interactions and referrals in the health record.

Patient Coaching With Nutrition

LEARNING OBJECTIVES

1. Describe metabolism.
2. Describe dietary nutrients, including carbohydrates, protein, fat, minerals and electrolytes, vitamins, water, and fiber. Also, define the function of dietary supplements.
3. Explain current dietary guidelines.
4. Describe how to read a food label.
5. Describe the different types of medically ordered diets.
6. Identify the special dietary needs for weight control, diabetes, cardiovascular disease, and hypertension.
7. Identify the special dietary needs for those with food allergies, celiac disease, and lactose intolerance.
8. Identify special dietary needs for those with various conditions, including pregnancy and lactation, epilepsy, infection with the human immunodeficiency virus (HIV), acquired immunodeficiency syndrome (AIDS), and cancer.
9. Instruct a patient on dietary changes while demonstrating awareness of others' concerns.

OUTLINE

▶ OPENING SCENARIO

Kayla Smith, registered medical assistant (RMA), has been working at Walden-Martin Family Medical (WMFM) Clinic for 4 years. She enjoys working with the patients and the providers. Her supervisor is impressed with Kayla's motivation, patient care skills, and attention to detail. Kayla was asked to mentor Tim Brown, a medical assistant student from a local college.

Tim has finished his courses and is now completing his practicum at the clinic. Tim has an interest in nutrition, because his mother is a registered dietitian. He is eager to see how Kayla works with patients who have dietary changes. He hopes he will have the opportunity to observe her and then assist with the teaching process before doing it by himself.

YOU WILL LEARN

1. To identify dietary nutrients, including carbohydrates, fat, protein, minerals/electrolytes, vitamins, fiber, and water.
2. To describe the function of dietary supplements.
3. To distinguish the special dietary needs of those with diabetes, cardiovascular disease, hypertension, cancer, and lactose sensitivity.
4. To identify the special dietary needs for a person with allergies or celiac disease.
5. To instruct a patient according to the patient's special dietary needs.
6. To show awareness of a patient's concerns regarding a dietary change.

INTRODUCTION

Nutrition is a field of study that examines the substances in food that help us grow and stay healthy. Nutrition can also be defined as the intake of food for the body's dietary needs. It is important to eat a healthy and balanced diet. *Nutrients* are the chemicals in food that the body uses for energy, growth, and development. Nutrients include water, protein, carbohydrate, fat, vitamins, and minerals.

A medical assistant helps the provider by coaching patients on dietary changes. It is important to be aware of nutrients and the different types of diets commonly ordered in the ambulatory care environment. This chapter discusses metabolism and the nutrients essential for growth and development. Dietary requirements, along with medically ordered diets, are also discussed.

METABOLISM

Metabolism is the process the body uses to obtain or make energy from the food eaten. Metabolism has two phases:

- *Catabolism*: The process of breaking down molecules into smaller molecules, resulting in energy being released.
- *Anabolism*: The process of smaller molecules being used to build larger molecules with the use of energy.

For example, you eat a piece of chocolate candy with peanuts. It is broken down by enzymes (EN zimes) in the intestines. The enzymes break down the proteins into amino (ah ME noe) acids, the fats into fatty acids, and the complex *carbohydrates* (KAAR bow hye drates) into simple sugars (e.g., glucose). These substances are absorbed by the blood and brought to the cells. In the cells, other enzymes catabolize, or break down, these substances, and energy is released. The energy released can be used or stored by the body. The small molecules created from catabolism are used to create larger molecules as the body repairs tissues and performs other functions. This process requires energy and is called *anabolism.* Every action of the body, involuntary or voluntary, requires energy.

Many times, metabolism is thought of as what influences our bodies to gain or lose weight. This is where calories come in. A *calorie* is a unit that measures how much energy is in a particular food. People use calories or the energy at different rates. Some people eat a lot of food and do not put on any weight, whereas others feel they look at food and gain weight. The number of calories a person burns each day is affected by the following factors:

- How much the person exercises
- The amount of fat and muscle on the person's body
- The person's *basal metabolic rate* (BMR), or the rate the body burns calories while the person is at rest

---

VOCABULARY

amino acids Found in protein-containing foods and released during the digestion process in the intestines; carried by the blood to cells, where they are used to make proteins. Used for growth, maintenance, and repair of cells; they also transport nutrients.

enzymes Special proteins that speed up chemical reactions in the body.

fatty acids Result when fats are broken down; used by the body for energy and tissue development.

glucose Results when carbohydrates are broken down; main sugar found in the blood and used as the main source of energy in the body.

metabolism The chemical process that occurs within a living organism to maintain life; the process the body uses to obtain or make energy from the food eaten.

Basal Metabolic Rate

The BMR can play a role in a person's tendency to gain weight. For example, two people eat and exercise the same amount, but they have two different BMRs. The person with the lower BMR would have a greater tendency to gain more weight. Remember, the body stores unused calories as fat.

Variables that affect the BMR include:

- *Genetics*: Some people are born with a higher metabolism.
- *Sex*: Males have a higher density of lean muscle mass with a lower body fat percentage. This causes a higher BMR.
- *Age*: BMR decreases with age.
- *Weight*: The heavier an individual, the higher the BMR.
- *Body surface area*: This relates to a person's height and weight. The larger the body surface area, the higher the BMR.
- *Body fat percentage*: The lower a person's body fat percentage, the higher the BMR.
- *Diet*: Starvation and low-calorie diets can reduce the BMR.
- *Body temperature*: A higher body temperature results in an increased BMR.
- *External temperature*: The colder the external temperature, the more the body has to provide additional heat to maintain the body's temperature. This increases the BMR.
- *Thyroxin*: Produced by the thyroid gland, thyroxin can increase the BMR.
- *Exercise and lean muscle tissue*: Exercise will create lean muscle tissue, which increases the BMR.
- *Drugs*: Certain drugs (e.g., caffeine) can increase the BMR.

DIETARY NUTRIENTS

Nutrients in food, such as carbohydrates, can provide energy. Nutrients can also supply materials to build and repair tissues (e.g., proteins and amino acids). Lastly, nutrients can regulate metabolic processes. Some nutrients have only one purpose, whereas others have several jobs in the body. A combination of different foods is necessary to promote health. With a little planning, all the body's needs can be met by a well-balanced diet.

Nutrients can be classified into two different groups. *Essential nutrients* cannot be made by the body and must be in the food eaten. *Nonessential nutrients* are created by the body and do not need to be in food. For example, vitamin D is created from sun exposure on the skin, so it does not need to be consumed. Foods can also be described as:

- *Nutrient rich* (also called *nutrient dense*): Foods high in nutrients (e.g., vitamins, minerals, complex carbohydrates, healthy fats, and lean protein) and low in calories.
- *Non–nutrient rich*: Foods lacking vitamins, minerals, and fiber. They provide "empty calories" and can cause people to gain weight.

Carbohydrate

Carbohydrate is a nutrient found in our diet. About 45% to 65% of our daily calories should come from carbohydrates. Carbohydrates are used for energy and to regulate protein and fat metabolism. This nutrient encompasses a broad range of simple sugars, starches, and fiber.

Simple Sugars. There are many types of simple sugars. Nutrient-rich foods containing simple sugars include:

- Fruits and vegetables, which contain fructose and glucose
- Milk and milk products, which contain lactose

Non–nutrient-rich foods and food additives containing simple sugars include desserts (cookies, cakes), candy, soda, syrups (including regular and high fructose corn syrups), white sugar (sucrose), honey, and molasses.

During digestion, most sugars (except lactose from milk) break down into fructose and glucose. Lactose breaks down into glucose and galactose. Simple sugars are rapidly absorbed and quickly raise blood glucose levels. They provide a quick source of energy.

Starches. Starches are called *complex carbohydrates*. Examples of food sources of complex carbohydrates include:

- *Nutrient-rich starches*: Legumes (e.g., split peas, beans [kidney, black, garbanzo, and pinto]), starchy vegetables (e.g., corn, green peas, and potatoes), and whole grains (e.g., oats, barley, quinoa [KEEN waah], seeds, and brown rice)
- *Non–nutrient-rich starches*: White bread, crackers, and white rice

Complex carbohydrates are digested in the intestine before being absorbed. They break down into simple sugars and become a source of energy. The glucose from the simple sugars and starches raises the blood glucose level. With the help of insulin (IN suh lin), glucose is moved out of the bloodstream and into cells; it is then used for energy. Some glucose is stored in the liver and muscles as *glycogen*. The body uses the stored glycogen in between meals and during strenuous exercise. As the blood glucose levels start to drop, glucagon works in the

---

liver to release the stored glycogen. Glycogen is released back into the blood and raises the blood glucose level.

It is important to remember that excessive carbohydrates can be converted into fat. The following are smart carbohydrate dietary choices:

- Eat a variety of whole grains, fruits, vegetables, legumes, and low-fat or nonfat dairy products.
- At least half of all grains eaten should be whole grains.
- Limit processed foods in your diet, especially those with added sugar, salt, and fat.
- Eat enriched refined grains, if eating refined grains (Box 42.1).

VOCABULARY

enriched Nutrients are added back into a food after they were lost during food processing.

glucagon A hormone produced by the alpha cells in the pancreas; works in the liver to release glycogen and thereby prevent dangerously low blood glucose levels.

insulin A hormone produced by the beta cells in the pancreas; moves glucose into the cells so it can be used for energy.

Glycemic index. The *glycemic index* (GI) is a numeric index used to indicate how much a carbohydrate food raises the blood glucose level. The foods are ranked from 0 to 100. Carbohydrates that are rapidly digested, absorbed, and considerably raise the blood glucose level are considered high GI foods (≥ 70). Low GI foods (≤ 55) produce a smaller change in the blood glucose level. The goal is to eat more low GI foods to reduce the risk of type 2 diabetes mellitus and heart disease. Low GI foods can also help maintain weight loss. Table 42.1 provides examples of the GI values of some common foods.

Fiber. Fiber is different from simple sugars and starches. It cannot be digested by the body and thus it does not raise the blood glucose level. Fiber helps a person feel full and can help with weight management. There are two types of fiber: soluble fiber and insoluble fiber.

Soluble fiber dissolves in water and forms a gel-like substance. Soluble fiber softens the stool. It lowers the blood glucose level by slowing sugar absorption. Soluble fiber lowers the low-density lipoprotein (or bad cholesterol) level by binding to fatty acids. Examples of soluble fiber foods include the following:

TABLE 42.1	Glycemic Index (GI) for Foods		
Per Serving	**GI**	**Per Serving**	**GI**
Bagel, white frozen	72	Skim milk	32
Bread, whole wheat	71	Apple	39
Tortilla, wheat	30	Banana	62
Gatorade	78	Watermelon	72
Instant oatmeal	83	Peanuts	7

- Nutrient-rich: Legumes, oats, barley, fruits (e.g., avocados, apples, and citrus fruits) and carrots
- Non–nutrient rich: Processed and refined goods

Insoluble fiber bulks up the stool and helps to prevent constipation. Examples of insoluble fiber include the following:

- Nutrient-rich: Whole grains (whole wheat and brown rice), vegetables (corn, broccoli, green beans, cauliflower, and potatoes with skins), nuts and seeds, popcorn, and prunes
- Non–nutrient rich: Processed and refined goods

Fiber supplements are usually taken to reduce constipation. They can help a person be "regular." The active ingredient in the supplements can vary between natural and synthetic soluble fiber. Consider the following:

- *Metamucil* (MET ah myoo sil) contains *psyllium* (SIL ee uhm) *husk*, a natural substance that contains about 70% soluble fiber and 30% insoluble fiber.
- Citrucel contains *methylcellulose* (METH ahl sel yuh lose), a semisynthetic soluble fiber.
- Fibercon contains calcium *polycarbophil* (pol ee KAHR bow fil), a synthetic soluble fiber.

It is important to drink plenty of water when taking fiber supplements. Some fiber supplements have been shown to lower blood pressure, blood glucose, and the risk of heart disease.

CRITICAL THINKING 42.1

Kayla wants to help Tim review carbohydrates. She asks him to list two foods from each category: simple sugars, starches, and fiber. What foods would you list?

Protein

Protein (PROE teen) is a nutrient in our diet. About 10% to 35% of our daily calories should come from protein. Proteins are broken down into amino acids. Amino acids can be used as a source of energy in the absence of carbohydrates. Amino acids are also used to make proteins to help the body:

- Break down food (e.g., enzymes)
- Grow and repair body tissues (e.g., connective tissue, hair, nails, muscles)
- Perform other functions (e.g., those related to hemoglobin, antibodies, and hormones)

Protein and amino acids are considered the building blocks of life. The body needs several amino acids in large enough amounts to maintain good health. Protein malnutrition is seen around the world and can lead to *kwashiorkor*. A lack of dietary protein can cause growth failure, loss of muscle mass, anemia, edema and potbelly, skin depigmentation and hair loss,

BOX 42.2   Omega-3 Fatty Acids

Omega-3 fatty acids are a group of polyunsaturated fatty acids found in fish (e.g., salmon, herring, halibut, and mackerel) and some nuts and seeds. These fatty acids play a role in reducing blood cholesterol, heart disease risk, inflammation, and depression. Omega-3 fatty acids also increase the effectiveness of anti-inflammatory and antidepressant drugs.

weakening of the circulatory and respiratory systems, decreased immunity, and death.

Amino acids are classified into three groups:

- *Essential amino acids*: Cannot be made by the body, thus must come from food eaten throughout the day
- *Nonessential amino acids*: Can be made by the body from essential amino acids or in the normal breakdown of proteins
- *Conditional amino acids*: Usually not essential except in times of illness and stress

Foods that have all the essential amino acids to support the body are called *complete proteins*. Foods that are considered complete proteins are fish, meat, poultry, dairy products, quinoa seeds, buckwheat, chia seeds, and eggs. Foods that do not contain all the essential amino acids are called *incomplete proteins*. Nuts, legumes, grains, and vegetables are examples of incomplete proteins.

Smart protein choices include the following:

- Choose lean or low-fat meat and poultry.
- Eat seafood rich in omega-3 fatty acids, such as salmon, trout, herring, Pacific oysters, and Atlantic and Pacific mackerel (Box 42.2).
- Limit processed meats (e.g., ham, sausage, and deli meats), which contain added salt (sodium).
- Eat unsalted nuts and seeds to keep sodium intake low.

MEDICAL TERMINOLOGY	
glyc/o	sugar, glucose
lip/o	fat
anti-	against
mal-	bad, poor
poly-	many, much, excessive, frequent

CRITICAL THINKING 42.2

Kayla wants to help Tim review proteins. She asks Tim to list six foods that contain proteins. What foods would you list?

Fat

Fat is an important nutrient in our diet. Fats provide 9 calories per gram, whereas carbohydrates and proteins provide only 4 calories per gram. About 20% to 35% of our daily calories should come from fats and less than 10% from saturated fatty acids. The body uses fat for:

- A source of energy. If glucose is not available for energy, the body will break down fat stores for energy. The process forms ketones, which can be seen in the urine and blood.

TABLE 42.2 Types of Fats

Type	Description	Impact on Cholesterol	Found in
Saturated fats	Solid at room temperature	Increase the LDL level	Butter, cheese, whole milk, ice cream, cream, fatty meats; processed coconut oil, palm oil
Unsaturated fats	Liquid at room temperature; two kinds: monounsaturated and polyunsaturated	Decrease the LDL level	Monounsaturated: olive and canola oil Polyunsaturated: safflower, sunflower, corn, and soy oil
Trans fatty acids	Also called *hydrogenated fats* and *trans fats*; created when hydrogen is added to vegetable oils during food manufacturing	Increase LDL and decrease HDL levels	Foods made with hydrogenated and partially hydrogenated oils; margarine, commercially prepared baked goods

HDL, High-density lipoprotein; *LDL*, low-density lipoprotein.

- Healthy skin and hair.
- Vitamin absorption. Vitamins A, D, E, and K are fat soluble.
- Insulation (cushion) for organs and to keep the body warm.
- Brain development, controlling inflammation, and blood clotting. Linoleic and linolenic acid, which are essential fatty acids, are used for these processes.

Fat is required in the diet. Table 42.2 describes the types of fats found in foods. Diets low in fats can cause cold sensitivity, increased infections, and amenorrhea in women. Long-term fat deficiency can lead to metabolic problems and fat-soluble vitamin deficiency.

Triglycerides. *Triglycerides* are another type of fat in the body. Our livers make triglycerides from the calories we do not use. Triglycerides are also found in foods. Triglycerides are stored in the fat cells and have the following characteristics:

- Used for energy when carbohydrates are limited
- Absorb vitamins and other nutrients
- Contain essential fatty acids, which are important for growth and development

A person's triglyceride level is usually checked with the cholesterol levels. High triglyceride levels increase one's risk for heart disease and stroke. There are other reasons for high triglyceride levels, including poorly controlled type 2 diabetes mellitus, liver disease, kidney disease, and hypothyroidism.

The best ways to lower triglyceride levels are to:

- Cut back on calories and lose weight.
- Avoid sugary and refined food; choose monounsaturated fats over saturated fats.
- Limit the amount of alcohol consumed and exercise daily.
- Take medications that can be ordered to help reduce the triglyceride level.

Cholesterol. *Cholesterol* (koh LES the rohl) is a waxy, fatlike substance. It is used to make hormones, vitamin D, bile acids, and cell membranes. Cholesterol is created in the liver, and dietary cholesterol is found in animal-based foods (e.g., egg yolks, meat, shellfish, and cheese). Cholesterol is carried in the blood by the following lipoproteins:

- *High-density lipoprotein* (HDL): Considered "good" cholesterol. It helps move the cholesterol from the tissues to the liver. The liver helps remove cholesterol from the body. A low level of HDL increases the risk of heart disease.

- *Low-density lipoprotein* (LDL): Considered "bad" cholesterol. It moves cholesterol to tissues, including arteries. Most of the cholesterol in the blood is LDL. The higher the LDL level in the blood, the greater the risk for heart disease. LDL can be lowered through diet, exercise, and medications. Eating unsaturated fats can also help lower the LDL level.

CRITICAL THINKING 42.3

Kayla wants to help Tim review the three types of fats. She asks Tim to describe unsaturated fats, saturated fats, and trans fatty acids. How would you describe them?

Minerals and Electrolytes

Minerals are naturally occurring inorganic substances (e.g., iron, zinc, and calcium). Minerals needed by the body are divided into two categories: major and trace. *Major minerals*, or *macrominerals*, are needed in larger amounts. *Trace minerals*, or *microminerals*, are needed in smaller amounts in the body.

Electrolytes are minerals in the body fluid that have an electrical charge. They are found in the blood, urine, and other body fluids. Electrolytes come from the foods we eat and fluids we drink (Table 42.3). Too little or too much water in the body, vomiting, diarrhea, sweating, and kidney problems can change our electrolyte levels. A provider will order laboratory tests to measure a patient's electrolyte levels.

VOCABULARY

antioxidant Synthetic or natural substance found in food and supplements; may prevent or delay some types of cell damage.

fortified The addition of one or more substances to a food to increase its nutrient density.

CRITICAL THINKING 42.4

Kayla asks Tim how he would explain the difference between minerals and electrolytes. How would you respond?

Vitamins

Vitamins are organic substances needed by the body in very small amounts for specific roles. There are 13 vitamins required

TABLE 42.3   Examples of Major and Trace Minerals

Category	Mineral	Role in the Body	Found in
Major minerals (macrominerals)	Calcium	For healthy teeth and bones; muscle and nerve function, blood clotting, blood pressure regulation, immune system health	Milk products, canned fish (e.g., salmon), fortified soy milk, greens (e.g., broccoli), and legumes
	Potassium	For proper muscle and nerve function, fluid balance	Milk, fresh fruits and vegetables, whole grains, legumes, meats
	Sodium	For proper muscle and nerve function, fluid balance	Table salt, processed foods, and condiments
	Chloride	For proper fluid balance; stomach acid	Table salt, processed foods, tomatoes, celery, and olives
	Phosphorus	For healthy teeth and bones; important in the acid-base balance system	Meat, poultry, fish, eggs, milk, processed foods, and soda pop
	Sulfur	Found in body proteins	Meats, poultry, fish, eggs, legumes, and nuts
	Magnesium	Needed to make proteins; for muscle and nerve function and immune system health	Nuts, legumes, seeds, seafood, chocolate, and leafy green vegetables
Trace minerals (microminerals)	Iron	Part of hemoglobin found in the red blood cell, used for energy metabolism	Meats, fish, poultry, shellfish, egg yolks, legumes, dark leafy greens, and iron-enriched or fortified foods
	Zinc	Used for making proteins, taste perception, wound healing, immune system health, production of sperm, normal growth	Vegetables, poultry, fish, and meats
	Iodine	Found in thyroid hormone, which is involved with metabolism, growth, and development	Seafood, iodized salt, and milk products
	Selenium	Antioxidant (AN tee ok si dahnt)	Seafood, grains, and meats
	Fluoride	Involved with healthy teeth and bones	Fish, tea, and drinking water
	Chromium	Used in the metabolism of carbohydrates and fats; also aids in insulin action and glucose metabolism	Brewer's yeast, beef, liver, eggs, chicken, wheat germ, and potatoes
	Copper	Helps to form red blood cells; involved with keeping the blood vessels, nerves, immune system, and bones healthy; aids in iron absorption	Shellfish, whole grains, beans, nuts, liver, dark leafy greens, dried fruits, yeast, and cocoa

by the body. It is important to get the recommended dietary allowance (RDA) of each vitamin. A deficit of a vitamin can lead to disease.

Vitamins are either water soluble or fat soluble (Table 42.4). Water-soluble vitamins dissolve in water. These include the B vitamins and vitamin C. Any unused water-soluble vitamins leave the body through the urine. Vitamin B_{12} is an exception because the liver stores the vitamin for years. Water-soluble vitamins need to be taken in daily. Fat-soluble vitamins are vitamins A, D, E, and K. These vitamins are absorbed more easily with the presence of fat in the diet. They can build up in the body, reaching toxic levels, so typically supplements are not needed (Box 42.3).

> **VOCABULARY**
> **recommended dietary allowance (RDA)** The average daily food intake needed to meet the nutrient requirements of most healthy people.

> **MEDICAL TERMINOLOGY**
> cheil/o   lip
> gloss/o   tongue
> hem/o   blood
> -emia   blood condition
> -itis   inflammation
> -lytic   pertaining to destruction
> an-   no, not, without

> **CRITICAL THINKING 42.5**
> Kayla and Tim are reviewing vitamins that patients commonly take. Tim asks Kayla to explain the difference between water-soluble and fat-soluble vitamins. How would you explain the difference?

Free Radicals and Antioxidants

Free radical molecules, or *free radicals,* are natural by-products of normal metabolic processes. A free radical is an atom that has one or more unpaired electrons, causing it to be especially reactive. The free radical seeks out and takes electrons from other molecules. This usually causes damage to the other molecules.

The production of free radicals in the body can increase due to lifestyle and environmental factors, including:

- Tobacco smoke and alcohol consumption
- Eating fried foods
- Exposure to toxins (e.g., pesticides) and air pollution
- Stress and excessive exercise

Free radicals play an important role in many cellular processes. They are involved in the inflammation process. Excessive free radicals can affect our health by attacking cells' deoxyribonucleic acid (DNA) and blood vessels, causing aging and illness. This increases the risk for cardiovascular disease, strokes, arthritis, cataracts, and other degenerative diseases.

Antioxidants protect cells from free radicals and limit the damage free radicals can do to the cells. Antioxidants are

TABLE 42.4 Fat- and Water-Soluble Vitamins

Category	Vitamin	Recommended Dietary Allowance for Adults	Role in the Body	Found in	Deficiency Causes	Toxic?
Fat-soluble vitamins	Vitamin A	700–900 mcg RAE (Retinol Activity Equivalents)	Antioxidant; helps form and maintain healthy teeth, bones, mucus membranes, soft tissue, and skin	Dark-colored fruits and leafy vegetables, egg yolks, fortified milk products, liver, beef, and fish	Night blindness	Yes, can cause liver toxicity
	Vitamin D	15–20 mcg (600–800 International Unit)	Bone growth; made by the body after being in the sun	Fatty fish (e.g., salmon, herring), fish liver oils, fortified cereals, and fortified milk products	Bone pain, muscle weakness	Yes, *hypercalcemia* (HYE per kal see mee ah) (elevated blood calcium levels) and kidney problems
	Vitamin E (tocopherol [toe KOF eh role])	15 mg	Antioxidant; helps form red blood cells and helps the body use vitamin K	Avocados, dark green and dark leafy vegetables (e.g. spinach, broccoli, and asparagus); safflower, corn, and sunflower oil; papaya, mango, wheat germ, seeds, and nuts	Hemolytic (hee moh LIH tick) anemia, neurologic deficits	Yes, hemorrhagic toxicity can occur with supplement use
	Vitamin K	90–120 mcg	Blood clotting; made in the intestine	Cabbage, cauliflower, cereals, dark green and dark leafy vegetables, fish, liver, eggs, and beef	Bleeding	No toxic effects reported
Water-soluble vitamins	Thiamine (THY ah min) (vitamin B1)	1.1–1.2 mg	Used for nervous system, muscle function, and carbohydrate metabolism	Egg, enriched flour, lean meats, legumes, nuts, seeds, organ meats, peas, and whole grains	Beriberi (BER ee ber ee) usually in alcoholics	No toxic effects reported
	Riboflavin (RYE bow flae vin) (vitamin B2)	1.1–1.3 mg	Works with other B vitamins; important for growth and red blood cell production	Milk, mushrooms, spinach, almonds, and lamb	Riboflavin deficiency	No toxic effects reported
	Niacin (NYE ah sin) (vitamin B3)	14–16 mg NE (niacin equivalents)	Used in digestive process and skin and nerve functions; treats low HDL and high LDL cholesterol and triglyceride levels	Avocados, eggs, enriched breads and cereals, lean meats, fish, poultry, legumes, nuts, and potatoes	Pellagra (pah LAG rah), digestive issues	Niacin-containing supplements should be taken as provider indicates
	Pantothenic acid (PAN toh then ik) (vitamin B5)	5 mg	Involved with metabolism and hormone and cholesterol production; needed for growth	Avocados, broccoli, egg yolks, legumes, milk, yeast, organ meats, potatoes, and whole grains	Vitamin B5 deficiency	No toxic effects reported
	Pyridoxine (PIR i dok seen) (vitamin B6)	1.3–1.7 mg	Helps form red blood cells and maintain brain function; also used for protein metabolism	Avocados, bananas, legumes, meat, nuts, poultry, and whole grains	Cracks around mouth, depression, rash	No toxic effects reported
	Biotin (BYE oh tin) (vitamin B7)	25–30 mcg	Used for fat and carbohydrate metabolism; also used in the production of hormones and cholesterol	Chocolate, legumes, milk, nuts, organ meats (e.g., liver, kidney) pork, egg yolk, and yeast	Hair loss, cheilitis (kye LYE tis), glossitis (glah SYE tis)	No toxic effects reported
	Folate (FOH late) (vitamin B9, folic acid)	400 mcg DFE (dietary folate equivalents)	Works with vitamin B12 to help form blood cells; important in pregnancy to prevent spina bifida	Asparagus, broccoli, beets, brewer's yeast, legumes, enriched breads and cereals, green leafy vegetables, oranges, and peanut butter	Anemia, diarrhea	Caution with high doses, limited data on toxicity
	Cobalamin (KOE bal ah min) (vitamin B12)	2.4 mcg	Important for protein metabolism, the formation of red blood cells, and the maintenance of the central nervous system	Meat, eggs, fortified foods, milk products, organ meats, poultry, and shellfish	Pernicious (pur NIH shush) anemia, confusion	No toxic effects reported
	Vitamin C (ascorbic [ah SKOOR bik] acid)	75–90 mg	Antioxidant; promotes healthy gums and teeth; helps absorb iron; maintains healthy tissue and promotes wound healing	Citrus fruits, tomatoes, broccoli, cabbage, cauliflower, potatoes, spinach, and strawberries	Scurvy (SKUHR vee)	Kidney stones, excess iron absorption, gastrointestinal disturbances

HDL, High-density lipoprotein; *LDL,* low-density lipoprotein; *mcg,* micrograms; *mg,* milligrams; *RDA,* recommended daily allowance.
Some information was obtained from the Vitamins Food and Nutrition Board, Institute of Medicine, National Academies. https://www.nal.usda.gov/sites/default/files/fnic_uploads//DRI_Vitamins.pdf.

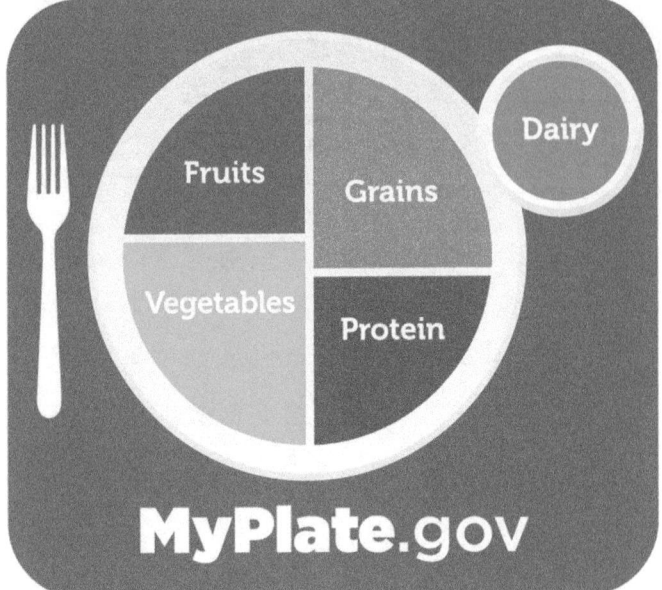

Fig. 42.1 Choose MyPlate. (From the US Department of Agriculture. www.myplate.gov.)

powerful and beneficial for us. Antioxidants include vitamins A, C, and E, beta-carotene, lycopene, lutein, and selenium.

Water

Drinking water every day is important for a person's health. Water is the basis for the fluids in the body. It makes up more than two-thirds of the body's weight. Without water, we would become dehydrated and die within a few days. All cells and organs need water to function and survive. Water plays important roles in the body, such as:

- Keeping the body temperature normal with perspiration
- Lubricating organs and cushioning joints (e.g., saliva, fluid around joints)
- Helping to prevent and relieving constipation by moving food through the intestines
- Protecting the spinal cord, brain, and other sensitive tissues
- Getting rid of waste products in the body through urine, sweat, and stools

Our need for water increases in hot weather, when we are more active, or when we have a fever, diarrhea, or vomiting. The recommended daily intake of water for healthy men is about 13 cups; the recommendation for healthy women is 9 cups. The individual need for water is based on a person's weight, age, activity level, and certain medical conditions.

Water and Diseases. Some patients are placed on fluid restrictions. This means they can only have a certain amount of fluids a day. The provider will indicate the maximum amount of fluids to be consumed daily. It is important to limit fluids that act as a diuretic (e.g., alcohol and caffeinated beverages), because they pull fluid from the body and increase the risk of dehydration. Conditions that may require fluid restrictions include:

- Heart problems, including congestive heart failure
- Kidney problems, such as those that might affect patients on dialysis and those with end-stage renal disease
- Adrenal insufficiency and corticosteroid treatment

Some diseases and conditions require more fluids/water to be consumed. People with postural orthostatic tachycardia syndrome (POTS) need to drink at least 2 to 3 liters of water a day to maintain their blood pressure. Other conditions, such as diabetes insipidus, diabetes mellitus, and Addison disease, may cause patients to excrete more urine and thus put them more at risk for dehydration.

FOOD GUIDES

For over a century, the US Department of Agriculture (USDA) has provided food guides to the public. Some of the more recent guides include:

- 1992: Food Guide Pyramid, which showed the five basic food groups arranged in a pyramid. The lower part of the pyramid consisted of the food groups that made up the majority of the daily diet. People were to eat less of the food groups at the top of the pyramid.
- 2005: MyPyramid Food Guidance System, which continued with the pyramid design but added physical activity and oils.
- 2011: MyPlate, which was introduced along with the 2010 Dietary Guidelines for Americans.

MyPlate

MyPlate focuses on making healthy food choices because everything eaten matters (Fig. 42.1). Some of the key messages with these dietary guidelines include:

- Fill half the plate with fruits and vegetables. Vary the colors and types of fruits and vegetables.
- Make half of the grains eaten each day whole grains.
- Vary the types of proteins eaten.
- Move to low-fat or fat-free milk and yogurt.
- Drink and eat less saturated fat, sodium, and added sugars.

TABLE 42.5 Food Groups With Serving Amounts for MyPlate

Food Group	What Counts?	Children 2–8*	Children 9–18*	Women 19–51+*	Men 19–51+*
Dairy	*1-cup equivalent:* 1 cup milk, yogurt, soymilk, almond milk, or coconut milk 1½ ounce (oz) natural cheese 2 oz processed cheese	2–2½ cups	3 cups	3 cups	3 cups
Proteins	*1-oz equivalent:* 1 oz meat, poultry, or fish ¼ cup cooked beans 1 egg 1 tablespoon peanut butter ½ oz nuts or seeds	2–4 oz	5–6½ oz	5–5½ oz	5½–6½ oz
Vegetables	*1-cup equivalent:* 1 cup raw or cooked vegetables or vegetable juice 2 cups raw leafy greens	½ cup	2–3 cups	2–2½ cups	2½–3 cups
Fruits	*1-cup equivalent:* 1 cup fruit or 100% fruit juice ½ cup dried fruit	1–1½ cups	1½–2 cups	1½–2 cups	2 cups
Grains	*1-oz equivalent:* 1 slice of bread 1 cup dry cereal ½ cup cooked rice, pasta, or cereal (at least half should be whole grains)	3–5 oz	5–8 oz	5–6 oz	6–8 oz

*Amount required is based on sex, age, and the amount of exercise. Ranges are indicated above, for more specific information, go to www.myplate.gov.

MyPlate consists of five food groups, along with oil (Table 42.5). Oil contains required nutrients, so the USDA addresses it. Oil is usually consumed in nuts, fish, cooking oil, and salad dressing. Most children need 3 to 6 teaspoons, and adults need 5 to 7 teaspoons daily, depending on sex and age.

The MyPlate website (www.myplate.gov) offers numerous online resources for individuals and professionals. Tip sheets, food plans, and other resources provide additional information. MyPlate is very flexible for cultural foods.

Dietary Guidelines

The USDA publishes Dietary Guidelines every 5 years. These guidelines are for individuals 2 years or older. The focus is on disease prevention and health promotion. The current dietary guidelines focus on overall eating patterns, health, and the risk of chronic disease.

Key recommendations from the 2020–2025 Dietary Guidelines for Americans include those listed with MyPlate, in addition to the following:
- Added sugars: Limit to less than 10% of calories per day starting at age 2. Avoid for infants and toddlers
- Saturated fat: Limit to less than 10% of calories per day starting at age 2. Examples of saturated fats include butter, whole milk, fatty meats, coconut oil, and palm oil.
- Sodium: Limit to less than 2,300 mg per day for age 14 and older.
- Alcoholic beverages: Men should limit intake to 2 drinks or less per day. Women should limit intake to 1 drink or less per day.

- Pay attention to portion sizes.
- Food choices should be rich in nutrients.

READING FOOD LABELS

Knowing how to read a food label is important when making healthy food selections. The food label contains the nutritional information and the ingredient list. The government has required food manufacturers to include certain information on the food label. The amounts for "Trans Fat" and "Added Sugars" are some of the newer additions to the food label.

Food labels provide nutritional facts. This information is presented in both the quantity (e.g., grams [g] or mg) and as a percentage. The percentage reflects the % Daily Value (DV). This is the percentage of the nutrient in a single serving in terms of the daily recommended amount based on a 2000-calorie diet. You will see this description at the bottom of the list of nutrition facts. Remember that if you are eating fewer than 2000 calories daily, these percentages will be different for you.

When reading the nutrition facts (Fig. 42.2), start at the top and work down:
- Check the calories per serving. If you eat the entire container and it consists of two servings, you need to double the calories.
- Check the amount of fat. Limit the saturated fat intake and avoid trans fats.
- The amounts listed for cholesterol, sodium, total carbohydrates, and added sugars are also numbers to consider. Choose foods with low amounts of these nutrients.

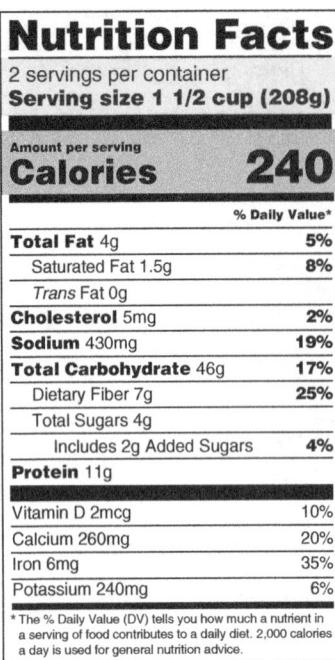

Nutrition Facts

2 servings per container
Serving size 1 1/2 cup (208g)

Amount per serving
Calories **240**

	% Daily Value*
Total Fat 4g	5%
Saturated Fat 1.5g	8%
Trans Fat 0g	
Cholesterol 5mg	2%
Sodium 430mg	19%
Total Carbohydrate 46g	17%
Dietary Fiber 7g	25%
Total Sugars 4g	
Includes 2g Added Sugars	4%
Protein 11g	
Vitamin D 2mcg	10%
Calcium 260mg	20%
Iron 6mg	35%
Potassium 240mg	6%

* The % Daily Value (DV) tells you how much a nutrient in a serving of food contributes to a daily diet. 2,000 calories a day is used for general nutrition advice.

Fig. 42.2 Nutrition Facts. (From the US Food and Drug Administration. https://www.fda.gov/Food/IngredientsPackagingLabeling/LabelingNutrition/ucm537159.htm.)

- Examine the dietary fiber, protein, vitamin D, calcium, iron, and potassium. Make sure you are getting enough of these beneficial nutrients.

Ingredient lists on foods are also important to understand (Fig. 42.3). The ingredients are listed in descending order, starting with the one that weighs the most and ending with the one that weighs the least. There are several reasons a person may look at the ingredient list:
- To look for trans fats: Even if the nutrition information indicates 0 grams trans fats, the product may still contain less than 0.5 gram of trans fats per serving. Look for ingredients such as "hydrogenated" or "partially hydrogenated oil." This indicates the presence of trans fats. So even if the nutrition information indicates 0 grams of trans fats, you may quickly reach your daily limit if you eat more than one serving.
- To avoid certain ingredients: Some people try to avoid ingredients such as high fructose corn syrup and certain food colorings.
- To identify allergens: More than 160 foods have been found to be allergens. The government has identified eight allergens that make up about 90% of all food allergy reactions. Laws regulating food labeling require manufacturers to indicate if any of these top allergens are in the food product. Advisory statements, such as "May contain peanuts" or "Made in a factory that also processes tree nuts," are optional and not required by law. (More information on allergens will be presented later in the chapter.)

MEDICALLY ORDERED DIETS

Patients may need to change their diet for a variety of reasons:
- Preparation for a procedure

Food Label #1	Food Label #2
Ingredients: semolina (wheat), durum flour (wheat), eggs, partially hydrogenated oil, niacin, ferrous sulfate, thiamin mononitrate, riboflavin. **Contains: Wheat, Eggs. Manufactured in a facility that uses tree nuts and eggs.**	**Ingredients:** grapes, corn syrup, high fructose corn syrup, fruit pectin, and citric acid.

Fig. 42.3 Ingredient List on Food Labels.

- Dental problems
- Illness
- A condition that requires dietary changes (e.g., allergy, hypertension)

If the dietary change is also a lifestyle change (e.g., for diabetes or hypertension), the provider may refer the patient to a registered dietitian (die eh TISH an). The registered dietitian can provide in-depth coaching and counseling on dietary changes.

For other dietary changes or to review a person's knowledge of a specific diet, the medical assistant may be involved. When the provider orders a specific test or a particular diet, the medical assistant may need to coach the patient on the new diet. As with other coaching, it is important for the medical assistant to provide the patient with a reference handout to take home. This will help guide the patient on the dietary changes. Learning about different medically ordered diets is important for the medical assistant.

> **VOCABULARY**
>
> **coaching** Providing information in a supportive environment that allows people to grow, change, or improve their situation.
>
> **registered dietitian** A credentialed healthcare professional who is trained in nutrition and is able to apply the information to the dietary needs of healthy and ill patients.

Clear Liquid Diet

A clear liquid diet is made up of foods and beverages that are liquid at room temperature. Clear means you need to see through the liquids. Examples of foods included on a clear liquid diet are:
- Water, tea, coffee, sport drinks, and clear soda
- Popsicles and juice without pulp
- Soup broth and gelatin (e.g., Jell-O)

Clear liquid diets are ordered for only a short time because they do not contain adequate nutrition. A clear liquid diet may be used when a person experiences diarrhea, vomiting, or nausea. It is commonly ordered after surgery and as part of the preparation for intestinal procedures. If a person is undergoing an intestinal procedure, red or pink clear liquids are not allowed because they could be mistaken for blood in the intestine.

Full Liquid Diet

A full liquid diet is made up of foods and beverages that are liquid at room temperature. Unlike the clear liquid diet, the full liquid diet includes milk products. Foods included in a full liquid diet are:

- Clear liquids (see previous section, Clear Liquid Diet)
- Strained creamy soups
- Milk, milkshakes, pudding, plain yogurt, custard, and ice cream
- Liquid supplements
- Sugar, honey, syrups, butter, margarine

Some providers will allow cooked, refined cereals (e.g., cream of rice), baby food strained meats, and potatoes pureed in soup on a full liquid diet. This diet is a step above a clear liquid diet and below a regular diet.

Full liquid diets are ordered for only a short time because they do not contain adequate nutrition. A full liquid diet may be used before or after surgery, as part of the preparation for tests or procedures, and if a person has difficulty chewing or swallowing.

VOCABULARY

regular diet The food and drink a person typically consumes when there are no dietary limitations.

CRITICAL THINKING 42.6

Kayla and Tim are working with Janine Butler. Janine needs to undergo an intestinal procedure and needs to be on clear liquids for 2 days. Janine states, "I was on a full liquid diet last year for a procedure. What is the difference between a clear liquid diet and a full liquid diet?" How would you answer this question?

Soft and Mechanical Soft Diets

A soft diet is a transition between a liquid diet and a regular diet. The foods on this diet are soft in texture, low in fiber, and easy for a person to digest. Foods on a soft diet include:
- Grains: soft breads, crackers, white rice, pasta
- Fruits and vegetables: soft cooked, canned (no skin)
- Milk products: milk, yogurt, cottage cheese, ice cream, pudding
- Protein: tender meat, poultry, and fish; eggs, tofu, smooth peanut butter

The soft diet eliminates foods that are hard to chew and swallow, including:
- Raw fruits and vegetables
- Chewy or crispy breads
- Tough meats, broccoli, cauliflower, nuts, and seeds
- Fried, greasy foods
- Highly seasoned or spicy foods

This diet is used for patients recovering from surgery or a lengthy illness. It can also be used for people with chewing or swallowing problems due to illness or dental issues.

Mechanical soft diets consist of foods that have been prepared for easier chewing and swallowing using household tools (e.g., grinder, blender, and knife). Typically, there are no limitations (e.g., spicy, gassy, and fried foods) to mechanical soft diets. Mechanical soft diets are used for:
- Those recovering from head, neck, or mouth surgery
- Those who have difficulty swallowing (*dysphagia* [dis FAY jee ah]), poor-fitting dentures, or no teeth
- Those who are too ill to chew

Bland Diet

A bland diet includes foods that are soft and low in fiber. This diet eliminates foods that are spicy, fried, or raw and beverages that contain caffeine or alcohol. Citrus juices and foods may also be eliminated. The foods included in a bland diet are similar to those incorporated into a soft diet. A bland diet is ordered to help treat gastroesophageal reflux disease (GERD), ulcers, nausea and vomiting, diarrhea, and gas. It can also be used after stomach or intestinal surgery.

Weight Control Diet

When trying to achieve or maintain a healthy weight, a person needs to find the balance between the number of calories eaten and the number used. Extra calories eaten and not used will result in a weight gain. For people to lose 1 to 2 pounds per week, they need to reduce their caloric intake by 500 to 1000 calories a day or increase their exercise to burn more calories. Identifying the calories consumed is an important step in achieving a healthy weight. Food diaries, apps, and trackers are available to help gauge food intake and activity.

Nutritional tips for patients trying to achieve a healthy weight include:
- Commit to a lifestyle change. Identify resources for information and support.
- Track foods eaten and beverages drunk, along with physical exercise.
- Set realistic goals, knowing that slips will occur.
- Eat healthy meals. They should be low in saturated fat, trans fat, cholesterol, salt, and added sugar. Eat lean meats, fish, poultry, beans, eggs, and nuts. Include fruits (especially whole fruits), vegetables, whole grains, and fat-free or low-fat milk products.
- Control portion sizes. *Portion size* is the amount of food we eat. *Serving size* is a standard measurement of food (e.g., 1 cup or 1 ounce [oz]). Many foods that come as a single portion actually contain multiple servings. For instance, a serving size of potato chips is 1 oz. The 3-oz potato chip bag is a single portion, but three servings. Another example is bread. You use two pieces of bread for a sandwich (portion size), but a serving is one slice. Most people overestimate serving sizes. It is best to measure the food or use a quick estimate method (Table 42.6 and Box 42.4).

CRITICAL THINKING 42.7

Kayla and Tim are working with Amma Patel. Kayla is explaining the weight control diet that Dr. Perez ordered for Amma. They are discussing serving size and portions. Amma states she is confused by the difference. How might you explain the difference between these two concepts? Provide an example for Amma.

Obesity. According to the Centers for Disease Control and Prevention (CDC), about 42.4% of adults were obese in 2017–2018, which is up from 10 years earlier. Obesity-related diseases (e.g., heart disease, type 2 diabetes, stroke, and certain types of cancer) are some of the leading causes of death in the US.

TABLE 42.6   Quick Methods to Estimate Portion Size

Amount of Food	Size of
3 ounces (oz) chicken and lean beef	Deck of cards
1 medium potato	A computer mouse
½ cup cooked pasta	Tennis ball
1 oz of cheese	Two dice
1 medium-sized fruit	Tennis ball
1 cup fruit or cooked vegetables	Baseball
1 oz of nuts	Handful
1 oz of chips or pretzels	Two handfuls (13–16 chips)
1 cup	Woman's fist
1 tablespoon (T.)	First joint of thumb
1 teaspoon (tsp.)	Fingertip

BOX 42.4   Portion Size and Obesity

In some cases, portion sizes and serving sizes are the same. Over the years many portion sizes have changed. Some experts attribute the growing obesity epidemic in the United States to this change. In the 1950s the dinner plate was 9 inches in diameter; today it is 11 to 12 inches. Some restaurants use even larger plates. With the plate change, the average portion of food also has increased. Restaurants have increased the amount of food they serve, and more Americans are eating out. With the increase in portions, *portion distortion* is occurring. The size of restaurant portions is causing Americans to rethink what the "normal" portions of food should be. Here are some examples of portion changes since the 1990s:

- Bagels have increased by 3 inches and added 210 calories.
- Muffins have increased by 3.5 ounces (oz) and added 290 calories.
- Cheeseburgers have increased in size and added almost 260 calories.
- Soda size has increased by 13.5 oz and added almost 170 calories.

As these examples show, the increase in portion sizes has led to an increase in the number of calories. Remember, the calories consumed and not used turn into fat.

Information from the National Heart, Lung, and Blood Institute. https://www.nhlbi.nih.gov/health/educational/wecan/eat-right/distortion.htm.

Childhood obesity remained stable over the past 10 years and affects about 18.5% of children. According to the CDC, about 13.7 million children and adolescents are obese. The prevalence of childhood obesity is higher in children after age 6 than in earlier years of life.

People are considered overweight or obese when they weigh more than what is considered a healthy weight for their height. The body mass index (BMI) is a screening tool for obesity. Chapter 33 discusses the BMI. If a person's BMI is less than 18.5, that person is considered underweight. A BMI higher than 18.5 but less than 25 is considered normal; a BMI higher than 25 but less than 30 is consider overweight; and a BMI of 30 or higher is considered obese.

Treatment for obesity includes:

- *Dietary changes*: Cutting calories, making healthier choices, restricting certain foods, and meal replacements.
- *Exercise and activity*: Exercising 150 to 300 minutes a week.
- *Behavior changes*: Trying to eliminate the obstacles to managing weight (e.g., high-risk situations). Recording diet and

exercise patterns. Counseling and support groups can be helpful.

- Prescription weight-loss medications (Table 42.7)
- *Vagal nerve blockade*: An implanted device sends electrical impulses to the vagus nerve, telling the brain when the stomach is empty or full.
- *Weight-loss surgery*: Also called *bariatric surgery*; it helps the person feel fuller sooner. Common weight-loss surgeries include:
  - *Gastric bypass surgery*: A small pouch is created at the top of the stomach, and the rest of the stomach is stapled shut. The small intestine is cut, with one end attached to the new pouch, thus bypassing the duodenum. The other end, which is attached to the stomach, is attached to another section of the intestine. Patients may have issues with iron and calcium absorption. Vitamin B_{12} supplements must be taken.
  - *Laparoscopic adjustable gastric* band (LAGB) surgery: A band is placed on the upper part of the stomach, creating a small pouch that helps to restrict food. A small port is implanted below the skin, and fluid can be injected into the band to adjust the size of the pouch outlet.
  - *Gastric sleeve surgery*: A small pouch is created in the stomach, and about 67% of the stomach is removed. The person feels full sooner.

Diabetic Eating Plans

People with diabetes mellitus need to monitor their carbohydrate intake. Remember that carbohydrates are broken down into glucose in the body. Insulin moves the glucose from the blood into the cells. For people with diabetes, the body either does not make enough insulin or does not respond to the insulin produced. As a result, their blood glucose levels are high. In the absence of insulin, the body metabolizes fat and uses ketones for energy. Ketones build up in the body. (Too many ketones can lead to ketoacidosis, a life-threatening condition.) See Chapter 7 for more information on the treatments for type 1 and type 2 diabetes.

Over the years, several different diabetic eating plans have been created for people with diabetes mellitus. You may hear of patients being on diet plans, such as the exchange list system. This diet plan grouped similar foods that had the same amount of carbohydrate, protein, fat, and calories. Each food item had a measurement (e.g., 1 cup) to indicate how much could be eaten for that exchange. Three main groups were given in the plan: carbohydrate, meat, and fat.

The American Diabetes Association (https://www.diabetes.org) encourages the following diabetes meal plans: the glycemic index approach, the Create Your Plate method, and carb counting. The GI was explained earlier in this chapter. Eating lower GI foods helps one to maintain a more stable blood glucose level.

The Create Your Plate method uses a 9-inch dinner plate (Fig. 42.4). To follow this meal plan, a person would:

- Fill half of the plate with nonstarchy vegetables (e.g., beans, broccoli, carrots, salad greens, and peppers).

TABLE 42.7 Weight Loss Medications

Medication	Class	Action	Common Side Effects
orlistat (OR li stat) (Xenical, Alli)	Lipase inhibitors	Prevents some of the fat consumed from being absorbed in the intestines	Oily spotting, loose stools, difficulty controlling stools, stomach pain, headache
phentermine (FEN ter meen) and topiramate (toe PYRE a mate) (Qsymia)	Anorectic (phentermine), anticonvulsants (topiramate)	Reduces appetite and causes a person to feel fuller longer after eating	Headache, dizziness, numbness and burning in hands and feet, decreased sensation, excessive tiredness, dry mouth, thirst
naltrexone (nal TREX one) and bupropion (byoo PROE pee on) (Contrave)	Opiate antagonist (naltrexone), antidepressant (bupropion)	Reduces hunger and helps control cravings	Drowsiness, anxiety, dry mouth, headache, stomach pain, vomiting, loss of appetite, excessive sweating, constipation
liraglutide (lir a GLOO tide) (Saxenda, Victoza)	Incretin mimetics	Helps the pancreas release the right amount of insulin when the blood glucose is high	Headache, constipation, heartburn, cough, tiredness, difficulty urinating

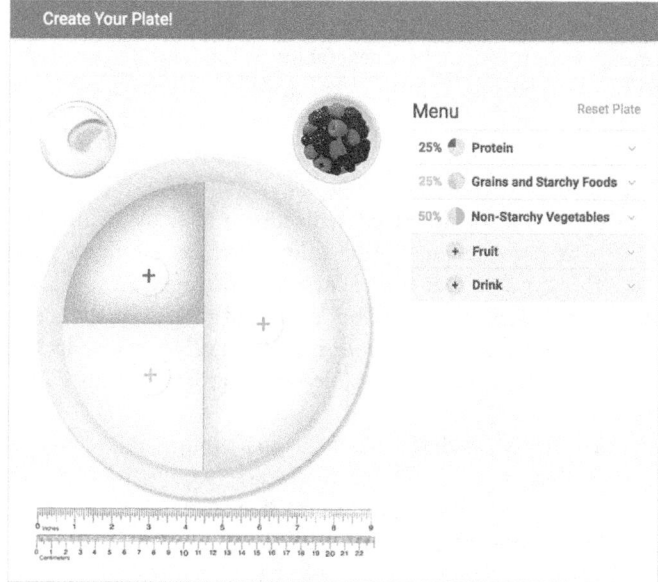

Fig. 42.4 Create Your Plate Method by the American Diabetes Association.

- Split the remaining unfilled side of the plate in half. Fill one half with a protein (e.g., lean meat, poultry, and fish) and fill the other half with a grain or a starchy vegetable (e.g., brown rice, potatoes, squash, green peas, and corn).
- Complete the meal with a serving of fruit, a serving of dairy (milk product), and a nonsweetened beverage.

Carb counting, or carbohydrate counting, is another meal planning tool used by people with diabetes mellitus. Using this method, a person keeps track of the amount of carbohydrates eaten each day. Carbohydrates are measured in grams. This system may give some people better control of their diabetes, but it is a learning process. The person needs to identify which foods contain carbohydrates and how to estimate the number of grams. The total grams are calculated over the day. Some people with type 1 diabetes may need to adjust the amount of insulin they take for a specific meal based on the amount of carbohydrates they will consume.

Low-Sodium Diet

Sodium is essential to our bodies because it helps to regulate fluid balance. The Food and Drug Administration (FDA) recommends that healthy adults consume no more than 2300 mg of sodium per day. Patients with high blood pressure, heart disease, or kidney disease are usually on reduced-sodium diets. Excessive sodium in a person's diet can lead to increased blood pressure, thus increasing the risk for heart disease and stroke.

If a patient is on a reduced-sodium diet, the provider will usually refer them to a registered dietitian. The dietitian will help educate the individual on the sources of sodium. Foods high in sodium include:

- Processed meats (e.g., deli meats, bacon, frankfurters, and sausage)
- Frozen dinners and ready-to-eat cereals
- Canned foods (e.g., soups, vegetables, and vegetable juice)
- Salted nuts and peanut butter
- Buttermilk, cheese, and processed cheese products
- Quick breads and salted crackers
- Prepackaged mixes for potatoes, rice, and pasta
- Olives, pickles, sauerkraut, pickled vegetables, and spaghetti sauce
- Soy sauce, seasoning salt, marinades, ketchup, mustard, and salad dressings
- Instant puddings and cakes
- Chips and pretzels

Typically, alternative lower sodium foods are discussed. Reading labels is also an important skill for those on reduced-sodium diets.

Dietary Approaches to Stop Hypertension. Dietary Approaches to Stop Hypertension (DASH) is a flexible eating plan recommended for those with hypertension and cardiovascular disease. The goal of the plan is to reduce blood pressure and LDL and triglyceride levels. Foods included in the DASH eating plan include:

- Fruits and vegetables
- Low-fat or fat-free dairy foods
- Whole grains
- Poultry and fish
- Beans, nuts, and vegetable oils
- Foods high in potassium, calcium, magnesium, protein, and fiber
- Foods low in salt (sodium)

Foods prohibited or limited on the DASH eating plan include:

- Foods high in saturated fat, total fat, and cholesterol
- Red meats
- Sugar-sweetened beverages and sweets
- High-salt (sodium) foods
- Full-fat dairy foods
- Tropical oils (coconut, kernel, and palm oil)

CRITICAL THINKING 42.8

Kayla and Tim are working with Al Neviaser, who has hypertension. Dr. Martin has ordered the DASH eating plan instructions for Mr. Neviaser. Tim explains to Mr. Neviaser that high-salt foods make the blood "salty" and more water is needed in the bloodstream to bring the "salty" level down. The extra water in the blood increases the blood pressure. Mr. Neviaser asks which foods he should stay away from. Give 10 foods that are high in salt (sodium).

Heart Healthy Diet

The diet and lifestyle recommendations of the American Heart Association (AHA) closely resemble the DASH diet and the MyPlate guidelines. The AHA incorporates a focus on exercise, along with a healthy diet. The following are the AHA's recommendations:

- Limit sugary drinks, sweets, fatty meats, and salty or highly processed foods.
- Read labels and select products with the lowest amounts of sodium, added sugar, and saturated fats. Eat fewer than 2400 mg of sodium a day to lower blood pressure. To lower the blood pressure even further, sodium can be reduced to 1500 or 1000 mg per day.
- Be physically active. Balance the calories you burn during exercise with the calories you consume to maintain your weight. Include 150 minutes of moderate physical activity or 75 minutes of vigorous physical activity or a combination of both each week. Break up exercise into 10-minute sessions if needed. To lower blood pressure or cholesterol, 40 minutes of aerobic exercise of moderate to vigorous intensity three to four times a week is recommended.
- Drink alcohol in moderation. Women should have only one drink and men should have only two drinks per day.
- Table 42.8 lists the adult servings for each food group. These are based on a 2000-calorie per day diet.

Low-Protein Diet

The body uses protein for tissue repair, growth, healing, and the ability to fight infection. When protein is broken down in the body, the waste products (e.g., urea and ammonia) are eliminated in the urine. People with liver and kidney disease are often prescribed a low-protein diet. They limit or restrict foods that contain high amounts of protein. Their bodies cannot clear the protein waste products. They can have nausea, headaches, fatigue, and a bad taste in their mouth. Eating a low-protein diet helps to prevent worsening of their disease. Remember, protein cannot be eliminated from the diet. It plays an essential role in the body.

Foods high in protein include milk products (e.g., yogurt and cheese), peanut butter, nuts (e.g., almonds, pistachios, and cashews), quinoa, legumes (e.g., lentils, soybeans, kidney beans, and chickpeas), meat, fish, poultry, and eggs. Foods with small amounts of protein include vegetables and starches (e.g., breads, cereals, and pastas). Fruits, sugars, and fats have trace amounts of protein.

High- and Low-Fiber Diets

A prior section of the chapter discussed fiber as a carbohydrate. The provider may order a low-fiber or restricted-fiber diet. This type of diet limits the types of vegetables, grains, and fruits eaten. Limiting fiber and food residue (e.g., peels, nuts, and seeds) makes stools smaller and lessens irritation on the intestinal lining. Possible reasons for a low-fiber diet include:

- Narrowing of the intestine due to a tumor
- A flare-up of an intestinal disease (e.g., irritable bowel syndrome, Crohn disease, and diverticulitis)
- After intestinal surgery
- Prior to an intestinal procedure (e.g., radiation and colonoscopy)

The provider can also order a high-fiber diet. This diet adds more bulk to the stools. High-fiber diets are used for:

- Reducing constipation and possibly lowering the risk of hemorrhoids
- Lowering cholesterol levels
- Controlling blood glucose levels
- Weight loss

TABLE 42.8   American Heart Association's Eating Healthy Recommendations

Food Group	Daily Amounts	Healthy Recommendations
Dairy	3 servings, or 3 cups	Use low-fat (1%) and fat-free options
Proteins	1–2 servings, or 5.5 ounces (oz)	Eat fish, skinless poultry, lean and extra lean meat, nuts, seeds, beans, and legumes; limit fatty or processed meats and red meats
Vegetables	5 servings, or 2.5 cups	Eat a variety of vegetables
Fruits	4 servings, or 2 cups	Eat a variety of fruits
Grains	3–6 servings, or 3–6 oz	Eat whole grains for at least half of the daily servings
Oils	3 tablespoons	Use polyunsaturated and monounsaturated oils; avoid hydrogenated oils and tropical oils

Data From: Information for these recommendations came from the American Heart Association, https://healthyforgood.heart.org/eat-smart/info-graphics/what-is-a-healthy-diet-recommended-serving-infographic. Accessed July 13, 2020.

Elimination Diet and Food Allergies

A food allergy occurs when the immune system overreacts to a protein in the food. The immune system makes IgE antibodies in response to the protein. This causes the person to quickly experience allergy symptoms. Symptoms may include itching, hives, nausea and vomiting, diarrhea, difficulty breathing (e.g., tightness in the throat or chest, coughing, wheezing), or anaphylaxis (AN ah fah lak sis).

As earlier indicated, eight allergies make up about 90% of the food allergy reactions. Sesame was added to the top eight allergies. These eight food allergens can be hiding in ingredient lists under other names. Some examples are listed here:

- Milk (e.g., cream, casein, ghee, galactose, lactalbumin, lactose, and whey)
- Eggs (e.g., albumin, eggnog, ovalbumin, and ovomucin)
- Fish (e.g., cod, bass, flounder)
- Crustacean shellfish (e.g., crab, lobster, shrimp)
- Tree nuts (e.g., almonds, cashews, filberts, hazelnuts, marzipan, nut meal)
- Peanuts (e.g., peanut butter, peanut flour)
- Wheat (e.g., emmer, einkorn, durum, kamut, modified wheat starch, wheat bran, wheat flour, wheat germ)
- Soybeans (e.g., edamame, miso, soya, tempeh, tofu)
- Sesame (a hidden ingredient in "spices" and "natural flavors")

It is important to realize that parts of these foods are used in other foods. For instance, milk proteins (e.g., whey and casein) and milk sugar (lactose) appear in some surprising food, medications, and hygiene products. Some examples include chicken broth, deli meats, hot dogs, French fries, shampoos and conditioners, and dry powder medication inhalers (e.g., Advair Diskus, Flovent Diskus, and Serevent Diskus). Reading ingredient lists is critical for those with allergies.

When people suspect a food allergy, the *elimination diet* can be used. People remove the allergy-potential foods from their diet. They may need to track what they eat and how they feel. Slowly, they may then add the suspicious foods back into their diet, one food at a time. This process helps identify the allergen. In some cases, a cross-reactivity may occur, and the person will have additional food allergies. An allergist can help identify additional food and environmental allergies.

> **VOCABULARY**
> **anaphylaxis** A rapidly progressing, life-threatening allergic reaction; characterized by hives, swelling of the mouth and airway, difficulty breathing, wheezing, and loss of consciousness.

Pollen-Food Syndrome. Another issue faced by those with food allergies is *cross-reactivity*. This means that the protein in the allergic food is similar to that in other foods. The person's immune system cannot tell the proteins apart and thus reacts to similar foods. Cross-reactivity can occur with foods and nonfood items. For instance, a person with a latex allergy could also be allergic to avocados, bananas, chestnuts, and kiwi.

Pollen-food syndrome (also called *oral allergy syndrome*) is caused by cross-reacting allergens found in pollens, raw foods, and tree nuts. Symptoms include itchy mouth and ears, scratchy throat, and swollen lips, mouth, tongue, and throat. Typically, the symptoms disappear when the food is out of the mouth. Some common cross-reactions include:

- Ragweed pollen: Cucumber, banana, melons, potatoes, and zucchini
- Grass pollen: Celery, melons, oranges, peaches, and tomatoes
- Birch pollen: Pitted fruit (e.g., plum, pear, peach, and apple), kiwi, carrot, celery, almond, and hazelnut

Alpha-gal Syndrome. Alpha-gal syndrome or allergy is an allergy to the alpha-gal sugar molecule found in mammals (except for people, apes, and monkeys). The alpha-gal sugar molecule can also be found in products made from mammals, including gelatin, some vaccines and medications, cosmetics, and milk products.

It is believed that the Lone Star tick carries this disease from animals to humans. Most cases occur in the southeastern and midwestern US and infect adults over age 50. Younger adults and children can also have it. Symptoms of alpha-gal syndrome include:

- Rash, hives, difficulty breathing, and wheezing
- Swelling of the lips, face, throat, and tongue
- Drop in blood pressure, dizziness, and faintness
- Nausea, vomiting, severe stomach pain

Symptoms can be life-threatening and commonly appear 3 to 6 hours after exposure (eating meat or using products). A skin test or a blood test can be used to diagnose alpha-gal syndrome. Treatment consists of avoiding foods and products that cause the reaction.

Celiac Disease. People with celiac disease are put on a gluten-free diet. (See Chapter 12 for additional information on celiac disease.) Gluten is a protein found in:

- Barley and malt products (e.g., flavoring and vinegar)
- Rye
- Triticale (wheat and rye crossbred hybrid)
- Wheat (e.g., durum flour, farina, graham flour, spelt, semolina, and kamut)

Gluten is commonly found in breads, cereals, pastas, cakes, cookies, and other foods. It causes inflammation in the small intestine of people with celiac disease. Removing gluten from the diet helps to control the symptoms.

The FDA regulates the gluten-free food labeling claim. This is a voluntary claim that manufacturers may opt to use. If they use the label, they are accountable for using the claim in a truthful way.

Lactose Intolerance Diet

Lactose intolerance, or sensitivity, is not an allergy. Lactose is the main sugar found in dairy products. Lactose is broken down by lactase, an enzyme created by the small intestine. If a person's small intestine does not produce enough lactase, the lactose moves into the large intestine. The bacteria in the large intestine break down the lactose, causing bloating, cramps, diarrhea, nausea, and gas. Treatment for lactose intolerance or sensitivity involves avoiding milk products or using an oral enzyme replacement supplement.

NUTRITIONAL NEEDS FOR VARIOUS POPULATIONS

Nutritional needs change throughout life. Our needs for calories, vitamins, minerals, and protein change as we grow and develop. With pregnancy and breastfeeding, the needs increase. With disease conditions, the needs change. We have already discussed different diets and conditions treated with those eating plans. Table 42.9 describes the nutritional needs by age groups. (Eating disorders are discussed in Chapter 15.)

Pregnancy and Lactation

During pregnancy, it is important to eat a healthy diet. The first trimester can be difficult with nutrition. Depending on the mother's morning sickness, eating a balanced diet can be tricky. Many providers recommend eating small, frequent meals to combat morning sickness. Dry crackers and toast are also encouraged. Eating low-odor protein foods can also help. Avoiding triggers such as spicy foods and certain smells are important in managing morning sickness.

Providers usually recommend a daily prenatal vitamin and mineral supplement to ensure adequate folic acid and prevent spina bifida. Consuming alcohol during pregnancy is not recommended. Despite the saying "eating for two," the daily caloric intake only needs to increase by 340 calories for the second trimester and about 450 calories for the third trimester.

Women who are pregnant or breastfeeding should avoid eating raw fish or fish high in mercury. Two to three servings of seafood per week are recommended during pregnancy and when breastfeeding. According to the FDA, examples of the best choices of seafood to eat include salmon, cod, tilapia, catfish, haddock, lobster, perch, squid, trout, shrimp, and light canned tuna. Mercury, which can be toxic to the nervous system, can be found in higher levels in marlin, orange roughy, bigeye tuna, swordfish, shark, king mackerel, and tilefish from the Gulf of Mexico. Consumption of locally caught fish and white albacore tuna intake should be limited to no more than 6 ounces per week.

With lactation, or breastfeeding, the mother needs to eat a healthy diet, and a vitamin supplement may be recommended.

It is important to get adequate vitamins and minerals, which are passed to the baby in the breast milk. The mother also needs to drink additional water to maintain her milk volume. During the first 6 months of breastfeeding, the mother should consume about 330 extra calories and 400 extra calories during the remaining 6 months of the first year.

Eating Disorders

Treatment for eating disorder includes psychological, behavioral, and nutritional therapies. (See Chapter 15 for additional information on eating disorders.) Some patients with eating disorders have medical complications from the malnutrition. Dietary needs for people with eating disorders are aimed at correcting nutritional imbalances and restore their weight. Nutritional plans focus on consuming a wide and balanced range of foods. Eating regularly spaced meals is also important.

Epilepsy

Some patients with epilepsy follow a ketogenic diet. This diet consists of very-low-carbohydrate, high-fat, and adequate protein foods. Some people have also used this type of diet to lose weight. Without carbohydrates, the body metabolizes fat, and the ketones are used for energy. It is important to monitor kidney function when a person is on a ketogenic diet.

HIV and AIDS

When a person has HIV infection or AIDS, it is important to eat a well-balanced diet. Making sure the immune system is nutritionally supported is critical. People with these diseases can struggle with several issues, including nausea, diarrhea, constipation, and poor appetite. The provider may order medications to help with the nausea. Drinking extra fluids will help with both diarrhea and constipation issues. Restricting milk products with diarrhea and increasing fiber intake with constipation can help. A poor appetite can cause weight and nutrient loss. Frequent small meals, nutritional supplements (e.g., Ensure), and light exercise may help. A provider may encourage a daily vitamin and mineral supplement. With unintended weight loss, additional "healthy" calories should be added to the diet.

TABLE 42.9	Nutritional Needs by Age Groups
Age	**Nutritional Needs**
Infancy to 2 years	Birth to 6 months of age: Breast milk or formula is given. If an infant cannot tolerate milk-based formulas, other types of formulas are available, including soy formula. Some formulas are available by prescription only. Six months of age: The child is started on soft, pureed solid foods. Usually, infant cereals, fruits, and vegetables are first introduced. One year of age: The child is transitioned to whole milk, and pureed foods are gradually replaced with easy-to-eat foods. It is important to offer foods from each food group.
2 to 12 years	Age 2: Children should eat several dairy products, fruits, vegetables, meats, breads, pasta, cereals, and beans. As children grow and develop, more foods can be added to their diet. Portion sizes also grow.
12 to adulthood	Adolescents experience rapid growth periods, which require more energy. Teens may need encouragement to consume dairy products (e.g., milk) instead of soda. The growth spurts require calcium for strong bones. Females who have started menstruating should eat foods high in iron to replace the iron lost in menstrual blood.
Older adults	As a person grows older, the metabolism decreases, and caloric needs also decrease. Special nutritional concerns of the older adult include: • Difficulty chewing and swallowing, which can be related to poor-fitting dentures • Decrease in eating due to changes in the senses (e.g., taste, smell) • Lack of a well-balanced diet (e.g., limited income, loneliness, and lack of initiative to cook for oneself)

Cancer

Patients undergoing radiation and chemotherapy can experience issues that affect eating. The treatments can harm fast-growing cells in the lining of the mouth, lips, and intestinal tract. Patients may have mouth sores that cause pain and swallowing problems. Taste and smell changes can occur. The treatments can cause appetite changes, diarrhea or constipation, fatigue, dry mouth, nausea, vomiting, and weight gain or loss. Good nutrition is critical for people to regain their strength and to heal after the treatments. A registered dietitian is commonly involved with the team of healthcare professionals caring for patients undergoing treatment. Nutritional tips for patients undergoing cancer treatments include the following:

- Eat a soft, bland diet.
- Eat six to eight small meals a day instead of three meals. Attempt to eat high-calorie, high-protein snacks (e.g., hard-cooked eggs, peanut butter, nuts, supplements, trail mix, and canned chicken).
- Take only sips of liquids during meals. Drink most liquids between meals. Drink 8 to 10 cups of liquid a day to prevent constipation. Water, prune juice, and warm liquids are helpful.
- To reduce mouth dryness and sores, limit caffeine and alcohol; keep the mouth clean using water or a mild mouth rinse; avoid tart, acidic or salty foods; eat lukewarm, cold, soft, and creamy foods; and use anesthetic rinses prior to eating.
- Avoid foods with strong odors and those that are overly sweet, spicy, greasy, or fried.
- Eat small bites and chew the food well. Eat dry foods (e.g., crackers, toast).
- In addition, use a straw and/or a small spoon, and puree food as needed. Suck on hard candies and ice chips to soothe the mouth and prevent mouth dryness.

CRITICAL THINKING 42.9

Kayla and Tim are working with Noemi Rodriguez, who is currently undergoing chemotherapy. She was not able to see her oncologist today, and she had a very sore mouth after the last treatment. List some nutritional tips for patients undergoing cancer treatments.

INSTRUCTING PATIENTS ON DIETARY CHANGES

When a patient needs a dietary change, the provider will give the order to the medical assistant. The provider will tell the medical assistant what type of diet the patient needs to be on. If the diet is only for a short period of time, the provider will indicate the time period. Sometimes the dietary change is related to a procedure. The provider will order the diagnostic procedure, and the medical assistant should be knowledgeable about the dietary changes required for that procedure.

Before meeting with the patient for coaching, it is important for the medical assistant to gather any brochures or information needed. Remember, it is a good idea to send the patient home with written instructions on dietary changes. If the patient does not understand English, use an interpreter service, and make sure brochures are in the patient's primary language.

Lastly, before meeting with the patient, the medical assistant should look over the brochure. It is important to be

BOX 42.5 Showing Awareness of a Patient's Concerns

Being aware means being alert and understanding what you are perceiving. When working with patients, you first need to be aware of the patient's concerns before you can show that you are aware. It is important to be accurate in your perception of the patient's concerns. If your perceptions are incorrect, you could speak or behave in a way that is insensitive to the patient.

Chapter 17 discusses therapeutic communication techniques. Let's review a few ways a medical assistant can show awareness of the patient's concerns:

- *Reflection:* The medical assistant puts words to the patient's emotional reaction, which acknowledges the person's feelings; for example, "It sounds like you are unsure of this new way of eating."
- *Restatement or paraphrasing:* The medical assistant rewords or rephrases a patient's statement to check the meaning and interpretation. This shows you are listening and understanding the patient. You might say, for example, "What I am hearing is that you really like your family traditions for holiday meals."
- *Summarizing:* This allows the medical assistant to recap and review what was said; for example, "If I understand how you feel about this new eating plan…"

Remember that a medical assistant can also show awareness by using positive and open, nonverbal behaviors. These nonverbal behaviors could be used when working with a patient on a dietary change:

- *Position:* The medical assistant should be at the level of the other person and angled toward the patient. For example, if the patient is sitting, then the medical assistant should be sitting also.
- *Arms and posture:* The medical assistant should be poised with their arms to the side. This is an open, positive nonverbal behavior that shows interest in the other person.
- *Facial expression:* The medical assistant should be smiling. Refrain from rolling your eyes, yawning, or frowning. These can be perceived as being bored or rude.
- *Gestures and touch:* The medical assistant should use small gestures and an appropriate light touch on the hand of the patient, depending on the situation.
- *Mannerisms:* The medical assistant should focus on the patient. It is not appropriate to look at your watch, phone, or the clock. This gives the patient the feeling you are bored or impatient.

knowledgeable about the content you are explaining to the patient. Reading the brochure aloud as a way of instructing the patient is not professional. The patient may feel you do not know what you are talking about.

When a medical assistant instructs a patient on a dietary change, it is important to know why people eat what they do and to understand how cultural dietary traditions relate to illness, as described in the following section. Box 42.5 provides a review of communication techniques and nonverbal behaviors that can show awareness of a patient's concerns. Procedure 42.1 details the process of coaching a patient regarding a dietary change.

AWARENESS OF OTHERS' CONCERNS

When you work with patients regarding a dietary change, it is important to understand the factors that can affect what they eat:

- *Cost:* How much money we have affects what foods we purchase. It can be expensive to purchase fresh fruits and vegetables, fish, and lean cuts of meat. Less expensive options are available, but they may not have the same taste or appeal.
- *Convenience:* With busy lifestyles, people sometimes choose what is easiest and quickest. This usually includes eating out or take-home meals.

- *Background*: Our background can influence the foods we eat. Some cultures have healthier diets than others. It can be helpful for people to modify cultural dishes by cutting the salt, fat, and sugar, without giving up the taste.
- *Emotional comfort*: Some people may eat when they are happy or when they are sad. Usually under these conditions, the food choices are not the healthiest. Some people stop eating when they are emotional.
- *Routine*: People eat what they always eat out of habit, personal preference, and availability. People may also eat with certain activities, like viewing a sports event, driving, or watching television. These habits are difficult to break.

It is important for the medical assistant to get to know what the patient is eating and why. This helps when coaching a patient on a dietary change. For instance, knowing your patient has a limited food budget is helpful when coaching them on healthier choices. You might be able to share ideas on healthy foods that are less costly or places to shop that are cheaper.

Cultural Diets

Medical assistants should be familiar with the diets of the various cultural groups in the area where they are practicing. This information can be helpful when coaching patients on specific diets ordered by the provider. General cultural diet information includes:

- Asian diets include whole grains (e.g., millet and rice), fruits, vegetables, legumes, nuts, and seeds. Fats are derived largely from vegetable oils (peanut or sesame oils). Dairy products are not traditionally eaten. Protein sources include broiled or stir-fried fish and seafood, egg whites, tofu, and nuts.
- Latin American diets include food from plant sources at each meal. This can include maize (corn), potatoes, fruits, vegetables, whole grains, beans, and nuts. Poultry, fish, and dairy typically are consumed daily. Meat and eggs are eaten weekly.
- Mediterranean diets include whole grains, fresh fruits and vegetables, and all types of legumes (e.g., beans, lentils, and peas) daily. Olive oil is used. Fish, poultry, and eggs are consumed weekly and meat monthly.
- Mexican diets include corn or flour tortillas, cabbage, legumes, squash, tomatoes, corn, and potatoes daily. Cheeses are eaten, but milk is not regularly consumed. Protein sources typically are fish, beef, poultry, lamb, and many types of beans.

CLOSING COMMENTS

Good nutrition is important for a person's health and well-being. For many people, changing their diet can be difficult and uncomfortable. It is important for the medical assistant to be sensitive to the change that the patient is asking about. Educating the patient about the benefits of making a dietary change may make the transition easier. Compliance with the diet increases if the person meets certain conditions:

- Can modify special foods and not give them up completely
- Has support from family and friends
- Can slowly transition to the new diet, though this might not always be possible

The medical assistant is an important team member when there is a need to help patients transition to a new diet. It is important for the medical assistant to be familiar with the dietary changes required for common procedures and diagnoses.

PATIENT-CENTERED CARE

As medical assistants work with patients from various cultures, it is important for them to know more about those cultures. Many cultures have dietary traditions that influence how they respond to illness. In some cultures, food is considered a cure for illness. For instance, in the Mexican culture, when people are sick, they are out of balance in that they have too much heat or cold. To correct this balance, the person needs to eat foods of the opposite quality. It is important to be sensitive to these cultural practices. If the dietary change conflicts with the cultural practice, it is important to talk with the provider. A referral to a registered dietitian may provide the patient with extra support and information.

BEING PROFESSIONAL

When you work with patients who are making dietary changes, it is important to be respectful of the patient. It is easy to tell a patient what to eat and what not to eat, but that might not be the best way to approach the situation. A medical assistant may want to start by finding out the patient's favorite foods. What foods does the patient typically eat at meals? Are any health beliefs related to that food? Learning about the patient's diet can then help the medical assistant coach the patient.

Role-play this scenario with a peer: You are a medical assistant and are coaching a patient on a low-fat diet, which was ordered by the provider. Practice being professional as you explore the patient's favorite foods and learn more about the patient's diet.

CHAPTER REVIEW

This chapter discussed nutrition and metabolism. Catabolism releases energy as the molecules are broken into smaller molecules. Anabolism uses energy to build larger molecules from smaller molecules. Nutrients include the following:

- Carbohydrates are used for energy and to regulate protein and fat metabolism. Simple sugars, starches, and fiber are carbohydrates.
- Proteins break down into amino acids; both are considered building blocks for the body.
- Fat provides a source of energy when carbohydrates are not available.
- Electrolytes are minerals in the body fluid that have an electrical charge.

- Vitamins can be either fat or water soluble. A deficit of a vitamin can lead to a disease.
- Water is the basis for the fluids in the body. Our bodies need water to function and survive.

Eating a well-balanced diet, low in saturated fat, trans fats, added sugars, and sodium, will help a person to get all the required nutrients.

There are many medically ordered diets that patients may be put on. Here are the diets that were discussed in this chapter:

- *Clear liquid diet*: Made up of foods and beverages that are liquid at room temperature.
- *Full liquid diet*: Made up of clear liquids and milk products.
- *Soft and mechanical soft diet*: Made up of foods soft in texture, low in fiber, and easy to digest. Mechanical soft diets are prepared for easier chewing.
- *Bland diet*: Consists of foods that are soft and low in fiber and eliminates foods that are spicy, fried, and raw. Citrus foods, caffeine, and alcohol are eliminated.
- *Weight control diet*: Can help people lose or maintain weight. Control of portion sizes is very important on the weight control diet.
- *Diabetic eating plans*: Used for people with diabetes, who need to monitor their carbohydrate intake. There are several diabetic eating plans, including the glycemic index approach, the "Create Your Plate" method, and carb counting.
- *Low-sodium diet*: Helps to lower the blood pressure and also used to address kidney disease. DASH is used for hypertension and cardiovascular disease.
- *Heart-healthy diet*: Consists of limiting sugary, salty, and highly processed foods. Limiting the consumption of saturated fats, trans fats, and added sugar is also important.
- *Low-protein diet*: Used for people with liver and kidney disease.
- *High- and low-fiber diets*: Limited or added fiber to the diet. A high-fiber diet helps with constipation and weight loss. Low-fiber diets are used during a flare-up of an intestinal disease.
- *Elimination diet*: Removes suspected allergens from the diet. Slowly they are reintroduced to find the exact allergens.
- *Gluten-free diet*: Used for people with celiac disease. Wheat, barley, and rye foods are removed from the diet.
- *Lactose intolerance diet*: Involves avoiding milk products or using oral enzyme replacement supplements.

Nutrient needs vary throughout the population and with different disease processes. For some situations, the provider may recommend dietary supplements to ensure that adequate vitamins and minerals are consumed.

SCENARIO WRAP-UP

Tim really enjoyed working with Kayla for his practicum. He learned a lot from her as she worked with patients. His favorite part of the experience was the patient education, in which he was able to observe and participate. Kayla also learned from Tim during the experience. Because of his interest in nutrition, Tim was able to share with Kayla what he knew about current dietary trends.

Tim hopes to obtain a medical assistant job in a practice like the one where he did his practicum. He feels that the family practice environment will allow him to use many of the skills he learned in school. He will also have a lot of experience talking to patients about dietary changes.

PROCEDURE 42.1   Instruct a Patient on a Dietary Change

Tasks

Instruct a patient regarding a dietary change related to a patient's special dietary needs. Show awareness of the patient's concerns regarding the dietary change. Document in the patient's health record.

Scenario

You are working with Dr. Angela Perez, a family practice provider. She just finished seeing Al Neviaser (date of birth [DOB] 6/21/19XX). Dr. Perez orders that the patient be given instructions on a heart-healthy diet.

Directions

Role play the scenario with a peer. You are the medical assistant, and the peer is the patient.

Equipment and Supplies

- Patient's health record
- Heart-healthy diet brochure

Procedural Steps

1. Assemble supplies needed for the provider's order. Ensure that the patient can read and understand the written materials. Verify the order if you have any questions.
   Purpose: Using written materials is helpful when instructing a patient on a dietary change.
2. Greet the patient. Identify yourself. Verify the patient's identity with the full name and date of birth. Explain the order from the provider. Answer any questions the patient may have.
   Purpose: It is important to identify the patient in two different ways to ensure that you have the correct patient. Explaining the order can make the patient feel more comfortable and helps to reduce anxiety.
3. Position yourself at the same level as the patient. Angle yourself toward the patient. Have a poised position.
   Purpose: This position shows positive nonverbal behaviors to the patient. Being at the same level as the patient and angling toward the patient show openness.
4. Accurately instruct the patient on the new diet. Use the written materials as you discuss the new eating plan.

Purpose: The information taught to the patient should match what is in the written materials. Any inaccuracies will confuse the patient.

5. Use words that the patient can understand. Refrain from jargon and medical terminology. Use professional verbal and nonverbal communication.
   Purpose: Jargon and medical terminology can confuse patients. Unprofessional nonverbal behaviors, such as rolling your eyes, checking the clock, or yawning, are disrespectful to the patient.
   Scenario update: After going over the heart-healthy eating plan, Mr. Neviaser states he is not sure this diet is for him. He likes his red meat and does not like to eat fish. He does not have a lot of money to buy expensive fresh fruits and vegetables.
6. Using therapeutic communication techniques (e.g., reflection, restatement, and summarizing), show the patient you are aware of his concerns.
   Purpose: By using therapeutic communication techniques, the medical assistant can show awareness of the patient's concerns.
7. Based on the patient's concerns, provide food alternatives that would meet the eating plan requirements.
   Purpose: The medical assistant can show awareness of the patient's concerns by providing alternative food choices that would meet the patient's requirements.
8. Evaluate the patient's understanding of the teaching by asking the patient to summarize the eating plan or describe a day's worth of meals. Answer any questions the patient may have.
   Purpose: It is important to check the patient's understanding of what was taught. Having the patient provide information back to the medical assistant is a better evaluation of understanding than asking, "Do you understand?"
9. Document the instruction in the patient's health record. Include the order, instruction given, written materials provided, and the patient's feedback.
   Purpose: Documenting indicates the instruction was provided to the patient.
   11/04/20XX 0923 Per Dr. Perez's order, the pt and his wife were instructed on a heart-healthy diet. Pt indicated he did not eat fish and was concerned about the cost of fresh foods. Alternative healthy proteins and inexpensive food options were discussed with the patient. The pt and his wife were able to describe a day's worth of heart-healthy meals. Pt was encouraged to call with any additional questions. _____ Kayla Smith, RMA

Patient Coaching With Rehabilitation

LEARNING OBJECTIVES

1. Describe how a medical assistant can assist with a patient's examination.
2. Explain how the range of motion measurements are obtained and muscle strength evaluations are performed.
3. Differentiate between splints, immobilizers, braces, ankle boots, and slings.
4. Apply a sling.
5. Describe cast care coaching, including what should be reported to the provider.
6. Differentiate between the effect of cold and heat therapy.
7. Apply cold and hot applications.
8. Differentiate between ultrasound, RICE, and exercise therapies.
9. Describe patient coaching for assistive devices, including fitting and using the device.
10. Coach a patient to use axillary crutches, a walker, and a cane.
11. Differentiate between types of complementary therapies.

OUTLINE

▶▶ OPENING SCENARIO

Tim Peterson, a certified medical assistant (CMA) (AAMA), has worked for Walden-Martin Family Medical (WMFM) Clinic for 2 years. Prior to being hired, Tim completed the medical assistant program at the local college. For his practicum, he spent part of the experience in family medicine and the remaining 100 hours in a local physical medicine and rehabilitation clinic. Tim enjoyed both experiences and realized he would eventually like to work in a physical medicine and rehabilitation clinic. He wanted to start his career in family medicine, to get comfortable with all of the various skills he learned in school.

One of the most interesting things Tim learned in practicum was how to remove a cast. Most people new to the experience were anxious about the procedure. Tim and his mentor took time to reassure the patients and showed them the equipment that they would use. Most of the patients were surprised that the cast saw did not have a sharp blade. That helped to reduce their anxieties.

YOU WILL LEARN

1. To assist with diagnostic procedures related to orthopedic conditions.
2. To apply a sling and cold and heat therapies.
3. To perform coaching as required for casts, cold and heat therapies, and RICE therapy.
4. To identify different types of assistive devices.
5. To perform coaching for assistive devices, including crutches, walkers, and canes.
6. To fit patients with assistive devices.

INTRODUCTION

Physical medicine and rehabilitation (PM&R) is also called *physiatry* (fiz ee AT ree) or *rehabilitation medicine*. PM&R uses therapies and physical agents (e.g., heat, electricity, and light) to diagnose, prevent, and treat disorders. This area of medicine is focused on improving and restoring a patient's ability and quality of life when the person has physical impairments. Such disabilities include conditions that impact the nervous, muscular, and skeletal systems. Goals of PM&R are to:

- Help the patient become as independent as possible with *activities of daily living* (e.g., grooming, walking, eating)
- Improve the person's quality of life (e.g., reduce pain, increase a person's ability to do activities)

A *physiatrist* (fi zee AT rist) is a physician who specializes in physical medicine and rehabilitation. A physiatrist diagnoses and prescribes treatments and therapies for the patient. As the patient undergoes rehabilitation, the physiatrist manages the patient's medical conditions. A physiatrist works closely with several therapies.

- *Physical therapy* (PT) focuses on improving a person's movement, strength, and mobility through the use of stretches, exercises, and other physical activities. A physical therapist works with patients to walk with assistive devices, such as walkers and canes.
- *Occupational therapy* (OT) focuses on improving a person's ability to perform activities of daily living, such as bathing, grooming, toileting, and eating. OT is focused on a patient's fine and gross motor skills.
- *Speech therapy* is involved with the diagnosis and treatment of patients with swallowing and communication (speech and language) difficulties.

Often medical assistants are hired to assist physiatrists with patient care. Medical assistants in other areas of ambulatory care also work with patients who have conditions that affect movement and mobility. Coaching patients how to use a sling, cold therapy, or assistive devices, such as crutches, is common in urgent care, orthopedics, and primary care settings. This chapter will address the medical assistant's role in assisting with the examination and treatments of conditions related to rehabilitation.

ASSISTING WITH THE EXAMINATION

When the medical assistant gathers a medical history on patients with a musculoskeletal concern, it is important to ask about the symptoms, the pain level, and the effect on their life. With the symptoms, information about the onset and what reduces or increases the symptoms should be obtained. The medical assistant can ask the patient to rate the pain using a 0 to 10 scale. Zero is no pain, and 10 is the worst pain ever. Another pain assessment tool is the Wong-Baker FACES Pain Rating Scale, which is described in Chapter 34. The medical assistant should explain the scale to patients, and then patients can state how they feel. This scale works well for children. The healthcare facility may also require a functional assessment to be done, which gathers information on the patient's mobility and ability to do activities of daily living (ADLs) (e.g., toileting, bathing, grooming, and eating).

When you work with a patient with an injury, assist the patient into a comfortable position and offer a pillow or folded blanket to support the extremity. For recent injuries, if ordered by the provider, apply a cold application to the injured area. (This procedure will be discussed later in the chapter.)

Patients may have limited mobility because of pain. The medical assistant may need to help patients change into the examination gown. Explain clearly what is happening and what the patient can expect.

During the exam, the provider may use inspection, palpation, range-of-motion (ROM) testing, and muscle testing to examine the major skeletal muscles and joints. Many times, the unaffected side is examined first and compared to the affected side. The provider may compare the size, position, and strength of the extremities. Depending on the concern, the provider may also perform a *gait analysis*, which means the provider observes the patient walking. Gait abnormalities may be the cause or the result of different musculoskeletal conditions.

If medical assistants are in the room for the exam, they may be responsible for taking notes, keeping the patient properly draped, and assisting by handing equipment to the provider. Always keep patient safety in mind, especially when the patient is transferring onto and off the exam table and changing positions.

> ### CRITICAL THINKING 43.1
> What is the advantage of using a pain scale when patients are experiencing pain?

COACHING FOR DIAGNOSTIC PROCEDURES

The medical assistant assists with diagnostic procedures by scheduling and preparing patients for procedures. If tests require restrictions of food or fluids, the medical assistant should address points with the patient after talking with the provider:

- Can the patient have water prior to the test?
- Which medications should the patient take prior to the test, or when can the patient resume the current medications?

Table 43.1 describes common diagnostic procedures used for musculoskeletal conditions. The medical assistant may need to screen the patient for specific allergies, medications, and so on prior to scheduling the procedure. For some procedures, a signed consent form is required. Patients should be notified of what they will experience during the procedure and any follow-up care required after the test.

> ### VOCABULARY
> **analgesic** A drug that reduces or eliminates pain.
> **anticoagulant** A substance (i.e., medication or chemical) that prevents clotting of blood.
> **cartilage** Flexible connective tissue that covers the ends of many bones at the joint.
> **ligaments** Supportive connective tissue that connects bones at a joint.
> **tendons** Connective tissue that attaches muscles to bone.

TABLE 43.1   Diagnostic Procedures for Musculoskeletal Conditions

Procedure	Description	Patient Preparation
Arthrogram	Provides visualization of the soft tissues in the joint (e.g., tendons [TEN duns], ligaments [LIH gah ments], cartilage [KAR tih lij]). A series of x-rays is taken of a joint after a contrast medium (e.g., dye) is injected into the joint.	Screen for pregnancy, anticoagulant (an tee koe AG yoo lant) use, and for allergy to contrast medium (iodine) or other medications used. Have patient sign a consent form. Patient may feel a sting when the medication is given. After the test, mild pain and swelling in the joint area may occur. Ice and analgesics (an ahl JEE zik) are typically ordered.
Bone scan	Imaging test used to diagnose bone disease, tumor, or cancer. A small amount of radiotracer is injected into the vein and collects in the bones and organs. A camera slowly scans the body and takes pictures of the radiotracer that collects in the bones.	Screen for pregnancy. Patient should not take any medication with bismuth (e.g., Pepto-Bismol) for 4 days before the test. Have the patient remove all metal items (e.g., jewelry). A small amount of pain is felt when the needle is inserted. The scan is painless. Depending on the condition, an initial scan may be done as the radiotracer is injected and then another in 3 to 4 hours after the radiotracer has collected in the bone.
Computed tomography (CT, CT scan)	Used to detect fractures, tumors, and other abnormalities. This imaging test takes cross-sectional pictures of the body. Contrast medium may be used.	Screen for pregnancy and for allergy to contrast medium (iodine). Patient should not eat or drink for 4 to 6 hours prior to the test if a contrast medium is used. Have the patient remove all metal items (e.g., jewelry) and put on a gown. When the contrast medium is given, the person may feel some burning and flushing and may have a metallic taste in the mouth.
Dual-energy x-ray absorptiometry (DEXA) scan	A bone density test used to measure the calcium and other minerals in the bone. Central DEXA requires the scanner to pass over the spine and hip. Peripheral DEXA measures the bone density in the wrist, fingers, legs, or heels.	Screen for pregnancy. Patient should not take calcium supplements for 24 hours before the test. Have the patient remove all metal items (e.g., jewelry). Test is painless. The test results are reported as a T-score (compares the bone density to that of a healthy woman) and Z-score (compares the bone density to other people of the same age, sex, and race).
Electromyography (EMG)	Checks the nerves and muscles. Thin needle electrodes are inserted through the skin into the muscle to pick up the electrical activity in the muscle.	Screen for anticoagulant use. No special preparation is required. The person may feel a little pain when the needles are inserted. The site may be tender or bruised for a few days after the test.
Myelogram	Uses fluoroscopy and contrast medium to evaluate the spinal cord and related structures.	Screen patient for pregnancy and allergy to iodine contrast medium. Anticoagulants should be stopped several days before the test. Patient may have food and liquid restrictions prior to the test. Patient will feel a brief sting when the medication is given. The table is moved into different positions as the images are taken.
Nerve conduction velocity (NCV)	Used with an EMG to test the speed of electrical signals through a nerve. Electrodes are placed on the skin. Each electrode gives off a mild electrical impulse that stimulates the nerve.	Screen the patient for a cardiac defibrillator or pacemaker. Patient should not wear lotion, perfume, or moisturizer. The impulse will feel like a small electric shock.

Range-of-Motion Measurement

Often orthopedic injuries severely affect the normal ROM of a joint. The *range of motion* is the normal movement allowed by the joint. Testing the ROM of specific joints is an objective measure of both the seriousness of an injury and the recovery progress. The joint may be evaluated with active and passive ROM. To determine the *active ROM* of a joint, the patient is asked to move the joint as far as possible. For evaluation of *passive ROM*, the provider moves the joint as far as possible.

A *goniometer* (go nee OHM eh ter) is the most common tool used to measure the ROM of a joint. Goniometers have calibration markings to indicate the measurement. A goniometer has two arms that are fixed together with a hinge joint at one end (Fig. 43.1A). Each of the arms is lined up with a bone on each side of the joint being tested (Fig. 43.1B). The degrees of motion are indicated on a scale on the hinged center of the nondigital instrument or on the digital display of the digital goniometer. All ROMs are measured in degrees. Usually, pain, tenderness, or crepitation (krep i TAY shun) is also noted during the procedure.

CRITICAL THINKING 43.2

How can Tim best assist Dr. Kahn in testing upper extremity ROM in a new patient? What equipment should Tim have ready? What patient position would best facilitate this examination? Why?

VOCABULARY
crepitation A dry, crackling sound or sensation.

Muscle Strength Evaluation

During the ROM evaluation, the provider also assesses each muscle group for strength. Normal muscle strength allows for complete voluntary ROM despite resistance. This resistance can be gravity, as when rising from a sitting to a standing position, or physical, as in pulling, pushing, or lifting an object. Muscle strength is bilaterally equal in normal conditions.

Hand grip strength can be measured with a *dynamometer* (die nah MOM eh ter) (Fig. 43.2A). Digital and nondigital dynamometers are available. A dynamometer provides an objective

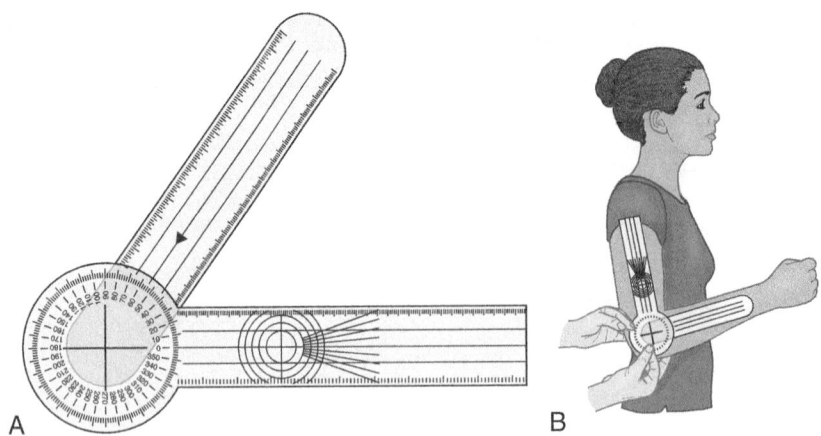

Fig. 43.1 A. Goniometer. B, Correct position of the goniometer on the arm. (From Niedzwiecki B, et al: *Kinn's the medical assistant*, ed 14, St. Louis, 2020, Elsevier.)

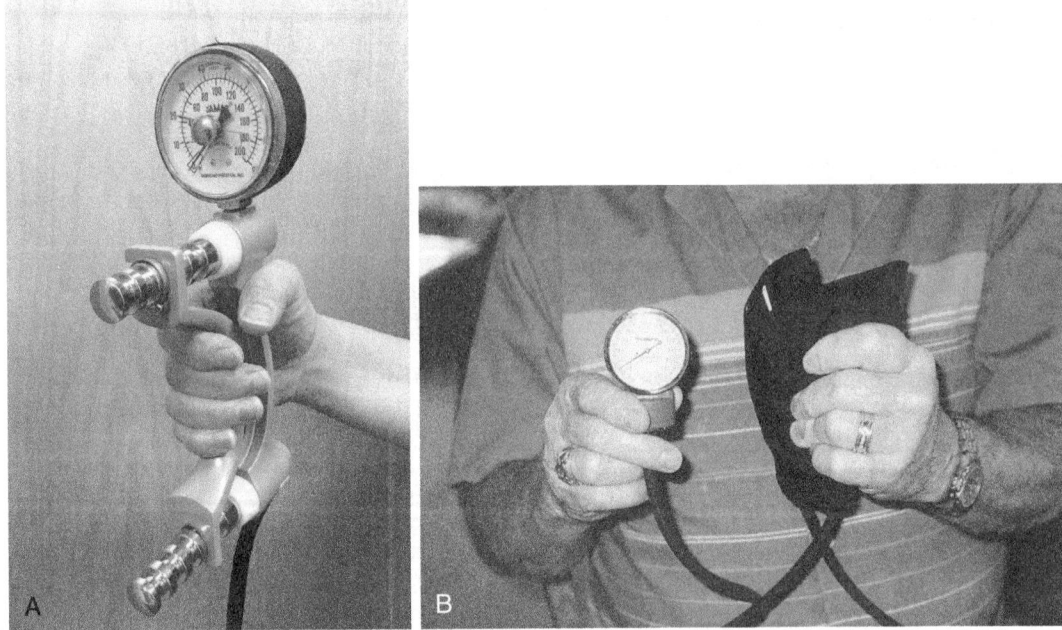

Fig. 43.2 A, Dynamometer. B, Assessing grip strength using a blood pressure cuff. (From Niedzwiecki B, et al: *Kinn's the medical assistant*, ed 14, St. Louis, 2020, Elsevier.)

measurement of hand grip strength. The patient holds the dynamometer in the hand being tested. Typically, the arm is at the side of the patient with the elbow bent at 90 degrees. Various arm and hand positions may be used for different assessments. If a dynamometer is not available, a blood pressure cuff can be used (Fig. 43.2B). Follow these steps to assess the hand strength:

1. Roll up an aneroid blood pressure cuff and have the patient hold it in one hand.
2. Inflate the cuff to 20 mm Hg of pressure and lock the valve.
3. Ask the patient to squeeze the cuff as tightly as possible.
4. Note the increase in pressure on the dial (a normal grip registers above 150 mm Hg).
5. Record the hand tested and the results of the test.
6. Repeat on the other hand.

COACHING FOR TREATMENTS

Splints

Splints are temporarily applied to immobilize joints and bones after injury or surgery. The splint can be adjusted as the swelling changes. It provides partial protection while the site heals.

A *splint* consists of a strip of rigid material that immobilizes an extremity. Custom-designed and ready-made splints are used in the ambulatory care environment. Custom-designed splints commonly use a strip of fiberglass as the rigid material. The fiberglass is held in place by elastic bandages (e.g., ACE bandages). The medical assistant can help the provider apply custom-designed splints. Ready-made splints usually have Velcro straps, which help when taking off or putting on the splints.

Immobilizers, Braces, and Ankle Boots

Immobilizers, braces, and ankle boots are used usually after an injury or surgery. Often the terms immobilizer and brace are used interchangeably, but they are different. An *immobilizer* keeps the joint from moving (Fig. 43.3). A *brace* provides stability and protection to the joint while allowing the joint to still function. Some knee braces have metal hinges that allow the knee to bend and straighten.

An *ankle boot* (also called a *moon boot* or *walker boot*) is a rigid, removable boot. It is used to protect and stabilize the ankle and lower leg after an injury or surgery. These boots can be used for partial, full, or non–weight-bearing extremities.

Slings

A *sling* is a device used to support and immobilize an injured part of the body, such as the arm, wrist, or shoulder. A sling is often used to help support the arm if a person has an arm casted (Procedure 43.1). A sling can help keep the hand elevated to reduce swelling in the hand and fingers. Slings come in adult and pediatric sizes.

If the sling is too loose, it may place stress and strain on the arm. The elbow should be kept at a 90-degree angle. If the sling is too tight, it can compromise or restrict circulation. The patient may have numbness, tingling, or swelling in the hand. The fingers and hand may be blue and cool to the touch.

Casts

Casts are applied to immobilize joints and bones after injury or surgery and provide additional protection. Casts are made from fiberglass or plaster. Fiberglass casts can be colorful, lightweight, durable, and porous. X-rays penetrate fiberglass casts better than plaster casts. Thus fiberglass casts do not need to be removed for x-rays. Plaster casts are cheaper and easier to shape. The medical assistant can help the provider apply the cast.

Casts applied in the ambulatory care facilities usually are either long or short casts.

- *Short arm cast* extends from the palm to just before the elbow.
- *Long arm cast* extends from the palm to the mid upper arm.
- *Short leg cast* extends from the foot to just before the kneecap (patella).
- *Long leg cast* extends from the foot to the mid-thigh (Fig. 43.4).

Extremity casts do not cover the fingers or toes because it is important to check circulation.

During the fiberglass cast application, the medical assistant helps the provider by assembling the supplies:

- Fiberglass bandage (available in a range of sizes; the width is determined by the width of the extremity)
- Room-temperature water
- Stockinette
- Cotton padding and cotton bandages
- Gloves for both the provider and medical assistant

The medical assistant applies the stockinette to the extremity being casted. The stockinette should extend beyond the casting material on both sides. A cast padding is then applied. This

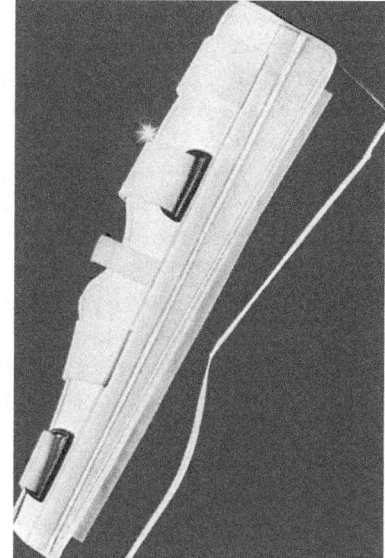

Fig. 43.3 Knee Immobilizer. (From Maher AB, Salmond SW, Pellino T, editors: *Orthopaedic nursing*, ed 3, Philadelphia, 2002, Saunders.)

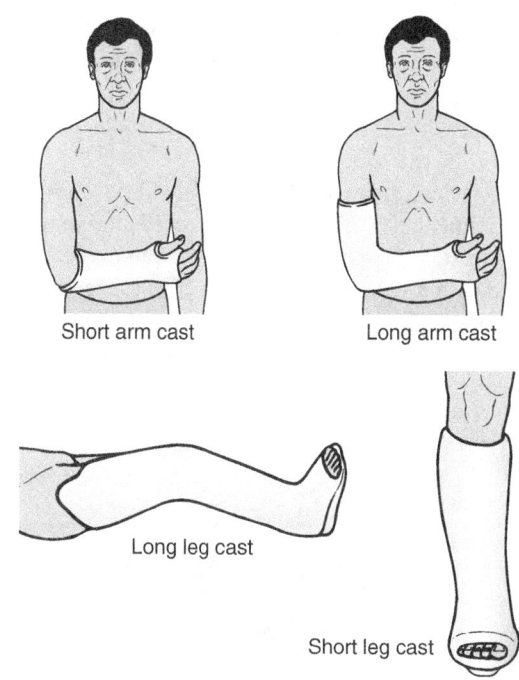

Short arm cast   Long arm cast

Long leg cast

Short leg cast

Fig. 43.4 Common Types of Casts. (From Harding M, et al: Medical-surgical nursing: assessment and management of clinical problems, ed 11, St. Louis, 2020, Elsevier.)

helps to protect the bony prominences. The stockinette is folded over the cast padding on both sides. The medical assistant holds the extremity in the position indicated by the provider. The fiberglass casting material can either be immersed in water or sprinkled with water. The provider wraps the extremity with the casting material, creating the cast. Over time, the fiberglass casting material dries and hardens.

CRITICAL THINKING 43.3

Describe the advantages of a fiberglass cast over a plaster cast.

Patient Coaching on CSMT. The medical assistant needs to provide cast care instructions to patients. It is important to teach patients about checking the CSMT (color, sensation, movement, and temperature) and comparing the casted extremity with the unaffected extremity. CSMT stands for:

- *Color*: The color of the extremity and nail beds should match those of the opposite extremity. It should be pink. The patient should contact the provider if the toes or fingers are bluish or pale.
- *Sensation*: Normal sensation should be intact. The person should be able to feel light touch on the fingers or toes. The patient should contact the provider if they notice:
  - An increased pain, burning, stinging, or numbness in the toes or fingers
  - A "sleeping" or pins-and-needles sensation
  - An inability to feel light touch on the toes or fingers
- *Motion*: Being able to move the toes and fingers of the casted extremity is normal. There should be no swelling. The patient should contact the provider if they are unable to move the toes or fingers or if swelling occurs in the fingers and toes.
- *Temperature*: The temperature of the toes or fingers on the casted extremity should match that of the opposite extremity. The fingers or toes should be warm. The patient should contact the provider if the fingers or toes are cooler than those of the opposite extremity.

Any suspicious abnormal findings should be reported to the provider immediately. If the extremity swells too much for the size of the cast, compartment syndrome can occur. The swelling of the casted extremity can cause damage to the muscles, blood vessels, and nerves. The damage can be permanent if not treated.

VOCABULARY

compartment syndrome A serious condition that involves increased pressure, usually in the muscles; it leads to compromised blood flow and muscle and nerve damage.

CRITICAL THINKING 43.4

In your own words, how would you explain CSMT to a patient, including signs and symptoms to report to the provider?

Patient Coaching on Cast Care. It is important for the patient to learn how to care for the cast and the extremity:

- Elevate and place dry cold packs on the casted extremity as indicated by the provider. Usually, this is done for the first 24 hours after an injury.
- Continue to move the fingers or toes, which helps return the blood to the heart and reduce the swelling.
- Keep the cast clean and dry. Contact the provider if the cast becomes smelly, moldy, or if drainage is noted.
- Cover the cast with a plastic bag prior to bathing or showering. If the fiberglass cast gets wet, use a hair dryer on a cool setting to dry it.

- Avoid putting weight or pressure on the cast.
- Do not put anything inside the cast, including sharp objects, powder, or lotion.
- A metal file can be used to smooth down rough sections of a fiberglass cast. Pad the rough areas to protect the skin.
- A sling can be used to help support a casted arm.

Removing Casts. The medical assistant can remove casts in the ambulatory care facility. To remove a cast, the medical assistant needs supplies and equipment:

- Cast cutter, which has a dull blade
- Cast spreader
- Large bandage scissors
- Basin of warm water, mild soap, a towel, and skin lotion (optional)

During the removal procedure, the medical assistant should provide adequate support for the extremity. Using the cast cutter, the medical assistant must make a cut on the medial and lateral sides of the long axis of the cast. Once the cuts have been made, the cast spreader can be used to pry apart the two halves. The stockinette and padding can be cut away with a large bandage scissors. Once the cast is off, the extremity should be washed with a mild soap and warm water, then dried. Skin lotion can be applied. This might be done in the ambulatory care facility or can be done at home.

The medical assistant must coach the patient prior to the cast removal that the extremity may look different. The skin may be dry and flaky. The extremity may be smaller and weaker than the other side. The patient may have some discomfort in the bones and joints that were immobilized. Sometimes patients will need physical therapy to help regain the strength and movement in the affected side.

Cold and Heat Therapy

Cold and heat therapeutic modalities (moe DAL i tee) or treatments are used for orthopedic injuries and infections. The applications can be:

- *Dry*: No moisture is left on the skin. Dry applications tend to pull moisture out of the skin.
- *Moist*: Moisture is left on the skin. Moist applications tend to increase tissue elasticity and allow heat or cold to penetrate deeper into the tissues.

When using hot or cold applications, the medical assistant should ask the patient if it feels too hot or too cold. The medical assistant should monitor the area being treated. Some patients are at higher risk for tissue injury with hot or cold applications:

- Younger children because of their thinner skin
- Older adults due to their reduced sensitivity to pain
- People with impaired circulation (e.g., those with peripheral vascular diseases and diabetes mellitus)
- People with altered sensitivity (e.g., those who are confused or have neurologic disorders, including diabetic neuropathy and spinal cord damage)
- Those for whom the application is placed on an open wound, broken skin, or stoma (this tissue is more sensitive)

- Those for whom the application is placed on edematous or scarred areas (scars and edema reduce sensitivity)

See Box 43.1 for patient education topics for cold and hot applications.

VOCABULARY

modalities Therapeutic treatments for a disorder.

stoma A temporary or permanent surgically created opening used for drainage (i.e., urine, stool).

vasoconstriction Contraction of the muscles that causes a narrowing of the inside tube of the blood vessel.

Cold Therapy. Cold therapy is typically used for sprains, strains, fractures, joint injuries, shin splints, and other injuries. In some facilities, it is a common practice to provide a cold pack to a patient who comes in with a recent injury.

A cold application causes vasoconstriction (VAY zoe kahn strik shuhn), which reduces blood flow to the area. As a result, tissue metabolism decreases, less oxygen is used, and less swelling occurs. The nerve endings in the area become numb. The blood viscosity increases, which can cause clotting. Cold therapy helps to reduce pain and inflammation and prevents edema (swelling) in the injured area. Table 43.2 describes common types of cold applications. Procedure 43.2 describes how to apply a cold pack.

BOX 43.1 Patient Education for Cold and Hot Applications

- Know what supplies are required and where they can be purchased.
- Use a protective covering between the skin and the application.
- Never fall asleep with an application on the skin.
- Never place an application over metal jewelry.
- Know the length of time for each application, the number of times a day ordered, and the number of days for treatment.
- Hot and cold therapy should be applied for 15 to 20 minutes. Additional time can harm the tissues.
- After the session, remove the application. Allow the skin to return to the normal temperature before applying again.
- Prolonged erythema or paleness, pain, swelling, and blisters should be reported to the provider.

Heat Therapy. Heat therapy can be used to relieve:

- Acute pain (e.g., back and menstrual) and chronic pain (e.g., arthritis)
- Sinus congestion
- Infection (e.g., localized abscesses)

Heat therapy can help with muscle relaxation. It can produce local vasodilation, which increases circulation. The increased blood supply to a local area helps to absorb the extra fluid (from edema). Table 43.3 discusses the types of hot applications. Additional types of heat therapy will be discussed. Procedure 43.3 describes how to apply a hot pack.

Paraffin bath therapy. Paraffin provides deep heat therapy. The heat can reduce pain and tenderness. It has been found to maintain muscle strength and increase mobility. Paraffin therapy is a common treatment for arthritis and other conditions that cause pain and stiffness.

A paraffin bath uses melted paraffin and mineral oil warmed to about 125°F (51.7°C). The patient bathes a foot or hand in the bath. Once the extremity is coated, the patient should lift it out and let it dry for a few seconds (Fig. 43.5). This process is repeated until the patient has 10 to 12 layers of wax built up on the extremity. The foot or hand is wrapped in plastic and then in a towel to retain the moisture and heat. After 20 minutes, it is unwrapped, and the wax is removed.

Heat lamp therapy. Two commonly used heat lamp therapies are red light therapy and near infrared light therapy. Red light therapy is used to treat skin conditions. Near infrared light therapy penetrates deeper, killing pathogens, healing tissue, improving circulation, and relieving pain.

Ultrasound Therapy

Ultrasound therapy has been used for a long time to treat pain and promote healing. The ultrasound transducer head produces sound waves. Ultrasound gel is applied to the skin. As the transducer head is moved over the skin, the gel helps with the transmission of sound waves into the soft tissue. There are two main types of ultrasound therapy: thermal and mechanical. The main difference between these types is the speed at which the sound waves penetrate the soft tissue. Ultrasound therapy must be done by a trained therapist. This treatment is often provided in chiropractic, sports medicine, physical therapy, and occupational therapy facilities.

TABLE 43.2 Types of Cold Applications

Type	Dry or Moist	Description	Uses
Cold compress	Moist	Washcloth or other soft cloth is dampened with a cold solution (e.g., water) and applied to the skin.	Usually used on the face and forehead for discomfort and pain.
Chemical cold pack	Dry	Comes in a variety of sizes. Stored at room temperature. Contains inner areas of a dry chemical and water. When activated, the water and chemical mix creates coldness.	Used to reduce inflammation, prevent edema, reduce bleeding, and decrease pain.
Ice bag	Dry	A bag with cubes or pieces of ice.	
Gel pack	Dry	Aqueous gel that freezes. Reusable. Stored in freezer.	
Bead pack	Dry	Little beads of gel conform to the site even when frozen. Similar to a frozen bag of peas. Reusable. Stored in freezer.	

TABLE 43.3   Types of Hot Applications

Type	Dry or Moist	Description	Uses
Hot soak/ whirlpool bath (Hydrotherapy)	Moist	Part of the body is submerged in warm water or a warm medicated solution. Should be warmed to 105°F to 110°F (40.6°C to 43.3°F).	Used to cleanse wounds. Helps to ease discomfort.
Hot compress	Moist	Washcloth or other soft cloth is dampened with a hot solution (e.g., water) and applied to the skin.	Can be used on many places on the body, including the face and eyes.
Heating pad	Dry	Electric pad that warms. Inspect for safety purposes.	Used for spasms and pain.
Chemical hot pack	Dry	Comes in a variety of sizes. Stored at room temperature. Contains inner areas of a dry chemical and water. When activated, the water and chemical mix, creating heat for a period of time.	
Gel pack	Dry	Aqueous gel that can be microwaved. Reusable.	
Bead pack	Dry	Little beads of gel that can be microwaved. Reusable.	

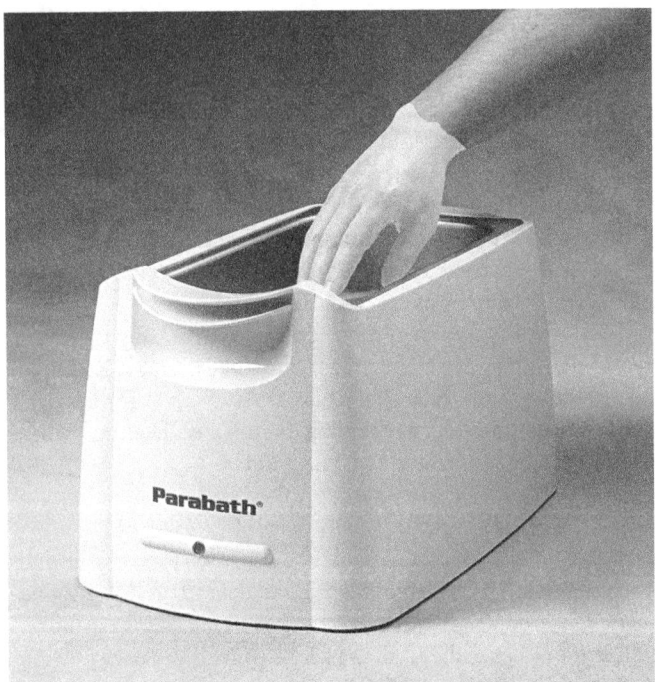

Fig. 43.5 A Paraffin Bath. (From Niedzwiecki B, et al: *Kinn's the medical assistant,* ed 14, St. Louis, 2020, Elsevier.)

RICE Therapy

For orthopedic injuries, RICE is commonly ordered as a treatment for usually the first 48 to 72 hours. After 72 hours, moist heat is prescribed. RICE stands for:

- *Rest*: Reduce activities for a period of time. Crutches can help an injured leg/ankle rest.
- *Ice*: Apply a cold pack to the injured area for 15 to 20 minutes, 4 to 8 times daily.
- *Compression*: Use elastic bandage (e.g., ACE Wrap) or splints to reduce swelling. It is important to monitor the CSMT of a wrapped extremity.
- *Elevation*: Elevate the injured extremity higher than the level of the heart to help reduce swelling.

CRITICAL THINKING 43.5

In your own words, how would you explain RICE to a patient?

Exercise Therapy

Often patients are encouraged to exercise to maintain their strength and joint mobility. Patients recovering from surgery (e.g., orthopedic, cardiac) may need to see a physical therapist or an occupational therapist. These therapists work with patients to help them regain their mobility and strength. Isometric, isotonic, and ROM exercises are encouraged to maintain strength, flexibility, and mobility.

Isometric (i so MEH trick) contractions do not change the muscle length, but they do increase the muscle tension. Isometric exercises help to maintain a person's strength. *Isotonic* (i so TON ick) contractions cause muscles to shorten and thicken, and movement at a joint. Isotonic exercises help restore movement after an injury and relieve stiffness and pain. ROM exercises help to maintain flexibility and joint mobility and reduce stiffness. *Active ROM exercises* are done by the patient, whereas *passive ROM exercises* are done by a caregiver or therapist. For patients who have had a stroke or other trauma that affects movement, daily ROM exercises are critical to prevent joints from freezing up. Frozen joints have limited to no movement.

CRITICAL THINKING 43.6

In your own words, describe isometric, isotonic, active ROM exercises, and passive ROM exercises.

Electrical Muscle Stimulation. A transcutaneous electrical nerve stimulation (TENS) unit is used for pain relief (Fig. 43.6). Electrodes are placed on the skin in specific locations. The adjustable low-voltage machine sends electrical current through disposable gel electrodes into the skin. The current stimulates specific nerves, producing a tingling or massaging sensation that reduces pain. TENS units have been used for passive exercise of muscles when a patient cannot exercise the extremity (e.g., due to injury or stroke). The electrical stimulation can prevent atrophy of normal muscles. TENS units are also used to treat the pain from muscle, joint, or other orthopedic conditions.

VOCABULARY

electrodes Adhesive patches that conduct electricity from the body to machine wires (e.g., electrocardiograph [ECG] and transcutaneous electrical nerve stimulation [TENS] unit).

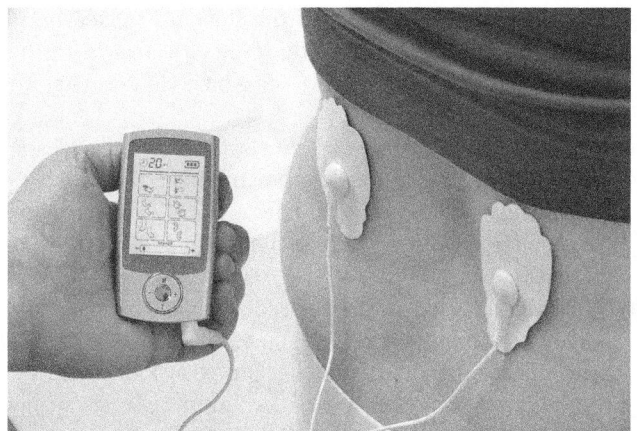

Fig. 43.6 A Transcutaneous Electrical Nerve Stimulation (TENS) Unit.

Assistive Devices

An assistive device is used to help a person perform a specific task, such as walking. Crutches, walkers, canes, and wheelchairs are considered assistive devices. Many times, these assistive devices can be purchased at pharmacies and medical supply stores. The medical assistant should know how to adjust the device to fit the patient. Medical assistants may also coach patients on the proper use of the assistive device. Improper use of assistive devices can lead to falls and injuries.

Crutches. Crutches are used to help a person walk. Crutches can be made out of aluminum or wood and can be adjusted for the patient. The more common crutches include:
- *Axillary crutches*: Most common type; used when recovering from a foot, ankle, or leg injury or surgery (Fig. 43.7).
- *Forearm crutches*: Also called *Lofstrand* or *elbow crutches*; require more upper body strength. An open elbow cuff fits around the patient's forearm (see Fig. 43.7). These crutches help with proper posture and body mechanics.
- *Extension crutches*: Also called *Canadian crutches*. These combine the underarm crutch with an elbow cuff, which provides extra support for the patient.
- *Platform crutches*: Also called *triceps crutches*. They have padded armrests with handgrips. These crutches are used when patients cannot straighten their arms to hold the handgrip of the crutch.
- *Hands-free crutch*: Straps to the thigh, and a platform supports the lower leg (Fig. 43.8A).
- *M+D crutches*: The hinged arm cradles the strap to the forearms, thus eliminating pressure in the axillae, wrists, and hands (Fig. 43.8B).

Axillary crutches need to be fitted correctly to allow for good body mechanics and to reduce the risk of injury. *Crutch palsy* can occur with poorly fitted crutches or if the patient rests on the top of the crutches while walking. The axillary nerves can be temporarily or permanently damaged. This can cause loss of hand strength and weakening of the wrist and forearm muscles.

When you fit axillary crutches, the patient must be wearing shoes. Have the patient stand straight up. Fit the crutches so they are 1 to 1½ inches (about 2 finger widths) below the armpit.

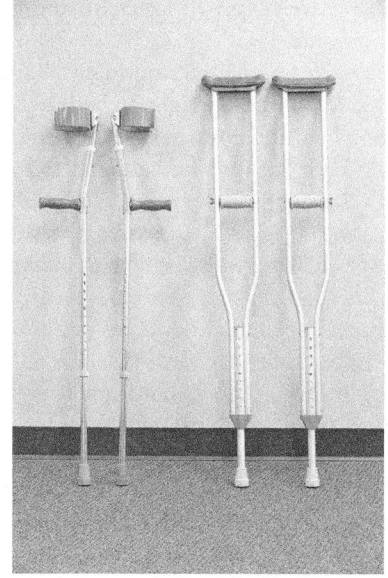

Fig. 43.7 *Left to right,* Forearm crutches and axillary crutches.

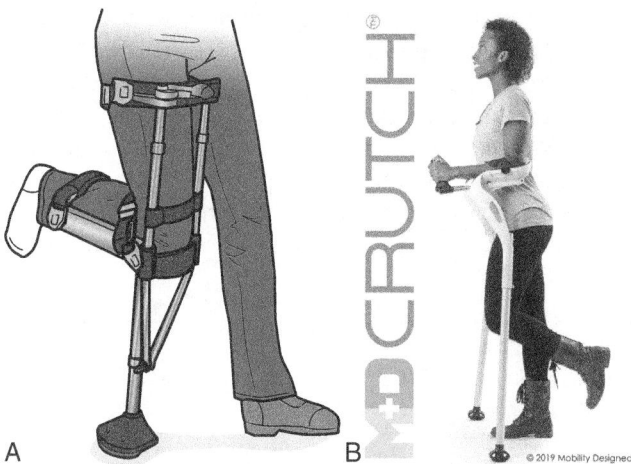

Fig. 43.8 A, Hands-free crutch. B, M+D crutches by Mobility Designed, Inc. (Courtesy Mobility Designed, Inc. https://www.mobilitydesigned.com/.)

The crutch should be about 4 to 6 inches to the side and front of each foot. Handgrips must be near the wrist and even with the top of the hip line. When the hands are on the handgrip, the elbow should be bent 15 to 30 degrees.

Providers will indicate the type of crutch, along with any limitations. Common limitations with crutches include:
- *Weight bearing as tolerated*: Patients can place more than half of their body weight on their "bad" or affected extremity if it is not painful.
- *Partial weight bearing*: The provider will indicate how much weight can be placed on the affected extremity.
- *Toe-touch weight bearing*: Patients can touch the ground with their toes on the affected side. The toe-touch helps with balance. No weight bearing is allowed on the affected extremity.
- *Non–weight bearing*: Patients cannot put weight on their affected extremity. This type of limitation would require the three-point crutch gait.

There are several gaits, or ways to walk, with crutches. The provider may also order the gait. The gait depends on whether the patient can put weight on the affected extremity. The following are common gaits.

- *Two-point crutch gait*: Mimics normal walking. The patient must be able to put some weight on both legs. From the tripod position (starting position) use this sequence: Move the right crutch with left foot forward and then move the left crutch with the right foot forward. There are two individual movements with this gait. Repeat this pattern (Fig. 43.9A).
- *Four-point crutch gait*: Must be able to put some weight on both legs. This gait is slower, but safer for those with generalized weakness. From the tripod position use this sequence: Move the right crutch forward, then the left foot forward, followed by the left crutch forward, and lastly bring the right foot forward. There are four individual movements with this gait. Repeat this pattern (see Fig. 43.9B).
- *Three-point crutch gait*: Used when partial weight bearing or non–weight bearing is indicated. From the tripod position, use this sequence: Move both crutches and the affected leg forward, then move the "good" or unaffected leg forward. Repeat this pattern (see Fig. 43.9C and Procedure 43.4).
- *Swing to crutch gait*: Must be able to put some weight on both legs. From the tripod position, use this sequence: Move both crutches forward, then swing the body so the feet are even with the line of the crutches. Repeat this pattern.
- *Swing-through crutch gait*: Must be able to put some weight on both legs. From the tripod position, use this sequence: Move both crutches forward, then swing the body so the feet land in front of the line of the crutches. Repeat this pattern (see Fig. 43.9D).

VOCABULARY

tripod position The standing position when using crutches; crutch tips are 4 to 6 inches to the side and front of each foot.

CRITICAL THINKING 43.7

Describe how a person would perform each of the five crutch gaits. Which gait(s) would be used for toe-touch weight bearing? Partial weight bearing? Non–weight bearing?

Walkers. Some patients use walkers after surgery. Many older adults use walkers for help with balance and support. Walkers provide more support than canes. A walker's wide base helps stabilize the gait of the patient and can support up to 50% of the body weight. Walkers have a metal frame and can easily be adjusted to fit an individual. They are lightweight, and several types can fold flat for storage and travel. Several types of walkers are available:

- *Hemi-walker*: Also called a *one-hand walker*. These walkers are used by patients who can only grasp the walker with one hand due to a stroke or arm/hand amputation (Fig. 43.10).
- *Standard walker*: A very common walker; it has four non-skid, rubber-tipped legs (see Fig. 43.10). A person needs to pick up the walker with every completed step. Sometimes tennis balls are inserted over the feet to help to move the walker easily across the floor.

- *Two-wheel walker*: Resembles the standard walker, but the front two legs have wheels. This type of walker is for those who need some help but not constant weight-bearing help (see Fig. 43.10).
- *Three-wheel walker* and *four-wheel walker*: Also called a *Rollator*. Each leg has a wheel, and many Rollators have brakes by the handles. Some models have a seat and a basket. These walkers are for people who do not need to lean on a walker for balance.
- *Knee walker*: A foot-propelled scooter that has a platform to rest the knee and lower leg (Fig. 43.11). This is commonly used instead of axillary crutches for leg or foot conditions.

When you fit a walker, the patient must be wearing shoes. Have the patient step into the walker and relax the arms at the sides of the body. The top of the walker grip should be near the crease in the wrist and even with the top of the hip line. With the shoulders relaxed and the hands on the grips, the elbows should be bent 15 degrees. Procedure 43.5 discusses fitting a walker and coaching a patient to use a walker.

Canes. A cane can provide extra assistance for a person who has a minor balance or stability problem. There are two basic types of canes but several different grips or handles. The basic types of canes are:

- Single-tipped cane: Provides minimal assistance with walking (Fig. 43.12).
- Four-tipped cane: Also called a *quad cane*. It provides greater stability for patients than the single-tipped cane (see Fig. 43.12).

When you measure a cane, the patient must be wearing shoes and have the arms relaxed at the sides of the body. The top of the cane should be near the crease in the wrist. With the shoulders relaxed and the hand on the cane, the elbow should be bent 15 degrees. Procedure 43.6 discusses measuring a cane and coaching a patient to use a cane. Tingling, numbness, or pain in the hand and fingers may indicate the handle is not appropriate for the person.

Wheelchairs. Wheelchairs provide mobility for patients who cannot walk or who are able to walk only short distances. With a regular wheelchair, the patient uses arm muscles for mobility. Motorized wheelchairs are also available. The patient is referred to a medical equipment store, where the appropriate wheelchair is fitted to the individual. It is important to encourage the patient to always lock the wheels before transferring into and out of a wheelchair.

CRITICAL THINKING 43.8

Put the assistive devices (wheelchair, cane, crutches, and walker) in order from the device that gives the most assistance to the device that gives the least assistance.

COMPLEMENTARY THERAPIES

Complementary therapies are used together with conventional medicine. For instance, massage and chiropractic care are considered complementary therapies. Sometimes people

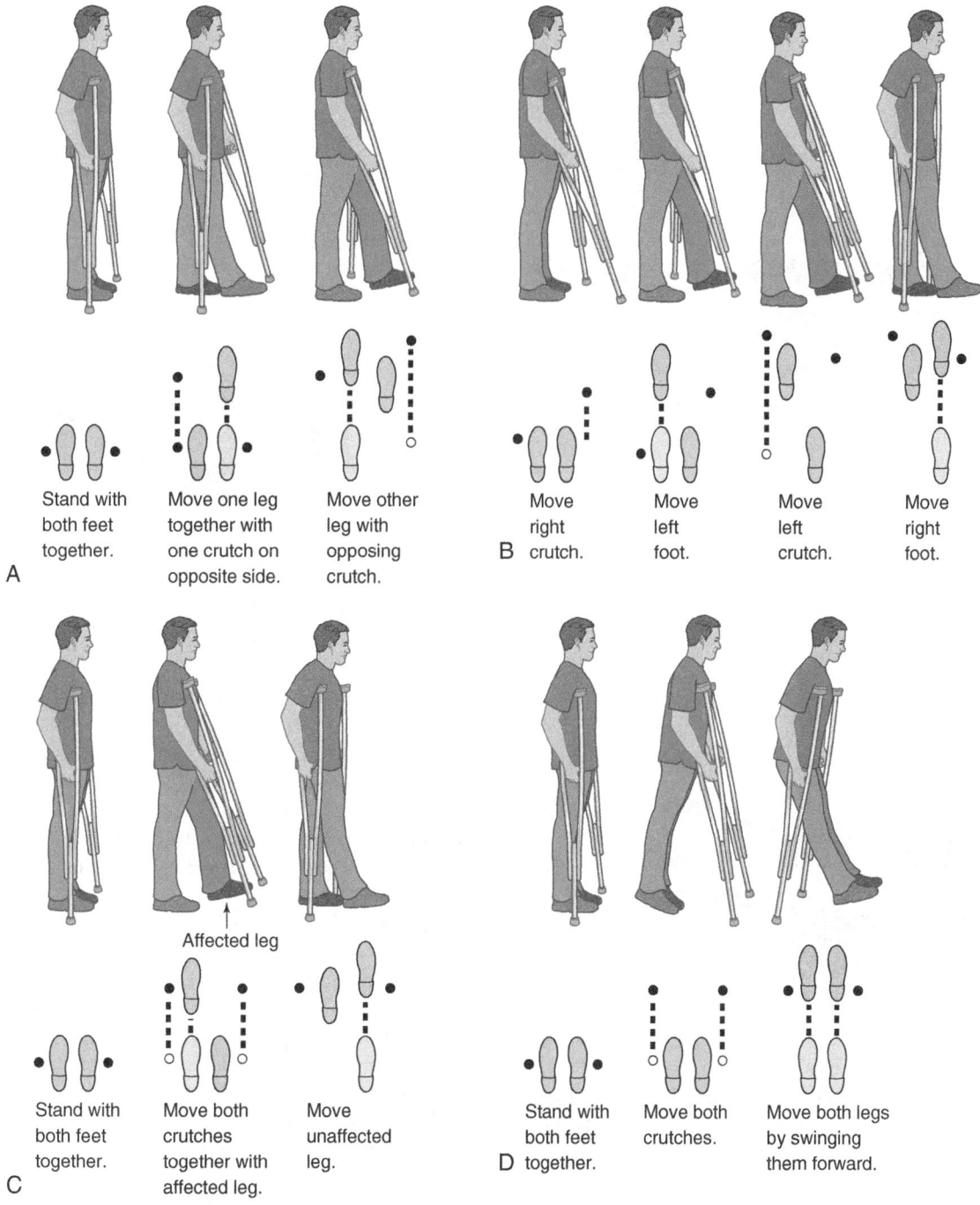

Fig. 43.9 Crutch Gaits. A, Two-point crutch gait. B, Four-point crutch gait. C, Three-point crutch gait. D. Swing-through gait. (From Niedzwiecki B, et al: *Kinn's the medical assistant*, ed 14, St. Louis, 2020, Elsevier.)

will use the term alternative, but that means the therapy is being used instead of conventional medicine. Most patients using complementary therapies will also see their healthcare provider.

Massage Therapy

Massage ranges from light stroking to deep rubbing. Pressure is applied to a person's skin and muscles. Studies have shown that massage reduces stress, pain, and muscle tension. Massage is performed by massage therapists, who are specially trained in the procedures. There are several types of massage:

- *Deep massage*: Used to help with muscle damage from injuries. Slower, more forceful massage is done to the muscles and connective tissues (e.g., tendons and ligaments).
- *Swedish massage*: Used to relax a person. Involves a gentle massage of long strokes and deep circular movements that can energize the individual.
- *Sports massage*: Used on athletes to help prevent or treat injuries. The technique is similar to Swedish massage.
- *Trigger point massage*: Used to help with muscle damage from injury or overuse. Involves a focused massage on tight muscles.

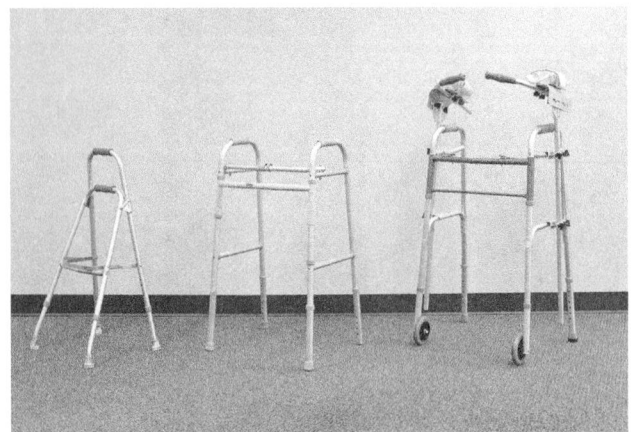

Fig. 43.10 *Left to right,* A hemi-walker, standard walker, and two-wheel walker with platform walker attachments.

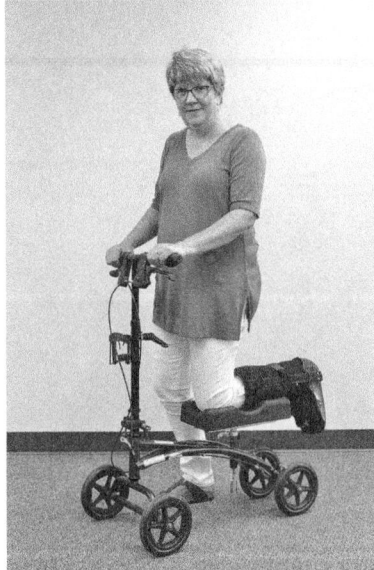

Fig. 43.11 Knee Walker.

Chiropractic Care

Chiropractic care focuses on the relationship between the spine and the function of the body. The goal is to correct alignment

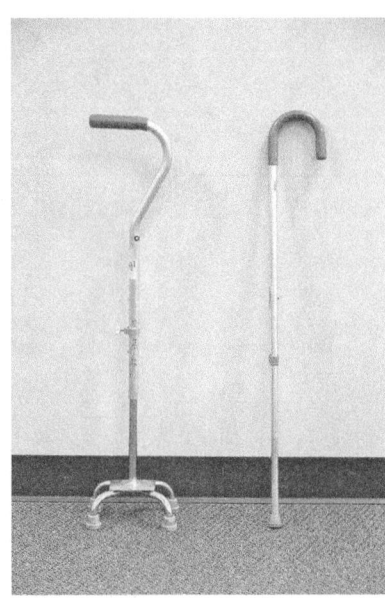

Fig. 43.12 *Left to right,* A four-tipped cane with an offset handle and a single-tipped cane with a tourist handle.

problems and thereby alleviate pain, improve function, and support the body's natural ability to heal itself. Spinal manipulation has been shown to be beneficial for low back pain, headaches, neck pain, whiplash-associated disorders, and upper and lower extremity joint conditions.

Chiropractic doctors have at least 4 years of additional training beyond a bachelor's degree. The training includes both classroom and direct patient care. The doctors must pass the national licensing exam. State law regulates their practice, and many state boards require continuing education to maintain the license.

Acupressure and Acupuncture

Both acupressure and acupuncture have been practiced for thousands of years. *Acupressure* involves applying firm pressure on specific points on the body. *Acupuncture* involves inserting fine needles into acupuncture points (specific sites on the body). The needles may be removed quickly or left in for longer periods of time. Acupressure and acupuncture are used to treat a wide range of symptoms, including pain, nausea, neuropathy, anxiety, depression, and sleep disturbance.

CLOSING COMMENTS

When doing a procedure on a patient, it is important to follow these guidelines:
- You must have a written order from the provider.
- You must follow the procedure precisely as it is ordered, without variation.
- Never advise the patient without permission.
- Make sure you know what instructions the provider gave the patient and reinforce them.

- If you have any concerns about a procedure, discuss them with the provider privately before proceeding.
- Do not perform a procedure if you are uncomfortable; get someone to help you.

Always remember – you are the assistant, and this is the provider's patient. The provider ultimately is responsible for every aspect of the patient's care. Always stay within the legal and ethical guidelines of the medical assisting profession in your state.

PATIENT-CENTERED CARE

When patients are using assistive devices, falls can occur. The medical assistant should teach patients how to prevent falls when using assistive devices. These instructions should include:

- Wear shoes with rubber or nonskid soles.
- Remove items in the walkway that can cause falls (e.g., throw or loose rugs, cords, and clutter). Small indoor animals may also cause falls if they are near the person's feet.
- Make sure that floors are clean and dry.
- When attempting to sit, back up until the seat touches the back of the legs. With a free hand, grab the seat or armrest and lower yourself into the chair or onto the toilet.
- To stand, scoot forward in the chair and use the free hand to push up from the seat to stand up. Make sure to get your balance before moving.
- Consider adding handrails inside the tub and by the toilet.

BEING PROFESSIONAL

Musculoskeletal injuries and disorders are commonplace in the ambulatory care setting. Because of this, patients may ask for your advice on how to manage their health problems. Remember that as the medical assistant, you should never diagnose or recommend treatment for a patient. That is the provider's responsibility. Responding professionally to inquiries and offering provider-approved educational materials and websites can be very helpful. Respectful and courteous behavior should be standard practice for medical assistants when they interact with patients and their families.

Role-play the following scenario with a peer: Your peer is Mrs. (or Mr.) James, a 70-year-old patient. She has arthritis and problems moving. The patient asks you what you take for pain, stating that might help her, too. How do you respond?

CHAPTER REVIEW

This chapter discussed the role of the medical assistant in coaching for diagnostic procedures and treatments. The medical assistant should ensure the patient knows how to prepare for procedures, including food, fluid, and medication restrictions. A provider may use a goniometer to measure the ROM of a joint. A dynamometer may be used to provide objective measurement of hand grip strength.

Splints, immobilizers, braces, ankle boots, slings, or casts may be used while a patient is recovering from an injury or surgery. The medical assistant should instruct the patient on the purpose of the device. If the device can be removed for periods of time, the medical assistant must coach the patient on how to apply and remove the device. Coaching regarding CSMT (color, sensation, movement, and temperature) is important to ensure adequate circulation to the affected extremity. For patients with casts, learning how to handle the cast is important.

Cold and heat modalities can be either dry or moist applications. Cold therapy is typically used for sprains, strains, fractures,

joint injuries, shin splints, and other injuries. Cold therapy helps to reduce pain and inflammation and prevents edema (swelling) in the injured area. Heat therapy is used to relieve pain, sinus congestion, and infection. It can relax muscles and produce local vasodilation. Heat therapy can reduce edema. Paraffin baths and heat lamp therapy are examples of heat therapy.

RICE therapy is used for the first 48 to 72 hours after an injury. RICE stands for rest, ice, compression, and elevation. After 72 hours, moist heat is prescribed. Isometric and isotonic exercises help patients maintain their strength and joint mobility.

Assistive devices are used to help a person perform a specific task, such as walking. This chapter discussed the different types of crutches, how to fit crutches, and the different crutch gaits. Walkers are used to help with balance and support. There are several types of walkers available for patients. Canes are used for minor balance or stability problems. Canes can be single tipped or four tipped. The handles or grips can vary. Wheelchairs provide mobility when a patient cannot walk.

SCENARIO WRAP-UP

Within the next few years, Tim hopes a full time clinical medical assistant position is posted at the physical medicine and rehabilitation clinic where he did his practicum. In the meantime, Tim enjoys assisting the WMFM Clinic providers. With

the wide variety of patients seen at WMFM Clinic, Tim knows he will learn a lot about patient care, diseases, and treatments. This information will be helpful when, hopefully, he moves into the physical medicine and rehabilitation clinic in the future.

PROCEDURE 43.1   Apply a Sling

Tasks

Apply a sling to a patient's arm. Document the procedure in the patient's health record.

Scenario

Dr. Kahn orders a commercial sling to be applied to a patient's left arm.

Equipment and Supplies

- Adult-sized sling
- Provider's order
- Patient's health record

Procedural Steps

1. Wash hands or use hand sanitizer.
   Purpose: Hand sanitization is an important step for infection control.
2. Read the provider's order. Assemble the equipment. Make sure to have the correct-sized sling for the patient.
   Purpose: It is important to know the provider's order before starting the procedure.
3. Greet the patient. Identify yourself. Verify the patient's identity with full name and date of birth. Explain the procedure to be performed in a manner that the patient understands. Answer any questions the patient may have about the procedure.
   Purpose: It is important to identify the patient in two different ways to ensure that you have the correct patient. Explaining the procedure can make the patient feel more comfortable and helps to reduce anxiety.

4. Gently place the arm and elbow in the sling. Support the arm on both sides of the injury. Make sure the sling fits comfortably around the elbow. The patient's hand should come to the end of the sling.
   Purpose: Having the correct-sized sling will help prevent complications. The sling should not be so snug that it is uncomfortable. The hand should be supported by the sling. If the hand hangs down at the wrist, the sling is too small for the patient.
5. Position the strap behind the elbow and pull the strap around the back of the neck. Make sure the strap does not rub against or cut into the skin on the neck. Secure the strap to the loops on the sling near the hand.
   Purpose: The strap should be comfortably positioned around the patient's neck and shoulder.
6. Adjust the straps so the hand and forearm are elevated about the level of the elbow.
   Purpose: This prevents swelling in the hand and wrist.
7. Check the CSMT of the fingers. Ask the patient if the fingers feel numb or asleep.
   Purpose: If the circulation is compromised, CSMT will indicate a problem, such as numb, blue, and cold fingers.
8. Document the procedure in the patient's health record. Include the provider's name, the order, what was taught, and how the patient responded.
   Purpose: It is important to document the procedure in the health record to show it was done.
   07/20/20XX 1505 Per Dr. Kahn's order, applied a commercial sling to the pt's left arm. Left hand and fingers elevated. CSMT normal. Pt's questions were answered. Pt was encouraged to call the department if they have additional questions or concerns. _____ Tim Peterson, CMA (AAMA)

PROCEDURE 43.2   Apply a Cold Pack

Tasks

Apply a cold pack (chemical, gel, or bead) to a body area to reduce pain and prevent further swelling per treatment plan. Document the procedure in the patient's health record.

Scenario

You are working with Dr. David Kahn. Johnny Parker (DOB 06/15/20XX) arrives holding his arm and crying. Another medical assistant brings the patient and parent to the exam room. The medical assistant comes out and updates you on Johnny. His parent states that Johnny fell off his bike an hour ago and has since been complaining of pain in his right wrist. The providers in the department have a standing order to apply a cold pack to orthopedic injuries if the patient does not arrive with one in place. The medical assistant asks you to apply the cold pack as he completes the vital signs and medical history on Johnny.

Equipment and Supplies

- Cold pack (chemical, gel, or bead)
- Towel or another type of protective covering for the cold pack
- Provider's order or standing order for orthopedic injuries
- Patient's health record

Procedural Steps

1. Wash hands or use hand sanitizer.
   Purpose: Hand sanitization is an important step for infection control.
2. Read the standing order or the provider's order. Assemble the equipment. If using a chemical cold pack, activate the pack by squeezing it.
   Purpose: It is important to know the provider's order or the standing order before starting the procedure.
3. Greet the patient. Identify yourself. Verify the patient's identity with full name and date of birth. Explain the procedure to be performed in a manner that the patient understands. Answer any questions the patient may have about the procedure.
   Purpose: It is important to identify the patient in two different ways to ensure that you have the correct patient. Explaining the procedure can make the patient feel more comfortable and helps to reduce anxiety.
4. Cover the cold pack with a towel or protective covering.
   Purpose: The cold pack must never be put directly on the skin. Place a towel or protective covering between the cold pack and the skin to prevent injuries.
5. Assist the patient to position the cold pack over the injured area (Fig. 1).
   Purpose: Some patients like to place the cold pack themselves on the injured area.

PROCEDURE 43.2 Apply a Cold Pack–cont'd

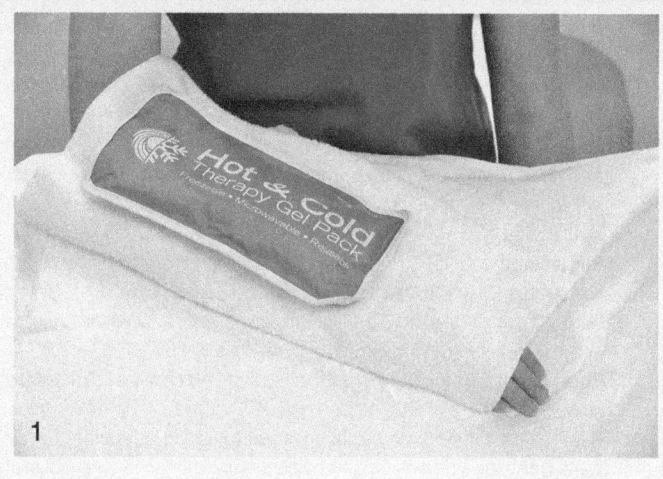

1

6. Coach the patient on the use of a cold pack. Advise the patient to leave the cold pack in place for 15 to 20 minutes or until the area feels numb, whichever comes first.
   Purpose: Cold applications are typically applied for 15 to 20 minutes or per the provider's order.
7. Wash hands or use hand sanitizer.
   Purpose: For infection control.
8. Document the procedure in the patient's health record. Include the provider's name, the order, what was taught, and how the patient responded.
   Purpose: It is important to document the procedure in the health record to show it was done.
   07/19/20XX 1505 Pt arrived holding right wrist and complaining of pain. Parent stated that he fell off his bike about 1 hour ago. Per Dr. Kahn's standing order, applied cold pack to pt's right wrist. Instructed pt and parent to keep the cold pack (covered with a towel) on the wrist for 15–20 minutes. Parent stated she would remove it at that time._____ Tim Peterson, CMA (AAMA)

PROCEDURE 43.3 Apply a Hot Pack

Tasks
Apply a hot pack (chemical, gel, or bead) to an infected wound. Document the procedure in the patient's health record.

Scenario
Dr. Kahn orders a hot pack to be applied to an infected wound for 15 minutes. He also orders coaching for the patient to continue the treatment at home four times a day for the next 3 days.

Equipment and Supplies
- Hot pack (chemical, gel, or bead)
- Towel or another type of protective covering for the hot pack
- Provider's order
- Patient's health record

Procedural Steps
1. Wash hands or use hand sanitizer.
   Purpose: Hand sanitization is an important step for infection control.
2. Read the provider's order. Assemble the equipment. If using a chemical hot pack, activate the pack by squeezing it. If the pack needs to be warmed, follow the manufacturer's directions.
   Purpose: It is important to know the provider's order or the standing order before starting the procedure.
3. Greet the patient. Identify yourself. Verify the patient's identity with full name and date of birth. Explain the procedure to be performed in a manner that the patient understands. Answer any questions the patient may have about the procedure.
   Purpose: It is important to identify the patient in two different ways to ensure that you have the correct patient. Explaining the procedure can make the patient feel more comfortable and helps to reduce anxiety.
4. Cover the hot pack with a towel or protective covering.
   Purpose: The hot pack must never be put directly on the skin. Place a towel or protective covering between the hot pack and the skin to prevent injuries.
5. Assist the patient to position the hot pack over the covered wound.
   Purpose: Some patients like to place the hot pack themselves on the area.
6. Coach the patient on the use of a hot pack. Advise the patient to leave the hot pack in place for 15 to 20 minutes per the provider's order or until the area feels warm, whichever comes first.
   Purpose: Hot applications are typically applied for 15 to 20 minutes or per the provider's order.
7. Wash hands or use hand sanitizer.
8. Document the procedure in the patient's health record. Include the provider's name, the order, what was taught, and how the patient responded.
   Purpose: It is important to document the procedure in the health record to show it was done.
   07/21/20XX 1505 Per Dr. Kahn's order, applied hot pack to pt's left lower arm. Instructed pt to keep the hot pack (covered with a towel) on the wound for 15 minutes. Instructed patient how to apply a hot pack at home. Instructed patient to apply a hot pack for 15 minutes, four times a day for the next 3 days. Pt's questions were answered. Pt was encouraged to call the department if they have additional questions or concerns. _____
   _____ Tim Peterson, CMA (AAMA)

PROCEDURE 43.4   Coach a Patient in the Use of Axillary Crutches

Tasks

Fit crutches to a patient. Coach the patient to use crutches properly, considering the patient's developmental life stage. Document your teaching in the patient's health record.

Scenario

You are working with Dr. David Kahn. He has ordered you to teach Daniel Miller (DOB 3/21/20XX) how to use axillary crutches. Daniel broke his left leg, and his treatment plan requires that he not bear weight on the left leg for 6 weeks. Daniel's bedroom is on the second floor, so he has to learn how to use crutches on the stairs also.

Equipment and Supplies

- Axillary crutches
- Handout on crutch walking (optional)
- Provider's order
- Patient's health record

Procedural Steps

1. Wash hands or use hand sanitizer.
   Purpose: Hand sanitization is an important step for infection control.
2. Read the provider's order. Assemble the equipment.
   Purpose: It is important to know the provider's order before starting the procedure.
3. Greet the patient. Identify yourself. Verify the patient's identity with full name and date of birth. Explain the procedure to be performed in a manner that the patient understands. Answer any questions the patient may have about the procedure.
   Purpose: It is important to identify the patient in two different ways to ensure that you have the correct patient. Explaining the procedure can make the patient feel more comfortable and helps to reduce anxiety.
4. Ensure the patient is wearing shoes and ask the patient to stand up straight. Assist as needed. Fit the crutches to the patient so they are 1 to 1½ inches (about 2 finger widths) below the armpit (Fig. 1). The crutch should be about 4 to 6 inches to the side and front of each foot.
   Purpose: Pressure in the axilla can cause crutch palsy. Adjust the length on the crutches as needed.

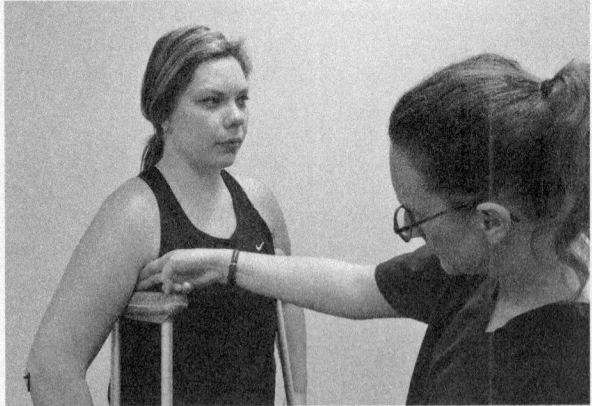

5. Adjust the handgrips so they are near the patient's wrist and even with the top of the hip line. This should allow for a 15- to 30-degree bend in the elbow when the patient's hands are on the handgrip.
   Purpose: This position allows for the most strength with the hands.
6. Coach the patient using strategies appropriate for the patient's developmental stage. Encourage discussion and questions. Use concrete terms when explaining the procedure. Show simple pictures.

Purpose: Coaching a child requires strategies that are simple and concrete. Encourage the child to ask questions, which helps to clear up any misconceptions. (See Chapter 17 for more information on communication and developmental life stage.)

7. Using age-appropriate language, instruct the patient to keep the injured leg as relaxed as possible. The knee should be slightly bent, and the patient should look forward when walking. Instruct the patient not to bear weight on the axilla.
   Purpose: For a child, it is important to keep your language simple and to demonstrate what you are saying.
8. Have the patient start in the tripod position and then move the crutches about 12 inches in front of the body (or less for a child).
   Purpose: For the three-point crutch gait, placing the crutches in front of the body is the first step.
9. Have the patient put their weight on the crutches and move the body forward. Finish the step by having the patient swing the "good" or unaffected leg forward. Do not place weight on the "bad" or affected leg. Continue with these steps.
   Purpose: Placing weight on the affected extremity may harm the leg.
10. To sit down: Instruct the patient to do the following: Back up to the chair, toilet, or bed until the seat touches the back of the legs. Move the "bad" or affected leg forward, balancing on the "good" or unaffected leg. Hold both crutches on the side with the "bad" or affected leg. Use the free hand to grab the seat or armrest. Slowly sit down.
    Purpose: Backing up until the seat touches the back of the legs is important to prevent falls.
11. To stand up: Instruct the patient to do the following: Move toward the front of the seat and move the "bad" or affected leg forward. Hold both crutches on the side with the "bad" or affected leg. Use the free hand to push up from the seat to stand up. Balance on the "good" or unaffected leg while placing a crutch in each hand. Balance is needed before moving.
    Purpose: If the person is unstable, the risk of falling is greater. Stand still until balance is achieved.
12. To go up the stairs: Instruct the patient to do the following: Step up with the "good" or unaffected leg first. Then bring the crutches up, one in each arm. Finally place weight on the "good" or unaffected leg and bring the "bad" or affected leg up.
    Purpose: It is important to go up the stairs starting with the "good" or unaffected leg.
13. To go down stairs: Instruct the patient to do the following: With a crutch in each hand, place the crutches on the first step. Then move the "bad" or affected leg forward and down. Lastly, follow with the "good" or unaffected leg.
    Purpose: When going down stairs, the crutches and then the "bad" or affected leg come first.
14. Instruct the patient and family on ways to prevent falls. Wash hands or use hand sanitizer.
    Purpose: It is important to also educate the patient on how to prevent falls.
15. Document the patient education in the patient's health record. Include the provider's name, the order, what was taught, how the patient responded, how the patient did the demonstration, and any handouts provided.
    Purpose: It is important to document the patient education in the health record to show it was done.

07/21/20XX 1423 Per Dr. Kahn's order, pt fitted with crutches and taught with his mother on the three-point crutch gait. They were told of the non–weight-bearing limitation on the left leg × 6 wk. Pt was able to correctly walk 20 feet using the three-point gait. He was able to walk up and down the stairs safely with crutches. Pt was also taught to sit down and get up from a chair. Pt demonstrated the techniques correctly. Pt's mother was given the crutch booklet. All their questions were answered, and the mother was given a follow-up number for additional questions.
—————————————————— Tim Peterson, CMA (AAMA)

PROCEDURE 43.5   Coach a Patient in the Use of a Walker

Tasks
Fit a standard walker to a patient. Coach the patient to use a standard walker properly, considering the patient's communication barrier and developmental life stage. Document teaching in the patient's health record.

Scenario
You are working with Dr. David Kahn. He has ordered you to teach Jana Green (DOB 5/1/19XX) how to use a standard walker. Jana needs the walker for extra stability. She has a hearing impairment. She can hear best with her right ear. She has no hearing in the left ear.

Equipment and Supplies
- Standard walker
- Walker handout (optional)
- Provider's order
- Patient's health record

Procedural Steps
1. Wash hands or use hand sanitizer.
   Purpose: Hand sanitization is an important step for infection control.
2. Read the provider's order. Assemble the equipment.
   Purpose: It is important to know the provider's order before starting the procedure.
3. Greet the patient. Identify yourself. Verify the patient's identity with full name and date of birth. Explain the procedure to be performed in a manner that the patient understands. Answer any questions the patient may have about the procedure.
   Purpose: It is important to identify the patient in two different ways to ensure that you have the correct patient. Explaining the procedure can make the patient feel more comfortable and helps to reduce anxiety.
4. Face the person when speaking. Position yourself so your voice is directed toward the patient's good ear. Use a low-pitched voice and speak clearly, slowly, and distinctly. Speak naturally. Limit medical terminology as you speak.
   Purpose: It is important to speak naturally; do not shout. Listen to the patient and follow what they state works the best with the impairment. (See Chapter 17 for more information on working with communication barriers.)
5. Use simpler language when talking. Speak clearly. Communicate with dignity and respect. Allow time for the patient to respond. Listen to the patient's concerns.
   Purpose: When working with older patients, it is important to show respect and to value their dignity. Listening is important.
6. Ensure the patient is wearing shoes and ask the patient to step into the walker. The top of the walker grip should be even with the top of the hip line and near the crease in the wrist when the arms are at the side of the body. Adjust as needed. Keeping the shoulders relaxed and the hands on the grips will ensure the elbows are bent at a 15-degree angle (Fig. 1).
   Purpose: For body mechanics, it is important to have the walker adjusted to fit the person. Using a walker that is too tall or too short can cause stress on the upper shoulders and back. A person should not lean over to walk because this increases the risk of falls.
7. Have the patient place the walker one step ahead of their body. Instruct the patient to use the "bad" or affected leg to step into the walker. The patient should not touch the front bar with the leg. Have the patient step forward with the other leg to complete the step. The patient will continue with this pattern while holding up the head and looking forward.
   Purpose: Being too close to the front bar can affect the patient's stability.

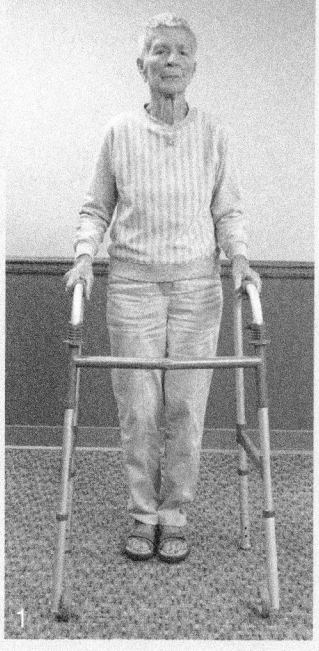

8. To sit down: Instruct the patient to back up to the chair, toilet, or bed until the seat touches the back of the legs. The patient can then use one hand to grab the seat or armrest and slowly sit down.
   Purpose: Backing up until the seat touches the back of the legs is important to prevent falls.
9. To stand up: Instruct the patient to move toward the front of the seat. Have the walker in front of the person. Have the patient use one hand to push up from the seat to stand up and then place hands on the walker. Remind patients to make sure they have their balance before moving.
   Purpose: If the person is unstable, the risk of falling is greater. It is important to stand still until balance is achieved.
10. Instruct the patient on ways to prevent falls. The walker should never be used on stairs or an escalator. If the patient will be using a bag on the front of the walker, instruct them to make sure not to overload it. Make sure to place all four legs of the walker on the ground before moving into the walker. Wash hands or use hand sanitizer.
    Purpose: It is important to educate the patient on how to prevent falls. Too much weight in the front of the walker may cause it to tilt and the patient to fall.
11. Document the patient education in the patient's health record. Include the provider's name, the order, what was taught, how the patient responded, how the patient did the demonstration, and any handouts provided.
    Purpose: It is important to document the patient education in the health record to show it was done.
    07/21/20XX 1423 Per Dr. Kahn's order, patient was fitted with a walker and instructed how to use it. Pt was able to walk using the walker correctly. Pt was also able to sit and stand while using the walker. Pt demonstrated techniques correctly and safely. Coached patient on safety issues with the walker and how to reduce the risk of falls. Pt was able to verbalize four ways to prevent falls when using the walker. All the pt's questions were answered. Pt was given the walker booklet to take home. _____ Tim Peterson, CMA (AAMA)

PROCEDURE 43.6   Coach a Patient in the Use of a Cane

Tasks

Fit a cane to a patient. Coach the patient in how to use a cane. Document teaching in the patient's health record.

Scenario

You are working with Dr. David Kahn. He has ordered you to teach Ella Rainwater (DOB 7/11/19XX) how to use a cane. Ella has left side weakness.

Equipment and Supplies

- Cane
- Handout on cane walking (optional)
- Provider's order
- Patient's health record

Procedural Steps

1. Wash hands or use hand sanitizer.
   Purpose: Hand sanitization is an important step for infection control.
2. Read the provider's order. Assemble the equipment.
   Purpose: It is important to know the provider's order before starting the procedure.
3. Greet the patient. Identify yourself. Verify the patient's identity with full name and date of birth. Explain the procedure to be performed in a manner that the patient understands. Answer any questions the patient may have about the procedure.
   Purpose: It is important to identify the patient in two different ways to ensure that you have the correct patient. Explaining the procedure can make the patient feel more comfortable and helps to reduce anxiety.
4. Ensure the patient is wearing shoes. The top of the cane should be near the crease in the wrist when the arms are at the side of the body. Adjust as needed. With the patient's shoulders relaxed and hand on the cane, ensure the elbows are bent at a 15-degree angle.
   Purpose: For body mechanics, it is important to have the cane fitted correctly.
5. Instruct the patient to hold the cane on the "good" or unaffected side. The patient should take a step moving the "bad" or affected leg and the cane forward at the same time and then step forward with the "good" leg. Instruct the patient to lean on the cane as needed.
   Purpose: The cane is held on the "good" or unaffected side so it can provide added support to the opposite leg.

6. To sit down: Instruct the patient to back up to the chair, toilet, or bed until the seat touches the back of the legs. The patient can then use a hand to grab the seat or armrest and slowly sit down.
   Purpose: Backing up until the seat touches the back of the legs is important to prevent falls.
7. To stand up: Instruct the patient to move toward the front of the seat and move the "bad" or affected leg forward. The patient can then use a hand to push up from the seat to stand up. Remind patients to make sure to get their balance before moving.
   Purpose: If the person is unstable, the risk of falling is greater. Instruct the patient to stand still until balance is achieved.
8. To go up the stairs: Instruct the patient to step up with the "good" or unaffected leg first while holding onto the rail. Then the patient should bring up the "bad" or affected leg to the same step. If there is no handrail, the cane and the "bad" leg should be placed on the stair at the same time.
   Purpose: It is important to go up the stairs starting with the "good" or unaffected leg.
9. To go down stairs: Instruct the patient to hold onto the rail and move the "bad" or affected leg down first. Then the patient should place the "good" or unaffected leg on the same step as the "bad" leg. When there is no handrail, instruct the patient to place the cane on the lower step, then place the "bad" or affected leg, and lastly place the "good" or unaffected leg next to the "bad" or affected leg.
   Purpose: When going down stairs, the cane and then the "bad" leg come down first, followed by the "good" leg.
10. Instruct the patient on ways to prevent falls. Wash hands or use hand sanitizer.
    Purpose: It is important to also educate the patient on how to prevent falls.
11. Document the patient education in the patient's health record. Include the provider's name, the order, what was taught, how the patient responded, how the patient did the demonstration, and any handouts provided.
    Purpose: It is important to document the patient education in the health record to show it was done.

07/25/20XX 1105 Per Dr. Kahn's order, pt was fitted with a cane and was instructed on walking with a cane, doing stairs, and sitting/standing. Pt was able to walk about 30 feet with a cane correctly. Pt was able to safely walk up and down and sit/stand while using the cane. Pt's questions were answered. Pt was given the Using a Cane booklet. _____ Tim Peterson, CMA (AAMA)

Pharmacology Basics

LEARNING OBJECTIVES

1. Describe the sources and uses of drugs.
2. Describe pharmacokinetics, including absorption, distribution, metabolism, and excretion.
3. Discuss drug action, including the factors that influence drug action, the therapeutic effects of drugs, and adverse reactions to drugs.
4. Explain drug legislation that is important in the ambulatory care setting.
5. Describe the four types of drug names.
6. Describe various methods of accessing drug reference information.
7. Identify the classifications of medications, including the indications for use, desired effects, side effects, and adverse reactions.
8. Discuss the terminology used in drug reference information, including describing the differences among biological half-life, onset, peak, and duration.
9. Discuss the solid, semisolid, and liquid forms of medication.
10. Discuss types of medication orders.
11. List the four parts of a prescription and the information required for all prescriptions.
12. Define commonly approved abbreviations.
13. Describe common requirements for scheduled substances.
14. Discuss over-the-counter (OTC) medications and herbal products.

OUTLINE

▶▶ OPENING SCENARIO

Gabe Garcia, a certified medical assistant (CMA) through the American Association of Medical Assistants (AAMA), has worked for Walden-Martin Family Medical (WMFM) Clinic for 7 years. He was hired right after he completed his medical assistant program. Gabe was asked to be Mark Allen's mentor for practicum. Mark has just completed all his medical assistant courses at the local college and now needs 160 hours of practicum. He is excited to be working with Gabe.

Gabe works with several of the WMFM Clinic providers. He spends 1 to 2 hours a day working with prescription refills. Gabe also rooms patients, obtains their vital signs and history, and assists with injections. Mark will have a lot of great experiences with Gabe.

YOU WILL LEARN

1. To identify the basics of drugs, including the sources, uses, pharmacokinetics, and action.
2. To describe drug legislation and how it impacts the medical assistant practice.
3. To list the four names a drug could have.
4. To describe common drug classifications and reference information terminology.
5. To prepare prescriptions for the provider to sign.

INTRODUCTION

Pharmacology (FAHR mah kol oh jee) is the study of the properties, actions, and uses of drugs. A *drug* is a chemical substance used to cure, treat, prevent, or diagnose disease. In the ambulatory care setting, medical assistants deal with medication, from history taking to administering medications. Medical assistants must have a general understanding of the classification of drugs. They need to know how to pronounce the medication names. They must know how to give medications, the dose to give, and typical side effects. New medications are continually being developed and released for patient treatment. Thus medical assistants must stay updated on medications.

PHARMACOLOGY BASICS

Medications have been around for a long time. The first medications came from natural products found in our ancestors' living environment. Today, with advancing technology, most medications are created in a laboratory setting. These sources and others will be explained along with the uses of medications.

In addition, a basic description of how medication enters, moves through, and exits the body will be given. This knowledge will help the medical assistant identify patients who may be at risk for medication issues because of their age or a disease process.

Sources of Drugs

Drugs are either created from natural sources or made synthetically in a laboratory. Plants, animals, minerals, and microbiological sources are natural sources of drugs.

Natural Sources of Drugs. Plants are the oldest source of drugs. Our ancestors found that different plants helped with different symptoms. Leaves, bark, stems, roots, and fruits have been used in medicinal preparations through the years. Some examples of medicinal plant sources include:

- Digitalis (DIJ i tal is), an antiarrhythmic (an tee ah RITH mik) medication, comes from the purple foxglove flower.
- Nicotine comes from tobacco leaves.
- Quinidine (KWIN i deen), an antimalarial (an tee mah LAR ee ahl) medication, comes from the bark of the cinchona tree.

Animals are also a source of medications. Natural substances are extracted from animal tissues and organs. *Heparin* (HEP ah

rin), an anticoagulant (AN tie koe ag yuh lahnt), comes from pig intestines. Lanolin is found in topical preparations used to protect the skin. It comes from the sebaceous glands of sheep. Other medications are developed with lactose and gelatin, which are from animals.

Minerals and microbiological substances are other natural sources of medications. Examples of minerals include:

- Iron is used to treat iron-deficiency anemia.
- Iodine is an antiseptic (an ti SEP tik).
- Zinc is used as a supplement and is found in topical pastes for wounds.

One microbiological source is *Penicillium chrysogenum*. This is a fungus that creates penicillin.

VOCABULARY

antiarrhythmic A drug that prevents or alleviates heart arrhythmias.

anticoagulant A substance (i.e., medication or chemical) that prevents the clotting of blood.

antimalarial A drug used to treat or prevent malaria.

antiseptic A substance that inhibits the growth of microorganisms on living tissue (e.g., alcohol and povidone-iodine solution [Betadine]).

side effects Unpleasant effects of a drug in addition to the desired or therapeutic effect.

Synthetic Sources of Drugs. Many medications originated in nature but have been recreated in the laboratory setting. For instance, insulin initially came from cattle and pigs. Many people developed allergies to the insulin. Now synthetic insulin is widely used. Biotechnology and genetic engineering techniques are continually being used to create new medications. With the help of technologic advances, individualized medications are also being produced. (Individualized medications will be discussed later in the chapter.) Synthetic medications are cheaper to produce because they are created in mass volumes. The quality of synthetic medications can also be controlled.

Uses of Drugs

When you are studying medications, it is important to identify the uses of drugs. Why are they being prescribed? What do they do in the body? Some medications may have more than one use. There are eight common uses of drugs:

- *Prevention*: Drugs used to prevent diseases. Example: Vaccines are given, and the body creates antibodies to protect against specific diseases.
- *Treatment*: Drugs that relieve the symptoms while the body fights off the disease. Example: Acetaminophen (a set a MEE noe fen), an *antipyretic* medication, brings down a fever while the body fights off a viral infection.
- *Diagnosis*: Drugs used to diagnose or monitor a condition. Example: Contrast medium (radiopaque dye) is given to highlight organs on x-rays.
- *Cure*: Drugs that eliminate the disease. Example: Amoxicillin (ah mox i SIL in), an antibiotic, is used to cure strep throat.
- *Contraceptive*: Drugs used to prevent pregnancy. Example: Depo-Provera (DEP oh proe VER ah) is an injectable contraceptive medication.

- *Health maintenance*: Medications used to maintain or enhance health. Examples: Vitamins and minerals.
- *Palliation* (PAL ee a shun): Drugs that do not cure or treat the disease but improve the quality of life. Example: Morphine (MOR feen), an analgesic, is commonly used by patients with cancer.
- *Replacement*: Drugs used to increase the blood levels of naturally occurring substances in the body. Example: Levothyroxine (lee voe thye ROX een) is used for patients with hypothyroidism.

CRITICAL THINKING 44.1

Gabe and Mark are discussing the basics of pharmacology and the eight common uses of medications. Gabe asks Mark which use would include taking an antihistamine for allergy symptoms. How would you answer this question?

Pharmacokinetics

Pharmacokinetics (FAHR mah koe ki net iks) is the study of drug absorption, distribution, metabolism, and excretion in the body. Through pharmacokinetics, we understand when a medication starts to work in the body. We know how it moves through the body and what organs metabolize and excrete the drug from the body. Some of the patients you will be working with will have greater risks of side effects and toxicity. Understanding the basics of pharmacokinetics will help you identify those at greater risk for problems.

VOCABULARY

toxicity The harmful and deadly effect of a medication that can develop due to the buildup of medication or by-products in the body.

Absorption. Drugs can be administered in many ways. *Route* is the means by which a drug enters the body. Where a drug enters the body is considered the *site of administration*. *Absorption* is the movement of drug from the site of administration to the bloodstream. The following are commonly used routes:

- *Oral* (po, PO): Taken by mouth.
- *Sublingual* (sub LIN gwal) (SL): Placed under the tongue to dissolve.
- *Buccal* (BUCK uhl): Placed between the cheek and the gums to dissolve and absorb quickly.
- *Intramuscular* (IM): Injected into the muscle.
- *Subcutaneous* (subcut): Injected just below the skin; moves into the capillaries or the lymphatic vessels and is brought to the bloodstream.
- *Intravenous* (IV): Injected directly into the bloodstream.
  The rate of absorption is influenced by the following factors:
- *Route*: Oral medications need to pass through the gastrointestinal (GI) tract. This takes time. IV medications are directly administered into the bloodstream and have virtually no absorption time. They start working faster than drugs given by other routes.
- *Blood flow to the absorption area*: The greater the number of blood vessels, the quicker the absorption. Medication given

by the sublingual and buccal routes is absorbed quickly into the bloodstream. These sites are rich with blood vessels. IM medications absorb quicker than subcut medications. The muscle tissue has more blood vessels than the subcutaneous tissue.

- *Ability of the medication to be absorbed*: Liquid medications are easier to absorb than solid medications. Solid medications need to be broken down before they absorb. Acidic medications are absorbed in the stomach. Base (or alkaline) medications are absorbed in the intestines.
- *Conditions at the site of the absorption*: Some medications must be taken with food, which can slow the absorption of the medication. Typically, medications taken on an empty stomach can be absorbed faster. The intestines provide more surface area than the stomach for the absorption of medications.

MEDICAL TERMINOLOGY

bucc/o	cheek
cutane/o	skin
lingu/o	tongue
muscul/o	muscle
thyroid/o	thyroid gland
ven/o	vein
hypo-	deficient
intra-	within
sub-	under
-al, -ar, -ous	pertaining to
-ism	condition

Distribution. Once the drug is absorbed into the blood, it rapidly circulates through the body (unless it must go through the liver) (Box 44.1). During this time, the drug is brought to the body tissues. The movement of absorbed drug from the blood to the body tissues is called *distribution*. The speed of the drug's movement from the blood to the tissues varies greatly. Some drugs bind with proteins in the blood and move slowly into tissues. Some drugs accumulate in certain tissues. These tissues act as *reservoirs*, slowly releasing the drug into the bloodstream and keeping the blood levels from decreasing too rapidly. This process prolongs

---

BOX 44.1 Routes Affect the Dose

Oral medications are absorbed in the stomach or in the intestines. The blood containing the absorbed digestive nutrients and drugs passes through the hepatic portal vein and the liver before it circulates to the rest of the body. In the liver, some of the drugs are chemically altered. Some of the active drug is lost during this first pass through the liver. This reduces the amount of drug in the circulating blood that can be used.

For instance, a person is having an allergic reaction and needs Benadryl. If the drug is to be taken orally, the person takes 50 mg. If it is to be given intravenously, 10 mg may be given. This is because all 10 mg gets into the bloodstream, whereas some of the 50 mg is lost as it passes through the liver before circulating through the body. It is important for a medical assistant to realize that doses (e.g., 10 mg) may vary based on the route used to give the medication.

the effect of the drug. Circulation issues (e.g., peripheral artery disease) can also slow the distribution of medication.

For the medication to move into certain organs, it must be able to pass through the tissues. The blood-brain barrier allows only certain fat-soluble medications to pass into the cerebrospinal fluid and the brain. In comparison, the placental membrane allows most drugs to pass through from the mother to the baby in utero. Therefore only certain medications are prescribed during pregnancy.

Metabolism. *Metabolism* is a series of chemical processes whereby enzymes change drugs in the body. Metabolism is necessary so that medications can be cleared from the body. Active forms of drugs may be converted into water-soluble compounds, which are eventually excreted.

Most drug metabolism occurs in the liver. Younger children, older adults, and those with liver disease may have problems metabolizing medications. These populations could be at risk for drug toxicity. To prevent toxicity, the dose of medication is adjusted for at-risk populations.

Prodrugs. Prodrugs (PROE drugs) are medications that are administered in an inactive form. Through the normal metabolic processes, the medication is changed into an active form of a drug. The liver and the intestines are sites that can convert prodrugs to active forms of drugs. For instance, sulfasalazine (sul fa SAL a zeen) (Azulfidine) is an anti-inflammatory drug that is used to treat ulcerative colitis. It is also a prodrug because it is ingested in an inactive form. Bacteria in the colon change the drug into an active drug that is used by the body.

Excretion. *Excretion* is the movement of metabolites (muh TAB uh lahyts) out of the body. Most drugs are excreted through the large intestine and kidneys. The large intestine excretes the undigested drug products in the stool. The kidneys excrete metabolites in the urine. Clinical Laboratory Improvement Amendments (CLIA)–waived urine drug screening tests can detect certain metabolites.

Drugs can also be excreted in breast milk. This is critical information to have when a mother is breastfeeding her baby. As with pregnancy, only a limited number of drugs are safe with breastfeeding. Most drug references indicate if medications pass into the breast milk. Other ways drugs can be excreted are through sweat, exhaled air, and saliva.

Young children, older adults, and those with kidney disease are at risk for the buildup of metabolic drug by-products in the body. These populations are at greater risk for symptoms of toxicity.

> **VOCABULARY**
> **metabolites** By-products of drug metabolism.

Drug Action

Drugs are chemicals that can cause changes in the cells. The four main drug actions are:

- *Depressing*: Slows down the cell's activity. For example, narcotic medications reduce the activity in the brain's respiratory center. This action slows the respiration rate.

- *Stimulating*: Increases the cell's activity. For instance, caffeine increases brain activity.
- *Destroying*: Kills cells or disrupts parts of cells. For example, chemotherapy medications destroy cancer cells.
- *Replacing substances*: Substances required by the body can be given as medications. For instance, patients with type 1 diabetes mellitus take insulin.

Factors Influencing Drug Action. One might think that a drug works the same for everyone. This is not so. Personal characteristics can cause minor differences in how a drug works from one person to another. Many factors influence drug action:

- *Age*: Infants and older adults have problems metabolizing and excreting medications. Their liver and kidneys are less effective. This can lead to possible drug accumulation and toxicity.
- *Body size*: A person's size affects the amount of drug needed. Children's dosages are calculated based on body weight. Thinner people require less medication than heavier people.
- *Sex*: Women have a higher proportion of body fat. Hormonal differences can affect metabolism. Women can react differently to some medications compared to men.
- *Genetics*: Genetic makeup can affect how a person responds to drugs. (This is discussed in more depth in the "Pharmacogenomics" section.)
- *Diseases*: Poor circulation, liver disease, and kidney disease can alter drug action.
- *Diet*: Certain foods can affect a drug's action. For instance, milk products can diminish the effects of tetracycline (tet ra SYE kleen), an antibiotic.
- *Drug dosage, route, and timing of administration*: The greater the amount of drug taken, the greater the effect will be. The route will also affect drug action. Drugs are absorbed, distributed, and metabolized differently based on the administration route. Some drugs work better when taken with food, whereas others do not.
- *Mental state*: People with positive attitudes tend to do better than those with negative attitudes.
- *Environmental temperature*: In hot weather, heat relaxes blood vessels. This can speed up the distribution of medication, thus speeding up the drug's action.

Pharmacogenomics. Most medications are dosed as "one size fits all." Each person's genetic makeup affects how that person responds to medications. *Pharmacogenomics* (FAHR mah koe jeh NOE miks) or *pharmacogenetics* (FAHR mah koe jeh net iks) is the study of how genetic factors influence a person's metabolic response to a specific medication. Pharmacogenomics testing usually requires a small blood or saliva sample. The sample is analyzed to determine if a specific medication will be an effective treatment for an individual. Testing can determine the best dose of medication and if the person could have serious adverse reactions (unexpected or life-threatening reactions) to the medication. A different test is required for each medication. Pharmacogenomics is largely used in cancer treatments, but it is becoming more common in other areas of medicine.

Therapeutic Effects. Medications can have local or systemic effects. Medication effects that are seen at the site of administration are *local effects*. Medication effects that are seen throughout the body are *systemic effects*. Each medication has one or more *therapeutic effects* or desired effects. This is the intended action of the medication. For instance, the therapeutic effect of a pain reliever is to reduce pain.

Sometimes multiple doses are needed to achieve the therapeutic effect. Other times just one dose of medication can achieve the therapeutic effect. For some medications, the provider may prescribe a higher initial dose, called a *loading dose*. This helps to quickly increase the medication level in the blood. A loading dose helps the person achieve the therapeutic range sooner. A *maintenance dose* is the amount of medication needed to keep the blood levels within the therapeutic range. If the blood levels go beyond the therapeutic range, the person can experience signs and symptoms of toxicity. This is considered a *toxic dose* of medication. A *lethal dose* is the amount of medication that could kill a person.

VOCABULARY

psychiatrists Medical doctors who have been specially trained to diagnose and treat patients with mental, emotional, and behavioral conditions.

therapeutic range The blood concentrations of a medication that are high enough to produce the drug's therapeutic effect.

CRITICAL THINKING 44.2

Gabe and Mark are discussing therapeutic effect and loading dose. Gabe shares that patients sometimes get confused on how much medication to take when they are given two amounts, a loading dose and the regular amount. How might a healthcare professional instruct a patient who needs to take a loading dose?

Adverse Reactions. Most of the time when a medication is correctly administered, the therapeutic effect occurs. However, sometimes issues arise, and the person has problems with the medication. The person can experience an unexpected or life-threatening reaction, which is called an *adverse reaction*. Table 44.1 lists common adverse reactions.

Many experts and drug reference information will include side effects with adverse reactions. They may divide these into mild, moderate, and severe reactions. The side effects usually fall into the mild category. Severe adverse reactions are those that can cause disability, hospitalization, death, or birth defects.

Other reference information separates adverse reactions/events and side effects. Adverse reactions or events would be those that are life-threatening and may cause disability or birth defects. *Side effects* would be unpleasant effects of the drug, in addition to the desired or therapeutic effect. They can be harmless or may cause injury. The most common side effects include symptoms of GI distress, such as nausea, vomiting, constipation, and diarrhea.

DRUG LEGISLATION AND THE AMBULATORY CARE SETTING

In the ambulatory care environment, medications can be prescribed, administered, and dispensed.

- *Prescribe* means to order a medication as a treatment for a condition. Doctors (MDs [including psychiatrists], DOs, and dentists) and advanced practice professionals, including physician assistants (PAs), nurse practitioners (NPs), and certified nurse midwives (CNMs), can prescribe medications. State prescribing laws can vary for advanced practice professionals.
- *Administer* means to give a prescribed dose of medication to a patient. Medical assistants, nurses, and providers can administer medications. State laws related to medication administration by medical assistants can vary.
- *Dispense* means to give a supply of medication that the patient will take later. In most scenarios, pharmacists dispense medications.

Federal and state legislation governs these three activities. The following sections will discuss these laws, the agencies responsible for overseeing the laws, and the laws' effect on medical assistants.

CRITICAL THINKING 44.3

At WMFM Clinic, pharmaceutical representatives drop off sample medications that are given to patients. Usually, the provider will give a few days' worth of samples to a patient to ensure the patient is tolerating the medication. If the patient has no issues, then they get the prescription filled. Mark sees the provider bag up a few samples and attach directions to the bag. The provider gives the bag to Gabe and asks him to give it to the patient. Mark asks Gabe, "Who is dispensing the medication?" How would you answer this question?

Food, Drug, and Cosmetic Act

The Food, Drug, and Cosmetic Act of 1938 is enforced by the Food and Drug Administration (FDA). The FDA is a federal agency in the Department of Health and Human Services (HHS). The FDA is responsible for the safety, effectiveness, security, and quality of drugs, cosmetics, and food. Some of the areas overseen by the FDA include:

- *Foods*: Dietary supplements, bottled water, food additives, infant formula, and other food products
- *Drugs*: Prescription drugs (brand name and generic) and nonprescription (over the counter) drugs
- *Biologicals*: Vaccines, blood, and blood products
- *Medical devices*: Medical equipment (from simple [tongue depressor] to complex [heart pacemaker]), dental devices, and surgical implants

Manufacturers must submit applications for new products to the FDA. Manufacturers must provide adequate data to show the safety and effectiveness of the product. The FDA must determine if drugs, devices, and products are safe and effective. Once this is determined, then the product is released to the general public.

The FDA monitors the safety of products released to the market. The FDA Adverse Event Reporting System (FAERS)

TABLE 44.1　Common Adverse Reactions

Adverse Reaction	Description
Allergy	Drug allergy occurs when a person develops antibodies against a specific drug. When the drug is taken, the antibodies attack the antigens from the drug. Tissues are damaged during this process, and histamines are released. Histamines cause the allergic reactions.
Anaphylaxis (AN ah fi LAK sis)	Extreme hypersensitivity to a specific drug (antigen) can cause life-threatening symptoms, including swelling of the mouth and airway, difficulty breathing (*dyspnea*), wheezing, loss of consciousness, and death.
Idiosyncrasy (ID ee oh sing kreh see)	A peculiar response to a certain drug. For instance, Benadryl causes drowsiness. However, when it is given to children, they often get extremely agitated.
Cumulative effect	For medications taken routinely, often the prior dose is not completely metabolized and excreted before the next dose is given. This can lead to a buildup of medication or by-products that can produce toxic effects.
Toxicity	The harmful and possibly deadly effects of a medication that can develop due to the buildup of medication or by-products in the body. People with liver or kidney disease, young children, older adults, and those who overdose are at risk for toxicity.
Drug interactions	When two or more drugs are taken, sometimes a drug-drug interaction can occur. The interactions can be helpful or harmful. Three types of drug interactions can occur: • *Antagonism* (an TAG o nizm): One drug reduces or blocks the effect of another drug. Example: Naloxone is given for narcotic overdosage. • *Synergism* (SIN er jizm): The combined effect of two drugs used together is greater than the sum of each drug's effect (e.g., 1 + 1 > 2). Example of a harmful interaction: Alcohol has a synergistic effect on antidepressants. • *Potentiation* (poe ten shee AE shun): A type of synergism; one drug increases the effect of the second drug. With L-dopa and carbidopa, one drug has no effect but increases the effect of the other drug (e.g., 0 + 1 > 1).
Tolerance	The need for a larger dose to get the same therapeutic or desired effect. Tolerance can be seen when narcotic pain medications are taken with anticonvulsants (an tee kahn VUL sahnt).
Drug dependence	Strong psychological or physical need to take a certain drug. Withdrawal symptoms can be experienced when a person stops using a drug. Drug dependence can occur with or without addiction.

is a computerized database that helps the FDA monitor drugs. It contains reports of adverse events reported to the FDA. MedWatch is the FDA's reporting program. It provides information on products overseen by the FDA. MedWatch is available to healthcare professionals (https://www.fda.gov/safety/medwatch-fda-safety-information-and-adverse-event-reporting-program).

If the FDA determines a medication is unsafe, it will recall the medication. The medical assistant should remove any recalled medications from the stock and sample cabinets. (*Sample medications* come from pharmaceutical companies and are used for patients.) Concerned patients may contact their providers. The provider will determine what action to take for each patient.

Controlled Substances Act

The Controlled Substances Act (CSA), Title II of the Comprehensive Drug Abuse Prevention and Control Act of 1970, is a federal law. The Drug Enforcement Agency (DEA) is a federal law enforcement agency under the US Department of Justice. The DEA enforces the CSA. The DEA oversees the manufacturing, importation, possession, use, and distribution of legal (or prescription) controlled substances. The DEA also handles illegal controlled substances, which cannot legally be manufactured, purchased, or sold in the US.

Under the CSA, controlled substances are divided into five schedules. These schedules are arranged from the greatest to the least abuse potential (Table 44.2). State statutes also address procedures related to scheduled medications. It is important for the medical assistant to know the schedule of commonly ordered medications. Some controlled substance prescriptions are handled differently. This will be discussed later in the chapter.

VOCABULARY

addiction A disease that occurs when a person cannot stop or limit the use of a drug, even after negative consequences have been experienced.

anticonvulsant A drug used to prevent or treat seizures.

controlled substances A behavior-altering or addictive drug or chemical substance whose possession and use are prohibited by or regulated under the federal Controlled Substances Act.

Compliance With the Controlled Substances Act. Providers prescribing controlled substances need a DEA registration number. Each provider has a unique number. The DEA number is good for 3 years. The medical assistant may need to assist the provider in renewing or obtaining a DEA number. This can be done at the DEA website at https://www.deadiversion.usdoj.gov/. Additional state requirements may need to be met before a provider can prescribe controlled substances.

Controlled substances have a paper trail. This record starts with the manufacturer and ends when the medication is dispensed or administered. In some healthcare facilities, the in-house pharmacy handles the controlled substances that are administered. The provider gives the medical assistant a prescription for a patient. The medical assistant gives the pharmacist the prescription and, in return, gets the medication.

TABLE 44.2 Schedules of Controlled Substances

Schedule	Psychological and Physical Dependence	Examples
I	Highest potential for abuse; drugs with no currently accepted medical use	• Heroin, lysergic acid diethylamide (LSD), ecstasy
II/IIN (2/2N)	High level of abuse; can lead to severe psychological or physical dependence	• Schedule II narcotics: hydromorphone (Dilaudid), methadone (Dolophine), oxycodone (OxyContin, Percocet), fentanyl (Duragesic), codeine, morphine • Schedule IIN stimulants: dextroamphetamine and amphetamine (Adderall), methamphetamine (Desoxyn), methylphenidate (Concerta, Ritalin LA)
III/IIIN (3/3N)	Moderate to low physical dependence or high psychological dependence	• Schedule III narcotics: acetaminophen with codeine (Tylenol #2 or #3), buprenorphine • Schedule IIIN non-narcotics: benzphetamine (Didrex), ketamine, anabolic steroids (e.g., Depo-Testosterone)
IV (4)	Low potential for abuse relative to substances in Schedule III	• Schedule IV substances: alprazolam (Xanax), carisoprodol (Soma), clonazepam (Klonopin), diazepam (Valium), lorazepam (Ativan), temazepam (Restoril)
V (5)	Lowest potential for abuse relative to substances listed in Schedule IV; contains limited quantities of certain narcotics	• Schedule V substances: Robitussin AC, ezogabine (Potiga)

(Please note that some state laws do not allow medical assistants to administer controlled substances.) With this scenario, the pharmacist is responsible for managing the paperwork for the controlled substances.

In healthcare facilities without pharmacies, providers must take the responsibility of ordering controlled substances from the manufacturer. The medical assistant must help the provider comply with the Controlled Substance Act. The following sections will discuss common compliance activities.

Storage. All controlled substances must be adequately safeguarded. They need to be kept in a locked cabinet or safe of substantial construction. Keys should be placed in a locked area accessible only to authorized persons. Store controlled substances in a different location than non-narcotic medications. Additional storage guidelines that apply to all medications include:

- Make sure all medications are kept in their original containers.
- Store medications in a cool, dry location. Keep medications away from light, heat, or moisture. Refer to package inserts for specific storage information.
- Do not combine or repackage medications with different lot numbers or expiration dates.
- Keep stock medications (purchased by department) separated from sample medications (given by pharmaceutical manufacturers for patients).
- Keep medications out of exam rooms. Lock medication cabinets at the end of the day.

Inventory Records. It is important to keep an ongoing log of controlled substances received from manufacturers and administered to patients. Medications are tracked by the manufacturer, lot number, and expiration date. This information is found on the package. When a patient needs a controlled substance, the medical assistant must complete the log. The log typically requires:

- The medication information (name, dose, lot number, and expiration date)
- The ordering provider's name

- Information on the patient receiving the medication (name, date of birth, address, health record number, and so on)
- The name or initials of the healthcare professional administering the medication

The log must be kept separate from the patient's health record. The medication must also be documented in the patient's health record after it is administered.

Periodic reconciling of the log with the actual inventory count is important to identify missing medications. An inventory of all controlled substances must be done at least annually, unless required more often by law. Some states have special requirements for the inventory. It is important for the medical assistant to be knowledgeable about the special state requirements. The controlled substance inventory and log records need to be kept for 2 years. The records may be inspected by individuals authorized by the state attorney general.

> **VOCABULARY**
> **reconciling** Comparing a document with another document to ensure that they are consistent.

Drug Destruction. Expired controlled substances are returned to the place from where they were received. For example, controlled substances that were sent by the manufacturer must be returned to the manufacturer, along with the required paperwork.

Sometimes a controlled substance must be destroyed in the healthcare facility. Examples of such situations are:

- Only part of the medication is used for the patient; the extra amount must be destroyed.
- The patient refuses the medication after it has been opened and prepared.
- The medication is accidentally contaminated before it can be administered.

In these situations, the controlled substance must be destroyed in the presence of two authorized persons (e.g., medical assistants, nurses). An entry on the waste log must be made. This information must include the date; the drug's name,

BOX 44.2   Discarding Medications in the Healthcare Facility

Discard medication that is expired, contaminated, unlabeled, or opened and not used. Some healthcare facilities have medication discarding programs to prevent medications from entering the city's water supply. Remember, if the medication is a controlled substance, two authorized employees must sign a waste log before the medication is discarded. Both employees must witness the disposal.

To discard medication, follow these steps if the facility has no other procedures in place:

- Return expired controlled substances to the place from which they were received (e.g., manufacturer), accompanied by the proper paperwork.
- Flush liquids down the sink.
- Flush pills down the toilet.
- Mix powdered medications with water and flush them down the toilet.
- Flush fluid from syringes down the sink and discard the syringe in a biohazardous sharps container.

strength, and quantity; the reason for destruction; and the signatures of both persons. Box 44.2 describes how to discard medications in the healthcare facility.

Theft and Diversion Reporting. *Diversion* of controlled substances means using the medication for personal reasons. If a medical assistant identifies that controlled substances are missing, it is important to notify the provider and supervisor. Many states and the DEA require any theft or loss to be reported to them within a given period. A report must be completed and filed by the deadline.

Medical Assistant's Role in Preventing Drug Abuse. By following these guidelines, the medical assistant can help prevent drug abuse.

- Carefully monitor patients who repeatedly call for prescription refills of controlled substances. Be aware that some patients will give aliases (false names).
- Request health records from other facilities for patients who report previous prescriptions for scheduled drugs.
- If the facility uses paper prescription pads, keep blank pads in a locked cabinet. They should be stored away from patient treatment areas.
- Never use prescription pads for notepads. Never use preprinted or presigned forms.
- Secure computers used for electronic health record (EHR) documentation to prevent patient access to prescription generation.
- Keep only a limited supply of controlled substances on hand.
- Keep accurate, complete records of controlled substances administered. Patients' records should contain information on prescribed and administered controlled substances.

DRUG NAMES

A single drug may have up to four names: chemical, generic, official, and brand. The drug is known by its chemical name until it receives FDA approval. The medical assistant should be familiar with the brand and generic names of common medications.

- *Chemical name*: Represents the drug's exact chemical formula. For example, the chemical name of ibuprofen is 2-(4-isobutylphenyl) propanoic acid.
- *Generic name*: Assigned by the US Adopted Names (USAN) Council. Similar medications are given similar-sounding generic names. All drugs need to have the generic name on the packaging. For example, ibuprofen is a generic name.
- *Official name*: Used to list the medication in the *United States Pharmacopeia and the National Formulary* (USP–NF). This book provides the standards (e.g., strength, purity, and so on) for drugs in the United States. In many cases, the official name is the same as the generic name. For example, ibuprofen is also the drug's official name.
- *Brand name* or *trade name*: The manufacturer assigns and registers the medication name. No other company can use that name. Usually the brand name begins with a capital letter and is followed by the registered sign (®). For example, brand names of ibuprofen include Advil and Motrin.

Generic versus Brand Name Medications

If you ever walk through the pain medication aisle at a local store, you will see many bottles of ibuprofen products. Generally, the more expensive products are name brands, and less expensive products are generic products.

The company that initially created the medication will market it using a brand name. That company has sole rights to manufacture the medication until the patent expires. During this time, it is not uncommon for the price to be higher. The manufacturer may have spent years developing the medication before it went to market. Once the patent expires, other companies may create their own version of the medication. Some will market the medication under a brand name and others will use generic names.

When a company creates a medication, the company determines the appearance of the medication (e.g., color, size, and shape). It also comes up with the *inactive ingredients* or additives. This might be a color, sweetener, flavor, fillers, binders, and so on. For the active ingredient of the medication (e.g., ibuprofen), the company must comply with the regulations of the Food and Drug Administration (FDA). The active ingredient must be of the same quality, purity, and amount as any other FDA-approved ibuprofen product of the same strength.

Most people do not notice a difference between generic and brand name medications. Other people do notice a difference. Their bodies may react to the inactive ingredients differently. This can affect their treatment for certain conditions. The provider can indicate if a generic medication can be used for prescriptions. This is important to keep in mind if you are assisting a provider by preparing prescriptions.

CRITICAL THINKING 44.4

Mark and Gabe are working with Janine Butler, a patient being seen for hypertension. While they are reviewing Janine's current medications list, she asks them what the difference is between generic and brand name medications. How might you answer this question?

DRUG REFERENCE INFORMATION

A medical assistant is obligated to become familiar with the drugs that are most frequently prescribed in the department. It is essential to know their indications, adverse reactions, administration routes, dosage, and storage. Using drug reference information can help the medical assistant learn about drugs. In the ambulatory care environment, drug reference information is available in both print and digital forms.

With each drug (including drug samples and stock medications), the manufacturer includes a package insert. The package insert provides information about the medication, side effects, administration techniques, dosages, storage, and so on.

Drug handbooks provide condensed, more common information on the drugs. Many of these books are organized by the generic names of drugs.

The *Prescribers' Digital Reference* (PDR) has replaced the *Physician's Desk Reference*. This digital product contains a comprehensive collection of package insert information. The PDR is available as an app and is also integrated with electronic health records. More information can be found on the PDR website (https://www.pdr.net/).

The digital drug reference information has a huge advantage over print information. Digital information can be updated more quickly and easily than the print information. The market for digital drug information has grown over the years. Digital drug reference information is available online, through apps, and with electronic health records.

- Online drug reference information is available from many sites. It is important for the medical assistant to use reliable websites. Government websites (e.g., https://medlineplus.gov/ and https://www.fda.gov/) contain updated, reliable information. Sites that patients use may contain older information and can include medications that are not available in the United States.
- When selecting an app for drug reference information, be sure it is routinely updated. Read the reviews and research the company providing the information. Only use reputable apps for drug reference information.
- Many EHR software programs incorporate drug reference information. This makes it easy for healthcare professionals to look up drug information.

Drug Classification

Drugs are grouped by classification or class. It is important for a medical assistant to be aware of the class of drugs. Oftentimes patients will ask what a specific medication is for, and the medical assistant can provide that information. Table 44.3 provides a list of classifications of medications with descriptions. (Appendix D, Medication Classifications, which can be found on the Evolve website, provides additional classification information. The appendix includes indications for use, desired effects, side effects, adverse reactions, and common generic and trade names of medications.)

TABLE 44.3	Examples of Medication Classifications	
Classification	**Pronunciation**	**Description**
Analgesic	(AN ahl jee zik)	Relieves pain
Anesthetic	(an es THET ik)	Produces local or general anesthesia
Antacid	(ant AS id)	Neutralizes stomach acid
Anti-Alzheimer	(AN tie AWLTZ hye mer) (*Note:* anti- can be [AN tie] or [AN tee])	Treats dementia (Alzheimer disease)
Antianxiety	(AN tie ang ZIE e tee)	Reduces anxiety and tension
Antiarrhythmic	(AN tie ah RITH mik)	Treats heart arrhythmias
Antibiotic	(AN ti bye OT ik)	Treats bacterial infections
Anticholinergic	(AN tie koe leh nuhr jik)	Reduces smooth muscle spasms
Anticoagulant	(AN tie koe ag yuh lahnt)	Reduces blood clotting ability
Anticonvulsant	(AN tie kohn vul sahnt)	Reduces the frequency and severity of seizures
Antidepressant	(AN tie di PRES ahnt)	Treats depression
Antiemetic	(AN tie e MET ik)	Reduces nausea and vomiting
Antifungal	(AN tie FUNG gal)	Treats fungal infections
Antigout	(AN tie GOUT)	Reduces the uric acid in the body
Antihistamine	(AN tie HIS tah meen [-min])	Relieves allergies by blocking the histamine action
Antihyperglycemic	(AN tie HYE per glye SEE mik)	Reduces the blood glucose level
Antihypertensive	(AN tie hye pehr ten siv)	Lowers blood pressure
Anti-inflammatory	(AN tie in FLAM ah tohr ee)	Reduces inflammation
Antimigraine	(AN tie MYE grain)	Treats or prevents migraine headaches
Antineoplastic	(AN tie NEE oh plaz tik)	Slows or stops the growth of cancer cells
Antiplatelet	(AN tie PLATE lit)	Prevents the function of platelets (formation of clots)
Antipsychotic	(AN tie sye KOT ik)	Alters the chemical actions in the brain
Antitussive	(AN tie TUS iv)	Suppresses coughs

Continued

TABLE 44.3   Examples of Medication Classifications—cont'd

Classification	Pronunciation	Description
Antiviral	(AN tie VIE rahl)	Treats viral infections
Bronchodilator	(BRONG koe die lay tohr)	Relaxes the smooth muscles of the bronchi
Cholesterol-lowering agent	(koh LES the rohl)	Reduces low-density lipoprotein and triglycerides in the blood while increasing the high-density lipoprotein
Contraceptive	(KON trah SEP tiv)	Inhibits conception (prevents pregnancy)
Corticosteroid	(KOHR ti koe STER oid)	Reduces inflammation
Decongestant	(DEE kohn JES tahnt)	Relieves nasal and sinus congestion
Diuretic	(DYE uh RET ik)	Increases urinary output and lowers blood pressure
Electrolyte	(ih LEK troh lite)	Maintains normal electrolyte level and proper functioning of the body systems
Erectile dysfunction agent	(ee REK tile)	Facilitates an erection
Expectorant	(ik SPEK tohr ahnt)	Thins bronchial secretions, making it easier to cough up the mucus
Hematopoietic	(HEE mah toe poi EE tik)	Promotes blood cell production
Hemostatic	(HEE moh STAT ik)	Clots blood
Hormone replacement	(HOHR mone)	Replaces hormones or compensates for hormone deficiencies
Laxative	(LAK sah tiv)	Promotes stools
Leukotriene receptor antagonist	(LOO koh TRY een, an TAG ah nist)	Blocks the action of substances that cause asthma and allergic rhinitis
Miotic	(mye OT ik)	Drains excessive fluid from the eye; used for glaucoma
Muscle relaxant	(re LAK sahnt)	Reduces pain
Mydriatic	(MID ree at ik)	Dilates the pupil; used for ophthalmic procedures
Osteoporosis agent	(OS tee oh poh roe sis)	Promotes bone mineral density; used to treat osteoporosis
Proton-pump inhibitor	(PROE ton, in HIB i tohr)	Reduces the acid produced in the stomach
Sedative-hypnotic	(SED ah tiv, hip NOT ik)	Slows brain activity, allowing sleep
Stimulant	(STIM yuh lahnt)	Stimulates the brain and body, makes the person more alert
Tumor necrosis factor (TNF) inhibitor	(neh KROE sis)	Blocks the action of TNF, preventing inflammation in autoimmune disorders

Drug Terminology

Regardless of how drug reference information is obtained, it is important for the medical assistant to understand the terminology. The following terminology is typically found in drug reference information.

- *Names*: Usually the generic name is listed with the trade names. Some references may indicate if the trade name found is in the United States or Canada.
- *Description*: Describes the medication and its general use.
- *Boxed warning*: Also referred to as a *black box warning*. It addresses serious or life-threatening risks. This information also appears on the drug's label.
- *Dosage*: Specifies the route, dose, and timing of the medication; usually corresponds to an indication (disease or condition). May provide information on doses for different age ranges. *Maximum dosage* indicates the greatest amount of medication a person should have within a 24-hour period.
- *Indications*: Conditions or diseases for which the drug is used.
- *Dosage considerations*: Indicates recommended changes in dosages for special populations (e.g., patients with hepatic impairment, renal impairment).
- *How supplied*: Lists the form (e.g., chewable tablets, capsules) and the strength (e.g., 250 mg)

- *Administration*: Provides information on how the medication should be administered. Includes important administration techniques, such as information on shaking the medication, if it needs to be taken with food, and so on.
- *Action*: How the drug provides therapeutic results in the body, or the use of the drug.
- *Adverse reactions*: Also called *side effects* in some information. This section describes known undesirable experiences associated with the medication. Reactions may be divided into severe (life-threatening, serious reactions), moderate, and mild.
- *Interactions*: Includes medications, foods, and beverages that interact with the medication. These products may either increase or reduce the medication level in the blood. They may also increase the risk of adverse reactions if taken together with the drug.
- *Contraindications* (KON trah IN di KAY shuns): Reasons or conditions that make administration of the drug improper or undesirable. For example, aspirin is contraindicated in patients with GI bleeding.
- *Precautions*: Indicates necessary actions or special care that needs to be taken when the patient is on the medication. May include information on laboratory tests, special populations (children and geriatric), pregnancy, breastfeeding, and so on. (More information will be discussed in the following section.)

- *Pharmacokinetics*: Provides information on the absorption, distribution, metabolism, and excretion of the medication. Information on when the drug is at its highest level in the body or when the drug starts working may be included. Important terms for understanding the pharmacokinetics of a drug include:
  - *Biological half-life*: The time it takes half of the drug to be metabolized or eliminated by normal biological processes.
  - *Onset*: The time it takes for the drug to produce a response.

- *Peak*: The time it takes for the drug to reach its greatest effective concentration in the blood.
- *Duration*: The time during which the drug is present in the blood at great enough levels to produce a response.

Table 44.4 provides drug information on the top commonly prescribed medications. Please use drug reference information for additional information on these products.

> **VOCABULARY**
>
> **form** The physical characteristics of a medication (e.g., tablet, suspension).

TABLE 44.4 Information on Commonly Prescribed Medications

Generic Name	Brand/Trade Name(s)	Class/Schedule	Medication Information
tamsulosin (tam SOO loe sin)	Flomax (FLOW maks)	Alpha blocker	*Indication:* Benign prostatic hyperplasia (BPH) *Desired effects/action:* Relaxes prostate and bladder muscles *Side effects:* Diarrhea, back pain, weakness, sleepiness, facial pain *Adverse reactions:* Painful erection lasting for hours, rash, itching, hives
hydrocodone/ acetaminophen (APAP) (hye droe KOE done, a set a MEE noe fen)	Vicodin (vye KOE din) Norco (NOHR koe) Lortab (LORE tab)	Analgesics (narcotic [opioids])/Schedule 2	*Indication:* Moderate to severe pain *Desired effects/action:* Changes the way the brain and nervous system respond to pain *Side effects:* Gastrointestinal (GI) intolerance, difficulty urinating, anxiety, fuzzy thinking *Adverse reactions:* Slowed breathing, chest tightness
oxycodone (ox i KOE done)	OxyContin (ox i KON tin)	Analgesics (narcotic [opioids])/Schedule 2	*Indication:* Moderate to severe pain *Desired effects/action:* Changes the way the brain and nervous system respond to pain *Side effects:* GI intolerance, flushing, headache, mood changes *Adverse reactions:* Slowed breathing, angina, hypersensitivity, seizures
tramadol (TRAH mah dole)	Conzip (KON zip)	Analgesics (narcotic [opioids])/Schedule 2	*Indication:* Moderate to severe pain *Desired effects/action:* Changes the way the brain and nervous system respond to pain *Side effects:* GI intolerance, insomnia, change in mood, dry mouth *Adverse reactions:* Hallucination, agitation, hypersensitivity, arrhythmias
alprazolam (al PRAY zoe lam)	Xanax (ZAN aks)	Antianxiety (benzodiazepines)/ Schedule 4	*Indications:* Anxiety and panic disorders *Desired effects/action:* Reduces abnormal excitement in the brain *Side effects:* Drowsiness, headache, dizziness, GI intolerance, dry mouth, weight changes *Adverse reactions:* Seizures, jaundice, depression, memory problems
clonazepam (kloe NA ze pam)	Klonopin (CLON uhh pin)	Antianxiety (benzodiazepines)/ Schedule 4	*Indications:* Seizures, panic attacks *Desired effects/action:* Reduces abnormal excitement in the brain *Side effects:* Drowsiness, coordination problems, joint pain, blurred vision, changes in sex drive *Adverse reaction:* Hypersensitivity
amoxicillin (ah mox i SIL in)	Amoxil (ah MUHHS il) Moxtag (MUHHS tag)	Antibiotics (Penicillin)	*Indication:* Bacterial infection (e.g., pneumonia, gonorrhea, ear, and throat) *Desired effects/action:* Stops bacterial growth *Side effect:* GI intolerance *Adverse reactions:* Hypersensitivity, seizures, jaundice
warfarin (WAR far in)	Coumadin (COU mah din) Jantoven (JAN to ven)	Anticoagulants	*Indication:* Prevents blood clots from forming *Desired effects/action:* Reduces clotting ability of the blood *Side effects:* GI intolerance, loss of hair, chills *Adverse reactions:* Hypersensitivity, infection, angina, jaundice, bleeding
gabapentin (GAH bah pen tin)	Neurontin (NOOR on tin) Horizant (huhh RI zant)	Anticonvulsants	*Indications:* Seizures, postherpetic neuralgia, restless legs syndrome (RLS) *Desired effects/action:* Reduces abnormal excitement in the brain; reduces seizures *Side effects:* Drowsiness, blurred vision, anxiety, memory problems, weakness, GI intolerance *Adverse reactions:* Hypersensitivity, seizures

Continued

TABLE 44.4   Information on Commonly Prescribed Medications—cont'd

Generic Name	Brand/Trade Name(s)	Class/Schedule	Medication Information
buropion (byoo PROE pee on)	Wellbutrin (Wel buo trin) Zyban (ZIE ban)	Antidepressant (atypical) and antismoking agent	*Indications:* Depression, seasonal affective disorder (SAD), smoking cessation *Desired effects/action:* Increases certain types of activity in the brain *Side effects:* Drowsiness, insomnia, dry mouth, stomach pain, weight loss *Adverse reactions:* Blisters, dyspnea, chest pain, seizures, hallucinations
duloxetine (doo LOX e teen)	Cymbalta (sim-BAL tuh)	Antidepressant (selective serotonin and norepinephrine reuptake inhibitors [SNRIs])	*Indications:* Major depressive disorder, generalized anxiety disorder, diabetic peripheral neuropathy, fibromyalgia, chronic pain *Desired effects/action:* Increases the amounts of serotonin and norepinephrine in the brain; helps to maintain mental balance and stop pain signals in the brain *Side effect:* Orthostatic hypotension *Adverse reactions:* Suicidal thoughts, hepatotoxicity, seizures, glaucoma, hyponatremia
venlafaxine (VEN la fax een)	(no brand names)	Antidepressant (selective serotonin and norepinephrine reuptake inhibitors [SNRIs])	*Indications:* Depression, generalized anxiety disorder (GAD), social anxiety disorder, panic disorder *Desired effects/action:* Increases serotonin in the brain *Side effects:* Drowsiness, weakness, headache, nightmares, dry mouth *Adverse reactions:* Chest pain, seizures, arrhythmias, bleeding, problems with coordination
citalopram (sye TAL oh pram)	Celexa (seh LEK suh)	Antidepressant (selective serotonin reuptake inhibitors [SSRIs])	*Indication:* Depression *Desired effects/action:* Increases the amount of serotonin in the brain; helps to maintain mental balance *Side effects:* GI intolerance, frequent urination, weakness, joint pain, weight loss *Adverse reactions:* Angina, shortness of breath, arrhythmias, hallucinating, coma, hypersensitivity, confusion, seizures, suicidal thoughts
escitalopram (es sye TAL oh pram)	Lexapro (LEK suh proh)	Antidepressant (selective serotonin reuptake inhibitors [SSRIs])	*Indications:* Depression, generalized anxiety disorder (GAD) *Desired effects/action:* Increases the amount of serotonin in the brain; helps to maintain mental balance *Side effects:* GI intolerance, increased sweating, change in sex drive, flulike symptoms *Adverse reactions:* Unusual excitement, hallucinations, confusion, arrhythmias, severe muscle stiffness, suicidal thoughts
fluoxetine (floo OX eh teen)	Prozac (PROW zak) Rapiflux (RAP i fluks)	Antidepressant (selective serotonin reuptake inhibitors [SSRIs])	*Indications:* Depression, obsessive-compulsive disorder (OCD), panic attacks *Desired effects/action:* Increases serotonin in the brain *Side effects:* Nervousness, anxiety, insomnia, diarrhea, heartburn *Adverse reactions:* Joint pain, dyspnea, seizures, abnormal bleeding
sertraline (SER tra leen)	Zoloft (ZOH loft)	Antidepressant (selective serotonin reuptake inhibitors [SSRIs])	*Indications:* Depression, OCD, panic attacks, posttraumatic stress disorder (PTSD) *Desired effects/action:* Increases the amount of serotonin in the brain; helps to maintain mental balance *Side effects:* GI intolerance, weight changes, insomnia, change in sex drive, excessive sweating *Adverse reactions:* Seizures, abnormal bleeding, arrhythmias, hypersensitivity, suicidal thoughts
trazodone (TRAZ oh done)	Oleptro (oh LEP troh)	Antidepressant (serotonin modulators)	*Indication:* Depression *Desired effects/action:* Increases the amount of serotonin; helps to maintain mental balance *Side effects:* GI intolerance, weakness, headache, confusion, sweating, decreased coordination *Adverse reactions:* Angina, fainting, seizures, coma, arrhythmias, suicidal thoughts
allopurinol (al oh PURE i nole)	Aloprim (AH low prim) Zyloprim (ZIE low prim)	Antigout (xanthine oxidase inhibitors)	*Indication:* Gout *Desired effects/action:* Reduces uric acid production *Side effects:* Upset stomach, diarrhea, drowsiness *Adverse reactions:* Dysuria, eye irritation, hematuria
glipizide (GLIP i zide)	Glucotrol (GLOO koe trohl)	Antihyperglycemics	*Indication:* Type 2 diabetes mellitus *Desired effects/action:* Lowers blood glucose by causing increased insulin production and usage *Side effects:* Flatus, diarrhea, dizziness, shaking, feeling jittery *Adverse reactions:* Jaundice, dark urine, light-colored stools, bleeding

TABLE 44.4 Information on Commonly Prescribed Medications—cont'd

Generic Name	Brand/Trade Name(s)	Class/Schedule	Medication Information
metformin (met FOR min)	Glucophage (gloo koe FAJE) Fortamet (for TAY met) Glumetza (gloo MET zah) Riomet (REE oh met)	Antihyperglycemics	*Indication:* Type 2 diabetes mellitus *Desired effects/action:* Reduces glucose absorption and increases body's response to insulin; controls the blood glucose level *Side effects:* GI intolerance, metallic taste in the mouth, flushing of the skin, nail changes *Adverse reactions:* Angina, rash
losartan (low SAR tan)	Cozaar (KOH zahr)	Antihypertensive (angiotensin II receptor antagonists)	*Indications:* Hypertension, heart failure *Desired effects/action:* Lowers the blood pressure *Side effects:* Headache, dizziness, diarrhea, muscle cramps and pain, nasal congestion, cough, upper respiratory infection, sinusitis *Adverse reactions:* Chest pain, difficulty swallowing, dyspnea, hoarseness
lisinopril (lyse IN oh pril)	(no brand names)	Antihypertensive (angiotensin-converting enzyme [ACE] inhibitors)	*Indications:* Hypertension, heart failure *Desired effects/action:* Causes vasodilation, reducing the blood pressure *Side effects:* Cough, dizziness, tiredness, GI intolerance, rash *Adverse reactions:* Angina, light-headedness, dyspnea, difficulty swallowing, hypersensitivity
atenolol (ah TEN oh lole)	Tenormin (TEN ore min)	Antihypertensive (beta-blockers)	*Indications:* Hypertension, angina *Desired effects/action:* Relaxes blood vessels and slows the heart rate, thus improving blood flow, and reduces blood pressure *Side effects:* Dizziness, tiredness, depression, GI intolerance *Adverse reactions:* Shortness of breath, swelling of legs and hands, weight gain, fainting
metoprolol (me TOE proe lole)	Lopressor (low PRES sohr) Toprol XL (TOE prohl)	Antihypertensive (beta-blockers)	*Indications:* Hypertension, angina *Desired effects/action:* Relaxes blood vessels and slows the heart rate, thus improving blood flow, and reduces blood pressure *Side effects:* Dizziness, tiredness, depression, GI intolerance *Adverse reactions:* Hypersensitivity, weight gain, arrhythmias
carvedilol (KAR ve dil ol)	Coreg (CORE ehg)	Antihypertensive (beta-blockers)	*Indications:* Heart failure, hypertension *Desired effects/action:* Relaxes blood vessels and slows the heart rate, thus improving blood flow, and reduces blood pressure *Side effects:* Hyperglycemia, tiredness, weakness, dizziness, visual changes, joint pain, insomnia *Adverse reactions:* Shortness of breath, swelling of arms and legs, arrhythmias
propranolol (proe PRAN oh lole)	Inderal LA, Inderal XL (in DER ahl)	Antihypertensive (beta-blockers)	*Indications:* Hypertension, arrhythmias *Desired effects/action:* Relaxes blood vessels, slows heart rate *Side effects:* Dizziness, light-headedness, tiredness, diarrhea, constipation *Adverse reactions:* Weight gain, arrhythmias, feeling faint, swelling of face and throat
amlodipine (am LOE di peen)	Norvasc (NOR vask)	Antihypertensive (calcium channel blockers)	*Indications:* Hypertension, angina *Desired effects/action:* Relaxes the vessels so the heart does not have to pump as hard *Side effects:* GI intolerance, headache, swelling of legs and arms, tiredness, flushing *Adverse reactions:* More frequent or severe angina, fainting, arrhythmias
meloxicam (mel OX i cam)	Mobic (MOW bik)	Anti-inflammatories (nonsteroidal anti-inflammatory drugs [NSAIDs])	*Indications:* Osteoarthritis, rheumatoid arthritis *Desired effects/action:* Reduces pain, tenderness, swelling, and stiffness *Side effects:* Diarrhea, constipation, flatus, sore throat *Adverse reactions:* Dyspnea, hives, blisters, tachycardia, jaundice
clopidogrel (kloh PID oh grel)	Plavix (PLAH viks)	Antiplatelets	*Indication:* Used to prevent clots after a stroke, heart attack, or severe angina *Desired effects/action:* Prevents platelets from collecting and forming clots *Side effects:* Excessive tiredness, GI intolerance, nosebleed, dizziness *Adverse reaction:* Hypersensitivity, bloody and tarry stools, coffee grounds–looking emesis, blood in urine, visual changes

Continued

TABLE 44.4 Information on Commonly Prescribed Medications—cont'd

Generic Name	Brand/Trade Name(s)	Class/Schedule	Medication Information
albuterol (al BYOO ter ole)	Ventolin HFA (ven TOE lin) Proventil HFA (PRO ven til) Proair (PRO air)	Bronchodilators	Indication: Bronchospasm (e.g., asthma) Desired effects/action: Relaxes bronchial muscles and increases airflow to lungs Side effects: Headache, dizziness, insomnia, cough, sort throat, nausea, vomiting, dry mouth Adverse reactions: Paradoxic bronchospasm, cardiovascular effects, hypersensitivity, hypokalemia
atorvastatin (a TORE va sta tin)	Lipitor (LIP ih tore)	Cholesterol-lowering agent	Indications: Hyperlipidemia, hypertriglyceridemia Desired effects/action: Slows production of cholesterol in the body; reduces low-density lipoprotein (LDL) and triglycerides; increases high-density lipoprotein (HDL) Side effects: GI intolerance, joint pain, memory loss, confusion Adverse reactions: Muscle pain, lack of energy, angina, weakness, hypersensitivity, dark-colored urine, jaundice
pravastatin (PRAH vah stat in)	Pravachol (PRAV ah kahl)	Cholesterol-lowering agent	Indications: Heart disease, hyperlipidemia, hypertriglyceridemia Desired effects/action: Slows cholesterol production Side effects: Heartburn, headache, memory loss, confusion Adverse reactions: Jaundice, extreme tiredness, dark-colored urine, unusual bleeding
rosuvastatin (roe soo vah STAT in)	Crestor (CRESS tor) Ezallor (EZ ah lor)	Cholesterol-lowering agent	Indications: Hyperlipidemia, hypertriglyceridemia Desired effects/action: Slows production of cholesterol in the body; reduces LDL and triglycerides; increases HDL Side effects: Headache, depression, muscle and joint pain, insomnia, GI intolerance Adverse reactions: Muscle damage leading to acute renal failure and liver damage
simvastatin (SIM va stat in)	Zocor (ZOE kore) Flolipid (Flow lip id)	Cholesterol-lowering agent	Indications: Hyperlipidemia, hypertriglyceridemia Desired effects/action: Slows production of cholesterol in the body; reduces LDL and triglycerides; increases HDL Side effects: GI intolerance, memory loss, confusion, headache Adverse reactions: Muscle pain, dark red urine, lack of energy, jaundice, hypersensitivity
ethinyl estradiol and norethindrone (ETH in il) (es tra DYE ole) (nor eth IN drone)	Loestrin (low ES trin) Leena (LEE nah) Microgestin (my kroe JES tin)	Contraceptive (oral)	Indication: Prevent pregnancy Desired effects/action: Estrogen and progestin prevent ovulation and pregnancy from developing Side effects: Headache, bloating, swelling, weight changes, breast tenderness Adverse reactions: Severe abdominal pain, dark urine, jaundice, heavy vaginal bleeding
fluticasone (floo TIK a sone)	Flonase allergy relief nasal spray (FLOW nase) Flovent HFA (FLOW vent) Flovent Diskus (FLOW vent DISK us)	Corticosteroid (nasal and inhaled)	Indications: Hay fever, allergies (nasal spray); asthma (inhaled) Desired effects/action: Reduces inflammation and allergy reaction Side effects: Headache, dryness in mouth, hoarseness or deepened voice Adverse reactions: Reduced bone marrow density, immunosuppression, adrenal suppression, glaucoma, cataracts, hypersensitivity in individuals with milk allergy (Diskus)
prednisone (PRED ni sone)	Sterapred (STER ah pred)	Corticosteroids (oral)	Indications: Severe allergic reaction, multiple sclerosis, lupus, and some types of arthritis Desired effects/action: Increases the levels of corticosteroid; reduces swelling and redness Side effects: Headache, dizziness, insomnia, personality and mood changes, slowed healing Adverse reactions: Vision problems, seizures, arrhythmias, confusion
furosemide (fyoor OH se mide)	Lasix (LAY siks)	Diuretics	Indication: Hypertension Desired effects/action: Causes the kidneys to increase the excretion of water and salt Side effects: Frequent urination, blurred vision, headache, constipation, diarrhea Adverse reactions: Ringing in the ears, loss of hearing, blisters, jaundice, hypersensitivity
hydrochlorothiazide (HCT) (hye droe klor oh THYE a zide)	Microzide (MYE kroe zide) Oretic (ORE eh tik)	Diuretics	Indication: Hypertension Desired effects/action: Causes the kidneys to increase the excretion of water and salt Side effects: Frequent urination, diarrhea, loss of appetite, headache, hair loss Adverse reactions: Joint pain, unusual bleeding, hypersensitivity, visual change

TABLE 44.4   Information on Commonly Prescribed Medications—cont'd

Generic Name	Brand/Trade Name(s)	Class/Schedule	Medication Information
potassium (poe TASS i um)	K-Tab (KAY tab) K-Dur (KAY duhr) Micro-K (MYE krow kay)	Electrolyte	*Indication:* Mineral supplement needed for certain diseases and medications (e.g., diuretic) *Desired effects/action:* Proper functioning of the body systems *Side effect:* GI intolerance *Adverse reactions:* Confusion, listlessness, gray skin, black stools
insulin glargine (IN su lin) (GLAR geen)	Lantus (LAN tus) Toujeo (to JAY oh)	Hormone replacement (insulin, long acting)	*Indications:* Type 1 and Type 2 diabetes mellitus *Desired effects/action:* Replaces insulin in the body *Side effects:* Redness and swelling at injection site, fever, cough, sore throat *Adverse reactions:* Tachycardia, hoarseness, sweating, wheezing
levothyroxine (lee voe thye ROX een)	Synthroid (SIN throid) Levoxyl (LEV ok sil)	Hormone replacement (thyroid hormone)	*Indications:* Hypothyroidism, pituitary thyroid-stimulating hormone (TSH) suppression *Desired effects/action:* Replacement hormone; regulates body's energy and metabolism *Side effects:* Reversible hair loss, dry skin, GI intolerance, headache, nervousness *Adverse reactions:* Cardiac arrhythmias, angina, myocardial infarction, heart failure
montelukast (mon te LOO kast)	Singulair (SING u lair)	Leukotriene receptor antagonists	*Indications:* Asthma, exercise-induced bronchospasms *Desired effects/action:* Blocks the action of substances that cause asthma and allergic rhinitis *Side effects:* Headache, dizziness, heartburn, stomach pain, tiredness *Adverse reactions:* Hypersensitivity, numbness in arms and legs, swelling of the sinuses
cyclobenzaprine (sye kloe BEN za preen)	Amrix (AM riks)	Muscle relaxant	*Indications:* Painful musculoskeletal conditions (e.g., strains, sprains, muscle injuries) *Desired effects/action:* Works on the brain and nervous system to allow muscle relaxation *Side effects:* GI intolerance, extreme tiredness, dry mouth *Adverse reactions:* Hypersensitivity, angina
omeprazole (oh MEE pray zol)	Prilosec (PRY low sek)	Proton-pump inhibitors	*Indications:* Gastroesophageal reflux disease (GERD), ulcers, *Helicobacter pylori (H. pylori)* infection *Desired effects/action:* Reduces stomach acid *Side effects:* GI intolerance, headache *Adverse reactions:* Hypersensitivity, dizziness, arrhythmias, muscle spasm
pantoprazole (pan TOE pra zole)	Protonix (pro TON iks)	Proton-pump inhibitors	*Indications:* GERD and esophagitis *Desired effects/action:* Reduces the amount of acid made in the stomach *Side effects:* Headache, nausea, vomiting, flatus, joint pain, diarrhea, dizziness *Adverse reactions:* Blistering, hives, dyspnea, difficulty swallowing, severe diarrhea
zolpidem (ZOL pi dem)	Ambien (am bee ehn) Edluar (ED loo ahr) Zolpimist (ZOL pi mist)	Sedative-hypnotics/ Schedule 4	*Indication:* Insomnia *Desired effects/action:* Slows activity in the brain, allowing sleep *Side effects:* Drowsiness, headache, dizziness, drugged feeling, unsteady walking, GI intolerance *Adverse reactions:* Jaundice, hypersensitivity, light-colored stools, angina, blurred vision
dextroamphetamine and amphetamine (dex troe am FET ah meen) (am FET ah meen)	Adderall (ADD er ahl)	Stimulants/Schedule 2	*Indications:* Attention deficit hyperactivity disorder (ADHD), narcolepsy *Desired effects/action:* Changes the amount of certain substances in the brain *Side effects:* Stomach pain, nausea, tachycardia, insomnia, weight loss *Adverse reactions:* Agitation, hallucination, mania, blurred vision, depression
methylphenidate (meth il FEN i date)	Concerta (con SERT ah) Ritalin LA (RIT ah lin el aye)	Stimulants/Schedule 2	*Indications:* ADHD, narcolepsy *Desired effects/action:* Changes certain substances in the brain, allowing a person to concentrate and focus *Side effects:* Nervousness, insomnia, GI intolerance, restlessness, muscle tightness *Adverse reactions:* Angina, arrhythmias, seizure, blurred vision
ergocalciferol (er goe kal SIF er ol)	Drisdol (DRIS dohl) Vitamin D2	Vitamin D	*Indication:* Hypoparathyroidism *Desired effects/action:* Helps the body use more calcium found in foods or supplements *Side effects:* Pale skin, tiredness *Adverse reactions:* Feeling tired, drowsiness, muscle aches, stiffness

Pregnancy and Lactation Labeling Rule. Since 1979 the Food and Drug Administration (FDA) has enforced the use of pregnancy risk categories. The A, B, C, D, and X categories indicate the risk to the baby in utero. In 2015 the Pregnancy and Lactation Labeling Rule (PLLR) replaced the pregnancy risk letter categories with more comprehensive information. The goal is to provide the provider and patient with pregnancy and lactation information. This information can be used when discussing the risks versus the benefits of a medication. The FDA created the new system to help with patient-specific counseling and informed decision making for pregnant and breastfeeding mothers who need medication therapies. The system consists of three subcategories with detailed information about the following:

- *Pregnancy*: Includes information on the risks during pregnancy for the mother and baby, in addition to data on the risk of adverse developmental outcomes.
- *Lactation*: Includes information on the presence of the drug in breast milk, the effects on a breast-fed child, and the impact on milk production.
- *Females and males of reproductive potential*: Includes information about when pregnancy testing or contraception is required during drug therapy and data that suggests drug-associated fertility effects.

FORMS OF MEDICATIONS

The form is the physical characteristics of the medication. Forms can be grouped into solids, semisolids, and liquids. Solid and semisolid medications are commonly prescribed and found in OTC products.

Solid Medication Forms

Examples of solid medication forms include the following:
- *Tablet*: Solid formed by compressed powdered medication; may be coated. Can come in various sizes and shapes (Fig. 44.1).
- *Chewable tablet*: Designed to be chewed prior to swallowing. Example: A chewable vitamin.
- *Caplet* (KAP lit): Coated, oval medication tablet.
- *Capsule* (KAP sul): Medication in a hard or soft gelatin shell.
- *Scored tablet*: A notched tablet, which can be split into half with a pill cutter or splitter (Fig. 44.2).
- *Enteric* (en TER ik) *coated tablets* or *capsules*: Coated to pass through the acidic environment of the stomach. Breaks down in the base environment of the intestines. These tablets should not be crushed, cut, or chewed because the protective property will be lost.
- *Buffered*: A solid medication containing the active medication and an antacid. The antacid neutralizes the stomach acid and thereby reduces stomach irritation. Example: Buffered aspirin.

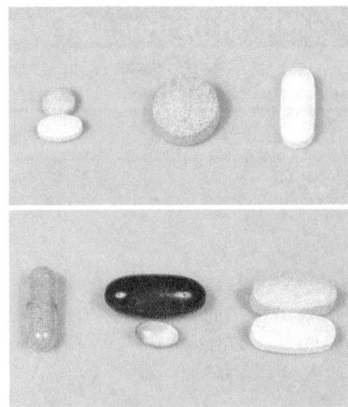

Fig. 44.1 *Left to right: Top row,* Tablets, chewable, and caplet. *Bottom row,* Hard-shelled capsule, soft-shelled capsules, and scored caplets.

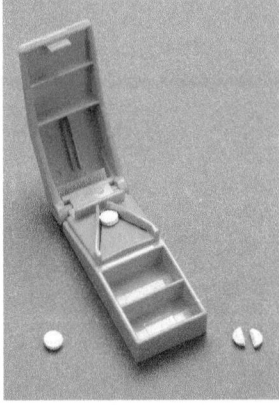

Fig. 44.2 Pill Cutter or Splitter. (From Niedzwiecki B, et al: *Kinn's the medical assistant,* ed 14, St. Louis, 2020, Elsevier.)

- *Fast-dissolving tablet* or *film strip*: Also called *oral disintegrating tablets.* Solid form of medicine that is placed on the tongue (or by the cheek [buccal]) and breaks down rapidly in the presence of saliva. Examples: Fasprin and acetaminophen.
- *Extended release tablet* or *capsule*: Designed to break down over time. These tablets should not be crushed, cut, or chewed because doing so may cause an overdose. Many acronyms are used (Box 44.3). Example: Calan SR.
- *Effervescent tablet*: Contains an acid substance and carbonate or bicarbonate. When placed in water, it releases carbon dioxide, creating a carbonated drink. Example: K-Lyte Effervescent Tablets.
- *Lozenge* (LOZ enj) (*troche* [TROE kee]): Flat, round form containing active medication and a sweetened flavoring; dissolves on the tongue. Used for local treatment of the mouth and throat. Example: Cough drop.
- *Powder*: Nonpotent powdered medication that must be mixed with a liquid before it can be taken. Example: Mira-LAX.

Some forms of medications can be crushed, whereas others cannot. Over the past few years, the FDA has approved new drug delivery systems or drug forms. This has provided additional options to those who cannot swallow pills. It is common for patients or parents to have concerns about swallowing pills.

BOX 44.4 Alcohol in Medications

Several forms of liquid medications contain alcohol. This is a concern for patients who are recovering alcoholics or have other health issues, such as diabetes. An internet search can provide lists of medications with their alcohol content. The drug reference information also provides information on the ingredients.

If patients mention that they are a recovering alcoholic, it is important for the medical assistant first to acknowledge the person's accomplishment. Then the medical assistant should communicate the information to the provider. This may make a difference in what medication the provider gives to the patient. Giving a patient a medication with alcohol may be harmful to the patient's success and health.

CRITICAL THINKING 44.6

What is an advantage of the fast-dissolving tablet or film strip? For what populations would this form be beneficial?

Semisolid Medication Forms

Examples of semisolid medication forms include:
- *Ointment* and *paste*: Semisolid, greasy drug preparations that are applied to the skin, rectum, or nasal mucosa. Pastes are thicker and less penetrating than ointments. Example: Nystatin Ointment.
- *Cream*: Semisolid drug preparation made of active medication, oil, and water. Example: Nystatin Cream.
- *Suppository* (su POZ i tore ee) and *pessary* (PES ah ree): Active medication mixed in an oil base (e.g., cocoa butter). Solid at room temperature but melts at body temperature. Suppositories are typically shaped like a small bullet and used in the rectum, urethra, or vagina. Pessaries are vaginal suppositories. Example: Dulcolax suppository.

Liquid Medication Forms

Liquid medications have various uses. They can be swallowed, rubbed on the skin, or instilled in the nose, eyes, or ears. Liquid medications are easily taken by children, older adults, and those with swallowing problems. With liquid medications, the active medication is mixed with water, alcohol, or both (Box 44.4).

If the active medication dissolves in the liquid, the medication is a *solution*. The following are examples of solutions:
- *Tincture* (TINGK chur): Very potent solution of alcohol or alcohol and water and the active medicine. Example: Iodine tincture.
- *Fluid extract*: Alcoholic plant source extractions; very concentrated and more potent than tinctures. Example: Belladonna fluid extract.
- *Spirit*: An alcoholic solution with substances that easily evaporate. Example: Aromatic ammonia spirit.
- *Elixir* (ee LIK sir): Clear sweetened liquid preparation that contains alcohol. Example: Digoxin elixir.
- *Syrup*: A sugar and water solution that contains flavoring and medicinal substance. Example: Cough syrup (some syrups contain alcohol).

If the active medication does not dissolve and becomes suspended in the liquid, it is called a *suspension*. Over time the suspended drug will settle to the bottom of the container. It is important to shake suspensions before pouring the medication. The following are examples of suspensions:
- *Emulsion* (ee MUL shun): A suspension of oil and water. Example: Ophthalmic cyclosporine.
- *Gel* and *magma* (MAG mah): Suspensions consisting of minerals and water. Gels are semisolids and contain finer particles than magmas. The minerals settle out with standing. Shake before using. Example: Milk of magnesia.
- *Liniment* (LIN uh mehnt): A suspension that is rubbed on the skin; used to reduce pain and stiffness. Example: Ben-Gay.
- *Lotion*: A water-based suspension that is applied to the skin. Example: Calamine lotion.
- *Aerosol* (ahr ah SOL): A suspension of medication in a gas, usually used for respiratory or sinus conditions. Example: Albuterol metered-dose inhaler.

CRITICAL THINKING 44.7

What forms of medication would not be helpful to people who are recovering from alcoholism?

TYPES OF MEDICATION ORDERS

A *medication order* refers to directions given by a provider for a specific medication to be administered to a patient. The medical assistant receives the information from the provider. The provider must give:
- Patient's name and health record number or date of birth (DOB) (e.g., Nancy Rodriguez DOB 11/04/1971)
- Medication name, dose, and route (e.g., Tylenol 1 g po)

The provider can give the order over the phone or in person. This type of order is called a *verbal order*. It is important for the medical assistant to write down the order and read it back to the provider. This process ensures the order was heard and recorded correctly. The provider can also give the medical assistant a *written order*. Usually, these are written on a prescription pad or in an electronic message. A written order only needs clarification from the provider if the medical assistant cannot read the order or has a question.

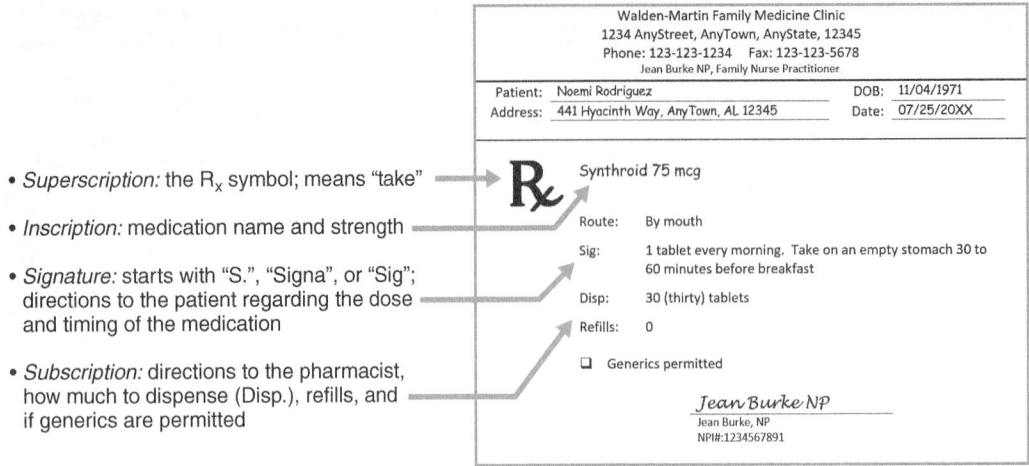

- *Superscription:* the R$_x$ symbol; means "take"
- *Inscription:* medication name and strength
- *Signature:* starts with "S.", "Signa", or "Sig"; directions to the patient regarding the dose and timing of the medication
- *Subscription:* directions to the pharmacist, how much to dispense (Disp.), refills, and if generics are permitted

Fig. 44.3 Parts of a Prescription.

In addition to describing how medication orders are given to the medical assistant, they can be described by the type of order. The following are five types of medication orders.

- *Routine order:* Medication taken at a regular interval until it is canceled or expired. (Most non-narcotic routine orders expire in 12 months.) Examples: "Vitamin B$_{12}$ 100 mcg IM monthly" and "Synthroid 75 mcg qam po."
- *Standing order:* Order applies to all patients who meet specific criteria. For departments, usually all providers agree collectively on standing orders and sign the order. Example: "For patients 18 years or older, with no allergy to acetaminophen and who have a temperature of 103°F or higher: give acetaminophen 650 mg po × 1 dose."
- *PRN order:* Medication that is given on an "as needed" basis for specific signs and symptoms. (It is important to indicate these symptoms when documenting the administered medication in the patient's health record.) Example: "Acetaminophen 325 mg, 2 tabs po q4–6h prn pain."
- *Single order* or *one-time order:* Medication is administered one time. Example: "Acetaminophen 650 mg po × 1 dose."
- *Stat order:* Medication is administered one time right now. Example: "EpiPen 0.3 mg IM stat."

Prescriptions

A *prescription* is a written order by a provider to the pharmacist. It tells the pharmacist what medication and how much should be dispensed to the patient. There are four parts to a prescription: superscription, inscription, signature, and subscription. Fig. 44.3 describes the four parts of a prescription.

Medical Assistant's Role. In some ambulatory care facilities, medical assistants prepare prescriptions for providers to sign. Some such scenarios may include:

- A patient may request refills while the medical assistant is rooming the patient. The medical assistant may prepare the prescriptions, so the provider just needs to sign for the refills.
- A patient may call the department and request a refill on a medication. Using a medication refill protocol,

the medical assistant needs to see if the patient can get a refill (Fig. 44.4). If the patient can, then the medical assistant prepares the prescription and has the provider sign it.

The prescription must be written in ink or be computer generated. A medical assistant can prepare prescriptions for the provider to sign. The provider is responsible for ensuring the prescription meets federal and state laws and regulations. All prescriptions need to include:

- Date of issue (when it was written)
- Patient information (name and address are required; date of birth is helpful)
- Provider's full name and address
- Drug name (e.g., amoxicillin)
- Drug strength (e.g., 500 mg)
- Dosage form (e.g., tablets)
- Quantity prescribed (e.g., 14 [fourteen]) – writing out the number prevents people from altering the prescription. This is especially important with controlled substances.
- Directions for use (e.g., Take 1 tablet q12h)
- Number of refills (e.g., Refills 0)
- National Provider Identifier (NPI) and signature of provider (a manual signature is required for controlled substances)
- Indicate if a generic is acceptable

> **VOCABULARY**
> **National Provider Identifier (NPI)** An identifier assigned by the Centers for Medicare and Medicaid Services (CMS) that classifies the healthcare provider by license and medical specialties.

If an electronic prescription is sent to the pharmacy and a paper copy is given to the patient, the copy should indicate that it is a copy ("Copy only – not valid for dispensing"). Procedure 44.1 indicates how to prepare prescriptions using a prescription refill procedure. Only facility-approved abbreviations should be used when preparing prescriptions and documenting in

Prescription Refill Protocol
Walden-Martin Family Medicine Clinic

Description: A Certified Medical Assistant (CMA) can refill current hypertensive medications that fall within the guidelines of this protocol.

Step 1	Step 2	
For medications to be refilled, the following points need to be addressed.	**Qualifying Medications**	**Prescription Refill**
• Has the person seen the provider within the last year? • Is the prescription for a hypertensive, hyperlipidemia, or hyperthyroidism medication a current prescription? • Is the person free of concerns or complications due to the medication? • Is it time for a refill? (The medical assistant must verify that it is time for a refill.) If the answers to the above questions are all YES, then proceed to Step 2. If any of the answers to the above questions are NO, then schedule the person for an appointment with the provider	amlodipine amlodipine/benazepril atenolol atenolol/Chlorthalidone benazepril captopril diltiazem enalapril felodipine fosinopril irbesartan isradipine lisinopril losartan nifedipine quinapril ramipril	Extend the current prescription for 6 months. Instruct patient that in 6 months: • A visit to the provider will be required • Blood pressure reading will be required • Lab work may be required

Fig. 44.4 Example of a Prescription Refill Protocol. The medical assistant uses a protocol to determine what action to take with prescription refill requests.

TABLE 44.5 Abbreviations Related Medications

Abbreviations Related to:	Abbreviations	Meaning	Abbreviations Related to:	Abbreviations	Meaning
Medication route	subcut	subcutaneous		lb	pound
	ID	intradermal		fl oz	fluid ounce
	IM	intramuscular		oz	ounce
	IV	intravenous		pt	pint
	NAS	nasal		qt	quart
	po, PO	by mouth		Tbs, tbsp	tablespoon
Medication form	tinct	tincture		tsp	teaspoon
	ung.	ointment	Timing	ac	before meals
	sol., soln	solution		pc	after meals
	cap	capsule		ad lib	as desired
	tab(s)	tablet(s)		d	day
Measurements	C	Celsius		AM, a.m.	morning
	F	Fahrenheit		PM, p.m.	afternoon
	m	meter		noc, noct	night
	cm	centimeter		h, hr	hour
	mm	millimeter		min	minute
	kg	kilogram		$\bar{p}$	after
	g	gram		prn	as needed
	mg	milligram		qh	every hour
	mcg	microgram		q(2,3,4,6,8)h	every (2, 3, 4, 6, 8) hours; (q2h = every 2 hours)
	L	liter			
	mL	milliliter		qid	four times a day
	gr	grain		tid	three times a day
	gtt(s)	drop(s)		bid	twice a day
				qam	every morning
				stat, STAT	immediately

Continued

TABLE 44.5   Abbreviations Related Medications—cont'd

Abbreviations Related to:	Abbreviations	Meaning	Abbreviations Related to:	Abbreviations	Meaning
Medications	ASA	aspirin	Miscellaneous	$\overline{aa}$	of each (used in prescriptions)
	APAP	acetaminophen		aq	water
	Fe	iron		$\overline{c}$	with
	HCT	hydrochlorothiazide		med	medicine
	K	potassium		NKA	no known allergies
	MOM	milk of magnesia		NKDA	no known drug allergies
	NS	normal saline		NPO	nothing by mouth
	NSAID	nonsteroidal anti-inflammatory drug		Pt, pt	patient
				qs	quantity sufficient
	OTC	over-the-counter (drugs)		Rx	take
	PPD	purified protein derivative (tuberculin skin test)		Sig	give the following directions
				$\overline{s}$	without
				VO	verbal order
				x	times

the patients' health records. Table 44.5 provides commonly approved abbreviations.

Once the prescriptions are prepared, they need to be given to the provider to sign. Either the provider or the medical assistant needs to document the refills in the patient's health record. The facility's policy will indicate who is responsible for the documentation.

Controlled Substance Prescriptions. For security reasons, the provider's DEA number should be used only on controlled substance prescriptions. It is not appropriate for the number to appear on non-narcotic prescriptions. The NPI is a national number that is unique to the provider. This number is found on prescriptions and may be used for tracking or treatment identification purposes.

The medical assistant needs to be aware of the special requirements for controlled substances. It is important for the medical assistant to stay updated on which frequently prescribed medications are controlled substances. Table 44.6 describes common requirements for scheduled substances.

CRITICAL THINKING 44.8

Mark and Gabe are working on prescription refills. A patient who has just started taking a Schedule 2 medication calls in for a refill. He says he is not happy that there were no refills on his original prescription. How might Gabe handle this type of call? What could he say to help the patient understand the situation?

OVER-THE-COUNTER MEDICATIONS AND HERBAL SUPPLEMENTS

OTC medications and herbal supplements can affect medication treatment. It is important for the medical assistant to obtain a list of the patient's current prescription and OTC medications,

TABLE 44.6   Special Requirements for Controlled Substances

Schedule	Prescription Specifics
I	Drugs with no currently accepted medical use.
II/IIN (2)	Written prescription manually signed by the provider or an electronic prescription that meets all Drug Enforcement Administration (DEA) requirements for electronic prescriptions for controlled substances. No refills. In some cases the prescription can be faxed to the pharmacy. The medication cannot be dispensed until the original prescription is given to the pharmacy.
III/IIIN and IV (3, 4)	Call-in prescriptions, written prescriptions, and electronic prescriptions are allowed. Faxed prescriptions must be manually signed by the provider prior to faxing. Prescription good for 6 months. No more than five refills are allowed.
V (5)	Phoned prescriptions, written prescriptions, e-prescriptions, and faxed prescriptions allowed. Prescription is good for 12 months (as with non-narcotic prescriptions). Refill quantity is up to the provider.

in addition to herbal supplements (Tables 44.7 and 44.8). Some patients may hesitate or may not want to share this information. They may not realize that OTC medications and herbal supplements can interfere with prescription medications. It is important for medical assistants to be professional and respectful when dealing with these situations. If they explain that sometimes the OTC medications and herbal supplements react with prescription medications, patients may be more willing to share information on what they take.

TABLE 44.7 Common Over-the-Counter (OTC) Medications

Generic Name	Brand/Trade Name(s)	Class/Schedule	Medication Information
acetaminophen (a set a MEE noe fen)	Tylenol (TIE len ohl)	Analgesics and antipyretics	Indications: Pain, fever Desired effects/action: Pain reliever and fever reducer Side effects: Nausea, vomiting Adverse reactions: Jaundice, stomach pain
diphenhydramine (dye fen HYE dra meen)	Benadryl (BEN ah dril)	Antihistamine	Indications: Hay fever, allergies, insomnia, motion sickness Desired effects/action: Blocks the action of histamine in the body Side effects: Dry mouth, dizziness, weakness, excitement (in children), constipation, nervousness Adverse reactions: Visual problems, difficulty urinating, painful urination
ibuprofen (eye BYOO proe fen)	Advil (AD vil) Motrin (MOE trin) Midol (MYE dohl)	Anti-inflammatory drugs (nonsteroidal [NSAIDs])	Indications: Osteoarthritis, rheumatoid arthritis, fever, pain Desired effects/action: Stops the body's production of substances that cause pain, fever, and inflammation Side effects: Gastrointestinal (GI) intolerance, ringing in the ears Adverse reactions: Weight gain, hypersensitivity, hoarseness, jaundice, bloody urine, stiff neck
naproxen (na PROX en)	Aleve (AH leev) Naprosyn (nah PRO sin)	Anti-inflammatory drugs (nonsteroidal [NSAIDs])	Indications: Osteoarthritis, rheumatoid arthritis, fever, pain Desired effects/action: Stops the body's production of substances that cause pain, fever, and inflammation Side effects: GI intolerance, ringing in the ears Adverse reactions: Weight gain, hypersensitivity, hoarseness, jaundice, bloody urine, stiff neck
dextromethorphan (dex troe meth OR fan)	(Many DM cough and cold formulas)	Antitussives	Indication: Cough Desired effects/action: Reduces coughs Side effects: Drowsiness, restlessness, light-headedness, stomach pain, dizziness Adverse reaction: Hives
pseudoephedrine (soo doe e FED rin)	Sudafed (SUE ah fed)	Decongestant	Indications: Colds, hay fever, sinus congestion Desired effects/action: Relieves nasal and sinus congestion Side effects: Restlessness, nausea, vomiting, weakness, headache Adverse reactions: Hypertension, vasospasm, arrhythmia, cerebrovascular accident
aspirin (ASA) (AS pir in)	Bufferin (BUFF er in) Ecotrin (ec OH trin) (many brand names)	Salicylates	Indications: Arthritis, fever, pain, heart attack prevention Desired effects/action: Relieves pain, fevers; increases clotting time Side effects: Nausea, stomach pain, heartburn, drowsiness, ringing in the ears Adverse reactions: Visual changes, tachycardia, wheezing, back pain, confusion

TABLE 44.8 Commonly Used Herbal Products

Name	Uses	Side Effects and Cautions
Acai	Weight loss and antiaging; antioxidant.	Little scientific information about the safety of acai; no scientific evidence to support use or any health-related purpose; might affect magnetic resonance imaging (MRI) results.
Aloe vera	Aloe gel is used for burns, frostbite, psoriasis, and cold sores. It can also be taken orally for osteoarthritis, bowel diseases, and fever.	Topical use of aloe gel is likely to be safe. More studies are needed to determine the safety of oral preparations. People with diabetes should be cautioned against using aloe, because it may lower blood glucose levels.
Black cohosh	Relieve symptoms of menopause; treat menstrual irregularities and premenstrual syndrome; induce labor.	Headaches, gastric complaints, heaviness in the legs, weight problems; safety unknown for pregnant women or those with breast cancer.
Echinacea	Treat or prevent colds, flu, and other infections; believed to stimulate the immune system.	Most studies indicate echinacea does not appear to prevent colds or other infections; some people experience allergic reactions, including rashes, increased asthma, and anaphylaxis; gastrointestinal (GI) side effects.

Continued

TABLE 44.8   Commonly Used Herbal Products—cont'd

Name	Uses	Side Effects and Cautions
Flaxseed	Flaxseed and flaxseed oil are used for constipation, diabetes, high cholesterol levels, cancer, and other conditions.	Few reported side effects; contains soluble fiber and is an effective laxative; both flaxseed and flaxseed oil can cause diarrhea. It is not recommended during pregnancy.
Garlic	Treat high cholesterol, heart disease, hypertension; prevent certain types of cancer, including stomach and colon cancer.	Some evidence indicates garlic can slightly lower blood cholesterol levels and may slow development of atherosclerosis; side effects include breath and body odor, heartburn, GI upset, and allergic reactions; acts as a mild anticoagulant (similar to aspirin); may increase the risk of bleeding; interferes with effectiveness of saquinavir, a drug used to treat human immunodeficiency virus (HIV) infection.
Ginger	Alleviate nausea associated with postoperative state, motion sickness, chemotherapy, and pregnancy; used for rheumatoid arthritis, osteoarthritis, and joint and muscle pain.	Short-term use can safely relieve pregnancy-related nausea and vomiting; also may help with chemotherapy nausea and vomiting. Side effects most often reported are gas, bloating, heartburn, and nausea.
Asian ginseng	Support overall health and boost immune system; improve mental and physical performance; treat erectile dysfunction, hepatitis C, and menopause symptoms; lower blood glucose and control blood pressure.	Limited information available, more studies needed. May affect blood glucose levels and blood pressure; thus patients should discuss this with their provider. May interact with certain medications such as anticoagulants.
Ginkgo biloba (GING koe BIL oh bah)	No conclusive evidence that it helps any health condition.	Side effects may include headache, stomach upset, and allergic skin reactions. Ginkgo may increase the risk of bleeding with pregnancy and in those taking anticoagulants.
Green tea	Improve mental alertness, relieve digestive symptoms and headaches, promote weight loss; may have protective effects against heart disease and cancer.	Safe in moderate amounts; possible complications include liver problems with concentrated green tea extracts but not when used as a beverage. A specific green tea extract ointment is a prescription drug used for treating genital warts.
St. John's wort (wohrt)	Treat mental disorders and nerve pain; kidney and lung diseases, insomnia, and wounds.	Some scientific evidence shows it helps treat mild to moderate depression; not effective in treating major depression. Side effects include photophobia (increased sensitivity to sunlight), anxiety, dry mouth, dizziness, GI symptoms, fatigue, headache, and sexual dysfunction. Can cause life-threatening reactions with certain medications. Drugs that can be affected include: • Antidepressants • Birth control pills • Cyclosporine (prevents rejection of transplants) • Digoxin (heart medication) • Some HIV and cancer medications • Warfarin and related anticoagulants

Modified from the National Center for Complementary and Alternative Medicine. https://nccih.nih.gov/health/herbsataglance.htm.

CLOSING COMMENTS

The magnitude of opioid abuse has increased dramatically, and it is currently considered a crisis. According to the Centers for Diseases Control and Prevention (CDC) (https://www.cdc.gov/), over 81,000 drug overdose deaths occurred in the US in a 12-month period ending in May 2020. Synthetic opioid overdoses increased 38.4% during this period compared to the prior year. With the frequency of opioid abuse, prescribing guidelines are changing. Many ambulatory care facilities have adopted procedures for specific controlled substance prescriptions. Before patients can get these prescriptions, they need to have a urine drug test. The urine drug test helps providers assess what drugs patients have taken. Providers expect the results to show the drug prescribed, but they check for other prescribed controlled substances and illicit drugs. In many cases, if the drug test shows evidence of illicit drug use or prescription-controlled substances not prescribed by the provider, the patient is referred for substance abuse counseling and treatment.

The CDC has published the document Guidelines for Prescribing Opioids for Chronic Pain (available at https://www.cdc.gov/drugoverdose/pdf/Guidelines_Factsheet-a.pdf). These guidelines help support providers who are working with patients with chronic pain. The provider may have the medical assistant coach patients on home care treatments. Opioids are not first-line or routine therapy for chronic pain. The medical assistant may need to coach the patient on the importance of using non-pharmacologic therapy and nonopioid pharmacologic therapy for chronic pain. For patients who receive opioid prescriptions, frequent follow-up is needed for the provider to evaluate the benefit and risk of the drug.

PATIENT-CENTERED CARE

Many healthcare facilities require that patients receive a printout of their current medications at the end of each visit. When patients are taking several medications, it is important for the medical assistant to encourage these patients to carry a current medications list in their wallet or purse. This can be helpful in an emergency or when the patient needs to see a different provider.

BEING PROFESSIONAL

When working with prescription refills, it is important for the medical assistant to process the refill in a timely fashion. If the medical assistant procrastinates and does not process the refill, the patient may not have the medication when they need it. Some medications need to be taken daily. If a dose is skipped, the patient may have serious consequences.

It is also important that the medical assistant honor what that patient was told. If the patient is told that the medication will be sent to a pharmacy by a specific time, it is important for the medical assistant to ensure this is done. If the medication is held up for some reason, the medical assistant should notify the patient about the delay.

Role-play this scenario: You and Vicki are medical assistants. You are completing the evening tasks, because the clinic has now closed. Vicki mentions that she forgot to process prescriptions. She states she promised the patients they would be sent to the pharmacy today. She tells you that she will do it in the morning when she gets time. Respond to Vicki in a respectful, professional manner regarding this situation.

CHAPTER REVIEW

This chapter covered the drug basics, including sources, uses, and pharmacokinetics. The sources of drugs include natural and synthetic. Natural sources include plants, animals, minerals, and microbiological sources. Synthetic medications are created in a laboratory setting. Medications are used for prevention, treatment, diagnosis, cure, contraception, health maintenance, palliative care, and replacement. Pharmacokinetics involves drug absorption, distribution, metabolism, and excretion. The very young, older adults, and those with kidney and liver disease are at risk for drug toxicity. Too much medication or metabolites in the body can cause harmful effects.

Drug action is influenced by many factors, including age, size, sex, disease, and diet. For the therapeutic or desired effect to occur, medication levels in the blood must be in the therapeutic range. If the level is beyond the therapeutic range, the person can experience symptoms of toxicity.

The Food, Drug, and Cosmetic Act enforced by the FDA and the Controlled Substance Act (CSA) imposed by the DEA impact the healthcare setting. The medical assistant is responsible for removing any recalled medications from the department. Compliance with the CSA is the responsibility of the medical assistant and the provider. The medical assistant needs to follow the storage, tracking, destruction, and theft reporting rules for controlled substances.

This chapter also covered the four names for medications: the chemical, generic, official, and brand names. Drug reference materials are critical for learning about medications. Terminology commonly found in reference information was discussed. Using drug reference information is common when you prepare prescriptions for the provider to sign. Remember, it is not within the medical assistant's scope of practice to order (sign) prescriptions. This falls within the provider's scope of practice. The provider is responsible for the accuracy of the prescription and for ensuring that it meets the state and federal laws.

SCENARIO WRAP-UP

Mark is enjoying working with Gabe. He is amazed at how much Gabe knows about medications that the providers commonly prescribe. Mark feels that he will never be as fluent with the medications as Gabe is. He even mentioned this to Gabe. His mentor laughed and said he felt the same way during his own practicum. Over the years, he has used drug reference materials to help him learn about medications. He has made it a practice to look up medications he does not know. This helped him become more fluent. He assured Mark that if he was willing to read up on medications, he, too, will become fluent with them.

Mark is looking forward to administering medications with Gabe. Now that he understands how to use the drug reference materials, he will be working hard to learn the medications he encounters.

PROCEDURE 44.1   Prepare a Prescription

Tasks

Prepare a prescription using a prescription refill protocol. Use approved abbreviations.

Scenario

You receive a call from Noemi Rodriguez (DOB 11/04/19XX). She is requesting refills on three of her prescriptions from Jean Burke, NP. She saw Jean Burke 10 months ago. Noemi has no known allergies (NKA). She is doing well with the prescriptions and has no concerns. You determine it is time for refills. Her prescriptions include Coumadin 5 mg, 1 tablet orally daily; Tenormin 50 mg, 1 tablet orally daily; and Plendil 5 mg, 1 tablet orally daily.

Directions

Prepare prescriptions for only the medications that are addressed by the protocol. The prescription should be for 30 days and include refills. Generic medication can be used.

Equipment and Supplies

- SimChart for the Medical Office (SCMO) or paper prescriptions and pen
- Prescription refill protocol (Fig. 44.4)
- Drug reference book or online resource

Procedural Steps

1. Using the scenario, look up the generic medication names using the drug reference book or online resource.

   Purpose: Generic names are typically used in the healthcare facility, though patients may give the brand name.

2. Read the prescription refill protocol. Compare the generic names to the list of medications given. Identify medications that meet the protocol.

   Purpose: All the criteria need to be met for the medical assistant to prepare prescriptions using the prescription refill protocol.

3. Prepare prescriptions for refill per the protocol using SCMO or paper prescriptions.

   - *SCMO:* Search for the patient. Verify the date of birth before selecting the patient. On the INFO PANEL, select Phone Encounter. Complete the fields on the Create New Encounter window and save. Check the box beside the No known allergy statement on the allergy screen and save. Select Order Entry from the Record dropdown list and select Add in the Out-of-office section (see the following figure).
   - *Paper prescriptions:* Add in the patient's complete name, date of birth, and address.

   Purpose: Most agencies using electronic health records require medical assistants to update the allergy screen when preparing refills. Prescriptions require the patient's name and address. If the DOB is available, add this to the prescription. An electronic health record will automatically add this information when it sends the prescription to the pharmacy.

4. Using the information in the scenario, complete the prescription information on either the paper prescription or in the SCMO fields. Use only approved abbreviations.

   Purpose: All information is required on the prescription for it to be accepted by the pharmacist and filled for the patient.

Add Order

WALDEN-MARTIN
FAMILY MEDICAL CLINIC
1234 ANYSTREET | ANYTOWN, ANYSTATE 12345
PHONE 123-123-1234 | FAX 123-123-5678

- James A. Martin MD — Internal Medicine — DEA #: 8D05034030
- Julie Walden MD — Internal Medicine — DEA #: 8D050305923
- Jean Burke NP — Family Nurse Practitioner — DEA #: 8D050303940

Diagnosis:
Drug:
☐ Generic Permitted   Pharmacy:
Strength: Form:
Route: Refills:
Directions:
Quantity: Issue Via: ○ Electronic transfer   ○ Paper
Days Supply:
Entry By: Date:
Notes:

[Print] [Send] [Save] [Cancel]

5. Complete any additional prescriptions as needed by the prescription refill protocol.

   Purpose: The patient requested refills on the medications indicated. Any medications that can be refilled should have prescriptions prepared for the provider.

6. Review the prescriptions for any errors. Void the prescription and redo if needed.

   Purpose: It is important to prepare accurate prescriptions. Any errors need to be fixed before giving the prescriptions to the provider. *Note:* After the provider signs the prescriptions and depending on the facility's policy, the medical assistant may need to document the refill in the health record. This cannot be done until the provider approves the prescriptions.

Pharmacology Math

LEARNING OBJECTIVES

1. Summarize the important parts of a drug label.
2. Discuss math basics, including writing numbers in healthcare and rounding numbers.
3. Define basic units of measure in the household system and the metric system and convert between measurement systems.

4. Convert between Fahrenheit and Celsius temperatures.
5. Perform pharmacology calculations, such as quantity needed for a specific time period, number of tablets per dose, liquid medication doses, and pediatric doses.
6. Read the calibration markings on various types of syringes.

OUTLINE

▶▶ OPENING SCENARIO

Gabe Garcia, a certified medical assistant (CMA) through the American Association of Medical Assistants (AAMA), has worked for Walden-Martin Family Medical (WMFM) Clinic for 3 years. During his first year at WMFM Clinic, Gabe worked almost exclusively with a family practice provider who cared for older patients. Once the provider retired, Gabe switched providers. He is now working with both children and adult patients. He finds himself administering more injections when working with the children than he does when working with the adults.

Gabe was asked to be Mark Allen's mentor for his clinical experience. Mark has just completed all of his medical assistant courses at the local college and now needs 160 hours of clinical experience. He is excited to be working with Gabe. This week, Gabe will be working with Mark to review reading syringes and applying the math used for medication calculations.

YOU WILL LEARN

1. To identify the parts of a drug label.
2. To identify the basic units of measure in the household system and the metric system.
3. To convert between different measurement systems.
4. To convert a temperature between Fahrenheit and Celsius.
5. To calculate medication doses.
6. To read calibration markings on syringes.

INTRODUCTION

Medical assistants are responsible for being absolutely certain that the medication they prepare and administer to a patient is exactly what the provider ordered. Although drugs often are delivered by the pharmacy or supplied by pharmaceutical representatives in unit-dose packaging, the dosage ordered may differ from the dosage on hand. In this case, the medical assistant must be prepared to calculate the correct dose accurately before dispensing and administering the medication. There is never a margin of error in drug calculations; even a minor mistake may result in serious complications for the patient. The medical assistant, therefore, must take meticulous care in calculating all drug dosages.

VOCABULARY

dosage The quantity of medication to be administered at one time.

exclusivity The sole right to market an approved medication granted by the FDA.

patent A grant from the government that gives a creator (or manufacturer) of an invention the sole right to produce, use, and sell the product for a set period of time.

unit-dose packaging Holds a specified quantity of medication in a single-use container.

DRUG LABELS

The first step in safely calculating a drug dosage is to accurately read the label of the drug on hand to determine whether the provider's order and the packaged drug are in the same system of measurement. The label shows the following information:

- *Trade* or *brand name*: The manufacturer's name for the drug (e.g., Cardizem) (Fig. 45.1). The brand name is capitalized

and typically in bold print. The brand name is copyright protected; therefore it is followed by an ® symbol that indicates the US government has granted a Federal Registration Certificate for the drug.

- *Generic name*: The drug name used by all manufacturers who make that specific medication (e.g., diltiazem HCl, cephalexin) (see Fig. 45.1). The name is printed in lowercase letters and usually appears under the brand name in smaller print. If the patent and exclusivity have expired, only a generic name may be present on the label (Box 45.1).

- *Strength*: The amount of drug in the unit dose (e.g., 200 mg, 180 mg/5 mL). In Fig. 45.1, each tablet of Cardizem is 120 mg. Cephalexin is a suspension (liquid), and the strength or unit dose is 250 mg (of powdered medication) per 5 mL (of liquid).

BOX 45.1 Patents and Exclusivity

A patent is granted on a drug for 20 years from the date of filing for the patent. Patents are granted at any point in time along the development of a drug.

Exclusivity is granted by the Food and Drug Administration (FDA) to give exclusive marketing rights to the manufacturers of the drug when it earns FDA approval. This exclusive marketing right can vary from 3 to 5 years. If a medication has been on the market longer than 20 years or after the exclusive rights to the drug have expired, the generic name may be the only one listed (e.g., meperidine instead of Demerol, diazepam rather than Valium).

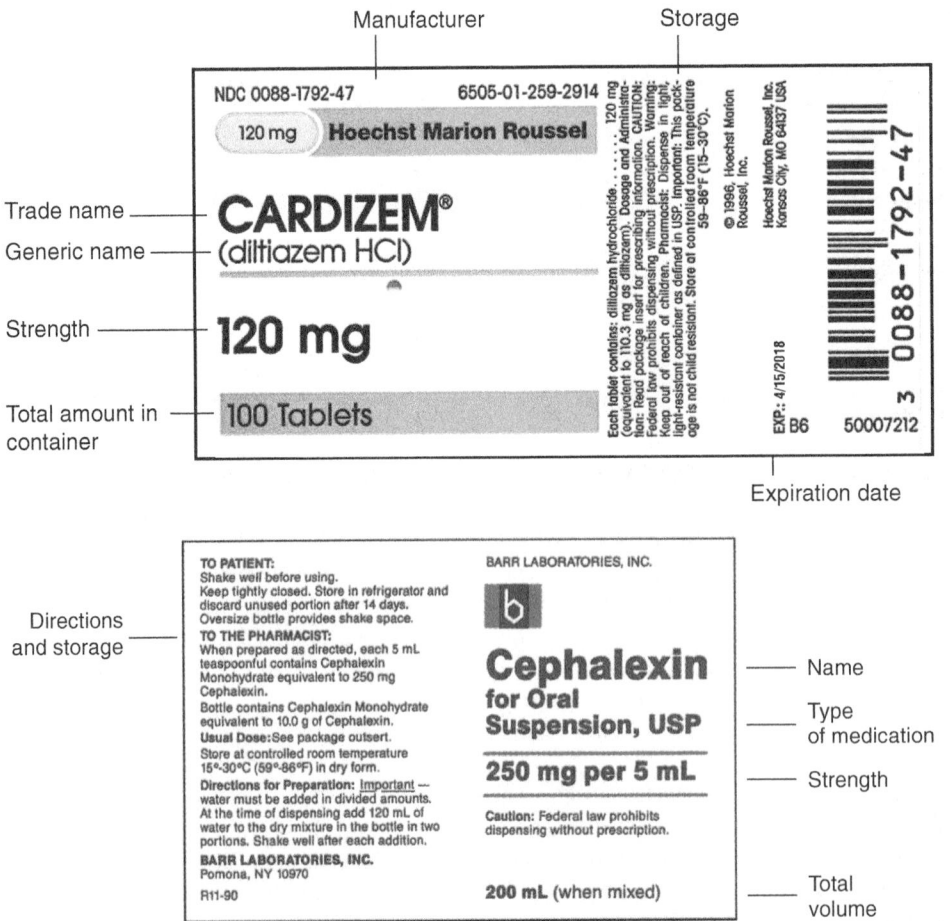

Fig. 45.1 Drug Labels. (From Brown M, Mulholland JM: *Drug calculations: process and problems for clinical practice*, ed 9, St. Louis, 2012, Mosby.)

- *Total amount* or *total volume*: Both liquid and solid medication labels indicate the amount of medication in the container.
- *Manufacturer*: The name of the manufacturer of the medication.
- *Directions and storage*: Instructions on how to take the medication and how to store the drug may be indicated on the label.
- *Expiration date*: Indicates when the drug can no longer be used.
- *Lot number*: Indicates the batch of drug the medication came from. The lot number is important to document when giving immunizations. Some agencies may require that lot numbers be documented for all medications administered.
- *National Drug Code (NDC)*: A unique 10-digit number indicating the product. The NDC is required by federal law to be on all prescription and nonprescription medication packages and inserts in the United States.

When the medical assistant prepares medications, it is important to compare the medication's name and strength with the provider's order. The medical assistant should also look at the expiration date. Preparing medications will be discussed in more detail in Chapter 46.

Critical Thinking 45.1

Gabe and Mark are discussing the labels on vaccines. Mark asks Gabe why the lot numbers are important on vaccine vials. How would you answer this question?

MATH BASICS

When working with math in healthcare, you need to thoroughly understand the addition, subtraction, multiplication, and division of fractions and decimals; the relationship of decimals and fractions; and how they are converted from one to the other.

Fractions

When you divide a whole unit into parts, you can create a fraction with a part. For instance, you cut a tablet into 2 parts; each part is $\frac{1}{2}$. If you cut a pizza into 8 slices, each slice is $\frac{1}{8}$.

The top number in a fraction is the *numerator*, and the bottom number is the *denominator*. In a *proper fraction*, the numerator is smaller than the denominator, such as $\frac{3}{4}$. In *improper fractions*, the numerator is equal to or greater than the denominator, such as $\frac{6}{5}$ and $\frac{5}{5}$. Improper fractions can be converted into whole numbers by dividing the numerator by the denominator. For example, if you had an improper fraction of $\frac{12}{3}$, you would divide the numerator by the denominator, or $12 \div 3 = 4$. Some improper fractions can be simplified. For example, $\frac{12}{5}$ would be $12 \div 5 = 2\frac{2}{5}$, which is considered a mixed number. A mixed number is a whole number with a proper fraction.

When multiplying fractions, you multiply the two numerators and the two denominators. Then you reduce the answer into the simplest form. Let us use this problem: $\frac{1}{6} \times \frac{2}{4}$. The two numerators are multiplied (1×2) and the two denominators are multiplied (6×4). The answer would be $\frac{2}{24}$. Now we must reduce the fraction to its lowest terms. Two is the largest number

that will divide equally into the 2 and 24. Therefore divide the numerator by 2 ($2 \div 2 = 1$) and the denominator by 2 ($24 \div 2 = 12$). Thus the final answer would be $\frac{1}{12}$.

To divide fractions, you must invert the *divisor* (the second fraction) and then multiply the numerators and denominators. Let us use this problem: $\frac{3}{5} \div \frac{3}{2}$. The divisor is $\frac{3}{2}$, and this needs to be inverted ($\frac{2}{3}$). Next, we rewrite the problem and multiply the numerators and the denominators: $\frac{3}{5} \times \frac{2}{3}$. Multiplying the numerators (3×2) would be 6, and multiplying the denominators (5×3) would be 15. The answer would be $\frac{6}{15}$, but it needs to be written in the simplest form. Three is the largest number that will divide equally into the 6 and 15. Therefore divide the numerator by 3 ($6 \div 3 = 2$) and the denominator by 3 ($15 \div 3 = 5$). Thus the final answer would be $\frac{2}{5}$. Box 45.2 contains practice problems.

Decimals

A decimal is similar to a fraction, but it is expressed in units of tenths (0.1), hundredths (0.01), and thousandths (0.001). To perform drug calculations, fractions first must be converted into decimals. To convert a fraction into a decimal, simply divide the numerator by the denominator.

For example, if a dose of medication is $\frac{2}{5}$ mL, the provider's order would be written in the decimal equivalent. To perform this math, you may need to add zeroes after the decimal point at the end of the numerator. The problem would be written: $2 \div 5$. The answer would be 0.4 mL. Box 45.3 provides practice problems.

Percentages

A *percentage* is a number expressed as part of 100. Decimal numbers can be converted to percentages by multiplying the number by 100 and adding a percent sign (%). Another way to

---

BOX 45.2 Fraction Practice Problems

Directions: Convert the improper fractions to mixed numbers. Write the answer in simplest form.

1. $\frac{22}{3} =$ _____
2. $\frac{17}{12} =$ _____
3. $\frac{52}{20} =$ _____
4. $\frac{25}{7} =$ _____
5. $\frac{15}{4} =$ _____
6. $\frac{62}{30} =$ _____

Directions: Solve these problems and write the answer in simplest form.

7. $\frac{1}{3} \times \frac{2}{3} =$ _____
8. $\frac{2}{5} \times \frac{6}{4} =$ _____
9. $\frac{4}{5} \times \frac{6}{8} =$ _____
10. $\frac{2}{3} \div \frac{5}{6} =$ _____
11. $\frac{12}{3} \div \frac{4}{7} =$ _____
12. $\frac{1}{3} \div \frac{2}{3} =$ _____

BOX 45.3 Decimal Practice Problems

Directions: Convert the fractions to decimals.

1. $\frac{3}{5} =$ _____
2. $\frac{6}{10} =$ _____
3. $\frac{2}{10} =$ _____
4. $\frac{5}{2} =$ _____
5. $\frac{4}{5} =$ _____
6. $\frac{5}{100} =$ _____

BOX 45.4   Percent Practice Problems

Directions: Convert the decimals to percentages.

1. 0.3 = _____   2. 1.03 = _____   3. 0.04 = _____
4. 0.52 = _____   5. 0.6 = _____   6. 0.32 = _____

---

convert the decimal is to move the decimal point two spaces to the right and add a percent sign (%). Examples:

$0.25 = {}^{25}/_{100} = 25\%$
$0.5 = {}^{5}/_{10} = 50\%$
$0.75 = {}^{75}/_{100} = 75\%$
$0.055 = {}^{55}/_{1000} = 5.5\%$

Box 45.4 provides practice problems.

MATH FOR MEDICATIONS

All medical assistants should be able to convert between units of measure. It is also important to be able to accurately calculate medication dosages. This section discusses different types of math problems that a medical assistant should be able to do. Please note that in some states, calculating medical dosages may be outside the legal scope of practice for medical assistants. State laws vary.

Math Basics for Medication

The following sections present guidelines for writing and calculating dosages. The medical assistant should always verify answers for dose calculations with a co-worker or the provider.

Healthcare Rules When Writing Numbers. With medications, it is important to be accurate in calculating and documenting amounts. There are four rules to follow when writing medication dosages in healthcare:

1. Follow the number with the correct abbreviation for the unit of measure. Leave a space between the number and the abbreviation. Do not use a period with the abbreviations.
   - Correct examples: 2 mg and 10 mL
   - Incorrect examples: mg2 and 10mL
2. Write a fraction of a dose as a decimal.
   - Correct examples: 0.2 mg and 0.5 mg
   - Incorrect examples: $\frac{1}{5}$ mg and $\frac{1}{2}$ mg
3. If the dose is less than 1, place a zero to the left of the decimal point. This reduces the risk of misreading the dose as a whole number.
   - Correct examples: 0.75 mcg and 0.2 mL
   - Incorrect examples: .75 mcg and .2 mL
4. Do not place a decimal point and a zero after a whole number. This can be easily misread, and the patient would be given an overdose of medication.
   - Correct examples: 2 mL and 5 mL
   - Incorrect examples: 2.0 mL and 5.0 mL

Rounding Numbers. When you calculate answers, sometimes the number needs to be rounded. The following steps describe the process for rounding a number.

BOX 45.5   Rounding Practice Problems

Directions: Round the following numbers to the nearest tenth. Write out as you would for a medication dose with a zero before the decimal point if the answer is less than 1 and no trailing zeros.

1. 2.467 = _____   2. .358 = _____   3. .98 = _____
4. 4.65 = _____   5. 45.234 = _____ 6. 7.788 = _____

---

1. Find the place value where you want to end up. (Most answers in this chapter will be rounded to the nearest tenth, or one place after the decimal point.)

Hundred	Ten	One		Tenth	Hundredth	Thousandth
7	5	1	.	3	5	7

2. Look at the number to the right of the place value. If the number is
   - *4 or below*, drop the number(s) to the right of the place value
   - *5 or above*, add 1 to the rounded place value and drop the number(s) to the right of the place value

   Let us practice rounding to the nearest tenth using the following examples:
   - First example: 569.365. In this example, 3 sits in the tenth-place value. The number to the right of the 3 is a 6. This means we need to add 1 to the 3, and then we can drop the 6 and 5. The answer is 569.4.
   - Second example: 339.926. In this example, 9 sits in the tenth-place value. The number to the right of the 9 is a 2. This means we just need to drop the 2 and 6. The answer is 339.9. Box 45.5 provides practice problems.

Roman Numerals. Sometimes a number might be written using Roman numerals. It is good for a medical assistant to be familiar with the following Roman numerals. In healthcare, you will see them written in lowercase letters. Sometimes a line may be written above the Roman numeral.

i = 1	vi = 6	$\overline{ss}$ = $\frac{1}{2}$ or 0.5 (For "$\overline{ss}$": write
ii = 2	vii = 7	out "one-half" in documen-
iii = 3	viii = 8	tation notes to avoid errors.)
iv = 4	ix = 9	*Examples:*
v = 5	x = 10	vss = 5½ or 5.5
		iiiss = 3½ or 3.5

Critical Thinking 45.2

Mark is confused by the numbers 5 and 10 in the Roman numeral system. Come up with a way to remember the difference between these two and share it with a classmate.

Measurement Systems

In healthcare, both the household and metric systems are used. For instance, we weigh patients in pounds and tell a mother to give her son 1 teaspoon of medication before meals. Using the metric system is more accurate. The provider will use a child's weight in kilograms (kg) to calculate a medication dosage. The pharmacist will show the mother that 1 teaspoon is really 5 mL on the oral syringe. The oral syringe and plastic medicine cup are more accurate for measuring medications than the spoons used in the kitchen.

Apothecary System. The apothecary (ah POTH i ker ee) system is the oldest measuring system for medications. Dry medications were measured based on a grain (gr), which equaled the weight of one grain of wheat. For liquid measurements, the basic unit of volume is a minim (MIN im). When writing numbers and abbreviations for the apothecary system, the abbreviation is written before the lowercase Roman numeral (e.g., gr v). Fractions are used for portions less than a full unit (e.g., gr ¼). Half of a unit can be expressed as ss (e.g., gr vss). The apothecary system has been replaced by the metric system. Medications should be calculated based on the metric system.

VOCABULARY

minim An apothecary unit of measurement for liquid; approximately equal to one drop.

product The number obtained by multiplying two or more numbers together.

Household System. Sometimes we need to work within the household system as we solve problems. Other times we need to use both the metric and household measurement systems. The following are common household measurement abbreviations.

gtt, gtts	drop, drops
tsp	teaspoon
Tbs or tbsp	tablespoon
fl oz	fluid ounce
oz	ounce
qt	quart
pt	pint
lb	pound

Box 45.6 shows the household and metric equivalents for weights and liquids. Some find remembering the following equivalents to be helpful: 1 oz = 2 Tbs = 6 tsp = 30 mL.

There are many ways to set up problems when converting between household and metric equivalents. The proportion method is one of the easiest techniques. In the proportion

method, the cross-products are equal. This approach is easy if you remember three things:

1. Keep the information separate. The problem information is on one side of the equals sign, and the equivalent information is on the other side.
2. Keep the labels in the same place. The labels should be in the exact same location on both sides of the equals sign.
3. Cross-multiply in the direction of the two numbers, then divide by the remaining number. You have your answer.

The following steps show how to solve household and metric problems. Box 45.7 provides practice problems.

Problem: 15 Tbs = _____ mL

***Solution for problem.* Step 1:** Turn the problem into a fraction. It does not matter which number is the *numerator* (top number in a fraction) and which is the *denominator* (bottom number in a fraction), just keep the label with the number. Use *x* for the unknown number.

Problem

$$\frac{15\ Tbs}{x\ mL}$$

Step 2: Add an equals sign and make a fraction on the opposite side. Fill in the labels. The labels need to be in identical locations on both sides of the equals sign.

Problem	**Equivalent**
$\dfrac{15\ Tbs}{x\ mL} =$	$\dfrac{\_\_\_\_\ Tbs}{\_\_\_\_\ mL}$

Step 3: Using Box 45.6, find the equivalent for Tbs and tsp. Fill in the numbers in the equivalent fraction. Make sure to put the right number in front of the correct label.

Problem	**Equivalent**
$\dfrac{15\ Tbs}{x\ mL} =$	$\dfrac{1\ Tbs}{15\ mL}$

Step 4: Now solve for the unknown.

Using a calculator: Multiply in the diagonal direction of the two numbers (15 × 15) and then divide by the number in the other direction (1); the answer is *x*.

Problem	**Equivalent**
$\dfrac{15\ Tbs}{x\ mL} =$	$\dfrac{1\ Tbs}{15\ mL}$

15 × 15 = 225 ÷ 1 = 225

BOX 45.6   Household and Metric Equivalents

Weight	Liquids	
2.2 lb = 1 kg	3 tsp = 1 Tbs	1 Tbs = 15 mL
16 oz = 1 lb	1 tsp = 60 gtt	1 oz = 2 Tbs
	1 oz = 30 mL	1 oz = 6 tsp
	1 tsp = 5 mL	

BOX 45.7   Household and Metric Practice Problems

Directions: Solve the following problems. Round your answers to the nearest tenth.

1. 11 oz = _____ lb
2. 90 mL = _____ oz
3. 8 tsp = _____ mL
4. 20 Tbs = _____ mL
5. 5.5 oz = _____ Tbs
6. 4 oz = _____ tsp
7. 23 lb = _____ kg
8. 28 kg = _____ lb
9. 56 oz = _____ lb

To solve without a calculator: Multiply diagonally and solve for *x*.

$$15 \times 15 = 1x$$
$$225 = 1x$$
$$\frac{225}{1} = \frac{1x}{1}$$
$$225 = x$$

Answer: 225 mL – *Always make sure to label your answer.*

Metric System. The metric system is commonly used in healthcare. We use it when measuring medications and wounds. A medical assistant should know how to use the metric system. Note these standards when using the metric system:

- Weight is measured in *grams* (g).
- Volume is measured in *liters* (L).
- Length is measured in *meters* (m).

Gram, liter, and meter are called *root words*. *Prefixes* are added to the front of root words to indicate the size of the unit. Fig. 45.2 lists the prefixes that can be added to the root words. Table 45.1 provides the metric measurements and equivalents commonly used in healthcare.

Remember that a person cannot convert from base unit to base unit (i.e., gram to liter or meter to gram). A person can only convert within a base unit (i.e., centimeter to millimeter). Fig. 45.3 provides a memory tool for solving metric problems. There are many ways to do so. The following steps show how to solve metric problems. Box 45.8 provides practice problems.

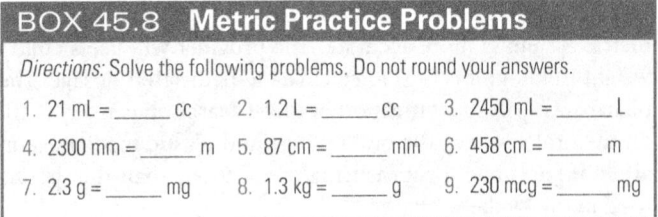

BOX 45.8   Metric Practice Problems

Directions: Solve the following problems. Do not round your answers.

1. 21 mL = _____ cc   2. 1.2 L = _____ cc   3. 2450 mL = _____ L
4. 2300 mm = _____ m   5. 87 cm = _____ mm   6. 458 cm = _____ m
7. 2.3 g = _____ mg   8. 1.3 kg = _____ g   9. 230 mcg = _____ mg

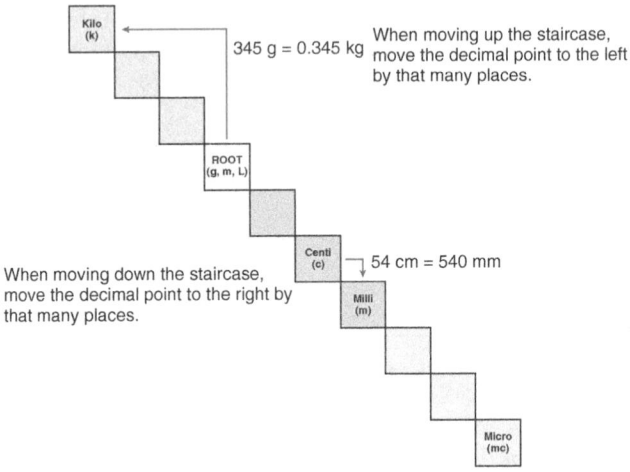

Fig. 45.3 Memory Tool for Solving Metric Problems.

Size of the unit of measure LARGE ↓ SMALL	Prefixes	Size	Or another way to look at it!	Larger than the base unit / Smaller than the base unit
	Kilo (k)	1000 base units	1 kilo = 1000 base units (Example: 1 kg = 1000 g)	Larger than the base unit
	BASE UNITS (Meter, Liter or Gram)			
	Centi (c)	0.01 unit	100 centi = 1 base unit (Example: 100 cm = 1 m)	Smaller than the base unit
	Milli (m)	0.001	1000 milli = 1 base unit (Example: 1,000 mL = 1 L)	
	Micro (mc)	0.000001	1,000,000 micro = 1 base unit (Example: 1,000,000 mcg = 1g)	

Fig. 45.2 Prefixes of Metric Measurements.

TABLE 45.1	Metric Measurements Used in Healthcare		
	Volume	**Length**	**Weight**
Units of measure with abbreviations	liter (L) milliliter (mL or ml) *(Note: 1 cc = 1 mL cubic centimeter [cc])*	meter (m) centimeter (cm) millimeter (mm)	gram (g) kilogram (kg) milligram (mg) microgram (mcg)
Equivalents commonly used	1 L = 1000 mL 1 L = 1000 cc 1 mL = 1 cc *(To avoid errors in documentation, use mL instead of cc.)*	1 m = 100 cm 1 m = 1000 mm 1 cm = 10 mm	1 g = 1000 mg 1 g = 1,000,000 mcg 1 kg = 1000 g 1 mg = 1000 mcg

Problem: 17 g = _____ mg

Solution for problem. **Step 1:** Turn the problem into a fraction. It does not matter which number is the numerator and which is the denominator, just keep the label with the number. Use *x* for the unknown number.

Problem

$$\frac{17g}{x\,mg}$$

Step 2: Add an equals sign and make a fraction on the opposite side. Fill in the labels. The labels need to be in identical locations on both sides of the equals sign.

Problem	Equivalent
$\frac{17g}{x\,mg}$ =	$\frac{\underline{\quad}\,g}{\underline{\quad}\,mg}$

Step 3: Using Table 45.1, find the equivalent for gram (g) and milligram (mg). Fill in the numbers in the equivalent fraction. Make sure to put the right number in front of the correct label.

Problem	Equivalent
$\frac{17g}{x\,mg}$ =	$\frac{1g}{1000\,mg}$

Step 4: Now solve for the unknown.

Using a calculator: Multiply in the diagonal direction of the two numbers (17 × 1000) and then divide by the number in the other direction (1); the answer is *x*.

Problem	Equivalent
$\frac{17g}{x\,mg}$ =	$\frac{1\,g}{1000\,mg}$

$$17 \times 1000 = 17,000 \div 1 = 17,000\ mg$$

To solve without a calculator: Multiply diagonally and solve for *x*.

$$17 \times 1000 = 1x$$
$$17,000 = 1x$$
$$\frac{17,000}{1} = \frac{1x}{1}$$
$$17,000 = x$$

Answer: 17,000 mg – *Always make sure to label your answer.*

Temperature Conversion

Fahrenheit (°F) and Celsius (°C) are used in healthcare. A medical assistant should be able to convert between these two units of measure. To remember the steps for temperature conversion, use the memory tool presented in Fig. 45.4.

The following steps show how to convert a Fahrenheit temperature to a Celsius temperature. Box 45.9 provides practice problems.

Problem: 102°F = _____ °C

Solution for problem. **Step 1:** Subtract 32 from the Fahrenheit temperature.

$$102 - 32 = 70$$

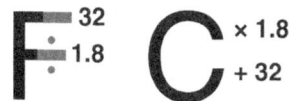

Fig. 45.4 Memory Tool for Temperature Conversions.

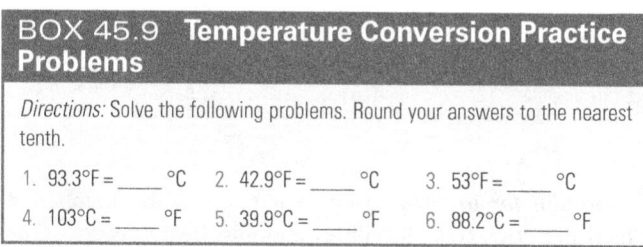

BOX 45.9 Temperature Conversion Practice Problems

Directions: Solve the following problems. Round your answers to the nearest tenth.

1. 93.3°F = _____ °C 2. 42.9°F = _____ °C 3. 53°F = _____ °C
4. 103°C = _____ °F 5. 39.9°C = _____ °F 6. 88.2°C = _____ °F

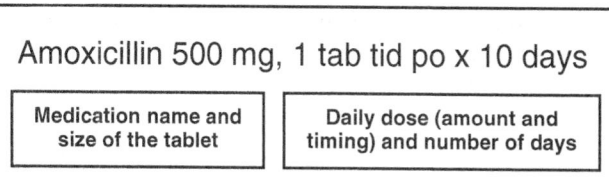

Fig. 45.5 Medication Order.

Step 2: Divide the answer by 1.8 and round to the nearest tenth.

$$70 \div 1.8 = 38.88889$$

Answer: 38.9°C

The following steps show how to convert a Celsius temperature to a Fahrenheit temperature.

Problem: 25°C = _____ °F

Solution for problem. **Step 1:** Multiply the Celsius number by 1.8

$$25 \times 1.8 = 45$$

Step 2: Add 32 to the answer.

$$45 + 32 = 77$$

Answer: 77°F

Solid Medication Doses

Number of Tablets Needed for Entire Course. It is not uncommon for patients to call their provider to request enough medication for a trip. It is important for the medical assistant to be able to calculate how many tablets a patient needs for a period of time.

Fig. 45.5 shows a medication order. The first part shows the name of the medication, along with the tablet size (strength of each tablet). The last part of the order shows:

- How many tablets to take *(dose)* (e.g., 1 tab [tablet])
- The route (e.g., po [oral])
- How many times to take the medication during the day (e.g., tid [three times a day])
- How long to take the medication (e.g., 10 days)

The following steps show how to calculate the number of tablets needed for the entire course of medication. Box 45.10 provides practice problems.

Problem: Amoxicillin 500 mg, 1 tab tid po × 10 days. How many tablets would the patient need for the entire course of medication?

BOX 45.10   Number of Tablets Needed for Entire Course Practice Problems

Directions: Calculate the number of tablets the patient will need for the entire time.
1. Prescription: XYZ medication 200 mg, 5 tabs tid × 6 days.
2. Prescription: XYZ medication 250 mg, 3 tabs qid × 14 days.
3. Prescription: XYZ medication 50 mg, 4 tabs bid × 10 days.
4. Prescription: XYZ medication 70 mg, 4 tabs tid × 13 days.
5. Prescription: XYZ medication 120 mg, 3 tabs tid × 12 days.

***Solution for problem.* Step 1:** Figure out the number of tablets per dose. (Use the abbreviation list if you need to. One tab equals 1 tablet.)

Step 2: Figure out the number of tablets taken throughout the day. Do this by multiplying the number of tablets per dose (1 tablet) by the number of times the medication is taken during the day (tid means 3 times a day).

1 tablet per dose × 3 times a day = 3 tablets per day

Step 3: Figure out the number of tablets needed. Multiply the number of tablets per day by the number of days.

3 tablets per day × 10 days = 30 tablets needed

Answer: 30 tablets needed

Number of Tablets per Dose. It is common for the provider to give medication orders without a tablet amount. For instance, the provider orders "Tylenol 975 mg po." The medical assistant must figure out how many tablets to give to the patient for each dose. To start, figure out the number of milligrams in each tablet, which will be indicated on the stock medication label. Once the tablet size is identified, the medical assistant can calculate the number of tablets required.

The following steps show how to calculate the number of tablets needed for the dose (Procedure 45.1). Box 45.11 shows the same problem solved using the formula method. Box 45.12 provides practice problems.

Problem: Order: Tylenol 975 mg po. Stock: Tylenol 325 mg per tablet. How many tablets should be given?

***Solution for problem.* Step 1:** Put the stock information into a fraction on one side. It does not matter the location of the numbers. Make sure to add the labels. (Remember: 325 mg per tablet really means 325 mg in each tablet.)

Stock

$$\frac{325 \text{ mg}}{1 \text{ tab}}$$

Step 2: Add an equals sign and make a fraction on the opposite side. Fill in the labels. The labels need to be in identical locations on both sides of the equals sign.

Stock   **Order**

$$\frac{325 \text{ mg}}{1 \text{ tab}} = \frac{\_\_\_ \text{ mg}}{\text{tab}}$$

BOX 45.11   Number of Tablets per Dose: Formula Method

Problem: Order: Tylenol 975 mg po. Stock: Tylenol 325 mg per tablet. How many tablets should be given?
   The set up for the formula method is the following:

$$\frac{D \text{ (desired)}}{H \text{ (on hand)}} \times V \text{ (vehicle [tablet or liquid])}$$

Step 1: D (desired) is 975 mg. H (on hand) is 325 mg. V (vehicle) is 1 tablet. Put the values into the formula method.

$$\frac{975 \text{ mg}}{325 \text{ mg}} \times V \text{ (vehicle [tablet or liquid])}$$

Step 2: Multiply the problem. Then divide 975 by 325 to figure out the tablet amount.

$$\frac{975 \text{ mg}}{325 \text{ mg}} \times 1 \text{ tablet} = \frac{975}{325}$$

Answer: 3 tablets

BOX 45.12   Number of Tablets per Dose Practice Problems

Directions: Calculate the number of tablets to give.
1. Order: ABC 120 mg po; stock: ABC 80 mg po scored tablet.
2. Order: ABC 150 mg po; stock: ABC 30 mg po scored tablet.
3. Order: ABC 105 mg po; stock: ABC 30 mg po scored tablet.
4. Order: ABC 65 mg po; stock: ABC 130 mg po scored tablet.
5. Order: ABC 210 mg po; stock: ABC 70 mg po scored tablet.

Step 3: Fill in the order information. You do not know the number of tablets, so that is the unknown *(x)*.

Stock   **Order**

$$\frac{325 \text{ mg}}{1 \text{ tab}} = \frac{975 \text{ mg}}{x \text{ tab}}$$

Step 4: Now solve for the unknown.

Using a calculator: Multiply in the diagonal direction of the two numbers (1 × 975) and then divide by the number in the other direction (325); the answer is *x*.

Stock   **Order**

$$\frac{325 \text{ mg}}{1 \text{ tab}} = \frac{975 \text{ mg}}{x \text{ tab}}$$
$$1 \times 975 = 975 \div 325 = 3$$

To solve without a calculator: Multiply diagonally and solve for *x*.

$$1 \times 975 = 325x$$
$$975 = 325x$$
$$\frac{975}{325} = \frac{325x}{325}$$
$$3 = x$$

Answer: 3 tablets

BOX 45.13   Liquid Medication Dose With Matching Labels: Formula Method

Problem: Order: ABC medication 1500 mg. Stock: ABC medication 1300 mg/2 mL. How much medication (in mL) should be given?

The setup for the formula method is the following:

$$\frac{D \text{ (desired)}}{H \text{ (on hand)}} \times V \text{ (vehicle [tablet or liquid])}$$

Step 1: D (desired) is 1500 mg. H (on hand) is 1300 mg. V (vehicle) is 2 mL. Put the values into the formula method.

$$\frac{1500 \text{ mg}}{1300 \text{ mg}} \times 2 \text{ mL}$$

Step 2: Multiply the problem. Then divide 975 by 325 to figure out the amount. Round the answer to the nearest tenth.

$$\frac{1500 \text{ mg}}{1300 \text{ mg}} \times 2 \text{ mL} = \frac{3000}{1300}$$

Answer: 2.3 mL

It is important to double-check your answers. If the order is larger than the stock tablet, then you will be giving more than 1 tablet. If the order is smaller than the stock tablet amount, then you will be giving less than a tablet.

> **VOCABULARY**
>
> **scored tablet** A tablet with a groove on the surface, used for splitting it in half.

Liquid Medication Doses

When preparing a liquid medication, you will see two different units of measure on the bottle label. These two units are the weight of the powdered medications and the volume of liquid. The units typically used include:

- Weight of the powdered medication: units, g, mg, or mcg
- Volume of liquid: cc or mL

For instance, a bottle label states "50 mg/2 mL." This means that there are 50 mg of powdered medication in every 2 mL of liquid. If you want 50 mg of medication, then you would need to give 2 mL of liquid. Another example is 1500 mg/mL. This means that there are 1500 mg of powdered medicine in each milliliter of liquid. Remember that sometimes 1 mL is indicated by just "mL."

Liquid Medication Dose With Matching Labels. If the unit label of ordered medication is the same as the stock medication, then the units are considered to match. For instance, in the following problem the ordered medication dose label is shown in milligrams (mg). The stock medication is 1300 mg/2 mL. The powdered medication label (mg) matches the label on the order.

The following steps show how to calculate the amount of medication needed for a dose when the labels match (see Procedure 45.1). Box 45.13 shows the same problem solved using the formula method. Box 45.14 provides practice problems.

BOX 45.14   Liquid Medication Dose With Matching Labels Practice Problems

Directions: Solve the following problems. Round your answers to the nearest tenth.
1. Order: ABC 3200 units; Stock: ABC 2800 units/mL. How many milliliters will you give?
2. Order: ABC 230 units; Stock: ABC 120 units/mL. How many milliliters will you give?
3. Order: ABC 10 mg; Stock: ABC 25 mg/3 mL. How many milliliters will you give?
4. Order: ABC 45 mg; Stock: ABC 125 mg/mL. How many milliliters will you give?
5. Order: ABC 120 mg; Stock: ABC 280 mg/mL. How many milliliters will you give?
6. Order: ABC 500 mg; Stock: ABC 1200 mg/2 mL. How many milliliters will you give?

Problem: Order: ABC medication 1500 mg. Stock: ABC medication 1300 mg/2 mL. How much medication (in mL) should be given?

Solution for problem. **Set up the problem:** Make sure the label information is on the stock side of the equation. The order is on the opposite side. Remember labels need to be in the same location on both sides of the equals sign.

Step 1: Put the stock information into a fraction. It does not matter the location of the numbers. Make sure to add the labels.

Stock

$$\frac{1300 \text{ mg}}{2 \text{ mL}}$$

Step 2: Put the order information on the other side. Make sure the labels are in the exact same location.

Stock		**Order**
$\dfrac{1300 \text{ mg}}{2 \text{ mL}}$	$=$	$\dfrac{1500 \text{ mg}}{x \text{ mL}}$

Step 3: Now solve for the unknown.

Using a calculator: Multiply in the diagonal direction of the two numbers (2 × 1500) and then divide by the number in the other direction (1300). Round your answer to the nearest tenth.

Stock		**Order**
$\dfrac{1300 \text{ mg}}{2 \text{ mL}}$	$=$	$\dfrac{1500 \text{ mg}}{x \text{ mL}}$

$$2 \times 1500 = 3000 \div 1300 = 2.3 \text{ mL}$$

To solve without a calculator: Multiply diagonally and solve for *x*. Round your answer to the nearest tenth.

$$1300x = 1500 \times 2$$
$$1300x = 3000$$
$$\frac{1300x}{1300} = \frac{3000}{1300}$$
$$x = 2.3 \text{ mL}$$

Answer: 2.3 mL

Liquid Medication Dose With Nonmatching Labels. Sometimes the stock medication's unit of measure does not directly match the order's unit of measure. For instance, the provider may want "ABC 500 mg" to be given. The stock vial indicates "1 g/mL." This might be confusing. The first step is to identify if there is a shared base unit between the order and the stock medication. In this example, they share the same base unit:gram. The second step is to change one of the shared unit labels (e.g., mg and gram) so it matches the other label. Remember that two of the labels need to match before you can solve the problem. Once the labels match, then the problem can be solved like the problems in the prior section.

The following steps show how to calculate the amount of medication needed for a dose when the labels do not match. Box 45.15 provides practice problems.

Problem: Order: ABC medication 1.5 g. Stock: ABC medication 1300 mg/2 mL. How much medication (in mL) should be given?

***Solution for problem.* Step 1:** Identify the two similar base unit labels. In this example, they are 1.5 g and 1300 mg. Essentially, a person could either convert the grams to milligrams or milligrams to grams. This example will show how to convert from grams to milligrams (1.5 g = _____ mg). Set up the problem and solve.

Problem	**Equivalent**
$\dfrac{1.5\ g}{x\ mg}$ =	$\dfrac{1\ g}{1000\ mg}$

$1.5 \times 1000 = 1500 \div 1 = 1500$ mg

Answer: 1500 mg (If it helps, cross out the 1.5 g and write in 1500 mg.)

Step 2: Put the stock information into a fraction. It does not matter the location of the numbers. Make sure to add the labels.

Stock

$$\frac{1300\ mg}{2\ mL}$$

Directions: Solve the following problems. Round your answers to the nearest tenth.
1. Order: ABC 2500 mg; Stock: ABC 2.8 g/2 mL. How many milliliters will you give?
2. Order: ABC 1800 mg; Stock: ABC 2 g/mL. How many milliliters will you give?
3. Order: ABC 1.2 g; Stock: ABC 2500 mg/2 mL. How many milliliters will you give?
4. Order: ABC 450 mg; Stock: ABC 1.2 g/2 mL. How many milliliters will you give?
5. Order: ABC 420 mg; Stock: ABC 1 g/2 mL. How many milliliters will you give?
6. Order: ABC 750 mg; Stock: ABC 1.2 g/2 mL. How many milliliters will you give?
7. Order: ABC 650 mg; Stock: ABC 1.8 g/3 mL. How many milliliters will you give?
8. Order: ABC 400 mg; Stock: ABC 3 g/2 mL. How many milliliters will you give?

Step 3: Put the order information on the other side. Make sure the labels are in the exact same location.

Stock	**Order**
$\dfrac{1300\ mg}{2\ mL}$ =	$\dfrac{1500\ mg}{x\ mL}$

Step 4: Now solve for the unknown.

Using a calculator: Multiply in the diagonal direction of the two numbers (2 × 1500) and then divide by the number in the other direction (1300). Round your answer to the nearest tenth.

Stock	**Order**
$\dfrac{1300\ mg}{2\ mL}$ =	$\dfrac{1500\ mg}{x\ mL}$

$2 \times 1500 = 3000 \div 1300 = 2.3$ mL

To solve without a calculator: Multiply diagonally and solve for *x*. Round your answer to the nearest tenth.

$$1300x = 1500 \times 2$$
$$1300x = 3000$$
$$\frac{1300x}{1300} = \frac{3000}{1300}$$
$$x = 2.3\ mL$$

Answer: 2.3 mL

Solutions

In the ambulatory care environment, many anesthetics used for minor surgeries come in a solution. For instance, a provider asks you to get the strongest Xylocaine vial in the cabinet. You see a 1% and a 2% vial. What does this mean?

When the manufacturer made the medication, the "recipe" called for powdered drug to be mixed with a liquid:

- A 1% solution means 1000 mg of powdered drug is mixed in 100 mL of liquid.
- A 2% solution means 2000 mg of powdered drug is mixed in 100 mL of liquid.

(The 100 mL of liquid always remains, regardless of the number in front of the percentage sign.) Going back to the provider's request, you would give the provider the 2% vial, because it is the strongest solution (or contains the most powdered drug).

Solution Dose. If a medical assistant needs to calculate a dose of medication using a stock solution vial, the process is similar to that used for the prior problems. The initial step would require the medical assistant to change the percent into a fraction. Using a 5% solution as an example, the fraction would be 5000 mg/100 mL. The remaining steps would be the same as for the previous problems.

The following steps show how to calculate the amount of medication needed for a dose when using a solution. Box 45.16 provides practice problems.

BOX 45.16   Solution Dose Practice Problems

Directions: Solve the following problems. Round your answers to the nearest tenth.

1. ABC 60 mg. Stock: ABC 4% solution. How many mL will you give?
2. ABC 80 mg. Stock: ABC 10% solution. How many mL will you give?
3. ABC 30 mg. Stock: ABC 4% solution. How many mL will you give?
4. ABC 70 mg. Stock: ABC 5% solution. How many mL will you give?
5. ABC 120 mg. Stock: ABC 11% solution. How many mL will you give?
6. ABC 50 mg. Stock: ABC 6% solution. How many mL will you give?

BOX 45.17   Pediatric Dose Practice Problems

Directions: Round to the nearest thousandth while solving, then round your answer to the nearest tenth.

1. Patient's weight: 40 lb; Order: ABC medication 0.3 mg/kg; Stock: ABC medication 2 mg/mL. How many milliliters will you give?
2. Patient's weight: 58 lb; Order: ABC medication 0.8 mg/kg; Stock: ABC medication 60 mg/2 mL. How many milliliters will you give?
3. Patient's weight: 145 lb; Order: ABC medication 2 mg/kg; Stock: ABC medication 80 mg/mL. How many milliliters will you give?
4. Patient's weight: 31 lb; Order: ABC medication 0.3 mg/kg; Stock: ABC medication 2 mg/mL. How many milliliters will you give?
5. Patient's weight: 60 lb; Order: ABC medication 0.8 mg/kg; Stock: ABC medication 50 mg/2 mL. How many milliliters will you give?
6. Patient's weight: 86 lb; Order: ABC medication 1.5 mg/kg; Stock: ABC medication 80 mg/2 mL. How many milliliters will you give?

Problem: Order: ABC medication 20 mg. Stock: ABC medication 2% solution. How much medication (in mL) should be given?

Solution for problem. **Step 1:** Change the 2% into a fraction. Tip: Take the number before the percentage sign. Add 3 zeros and mg after it. Then put it over 100 mL.

$$2\% = \frac{2000 \text{ mg}}{100 \text{ mL}}$$

Step 2: Use the fraction created in step 1 as the stock medication.

Stock

$$\frac{2000 \text{ mg}}{100 \text{ mL}}$$

Step 3: Put the order information on the other side. Make sure the labels are in the exact same location.

Stock   **Order**

$$\frac{2000 \text{ mg}}{100 \text{ mL}} = \frac{20 \text{ mg}}{x \text{ mL}}$$

Step 4: Now solve for the unknown.

Using a calculator: Multiply in the diagonal direction of the two numbers (100×20) and then divide by the number in the other direction (2000). Round your answer to the nearest tenth.

Stock   **Order**

$$\frac{2000 \text{ mg}}{100 \text{ mL}} = \frac{20 \text{ mg}}{x \text{ mL}}$$
$$100 \times 20 = 2000 \div 2000 = 1 \text{ mL}$$

To solve without a calculator: Multiply diagonally and solve for *x*. Round your answer to the nearest tenth.

$$2000x = 100 \times 20$$
$$2000x = 2000$$
$$\frac{2000x}{2000} = \frac{2000}{2000}$$
$$x = 1 \text{mL}$$

Answer: 1 mL

Pediatric Dose

As with all medication calculations, it is important to be accurate for the safety of the patient. It is recommended that two

people calculate a dose just to be sure of the accuracy. Know the facility's policies and procedures regarding calculating pediatric doses, because variations may be seen.

Medication dosages for children are typically based on the child's weight. For this type of problem, the medical assistant needs the child's weight, the drug order, and the information on the stock medication label. For instance, a child's weight is 33 pounds (lb), the drug order is ABC medication 0.1 mg/kg, and the stock medication label states "ABC medication 1 mg/mL." Notice that the child's weight is in pounds, and the order is 0.1 mg per every kilogram of weight. The unit of measure for weight is different, one being pounds and the other kilograms.

Step 1: Convert the patient's weight to kilograms. This goes back to converting between the household and metric systems that was discussed earlier in the chapter.

Step 2: Calculate the number of milligrams of medication the child needs. Imagine this scenario: A person tells you that you can have two chocolate bars for each kilogram you weigh. How would you figure it out? A simple way is to multiply the number of kilograms you weigh by 2 ($68 \times 2 = 136$ bars). You can use this same method to calculate the medication order – multiply the kilograms by the order.

Step 3: Calculate the liquid medication dose or the number of milliliters you will give. An example of this step was shown in the Liquid Medication Dose with Matching Labels section.

The following steps show how to calculate the amount of medication for a pediatric patient (see Procedure 45.1). You can modify the steps and use the formula method if you like. Box 45.17 provides practice problems.

Problem: Patient's weight: 33 lb. Order: ABC medication 0.1 mg/kg. Stock: ABC medication 1 mg/mL. How much medication (in mL) should be given?

Solution for problem. **Tip on solving the problem:** There are three main steps to this problem. When you complete a step, round two places beyond your answer. For instance, if your answer is to be in tenths, then during the problem, round to the thousandth (3 places after the decimal). This will ensure accuracy in the answer.

Step 1: Convert the patient's weight into kg. This can be done several ways. Use your favorite method or follow the example and solve for the unknown.

Problem: 33 lb = _____ kg

Problem	Equivalent
$\dfrac{33 \text{ lb}}{x \text{ kg}} =$	$\dfrac{2.2 \text{ lb}}{1 \text{ kg}}$

Using a calculator: Multiply in the diagonal direction of the two numbers (33 × 1) and then divide by the number in the other direction (2.2). Round your answer to the nearest tenth (if needed).

To solve without a calculator: Multiply diagonally and solve for *x*. Round your answer to the nearest tenth (if needed).

$$33 \times 1 = 2.2x$$
$$33 = 2.2x$$
$$\frac{33}{2} = \frac{2.2x}{2}$$
$$15 = x$$

Step 2: Calculate the number of mg of medication needed. Again, there are several ways. The easiest is to multiply the weight by the order (15 kg × 0.1 mg), or you can set it up like the example and solve it. Because this is in the middle of the problem, round to the nearest thousandth (if needed).

Order	Weight
$\dfrac{0.1 \text{ mg}}{1 \text{ kg}} =$	$\dfrac{x \text{ mg}}{15 \text{ kg}}$

$$0.1 \times 15 = 1.5 \div 1 = 1.5 \text{ mg}$$

Updated order: ABC medication 1.5 mg

Step 3: Calculate the liquid medication dose. Put the stock information into a fraction. Put the order information on the other side. Make sure the labels are in the exact same location.

Stock	Order
$\dfrac{1 \text{ mg}}{1 \text{ mL}} =$	$\dfrac{1.5 \text{ mg}}{x \text{ mL}}$

Using a calculator: Multiply in the diagonal direction of the two numbers (1.5 × 1) and then divide by the number in the other direction (1). Round your answer to the nearest tenth (if needed).

To solve without a calculator: Multiply diagonally and solve for *x*. Round your answer to the nearest tenth (if needed).

$$1x = 1 \times 1.5$$
$$1x = 1.5$$
$$\frac{1x}{1} = \frac{1.5}{1}$$
$$x = 1.5 \text{ mL}$$

Answer: 1.5 mL

Using Drug Labels

Now that you have learned how to calculate medications, use the labels to identify how the medication comes and the amount of medication to give.

Problem 1.
Order: Crestor 20 mg po daily.
Available drug (Fig. 45.6):
- How does the medication come?
- How many tablets would you give?

Problem 2.
Order: Amoxicillin 875 mg po
Available drug (Fig. 45.7):
- How does the medication come?
- How many milliliters would you give?

Problem 3.
Order: cefaclor 262 mg po
Available drug (Fig. 45.8):
- How does the medication come?
- How many milliliters much would you give?

Problem 4.
Order: cefprozil 75 mg po
Available drug (Fig. 45.9):
- How does the medication come?
- How many milliliters would you give?

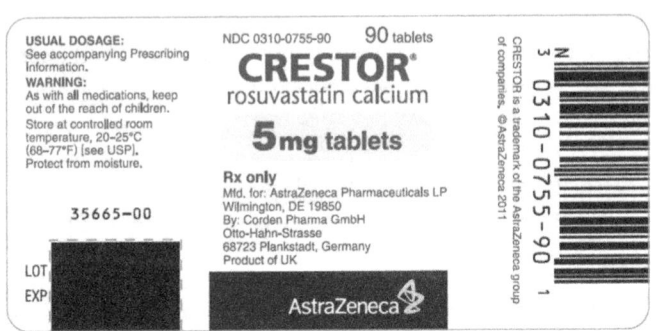

Fig. 45.6 Crestor 5 mg Tabs. (From Kee JL, Marshall SM: *Clinical calculations,* ed 8, St. Louis, 2017, Elsevier.)

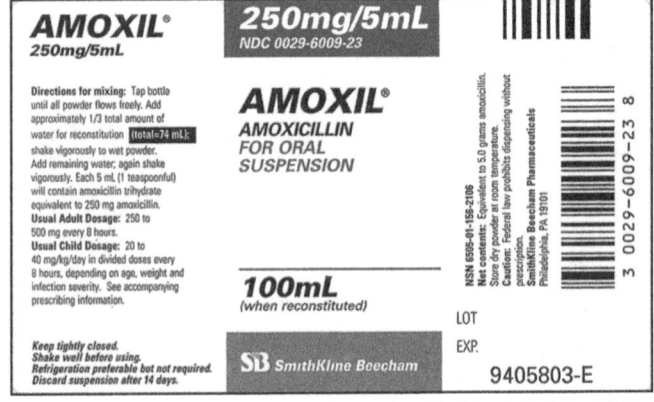

Fig. 45.7 Amoxil 250 mL/5 mL. (From Kee JL, Marshall SM: *Clinical calculations,* ed 8, St. Louis, 2017, Elsevier.)

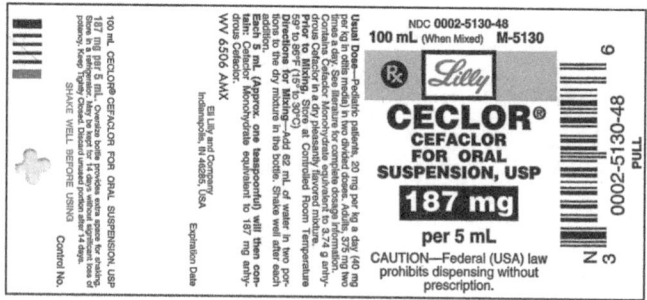

Fig. 45.8 Ceclor 187 mg/5 mL. (From Kee JL, Marshall SM: *Clinical calculations*, ed 8, St. Louis, 2017, Elsevier.)

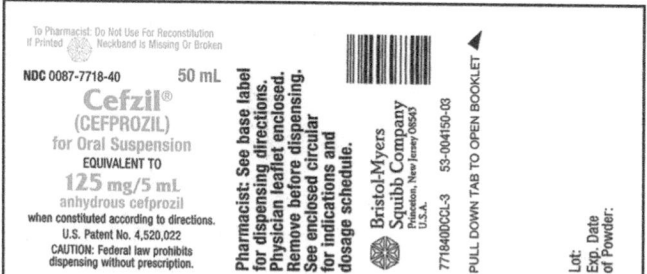

Fig. 45.9 Cefzil 125 mg/5 mL. (From Kee JL, Marshall SM: *Clinical calculations*, ed 8, St. Louis, 2017, Elsevier.)

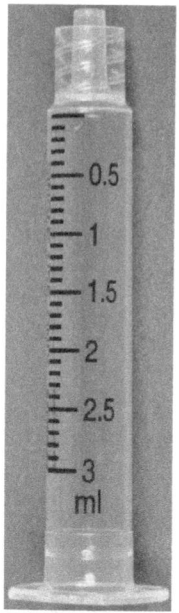

Fig. 45.10 A 3-mL Syringe. (From Niedzwiecki B, et al: *Kinn's the medical assistant*, ed 14, St. Louis, 2020, Elsevier.)

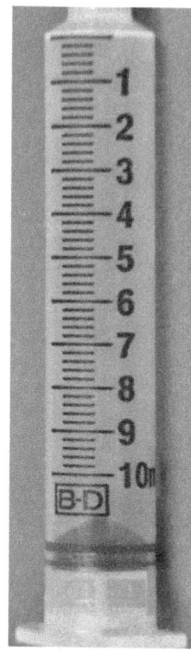

Fig. 45.11 A 10-mL Syringe. (From Niedzwiecki B, et al: *Kinn's the medical assistant*, ed 14, St. Louis, 2020, Elsevier.)

READING SYRINGES

For the safety of patients, it is important that medical assistants be accurate when measuring medications in syringes. Syringes have calibrations printed on the barrel. These markings are used when measuring the medication prior to administration. The calibration markings include longer or darker lines and shorter lines. The first step in reading a syringe is to identify the amount of each calibration line. With many types of syringes, a person should count the number of lines for 1 mL or for 0.1 mL, depending on the syringe.

Fig. 45.10 shows a 3-mL syringe, the most commonly used syringe in ambulatory care. The maximum amount that the syringe can hold is indicated at the bottom of the syringe. To identify what each line is worth, count the lines for 1 mL. For this syringe, there are 10 lines for 1 mL, which means each line is equal to 0.1 mL. Medication amounts to the nearest tenth (one place after the decimal point) can be measured using this syringe.

Fig. 45.11 shows a 10-mL syringe. The calibration markings on this syringe are the same as on most 5-, 6-, 10- and 12-mL syringes. For this syringe, there are 5 lines for 1 mL, which means each line is equal to 0.2 mL. Syringes with this type of calibration can only measure medication ordered in even numbers (e.g., 1.2 mL, 2 mL, 3.6 mL).

Fig. 45.12 shows a 60-mL syringe. The calibration markings are different with this type of syringe. Unlike prior syringes, the numbers labeled are in increments of 5 (e.g., 5, 10, 15). Each line is equal to 1 mL. Syringes with this type of calibration can only measure whole number amounts (e.g., 5, 9,

11). This type of syringe may be used in ambulatory care for irrigation.

Fig. 45.13 shows a 1-mL syringe. The numbers on this syringe are tenths (e.g., .1, .2). For this syringe, there are 10 lines for 0.1 mL, which means each line is equal to 0.01 mL. Syringes with this type of calibration can measure to the hundredth place (e.g., 0.08, 0.09, 0.15). The most common use of these syringes is for tuberculin (TB) skin tests.

If a medication order indicates that 0.14 mL is to be given, the medical assistant should find the calibration marking for 0.1. A trick is to think of 0.1 as 0.10. The next small line would be 0.11, then 0.12, and so on. If a medication order indicates

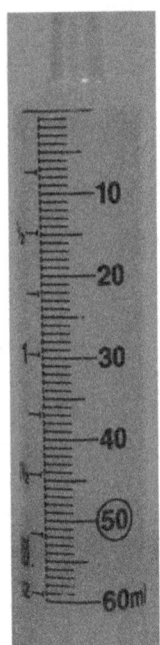

Fig. 45.12 A 60-mL Syringe. (From Niedzwiecki B, et al: *Kinn's the medical assistant*, ed 14, St. Louis, 2020, Elsevier.)

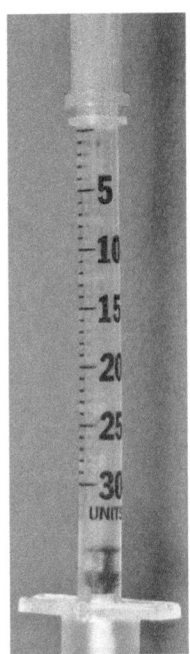

Fig. 45.14 U-100 Insulin Syringe. (From Niedzwiecki B, et al: *Kinn's the medical assistant*, ed 14, St. Louis, 2020, Elsevier.)

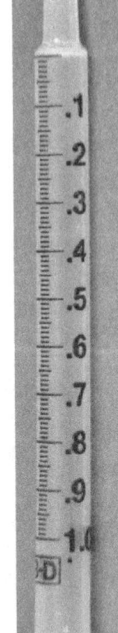

Fig. 45.13 A 1-mL Syringe. (From Niedzwiecki B, et al: *Kinn's the medical assistant*, ed 14, St. Louis, 2020, Elsevier.)

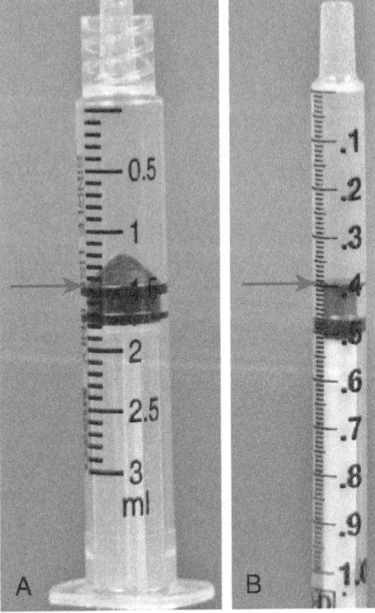

Fig. 45.15 A, The rubber stopper is pointed. B, The rubber stopper is flat.. (From Niedzwiecki B, et al: *Kinn's the medical assistant*, ed 14, St. Louis, 2020, Elsevier.)

that 0.04 mL is to be given, the medical assistant should find the large line at the top of the syringe. This would be 0, and the next little line would be considered 0.01, followed by 0.02, and so on.

Fig. 45.14 shows an insulin syringe. Insulin is measured in units. The calibration markings on this type of insulin syringe are similar to those of the 60-mL syringe. The numbers labeled are in increments of 5 (e.g., 5, 10, 15). Each line is equal to 1 unit. Syringes with this type of calibration can only measure whole number amounts (e.g., 5, 9, 11). This type of syringe may be used in ambulatory care for U-100 insulin administration.

When you use a syringe, the rubber stopper on the plunger indicates the amount in the syringe. Some rubber stoppers are pointed (Fig. 45.15A), and others are flat (Fig. 45.15B). The top of the rubber stopper that touches the barrel is used for measuring. That part of the rubber stopper should be right on the correct calibration mark. The red arrow indicates this location on both rubber stoppers.

CLOSING COMMENTS

Not all states allow medical assistants to calculate medication dosages. It is important for the medical assistant to review the state's scope of practice laws. Some agencies may also have policies and procedures for calculating medication dosages. The medical assistant must follow both the state's scope of practice laws and the agency's policies and procedures.

PATIENT-CENTERED CARE

In some cases, the medical assistant needs to teach patients and parents how to read oral medical syringes. These syringes are used to draw up and administer oral medications, usually to young children. When coaching a patient or parent on using an oral syringe to measure medications, it is important for the medical assistant to refer to the provider's order. If the order states 1 teaspoon, the medical assistant should coach the person that this is the same as 5 mL. Prior to finishing the coaching session, the medical assistant should have the patient or parent draw up (with air) the dose ordered to determine if the person understands the procedure.

BEING PROFESSIONAL

If a medical assistant needs to calculate a medication dosage, it is important to have another qualified staff person recheck the calculations. If a medical assistant forgets how to calculate a medical dosage or has questions regarding the procedure, the medical assistant must talk with the provider for clarification.

Role-play this scenario with a peer: Both of you are medical assistants, and the provider has ordered the following medication to be given to a child:

Patient's weight: 76 lb; Order: ABC medication 1.3 mg/kg; Stock: ABC medication 70 mg/2 mL. How many milliliters will you give? You need to use a 3-mL syringe.

Both you and your peer should solve the problem, and then compare your answers.

CHAPTER REVIEW

Medication labels show the brand name, generic name, strength, total amount or total volume, manufacturer, directions and storage, expiration date, lot number, and the National Drug Code. When preparing medications, the name, strength, and expiration date are important.

Important healthcare rules when writing numbers include the following:

- Follow the number with the correct abbreviation for the unit of measure. Leave a space between the number and the abbreviation. Do not use a period with the abbreviations.
- Write a fraction of a dose as a decimal.
- If the dose is less than 1, place a zero to the left of the decimal point.
- Do not place a decimal point and a zero after a whole number.

When rounding, remember the following:

- 4 or below: drop the number(s) to the right of the place value
- 5 or above: add 1 to the rounded place value and drop the number(s) to the right of the place value.

The household and metric equivalents were discussed, along with temperature conversions. Examples of different types of problems were discussed, including the quantity needed for a specific time period, number of tablets per dose, liquid medication dose with matching labels, liquid medication dose with nonmatching labels, solution dose, and pediatric dose.

When reading syringes, the first step is to identify how much each calibration line is worth.

- If there are 10 lines per 1 mL, each line is equal to 0.1 mL.
- If there are 5 lines per 1 mL, each line is equal to 0.2 mL.
- If there are 10 lines per 0.1 mL, each line is equal to 0.01 mL.
- Insulin syringe calibration lines are usually measured in 1-unit increments.

SCENARIO WRAP-UP

Mark is enjoying working with Gabe. Mark was able to review the different types of commonly used math problems in ambulatory care. Besides working on calculations, Mark and Gabe reviewed syringes. The WMFM Clinic carries 1-mL and 3-mL syringes for medication administration, 5-mL and 10-mL syringes for medication mixing procedures, and 60-mL syringes for wound irrigation procedures. A small box of insulin syringes is also available in case a patient needs insulin administration directions. It took Mark a couple of days to get comfortable measuring medications using the various syringes, but he realized that being accurate when measuring medications is critical to patients' safety.

PROCEDURE 45.1   Calculate Medication Dosages

Tasks

Calculate dosages for oral medication, injectable medication, and children.

Orders

- Order 1: Dr. Martin orders ABC medication 135 mg. Stock bottle reads: 45 mg scored tablets
- Order 2: Dr. Martin orders ABC medication 650 mg. Stock bottle reads: 1300 mg scored tablets
- Order 3: Dr. Martin orders XYZ medication 430 mg IM. Stock vial reads: 1000 mg/2 mL
- Order 4: Dr. Martin orders XYZ medication 680 mg IM. Stock vial reads: 1200 mg/mL
- Order 5: Dr. Martin orders MNO medication 3 mg/kg IM. Child weighs 53 pounds. Stock vial reads: 125 mg/mL
- Order 6: Dr. Martin orders MNO medication 5 mg/kg IM. Child weighs 71 pounds. Stock vial reads: 225 mg/mL

Equipment and Supplies

- Provider's order
- Paper and pencil
- Calculator (optional per instructor)

Procedural Steps

1. Using Order 1, calculate the number of tablets to give the patient. Label your answer.

    Purpose: It is important to label your answer to avoid any mistakes in the dosage.

2. Using Order 2, calculate the number of tablets to give the patient. Label your answer.

3. Using Order 3, calculate the amount in milliliters to give the patient. Round your answer to the nearest tenth. Label your answer.

    Purpose: Most injections are measured in tenths of a milliliter.

4. Using Order 4, calculate the amount in milliliters to give the patient. Round your answer to the nearest tenth. Label your answer.

5. Using Order 5, calculate the amount in milliliters to give the patient. Round your answer to the nearest tenth. Label your answer.

    Note: When working through the problem, round your answer two places beyond your answer. In this situation, round your answers as you work to the thousandth place (or three places after the decimal point).

6. Using Order 6, calculate the amount in milliliters to give the patient. Round your answer to the nearest tenth. Label your answer.

7. Double-check your answers to ensure the correct dose will be given.

    Purpose: When calculating medications, it is important to recheck the work to ensure your answer is correct.

Administering Medication

▶▶ OPENING SCENARIO

Gabe Garcia, CMA (AAMA), has worked for the Walden-Martin Family Medical (WMFM) Clinic for 7 years. He is currently Mark Allen's mentor for practicum. Mark has been working with Gabe for a couple of days. He has learned how Gabe handles prescriptions from the providers. As Mark advances in his practicum, he will be working with Gabe to administer medications to patients. Mark enjoyed practicing injections on his peers in school and looks forward to improving his skills during practicum.

YOU WILL LEARN

1. The nine rights of medication administration.
2. The routes of medications commonly used in the ambulatory care setting.
3. To handle syringes and needles, including uncapping, recapping, and switching needles.
4. To prepare parenteral medications, including using an ampule, prefilled sterile cartridge, and vials; also, reconstituting medication and mixing insulins.
5. Administration techniques for intradermal, subcutaneous, and intramuscular injections.
6. To locate the sites for intradermal, subcutaneous, and intramuscular injections.
7. To administer intradermal, subcutaneous, and intramuscular injections.

INTRODUCTION

Chapter 44 discussed the basics of pharmacology. Chapter 45 discusses pharmacology-related math problems and reading syringes. You will use these skills when administering medications. This chapter discusses administration safety techniques, along with medication forms and routes. The techniques of preparing and administering medications will be the primary focus.

It is important to remember that medications can cause serious harm to patients. It is critical to pay attention to the details when you prepare and administer medications. Preventing errors and providing superior patient care are goals each time medication is given. Administering medication is an important responsibility for healthcare professionals.

State laws vary regarding whether or not medical assistants may administer medications. In some situations, the state law allows medical assistants to administer medications, but the facility's policies do not. It is important for medical assistants to know their state's laws and the facility's policies on medication administration.

NINE RIGHTS OF MEDICATION ADMINISTRATION

Throughout this chapter, administration procedures for various routes will be given. Before learning how to give medications, it is important to understand medication safety rights. Over the

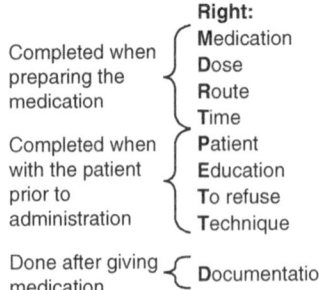

Mnemonic: **M**aybe **D**ogs **R**eally **T**alk, **PET**s **T**ruly **D**o.

Fig. 46.1 Mnemonic for the Nine Rights of Medication Administration.

years the guidelines have grown to include additional steps to address patient education and the right to refuse the medication.

Each time you prepare and give medication, it is important that you follow the nine rights of medication administration. These rights are designed to help you look at the details and avoid making errors during the procedure (Fig. 46.1).

Right Medication

A prescription (or an order) from a provider is required before a medication can be given. As discussed in a prior chapter, orders can be written or verbal. For all verbal orders, make sure to write down the order and read it back to the provider. This helps to ensure the accuracy of the order. The order requires several factors, including the medication's name and *form*. The form is the physical characteristics of a medication, such as a tablet or suspension.

With the order in hand, the medical assistant must prepare the medication. This requires finding the correct medication. Use drug reference information if you are not familiar with the medication listed on the order. Sometimes the provider will give a brand name, but the stock medication will indicate only a generic name. Make sure you have the correct medication, which includes the correct form (e.g., tablet, suppository, suspension).

You will need to check the medication order against the label three times during the preparation process to ensure that you have the correct name and form of medication. You check the label:

- When you get the medication from the storage area (e.g., cabinet, freezer, or refrigerator)
- Before preparing the medication
- Before you return the medication to the storage area

It is important that you do an activity between each check. For instance, after you do the first check, assemble the supplies you need to prepare the medication. Then do the second check. As you clean up your area, you do the third check. Too often we reach for something based on the color, size, or location of the object. We may look at the label and think we see what we want to see. Checking the label three times, with activities between, helps to ensure that you have the right medication.

Right Dose

The dose of medication is on the order. The provider may have written the order in two different ways, even though the amount is the same. For example, both of these orders give the patient 1000 mg:

- Acetaminophen 500 mg, 2 tabs po × 1 dose
- Acetaminophen 1000 mg po × 1 dose

The first order shows the tablet strength (e.g., 500 mg) and the number of tablets (e.g., 2) to give. If the stock medication comes in 500-mg tablets, the medical assistant has no calculations to do. The second order just shows the number of milligrams to give (e.g., 1000 mg). The medical assistant would need to calculate how many tablets to give. (This procedure was discussed in Chapter 45.)

Right Route

Besides checking the label for the name and form of the medication, it is also important to check the route. The *route* is the means by which a drug enters the body. The route of the medication must match the provider's order. The route should be checked, along with the name and form, three times before the medication is given.

Right Time

Medications need to be given at the right time. For most medication orders, the time is part of the order. Some orders are STAT, whereas others are every month. Vaccines are a little different.

Vaccines. There are several types of vaccines:

- *Inactivated vaccines*: The microorganism is dead. Examples of inactivated vaccines include hepatitis A, (injectable) influenza, (injectable) polio, and rabies.
- *Live-attenuated vaccines:* The microorganism is alive but *attenuated* (weakened) in the laboratory. Examples of live virus vaccines include MMR (measles, mumps, and rubella), smallpox, varicella (chickenpox), and yellow fever. Live virus vaccines need to kept cool. Patients may not receive a live-virus vaccine if:
  - They were vaccinated with another live-virus vaccine less than 28 days earlier.
  - They are pregnant or may become pregnant in the next month.
  - They are immunocompromised (e.g., cancer, leukemia, human immunodeficiency virus [HIV] infection).
  - They are receiving chemotherapy or high-dose steroid therapy.
  - They recently received a blood transfusion, immune (gamma) globulin, or antiviral medication.
- *Messenger RNA (mRNA) vaccines:* According to the Centers for Disease Control and Prevention (CDC), the mRNA vaccines cause the cells to make a protein that triggers the immune response, which then causes antibodies to be produced. These antibodies protect the body when it is exposed to the disease. The mRNA COVID-19 vaccines are examples of this type of vaccine (Box 46.1).
- *Subunit, recombinant, polysaccharide, and conjugate vaccines:* Use specific pieces of the microorganism, which creates a very strong immune response. Examples of these types of vaccines include Hib (Haemophilus influenzae type b), hepatitis B, HPV (human papillomavirus), pertussis, pneumococcal,

meningococcal, and shingles (Shingrix). These vaccines can be used by people with weakened immune systems. HPV is contraindicated with pregnancy.

- *Toxoid vaccines:* Use the toxin made by the microorganism. Examples of toxoid vaccines include diphtheria and tetanus.
- *Viral vector vaccines*: Use a modified version of a different virus as a vector to deliver protection. The COVID-19 vaccine is an example of this type of vaccine (see Box 46.1).

Timing for vaccines may not be written on the provider's order, but the medical assistant should ensure that it is the correct time for a vaccine to be given. The timing of a vaccine is based on the patient's vaccination history and the person's age. Using immunization schedules or the immunization tables in electronic health records (EHRs), the medical assistant can determine what vaccines are due. The immunization schedule indicates the person's age and the timing between doses. If a vaccination is administered too early or before the patient reaches a specific age, the patient will have to be revaccinated.

The provider will postpone vaccinations when patients have a moderate or severe acute illness. Specific vaccines are not given if a person has had a severe allergic reaction to a vaccine component, to latex, or to a prior dose.

Consult the CDC website for information on vaccine schedules and catch-up schedules (https://www.cdc.gov/vaccines/index.html). The CDC also offers a free app that provides vaccine information.

BOX 46.1 Vaccines to Prevent COVID-19

In December 2020, the U.S. Food and Drug Administration (FDA) issued an Emergency Use Authorization (EUA) to permit the emergency use of two unapproved messenger RNA (mRNA) vaccines for COVID-19. In February 2021, the FDA issues an EUA for a third vaccine, a viral vector vaccine. This vaccine uses an adenovirus to help the body create antibodies to protect against the disease. In 2021, the FDA approved Comirnaty (koe MIR na tee), a vaccine to prevent COVID-19.

Pfizer-BioNTech COVID-19 Vaccine: This mRNA vaccine is given as an intramuscular (IM) injection. The series consists of 2 doses spaced 3 weeks apart. The vials are frozen and must be thawed and stored in the refrigerator before use. The vaccine must be diluted with 0.9% Sodium Chloride Injection, USP prior to administration. Do not use bacteriostatic 0.9% Sodium Chloride injection or any other diluent. The vials should be protected from direct sunlight and ultraviolet light. The vaccine will be an off-white suspension. Do not use if the vaccine is discolored or contains particulate matter.

Moderna COVID-19 Vaccine: This mRNA vaccine is given as an intramuscular (IM) injection. The series consists of 2 doses spaced 1 month apart. The vials are frozen and must be thawed before administering. The thawed vials are refrigerated before use, and the vial should stand at room temperature for 15 minutes before administering. The suspension is whitish in color and may contain white or translucent particulates. Do not give the vaccine if the suspension or particulates are discolored.

Janssen COVID-19 Vaccine: This viral vector vaccine is given as a single intramuscular dose. The vaccine is refrigerated and should not be frozen. Protect the vials from light. The vaccine is clear, colorless to slightly yellow. Do not administer the vaccine if it is discolored or contains particulate matter.

See package inserts for more information on storage, administration, dosage, contraindications, and adverse effects of the vaccine. Clinical research continues with these vaccines. For the latest information, see: https://www.fda.gov/consumers/consumer-updates/learn-more-about-covid-19-vaccines-fda.

Right Patient

Before you administer the medication, it is important to correctly identify the patient. Ask patients or parents/guardians to state their full name and date of birth. Some agencies require patients to spell their last names. Verify the information against the order and the patient's health record. All three must match. Any differences must be resolved before the medication is given.

In some agencies, patients are given identification bracelets that are scanned before medication is given. The medication is also scanned. An automatic entry is made in the EHR. This is a common practice in hospitals and is starting to be used in ambulatory care facilities. The identification process with bracelets still requires asking the patient's name and date of birth. The information is checked against the bracelet and the order.

CRITICAL THINKING 46.1

Gabe is introducing Mark to the facility's medication procedures. Gabe encourages Mark to have the patients give their complete name and date of birth. He also tells Mark it is a good idea to have the patients spell their last names. Why is spelling the last name an important safety check?

Right Education

Before administering the medication to the patient, the medical assistant must:

1. Give the patient the name of the medication and who ordered it. For example, "Dr. Martin ordered acetaminophen for your fever."
2. Explain the desired effect or action of the medication. For example, "The acetaminophen will bring down your fever."
3. Describe common side effects of the medication. For example, "The acetaminophen may cause nausea, rash, and a headache."
4. Verify the patient's allergies.

If the patient is receiving a vaccination, the facility may require a questionnaire to be completed. The medical assistant may need to give a Vaccine Information Statement (VIS) prior to administering the vaccine. The VIS provides important information to the patient about the vaccine and common and uncommon side effects. The National Childhood Vaccine Injury Act requires that all patients (or parents/guardians) get the appropriate VIS prior to every dose of vaccine administered, regardless of the age of the patient. The specific list of vaccines that require the VIS are listed on the website of the CDC: https://www.cdc.gov/vaccines/hcp/vis/about/facts-vis.html.

The VIS can be displayed on a computer screen or as a laminated copy that the patient can read prior to administration of the vaccine. Copies of the VIS can be given to the patient or parent/guardian to take home. The provider must offer the information; however, the patient or parent/guardian has the right to decline to take the document. If the patient cannot read, the medical assistant should review the VIS with the patient. VISs can be downloaded in about 40 different languages for patients who do not speak English.

Besides giving the patient or parent/guardian the VIS prior to the vaccination, the medical assistant must document the following in the patient's health record:

- The edition date of the VIS. This is found on the back of the document in the bottom right corner. Make sure to have the latest edition of the VIS.
- The date the VIS was provided and the date the vaccine was administered (usually the two are done on the same day).
- The office address, name, and title of the person who administered the vaccine.
- The vaccine's manufacturer and lot number.

CRITICAL THINKING 46.2

Part of the WMFM Clinic's policy is to explain to patients what was ordered and why they are getting it. Why is it important to tell patients the name of a medication or procedure and the reason it has been prescribed? How might this add to patient-centered care?

Right to Refuse

The patient or the person legally responsible for the patient (e.g., parent, guardian) has a right to refuse any medication. If a patient refuses the medication, the medical assistant should respect the patient's wishes. Do not pressure the patient. Notify the provider that the ordered medication was refused and specify the reason if it was shared. Document the refusal of the medication and identify the provider who was informed. The provider will talk with the patient regarding other options.

Right Technique

When administering the medication, the medical assistant must give it in the right way. This may include an assessment before the medication is administered. Examples of right technique include:

- Obtain vital signs before giving a specific medication. For instance, digoxin must be withheld if an adult's pulse is under 60.
- Obtain information about the patient's pain level before giving an analgesic medication. The medical assistant can ask the patient to rate the pain using a 0 to 10 scale. Zero is no pain, and 10 is the worst pain ever. Another pain assessment tool is the Wong-Baker FACES Pain Rating Scale, which is discussed in Chapter 34. The medical assistant should explain the scale to patients. Then patients can indicate how they feel. This scale works well for children.
- Some medications must be taken with food and others with a full glass of water. Medications that need to be taken on an empty stomach need to be taken 1 hour before meals or 2 hours after meals.

Information regarding the techniques to use when administering the medication can be found in drug reference information.

Right Documentation

After giving a medication, the medical assistant must document it in the patient's health record. If the medication is not documented, it will appear to others as though it were not given. The documentation will vary based on what the patient received. Some documentation is done in narrative form, whereas vaccines are documented on paper or in electronic vaccination forms. Elements that should be in the documentation include:

- Provider ordering the medication
- Assessment done (e.g., vital signs or pain level)
- Allergies
- Coaching/instructions given to patient (includes the edition date of the VIS for vaccine teaching)
- Name of medication (e.g., acetaminophen)
- Dose given (e.g., 650 mg)
- Route given (e.g., po)
- Lot number, expiration date, and manufacturer (usually only required for vaccines and controlled substances)
- How the patient tolerated the medication
- Additional information as needed (e.g., patient is resting on exam table)
- Signature if the note is handwritten (an EHR uses automatic signatures for documentation entries)

ROUTES OF MEDICATIONS

For drug administration, the route is how a drug enters the body. As discussed in a prior chapter, the dose of medication can differ based on the route. The following sections discuss common routes of medication. There are many other routes that are not commonly used in the ambulatory care environment.

Oral Route

Medications taken by the oral route (po) are those we take by mouth (Procedure 46.1). Special administration techniques may be required for oral medications. These may include:

- Oral medications that coat the mouth or throat should not be immediately followed with water.
- Oral medications that require water for swallowing call for more than a sip. Some medications require a glass of water after taking the medication.
- A straw should be used for liquid medications that stain the teeth.
- Liquid medications should be measured only with a plastic medication cup or an oral medication syringe. Household measuring devices, such as spoons, are not accurate.

It is important to notify the provider if the patient is unable to take the medication due to nausea, vomiting, or problems swallowing. Do not attempt to see if the patient can swallow the pill. It is better to talk with the provider if the patient is concerned. Some medications can be crushed safely, whereas others cannot. The following discussion covers crushing medications.

Crushing Medication. Children, older adults, and others may have problems swallowing solid medications. Crushing medications is sometimes an option. The medication should be placed in a small amount of food or liquid (e.g., pudding or jam). It is important to eat or drink all the food or liquid to get the entire dose of medication.

Solid medications typically have an unpleasant taste. It is important to share with parents that children sometimes shy away from foods with an unpleasant taste. For instance, if a parent mixes the medication with the milk in a bottle, the baby may not want to drink the milk. This can be a problem if the baby drinks only milk.

Medications that cannot be crushed include:

- *Slow-* or *extended-release tablets*: Crushing, chewing, or cutting the tablet can cause a person to get the dose faster than they should, resulting in an overdose.
- *Enteric-coated tablets*: Crushing, chewing, or cutting the tablet causes the protective nature of the coating to be lost. The person could have more stomach distress.

CRITICAL THINKING 46.3

Gabe and Mark are working with Charles Johnson, who has a temperature of 103.4°F (39.7°C). The provider orders acetaminophen 500 mg, 2 tabs po for the patient. Mr. Johnson tells Gabe and Mark that he cannot swallow pills. Can they give him liquid acetaminophen, or must they talk with the provider first about the situation?

Sublingual and Buccal Routes

Sublingual (sub LING gwehl) (SL) medications are placed under the tongue. *Buccal* (BUK ahl) medications are placed between the cheek and the gums. Both mucous membrane areas are rich in blood vessels. The medication is absorbed rapidly into the bloodstream. Special administration techniques may be required for SL and buccal medications. These may include:

- Do not eat or smoke prior to taking SL and buccal medications.
- Do not chew or swallow SL or buccal medications.
- Water can be taken prior to the medication to wet the mouth. No liquids can be taken until the medication has dissolved.
- Alternate cheeks used for buccal medication to avoid mucosal irritation.

Transdermal Route

Transdermal (trans DUHR mahl) *medications* are placed on the skin and absorbed into the bloodstream. Transdermal medications are different from topical medications, which provide a local action. Transdermal medications provide a systemic action. The transdermal drug delivery system uses patches that adhere to the skin (Fig. 46.2). Medication in the patch is slowly absorbed through the skin. Depending on the medication, the patch may be worn for a part of a day to many days.

When replacing a patch or teaching a patient to use transdermal patches, follow these steps:

1. Write the date and time on the new patch.
2. Wear disposable gloves if changing a patch on another person.
3. Remove the old patch. Fold the sticky sides together and discard. If the old patch is not removed, the person may be at risk for an overdose.
4. Remove any residual medication from the skin using a tissue.
5. Decide where to apply the new patch. Select a different location. Depending on the medication, it may be on the shoulder, back, upper arm, lower abdomen, or hip. Clean and dry the new site.

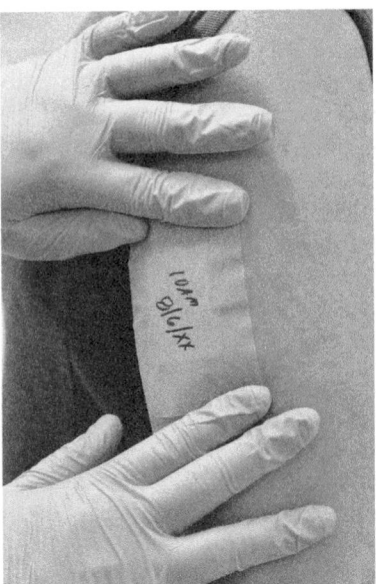

Fig. 46.2 Transdermal Patch.

6. Remove the protective liner on the patch. Do not use torn patches. Do not touch the sticky side of the patch.
7. Place the patch's sticky side on the skin. Press down on the patch to ensure it adheres to the skin. Make sure the patch is smooth, without folds.

MEDICAL TERMINOLOGY	
sub-	under
trans-	through
-al	pertaining to

> **VOCABULARY**
> **local** Affecting the area where applied.
> **systemic** Affecting the entire body.

Inhalation Route

Medications for the nose, throat, and lungs can be inhaled. The small particles of medication are aerosolized (AR oh sol eye zed) in a fine mist. The medication is inhaled and reaches the mucous membrane or alveoli in the lungs, where it is absorbed. Metered-dose inhalers (MDIs) and nebulizers (NEB you lize ehrs) are common devices for inhaled drugs. Many nebulized medications come in a premixed solution. If the medication is not premixed, normal saline is usually recommended to dilute the medication. (Chapter 48 discusses MDIs and nebulizers.)

Topical Route

Applying a drug to a mucous membrane or the skin is considered use of the *topical route*. Absorption through the mucous membrane is usually faster than through the skin. Topical medications provide a local effect.

Many times, when a drug is ordered to be applied "topically," it means that it should be applied to the skin. Topical drugs may also be administered by other routes. The provider will indicate a more specific route, such as rectal, vaginal, ophthalmic, nasal, or optic, for these medications.

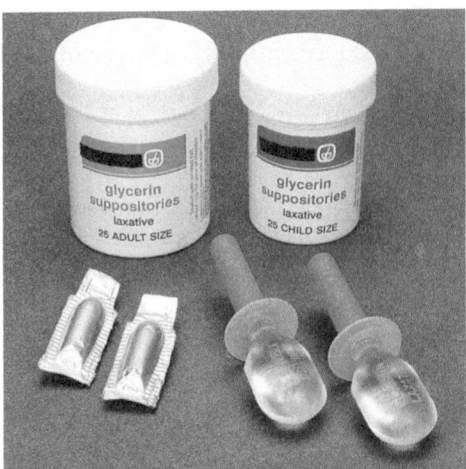

Fig. 46.3 Rectal Suppositories and Enemas.

When the medical assistant applies a topical medication to a patient's skin, it is important to:
- Wear gloves.
- Use a sterile applicator (tongue blade or swab) to remove medication from the container. To keep the container sterile, a new sterile applicator must be used each time.
- Rub creams gently into the skin, pat lotions onto the skin, and apply ointment using a sterile applicator.
- Liniments must be rubbed into the skin.
- For aerosol topical sprays, hold the bottle 3 to 6 inches from the skin and spray.

Vaginal Route

The vaginal route is used to insert suppositories, tablets, creams, and foams into the vagina. Typically, vaginal medications are used to treat local infections. Most medications can be inserted using the accompanying applicator. If no applicator is available, the patient should insert medications as is done with suppositories, using a finger. Usually, the medication must be inserted about 3 to 4 inches.

Vaginal instillation is most effective if the patient remains lying down after administration to prevent leakage. Many medications are intended to be used at bedtime. The patient may need to wear a pad to absorb drainage.

Rectal Route

Rectal medications are inserted into the rectum. Suppositories and enemas are the most common forms of rectal medications (Fig. 46.3). The medication is absorbed slowly and irregularly through the rectal mucous membrane. This route is useful when a patient cannot tolerate oral medications or if the patient is constipated. It is important for the medical assistant to remind patients to give both the enema and suppository time to work before using the bathroom.

Sometimes a medical assistant needs to teach a patient about inserting suppositories. It is helpful for the patient to know what supplies are needed and where the supplies can be purchased. Supplies required include the suppository, disposable gloves, and water-soluble jelly (KY jelly). Encourage the patient to review the storage directions for the suppositories. The following tips are helpful for inserting a suppository:

- Remove the wrapping from the suppository.
- Lubricate the pointed part of the suppository with water-soluble jelly.
- Be in the side-lying position, with the knee drawn up toward the chest.
- Carefully insert the suppository pointed side first.
- For adults and older children: Use the gloved index finger to push the medication in. Both vaginal and rectal suppositories should be inserted about 3 to 4 inches. Have the person slowly breathe to help with the discomfort.
- For small children: Use the gloved little finger to insert the medication. Rectal suppositories should be advanced about 2 inches.

> ### CRITICAL THINKING 46.4
>
> Gabe and Mark are working with Jana Green. She needs to have an intestinal procedure performed. To prepare, she needs to give herself an enema at home prior to the procedure. Why is it important for Gabe and Mark to provide her with information on how to do the procedure and where to purchase the supplies?

Nasal Route

Drugs given via the nasal route are breathed in through the nose. The medication is absorbed through the nasal mucous membrane. The medication can have local or systemic effects. If the medical assistant is administering the nasal medication, it is important to wear gloves. Patients should blow their nose prior to receiving the medication. They should sit in an upright position. The patient should sniff when the medication is given. Intranasal medications should be charted as "intranasal."

Ocular Route

Medication may be *instilled* (poured drop by drop) into the eye to treat an infection, soothe irritation, anesthetize the eye, or dilate the pupils before examination or treatment. Ophthalmic (of THAL mik) medications are available in different forms. Liquid drops usually are supplied in small squeeze bottles. The tip allows one drop at a time to be administered. Other bottles may have a dropper that is used to administer the medication. Eye ointments come in small metal or plastic tubes. The tip allows a small ribbon of ointment to be administered along the inner lower eyelid margin (Procedure 46.2).

When instilling eye medications, avoid injuring the eye. Do not touch the eye with the tip or applicator. Always keep the tip or applicator sterile. If it gets contaminated, discard the container.

Otic Route

Ear conditions can cause pain and make hearing difficult. Medication may be instilled into the ear to treat infection or inflammation or to soften cerumen. Procedure 46.3 describes how to administer ear drops. It is important to ensure that the ear drops get into the external canal.

Irrigation Route

As recommended by the Food and Drug Administration (FDA), irrigation is also a route of administration. *Irrigation* means to bathe or flush open wounds or body cavities. Irrigation can be used to remove foreign bodies or debris. It can also be used to bathe the area with medication. Wound, eye, and ear irrigations are commonly seen in ambulatory care settings.

Eye irrigation is done to remove foreign bodies or to flush irritants (e.g., chemicals) from the eye (Procedure 46.4). Irrigation equipment can vary and may include a normal saline intravenous (IV) bag and tubing, prepackaged eye irrigation, or a bulb syringe and sterile normal saline fluid.

Irrigation of the external auditory canal will do the following:

- Remove excessive or impacted cerumen (Procedure 46.5). Often ear drops are used to soften impacted cerumen. Softening the cerumen usually means that less time will be needed for irrigating, which lessens the patient's discomfort.
- Remove a foreign body (contraindicated if the item will absorb fluid, such as a bean, pea, or corn kernel).
- Treat the inflamed ear with an antiseptic solution.

Irrigation of the ear can be difficult for some patients to experience. Use sterile irrigation fluid to reduce the risk of infection. Warm the fluid to body temperature. Studies have shown that lukewarm fluid is better tolerated than room temperature fluid. Monitor the patient during the procedure. Should the patient have problems, stop the procedure and talk with the provider. Ear irrigation should not be done if the tympanic membrane is perforated or if an infection or tympanic tube is present.

There are several ear irrigation systems on the market. Ear irrigation equipment can include:

- A large syringe and a container of fluid; it is important to regulate the flow of solution into the ear. Too much air or solution from the syringe can cause discomfort for the patient.
- Systems that connect to a faucet and have flow regulators.
- A spray bottle system (e.g., the Elephant Ear Wash System) and similar systems, which are economical and safe (Fig. 46.4).

> ### CRITICAL THINKING 46.5
>
> Aaron Jackson comes in with a dried pea stuck in his ear. Mark is excited to do an ear irrigation, but Gabe tells Mark that the provider may not order irrigation. Why might irrigation not be ordered for foreign bodies that can absorb fluid?

Parenteral Route

The *parenteral* (pa REN tehr ahl) *route* involves administration by infusion, injection, or implantation. In the ambulatory care environment, injections and infusions are common. Vaccine administration in primary care settings (e.g., family practice and internal medicine) is a frequent duty of medical assistants. Types of injections performed by medical assistants include the following:

- *Intramuscular* (IM): Administration within a muscle
- *Subcutaneous* (subcut): Administration beneath the skin
- *Intradermal* (ID): Administration within the dermis

The rest of the chapter will focus on the parenteral route. The following topics are discussed: injection supplies, medication preparation, site location, and medication administration.

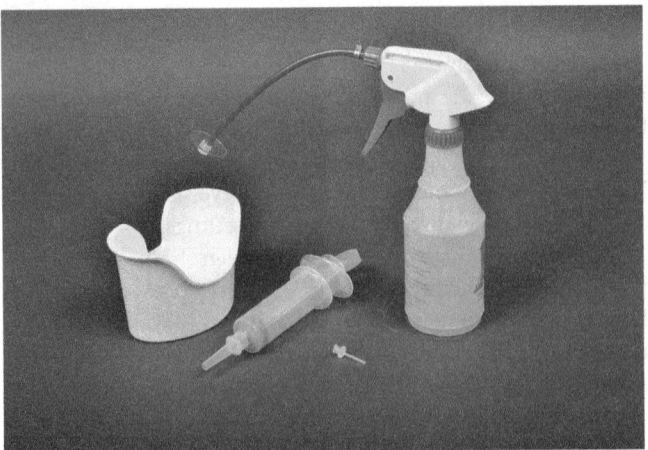

Fig. 46.4 *Left to right:* Ear basin, large syringe, and spray bottle system (disposable tip and spray bottle).

Chapter 47 discusses intravenous (IV) infusions and the role of the medical assistant. An *intravenous infusion* means fluid and medications are administered into a vein.

MEDICAL TERMINOLOGY	
derm/o, cutane/o	skin
hypo	under
muscul/o	muscle
ven/o	vein
intra-	within
-ic, -ous, -al	pertaining to

NEEDLES AND SYRINGES

Hypodermic Needles

A hypodermic needle attaches to a hypodermic syringe. Hypodermic needles come with syringes or are packaged separately. The entire needle needs to remain sterile for the injection. It is important for the medical assistant to know the parts of the needle (Fig. 46.5). The parts of a hypodermic needle include:
- *Hub*: Attaches or screws onto the syringe
- *Hilt*: Where the needle attaches
- *Bevel*: Slanted end of the shaft
- *Lumen* (LOO muh n): Hollow space inside the needle; the size is indicated by the *gauge* (geyj) number

Gauge and Length. Each needle has two measurements: the gauge (G) and the length. The lumen size is indicated by the gauge and is given a numeric value. The higher the gauge number, the smaller the lumen. The thickness of the needle wall increases along with the lumen size. This means that an 18 G needle makes a larger hole than a 25 G needle. The 18 G needle has a thicker wall than the 25 G needle. As the gauge number increases, the needles bend more easily. Thicker-walled needles (smaller gauge numbers) are used for deeper injections. Thinner-walled needles (larger gauge numbers) are used for more superficial injections.

The medication's viscosity (vi SKOS i tee) is also an important factor when selecting the gauge of the needle. A medication

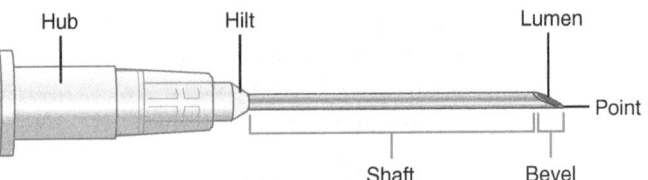

Fig. 46.5 Parts of a Hypodermic Needle. (From Niedzwiecki B, et al: *Kinn's the medical assistant*, ed 14, St. Louis, 2020, Elsevier.)

with a syrupy thickness (high viscosity) would be harder to push out of a needle compared with a medication as thin as water. Using a wider lumen needle (smaller gauge number) would be better for thicker medications. Using a finer lumen needle (a larger gauge number) would be more appropriate for watery medications.

The needle length refers to the length of the shaft. The needle length used is dependent on the type of injection given and the size of the patient. The length of the needle for an intradermal injection is smaller than that used for an intramuscular injection. The length of an intramuscular injection needle for a 300-pound person would be longer than that for a 100-pound person. Knowing the length and gauge required for an injection are important information for the medical assistant.

> **VOCABULARY**
> **viscosity** Resistance to flow; the thicker the liquid, the higher the viscosity.

Safety Needles. Due to the Needlestick Safety and Prevention Act, safety needles are common in the ambulatory care setting. Safety needles are designed to reduce the risk of needlesticks after an injection. A *passive safety needle* is designed so that the needle is automatically covered after the injection. Passive safety needles are currently used with insulin pens (e.g., the BD AutoShield Duo pen needle). An *active safety needle* requires the healthcare professional to activate the safety device. These are most common for injections. Current active safety needles fall into two groups:
- *Protective sheaths and hinged needle shields*: The safety device is a sleeve over the syringe barrel or a hinged needle shield (Fig. 46.6). These devices are moved over the needle after the injection. Once they are in place, the needle cannot be uncovered. The risk of needlesticks decreases if the safety device is activated with the hand holding the syringe.
- *Retractable needles*: After the injection, the healthcare professional activates a device that retracts the needle either into the syringe or into another chamber (Fig. 46.7).

Hypodermic Syringes

Hypodermic syringes attach to needles and hold the medication for the injection. They come in many sizes (e.g., 1, 3, 5, 6, 10, and 12 mL), but usually the facility only stocks three or four sizes (Fig. 46.8). Fig. 46.9 shows the parts of the syringe. Syringes can have either a Luer-Lok tip or a slip tip (Fig. 46.10). Calibration marks are on the barrel of the syringe. It is important for the medical assistant to be able to read medication amounts in syringes.

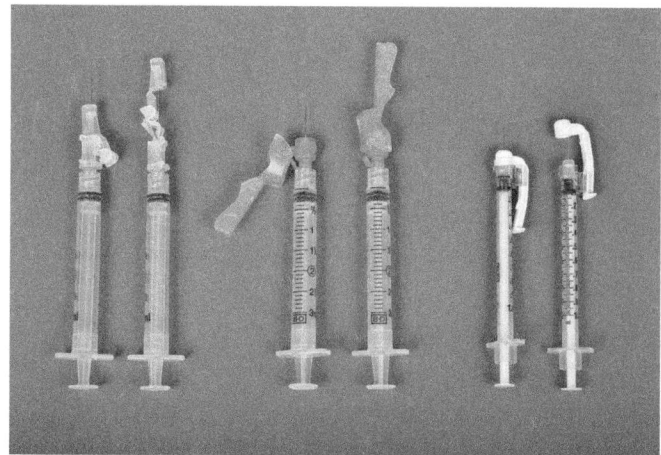

Fig. 46.6 Protective sheaths and hinged needle shields must be activated by the healthcare professional. Each type of needle is shown before the injection and after the safety device has been activated.

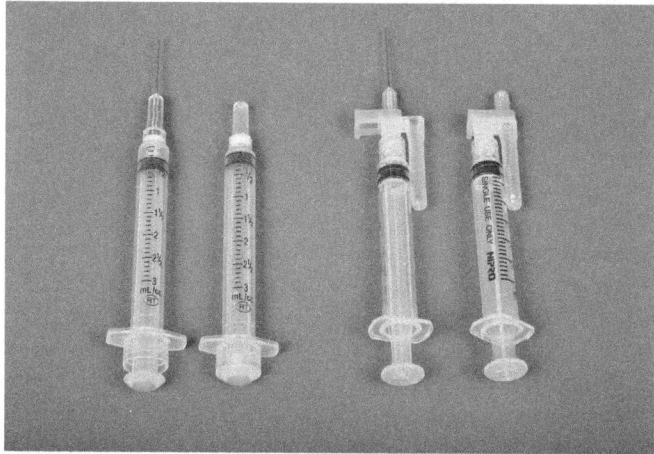

Fig. 46.7 With retractable needles, the needle is retracted into the syringe or another chamber. Each type of needle is shown before the injection and after the needle has been retracted.

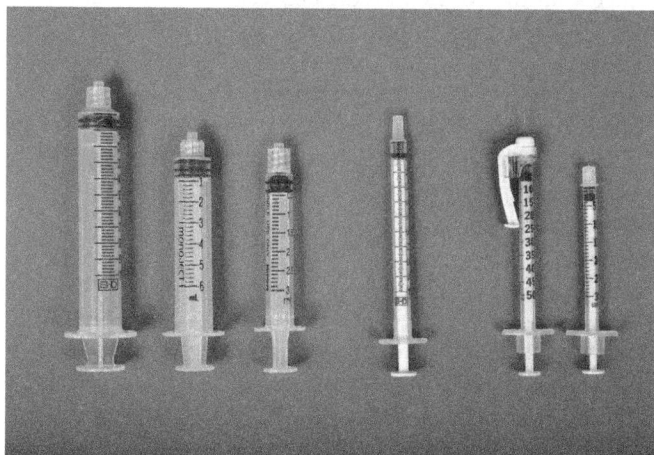

Fig. 46.8 Syringes come in various sizes. Some come with the needles attached.

Working With the Needle and Syringe

Syringes come packaged in different ways:

- A syringe can be packaged by itself. A needle must be added to the syringe when giving an injection.

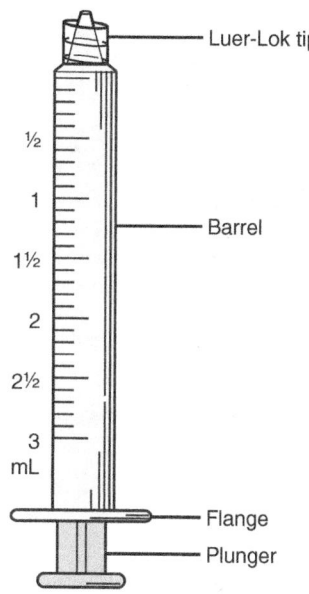

Fig. 46.9 Parts of a Syringe. (From Niedzwiecki B, et al: *Kinn's the medical assistant,* ed 14, St. Louis, 2020, Elsevier.)

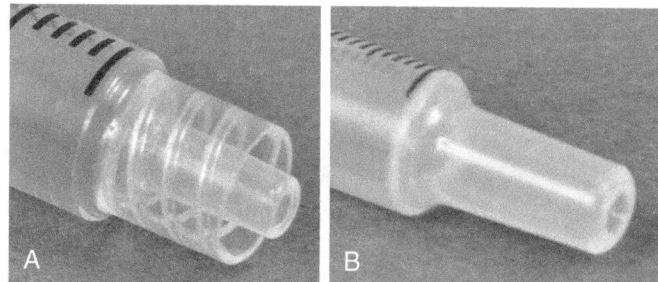

Fig. 46.10 A, Luer-Lok. B, Slip tip.

- A syringe may be packaged with a needle. The unit must be assembled.
- A syringe and needle unit may come preassembled. Always tighten the needle on the syringe before using the unit.

The needle and syringe can be assembled with clean, ungloved hands.

When a syringe is packaged by itself, first open the syringe. When removing the syringe from the packaging, it is important not to touch the syringe tip to anything (Fig. 46.11A). The tip needs to remain sterile because it attaches to the needle. The syringe should be held until the needle is attached. As you are holding the syringe, use your fingers to open the needle package (Fig. 46.11B). It is important to hold down the packaging flaps to prevent contamination of the needle. Attach the syringe to the needle and lift the needle out of the package (Fig. 46.11C). The needle and syringe unit can be placed on the counter. The needle cover should remain on to protect the sterility of the needle.

When the needle and syringe are packaged together but not assembled, carefully open the packaging. Hold down the packaging flaps. Angle the contents so the syringe can be grasped without going over or touching the needle (Fig. 46.12A). Remove the syringe, then attach it to the needle

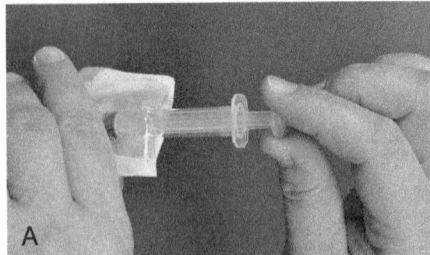
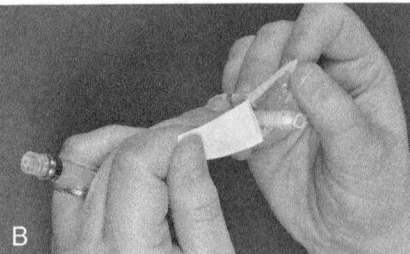
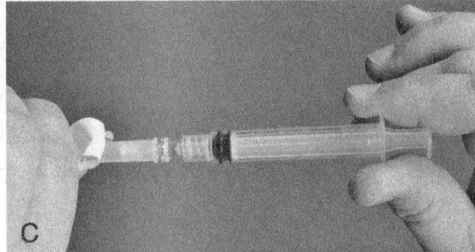

Fig. 46.11 A, When removing the syringe from the packaging, touch only the flange or barrel. B, Place the syringe between your fingers with the tip facing away from your fingers. Then open the needle package. C, Hold down the packaging flaps to prevent contamination of the needle. Attach the syringe.

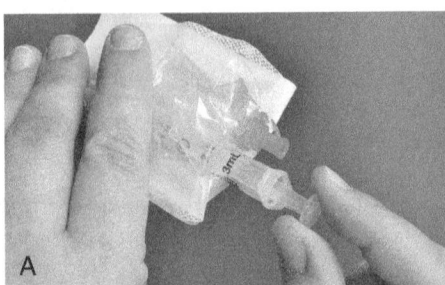
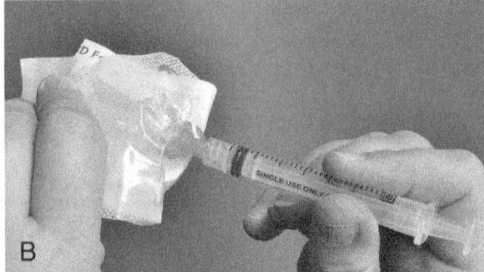

Fig. 46.12 A, Remove the syringe without touching the needle. B, Continue to hold down the packaging flaps and attach the needle to the syringe.

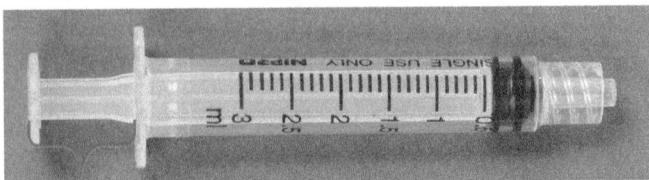

Fig. 46.13 Touch only the part of the plunger that is outside of the barrel.

(Fig. 46.12B). Remove the needle from the packaging. Once the syringe and needle are assembled, the unit can be placed on the counter.

When working with the plunger, only touch the section that remains outside of the syringe when the plunger is completely pushed in (Fig. 46.13). Touching the plunger that goes inside the barrel could potentially contaminate the medication.

Uncapping and Recapping Needles. Never recap a needle that has been used on a patient. Needles can be recapped until they are used on a patient. As you prepare medication, you will need to uncap and recap the needle. It is important to maintain the sterility of the needle. If there is any doubt, consider the needle contaminated and replace it with a new one.

- *To uncap*: Hold the cover between the fingers and thumb of your nondominant hand. Hold the syringe with the fingers and thumb of your dominant hand. Pull your hands apart horizontally (side to side) in a smooth continuous motion (Fig. 46.14A).
- *To recap*: Use the one-handed scoop technique. Place the cover on a firm, flat surface. If the cover rolls, place a finger of your nondominant hand at the far end of the cover. This will keep the cover in place. Carefully insert the needle into the cover. If the needle touches the outside surface of the

cover or any other surface, it is contaminated and must be replaced. Scoop up the cover and secure the cover onto the needle (Fig. 46.14B).

Switching Needles. When switching needles, it is important not to give yourself a needlestick and to protect the sterility of the new needle. Several methods are used to switch needles. One method includes opening the new needle package. Hold the packaging flaps down with the index finger and thumb of your nondominant hand. With your dominant hand, place the syringe with the covered needle between the middle and ring fingers of your nondominant hand (Fig. 46.15A). Firmly grasp the covered needle in your palm. The syringe should be above the top of your hand. With your dominant hand, remove the syringe from the old needle and attach it to the new needle (Fig. 46.15B–C). Your nondominant hand should be holding both needles the entire time. Discard the old needle into the biohazardous sharps container.

PREPARING PARENTERAL MEDICATIONS

As with all medication preparation, it is important to be in a well-lit room and to be free from distraction. The medical assistant must be focused on the procedure to reduce the risk of errors. For all parenteral medications:

- If the medication looks abnormal in color or clarity, discard it.
- Some medications will have precipitate (pri SIP i tate) at the bottom of the vial. If this is normal for that medication, make sure to mix it prior to withdrawing medication. If the precipitate is abnormal, a chemical reaction may have occurred. The vial needs to be discarded.

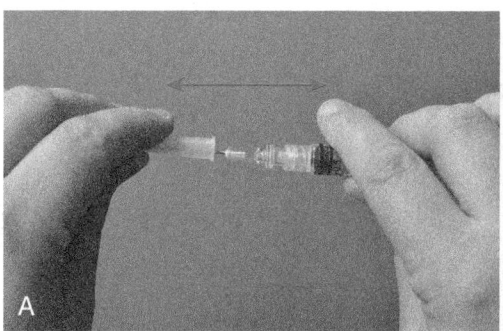
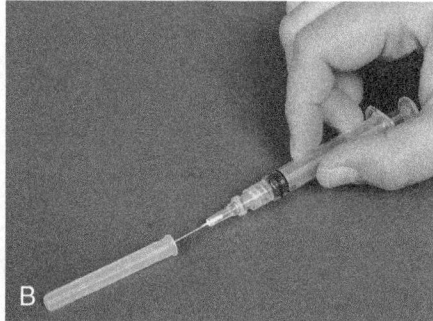

Fig. 46.14 A, Uncapping a needle. B, One-handed scoop technique.

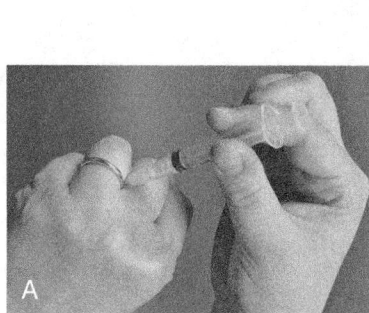
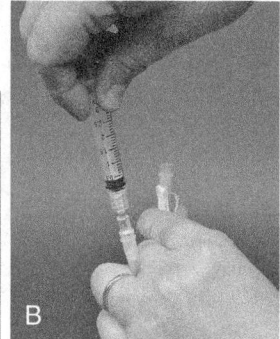
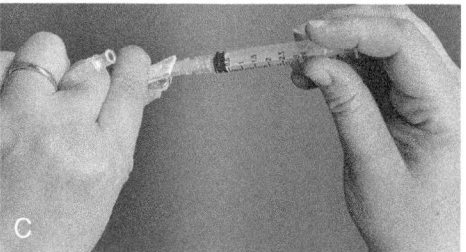

Fig. 46.15 A, Place the syringe unit between the fingers of your nondominant hand and firmly grasp the covered needle. B, Hold the old covered needle securely as you detach it from the syringe. C, Attach the new needle while holding the old needle between your fingers.

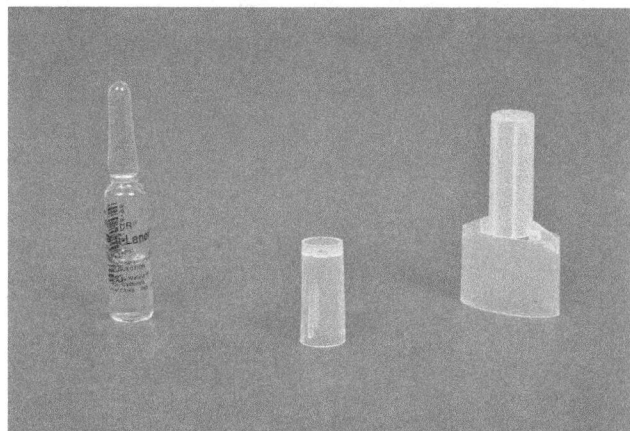

Fig. 46.16 An Ampule With Two Different Ampule Openers/Breakers. (From Niedzwiecki B, et al: *Kinn's the medical assistant,* ed 14, St. Louis, 2020, Elsevier.)

- If the medication has expired, discard it.
- If the medication is no longer sterile, discard it.

Using an Ampule

Ampules (AM pools) contain a single dose of medication. They may contain more than the patient needs. The extra medication is wasted. Medications in ampules react to other substances and require the all-glass environment to remain stable. An ampule has a prescored neck, which is snapped off during the preparation process. An ampule opener or breaker is a safety device used to snap off the top of the ampule (Fig. 46.16). A filter needle on a syringe is used to aspirate (AS pi rate) the medication into the syringe. This

needle has a small filter that catches glass particles before they enter the syringe barrel. The filter needle must be removed before the injection is given to the patient. Procedure 46.6 describes the steps required to prepare medication from an ampule.

> **VOCABULARY**
> **aspirate** To withdraw fluid using suction.
> **precipitate** Solid particles that settle out of a liquid.

Using a Prefilled Sterile Cartridge

A prefilled, sterile cartridge comes filled with a single dose of medication. It is not uncommon for the medication in the syringe to be more than what the provider ordered. The cartridge may come with or without a needle. A safety needle can be attached to the Luer-Lok on the prefilled cartridge. A reusable cartridge holder (e.g., Carpuject or Tubex) is needed to dispense the medication (Fig. 46.17). The medical assistant must assemble the cartridge and the reusable cartridge holder prior to administering the medication. Procedure 46.7 describes how to use a Carpuject holder and prepare the medication.

Specialty Syringe Units

Specialty syringe units are designed so that patients can administer their own medication. Different types of syringe units are available. Fig. 46.18 shows an insulin pen. The dose of insulin required can be set by the dial. The patient needs to change the needle with each dose. Insulin pens cannot be shared between patients.

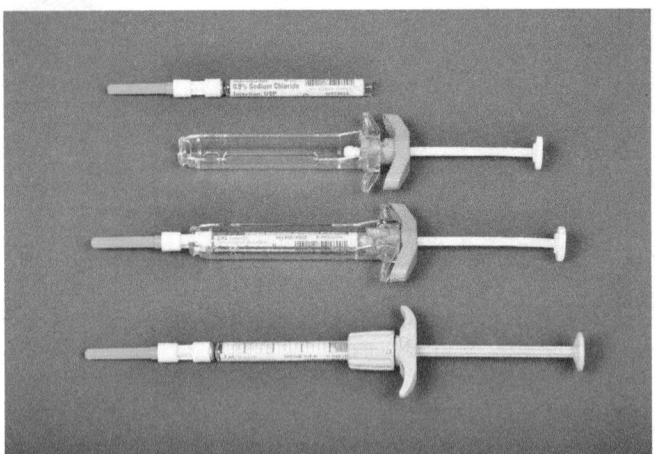

Fig. 46.17 *Top to bottom:* Prefilled syringe, Carpuject holder, prefilled syringe in a Carpuject holder, and a prefilled syringe in a Tubex cartridge holder.

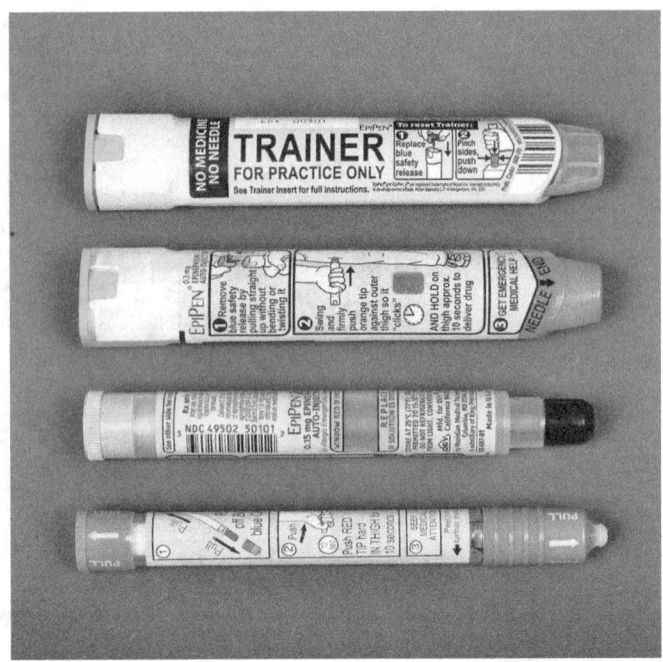

Fig. 46.19 *Top to bottom:* EpiPen trainer, Epipen for older children and adults, EpiPen Jr for children, and a generic epinephrine pen.

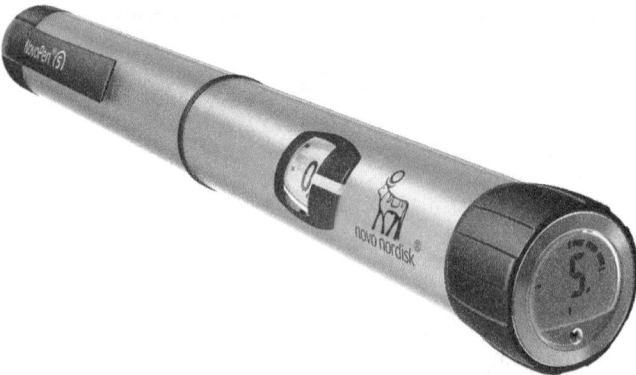

Fig. 46.18 NovoPens use insulin cartridges. Patients change the cartridges and retain the pen. (From Niedzwiecki B, et al: *Kinn's the medical assistant,* ed 14, St. Louis, 2020, Elsevier.)

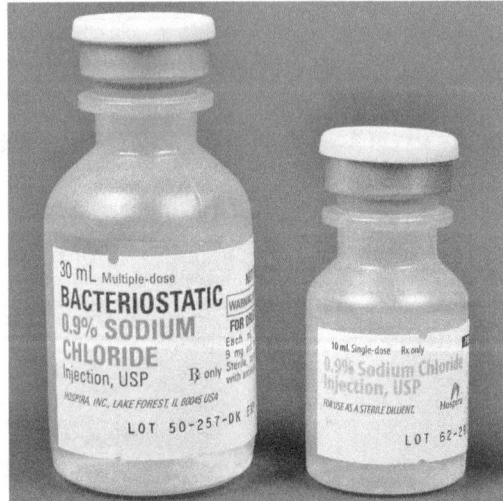

Fig. 46.20 Multidose and Single-Dose Vials.

The EpiPen and other epinephrine pens are automatic injector systems (Fig. 46.19). The pens are dosed for adults or children. People at risk for anaphylactic reactions (e.g., from food allergens, bee stings) should carry epinephrine pens to prevent a fatal reaction. Simulators can accompany some of the injector systems. These are useful when teaching patients how to give their own injections.

Using a Vial

A vial is a plastic or glass container with a rubber stopper that is covered by a cap. Vials contain powdered or liquid medications. Liquid medication is more common. The liquid can be a parenteral medication, sterile *normal saline* (0.9% sodium chloride), or sterile water. Vials come in single dose or multidose (Fig. 46.20). Single-dose or single-use vials are only good for a single patient and a single injection procedure. If the vial needs to be entered more than once for a single patient as part of a single procedure, then a new needle and syringe must be used. Discard the vial after the procedure. Single-dose vials do not contain any ingredients that would prohibit microorganism growth. Thus they are only good for a single use.

Multidose vials contain many doses of medication. The label will clearly state that the vial is a multidose vial. These vials contain an antimicrobial preservative that prevents the growth of bacteria. The preservative does not help protect the fluid against viruses and other sources of contamination if safe injection practices are not followed. When multidose vials are opened (the cap is removed or the stopper is punctured), they are only good for 28 days (unless the manufacturer states otherwise). The new expiration date should be written on the label. If the manufacturer's expiration date comes sooner than the 28 days, then the earlier date must be used.

Each time the multidose vial is entered, the rubber stopper must be disinfected, and a sterile needle and syringe must be used. The vial is under pressure. You need to add air into the vial before you draw out the amount of liquid you need. The amount of air added should equal the amount of liquid you draw out. Always make sure you have the correct amount of medication

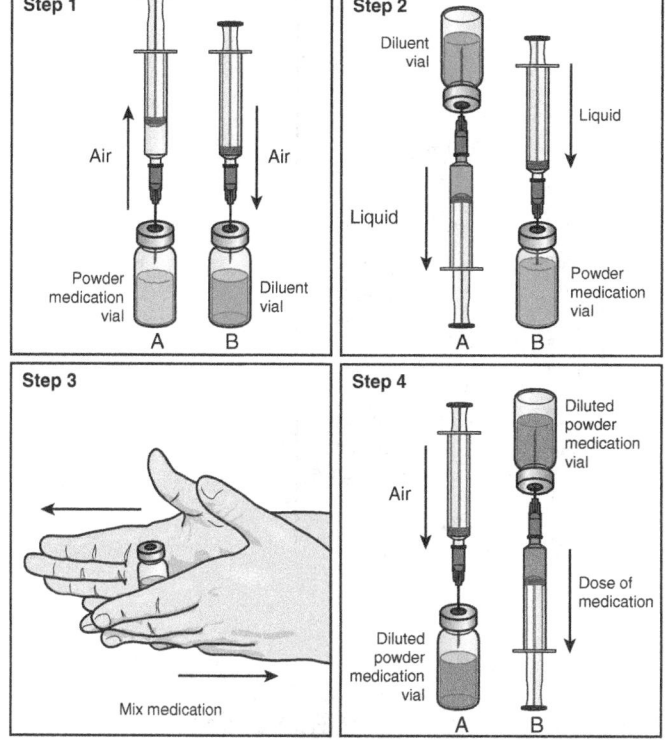

Fig. 46.21 Steps for Reconstituting Medication and Withdrawing a Dose of Medication.

in your syringe before you withdraw the needle. Never inject unneeded medication back into the vial once the needle has been removed. Procedure 46.8 describes how to prepare medication from a vial.

Reconstituting Powdered Medication

As previously mentioned, vials can contain powdered medication. A powdered medication needs to be mixed with a diluent (DIL yoo ehnt). Typically, sterile normal saline or sterile water is used as a diluent, although other medications may also be used (according to the provider's order and the manufacturer's directions). The most common powdered medications in primary care are live-virus vaccines. These need to be reconstituted (ree KON sti toot ed) (Procedure 46.9).

If the vial is a multidose vial, it is important to write the expiration date on the label. The expiration dates for reconstituted medications will vary. See the manufacturer's insert for the length of time that the medication will remain stable after reconstitution. Besides the expiration date, include your initials and the fluid that was used to reconstitute the medication. These three pieces of information need to be on the multidose label.

There are four major steps in reconstituting powdered medication and withdrawing a dose of the medication (Fig. 46.21):

Step 1: Remove air from the powdered medication vial and put air into the diluent vial.

Step 2: Withdraw liquid from the diluent vial and add it to the powdered medication vial.

Step 3: Mix the liquid with the powdered medication.

Step 4: Add in air and withdraw the dose needed.

CRITICAL THINKING 46.6

Mark struggles to remember the steps to reconstitute powdered medication. What are the steps?

Mixing Insulins

Patients with diabetes may use insulin to help manage their disease. Taking insulin requires about four injections a day. Some patients may need two different insulins at the same time. Many premixed insulins are available for patients. However, for some individuals the premixed insulins are not an option, and they must mix the two insulins in one syringe. During this combination process, it is important that the vials do not become contaminated with another type of insulin. If by chance contamination occurs, it is better for the rapid-acting or short-acting insulin (Regular insulin) to be mixed in the intermediate-acting insulin vial (e.g., NPH insulin). This means that Regular insulin must be drawn up in the syringe first and then NPH is added (Fig. 46.22). Procedure 46.10 describes the steps for mixing two insulins in one syringe.

Depending on state laws and facility policies, administering insulin may be within the medical assistant's scope of practice. Understanding how to mix two insulins in the same syringe is important. Not all insulins can be mixed. Use drug reference information to ensure that the two insulins ordered can be mixed.

As discussed earlier, insulin is measured in units. Special insulin syringes are available to measure small or large insulin dosages. Insulin is typically stored in the refrigerator and should be warmed to room temperature prior to administration. Cloudy insulins (e.g., NPH) are suspensions and need to be mixed before drawing up the insulin. Mix cloudy insulins by gently rolling the vial between your hands. Clear insulin (e.g., Regular insulin) does not need to be mixed or rolled in your hand.

Patients receiving insulin must rotate their injection sites. This prevents tissue damage and absorption issues with the insulin. It might be helpful for patients to mark the site of the last injection with a spot bandage or a piece of tape. The easiest way to rotate sites is to give subsequent injections in a circular pattern around the first injection site in a specific location. The goal is to avoid using the same location again for another month.

CRITICAL THINKING 46.7

Mark struggles to remember the order for drawing up insulin. What might be a few good ways to remember the process of drawing up two insulins in the same syringe?

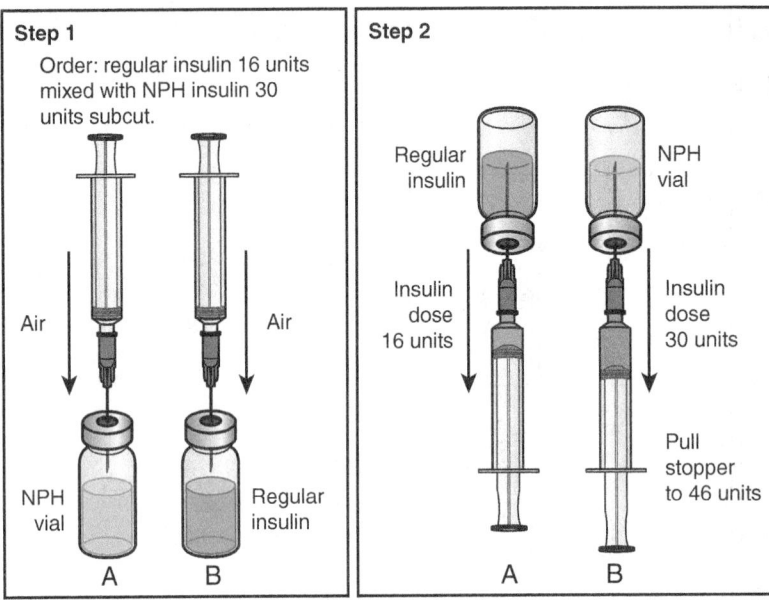

Fig. 46.22 Mixing Two Insulins.

GIVING PARENTERAL MEDICATIONS

Some medications can be given by several routes. Other medications can only be given by injection. Parenteral medication administration has several advantages:

- It is useful when the patient has gastrointestinal distress or is unconscious.
- It offers good absorption compared with other routes, such as the oral route.
- The *onset* (time medication starts working) is more rapid than with other routes.
- Some types of parenteral medications have a longer *duration time* (time the medication works in the body).

Pain with the injection and a risk of infection due to the injection are disadvantages of parenteral medications. Another disadvantage is an unpredictable absorption rate for those with poor circulation (e.g., patients with peripheral artery disease, diabetes, obesity, or Raynaud disease).

When it comes to giving injections, over time you will gain confidence and it will become easy. Always do the following:

- Follow the nine rights of medication administration.
- Check the medication's label against the order three times.
- Know about the medication you are giving. (What is it, why is it being ordered, how is it given, and what are the common side effects?)
- Label all syringes with the name of the medication they contain.
- Follow medical asepsis and the Bloodborne Pathogens Standard established by the Occupational Safety and Health Administration (OSHA).
- Ensure that the needle is not directed at your hand holding the patient when giving an injection. Slight movement may cause a needlestick.

Following these guidelines will help you to perform injections safely and protect your patient from medication errors.

Guidelines for Parenteral Medications

Prepare and store medications in a separate area, away from the exam rooms. Medications can be prepared without the use of gloves. Ensure that all needles are tightly covered and placed on a tray when carrying them to the exam room. Never transport medication in your pockets. Bring only one patient's medication at a time to avoid confusion and error.

Follow these guidelines when selecting an injection site:

- Never give an injection near bones or blood vessels.
- Avoid scar tissue, a change in skin pigmentation or texture, or abnormal growth (e.g., mole or wart).
- Avoid abrasions, lesions, wounds, bruises, and edematous areas.
- Select a site that is large enough to hold the amount of medication injected.
- Avoid sites recently used (within the last month).

According to the Immunization Action Coalition (https://www.immunize.org), it is safe to give subcut and IM vaccines into a tattoo. However, it is not a good idea to inject into a newly tattooed area. If you must inject into a tattooed area, attempt to use a lighter pigmented area. All injections pose the risk of a reaction or an infection at the injection site. Dark pigments may mask a reaction or an infection.

Reducing Pain and Anxiety

To minimize pain with injections, insert subcut and IM needles swiftly. Inject the medication at the rate of 10 seconds per 1 mL to avoid unnecessary discomfort. Remove the needle quickly, using the same angle as for entry.

Various techniques can be used to reduce a patient's pain and anxiety about injections:

- Give a sugar-coated pacifier or sugar water (must be ordered by the provider), which helps to soothe children under age 1 year after injections.

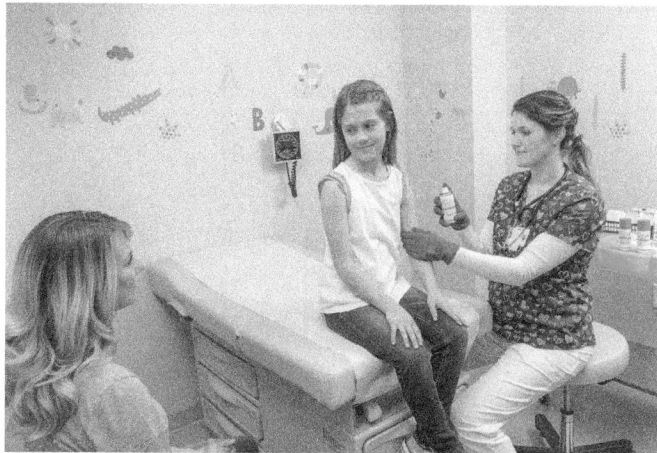

Fig. 46.23 Topical Anesthetic Skin Refrigerant Spray. (Courtesy Gebauer-Tri-Point-Medical, Cleveland, OH.)

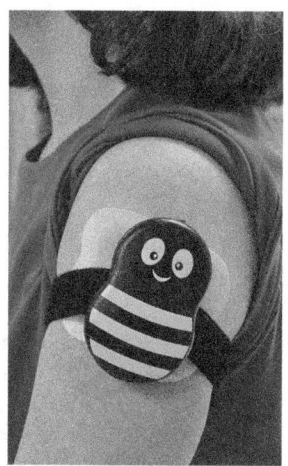

Fig. 46.24 Buzzy helps reduce pain naturally by overwhelming the nerves with vibration and cold sensations.

- Apply a topical anesthetic skin refrigerant (e.g., Pain Ease), which works immediately (Fig. 46.23).
- Apply a topical anesthetic (e.g., EMLA cream) at the injection site, which works in about 30 to 40 minutes.
- Talk with the patient to distract them from the procedure.
- Have patients move their toes or fingers on the extremity receiving the IM injection. (Have a patient "play the piano" with their fingers when giving a deltoid injection.)
- Administer the most painful injection last.
- Use products that provide cold and vibration sensations (e.g., Buzzy), which overwhelm the nerves affected by the injection (Fig. 46.24).

CRITICAL THINKING 46.8

Gabe talks with Mark about distractions to use when giving IM injections. He mentions having patients wiggle their toes or move their fingers when an injection is given on that extremity. He explains that he tells the patient about the movement prior to starting the injection. Gabe reminds the patient when he is aspirating, just prior to injecting the medication. What might be the benefit of reminding the patient when aspirating?

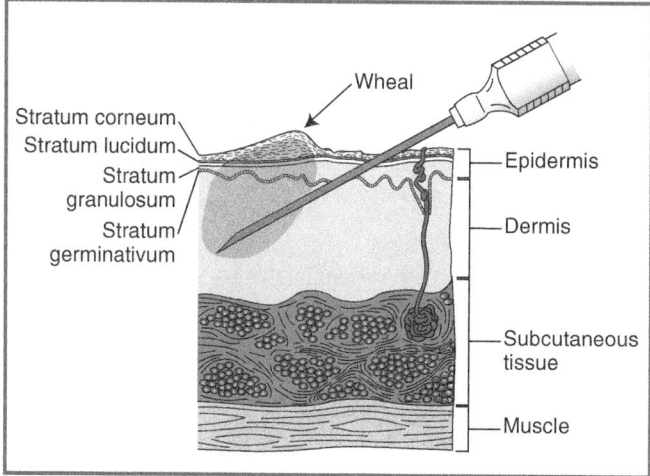

Fig. 46.25 The intradermal (ID) injection is administered just under the epidermis. Because the drug is dispersed in an area where many nerves are present, it causes momentary burning or stinging. Small amounts of medication are injected. (From Niedzwiecki B, et al: *Kinn's the medical assistant*, ed 14, St. Louis, 2020, Elsevier.)

Special Situations

Even if the procedure was done correctly, sometimes things can go wrong. It is important for the medical assistant to know what to do in those situations.

If a needle breaks during an injection or if the needle separates from the syringe, pull out the needle if it is visible. Discard the needle in the biohazardous sharps container. If the needle breaks off and it is not visible, mark the spot with a pen and yell for help. If the injection was given in the arm, place a tourniquet above the spot to prevent the needle from moving in the body. Notify the provider immediately.

With intramuscular injections, sometimes the bone can be hit during the procedure. If this occurs, pull the needle out about ¼ inch and give the medication.

With any medication, a patient can experience an anaphylactic reaction. *Anaphylaxis* (AN ah fi LAK sis) is a severe allergic reaction that can be life-threatening. Having the patient wait 15 minutes after an injection allows you to monitor for unusual symptoms. Symptoms include:

- Warm feeling, flushing, throat tightening, difficulty swallowing, and cough
- Shortness of breath, *dyspnea* (DISP nee uh) (difficulty breathing), and wheezing
- Anxiety, loss of consciousness, and shock
- Pain or cramping, vomiting, diarrhea, palpitations, and dizziness

If the patient is experiencing any unusual symptoms, it is important to tell the provider immediately. The first-line medication for anaphylaxis is epinephrine.

INTRADERMAL INJECTIONS

Intradermal (ID) injections are given just under the epidermis (Fig. 46.25). Because the drug is dispersed in an area where many nerves are present, it causes momentary burning or stinging. Small amounts of medication are injected. Fig. 46.26 show sites

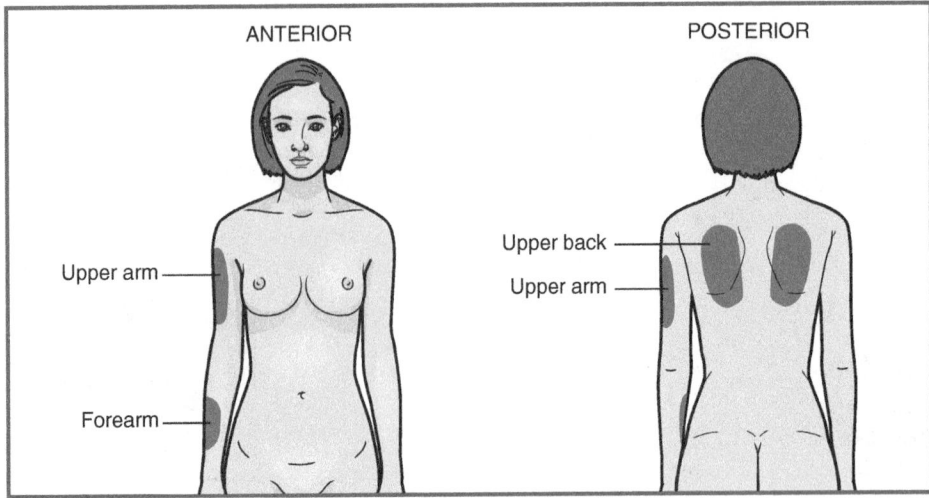

Fig. 46.26 Sites Recommended for Intradermal Injections.

TABLE 46.1	Quick Summary of Intradermal Injections
Syringe used	1 mL (tuberculin syringe)
Needle size	¼ to ½ inch; 25–27 gauge
Angle of entry	5–15 degrees with bevel facing upward
Maximum volume	0.1 mL
Common sites	Forearm, upper arm, and middle of the back
Additional sites	Separate by at least 2 inches
Patient position	Sitting with arm extended
Administration	Pull skin taut at injection site

recommended for intradermal injections. Table 46.1 contains a summary of intradermal injection information. In ambulatory care, the following intradermal injections may be given:

- Mantoux tuberculin skin test (TST)
- Allergy testing

Tuberculin Testing

Two types of tuberculin tests have been approved by the FDA: the skin test and the blood test. The TST is used to determine whether a patient is infected with *Mycobacterium tuberculosis*. It is important for the medical assistant to be knowledgeable about and skilled at administering and reading the test.

The TST can be given to most patients, including infants, pregnant women, patients infected with the human immunodeficiency virus (HIV), and those vaccinated with bacillus Calmette-Guérin (BCG). Patients with a history of BCG vaccination may have a positive reaction to the TST. If a patient mentions a history of receiving BCG vaccine, it is important for the medical assistant to inform the provider before performing the skin test. The provider may opt to have the patient undergo the blood test instead.

The TST is contraindicated in patients who had:

- A severe reaction to a past TST (e.g., necrosis, ulcers, blisters, or anaphylaxis)

- A history of a positive TST result
- A live-virus vaccine less than 4 to 6 weeks earlier (A TST and a live-virus vaccine can be given on the same day, or the TST can be given 4 to 6 weeks after the vaccine.)

Tuberculin Skin Test Procedure and Reading. To perform the TST, tuberculin purified protein derivative (PPD) 0.1 mL is given ID into the inner surface of the forearm (Procedure 46.11). A tuberculin syringe and needle, with the bevel facing upward, is used to slowly inject the PPD, creating a tense, pale wheal. The wheal must measure 6 to 10 mm in diameter, or the test must be repeated.

The patient returns within 48 to 72 hours to have the test read. Reading before or after this time invalidates the results. When reading the test, palpate the site to check for a raised, hardened area, called an *induration* (IN duh RAY shuhn). If an induration is felt, measure the raised area across the forearm (perpendicular to the bone). The *erythema* (redness) is not measured. The diameter of the induration is read in millimeters (mm) and must be noted in the health record. The medical assistant can never state that the test result is positive or negative. The provider uses the test results and the patient history to determine if the patient has tuberculosis (TB). A TST reading between 5 and 15 mm can be positive for different populations. Table 46.2 describes the different populations.

> **VOCABULARY**
> **wheal** A raised mark on the skin.

Incorrect tuberculin skin test readings. At times, the TST reading may be incorrect. A *false-positive reaction* means the person reacted to the test even though no *M. tuberculosis* is present. Reasons for false-positive reactions with TST include:

- Lung infection with nontuberculous mycobacteria (NTM). This organism is found in the water and soil and is inhaled.
- Previous vaccination with BCG vaccine. Many foreign-born patients from countries with a high risk of TB may have

TABLE 46.2 Tuberculin Skin Reaction Categories

Induration ≥5mm considered positive in patients with:	Induration ≥10mm considered positive in patients with:	Induration ≥15mm considered positive in patients with:
• Human immunodeficiency virus (HIV) infection • Organ transplant • Immunosuppression • Recent contact with a person with tuberculosis (TB) • Fibrotic changes on a chest x-ray consistent with prior TB	• Recent immigrants (<5 years) from high-risk areas • Injection drug users • People living or working in high-risk areas (e.g., living in a group setting [jail, nursing home]; employees in a clinical position with a high risk of TB exposure) • Children < 4 years of age or children exposed to high-risk adults	• No known risk for TB

From the Centers for Disease Control and Prevention (CDC). https://www.cdc.gov/tb/topic/treatment/decideltbi.htm.

received BCG abroad. The BCG vaccine has been approved by the FDA, but it is used in very limited situations.

• Incorrect administration or reading of the TST.

A *false-negative reaction* means the person may not have reacted to the test, even though the patient is infected with *M. tuberculosis*. Reasons for false-negative results with TST include:

• Weakened immune system
• Exposure to TB infection within previous 8 to 10 weeks
• Very old TB infection
• Patient is younger than 6 months old
• Recently received a live-virus vaccine (e.g., measles, yellow fever, chickenpox), or had a viral infection (e.g., influenza), or received corticosteroids or immunosuppressive medications (a false reaction may occur up to 5 to 6 weeks afterward)
• Incorrect administration or reading of TST

Two-Step Testing. In some patients who have had a TB infection, the body "forgets" to react to the TST. This can occur if the infection was many years before. The initial TST may be negative, and the person may have a false-negative reaction. Receiving a second TST can help the body "remember" the infection, thus causing a more accurate (positive) reading. This is called the *booster effect* or *booster phenomenon*. The second TST can be done 1 to 3 weeks after the initial test was read.

New residents in long-term care facilities (e.g., nursing homes) usually have a two-step TST done. Healthcare students and professionals also need to have a two-step TST. Once the two-step TST has been completed, they need yearly TSTs. If the time since the last TST exceeds 1 year, they may need to complete another two-step TST. Fig. 46.27 shows what occurs if the initial test result is positive or negative.

CRITICAL THINKING 46.9

Gabe and Mark are working with Julia Berkley, who has come in for a physical prior to starting college. She is going into the healthcare field, and her paperwork indicates that she needs a two-step TB skin test. Julia asks what this means. How might you explain a two-step TB skin test?

Tuberculin Blood Tests. The FDA has approved two tuberculin blood tests: the QuantiFERON-TB Gold In-Tube test (QFT-GIT) and the T-SPOT TB test (T-Spot). If a patient has had the

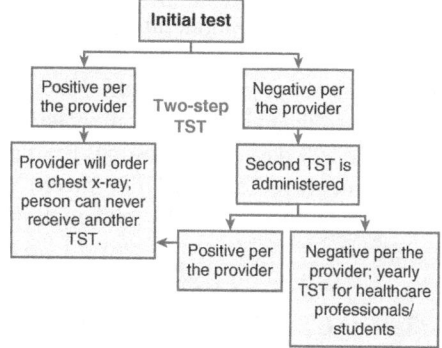

Fig. 46.27 The Process With the Two-Step Tuberculin Skin Test (TST).

BCG vaccine or is unable to return for the skin test reading, the blood test is preferred. The blood test replaces the skin test. A healthcare professional or student only needs one blood test initially, unlike the two-step skin test. After the initial test, a yearly skin or tuberculin blood tests is required.

After the medical assistant draws a patient's blood, it is sent to the laboratory for analysis. The error rate with a blood test is much lower than with the palpated, measured reading of the TST. The next step will depend on whether the TB blood test result is positive or negative:

• *Positive*: The person has been infected with TB. The provider will order additional tests to determine if the person has a latent TB infection or TB disease. (See Chapter 11 for more information on these two diseases.)
• *Negative*: It is unlikely the person has TB.

Allergy Testing

Allergy testing is done to identify a patient's food, medication (e.g., penicillin), or environmental allergies. There are three direct skin tests commonly used:

• *Skin prick/puncture test*: A small amount of diluted allergen is applied to the skin. A small disposable plastic device pricks or punctures the skin, allowing the allergen to go under the skin's surface. Several allergens can be tested at the same time. Once the test is given, the patient is monitored. After 15 minutes the medical assistant measures the erythema (redness) and the induration at each site.
• *Intradermal skin test*: Involves giving small amounts of the allergen using the intradermal route. This is used for bee

venom and penicillin allergy testing. It can also be used if the skin prick test was negative and the provider still believes the patient has the allergy.

- *Patch test*: Involves taping possible allergens to the skin for 48 hours (Fig. 46.28). The test results are measured in 72 to 96 hours.

Patient Education for Direct Skin Testing. Prior to the appointment, it is important that patients stop medications that may mask or hide allergies. Typically, guidelines include:

- Stop long-acting antihistamines for 5 days before the testing. Examples include cetirizine (se TI ra zeen) (Zyrtec), desloratadine (des lor AT a deen) (Clarinex), fexofenadine (fex oh FEN a deen) (Allegra), and loratadine (lor AT a deen) (Claritin, Alavert).
- Stop all over-the-counter (OTC) cold, sleep, and allergy medications; prescribed allergy medication; and specific acid reflux medications 3 days before testing. Examples include diphenhydramine (dye fen HYE dra meen) (Benadryl), meclizine (MEK li zeen) (Antivert), and famotidine (fa MOE ti deen) (Pepcid).

Direct Skin Testing Guidelines. It is important that the patient prepare for the test. After meeting with the patient and reviewing the allergy symptoms and medical history, the provider will determine what allergies should be tested.

- Select an appropriate testing site. Sites should be at least 1 inch apart so reactions are independent from each other. Usually sites are numbered to indicate the allergens.
- Put on gloves and cleanse sites with an alcohol wipe prior to the test.
- Perform the direct skin test.
- After the proper waiting time, measure the length and width of the wheal and flare using millimeters (mm). The wheal is

red and itchy. The larger the wheal and flare, the greater the sensitivity. Document the measurements.

- Monitor the patient for 30 minutes after administration of the tests for severe allergic reactions.
- After the testing, the pen marks can be removed with alcohol wipes. Some providers will order diphenhydramine cream to be applied to the sites. This will reduce the erythema, itchiness, and indurations.
- A positive and negative control test will also be done with the direct skin test to ensure the accuracy of the results. The negative test usually uses normal saline. Some patients will have a minor reaction at the injection site due to the needle entry. The positive test usually uses a histamine that should cause a 3 mm induration reaction with surrounding erythema.

> **VOCABULARY**
> **flare** An area of redness on the skin that surrounds the wheal.

Serum Antibody Tests for Allergies. Sometimes the provider will order a blood test for certain allergens instead of doing the direct skin test. A serum antibody test (blood test) is required. Specific immunoglobulin E antibodies are increased in people with allergies. In the past the tests were called RASTs (radioallergosorbent test). The RASTs used radioactivity to detect the antibodies, but current tests do not. A *multiple-antigen simultaneous test* (MAST) is a blood test that can examine multiple antigens at the same time. The blood tests are not affected by antihistamines taken by the patient, unlike the skin tests. The results are available in a few days.

SUBCUTANEOUS INJECTIONS

Subcutaneous (subcut) injections involve placing medication into the subcutaneous layer, under the dermis (Fig. 46.29). The subcutaneous layer has fewer blood vessels than the muscles

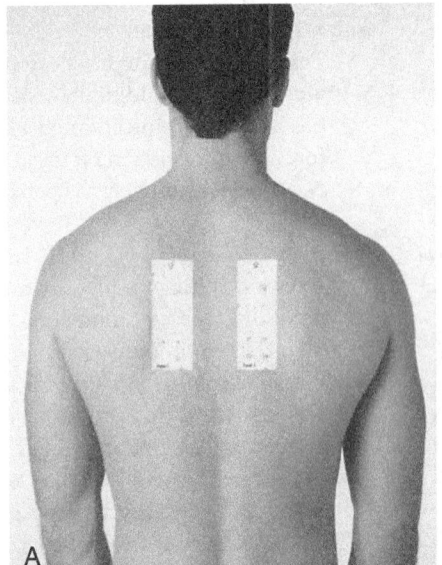
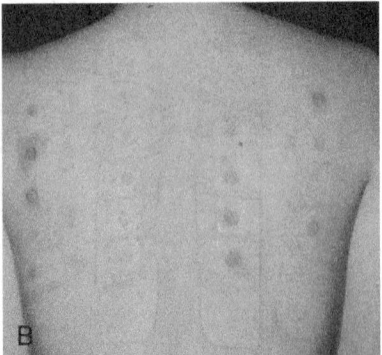

Fig. 46.28 A, For the allergen patch test, a patch impregnated with individual allergens is applied to the patient's back. B, Positive allergy reactions of varying intensity. (From Habif TP: Clinical *dermatology*, ed 5, St, Louis, 2010, Mosby.)

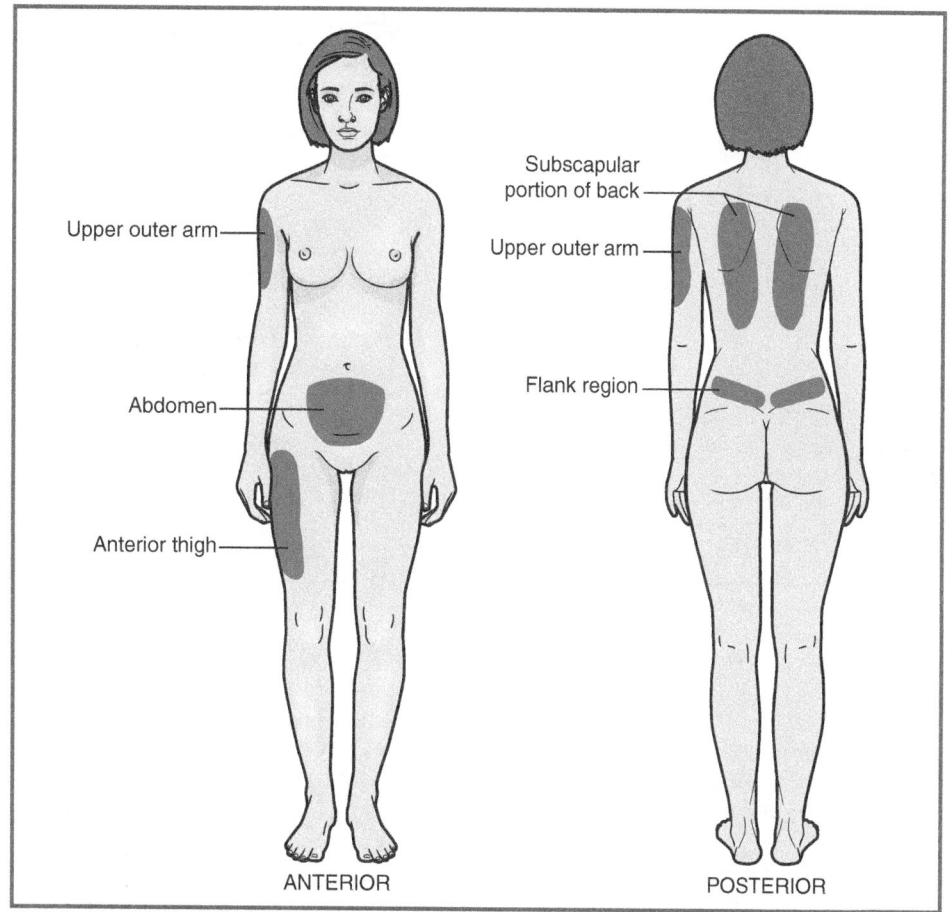

Fig. 46.29 The subcutaneous (subcut) injection sites commonly used include the outer posterior aspect of the upper arm, the lower abdomen, and the anterior aspect of the thigh. The subscapular portion of the back and the flank region are other subcut sites.

do. The medication absorbs more slowly in the subcutaneous layer compared with medications injected into the muscles. The patient may complain of discomfort or pain with a subcutaneous injection. Subcutaneous tissue contains pain receptors.

Common medications given via the subcutaneous route include several vaccines (e.g., MMR, varicella, and polio), enoxaparin (Lovenox), heparin, and insulin. Box 46.2 discusses the abbreviations used for subcutaneous injections.

Administration Techniques

When a subcut injection is given, the angle depends on the needle length. If a ⅝-inch needle is used, then the medical assistant should use a 45-degree angle (Fig. 46.30). If a ½-inch needle is used, then a 90-degree angle should be applied. It is important to pinch up the tissue with the index finger and thumb of the nondominant hand. This ensures that the injection is given into the subcutaneous tissue. Table 46.3 contains a summary of subcutaneous injection information.

Aspiration. Aspiration is used to check if the needle is in a blood vessel. This is done once before the medication is given. (The aspiration technique will be discussed in detail in the "Intramuscular Injections" section, presented later in the chapter.) With subcut injections, the aspiration should be done if

---

BOX 46.2   Abbreviations for Subcutaneous Injections

There have been many abbreviations for subcutaneous injections over the years. Some may still be used in practice, although they are not recommended. The Institute for Safe Medication Practices (ISMP) discourages the use of: SC, SQ, and sub q. Healthcare professionals should use "subcut" or "subcutaneously." For more information, refer to the ISMP website: https://www.ismp.org/recommendations/error-prone-abbreviations-list.

---

the medication manufacturer recommends it. It should also be done if it is part of the facility's policy.

Insulin is not aspirated. Subcut immunizations do not need to be aspirated, as recommended by the CDC. Anticoagulants, such as enoxaparin and heparin, are administered in the abdomen (Box 46.3). They are not aspirated, as specified by the manufacturers.

Subcutaneous Sites

Typically, three subcut sites are used in ambulatory care:
- *Abdominal site*: Have the patient remove the clothing in that area. Provide a drape sheet if needed to protect the patient's modesty. The site is located below the costal margins to the iliac crests. Stay 2 inches away from the umbilicus. It is

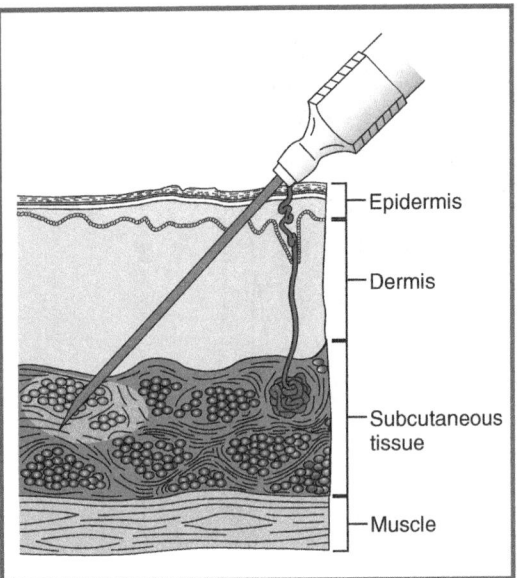

Fig. 46.30 The subcutaneous (subcut) injection is administered in the subcutaneous layer. This method is used for small amounts of nonirritating medications in aqueous solution. (From Niedzwiecki B, et al: *Kinn's the medical assistant,* ed 14, St. Louis, 2020, Elsevier.)

TABLE 46.3 Quick Summary of Subcutaneous (Subcut) Injections

Syringe used	3 mL most common; 1 mL could be used
Needle size and angle of entry	23-27 gauge; ½ inch with a 90-degree angle of entry, or 5/8 inch with a 45-degree angle of entry. The bevel position does not matter.
Maximum volume	0.5–1.5 mL (0.5 mL in children)
Common sites	Lower abdomen, anterior thigh, and upper outer arm (see Fig. 46.29)
Sites for vaccines	<1 yr: anterior thigh >1 yr: upper outer arm or anterior thigh
Additional sites	Separate sites by 1 inch
Patient position	Sitting
Administration technique	Pinch site. If 2 inches of tissue can be pinched, insert the needle at a 90-degree angle. If 1 inch of tissue can be pinched, insert the needle at a 45-degree angle. Rotate sites.

important to stay away from the waistline and any scars. The patient may have more discomfort if the injection is given at the waistline due to the rubbing of clothing.

- *Outer posterior aspect of the upper arm*: Expose the arm. The outer posterior site extends from 3 inches above the elbow to about 3 fingerbreadths below the acromion process. It is important to stay away from the shoulder area.
- *Anterior aspect of the thigh*: Place one hand above the knee and the other hand below the greater trochanter. The site is the middle one-third of the thigh. The site extends from the front midline to the back midline, wrapping around the outer thigh. Usually only the middle one-third—from the front midline to the outer thigh—is used. Injections are not done on the back of the leg, because sitting would irritate the injection site.

Procedure 46.12 describes the steps to follow when giving a subcutaneous injection.

INTRAMUSCULAR INJECTIONS

Intramuscular injections involve placing medication into the muscle (Fig. 46.31). There are more blood vessels in the muscles; thus absorption is faster than in the subcutaneous layer. For medications given by IM injection, *aqueous* (watery) medications should be given with a higher gauge needle than that used for oil-based medications. Table 46.4 contains a summary of intramuscular injection information. Common medications given via the intramuscular route include:

- Several vaccines (e.g., hepatitis A and B, tetanus-diphtheria (Td) or with pertussis (TDaP), influenza, and meningococcal)
- Antibiotics and medroxyprogesterone (me DROX ee proe JES te rone) (Depo-Provera)

Administration Techniques

As with all injections, it is important to do the procedure safely. The medical assistant must identify the correct site and follow the guidelines for medical asepsis. When administering an IM injection, it is important to use a 90-degree angle for entry. The skin should be flattened or stretched over the site with the non-dominant hand. Administration techniques for IM injections consist of being safe, minimizing pain, and finding the correct site. The following sections address these three goals.

Aspiration. When giving an intramuscular injection, it is important to aspirate prior to injecting the medication. Once the needle is in the site, the medical assistant should pull back on the plunger for 5 seconds and check the barrel of the syringe. Lack of blood in the barrel means the needle is not in a blood vessel, so it is safe to inject the medication. If blood appears in the barrel, remove the needle, discard the syringe, and restart the procedure. Immunizations do not need to be aspirated, according to the CDC.

Air Lock Technique. When an IM injection is given, the air lock technique can be used. Remove the bubbles in the syringe and measure the exact amount of medication needed. Once these steps have been done, add 0.2 to 0.5 mL of air into the syringe. This is the known as the *air lock technique*. When the IM injection is given, the medication is pushed in first, followed by the air. When the needle is withdrawn, the air creates a "lock," keeping the medication in the muscle. The air fills in the needle hole. The air lock prevents the irritating medication from tracking back up the tissues to the skin, creating pain for the patient.

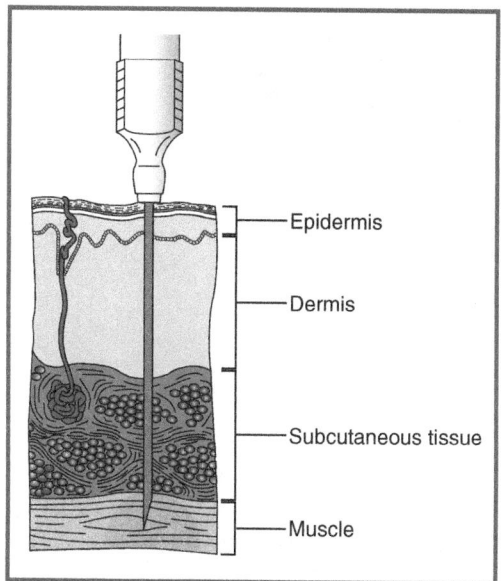

Fig. 46.31 Anatomical Illustration of the Intramuscular (IM) Injection. Note that the needle is inserted at a 90-degree angle, which deposits the medication into the large central part of the muscle. (From Niedzwiecki B, et al: *Kinn's the medical assistant*, ed 14, St. Louis, 2020, Elsevier.)

Z-track Technique. The Z-track technique is another injection method that can reduce pain and discomfort for the patient. Like the air lock technique, this method prevents the medication from tracking back through the subcutaneous tissue. The medication is sealed in the muscle, thus minimizing discomfort for the patient.

The Z-track technique should be used for irritating medications. The ventrogluteal site is the recommended site for injections of irritating medications. For the Z-track technique, the skin is pulled laterally with the medical assistant's nondominant hand. The site is cleansed, and the injection is given (Fig. 46.32A–B). As the needle is withdrawn, the skin is released (Fig. 46.32C).

Intramuscular Sites

Deltoid Site. The deltoid is a triangular-shaped muscle located near the shoulder and upper arm (Fig. 46.33). This muscle site is used to give a small volume of aqueous medications, such as vitamin B_{12} and vaccines. The CDC recommends this site be used when vaccines are given to teens and adults. To find the site, expose the upper arm. Make sure the sleeve does not act as a tourniquet. If the sleeve is tight, have the patient slip the arm out of the shirt.

Palpate the acromion process. Place a finger on the acromion process and then 2 fingers below that. The top of the site is 1 to 2 inches (or 2 fingerbreadths) below the acromion process. The bottom of the site is at the anterior axillary fold (top of the axilla). The injection site should be somewhere between the top and the bottom of the site. Once the medical assistant finds the

TABLE 46.4 Quick Summary of Intramuscular (IM) Injections

	Deltoid	Vastus Lateralis	Ventrogluteal
Syringe used	3 mL		
Needle length (determined by the patient's size)	*1–11 yr:* 5/8–1 inch *Adults:* 5/8–1½ inch *By weight:* • <130 lb: 5/8 inch • 130–152 lb: 1 inch • Females 152–200 lb/males 152–260 lb: 1–1½ inch • Females >200 lb/males >260 lb: 1½ inch	*Birth–28 days:* 5/8 inch *1–12 mo:* 1 inch *1–18 yr:* 1–1½ inch *18+ yr:* 1–1½ inch	*Birth–28 days:* 5/8 inch *1 mo–12 yr:* 1 inch *12+ yr:* 1–1½ inch
Needle gauge (G) (determined by the medication)	22–25 G	*Children:* 22–25 G *Adults:* oil-base: 18–21 G; aqueous: 20–25 G	
Angle of entry	90 degrees (bevel does not matter)		
Maximum volume	1 mL for teens and adults	*Birth–1 yr:* 1 mL *1–11 yr:* 2 mL *12+ yr:* 3 mL	
Sites for vaccines per Centers for Disease Control and Prevention (CDC)	*1–3 yr:* Only if muscle mass is adequate *3+ yr:* Can be used	*Birth–1 yr:* required *1–3 yr:* Preferred *3+ yr:* Can be used	
Additional sites	Separate sites by 1 inch		
Patient position	Sitting	Sitting, supine	Side lying
Administration technique	Stretch the skin over the injection site. Use a 90-degree angle of entry.		
Possible complications	Necrosis, hematoma, ecchymosis (bruising), abscess, pain, and vascular and nerve injuries		

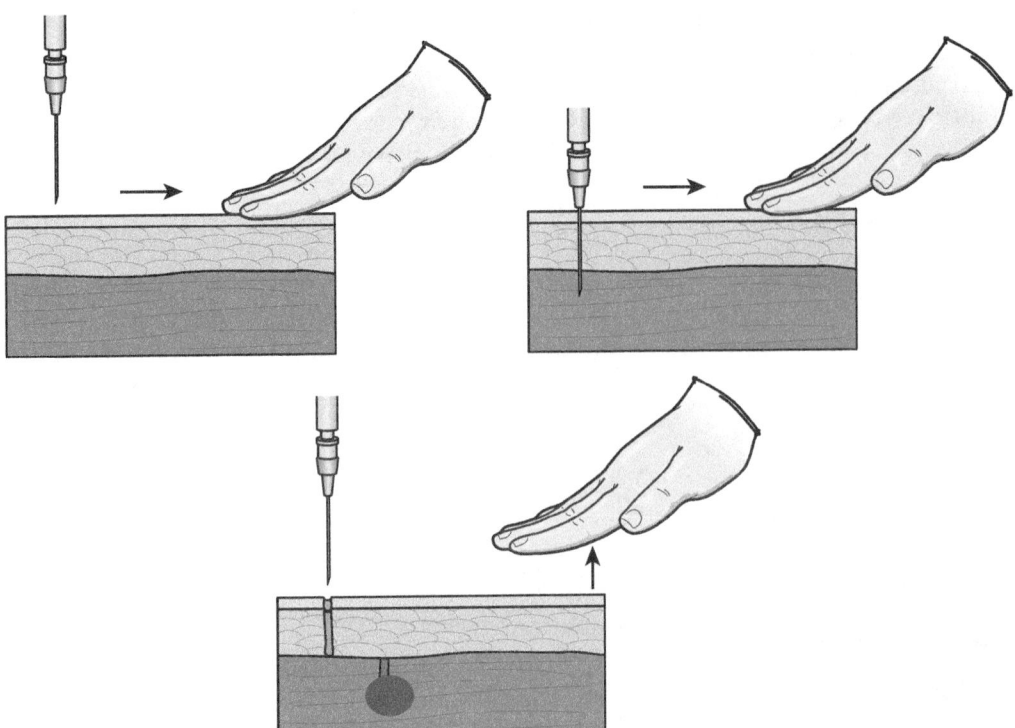

Fig. 46.32 Z-Track Technique. A, Displace and then cleanse the skin. B, Inject the medication. C, Release the skin and pull the needle out at the same time. The medication is locked in the muscle.

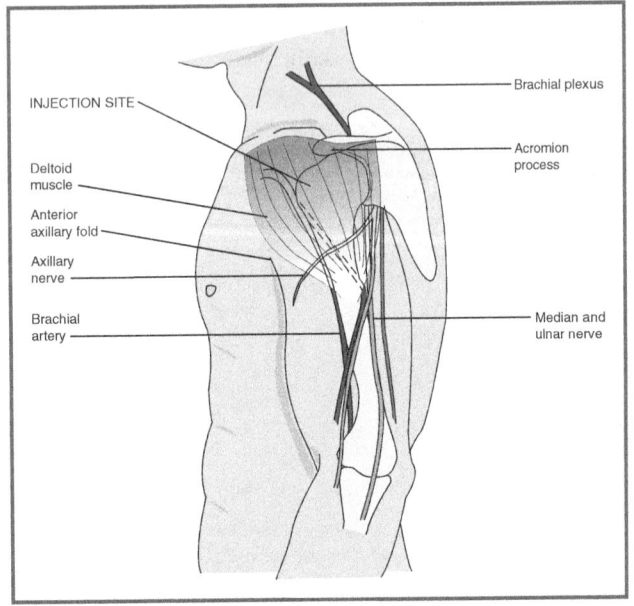

Fig. 46.33 **Deltoid Site.** (From Niedzwiecki B, et al: *Kinn's the medical assistant*, ed 14, St. Louis, 2020, Elsevier.)

site, it is a good idea to have the patient lift their arm. The medical assistant can find the bulk (biggest part) of the deltoid muscle. The injection should be given into the bulk of the deltoid muscle.

Vastus Lateralis Site. The vastus lateralis (VAS tuhs LAT her ray lis) site is used on patients from birth through adulthood.

This site uses a thick, well-developed muscle. The CDC recommends this site until the deltoid muscle is the appropriate size for vaccines (after the patient is 1 year or older). Have patients remove the clothing over the thigh. Remember to give patients a drape sheet to protect their modesty during the procedure.

To find the site, you will need to create a rectangle. Think about dividing the thigh into three sections. With adults, each of your hands will cover one-third of the thigh. Place one hand above the knee and the other hand below the greater trochanter (Fig. 46.34A). This creates the top and bottom borders of the rectangle (or the vastus lateralis site). The middle one-third is used for the injection site. Next, find the midline of the thigh (remember, the midline creates equal right and left sides). That is the inner border of your rectangle. The final border is created by the midline of the outer thigh (i.e., it creates equal front and back sections of the thigh). Once the site is identified, the medical assistant should have the patient slightly lift the thigh. This allows the medical assistant to see if the injection site is in the bulk of the muscle, which is the goal (Fig. 46.34B). Procedure 46.13 describes the procedure for giving an intramuscular injection.

Ventrogluteal Site. The ventrogluteal site is an excellent site for oil-based medications and irritating medications. This site is being used more often, because the dorsogluteal site is no longer a recommended site for IM injections due to the risk of injury. To administer an injection in the ventrogluteal site, it is important to have patients remove clothing from this area. Offering a drape sheet to protect their modesty is important. For this injection, the patient needs to be in a side-lying position.

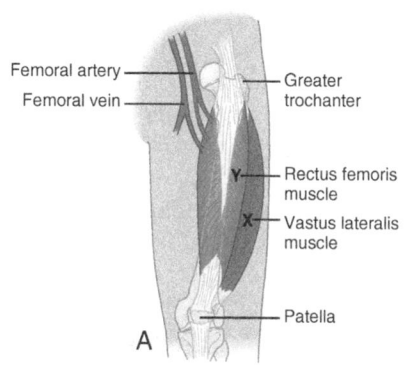
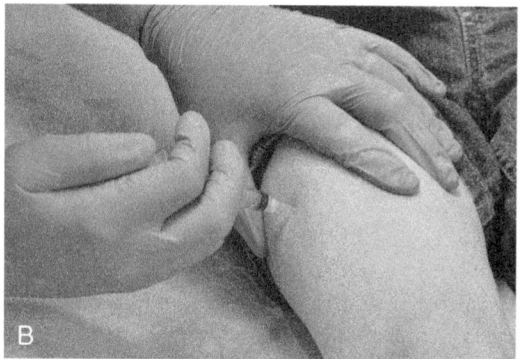

Fig. 46.34 A, Vastus lateralis site. The vastus lateralis muscle is typically used in ambulatory care. The rectus femoris muscle is used more by patients for intramuscular (IM) injections than by healthcare professionals. B, The vastus lateralis site is the recommended site for IM injections in infants and young children. (From Niedzwiecki B, et al: *Kinn's the medical assistant*, ed 14, St. Louis, 2020, Elsevier.)

The most complex part of using the ventrogluteal site is to ensure that the correct hand is used to find the site. Remember to use the hand opposite the injection site. For instance, if the injection site is on the patient's left side, then use your right hand. Follow these steps to find the site:

1. Place the palm of your hand on the patient's greater trochanter.
2. Your fingers need to point toward the patient's head, and your thumb to the patient's groin. (If your thumb is facing the patient's back side, you are using the wrong hand!)
3. Place your index finger on the anterior superior iliac spine. If your fingers are short or if the patient is tall, point your index finger toward the anterior superior iliac spine.
4. Move your middle finger back along the iliac crest toward the patient's buttock (Fig. 46.35).

The positioning of your index and middle fingers forms a triangle. The injection point is at the center of the triangle. Remember, if you are giving an irritating medication, use the Z-track method to reduce pain. Procedure 46.14 describes the steps of the Z-track technique.

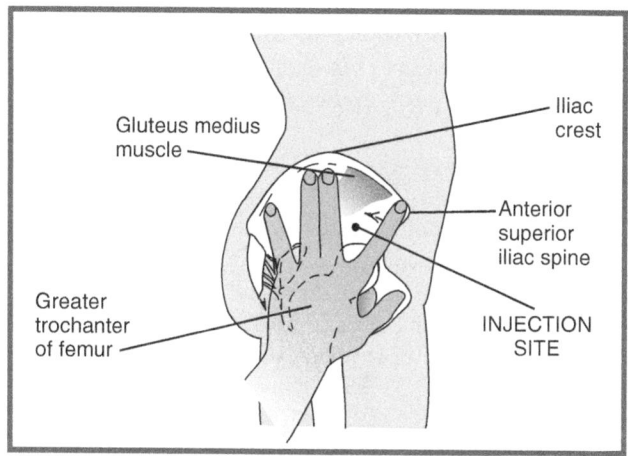

Fig. 46.35 Ventrogluteal Site.

CLOSING COMMENTS

The medical assistant's scope of practice regarding injections differs across the nation. It is important for medical assistants to know their scope of practice in their state. Agencies may also have limitations on what medical assistants can do. For instance, if a scope of practice in the state allows medical assistants to give injections but the agency does not allow it, medical assistants must abide by the agency's policies and procedures.

PATIENT-CENTERED CARE

For injections given to small children, the subcut and IM sites in the thigh are in the same location. It is helpful to have the parent/guardian hold the child's upper body and hands (however, the medical assistant should anticipate that the adult may not hold securely). If another staff member is available, having them hold the lower extremities is helpful. Many times, children may need more than one injection. For this scenario, it is helpful to have two medical assistants each give an injection at the same time.

The medical assistant should hold the joint above the injection site with their nondominant hand. The child's lower leg can be carefully bent off the table and held between the side of the table and the medical assistant's body. If you use this technique, be careful not to hurt the child's leg. Injections for children need to be done using the one-handed technique, because the other hand is holding near the site.

BEING PROFESSIONAL

The medical assistant has an important role in administering medications. Paying attention to details is critical. If a medication error occurs, the medical assistant must act immediately to notify the provider. The provider will identify what steps need to be taken. The medical assistant needs to also complete an incident report. (Incident reports are discussed in Chapter 19.) The supervisor needs to also be notified. In most cases the supervisor will ensure that the patient is not charged for the medication given in error. The supervisor may also need to complete a state or federal report on the medication error.

Role-play this scenario: You and Vicki are medical assistants. Vicki just came to you and stated she made a mistake with a vaccine. She gave the wrong one. This is the third time it has happened to her. She is worried about reporting it and states she thinks she might be fired. Respond to Vicki in a respectful, professional manner regarding this situation.

CHAPTER REVIEW

This chapter covered the nine rights of medication administration: the right medication, dose, route, time, patient, education, technique, and documentation, and the right to refuse. Comparing the label with the order three times is important before giving the medication.

The form is the physical characteristics of a medication, and the route is how the medication gets into the body. Routes discussed include oral, sublingual (under the tongue), buccal (in the cheek), transdermal, inhalation, topical, vaginal, rectal, nasal, ocular, otic, irrigation, and parenteral.

The gauge and length of needles are important considerations when giving injections. The gauge is selected based on the thickness of the medication. The length is based on the size of the patient and the type of injection. Safety needles help prevent needlesticks. Most safety needles require the medical assistant to activate the safety device after the injection.

When you are preparing medication using an ampule, it is important to use a filter needle to withdraw the medication. Single-dose or multidose vials are available. It is important to add the expiration date to the multidose vials. Reconstituting powdered medications requires the correct diluent, as indicated by the manufacturer. All the medication powder needs to be dissolved before the dose can be withdrawn. When you measure medications, it is important to get the bubbles (air) out of the syringe before measuring the correct dose.

Common intradermal sites include the forearm, upper arm, and back. TST and allergy tests are common ID injections. Tuberculosis testing can include either a skin test or a blood test. The two-step TST helps to ensure that the test results are accurate.

Insulin and several vaccines are given by a subcut injection. The subcutaneous sites include the abdomen, posterior outer upper arm, and middle third of the thigh. Medication administered by subcut injection absorbs more slowly than that given by IM injection.

The deltoid, vastus lateralis, and ventrogluteal muscles are the common sites used for IM injections. The Z-track technique can be added to the procedure to help minimize discomfort with irritating medications. The air lock technique can also be used. It is important to aspirate prior to injecting the medication.

SCENARIO WRAP-UP

Gabe and Mark continued to work together for the remaining weeks of the practicum. Mark had the opportunity to give several TSTs. He was able to do subcut and IM injections also. Mark learned the importance of distracting patients during injections; they seemed to tolerate the injection much better.

One of the other medical assistants had a medication error. The medication was given to the wrong patient. This error really impressed upon Mark the importance of the nine rights of medication administration. He is adamant that he will never forget to follow each right each time he gives medications. He does not want to deal with a medication error.

PROCEDURE 46.1   Administer Oral Medications

Tasks
Calculate the dose to give. Prepare a liquid and a solid medication and administer medications to a patient. Document medication administration.

Equipment and Supplies
- Provider's orders
- Patient's health record
- Drug reference information
- Liquid medication and a solid medication
- Paper cup
- Plastic medication cup
- Marker

- Medication tray
- Glass of water
  Orders: Diltiazem 240 mg po and Cephalexin Oral Suspension 375 mg po.

Procedural Steps
1. Using the drug reference information and the orders, review the information on the medications.
   Purpose: The medical assistant must know about the medication that is being given.
2. Using the orders and the labels in Fig. 1, calculate the amount of medication you need to give. Verify the right doses with the instructor. Verify if it is the right time for the order if that applies.

PROCEDURE 46.1   Administer Oral Medications—cont'd

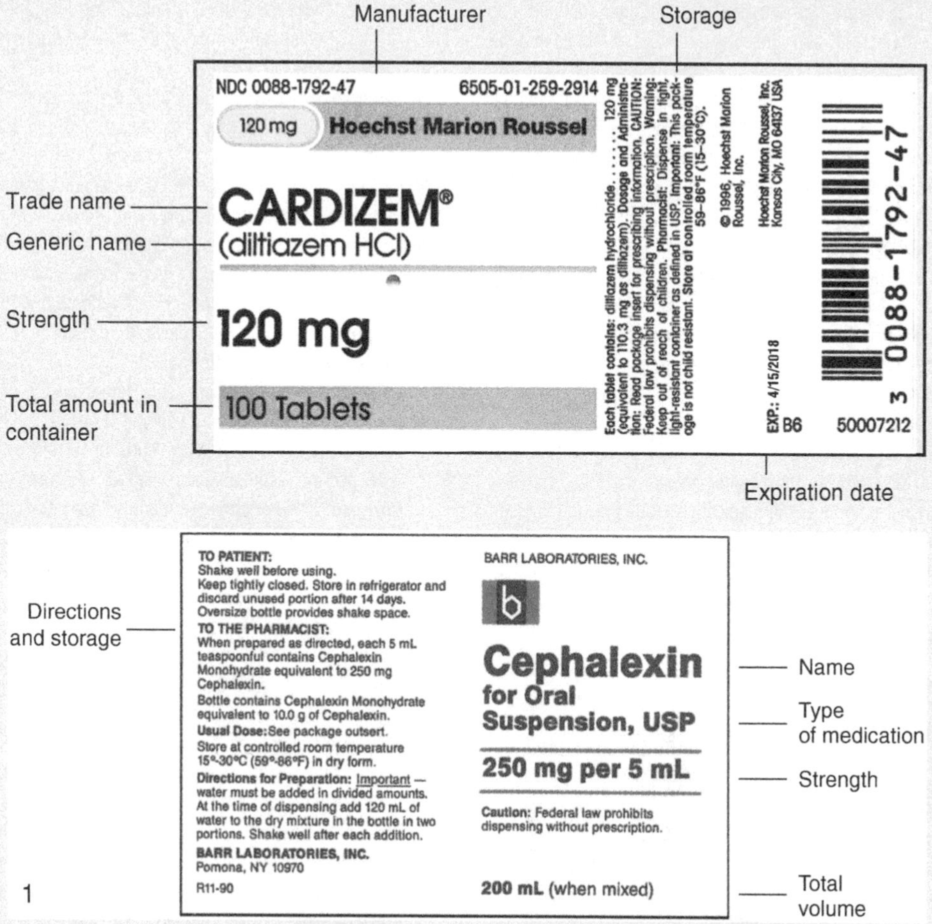

Manufacturer   Storage

NDC 0088-1792-47   6505-01-259-2914

120 mg   **Hoechst Marion Roussel**

Trade name —— **CARDIZEM®**

Generic name —— (diltiazem HCl)

Strength —— **120 mg**

Total amount in container —— **100 Tablets**

Each tablet contains: diltiazem hydrochloride........ (equivalent to 110.3 mg as diltiazem). Dosage and Administration: Read package insert for prescribing information. CAUTION: Federal law prohibits dispensing without prescription. Warning: Keep out of reach of children. Pharmacist: Dispense in tight, light-resistant container as defined in USP. Important: This package is not child resistant. Store at controlled room temperature 59°–86°F (15°–30°C).

120 mg

© 1996, Hoechst Marion Roussel, Inc.

Hoechst Marion Roussel, Inc. Kansas City, MO 64137 USA

EXP: 4/15/2018

EXP: B6   50007212

0088-1792-47

Expiration date

Directions and storage ——

TO PATIENT:
Shake well before using.
Keep tightly closed. Store in refrigerator and discard unused portion after 14 days.
Oversize bottle provides shake space.
TO THE PHARMACIST:
When prepared as directed, each 5 mL teaspoonful contains Cephalexin Monohydrate equivalent to 250 mg Cephalexin.
Bottle contains Cephalexin Monohydrate equivalent to 10.0 g of Cephalexin.
Usual Dose: See package outsert.
Store at controlled room temperature 15°–30°C (59°–86°F) in dry form.
Directions for Preparation: Important — water must be added in divided amounts. At the time of dispensing add 120 mL of water to the dry mixture in the bottle in two portions. Shake well after each addition.
BARR LABORATORIES, INC.
Pomona, NY 10970

R11-90

1

BARR LABORATORIES, INC.

Cephalexin
for Oral
Suspension, USP

—— Name

—— Type of medication

250 mg per 5 mL

—— Strength

Caution: Federal law prohibits dispensing without prescription.

200 mL (when mixed)

—— Total volume

(From Brown M, Mulholland JM: *Drug calculations: process and problems for clinical practice*, ed 9, St. Louis, 2012, Mosby.)

Purpose: The orders do not specify the number of tablets or the amount of liquid (mL) to give. The medical assistant must calculate both. It is important to check your answer with a peer in the workplace before preparing the medication. This ensures that the right dose is being given.

3. Wash your hands or use hand sanitizer. Select the right medications from the storage area. Check each medication label against the order. Check for the right name, form, and route. Check the expiration date to make sure the drug is not expired.

Purpose: It is important to do the first check of the label when getting medications from the cabinet. Do not administer expired medications.

4. Assemble the supplies required to prepare the medications. Using the marker, write the medication name and dose on the appropriate cups (Fig. 2).

Purpose: The paper cup will be used for the tablets, and the plastic cup will be used for the liquid. Make sure not to write over the measurement markings on the plastic cup. Labeling the cups is a safety measure. All medications prepared need to be labeled. Writing an assessment reminder on the cup is optional and can be helpful when the medical assistant needs to do an assessment (e.g., blood pressure) prior to the administration.

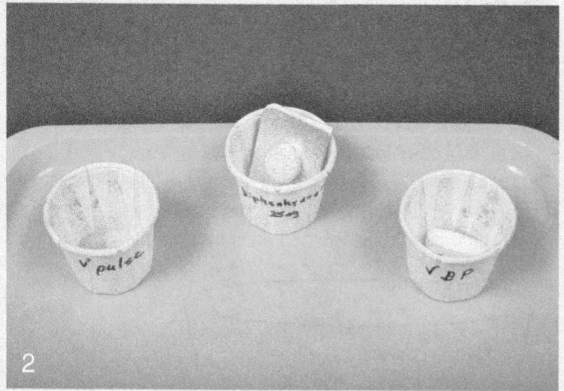

2

5. Perform the second medication check. Check each medication label against the order. Check for the right name, form, and route.

Purpose: It is important to do the second check of the label before pouring the medications into the cups.

Continued

PROCEDURE 46.1   Administer Oral Medications—cont'd

6. For the solid medication: Remove the cover of the container and hold it so the inside is facing up. Carefully pour the correct number of tablets into the cover. If you pour too many into the cover, pour the extra tablets back into the bottle. When you have the correct number of tablets in the cover, pour them from the cover into the paper cup. Place the cover on the container. Make sure not to contaminate the inside of the container or the cover.

   Purpose: Inside the medication container and the cover are sterile. You can pour the tablets back and forth between these two sites until you have the correct number of tablets in the cover. Once you pour the tablets into the paper cup, they are no longer sterile. They cannot be put back into the sterile medication container. If using *unit dose* (individual packaged tablets [blister packs]), tear off the number of tablets needed and place in the paper cup. Do not open until you are with the patient. If the patient refuses the medication, the unopened unit dose medications can be returned to the original box.

7. For the liquid medication:

   a. Place the plastic medication cup on a high, even surface. Uncover the bottle and place the cover on the counter, making sure the inside is facing up. Place your palm over the medication label. Position yourself so you are eye level with the medication cup (Fig. 3).

   Purpose: The cup needs to be on an even surface. Read the amount at eye level to ensure the accuracy of the measurement. Palming the label keeps the label clean as you pour the medication.

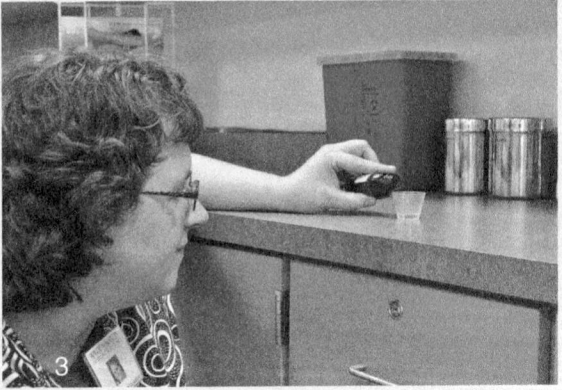

   b. Pour the medication into the cup until the lowest point of the meniscus is at the measurement needed (Fig. 4).

   Purpose: When liquid is poured into a container, it is higher at the edges than in the middle. This is called the *meniscus* (meh NIS kuhs). The liquid must be measured at the lowest point of the meniscus.

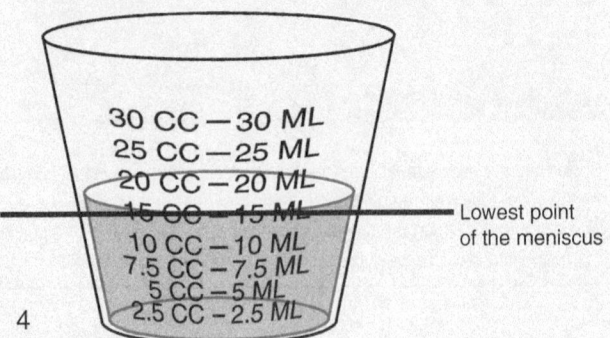

30 CC — 30 ML
25 CC — 25 ML
20 CC — 20 ML
15 CC — 15 ML — Lowest point of the meniscus
10 CC — 10 ML
7.5 CC — 7.5 ML
5 CC — 5 ML
2.5 CC – 2.5 ML

4

   c. If too much medication is poured into the cup, flush the extra down the sink. Replace the cover on the bottle without contaminating the inside of the cover or bottle.

   Purpose: Any extra medication in the cup cannot be poured back into the sterile medication bottle. The medication in the bottle and the inside cover need to remain sterile.

8. Place the medication cups on the medication tray. Clean up the area.

   Purpose: It is important for the medical assistant to clean up the work area.

9. Perform the third medication check. Check each medication label against the order. Check for the right name, form, and route. Verify that the amount of medication in each cup is correct according to the order.

   Purpose: It is important to do the third check of the label before placing the medications back into the cabinet.

10. Prior to entering the exam room, knock on the door and wait a moment. Greet the patient. Identify yourself. Verify the patient's identity with full name and date of birth. Make sure the patient's information matches the order and the record. Explain what you are going to do.

    Purpose: It is important to identify the patient in two different ways to ensure that you have the correct patient. Explaining the procedure can make the patient feel more comfortable and helps to reduce anxiety.

11. Provide the right education to the patient. Explain the medication ordered, the desired effect, and common side effects, and identify the provider who ordered it. Answer any questions the patient may have. Use language the patient can understand. Ask the patient if they have any allergies. If the patient refuses the medication, notify the provider.

    Purpose: The patient needs to be aware of what you are giving, the action, side effects, and who ordered it. It is also important to double-check the patient's allergies before administering the medication.

12. Perform the right technique. Do any assessments required prior to giving the medication. If the patient can have water with the medication, have water available.

    Purpose: Some medications require assessments prior to administration.

13. Allow patients to take the medication in their hand or to use the cup. Stay with the patient until the medication has been taken.

    Purpose: The medical assistant needs to ensure that the medication is taken.

14. Document the procedure in the health record. Include assessments done; allergies; teaching or instructions provided; the name of the provider who ordered the medication; the medication's name, dose, and route; and how the patient tolerated the medication. For vaccines and controlled substances, add the lot number, the expiration date, and the manufacturer's number.

    Purpose: The medications given need to be documented to indicate that they were given.

Documentation Example

10/30/20XX 0936 BP 162/92 left arm, sitting, adult cuff. NKA. Per Dr. Martin's order, administered diltiazem 120 mg, 2 tabs po and cephalexin suspension 250 mg/5 mL, 375 mg po. Medication action and side effects discussed with patient prior to administration. Pt had no questions and verbalized understanding. Pt tolerated the medications without problems. _____ Gabe Garcia CMA (AAMA)

PROCEDURE 46.2   Instill an Eye Medication

Tasks
Instill an eyedrop or ointment and document medication administration.

Equipment and Supplies
- Provider's order
- Patient's health record
- Drug reference information
- Sterile ophthalmic eyedrops or ointment
- Sterile gauze
- Gloves

Order 1: Atropine Sulfate Ophthalmic Solution 1% 1 drop in both eyes.
Order 2: Neosporin Ophthalmic Ointment to left eye.

Procedural Steps
1. Wash your hands or use hand sanitizer.
   Purpose: Hand sanitization is an important step for infection control.
2. Select the right medication from the storage area. Check the medication label against the order. Check for the right name, form, and route. Check the expiration date to make sure the drug is not expired. Verify the right dose and the right time.
   Purpose: It is important to do the first check of the label when getting the medication from the cabinet. Do not administer expired medications.
3. Using the drug reference information and the order, review the information on the medication.
   Purpose: The medical assistant must know about the medication that is being given.
4. Perform the second medication check. Check the medication label against the order. Check for the right name, form, dose, and route.
   Purpose: It is important to do the second check of the label before continuing with the procedure.
5. Assemble the supplies required for the procedure.
   Purpose: You need to have the supplies ready before going to the exam room.
6. Perform the third medication check. Check each medication label against the order. Check for the right name, form, dose, and route.
   Purpose: It is important to do the third check of the label before seeing the patient.
7. Prior to entering the exam room, knock on the door and wait a moment. Greet the patient. Identify yourself. Verify the patient's identity with full name and date of birth. Make sure the patient's information matches the order and the record. Explain what you are going to do.
   Purpose: It is important to identify the patient in two different ways to ensure that you have the correct patient. Explaining the procedure can make the patient feel more comfortable and helps to reduce anxiety.
8. Provide the right education to the patient. Explain the medication ordered, the desired effect, common side effects, and identify the provider who ordered it. Answer any questions the patient may have. Use language the patient can understand. Ask the patient if they have any allergies. If the patient refuses the medication, notify the provider.
   Purpose: The patient needs to be aware of what you are giving, its action, side effects, and who ordered it. It is also important to double-check the patient's allergies before administering the medication.
9. Assist the patient into a sitting or supine position. Ask the patient to tilt the head backward and look up.
   Purpose: These positions allow the medical assistant to instill the medication.
10. Put on gloves. If crusting or drainage is present on the eyelid, gently wash the area from the inner to outer canthus (KAN thus) (Fig. 1). Discard the gauze after each wipe. Dry the area.

Purpose: Gloves are used for infection control purposes. Washing and drying the eye prepares the area for the medication. The *canthus* is the angular junction of the eyelids at either corner.

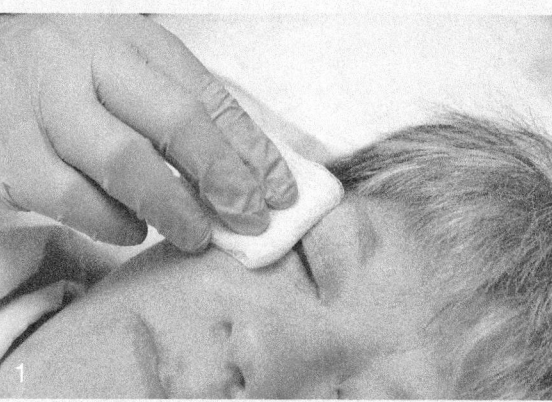

11. Perform the right technique. With your nondominant hand holding a sterile gauze, pull the lower conjunctival sac downward, creating a pocket for the medication (see the following figure). Instruct the patient to look up.
    a. *For eyedrops:* With your dominant hand, hold the bottle or the dropper ¾ inch away from the conjunctival sac. Drop the required number of drops into the pocket (Fig. 2). If the drop misses the eye or the patient blinks, wipe the liquid on the skin and repeat the drop. Have the person keep the eye closed for 2 to 3 minutes after the administration of the drop. Have the person gently press against the inner corner of the eye and the nose bone for 2 to 3 minutes.

Purpose: Pressing in the corner after the drops keeps the medication from draining into the tear ducts and nose. This helps to reduce the systemic effects of the medication.
Note: For patients who struggle with eyedrop administration, some practices allow patients to close their eyes. The drops are placed in the inner canthus. Then the patient must open their eyes. The drops spread across the eyes when they are opened.

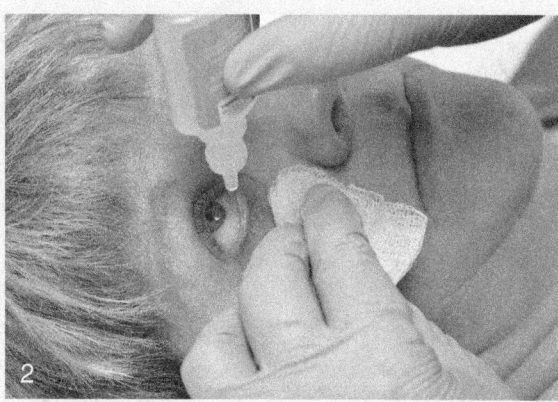

    b. *For eye ointment:* With the dominant hand, hold the ointment container above the lower lid. Working from inner to outer canthus, apply a small strip (about ½ inch) of ointment along the inner lower lid margin (Fig. 3). Have the patient look down and then close the eye for 1 to 2 minutes to allow the medication to be absorbed. Wipe up any extra ointment from the eyelid.

Continued

PROCEDURE 46.2   Instill an Eye Medication—cont'd

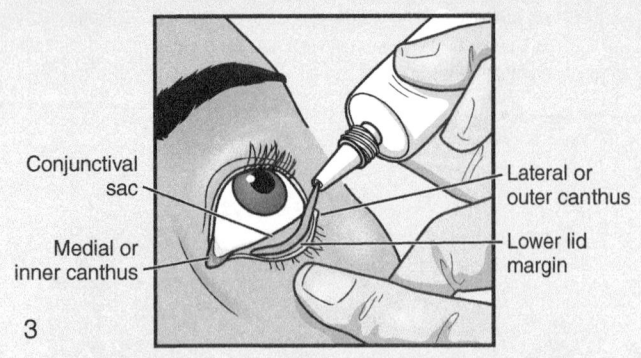

Conjunctival sac

Medial or inner canthus

Lateral or outer canthus

Lower lid margin

3

12. Help the patient into a comfortable position. Clean up the area. Remove your gloves and wash your hands or use a hand sanitizer.

Purpose: It is important for the patient to be comfortable.

13. Document the procedure in the health record. Include allergies, teaching or instructions provided; the name of the provider who ordered the medication; the medication's name, dose, and route; and how the patient tolerated the medication.

Purpose: The medication given needs to be documented to indicate it was given.

Documentation Example

10/30/20XX 1136 NKA. Per Dr. Martin's order, administered Neosporin Ophthalmic Ointment to left eye. Medication action and side effects discussed with patient prior to administration. Pt had no questions and verbalized understanding. Pt tolerated the medication without problems._____
_____ Gabe Garcia, CMA (AAMA)

PROCEDURE 46.3   Instill Ear Drops

Tasks

Instill ear drops and document medication administration.

Equipment and Supplies

- Provider's order
- Patient's health record
- Drug reference information
- Otic drops
- Gauze
- Gloves

Order: Ciprodex Otic 0.1% 4 drops in left ear.

Procedural Steps

1. Wash your hands or use hand sanitizer.
   Purpose: Hand sanitization is an important step for infection control.
2. Select the right medication from the storage area. Check the medication label against the order. Check for the right name, form, and route. Check the expiration date to make sure the drug is not expired. Verify the right dose and the right time.
   Purpose: It is important to do the first check of the label when getting medications from the cabinet. Do not administer expired medications.
3. Using the drug reference information and the order, review the information on the medication.
   Purpose: The medical assistant must know about the medication that is being given.
4. Perform the second medication check. Check the medication label against the order. Check for the right name, form, dose, and route.
   Purpose: It is important to do the second check of the label before continuing with the procedure.
5. Assemble the supplies required for the procedure.
   Purpose: You need to have the supplies ready before going to the exam room.
6. Perform the third medication check. Check the medication label against the order. Check for the right name, form, dose, and route.
   Purpose: It is important to do the third check of the label before seeing the patient.
7. Prior to entering the exam room, knock on the door and wait a moment. Greet the patient. Identify yourself. Verify the patient's identity with full

name and date of birth. Make sure the patient's information matches the order and the record. Explain what you are going to do.
   Purpose: It is important to identify the patient in two different ways to ensure that you have the correct patient. Explaining the procedure can make the patient feel more comfortable and helps to reduce anxiety.
8. Provide the right education to the patient. Explain the medication ordered, the desired effect, and common side effects, and identify the provider who ordered it. Answer any questions the patient may have. Use language the patient can understand. Ask the patient if they have any allergies. If the patient refuses the medication, notify the provider.
   Purpose: The patient needs to be aware of what you are giving, its action and side effects, and who ordered it. It is also important to double-check the patient's allergies before administering the medication.
9. Assist the patient into a sitting position, or into a side-lying position on the unaffected side.
   Purpose: These positions allow the medical assistant to instill the medication.
10. Warm the medication bottle with your hands if needed. The drops should be at room temperature. Shake the medication if needed. Put on gloves.
    Purpose: If the drops are too hot or too cold, the patient may experience nausea and vertigo. Gloves are used for infection control purposes.
11. Perform the right technique. Have patients tilt their head so the affected ear is upward. If cerumen or drainage is blocking the canal, gently remove it with a cotton-tipped applicator.
    Purpose: The canal must be opened to instill the drops.
12. Remove the cover of the bottle. With your nondominant hand, gently pull the pinna up and back if the patient is older than age 3. This straightens the external auditory canal. For patients younger than 3, pull the pinna down and back.
    Purpose: Straightening the canal allows the medication to flow down it.
13. Hold the dropper firmly in your dominant hand. Place the tip of the dropper about ½ inch above the ear canal (Fig. 1). Be sure not to contaminate the dropper by touching it to the patient. Carefully drop the required number of drops in the patient's ear. Replace the cover.
    Purpose: If the bottle tip gets contaminated, the bottle needs to be discarded.

PROCEDURE 46.3 Instill Ear Drops—cont'd

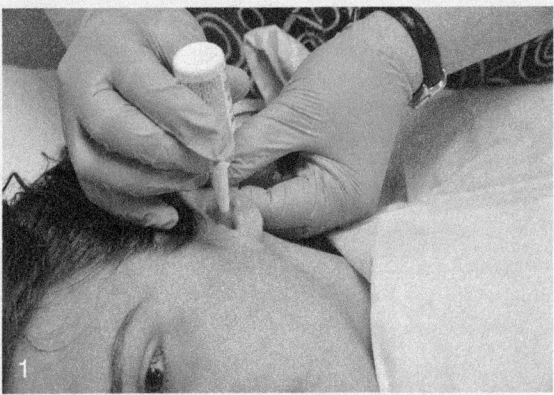
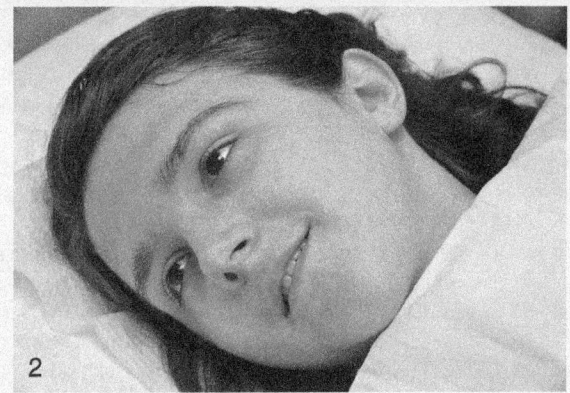

14. Have the patient keep the ear facing up for 3 to 5 minutes, depending on the medications (Fig. 2).
    Purpose: This allows the medication to move throughout the canal.

15. Help the patient into a comfortable position. Clean up the area. Remove your gloves and wash your hands or use hand sanitizer.
    Purpose: It is important for the patient to be comfortable.

16. Document the procedure in the health record. Include allergies, teaching or instructions provided; the name of the provider who ordered the medication; the medication's name, dose, and route; and how the patient tolerated the medication.
    Purpose: The medication given needs to be documented to indicate it was given.

Documentation Example

11/02/20XX 1526 NKA. Per Dr. Martin's order, administered Ciprodex 0.1% 4 gtts to left ear. Pt kept left ear facing up for 5 minutes. Medication action and side effects discussed with patient prior to administration. Pt had no questions and verbalized understanding. Pt experienced slight dizziness when drops were instilled. Dizziness went away within a few minutes. Pt states they are feeling fine._____Gabe Garcia CMA (AAMA)

PROCEDURE 46.4 Irrigate a Patient's Eye

Tasks

Irrigate a patient's eye and document patient care.

Equipment and Supplies

- Provider's order
- Patient's health record
- Drug reference information
- Sterile ophthalmic irrigation solution and supplies
- Disposable waterproof pad and towels
- Basin
- Sterile gauze
- Gloves

Order: Irrigate right eye with 1 L Normal Saline.

Procedural Steps

1. Wash your hands or use hand sanitizer.
   Purpose: Hand sanitization is an important step for infection control.

2. Select the right medication (fluid) from the storage area. Check the medication label against the order. Check for the right name, form, and route. Check the expiration date to make sure the fluid is not expired. Verify the right dose and the right time.
   Purpose: It is important to do the first check of the label when getting medications from the cabinet. Do not administer expired medications or fluids.

3. Using the drug reference information and the order, review the information on the medication.
   Purpose: The medical assistant must know about the medication that is being given.

4. Perform the second medication check. Check the medication label against the order. Check for the right name, form, dose, and route.
   Purpose: It is important to do the second check of the label before continuing with the procedure.

5. Assemble the supplies required for the procedure.
   Purpose: You need to have the supplies ready before going to the exam room.

6. Perform the third medication check. Check the medication label against the order. Check for the right name, form, dose, and route.
   Purpose: It is important to do the third check of the label before seeing the patient.

7. Prior to entering the exam room, knock on the door and wait a moment. Greet the patient. Identify yourself. Verify the patient's identity with full name and date of birth. Make sure the patient's information matches the order and the record. Explain what you are going to do.
   Purpose: It is important to identify the patient in two different ways to ensure that you have the correct patient. Explaining the procedure can make the patient feel more comfortable and helps to reduce anxiety.

Continued

PROCEDURE 46.4   Irrigate a Patient's Eye—cont'd

8. Provide the right education to the patient. Explain the procedure ordered, the desired effect, and common side effects, and identify the provider who ordered it. Answer any questions the patient may have. Use language the patient can understand. Ask the patient if they have any allergies. If the patient refuses the procedure, notify the provider.

   Purpose: The patient needs to be aware of the procedure you will be performing, its action and side effects, and who ordered it. It is also important to double-check the patient's allergies before starting the procedure.

9. Using room temperature fluid, set up the equipment. If using an intravenous (IV) bag, prime or run fluid through the tubing. If using a prepackaged solution, remove the cover. If using a bulb syringe, pour the required fluid into a basin – remember to palm the label. Draw the solution into the bulb syringe.

   Purpose: Having the fluid ready for the irrigation is important before you hold the eye open.

10. Assist the patient into a sitting or supine position. Have the patient remove glasses or contact lens. Ask the patient to turn the head toward the side of the affected eye. Place the disposable waterproof pad over the patient's neck and shoulder. Place or have the patient hold the drainage basin next to the affected eye.

    Purpose: Protecting the unaffected eye from the solution is important so it does not also get contaminated. The basin will collect the irrigation fluid from the eye.

11. Put on gloves. Moisten a gauze pad with the irrigation fluid. Using the gauze, clean the eyelid from the inner to outer canthus (Fig. 1). Discard the gauze after each wipe.

    Purpose: Debris on the eyelid must be removed before the irrigation can be done.

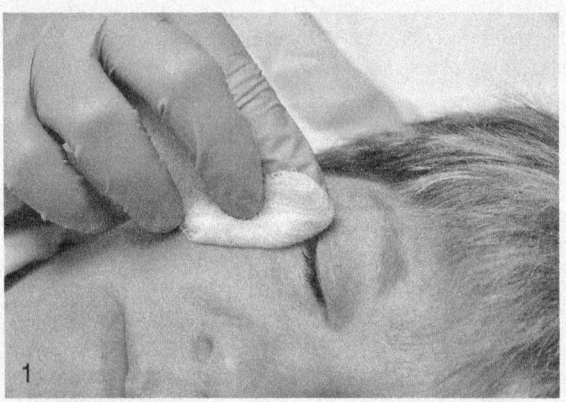

12. Perform the right technique. With your nondominant hand, separate and hold the eyelids using the index finger and thumb. With the dominant hand, hold the irrigation equipment on or near the bridge of the nose (Fig. 2).

    Purpose: Using the nose to help steady the irrigation will help to provide a steady flow of fluid going into the eye.

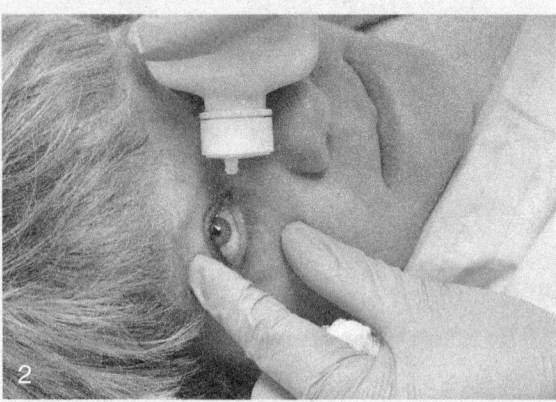

13. Direct the solution toward the lower conjunctiva of the inner canthus. Allow a steady flow of solution to slowly flush the eye from the inner to the outer canthus. Do not touch the tip of the irrigation equipment to the eye.

    Purpose: Touching the eye with the irrigation equipment could lead to an eye injury.

14. Continue until the ordered amount of fluid has flushed the eye. Dry the eyelid with sterile gauze, moving from the inner to outer canthus.

    Purpose: It is important to follow the exact order of the provider.

15. Help the patient into a comfortable position. Clean up the area. Remove your gloves and wash your hands or use hand sanitizer.

    Purpose: It is important for the patient to be comfortable.

16. Document the procedure in the health record. Include allergies, teaching or instructions provided; the name of the provider who ordered the irrigation; the fluid used for the irrigation, the amount used, the site; and how the patient tolerated the procedure.

    Purpose: The irrigation performed needs to be documented to indicate that it was done.

Documentation Example

10/30/20XX 1440 NKA. Per Dr. Martin's order, irrigated right eye with 1 liter of normal saline IV fluid. Purpose of irrigation and side effects discussed with patient prior to procedure. Pt had no questions and verbalized understanding. Pt tolerated the procedure without problems._____
_____ Gabe Garcia CMA (AAMA)

PROCEDURE 46.5   Irrigate a Patient's Ear

Tasks

Irrigate a patient's ear and document patient care.

Equipment and Supplies

- Provider's order
- Patient's health record
- Ear wash basin
- Elephant ear wash system (or other ear wash system)
- Disposable waterproof pad and towels
- Thermometer (optional)
- Otoscope and disposable speculum (optional)
- Gauze
- Gloves

- Sterile water or saline
- Waste container

   Order: Irrigate left ear with warm sterile water.

Procedural Steps

1. Wash your hands or use hand sanitizer.

   Purpose: Hand sanitization is an important step for infection control.

2. Select the right medication (fluid) from the storage area. Check the medication label against the order. Check for the right name and route; check the expiration date.

   Purpose: It is important to do the first check of the label when getting the medications from the cabinet.

PROCEDURE 46.5 Irrigate a Patient's Ear—cont'd

3. Assemble the equipment and supplies needed. Perform the second medication check. Check the medication (fluid) name and route against the order.
   Purpose: You need to have the supplies ready before going to the exam room.
4. Clean up the work area and perform the third medication check. Check the medication (fluid) name and route against the order,
   Purpose: It is important to do three checks before using the fluid.
5. Prior to entering the exam room, knock on the door and wait a moment. Greet the patient. Identify yourself. Verify the patient's identity with full name and date of birth. Make sure the patient's information matches the order and the record. Explain what you are going to do.
   Purpose: It is important to identify the patient in two different ways to ensure that you have the correct patient. Explaining the procedure can make the patient feel more comfortable and helps to reduce anxiety.
6. Provide the right education to the patient. Explain the procedure ordered, the desired effect, and common side effects of ear irrigations; also identify the provider who ordered the procedure. Answer any questions the patient may have. Use language the patient can understand. If the patient refuses the procedure, notify the provider.
   Purpose: The patient needs to be aware of the procedure you will be performing, its action and side effects, and who ordered it.
7. Prepare the equipment. Warm the irrigating solution to body temperature (98.6°F [check with a thermometer]) or until it is lukewarm. Lukewarm is neither hot nor cold. Fill the spray bottle with the fluid. Attach the disposable tip to the nozzle on the hose. If another type of ear wash system is being used, prepare the equipment and the fluid.
   Purpose: Having the fluid ready for the irrigation is important before holding the ear. Sterile irrigating fluid is recommended.
8. Assist the patient into a sitting position. Wrap a waterproof pad around the person's shoulder, protecting the clothing. Have a towel available for the patient if needed. Have the patient tilt the head toward the affected ear. Have the patient hold the ear wash basin under the affected ear.
   Purpose: It is important to protect the patient's clothing from the irrigating fluid.
9. Put on gloves. Using gauze, wipe any debris from the outer ear.
   Purpose: Debris on the outer ear must be removed before the irrigation can be done.
10. Insert the disposable tip gently into the ear (Fig. 1). Do not insert it too far because it could injure the canal. If possible, gently pull the pinna up and back if the patient is older than age 3. For patients younger than 3, pull pinna down and back.
    Purpose: If using the spray bottle irrigation system, you will not be able to pull the pinna. One hand is holding the tip, and the other hand is squeezing the trigger. Other systems may allow you a free hand to position the pinna to open the canal.

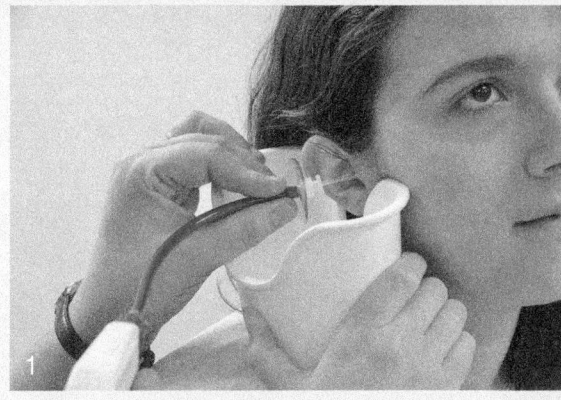

11. Keeping the tubing straight, spray the fluid into the ear canal. Aim the fluid toward the top of the ear canal.
    Purpose: Aiming the fluid toward the top of the canal helps prevent injury to the tympanic membrane. It can also make the procedure more comfortable for the patient.
12. Continue irrigating until the solution is used up, the maximum time has been reached, the desired result is achieved, or the patient has problems with the procedure. Empty the ear wash basin when it fills. Observe the fluid for any substances (e.g., cerumen).
    Purpose: The provider's order or the facility's procedures will indicate the amount of irrigation fluid to use or when to stop the irrigation.
13. Dry the outside of the ear with gauze. If the facility's procedure indicates, use an otoscope to observe the canal. Attach the speculum to the otoscope. Straighten the ear canal by pulling in the appropriate direction on the pinna. Gently insert the otoscope and observe the canal.
    Purpose: Observing the canal helps you check the results of the irrigation.
14. Place a clean, absorbent towel on the examination table. Have the patient rest quietly with the head turned to the irrigated side while you wait for the provider to return to check the affected ear.
    Purpose: This allows the fluid in the canal to drain out.
15. Clean up the work area. Remove your gloves and dispose in the waste container. Sanitize your hands.
    Purpose: Hand sanitization is an important step for infection control.
16. Document the procedure in the health record. Include teaching or instructions provided; the name of the provider who ordered the irrigation; the fluid used for the irrigation, the amount used, the site; and how the patient tolerated the procedure.
    Purpose: The irrigation performed needs to be documented to indicate that it was done.

Documentation Example

11/04/20XX 1540 Per Dr. Martin's order, irrigated left ear with lukewarm sterile water for 15 min. Flushed out moderate amount of brown cerumen. Pt had slight dizziness initially with irrigation, which resolved quickly. Pt rested on exam table.
_____ Gabe Garcia CMA (AAMA)

PROCEDURE 46.6   Prepare Medication From an Ampule

Task
Prepare medication from an ampule.

Equipment and Supplies
- Provider's order
- Ampule of medication
- Gauze or ampule breaker
- Alcohol wipes
- Filter needle and hypodermic safety needle
- 3-mL syringe
- Biohazardous sharps container
- Waste container
- Drug reference information
- Marker

Order: 0.9% Sodium Chloride 0.7 mL IM

Procedural Steps

1. Wash your hands or use hand sanitizer. Using the drug reference information and the order, review the information on the medication if needed. Clarify any questions you have with the provider.
   Purpose: Hand sanitization is an important step for infection control. It is important to be knowledgeable about the medication you are giving.

2. Select the right medication from the storage area. Check the medication label against the order. Check for the right name, form, and route. Check the expiration date to make sure the drug is not expired. Verify the right dose and the right time.
   Purpose: It is important to do the first check of the label when getting medications from the cabinet. Do not administer expired medications.

3. Assemble the supplies required for the procedure.
   Purpose: Remember to split up the three medication checks with activities between each check.

4. Perform the second medication check. Check the medication label against the order. Check for the right name, form, dose, and route.
   Purpose: It is important to do the second check of the label before continuing with the procedure.

5. Attach the filter needle to the syringe without contaminating the unit. Using a marker, label the syringe with the medication name.
   Purpose: You will use the filter needle first during the procedure.

6. Gently tap the medication from the head of the ampule or hold the ampule securely, upright in your hand (Fig. 1). Quickly move your hand downward. After all the medication has drained into the body of the ampule, wipe the neck with an alcohol wipe.
   Purpose: Any medication left in the head will be lost after it is snapped off. Tapping or quickly bringing the ampule down will drain the medication into the body.

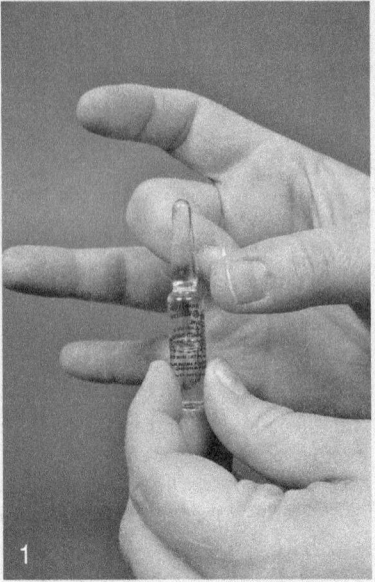

1

7. Place the ampule breaker over the head of the ampule (following the directions from the manufacturer) or wrap the neck with gauze (Figs. 2–4). Hold the body with your nondominant hand. With your dominant hand, firmly hold the head (or breaker) between your first two fingers and thumb. Quickly snap off the head of the ampule, making sure it breaks away from your body and others (see the third following figure).
   Purpose: It is important to protect your fingers from the broken glass.

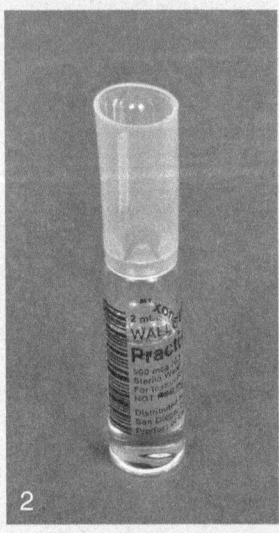

2

PROCEDURE 46.6 Prepare Medication From an Ampule—cont'd

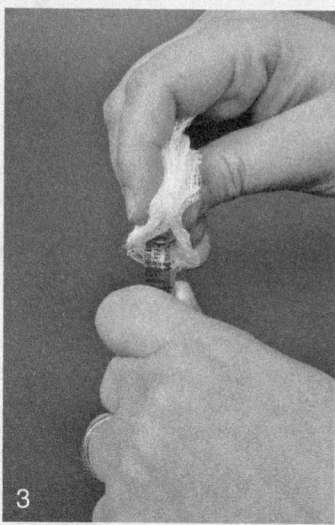

3

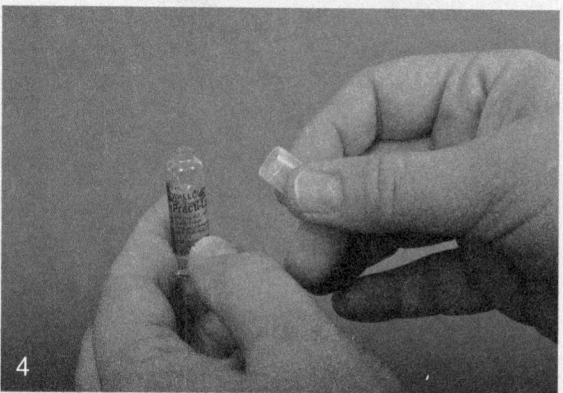

4

8. Discard the breaker or gauze with the ampule head in a biohazardous sharps container.

Purpose: It is important to discard the head immediately to protect yourself.

9. Place the ampule on a flat surface. Uncover the filter needle and insert the needle into the ampule without contaminating the needle. Keeping the bevel in the medication, pull the plunger upward, aspirating the medication into the syringe. Tilt the ampule as you remove all the medication.
   Purpose: Keeping the bevel in the medication will prevent air being aspirated into the syringe.

10. Recap the needle using the one-handed scoop technique. Perform the third medication check. Check the medication label against the order. Check for the right name, form, and route. Discard the ampule in the biohazardous sharps container.
    Purpose: It is important to do the third check of the label before seeing the patient.

11. Remove the filter needle and attach a new needle without contaminating the unit. Discard the filter needle in the biohazardous sharps container.
    Purpose: The filter needle needs to be removed before the injection is given.

12. Hold the syringe in a vertical position with the uncapped needle pointed upward. Tap the barrel carefully with the fingertips or a pen to move the air bubbles up to the top of the barrel. Once all the air bubbles are at the top, push the plunger slowly to the correct calibration marking for the ordered dose. Recap the needle.
    Purpose: The air needs to be at the top of the syringe before you measure the correct amount of medication.

13. Double-check the dose of medication measured against the order. Make sure no air bubbles are in the syringe.
    Purpose: Air bubbles take up space. If air bubbles are present, then the correct dose will not be given.

14. Maintain sterility of the medication and the needle throughout the procedure.
    Purpose: The needle and medication need to be sterile for the injection.

15. Clean up the work area. Packaging and other waste should be discarded in the waste container.
    Purpose: It is professional to clean up after yourself. Never fill a biohazardous sharps container with uncontaminated waste (e.g., packaging).

PROCEDURE 46.7 Prepare Medication Using a Prefilled Sterile Cartridge

Tasks

Prepare medication using a prefilled sterile cartridge. Discard a prefilled sterile cartridge while keeping the reusable holder.

Equipment and Supplies

- Provider's order
- Prefilled sterile cartridge
- Hypodermic safety needle (if needed)
- Carpuject cartridge holder
- Biohazardous sharps container
- Waste container
- Drug reference information
  Order: 0.9% Sodium Chloride 1.6 mL IM

Procedural Steps

1. Wash your hands or use hand sanitizer. Using the drug reference information and the order, review the information on the medication if needed. Clarify any questions you have with the provider.
   Purpose: Hand sanitization is an important step for infection control. It is important to be knowledgeable about the medication you are giving.

2. Select the right medication from the storage area. Check the medication label against the order. Check for the right name, form, and route. Check the expiration date to make sure the drug is not expired. Verify the right dose and the right time.
   Purpose: It is important to do the first check of the label when getting the medication from the cabinet. Do not administer expired medications.

3. Assemble the supplies required for the procedure.
   Purpose: Remember to split up the three medication checks with activities between each check.

4. Perform the second medication check. Check the medication label against the order. Check for the right name, form, dose, and route.
   Purpose: It is important to do the second check of the label before continuing with the procedure.

5. Break the seal. With one hand on the needle cover and the other on the barrel of the prefilled cartridge, move your hands together until you hear a pop. If needed, remove the cover on the cartridge and attach a covered safety needle.
   Purpose: The seal needs to be broken before the cartridge is used.

Continued

PROCEDURE 46.7   Prepare Medication Using a Prefilled Sterile Cartridge—cont'd

6. Hold the Carpuject holder so the opening (for the barrel) is facing up. Pull the plunger rod out until it clicks. Turn the blue lock until it clicks. This should increase the space between the blue lock and the flange (Fig. 1).

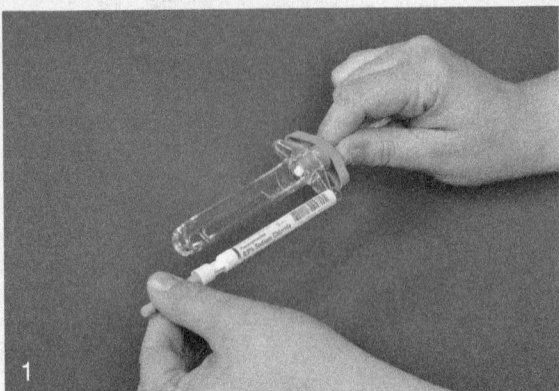

Purpose: The Carpuject holder needs to be opened before the cartridge can be placed in it.

7. Insert the cartridge into the Carpuject holder (Fig. 2). To secure the cartridge, turn the blue lock on the Carpuject holder until it clicks. The space between the blue lock and the flange should decrease. Turn the white plunger rod until it screws onto the rubber stopper (Fig. 3).
   Purpose: The cartridge must be secured in the Carpuject holder.

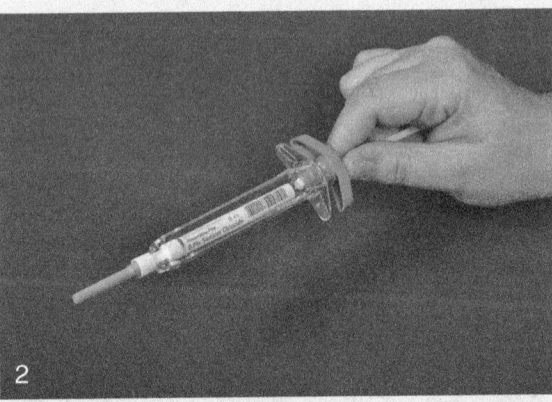

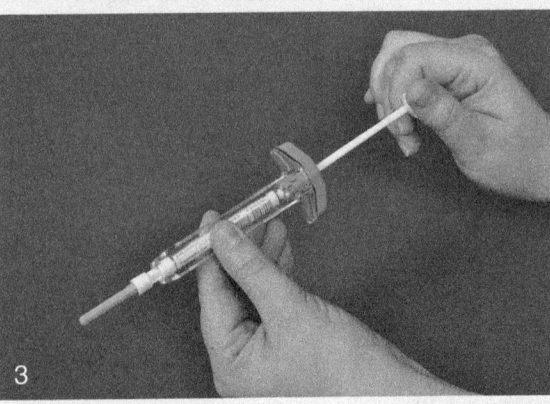

8. Remove the cover. Hold the syringe unit in a vertical position with the uncapped needle or tip pointed upward. Tap the barrel carefully with the fingertips or a pen to move the air bubbles up to the top of the barrel. Once all the air bubbles are at the top, push the plunger slowly to the correct calibration marking for the ordered dose.
   Purpose: The air needs to be at the top of the syringe before you measure the correct amount of medication.

9. Recap the needle using the one-handed scoop technique. Perform the third medication check. Check the medication label against the order. Check for the right name, form, and route.
   Purpose: It is important to do the third check of the label before seeing the patient.

10. Double-check the dose of medication measured against the order. Make sure no air bubbles are in the syringe.
    Purpose: Air bubbles take up space. If air bubbles are present, then the correct dose will not be given.

11. Maintain sterility of the medication and the needle throughout the procedure.
    Purpose: The needle and medication need to be sterile for the injection.

12. After giving the injection, unscrew the plunger rod and pull out until it clicks. Turn the blue lock until it clicks. The space between the blue lock and the flange should increase in size.
    Purpose: The Carpuject holder needs to be opened to remove the used cartridge.

13. Carefully invert the Carpuject holder over a biohazardous sharps container to discard the cartridge (Fig. 4). Hold the Carpuject holder firmly so it does not end up in the sharps container.
    Purpose: Only the cartridge should be discarded.

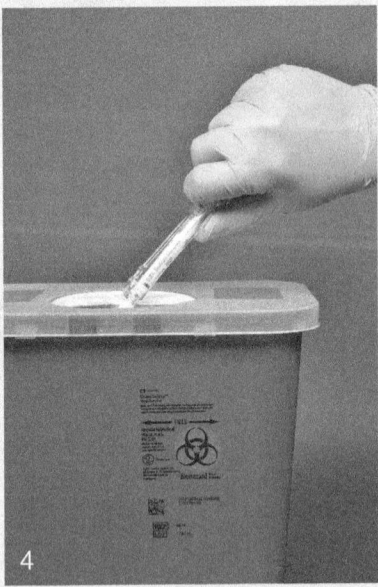

14. Disinfect the Carpuject holder. Clean up the work area. Waste should be put in the waste container.
    Purpose: Disinfection is an important step for infection control.

PROCEDURE 46.8 Prepare Medication From a Vial

Task
Prepare medication from a vial.

Equipment and Supplies
- Provider's order
- Vial of medication
- Alcohol wipes
- Hypodermic safety needle and 3 mL syringe or needle/syringe unit
- Biohazardous sharps container
- Waste container
- Drug reference information
- Marker

Order: 0.9% Sodium Chloride 1.2 mL IM

Procedural Steps

1. Wash your hands or use hand sanitizer. Using the drug reference information and the order, review the information on the medication if needed. Clarify any questions you have with the provider.
   Purpose: Hand sanitization is an important step for infection control. It is important to be knowledgeable about the medication you are giving.
2. Select the right medication from the storage area. Check the medication label against the order. Check for the right name, form, and route. Check the expiration date to make sure the drug is not expired. Verify the right dose and the right time.
   Purpose: It is important to do the first check of the label when getting medications from the cabinet. Do not administer expired medications.
3. Assemble the supplies required for the procedure.
   Purpose: Remember to split up the three medication checks with activities between each check.
4. Perform the second medication check. Check the medication label against the order. Check for the right name, form, dose, and route.
   Purpose: It is important to do the second check of the label before continuing with the procedure.
5. Open the syringe and needle. Tighten the preassembled syringe and needle unit or attach the needle to the syringe. Using a marker, label the syringe with the medication name.
   Purpose: Labeling the medication is critical for medication safety.
6. Mix the medication by rolling it with your hands if needed (Fig. 1). Remove the cap on the vial (if present). Clean the rubber stopper with an alcohol wipe (Fig. 2). Let the stopper dry.
   Purpose: The rubber stopper must be disinfected each time you enter the vial with a needle.

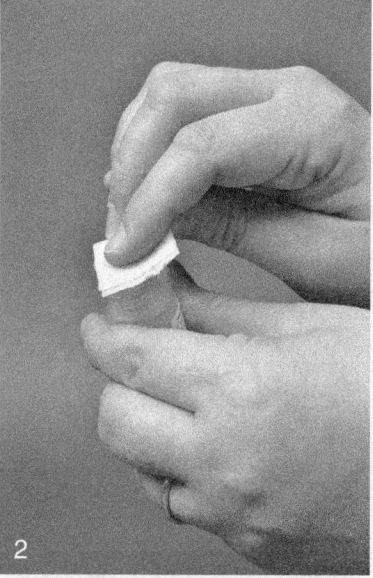

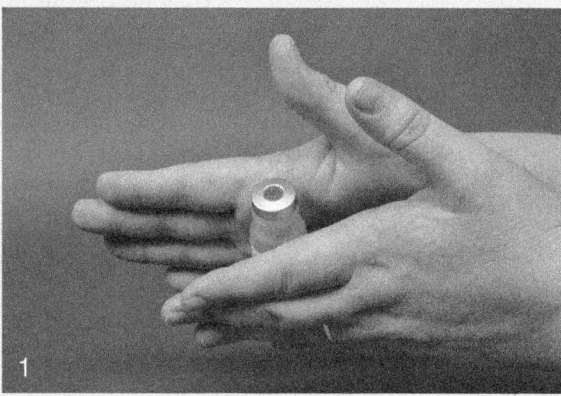

7. With the syringe in a vertical position, pull the syringe plunger down. Draw up an amount of air equal to the amount of medication ordered.
   Purpose: The vial is under pressure. When fluid is taken out, air must be added in. Not enough replaced air makes it difficult to withdraw the medication. Too much air causes the pressure to increase in the vial. The extra pressure causes the medication to be forced into the syringe without the plunger being pulled.
8. Hold the vial firmly against a flat surface. Insert the needle into the center of the dried rubber stopper. Inject the aspirated air above the fluid in the vial (Fig. 3).
   Purpose: Adding the air into the fluid will increase the bubbles.

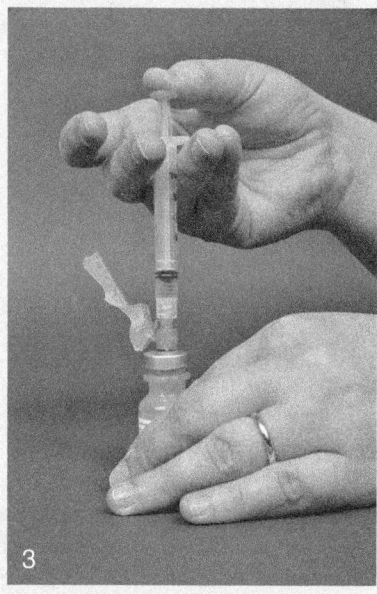

9. With the palm of your nondominant hand facing upward, grasp the vial between your middle and index fingers. Keeping the syringe unit in the vial, pick up and invert them. Use your thumb and the ring and little fingers of your nondominant hand to stabilize the syringe in the vial (Fig. 4).

Continued

PROCEDURE 46.8 Prepare Medication From a Vial—cont'd

Purpose: It is important to stabilize the syringe, so the needle does not bend.

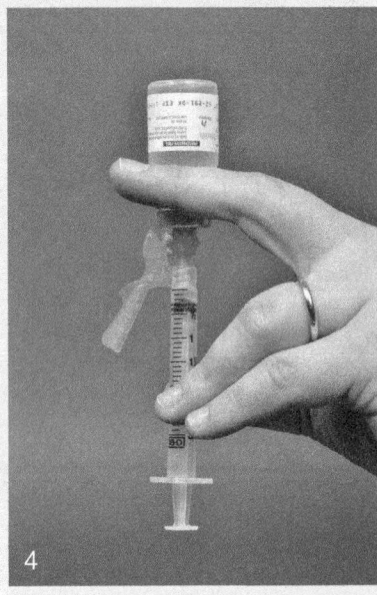

4

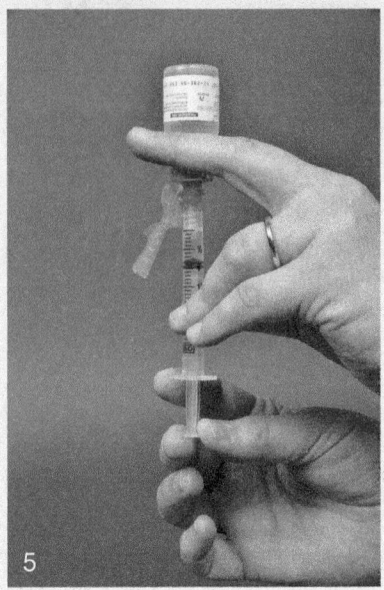

5

10. With the syringe at eye level, pull the plunger down using your dominant hand. Fill the syringe with more medication than what was ordered (Fig. 5).
    Purpose: Air bubbles will need to be ejected back into the vial. The extra medication helps with this process.

11. Continue to hold the vial/needle/syringe unit in a vertical position (with the needle pointing upward) with your nondominant hand. With your dominant hand, either use your fingers or a pen to tap the bubbles to the top of the barrel.
    Purpose: Bubbles rise to the top. With the syringe pointing straight up, the bubbles tend to move to the top of the barrel near the needle.

12. Once all the air bubbles are at the top, push the plunger slowly to the correct calibration marking for the ordered dose.
    Purpose: The air needs to be at the top of the syringe before you measure the correct amount of medication.

13. Double-check that no air bubbles are in the syringe and the right dose was measured. If everything is correct, remove the vial from the syringe/needle unit.
    Purpose: Air bubbles take up space. If air bubbles are present, then the correct dose will not be given.

14. Use the one-handed scoop technique to cover the needle. Perform the third medication check. Check each medication label against the order. Check for the right name, form, and route.
    Purpose: It is important to do the third check of the label before seeing the patient.

15. Maintain sterility of the medication and the needle throughout the procedure.
    Purpose: The needle and medication need to be sterile for the injection.

16. Clean up the work area.
    Purpose: It is professional to clean up after yourself.

PROCEDURE 46.9 Reconstitute Powdered Medication

Tasks
Reconstitute powdered medication and prepare the dose of medication.

Equipment and Supplies
- Provider's order
- Vial of powdered medication
- Vial of diluent
- Alcohol wipes

- 2 hypodermic syringes (a 3-mL and a larger syringe)
- 2 hypodermic safety needles
- Biohazardous sharps container
- Biohazardous waste container
- Waste container
- Drug reference information
- Marker

Order: (Powdered medication name) 0.5 mL IM

PROCEDURE 46.9 Reconstitute Powdered Medication—cont'd

Procedural Steps

1. Wash your hands or use hand sanitizer. Using the drug reference information and the order, review the information on the medication if needed. Clarify any questions you have with the provider.
Purpose: Hand sanitization is an important step for infection control. It is important to be knowledgeable about the medication you are giving.

2. Select the right medication from the storage area. Check the medication label against the order. Check for the right name, form, and route. Check the expiration date to make sure the vials are not expired. Verify the right dose and the right time. Read the medication label to determine the correct diluent. Obtain the diluent and check the name, route, and expiration date.
Purpose: It is important to do the first check of the label when getting the medications from the cabinet. The label of the powdered medication will indicate the diluent to use. The diluent label must also be checked.

3. Assemble the supplies required for the procedure. If needed, calculate the dose of medication required.
Purpose: Remember to split up the three medication checks with activities between each check.

4. Perform the second medication check. Check the medication labels against the order and directions for reconstituting the powder. Check for the right name, form, and route.
Purpose: It is important to do the second check of the label before continuing with the procedure.

5. Open and assemble the syringes and needles. Using a marker, label the 3-mL syringe with the medication name.
Purpose: It is important to keep the needle sterile. If contamination occurs, discard the equipment and start over.

6. Remove the caps on the vials. Clean the rubber stoppers with an alcohol wipe. Let the stoppers dry.
Purpose: The rubber stopper must be disinfected each time you enter the vial with a needle.

7. With the powdered medication vial on a firm surface, insert the needle of the largest volume syringe unit. Make sure the tip stays out of the powder. Pull back on the plunger and withdraw air equal to the amount of diluent that must be added. Pull the needle/syringe out of the stopper.
Purpose: The vial is under pressure. When liquid is put in, the same volume of air must be removed to keep the pressure equal.

8. Using the syringe with the aspirated air (equal to the amount of diluent needed), insert the needle into the center of the dried rubber stopper of the diluent vial. Push the air into the vial, but do not force the air into the vial. Make sure the needle is not in the fluid.
Purpose: Adding the air into the fluid will increase the bubbles. Forcing the air into the vial may cause the vial to have too much pressure.

9. With the palm of your nondominant hand facing upward, grasp the vial between your middle and index fingers. Keeping the syringe unit in the vial, pick up and invert them. Use your thumb and the ring and little fingers of your nondominant hand to stabilize the syringe in the vial. Pull down on the plunger until you have more diluent than what you need.
Purpose: It is important to stabilize the syringe, so the needle does not bend.

10. Continue to hold the vial/needle/syringe unit in a vertical position (with the needle pointing upward) with your nondominant hand. With your dominant hand, either use your fingers or a pen to tap the bubbles to the top of the barrel.
Purpose: Bubbles rise to the top. With the syringe pointing straight up, the bubbles tend to move to the top of the barrel near the needle.

11. Once all the air bubbles are at the top, push the plunger slowly to the correct calibration marking for the ordered dose. Keep the syringe at eye level.
Purpose: The air needs to be at the top of the syringe before you measure the correct amount of medication.

12. Double-check that no air bubbles are in the syringe and the right dose was measured. If everything is correct, remove the vial from the syringe/needle unit.

Purpose: Air bubbles take up space. If air bubbles are present, then the correct dose will not be given.

13. Using an alcohol wipe, clean the rubber stopper of the powdered medication vial. With the vial flat on a hard surface, insert the needle into the dried stopper. Push the diluent into the vial. If resistance is met, take your finger off the plunger and allow air to fill in the syringe. Gradually work all the diluent into the vial. Withdraw the needle from the vial and discard the needle and syringe in the biohazardous sharps container.
Purpose: Forcing the diluent into the vial may cause the vial to "explode" at the weakest point.

14. Gently mix the vial by rolling it in your palms. Mix the medication until all the powder is dissolved.
Purpose: The powder needs to be totally dissolved so the correct dose is given.

15. Clean the rubber stopper of the powdered medication vial with an alcohol wipe. Let the stopper dry. With the second syringe in a vertical position, pull the syringe plunger down. Draw up an amount of air equal to the amount of medication ordered.
Purpose: Think of this step as starting over. Air needs to be inserted into the diluted powder vial to draw up the correct amount of medication.

16. Hold the vial firmly against a flat surface. Insert the needle into the center of the dried rubber stopper. Inject the aspirated air above the fluid in the vial.
Purpose: Adding the air into the fluid will increase the bubbles.

17. With the palm of your nondominant hand facing upward, grasp the vial between your middle and index fingers. Keeping the syringe unit in the vial, pick up and invert them. Use your thumb and the ring and little fingers of your nondominant hand to stabilize the syringe in the vial.
Purpose: It is important to stabilize the syringe, so the needle does not bend.

18. With the syringe at eye level, pull the plunger down using your dominant hand. Fill the syringe with more medication than what was ordered.
Purpose: Air bubbles will need to be ejected back into the vial. The extra medication helps with this process.

19. Continue to hold the vial/needle/syringe unit in a vertical position (with the needle pointing upward) with your nondominant hand. With your dominant hand, either use your fingers or a pen to tap the bubbles to the top of the barrel.
Purpose: Bubbles rise to the top. With the syringe pointing straight up, the bubbles tend to move to the top of the barrel near the needle.

20. Once all the air bubbles are at the top, push the plunger slowly to the correct calibration marking for the ordered dose.
Purpose: The air needs to be at the top of the syringe before you measure the correct amount of medication.

21. Double-check that no air bubbles are in the syringe and the right dose was measured. If everything is correct, remove the vial from the syringe/needle unit.
Purpose: Air bubbles take up space. If air bubbles are present, then the correct dose will not be given.

22. Use the one-handed scoop technique to cover the needle. Perform the third medication check. Check each medication label against the order. Check for the right name, form, and route.
Purpose: It is important to do the third check of the label before seeing the patient.

23. Maintain sterility of the medication and the needle throughout the procedure.
Purpose: The needle and medication need to be sterile for the injection.

24. If the medication is in a multidose vial, label the vial with the expiration date, diluent added, and your initials. Clean up the work area. Put the packaging and other waste in the waste container. Discard the vial(s) in the biohazardous waste container.
Purpose: It is professional to clean up after yourself.

PROCEDURE 46.10   Mix Two Insulins in One Syringe

Task
Mix two insulins in one syringe.

Equipment and Supplies
- Provider's order
- Regular insulin vial
- NPH insulin vial
- Alcohol wipes
- U100 insulin needle and syringe unit insulin
- Biohazardous sharps container
- Waste container
- Drug reference information
- Marker

Order: Regular insulin 16 units mixed with NPH insulin 30 units subcut.

Procedural Steps

1. Wash your hands or use hand sanitizer. Using the drug reference information and the order, review the information on the medication if needed. Clarify any questions you have with the provider.
   Purpose: Hand sanitization is an important step for infection control. It is important to be knowledgeable about the medication you are giving.

2. Select the right medications from the storage area. Check the medication labels against the order. Check for the right name, form, and route. Check the expiration date to make sure the vials are not expired. Verify the right dose and the right time.
   Purpose: It is important to do the first check of the label when getting the medications from the cabinet.

3. Assemble the supplies required for the procedure. If the insulin is cold, roll the vials in your hands to warm the medication.
   Purpose: Remember to split up the three medication checks with activities between each check.

4. Perform the second medication check. Check the medication labels against the order. Check for the right name, form, and route.
   Purpose: It is important to do the second check of the label before continuing with the procedure.

5. Open and assemble the syringe and needle. Using a marker, label the syringe with the medication name. Mix the NPH insulin by rolling the vial in your hands. If present, remove the metal or plastic caps on the vials. Clean the rubber stoppers with an alcohol wipe. Let the stoppers dry.
   Purpose: The rubber stopper must be disinfected each time you enter the vials with a needle.

6. With the syringe in a vertical position, pull the syringe plunger down. Draw up an amount of air equal to the amount of NPH insulin ordered. With the NPH vial on a firm surface, insert the needle in the rubber stopper. Inject the air into the NPH vial, keeping the needle tip out of the medication. Withdraw the needle from the stopper.
   Purpose: The vial is under pressure. Adding air is required before removing medication.

7. With the syringe in a vertical position, pull the syringe plunger down. Draw up an amount of air equal to the amount of Regular insulin ordered. With the Regular vial on a firm surface, insert the needle into the rubber stopper. Inject the air into the Regular vial, keeping the needle tip out of the medication.
   Purpose: The vial is under pressure. Adding air is required before removing medication.

8. With the palm of your nondominant hand facing upward, grasp the vial between your middle and index fingers. Keeping the syringe unit in the vial, pick up and invert them. Use your thumb, ring, and little fingers of your nondominant hand to stabilize the syringe in the vial. Pull down on the plunger until you have more Regular insulin than what you need.
   Purpose: It is important to stabilize the syringe, so the needle does not bend.

9. Continue to hold the vial/needle/syringe unit in a vertical position (with the needle pointing upward) with your nondominant hand. With your dominant hand, either use your fingers or a pen to tap the bubbles to the top of the barrel.
   Purpose: Bubbles rise to the top. With the syringe pointing straight up, the bubbles tend to move to the top of the barrel near the needle.

10. Once all the air bubbles are at the top, push the plunger slowly to the correct calibration marking for the ordered dose. Keep the syringe at eye level.
    Purpose: The air needs to be at the top of the syringe before you measure the correct amount of medication.

11. Double-check that no air bubbles are in the syringe and the right dose was measured. If everything is correct, remove the vial from the syringe/needle unit.
    Purpose: Air bubbles take up space. If air bubbles are present, then the correct dose will not be given.

12. Using an alcohol wipe, wipe the rubber stopper of the NPH vial. Calculate the total amount of insulin that needs to be given.
    Purpose: This total represents the calibration marking where the rubber stopper of the plunger needs to be pulled down to when withdrawing the NPH insulin.

13. With the NPH vial flat on a hard surface, insert the needle into the dried stopper. With the palm of your nondominant hand facing upward, grasp the vial between your middle and index fingers. Keeping the syringe unit in the vial, pick up and invert them. Use your thumb and the ring and little fingers of your nondominant hand to stabilize the syringe in the vial. Pull down on the plunger until the rubber stopper reaches the calibration mark required. Do not withdraw any extra NPH insulin.
    Purpose: If any additional NPH insulin is drawn up, the syringe must be discarded in the biohazardous sharps container. No insulin can be injected into the NPH vial.

14. Double-check that no air bubbles are in the syringe and the right dose was measured. If everything is correct, remove the vial from the syringe/needle unit.
    Purpose: Air bubbles take up space. If air bubbles are present, discard the syringe and start over.

15. Use the one-handed scoop technique to cover the needle. Perform the third medication check. Check each medication label against the order. Check for the right name, form, and route.
    Purpose: It is important to do the third check of the label before seeing the patient.

16. Maintain sterility of the medication and the needle throughout the procedure.
    Purpose: The needle and medication need to be sterile for the injection.

17. Clean up the work area. Put the packaging and other waste in the waste container. Place the insulin vials back in their storage location.
    Purpose: It is professional to clean up after yourself.

PROCEDURE 46.11 Administer an Intradermal Injection

Tasks
Prepare medication from a vial, administer an intradermal injection, read the tuberculin skin test, and document in the health record.

Equipment and Supplies
- Provider's order
- Patient's health record
- Vial of medication
- Alcohol wipes
- 1-mL syringe with ¼- to ½-inch, 25- to 27-gauge safety needle
- Bandage (if per facility's policy)
- Medication tray
- Biohazardous sharps container
- Waste container
- Drug reference information
- Gloves
- Marker and pen
- Millimeter ruler

Order: Tuberculin purified protein derivative (PPD) (5 tuberculin units) 0.1 mL ID.

Procedural Steps
1. Draw medication up from a vial (see Procedure 46.8).
2. Prior to entering the exam room, knock on the door and wait a moment. Greet the patient. Identify yourself. Verify the patient's identity with full name and date of birth. Make sure the patient's information matches the order and the record. Explain what you are going to do.
   Purpose: It is important to identify the patient in two different ways to ensure that you have the correct patient. Explaining the procedure can make the patient feel more comfortable and helps to reduce anxiety.
3. Provide the right education to the patient. Explain the medication ordered, the desired effect, and common side effects; also identify the provider who ordered it. Answer any questions the patient may have. Use language the patient can understand. Ask the patient if they have any allergies. If the patient refuses the medication, notify the provider.
   Purpose: The patient needs to be aware of what you are giving, its action and side effects, and who ordered it. It is also important to double-check the patient's allergies before administering the medication.
4. Perform the right technique. Ask the patient:
   - Can you return in 48 to 72 hours for the reading?
   - Have you ever had BCG?
   - Have you ever had a TB skin test? If yes, did you have a reaction to it?
   Purpose: These questions are important to determine if the patient should get the test or if the medical assistant should talk with the provider.
5. Use hand sanitizer and put on gloves.
   Purpose: Hand sanitization is an important step for infection control.
6. Have the patient extend a forearm. With the palm facing upward, identify an appropriate site for an injection. The site should be 2 to 4 inches below the elbow. Loosen the cap on the needle, but still protect the needle from contamination. Open the alcohol wipes.
   Purpose: The site should be free from veins, scars, wounds, abrasions, and so on. If the person has a reaction, having the site away from the elbow does not limit its motion. Loosening the cap prior to starting allows you to remove the cap with one hand during the procedure.
7. Place your nondominant hand to the side of the site, pulling the skin taut (Fig. 1). *Option:* Place your nondominant hand on the back of the patient's forearm, pulling the skin taut (Fig. 2).
   Purpose: The skin needs to be taut to insert the needle.

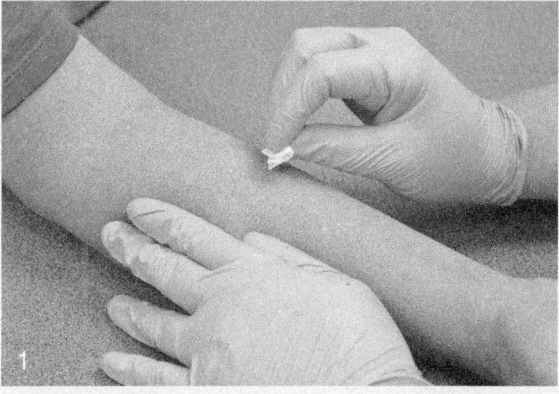

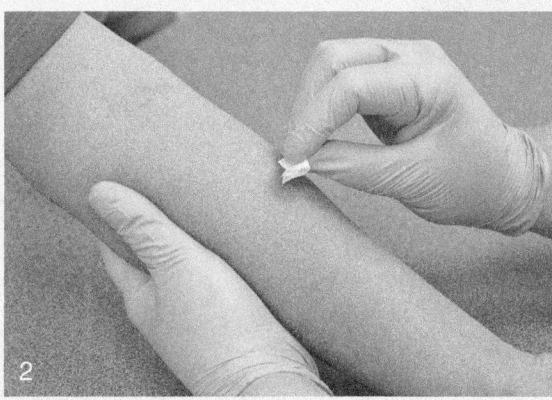

8. Cleanse the site with an alcohol wipe using a circular motion. Move from the center outward, using some friction to help clean the site. Create about a 2-inch circle at the site. Let the site dry while continuing to hold the area.
   Purpose: Cleaning from the inside to the outside prevents contamination of the cleaned area. Avoid waving over or blowing on the alcohol, which contaminates the site.
9. Pick up the syringe and tip it to remove the cover. Grasp the syringe in your dominant hand, using your thumb and index finger. Make sure to have no fingers under the syringe. Ensure that the bevel is up.
   Purpose: The syringe needs to be lowered to the skin after it is inserted. Having fingers under the syringe changes the angle and can affect the administration.
10. At a 5- to 15-degree angle, slowly insert the needle until the bevel is covered with skin (Fig. 3). Carefully lower the syringe to the skin and hold it steady with your dominant hand (Fig. 4).
    Purpose: If a greater angle is used or if more of the needle is inserted, the injection may be given deeper than it should be. Holding the syringe against the skin helps support it during the injection.

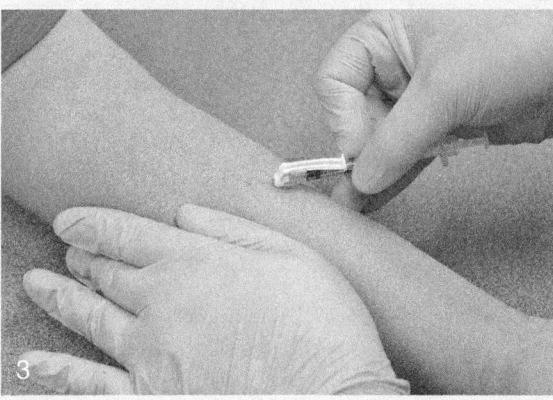

Continued

PROCEDURE 46.11   Administer an Intradermal Injection—cont'd

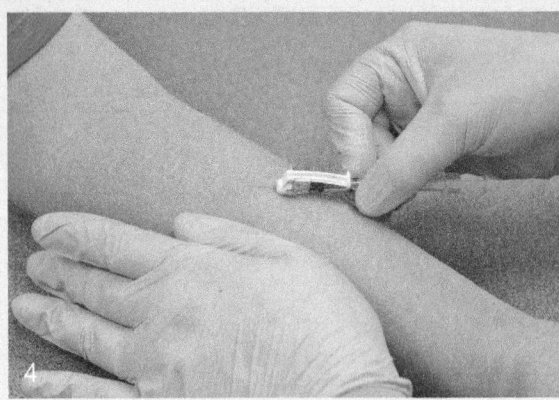

11. Carefully move your nondominant hand to the plunger. Slowly and steadily inject the medication by pressing on the plunger (Fig. 5). If a 6- to 10-mm wheal does not appear, repeat the test at least 2 inches from the site (Fig. 6).
    Purpose: Any movement of the needle/syringe can dislodge the needle from the site.

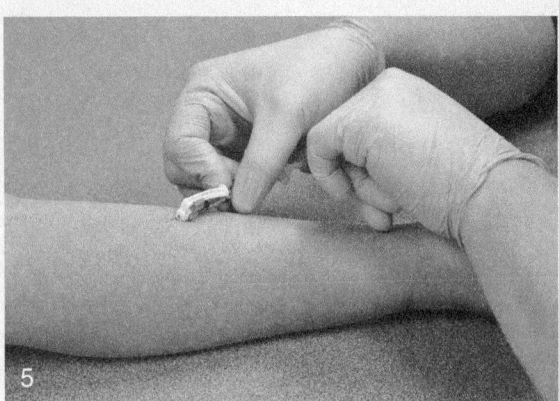

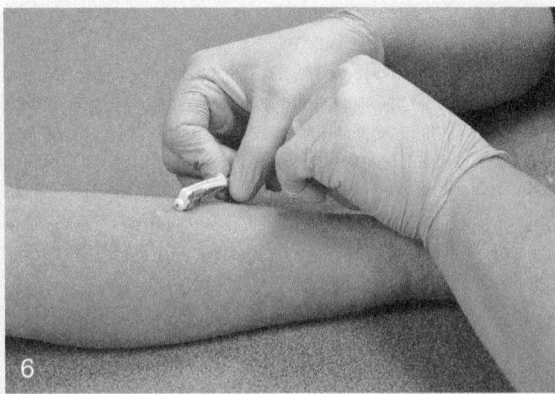

12. Double-check the barrel of the syringe to make sure all the medication was administered. Withdraw the needle. Activate the needle's safety device with one hand.
    Purpose: It is important to administer all the medication. Using more than one hand to activate the safety device increases the risk for needlestick injuries.
13. Discard the needle/syringe in a biohazardous sharps container. Make sure to put the needle in first.
    Purpose: Safely discarding the needle/syringe will help prevent needlestick injuries.

14. Do not massage the area. Per the facility's policy, if the person has a light-colored shirt with long sleeves, offer a bandage. Place the bandage on very loosely to just absorb any blood from the site.
    Purpose: It is very important that the bandage not be put on snugly, because some of the medication could be lost at the site. If a bandage is used, it needs to be very loosely applied. Some agencies will not allow the use of a bandage.
15. Observe the patient for any adverse reactions. Clean up the area. Discard the waste in the waste container. Sanitize your hands.
    Purpose: It is important to monitor the patient and clean up the work area.
16. Document the procedure in the health record. Include assessments done, allergies, teaching or instructions provided; the medication name, dose, and route; the name of the provider who ordered the medication; and how the patient tolerated the medication. Also include the manufacturer, the lot number, and the expiration date of the vial.
    Purpose: Medications given need to be documented to indicate they were given.
    Scenario update: The patient returns for the reading.
17. Check the health record to identify the location of the test. Greet the patient. Identify yourself. Verify the patient's identity with full name and date of birth. Make sure the patient's information matches the order and the record. Explain what you are going to do.
    Purpose: It is important to identify the patient in two different ways to ensure that you have the correct patient. Explaining the procedure can make the patient feel more comfortable and helps to reduce anxiety.
18. Palpate the site for an induration. If an induration is felt, ask patients if you can write on their arm. Using a ball point pen, draw a line toward the induration from the outer edge of the arm. Repeat on the other side (Fig. 7).
    Option: Palpate the induration to find the edge and then mark it with a pen. Repeat on the other side. Using a millimeter ruler, accurately measure the distance between the two points.
    Purpose: The ball point pen will stop at the edge of the induration. This provides you with two visible points to measure the size of the induration.

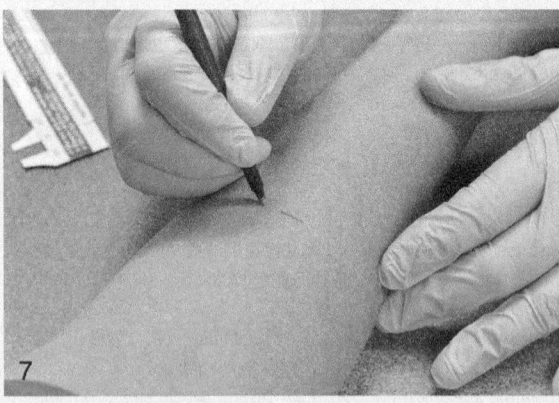

19. Document the reading in the patient's health record. Include the reason for the patient's visit, the test site, the size of the induration in millimeters, and the name of the provider who was notified.
    Purpose: The medical assistant must document the size of the induration if one is present. If no induration is present, then document 0 mm. The provider will determine if the test is negative or positive.

Documentation Example 1

11/1/20XX 0805 NKA. No prior history of TST. Per Dr. Martin's order, administered: Tuberculin purified protein derivative (PPD) 0.1 mL (5 tuberculin units) ID left forearm. (Vial: ABC Manufacturer, Lot#1345, Expires 10/20XX). Pt tolerated test without a problem. Test side effects discussed with pt prior to

PROCEDURE 46.11   Administer an Intradermal Injection—cont'd

administration. Pt instructed to return between 48 and 72 hours, and follow-up appointment was made. Pt had no questions and verbalized understanding of instructions._____Gabe Garcia CMA (AAMA)

Documentation Example 2

11/3/20XX 1005 Pt returned for TST reading. Left forearm induration measured 4 mm. Dr. Martin was notified._____Gabe Garcia CMA (AAMA)

PROCEDURE 46.12   Administer a Subcutaneous Injection

Tasks

Prepare medication from a vial, administer a subcutaneous injection, and document the medication administration in the health record.

Scenario

Dr. Martin orders polio vaccine (IPV) 0.5 mL subcut for Johnny Parker (DOB 06/15/20XX). (Vial information: ABC Manufacturer, Lot #1234, expires 1 year from today)

Equipment and Supplies

- Provider's order
- Patient's health record
- Vial of medication
- Alcohol wipes
- 3-mL syringe with ⅝-inch or ½-inch, 23 to 27-gauge safety needle
- Gauze
- Bandage
- Medication tray
- Biohazardous sharps container
- Waste container
- Drug reference information
- Vaccine Information Statement (VIS) for polio vaccine (IPV) (optional)
- Gloves
- Marker

Procedural Steps

1. Draw the medication up from a vial (see Procedure 46.8).
2. *(Peer will play the parent.)* Prior to entering the exam room, knock on the door and wait a moment. Greet the parent/patient. Identify yourself. Verify the patient's identity with full name and date of birth. Make sure the patient's information matches the order and the record. Explain what you are going to do.
   Purpose: It is important to identify the patient in two different ways to ensure that you have the correct patient. Explaining the procedure can make the patient feel more comfortable and helps to reduce anxiety.
3. Provide the right education to the parent/patient. Explain the medication ordered, the desired effect, and common side effects; also identify the provider who ordered it. Answer any questions the parent/patient may have. Use language the parent/patient can understand. Ask if the patient has any allergies. If the parent/patient refuses the medication, notify the provider.
   Purpose: The patient needs to be aware of what you are giving, its action and side effects, and who ordered it. It is also important to double-check the patient's allergies before administering the medication.
4. Use hand sanitizer and put on gloves.
   Purpose: Hand sanitization is an important step for infection control.

5. Loosen the cap on the needle, but still protect the needle from contamination. Open the alcohol wipes. Have gauze and a bandage available.
   Purpose: Loosening the cap prior to starting allows you to remove the cap with one hand during the procedure. You should never remove the cap with your teeth.
6. Find the injection site.
   Purpose: It is important to find the correct location for the injection.
7. Cleanse the site with an alcohol wipe using a circular motion (Fig. 1). Move from the center outward, using some friction to help clean the site. Create about a 2-inch circle at the site. Let the site dry.
   Purpose: Cleaning from the inside to the outside prevents contamination of the cleaned area.

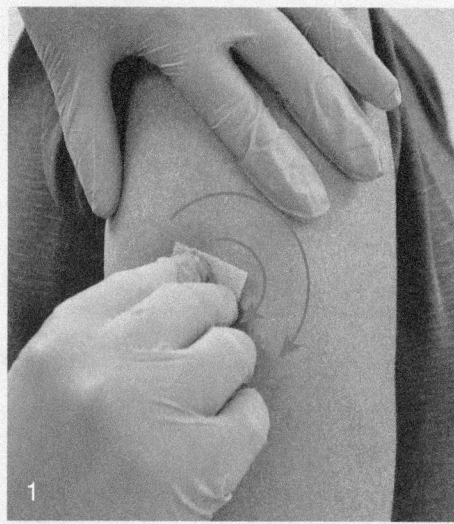

8. Avoid waving over or blowing on the alcohol, which contaminates the site.
9. Perform the right technique. Place a gauze between the index and middle fingers of your nondominant hand. With that hand, use your index finger and thumb to pinch up at the cleansed area.
   Purpose: The site needs to be pinched for a subcut injection.
10. Pick up the syringe and tip it to remove the cover. Hold the syringe between the thumb and index finger of your dominant hand (Fig. 2). Quickly and smoothly insert the needle into the site at a 45- or 90-degree angle, depending on the needle size. Insert the entire needle. Make sure the needle tip is not pointed toward your nondominant hand.
    Purpose: Ensuring that the tip is not pointed toward your hand will lessen the needlestick risk. Aspiration for subcut injections is based on the facility's policy and the recommendation from the manufacturer.

Continued

PROCEDURE 46.12 Administer a Subcutaneous Injection—cont'd

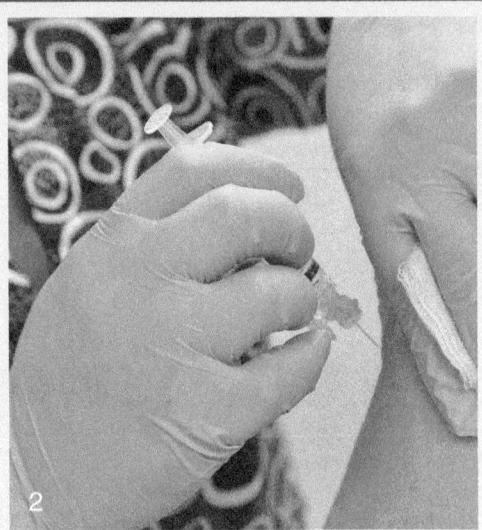

11. *One-handed option:* Continue to pinch the site. Securely grasp the syringe between your fingers of your dominant hand. With your dominant hand, aspirate if required, and then push the plunger to inject the medication. *Two-handed option:* Release the pinch and with the nondominant hand, aspirate if required, and then push the plunger to inject the medication.
    Purpose: Follow the facility's policy on whether to use the one- or two-handed option.

12. Inject the medication at a rate of 1 mL over 10 seconds. Ensure that all the medication has been injected before pulling out the needle at the same angle used for entry. Release the pinch if using the one-handed option.
    Purpose: Injecting the medication too slowly or too quickly can be uncomfortable for the patient.

13. Activate the needle's safety device with one hand while using the other hand to cover the site with gauze. Gently apply pressure at the site to stop any bleeding. Apply a bandage if the patient requests it.
    Purpose: Ask the patient if they would like a bandage if the site has stopped bleeding. Remember that some bandages may contain latex, which can be an allergen to some people. Some people may be allergic to the adhesive.

14. Discard the needle/syringe in a biohazardous sharps container. Make sure the needle goes into the sharps container first.
    Purpose: Safely discarding the needle/syringe will help prevent needle-stick injuries.

15. Observe the patient for any adverse reactions. Clean up the area. Discard the waste in the waste container. Sanitize your hands.
    Purpose: It is important to monitor the patient and to clean up the work area.

16. Document the procedure in the health record. Include assessments done, allergies, teaching or instructions provided; the name of the provider who ordered the medication; the medication's name, dose, and route; and how the patient tolerated the medication. Also include the manufacturer, the lot number, and the expiration date for vaccines and controlled substances. Fig. 3 shows the documentation using an electronic health record.
    Purpose: Medications given need to be documented to indicate they were given.

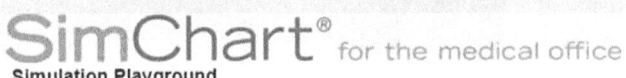

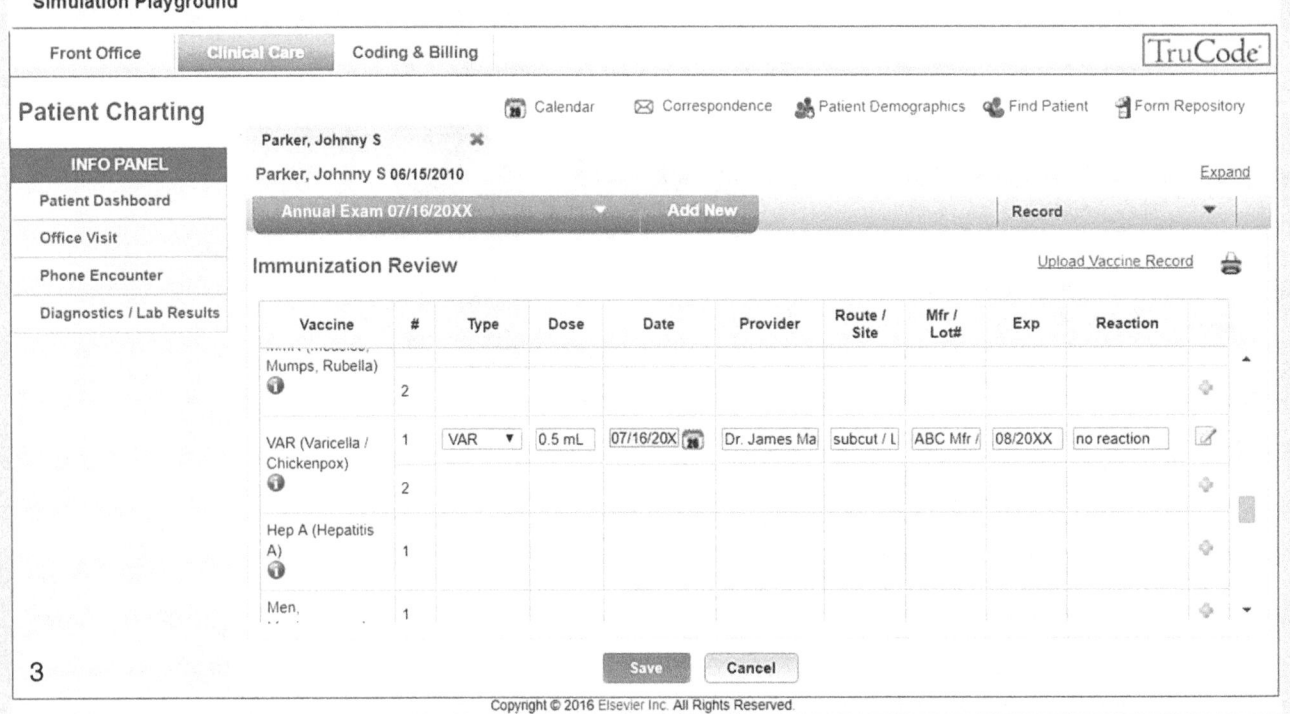

Vaccine	#	Type	Dose	Date	Provider	Route / Site	Mfr / Lot#	Exp	Reaction	
Mumps, Rubella)	2									
VAR (Varicella / Chickenpox)	1	VAR ▼	0.5 mL	07/16/20X	Dr. James Ma	subcut / L	ABC Mfr /	08/20XX	no reaction	✎
	2									
Hep A (Hepatitis A)	1									
Men,	1									

3

PROCEDURE 46.13 Administer an Intramuscular Injection

Tasks
Prepare medication from a vial, administer an intramuscular injection, and document the medication administration in the health record.

Scenario
Dr. Martin orders Influenza vaccine (IIV) 0.5 mL IM for Erma Willis (DOB 12/09/19XX). (Vial information: MN Manufacturer, Lot #7845, expires 1 year from today).

Equipment and Supplies
- Provider's order
- Patient's health record
- Vial of medication
- Alcohol wipes
- 3-mL syringe
- 22–25 gauge, 5/8–1½-inch needle
- Gauze
- Bandage
- Medication tray
- Biohazardous sharps container
- Waste container
- Drug reference information
- Vaccine Information Statement (VIS) for influenza vaccine (optional)
- Gloves
- Marker

Procedural Steps
1. Draw the medication up from a vial (see Procedure 46.8).
2. Prior to entering the exam room, knock on the door and wait a moment. Greet the patient. Identify yourself. Verify the patient's identity with full name and date of birth. Make sure the patient's information matches the order and the record. Explain what you are going to do.
   Purpose: It is important to identify the patient in two different ways to ensure that you have the correct patient. Explaining the procedure can make the patient feel more comfortable and helps to reduce anxiety.
3. Provide the right education to the patient. Explain the medication ordered, the desired effect, and common side effects; also identify the provider who ordered the medication. Answer any questions the patient may have. Use language the patient can understand. Ask the patient if they have any allergies. If the patient refuses the medication, notify the provider.
   Purpose: The patient needs to be aware of what you are giving, its action and side effects, and who ordered it. It is also important to double-check the patient's allergies before administering the medication.
4. Use hand sanitizer and put on gloves.
   Purpose: Hand sanitization is an important step for infection control.
5. Loosen the cap on the needle, but still protect the needle from contamination. Open the alcohol wipes. Have gauze and a bandage available.
   Purpose: Loosening the cap prior to starting allows you to remove the cap with one hand during the procedure. You should never remove the cap with your teeth.
6. Find the site using the landmarks.
   Purpose: It is important to find the correct location for the injection.
7. Cleanse the site with an alcohol wipe using a circular motion. Move from the center outward, using some friction to help clean the site. Create about a 2-inch circle at the site. Let the site dry.
   Purpose: Cleaning from the inside to the outside prevents contamination of the cleaned area. Avoid waving over or blowing on the alcohol, which contaminates the site.

8. Perform the right technique. Place a gauze between the index and middle fingers of your nondominant hand. With that hand, stretch or flatten the site. Hold the site.
   Purpose: The site needs to be flattened or stretched for an intramuscular injection.
9. Pick up the syringe and tip it to remove the cover. Hold the syringe like a dart with your dominant hand (Fig. 1). Quickly and smoothly insert the needle into the site at a 90-degree angle. Insert the entire needle.
   Purpose: Inserting the needle quickly is important to minimize pain.

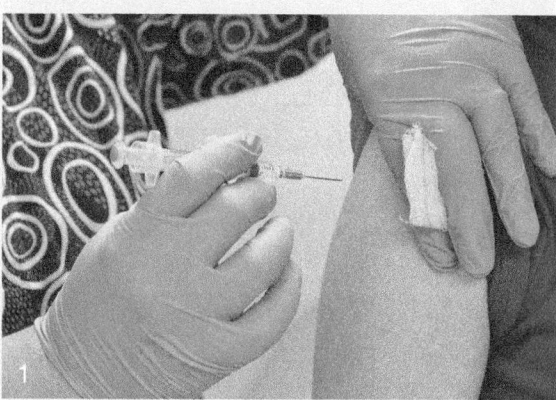

10. *One-handed option:* Continue to hold the site. Securely grasp the syringe between the fingers of your dominant hand. Place your thumb under the plunger edge and push the plunger out farther to aspirate (Fig. 2). *Two-handed option:* Move the nondominant hand to the plunger. Pull the plunger out farther to aspirate.
    Purpose: It is important to aspirate before giving an IM injection. Follow the facility's policy on whether to use the one- or two-handed option.

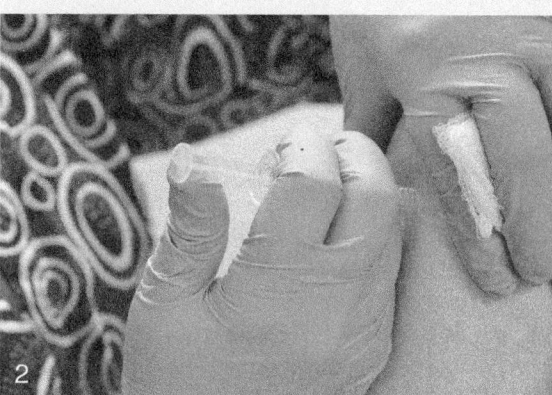

11. Aspirate for 5 seconds and check the barrel for blood. If blood is seen, pull out the needle and discard. Restart the procedure. If no blood is seen, inject the medication at a rate of about 10 seconds per milliliter. Ensure that all the medication has been injected before pulling out the needle at the same angle used for entry.
    Purpose: It is important not to give the injection if the needle is in the bloodstream.
12. Activate the needle's safety device with one hand while using the other hand to cover the site with gauze. Gently apply pressure at the site to stop any bleeding. Apply a bandage if the patient requests it.
    Purpose: Ask the patient if they would like a bandage if the site has stopped bleeding. Remember that some bandages may contain latex, which

Continued

PROCEDURE 46.13   Administer an Intramuscular Injection—cont'd

can be an allergen to some people. Some people may be allergic to the adhesive.

13. Discard the needle/syringe in a biohazardous sharps container. Make sure to put the needle in first.

    Purpose: Safely discarding the needle/syringe will help prevent needle-stick injuries.

14. Observe the patient for any adverse reactions. Clean up the area. Discard the waste in the waste container. Sanitize your hands.

    Purpose: It is important to monitor the patient and clean up the work area.

15. Document the procedure in the health record. Include assessments done, allergies, teaching or instructions provided; the name of the provider who ordered the medication; the medication's name, dose, and route; and how the patient tolerated the medication. Also include the manufacturer, lot number, and expiration date for vaccines and controlled substances. Fig. 3 shows the documentation using an electronic health record.

    Purpose: Medications given need to be documented to indicate they were given.

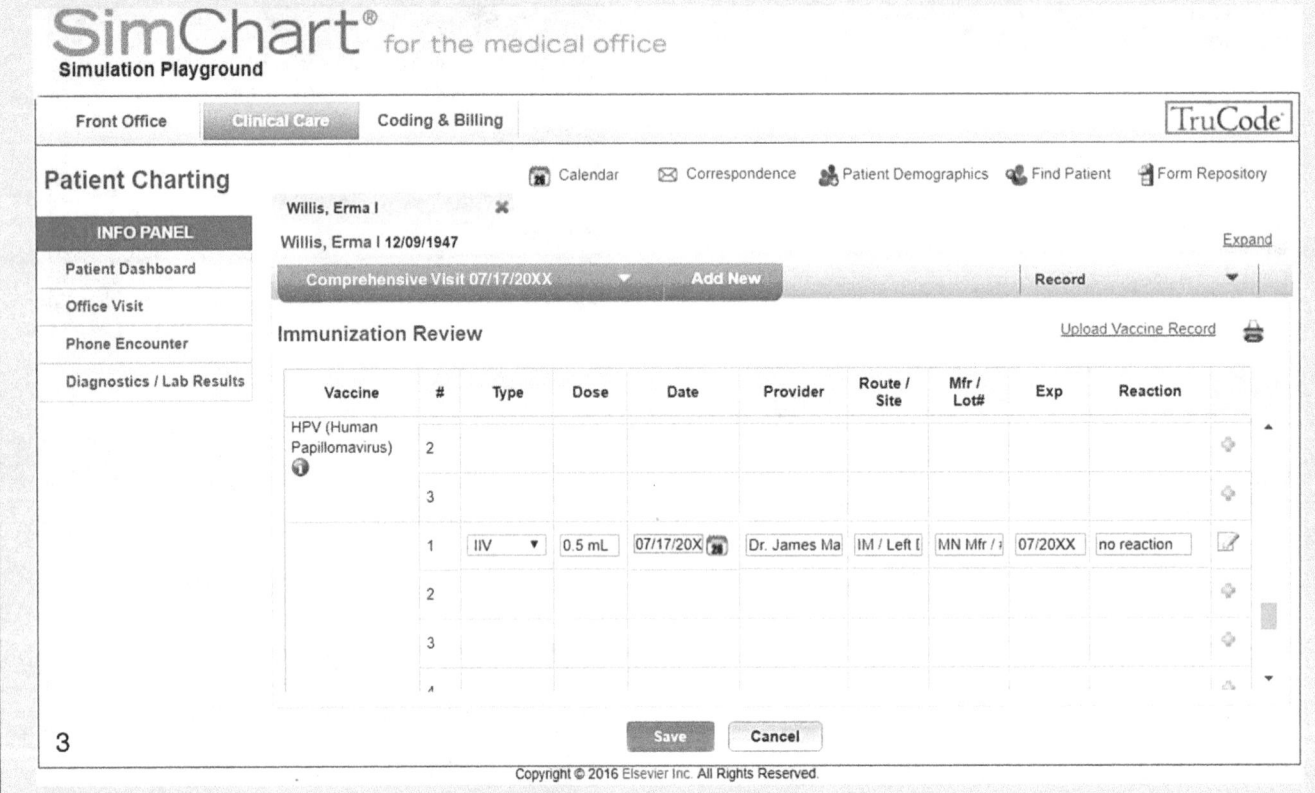

3

PROCEDURE 46.14   Administer an Intramuscular Injection Using the Z-Track Technique

Task

Prepare medication from a vial, administer an intramuscular injection, and document the medication administration in the health record.

Scenario

Dr. Martin orders Iron Dextran 0.5 mL IM for Erma Willis (DOB 12/09/19XX). (Vial information: FE Manufacturer, Lot #625, expires 1 year from today)

Equipment and Supplies

- Provider's order
- Patient's health record
- Vial of medication
- Alcohol wipes
- 3-mL syringe
- 18–21 gauge, 1½-inch needle
- Gauze
- Bandage
- Medication tray
- Biohazardous sharps container
- Waste container
- Drug reference information
- Gloves
- Marker

Procedural Steps

1. Draw the medication up from a vial (see Procedure 46.8).

2. Prior to entering the exam room, knock on the door and wait a moment. Greet the patient. Identify yourself. Verify the patient's identity with full name and date of birth. Make sure the patient's information matches the order and the record. Explain what you are going to do.

   Purpose: It is important to identify the patient in two different ways to ensure that you have the correct patient. Explaining the procedure can make the patient feel more comfortable and helps to reduce anxiety.

3. Provide the right education to the patient. Explain the medication ordered, the desired effect, and common side effects; also identify the provider who ordered the medication. Answer any questions the patient may have. Use language the patient can understand. Ask the patient if they have any allergies. If the patient refuses the medication, notify the provider.

PROCEDURE 46.13   Administer an Intramuscular Injection Using the Z-Track Technique—cont'd

Purpose: The patient needs to be aware of what you are giving, its action and side effects, and who ordered it. It is also important to double-check the patient's allergies before administering the medication.

4. Use hand sanitizer and put on gloves.

Purpose: Hand sanitization is an important step for infection control.

5. Loosen the cap on the needle, but still protect the needle from contamination. Open the alcohol wipes. Have gauze and a bandage available.

Purpose: Loosening the cap prior to starting allows you to remove the cap with one hand during the procedure. You should never remove the cap with your teeth.

6. Find the site using the landmarks.

Purpose: It is important to find the correct site.

7. Perform the right technique. Place a gauze between the index and middle fingers of your nondominant hand. With that hand, displace the tissue.

Purpose: The tissue needs to be displaced before you cleanse the site.

8. Cleanse the site with an alcohol wipe using a circular motion. Move from the center outward, using some friction to help clean the site. Create about a 2-inch circle at the site. Let the site dry while continuing to hold the area.

Purpose: Cleaning from the inside to the outside prevents contamination of the cleaned area. Avoid waving over or blowing on the alcohol, which contaminates the site.

9. Pick up the syringe and tip it to remove the cover. Hold the syringe like a dart with your dominant hand. Quickly and smoothly insert the needle into the site at a 90-degree angle. Insert the entire needle.

Purpose: Inserting the needle quickly is important to minimize pain.

10. Continue to hold the site. Securely grasp the syringe between the fingers of your dominant hand. Place your thumb under the plunger edge and push the plunger out farther to aspirate.

Purpose: It is important to aspirate before giving an IM injection. Follow the facility's policy on whether to use the one- or two-handed option.

11. Aspirate for 5 seconds and check the barrel for blood. If blood is seen, pull out the needle and discard. Restart the procedure. If no blood is seen, inject the medication at a rate of about 10 seconds per mL. Ensure that all the medication has been injected. Wait 10 seconds before withdrawing the needle and letting go with your nondominant hand.

Purpose: It is important not to give the injection if the needle is in the bloodstream. Waiting 10 seconds allows the medication to start absorbing.

12. Activate the needle's safety device with one hand while using the other hand to cover the site with gauze. Gently apply pressure at the site to stop any bleeding. Apply a bandage if the patient requests it.

Purpose: Ask the patient if they would like a bandage if the site has stopped bleeding. Remember that some bandages may contain latex, which can be an allergen to some people. Some people may be allergic to the adhesive.

13. Discard the needle/syringe in a biohazardous sharps container. Make sure to put the needle in first.

Purpose: Safely discarding the needle/syringe will help prevent needle-stick injuries.

14. Observe the patient for any adverse reactions. Clean up the area. Discard the waste in the waste container. Sanitize your hands.

Purpose: It is important to monitor the patient and also clean up the work area.

15. Document the procedure in the health record. Include assessments done, allergies, teaching or instructions provided; the name of the provider who ordered the medication; the medication's name, dose, and route; and how the patient tolerated the medication. Also include the manufacturer, lot number, and expiration date for vaccines and controlled substances.

Purpose: Medications given need to be documented to indicate they were given.

Documentation Example

11/1/20XX 1420 NKA. Per Dr. Martin's order, administered Iron Dextran 0.5 mL IM in left ventrogluteal site using Z-track method. Pt stated she had pain initially but is feeling better. Side effects were discussed with pt prior to administration. Pt had no questions and verbalized understanding of instructions._____Gabe Garcia CMA (AAMA)

47

Intravenous Procedures

LEARNING OBJECTIVES

1. Discuss the reasons for intravenous (IV) therapy in ambulatory care.
2. List common isotonic, hypotonic, and hypertonic IV solutions used in ambulatory care.
3. Describe the action of isotonic IV solution in the body and potential complications that can occur.
4. Describe the action of hypotonic IV solution in the body and potential complications that can occur.
5. Describe the action of hypertonic IV solution in the body and potential complications that can occur.
6. Describe parts of a primary infusion set.
7. Discuss the difference between macro-drip and micro-drip infusion sets when doing a gravity infusion.
8. Describe the supplies needed to start an IV.
9. Calculate the infusion rate (mL/hr).
10. Calculate the flow rate for gravity infusions.
11. Demonstrate how to prime the infusion set, administer IV fluids, change an IV bag, and remove an IV catheter.
12. Describe infiltration, phlebitis, extravasation, hypersensitivity, local and systemic infections, pulmonary edema, and air embolism and the signs and symptoms that may occur.

OUTLINE

⯈ OPENING SCENARIO

Gabe Garcia, CMA (AAMA), works at Walden-Martin Family Medical (WMFM) Clinic. Recently, state statutes were updated, and medical assistants now can insert and monitor intravenous (IV) fluid infusions. The statute stipulates that a medical assistant must pass a training course and the provider must be present at all times during the IV fluid therapy.

After talking with the providers, Gabe took a training course at the local college. He learned about the different types of IV fluids available, complications that can occur, and how to insert the

IV catheter. During the training course, Gabe practiced giving IV fluid therapy. He learned how to prepare the equipment and supplies. Gabe practiced on an IV arm and then was able to insert an IV on his partner. By the end of the training course, Gabe was feeling more confident with IV fluid therapy. He is excited to assist the providers with IV fluid therapy at WMFM Clinic.

YOU WILL LEARN

1. Reasons for IV therapy in ambulatory care.
2. The differences between isotonic, hypotonic, and hypertonic IV solutions, including potential complications with infusions.

3. To calculate the infusion rate and the flow rate.
4. To prime the infusion set, administer IV fluid, change an IV bag, and remove an IV catheter.
5. To identify issues related to IV infusions.

INTRODUCTION

The administration of intravenous (in TRAH vee nus) (IV) fluids, medications, nutritional supplements, and blood components is common in the hospital setting. Over the years, more intravenous therapy has occurred in ambulatory healthcare facilities. Ambulatory care providers usually order IV therapy for the following reasons:

- *To replace fluids and electrolytes*: Used as a treatment for dehydration due to a reduced fluid intake, diarrhea, or vomiting. IV fluids (also called IV solutions) are given.
- *To treat infections*: IV antibiotics provide a quicker response than oral medications.
- *To treat cancer*: Some chemotherapy medications are given intravenously.
- *For diagnostic tests*: IV contrast media can be given for some diagnostic tests, including computerized axial tomography (CT) scans and intravenous pyelograms.

Providing IV therapy in ambulatory care facilities is an inexpensive option compared to hospitalizing patients.

State laws vary on the role of medical assistants regarding starting and monitoring IV fluid infusions and administering IV contrast media. It is important for medical assistants to know the state laws and the healthcare facility's policies before working with IVs. In this chapter, the techniques for preparing and administering IV fluids will be the primary focus. Administering IV medications, such as chemotherapy and antibiotics, is outside the medical assistant's scope of practice.

In previous chapters, you learned the basics of pharmacology and how to prepare and administer injections. To administer IV fluid therapy, you will need to apply the nine rights of medication administration you learned in the prior chapter.

IV SUPPLIES

IV Solutions

IV solutions should be treated like medications. The medical assistant must follow the nine rights of medication administration. As part of these rights, the name of the IV solution must be checked three times before the IV therapy is started on the patient (Box 47.1). The IV solution type, the amount of fluid in the bag, and the expiration date are all labeled on the bag and must be checked.

IV solutions come in plastic bags and are then connected to IV infusion sets. The IV solution bag has a hole at the top that is used to hang it from an IV pole or wall hook. Markings on the bag can help indicate the amount of fluid left. The *medication port* (also called the *injection port*) is located at the bottom of the bag and is used to inject medication into the IV fluid bag. (Injecting a medication into an IV solution bag is

---

> ### BOX 47.1 Safety With IV Solutions
>
> The IV solution should be discarded if the fluid:
> - Contains *precipitate* (solid particles) or looks cloudy
> - Has expired
> - Has become contaminated
> - Is no longer needed or the patient's IV therapy has been completed

beyond the scope of a medical assistant.) The *IV tubing port* is located next to the medication port and is used to attach the IV infusion set. Once the IV bag is punctured by the infusion set, it is only good for 24 hours (unless otherwise stated by the healthcare facility).

When a patient requires IV fluid therapy in ambulatory care, the patient receives a *crystalloid* (KRIS tah loid) *solution*. Solutes such as electrolytes or dextrose (DEK strose) are dissolved in a fluid, or solvent, creating a crystalloid solution. Crystalloid solutions can pass through semipermeable membranes, such as blood vessel walls and move into cells and tissues. Crystalloid solutions can be isotonic, hypotonic, or hypertonic.

> ### VOCABULARY
> **dextrose** A glucose solution administered intravenously.
> **interstitial fluid** Liquid found between the cells of the body.
> **intravenous** Through a vein; fluids and medications can be given through a vein.
> **intravenous therapy** Administration and monitoring of fluid and medication by intravenous infusion.
> **solute** A substance that is dissolved in a solvent (liquid) to form a solution.
> **solvent** A liquid that is able to dissolve other substances.

> ### CRITICAL THINKING 47.1
> Describe the difference between a solute and a solvent.

Isotonic Solutions. *Isotonic solutions* and plasma have a similar dissolved particle concentration. When an isotonic solution is administered, it is distributed between the bloodstream, the interstitial fluid, and cells. Isotonic solutions are typically ordered when a patient is dehydrated due to vomiting or diarrhea. Types of isotonic IV solutions include:

- 0.9% sodium chloride (also called 0.9% NaCl, normal saline, and NS)
- Lactated Ringer Solution (also called LR and Ringer Lactate)
- 5% dextrose in water (or D5W)
- Ringer Solution

Prior to starting the IV fluid infusion, the medical assistant should obtain the patient's vital signs. During the infusion, the patient's vital signs should be monitored. Isotonic solutions can cause *hypervolemia,* or fluid volume overload. Signs and symptoms of hypervolemia include hypertension, pulmonary crackles, dyspnea, shortness of breath, and peripheral edema. If the patient experiences any of these, the medical assistant must immediately notify the provider.

Hypotonic Solutions. *Hypotonic solutions* have a lower concentration of dissolved particles than plasma. This causes the fluid to move out of the blood vessels and into the interstitial fluid and cells. Hypotonic solutions are typically ordered for patients with diabetic ketoacidosis. Types of hypotonic IV solutions include:

- 0.45% sodium chloride (also called 0.45% NS and ½ NS)
- 0.33% sodium chloride (or 0.33% NS)
- 2.5% dextrose in water (or D2.5W)

Prior to starting the IV fluid infusion, the medical assistant should obtain the patient's vital signs. During the infusion, the patient's vital signs should be monitored. Because the hypotonic fluid moves out of the bloodstream, the patient has to be monitored for hypovolemia. Signs and symptoms of hypovolemia include hypotension, dizziness, and confusion. If the patient experiences any of these, the medical assistant must immediately notify the provider.

CRITICAL THINKING 47.2

Describe why hypotonic solutions cause hypotension.

Hypertonic Solutions. *Hypertonic solutions* have a higher concentration of dissolved particles than plasma. This causes fluid from the cells to move into the bloodstream, increasing the blood volume and thus the blood pressure. Hypertonic solutions are typically ordered for patients with hypotension and *hyponatremia* (low sodium). Types of hypertonic IV solutions include:

- 3% sodium chloride (or 3% NS) and 5% sodium chloride (or 5% NS)
- Dextrose 5% in 0.45% sodium chloride (also called D5.45NS, D5 ½ NS, Dextrose 5% in 0.45% NaCl)
- Dextrose 5% in 0.9% sodium chloride (also called D5NS, Dextrose 5% in 0.9% NaCl)
- Dextrose 5% in Lactated Ringer (or D5LR)
- 10% dextrose in water (or D10W)

Prior to starting the IV fluid infusion, the medical assistant should obtain the patient's vital signs. During the infusion, the patient's vital signs should be monitored. Because the hypertonic solutions pull fluids into the bloodstream, the patient has to be monitored for hypervolemia. Signs and symptoms of hypervolemia include hypertension, pulmonary crackles, dyspnea, shortness of breath, and peripheral edema. If the patient experiences any of these, the medical assistant must immediately notify the provider.

CRITICAL THINKING 47.3

Describe why hypertonic solutions cause hypertension.

IV Tubing

A *primary infusion set* is also called an *infusion set* or a *primary infusion administration set*. The primary infusion set connects to the IV solution bag. The infusion set can be either a macro-drip or a micro-drip set. The difference between these two sets is the drop factor. The *drop factor* is the number of drops (gtt) per milliliter (mL) of fluid. The drop factor (gtt/mL) is listed on the infusion set packaging.

The macro-drip infusion set creates larger drops and comes in a variety of sizes, such as 10, 12, 15, or 20 gtt/mL. Macro-drip infusion sets are the most common type of set to use for routine IV therapy in adults. These infusion sets are used when delivering a larger volume of fluid in an hour.

Micro-drip infusion sets create smaller drops and deliver 60 gtt/mL. These sets can deliver smaller amounts of fluid over a given time frame. Micro-drip infusion sets are used for pediatric patients and for an adult who needs a smaller volume of fluid (e.g., 40 mL/hr).

The primary infusion set consists of the following parts.

- *Spike*: A sterile spike that is inserted into the IV bag using the IV tubing port.
- *Drip chamber*: Used to count the drip rate of the IV if an IV pump is not used. Counting the drips over 1 minute helps determine the flow rate of the IV fluid. The drip chamber needs to be one-third to one-half full of IV fluid at all times. If the drip chamber is too full, the drip rate cannot be counted. If the drip chamber is not full enough, air can get into the IV tubing and can be dangerous for the patient.
- *Roller clamp*: Used to control the rate at which the IV flows with a gravity infusion. If the roller clamp is moved down, the tubing is pinched, stopping the flow of fluid (Fig. 47.1). As the roller clamp is moved towards the opposite side, the solution starts flowing. If the roller clamp is opened up completely, the IV solution flows quickly into the patient, which can be dangerous if not ordered at that rate.
- *Slide clamp*: Used to completely stop the IV infusion. The slide clamp pinches off the tubing, stopping the solution flow. It can be helpful to use the slide clamp when the infusion must be stopped for a few minutes. It prevents having to readjust the flow rate with the roller clamp with gravity infusions.
- *Luer lock*: Found at the end of the infusion tubing. The luer lock connects the infusion set to the IV catheter or extension tubing.

VOCABULARY

flow rate The number of drops (gtt) in 1 minute required to infuse the ordered solution; also called the drip rate.

In addition to these parts, some primary infusion sets may also have:

- *Backcheck valve*: Prevents fluid or medications from traveling up the IV tubing and into the IV bag.
- *Injection ports*: Used to infuse IV medication. If the patient needs an IV medication, the medication can be infused either using a second IV solution bag or by IV push using a syringe. The injection port closest to the drip chamber is used to connect the secondary infusion set and bag. The injection port closer to the luer lock and patient is used for IV push medications. Administering IV medications is outside the scope of practice for medical assistants and is usually done by the registered nurse (RN) or provider.

- *Buretrol*: A cylinder holding device that limits the amount of IV solutions given; may be used in pediatrics.

A secondary infusion set is used to give IV medications. The secondary infusion set has fewer features than the primary infusion set, and the tubing is shorter. The secondary infusion set has a sterile spike, drip chamber, roller clamp, and a luer lock used to connect into the primary infusion set's injection port. When a secondary infusion set is used, the IV bag on the primary infusion set (or the primary IV bag) is hung lower. The secondary infusion bag is hung higher or "piggybacked" on the primary IV bag. The higher position creates greater gravitational pressure on the secondary IV bag, and it will infuse first. After the secondary IV bag is empty, the primary IV bag infuses.

An extension tubing can be used to connect the IV catheter with the primary infusion set. The extension tubing has a slide clamp, a male luer connector on one end, and a female luer connector on the other end. The male luer connector connects with the primary infusion set, and the female connecter connects with the IV catheter. The length of the extension tubing can vary.

IV Catheters

Intravenous access can be done as either peripheral or central access. Commonly in ambulatory care, short peripheral IV catheters are inserted into a peripheral vein in the hand or arm. If

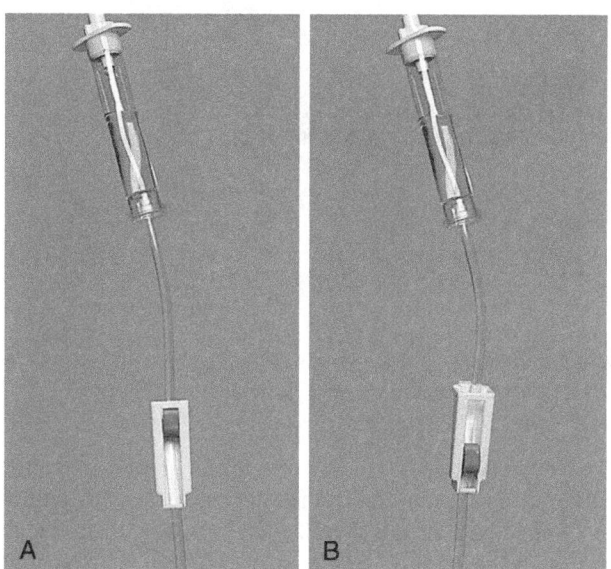

Fig. 47.1 A, Roller clamp in open position. B, Roller clamp in closed or off position. (From Potter P, Perry A: *Basic nursing*, ed 7, St. Louis, 2011, Mosby.)

allowed by the state laws and the agency's policy, this is the type of IV a medical assistant can insert. Table 47.1 describes the different types of IV access devices that may be seen in ambulatory care.

Usually catheters 20 to 24 gauge are used for adult infusions in ambulatory care. For pediatric and older adult patients, 22- to 24-gauge catheters may be used. Catheters with a larger gauge than 20, such as 16 and 18, can increase the risk of phlebitis (fle BYE tis). The medical assistant should select the shortest and smallest catheter possible to reduce the risk of phlebitis.

> **VOCABULARY**
> **patency** Open condition of a body cavity or canal.
> **phlebitis** Inflammation of a vein.

The IV safety needle is beveled. The needle is covered with a *catheter*, a thin plastic tube. A clear flashback chamber behind the needle fills with blood when the needle enters the vein. Once the IV safety needle is inserted, the catheter is pushed into the vein, and the needle is withdrawn. The catheter is attached to extension tubing or the IV infusion set.

Two types of IV catheters seen in ambulatory care are straight and winged hub safety catheters. The wings vary in size and can be used to insert the needle and stabilize the catheter (Fig. 47.2). Various features are available with IV catheters that improve the insertion success and the safety of the procedure.

The IV safety needles are passive or active. *Passive IV safety needles* are designed so the needle is automatically covered after use. Many IV needles are covered as the user pulls the needle from the catheter. The safety clamps onto the needle and protects against accidental needlesticks. *Active IV safety needles* require the healthcare professional to activate the safety device. Several active IV safety needles have buttons that retract the needle into the needle guard (Fig. 47.3).

With the design of traditional IV catheters, blood backflows out of the catheter onto the patient's skin when the needle is removed. This causes a risk of contamination to the medical assistant. Newer IV safety catheters prevent blood from backflowing out of the catheter. Some catheters have a septum that closes as the needle is retracted, preventing blood from backflowing. The septum opens when the luer lock is connected to the catheter. Some winged hub catheters have preattached extension tubing that prevents blood from backflowing. With the wide variety of IV safety needle/catheter units on the market, the medical assistant needs to be trained on the types available in the facility before using them on patients.

TABLE 47.1 IV Access Devices

Types	Placement	Left in Place for:	Uses
Peripheral IV line (PIV or IV)	Short catheter is placed in the hand or forearm.	3–4 days, depending on agency's policy; must be kept dry.	Fluid and medication infusion; harsh medications can cause phlebitis and irritation.
Peripherally inserted central line catheter (PICC)	Longer catheter is placed in the upper arm.	Weeks to months; must be kept dry and requires regular cleaning and maintenance to maintain patency (PAT en see).	Usually requires a registered nurse to start the IV therapy, perform blood draws, and maintain the catheter.
Central venous catheter (CVC)	Like the PICC but placed in the chest or neck.		
Port	Catheter is surgically implanted under the skin in the chest; type of central line.	Years; requires limited maintenance. No limitation with showering or swimming.	

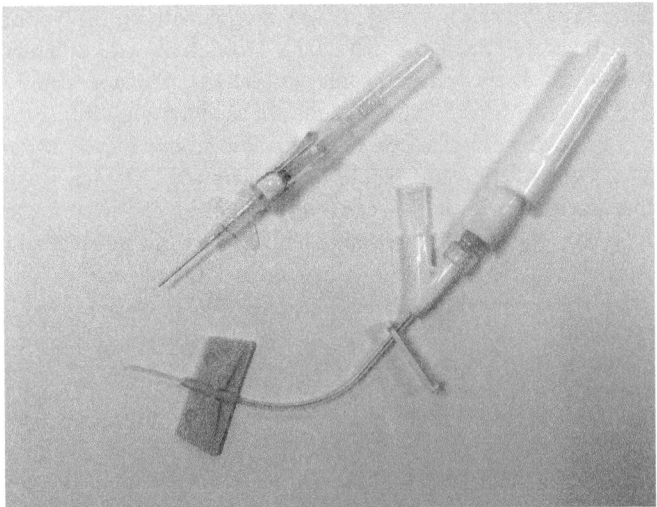

Fig. 47.2 Examples of Winged Hub Safety Needles.

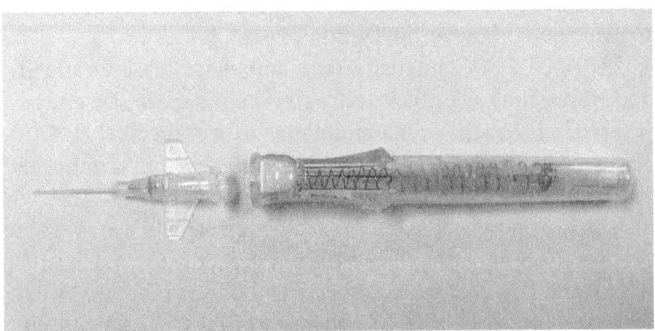

Fig. 47.3 BD Insyte Autoguard Intravenous Catheter. When a button is pushed, the needle retracts into the needle guard.

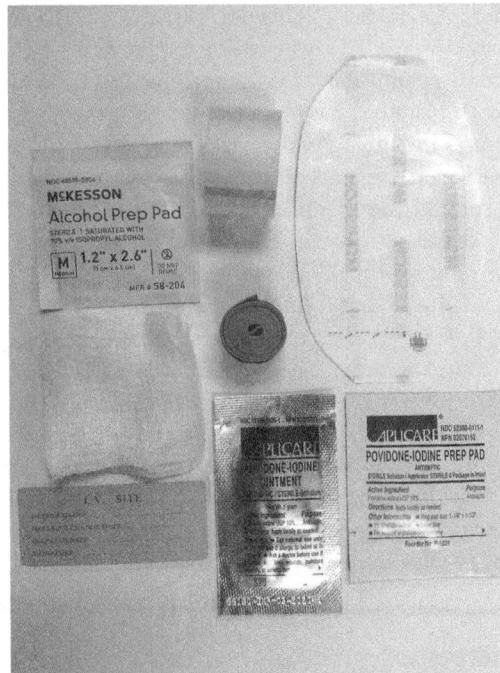

Fig. 47.4 Intravenous Start Kit.

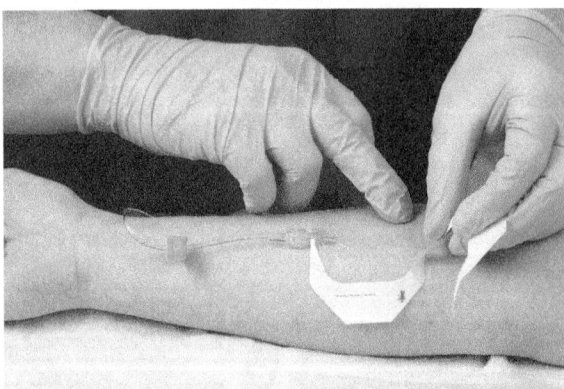

Fig. 47.5 Applying a Transparent Dressing. (From Potter PA, Perry AG: *Fundamentals of nursing*, ed 9, St. Louis, 2017, Elsevier.)

CRITICAL THINKING 47.4

Describe the safety features typically found in today's IV needle/catheter units. Why would these features be important for the medical assistant?

Additional Supplies

Some ambulatory care facilities use IV start kits, which contain supplies needed to insert an IV. IV start kits may include (Fig. 47.4):

- *A tourniquet*: To help engorge the vein during the insertion procedure.
- *Antiseptic swabs or applicators*: Chlorhexidine, Betadine, or alcohol is used to clean the insertion site prior to the catheter insertion.
- *Sterile gauze*: Used to apply pressure to the site if the insertion is unsuccessful. It can also be used to clean up any blood at the site when the needle is removed.
- *A transparent dressing*: Typically, a semipermeable membrane dressing. Used to cover the insertion site (Fig. 47.5).
- *Sterile tape*: Used to secure the catheter and tubing to the skin.

A topical anesthetic or vapocoolant may be ordered by the provider prior to the IV catheter cinsertion. This medication helps minimize the discomfort felt during the IV catheter insertion. Depending on the state law and the healthcare facility's policies and procedures, the medical assistant may be able to administer the medication. Prior to administration, always check the patient's allergies and be familiar with the medication – the action, side effects, and administration techniques.

To administer IV fluids, an IV pole or hook must be used to keep the IV bag higher than the patient. The IV tubing drip chamber should be about 3 feet about the level of the catheter insertion site. An infusion pump may also be used for IV infusions.

IV INFUSIONS

During the IV infusion, the goal is to deliver the solution at the rate ordered by the provider. The IV solution can be delivered by an infusion pump or by gravity.

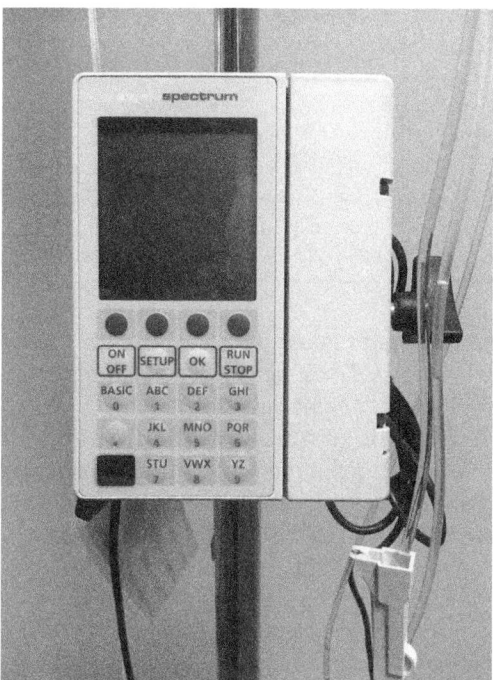

Fig. 47.6 An Example of an Infusion Pump. Many infusion pumps are available on the market.

Infusion Pump Delivery

Using an IV infusion pump is safer than a gravity infusion for IV fluids. Most infusion pumps have built-in safety features that prevent an accidental infusion of extra fluid. The pump regulates the amount of fluid the patient gets (Fig. 47.6). The total amount of fluid infused, and the rate of infusion are shown on the pump's screen. Locking mechanisms prevent unauthorized changes in the infusion rate. Most infusion pumps allow for dual programming, a rate for the primary IV bag and another rate for a secondary IV medication bag. IV infusion pumps require specific infusion sets. If an IV pump is used, the medical assistant should be familiar with how to use the pump and troubleshooting issues.

VOCABULARY

infusion rate The volume of fluid infused per hour; written as mL/hr.

Calculations for Infusion Pump Delivery. Most IV infusion pumps require the healthcare professional to enter:
- The amount of fluid to be infused.
- The infusion rate or volume (mL) of fluid to be infused per hour (mL/hr).

Many times, the provider's order includes both the rate and the volume to be infused. Sometimes the medical assistant must calculate the rate when the provider indicates the volume of fluid to infuse over a set period of time.

The provider may write the IV order as:
- 0.9% NS IV 125 mL/hour for 4 hours
- 0.9% NS IV 500 mL over 4 hours

The first example provides the medical assistant with the rate (125 mL/hr). The medical assistant would program the pump to administer 125 mL per hour. In the second example, the

provider wants 500 mL to be given over a period of 4 hours. In this example, the medical assistant must calculate the infusion rate or number of mL to give over 1 hour. We will use the following formula to determine the infusion rate.

Order: 0.9% NS IV 500 mL over 4 hours
Formula: Total amount (mL) ÷ hours = mL per hour (infusion rate)
Solution: 500 mL ÷ 4 hours = 125 mL per hour

In both examples, the patient receives 125 mL per hour for 4 hours.

In some cases, the medical assistant might receive an order for the IV solution to be infused in less than 1 hour. Infusions less than 1 hour are more common with IV medications than IV fluids. A medical assistant performing IV fluid administration should be familiar with calculating infusion rates for infusions less than 1 hour. The following example demonstrates how to calculate the infusion rate.

Order: 0.9% NS IV 100 mL over 30 minutes

Formula: $\dfrac{\text{Total amount (mL)} \times 60 \text{ minutes}}{\text{Time (minutes)} \times 1 \text{ hour}}$

Solution: $\dfrac{100 \text{ mL} \times 60 \text{ minutes}}{30 \text{ minutes} \times 1 \text{ hour}} = \dfrac{6000 \text{ mL}}{30 \text{ hour}} = \dfrac{200 \text{ mL}}{1 \text{ hour}}$

With this type of problem, you need to multiple the two *numerators* (the top numbers) and then multiple the two *denominators* (the bottom number). The minute labels cancel out, and your label is mL/hour. Box 47.2 provides practice problems for calculating the infusion rate.

Gravity Infusions

When an IV is delivered by gravity, the medical assistant must use the roller clamp to regulate the IV flow. The roller clamp is used to adjust the rate of drops falling in the drip chamber. The speed of the drops relates to the amount of fluid delivered. The faster the drops fall in the drip chamber, the more fluid is being delivered. It is important that the IV solution be infused at the rate ordered, and the medical assistant should frequently check the IV flow rate. IV solution delivered too quickly or giving too much fluid, can cause harm to the patient.

Calculations for Gravity Infusions. The flow rate (drip rate) is the number of drops (gtt) in 1 minute required to infuse the ordered

---

BOX 47.2   Practice Problems: Calculating Infusion Rates

Find the infusion rate (mL/hr). Round to the nearest mL.
1. 0.9% NS IV 500 mL over 8 hours.
2. 0.9% NS IV 250 mL over 5 hours.
3. LR IV 1000 mL over 8 hours.
4. LR IV 500 mL over 6 hours.
5. 0.9% NS IV 250 mL over 2.5 hours.
6. 0.9% NS IV 100 mL over 30 minutes.
7. 0.9% NS IV 50 mL over 20 minutes.
8. LR IV 75 mL over 30 minutes.
9. LR IV 50 mL over 30 minutes.
10. 0.9% NS IV 50 mL over 40 minutes.

solution. The flow rate is determined by the infusion rate and the infusion set drop factor. Once the flow rate is determined, the medical assistant must adjust the roller clamp so the drops falling in the drip chamber for 1 minute match the flow rate. Usually, the drops are counted for 30 seconds and multiplied by 2.

To calculate the flow rate, the medical assistant must have the infusion set drop factor and the amount of fluid to infuse over x number of minutes. For example, let us take the following order and find the flow rate:

Order: 0.9% NS IV 50 mL over 30 min
Infusion set: Drop factor of 20 gtt/mL

Formula: $\dfrac{\text{Volume to infuse (mL)} \times \text{drop factor (gtt)}}{\text{Time (min)} \times \text{(mL)}} = \dfrac{\text{gtt (flow rate)}}{\text{min}}$

Solution: $\dfrac{50\text{ mL} \times 20\text{ gtt}}{30\text{ min} \times 1\text{ mL}} = \dfrac{1000\text{ gtt}}{30\text{ min}}$
$= 33.3 = 33$ gtt/min (flow rate)

With this type of problem, you need to multiple the two numerators and then multiple the two denominators. The mL labels cancel out, and your label is gtt/min. The medical assistant would need to regulate the roller clamp so that 33 drops fall in the drip chamber in 1 minute.

If the medical assistant does not have the number of minutes for the infusion, this can be calculated using the formula discussed earlier. For example, let us take the follow order, find the number of minutes for the infusion, and then find the flow rate:

Order: 0.9% NS IV 150 mL over 2 hours
Infusion set: Drop factor of 15 gtt/mL.

Step 1: Find the volume to infuse (mL) in 1 hour (the infusion rate)
Formula: Total amount (mL) ÷ hours = mL per hour
Solution: 150 mL ÷ 2 hours = 75 mL per hour
Step 2: Switch 1 hour to 60 minutes (75 mL/60 min)
Step 3: Find the flow rate.

Formula: $\dfrac{\text{Volume to infuse (mL)} \times \text{drop factor (gtt)}}{\text{Time (min)} \times \text{(mL)}} = \dfrac{\text{Flow Rate (gtt)}}{\text{(min)}}$

Solution: $\dfrac{75\text{ mL} \times 15\text{ gtt}}{60\text{ min} \times 1\text{ mL}} = \dfrac{1125\text{ gtt}}{60\text{ min}} = 18.75 = 19$ gtt/min

With this type of problem, you need to multiple the two numerators and then multiple the two denominators. The mL labels cancel out, and your label is gtt/min. The answer is rounded to the nearest drop. Box 47.3 provides practice problems for calculating the flow rate.

INITIATING IV INFUSIONS

Priming the Primary Infusion Set

The preparation begins with an order from the provider. The order must include:
- Patient's name and date of birth (DOB)
- Type of IV solution

> **BOX 47.3** **Practice Problems: Calculating the Flow Rate**
>
> Find the infusion rate and the flow rate. Round to the nearest gtt.
> 1. 0.9% NS IV 500 mL over 7 hours. Infusion set: drop factor of 10 gtt/mL.
> 2. 0.9% NS IV 250 mL over 5 hours. Infusion set: drop factor of 60 gtt/mL.
> 3. LR IV 1000 mL over 8 hours. Infusion set: drop factor of 10 gtt/mL.
> 4. LR IV 500 mL over 6 hours. Infusion set: drop factor of 20 gtt/mL.
> 5. 0.9% NS IV 250 mL over 2.5 hours. Infusion set: drop factor of 10 gtt/mL.

- Amount of fluid to infuse over a specific time period (e.g., 500 mL over 4 hours) or the rate of the infusion for a specific time period (e.g., 125 mL/hr × 4 hours)

As described earlier, IV orders may vary. The medical assistant must follow the nine rights of medication administration described in Chapter 46. The IV label must be compared to the order three times prior to the start of the infusion. The expiration date on the bag of fluid must also be checked.

The primary infusion set must be primed with the IV solution just before it is used. *Priming* means to run IV fluid through the tubing to remove all of the air. This procedure prevents air from entering the patient's circulatory system, which can cause an air embolism. Deaths have been attributed to as little as 10 mL of air. Procedure 47.1 describes how to prime the infusion set.

As the medical assistant prepares the IV supplies, it is important to use sterile technique. The sterile spike, which is used to spike the IV bag, must remain sterile. The luer lock, found on the opposite side of the infusion set, also must remain sterile.

Identifying a Vein

In ambulatory care, a peripheral IV is usually inserted in an upper extremity. When looking for a potential insertion site, the medical assistant should start distally and work up the hand and arm (Fig. 47.7). If an IV attempt is unsuccessful, all future sites must be more proximal to that site. In other words, the medical assistant should start looking for a vein on the top of the hand and move up the arm. If a site on the arm is unsuccessful, the medical assistant cannot attempt a site more distal, such as on the hand. The IV catheter should not be inserted:
- in an area that is painful, tender, infected, burned, or compromised (e.g., lymphedema).
- in an area with an open wound.
- in an extremity that is paralyzed or affected by a stroke, contains a dialysis fistula, or on the same side of a mastectomy.
- distal to a previous IV site or infiltrated site.
- in a fragile vein.

The medical assistant should avoid inserting the catheter in areas of flexion. Inserting the catheter in the antecubital site, on the inside of the wrist (ventral surface), or the cephalic vein at the wrist can increase the risk for nerve damage.

Typically, the IV catheter is inserted and removed during the same visit. If the patient needs the IV catheter to remain in for a longer period of time, the medical assistant must consider the following:
- If possible, use the nondominant hand/arm.
- Avoid inserting the catheter in the hand if the patient is using an assistive device, such as a walker or cane.

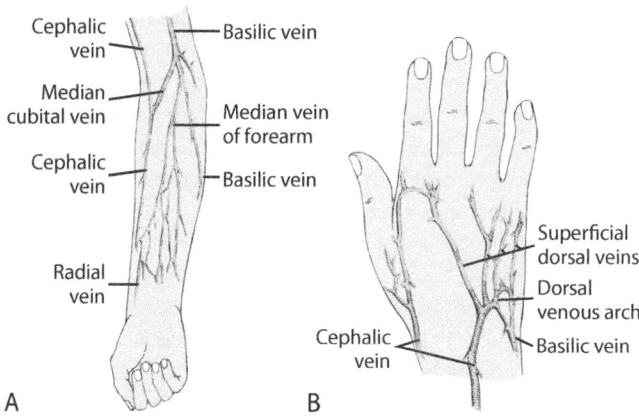

Fig. 47.7 **Common IV Sites in Adults.** A, Inner arm. B, Dorsal surface of hand. (From Potter PA, Perry AG: *Fundamentals of nursing,* ed 9, St. Louis, 2017, Elsevier.)

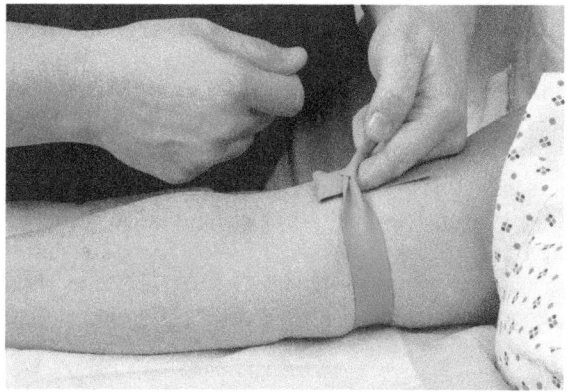

Fig. 47.8 **Tourniquet Placed on Arm for Initial Vein Selection.** (From Potter P, Perry A: *Basic nursing,* ed 7, St. Louis, 2011, Mosby.)

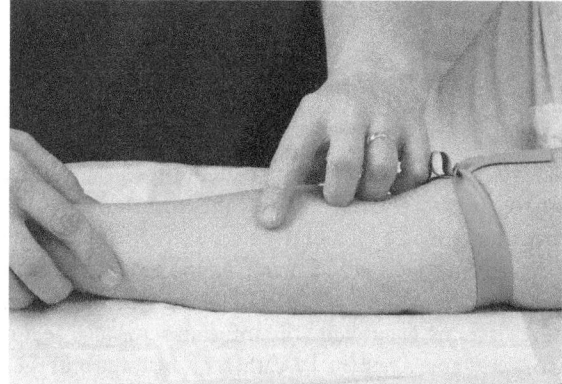

Fig. 47.9 **Palpating Vein.** (From Potter P, Perry A: *Basic nursing,* ed 7, St. Louis, 2011, Mosby.)

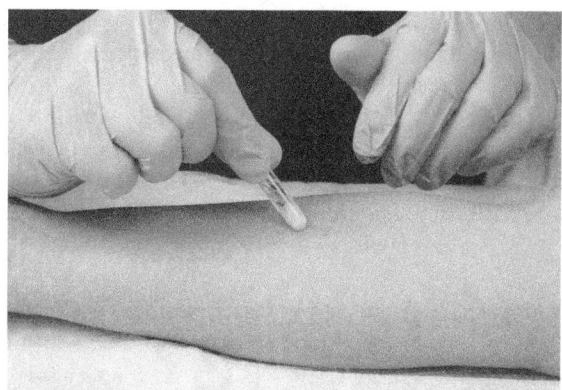

Fig. 47.10 **Cleansing Site With Chlorhexidine.** (From Potter PA, Perry AG: *Fundamentals of nursing,* ed 9, St. Louis, 2017, Elsevier.)

- Avoid inserting the catheter in a flexible area, such as near the wrist or elbow.

The medical assistant should look for a straight, nonbranched vein (Procedure 47.2). The tourniquet can be placed about 4 to 6 inches proximal to the site to help the vein engorge with blood (Fig. 47.8). When using the tourniquet, the medical assistant must check the patient's radial pulse on the side with the tourniquet. If the radial pulse is diminished or absent, loosen the tourniquet. Other strategies to help engorge the vein include:
- Stroking the vessel
- Applying a warm pack to the site for a few minutes
- Having the patient open and close the hand, making a fist

When the medical assistant palpates the vein, it should feel spongy (Fig. 47.9). If the vessel is pulsing, it is likely to be an artery and should not be used. Some facilities use technology to help find a vein for catheter placement. Visible light devices transilluminate the vessel, and near infrared and ultrasound can also be used. Once the insertion site is determined, the tourniquet is removed.

Site Preparation

If the patient's skin is visibly soiled, it should be washed with soap and water and dried. If hair needs to be removed from the site, a disposable-head electric shaver can be used. Shaving is usually done for IVs that will remain in for a long period of time.

The skin can be cleansed using several different antiseptics. Always check the patient's allergies before starting the procedure. The most common antiseptics include chlorhexidine, povidone-iodine (Betadine), and alcohol. Chlorhexidine is the preferred antiseptic. When using chlorhexidine, place the applicator to the skin and do a friction scrub (Fig. 47.10). Scrub back and forth and up and down for 30 seconds. Allow the product to dry on the skin for at least 30 seconds. If using Betadine or alcohol, place the applicator at the intended site of insertion and work outward in a circular pattern, making larger circles as the area is cleaned. Betadine must dry before starting the catheter insertion. The drying process kills the microorganisms. If the skin is touched with gloves or ungloved hands, the cleansing process needs to be repeated.

Inserting the IV Catheter

Once the antiseptic is dried, the tourniquet is reapplied. Using the dominant hand, grasp the IV needle/catheter unit and place it parallel to the vein. Using the nondominant hand, hold the skin taut. The thumb should stabilize the vein in place during the insertion process.

With the bevel facing up, insert the needle/catheter unit using a 10- to 30-degree angle. Superficial veins require a lesser angle of insertion, whereas a deeper vein requires a greater angle. Once the needle enters the vein, a blood flashback is seen in the clear flashback chamber. The needle should be advanced a bit further. Then the catheter is pushed off the needle and advanced into the vein until the hub reaches the insertion site. A blood flashback may also be seen in the catheter as the catheter enters the vein. The needle is withdrawn, and the tubing is attached to the catheter. The catheter is taped to the arm, and a transparent or gauze dressing is applied. The infusion set is also secured to the arm with tape. After the IV catheter is inserted and the solution is infusing, the medical assistant should observe the site for a few minutes to ensure no complications are occurring.

If the patient experiences tingling or numbness during the insertion process or during the infusion, the medical assistant should pause the infusion and notify the provider. This type of pain can indicate nerve damage.

If the medical assistant is unsuccessful with the insertion attempt, the entire cleansing process must be repeated in another location proximal to the attempted site. A new catheter must be used. The standard is two insertion attempts per person with a total of four attempts.

CRITICAL THINKING 47.6

When inserting an IV, Gabe warns the patient, "You will feel a poke" just before he inserts the IV. Is this a good practice? Why or why not?

Documentation

After completing the catheter insertion and starting the IV infusion, the medical assistant must document the procedure. The documentation should include:
- Date and time
- Ordering provider's name
- IV order, which includes the IV solution, amount, and rate per hour or over the number of hours
- Type and size of catheter inserted
- Location of insertion site
- Any issues with the insertion process, including the number of insertion attempts
- Type of IV fluid being infused and the infusion rate
- Name and credentials (e.g., RMA) of the person who inserted the catheter
- Any other documentation required by the facility

Monitoring IVs

The patient should be checked at least every 30 to 60 minutes, depending on the situation and the facility's policy. The medical assistant should check on the patient and the site for complications. If a gravity infusion is used, the flow rate must be checked.

Even though a medical assistant sets the flow rate, frequent checking of the flow rate is critical to the safety of the IV infusion. If the IV catheter is inserted near an area of flexion, the flow rate can change if the patient bends the area. Sometimes the patient changes their position, which can speed up or slow

down the infusion rate. The hand and arm should be below the heart level. If raised above the heart, the flow rate can change. If the tubing becomes kinked, the infusion rate slows down. In some situations, the patient or family member may "adjust" the roller clamp, changing the flow rate. The patient should be instructed not to touch the roller clamp. Frequent checks can help prevent infusion issues.

Maintaining IVs

Many times, a patient receives a one-time treatment of IV solution. The catheter is inserted, the IV therapy is performed, and the catheter is removed. In some causes the patient may need to return to the ambulatory care facility for additional infusions. In those cases, the medical assistant must know the guidelines for flushing the IV catheter and when to change the IV site, tubing, and IV solution bags. The following strategies are used to reduce the risk of complications.
- Use sterile technique when changing IV solution bags or priming IV tubing.
- IV tubing and the site are changed every 72 to 96 hours or per the healthcare facility's policies.
- The IV catheter is removed if the insertion site has any tenderness, redness, swelling, or drainage.
- If the IV catheter remains in for an extended period of time, the transparent semipermeable membrane dressing should be changed every 5 to 7 days. Gauze dressings should be changed every 2 days.
- IV solution bags are changed every 24 hours (Procedure 47.3).
- IV catheter and extension tubing not in use need to be flushed every 12 hours with 3 to 5 mL of sterile normal saline. This maintains the patency of the catheter. (Flushing IV catheters may be outside the medical assistant's scope of practice in some states.)

COMPLICATIONS OF IV THERAPY

Complications that can arise from IV therapy include infiltration, phlebitis, extravasation, hypersensitivity, local and systemic infections, pulmonary edema, and air embolism. With any suspicion of a complication, the medical assistant should notify the provider. If the medical assistant is helping the RN monitor the infusion, any suspicion of complications should be reported to the RN immediately.

Infiltration

Infiltration occurs when the IV solution leaks or is administered into the surrounding tissues. It is caused when the IV catheter is placed improperly, slips out of the blood vessel, or punctures through the blood vessel. Usually, patient movement and/or a poorly secured catheter can lead to the catheter moving out of the vessel. Signs and symptoms of infiltration include:
- Swelling, discomfort, or pain at the site
- Coolness, blanching, and tightness of the skin at the site
- Slowed or stopped flow rate; an alarm on the IV infusion pump may go off

If infiltration is suspected, the medical assistant needs to stop the infusion and remove the IV catheter. Elevating the extremity and applying a warm compress can help reduce the swelling. The medical assistant can prevent infiltration by avoiding joint areas when inserting an IV and properly securing the catheter. The site should be checked for infiltration when the IV infusion starts. Infiltration can occur at any time during the infusion; thus, the medical assistant must frequently check the site.

Phlebitis

Phlebitis is inflammation of a vein. It is caused when the IV catheter rubs on the walls of the vein; with prolonged use of a site; or by trauma during the insertion process. Phlebitis can also be caused by the IV solution or medication, especially if it is acidic, alkaline, or hypertonic. Signs and symptoms of phlebitis include redness, tenderness or pain, heat, or swelling at the insertion site and tracking up the vein.

If phlebitis is suspected, the medical assistant must stop the infusion and remove the catheter. The extremity should be elevated above the heart level, and a warm compress can be applied. To help prevent phlebitis, the medical assistant should change the IV site according to the ambulatory care facility's policy. Frequent checks of the site during the IV infusion are important.

CRITICAL THINKING 47.7

Describe the difference between the signs and symptoms of an infiltrated site and phlebitis.

Extravasation

Extravasation (eks trav ah SAY shun) occurs when medication leaks into and damages the surrounding tissues. Vesicant (VES i kant) medications (e.g., certain types of antineoplastic drugs) can cause extravasation. In most cases, administering vesicant medications is outside the medical assistant's scope of practice. However, the medical assistant may help the RN monitor infusions and thus should be aware of extravasation. Signs and symptoms of extravasation include blanching, burning, tenderness or pain, cool skin, and swelling at the IV site. Blistering can be seen.

If extravasation is suspected, the medical assistant should stop the IV flow and notify the provider and/or RN. The catheter should remain in if an antidote will be administered. The arm should be elevated. Warm or cold compresses per the medication manufacturer should be applied. To prevent extravasation, larger veins should be used when a vesicant medication is given.

VOCABULARY

vesicant medication A medication that can damage tissue and can produce blisters.

Hypersensitivity

The risk of hypersensitivity is higher when IV medications are given compared to IV solutions. Thus the medical assistant should be aware of hypersensitivity if they are helping to monitor medication infusions. *Hypersensitivity* is an immune response that causes the body to react with an exaggerated response to a foreign agent or antigen. A hypersensitivity reaction occurs when the patient is allergic to the medication being infused. The signs and symptoms of hypersensitivity include fever, bronchospasm, difficulty breathing, wheezing, rash, and urticaria.

If a hypersensitivity reaction is suspected, the medical assistant should stop the infusion and notify the provider and/or RN. The patient's vital signs should be monitored. Treatments ordered by the provider should be administered, such as epinephrine or diphenhydramine. To prevent hypersensitivity, a patient's allergy history should be obtained. The patient should be monitored closely during the first 10 minutes of a medication infusion for signs of a hypersensitivity reaction. The medical assistant should remember that a hypersensitivity reaction can occur at any time during and after the infusion.

Local and Systemic Infections

A local infection at the IV insertion site may occur 2 to 3 days after the IV catheter is placed. The site may become tender and red; purulent drainage may be present. With a systemic infection *(sepsis)*, the patient may experience a fever. Microorganisms may enter the blood through the insertion site or from contaminated IV tubing or solution.

If the IV catheter is in the extremity, it should be removed. The provider should be notified of the patient's symptoms. A blood culture and antibiotics may be ordered. To prevent a local or systemic infection, the medical assistant should:
- Wash their hands or use hand sanitizer before putting on gloves to start an IV.
- Use aseptic technique during IV insertion.
- Use sterile technique when priming the IV tubing and attaching the tubing to the catheter.
- Perform dressing, site, and tubing changes as indicated by the facility's policies.

Pulmonary Edema

Pulmonary edema (also called *circulatory* or *fluid overload*) is caused by fluid accumulation in the lungs. This condition can occur if IV fluids are given too quickly, or the patient receives too much fluid. Signs and symptoms of pulmonary edema include:
- Shortness of breath and dyspnea
- Restlessness
- Productive cough and wheezing
- Labored and rapid breathing, rapid pulse, and a decreased blood pressure

If the patient experiences signs and symptoms of pulmonary edema, the medical assistant should notify the provider immediately. Typical treatments for pulmonary edema include having the person sit up, oxygen therapy, and monitoring of vital signs. The provider may order additional treatments. To prevent pulmonary edema, the medical assistant must ensure the IV infusion is done at the ordered rate. Frequent checking on the patient may help to identify early signs and symptoms of pulmonary edema.

Air Embolism

An air embolism occurs when air is introduced into the circulatory system and can block small arteries. Small air bubbles are usually tolerated by patients, but 10 mL of air or more can lead to an air embolism and possible death. Signs and symptoms of an air embolism include:

- Dyspnea, shortness of breath, wheezing, and coughing
- Shoulder, neck, or chest pain
- Light-headedness, agitation, confusion, and loss of consciousness
- Hypotension and tachycardia

If the patient experiences any of these signs or symptoms, the medical assistant should stop the entry of air and notify the provider immediately. Treatment includes oxygen therapy and monitoring of vital signs. To prevent an air embolism, the medical assistant must ensure all air is out of the tubing during the priming process. All connections should be tight.

DISCONTINUING THE IV

When the provider orders the IV to be discontinued, the medical assistant must stop the IV fluid infusion. Procedure 47.4 describes how to remove the catheter. The medical assistant must check the catheter tip to ensure it is intact. If a small part of the catheter breaks off, it can flow into the circulatory system, causing a catheter embolism. If the catheter is broken when removed, the provider should be notified immediately.

CLOSING COMMENTS

Inserting an IV catheter and managing IV fluid infusions are skills the medical assistant needs to practice to become confident and to provide these services safely. Continuing education on IV fluid therapy is important if the medical assistant's duties include IV insertion and fluid infusion. A medical assistant should always be watchful of complications of IV therapy, regardless of the age of the patient. Skill refreshers and continuing education can help the medical assistant remain competent and confident with these skills.

PATIENT-CENTERED CARE

Providing patient-centered care includes providing education, emotional support, and assisting with the patient's physical comfort. When performing IV fluid therapy, the medical assistant needs to coach the patient on what to expect, the length of time for the infusion, and signs and symptoms of complications. This can help the patient understand what is occurring and reduce the anxiety they may be feeling. Because the infusion can take several hours, the medical assistant must:

- Ensure the patient is comfortable.
- Provide something for the patient to do, such as watch television or read a magazine.
- Have blankets available if the patient becomes chilled, which is common during the therapy.
- Ensure the patient has something to drink if allowed by the provider.

BEING PROFESSIONAL

When administering IV fluids, the medical assistant must be under the direct supervision of a provider. The provider needs to be present in the facility when the procedure is being done.

Role-play this situation with a peer: You are a medical assistant, and your peer is Mrs. (or Mr.) Johnson. By state law, you can administer IV therapy under the supervision of a provider. Mrs. Johnson needs to come in for an IV fluid infusion. She is insistent that the infusion occur at 8 a.m. tomorrow. The provider has ready ordered the IV for the patient, but the provider will not be in the office until 9 a.m. Respond to the patient's request in a respectful and professional manner.

CHAPTER REVIEW

Intravenous therapy is done in ambulatory care to replace fluids and electrolytes, as a treatment for infections or cancer, and for diagnostic tests. State laws vary on the role of the medical assistants with starting and monitoring IV fluid infusion, along with administering IV contrast media.

IV solution should be treated as a medication. The medical assistant must follow the nine rights of medication administration with IV therapy. The following are three types of IV fluids:

- *Isotonic solutions*: Have a similar dissolved particle concentration as plasma. This means that isotonic solutions are distributed between the bloodstream, the interstitial fluid, and cells.
- *Hypotonic solutions*: Have a lower concentration of dissolved particles than plasma. This causes the fluid to move out of the blood vessels and into the interstitial fluid and cells.
- *Hypertonic solutions*: Have a higher concentration of dissolved particles than plasma. This causes fluid from the cells to move into the bloodstream, increasing the blood volume and thus the blood pressure.

The primary infusion set can be either a macro-drip or a micro-drip set. The drop factor is the number of drops (gtt) per milliliter (mL) of fluid. The drop factor (gtt/mL) is listed on the infusion set packaging. The primary infusion set consists of a spike, drip chamber, roller clamp, slide clamp, and luer lock. A secondary infusion set is used to give IV medications. An extension tubing can be used to connect the IV catheter with the primary infusion set. Straight and winged hub safety catheters are the types of catheters used.

When using an infusion pump, the medical assistant must know the infusion rate. The flow rate is used when doing a gravity infusion. Procedure 47.1 describes how to prime the primary infusion set. When inserting an IV catheter in an adult, the medical assistant uses a site on an upper extremity. Procedure 47.2 details the steps involved in inserting a catheter. Procedure 47.3 describes how to switch IV bags, and Procedure 47.4 describes how to discontinue an IV infusion.

The medical assistant should monitor the patient for complications. Common complications that can arise from IV therapy include infiltration, phlebitis, extravasation, hypersensitivity, local and systemic infections, pulmonary edema, and air embolism. With any suspicion of a complication, the medical assistant should notify the provider.

■ SCENARIO WRAP-UP

Gabe has had the opportunity to insert several IV catheters and perform IV fluid infusions. He is gaining more confidence with the insertion procedure. Gabe has worked with the providers to purchase an IV infusion pump and the required primary infusion sets. A representative from the company provided an in-service session on using the pump and troubleshooting issues. Gabe has found the pump to be easy to use and likes that

it provides extra safety for IV infusions. Because the patients are in the facility for several hours for the infusions, Gabe has also worked with the providers to create a special room for IV infusions. The room includes a recliner, television, a few Mayo stands, and the infusion pump. Gabe is excited to continue to assist with IV therapy.

PROCEDURE 47.1   Prime an IV Infusion Set

Tasks
Prime an IV infusion set with IV solution.

Scenario
Dr. Martin ordered LR 500 mL over 5 hours for Celia Tapia (DOB 05/18/19XX). You need to administer the IV infusion.

Equipment and Supplies
- Provider's order
- Patient's health record
- Primary IV infusion set
- IV fluid (LR 500 mL)
- Time label and marker or pen
- Waste container
- Sink or basin

Procedural Steps
1. Wash your hands or use hand sanitizer. Review the order. Clarify any questions you have with the provider.
   Purpose: Hand sanitization is an important step for infection control. It is important to be knowledgeable about the medication you are giving.
2. Select the IV solution bag from the storage area. Check the IV solution label against the order. Check for the right name, form, and route. Check the expiration date to make sure the IV solution is not expired. Verify the right dose and the right time.
   Purpose: It is important to do the first check of the label when getting the IV solution bag from the cabinet.
3. Assemble the supplies required for the procedure. Remove the IV solution from the outer plastic packaging if present.
   Purpose: Remember to split up the three medication checks with activities between each check.
4. Check the IV bag for leaks. Check the IV fluid for unusual color, precipitate, or cloudiness.
   Purpose: Do not use an IV bag that has a leak or IV fluid that is cloudy or a different color than normal.

5. Remove the primary IV tubing from the packaging. Position the roller clamp about 1 inch below the drip chamber. Close the roller clamp. Keep the spike and luer lock sterile.
   Purpose: Closing the roller clamp, prevents fluid from moving beyond the roller clamp.
6. Perform the second medication check. Check the IV solution label against the order. Check for the right name, form, and route.
   Purpose: It is important to do the second check of the label before continuing with the procedure.
7. Remove the covers from the IV solution port and the IV tubing spike (Fig. 1). Maintain the sterility of both during the removal process.

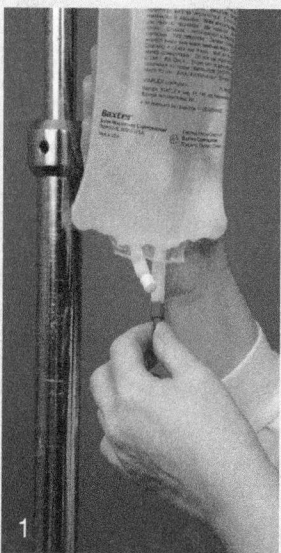

(From Potter P, Perry A: *Basic nursing,* ed 7, St. Louis, 2011, Mosby.)

8. Insert the IV tubing spike into the IV solution port, using a twisting motion (Fig. 2). Hang the IV solution bag on the IV pole or hook. Hold the luer lock end of the IV tubing.

Continued

PROCEDURE 47.1   Prime an IV Infusion Set—cont'd

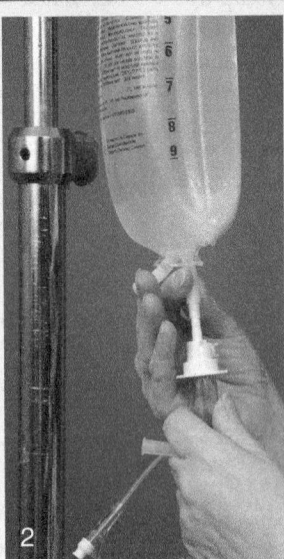

(From Potter P, Perry A: *Basic nursing,* ed 7, St. Louis, 2011, Mosby.)

Purpose: The IV solution bag must be higher than the patient for the fluid to infuse.

9. Gently squeeze the drip chamber so it fills about half full (Fig. 3).

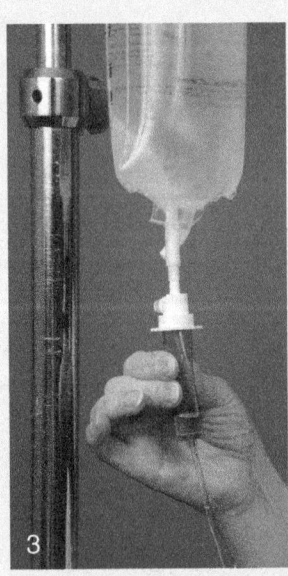

(From Potter P, Perry A: *Basic nursing,* ed 7, St. Louis, 2011, Mosby.)

10. Slowly open the roller clamp to prime the tubing. Invert the ports and any valves as the fluid passes. Tap the air out of the ports and valve (Fig. 4). Remove the cover on the luer lock and keep end sterile. Hold the luer lock end over a sink or basin and allow a small amount of fluid to drain out of the tubing.

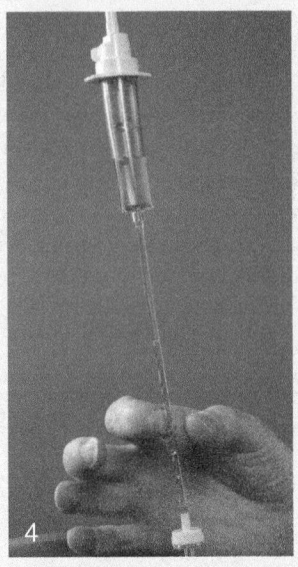

(From Potter P, Perry A: *Basic nursing,* ed 7, St. Louis, 2011, Mosby.)

Purpose: The air must be removed from the tubing to prevent an air embolism.

11. Close the roller clamp. Check the tubing for air. If air is found, reposition the tubing as needed to help move the air either to the drip chamber or out through the luer lock. Slowly open the roller clamp and allow a small amount of fluid to drain to remove the air. When the tubing is free of air, cover the luer lock end with the sterile cover.
    Purpose: Air must be removed from the tubing to prevent an air embolism.
12. Place the tubing on the IV hook or pole. Perform the third medication check. Check the IV solution label against the order. Check for the right name, form, and route.
    Purpose: Placing the tubing on the pole or hook helps to protect the tubing from touching the ground.
13. Following the healthcare facility's policy, complete the IV bag label with a pen or marker and place label on the solution.
    Purpose: The label provides important information needed when checking the infusion rate.
14. Clean up the work area. Packaging and other waste should be discarded in the waste container.
    Purpose: It is professional to clean up after yourself. Never fill a biohazardous sharps container with uncontaminated waste (e.g., packaging).

PROCEDURE 47.2   Administer IV Fluids

Tasks
Insert an IV catheter, attach the primed IV tubing with the IV solution, and document in the patient's health record.

Scenario
Dr. Martin ordered LR 500 mL over 5 hours for Celia Tapia (DOB 05/18/19XX). You need to administer the IV infusion.

Equipment and Supplies
- Provider's order
- Patient's health record
- Primed IV infusion set attached to the IV solution bag with an IV stand or hook
- Infusion pump (optional)
- Short extension tubing with syringe containing 1 to 3 mL of 0.9% sodium chloride (optional)

PROCEDURE 47.2 Administer IV Fluids—cont'd

- IV safety catheter
- IV start kit
- Gloves
- Biohazardous sharps container
- Waste container

Procedural Steps

1. Wash your hands or use hand sanitizer. Review the order. Clarify any questions you have with the provider.

   Purpose: Hand sanitization is an important step for infection control. It is important to be knowledgeable about the medication you are giving.

2. Calculate the infusion rate. Calculate the flow rate if needed.

   Purpose: The infusion rate is needed for the infusion pump. The infusion rate and the flow rate are needed if doing a gravity infusion.

3. Gather the supplies and equipment needed, including the primed IV tubing with the IV solution and the IV pole or hook (see Procedure 47.1). If using a short extension tubing, remove any protective covers, prime with the 0.9% sodium chloride, and replace protective cover to maintain the sterility of the tubing.

   Purpose: Having all of the needed supplies and equipment is necessary before starting the procedure.

4. Prior to entering the exam room, knock on the door and wait a moment. Greet the patient. Identify yourself. Verify the patient's identity with full name and date of birth. Make sure the patient's information matches the order and the record. Explain what you are going to do.

   Purpose: It is important to identify the patient in two different ways to ensure that you have the correct patient. Explaining the procedure can make the patient feel more comfortable and helps to reduce anxiety.

5. Provide the right education to the parent/patient. Explain the medication ordered, the desired effect, and common side effects; also identify the provider who ordered it. Answer any questions the parent/patient may have. Use language the parent/patient can understand. Ask if the patient has any allergies. If the parent/patient refuses the medication, notify the provider.

   Purpose: The patient needs to be aware of what you are giving, its action and side effects, and who ordered it. It is also important to double-check the patient's allergies before administering the medication.

6. Use hand sanitizer and put on gloves.

   Purpose: Hand sanitization is an important step for infection control.

7. Ask the patient which arm they prefer. Apply the tourniquet about 4 to 6 inches above the intended site. Do not apply the tourniquet too tight to avoid injuring the tissue. Check for a radial pulse. If the radial pulse is absent, loosen the tourniquet.

   Purpose: Some patients may have reasons for preferring certain arms. If a patient has lymphedema or had a recent mastectomy (under 3 years), the opposite arm should be used for the IV infusion if possible. A radial pulse should be present.

8. Palpate the vein with your index finger. Select a straight, well-dilated vein that is large enough for the IV catheter. Stroke the vessel or have the patient open and close their hand, making a fist.

   Purpose: A well-dilated vein is needed to insert the catheter.

9. Release the tourniquet.

   Purpose: The tourniquet needs to be released to prevent tissue damage.

   Note: If a topical anesthetic needs to be applied, it can be applied once the tourniquet is released.

10. Clean the intended site with the antiseptic swab or applicator as indicated by the facility's policies. If chlorhexidine is used, do a 30-second friction scrub back and forth and up and down at the site. Let the site dry.

11. Rotate the needle in the catheter 360 degrees.

    Purpose: This ensures the needle will separate from the catheter.

12. Using the dominant hand, firmly grip the catheter on each side of the hub. Align the catheter parallel with the vein. Use the nondominant hand to apply distal traction on the vein and hold the skin tautly. Anchor the vein with the thumb.

    Purpose: Applying traction helps to stabilize the vein, and holding the skin tautly helps with a smooth insertion of the needle.

13. With the bevel up and using a 10- to 30-degree angle, insert the needle through the skin. Aim toward the vein and slowly advance it until blood flashback is seen in the clear flashback chamber (Fig. 1A).

    Note: If a drop of blood appears in the chamber, insert about 1 to 2 mm until the flash of blood is seen.

14. Advance the cannula over the needle until the hub sits on the skin (Fig. 1B).

15. Loosen the tourniquet. Depending on the device used, stabilize the catheter. With the dominant hand, withdraw the needle and activate the safety device if needed. Depending on the type of device used, apply pressure over the vein if needed.

    Purpose: The pressure occludes the vessel, preventing the blood from spilling out of the catheter as the tubing is connected.

16. Connect the luer lock on the tubing to the catheter hub without contaminating the hub. If the extension tubing is used, occlude the tubing with the slide clamp, remove the syringe, and connect the extension tubing to the primary infusion set.

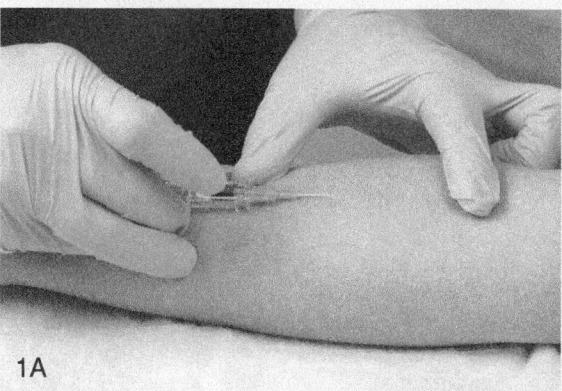
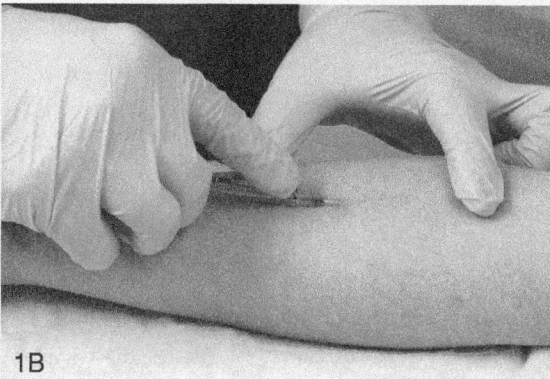

1A 1B

(From Potter PA, Perry AG: *Fundamentals of nursing,* ed 9, St. Louis, 2017, Elsevier.)

Continued

PROCEDURE 47.2 Administer IV Fluids—cont'd

17. Tape the catheter hub to the skin (Fig. 2). Per the facility's policy, place the transparent dressing over the insertion site or place a 2 × 2-inch gauze dressing over the insertion site and the hub (Fig. 3).

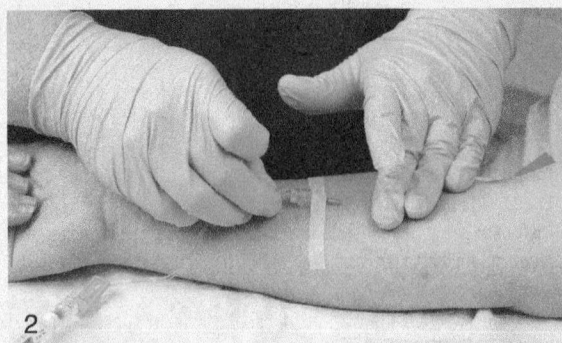

(From Potter PA, Perry AG: *Fundamentals of nursing,* ed 9, St. Louis, 2017, Elsevier.)

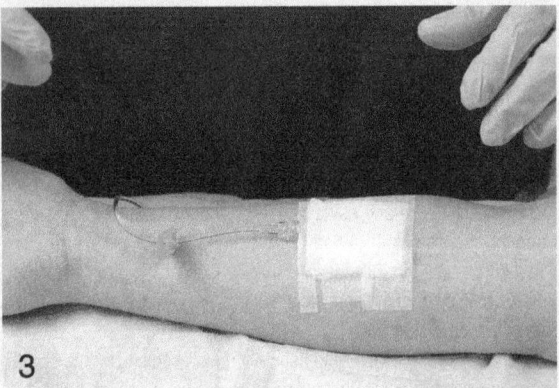

(From Potter PA, Perry AG: *Fundamentals of nursing,* ed 9, St. Louis, 2017, Elsevier.)

Purpose: Taping the hub prevents the catheter from being dislodged.

18. Create a loop with the IV tubing and secure the tubing to the skin with tape (Fig. 4). If using extension tubing, connect it to the IV infusion set.

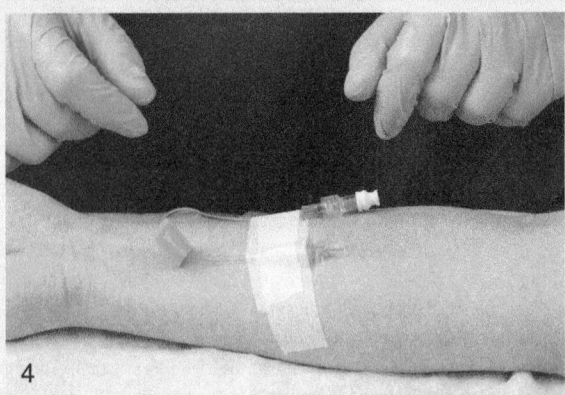

(From Potter PA, Perry AG: *Fundamentals of nursing,* ed 9, St. Louis, 2017, Elsevier.)

Purpose: Taping the tubing to the skin helps secure the IV and prevents the catheter from being dislodged.

19. Set the infusion rate if using a pump and ensure the clamps are opened. If using gravity infusion, count the drops and adjust the roller clamp to get the flow rate.

20. Observe the site for swelling during the infusion of the fluid.

    Purpose: If the site is infiltrated, the swelling will occur as the fluid infuses.

21. Discard the needle in the biohazard sharps container. Clean up the area. Discard the supplies per the facility's policy. Remove gloves and wash or sanitize hands.

22. Document the procedure, including the ordering provider's name, IV order, the type and size of catheter inserted, number of attempts, IV solution, and the infusion rate.

    05/26/20XX 10:10 a.m. Per Dr. Martin's order, LR 500 mL over 5 hours started. Insyte Autoguard 20G 1-inch catheter inserted in right hand on first attempt. LR 100 mL/hr infusing per infusion pump. Patient tolerated the procedure without concerns. Patient resting in recliner. BP 112/72 right arm, sitting (adult cuff); P: 82 regular, 1+; R: 18, regular, normal. _____

    _____ Gabe Garcia, CMA (AAMA)

PROCEDURE 47.3 Change an IV Bag

Task

Change an IV bag.

Scenario

Dr. Martin ordered LR 500 mL over 5 hours for Celia Tapia (DOB 05/18/19XX). The first bag you hung was 250 mL, and now you need to switch bags to give the other 250 mL.

Equipment and Supplies

- Provider's order
- IV bag

Procedural Steps

1. Wash your hands or use hand sanitizer. Review the order. Clarify any questions you have with the provider.

   Purpose: Hand sanitization is an important step for infection control.

2. Select the IV solution bag from the storage area. Check the IV solution label against the order. Check for the right name, form, and route. Check the expiration date to make sure the IV solution is not expired. Verify the right dose and the right time.

   Purpose: It is important to do the first check of the label when getting the IV solution bag from the cabinet.

3. Remove the IV solution from the outer plastic packaging if present. Check the IV bag for leaks. Check the IV fluid for unusual color, precipitate, or cloudiness.

   Purpose: Do not use an IV bag that has a leak or IV fluid that is cloudy or a different color than normal.

4. Perform the second medication check. Check the IV solution label against the order. Check for the right name, form, and route.

   Purpose: It is important to do the second check of the label before continuing with the procedure.

5. Prior to entering the exam room, knock on the door and wait a moment. Greet the patient. Identify yourself. Verify the patient's identity with full

PROCEDURE 47.3   Change an IV Bag–cont'd

name and date of birth. Make sure the patient's information matches the order and the record. Explain what you are going to do.

Purpose: It is important to identify the patient in two different ways to ensure that you have the correct patient. Explaining the procedure can make the patient feel more comfortable and helps to reduce anxiety.

6. Perform the third medication check. Hang the new IV solution bag on the IV pole.

7. Pause the IV infusion pump or close the roller clamp if giving the IV by gravity.

Purpose: Pausing the pump or clamping the tubing prevents air from getting into the IV tubing.

8. Remove the protective plastic cover over the tubing port. Remove the old IV bag from the pole and turn the bag upside down. Using a twisting motion remove the IV tubing spike from the IV bag (Fig. 1A). Using a twisting motion, insert the spike in the new IV bag at using the tubing port (Fig. 1B). Keep the spike sterile during this procedure.

Purpose: The spike must be kept sterile so the fluid does not become contaminated.

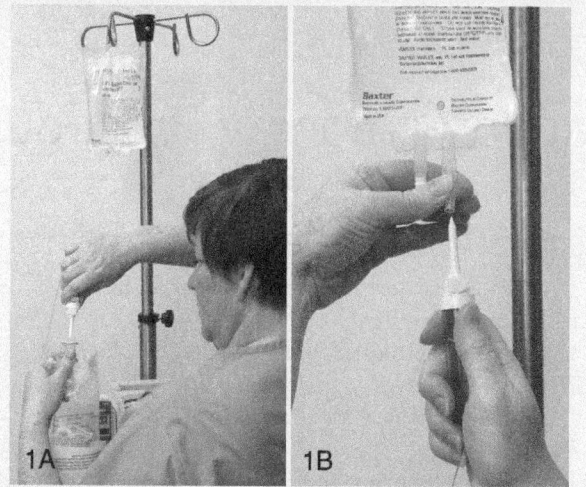

(From Potter PA, Perry AG: *Fundamentals of nursing*, ed 9, St. Louis, 2017, Elsevier.)

9. If the drip chamber is less than one-third to one-half filled, squeeze the drip chamber to fill it to this level. Check for air in the tubing before restarting the infusion pump or opening and regulating the roller clamp.

10. Label the bag per the healthcare facility's policy. If the facility requires documentation when administering a new bag of fluid, document at this time.

PROCEDURE 47.4   Remove an IV Catheter

Tasks

Remove an IV catheter and document the patient care.

Scenario

Dr. Martin ordered LR 500 mL over 5 hours for Celia Tapia (DOB 05/18/19XX). The fluid has been infused, and the IV needs to be discontinued or removed.

Equipment and Supplies

- Provider's order
- Sterile gauze (e.g., 2 × 2s)
- Gloves
- Tape or bandage (e.g., Band-Aid)
- Patient's health record

Procedural Steps

1. Wash your hands or use hand sanitizer. Review the order. Clarify any questions you have with the provider.

   Purpose: Hand sanitization is an important step for infection control.

2. Gather the supplies needed.

   Purpose: Having all of the needed supplies and equipment is necessary before starting the procedure.

3. Prior to entering the exam room, knock on the door and wait a moment. Greet the patient. Identify yourself. Verify the patient's identity with full name and date of birth. Make sure the patient's information matches the order and the record. Explain what you are going to do.

   Purpose: It is important to identify the patient in two different ways to ensure that you have the correct patient. Explaining the procedure can make the patient feel more comfortable and helps to reduce anxiety.

4. Put on gloves. Open the supplies. If an IV is infusing, stop the flow.

5. Remove the tape that secured the tubing to the skin. Hold the IV catheter with one hand. With the other hand, start to remove the transparent dressing by loosening one side and stretching the dressing. Then loosen and stretch the dressing on the opposite side. Completely remove the transparent dressing.

   Purpose: Holding the catheter prevents additional tissue trauma when removing the dressing.

6. Hold the sterile gauze above the insertion site. Pull the IV catheter back and straight out.

7. Once the catheter is removed, place the sterile gauze over the site and hold pressure until the bleeding has stopped, which may be 2 to 3 minutes.

   Note: If a patient is taking an anticoagulant, it may take longer than 3 minutes to stop the bleeding.

8. Inspect the catheter tip for any breakage. Discard the catheter in the biohazardous sharps container.

   Purpose: If the tip of the catheter breaks off, it can cause a catheter embolism. The medical assistant must always inspect the catheter tip to ensure the end is intact before discarding the catheter into the biohazardous sharps container.

9. Once the bleeding has stopped, replace the gauze with a new piece of sterile gauze. Apply tape over the gauze.

10. Clean up the area. Discard the supplies per the facility's policy. Remove your gloves and wash or sanitize your hands.

11. Document the IV catheter removal. Include the ordering provider's name, the order, the amount of fluid infused, and the appearance of the catheter tip.

   05/26/20XX 3:20 p.m. Per Dr. Martin's order, the IV was discontinued. Catheter removed and tip intact. LR 500 mL infused. Patient stated she "feels better."

   _____ Gabe Garcia, CMA (AAMA)

48

Cardiopulmonary Procedures

LEARNING OBJECTIVES

1. Review the structures and functionality of the cardiovascular system.
2. Use correct electrocardiography (ECG) terminology.
3. Discuss ECG waves, segments, and intervals.
4. Describe the medical assistant's role in a resting 12-lead ECG.
5. Describe the bipolar (standard) leads, augmented leads, and chest (precordial) leads.
6. Prepare a patient for an ECG and obtain an electrocardiogram.
7. Troubleshoot artifacts in an ECG.
8. Identify abnormal rhythms in an ECG tracing.
9. Discuss additional ECG testing, including exercise stress tests, nuclear stress tests, Holter monitors, cardiac event recorders, implantable loop recorders, transtelephonic monitoring, and portable handheld ECG monitors.
10. Discuss the respiratory system, measure the peak flow rate, and perform spirometry.
11. Describe pulmonary treatments, including metered-dose inhalers, nebulizer treatments, and oxygen therapy.

OUTLINE

▷▷ OPENING SCENARIO

Renee Thomas, CMA (AAMA), is a certified medical assistant at Walden-Martin Family Medical (WMFM) Clinic. According to her manager, over the time that she has been at WMFM Clinic, she has excelled. Because of Renee's professionalism and attention to detail, her manager, Sue, has asked her to mentor a new employee, Eva Ning.

Eva Ning, RMA, just graduated from a local medical assistant program. She really enjoyed the hands-on learning with the skills. During her clinical experience for school, she worked in a cardiology department for 6 weeks and really enjoyed the experience. Now that she has graduated, she looks forward to learning on the job.

Eva and Renee will spend a month with each provider. This month they are working with Dr. David Kahn, who sees many older patients. Renee tells Eva that they will be doing a lot of cardiac tests and treatments. Eva looks forward to learning from Renee and Dr. Kahn.

YOU WILL LEARN

1. To describe the components of the ECG tracing.
2. To obtain a clear ECG and to reduce artifacts in a tracing.
3. To describe other types of ECG tests.
4. To perform pulmonary testing procedures, including peak flow reading and spirometry.
5. To perform pulmonary treatments, including nebulizer treatments and oxygen therapy.

INTRODUCTION

Heart disease is the leading cause of death in the United States. Medical assistants in primary and specialty areas often care for patients with heart disorders. All medical assistants must:
- Understand the cardiovascular system
- Recognize early symptoms of potential disorders
- Coach patients on cardiac tests and treatments ordered by providers
- Accurately perform cardiac tests
- Identify and troubleshoot problems when performing tests

The heart is a complex organ. Electrical impulses move through the heart, and the cells react by contracting. The contracting cells result in contraction of the chambers. The contractions cause the blood to move through the heart and out to the arteries. To monitor the heart's function, both the electrical and mechanical activities of the heart can be assessed. When a provider needs to assess the electrical activity of the heart, an electrocardiogram (ee leck troh kar dee AH gram) is commonly ordered.

Electrocardiography is a painless test. Electrodes are placed on the body, and wires connect the electrodes to the ECG machine (electrocardiograph). Electrical impulses from the heart make their way to the surface of the skin. Think of what occurs when you throw a rock into a lake. Waves are created, and they eventually make their way to the shore. The electricity from the heart eventually makes its way to the surface of the skin. The electrodes pick up the electricity, and the electricity moves into the machine. The electrocardiograph creates a record of the impulses, which is called an electrocardiogram (ECG, EKG).

A medical assistant performs the electrocardiography. The provider reads and interprets the ECG to identify any abnormalities in the electrical conduction in the heart. It is important that the medical assistant should:
- Know the normal function of the heart
- Perform the procedure accurately
- Identify problems during the ECG procedure and take appropriate actions

Besides ECGs, the medical assistant is responsible for pulmonary testing, including measuring the peak flow rate and performing spirometry (spi ROM e tree) testing. The medical assistant can administer nebulizer treatments and oxygen therapy, as ordered by the provider.

In this chapter, ECGs, pulmonary tests, and pulmonary treatments are discussed. The chapter begins with a review of the cardiovascular system. The components of the ECG and the process of obtaining an ECG follow the review. The chapter concludes with a discussion about pulmonary testing and treatments.

VOCABULARY

echocardiography (ECHO) The use of ultrasonic waves directed through the heart to study the structure and motion of the heart. The visual record produced is called an *echocardiogram*.

electrocardiogram (ECG, EKG) A record or recording of electrical impulses of the heart as produced by an electrocardiograph.

electrodes Adhesive patches that conduct electricity from the body to the ECG machine wires.

CARDIOVASCULAR SYSTEM REVIEW

Heart Structure

The heart is divided into four chambers. Two atrial chambers receive blood from the body. Two ventricular chambers pump blood out to the body. The septum (SEP tum) divides the right and left sides of the heart.

The tricuspid (try KUSS pid) valve is found between the right atrium and the right ventricle (Fig. 48.1). The pulmonary valve is between the right ventricle and the pulmonary artery. The bicuspid (bye KUSS pid), or mitral (MYE trul), valve is found between the left atrium and left ventricle. The aortic (AE ore tik) valve is between the left ventricle and the aorta. When the valves open, blood moves to the next chamber, or out of the heart through the arteries. The mechanical action of the heart and valves can be assessed by echocardiography (eck oh KAR dee ah gruh fee) (ECHO).

The heart wall has three layers: the epicardium (eh pee KAR dee um), the myocardium (mye oh KAR dee um), and the endocardium (en doh KAR dee um). Cardiac muscle fibers in the myocardium are electrically linked together, forming "one unit." A myocardial cell forms a strong connection to the next cells through special junctions called *intercalated discs*. These discs allow electricity to flow freely from one cell to the next. The intercalated discs are responsible for the cell-to-cell communication that is required for coordinated muscle contraction. The intercalated discs help the muscle fibers form one unit that contracts all at once, instead of a little at a time. The one-unit approach is important, because the atria and ventricles need to contract in an appropriately timed and coordinated effort.

Blood Flow

The right atrium receives deoxygenated blood from these structures:
- Superior vena cava (blood comes from the head, neck, chest, and upper extremities)
- Inferior vena cava (blood comes from the abdomen, pelvis, and lower extremities)
- Coronary sinus (blood from the coronary veins in the heart muscle)

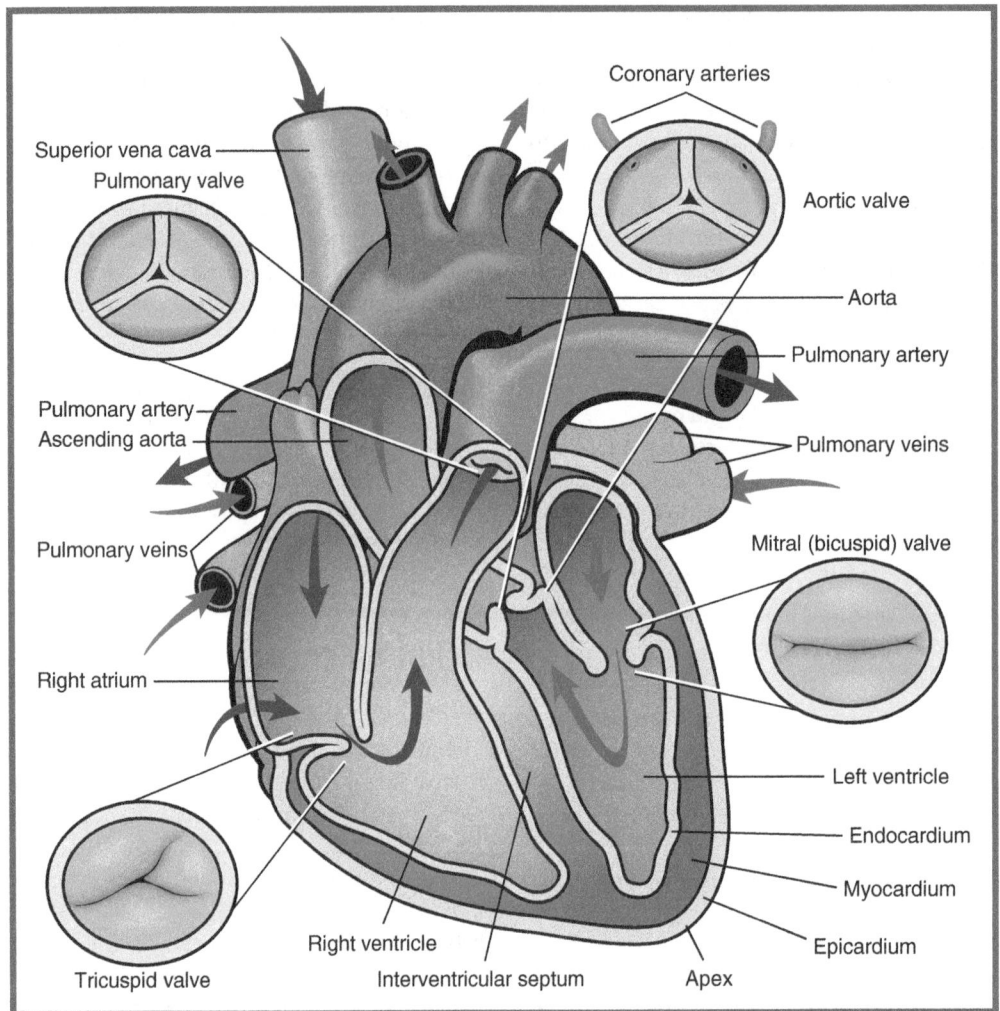

Fig. 48.1 Chambers and Valves of the Heart. (From Damjanov I: *Pathology* for *the health-related professions,* ed 4, St. Louis, 2012, Saunders.)

When the right atrial chamber contracts, the tricuspid valve (atrioventricular [AV] valve) opens. Blood empties from the right atrium into the right ventricle. When the ventricles contract, the deoxygenated blood in the right ventricle passes through the opened pulmonary valve (semilunar [SL] valve) and moves into the pulmonary artery. The pulmonary artery brings the blood to the lungs. In the lungs, the blood picks up oxygen (O_2) and gives up carbon dioxide (CO_2). The pulmonary vein brings the oxygenated blood back to the left atrium. When the left atrial chamber contracts, the blood is pushed past the opened mitral (or bicuspid) valve (AV valve). The blood empties into the left ventricle. When the ventricles contract, the blood in the left ventricle moves through the opened aortic valve (SL valve) and into the aorta. The aorta transports oxygenated blood to the body. The first arteries to split off the aorta are the left and right coronary arteries. These arteries bring the oxygenated blood to the heart muscles.

A complete heartbeat, or cardiac cycle, can be divided into diastole and systole phases. During the *diastole phase*, the heart is at rest and the atria fill with blood. The *systole phase* occurs when the heart is contracting.

MEDICAL TERMINOLOGY

atri/o	atrium
cardi/o	heart
endocardi/o	endocardium
myocardi/o	myocardium
sept/o	septum
ventricul/o	ventricle
echo-	sound
electro-	using electricity
epi-	above, on top of
-gram	record, recording
-graphy	process of recording
atrium (singular), atria (plural)	
septum (singular), septa (plural)	

CRITICAL THINKING 48.1

Renee wants to help Eva review the cardiovascular structures before they see their first patient of the day. She asks Eva to describe the blood flow through the heart, starting with the superior vena cava and the inferior vena cava. Describe the blood flow.

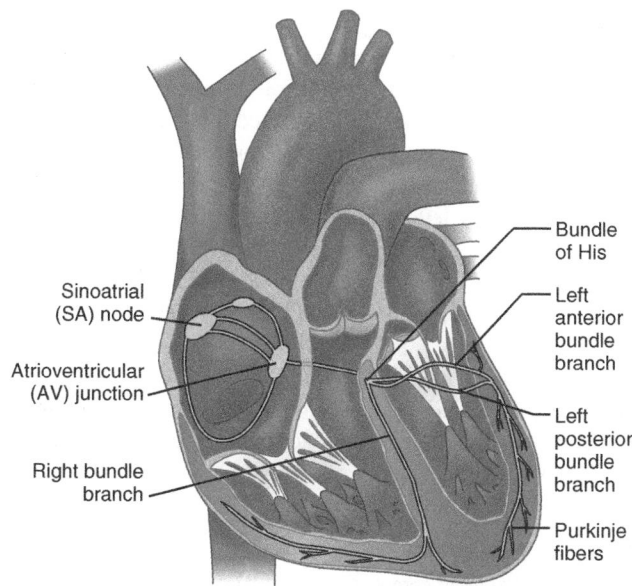

Fig. 48.2 Cardiac Conduction System. (From Niedzwiecki B, et al: *Kinn's the medical assistant,* ed 14, St. Louis, 2020, Elsevier.)

Heart's Conduction System

The electrical cells make up the conduction system of the heart. These cells are found throughout the myocardium. They can respond to and transmit electrical impulses to neighboring cells. The conduction system is composed of five structures.

- *Sinoatrial* (SIE noe ae tree el) *(SA) node:* The SA node is called the "pacemaker of the heart" (Fig. 48.2). It is located in the posterior superior wall of the right atrium. The cardiac cells in the SA node generate the impulse. An impulse from the SA node starts each heartbeat. When the SA node discharges the impulse, it travels in many directions through the heart muscle. Nearby atrial cardiac cells slowly pick up the impulse. The impulse also moves quickly across special bands of tissue called *intermodal tracts.* The *Bachmann bundle,* a specialized intermodal tract, takes the impulse to the left atrium. Other intermodal tracts take the impulse quickly to the AV node.
- *Atrioventricular (AV) node:* The AV node is located at the base of the interatrial septum. When the impulse reaches the AV node, it moves very slowly through the node. This slowdown allows the atrial chambers to finish contracting, moving the blood into the ventricular chambers.
- *Bundle of His* (or *AV bundle*): The bundle of His is located in the upper interventricular septum. When the impulse leaves the AV node, it moves to the bundle of His.
- *Right and left bundle branches:* The bundle branches are located in the lower interventricular septum. After the impulse passes through the bundle of His, it enters the right and left bundle branches. The right bundle branch brings the impulse to the right ventricle. The left bundle branch brings the impulse to the left ventricle.
- *Purkinje* (pur KIN jee) *fibers:* The bundle branches split into many Purkinje fibers. The Purkinje fibers transmit the impulse quickly and efficiently to the ventricular cardiac cells. This helps the ventricular chambers to contract.

The cardiac cells cycle through three states, or steps, in the same sequence for each impulse.

- *Polarized state:* Before the impulse hits the cardiac cell, the cell is in the resting state, or resting potential. The inside of the cardiac cell is negatively charged. Outside of the cell is positively charged. There is no electrical activity seen on the ECG during the polarized state.
- *Depolarized state:* When the impulse hits the cardiac cell, large numbers of positively charged sodium ions (AHY ons) move into the cell. A small number of potassium ions moves outside the cell. The movement of sodium and potassium changes the cell's charge to positive. The change, also called *action potential,* allows the impulse to move through the cell. *Depolarization* (when the impulse hits the cell) causes electrical activity on the ECG.
- *Repolarized state:* After the impulse passes over the cell, the sodium and potassium ions move back to their original locations. This causes the cell's charge to change back to a negative charge. This recovery phase is called the *repolarized state.* Electrical activity (less than the depolarized state) can be recorded during the repolarized state.

Remember that the impulse occurs first and very soon after the contraction starts. These are two very distinct activities yet appear very closely together. The electrical activity from the depolarized state and the repolarized state is recorded on the ECG. The contractions are mechanical actions and are not recorded on the ECG. An echocardiogram (ECHO) can be used to gather information on the mechanical action of the heart, such as the valves opening and closing.

CRITICAL THINKING 48.2

Renee, knowing they have ECGs scheduled for today, asks Eva to list the conduction system structures in order and briefly describe polarization, depolarization, and repolarization. List the conduction system structures in order and then describe polarization, depolarization, and repolarization.

VOCABULARY

ion An electrically charged atom, or the smallest component of an element.

✳ STUDY TIP

Think of the three states as:
- Polarized state – resting state
- Depolarized state – discharge (impulse) state
- Repolarized state – recovery state
  Remember when discussing these three states that the cardiac chamber comes before the word (e.g., atrial polarization).

ECG TRACING

The medical assistant performs the ECG procedure. The ECG is read or interpreted by the provider. It is important for the medical assistant to understand the components of the ECG tracing. A medical assistant must be able to identify artifact in the recording. If artifact is seen, corrective action needs to be taken to get a clear ECG tracing. The medical assistant will also need to know how to identify life-threatening rhythms. When these are seen, it is important that the medical assistant get immediate help. Artifact and life-threatening rhythms will be discussed later in the chapter.

> **VOCABULARY**
>
> **artifact** A substance, structure, or event that does not naturally occur in a situation. Examples include interference, or electrical "garbage," on an ECG, or crystals, lint, or contamination of a staining technique.

ECG Terminology

To understand the ECG tracing, it is important to understand the common terminology used:

- *Isoelectric line*: A straight line that is also called the *baseline*. It represents a period of time with no electrical activity.
- *Deflection*: Any movement away from the baseline in the tracing. The deflections reflect the heart's electrical flow. Upward movement is called a *positive deflection*. Downward movement is a *negative deflection*.
- *Wave*: A deflection from the baseline.
- *Complex*: A form made up of many waves (e.g., QRS complex).
- *Segment*: A part of a line between two points (e.g., the ST segment starts at the end of the S wave and ends at the start of the T wave).
- *Interval*: A period of time between two points or events. During an interval, many waves can occur.

Each deflection in the ECG tracing corresponds to a part of the cardiac cycle. The ECG cycle consists of waveforms that are labeled: P, Q, R, S, T, and U (Fig. 48.3). The Q, R, and S waves are usually grouped together and called the *QRS complex*. In the next section, each part of the ECG is discussed in more detail.

ECG Waves and Segments

The *P wave* is the first deflection in the tracing. It is created from the electrical impulses moving through the right and left atria. The P wave appears as a small, rounded hill. The first part of the P wave reflects the impulse moving from the SA node to the AV node in the right atrium. The second part of the P wave reflects the impulse in the left atrial chamber. Electricity given off when the atrial cells are depolarized creates the P wave. Thus the P wave represents *atrial depolarization*. During the P wave, the atrial chambers contract and the blood moves into the ventricles (Table 48.1).

The *PR segment* follows the P wave and appears as an isoelectric line. The electrical impulse moves slowly through the AV node. This electricity is not picked up on the ECG tracing. The PR segment is the time between the end of the *atrial*

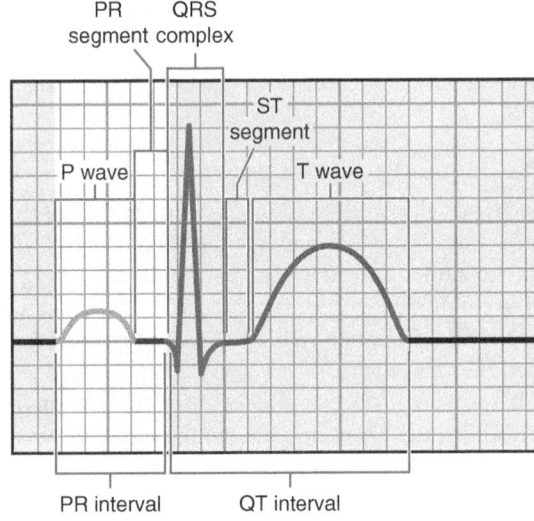

Fig. 48.3 Electrocardiogram Cycle.

TABLE 48.1 Summary of ECG Waves and Segments

Waves	Appearance	Summarized	Conduction System	Mechanical Action
P wave	Small "hill" (positive deflection seen on lead II)	Atrial depolarization	Impulse moves from the SA node (pacemaker) to the AV node.	Atrial chambers contract; blood moves into the ventricles.
PR segment	Isoelectric line		Impulse moves slowly through AV node; electricity is not picked up on tracing.	
QRS complex	(See below)	Ventricular depolarization; interventricular septal depolarization; and atrial repolarization (hidden)	AV node to the bundle of His to the right and left bundle branches to the Purkinje fibers.	Ventricular chambers contract, pushing blood out of the heart.
Q wave	Negative deflection	Interventricular septal depolarization		
R wave	Positive triangular deflection	Ventricular depolarization; atrial repolarization (hidden)		
S wave	Any downward deflection following the R wave			
ST segment	Isoelectric line			
T wave	Positive deflection (upright and rounded in lead II)	Ventricular repolarization		
U wave	Usually not seen	Purkinje fibers are repolarized		

AV, Atrioventricular; *SA*, sinoatrial.

depolarization and the start of the ventricular depolarization. During the PR segment, the atrial chambers finish contracting.

The *QRS complex* is the next wave in the tracing. The impulse moves from the AV node through the remaining conduction system structures. The electricity given off from the impulse moving down the septum and around the outer walls of the ventricles creates the QRS complex. The electricity from the activity in the ventricles masks the repolarization electricity given off from the atrial cells as they recover. The QRS complex activity can be summarized as *ventricular depolarization* and *atrial repolarization*. During the QRS complex, the ventricles start contracting and the blood moves into the arteries.

Each wave in the *QRS complex* is different. The Q wave is a negative deflection and represents *interventricular septal depolarization*. The large, triangular-shaped R wave reflects the depolarization of most of the ventricular walls. The S wave is the final depolarization of the ventricular walls. Not all of these three waves may be seen. The positive and negative deflections of these waves can be different in the 12 leads, or pictures, of the ECG.

The *ST segment* follows the last wave in the QRS complex and ends at the start of the T wave. The *J point* is the point where the QRS complex ends and the ST segment starts. The ST segment is an isoelectric line. There is no electrical activity in the heart during this segment. (Remember, the impulse moving through the conduction system finished in the QRS complex.) During the ST segment, the ventricles finish contracting.

Repolarization causes electrical activity that creates the remaining waves. The T wave follows the ST segment and appears as a smooth, rounded, asymmetric waveform. The electrical activity from *ventricular repolarization* creates the T wave.

The U wave may follow the T wave, but in many cases it is not seen. The U wave is created from the repolarization of the Purkinje fibers. A U wave may also appear if the patient has hypercalcemia, hypokalemia, or digoxin toxicity.

☀ STUDY TIP

Summary of the Tracing

- P wave: Atrial depolarization (the impulse moves through the atria)
- QRS complex: Ventricular depolarization (the impulse moves through the ventricles) and atrial repolarization (atrial cells are in a recovery state)
- T wave: Ventricular repolarization (ventricular cells are in a recovery state)
  The atria are always one stage ahead of the ventricles until both are in the polarized state. For instance, atrial polarization occurs with ventricular repolarization.

CRITICAL THINKING 48.3

Before doing the ECGs scheduled for today, Renee reviews the waveforms with Eva. She asks Eva the following questions regarding the ECG tracing:
- What shows atrial depolarization?
- What shows ventricular depolarization?
- What shows ventricular repolarization?

ECG Intervals

An *interval* is a period of time from a start point to an end point. It is not a wave. If you need to define what occurs during an interval, you will simply summarize the activities that happen for each wave and segment during the interval period of time.

The PR interval starts at the beginning of the P wave and ends at the start of the Q wave. It represents atrial depolarization. The QT interval starts at the beginning of the Q wave and extends to the end of the T wave. During the QT interval, the atrial chambers move from repolarization to the polarized state. The ventricular chambers depolarize and then move into the repolarized state.

CRITICAL THINKING 48.4

Eva is confused about the PR interval and the QT interval. How might Renee describe these two intervals?

12-LEAD ECG

One of the most common ECG procedures in the ambulatory care setting is a resting 12-lead ECG. The medical assistant is responsible for:
- Assembling the supplies and equipment needed
- Preparing the patient for the test
- Performing the test

Before the medical assistant finishes the procedure, the ECG tracing must be examined for artifact. If any artifact is present on the tracing, the medical assistant must problem-solve the situation. Ultimately, the goal is to give the provider a clear ECG.

For a resting 12-lead ECG, the patient rests on the exam table. Ten electrodes are placed on the body. Lead wires attach to the electrodes and connect to the ECG machine (electrocardiograph). The 10 electrodes and lead wires pick up the electrical impulse from the surface of the body and carry it to the ECG machine (Fig. 48.4). The machine creates the ECG tracing.

A more in-depth discussion of electrode placement and artifact is presented later in the chapter. For now, it is important to have an idea of where the electrodes are placed on the body. An electrode is placed on each of the arms and legs. The right leg electrode is considered the ground electrode and is required for a clear ECG tracing. Six electrodes are placed on the chest.

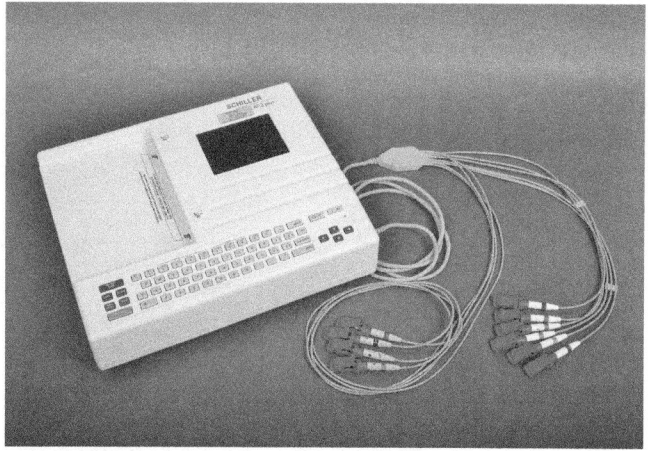

Fig. 48.4 Electrocardiogram Machine. (From Niedzwiecki B, et al: *Kinn's the medical assistant,* ed 14, St. Louis, 2020, Elsevier.)

Using the 10 electrodes and lead wires, the ECG machine creates 12 images, or pictures, that are called *leads*. Each lead picture looks different. Think of a photographer moving around a person, taking 12 pictures. Each picture looks different because of the change of the photographer's angle. For each lead, the picture is created differently. It is important for the medical assistant to know what electrodes and lead wires create the leads when troubleshooting unclear tracings. The three types of leads —bipolar, augmented, and precordial—are discussed in the following sections.

CRITICAL THINKING 48.5

Robert Caudill is scheduled for an ECG today. When he arrives, Eva discusses the procedure. Robert asks what "12 lead" stands for. How would you answer his question?

Bipolar (or Standard) Leads

The bipolar or standard leads are named leads I, II, and III. They use the arm electrodes and the left leg electrode to create pictures of the vertical (or frontal) plane of the heart. (Remember, the right electrode is used as a ground and is important for all leads.)

The bipolar leads are created from a measurement of current traveling from a negative pole to the positive pole (Fig. 48.5A):
- Lead I: Right arm (RA) to left arm (LA)
- Lead II: Right arm (RA) to left leg (LL)
- Lead III: Left leg (LL) to left arm (LA)

If you join the end points (positive poles) of these three leads, you get a triangle. This triangle is known as the *Einthoven triangle*.

It is important to know which two electrodes create each lead when troubleshooting problems with the ECG tracing. If a lead has artifact, the medical assistant must check the two electrodes and the lead wires that create the lead.

VOCABULARY

bipolar Having two poles or electrical charges.
unipolar Having one pole or electrical charge.

CRITICAL THINKING 48.6

As Eva and Renee perform an ECG, they find artifact on a few leads. For the following leads, which electrodes should be checked in each situation?
- Lead II is unclear.
- Leads I and III are unclear.
- Leads II and III are unclear.

Augmented Leads

Augmented leads (see Fig. 48.5B) also provide information on the vertical (frontal) plane of the heart. These unipolar leads are *augmented*, or increased in size, on the tracing. Augmented leads use the right arm (RA), left arm (LA), and left leg (LL) electrodes.

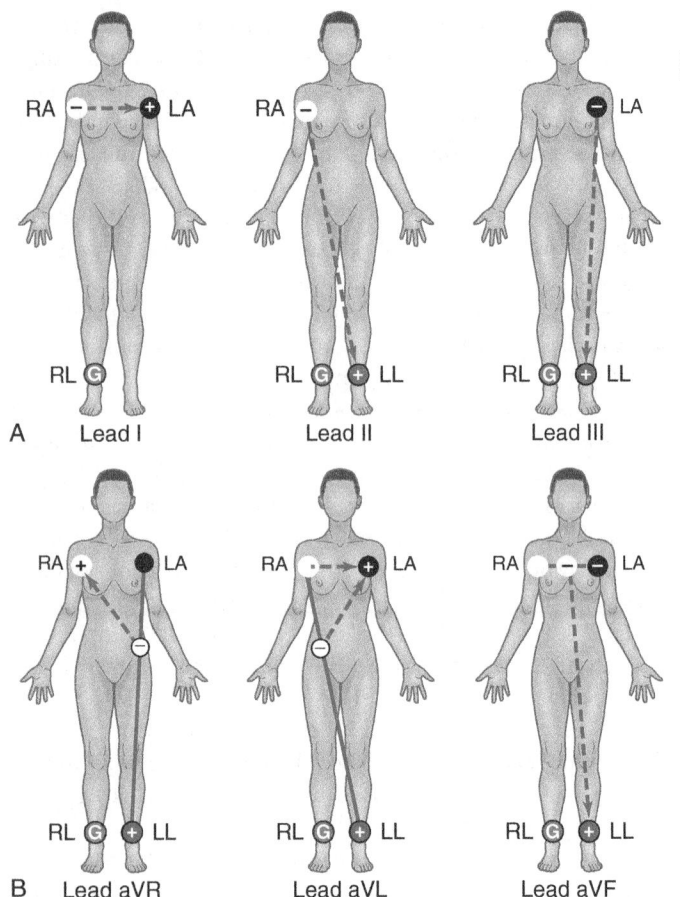

Fig. 48.5 Bipolar or standard (A) and augmented (B) limb leads. *aVF,* Augmented vector foot; *aVL,* augmented vector left; *aVR,* augmented vector right; *LA,* left arm; *LL,* left leg; *RA,* right arm, *RL,* right leg. (From Niedzwiecki B, et al: *Kinn's the medical assistant,* ed 14, St. Louis, 2020, Elsevier.)

Each augmented lead uses all three extremity electrodes (RA, LA, and LL) to create the picture. Midpoint between two of the electrodes is the negative pole. The current is measured as it moves from the negative pole to the positive pole.
- Lead aVR (augmented Vector Right) records current traveling between the right arm and the central point between the left arm and left leg.
- Lead aVL (augmented Vector Left) records current traveling between the left arm and the central point between the right arm and left leg.
- Lead aVF (augmented Vector Foot) records current traveling between the left leg electrode and the central point between the left and right arms.

If the medical assistant identifies artifact on the aVR lead, all three electrodes and lead wires should be checked. (Check the RA, LA, and LL electrode and lead wires.)

Chest (or Precordial) Leads

The chest (precordial) leads are also unipolar leads. Each is a positive pole. The precordial leads provide information on the horizontal (front to back) plane of the heart. The six precordial leads are labeled V_1, V_2, V_3, V_4, V_5, and V_6 (Fig. 48.6).

The six leads are numbered the same as the precordial lead wires (i.e., V_1 through V_6). If one of the leads is unclear, the medical assistant should refer to the related lead wire and

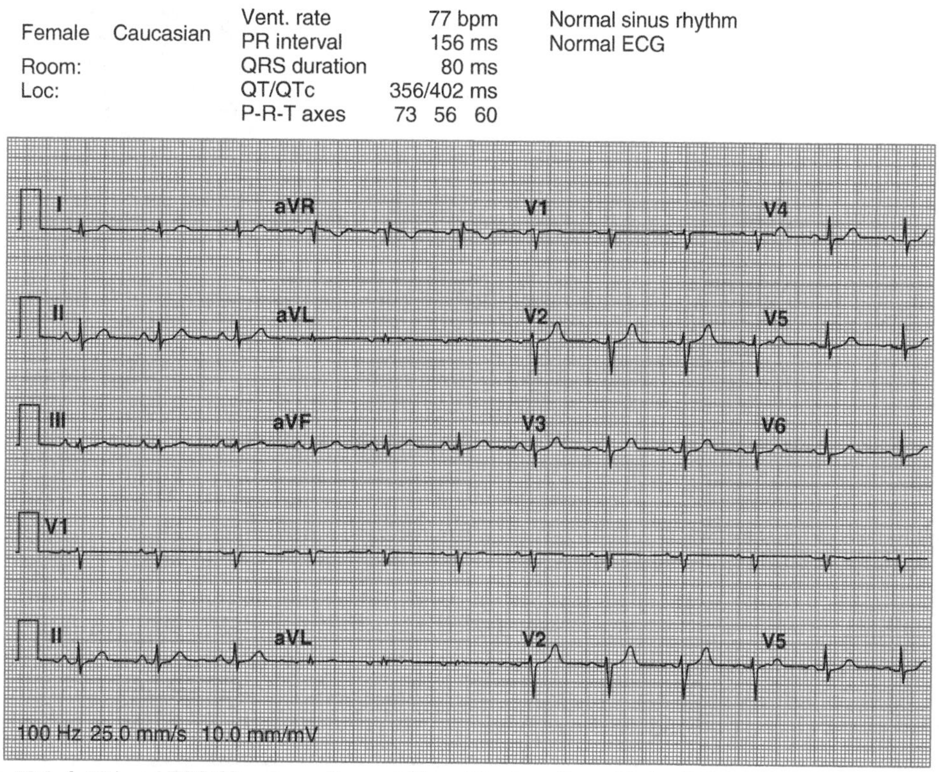

Female   Caucasian   Vent. rate   77 bpm   Normal sinus rhythm
Room: PR interval   156 ms   Normal ECG
Loc: QRS duration   80 ms
                        QT/QTc   356/402 ms
                        P-R-T axes   73 56 60

Fig. 48.6 A 12-Lead ECG Showing a Normal Sinus Rhythm. (From Phalen T, Aehlert BJ: *The 12-lead ECG in acute coronary syndromes,* ed 3, St. Louis, 2012, Mosby.)

electrode. For instance, with artifact on V_4, the medical assistant will check the V_4 electrode and lead wire.

ECG SUPPLIES AND EQUIPMENT

The medical assistant needs to be familiar with the supplies and equipment used for ECGs. It is important to monitor the expiration dates of ECG supplies. Using expired supplies can cause unclear ECG tracings.

Thermal ECG Paper

ECG machines with printers use special ECG paper. The paper can be either Z-fold paper or 8.25 × 11-inch paper. A special heat-sensitive coating on the paper allows the tracing to be "burnt" onto the paper. Tips for handling the ECG paper include:

- Store in a dry, cool, dark location.
- Do not expose to heat, bright light, or an ultraviolet (UV) light source.
- Do not expose to alcohol, adhesives, cleaners, or solvents.
- Do not store with vinyl, shrink wrap, or plastics.

The ECG paper is universally created with small and large boxes. The small box is 1 × 1 mm, and the large box is 5 × 5 mm. The large box is made up of 25 small boxes (5 rows and 5 columns) (Fig. 48.7). It has a thicker border than the small boxes. When the provider analyzes the tracing, the height and the width of the wave forms are measured with a caliper (Fig. 48.8). The small and large boxes can help in the interpreting process.

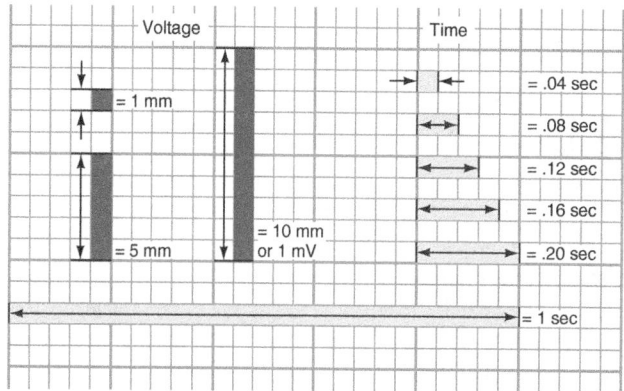

Fig. 48.7 Electrocardiogram Paper. (From Niedzwiecki B, et al: *Kinn's the medical assistant,* ed 14, St. Louis, 2020, Elsevier.)

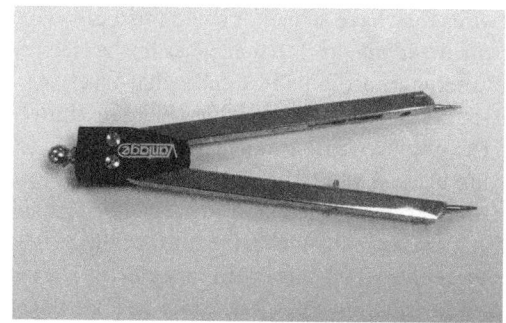

Fig. 48.8 Caliper.

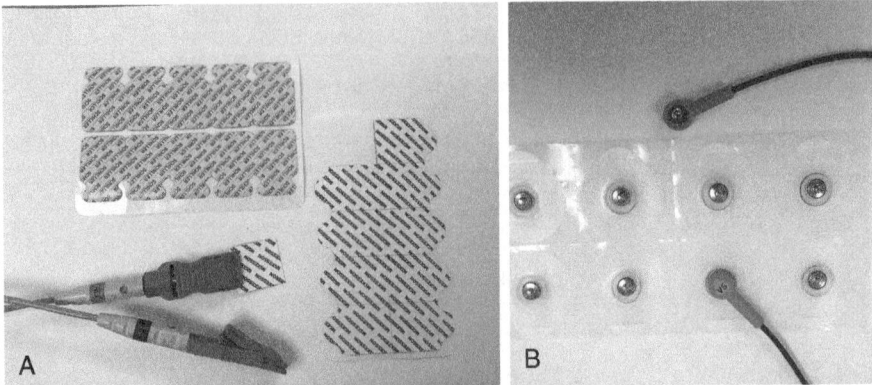

Fig. 48.9 A, The appearance of tab electrodes can vary, depending on the manufacturer. Alligator clips on the lead wires attach to the tab electrodes. B, Snap electrodes use the snap adaptors on the lead wires.

The vertical lines measure the amplitude, or *voltage*, of the waveforms. Each small box is 0.1 mV (millivolt), and each large box is 0.5 mV. To determine the amplitude, count the small boxes vertically, starting at the baseline, to the highest/lowest point of the wave.

The horizontal lines measure the time. When the paper speed *(chart speed)* is set at 25 mm/second, each small box is 0.04 second and each large box equals 0.2 second. To determine the width and time of the waveform, count the small boxes horizontally from the start to the finish of the wave. Multiply the number of small boxes by 0.04 to find the time.

VOCABULARY

caliper A pocket-sized tool used for measuring the height and width of the ECG waves and intervals.

Electrodes

Electrodes are single-use disposable adhesive tabs that are placed on the skin. The skin is a poor conductor of electricity. The electrodes contain an electrolyte gel that helps pick up the electrical impulses. As the impulses make their way to the surface of the body, the electrolyte gel helps to conduct the impulses into the lead wires. For a resting 12-lead ECG, the most common type of electrode is the tab variety (Fig. 48.9A). The snap electrode is used more often for exercise stress tests and in hospital settings (Fig. 48.9B).

It is important to check the expiration date of the electrodes. If they are expired, the gel may be dried out and the conduction will be poor. Many operators' manuals for ECG machines recommend not mixing different manufacturers' electrodes.

Electrocardiograph

The lead wires may have a snap or a clip (also called an *alligator clip*; *patient end adaptor*) that attaches to the electrode. The lead wires merge into the patient cable that takes the electrical impulses to the electrocardiograph (ECG machine). In the machine, the impulses pass through an amplifier, which magnifies the impulses. A digital converter changes the analog signal into a digital signal. The digital signal can be printed off on special ECG paper, which will be discussed in the next section.

The features of ECG machines can vary greatly. The two types of ECG devices in ambulatory healthcare facilities include the box model and computer-based models. The box model ECG

machine usually has an LCD screen. The computer-based ECG may have a touch screen and stress testing features. The software can be preloaded onto its own computer, or the facility can purchase software to be added to any laptop computer. Additional features commonly seen in both types of ECG devices are:

- Interpretive software: Assists providers with reading the tracing.
- Bluetooth or Wi-Fi capacity: Allows the ECG to be sent to providers and printers and to be uploaded into an electronic health record (EHR).
- Thermal printers
- Spirometer

Settings and Calibration. ECG machines have settings that can be useful for obtaining a tracing. Many machines have filters to block disturbances. Filters can help to create a clearer tracing. Refer to the operators' manual when changing settings. Table 48.2 presents common settings. It is important to indicate on the tracing if any of the default settings were changed. Changes to the default settings will affect how the provider measures and interprets the tracing.

Most ECG machines automatically complete a self-test when the machine is turned on. Typically, the self-test examines the battery and the memory. Like many machines used in the healthcare setting, the ECG machine needs to be calibrated daily or per the facility's policy. The calibration results should be documented on the log flow sheet.

When ECG machines are calibrated, the *sensitivity* (also called *gain*) should be checked. The machines usually print a calibration marking either at the beginning or at the end of the tracing. This marking is called the *standardization mark*. If the machine is set at 10 mm/mV, the standardization mark will be an upward rectangle that is 10 small boxes tall. If the gain is doubled, then the standardization mark also will be doubled in size (Fig. 48.10).

CRITICAL THINKING 48.7

The next day, Eva prepares to do an ECG on Charles Johnson. She turns on the machine to check to see if it has been set up correctly. She sees the following:

- Chart speed: 10 mm/s
- Gain: 10 mm/mV

Which of these settings is normal and which needs to be changed prior to the next ECG?

TABLE 48.2 Common ECG Settings

Setting	Description	Normal Default	Reason to Change Setting
Chart speed	Regulates the speed of the paper during the recording. *Example:* 25 mm/s means 25 millimeters (25 small blocks) of tracing is printed in 1 second.	25 mm/s (second)	*For very fast rates:* Increase speed to 50 mm/s to get more defined waveforms. *For very slow rates:* Reduce rate to 5 or 10 mm/s to capture more waveforms on the paper.
Gain or sensitivity	Regulates the height (amplitude) of the tracing. *Example:* 10 mm/mV means 1 mV (millivolt) of electricity causes the recorder to move up 10 millimeters (10 small blocks).	10 mm/mV	*For very short waveforms:* Increase to 20 mm/mV, which doubles the height of the waves. *For very tall waveforms:* Reduce to 5 mm/mV, which reduces the wave height by half.

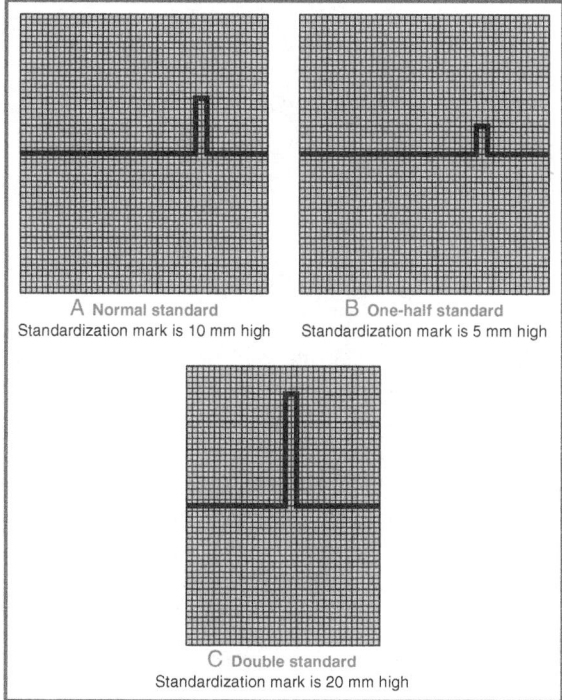

A Normal standard
Standardization mark is 10 mm high

B One-half standard
Standardization mark is 5 mm high

C Double standard
Standardization mark is 20 mm high

Fig. 48.10 Sensitivity Standards. (From Niedzwiecki B, et al: *Kinn's the medical assistant,* ed 14, St. Louis, 2020, Elsevier.)

ECG PROCEDURE

Patient Preparation

Before the procedure is started, it is always important for the medical assistant to coach the patient on the procedure and the preparation required. The medical assistant should prepare the patient for an ECG by explaining these points:

- Ten electrodes and wires are placed on the body.
- The machine will take 12 pictures of the electrical activity of the heart.
- The procedure is painless.
- The patient must be still and not talk during the time the pictures are being made (during the actual tracing).
- Patients should not use their cell phone or other electronic device during the procedure.
- The provider will need to look at the ECG pictures and then the patient will be notified of the results. (Remember, the medical assistant cannot tell the patient if it is normal or abnormal.)

The patient needs to remove all clothing above the waist and wear a gown that opens in the front. Cloth gowns or paper capes can be used. An electrode must be placed on each lower leg, so tights or pantyhose also must be removed. Socks and pants can be moved to allow application of the electrodes, so they can usually stay on (Procedure 48.1).

The patient should be in the supine position on the exam table. A pillow can be placed under the patient's head. The patient's legs and arms need to be supported on the table. It is important for the patient to be relaxed and comfortable during the procedure. If the patient is having chest pain or problems breathing, the head of the exam table may be elevated. Any change of position from the supine position must be noted on the ECG tracing. Any position change can create a change on the leads (pictures). The provider needs to be aware of it when reading the tracing.

Before placing the electrodes on the skin, it is important to prepare the skin. This helps the electrodes adhere and minimizes artifact, thus producing an accurate tracing. There are several techniques used to prepare the skin:

- Wipe the area with an alcohol pad to clean it. This helps to remove sweat and lotion that may prevent the electrodes from adhering to the skin.
- Use a razor to shave chest hair. Obtain the patient's verbal consent before shaving the chest.
- Gently abrade the skin, using a gauze sponge, special gel, or special fine sandpaper tape (Fig. 48.11)

Applying Electrodes and Lead Wires

Apply electrodes to both arms and legs. The electrodes on the lower legs should be placed on the inner side, just above the ankles. If tab electrodes are used, have the tabs on the leg electrodes point toward the center of the person. All the other tabs can be facing the feet.

The placement of the arm electrodes may vary, depending on the ECG machine and manufacturer. For instance, many Schiller ECG machines indicate that the electrodes should be placed just above the wrists. Other machines indicate placement on the upper arms. Check the users' guide for correct placement of the arm electrodes. Table 48.3 describes where to place the electrodes on the limbs and the chest (Fig. 48.12).

The lead wires are typically color coded and include an abbreviation on each wire. Colors may vary from manufacturer to manufacturer. It is important to know and to use the abbreviations. One of the most common errors is to mix up the right

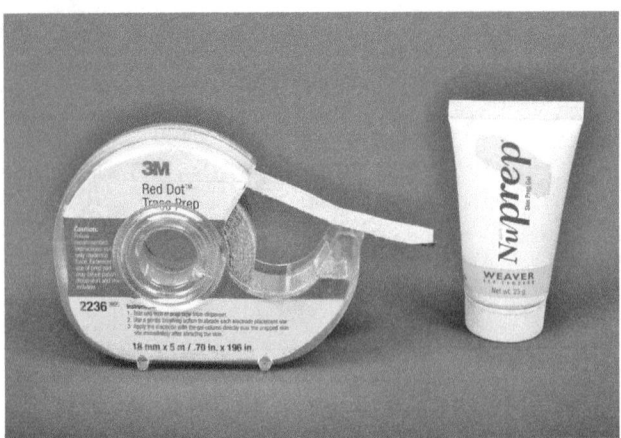

Fig. 48.11 Special fine sandpaper tape and Nuprep Skin Prep Gel are used to abrade the skin. This provides a better electrocardiogram tracing.

TABLE 48.3	Electrode and Lead Wire Placement	
Electrode	**Lead Wire Abbreviation and Color**	**Placement**
Right arm	RA (white)	Just above the wrist or upper arm, as indicated in the users' guide
Left arm	LA (black)	
Right leg	RL (green)	Inner lower leg, just above the ankle
Left leg	LL (red)	
Chest V₁	V1 (red)	Fourth intercostal space at the right sternal edge
Chest V₂	V2 (yellow)	Fourth intercostal space at the left sternal edge
Chest V₃	V3 (green)	Midway between V_2 and V_4
Chest V₄	V4 (blue)	Fifth intercostal space on the midclavicular line
Chest V₅	V5 (orange)	Same horizontal plane as V_4 at the left anterior axillary line or the midpoint between V_4 and V_6
Chest V₆	V6 (purple)	Same horizontal plane as V_4 at the midaxillary line

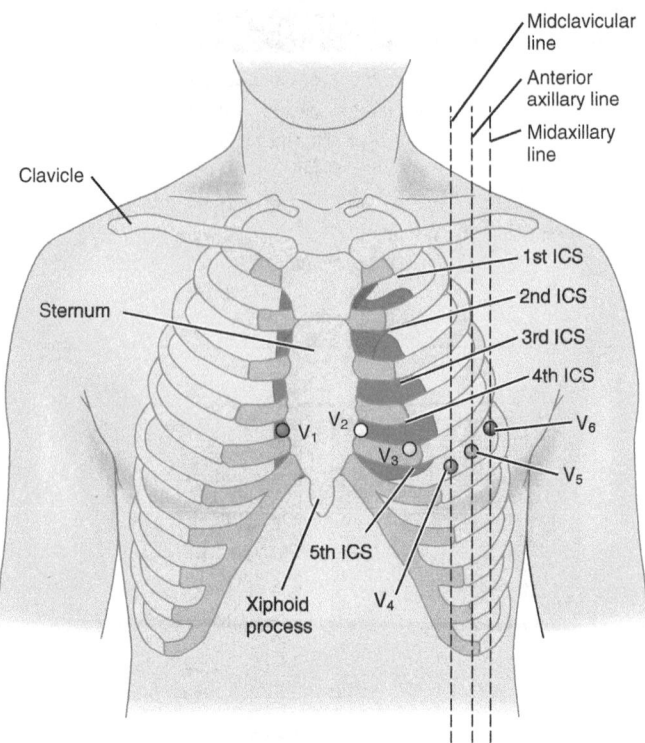

Fig. 48.12 Chest Leads. *ICS,* Intercostal space. (From Niedzwiecki B, et al: *Kinn's the medical assistant,* ed 14, St. Louis, 2020, Elsevier.)

It is important to note on the ECG tracing any electrode placement deviation from the normal location. The provider reading the tracing needs to take the placement into consideration.

> **VOCABULARY**
> **dextrocardia** The condition in which the heart is located on the right side of the chest, and the apex is pointing to the right.

Running the ECG Tracing

Once the lead wires are attached to the electrodes, the medical assistant enters the patient information into the ECG machine. In some facilities this may be done prior to bringing the patient into the room for the ECG. Typically, the patient's name, date of birth, and medical record number are entered. Facilities will have additional information that they require to be entered, such as the ordering provider's name and the provider reading the ECG.

After the information is entered, the medical assistant should remind the patient to remain still and not to talk during the procedure. It usually takes a minute or less for the tracing to be created with a multichannel machine (Box 48.1). Talking and movement will create artifact. If the patient is cold, a blanket can be used to cover them.

Prior to running the tracing, double-check that all the electrodes are attached and the lead wires are in the correct location. If the ECG machine has a screen, check the digital picture of the leads. Are they clear (without artifact)? If not, is the filter(s) on? Are the leads (pictures) an equal distance from each other? Is the baseline horizontal, or is it moving up and down like a roller coaster? Do not run the tracing until it is clear and the baseline is horizontal. Problem-solve and fix the issue before running the

and left limb lead wires. This can cause abnormal leads (pictures) and result in additional patient workup before the mistake is discovered. It is important to always double-check the placement of the lead wires.

In some cases the electrodes may need to be placed in alternative locations, such as with the following:

- Dextrocardia (dek stro KAHR dee ah): Place the chest electrodes on the right side of the chest using the same intercostal spacing and landmarks. Switch the right and left limb lead wires (e.g., LA would be attached to the right arm electrode).
- *Amputated limb*: Place the electrode on the remaining part of the limb. Place the electrode on the opposite limb in the same location.
- *Casted limb*: Place the electrode above the cast on the limb. Place the electrode on the opposite limb in the same location.
- *New surgical incision or wound*: Place the electrodes near the correct area, but not on the incision or wound.

ECG machines can be single-channel or multichannel. In *single-channel* models, the machine contains one amplifier channel and one recording stylet. The single-channel machines record one lead (picture) at a time. The medical assistant must manually switch to the next lead until the procedure is done. When these machines are used, the process of recording a tracing takes up to 3 to 5 minutes. Single-channel machines can use paper rolls or Z-fold paper. These small strips of paper need to be mounted (see the section "Finishing the ECG").

Multichannel machines monitor all 12 leads. This model has several stylets that allow for four groups of three leads to be traced every few seconds. With some machines, a fourth stylet traces one lead for the entire width of the page. Typically, the multichannel machines print the tracing on 8.25 × 11-inch paper or Z-fold paper.

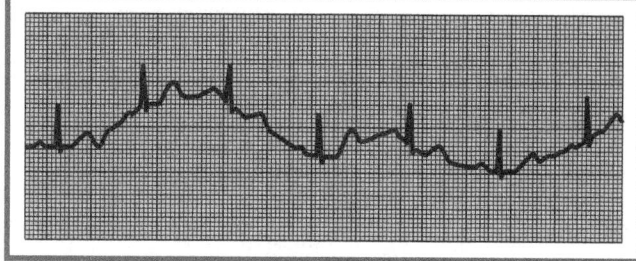

Fig. 48.13 Wandering Baseline Artifact. (From Niedzwiecki B, et al: *Kinn's the medical assistant,* ed 14, St. Louis, 2020, Elsevier.)

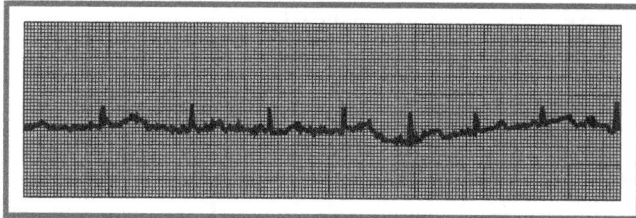

Fig. 48.14 Somatic Tremor Artifact. (From Niedzwiecki B, et al: *Kinn's the medical assistant,* ed 14, St. Louis, 2020, Elsevier.)

tracing or redo the tracing if it was printed. Additional problem-solving strategies will be discussed later in this chapter. Once the tracing looks good on the screen, print it.

Troubleshooting Artifact

Artifact is signal distortion or unwanted, erratic movement of the stylus caused by outside interference. The medical assistant needs to identify the type of artifact and then take actions to prevent the artifact. The leads can be viewed on the screen or after printing the ECG tracing. Carefully look for artifact. The following sections discuss the appearance and causes of the common types of artifact and ways to prevent them.

Wandering Baseline. *Wandering baseline* artifact is an upward and downward movement of the waveform (Fig. 48.13). The isoelectric lines shift locations. This artifact can be the result of:
- *Poor skin preparation*: The patient has oily skin or used lotion. The electrodes are falling off.
- *Old electrodes*: The electrodes are dirty or expired, or the gel on the electrodes is dried.
- *Placement of electrodes*: The electrodes are placed on bony areas.
- *Movement*: The movement of breathing can also be the cause of this artifact.
The medical assistant should:
- Clean the skin with alcohol and allow it to dry. Slightly abrade the skin with a gauze pad or fine sandpaper tape to help the electrodes stick to the skin.
- Replace the electrode with a new one. Ensure the electrodes are not expired and the gel is not dried.
- Make sure all electrodes and lead wires are firmly attached.
- Make sure the baseline filter is turned on (if it is a feature of the machine).

Somatic Tremor. *Somatic tremor artifact* appears as jagged peaks with irregular heights and spacing (Fig. 48.14). The causes include:
- *Involuntary movement*: Tremors from disease conditions (e.g., Parkinson disease), shivering due to coldness
- *Voluntary movement*: Talking, chewing gum, supporting arms or legs because table is too small for the person
The medical assistant should:

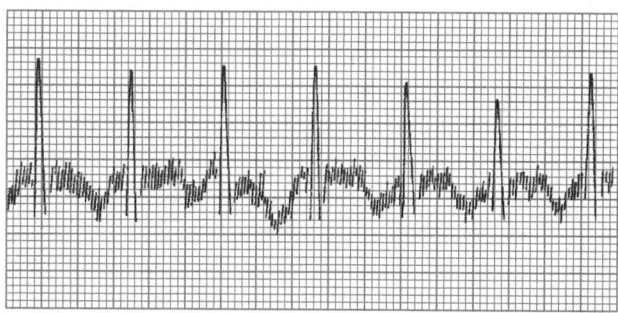

Fig. 48.15 AC Interference Artifact. (From Urden L, Stacy K, Lough M: *Thelan's critical care nursing: diagnosis and management,* ed 7, St. Louis, 2014, Mosby.)

- Help the patient relax. Cover the patient with a blanket if they are cold.
- Remind the patient to not move or talk during the tracing.
- Watch to see if there is a pattern with involuntary movements. Take the tracing when the movements lessen.
- Use a larger exam table for the procedure.
- If the machine has a muscle tremor filter, make sure it is turned on.

AC Interference. *AC interference artifact* appears as a series of small spikes that creates a thick-looking tracing (Fig. 48.15). The cause includes:
- *Electrical interference*: There are too many electrical devices in the area; the patient cable and lead wires are wrapped closely together; an electrical cord is under the exam table; and an electrical outlet is improperly grounded. A cell phone in a patient's pocket or a smart watch may also cause interference.
The medical assistant should:
- Unplug the ECG machine.
- Unplug or remove nearby electrical devices (e.g., laptops, pagers, cell phones).

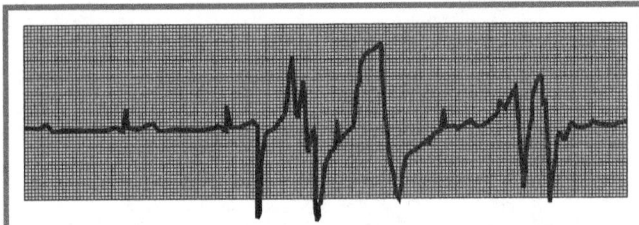

Fig. 48.16 Interrupted Baseline Artifact. (From Niedzwiecki B, et al: *Kinn's the medical assistant*, ed 14, St. Louis, 2020, Elsevier.)

- Separate the lead wires so they do not overlap.
- Move the table away from the wall or move to another room for the procedure.
- Ensure cell phones are not near the procedure area.

Interrupted Baseline. *Interrupted baseline artifact* (also called *intermittent signal artifact*) occurs when the tracing looks normal at the beginning but then disappears or goes all over when the electrical connection is interrupted (Fig. 48.16). The causes include:
- *Electrical connection is interrupted*: Due to a loose cable or lead wire, or a broken cable, clip, or lead wire.
  The medical assistant should:
- Check that all electrodes and lead wires are attached.
- If a broken wire is suspected, a new cable will be needed.

Evaluating an ECG Tracing

The provider reads the ECG, but the medical assistant must be able to determine abnormal rates and rhythms that might be life-threatening. This section will discuss how to determine the heart rate, evaluate the ECG tracing, and identify abnormal rhythms.

Rate. Many machines indicate the heart rate. The medical assistant can also calculate the rate from the ECG tracing. Methods used to calculate a regular heart rate when the paper speed (chart speed) is 25 mm/second include:
- *Six-second method*: Count the number of P waves in a 6-second strip (30 large boxes) and multiply by 10 (least accurate method).
- *1500 method*: Count the number of small boxes between two R waves or the two P waves. Divide the number into 1500.
- *Sequence method*: Count the number of large boxes between the R waves. By memorizing the numbers in Table 48.4, you will have a quick method to calculate the heart rate.

Analyzing an ECG Tracing. For most medical assistants, their job description states that they need to be able to perform ECGs. For some medical assistants, they may work as an ECG technician. In this position they may need to analyze an ECG tracing.

TABLE 48.4 **Sequence Method**	
Number of Large (5 mm) Boxes Between R Waves	**Heart Rate**
1	300
2	150
3	100
4	75
5	60
6	50
7	43
8	37

The ECG rhythm strip (lead II view) is evaluated from left to right. The following should be assessed:
- *Rate:* What is the rate?
- *Rhythm:* Is it regular or irregular? An irregular rhythm on an ECG tracing will have time differences between cardiac cycles. With a regular rhythm, each cardiac cycle occurs the same length of time apart.
- *Appearance of the segments, waves, and intervals:* Table 48.5 lists questions to consider when analyzing a tracing.

Identifying an Abnormal Rhythm. When performing an ECG, the medical assistant must identify if the patient has an arrhythmia (ah RITH mee ah) that requires immediate care by the provider. If the medical assistant identifies a life-threatening arrhythmia, it is important to keep the patient hooked up to the ECG machine and to immediately get the provider.

VOCABULARY
arrhythmia An abnormal heart rate or rhythm.

Sinus arrhythmias. A sinus rhythm is considered normal. The electrical activity begins in the SA node and goes through the rest of the conduction system. Atrial and ventricular depolarizations occur. With sinus arrhythmias, the electrical pathway is normal. The rate or rhythm of the heartbeat is altered. The alteration may result from the SA node firing too slowly or too quickly.
- *Sinus bradycardia*: The adult heart rate is below 60 beats per minute. This is a normal finding in well-conditioned athletes. It is abnormal in other individuals.
- *Sinus tachycardia*: The adult heart rate is above 100 beats per minute. This is normal in a person doing aerobic exercise. It is abnormal in a resting individual.

Atrial arrhythmias. Atrial arrhythmias occur when there is a problem with the SA node starting the impulse. They can also occur due to a conduction problem in the atria.
- *Premature atrial contractions (PACs)*: Occur when the atria contract sooner than they should. The P wave can be abnormally shaped, or an extra P wave can be seen. PACs can be seen in people who smoke or consume large amounts of caffeine. An occasional PAC is not abnormal. More than six PACs in a minute is considered abnormal.

TABLE 48.5 Analyzing an ECG Tracing

	Normal	Questions to Address	Timing (Horizontal – Length)
P wave	Largest in lead II Upright in all leads except aVR Voltage (vertical – height): less than 2.5 small boxes (0.25 millivolts)	• Is there one P wave before each QRS complex? • Is each P wave a positive deflection? • Are all the P waves similar in size and shape? • Is there more than one P wave per cardiac cycle?	>0.11 seconds
PR interval	From start of P wave to start of QRS complex	• Are the PR intervals the same size throughout the tracing?	0.12–0.2 seconds
QRS complex	Largest in lead II compared to leads III and I	• Is there a QRS complex without a previous P wave?	0.06–0.12 seconds
ST segment	On the baseline	• Is the ST segment lower or higher than the baseline? (Could be an indication of infarction or ischemia.)	Not usually measured
QT interval	From start of Q wave to end of T wave	• Are the QT intervals the same size throughout the tracing?	0.40 seconds

• *Atrial flutter*: Occurs when the atria contract faster than the ventricles (up to 300 beats per minute). They become out of sync with the ventricles. Extra P waves are seen with regular QRS complexes. Atrial flutter can be caused by alcohol and stimulants (cocaine, caffeine, diet pills, and cold medications). It can also be caused by coronary heart disease, hypertension, cardiomyopathy, heart valve diseases, hyperthyroidism, obstructive pulmonary disease, and pulmonary embolism diseases. Atrial flutter is reversed with medication to slow the heart or with cardioversion (electrical shock).

Heart block. A heart block occurs when there is a disruption or slowing of the electrical impulse through the heart. Heart block can be congenital or acquired. Heart disease, surgery, or medications can cause acquired heart block. There are three types of heart block, with third degree being the most severe:

• *First-degree heart block*: The impulse slows as it moves from the atria to the ventricles. This creates a longer PR segment. First-degree heart block may not cause symptoms. It may not require treatment.

• *Second-degree heart block*: The impulse slows or is blocked as it moves into the ventricles. When blocked, there is no QRS complex after the P wave, and the ventricles do not contract. When the impulse slows, the PR segment is longer. This arrhythmia requires a pacemaker to help maintain the heart rate. Pacemakers will be discussed in a later section of this chapter.

• *Third-degree heart block*: The impulse does not reach the ventricles. As a backup system, special ventricular cells create an impulse that causes the ventricles to contract. On the ECG tracing, the P wave is faster than normal and the QRS complex is not coordinated with the P wave. This is a life-threatening arrhythmia and requires emergency treatment and a pacemaker.

Ventricular arrhythmias. Ventricular arrhythmias are abnormalities in the ventricles. Most of the ventricular arrhythmias discussed are life-threatening rhythms.

• *Premature ventricular contractions (PVCs)*: Occur when the ventricles contract sooner than they should. An impulse originating in the ventricles creates this abnormality. The QRS complex appears before a P wave. The P wave can also be absent. The T wave can be abnormally shaped, and a widened QRS complex can be seen (Fig. 48.17A–B). PVCs can be caused by tobacco, alcohol, epinephrine, and anxiety. They can also be caused by hypertension, coronary artery disease, and lung disease. Infrequent PVCs can be normal. More than six PVCs in a minute is abnormal and can lead to a life-threatening condition.

• *Ventricular tachycardia (V-tach)*: Occurs when the ventricles beat at a rapid rate (up to 250 beats per minute). It may be seen with multiple PVCs in a row. It may be a short run of fast beats or may last longer than 30 seconds (see Fig. 48.17C). V-tach is a life-threatening condition. If it is not reversed with drugs and/or cardioversion, it can become ventricular fibrillation.

• *Ventricular fibrillation (V-fib)*: Occurs when the ventricles quiver uncontrollably (see Fig. 48.17D). They are essentially ineffective at pumping any blood. The patient has no pulse, is not breathing, and is unresponsive. This is the most critical, life-threatening arrhythmia. Cardioversion with a defibrillator is necessary to restore normal function of the electrical conduction system.

• *Asystole*: Results in the absence of a heartbeat. A flat line appears on the tracing (see Fig. 48.17E.)

Implantable device rhythms. Implantable devices (e.g., pacemaker and implantable cardioverter-defibrillator) create abnormal waveforms on the ECG tracing. A pacemaker is used to treat some types of arrhythmias. It uses low-energy electrical pulses to assist the heart to beat at a normal rate. Pacemakers can change the ECG tracing. Fig. 48.18 shows a pacemaker rhythm strip. There are two types of pacemakers:

• *Temporary pacemaker:* Used in an emergency until the permanent pacemaker can be placed; also used for temporary conditions (e.g., heart attack and medication overdose).

• *Permanent pacemaker:* Surgically inserted into the chest or abdomen. Patients can use technology (e.g., smart phones) to transmit their pacemaker data to their provider.

An implantable cardioverter-defibrillator (ICD) can provide low-energy electrical pulses and high-energy pulses (Fig. 48.19). The high-energy pulses can treat life-threatening arrhythmias. ICDs are surgically implanted in the chest or abdomen. The

ICD is programmed to meet the needs of the patient. Some ICD functions can be checked using technology such as pacemakers. ICD batteries can last 5 to 7 years.

Finishing the ECG

If the ambulatory care facility uses an EHR system and the ECG machine interfaces with the EHR software, then follow the procedure and upload the tracing to the patient's health record. The provider will read the tracing once it is uploaded.

An ECG must be read by the provider before it is filed in the paper medical record. If the tracing was done on small strips of ECG paper, the strips need to be mounted per the facility's procedures. Special 8.5 × 10-inch paper with adhesive strips is used to stick the ECG tracing strips. Once the strips are mounted, they can be given to the provider to read. If the ECG prints on 8.5 × 10-inch paper, it does not need to be mounted. It can be given to the provider immediately.

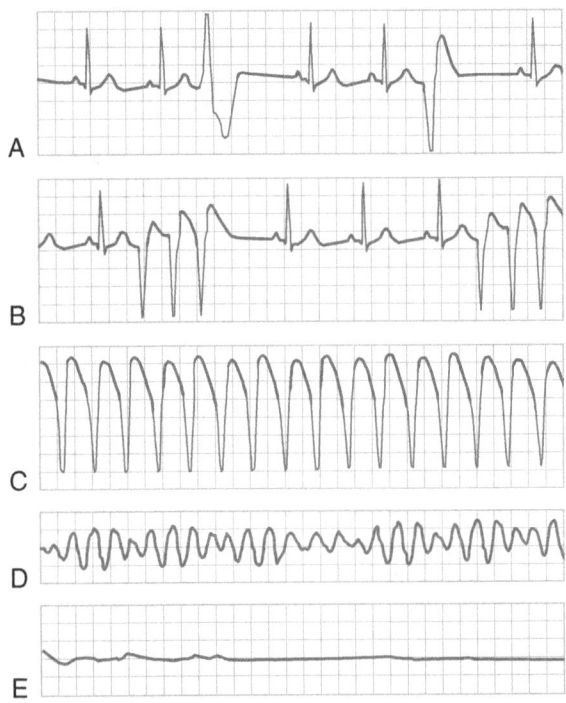

Fig. 48.17 A, Premature ventricular contraction (PVC). B, Three PVCs in a row. C, Ventricular tachycardia (V-tach). D, Ventricular fibrillation (V-fib). E, Asystole. (From Niedzwiecki B, et al: *Kinn's the medical assistant,* ed 14, St. Louis, 2020, Elsevier.)

Maintenance of the Electrocardiograph

After the ECG is obtained and the patient has left, the medical assistant must clean the room and the electrocardiograph. Maintenance of the machine includes these steps:

- Clean the lead wires as indicated in the users' guide. The lead wires are not disposable.
- Handle the lead wires and patient cable with care. They should be stored in a loose coil. Tight coils or bending of the wires and cable can result in breakage of the fine wires inside the unit. This will cause artifact on the ECG and requires replacement of the cable.
- Clean the tracing stylus and the machine casing as indicated in the users' guide.

ADDITIONAL ECG TESTING

Exercise Stress Test

An exercise stress test records the ECG while the patient is exercising. The patient either walks on a treadmill with an incline or uses an exercise bike (Fig. 48.20). During the test, a continual ECG is recorded, and the blood pressure is monitored.

The test may be ordered for these reasons:

- The patient is starting an exercise program.
- The patient has angina that is getting worse.
- To evaluate the patient's heart after an angioplasty or bypass surgery.
- To evaluate heart rhythm changes with the stress of exercise. Preparation for the test includes the following:
- The patient should wear clothes and shoes for exercising.
- The provider will indicate what daily medications should be taken prior to the test.
- The patient should not take a dose of Viagra, Cialis, or Levitra for erectile dysfunction 48 hours before a stress test.
- The patient should not smoke or consume caffeine or alcohol 3 hours before the test.
- The patient signs a consent form prior to the test.

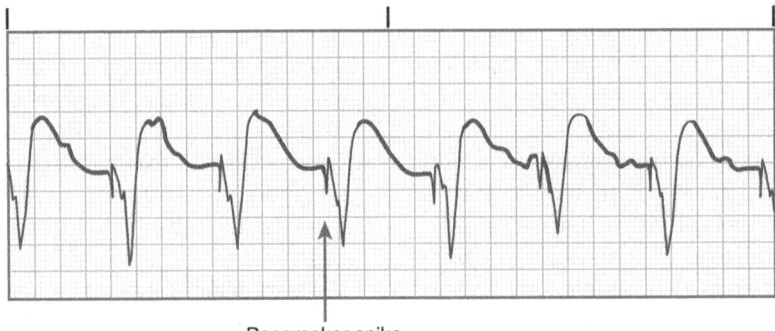

Pacemaker spike

Fig. 48.18 Pacemaker Rhythm Strip. (From Lewis S, et al: *Medical-surgical nursing,* ed 9, St. Louis, 2014, Mosby.)

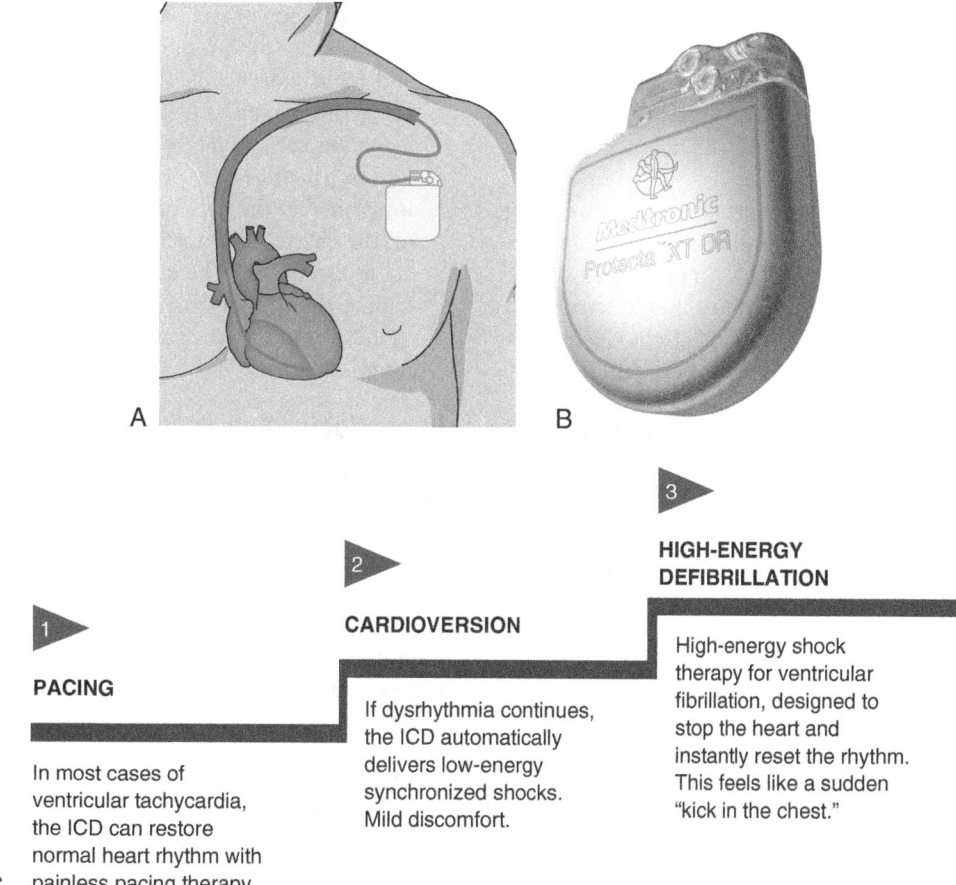

A   B

3 ▶

**HIGH-ENERGY
DEFIBRILLATION**

2 ▶

CARDIOVERSION

High-energy shock
therapy for ventricular
fibrillation, designed to
stop the heart and
instantly reset the rhythm.
This feels like a sudden
"kick in the chest."

1 ▶

PACING

If dysrhythmia continues,
the ICD automatically
delivers low-energy
synchronized shocks.
Mild discomfort.

In most cases of
ventricular tachycardia,
the ICD can restore
normal heart rhythm with
C   painless pacing therapy.

Fig. 48.19 Implanted Cardioverter-Defibrillator (ICD). (From Urden L, Stacy K, Lough M: *Thelan's critical care nursing: diagnosis and management*, ed 7, St. Louis, 2014, Mosby.)

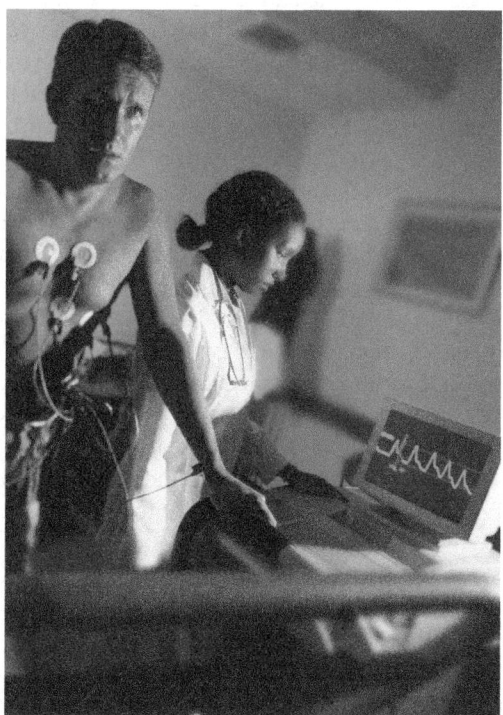

Fig. 48.20 Exercise Stress Test. (Courtesy Stockbyte/Thinkstock.)

During the test:

- Electrodes and lead wires will be placed on the patient. A blood pressure cuff will be applied to the patient's arm.
- The patient will begin to exercise slowly, and gradually the exercise difficulty will increase.
- The provider should always be present during the test. If the patient has chest discomfort, dizziness, palpitations, or shortness of breath, the test will stop. Emergency supplies or a crash cart should be kept nearby in case of an emergency.

Nuclear Stress Test

The nuclear stress test shows the blood flow into the heart muscle during rest and activity. A radioactive substance (e.g., thallium or sestamibi) is injected into a vein using an intravenous line (IV). After the patient has rested for 15 to 45 minutes, a gamma camera is used to take images of the blood flow in the heart. Then the person either exercises or is given a vasodilating medication to dilate the coronary arteries. The radioactive substance is again injected, and the person rests. After the required rest period, the gamma camera is used to take additional images of the blood flow through the coronary vessels. Throughout the test, the blood pressure and ECG are monitored.

Holter Monitor

A Holter monitor is used to monitor the heart over a 24- to 48-hour period while patients go about their normal activities. Sometimes patients experience a heart issue that cannot be picked up on a resting 12-lead ECG. Having a longer monitoring period can capture the abnormalities.

When placing electrodes for a Holter monitor, consult the users' guide. There are many configurations for electrode placement. Different monitors use varying numbers of electrodes. Holter monitors typically use three to seven chest electrodes. As with the resting 12-lead ECG, lead wires attach the electrodes to the small Holter monitor. The monitor runs on batteries and is small enough to fit into a pocket.

The following are patient education points for a Holter monitor test:

- Wear the monitor continuously. The monitor will be removed during your appointment in 24 to 48 hours.
- While wearing the Holter monitor, avoid metal detectors, large magnets, high-voltage areas, x-rays, and electric blankets. Do not get the monitor wet (e.g., no bathing, showering, or swimming).
- Keep a detailed journal of the symptoms experienced. These symptoms could include chest pain, shortness of breath, palpitations or changes in the heartbeat, dizziness, or fainting. Document the date, time, symptoms experienced, and the activity being done at the time. (Many facilities provide patients with a journal for the documentation.)
- At the return visit, the provider will look at the tracing for abnormalities. The journal of timed activities will help the provider identify what is occurring.
- What to do if the electrodes or lead wires fall off.
- Who to contact in case of questions or if problems occur.

Procedure 48.2 describes the steps in applying a Holter monitor to a patient.

Cardiac Event Recorder

The cardiac event recorder is a portable, battery-powered ECG device. The recorder is activated by the patient when symptoms occur, and it records the ECG. Patients may wear a cardiac event recorder for 30 days. When symptoms occur only occasionally, it is difficult to capture the abnormality on a resting 12-lead ECG or a Holter monitor. The patient may also be asked to keep a journal, as with the Holter monitor. With the cardiac event recorder, patients go about their daily activities. The monitor can be removed during bathing and showering or swimming.

When patients experience symptoms, they push the recorder's activation button. An ECG is recorded and stored. The ECG can be sent to the provider via a phone or other technology. A provider will review the tracing. If there is an emergency, the patient will be called and told to go to the nearest emergency department.

There are two types of cardiac event recorders:

- *Looping memory monitor* (also called a *cardiac loop recorder*): A pager-sized monitor that connects to two chest electrodes by wires. The monitor continuously records the ECG. When the memory is full, it overwrites from the beginning (i.e.,

continues loop of recording). When a patient has symptoms, they activate the monitor. The ECG from prior to, during, and for a short while after the event is stored. It does not overwrite the stored ECGs.

- *Symptom event monitor* (also called a *post-event monitor*): Can be a handheld device or worn on the wrist. When symptoms are felt, the patient activates the monitor and places it on the chest. Small metal disks on the back of the monitor act as electrodes. The current ECG is recorded and stored. Unlike the looping memory monitor, the symptom event monitor cannot record and store the ECG prior to the symptoms.

Implantable Loop Recorder

The implantable *loop recorder* (also called a *loop recorder implant*) is a small recorder (under 2 inches) that looks like a flash drive. It is surgically implanted just under the skin in the upper left chest. It can be implanted in an ambulatory care facility.

Often the device is used for patients who have episodes of fainting, seizures, and palpitations, and other ECG tests have not been able to detect the abnormality. It also catches infrequent arrhythmias that can be missed with traditional ECG monitoring.

The device continuously records the ECG for 2 to 3 years. It records the ECG if the heart rate falls below or rises above the preset limits (set by the provider). The patient can also record the ECG if symptoms are experienced. The provider can download the saved ECG data at the next appointment.

Transtelephonic Monitoring

A *transtelephonic monitor* (TTM) is a small device that records a patient's ECG when the patient pushes the activation button. The TTM has four electrodes on the back of the device that can record a single lead. The ECG data is sent via phone to the base station at the provider's office. The signal is converted to a readable tracing that can be displayed on a monitor or printed out. There are two types of TTMs:

- *TTM with internal memory*: The ECG is recorded and stored when the patient pushes a button. The data can be transmitted by phone to the provider. This type of TTM is used for patients with infrequent arrhythmias.
- *TTM with no internal memory*: The TTM is placed over the heart, and the phone receiver is placed over the TTM. Once the activation button is pushed, the TTM records and immediately sends the live ECG to the provider via the phone line. The data is not saved in the device. This type of TTM is used for patients with pacemakers and internal cardioverter-defibrillators. It allows the provider to monitor the patient remotely.

Portable Handheld ECG Monitors

There are a variety of portable handheld ECG monitors on the market. Many produce a single lead. The ECG data can then be transferred to other devices using software, Bluetooth, smart phones, or USB ports. These devices are marketed to be used at home. A person can use the device and save ECG tracings. The tracings can then be reviewed by the person's provider at the next visit. The machines work differently; some having several electrode options. Finger contact, chest contact (bare skin just below the nipple), and regular chest electrodes can be used to create an ECG tracing.

RESPIRATORY SYSTEM

In addition to cardiac testing, pulmonary testing is done in the ambulatory care facility. For the rest of the chapter, pulmonary testing, including measuring the peak flow rate and performing spirometry (spi ROM e tree) testing, will be examined. In addition, pulmonary treatments, including medication administration (nebulizers [NEB uh lize er] and metered-dose inhalers) and oxygen administration, will be explained.

Pulmonary Function Tests

Pulmonary function tests (PFTs) measure the patient's lung function, or how well the lungs work. Some PFTs can measure airflow, and others measure lung size. Table 48.6 reviews PFTs. The following sections provide additional information.

Peak Flow Rate. The peak flow meter measures the amount of air exhaled. A peak flow rate is measured using a manual or digital peak flow meter in an ambulatory care or home

setting (Fig. 48.21). It is used to diagnose acute conditions and to manage chronic diseases, such as asthma. Procedure 48.3 describes the steps to take when measuring a peak flow rate. When a patient is performing a peak flow rate test, it is important that the medical assistant obtain three adequate readings.

Spirometry. Spirometry evaluates lung function as it is affected by respiratory, cardiac, and neuromuscular diseases. It can be ordered if the provider identifies abnormalities in the respiratory system. A spirometer can evaluate the amount of air you exhale and inhale. It looks at how quickly the air is exhaled and the rate at which air is breathed in. Several different tests can be done with spirometry (Table 48.7).

With spirometry testing, it is important that the medical assistant enter accurate patient data into the spirometer computer (Fig. 48.22). Besides the patient's name, medical record

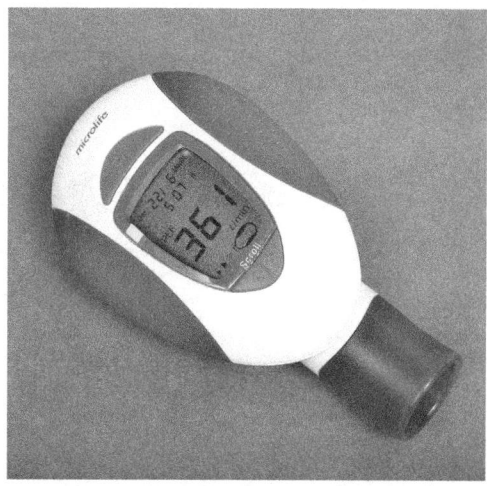

Fig. 48.21 Digital Peak Flow Meter. (From Niedzwiecki B, et al: *Kinn's the medical assistant,* ed 14, St. Louis, 2020, Elsevier.)

TABLE 48.6	Pulmonary Function Tests	
Test	**Measures**	**Procedure and Patient Preparation**
Peak flow monitor	Measures the exhaled air.	• Handheld device used in ambulatory care facility and at home to manage chronic respiratory conditions (e.g., asthma). • Need to loosen any restrictive clothing. Gum and loose dentures should be removed. Instruct patient on how to perform the test.
Spirometry	Measures the volume of inhaled and exhaled air and the time required for each one.	• Patient breathes multiple times through a tube that is connected to a computer. • Patient will need instructions regarding taking or holding respiratory medications. Need to loosen any restrictive clothing. Gum and loose dentures should be removed. Instruct patient on how to perform the test.
Lung volume tests	Determines lung volume after inhalation and exhalation. Also called *plethysmography* (PLETH iz MOG rah fee).	• One method: Patient sits in a clear box and breathes in and out of a mouthpiece of the plethysmograph (ple THIZ ma GRAF).
Lung diffusion capacity	Determines how effectively gas travels from the lungs to the bloodstream.	• Patient breathes in a *tracer gas* (harmless gas), and the concentration of the gas is measured in the exhaled air.
Arterial blood gas test	A test that measures the pH, carbon dioxide (CO_2), and oxygen (O_2) content of the blood.	• Typically done in hospital settings but may be done in clinics. Blood is taken from a wrist artery.
Pulse oximetry (ok SIM e tree)	Measures the oxygen saturation of the blood.	• A probe is placed on the finger or on skin in other locations. (See Chapter 33 for more details.) • Remove nail polish or artificial nails to get an accurate reading.

TABLE 48.7   Spirometry Tests

Test	Description	Patient Coaching
Tidal volume (TV)	Volume of air inhaled and exhaled during a normal respiration	Breathe in and out normally with lips pursed around the mouthpiece.
Forced vital capacity (FVC)	Amount of air that can be forcefully exhaled from a maximum inhalation	Inhale as deeply as possible, then quickly forcibly exhale as much as possible.
Forced expiratory volume in 1 second (FEV1)	Volume of air exhaled in the first second of the FVC	
Expiratory reserve volume (ERV)	Maximal volume of air exhaled after normal exhalation	Breathe in and out normally, then exhale forcibly at the end of the TV.
Inspiratory reserve volume (IRV)	Maximal volume of air inhaled after normal inhalation	Breathe in normally, then forcibly inhale.
Vital capacity (VC)	Maximum amount of air that can be exhaled during a normal or slow exhalation after maximum inhalation	Inhale deeply and exhale completely.
Inspiratory capacity (IC)	Maximum amount of air that can be inhaled after a normal exhalation	Breathe in and out normally, then forcibly inhale at the end of the TV.
Functional residual capacity (FRC)	Amount of air remaining in the lungs at the end of a normal exhalation	
Residual volume (RV)	Volume of air remaining in the lungs after a forced exhalation	
Total lung capacity (TLC)	Maximum amount of air in the lungs with maximum inhalation	
Maximum voluntary ventilation (MVV)	Maximum volume that is breathed in and out in 1 minute	Breathe in and out as deeply and as frequently as possible for 15 seconds.

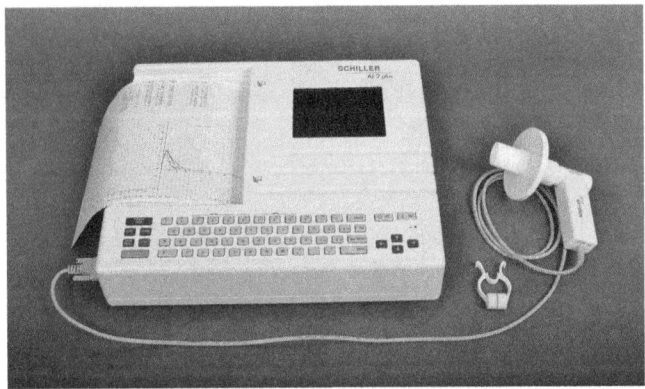

Fig. 48.22 Spirometer. (From Niedzwiecki B, et al: *Kinn's the medical assistant*, ed 14, St. Louis, 2020, Elsevier.)

- Make sure to follow the operators' manual for the machine you are using.
- Be encouraging yet respectful of the patient when coaching them through the procedure.

MEDICAL TERMINOLOGY	
nas/o	nose
ox/o, ox/i	oxygen
pulmon/o	lung
spir/o	breathing
-metry	process of measurement

CRITICAL THINKING 48.11

Eva's last patient of the day is Janine Butler, who is seeing the provider because of her asthma. After the provider sees Ms. Butler, he orders a spirometry test. Eva prepares the equipment and brings Ms. Butler into the testing room. However, she refuses to have her height and weight measured. How might Eva explain to Ms. Butler the importance of getting an accurate height and weight?

number, and date of birth, the medical assistant may need to enter the person's sex, age, race, height, and weight. The patient's current height and weight need to be obtained prior to the spirometry. The computer then pulls stored data and creates a "normal" person for those characteristics. After the patient has completed the test, the computer will print out the patient's results compared with the "normal" person's results. This helps the provider identify areas of concern.

Procedure 48.4 describes the spirometry procedure. When performing the spirometry procedure, the following steps should be taken:

- Adults should exhale 6 seconds and children should exhale 3 seconds for the forced vital capacity (FVC). For patients with obstructive breathing patterns, the FVC may take up to 15 seconds.
- Give the patient at least 30 seconds between blows. Have the patient indicate when they are ready for the next blow.
- Do a minimum of three blows and a maximum of eight blows (unless otherwise indicated by the facility's protocols).

Pulmonary Treatments

In the ambulatory care facility, common respiratory treatments include medication administration and oxygen therapy. Depending on the state's statutes and the facility's policies, the medical assistant may be able to administer nebulizer treatments and oxygen therapy when ordered by the provider. The medical assistant may also instruct patients on how to use metered-dose inhalers. The following sections cover metered-dose inhaler education, nebulizer treatments, and oxygen therapy.

Metered-Dose Inhalers. A metered-dose inhaler (MDI) provides aerosol medication that is breathed into the lungs. MDIs

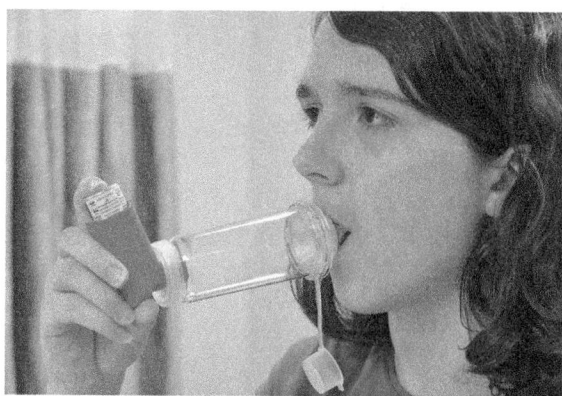

Fig. 48.23 Using a Metered-Dose Inhaler With a Spacer.

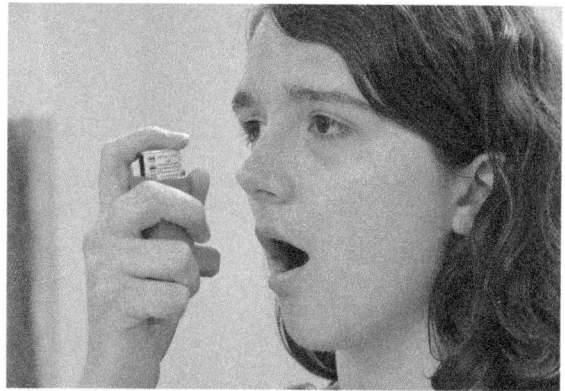

Fig. 48.24 Using a Metered-Dose Inhaler Without a Spacer.

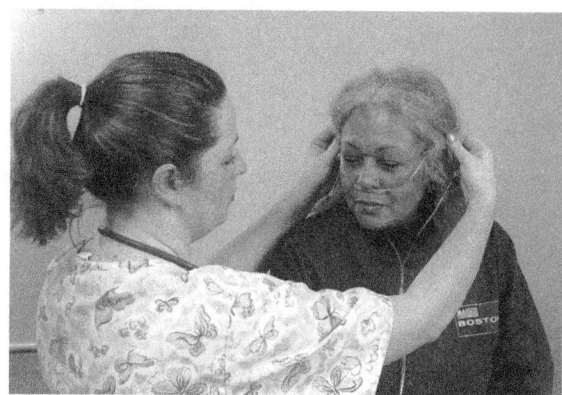

Fig. 48.25 Applying a Nasal Cannula. (From Niedzwiecki B, et al: *Kinn's the medical assistant,* ed 14, St. Louis, 2020, Elsevier.)

are typically ordered for conditions such as asthma and chronic obstructive pulmonary disease (COPD).

In many cases the provider will order an MDI with a *spacer*. A spacer is a long tube that is attached to the mouthpiece of an MDI (Fig. 48.23). Spacers slow the delivery of medication from MDIs. Without a spacer, the MDI blasts the medication to the back of the throat and mouth. With inhaled corticosteroids, this can cause irritation and infections over time. When a spacer is used, the medication is blasted into the tube and over several breaths is pulled into the lungs. In an ambulatory care facility, the medical assistant may need to instruct the patient on the proper use of an MDI.

Using a metered-dose inhaler. When teaching a patient to use an MDI, the medical assistant should instruct the patient to shake the MDI three or four times. Then remove the cover from the mouthpiece. If using a spacer, the patient should:

- Attach the spacer. Breathe out. Place the mouthpiece between the lips and close the lips around it.
- Press the top of the canister on the MDI.
- Breathe in very slowly, taking a full breath in. Some spacers will produce a whistlelike sound if the person is breathing in too fast.

If the patient is not using a spacer, the patient should:

- Breathe out. Place the inhaler 1 to 2 inches (about 2 finger widths) in front of your opened mouth (Fig. 48.24).
- Press the top of the canister on the MDI.
- Breathe in very slowly, taking a full breath in.

After taking the medication, patients should hold their breath for 10 seconds (or count to 10), and then breathe out. When using an inhaled, quick-relief medication (beta-agonists), the patient should wait 1 minute between puffs. These steps should be repeated until the dose is completed.

Patients should be instructed to periodically clean the spacer and the MDI:

- Take the spacer apart. Clean the spacer with mild soap and allow it to air dry.
- Remove the medication canister and the mouthpiece cover from the MDI. Let warm water flow over the top and bottom of the MDI inhaler for about 30 seconds. Shake off and let air dry overnight. When assembling the device, spray twice in the air before taking a dose. Clean the MDI weekly to prevent medication from building up and blocking the sprayer.

Cleaning techniques can vary with medication products. Patients should be encouraged to check the product's website for directions.

Nebulizer Treatment. Inhaled medication for asthma, COPD, and other lung diseases can be given using a nebulizer. A nebulizer treatment can be done in the ambulatory care setting and in the home. A nebulizer is a small machine that turns liquid medication into a fine spray that can be inhaled. Typically, the medication used for nebulizers is much stronger than the same medication found in an MDI. Procedure 48.5 describes the steps for administering a nebulizer treatment.

Oxygen Therapy. When a patient comes to the ambulatory care facility with a cardiac or respiratory condition, the provider may order oxygen to be administered. Oxygen should be treated as a medication. The medical assistant must get the order from the provider for how much oxygen to administer and how to administer it. In the ambulatory care facility, oxygen may be available in the room by means of a wall-mounted flow meter or oxygen cylinders (portable tanks).

Room air is about 21% oxygen. Oxygen devices increase the concentration of oxygen for the patient to breathe in. Typically, a nasal cannula (NC) or a simple mask is used in the ambulatory care setting (Fig. 48.25). Other masks that deliver higher oxygen concentrations may also be available (Fig. 48.26). Table 48.8 provides information on the more common oxygen delivery devices used in the ambulatory care setting. Procedure 48.6 presents the steps for administering oxygen.

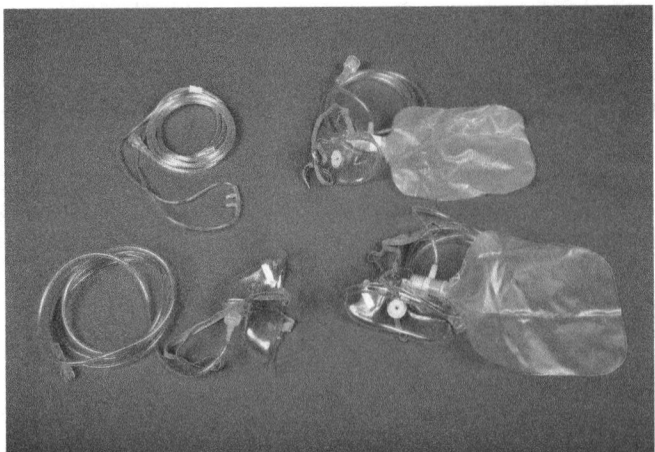

Fig. 48.26 *Top left to right:* Nasal cannula and child non-rebreather mask. Non-rebreather masks have one-way valves (e.g., yellow circle on the mask). *Bottom left to right:* Simple face mask and adult non-rebreather mask.

TABLE 48.8   Common Oxygen Delivery Devices

Type	Flow Range (liters/minute [LPM])	Oxygen Delivered	Descriptions
Nasal cannula	1–2 2–4 4–6	24%–28% 28%–34% 34%–44%	• Soft tube with prongs that are placed in the nose; make sure prongs curve downward. • A humidification device is used if flow is over 4 L/min. • Allows patient to talk, drink, and eat. • Cannot be used with upper respiratory obstructions (e.g., nasal polyps); not helpful for mouth breathers.
Mask	5–10	30%–60%	• Used for strictly mouth breathers. • Best used for short-term situations (e.g., ambulatory care). • Restrictive for communication, coughing, and eating. • Requires 5–6 L/min to avoid carbon dioxide (CO_2) accumulation in the mask.
Partial rebreathing mask	6–10	40%–70%	• Oxygen feeds into a reservoir bag attached to a mask. • About one-third of expired air enters reservoir bag, and the rest exits mask through exhalation ports.
Non-rebreathing face mask	10–15	Up to about 90%	• Mask with a reservoir bag and one-way valves. • One-way valve allows patient to inhale oxygen from the reservoir bag but prevents expired air from entering the bag. • Before applying to patient, occlude valve and allow reservoir bag to fill with oxygen.

CLOSING COMMENTS

In many ambulatory care facilities the providers will order some type of cardiopulmonary testing. Knowing how to produce a clear ECG tracing is critical. Putting the electrodes on incorrectly or switching the lead wires can lead to many problems for the patients, because they may be wrongly diagnosed with cardiac disease.

Besides knowing how to perform an ECG, the medical assistant should be knowledgeable about other ECG tests, pulmonary testing, and pulmonary treatments. The medical assistant should also be familiar with the medical terminology associated with the cardiovascular and respiratory systems.

CHAPTER REVIEW

This chapter reviewed the cardiovascular anatomy, including the heart structures, blood flow, and conduction system. The components of the ECG tracing are:
• P wave: Shows atrial depolarization; atrial chambers contract, and the blood is pushed to the ventricles.

• PR segment: Isoelectric line; allows the atria to finish contracting.
• QRS complex: Shows ventricular depolarization; atrial repolarization also occurs during this time, though it is hidden. The ventricles contract, pushing blood out of the heart.

- ST segment: Isoelectric line; allows the ventricles to finish contracting.
- T wave: Ventricular repolarization and atrial polarization.

After the T wave or U wave, ventricular polarization occurs.

For a resting 12-lead ECG, three leads are bipolar, three are augmented, and the remaining six are precordial. Ten electrodes are used for the 12-lead ECG. One electrode is placed on each of the extremities, with the right leg (RL) being the ground. Six electrodes are placed on the chest. Lead wires are attached to the electrodes. If the electrocardiograph is set at 10 mm/mV, the standardization mark will be an upward rectangle that is 10 small boxes tall. The chart or paper speed should be set at 25 mm per second. Both settings can be changed, but the change needs to be indicated on the ECG for the provider.

The medical assistant should examine the ECG tracing for artifact. If artifact is seen, steps should be taken to problem-solve the situation. Then a new tracing should be run. If a life-threatening rhythm is seen on the tracing, the medical assistant needs to notify the provider immediately.

There are several ECG tests besides the 12-lead ECG. Some require testing at the ambulatory care facility, whereas others monitor the ECG while patients go about their daily activities. Tests such as the Holter monitor and the cardiac event record require patients to keep a journal of their symptoms and activities.

Pulmonary function tests provide information on the function and size of the lungs. The medical assistant can perform the peak flow and spirometry tests. A medical assistant can also perform pulmonary treatments, including nebulizer treatments and oxygen therapy.

PATIENT-CENTERED CARE

When a patient is undergoing cardiac testing to rule out or rule in a heart condition, it can be a stressful experience. It is important for the medical assistant to be sensitive to the patient's concerns and feelings. Questions from the patient and family members should be addressed, and any questions outside the medical assistant's scope of practice should be directed to the provider.

The medical assistant should provide the patient with clear directions on the cardiac procedure being done. After the procedure, the medical assistant should let the patient know who will contact them about the test results. If possible, give the patient the timeline of when to anticipate the notification.

BEING PROFESSIONAL

Many times, patients may think that the medical assistant can read ECGs. They may ask the medical assistant if everything looks all right or if the ECG is normal. It is outside the medical assistant's scope of practice to read ECGs. This is the role of the provider. The medical assistant should explain to the patient that the provider will read the ECG and the patient will be informed of the results. The medical assistant should take care not to add in false hope comments, such as "I am sure the ECG will be normal." These types of comments may give the patient a false impression of the results, and the medical assistant's behavior is unprofessional.

Role-play this scenario: You are a medical assistant. Dr. Walden has ordered an ECG on Peter Smith. Peter is your peer. During the ECG, Peter tells you he is nervous about the results. After you complete the ECG, Peter asks you if the ECG is normal. Respond to his question.

SCENARIO WRAP-UP

Renee is enjoying working with Eva. They have seen many different cardiac tests while working with Dr. Kahn's patients. Renee has found herself learning new things. If she does not have the answers to Eva's questions about cardiac tests, she looks up the information. She finds herself learning new information as a result.

Eva is really enjoying working with Renee and Dr. Kahn. She is feeling so much better performing ECGs. Her understanding of the ECG tracing and how to resolve artifact has greatly improved. She is also feeling more confident performing cardiac testing. She is hoping to be able to work with Dr. Kahn in the future, because she enjoys doing ECGs so much!

PROCEDURE 48.1   Perform Electrocardiography

Tasks

Perform electrocardiography and routine maintenance on the machine. Document the procedure in the patient's health record. Show awareness of a patient's concerns and incorporate critical thinking skills when performing patient care.

Equipment and Supplies

- ECG machine
- Disposable electrodes
- ECG paper
- Alcohol pads
- Razor (optional)
- Gauze pads (optional)
- Patient gown or paper cape
- Tissue
- Disinfecting wipes
- Gloves
- Waste container
- Patient's health record

Procedural Steps

1. Wash your hands or use hand sanitizer.

   Purpose: Hand sanitization is an important step for infection control.

2. Assemble equipment and supplies needed for the ECG procedure. Plug in and turn on the ECG machine. Verify that the standardization and chart/paper speed are correct.

   Purpose: Having the equipment ready helps reduce the patient's wait time.

3. Greet the patient. Identify yourself. Verify the patient's identity with full name and date of birth. Make sure the patient's information matches the order and the record. Explain the procedure in a manner that the patient understands. Answer any questions the patient may have about the procedure.

   Purpose: It is important to identify the patient in two different ways to ensure that you have the correct patient. Explaining the procedure can make the patient feel more comfortable and helps to reduce anxiety.

   Scenario update: The patient states that she is really worried that something is wrong with her heart. She states that she is really nervous about having an ECG.

4. Using therapeutic communication techniques (e.g., reflection, restatement, and summarizing), show the patient you are aware of her concerns.

   Purpose: Using therapeutic communication techniques can be helpful to show patients you hear their concerns. It also always helps the medical assistant to clarify the patient's concerns.

5. Ask the patient to remove all clothing from the waist up, including undergarments, and put on the gown/cape so that the opening is in the front. Ask the patient if assistance is needed. If so, provide help. If not, leave the room and allow the patient time to change. When reentering the room, provide a courtesy knock on the door.

   Purpose: The patient needs to be undressed from the waist up for you to place the electrodes. Patients require privacy to change.

6. Assist the patient into a comfortable supine position on the exam table. Provide support for the legs and arms.

   Purpose: To reduce artifact on the tracing, the patient must be comfortable, and the extremities need to be supported.

7. Identify the locations for the ECG electrodes on the chest. Prepare the skin. If the patient has a hairy chest, get the person's permission prior to shaving the areas (optional). Wipe each spot with alcohol and allow it to dry. Fold the gauze pad over your index finger and briskly rub the site to abrade the skin (optional) (Fig. 1).

Purpose: The alcohol will prepare the skin and help the electrode adhere to the skin.

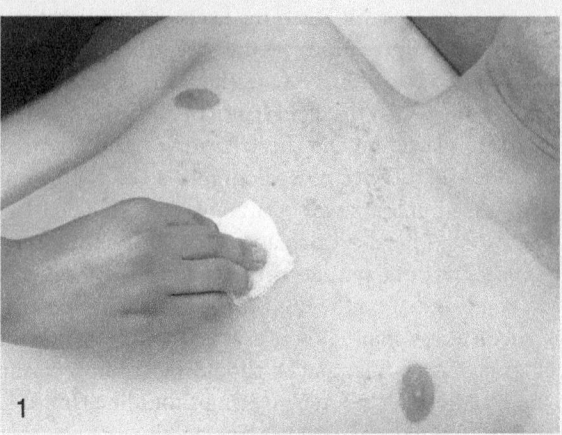

1

8. Correctly apply the six chest electrodes. If tab electrodes are used, the tabs should be pointed toward the waist.

   Purpose: Having the tabs face the core of the body will help reduce the tension on the lead wires when they are attached.

9. Identify the locations for the ECG electrodes on the extremities. Refer to the users' guide for arm electrode position if needed. Wipe each spot with alcohol and allow it to dry. Correctly apply the four limb electrodes to non-bony areas. If using tab electrodes, the lower leg tabs should point toward the waist. The arm/wrist tabs should be pointed toward the fingers.

   Purpose: The alcohol will prepare the skin and help the electrode adhere to the skin.

10. Attach the correct lead wire to each of the electrodes. The wires should follow the natural contour of the body and not overlap.

    Purpose: Overlapping wires can cause artifact.

11. Enter the patient's data into the ECG machine. Identify any changes with the default settings, electrode position, or patient's position.

    Purpose: The ECG tracing needs to be labeled with the patient's identifying information. The provider must be aware of any changes in the procedure. Electrode position changes, chart/paper speed, and so on can change the appearance of the tracing.

12. Double-check that the lead wires are in the correct position and attached to the electrodes. Make sure each electrode is attached to the skin. Take any corrective action necessary.

    Purpose: The lead wires and electrodes must be in the correct spot and attached for the tracing to be accurate.

13. Instruct the patient to lie still and not to talk during the tracing. Tell the patient how long the tracing will take.

    Purpose: Talking and moving during the tracing will create artifact.

14. Verify that the filter(s) are on. Check the leads on the screen or monitor. Based on what you observe, use critical thinking skills and take any corrective action necessary. Run the tracing when the leads look clear and without artifact.

    Purpose: The filters will minimize the artifact. Checking the appearance of the leads helps to identify if corrective action is needed to minimize artifact.

15. Check the tracing for clarity, artifact, and abnormal life-threatening rhythms. Based on what you observe, use critical thinking skills and take any corrective action necessary.

    Purpose: The provider will need a clear tracing. Life-threatening rhythms need to be identified, and the provider needs to be told immediately.

Continued

PROCEDURE 48.1 Perform Electrocardiography—cont'd

16. Disconnect the lead wires and remove the electrodes. Wipe any reside from the patient's skin. Wash your hands or use hand sanitizer. Instruct the patient to get dressed. Ask the patient if assistance is needed. If so, help the patient to dress.

    Purpose: The medical assistant must be the one to remove the wires and electrodes.

17. Provide the patient with information about following up with the provider. Complete any necessary actions with the ECG (e.g., upload to the electronic health record, mount, and route to the provider).

    Purpose: After tests, patients will want to know what the results are. The provider will need to read the tracing before any results are given to the patient.

18. Document accurately in the patient's health record. Indicate the name of the provider ordering the test, what test was performed, how the patient tolerated the test, and what you did with the ECG tracing. You can also add any instructions you provided to the patient regarding follow-up.

    Purpose: Indicating who ordered the test and what was done is important for insurance reimbursement and for legal reasons.

    Scenario update: Perform routine machine maintenance by adding paper to the ECG machine or printer.

19. Review the users' guide on how to change the paper. Gather the new ream or roll of ECG paper.

    Purpose: The users' guide will indicate how the paper should be added to the machine.

20. Open the machine. Remove the remaining paper and add the new paper per the steps in the guide.

    Purpose: It is important to remove the last few sheets of the old paper to make room for the new ream.

21. Put on gloves and disinfect the lead wires per the users' guide. Disinfect the exam table. Clean up the work area. Remove your gloves and dispose of them in the waste container. Wash your hands or use hand sanitizer.

    Purpose: For infection control purposes, it is important to disinfect the lead wires and exam table between each use.

Documentation Example

08/06/20XX 1423 Per Dr. James Martin's order, a resting 12-lead ECG was performed. Pt tolerated the procedure well. Pt was instructed to call the clinic tomorrow for the ECG results. The ECG tracing was routed to Dr. Martin
_____Eva Ning, RMA

PROCEDURE 48.2 Apply a Holter Monitor

Tasks

Apply a Holter monitor and coach a patient on the procedure. Document the procedure in the patient's health record.

Equipment and Supplies

- Holter monitor, new batteries, flash memory card (if required), carrying case, and users' guide
- Disposable electrodes
- Razor
- Sharps container
- Alcohol pads
- Gauze pads (optional)
- Cloth nonallergenic tape (optional)
- Journal
- Waste container
- Patient's health record

Procedural Steps

1. Wash your hands or use hand sanitizer.

   Purpose: Hand sanitization is an important step for infection control.

2. Assemble the equipment and supplies needed for the procedure. Insert a flash memory card if required. Insert new batteries into the monitor (Fig. 1). Consult the users' guide for the required number and placement of electrodes.

   Purpose: Having the equipment ready helps reduce the patient's wait time. New batteries will ensure accurate functioning.

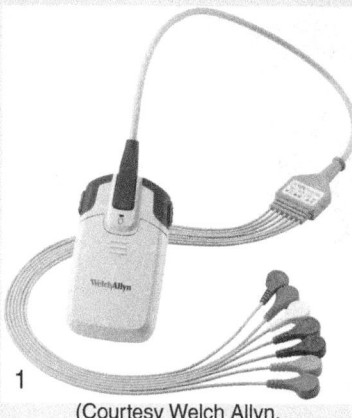

1

(Courtesy Welch Allyn,
Skaneateles Falls, NY.)

3. Greet the patient. Identify yourself. Verify the patient's identity with full name and date of birth. Make sure the patient's information matches the order and the record. Explain the procedure in a manner that the patient understands. Answer any questions the patient may have about the procedure.

   Purpose: It is important to identify the patient in two different ways to ensure that you have the correct patient. Explaining the procedure can make the patient feel more comfortable and helps to reduce anxiety.

4. Ask the patient to remove clothing from the waist up and to sit at the end of the exam table. Ask the patient if assistance is needed. If so, help. If not, leave the room and allow the patient time to change. When reentering the room, provide a courtesy knock on the door.

   Purpose: The patient needs to be undressed from the waist up for you to place the electrodes. Patients require privacy to change.

Continued

PROCEDURE 48.2   Apply a Holter Monitor—cont'd

5. Identify the locations for the electrodes and prepare the skin for the electrodes. Shave the area if the patient has a hairy chest. Wipe the area with the alcohol pad and allow it to dry. Fold the gauze pad over your index finger and briskly rub the site to abrade the skin.

   Purpose: These techniques help the electrodes to better adhere to the skin, which creates a better tracing.

6. Snap the lead wire onto the electrode. Apply the electrodes to the sites as indicated by the manufacturer. Press firmly and make sure the entire electrode adheres completely to the skin (Fig. 2).

   Purpose: Secure electrode attachment is necessary to produce an accurate tracing.

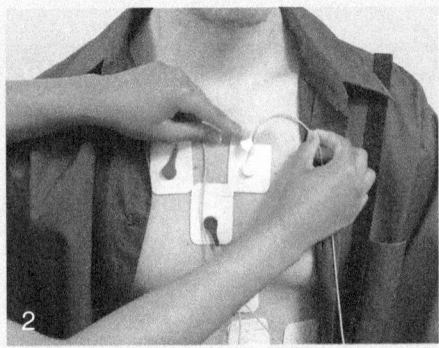

7. Loop and tape down the wires on the chest.

   Purpose: The tape will hold the wires in place and reduce the tension on the electrodes.

8. Attach the patient cable to the monitor if required. Turn on the recorder and set as indicated by the manufacturer. Enter the patient data as indicated.

   Purpose: Each manufacturer will have directions for operating the monitor.

9. Have the patient get dressed. Assist as needed.

   Purpose: Some patients may require assistance when hooked up to the monitor.

10. Coach the patient about making journal entries while wearing the monitor (Fig. 3). Provide the required patient education.

    Purpose: It is important for the patient to keep a diary of what they are doing. The provider will check the ECG for abnormalities and then check what the patient was doing during the event.

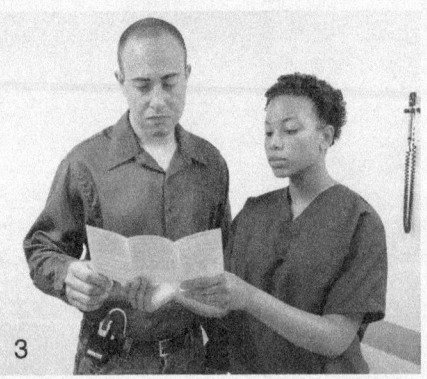

11. Assist the patient in scheduling a return appointment in 24 hours. Provide the patient with contact information should a question arise.

    Purpose: The patient will need to return in 24 hours for the monitor to be removed. Providing contact information will help reduce the patient's anxiety.

12. Document accurately in the patient's health record. Indicate the name of the provider ordering the test, the procedure done, patient education provided, and return appointment.

    Purpose: Indicating who ordered the test and what was done is important for insurance reimbursement and for legal reasons.

Documentation Example

08/06/20XX 1423 Per Dr. James Martin's order, a Holter monitor was applied. Pt was instructed how to complete the diary, and a contact number was provided if pt has additional questions. Pt verbalized what he was to write in the diary. Appointment was made for 08/07/20XX to remove the monitor. _____

_____Eva Ning, RMA

PROCEDURE 48.3   Measure the Peak Flow Rate

Tasks

Perform a peak flow measurement. Document the procedure in the patient's health record.

Equipment and Supplies
- Peak flow meter
- Disposable mouthpiece
- Disinfection wipes
- Gloves
- Waste container
- Paper towel or denture cup (optional)
- Patient's health record

Procedural Steps

1. Wash your hands or use hand sanitizer.
   Purpose: Hand sanitization is an important step for infection control.
2. Assemble the equipment and supplies needed for the peak flow procedure. Place the mouthpiece on the peak flow meter. Move the indicator to the bottom of the calibration scale (if not using a digital meter).
   Purpose: Having the equipment ready helps reduce the patient's wait time. The indicator needs to be at the bottom of the scale before the test to get an accurate reading.
3. Greet the patient. Identify yourself. Verify the patient's identity with full name and date of birth. Make sure the patient's information matches the order and the record. Explain the procedure in a manner that the patient understands. Answer any questions the patient may have about the procedure.
   Purpose: It is important to identify the patient in two different ways to ensure that you have the correct patient. Explaining the procedure can make the patient feel more comfortable and helps to reduce anxiety.
4. Ask the patient to loosen any restrictive clothing. Have the patient remove any gum and loose dentures. Make sure to provide a paper towel or denture cup if needed.
   Purpose: To get the most accurate results, the patient needs to be able to take a large breath in before the test. Normally, dentures can be left in the mouth, but loose-fitting dentures may affect the results of the test and must be removed.
5. With patients in the seated position, ensure that their feet are flat on the floor and the legs are uncrossed. The patient should sit straight up and against the back of the chair.
   Purpose: It is important for the patient to be in a position in which the lungs can fully expand.
6. Describe how the patient should do the test. "Take the deepest breath possible. Seal your lips around the mouthpiece. Blow as hard and as fast as you can." Encourage the patient to state when they are ready to start the test. Tell patients to seal their lips around the mouthpiece (Fig. 1).

Purpose: Clear directions will help the patient understand what to do.

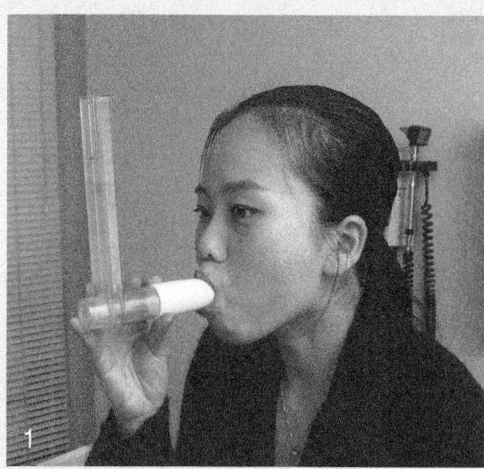

7. Coach the patient during the test. After the patient has blown through the meter, read the number next to the indicator. Write the number down. Reset the indicator to the bottom of the scale (if it is not a digital meter).
   Purpose: If the patient has breathing problems, it is important to allow the patient to indicate when they are ready.
8. Make any adjustments as needed. Repeat the test two additional times. Write down the last two numbers.
   Purpose: Three acceptable readings are needed for the peak flow procedure.
9. Put on gloves and remove the mouthpiece. Discard the mouthpiece in the waste container. Disinfect the peak flow meter. Remove your gloves and dispose of them in the waste container. Wash your hands or use hand sanitizer.
   Purpose: Wearing gloves and disinfecting the peak flow meter are important for infection control.
10. Notify the provider of the readings and document the readings in the patient's health record. Indicate the name of the provider who ordered the test, the procedure done, the results of the test, and how the patient tolerated the test.
    Purpose: Indicating who ordered the test and what was done is important for insurance reimbursement and for legal reasons.

Documentation Example

08/07/20XX 1423 Per Dr. Angela Perez's order, a peak flow was performed. Pt stated she was "a little short of breath" on the third test. Peak flow readings: 260, 230, and 200 L/min. Dr Perez was notified of results and patient's SOB complaint._____Eva Ning, RMA

PROCEDURE 48.4 Perform Spirometry Testing

Tasks

Perform a spirometry test. Document the procedure in the patient's health record.

Equipment and Supplies

- Spirometry machine with paper (and users' guide if applicable)
- Disposable mouthpiece and tubing (if applicable)
- Nose clip
- Calibration equipment
- Disinfection wipes
- Gloves
- Waste container
- Paper towel or denture cup (optional)
- Patient's health record
- Scale (if no height or weight measurements were taken earlier that day)

Procedural Steps

1. Wash your hands or use hand sanitizer.
   Purpose: Hand sanitization is an important step for infection control.
2. Assemble the equipment and supplies needed for the spirometry procedure. Calibrate the machine according to the users' guide and the facility's procedures.
   Purpose: It is important to calibrate per the facility's procedures. Calibration ensures that the results are accurate and reliable.
3. Greet the patient. Identify yourself. Verify the patient's identity with full name and date of birth. Make sure the patient's information matches the order and the record. Explain the procedure in a manner that the patient understands. Answer any questions the patient may have about the procedure.
   Purpose: It is important to identify the patient in two different ways to ensure that you have the correct patient. Explaining the procedure can make the patient feel more comfortable and helps to reduce anxiety.
4. Enter the patient's name, medical record number, age (or date of birth), race, sex, weight, and height into the machine. Enter any additional required information.
   Purpose: The information used for the spirometry calculations is current weight, height, age, race, and sex.
5. Ask the patient to loosen any restrictive clothing. Have the patient remove gum and loose dentures (if applicable). Make sure to provide a paper towel or denture cup if needed.
   Purpose: To get the most accurate results, the patient needs to be able to take a large breath in before the test. Loose-fitting dentures can affect the results of the test.
6. With the patient in the seated position, ensure that the feet are flat on the floor and the legs are uncrossed. The patient should sit straight up and against the back of the chair.
   Purpose: The patient may get dizzy during the test, so standing can be problematic. The seated position provides the maximum lung expansion for the test.
7. Describe how the patient should do the test. "Take the deepest breath possible. Seal your lips around the mouthpiece. Blow as hard and as fast as you can. Blow until you empty the air from your lungs."

Purpose: Clear directions will help the patient understand what to do.

8. Attach the mouthpiece to the machine. Explain the purpose of the nose clip to the patient. Apply the nose clip to the patient (Fig. 1). Have the patient state when they are ready to start. Start the test as directed by the users' guide.
   Purpose: The nose clip prevents air from leaking out through the nose. It provides a more accurate reading.

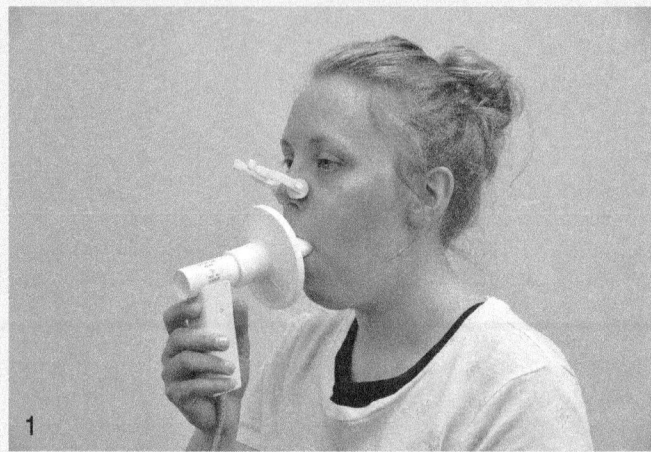

9. During the test, encourage the patient to empty the lungs. Repeat until three acceptable tests have been done. Allow the patient to rest between tests, if needed, and to indicate when they are ready for next test.
   Purpose: Usually three tests results are needed for comparison. If the patient is struggling and having difficulty breathing, ask the provider if three tests need to be done.
10. Put on gloves and remove the mouthpiece. Discard the mouthpiece in the waste container. Disinfect the spirometer as indicated in the users' guide. Remove your gloves and dispose of them in the waste container. Wash your hands or use hand sanitizer.
    Purpose: Wearing gloves and disinfecting the equipment is important for infection control.
11. Document that the test was performed. Indicate the name of the provider who ordered the test, the name of the test, how the patient tolerated the test, and what you did with the test results. Any patient instructions regarding follow-up can also be documented.
    Purpose: Indicating who ordered the test and what was done is important for insurance reimbursement and for legal reasons.

Documentation Example

08/08/20XX 1423 Per Dr. James Martin's order, a spirometry test was performed. Pt stated she felt dizzy during the third attempt. The dizziness cleared within 5 minutes, and she stated she felt better. Pt was instructed to call the clinic tomorrow for the spirometry results. The spirometry results were given to Dr. Martin. _____Eva Ning, RMA

PROCEDURE 48.5 Administer a Nebulizer Treatment

Tasks

Administer a nebulizer treatment. Document the medication administration in the patient's health record.

Equipment and Supplies

- Nebulizer machine
- Disposable nebulizer patient kit (tubing, medication cup, mouthpiece or mask, flexible tube, and tee)
- Medication as ordered
- Normal saline (as ordered or per facility's protocol)
- Provider's order
- Disinfection wipes
- Gloves
- Waste container
- Patient's health record

Order: Levalbuterol 0.63 mg by nebulization.

Procedural Steps

1. Wash your hands or use hand sanitizer. Using the drug reference information and the order, review the information on the medication if needed. Clarify any questions you have with the provider.

   Purpose: Hand sanitization is an important step for infection control. It is important to be knowledgeable about the medication you are giving.

2. Select the right medication from the storage area. Check to see if the medication is concentrated and requires normal saline to dilute it. Check the medication label (and normal saline label, if used) against the order. Check for the right name, form, and route. Check the expiration date to make sure the drug has not expired. Verify that it is the right dose and time.

   Purpose: A provider's order is required for the nebulizer treatment. The medication needs to be verified three times before it is given. The nine rights of medication administration also need to be followed.

3. Assemble the equipment and supplies needed for the nebulizer treatment.

   Purpose: Having the equipment ready helps reduce the patient's wait time.

4. Perform the second medication check. Check the medication and normal saline label(s) against the order. Check for the right name, form, and route.

   Purpose: It is important to do the second check of the label(s) before pouring the medication into the medication cup.

5. Add the medication and, if required, the normal saline to the medication cup (Fig. 1). Secure the cover on the cup.

   Purpose: The medication cup holds the medication during the treatment.

6. Perform the third medication check. Check the medication label and normal saline label (if used) against the order. Check for the right name, form, and

route. Verify that the amount of medication in the cup is correct according to the order. Clean up the area.

   Purpose: It is important to do the third check of the label before giving the medication.

7. Prior to entering the exam room, provide courtesy knock on the door. Greet the patient. Identify yourself. Verify the patient's identity with full name and date of birth. Make sure the patient's information matches the order and the record.

   Purpose: It is important to identify the patient in two different ways to ensure that you have the correct patient. Explaining the procedure can make the patient feel more comfortable and helps to reduce anxiety.

8. Provide the right education to the patient. Explain the medication ordered, the desired effect, and common side effects; also identify the provider who ordered it. Explain the procedure in a manner that the patient understands. Answer any questions the patient may have about the procedure. Ask the patient if they have any allergies. If the patient refuses the medication, notify the provider.

   Purpose: The patient needs to be aware of what you are giving, the action and side effects, and who ordered it. It is also important to double-check the patient's allergies before administering the medication.

9. Attach the mouthpiece (or mask). Attach the tubing to the medication cup and the machine.

   Purpose: Use a mask if ordered by the provider.

10. Perform the right technique. The patient should be sitting upright on a chair. Instruct the patient to hold the mouthpiece between the teeth and seal the lips around the mouthpiece. Encourage the patient to take slow, deep breaths through the mouth. The patient should hold each breath 2 to 3 seconds before exhaling.

    Purpose: Sitting upright allows for total lung expansion. If patients breathe too deeply and too fast, they will become dizzy and may hyperventilate. Holding the breath in allows the medication to disperse through the lungs.

11. Turn on the nebulizer and give the medicine cup and mouthpiece to the patient to start the treatment. Instruct patients to put it into their mouth. If using a mask, position it securely and comfortably over the patient's nose and mouth.

    Purpose: It is important to make sure the mask is comfortable over the patient's face. If it is not comfortable, the patient may not tolerate the treatment.

12. Continue the treatment until the mist has stopped (approximately 10 minutes) (Fig. 2). Turn off the nebulizer. Encourage the patient to take several deep breaths and cough.

    Purpose: After the treatment, it is common that patients will need to cough. Ensure that tissue is available if the patient needs it.

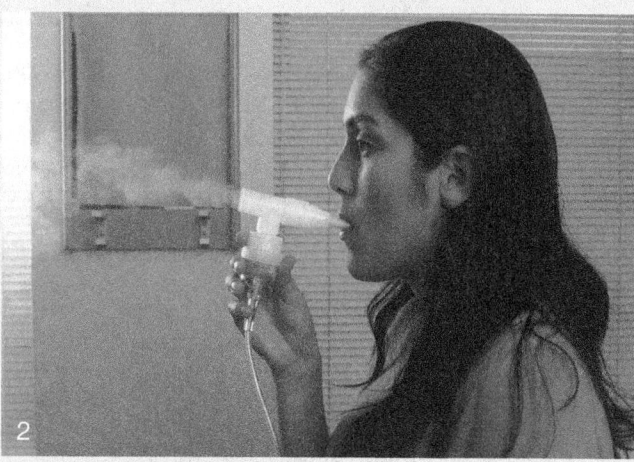

PROCEDURE 48.5   Administer a Nebulizer Treatment—cont'd

13. Put on gloves and dispose of the used supplies. Disinfect the nebulizer machine. Remove your gloves and dispose of them in the waste container. Wash your hands or use hand sanitizer.

    Purpose: To ensure infection control.

14. Document in the patient's health record. Include the name of the provider ordering the treatment, what was administered, how the patient tolerated the medication, and any follow-up assessments (e.g., vital signs).

Purpose: Documentation is the last of the nine rights of medication administration.

Documentation Example

08/06/20XX 1120 P: 76 regular, 1+ ; R: 26 regular, shallow. Per Dr. Angela Perez's order, Levalbuterol 0.63 mg administered by nebulizer. Pt stated she felt a little shaky after the treatment and her lungs feel less tight. Pt is resting on the exam table. P: 86 regular, 1+; R: 20 regular, normal. Dr. Perez notified._____Eva Ning, RMA

PROCEDURE 48.6   Administer Oxygen Per Nasal Cannula or Mask

Tasks

Administer oxygen per nasal cannula or mask. Document the oxygen administration in the patient's health record.

Equipment and Supplies

- Oxygen cylinder with oxygen regulator or oxygen flow meter (wall unit)
- Adult nasal cannula or simple mask
- Provider's order
- Patient's health record
- Mannequin (optional)

Order 1: Administer 2 L/min of oxygen per nasal cannula.

Order 2: Administer 6 L/min of oxygen per simple mask.

Procedural Steps

1. Wash your hands or use hand sanitizer.

    Purpose: Hand sanitization is an important step for infection control.

2. Assemble the equipment and supplies needed for the provider's order. If an oxygen cylinder is used, identify the amount of oxygen left in the cylinder.

    Purpose: The order will include the amount to give and the device (e.g., cannula) to use for the administration. It is important to make sure the cylinder has enough oxygen for the patient.

3. Verify the order if you have any questions.

    Purpose: A provider's order is required for the oxygen administration.

4. Greet the patient. Identify yourself. Verify the patient's identity with full name and date of birth. Make sure the patient's information matches the order and the record. Explain the procedure in a manner that the patient understands. Answer any questions the patient may have about the procedure.

    Purpose: It is important to identify the patient in two different ways to ensure that you have the correct patient. Explaining the procedure can make the patient feel more comfortable and helps to reduce anxiety.

5. Connect the nasal cannula or mask to the regulator or flow meter. Turn on the oxygen and adjust the flow rate to the correct amount per the provider's order. The ball should be centered on the number of liters ordered.

    Purpose: Oxygen needs to be flowing through the tubing before the cannula is applied to the patient.

6. Apply the mask or nasal cannula.

    a. Place the mask over the patient's nose, mouth, and chin. Place the elastic over the head. Adjust the elastic strap to tighten the mask on the face. Adjust the metal nasal bridge clamp, making sure it fits without obstructing the nose. Ensure that the mask fits tightly on the face.

    Purpose: A poorly fitting mask can cause oxygen to be directed into the eyes, causing additional problems.

b. Insert the tips of the cannula into the nostrils. If the tips are curved, the curves face downward toward the bottom of the nose (Fig. 1). Adjust the tubing around the back of the ears and then under the chin. Encourage the patient to breathe through the nose with the mouth closed.

    Purpose: The cannula needs to be inserted correctly into the nostrils. The cannula tips may be blocked by the top of the nostrils if they are inserted incorrectly. Breathing through the mouth when using a cannula is not as beneficial as breathing through the nose.

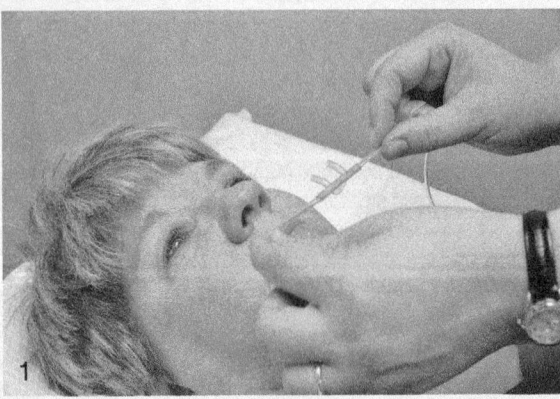
1

7. Make sure the patient is comfortable. Answer any questions they may have. Sanitize your hands.

    Purpose: Unanswered questions can cause anxiety. With breathing problems, it is important for the patient to be comfortable and calm.

8. Document the procedure. Include the name of the ordering provider, the number of liters of oxygen administered, the device used for administering the oxygen, and the patient's condition.

    Purpose: Indicating who ordered the oxygen and what was administered is important for insurance reimbursement and for legal reasons.

Documentation Examples

08/07/20XX 1540 R: 28 regular, shallow. Per Dr. Angela Perez's order, 2 L/min of oxygen administered via nasal cannula. Pt resting on exam table._____Eva Ning, RMA

08/07/20XX 1555 R: 20 regular, normal. Pt stated she is "feeling better" with the oxygen and has less SOB. Dr. Angela Perez was notified._____Eva Ning, RMA

49

Medical Emergencies

LEARNING OBJECTIVES

1. Discuss emergencies in healthcare settings and possible roles each team member has during an emergency.
2. Describe emergency equipment and supplies.
3. Explain first aid procedures for environmental emergencies, including temperature-related emergencies, burns, poisonings, chemical exposures, anaphylaxis, bites and stings, and foreign bodies in the eyes.
4. Discuss diabetic emergencies and provide first aid for a patient with insulin shock.
5. Discuss musculoskeletal and neurologic emergencies and provide first aid for a patient with seizure activity.
6. Discuss respiratory emergencies and provide first aid for a choking patient.
7. Discuss cardiovascular emergencies and provide first aid for a patient with a bleeding wound, fracture, or syncope; a patient in shock; and a patient in need of rescue breathing or cardiopulmonary resuscitation (CPR).

OUTLINE

⟫ OPENING SCENARIO

Gabe Garcia, CMA (AAMA), has worked for Walden-Martin Family Medical (WMFM) Clinic for 7 years. He was hired right after he completed his medical assistant program. Gabe has learned a lot through the years. He has impressed his supervisor with his dedication, attention to detail, punctuality, and patient care skills. Gabe was just promoted to a medical assistant lead position. In this new position, Gabe has additional responsibilities. He will now oversee the crash carts in the clinic, and he will train staff on emergency procedures.

The current emergency procedures need to be revised, and the crash cart procedures need updating. Gabe is excited to take over his new responsibilities. He looks forward to what he will learn in this new role.

YOU WILL LEARN

1. To handle emergencies in ambulatory care settings.
2. To use emergency equipment and supplies in ambulatory care settings.
3. To apply first aid for environmental emergencies, including cold and heat illnesses, burns, poisonings, anaphylaxis, bites, and foreign bodies in the eye.
4. To apply first aid for diabetic and musculoskeletal emergencies.
5. To apply first aid for neurologic emergencies, including vertigo, concussion, seizure, and stroke.
6. To apply first aid for respiratory emergencies, including hyperventilation, asthma attack, and choking.
7. To apply first aid for cardiovascular emergencies, including syncope, bleeding, shock, and heart attack.

INTRODUCTION

Emergencies happen everywhere. As a medical assistant, it is important for you to know how to handle emergencies because you may need to respond to one:

- *Outside of your job, in the community.* You may be one of the first people on the scene and need to provide first aid to the victims.
- *In the healthcare setting.* You may need to provide first aid as the provider assesses the injured person. Additional treatments, such as oxygen and medications, are provided in the healthcare setting.
- *Over the phone.* You may need to obtain information from someone involved in an emergency and provide first aid coaching. The medical assistant asks screening questions and provides the information to the provider. The provider instructs the medical assistant what to tell the caller.

This chapter starts by discussing emergencies in the healthcare setting and the medical assistant's role. Next, common emergency medical equipment, supplies, and medications are explained. Lastly, emergency conditions are described, along with the first aid procedures to perform.

EMERGENCIES IN HEALTHCARE SETTINGS

Every employee in a healthcare setting should know how to get help in an emergency. This process will vary. Healthcare facilities use special phrases for emergencies. For instance, "Code Blue Urgent Care" may indicate that an emergency is occurring in Urgent Care. Sometimes the code words indicate the age of the person. For instance, "Code Pink Family Practice" may mean that an emergency is occurring in Family Practice and "pink" indicates a child.

Once the call goes out for help, staff members respond to the scene. In small settings, most members of the staff may be needed. In large facilities, only certain staff members respond. Usually, medical assistants, licensed practical nurses (LPNs), registered nurses (RNs), and providers attend the emergency. Possible roles for each team member include:

- *Provider*: Assesses the patient, orders treatments and procedures, performs advanced procedures, may administer intravenous (IV) medications, and indicates when 911 needs to be called.
- *Nurse*: Registered nurses (RNs) IV medications and fluids. Licensed practical nurses (LPNs) may do the same if permitted by the state's scope of practice. RNs and LPNs assist with treatments and procedures, perform cardiopulmonary resuscitation (ri sus i TAY shun) (CPR), call 911, and document the code activities as they occur.
- *Clinical medical assistant*: Assists with treatments and procedures, performs CPR, documents the code activities as they occur, and calls 911. They may hand supplies to staff members and assist with caring for the family (moving them to a private area away from the emergency).
- *Administrative medical assistant*: Performs CPR and hands supplies to the staff (in small agencies), calls 911, escorts the emergency responders to the patient, and assists with caring for the family.

Importance of Documentation

In a code situation, it is important that at least one team member document everything that occurs. This is a stressful job because many things are occurring during an emergency. There are several reasons why accurate documentation is critical.

- The information is used during the code. For instance, CPR was started, and the team member documented "1413 CPR initiated." As the code progresses, the provider may want to know when the CPR was started.
- Emergency responders will need to know what occurred during the code. (What medications were given? When were they given? How much was given?)
- The documentation will provide evidence that the standard of care was met in the treatments given to the patient. Many lawsuits have originated from emergencies. The lawyers review the documentation. They look for delays in emergency care and lack of appropriate treatment. Complete and accurate documentation may make a difference between a lawsuit surviving and being dismissed in favor of the healthcare team.

If you are new to codes and if given the option, perform a role other than documenting. Observe what occurs during a code as you complete your task. Study the code documentation form during noncode times. As you become more comfortable with codes, assist the documenter if you can. A second pair of eyes is always helpful. Lastly, become the documenter and have a seasoned team member assist you.

VOCABULARY

cardiopulmonary resuscitation (CPR) The application of manual chest compressions and ventilations (also called *rescue breathing*) to patients who are not breathing or do not have a pulse; also known as *basic life support* (BLS).

code A term used in healthcare settings to indicate an emergency situation and to summon the trained team to the scene.

standard of care The level and type of care an ordinary, prudent healthcare professional with the same training and experience in a similar practice would have provided under a similar situation.

CRITICAL THINKING 49.1

Currently, the clinic does not have a procedure for documenting during code situations. The provider documents after the emergency. Gabe would like to discuss using a standard code form for all emergencies. A team member would be responsible for documenting during the code. Discuss the pros and cons of documenting during the code.

EMERGENCY EQUIPMENT AND SUPPLIES

The emergency supplies available at healthcare facilities will vary based on the size and location of the facility. Some practices have a small box that contains a few supplies and medications. Other practices place many crash carts throughout the building (Fig. 49.1A). A *crash cart* is a rolling supply cart that contains emergency equipment.

The crash cart should be checked monthly. This can be done by the supervisor or by two qualified employees (e.g., medical assistants, LPNs, or RNs). Expiration dates on the supplies are checked. Old supplies are replaced with new supplies. All the equipment and supplies are inventoried. When the inventory is completed, a plastic lock (or locking tag) is placed on the cart (Fig. 49.2). The crash cart is used only in emergencies. You should never break the lock and use something from the crash cart unless it is an emergency. The plastic locks should be kept safe and used only when the cart is inventoried monthly or after an emergency. Many of the locks are numbered, and the number is written on the inventory document. Keeping the locks safe minimizes the number of people going into the crash cart for nonemergency reasons.

This section will focus on the equipment and supplies typically found on a crash cart. The medical assistant should be familiar with the supplies and their location on the crash cart.

Oxygen and Airway Supplies

Oxygen and airway supplies are common items found on crash carts. If the patient needs oxygen, the provider will order oxygen to be applied via a mask or a nasal canula (CAN you lah). (Refer to Chapter 48 for additional information on oxygen delivery systems.)

If the patient has difficulty breathing or if an airway constriction may be occurring, the provider will insert a naso-pharyngeal (NAE zoe fah RIN jee ahl) airway (NPA) or an endotracheal (EN doe TRAY kee al) (ET) tube to create a patent (PAY tent) airway (Fig. 49.3). Providers maintain airways using:

VOCABULARY

endotracheal (ET) tube A catheter that is inserted into the trachea through the mouth; provides a patent airway.
nasopharyngeal airway (NPA) A soft flexible tube that is inserted in the nose and provides a patent airway; also known as a *nasal trumpet.*
patent Open.

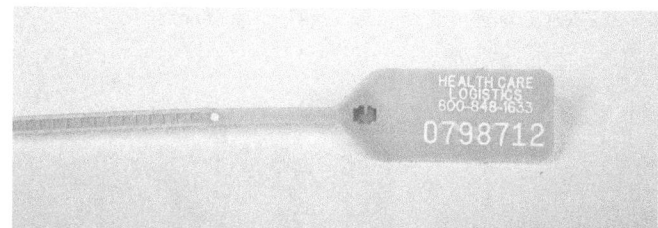

Fig. 49.2 A plastic lock is placed on the inventoried crash cart. The number is written on the inventory form for tracking purposes. These locks are easy to break in emergencies.

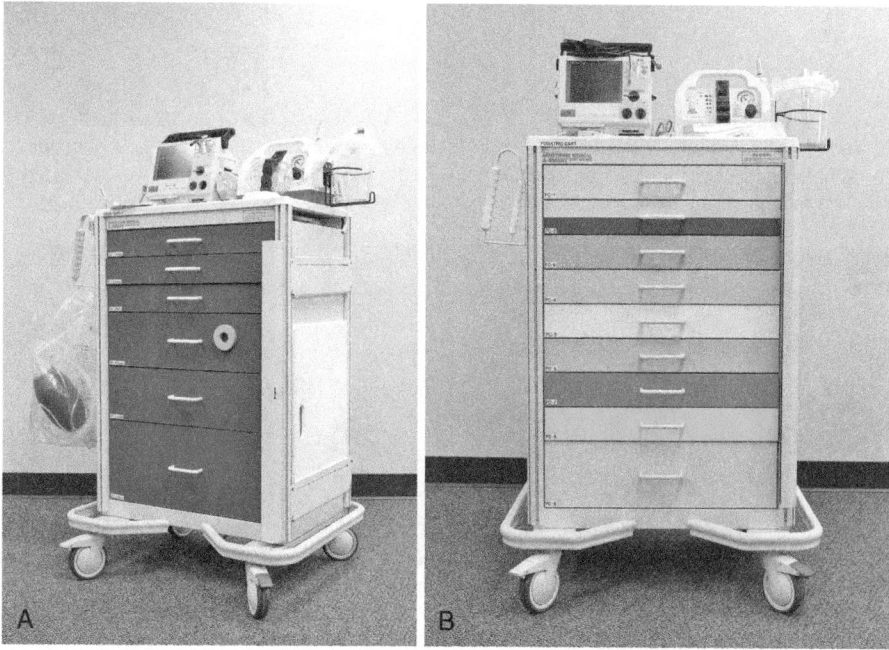

Fig. 49.1 A, Crash carts are used in an emergency. Having the drawers labeled allows for the speedy retrieval of supplies. B, The Broselow ColorCode cart is a crash cart for children. Each drawer is color coded for a certain-sized child.

- *Esophageal tracheal tubes*, which are placed in the trachea or esophagus
- *Laryngeal mask airways*, which are inserted through the mouth and advanced to the hypopharynx
- *Laryngeal tubes*, which are also inserted through the mouth and placed in the hypopharynx

Endotracheal Tube Intubation. The medical assistant should be aware of the equipment required during an ET tube intubation. During an endotracheal intubation, the provider will need:
- Laryngoscope with either a curved (MacIntosh) or a straight (Miller) blade. The sizes of blades are indicated on the side or back of the blade (Fig. 49.4A). The medical assistant must hand the laryngoscope with the blade attached to the provider (Fig. 49.4B).
- ET tube in the appropriate size. Cuffed ET tubes come in a variety of sizes for adults and older children (e.g., 7.5, 8, and 8.5). Uncuffed ET tubes come in a variety of sizes for children (e.g., 2.5, 3, and 3.5) (Fig. 49.5A). A syringe is used to inflate the cuff with air once it is in place.
- Stylet is a metal or flexible plastic wire inserted into the ET tube to create a firm, curved tube (see Fig. 49.5A). After the ET tube is in place, the stylet is removed.
- Ambu bag, which is attached to the ET tube and used to administer room air or oxygen (Fig. 49.5B). An Ambu

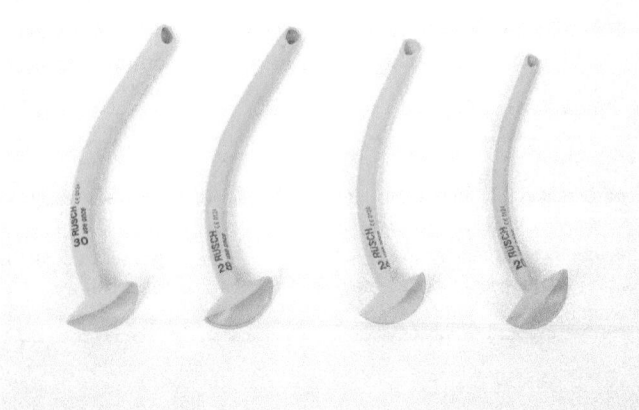

Fig. 49.3 Nasopharyngeal airways come in a variety of sizes.

> **VOCABULARY**
>
> **Ambu bag** A self-refilling bag-valve-mask unit used for artificial respiration that is effective for ventilating and oxygenating intubated patients.

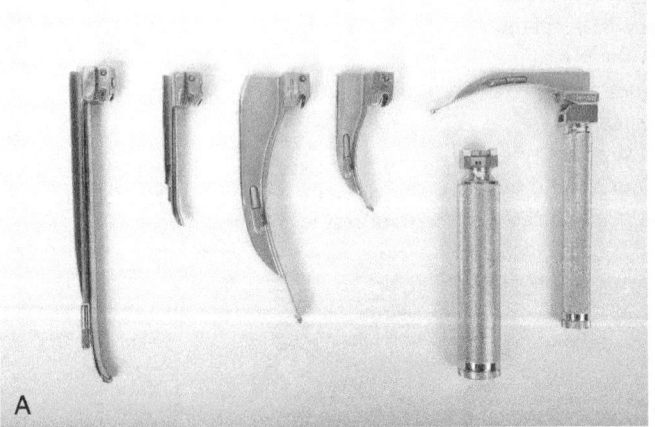
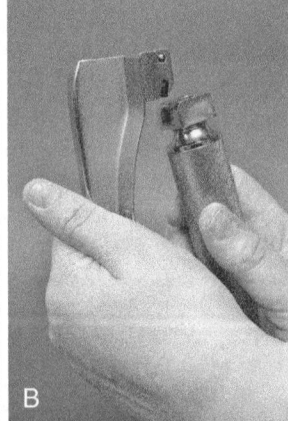

Fig. 49.4 A, *Left to right:* Two different sizes of straight blades and curved blades; adult laryngoscope handle and an assembled pediatric laryngoscope. A curved or straight blade must be attached to the laryngoscope handle. B, To attach the blade, hold the blade parallel to the handle and attach.

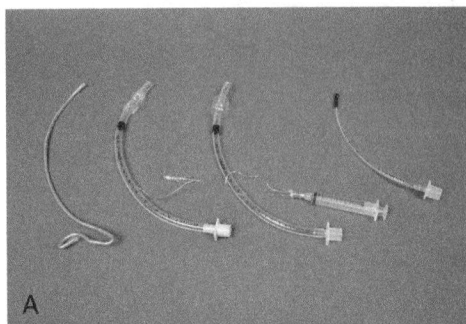
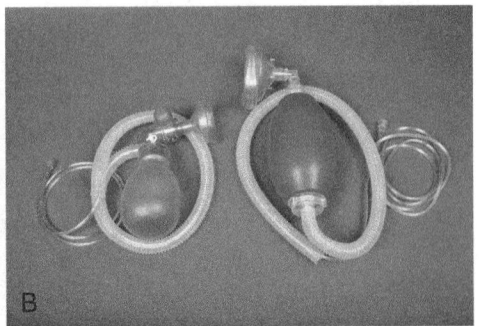

Fig. 49.5 A, *Left to right:* A stylet is threaded into the endotracheal (ET) tube to help maintain the tube's curve. ET tubes for adults are cuffed (or have a balloon that is inflated using a syringe). ET tubes for children are uncuffed *(far right picture)*. ET tubes come in a variety of sizes. B, *Left to right:* Pediatric and adult Ambu bags. An Ambu bag can cover the mouth or can be attached to an airway tube (e.g., endotracheal tube). Ambu bags can come with oxygen tubing attached. The tubing can be connected to an oxygen tank. Oxygen can be administered during the ventilation.

bag, which is a bag-valve-mask unit, can cover the mouth or can be attached to an airway tube (e.g., endotracheal tube). Ambu bags can come with oxygen tubing attached, which can be connected to an oxygen tank. Oxygen can be administered during the ventilation.

- Stethoscope. Once the tube is in place, a team member will provide ventilation with the Ambu bag. The provider must ensure the ET tube is in the correct location by listening over the lung field for air movement. If the ET tube is in the wrong location, the abdomen will become bloated with air; the patient is not being ventilated. (A provider will usually state that breath sounds are heard bilaterally. This is important to document on the code form. This verifies the ET tube is in the correct location.)

Defibrillator

A *defibrillator* (dee FIB rah LAE tohr) is a device that delivers an electrical shock to the heart muscle in an attempt to restore a normal heartbeat. The defibrillator's shock causes the heart to momentarily stop. When it restarts, the hope is the heart will beat at a normal rhythm. The quicker a defibrillator can be used, the better the person's chances of survival.

Typically, a defibrillator or an automated external defibrillator (AED) is used in healthcare facilities.

- A defibrillator consists of two handheld paddles that are placed on gel pads located on the patient's chest (Fig. 49.6A). Gel pads are required to prevent burns. They provide better electricity conduction from the paddles to the patient. The provider indicates how many joules at which to set the machine, and someone announces "All clear" to ensure no one is touching the patient. The provider pushes the button to give the shock.
- An *automated external defibrillator* is a portable, lightweight machine (see Fig. 49.6B). Sticky pads that contain electrodes (sensors) are attached to the patient's chest. The AED checks the heart rate and determines if a shock is required. If a shock is needed, the AED gives audible directions to the user to administer a shock.

Medications

The medications in crash carts can vary. Common medications used in emergencies are listed in Table 49.1. Most crash carts and emergency supply boxes include IV supplies. An IV line is usually inserted into the hand, wrist, or arm of the patient. If an IV line cannot be inserted, the provider may insert an intraosseous (in tra OS ee us) needle that can be used to give IV fluids and medications (Fig. 49.7). The intraosseous needle can be inserted into the humerus, tibia, femur, sternum, or iliac crest. The provider must be specially trained to insert the intraosseous needle.

Administering IV medications is outside the scope of practice for the medical assistant. In many states, inserting an IV

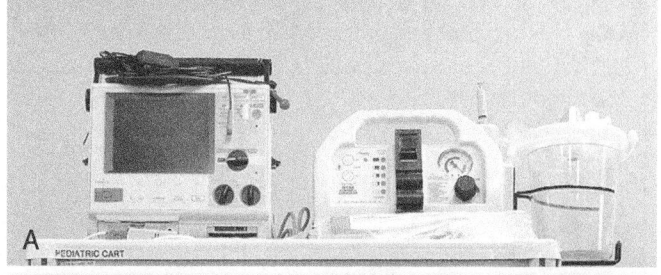
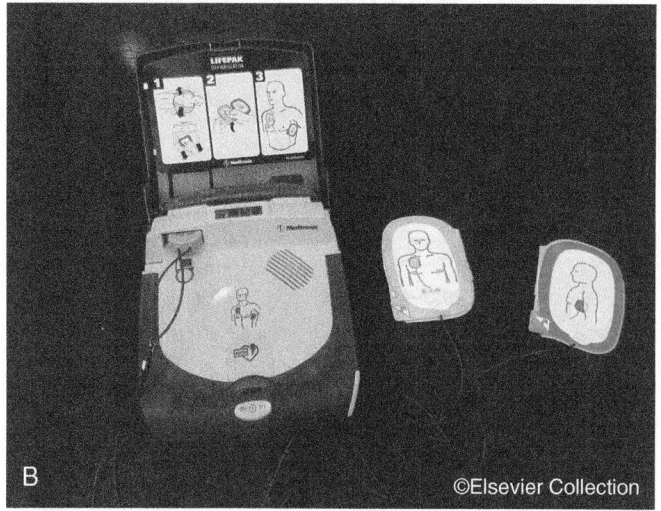

©Elsevier Collection

Fig. 49.6 A, *Left to right:* The defibrillator usually sits on top of the crash cart. Other equipment, such as a suction machine, can also be found on the top of the crash cart. *B,* Automated external defibrillator.

line and giving IV fluids are also outside the medical assistant's scope of practice. The medical assistant may help by getting the required supplies and documenting what was given.

MEDICAL TERMINOLOGY	
calc/o	calcium
epiglott/o	epiglottis
gluc/o, glyc/o	glucose, sugar
kal/i	potassium
laryng/o	voice box (larynx)
nas/o, rhino/o	nose
pharyng/o	pharynx
rhythm/o	rhythm
steth/o	chest
ventricul/o	ventricle
a-	without
brady-	slow
endo-	within
hyper-	excessive, above
hypo-	under, below
tachy-	rapid
-ar	pertaining to
-cardia	heart condition
-emia	blood condition
-ia	condition
-scope	instrument to view

VOCABULARY

intraosseous Within bone; route for delivery of fluids and medications through a needle inserted into the marrow of certain bones (e.g., humerus, tibia, and femur).

TABLE 49.1 Common Medications Used in Emergencies

Medications	Action	Used for
amiodarone (Cordarone, Pacerone) (ah mee OH dah rone)	Slows the heart rate and allows blood to fill the ventricular chambers.	Ventricular tachycardia (tack ee KAR dee ah), ventricular fibrillation (fibrill LAY shun)
Atropine (AT roe peen)	Increases the heart rate.	Bradycardia (brad dee KAR dee ah)
calcium chloride (KAL see uhm KLOR ide)	Increases the calcium levels in the serum.	Hyperkalemia and *hypocalcemia* (hye poe kal SEE mee ah) (too little calcium in the blood)
diazepam (Valium) (dye AZ ee pam)	Affects the chemicals in the brain.	Seizures (see zhurs), agitation
diphenhydramine (Benadryl) (DIE fen HYE dra meen)	Antihistamine that reduces the effects of histamine.	Allergic reactions, second-line drug for anaphylaxis (used after epinephrine has been given)
dopamine (Intropin) (DOE pah meen)	Increases the stimulation of the heart muscle.	Hypotension, heart failure
epinephrine (Epipen, Adrenalin) (EP i NEF rin)	Increases the stimulation of the heart muscle; vasoconstrictor and bronchial relaxant.	Anaphylaxis, cardiac arrest, severe asthma, bronchospasms
Glucagon (GLUE kah gon)	Hormone that stimulates the liver to release glucose into the blood.	*Hypoglycemia* (hye poh gly SEE mee ah) (too low glucose in the blood)
Lidocaine (LIE dah kane)	Helps to restore the regular heart rhythm.	Ventricular arrhythmias (ah RITH mee ah)
magnesium (mag NEE zee um)	Electrolyte that helps maintain a normal heart rhythm.	Arrhythmias (ah RITH mee ahs)
naloxone (Evzio, Narcan) (nal OX one)	Blocks or reverses the opioid medication effects.	Opioid (narcotic) overdose
nitroglycerin (nye troe GLI ser in)	Vasodilator.	Congestive heart failure, angina (an JYE nuh)
sodium bicarbonate (SOE dee uhm bye KAHR bah nate)	Reduces the pH of the serum.	Metabolic acidosis, *hyperkalemia* (hye per kuh LEE mee ah) (excessive potassium in the blood)

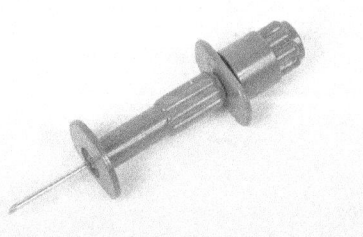

Fig. 49.7 An intraosseous needle maybe used to give intravenous fluids and medications in an emergency.

Other Supplies

Various other supplies can be found in the crash cart. Some items not already mentioned include:

- Personal protective equipment (PPE), such as gloves, a sharps disposal container, and a pocket face mask
- *Algorithms* (AL guh rith uhms), or step-by-step instructions, for reference
- Clipboard with documents for charting the code
- Backboard, which is placed under the patient to provide a firm surface for compressions
- Extra batteries for the laryngoscope

> **VOCABULARY**
> **pocket face mask** A device used to deliver a rescue breath.

Pediatric Supplies

In the 1980s, James Broselow, a family practice doctor working in an emergency department, came up with an idea for simplifying how to determine pediatric medication doses administered during emergencies. Medications for children are based on weight. Rescue personnel spent critical moments during emergencies calculating medication doses for children. Broselow's idea was to measure the child's length and come up with a suggested dose. After much research, the Broselow tape was created (Fig. 49.8A).

A healthcare professional measures a child using the tape. The tape is placed from the top of the head to the child's heel. The length is measured as a specific color (see Fig. 49.8B). Based on the "color" of the child, the tape lists common medication dosages and emergency equipment sizes that should be used for that size of child. This system has sped up the response time for treating children during emergencies. It eliminates the use of reference guides and calculators for medication dosages.

Many ambulatory care settings that routinely see sick children use the Broselow tape. In addition to the tape, pediatric crash carts (e.g., Broselow ColorCode Cart) have been created

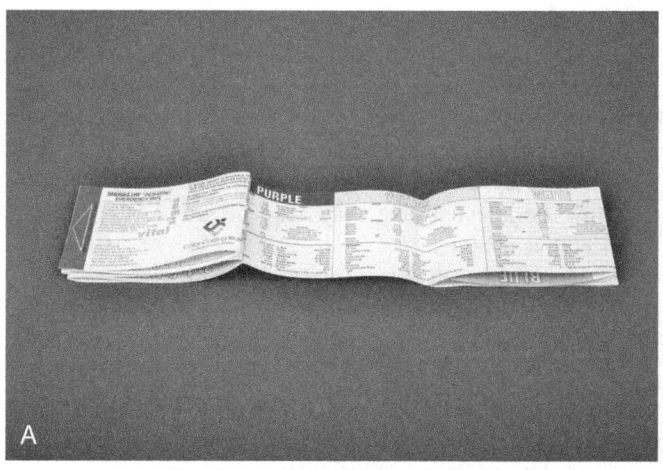
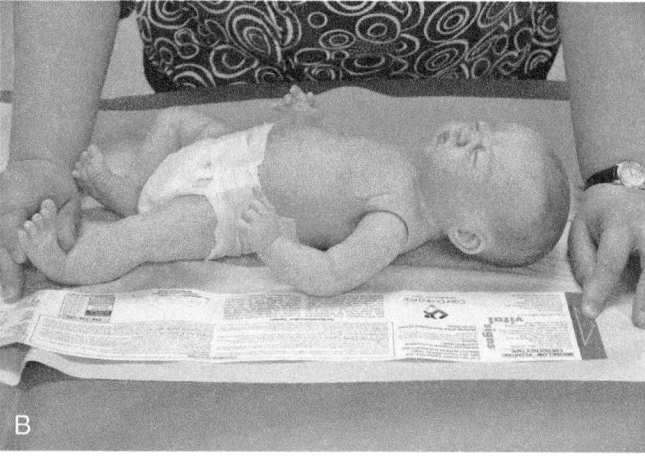

Fig. 49.8 A, Broselow tape. B, Measure the child with the Broselow tape. Measure from the head to the heel and identify the color by the child's heel. This is the color to use during the emergency.

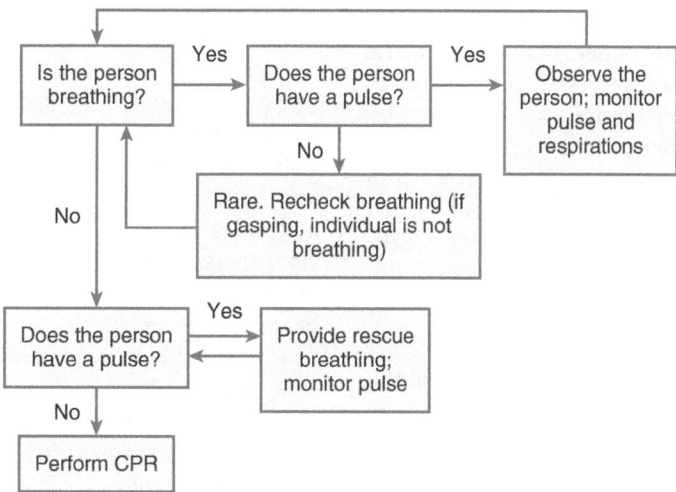

Fig. 49.9 Example of a Flow Map. Similar flow maps can be used when triaging or treating emergencies. *CPR,* Cardiopulmonary resuscitation.

(see Fig. 49.1B). Each color on the tape has a matching drawer. Each drawer contains the right-sized equipment for that size of child.

HANDLING EMERGENCIES

In the ambulatory care setting, many different types of emergencies can occur. Some of the more common emergencies include:

- A patient who is being seen and treated has a life-threatening occurrence (e.g., an allergic reaction to a medication).
- A person (e.g., employee, visitor, or patient) has an accident or health issue that results in an emergency.
- A *walk-in patient* (a patient without an appointment) comes to the facility with a critical health issue.
- An individual calls about an emergency.

How these are handled can differ greatly among ambulatory care facilities. Factors that affect how emergencies are handled include:

- Facility's size and distance from emergency medical services
- Available equipment and supplies
- Providers' training and scope of practice

- Number and type of clinical care employees (medical assistants, licensed practical nurses, and registered nurses) and their scopes of practice

Some facilities only have minimal staff, whereas others have specific employees who respond to emergencies.

In small facilities, the medical assistant may be responsible for screening emergency calls and walk-in patients. The medical assistant must follow the facility's screening protocols. They cannot assess the patient or give advice. The information collected must be reported to the provider. The provider tells the medical assistant what should be done. Examples of screening questions are provided later in the chapter.

In larger facilities, registered nurses (sometimes called triage [tree AHZH] nurses) gather information from walk-in patients and emergency calls. Using a triaging flow map or triaging software, the nurse identifies how quickly the patient needs to be seen and where the patient needs to be seen (Fig. 49.9).

VOCABULARY

triage To sort out and classify the injured; used in the military and emergency settings to determine the priority of a patient to be treated.

triaging flow map A written flow map to make triage decisions; based on answers to questions, the person moves through the map until a triage decision is made.

Sometimes patients come to the ambulatory healthcare setting with life-threatening conditions. The provider sees these patients immediately and assesses their conditions. The provider will order 911 to be called if needed. Treatment is provided as the team waits for the emergency responders to transport the patient to the emergency department. The following sections explain the first aid given for different types of emergencies.

CRITICAL THINKING 49.3

Gabe knows that there are times when medical assistants need to screen phone calls. This can be intimidating for new medical assistants. What procedures would Gabe put in place to help medical assistants screen emergency calls accurately yet minimize their feelings of intimidation?

ENVIRONMENTAL EMERGENCIES

Environmental emergencies arise from an exposure to a harmful environmental agent rather than a traumatic injury or medical condition already present in the patient. For instance, the outdoor temperature can cause a life-threatening condition. A bite from certain reptiles can cause death if not treated immediately. A flying piece of metal in a factory can cause blindness. Many environment-related emergencies are severe enough that the affected person seeks medical care.

Temperature-Related Emergencies

Overexposure to hot or cold temperatures can cause mild to life-threatening issues. Environmental temperatures affect the body's temperature.

Cold-Related Conditions. Cold-related conditions include frostbite and hypothermia. In cold weather, our bodies tend to lose heat faster than we can produce it. This results in a lowered body temperature. Uncovered skin can result in injuries faster than covered skin. It does not take long for frostbite to occur. For instance, with a 10 mile per hour (mph) wind speed and a temperature of −5°F (−20.6°C), a person can get frostbite in 30 minutes. With the same wind speed and a temperature of −25°F (−31.7°C), a person can get frostbite in 5 minutes. Risk factors for cold-related conditions include:

- Smoking or taking a beta-blocker medication (e.g., atenolol)
- Having diabetes or poor blood circulation
- High winds, wet clothes
- Dehydration and exhaustion

Possible screening questions for cold-related conditions include:

- What is the person's age?
- How long was the person exposed to the cold temperature?
- What symptoms does the person have? What color is the exposed skin?
- What is the person's medical history?

Frostbite. Frostbite occurs when the skin and body tissues are exposed to cold temperatures. Susceptible areas include cheeks, nose, ears, fingers, toes, and chin. Frostbite is caused by exposure to cold temperatures. The person may experience a pins and needles sensation followed by numbness in the frostbitten area. The skin is hard, pale, and cold; blisters may occur. The affected area may ache or lack feeling. First aid procedures include:

- Move the person to a warmer location.
- Remove all wet clothing and cover with warm dry clothing.
- Observe for signs of hypothermia.
- Seek medical care; if it is not available, then rewarm the area by soaking it in warm water (104°F to 108°F [40°C to 42.2°C]) for 20 to 30 minutes. Do not rub the area. Apply a sterile dressing to the area.
- Give the person a warm drink to replace lost fluids; do not give alcohol.

Hypothermia. With hypothermia, the core body temperature drops below 95°F (35°C). In severe hypothermia, the body temperature drops below 82°F (27.8°C), causing a life-threatening condition and arrhythmias. Hypothermia is caused by exposure to cold temperatures or immersion in cold water for a long period of time. A person with hypothermia may experience slurred speech and slow, shallow breathing and weak pulse. Additional signs and symptoms include clumsiness, drowsiness, confusion, and a loss of consciousness. With infants, the skin may be bright red and cold. First aid procedures include:

- Move the person to a warmer location.
- Remove all wet clothing and cover with warm dry clothing.
- Seek medical care.
- Give the person a warm drink to replace lost fluids; do not give alcohol.

Warming a patient with hypothermia too quickly can also lead to cardiac issues and additional tissue damage. Because of this, the emergency department gradually warms all patients with hypothermia.

Heat-Related Conditions. Heat-related conditions include heat cramps, exhaustion, and stroke. Heat injuries occur most often on hot, humid days and are caused by prolonged heat exposure. With high humidity, sweat, which cools the skin, does not evaporate as quickly. Risk factors for heat injuries include:

- Age (older adults and children age 4 and younger)
- Dehydration, heart disease, and poor blood circulation
- Fever and sunburn
- Mental illness
- Using alcohol and taking certain prescription drugs, such as antidepressants, anticonvulsants, antipsychotics, and diuretics

Possible screening questions for heat-related conditions include:

- What is the person's age?
- How long was the person exposed to the hot temperature?
- What symptoms does the person have? Is the person sweating? What does the skin look like? Is the person alert or confused?

It is important to treat heat-related illnesses immediately. An untreated condition can progress to become a more severe situation. An effective way to lower the person's temperature is to apply cool, wet cloths and then fan the moist skin. This will lower the person's body temperature by the evaporation process.

Heat Cramps. Heat cramps are a mild heat-related illness that causes muscle pain and spasms due to electrolyte imbalance. It usually occurs with strenuous activities or in those who sweat a lot. The person may experience muscle pains or spasms in the abdomen, arms, or legs. First aid measures include:
- Rest for several hours in a cool place.
- Drink cool electrolyte (sports) beverages to replace electrolytes lost.

Heat Exhaustion. Heat exhaustion is a milder form of a heat-related illness. It is caused by exposure to high temperatures and inadequate fluid and electrolyte replacement. A person with heat exhaustion may experience:
- Heavy sweating, muscle cramps, nausea, and vomiting
- Pale, cool, moist skin
- Fast, weak pulse and fast, shallow respirations
- Tiredness, weakness, dizziness, headache, and fainting

First aid procedures for heat exhaustion include:
- Move to a shady or air-conditioned area and rest.
- Drink cool sports beverages.
- Do not drink caffeinated or alcoholic beverages.
- Take a cool shower or sponge bath.

Heat Stroke. Heat stroke is a serious heat-related illness. The body is unable to sweat and thus cannot cool down. The body temperature over 103°F (39°C). The skin is red, hot, and dry. The person may have a rapid, strong pulse. Dizziness, a throbbing headache, nausea, confusion, and eventually loss of consciousness can occur.

First aid procedures include:
- Move the person to a shady or air-conditioned area.
- Spray or sponge down the person with cool water.
- Seek medical attention immediately.

Burns

Heat, freezing cold temperatures, chemicals, sunlight, radiation, and electricity can cause burns to the body tissues. Hot liquids, fires, and flammable products are the most common causes of burns. Breathing in smoke can cause inhalation injuries.

Possible screening questions for burns include:
- What occurred? What caused the burn?
- Where was the person burned?
- What symptoms does the person have? What does the person's skin look like?
- If the burn affects the face or chest, is the person experiencing any breathing issues?

Table 49.2 describes the different degrees of burns. Providers estimate the percent of total burn surface area (%TBSA) by using the Rule of Nines diagram (Fig. 49.10). Table 49.3 shows the difference between the Rule of Nines for an adult and for a child.

Poisonings

Poison can enter the body through swallowing, inhaling, injecting, or absorbing it through the skin. Common poisons include:
- Medications (prescription or over the counter) taken in high doses
- Overdoses of illegal drugs
- Household products, such as laundry detergent, furniture polish, and cleaning products
- Indoor and outdoor plants
- Pesticides and fertilizers
- Metals, such as mercury and lead

The American Association of Poison Control Centers is a national poison resource with 55 centers around the country. This resource is available online (https://poisonhelp.org/) and via a hotline (1-800-222-1222). Medical assistants should have the phone number and website available for reference. If the medical assistant receives a call regarding a poisoning, the call must be handled according to the facility's protocols. Many times, the medical assistant must contact Poison Control while keeping the patient on the phone. The medical assistant then relays the information from Poison Control to the patient.

Signs and symptoms of poisoning can develop over time. They can also vary based on the poison. Some examples of symptoms include:
- Bluish lips, cough, and difficulty breathing
- Heart palpitations and chest pain

TABLE 49.2	Types of Burns			
Condition	First-degree burn	Second-degree burn	Third-degree burn	Fourth-degree burn
Also known as	Superficial burn	Partial-thickness burn	Full-thickness burn	Deep full-thickness burn
Description	Damage to epidermis.	Damage to the epidermis and part of the dermis	Damage to the epidermis, dermis, and subcutaneous tissue	Damage beyond the subcutaneous tissue into the muscle and bone (not universally accepted)
Signs and symptoms	Redness (*erythema*), tenderness, physical sensitivity. No scar development.	Redness, blisters, and pain. Possible scar development.	No pain because nerve endings are destroyed. Skin appears deep red, pale gray, brown, or black. Scar formation is likely.	
First aid procedures	For minor burns: • For unbroken skin, soak in cool water (not ice water) for at least 5 minutes. • Cover with sterile dressing. (For second-degree burns 3 inches or larger or located on the hands, feet, groin, buttock, or over a joint, treat as major burn.)		For major burns: • Seek immediate medical attention (call 911). • Do not remove burned clothing stuck to skin. • Monitor breathing. Perform rescue breathing or cardiopulmonary resuscitation (CPR) as needed. • Raise burned body part above the heart level. • Separate burned fingers or toes with a dry, sterile dressing.	

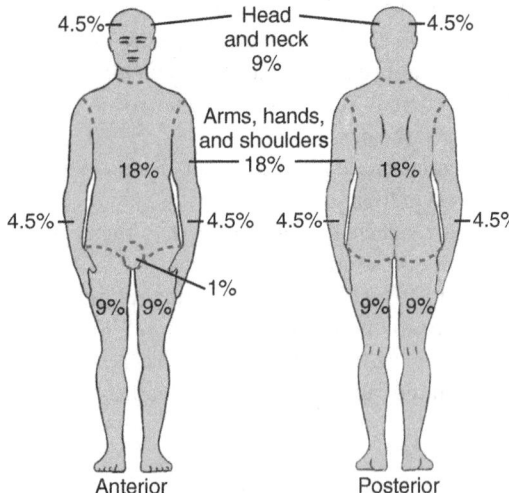

4.5% — Head and neck 9% — 4.5%

Arms, hands, and shoulders 18%

18% 18% 18%

4.5% 4.5% 4.5% 4.5%

1%

9% 9% 9% 9%

Anterior   Posterior

Fig. 49.10 Rule of Nines for Adults. (From Callen JP, Greer KE, Saller AS, et al: *Color atlas of dermatology*, ed 2, St. Louis, 2000, Mosby/Elsevier.)

TABLE 49.3 Rule of Nines for Adults and Children

	Adult	Child
Head and neck	9%	18%
Front of torso	18%	18%
Back	18%	18%
Arm, hand, and shoulder	9% (LA) 9% (RA)	9% (LA) 9% (RA)
Leg and foot	18% (LL) 18% (RL)	13.5% (LL) 13.5% (RL)
Genital	1%	1%
Total	100%	100%

LA, Left arm; *LL*, left leg; *RA*, right arm; *RL*, right leg.

- Nausea, vomiting, and abdominal pain
- Numbness, tingling, dizziness, weakness, double vision, drowsiness, irritability, and headache
- Unusual odor
- Confusion, seizures, stupor, and unconsciousness

First aid includes checking and monitoring the person's airway, breathing, and pulse. If required, rescue breathing and CPR are provided. Call 911 for medical help. If the person vomits, clear the airway. Monitor the person until help arrives. If poisoning is suspected, it is important to identify what the toxin is, and the amount taken (Box 49.1).

Do not have the person vomit unless you are instructed to do so by the Poison Control staff. If the person has swallowed a corrosive substance, it will cause additional injury as it is vomited. In this type of situation, a tube must be passed into the stomach to remove the substance. This is usually done in the emergency department.

CRITICAL THINKING 49.4

Where might Gabe post the Poison Control numbers around the clinic? Describe places where this number will be useful.

BOX 49.1 Poisoning Facts

- Children younger than 6 years of age make up about half of the poisoning exposures reported.
- Children ages 1 to 2 have the greatest risk of poisoning.
- Cosmetics and personal care products, followed by cleaning products, are the most common substances involved in childhood poison exposures.
- About 22% of adult poisonings and 48% of teen poisonings are suspected suicides.
- Analgesics, followed by sedative/hypnotics/antipsychotic medications, are the top substances in adult poisonings.

From Poison Control. https://www.poison.org/poison-statistics-national.

Chemical Exposures

Chemical exposures can cause burns or be absorbed through the skin or lungs. Information on treatments for chemical exposures can be obtained from products' Safety Data Sheet (SDS) or by contacting the Poison Control Center.

Follow the information for first aid from the SDS or the Poison Control Center. Typical first aid for chemical exposures involves:

- Removing the person from the source of exposure, while protecting yourself from exposure. If the chemical is on the person's clothing, the clothing should be removed. If the chemical is airborne, bring the person to fresh air.
- For chemical exposures affecting the lungs, bring the person to fresh air.
- For chemical exposures of the eye, flush the eye with cool water for 15 minutes while protecting the other eye from an accidental exposure.

Patients with symptoms of shock, trouble breathing, or burns call 911 and be seen in the emergency department. While waiting for help, provide rescue breathing or CPR as needed.

Anaphylaxis

Anaphylaxis (AN ah fi LAK sis) is a severe allergic reaction that can be life-threatening. The most common allergens include:

- Animal dander
- Insect bites and stings (especially bee stings)
- Medicines
- Plants and pollens
- Foods: Eggs, fish, milk, tree nuts (hazelnuts, walnuts, almonds, Brazil nuts), peanuts (groundnuts), shellfish (crab, mussels, shrimp), soy, and wheat

Anaphylaxis signs and symptoms include:

- Anxiety, warm feeling, and flushing
- Shortness of breath (SOB), *dyspnea* (difficulty breathing), wheezing, and cough
- Throat tightening, difficulty swallowing
- Pain or cramping, vomiting, and diarrhea
- Palpitations, dizziness, shock, and loss of consciousness

Allergic reactions that affect breathing are life-threatening. First aid for severe allergic reactions includes:

- Do the 3Cs: Check the scene for safety. Call 911. Care for the victim (Box 49.2).

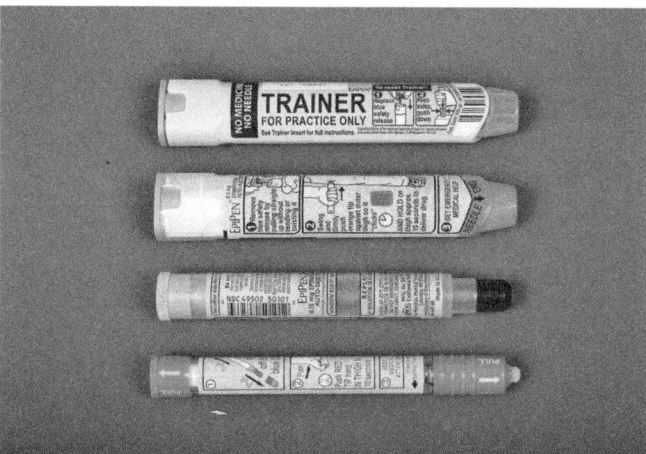

Fig. 49.11 *Top to bottom:* Trainer that comes with the EpiPen, adult EpiPen, EpiPen Jr., and a generic adult epinephrine pen.

- Give epinephrine (e.g., EpiPen) if the person has it available (Fig. 49.11).
- Stay with the individual and try to keep the person calm.
- If the person has a bee sting, scrape the stinger off the skin if it is visible. Use a fingernail or credit card to scrape it. Do not use tweezers, which can squeeze the stinger, releasing more venom.
- Monitor the individual's airway, breathing, and pulse. Perform rescue breathing or CPR if needed.
- Have the person lie flat and raise the feet 12 inches. Keep the person warm. This will help to prevent shock.

In the ambulatory care facility, if the medical assistant suspects the patient is starting to have an allergic reaction, they should immediately notify the provider. The provider will order epinephrine and oxygen to be administered. Research has shown that epinephrine administered intramuscularly (IM) into the vastus lateralis absorbs quicker than that given IM in the deltoid or subcutaneously in the arm. If ordered, repeat every 5 to 10 minutes. Do not administer repeated injections in the same site, because vasoconstriction may cause tissue necrosis (neck KROH sis). The typical dose of epinephrine injectable solution (1 mg/mL) for anaphylaxis is:

- Children and adults (66 lb [30 kg] or more): 0.3 to 0.5 mg (0.3–0.5 mL)
- Children (under 66 lb [30 kg]): 0.01 mg/kg (0.01 mL/kg) with a maximum dose per injection of 0.3 mL

VOCABULARY

necrosis Tissue death.

pruritus Itching.

vasoconstriction Contraction of the muscles, causing narrowing of the inside tube of the vessel.

Insect Bites and Stings

Insect bites and stings can cause immediate skin reactions, including pain, burning, erythema, numbness, swelling, and *pruritus* (proo RIE tuss). In some cases, the venom can cause severe illness and death. Some people have anaphylactic reactions to stings and bites (e.g., bee stings). Anaphylaxis symptoms were addressed in the prior section. If the medical assistant receives a phone call regarding a bite or sting, it is important to gather additional information for the provider, such as:

- What bit you?
- Do you have any allergies?
- How does the wound look? Describe the wound to me.
- Are you having any problems breathing? Any wheezing, shortness of breath, or difficulty breathing?
- Is there any swelling in the mouth or lips?

First aid for severe reactions includes all the steps indicated in the anaphylaxis section. Additional steps include removing any nearby constricting items, such as rings and clothing. The affected area may swell, and constricting items can cause additional problems. First aid for mild reactions includes:

- Move to a safe location.
- Remove the stinger if it is visible.
- Wash the affected area with soap and water.
- To reduce pain and swelling, apply a cool cloth and elevate the extremity.
- For pain, apply hydrocortisone (HIE drah KOHR ti zone) or lidocaine cream to the area. An over-the-counter pain reliever can also be taken.
- *Calamine* (KAL ah min) lotion or a similar product can be applied to the area to reduce the pruritus.

Patients may also call for advice on removing ticks. Ticks can spread diseases, including Rocky Mountain spotted fever, Powassan virus, Babesia infection, Lyme disease, and ehrlichiosis. If a person has a tick embedded, it needs to be removed. Wear gloves and use a fine-tipped, pointed tweezers. Get as close to the head as possible. Do not squeeze the abdomen, because it may inject secretions into the person's body. Slowly pull the head out. Do not twist. Do not burn it or use petroleum jelly or nail polish. Once the tick is removed, place it in a container of rubbing alcohol to kill it. Clean the site with antiseptic soap and water. Apply an antibiotic ointment. Monitor the site for infections or other complications.

CRITICAL THINKING 49.5

Gabe realized that there were no patient education pamphlets in the exam rooms. He would like to talk with his supervisor about getting brochure racks for each room. His thought was to include procedures on home emergencies/first aid for patients. If you were Gabe, describe the talking points you could make to your supervisor in favor of placing patient education materials in the exam rooms.

Animal Bites

Patients who have animal bites will typically seek care or call their providers. It is important for the medical assistant to ask some screening questions before talking with the provider, such as:

- What type of animal bit you? Do you know the animal? If so, are the shots up to date?
- How does the wound look? Is it bleeding, dirty, or deep? Was it a puncture wound?
- Have you had the rabies vaccine series?
- When was your last tetanus vaccine?

Frequently, the bites are caused by domestic pets (e.g., dogs and cats). First aid for minor bites that only break the skin includes washing the area with soap and water. Then the person should apply over-the-counter antibiotic cream and cover the area with a clean bandage.

It is important to seek medical attention in the following situations:

- *For fang punctures*: For instance, cat bites. Bacteria are left deep in the puncture wound. Initially the wound may not look bad, but in a few hours the entire area could be hot and swollen.
- *For bleeding wounds*: Apply pressure with a clean cloth or bandage and seek help.
- *For dirty or deep wounds*: The person may require a tetanus vaccine booster if the last injection was given 5 or more years earlier.
- *For wounds that look infected*: The wound may look swollen, red, painful, or oozing.
- *For questions about the rabies risk*: Any wild or domestic mammal can get rabies and pass it on to people. Animals commonly seen with rabies include raccoons, skunks, bats, woodchucks (groundhogs), foxes, coyotes, cats, dogs, and cattle.

In the ambulatory care facility, the wound is examined, cleaned, and bandaged. The medical assistant should gather information on the patient's last tetanus booster. A tetanus immunization may be given. If there is a chance of rabies exposure, the provider will discuss the treatment options. Treatment for rabies can be costly, and the treatment time window is narrow. Table 49.4 describes the medications that can be given as treatment.

Foreign Body in the Eye

It is common for people with "something in the eye" to call or visit the ambulatory healthcare facility. This condition is known as a foreign body in the eye.

First aid for a foreign body in the eye is eye irrigation. Washing your hands before starting is important. Flush the eye with clean, warm water or with saline eyedrops. Saline eyedrops will be less irritating than water. If the foreign body cannot be removed through irrigation, the person should seek immediate medical care. It is important not to rub the eye, which may cause further damage.

In the ambulatory care facility, the medical assistant needs to ask the patient how the injury occurred. Further irrigation may be ordered after the provider examines the patient. It is important to check the date of the patient's last tetanus booster. The provider may order an updated tetanus booster, along with additional treatments.

DIABETIC EMERGENCIES

Diabetic emergencies occur when the person's blood glucose level is too low or too high. When a person eats carbohydrates (starches and sugars [e.g., breads, candy]), the blood glucose level rises. Insulin from the pancreas or insulin injections help bring down the blood glucose level. Insulin is the only thing that moves the glucose out of the blood and into the cells, where it is used for energy. Without enough insulin, the blood glucose level rises. With too much insulin, the blood glucose level drops (Table 49.5).

If the blood glucose gets too high (*hyperglycemia*) or too low (*hypoglycemia*), the person can go into a diabetic coma. Permanent brain damage and death can occur. If you come across an unresponsive person, check to see if the individual has a medical alert bracelet or necklace. (Some individuals have tattoos instead of wearing the medical alert jewelry.) The medical alert information may provide clues to what is occurring.

First aid for hypoglycemia includes:

- Test the blood glucose level if possible.
- If the individual is conscious and able to swallow: Give 4 ounces of fruit juice or regular (not diet) soda or three glucose tablets. Test the blood glucose every 15 minutes. If the

TABLE 49.4	**Rabies Postexposure Treatment for Nonimmunized Individuals**	
Medication	**Purpose**	**Administration**
Rabies immune globulin (RIG)	Antibodies specifically for rabies. Provides rapid (immediate) passive immune protection against rabies.	Dose based on weight. Administer only once between day 0 (day of the bite) and day 7. Provider injects RIG around the bite wound if present. Remaining RIG is administered intramuscularly (IM) in the vastus lateralis or deltoid muscle (most distant from the wound). *If required, live-virus vaccines (varicella, measles) must be either given with or spaced out 4 months after RIG.*
Rabies vaccine	Helps to provide long-term active immune protection against rabies.	Administer 1 mL IM in the deltoid muscle for adults and the vastus lateralis for children. Administer one dose on days 0, 3, 7, and 14. A fifth dose may be recommended on day 28 for immunocompromised individuals.

TABLE 49.5   Diabetic Emergencies

	Insulin shock	Diabetic ketoacidosis (DKA)
Alternative names	Severe *hypoglycemia* (low blood glucose); insulin reaction	Severe *hyperglycemia* (high blood glucose)
Why does it occur?	Imbalance between insulin and blood glucose. Too little glucose is in the blood because the individual: • Took too much insulin • Ate too few carbohydrates • Engaged in too much physical activity • Drank alcohol (may occur up to 2 days after drinking)	Imbalance between insulin and blood glucose. Too much glucose is in the blood because the individual: • Took too little insulin • Ate too many carbohydrates • Is ill, has an infection, trauma, or surgery • Used an illegal drug (e.g., cocaine, ecstasy)
Symptoms	**Hypoglycemia** • Double or blurry vision • Fast pulse, palpitations • Irritable, aggressive, nervous • Headache, unclear thinking • Shaking, tired • Sweaty, cold skin • Hunger **Severe Hypoglycemia** • Disorientation, unconsciousness • Seizures • Shock • Diabetic coma and death	**Hyperglycemia** • Thirsty, hungry, stomach pain • Nausea, vomiting • Frequent urination • Fatigue • Shortness of breath • Very dry mouth • Rapid pulse **Diabetic Ketoacidosis** • Fruity odor on breath • Diabetic coma and death

blood glucose is under 70, give additional glucose. Continue until the glucose level is 70 or above (Procedure 49.1).

• If the individual is unconscious: Place the patient in the recovery position (Fig. 49.12 and Box 49.3). Call 911 and get medical help. Monitor the airway and pulse. Perform rescue breathing and CPR as needed. For an unconscious adult patient, glucagon 1 mL is given subcutaneously or IM (Fig. 49.13). Repeat the dose in 15 minutes if the patient is unconscious. (Children younger than 6 years of age get 0.5 mL.) Monitor the blood glucose. Once the patient is alert and able to swallow, give additional food (e.g., a sandwich).

First aid for hyperglycemia includes:

• Call 911 and get medical help. Monitor the airway and pulse. Perform rescue breathing and CPR as needed.
• The patient will need IV fluids, insulin, and monitoring to bring down the blood glucose level.

VOCABULARY

recovery position A position on the person's side that helps to keep the airway open and clear.

MUSCULOSKELETAL EMERGENCIES

Without a diagnosis, it is hard to tell if an injury is a strain, sprain, fracture, or dislocation. It is important always to treat the injury as a fracture until the provider diagnoses the injury. A few symptoms will indicate if the injury is more severe (e.g., dislocation), including:

• The person has difficulty moving the extremity normally or is not able to do so.
• The extremity is deformed.
• Bone is exposed through the skin.
• There is heavy bleeding.

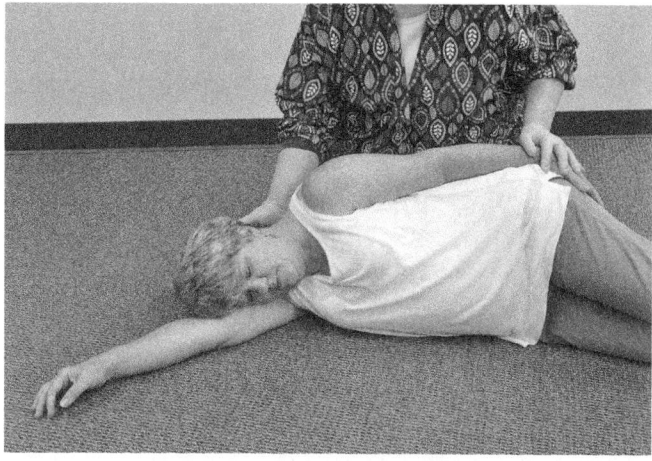

Fig. 49.12 Recovery Position.

BOX 49.3   Placing a Person in the Recovery Position

• While kneeling at the person's side, place the lowermost arm next to the head with the palm facing up. Take the other arm and place it next to the person's side.
• Bend the lowermost leg up.
• You want to roll the person as one unit in case of head, neck, or spinal injuries. To do this, carefully slide one arm under the person's shoulder closest to you and the other under the arm and hip. Roll the person away from you and onto their side.
• Bend the top leg at the knee and place on top of the other knee. Place the upper arm near the person's hip.

If a person has any of these symptoms or the injury was related to major trauma, call 911 and get medical help. Additional first aid steps involve:

• *For bleeding*: Apply pressure to the wound with a clean cloth or sterile bandage.
• *Immobilize the injured area*: Do not push the bone back. Do not move the area affected by the injury. Apply a splint beyond

the joint above and the joint below the injury (Fig. 49.14 and Box 49.4).

- *To limit swelling*: Apply a cold pack to the area. Make sure to cover the cold pack with a towel. Do not apply the cold pack directly on the skin (Fig. 49.15).
- *If the person is going into shock*: Make sure the person is lying down with the head slightly lower than the abdomen and elevate the legs. Monitor the person's breathing and pulse rate. Provide rescue breathing and CPR if needed.

Many times, patients will contact their provider regarding musculoskeletal injuries. The medical assistant should screen the patient and relay the information to the provider. Possible screening questions for musculoskeletal emergencies include:

- What happened?
- What does the injured body part look like? Is it deformed? Is it bleeding?
- Can the person move the injured part? Is there pain?
- How does the skin look over and near the injury?

Typically, the provider will need to examine the patient; then an x-ray will be taken before a final diagnosis is made. Depending on the diagnosis, the medical assistant may need to help apply a splint, cast, sling, or another device. Good patient education is required. The medical assistant should coach the patient on checking the circulation on the affected extremity. Coaching the patient on how to handle the protective device (e.g., cast, splint) while doing basic hygiene activities (e.g., showering) is important. Typically, musculoskeletal injuries require **r**est, **i**ce, **c**ompression, and **e**levation (RICE).

NEUROLOGIC EMERGENCIES

Neurologic emergencies can range from minor conditions, such as dizziness, to serious conditions, such as stroke. The medical assistant should know how to handle neurologic emergencies.

Vertigo and Dizziness

Vertigo (VUR tih goh) is a false sensation that you or your environment is spinning or moving. *Peripheral vertigo* is caused by a problem in the inner ear (i.e., vestibular labyrinth, semicircular canals, and vestibular nerve). This issue affects the sense of balance. *Central vertigo* is caused by a brainstem or cerebellum disorder. It can be caused by certain drugs (e.g., aspirin, anticonvulsants, and alcohol), migraines, multiple sclerosis, stroke, and tumors.

With dizziness, people may feel light-headed or lose their balance. Many people get dizzy if they move too quickly from a sitting or lying position to a standing position. Their blood pressure drops, causing dizziness. People may feel as if they will

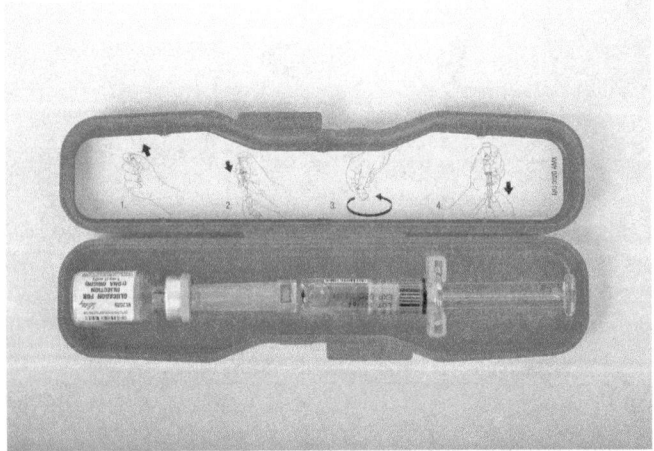

Fig. 49.13 Glucagon is given to unconscious patients with diabetes. This hormone stimulates the liver to release glucose into the bloodstream, thus increasing the blood glucose level.

BOX 49.4   Applying a Splint

- Splint the body part in the position it is in. Do not attempt to readjust the area or straighten it.
- Use a commercial splint or create a splint. Use sticks, a board, or rolled up magazines, newspaper, or clothing as a splint.
- Make sure the splint extends below and above the injury.
- Secure the splint with ties (e.g., belt, cloth strips).
- Check the injured area for swelling, paleness, or numbness, which may indicate the ties are too tight. Loosen ties if needed.

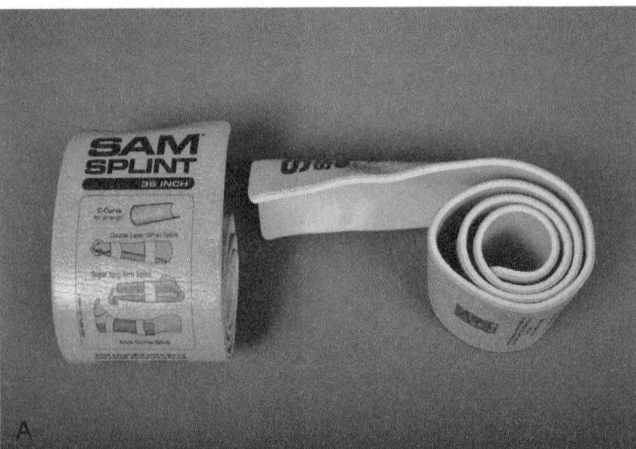

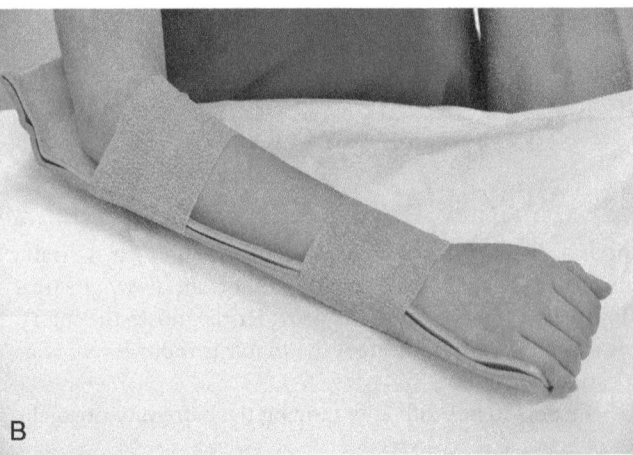

Fig. 49.14 A, A SAM Splint is a reusable splint that can conform to the extremity affected by the injury. B, Splint beyond the joint above and below the injury.

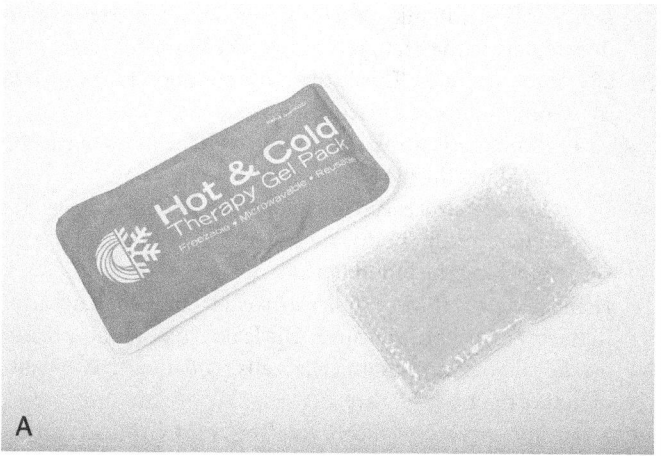 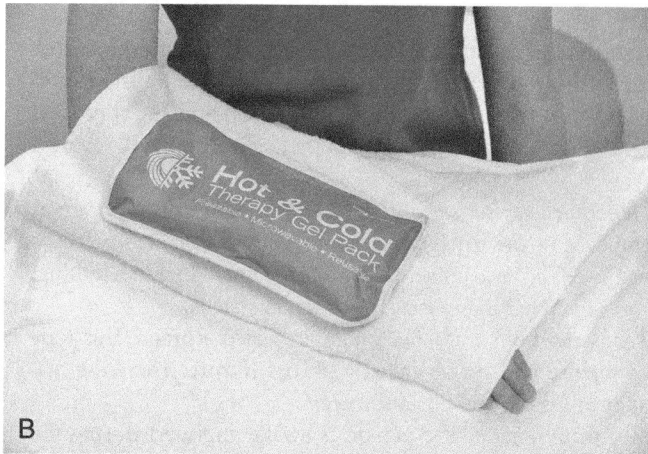

Fig. 49.15 A, Some reusable packs can be either cold or hot packs. B, A cold or hot pack cannot be applied directly to the skin. Place a towel between the pack and the skin.

pass out. Usually dizziness resolves on its own, but it could be a symptom of another disorder.

First aid for vertigo and dizziness involves sitting or lying down. The affected person should gradually resume activities when the episode passes. In addition, they should avoid sudden position changes and bright lights and should drink more fluids. The patient should contact the provider if any of the following apply:

- This is the first episode of vertigo or dizziness.
- The episodes are increasing in number.
- The episodes are getting worse.

Concussion

A *concussion* (kahn KUSH ehn) is a traumatic brain injury caused by a blow to the head. Violently shaking the head can also cause a concussion. Concussions can occur with sports injuries, falls, physical assaults, and traffic accidents. Concussion symptoms may be slow to develop and could last for weeks. Symptoms include:

- Head pressure or headache
- Temporary loss of consciousness right after the incident
- Confusion, amnesia, disorientation, irritability, and personality changes
- Dizziness and ringing in the ears
- Nausea and vomiting; taste and smell issues
- Slurred speech and delayed response to questions
- Listlessness, tiredness, sleep disturbances, and concentration and memory problems
- Loss of balance and unsteady gait (walk)

First aid for moderate to severe head injuries involves immediately calling 911. Monitor the person until help arrives. Check the breathing and pulse. Provide rescue breathing and CPR as needed. If the person is breathing and has a pulse, treat the condition as a spinal injury. Stabilize the head and neck by placing your hands on both sides of the person's head. Prevent any movement of the head and keep the head in line with the spine until help arrives. If the person vomits, roll the person to the side, and move the head, neck, and body as one unit.

Moderate to severe head injuries are often seen in the emergency department.

Patients will call or come to ambulatory care facilities if they have a possible concussion or a mild head injury (Procedure 49.2). Possible screening questions include:

- What happened?
- Did the person lose consciousness? If so, for how long?
- Any bleeding? Any vomiting?
- How is the person doing?
- Are the pupils dilated, or is one larger than the other?
- Does the person remember what happened? Is the person confused or slurring their speech?

For mild head injuries, usually a person should seek medical treatment with the occurance of:

- Loss of consciousness lasting longer than 30 seconds after the initial injury
- Repeated vomiting
- Worsening headache
- Changes in behavior or coordination (irritable, stumbling, or falling)
- Changes in orientation and speech (disoriented, confused, or slurred speech)
- Neurologic changes (seizures, visual disturbance, recurrent dizziness, difficulty with concentration, and one pupil larger than the other or both pupils dilated)

The patient may need to undergo radiologic testing to check for skull fractures and internal bleeding. If there are no fractures, the provider will educate the patient about other symptoms that would require follow-up and postconcussion care. Athletes need to refrain from playing sports until the concussion symptoms are gone. Another hit on the head can cause additional damage.

> ### CRITICAL THINKING 49.6
>
> Gabe has a 12-year-old son who plays middle school football. Before the season started, Gabe and his wife had to sign an acknowledgment form discussing concussions. What are the benefits of informing parents of school athletes about concussion symptoms?

Seizures

A seizure is a sudden increase of electrical activity in one or more parts of the brain. Epilepsy is a disorder that causes recurring seizures. Seizures are classified based on how the abnormal brain activity begins. The three major classifications of seizures are:

- *Generalized onset seizure*: Affects both sides of the brain at the same time. Includes several types of seizures, such as tonic-clonic and absent. Symptoms may include jerking, rigid or twitching muscles, and staring spells.
- *Focal onset seizure*: Affects one area of the brain. This type of seizure used to be called a partial seizure. There are two subgroups of focal onset seizures:
  - *Aware seizure*: The person is awake and alert during the seizure.
  - *Impaired awareness seizure*: The person is confused during the seizure. This type of seizure was known as a complex partial seizure.
- *Unknown onset seizure*: When the seizure began is not known.

In most situations, seizures last 30 seconds to 2 minutes. Usually, they do not cause lasting issues. It is a medical emergency if the seizure lasts longer than 5 minutes or if a person has multiple seizures without becoming conscious between them.

Parents commonly call when their child has had a seizure. According to the facility's protocol, the medical assistant may need to ask some screening questions and relay the information to the provider. Possible screening questions for musculoskeletal emergencies include:

- What did the patient do during the seizure? How long was the seizure?
- Did the person lose consciousness?
- How is the patient now after the seizure?

If a person has a seizure in the healthcare facility, the medical assistant must also notify the provider immediately (Procedure 49.3). First aid for seizures focuses on the safety of the individual:

- Move the person to the floor and place the patient in the recovery position. Gently raise the chin to tilt the head back slightly to open the airway. Monitor the person's breathing and pulse. Perform rescue breathing after the seizure has stopped if the patient does not resume breathing. Provide CPR if needed.
- Protect the patient from harm. Clear the area of anything hard or sharp. Place a soft, folded towel under the head.
- Do not place anything in the patient's mouth.
- Remove any glasses and loosen any constrictive clothing around the neck (e.g., ties).
- Time the length of the seizure. Call 911 if the seizure lasts longer than 5 minutes.
- Stay with the person until they are fully awake and alert.

Cerebrovascular Accident

A cerebrovascular (she ree broh VAS kyoo lur) accident (CVA), also called a *stroke,* is a medical emergency. There are three types of strokes:

- *Ischemic* (I SKEE mik) *stroke*: Occurs when the arterial blood flow to part of the brain is blocked. The brain cells start to die after a few minutes. This is the most common type of stroke. Two common types of ischemic stroke are:
  - *Thrombotic stroke*: A blood clot forms in an artery, blocking the blood flow to part of the brain.
  - *Embolic stroke*: A blood clot or other debris forms elsewhere in the body and moves into the brain arteries, blocking the blood flow.
- *Hemorrhagic* (HEM or aj ik) *stroke*: Occurs when an artery in the brain leaks or ruptures. The leaked blood puts pressure on the surrounding brain cells, causing damage. Two causes of hemorrhagic stroke are:
  - *Intracerebral hemorrhage*: The most common type of stroke; it occurs when a cerebral aneurysm ruptures.
  - *Subarachnoid hemorrhage*: Bleeding occurs in the subarachnoid space, usually as a result of small aneurysms.
- *Transient ischemic attack* (TIA): Also called a "mini-stroke" because it lasts for only a few minutes. The blood supply to a part of the brain is briefly blocked. Symptoms are similar to stroke symptoms but do not last as long (e.g., 1 to 24 hours).

The symptoms of a CVA relate to the part of the brain affected. The individual may not have all the symptoms. Possible symptoms of CVAs include:

- Confusion or mental changes; sudden severe headache
- Speech problems (difficulty forming words, difficult to understand, or using words that do not make sense)
- Numbness of the face, arm, or leg, usually on one side of the body
- Problem seeing in one or both eyes; facial drooping
- Trouble walking, lack of coordination or balance, or arm weakness

First aid for stroke-type symptoms involves getting help (calling 911) immediately (Box 49.5). The emergency department (ED) is the best place for a patient to go. There is a small window of time during which clot-dissolving medications (e.g., a tissue plasminogen activator) can be given to help the body break down the clot that is blocking the artery. If a bleeding artery has caused the stroke, the ED providers can detect this on radiologic studies.

If a patient comes to the ambulatory care facility with stroke-like symptoms, it is important for the provider to see the patient immediately. Be ready to call 911 when the provider orders you to do so. Also, monitor the patient's vital signs for changes.

MEDICAL TERMINOLOGY	
cerebr/o	cerebrum
vascul/o	vessel
-ar	pertaining to

RESPIRATORY EMERGENCIES

Respiratory emergencies can create a number of different signs and symptoms. For example:

- Skin: Unusually moist, flushed, pale, bluish, or ashen
- Respirations: Slow, rapid, deep, or shallow; trouble breathing or no breathing
- Audible breathing sounds: Gasping, gurgling, high-pitched noises (e.g., whistling sound), wheezing
- Patient complaints: Shortness of breath, dizziness, light-headedness, chest pain, tingling in the extremities, a sense of fearfulness

It is important to get help immediately with respiratory emergencies. After calling 911, help the conscious individual into a comfortable position and monitor the respirations and pulse. Be ready to provide rescue breathing and CPR if required.

Common respiratory emergencies are discussed in the following sections. It is important for the medical assistant to recognize when a patient is having a respiratory emergency and get help immediately.

Hyperventilation

Hyperventilation, or overbreathing, is rapid and deep breathing. This leads to a low carbon dioxide level in the blood. This gas imbalance creates symptoms that can mimic those of a heart attack, thus increasing the person's anxiety, in addition to the hyperventilation. Symptoms of hyperventilation include:

- Dry mouth, belching, and bloating
- Light-headedness, weakness, dizziness, and difficulty concentrating
- Shortness of breath and breathlessness
- Chest pain and heart palpitations
- Numbness and tingling in the arms or around the mouth
- Muscle spasms

Hyperventilation can be caused by many things, including panic attacks, stress, anxiety, bleeding, heart attack, drugs, and infections.

First aid treatments focus on raising the carbon dioxide level in the blood. This can be done by relaxing and using pursed lip breathing or slowly blowing out through the lips. A person should seek medical care if the hyperventilation episodes get worse. After diagnosing the condition, the provider may have the patient breathe slowly into a paper bag. This helps to restore the carbon dioxide and oxygen balance in the blood.

Asthma Attack

Asthma affects the airway and the lungs. During an asthma attack, the airway constricts, reducing the air moving into and out of the lungs. Mucus clogs up the airway, making airflow more difficult. Asthma causes wheezing, breathlessness, chest tightness, and coughing. Typically, asthma attacks occur at night or in the early morning hours.

If a patient or family member calls about an asthma attack, it is important to gather information quickly and talk with the provider. Possible questions to ask include:

- What symptoms is the person experiencing?
- Was medication given? What was the medication, and how much was administered?
- Did the medication ease the symptoms?
- Is the person having severe respiratory distress (e.g., unable to talk, blue lips, or retractions [re TRAK shuns])? (This would be a medical emergency and calling 911 is critical.)

In the ambulatory healthcare setting, an asthma attack is an emergency. The provider needs to see the patient immediately. First aid actions for an asthma attack include:

- Helping the person into a comfortable sitting position. Usually sitting upright allows for easier breathing.
- Giving short-acting inhalers (e.g., albuterol), which will lessen the asthma attack within minutes.
- Monitoring the pulse oximetry and vital signs.

> **VOCABULARY**
>
> **retractions** The sucking in of tissues between the intercostal spaces and neck due to respiratory distress; classic sign of severe asthma.

Choking

Choking can occur in all age groups. Most choking cases relate to swallowing large pieces of food or doing an activity (e.g., running) while eating. Other causes are denture-related issues and eating too fast. Children under age 5 tend to choke on candy, grapes, and large pieces of food. They are also more likely to put nonfood items in the mouth. Plastic, balloon pieces, coins, and buttons are extremely dangerous to children. Objects smaller than 1.75 inches (the diameter of a golf ball) can be caught in the throat and cause choking.

Any object caught in the throat is considered a foreign body obstruction. Signs of a partial airway obstruction include:

- Can still speak
- Forceful or weak coughing
- Labored, noisy, or gasping breathing
- Panicked appearance, extreme anxiety, or agitation

Signs of a total airway obstruction include:

- Clutching the throat with one or both hands
- Unable to breathe, cry, cough, or speak
- Bluish skin color (e.g., lips)

Do not give the person any liquids until the obstruction is cleared.

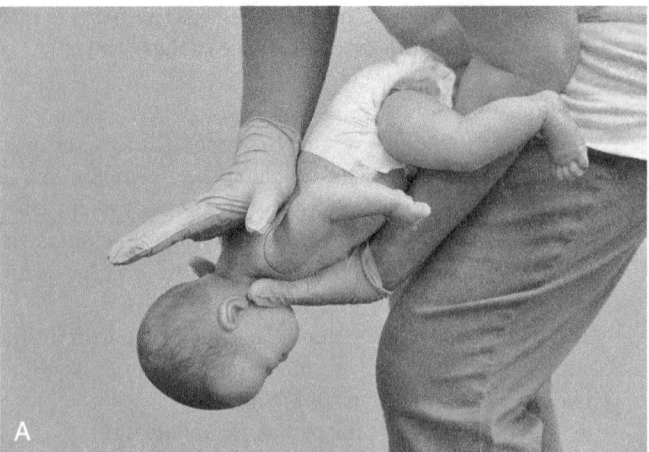
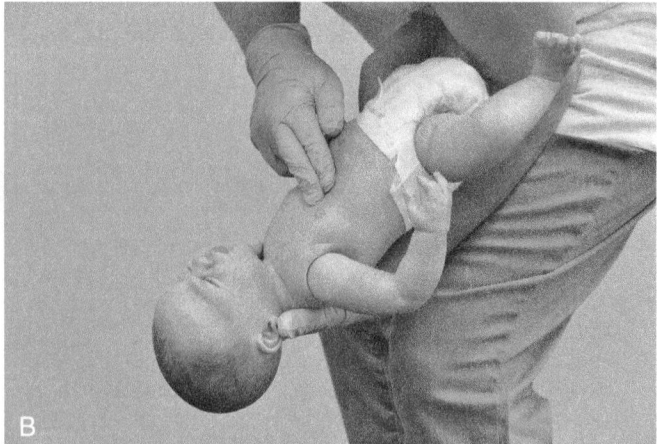

Fig. 49.16 A, Support the infant with your arm and thigh while giving back blows. B, Chest thrusts are administered in the same position as for cardiac compressions.

First aid for an adult or child over 1 year of age for choking includes asking people if they are choking. If the person is forcefully coughing, stand by and see if the person can clear the airway without assistance. Procedure 49.4 describes the abdominal thrusts used on a conscious adult with a total airway obstruction. If a person is pregnant or obese, wrap your arms around the person's chest. Place your fist in the middle of the breastbone between the nipples. Give firm, backward thrusts.

First aid for a conscious choking infant includes:

- Do the 3 Cs after gaining consent from the parent or guardian; check the scene, have someone call 911, and care for the infant. (If you are alone and have a cell phone, call 911. If you are alone without a cell phone, it is recommended that you attempt to clear the airway or provide rescue breathing or CPR for 1 minute to children under 8 years of age before calling 911. Most cardiopulmonary arrest in young children is related to airway issues.)
- Hold the child with the head below the chest for the entire procedure. This allows gravity to help move the obstruction. Support the chin with your hand and the infant's body with your arm.
- Have the child facing downward and give 5 back blows between the shoulder blades with the heel of your hand (Fig. 49.16A).
- Flip the infant and place two or three fingers below the nipple line on the chest. Give 5 chest thrusts (see Fig. 49.16B).
- Do a mouth check and insert a finger only to pull a loose object out. Doing a finger sweep is not recommended because it can push the item in farther.
- Continue until the object is out or the child becomes unconscious. If the child is unconscious, place the child on a hard surface and begin CPR, starting with chest compressions. Make sure 911 was called.

CARDIOVASCULAR EMERGENCIES

Syncope

Syncope (SING kuh pee) means fainting, passing out, or having a temporary loss of consciousness. When people are about to faint, they may feel dizzy, nauseous, or light-headed. The skin may be cold and clammy. People may experience a "black out" or "white out" in their visual field. Muscle control is lost. Fainting occurs when the blood pressure drops suddenly and the blood flow to the brain is reduced. Possible causes of syncope include:

- Being dehydrated or too hot.
- Using alcohol.
- Standing up too quickly.
- A drop in blood glucose.
- Using certain medications, such as diuretics, antihistamines, levodopa, calcium antagonists, angiotensin-converting enzyme (ACE) inhibitors, nitrates, antipsychotics, and narcotics.
- Having a heart condition.
- Having a neurologic condition, such as Parkinson disease, postural orthostatic tachycardia syndrome (POTS), and diabetic neuropathy.
- Vasovagal syncope caused by emotional stress, trauma, pain, reaction to the sight of blood, or prolonged standing.
- Carotid sinus syncope caused by constriction of the carotid artery in the neck, which can occur with turning the head, shaving, or wearing tight clothing around the neck.
- Situational syncope, which occurs during defecation, urination, and coughing.

First aid actions for people who feel faint include having them sit and place their head between their knees (Fig. 49.17). For people who faint, position them on their back. Check their airway and make sure it is clear. Check for a pulse. If the pulse is not present, start CPR.

Additional first aid actions include:

- Loosen any constrictive clothing.
- Raise the legs above the heart level (about 12 inches) (Fig. 49.18).
- Get help/call 911 if the person does not regain consciousness within 1 minute.

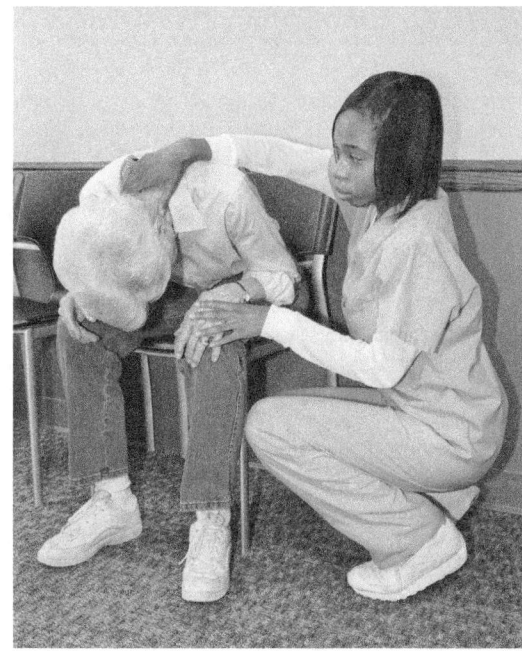

Fig. 49.17 Placing the head between the legs helps to reduce the faint feeling. (From Niedzwiecki B, et al: *Kinn's the medical assistant*, ed 14, St. Louis, 2020, Elsevier.)

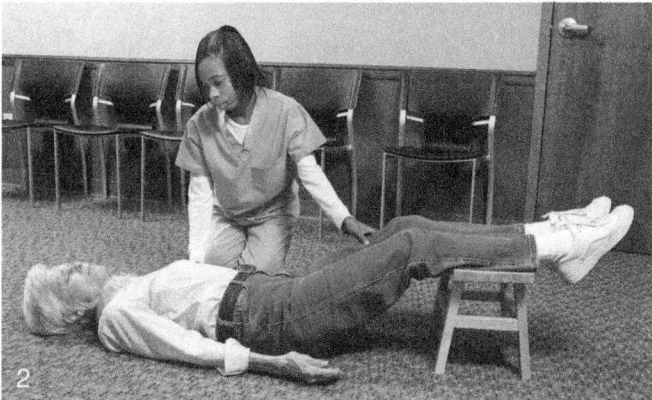

Fig. 49.18 Elevate the legs about 12 inches using pillows, blankets, or a small stool. (From Niedzwiecki B, et al: *Kinn's the medical assistant*, ed 14, St. Louis, 2020, Elsevier.)

Bleeding

Bleeding can occur with and without trauma. First aid for bleeding involves stopping the bleeding and calling for help (Procedure 49.5). Nosebleeds are common in certain people. If a person has a nosebleed, have them sit upright and lean forward to prevent the person from swallowing the blood. Pinch the nostrils for 5 to 10 minutes, which helps to stop the bleeding. Continue to pinch the nostrils until the bleeding stops. The individual should refrain from blowing the nose for several hours to prevent rebleeding.

In the ambulatory care facility, always wear gloves and the required PPE before assisting patients. Follow these steps to stop the bleeding:

- For bleeding wounds, remove any obvious debris. Do not remove any large objects embedded in the wound.
- Place a sterile gauze or clean cloth over the wound and press firmly to control the bleeding. Do not put direct pressure over an embedded object, an eye, or displaced organs.
- For severe bleeding, help the person lie down and cover them with a blanket. This will keep the person warm and conserve body heat.
- If the bleeding seeps through the gauze, apply another layer on top of the initial gauze. Do not move the initial gauze.
- To slow the bleeding or if the bleeding is spurting from an artery:
  - Elevate the bleeding extremity above the heart level.
  - Hold direct pressure over the site.
  - If the bleeding does not stop with the elevation and direct pressure, apply pressure to the artery above the wound by pushing the artery against a bone. Continue to apply direct pressure on the wound.
  - To see if the bleeding has stopped, slowly lift your fingers from the pressure point over the artery. Check to see if the wound is still bleeding. If so, continue to apply pressure.
  - Do not hold pressure at the pressure point for longer than 5 minutes after the bleeding stops.

Shock

Shock occurs when the body is not getting enough blood flow. The vital organs (e.g., heart, brain) do not get enough oxygen and nutrients for the cells to function properly and survive. Organ damage can occur. Shock is a life-threatening condition. There are many types of shock, such as:

- *Cardiogenic* (KAR dee oh JEN ik) *shock*: Due to heart muscle damage caused by a myocardial infarction (also known as MI or heart attack); the heart cannot pump enough blood to the other organs.
- *Hypovolemic* (HYE poe voe LEE mik) *shock*: Due to heavy bleeding (i.e., accident or internal bleeding) or dehydration; blood volume is too low to provide nutrients and oxygen to the organs.
- *Anaphylactic shock*: Caused by a severe allergic reaction (anaphylaxis); blood pressure drops and the airway narrows. Not enough blood gets to the vital organs, and the narrowed airway prevents adequate oxygenation.
- *Septic* (SEP tik) *shock*: Caused by a severe infection (severe sepsis) that affects the functioning of vital organs (e.g., heart, brain, kidneys). The blood pressure falls, and major organs can fail.
- *Neurogenic* (NOO roe JEN ik) *shock*: Due to a central nervous system injury (e.g., spinal cord injury). Leads to vasodilation (not enough blood can return to the heart) and low blood pressure.

Possible signs and symptoms of shock include:

- Anxiety, agitation, dizziness, feeling faint, lightheadedness, confusion, and unconsciousness
- *Cyanosis* (blue lips, fingernails) and shallow respirations
- Chest pain and a rapid, weak pulse
- Moist skin and *diaphoresis* (profuse sweating)
- Poor or no urine output

Shock requires immediate treatment for the person to have a chance of survival. First aid actions for shock include calling

911 immediately. Check the person for responsiveness. Monitor the airway, breathing, and pulse. If needed, perform rescue breathing and CPR. If the person is breathing and has a pulse, monitor the vital signs at least every 5 minutes. If the person does not have any injuries to the head, neck or back, or legs, raise the legs 12 inches. This helps the blood to move back to the vital organs of the body. If the person has pain with raising the legs, keep them flat. Make sure the person's head is flat. Loosen clothing and provide the appropriate first aid for the person's injuries (Procedure 49.6).

If a person goes into shock in the ambulatory healthcare facility, the provider will order that 911 be contacted. Oxygen and IV fluids are given. The vital signs are monitored, and the person's legs are elevated. Based on the medications available and the person's blood pressure, the provider may give IV medications that will increase the blood pressure. The goals are to keep the blood pressure high enough to sustain life, and to get the patient to the emergency department as quickly as possible.

Myocardial Infarction

Myocardial infarction (MI) is more commonly known as heart attack. Coronary arteries that bring blood to the heart muscle are blocked by a clot or narrowed by plaque. When the blood flow to an area of the heart is limited or stopped, the heart cells die and an MI occurs. Chest pain (angina pectoris), cold sweats, and heartburn are the most common symptoms. Chest pain can be described as mild or severe; sharp, burning, heaviness, squeezing, pressure; and constant or intermittent (comes and goes). Additional symptoms include:

- Upper body discomfort or pain in one or both arms, shoulders, neck, jaw, upper part of the abdomen, or back
- Arrhythmia, palpitations, tiredness without a reason, nausea, and vomiting
- Shortness of breath with activity or rest, cold sweats, dizziness, and light-headedness
- Back pain in women

First aid for a heart attack includes these measures:

- Have the person sit down and rest. Keep the individual calm and loosen any tight clothing on the chest and neck area.
- Have the person take nitroglycerin if prescribed (Box 49.6).
- Call 911 within 5 minutes of the onset of pain.
- Have the person chew an aspirin (if not allergic).
- Monitor the person's respirations and pulse. Perform rescue breathing and CPR if needed (Figs. 49.19 to 49.21, Table 49.6, and Procedure 49.7).

If a patient arrives at the ambulatory care facility with chest pain or other MI-type symptoms, bring the patient to a procedure or exam room immediately. Notify the provider at once. Usually the provider will give these orders:

- One aspirin chewed and nitroglycerin administered sublingually.
- Call 911.
- Obtain vital signs, pulse oximetry, and an electrocardiogram (ECG) and administer oxygen while waiting for the ambulance.

The goals are to limit the damage to the heart muscle and transport the patient to the emergency department.

BOX 49.6   Nitroglycerin and Angina

Nitroglycerin is used for angina (chest pain). It dilates the coronary arteries, allowing more blood to move into the heart muscle. Nitroglycerin can be given as an oral spray, a sublingual (SL) powder, or sublingual tablets.

- Do not shake the spray. Prime (or release a test spray) 5 to 10 times for new bottles, up to 5 times for bottles not used within 3 months, and 1 to 2 times for bottles that have not been used in more than 6 weeks. Prime the bottles away from everyone. When administering the dose, spray onto or under the tongue. One or two sprays can be taken at the start of the pain. Then, if the pain is not relieved in 5 minutes, give the third spray. Call 911 if the pain continues for an additional 5 minutes.
- Empty the pack of powder under the tongue. Allow the powder to dissolve without swallowing. Make sure the patient does not eat or rinse the mouth for 5 minutes.
- Tablets cannot be chewed or swallowed. Place a tablet under the tongue and let it dissolve. Usually it starts providing relief within 1 to 5 minutes. If the pain is not relieved in 5 minutes, give another tablet. If the pain continues after 5 minutes, give a third tablet. Call 911 if the pain is not relieved 5 minutes after taking the third tablet. (Do not give more than three tablets within 15 minutes.)

Nitroglycerin works fast. The patient may feel dizzy, light-headed, or faint after taking the medication.

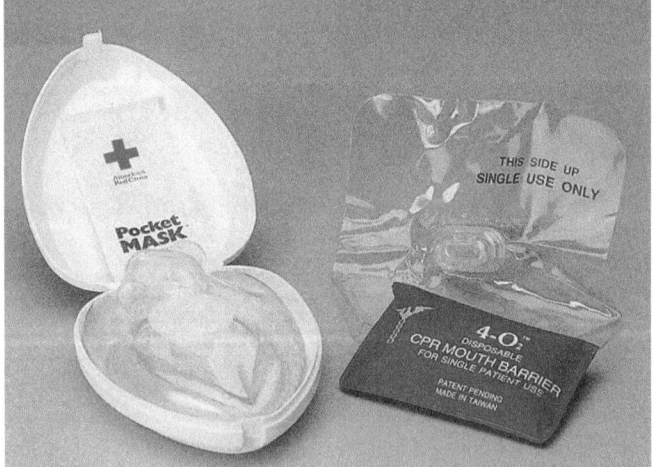

Fig. 49.19 Rescue Breathing Mouth Barriers. (From Niedzwiecki B, et al: *Kinn's the medical assistant*, ed 14, St. Louis, 2020, Elsevier.)

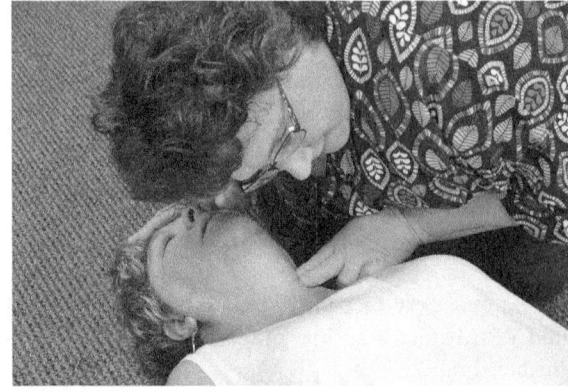

Fig. 49.20 Use the head-tilt position to open an adult's airway while checking the carotid pulse.

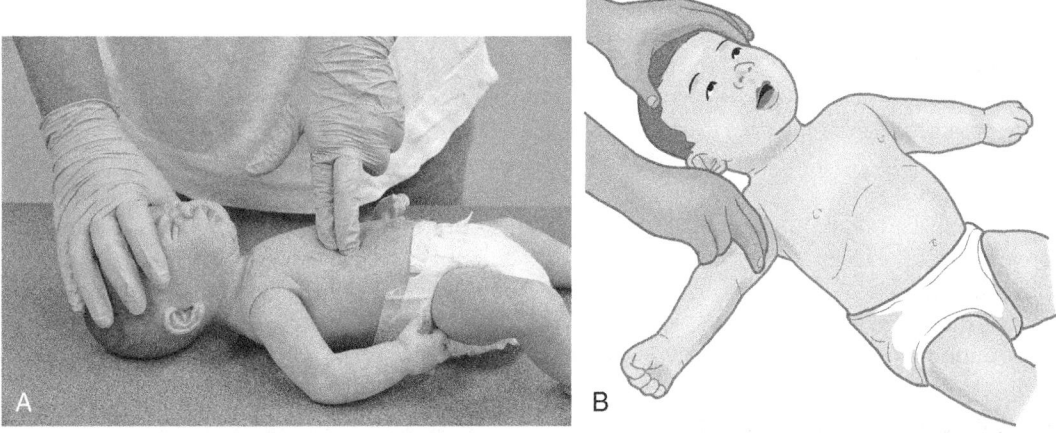

Fig. 49.21 A, Open an infant's airway by tilting the head to a neutral position. For chest compressions, place two fingers below the nipple line. B, In an infant, check for a brachial pulse. (**B** from Niedzwiecki B, et al: *Kinn's the medical assistant*, ed 14, St. Louis, 2020, Elsevier.)

TABLE 49.6	**Summary of Rescue Breathing and Cardiopulmonary Resuscitation Differences**		
	Adult	**Child**	**Infant**
Age	**8+ years old**	**1-8 years old**	**Less than 1 year**
Check responsiveness	Shout, "Are you all right?"		Tap the foot.
Open airway	Head-tilt or if spinal injury is suspected, use the jaw thrust without head extension (see Fig. 49.20).	Tilt head slightly past the neutral position.	Tilt head to the neutral position (see Fig. 49.21A).
Assess pulse	Feel for a carotid pulse near the middle of the throat (see Fig. 49.20).	Feel for the carotid pulse. If pulse is less than 60 beats/minute with signs of poor perfusion (such as skin color changes), start CPR.	Feel for a brachial pulse on the inside upper arm (see Fig. 49.21B)
Give rescue breathing (ventilation) only	One rescue breath every 5–6 seconds. About 10-12 breaths per minute. Deliver each breath for 1 second.	One breath every 2-3 seconds or about 20-30 breaths per minute.	
Chest compression hand position	Heel of a hand is placed on the lower part of the chest (below the nipple line), and the other hand is placed on top, so it overlaps the first hand.		Place two fingers just below the nipple line (see Fig. 49.21A)
Compressions	2–2.4 inches deep; 100 per minute.	2 inches deep; 100–120 per minute.	1.5 inches deep with 2 fingers; 100–120 per minute.
Compression to ventilation ratio	One or two rescuers: 15 compressions and 2 ventilations.	One rescuer: 30 compressions and 2 ventilations. Two rescuers: 15 compressions and 2 ventilations.	
Automated external defibrillator (AED) pads	Use only adult pads. Place one pad on the upper right chest and the second on the left side of the chest.	Use pediatric pads for children younger than 8 years; if not available, use adult pads. If pads touch, place one on the back between the shoulder blades.	Use pediatric pads; if not available, use adult pads. Place one pad on the chest and the other on the back.

Medical Terminology

cyan/o	blue
myocardi/o	heart muscle
pector/o	chest
-is	structure
-osis	abnormal condition

CRITICAL THINKING 49.7

Gabe is thinking of having a rescue breathing mouth barrier in each exam room and procedure room. He is also thinking of adding one to each of the first aid kits located in other parts of the clinic. Why is it important to make mouth barrier devices more available in the clinic?

CLOSING COMMENTS

A variety of emergencies can occur in the healthcare facility. It is important for the medical assistant to know which first aid actions to take. Knowing where the equipment and supplies are located is also vital in emergencies. Many agencies have mock codes to help prepare staff. These are training events that allow staff members to practice their skills. Often after mock events, the supervisors assess how the training went. They identify processes and procedures that need refinement and additional training.

Another method of improving processes comes after a real-life code situation. Usually a few days after a code, the staff involved will gather to debrief or discuss what occurred. They will usually talk about the following:

- How the code progressed, from the time the patient had symptoms to the time the patient was transported to the emergency department
- What went well and what was not so smooth
- Where more training is needed

These debriefings are extremely important after an emergency. Code situations can be anxiety inducing and stressful for staff members. It is important to talk through what occurred while taking confidentiality into account. Besides talking, it is critical to manage one's stress by maintaining a healthy diet and getting adequate sleep and exercise.

An employee assistance program (EAP) is also helpful after stressful code situations. EAP is a work-based program designed to help employees resolve issues. These issues can be personal (e.g. financial, marital, or involving substance abuse) and professional (e.g., communication issues with co-workers and stress-related issues). The EAP services are confidential and designed to help the employee's work performance. EAP counselors help employees to deal with the aftereffects of an emergency.

PATIENT-CENTERED CARE

Medical emergencies are scary for patients and their families. We may be focused on providing emergency care, but we need to remember to communicate with the patient. Being sensitive to what patients are feeling is important. Remember to explain what you are doing. Ask the patient how they are doing.

Families of patients are often forgotten. In emergencies, often the family is moved to another room to allow more room for those helping with the code. It is helpful for the family to have a staff person wait with them. If this is not possible, then a staff person needs to report to the family and provide updates. It is important to remember that the rules of the Health Insurance Portability and Accountability Act (HIPAA) still apply in emergency situations.

BEING PROFESSIONAL

New medical assistants should actively take part in learning the emergency procedures of the ambulatory care facility. Inventorying the crash cart and attending mock codes can help new healthcare workers become more familiar and comfortable with codes.

Role-play this scenario with a peer: You and Pat (your peer) are medical assistants in a primary care department. Pat, who is a new CMA, confides in you that he (or she) is nervous about the emergency procedures and codes and the emergency equipment on the crash cart. Respectfully address Pat's concerns.

CHAPTER REVIEW

This chapter covers basic first aid in and out of the healthcare setting. In the healthcare setting, emergencies are communicated using special phrases (e.g., Code Blue). The healthcare team must respond immediately to the emergency and gather the crash cart and other required supplies. The first to respond to the emergency should initiate first aid. After the provider examines the patient, additional treatments may be done.

Many patients with environmental emergencies will contact or come to the ambulatory healthcare setting. In some cases, the most appropriate location for care is the emergency department. Hypothermia, heatstroke, full-thickness burns, and certain bites can be life-threatening. These conditions are best treated in the emergency department. Heat cramps and heat exhaustion require electrolyte drinks and a cooler environment to bring down the body temperature. For minor burns, soaking the area in cool water immediately is important.

Diabetic emergencies occur when the blood glucose level is too high or too low. Insulin will bring down elevated glucose levels, whereas carbohydrates (sugars and starches) will increase glucose levels.

Musculoskeletal emergencies are usually treated as fractures until the provider gives a diagnosis. First aid requires splinting the injured area. Applying pressure to stop bleeding and using ice packs to limit swelling are also steps to take.

Neurologic emergencies range from minor to serious conditions. Frequently, patients can feel dizzy during or after procedures. Encouraging people to put their head between their legs will help relieve the dizzy or faint feeling. Having patients recline in a supine position and elevating their legs 12 inches will also help. With seizures, it is important to protect the patient from harm and get a provider immediately. Remember to time the length of a seizure. Strokes or CVAs can present with different symptoms. It is vital for the provider to see patients who have strokelike symptoms immediately so treatment can begin.

Respiratory emergencies can also be life-threatening. As with other life-threatening conditions, monitoring the airway, breathing, and pulse is important. Be ready to provide rescue breathing and CPR if it is required. With asthma attacks, help the person into a comfortable sitting position and give short-acting inhalers or nebulizer treatments.

Cardiovascular emergencies also range from minor to life-threatening. With bleeding, apply direct pressure over the wound. Elevating the area and applying pressure over the artery between the wound and the heart can reduce the bleeding. Shock conditions require immediate medical attention. Managing the blood pressure and treating the condition that led to shock are important. The goal is to get the patient to the hospital for additional treatments. Myocardial infarction or heart attack requires early detection and treatment.

SCENARIO WRAP-UP

Gabe has been in his new position for only 2 weeks. Already he has a list of concerns and possible solutions he wants to address with his supervisor. Gabe also wants to discuss forming an emergency response team. This team would respond when a code is called throughout the building.

He hopes to begin quarterly mock codes within the next 3 months. He wants to rotate the types of emergencies addressed by the mock codes. Gabe hopes that with additional training and more exposure to emergency supplies, the medical assistants will feel more comfortable with emergencies.

PROCEDURE 49.1   Provide First Aid for a Patient With an Environmental Emergency and Insulin Shock

Task
Provide first aid to an individual with who has a dog bite and hypoglycemia.

Background Information
With hypoglycemic symptoms, test the blood glucose level. If the blood glucose is under 70 and the patient is conscious and able to swallow, give 4 ounces of fruit juice or regular soda or 3 glucose tablets. Test the blood glucose in 15 minutes. Continue with these steps until the glucose level is 70 or above.

Scenario
You are working with Dr. Martin, a family practice provider. Maude Crawford (date of birth [DOB} 12/22/19XX) is being seen for a dog bite on her left arm. The wound is still bleeding.

Directions
Role-play the scenario with a peer, who will be the patient, and you are the medical assistant.

Equipment and Supplies
- Gloves and sterile gauze
- Sugary drink (4 ounces of fruit juice or regular soda) or three glucose tablets
- Patient's health record

Procedural Steps
1. Wash your hands or use hand sanitizer.
2. Greet the patient. Identify yourself. Verify the patient's identity with full name and date of birth.
3. Apply gloves. Place sterile gauze over the wound and apply direct pressure to control the bleeding.

4. Identify when the patient had her last tetanus booster.
   Scenario update: Mrs. Crawford has diabetes and states that she thinks she has low blood sugar. She has blurry vision, tremors, and a headache. She asks you for something to eat. According to the facility's policy, you check her blood glucose level, and it is 48 mg/dL.
5. Obtain a sugary drink or glucose tablets. Indicate how much to give to the patient.
   Purpose: Consuming a sugary food or drink will help to increase the blood glucose.
   Scenario update: After 15 minutes, her blood glucose level is 59 mg/dL. You notify the provider while a co-worker stays with the patient.
6. Describe follow-up care for the patient. (See the background information.)
   Purpose: A blood glucose test should be done to find out how low the patient's level is. After 15 minutes of her eating/drinking the sugary food, the glucose test should be done. If her level is below 70 mg/dL, give her additional sugary food/drink and repeat the glucose test in 15 minutes. Continue until the blood glucose level is 70 or higher.
   Scenario update: After 15 minutes, her blood glucose level is 82 mg/dL. You notify the provider.
7. Document the situation. Include the blood glucose levels, your actions, the provider who was notified, and the patient's response.

10/04/20XX 1023 Sterile gauze and pressure applied to wound. Pt c/o blurry vision, tremors, and a headache. She stated she thought she had low blood sugar. Four oz. of orange juice given to pt. After 15 minutes her blood glucose was 59 mg/dL. Dr. Martin notified and ordered additional orange juice and to recheck blood glucose until 70 mg/dL or more. Four oz. of orange juice given and after 15 minutes her blood glucose was 82 mg/dL. Provider notified.
_____ Gabe Garcia, CMA (AAMA)

PROCEDURE 49.2   Incorporate Critical Thinking Skills When Performing a Patient Assessment

Task
Use critical thinking skills while performing a patient assessment regarding a neurologic emergency.

Scenario
You are working with Dr. Martin, a family practice provider. Maude Crawford's daughter calls concerned about her mother. The daughter stated that Maude Crawford (DOB 12/22/19XX) fell and hit her head.

Directions
Role-play the scenario with a peer. The peer will be the daughter, and you will be the medical assistant. The peer can make up information regarding the scenario. Your instructor will be the provider.

WMFM Neurological Emergency Phone Protocol
Obtain the patient's name, date of birth, signs/symptoms, and the history of the situation. After call, document situation, symptoms, and action in the patient's health record.
  With the following neurologic concerns, send the patient to the emergency department via the ambulance immediately.
- Seizure or seizure like symptoms lasting 3 or more minutes
- Passing out or fainting; dizziness or weakness that does not go away
- Sudden or unusual headache that starts suddenly
- Unable to see or speak, sudden confusion
- Neck or spine injury
- Injuries that cause loss of feeling or inability to move
- Head injury with passing out, fainting, or confusion
- Facial drooping or sudden speech difficulties or visual problems

Continued

PROCEDURE 49.2 Incorporate Critical Thinking Skills When Performing a Patient Assessment–cont'd

With the following concerns, schedule a visit for the same day. If no appointments are available, consult the triage nurse or the provider regarding the situation.

- Headache/migraine
- Nonemergent neurologic concern, such as muscle stiffness or rigidity that is progressively getting worse, insomnia, or a history of blurry or double vision.

Equipment and Supplies
- Patient's health record
- Paper and pen
- Emergency Phone Protocol for clinic

Procedural Steps
1. Obtain the patient's name and date of birth.
   Purpose: Obtaining the patient's information is important for any patient-related phone call.
2. Using critical thinking skills, ask appropriate questions to obtain information about the patient's condition. Write down the patient's issues or concerns or the situation.

Purpose: Writing down the information will help when you discuss the situation with the provider and when you document the call. Thoughtful questions related to the situation and the patient's condition must be asked to gather the appropriate information.

Scenario update: The daughter stated that Maude was "knocked out" for about a minute. She has been acting differently since the fall. You realize you need to complete the Neurological Emergency Phone Protocol.

3. Complete the protocol and determine what actions to take.
   Purpose: Protocols are approved and signed by the providers. They need to be followed by the staff.
4. Instruct the caller on what should be done based on the protocol. Talk with the provider if needed
   Purpose: The caller needs clear directions on what to do.
5. Document the call in the patient's health record. Include the caller's name, the patient's condition (e.g., signs, symptoms, and concerns), name of the protocol used, information given to the caller, and the provider who was notified.
   Purpose: Legally it is important to document all patient interactions.

PROCEDURE 49.3 Provide First Aid for a Patient With a Stroke and Seizure Activity

Tasks
Provide first aid to an individual having a stroke and seizure activity. Document care in the health record.

Scenario
You are working with Dr. Martin, a family practice provider. Walter Biller (DOB 1/4/19XX) arrives for his appointment.

Directions
Role-play the scenario with a peer, who will be the patient, and you are the medical assistant.

Equipment and Supplies
- Watch, stethoscope, and sphygmomanometer
- Folded towel, blanket, or coat
- Patient's health record
- Gloves and other personal protective equipment (as required)

Procedural Steps
1. Wash your hands or use hand sanitizer.
2. Greet the patient. Identify yourself. Verify the patient's identity with full name and date of birth.
   Scenario update: As you room Mr. Biller, you notice that he seems to be dragging his left leg when walking, the left side of his face is drooping, and he states his left arm is weak. You suspect that he might be having a stroke. He asks for a drink of water when you get to the exam room.
3. You call for help and assist the patient onto the examination table. Place the patient in the recovery position with his head slightly raised.
4. Monitor the patient's airway. Obtain the patient vital signs.
5. Speak calmly to the patient. Do not give the patient anything to drink.
   Purpose: The patient may be at risk for choking.

Scenario update: While you are waiting for the provider, Mr. Biller starts to jerk his arms and he becomes unresponsive.

6. Keep the patient in the recovery position. Note the time when the seizure started. Gently raise the chin to tilt the head back slightly to open the airway. Yell for help if help has not arrived.
   Purpose: The recovery position will help to open up the person's airway. Yelling for help in the ambulatory care facility is reserved for emergencies.
7. Continue to monitor his pulse rate and respiration rate. Put on gloves and other personal protective equipment as needed.
   Purpose: Wearing personal protective equipment will protect you if the patient vomits or becomes incontinent of urine or stool during the seizure.
8. Clear any hard or sharp items away from the patient. Place a soft, folded towel, blanket, or coat under the patient's head.
   Purpose: It is important to protect the patient from harm.
9. Remove the patient's glasses (if on) and loosen any constrictive clothing around the neck. Stay with the person until they are fully awake and continue to monitor the respiration and pulse rates.
   Purpose: Tight clothing can restrict breathing.
10. Document the first aid measures you provided in the order that they occurred. In addition, document the seizure activity you witnessed, the length of the episode, and the provider notified.
    Purpose: Specifying the care provided, along with details of the seizure activity, will help the provider.

10/05/20XX 1423 Patient appeared to be dragging his left leg when walking, the left side of his face was drooping, and he stated his left arm was weak. Pt was placed in the recovery position on the examination table. Provider was called. Patient started to jerk his arms and he became unresponsive. P: 86 regular, 1+; R: 18 regular, normal. Dr. Martin arrived. Pt's clothing was loosened. The seizure activity lasted for 4.5 minutes. _____
_____ Gabe Garcia, CMA (AAMA)

PROCEDURE 49.4   Provide First Aid for a Choking Patient

Tasks

Provide first aid to a conscious adult who is choking. Document it in the health record.

Scenario

You are working with Dr. Martin, a family practice provider. As you return from lunch, you notice that an adult visitor is having an issue. It appears that she had been eating fast food, and now she is holding her neck with both hands. She appears to be panicking.

Directions

Role-play the scenario with a peer. The peer will be the visitor, and you will be the medical assistant

Equipment and Supplies

- Patient's health record
- Gloves
- Mannequin

Procedural Steps

1. Approach the person and ask, "Are you choking?"

   Purpose: If the person can speak and is coughing forcefully, then let her cough and try to dislodge the obstruction. If the person is not able to speak, then assist the patient.

   Scenario update: She nods her head yes but cannot speak. She is standing.

2. Yell for help. Put on gloves if available. Stand behind the victim with your feet slightly apart. Reach your arms around the person's waist.

   Purpose: With an obstructed airway, the person may lose consciousness at any time. The rescuer must be prepared to lower the unconscious individual to the floor safely. If the person in distress is a child, the rescuer may need to kneel when providing assistance.

3. Make a fist and place it just above the person's navel. Make sure your thumb side is next to the person. Grasp the fist tightly with your other hand (Fig. 1).

   Purpose: Correct hand position is important as you do abdominal thrusts.

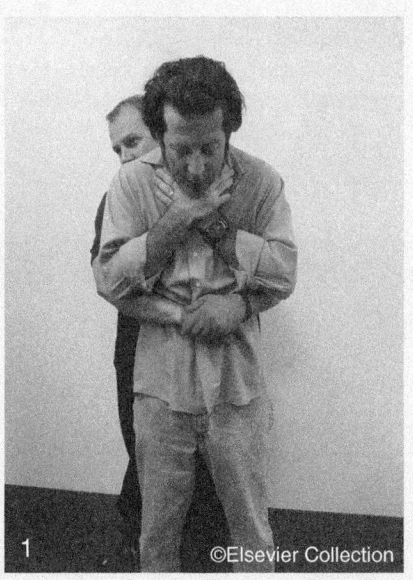

Scenario update: The next steps must be done on a mannequin.

4. With the correct hand position, make quick, upward and inward thrusts with your fist. Do 5 abdominal thrusts before doing back blows.

   Purpose: The fist should be placed in the soft tissue of the abdomen to avoid injury to the sternum or rib cage. If the person is supine, straddle and face the person's head. Push your grasped fist upward and inward.

5. Stand behind the person and wrap one arm around the person's upper body. Position the person so they are bent forward with the chest parallel to the ground.

   Purpose: This position helps objects to dislodge.

6. Use the heel of your other hand to give a firm blow between the shoulder blades. Check to see if the object dislodges. If not, continue by giving another 4 back blows.

   Purpose: Back blows can help dislodge the item.

7. Continue to give 5 abdominal thrusts followed by 5 back blows until the object is dislodged or the person loses consciousness.

   Purpose: Repeated abdominal thrusts and back blows can help dislodge the item.

   Note: If the person faints or loses consciousness, lower the person to the floor. Call 911 (or the local emergency number) or have someone else call. Begin CPR, starting with chest compressions. Check to see if the item is in the airway. Remove it only if it is loose.

   Scenario update: After two sets of abdominal thrusts and back blows, the woman coughs out a piece of food. She can now talk.

8. Arrange for the person to be seen by the provider. Document the first aid measures you provided in the order that they occurred.

   Purpose: Specifying the care provided, along with details of the situation, will present the provider with a full picture of what happened.

   10/06/20XX 1223 Pt was found in reception room with her hands on her throat. She appeared to be panicky. She could not speak but indicated with a nod of her head that she was choking. After being given 2 sets of back blows and abdominal thrusts, she was able to cough out some undigested food. R: 22 regular, normal. Pt is alert. She agreed to see Dr. Martin immediately. _____

   _____ Gabe Garcia, CMA (AAMA)

PROCEDURE 49.5 Provide First Aid for a Patient With a Bleeding Wound, Fracture, and Syncope

Tasks
Provide first aid to an individual with a suspected fracture, a bleeding wound, and syncope. Document the first aid you provide.

Scenario
You are returning from lunch and see a person fall at the entrance of the healthcare facility. He is an older man and complains of pain in his right lower arm. His arm looks deformed and is bleeding. You call for help. A provider comes, and co-workers bring supplies. The provider tells you to care for the wound and splint the arm before moving the individual. You have a co-worker helping you.

Directions
Read the scenario and role-play the situation with two peers. One peer will be the patient and the other peer will be a co-worker. You will be the medical assistant.

Equipment and Supplies
- Gloves
- Sterile gauze
- Bandage
- Splinting material (e.g., SAM splint)
- Coban wrap or gauze roll

Procedural Steps
1. Wash your hands or use hand sanitizer if possible. Identify yourself to the patient. Obtain the patient's name and date of birth as you put on gloves.
   Purpose: It is important to wear gloves when working with a wound. Obtaining the patient's name is important because the patient will be seen, and you need to document the first aid provided.
2. Using sterile gauze, apply direct pressure over the wound to stop the bleeding. Make sure to immobilize the injured arm as you apply pressure. If possible, elevate the arm to help slow the bleeding. If the blood seeps through the gauze, apply another layer of gauze on the initial one. Continue with the direct pressure until the bleeding stops.
   Purpose: Applying pressure and elevating the arm will slow the bleeding.
3. Once the bleeding has stopped, cover the dressing with a bandage. Remember to immobilize the injured arm as you work.

Purpose: It is important to cover the wound with a bandage in case the bleeding restarts. Immobilizing a suspected arm is important until the splint can be applied.
   Scenario update: As you apply the bandage to the injured arm, the patient states he does not feel good. He says he feels dizzy and thinks he is going to pass out. Your peer takes over by supporting his arm, and the man faints. He is still breathing and has a pulse.
4. Position the patient on his back. Continue to check his respirations and pulse rates.
   Purpose: If the patient is not breathing or does not have a pulse, administer rescue breathing and begin CPR.
5. Loosen any constrictive clothing around the neck and chest. Raise the legs above the heart level (about 12 inches).
   Purpose: Raising the legs allows the blood to return to the vital organs.
   Scenario update: After a few minutes, he starts to come around. He jokes that blood makes him faint. As he is lying on his back talking with you, you need to splint his injured arm.
6. Use the splint material and shape it to the injured arm. Do not straighten the arm. Apply the splint beyond the joint above and the joint below the injury.
   Purpose: It is important to keep the arm in the same position until the provider examines the arm and x-rays are taken.
7. Use Coban or a gauze roll to secure the splint in place. Encourage the patient to hold the injured arm against his chest as he moves.
   Purpose: If the patient can hold the arm, this will reduce the pain.
8. Document the first aid measures you provided in the order they occurred. Note that the provider was at the scene.
   Purpose: Specifying the care provided, along with details of the seizure activity, will help the provider.
   10/07/20XX 1215 Pt fell at the clinic entrance. He c/o pain in his lower right arm. Dr. Martin ordered wound care and splinting of the arm before moving the pt. Using sterile gauze, applied direct pressure over the wound until the bleeding stopped. Wound was covered with a bandage while arm was manually immobilized. Pt stated he felt dizzy and fainted. P: 68 regular, 1+; R: 16 irregular, normal. Pt was positioned on his back with his feet elevated. Within a few minutes patient came to and started talking. SAM Splint applied to right arm and Coban applied to hold the splint. Pt held arm while transferring into wheelchair. Pt to see Dr. Martin immediately. _____ Gabe Garcia, CMA (AAMA)

PROCEDURE 49.6 Provide First Aid for a Patient in Shock

Tasks
Provide first aid to an individual with who is in shock. Document the first aid you provide.

Scenario
You are working with Dr. Julie Walden. The administrative medical assistant at the reception desk notifies you that Robert Caudill (date of birth [DOB] 10/31/19XX) is here and looks very ill. You bring the patient and his wife immediately back to the procedure room because it is the only available room. He asks to move to the exam table, and you assist him as he transfers to the table. You obtain his vital signs, which are P: 92, R: 26, BP 72/48, and T: 103.2.

Directions
Role-play the scenario with two peers. One peer will be the patient and the other will be the wife. You will be the medical assistant.

Equipment and Supplies
- Stethoscope
- Watch
- Pen
- Sphygmomanometer (blood pressure cuff)
- Pillows, blankets, or small stool to help elevate the feet
- Exam table

Procedural Steps
1. Call for help. Monitor the patient's breathing and pulse until the provider arrives.
   Purpose: It is important to have the provider see the patient immediately.
   Situation update: The provider examines the patient and suspects septic shock. You administer 2 L of oxygen per nasal canula as the provider ordered. The triage RN inserts an IV and administers IV fluids. The provider directs another medical assistant to call 911.

PROCEDURE 49.6   Provide First Aid for a Patient in Shock—cont'd

2. Raise the patient's legs 12 inches.
   Purpose: Raising the person's legs helps the blood to return to the heart. Some tables will allow you to elevate the foot section. If this is not possible, use things such as pillows, blankets, or a small stool.
3. Make sure the patient's head is flat on the bed.
   Purpose: This helps the blood to flow to the head.
4. Loosen the person's clothing. Make sure the clothing does not restrict the neck and chest area.
   Purpose: Clothing that is tight can affect the breathing.
5. Obtain a pulse rate, respiration rate, and blood pressure. Continue to monitor the patient's airway, pulse rate, and respiration rate.
   Purpose: Monitor the patient's vital signs. If the person is not breathing, provide rescue breathing. If the person has no pulse, start CPR.
6. While monitoring the patient, speak calmly with him. Use a gentle tone of voice. Demonstrate calming body language (e.g., do not appear scared, rushed, or out of control).
   Purpose: It is important to keep the patient calm during the crisis. Anxiety can be a symptom of shock.

7. Talk calmly with the patient's wife and explain what is occurring. Answer any questions the wife may have.
   Purpose: In an emergency, it is important to keep the family in the room updated on what is occurring. Depending on the emergency, sometimes a staff person will take the family members to another room.
8. Document the first aid measures you provided in the order they occurred. Indicate which provider examined the patient. In addition, document the administration of oxygen and the vital signs obtained.
   Purpose: Specifying the care provided, along with the vital signs, will help the provider and the emergency responders.

   10/07/20XX 1525 P: 92 irregular, 1+; R: 26 regular, shallow; BP: 72/48 RA lying; T: 103.2 (TA). Notified Dr. Walden. Pt resting on table with his wife at his side. _____ Gabe Garcia, CMA (AAMA)

   10/07/20XX 1535 Administered 8 L of oxygen per mask per Dr. Walden's order. Raised legs about 12 inches, and head is flat. P: 98 irregular, 1+; R: 32 regular, shallow; BP: 70/42 RA lying. _____ Gabe Garcia, CMA (AAMA)

PROCEDURE 49.7   Provide Rescue Breathing and Cardiopulmonary Resuscitation (CPR) and Use an Automated External Defibrillator (AED)

Tasks
Perform rescue breathing and CPR. Use the AED machine.

Scenario
You are in the healthcare facility parking lot and find a person on the ground. No one is around.

Directions
Role-play the scenario with two peers. One peer will be the person on the ground. You will be the medical assistant.

Equipment and Supplies
- AED machine with adult pads
- Barrier ventilation device
- Mannequin
- Gloves (if available)

Procedural Steps
1. Check the scene for safety. Is it safe to approach and provide help to the victim?
   Purpose: It is important to look for toxic or electrical hazards. Also, look for other hazards that make the scene unsafe for you. If you find something, call 911 and wait for the emergency responders.
2. Check the person's response. Tap the individual on the shoulder and shout, "Are you all right?" Pause for a few moments for a response.
   Purpose: If the patient is responsive, the individual will talk, moan, move, or do something that indicates responsiveness.
   Scenario update: There is no response from the individual. A bystander comes up and you direct that person to find an AED machine.
3. Call 911 and answer the questions from the dispatcher.
   Purpose: The dispatcher needs to know what is occurring and where the emergency is located.

4. Put on gloves if available. Roll the person over if the person is face down. Roll the person as an entire unit, supporting the head, neck, and back. Open the airway and assess the respirations and the pulse for 10 seconds.
   Note: Occasional gasping is not considered breathing.
   a. *Breathing, has a pulse:* Monitor the person until the emergency responders arrive. If needed and if no head, neck, or spinal injury is suspected, then place the patient in the recovery position.
   b. *No normal breathing, has a pulse:* Give 1 breath every 5-6 seconds. Check the pulse every 2 minutes. If pulse remains, continue with rescue breathing. If pulse is absent, start CPR.
   c. *Not breathing, no pulse:* Give CPR, starting with compressions. Give 15 compressions and 2 breaths.
   Purpose: Before you initiate rescue breathing or CPR, you need to know if the person is breathing or has a pulse.
   Scenario update: The individual has a weak pulse and is not breathing. (Use a mannequin for the following steps.)
5. Use a barrier device if available. Pinch the person's nose and give each rescue breath over 1 second. Watch for the chest to rise. Give the appropriate amount of ventilations for the person's age (see Table 49.6). Continue to monitor the pulse as you give rescue breaths.
   Note: If the person had been choking, look in the mouth before giving a rescue breath. If you see the object, sweep it out with your finger. You can also provide nose ventilation if the mouth is injured. Stoma ventilation must be done if the person has a stoma (in the throat area).
   Purpose: Adults get a rescue breath every 5 to 6 seconds. Children and infants get one every 2 to 3 seconds. If the chest does not rise, reposition, and open the airway. *Scenario update:* When you check the pulse again, there is no pulse.
6. Place your hands at the correct location on the chest (Fig. 1). Bring your shoulders directly over the victim's sternum as you compress downward. Keep your elbows locked (Fig. 2).
   Purpose: The correct position will allow you to do the compressions at the necessary depth.

Continued

PROCEDURE 49.7 Provide Rescue Breathing and Cardiopulmonary Resuscitation (CPR) and Use an Automated External Defibrillator (AED)—cont'd

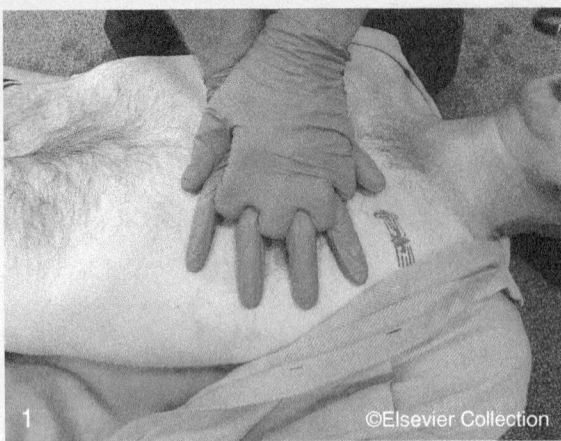

©Elsevier Collection

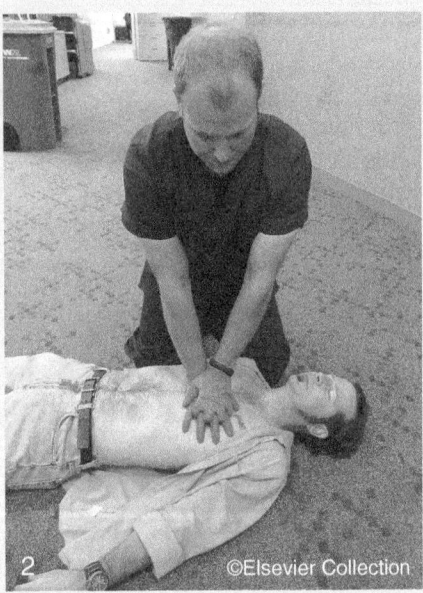

©Elsevier Collection

7. Give 15 compressions at the appropriate depth (see Table 49.6). Give two ventilations and watch for the chest to rise. Continue with the cycle. Give approximately 100 compressions per minute to an adult.

Purpose: The appropriate depth is required to help compress the chambers of the heart. It is important to continue to provide ventilations and compressions until you are too exhausted, the person is breathing, an AED arrives, or emergency responders arrive.

Scenario update: After two cycles, a bystander brings an AED but does not know how to use it. The bystander also does not know CPR. You need to stop the CPR and use the AED.

8. Turn on the AED and follow the directions. Attach the AED pads to the individual's bare dry chest (see Table 49.6 and Fig. 3). Attach the pads to the machine if required.

Note: Make sure to remove any medication patches and medication residue from the chest before applying the pads.

Purpose: The pads need to be placed on the bare, dry chest for the AED to work correctly.

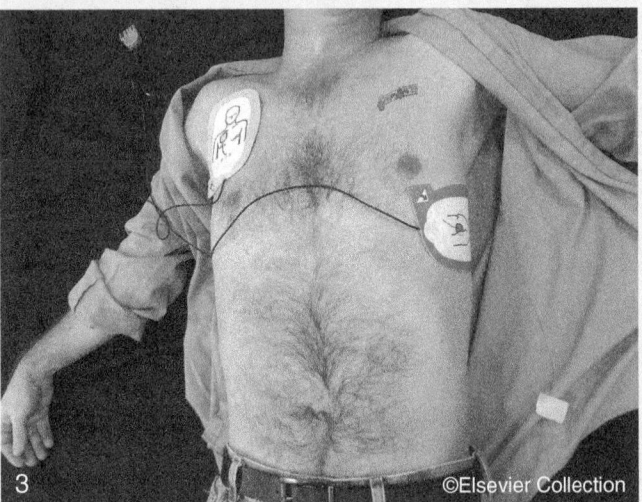

©Elsevier Collection

9. Have everyone stand back from the patient by announcing, "Stand clear." Push the analyze button and allow the machine to analyze the heartbeat.

Purpose: "Stand clear" tells everyone to not touch the patient during this step.

10. Follow the prompts on the AED machine.

   a. *Shock advised:* Announce, "Stand clear" and make sure no one is touching the individual. Press the shock button. After the shock, do CPR for 2 minutes, starting with compressions. Continue following the prompts until the emergency responders arrive.

   b. *Shock not advised:* Continue doing CPR for 2 minutes, starting with compressions. Continue following the prompts until the emergency responders arrive.

Purpose: The AED will prompt you as to what to do next.

50

Assisting With Radiology

LEARNING OBJECTIVES

1. Describe how x-rays are produced.
2. Explain the radiation field and the central ray.
3. Describe how different tissue densities appear on x-ray images.
4. Describe the three things that can occur when radiation enters the body.
5. Describe the difference between computed radiography and digital radiography.
6. Explain the importance of PACS and DICOM with radiography.
7. Describe the x-ray room and equipment.
8. Explain how density, contrast, distortion, and spatial resolution affect the x-ray image.
9. Discuss the risks associated with radiation, including radiosensitive tissues and short-term and long-term effects of radiation exposure.
10. Describe radiation safety measures and the significance of the ALARA (as low as reasonably achievable) principle.

OUTLINE

OPENING SCENARIO

Taylor Jones, CMA (AAMA), is a certified medical assistant who works at the Walden-Martin Family Medical (WMFM) Clinic. WMFM Clinic has recently received funding to build an x-ray suite within the clinic. Although there are individuals at the clinic who can take x-rays, Taylor has been asked to take a course in limited scope radiography. He will also need to pass the state examination before he can perform x-rays independently. Taylor was a bit surprised, because he did not realize that medical assistants could receive such training and take x-rays. He is now very excited, but a little nervous, to receive this additional training.

YOU WILL LEARN

1. To describe how x-rays are produced.
2. To distinguish between the effect of different tissue densities on x-ray images.
3. To describe what occurs when radiation enters the body.
4. To distinguish between computed radiography and digital radiography.
5. To identify x-ray equipment.
6. To identify factors that affect the x-ray image.
7. To discuss radiation health risks and safety measures.

INTRODUCTION

Radiography is the process of creating an x-ray image to examine internal structures of the body. In 1895, Wilhelm Konrad Roentgen accidentally discovered the first x-ray during an experiment at a German university. Traditional x-rays captured images of the internal structures on film. With advances in technology, digital radiology was developed and is more efficient and cost-effective. With digital radiology, the patient has less radiation exposure compared to traditional x-rays.

Today, more ambulatory care facilities have digital radiology available. Medical, chiropractic, and dental facilities use digital radiology. In medical facilities, x-rays are used to help diagnose fractures, pneumonia, arthritis, dislocated joints, and many other conditions.

Depending on the state laws and the facility's size, the person taking the x-rays and the person interpreting or "reading" the x-rays vary. Larger ambulatory care facilities hire radiology technicians to take x-rays, and a radiologist interprets the x-rays. Smaller facilities may only do limited radiography. The limited radiographer may be a medical assistant with a limited scope license, and the provider may read the x-rays (Box 50.1).

VOCABULARY

limited radiography A simplified role in radiography, usually in an outpatient setting; also called *practical radiography*. The limited radiographer may be referred to as a *limited operator* or *basic machine operator*.

radiography The process of creating an x-ray image to examine internal structures of the body.

radiologist A physician who specializes in medical imaging or therapeutic applications of radiation.

MEDICAL TERMINOLOGY

radi/o	rays
therm/o	heat, temperature
-graphy	process of recording

CRITICAL THINKING 50.1

In the small ambulatory care facilities with limited employees, what is the benefit of having a medical assistant who is also training in limited radiography perform x-rays?

HOW X-RAYS ARE PRODUCED

X-rays are a type of electromagnetic radiation, just like the sunlight that we see. X-rays and sunlight share similar characteristics.

BOX 50.1   American Registry of Radiologic Technologists (ARRT)

States have different requirements for radiologic operators of x-ray equipment. Many states require radiologic technicians or technologists to be licensed. Other states do not require the radiologic operator to be licensed or certified. The American Registry of Radiologic Technologists (AART) developed and administers the Limited Scope of Practice in Radiography Examination for certain states. The exam scores are sent from AART to the states. If a person meets the state's requirements, such as the exam score, the person obtains a limited scope license and can perform certain radiology procedures. Medical assistants with training in radiology can take the examination. For information specific to your state, please see your state Department of Occupational Licensing. Information on the examination can be found on the AART website (https://www.arrt.org/).

They both travel in a straight line, at the same speed, and have an effect on living organisms. For example, a high exposure to x-rays and to sunlight can both cause burns to the skin. X-rays are also different from sunlight. They are not visible to the eye, and they produce more energy than sunlight. This extra energy allows x-rays to be strong enough to pass through the body.

Within the x-ray machine, an x-ray tube (also called a *vacuum tube*) is where x-rays are created. The x-ray tube is like a magnet. One end has a negative charge and is called the *cathode* (KATH ode). The opposite end, the *anode* (AN ode), has a positive charge. The anode is commonly made of tungsten and is sometimes referred to as the "tungsten anode." Tungsten is a metal with a high melting point, which means it can withstand very high temperatures.

When the x-ray tube is activated, the cathode gets very hot. Electrons (ee LEK trons) are released from the heated metal (cathode) through a process called thermionic (THER mie on ik) emission (ee MISH un). The electrons are released into the vacuum tube. The electrons are attracted to the tungsten anode. They move very quickly to the anode and then are immediately stopped. This process forces the electrons to release their energy. This energy is released as heat and x-rays, which is called bremsstrahlung (BREMZ strah lung). The heat is absorbed into the anode, and the x-rays are channeled through a focal spot on the lower part of the anode. This allows the x-ray to be focused and creates a *primary (x-ray) beam*. Most x-ray tubes have two focal spots, one larger and one smaller. The focal spot used will depend on the specific x-ray being taken. (Once the x-ray tube is turned off, the electrons return to their atom and once again start circling it, building up energy that can be used the next time an x-ray is needed.)

When x-rays are created, some have higher energy than others. The high-energy rays are most effective for creating an image. The low-energy rays are not as effective and are more likely to be absorbed by the patient. This causes higher levels of radiation exposure. To limit the low-energy rays, a filter is placed below the focal spot. This filter absorbs the low-energy rays and allows the more useful high-energy rays to pass.

As with a flashlight beam, when x-rays emerge from the machine, they create a beam in a conelike field that enlarges as it moves farther from the energy source. In radiography, the beam of x-rays is called the *radiation field* (Fig. 50.1A). Only

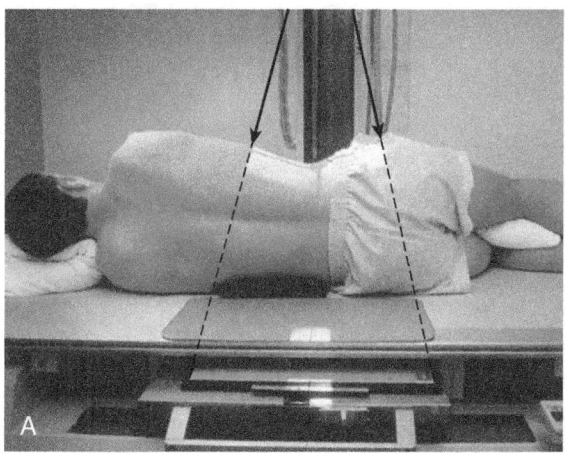

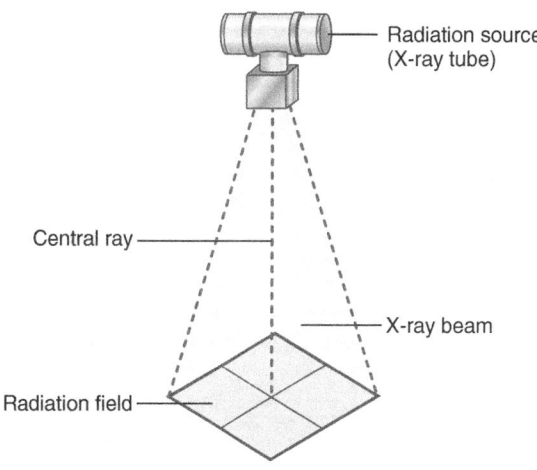

Fig. 50.1 A, The collimator's light beam demonstrates the radiation field and aids alignment of the image receptor. As does the x-ray beam, the conelike shape of the light becomes larger and less concentrated as it gets farther from the x-ray tube. B, The primary x-ray beam leaves the x-ray tube. The useful part of the beam is called the *radiation field*. The center of the beam is called the *central ray*. (**A** from Bontrager KL, Lampignano J: *Textbook of radiographic positioning and related anatomy,* ed 7, St. Louis, 2009, Mosby. **B** from Proctor D, et al: *Kinn's the medical assistant,* ed 13, St. Louis, 2017, Elsevier.)

body structures placed within this field can be imaged. The very center of this field is called the *central ray (CR)* (Fig. 50.1B). Because it is the most concentrated point of radiation, the structure to be imaged is placed in this area.

Densities Seen on X-Rays

The primary beam travels in a straight line. To take an x-ray image, the body part must be directly below the x-ray tube within the primary beam. Depending on the density of the tissue, varying amounts of radiation will be absorbed by the body. The remaining radiation not absorbed by the body will exit the body and come into contact with the image receptor (IR), which is placed behind the body. The image created on the IR is called the latent image (Fig. 50.2).

The darkness of the image will increase as more x-rays reach the image receptor (and thus less is absorbed by the body). The fewer the x-rays that exit the body and hit the IR, the lighter the image. The tissue density affects the amount of x-rays absorbed by the body. For example, dense tissue,

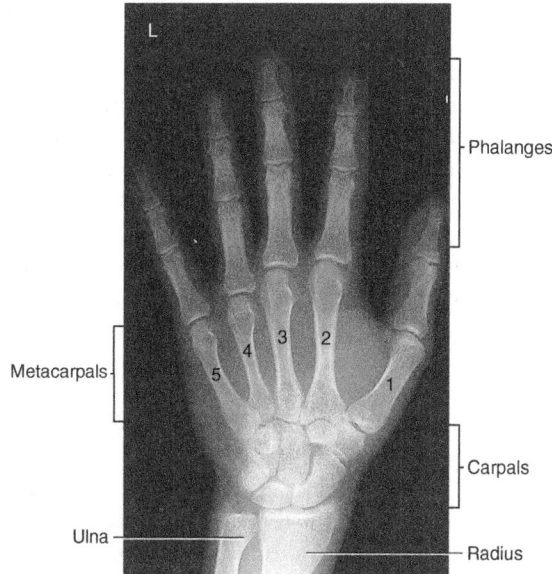

Fig. 50.2 Posteroanterior (PA) Projection of the Hand. The bones block x-rays from reaching the film, creating a white shadow. (From Long BW, Frank ED, Ehrlich RA: *Radiography essentials for limited practice,* ed 4, Philadelphia, 2013, Saunders.)

such as bones, absorb more x-rays and appear white on the image. Fluid and soft tissue, such as blood and muscles, are less dense than bones. They absorb less x-rays, creating a darker image. Fat appears darker than soft tissue on the image. Air absorbs the least x-rays and thus the image is the darkest. The lungs are an example of an area where the image is the darkest.

VOCABULARY

bremsstrahlung The radiation produced when an electron decelerates (or slows down).

electron A tiny particle of matter with a negative charge, which circles around the center of an atom.

filter A device placed below the focal spot that absorbs low-energy radiation and reduces the total radiation exposure to the patient.

focal spot A point on the bottom of the anode used to allow the x-ray beam to be focused.

image receptor (IR) A cassette or digital image receptor that receives the energy from the remnant radiation and forms the image; found in the Bucky.

latent image An invisible or a hidden image, created by x-rays, that is made visible through processing.

thermionic emission The release of free electrons from the tungsten filament of a cathode that is heated by an electric current passing through it.

tissue density How dense or solid a body part is.

CRITICAL THINKING 50.2

Think about a chest x-ray. What areas would you expect to be darker? What areas would you expect to be lighter?

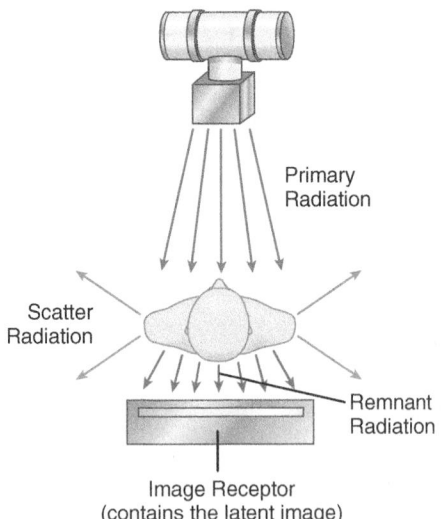

Fig. 50.3 X-Ray Beam. (From Proctor D, et al: *Kinn's the medical assistant*, ed 13, St. Louis, 2017, Elsevier.)

Types of Radiation

When an x-ray beam leaves the machine, it is called the *primary radiation* (Fig. 50.3) or direct beam radiation. The primary radiation can either penetrate the body or be absorbed by the body. When radiation enters the body, three things can occur:

- *Remnant radiation*: When the primary radiation penetrates the body, radiation exiting the body is called *remnant radiation*. When the remnant radiation comes in contact with the IR, the latent image is created. This is the main goal in radiography.
- *Photoelectric effect*: Also called *photoelectric absorption*. This occurs when the primary radiation is totally absorbed by the body. The radiation absorbed by the body is known as the *absorbed dose* and is measured in milligray (mGy) (Box 50.2).
- *Compton effect*: Primary radiation interacts with substances, such as the table, wall, or a body structure (when absorbed by the body). The reaction causes radiation to scatter in all directions. This radiation is called *scatter radiation* or *scatter* and has less energy than the primary radiation. Scatter radiation in the body can affect other structures in the body and also create a cloudiness on the image. Shielding has been used to help with scatter radiation from the environment and will be discussed later in the chapter.

CRITICAL THINKING 50.3

In your own words, describe the three things that can occur when radiation enters the body.

TYPES OF RADIOGRAPHY

With changes in technology over the years, computed radiography (CR) became more popular than the old film radiography. Digital radiography (DR) has now become more popular than CR.

Computed radiography uses a cassette (called a *phosphor storage plate* [PSP]) to capture the image. After the image is taken, the radiographer must remove the cassette from the Bucky and

---

BOX 50.2 **Radiation Dose**

There are three types of radiation doses, and each has its own unit of measure:

- *Absorbed dose*: The amount of energy absorbed by the body. When the radiation enters the body, it will either be absorbed or will penetrate and exit the body. The absorption of radiation means the energy from the radiation is transferred to the body structures. The absorbed energy is measured in milligray (mGy).
- *Equivalent dose*: The damage that the absorbed radiation dose will have on the tissues. Types of radiation differ, and the equivalent dose addresses how the different types of radiation impact the body. The equivalent dose is measured in millisievert (mSv). For diagnostic x-rays, the risk of harm is low. Thus the equivalent rate is the same (numerically) as the absorbed rate. The units are just different between the two rates.
- *Effective dose*: The sum of the equivalent doses the person has received and factors in the harm level of the radiation and the radiosensitive nature of the organs. Measured in mSv.

place it in the scanner. The scanner uses a laser beam to read the latent image on the plate, and a digital image is created in about 1 to 3 minutes. The cassette is erased, preparing it for another image. The digital image is displayed on a computer monitor or can be printed. This process can take valuable time in a busy healthcare environment. The digital image can be digitally archived. An advantage of the CR system is that the initial investment costs are lower, because the system can be used with older film radiology systems.

Digital radiography uses a digital image detector (a flat x-ray–sensitive plate or panel) to capture the image. The image is then transferred to the computer system without the use of any cassettes (which are used with CR). The computer produces the digital image. With digital radiography, all the computer components are connected, and it takes seconds to produce the final digital image. There is less radiation exposure compared to CR systems. The image produced has a better quality than CR images. The DR system costs more for the initial investment and requires new equipment.

There are several advantages to digital images from the CR and DR systems. Digital images are stored on the facility's network or cloud storage, thus freeing up valuable physical space. Multiple providers can view the image at the same in various locations. Digital images can be enlarged to help identify abnormalities. The image can also be adjusted digitally, without having the patient undergo multiple x-rays.

Conventional radiographs can be added to the electronic system by scanning them with a laser device called a *film digitizer*; however, both the quality of the images and the ability to adjust them are limited.

VOCABULARY

Bucky Contains a moveable grid device that absorbs scatter radiation and also contains the image receptor.

CRITICAL THINKING 50.4

Describe the difference between the CR and the DR systems. What are the advantages and disadvantages of both systems?

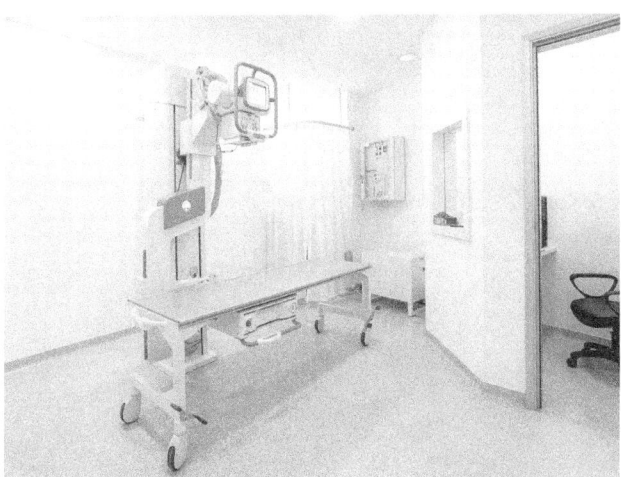

Fig. 50.4 Control Station. (jazzIRT/iStock.com)

PACS and DICOM

Picture archiving and communication system (PACS) is technology that allows digital images in healthcare to be stored, retrieved, managed, transmitted, and viewed. Digital Imaging and Communications in Medicine (DICOM) is the universal clinical messaging format used to exchange images between medical equipment and information systems (e.g., the computer network). Using this system, digital images are transmitted into the electronic health record (EHR). *DICOM* is a set of rules or standards used to ensure that the quality of an image stays the same, regardless of the equipment used to take, view, or store it. Standards are critical because the slightest difference in a radiographic image can have a significant impact on the patient's diagnosis and care.

X-RAY ROOM AND EQUIPMENT

When an x-ray room and a control station are built, state and local regulations must be followed. Some regulatory agencies require lead-lined walls, which will not allow x-rays to pass out of the room.

Control Station

A control station is a separate area or room where the radiographer can remain safe from radiation while operating the equipment and obtaining the image (Fig. 50.4). It is protected by a special wall and/or window lined with lead.

In the control station, the limited radiographer or radiographer can use the control console and/or the computer to prepare to take the image. The radiographer can adjust the primary settings, which include kilovoltage (kVp), milliamperage (mA), and exposure time in seconds (s). After the image is obtained, patient information is typed into the computer and superimposed on a corner of the image, identifying the image as that patient's image.

X-Ray Machine

The x-ray machine is most commonly supported by a ceiling mount or a tube stand (also called a *floor-mounted tube*). The

tube supports the x-ray machine and makes it easily mobile in order to correctly position the primary x-ray beam. The ceiling-mounted support, also called a *ceiling crane* or *tube hanger,* is connected to tracks that run along the ceiling (Fig. 50.5). This allows the x-ray machine to be moved to different locations throughout the room. A *tube stand* is a column with an arm that holds the x-ray machine over the x-ray table. The x-ray stand can generally move back and forth along a track but is not as flexible in movement as the ceiling-mounted support.

An x-ray machine is made up of the x-ray (vacuum) tube and a covering called the *tube housing,* which is lead lined. The *collimator* (KOL ah mae tohr), a boxlike device with controls, is found on the x-ray machine. The collimator is used to adjust the size of the x-ray beam. The x-rays exit the machine through the tube port.

Portable X-Ray Machine. Some ambulatory care facilities do not have a dedicated x-ray room with a permanent control station. In these situations, a portable x-ray machine can be used. The control panel on the portable x-ray machine is attached to the portable mount. A remote can be used to activate the x-ray machine.

Scatter radiation is a concern with portable x-ray machines. The radiographer should stand at least 6 feet back. The examination rooms in an ambulatory care facility are not lead lined, thus radiation safety is a concern. Portable x-ray machines are not as common in ambulatory care facilities as they are in the hospital setting.

CRITICAL THINKING 50.5

Why are portable x-ray machines used more in in-patient and emergency facilities?

Radiographic Table

If the patient needs to lie down or an extremity needs to be imaged, the radiographic table is used. The radiographic table is generally mounted to the floor. The moving tabletop, known as a *floating tabletop,* can move in all directions, which helps when positioning the patient. If the table is to be tilted, the patient must be secured to the table to prevent sliding.

CRITICAL THINKING 50.6

Taylor's manager does not understand why the clinic would need to purchase an x-ray table when it already has examination tables. How could Taylor explain the need for a specific x-ray table, and why would a normal examination table not be ideal for taking x-rays?

Bucky

The Bucky contains a grid, which is a device that absorbs scatter radiation. With many units, the grid is moveable. The Bucky also contains a tray where the image receptor (cassette) is placed. For digital radiography, the digital image receptor is built into the

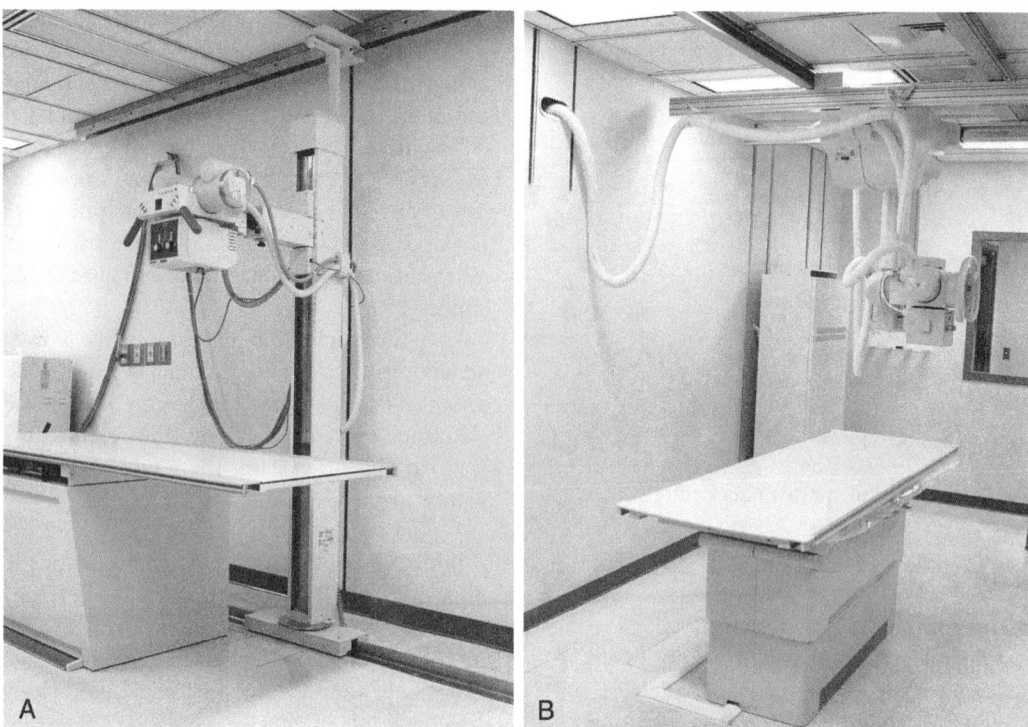

Fig. 50.5 Tube Mounts. A, Tube stand. B, Ceiling mount. (From Johnston J: *Essentials of radiographic physics and imaging*, ed 3, St. Louis, 2020, Elsevier.)

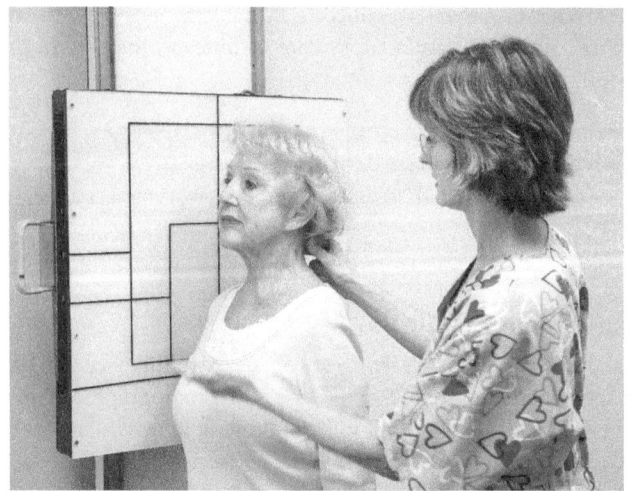

Fig. 50.6 A wall-mounted upright Bucky is behind the patient. The handles on the Bucky allow the radiographer to position the unit with ease. (lisafx/iStock.com)

Bucky. The upright Bucky is mounted on the wall or on a floor-mounted tube (Fig. 50.6). The Bucky is adjustable, so it can be placed behind the body structure being imaged. Body parts less than 10-cm thick produce relatively less scatter radiation and do not require a Bucky. In this instance, an image receptor would be placed on top of the table with the body part directly on top of it.

Markers

When a patient is positioned for an x-ray image, it is important to align the image receptor, grid, and x-ray beam, with the central ray at the center of the body part to be evaluated. Radiopaque (RAE dee oh PAKE) anatomic markers are then used to indicate which side of the body is being imaged. Markers are small squares of plastic with a metal letter in the center that are captured on the image when placed in the radiation field. Right (R) and left (L) are used to indicate the side of the body according to anatomic position (i.e., from the patient's viewpoint). An R or L marker is placed within the radiation field and appears on the image; this helps the viewer identify which part is being viewed. Some healthcare facilities may digitally annotate an R or L on the x-ray image instead of using a radiopaque anatomic marker.

> **VOCABULARY**
> **radiopaque** Not allowing the passage of x-rays or other radiation.

> **CRITICAL THINKING 50.7**
>
> Why is it important to use markers when taking an x-ray image? What could happen if the medical assistant places the incorrect marker on the field? (For instance, places a left marker instead of a right marker.)

IMAGE QUALITY

In the production of the x-ray, a number of factors can be controlled to change how the final image looks.

- Tube current (mA): The total number of electrons in the x-ray tube traveling from the cathode to the anode, which creates the total amount of x-rays produced. It can be changed by adjusting the amount of heat entering the cathode. The greater the x-ray amount, the easier it is for them to move through the body, causing a lighter final image. Tube current affects the image density.

- **Electron energy (kVp):** More energy in the electrons causes more energy in the x-ray. This increased energy causes the x-rays to react more strongly when they come in contact with a body structure. By adjusting the strength of the positive charge emitted by the anode, the amount of energy can be changed. This will affect the image contrast.
- **Source–image receptor distance (SID):** The shorter the distance, the smaller the image is and the more intense the radiation becomes. The greater the distance, the larger the image becomes but the quality lessens. SID can also cause image distortion.

These factors influence the density, contrast, distortion, and spatial resolution of the final image. All of these are important in order to have a clear image that the provider can use to determine a diagnosis. It is important for the medical assistant to adjust the mA, kVp, and SID to ensure the final image is as clear as possible.

VOCABULARY

contrast The difference between the light areas and dark areas in an x-ray that allows detail to be seen.

density Overall darkness or lightness of the radiographic image related to the number of x-rays that pass through the tissue.

distortion The difference between the actual subject and the radiographic image.

electron energy (kVp) The speed at which the electrons travel, or the total energy of those electrons.

source–image receptor distance (SID) The distance between the x-ray tube and the receptor.

tube current (mA) The total number of electrons in the x-ray tube traveling from the cathode to the anode.

CRITICAL THINKING 50.8

What could happen if the provider tries to determine a diagnosis from an unclear x-ray?

Density

Density, or brightness, is the overall darkness or lightness of the radiographic image. This is generally a reflection of the number of x-rays that pass through the tissue. If the energy of the x-rays is too high or the exposure time is too long, too many x-rays pass through the tissue. This causes the final image to be too dark. When this happens, it is called *overexposure*. If there is too little energy or the exposure time is too short, the final image will be too light. When this happens, the image is said to be *underexposed*. If the image is overexposed or underexposed, the provider may have difficulty seeing the details in the final picture. Often the term "brightness" is used in place of density, specifically when using digital imaging. Density of the image should not be confused with tissue density, which was described at the beginning of the chapter (Fig. 50.7).

Contrast

Contrast is the overall difference between the light areas and dark areas in an image. High contrast will give the final image more black and white tones. Low contrast will cause the final image to have more gray tones. Correct contrast levels will allow the provider to see details in the image. In some cases, contrast is affected by the body itself. For example, an abdominal x-ray involves many organs with similar tissue density. This will cause a cloudy appearance (or low contrast) in the final x-ray. On the other hand, a chest x-ray includes a lot of open space (within the lungs), causing a much higher contrast. Low levels of kVp, inappropriate focus of the x-ray beam, and very overweight patients can also cause low contrast.

Fig. 50.7 is an example of how contrast can affect the final image. Note that image A has more gray tones in the final image. Image B is mostly black and white. Both high and low contrast highlight different aspects of the area being x-rayed. The contrast is often changed based on what the provider wants to see in the final x-ray. The medical assistant must be familiar with how changing the contrast will affect the final image. Using the correct contrast will ensure the provider can clearly see what is needed to make the diagnosis (Fig. 50.8).

Distortion

Distortion refers to the difference between the actual subject and the radiographic image. Size distortion and shape distortion are the two main types of distortions seen in an x-ray image.

Size distortion occurs when there is too much space between the patient and the image receptor (Fig. 50.9). The created image appears larger but less clear. To help understand this concept, imagine using a magnifying glass to look at an object. As you move the magnifying glass farther away, the object looks larger but less clear. It is harder to see the details of the object. To prevent size distortion, the patient must be placed as close as possible to the image receptor. This will create an accurate image both in terms of size and clarity.

Shape distortion also relates to magnification. *Shape distortion* can make a body part appear longer or shorter than it really is, depending on the angle of the x-ray beam to the body part (Fig. 50.10). To help understand this concept, think of using a magnifying glass to look at the text in a book. If you were to angle it so one side was close to the book and one side was farther away, what would the text look like? The text closer to the magnifying glass would be small but clear. The text farther away would be larger and not as clear. Shape distortion occurs when the body part imaged is not set parallel to the receptor and one part is farther away than the other. The body part farther away will appear larger than it really is on the final image.

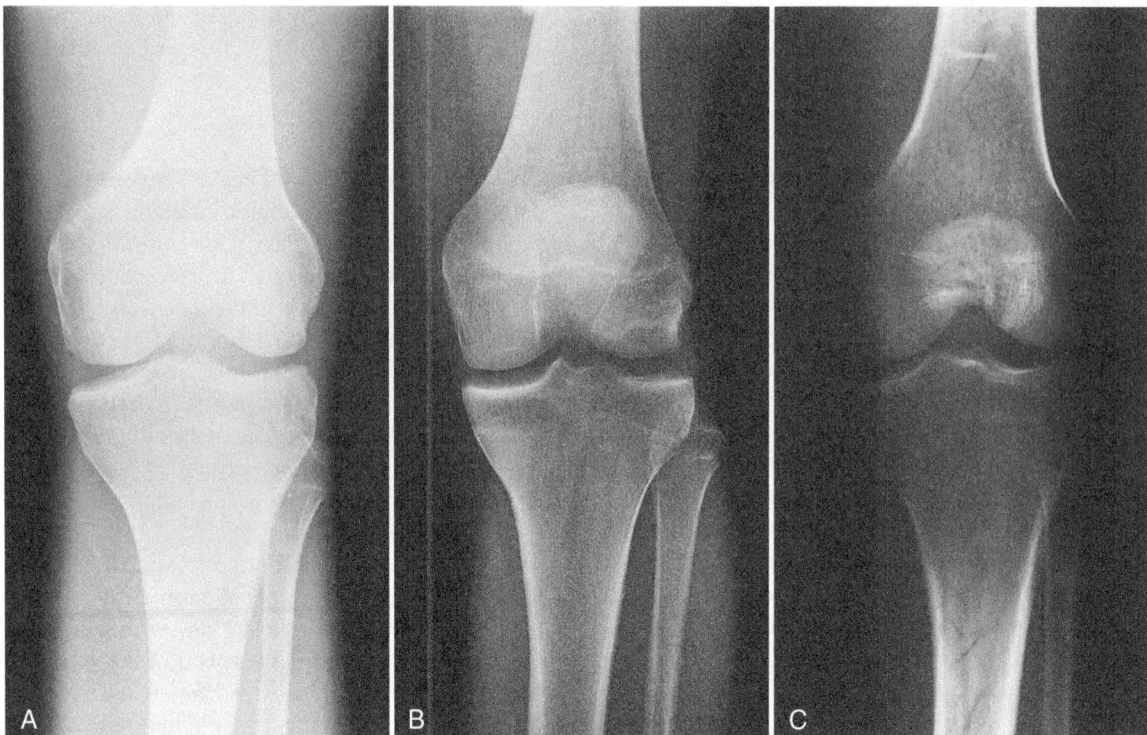

Fig. 50.7 X-Ray Density. Proper x-ray density is needed to make a diagnosis. A, Too little density, or overexposed. It is too light to make a diagnosis. B, Proper density. C, Too much density, or underexposed. It is too dark to see the structures and make a proper diagnosis. (From Long, B: *Radiography essentials for limited practice,* ed 5, St. Louis, 2017, Elsevier.)

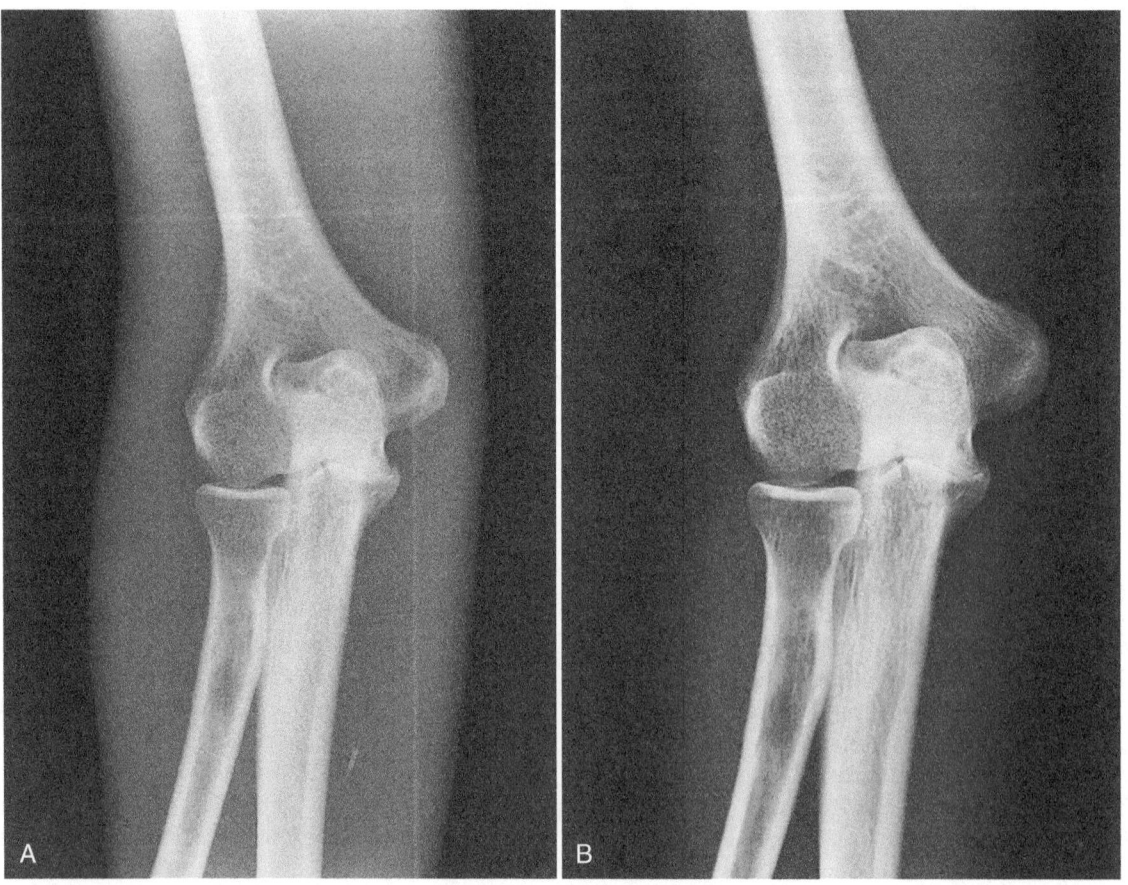

Fig. 50.8 X-Ray Contrast. A, An elbow x-ray with low contrast. B, An elbow x-ray with high contrast. (From Long, B: *Radiography essentials for limited practice,* ed 5, St. Louis, 2017, Elsevier.)

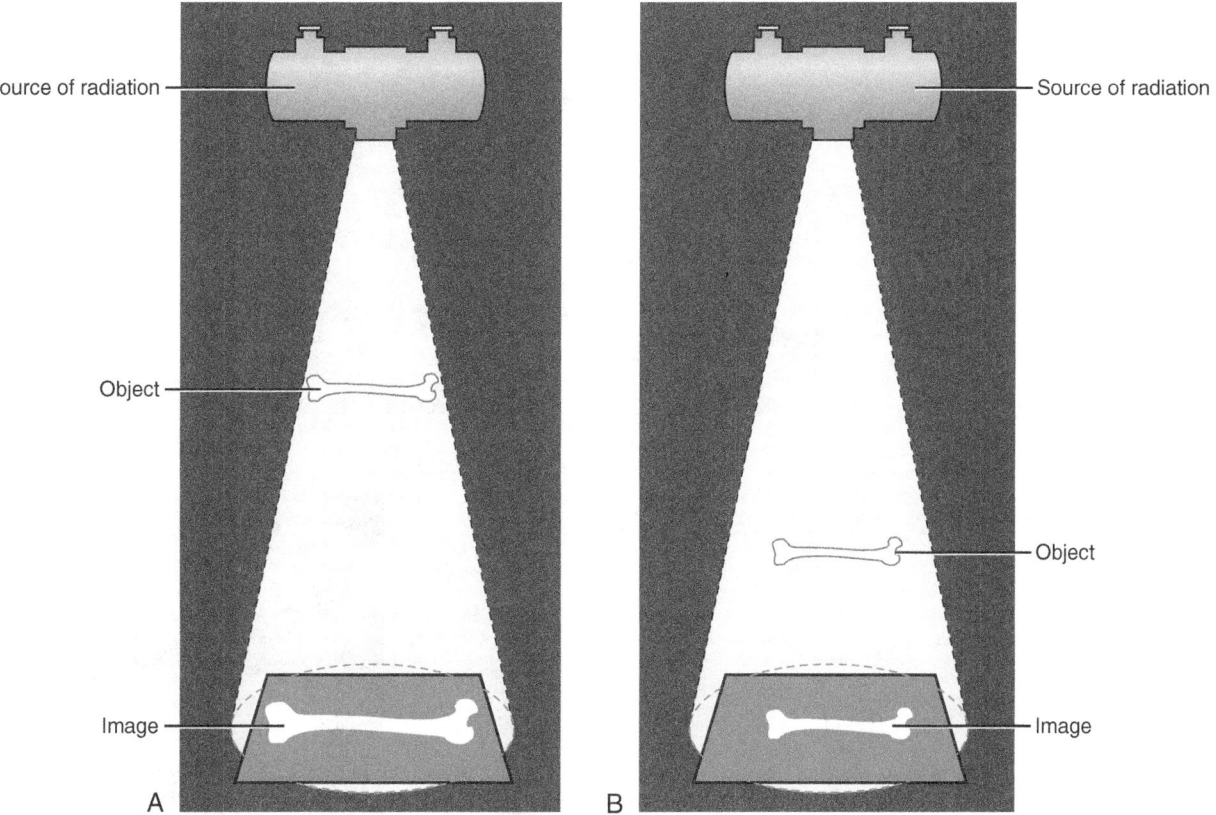

Fig. 50.9 Size Distortion. (From Johnston J: *Essentials of radiographic physics and imaging,* ed 3, St. Louis, 2020, Elsevier.)

Spatial Resolution

Spatial resolution is also referred to as *recorded detail, resolution, sharpness, definition,* or *detail.* Whatever the name, spatial resolution refers to the amount of detail that can be seen in the produced x-ray image. When the image is more detailed, it is easier for the provider to make a diagnosis based on the image. There are four factors that affect spatial resolution, each of which can be adjusted to ensure a very clear image.

1. *Distance between the focal spot and the image receptor.* The further the image receptor is from the focal spot, the wider the beam and the less focused the x-ray. This causes the images to be less clear.
2. *Distance between the object being x-rayed and the image receptor.* As discussed with size distortion, the further an object is from the image receptor, the less clear the image tends to be.
3. *The size of the focal spot.* There are generally two settings for the focal spot:
   - Small focal spot setting: Leads to a more focused x-ray beam and more detail. The x-rays will cover a smaller area but tend to provide more detail in the final image. Depending on the size of the structure being imaged, a small focal spot setting may be too small.
   - Large focal spot setting: More electrons are emitted and a larger area can be imaged, but the final image will be less detailed. The larger focal spot is often necessary for very dense body parts or obese patients.
4. *Movement.* Any movement, including breathing, can cause blurriness of the final image. Prior to the procedure, the patient should be instructed not to move. Depending on the type of x-ray ordered by the provider, the medical assistant must address if the patient needs to exhale or inhale before holding the breath. If possible, involuntary movements, such as tremors, need to be minimized. The medical assistant should observe the patient to check for patterns of tremors. If a pattern exists, the image should be captured when the tremors are less. Other strategies involve using the shortest exposure time necessary and applying a weight, such as a sandbag, to the extremity.

> **VOCABULARY**
> **spatial resolution** The amount of detail that can be seen in the produced x-ray image.

IMAGE PROCESSING AND DISPLAY

There are many considerations and adjustments that can be made to ensure a clean x-ray image with minimal radiation exposure. Every patient is different, and there are different things to keep in mind for each body part being x-rayed. To make this process easier, most facilities provide a *technique chart.* A technique chart is a list of the most common x-ray images ordered in the facility. The list contains the settings for each type of image based on the size of the body part being x-rayed. Table 50.1 is an example of what this may look like. Notice that the chart states the mA and kVp settings, along with the exposure time (in seconds) based on how wide the body part is.

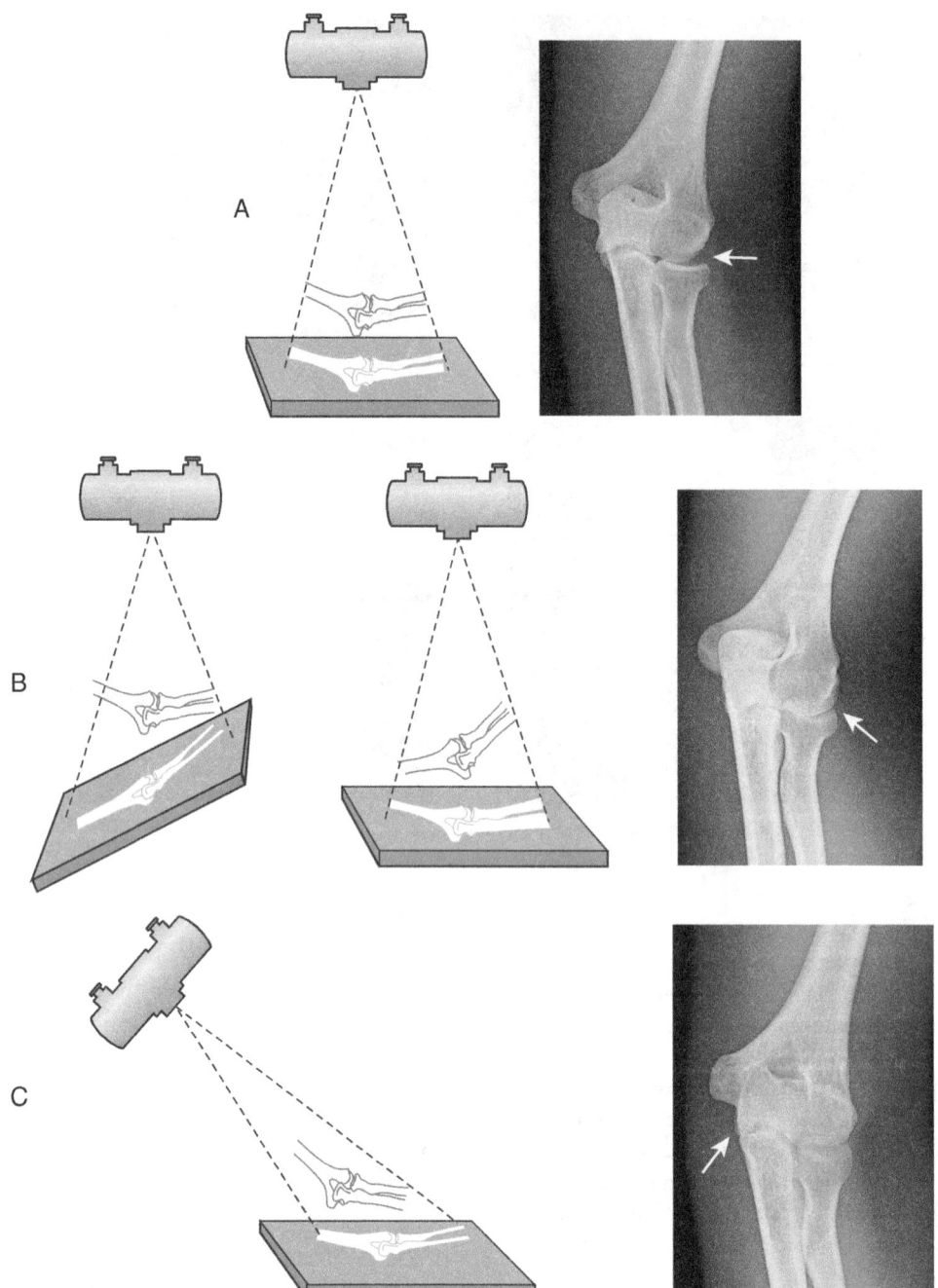

Fig. 50.10 Misalignment and Shape Distortion. A, Proper alignment among the x-ray tube, part, and image receptor. The image is a quality image with minimal distortion. B, Improper alignment among the x-ray tube, part, and image receptor. The illustration on the left shows the image receptor misaligned to the part and the one on the right shows the part not parallel to image receptor. The image has shape distortion due to misalignment of the part and image receptor. C, Improper alignment among the x-ray tube, part, and image receptor. The image has shape distortion due to the central ray not perpendicular to the part. Note the elongation of the olecranon process. (From Johnston J: *Essentials of radiographic physics and imaging*, ed 3, St. Louis, 2020, Elsevier.)

Body parts should be measured through the center of the image, where the central part of the primary x-ray will pass. The medical assistant must measure the body part using an x-ray caliper. The x-ray caliper looks like a large letter F with the center line moving back and forth. The back side of the caliper lists measurements in centimeters. When using the caliper, place the top on one side of the body part. The middle part is moved to the other side of the body part, and the distance from front to back is read on the side (Fig. 50.11).

VOCABULARY

x-ray caliper A device used to measure the size of a body part to assist in determining proper x-ray settings.

TABLE 50.1 Example of Technique Chart for Lumbar Spine

	LUMBAR SPINE					
	AP AND OBLIQUE 40-INCH SIT BUCKY			LATERAL 40-INCH SID BUCKY		
cm	mA	Sec	kVp	mA	Sec	kVp
18–19	200	.04	86			
20–21	200	.05	86			
22–23	200	.06	86			
24–25	200	.08	86	200		96
26–27	200	.1	90	200	.15	96
28–29	200	.15	90	200	.2	96
30–31	200	.2	90	200	.25	96
32–33	200	.25	90	200	.37	96
34–35	200	.37	95	200	.5	102
36–37	200	.5	95	200	.65	102
38–39	200	.65	95	200	.85	102
40–41	200	.85	95	200	1.2	102

From Long B: *Radiography essentials for limited practice*, ed 5, St. Louis, 2013, Elsevier.

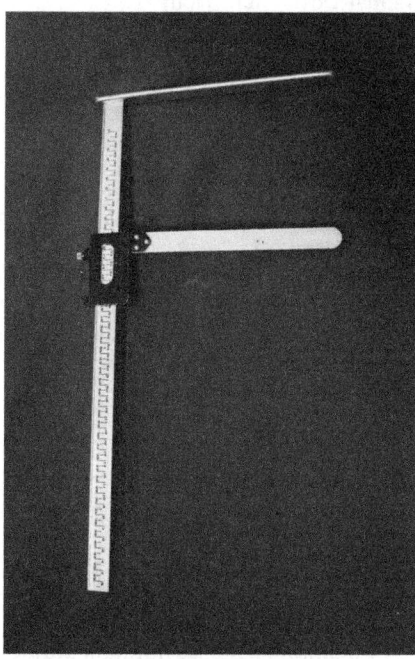

Fig. 50.11 X-Ray Caliper. (From Johnston J: *Essentials of radiographic physics and imaging*, ed 3, St. Louis, 2020, Elsevier.)

RISKS ASSOCIATED WITH RADIATION

Radiation doses are measured in millisieverts (international units) or rem (US units). The dose can be based on a lifetime of exposure or just one dose of radiation.

Radiosensitive Tissues

Different cells and tissues in the body are considered *radiosensitive*, which means they are at higher risk of injury from radiation. Many of these cells have a high division rate or a high metabolic rate. Highly radiosensitive tissues and organs include:

- Bone marrow and blood: Serious changes can occur with these cells.

- Intestines and lymphoid organs, such as the spleen, thymus gland, and lymph node.
- Gonads, such as the testes and ovaries. Permanent damage can occur that results in genetic mutations and sterility. Genetic mutations can be passed to offspring.

Organs and tissues that have a middle-range radiosensitivity include the epidermis, hair, eye lens, lungs, thyroid gland, liver, and kidneys. Tissues with lower radiosensitivity include muscles, bones, nerves, and blood vessels.

Short-Term Health Effects of Radiation Exposure

Acute Radiation Syndrome. Acute radiation syndrome (ARS), or radiation sickness, can occur when a person is exposed to a high dose of radiation over a short period of time, such as within minutes. The entire body was exposed, and the radiation reached the person's internal organs.

The signs and symptoms of ARS include nausea, vomiting, headache, and diarrhea. These symptoms may occur within minutes to days of the exposure and may be intermittent for several days after the exposure. The person may feel better for a period of time before getting sick again. The symptoms are more severe and can include loss of appetite, fatigue, nausea, fever, vomiting, diarrhea, seizures, and coma. These symptoms may last for hours to months.

The person's skin may also be affected by the radiation. Initially, the damage may appear to be similar to a severe sunburn. It may include swelling, itching, redness, blisters, and ulcers. Temporary hair loss may also occur. The symptoms may resolve for a period of time and then return. Complete healing may take several weeks to a few years.

Treatment includes treating burns and infections and maintaining hydration. Death can occur due to infections and internal bleeding.

Cutaneous Radiation Injury. Cutaneous radiation injury (CRI) occurs when a large dose of radiation causes skin injury. Usually, CRI is diagnosed when a person has a burn without being exposed to a chemical or heat source. Symptoms of CRI can appear hours to days after the exposure to the radiation. The person can experience itchiness, tingling, erythema, and edema. First aid treatment involves rinsing the area with water and keeping the site clean and dry. Seeking medical attention is important.

Long-Term Health Effects of Radiation Exposure

Cancer. Exposure to low levels of radiation does not cause immediate health concerns. Over time it can cause a small increase in the risk of cancer. Studies have shown that the risk declines as the dose falls. So a lower dose means a lower risk. People who have received high doses of radiation have a greater risk of developing cancer later in their life.

Prenatal and Child Exposure

Children and fetuses (babies in utero) are more sensitive to radiation exposure. During weeks 2 through 18 of pregnancy, babies in utero are particularly sensitive to the radiation. The sensitivity is due to the rapid growth. The radiation can disrupt the cell division process and cause cell damage. Potential health concerns include stunted growth, deformities, abnormal brain function, and cancer later in life. Radiation exposure during pregnancy can also cause miscarriage.

RADIATION SAFETY

When a provider considers ordering an x-ray for a patient, they must judge that the x-ray will do more good than harm to the patient. X-rays should only be performed when needed to answer a medical question, treat a condition, or guide a procedure. The patient's history and clinical need should be carefully considered before the x-ray is ordered. Although x-rays that are used in the outpatient setting generally use very small amounts of radiation, every effort should still be made to limit the total exposure to both patient and the limited scope radiographer. This is so important it has been identified as a specific radiology principal known as the ALARA principle. *ALARA* stands for "as low as reasonably achievable." This principle needs to be used to remind healthcare professionals to limit radiation to the lowest levels possible to achieve a clear x-ray image. It also is used to eliminate radiation doses that have no direct benefit.

Sources of Radiation

Radiation exposure can occur from primary and secondary radiation. *Primary radiation* comes from the primary beam, from the x-ray machine, and the remnant radiation, which exits the body. *Secondary radiation* comes from the following:

- *Leakage radiation*: Radiation leaks from the x-ray tube housing, though it does not add significantly to the medical assistant's radiation dose. This radiation can be reduced by having the x-ray machine on as minimally as needed.
- *Scatter*: Occurs from the Compton effect in the patient. The amount of scatter depends on the size of the patient and radiation field. The quality of the primary beam also influences the amount of scatter. For instance, an increase in exposure time, increase in energy, and the larger the area x-rayed affect the amount of scatter. Scatter significantly contributes to the medical assistant's radiation dose. Using the grid and

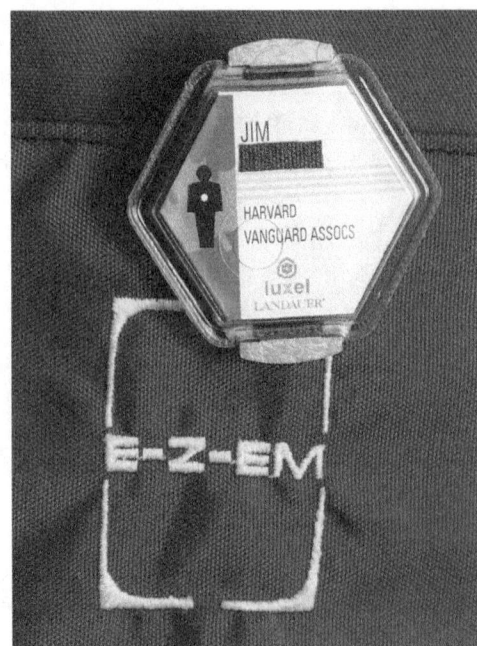

Fig. 50.12 Personal Dosimeter. (From Proctor D, et al: *Kinn's the medical assistant,* ed 13, St. Louis, 2017, Elsevier.)

BOX 50.3   Dosimeters

A dosimeter is worn by an individual and records the amount of external radiation exposure the person receives. Dosimeters provide legal records of the individual's work-related radiation exposure over a lifetime. The dosimeter is a personal device and should not be shared among individuals.

There are several types of dosimeters. It is recommended that badge dosimeters be worn at the collar. If a female is pregnant, the fetal badge must be worn near the waist and under a lead apron if worn. Ring dosimeters should be placed on a finger on the hand that has the most exposure. The dosimeter on the hand should be under the lead-lined glove, if worn. The dosimeters usually are used for 3 to 4 months and then sent to a commercial laboratory for processing. Reports are given to the healthcare agency indicating the radiation exposure for each dosimeter (or each individual). These records are kept on file.

When the dosimeter is not in use, it should be kept in a safe place, away from radiation, heat, or sunlight. The dosimeter should not be crushed, compressed, punctured, or damaged.

---

ensuring the radiation field is as minimal as possible for the area imaged are ways to reduce scatter.

Protecting the Radiographer

The Occupational Safety and Health Administration (OSHA) recommends the development and implementation of a radiation protection program to help protect healthcare workers. In larger healthcare organizations, a radiation safety officer (RSO) manages the radiation protection program. OSHA recommends as part of the radiation protection program:

- Training programs on radiation protection.
- Emergency procedures to identify and respond to radiologic emergency situations.
- Dosimetry program, which monitors the personal radiation exposure of healthcare workers (Fig. 50.12 and Box 50.3).
- Record keeping and reporting programs, including providing dosimetry reports as required by state and federal agencies.

The medical assistant should remember "time, distance, and shielding" when working in radiology. This includes:

• *Minimizing the exposure time to the radiation*: This reduces the personal radiation dose.

• *Maximizing the distance from the sources of radiation*: The radiation intensity is inversely proportional to the square of the distance from the source. This is called the *inverse square law*. This means that by increasing the distance by a factor of 2, the dose rate decreases by a factor of 4. The farther away the medical assistant is from the source, the more the dose lessens.

• *Using shielding* for the radiation source: The medical assistant should use lead or concrete as a shield from the radiation source. For instance, standing behind a concrete or lead-lined wall will help reduce the radiation exposure. Using personal protective equipment (PPE) that contains shielding materials (e.g., lead) will help reduce the radiation exposure. The following PPE can be used:

• Lead aprons or vests: Visual and tactile inspections of the aprons and vests should be done to check for damage or prior misuse that would put the employee at additional risk (Fig. 50.13).

• Lead thyroid collar: Offers protection to the thyroid gland in the neck.

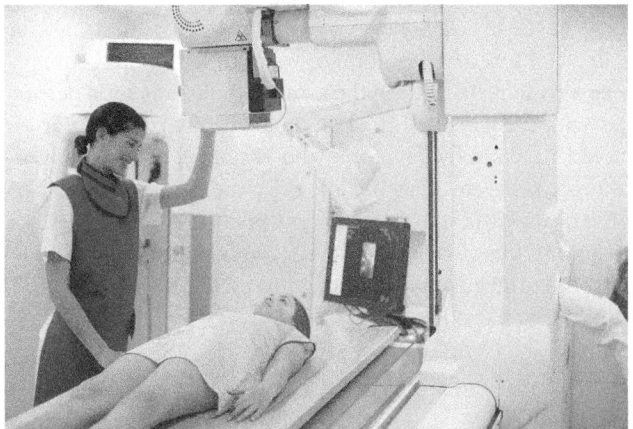

Fig. 50.13 The medical assistant is wearing an apron and a thyroid collar around her neck. (Tempura/iStock.com)

• Lead gloves: Should be used if the medical assistant will have possible exposure to the primary beam.

• Safety goggles: Leaded eyewear or opaque safety goggles can protect the eyes.

Ambulatory care facilities should have policies on how pregnant females working in radiology can report the pregnancy. Extra measures, such as a fetal badge and lead apron, are usually encouraged to help protect the unborn baby, which is more sensitive to radiation than adults.

Protecting the Patient

As discussed in a prior section, the principle of *ALARA* is focused on minimizing the radiation exposure to the patient. The radiographer can help protect the patient from radiation by:

• Using the recommended filters.

• Minimizing metal assistive devices in the x-ray room during the procedure.

• Using the smallest radiation dose possible.

• Using the smallest primary beam possible.

• Ensuring that the patient's position and the central ray position are correct prior to taking the image. This will help limit the need for repeated attempts.

• Using shielding as indicated by the healthcare facility's policies and procedures. Shielding is used to protect radiosensitive tissues, such as the gonads, thyroid gland, and eyes, from primary radiation (Figs. 50.14 and 50.15). Fetal shielding can also be used for patients who are pregnant or could be pregnant.

Fetal and gonadal shielding has been an important practice in radiology since the 1950s. In recent years, the American Association of Physicists in Medicine recommended that providers stop using fetal and gonadal shielding during diagnostic x-rays. Several groups, including the American College of Radiology, support their recommendation. Research has shown that routine diagnostic imaging exams do not expose an unborn baby or a patient to harmful levels of radiation. Studies have shown that often shields are placed inappropriately and larger doses of x-rays are used, or repeated x-rays are needed because the shield blocks important structures. The medical assistant should be aware of the controversy over the use of shielding with patients but must know that shielding is required for employees. When using

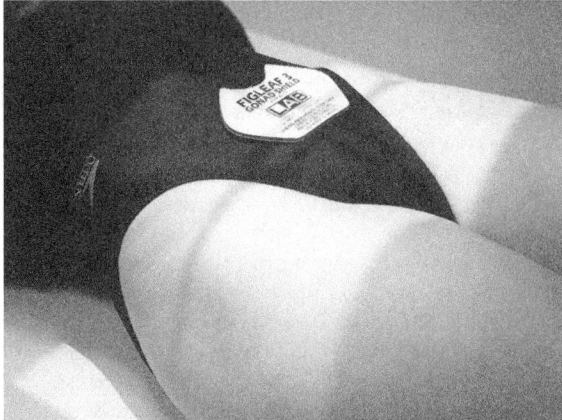

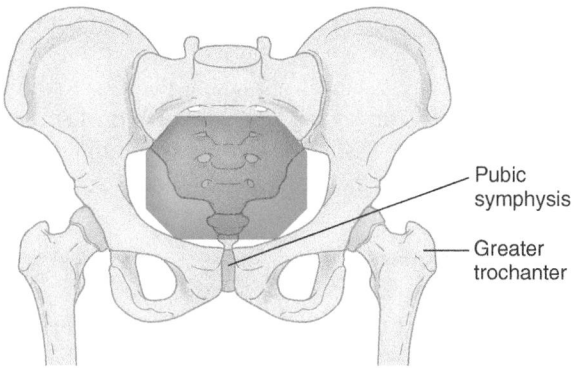

Pubic symphysis

Greater trochanter

Fig. 50.14 When precise gonad shielding is required for female patients, place the lower margin of the shield on the upper margin of the pubic symphysis. (Bontrager KL, Lampignano J: *Textbook of radiographic positioning and related anatomy*, ed 8, St. Louis, 2014, Mosby.)

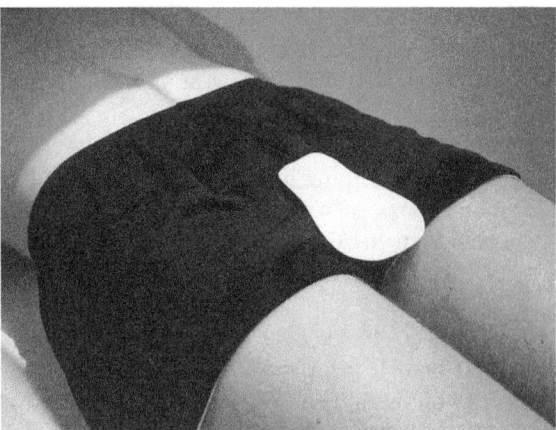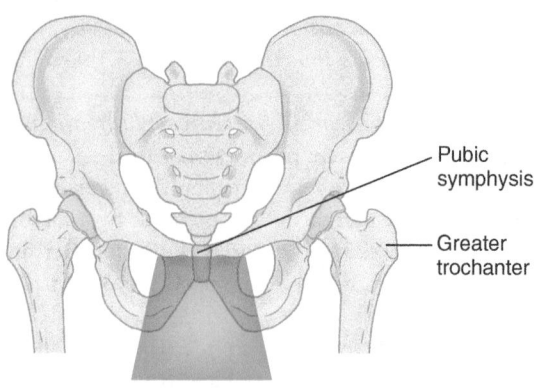

Pubic
symphysis

Greater
trochanter

Fig. 50.15 When precise gonad shielding is required for male patients, place the upper margin of the shield 1 inch below the pubic symphysis. (Bontrager KL, Lampignano J: *Textbook of radiographic positioning and related anatomy*, ed 8, St. Louis, 2014, Mosby.)

shielding for patients, the medical assistant must follow the policies and procedures of the healthcare facility. Shielding should be used if it offers psychological benefits to the patient.

Working With Children. Getting children to stay in position and not move can be challenging. The parent or guardian can accompany the child into the room. Restraints may be used, with parental or guardian consent, to hold the child or an extremity still during the procedure. Explaining the use of the restraint is important. Restraints used allow x-rays to penetrate the area and should only be placed for the shortest time possible.

In some cases, children may simply need some comfort when left alone in an x-ray area. It is appropriate to allow individuals to keep items with them that will help comfort them, as long as they will not interfere with the x-ray. Such items may include a blanket or small stuffed animal for children. Because of the increased risk of scatter, items containing metal should not be near the x-ray beam when it is activated. Many facilities also discourage or do not allow the use of cellphones or other technology in the x-ray room.

If a comfort item and/or a restraint device are not enough to keep a patient still during the x-ray, it is possible for a person to stay with the patient. This should only be done if necessary and should be done by someone who is not regularly involved in taking x-rays. This may include the patient's family member or a medical assistant. It is important to ensure this person is not pregnant. This person should also wear appropriate radiology personal protective equipment to reduce their exposure to the secondary radiation.

CLOSING COMMENTS

Limited radiography involves taking x-rays in the ambulatory care center. In this setting it is common for medical assistants to be involved in patient care, patient support, and in some cases in taking the x-ray. Medical assistants who will be taking x-rays need specialized training and may need licensing or additional certification.

Even if the medical assistant is not taking the actual x-ray image, it is important to understand the process and what can be done to keep the patient safe. It also is important to understand what is happening during the x-ray in order to help ensure

the best image is captured. This will not only prevent the patient from needing to repeat the x-ray, getting unnecessary radiation exposure, but it also will allow the provider to have the best information possible from which to make a diagnosis.

CHAPTER REVIEW

X-rays are a type of electromagnetic radiation. X-rays are created within the vacuum tube in the x-ray machine. When x-rays emerge from the machine, they create a beam in a conelike radiation field that enlarges as it moves farther from the energy source. The very center of this field is called the *central ray*.

The primary beam travels in a straight line. To take an x-ray image, the body part must be directly below the x-ray tube within the primary beam. Depending on the density of the tissue, varying amounts of radiation will be absorbed by the body. The remaining radiation not absorbed by the body will exit the body, come into contact with the image receptor (IR), and create a latent image. The darkness of the image will increase as more x-rays reach the image receptor, thus less is absorbed by the body. When fewer x-rays exit the body and hit the IR, the image is lighter. When radiation enters the body, remnant radiation, photoelectric effect, and the Compton effect occur.

With the changes in technology over the years, computed radiography (CR) became more popular than the old film radiography; then digital radiography (DR) become more popular than CR. Picture archiving and communication system (PACS) is technology that allows digital images in healthcare to be stored, retrieved, managed, transmitted, and viewed. Digital Imaging and Communications in Medicine (DICOM) is the universal clinical messaging format used to exchange images between medical equipment and information systems (e.g., the computer network).

The medical assistant should be familiar with the x-ray room and equipment used. When the medical assistant takes the x-ray image, different factors influence the quality of the image, including density, contrast, distortion, and spatial resolution.

Radiation can cause changes to the tissues. Radiosensitive tissues are at higher risk of injury from radiation. Short-term health effects of radiation include acute radiation syndrome and cutaneous radiation injury. Long-term health effects include cancer and changes in the growth and development of children and babies in utero. The medical assistant must follow the ALARA principle and minimize the exposure of radiation to the patient and to themself. The medical assistant should remember "time, distance, and shielding" when working in radiology. Lead-lined PPE, shielding, and dosimeters are used. Shielding for patients has become controversial recently, and the medical assistant must follow the healthcare facility's policy and procedures.

SCENARIO WRAP-UP

Taylor enjoyed his training in limited scope radiography. He now has a clear understanding of the role of x-rays in ambulatory care and how to ensure his patients' safety, and his own, while using this valuable tool. He currently assists with x-rays as he prepares to take his exam, which will enable him to perform them independently. With each x-ray he reminds himself of ALARA and double-checks all aspects of the x-ray and room to make sure the patient is getting the lowest radiation dose possible that produces a clear image. He also follows his technique charts carefully to make sure that the x-ray does not need to be repeated. Taylor is developing habits that will make him a safe and effective limited scope radiographer.

51

Radiologic Positioning

LEARNING OBJECTIVES

1. Describe the anatomic position and the planes of the body.
2. Describe the anteroposterior and posteroanterior projections.
3. Explain the positioning for the left and right lateral projections.
4. Describe the different types of oblique positions.
5. Describe the cephalad axial, caudad axial, and tangential projections.
6. Describe patient preparation and positioning for chest x-rays.
7. Explain the types of spinal x-rays and the positioning for each.
8. Describe the types of x-rays done for shoulder and upper extremity conditions.
9. Describe the types of x-rays done for lower extremity conditions.
10. Position and shield a patient for a posteroanterior chest x-ray and an extremity x-ray.

OUTLINE

▶▶ OPENING SCENARIO

Taylor Jones, CMA (AAMA), is a certified medical assistant who works at Walden-Martin Family Medical (WMFM) Clinic. Taylor has been training to take x-rays in his clinic. He is excited to take his limited radiography certification exam, which will allow him to take the x-ray images. In the meantime, he has been assisting in the radiology suite, specifically positioning patients and answering their questions about the x-rays.

YOU WILL LEARN

1. To recognize the different radiologic projection positions.
2. To prepare and position a patient for a chest x-ray.
3. To describe types of spinal x-rays and the positioning for each.
4. To describe the types of x-rays done for shoulder and upper extremity conditions.
5. To describe the types of x-rays done for lower extremity conditions.

INTRODUCTION

Even though some states and/or healthcare facilities do not allow medical assistants to take radiologic images (x-rays), it can be helpful for medical assistants to learn about radiology. In smaller clinics, the medical assistant may be asked to assist the radiographer with children and adults who are having difficulty moving. In these situations, the medical assistant must follow the radiographer's directions.

When a medical assistant can work as a limited scope radiographer, proper positioning is important and will help create a clear x-ray image for the provider. It is the responsibility of the radiographer to position the patient for the x-ray. The patient also needs to be able to hold still during the x-ray so movement does not cause the final image to appear blurry. Helping patient get into the position required and to be comfortable are critical for the success of the procedure.

Proper understanding of body mechanics, as discussed in Chapter 35, is also important in assisting patients in radiologic procedures. The medical assistant may need to help patients move between the radiologic table and a wheelchair. The patient's position on the table may need to be adjusted. Medical assistants must use proper body mechanics, to prevent injury to themselves and patients when positioning for x-rays.

Assistive devices used by patients, such as wheelchairs, walkers, and canes, need to be removed once the patient is positioned on the table. These objects can cause radiation to scatter even more in the room, possibly leading to overexposure to the image. Drapes, restraints, and supports approved for use in radiologic procedures may also be used to ensure patient security and privacy.

REVIEW OF THE ANATOMIC POSITION, PLANES, AND DIRECTIONAL TERMS

A medical assistant performing limited scope radiology must be knowledgeable about body positions, planes, and directional terms. The *anatomic position* is a standard frame of reference. This means the body stands erect with the face forward, arms at the sides, palms forward, and toes pointed forward. Using the anatomic position, the body can be divided into planes:

- *Coronal* (koh ROH nul) *plane* or *frontal plane*: Divides the body into front and back portions. The front of the body is referred to as the *anterior* or *ventral*. The back of the body is referred to as the *posterior* or the *dorsal*.
- *Midsagittal* (mid SAJ ih tul) *plane* or *median plane*: Separates the body into equal right and left halves. The *medial line* or *midline* starts at the top of the head (cranium) and continues down the body to between the legs to the ground. Closer to the midline is referred to as *medial*, and farther away from the midline is called *lateral*.
- *Transverse plane* or *horizontal plane*: Divides the body horizontally into upper and lower sections. The area above the plane is called *superior* (pertaining to upward) or *cephalad* (towards the head). The area below the plane is called *inferior* (pertaining to downward) or *caudad* (towards the tail).

Additional positional and directional terms used in radiology include:

- *Proximal* (PROCK sih muhl): Pertains to near the origin or towards the trunk of the body.
- *Distal* (DISS tuhl): Pertains to far from the origin or farthest from the trunk of the body.
- *Supine* (SOO pine) *position*: A person is lying face up.
- *Prone* (PROHN) *position*: A person is lying face down.
- *Lateral* (LAT er uhl) *position*: Lying on one's side.

MEDICAL TERMINOLOGY	
anter/o	front
caud/o	tail
cephal/o	head
dist/o	far
dors/o	back
front/o	front
infer/o	downward
later/o	side
medi/o	middle
poster/o	back
proxim/o	near
super/o	upward
ventr/o	belly

VOCABULARY

anteroposterior (AP) projection The central ray passes from the front of the patient to the back of the patient.

oblique projection The patient is placed in such a way that the central ray passes through the transverse plane of the body at an angle.

planes Imaginary cuts or sections through the body.

posteroanterior (PA) projection The central ray passes from the back of the patient to the front of the patient.

RADIOGRAPHIC PROJECTIONS

Body positioning in radiographic procedures depends on the path the x-ray will need to take through the body to get the best image. Think of an x-ray like taking a picture. It is much easier to see the details of people's faces if they are facing the camera. It is much more difficult to get a clear idea of what people look like if they are not facing the camera. This is the same with x-ray images. The patient needs to be positioned so that the area that needs to be shown on the image is facing the "camera" or in this case the x-ray tube. To better understand how the patient needs to be faced in relation to the x-ray tube, we use terms to indicate the path of the x-ray based on the patient's anatomy. It is important that the medical assistant have a clear understanding of anatomic terms, specifically directions and planes of the body (Fig. 51.1).

Anteroposterior and Posteroanterior Projections

With the anteroposterior (AP) projection, the primary x-ray beam passes from the front (*anterior surface*) to the back (*posterior surface*). With an AP view of the hand, the x-ray is taken from the palm side. With an AP projection for a chest x-ray, the patient is supine or facing the x-ray tube (Fig. 51.2). The x-ray beam leaves the tube, passes through the front of the patient, and exits through the patient's back to reach the image receptor (IR). Anytime the x-ray beam passes through the anterior portion of the body and moves to the posterior portion, this is considered an AP projection.

The posteroanterior (PA) projection is the exact opposite of the AP projection. In PA projections the x-ray beam passes from the back (posterior surface) to the front (anterior surface) to reach the image receptor. For a PA projection of the chest, the patient would be prone or facing the image receptor (Fig. 51.3).

CRITICAL THINKING 51.1

Describe the PA and the AP views in your own words.

Lateral Projections

With the *lateral projection*, the primary x-ray beam passes from one side of the person to the other side of the person. The position is named for the side of the patient nearest to the image receptor. With the *left lateral projection*, the patient's left side is on the image receptor. The x-ray beam enters the right side of the body and exits the left as it enters the image receptor (Fig. 51.4). With the *right lateral projection*, the patient's right side is on the image receptor. The x-ray beam enters the left side and exits the right side of the body.

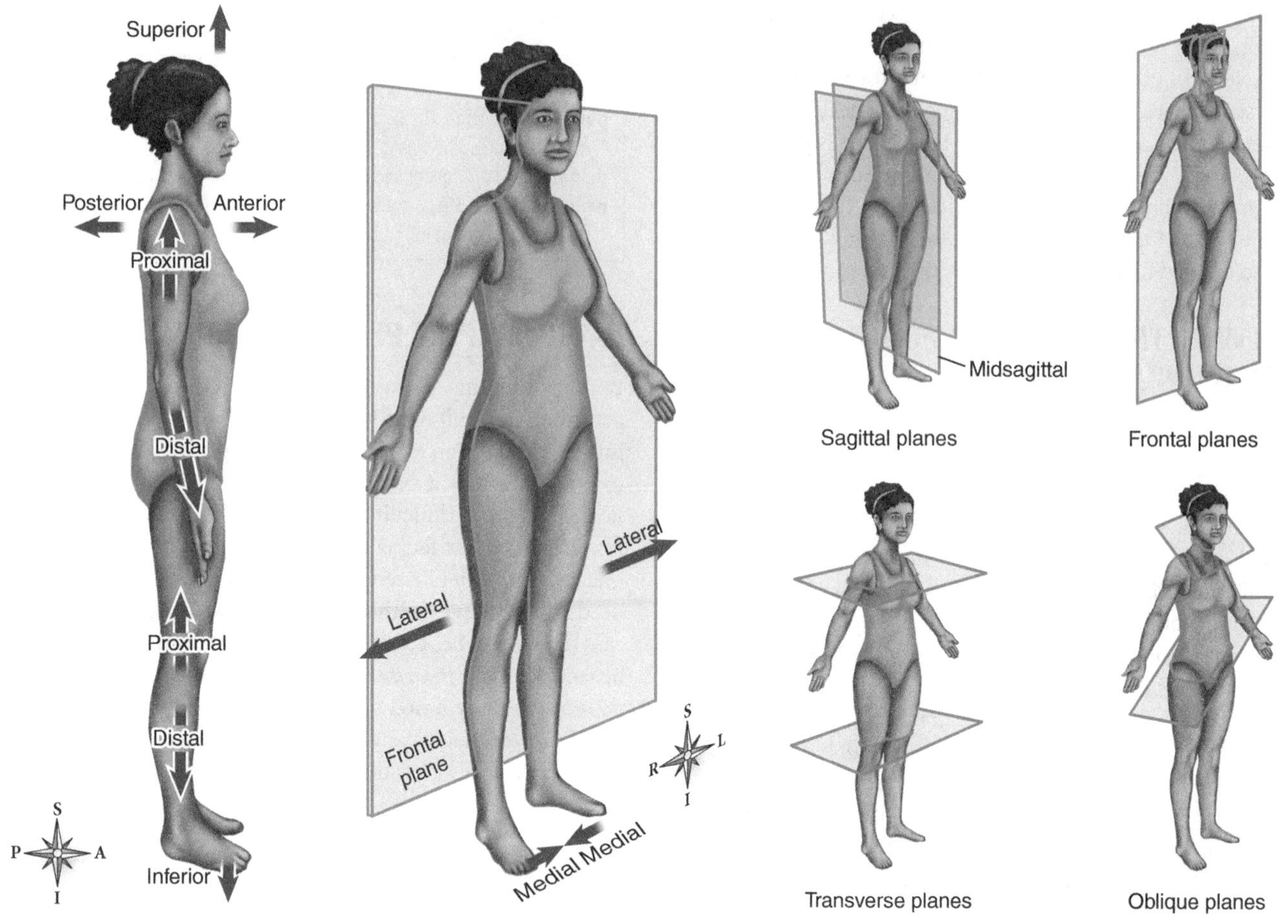

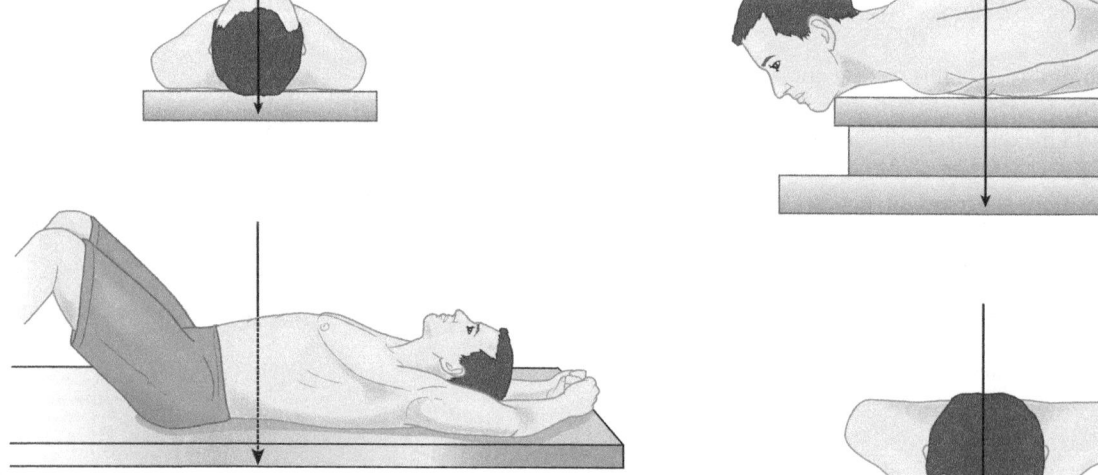

Fig. 51.1 **Directions and Planes of the Body.** (Redrawn from Muscolino JE: *Know the body: muscle, bone, and palpation essentials,* St. Louis, 2012, Mosby.)

Fig. 51.2 **Anteroposterior Projection.** (From Proctor D, et al: *Kinn's the medical assistant,* ed 13, St. Louis, 2017, Elsevier.)

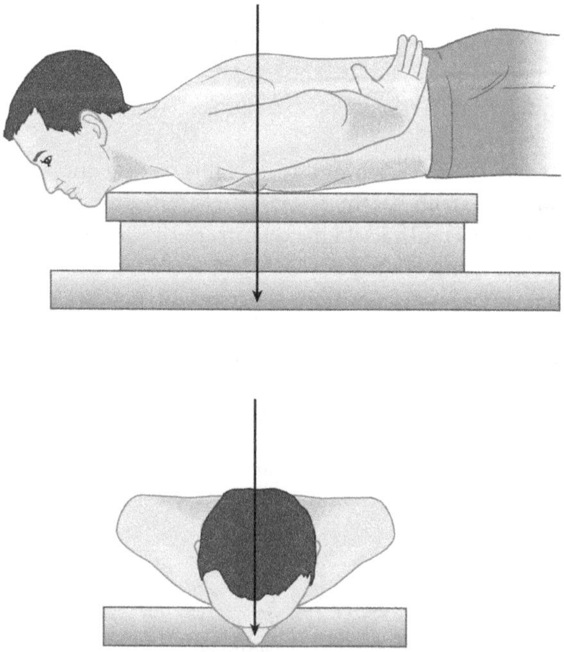

Fig. 51.3 **Posteroanterior Projection.** (From Proctor D, et al: *Kinn's the medical assistant,* ed 13, St. Louis, 2017, Elsevier.)

Oblique Projections

With the oblique projection, the x-ray beam passes through the body at an angle or a slant. With some x-ray views, some structures may hide other body structures. With the oblique projection, the hidden structures are seen. The position is always named for the side of the body nearest to the image receptor:

- *Right anterior oblique (RAO) position*: The patient's right side is on the image receptor. The anterior (front) side of the body leans towards the image receptor (Fig. 51.5A).

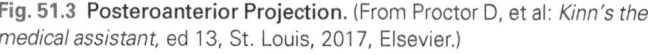

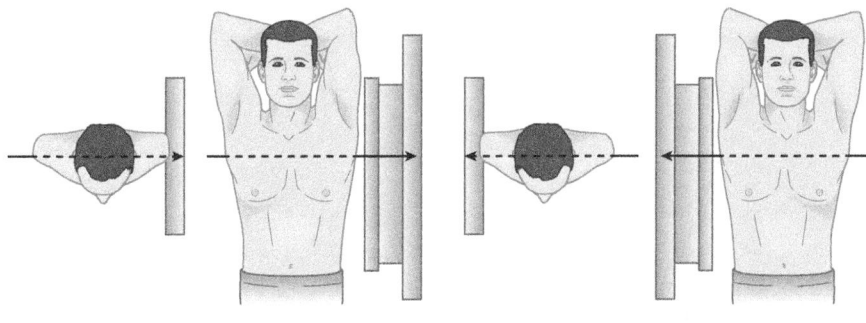

Left lateral   Right lateral

Fig. 51.4 Lateral positions are named for the side of the body nearer the image receptor. (From Proctor D, et al: *Kinn's the medical assistant*, ed 13, St. Louis, 2017, Elsevier.)

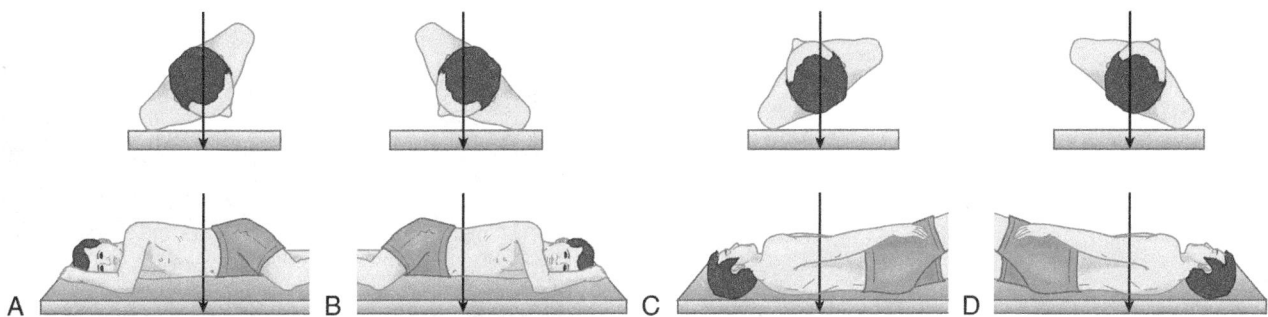

A   B   C   D

Fig. 51.5 **Oblique Projections.** A, Posteroanterior (PA) oblique projection, right anterior oblique position. B, PA oblique projection, left anterior oblique position. C, Anteroposterior (AP) oblique projection, left posterior oblique position. D, AP oblique projection, right posterior oblique position. (From Proctor D, et al: *Kinn's the medical assistant*, ed 13, St. Louis, 2017, Elsevier.)

- *Left anterior oblique (LAO) position:* The patient's left side is on the image receptor. The anterior side of the body is leaning towards the image receptor (Fig. 51.5B).
- *Left posterior oblique (LPO) position:* The patient's left side is on the image receptor. The posterior (back) side of the body is leaning towards the image receptor (Fig. 51.5C).
- *Right posterior oblique (RPO) position:* The patient's right side is on the image receptor. The posterior side of the body is leaning towards the image receptor (Fig. 51.5D).

CRITICAL THINKING 51.2

Describe the RAO, LAO, LPO, and RPO positions in your own words. How might you remember these projections?

Axial and Tangential Projections

Axial and tangential (tan JEN chl) projections also require the primary x-ray beam to pass through the body at an angle. This is done by having the patient lie on the table or stand. The x-ray tube and the receptor are placed in a way to create the angle. The angle differs between the axial and tangential projections. An axial projection has a narrow angle. The tangential projection has a steeper angle. The machine is placed in a way that the x-ray just skims the surface of the body.

Axial projections are further defined by the way the beam is angled. If it is angled toward the head, it is called a *cephalad*

axial projection. If it is angled toward the feet, it is called a *caudad axial projection* (Fig. 51.6). Axial projections can cause shape distortion; thus they are uncommon in ambulatory care facilities.

Tangential projections also cause shape distortion and are not commonly ordered. The exception to this is an x-ray of the patella (kneecap). A tangential projection of the knee shows the joint space and space below the kneecap. The provider can clearly view the patella and bones within the knee joint. This position is called the *sunrise position* because the patella looks like the sun just rising above the horizon (Fig. 51.7).

It can be difficult to clearly view all of the needed structures in one x-ray, regardless of the projection used. Because of this, when an x-ray is needed, it is very common for the provider to order a series. A *series* is a set of x-rays taken together to see a particular bone, or set of bones, from different angles. The knee is a good example; generally when the knee needs to be x-rayed, a series is ordered that includes PA, lateral, and sunrise positioning.

VOCABULARY

axial projection The central ray passes through the long axis of the body at an angle.

tangential projection A type of axial projection; the angle at which the central ray passes through the patient is very small. The central part of the beam skims the surface.

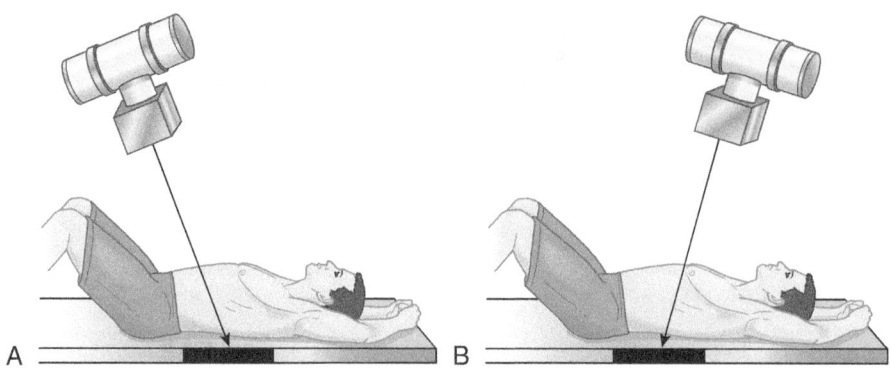

Fig. 51.6 In axial projections, the x-ray tube is angled to direct the central ray along the long axis of the body or part. A, Anteroposterior (AP) projection with a cephalic angulation. B, AP projection with a caudal angulation. (From Proctor D, et al: *Kinn's the medical assistant*, ed 13, St. Louis, 2017, Elsevier.)

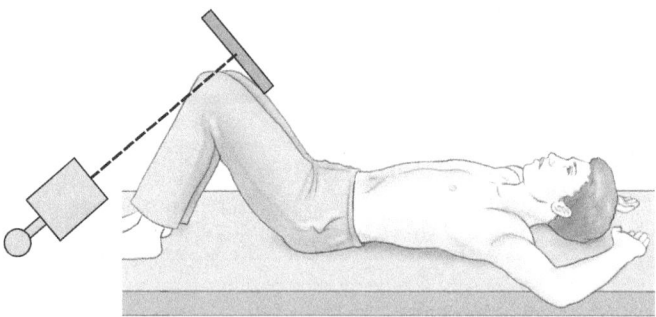

Fig. 51.7 Tangential Projection. Central ray "skims" the profile of the subject. (From Long B, Frank E, Ehrich A: *Radiography essentials for limited practice*, ed 5, St. Louis, 2017, Elsevier.)

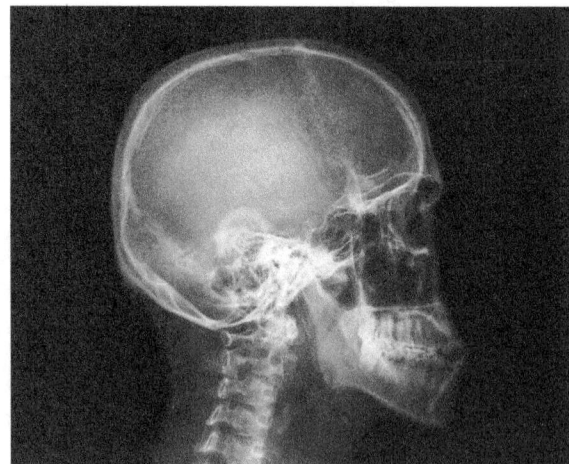

Fig. 51.8 Skull and Cervical Spine, Lateral View. (stockdevil/iStock.com.)

TYPES OF X-RAYS

With limited scope radiology, only specific types of x-rays can be taken. The following sections discuss common x-rays taken in the ambulatory care facility.

Head X-Rays

X-rays of the head are most commonly used in dental procedures and to view fractures or defects within the bony structures of the skull. These are not as common in the ambulatory care setting except for specialty centers (e.g., ear, nose, and throat [ENT] and plastic surgery centers). These departments use x-rays of the head to look for deformities in the sinuses and other issues that will need to be surgically corrected.

When x-rays of the head are ordered, they tend to focus on the area of concern. The head has many bones and other dense tissue (e.g., teeth), which can affect the clarity of the image. In facilities where head x-rays are common, such as a dental office, there will be equipment specifically designed to get clear images of the areas of concern. This specialty equipment is not often seen in general ambulatory care. If a head x-ray is ordered, patient positioning becomes even more important to ensure a clear image (Fig. 51.8).

Chest X-Rays

Unlike x-rays of the head, x-rays of the chest are very common in the ambulatory care setting. (Procedure 51.1) The two most

common reasons for a chest x-ray (CXR) to be ordered are to view a rib fracture and to view pathologic conditions within the lungs. The lungs have a very low tissue density, and because of this, they generally do not show on x-ray. Some diseases, such as pneumonia, emphysema, cystic fibrosis, and tuberculosis, can be seen in the lungs on x-ray. Chest x-rays are commonly taken in the AP, PA, and lateral views.

For chest x-rays, patients are instructed to remove all clothing and jewelry above the waist. They are given a gown to wear with the opening in the back. For routine PA and left lateral projections, the patient stands. With the AP projection, the patient can be sitting or in a supine position. With the PA projection, it is important to get a clear view unobstructed by the scapulae. To do this, the person stands facing the image receptor. The tops of patients' hands should be placed near their waist, and the shoulders should be moved forward (Fig. 51.9A). With the lateral view, the left lateral side of the patient is next to the image receptor. Patients need to raise their arms over the head; each hand could hold the opposite elbow (Fig. 51.9B). The chin needs to be raised and out of the image field. The central ray should be at the level of T7 for both the PA and lateral projections. As with all x-ray procedures, the patient should be instructed not to move during the x-ray. When taking a chest x-ray, it is important to have the patient take a deep

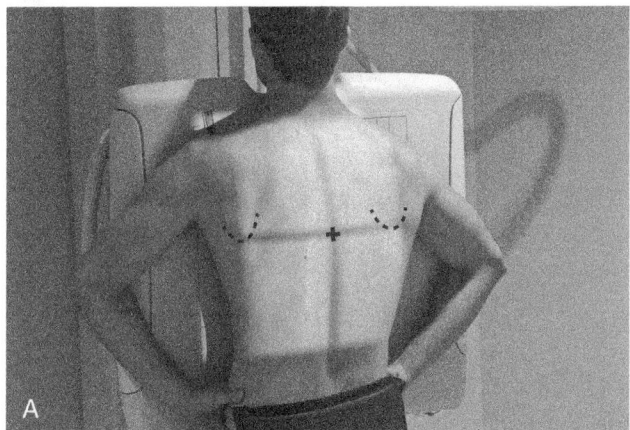

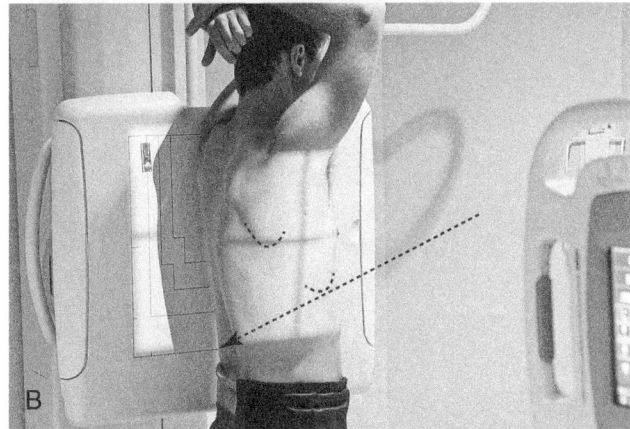

Fig. 51.9 A, Posteroanterior chest position. B, Left lateral chest position. (From Lampignano J, Kendrick L: *Bontrager's textbook of radiographic positioning and related anatomy,* ed 9, St. Louis, 2018, Elsevier.)

breath, release it, and then take a second deep breath and hold it as the x-ray is taken (Fig. 51.10).

CRITICAL THINKING 51.3

Taylor needs to take a chest x-ray (AP view). Describe how he should position the patient.

Rib X-Rays

The rib cage is made up of the sternum and the ribs. The sternum, or breastbone, is made up of the manubrium, body, and xiphoid process. There are seven pairs of *true ribs,* which attach to the sternum by costal cartilage. There are five pairs of *false ribs.* The first three pairs of false ribs attach to the seventh rib and indirectly to the sternum by costal cartilage. The last two pairs of false ribs are called *floating ribs,* because they are not attached in the front of the body. Rib x-rays are usually taken to help diagnose rib fractures.

An AP projection shows the posterior portion of the ribs. A PA projection shows the anterior portion of the ribs. Ribs in the axillary area are seen using an oblique projection, with the RPO position being used for the right ribs and the LPO position for the left ribs. X-rays are usually taken when the patient is

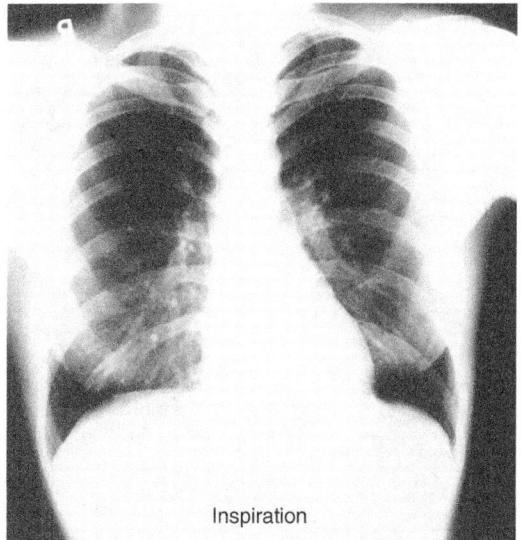

Inspiration

Fig. 51.10 Chest X-Ray. Good inspiration on a chest x-ray makes the hemidiaphragms come down to about the level of the posterior tenth or eleventh rib. (From Mettler F: *Essentials of radiology,* ed 4, Philadelphia, 2019, Elsevier.)

standing or in the recumbent position. The center ray should be at the level of the axillary fold.

Spinal X-Rays

An x-ray of the spine or vertebral column is made up of 24 bones or vertebrae. A spinal x-ray is used to check for damage to a vertebra or multiple vertebrae. A spinal x-ray is also used to assess for degeneration of the vertebral disks and the progression of arthritis. Each vertebra is identified by a letter and number, indicating its location. The vertebra serves to protect the spinal cord and also many large nerves. Damage to the spine or any individual vertebra can lead to pain and tingling or numbness in the body. X-rays of the spine are often ordered when these symptoms are present. The area of the pain and tingling or numbness will determine what area of the spine needs to be imaged. The vertebral column consists of sections:

- *Cervical spine*: Located at the top of the vertebral column. Consists of 7 vertebrae, numbered C1 to C7 (see Fig. 51.8). C1 is also called the *atlas,* and C2 is the *axis.* The cervical spine supports the head and structures of the neck. Damage to the cervical spine and nerves connected to the cervical spine can cause pain, weakness, or numbness in the neck and arms.
- *Thoracic spine*: Located just below the cervical spine. Consists of 12 vertebrae (T1–T12). The thoracic vertebrae are shaped slightly differently than the cervical vertebrae and serve as an attachment point for the ribs (Fig. 51.11). Injury to the vertebrae and nerves in this section can affect the chest and abdomen.
- *Lumbar spine*: Lies directly below the thoracic vertebrae. The 5 lumbar vertebrae are numbered L1 to L5. The lumbar vertebrae are larger in size and have a heavy weight-bearing responsibility in the body. Damage to the structures in the lumbar spine are felt in the lower back, hips, buttocks, and legs.

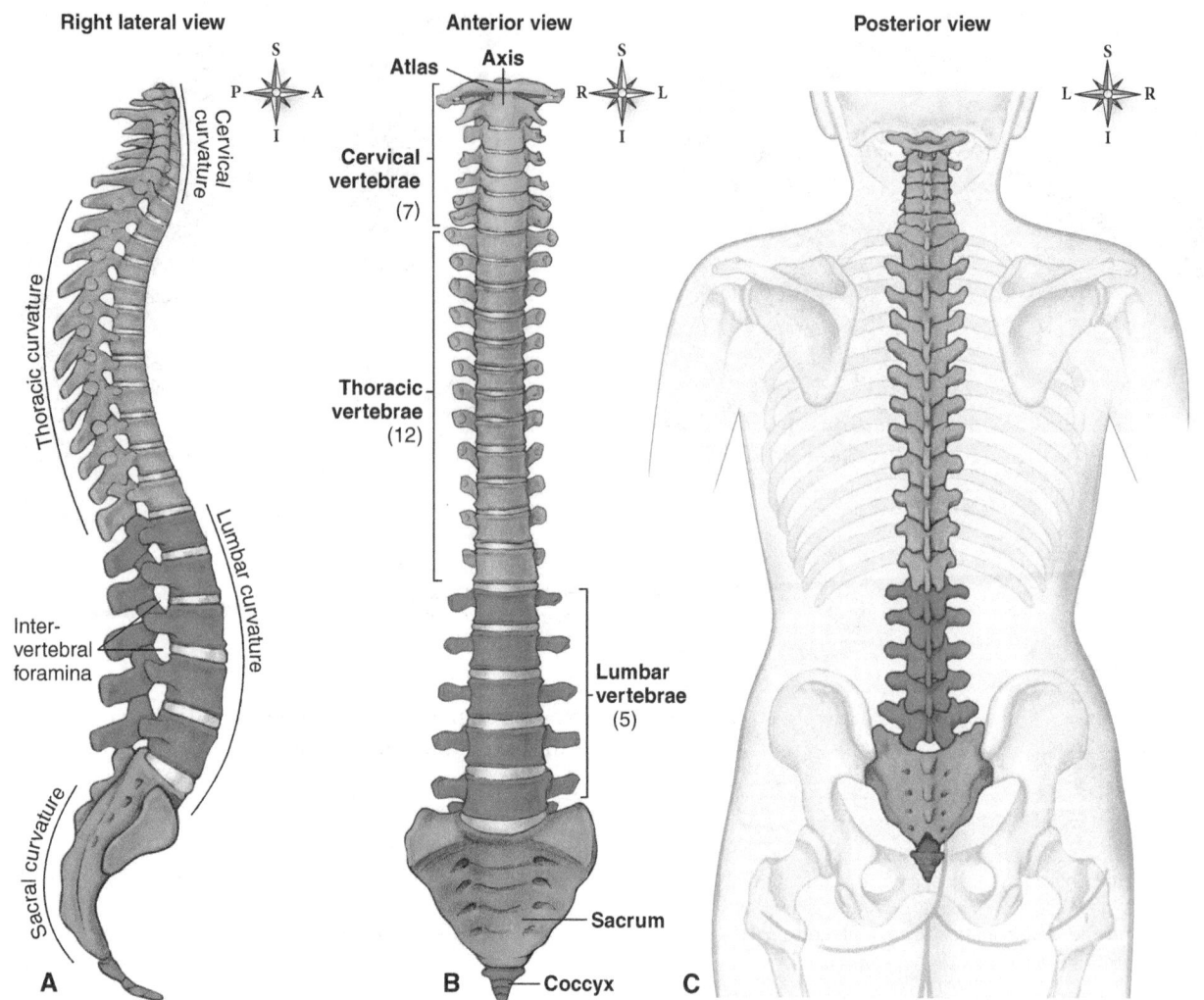

Fig. 51.11 Vertebral Column. (From Patton KT, Thibodeau GA: *The human body in health and disease,* ed 7, St. Louis, 2018, Elsevier.)

- *Sacrum*: Lies below the lumbar spine and consist of 5 vertebrae (S1–S5). Around age 25 to 33, these 5 bones fuse together in most people. The sacrum sits in the middle of the 2 iliac bones. The sacroiliac joint (SIJ) is the location where the sacrum and the iliac bones join. This joint connects the pelvis and the spine. Very little movement occurs at this joint.
- *Coccyx*: Lies below the sacrum and is often referred to as the "tailbone." The coccyx consists of 3 to 5 bones that fuse by early adulthood.

Positioning. Capturing the cervical vertebrae on x-rays requires two different positions. C3 through C7 are seen with an AP axial projection, but an AP projection taken through an open mouth is required to see C1 and C2 (Fig. 51.12). Prior to a cervical x-ray, the patient should be instructed to remove all jewelry on the neck, face, and ears. All metal products, including hearing aids, dentures, hair accessories, glasses, and clothing with metal fasteners, need to be removed. The patient should not move or breathe while the x-ray is taken.

CRITICAL THINKING 51.4

Describe the two types of x-rays required to view the cervical vertebrae.

For a thoracic spinal x-ray, the patient can be in the recumbent position, standing, or sitting. AP and lateral projections are done. For the AP projection, the center ray should at the midpoint of the sternum and at the level of T7 for the lateral projection (Fig. 51.13A). The patient should remove all clothing above the waist and wear a gown with the opening in the back. Just before the x-ray is taken, the patient should exhale and then pause with breathing as it is taken.

Shielding should be applied to the sensitive areas. These patient instructions and shielding requirements also apply for the next two types of spinal x-rays.

AP, PA, and lateral projections can be taken with the lumbar spine. The patient can be standing or in the recumbent position. When standing, the feet should be shoulder-width apart with equal weight placed on both feet. The person's torso

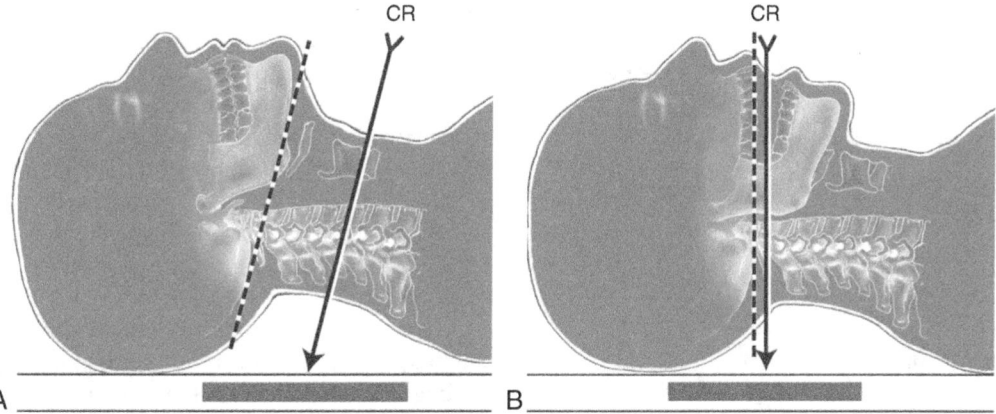

Fig. 51.12 A, Head position for anteroposterior (AP) axial projection of lower cervical spine. Chin is projected over base of skull. Angled x-ray beam is parallel to cervical disk spaces. B, Head position for AP projection of upper cervical spine. With mouth wide open, upper teeth are projected over base of skull, with atlas and axis projected between upper and lower teeth. *CR,* Central ray. (From Long B, Frank E, Ehrich A: *Radiography essentials for limited practice,* ed 5, St. Louis, 2017, Elsevier.)

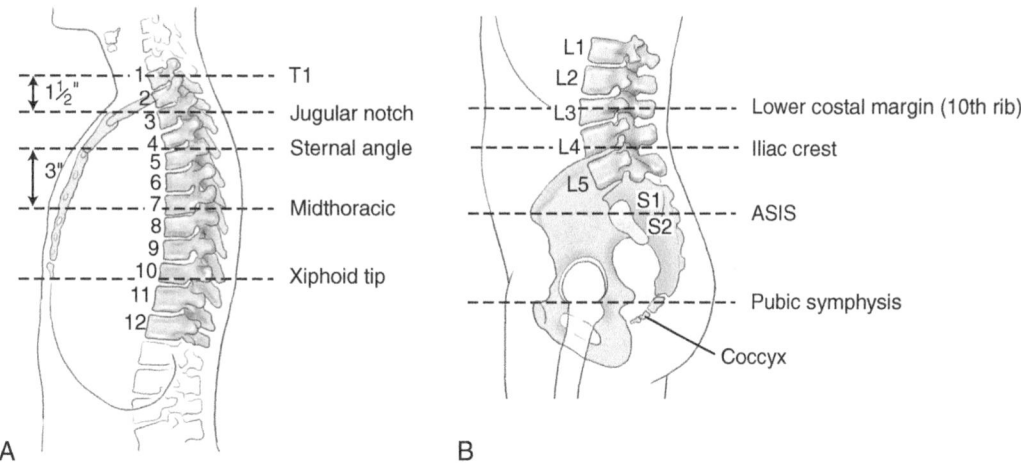

Fig. 51.13 Palpable Landmarks for Spine Positioning. A, Thoracic region. B, Lumbar region. *ASIS,* Anterior superior iliac spine. (From Long B, Frank E, Ehrich A: *Radiography essentials for limited practice,* ed 5, St. Louis, 2017, Elsevier.)

should be centered against the image receptor. In addition, with the lateral projection, the arms are crossed over the chest and the hands are on the opposite shoulders. The center ray should be at the level of the iliac crest (see Fig. 51.13B). For the AP and PA projections the center ray is at the midline, and with the lateral projection the center ray is at the midaxillary line.

X-rays of the sacrum can include AP axial and lateral projections. The patient can be in the supine or recumbent position for the AP axial projection. The knees are flexed and must be elevated and supported with a bolster. The central ray should be at the midline about an inch below the anterior superior iliac spine (see Fig. 51.13B). With the lateral projection, the patient is in the recumbent position with a towel or pad between the flexed knees. The central ray should enter about 3.5 inches posterior to the anterior superior iliac spine.

At times it may be necessary to get an x-ray image of the full spine. The most common example of this is if there is a suspicion that the patient may have a structural problem of the back, such as scoliosis. Taking an x-ray image of the full spine has some unique challenges:

- There are significant differences in tissue density between the area of the cervical spine and the area of the lumbar spine.
- The larger area required will lead to a wider spread of x-rays and increased presence of secondary radiation.
- Many highly sensitive tissues will have an increased chance of exposure to radiation, including the breasts, thyroid gland, gonads, and eyes.

Because of these unique challenges, specialized filters need to be used to allow for even density throughout the entire image and reduced scatter. Also, special care needs to be taken to shield all sensitive tissue possible while still obtaining a clear image.

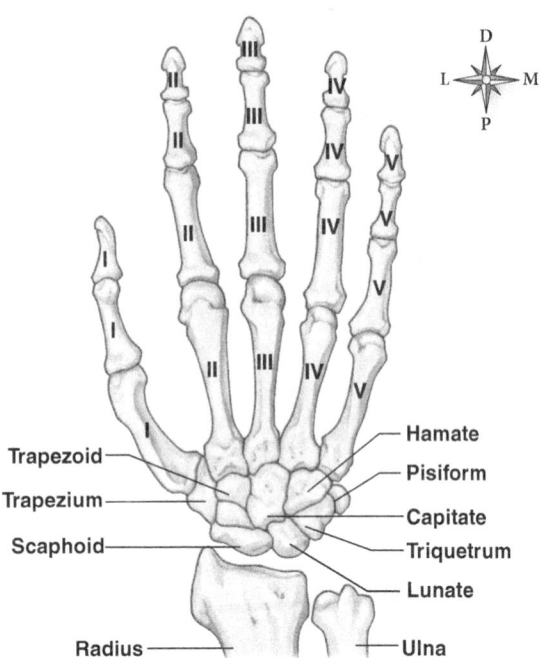

Fig. 51.14 Right Hand and Wrist (Posterior View). (From Patton KT, Thibodeau GA: *The human body in health and disease,* ed 7, St. Louis, 2018, Elsevier.)

CRITICAL THINKING 51.5

Describe the views of x-rays that can be done for the thoracic, lumbar, and sacral spine.

Extremities

Commonly, x-rays are taken of the extremities to help evaluate damage from trauma, such as sports injuries and falls. X-ray series of these areas are common. This allows the provider to see the injured area from multiple angles to be sure that a nondisplaced or incomplete fracture is not missed (Procedure 51.2). The following sections will discuss x-rays of the upper and lower extremities.

Upper Extremities. The upper extremities are made up of:
- Clavicle (collarbone), scapula (shoulder blade), and humerus (upper arm bone).
- Radius and ulna (lower arm bones). The radius is the bone on the thumb side, and the ulna is the little finger side of the forearm.
- Carpals (wrist bones), metacarpals (in the palm of the hand), and the phalanges (finger bones) (Fig. 51.14).
  Positioning. With the shoulder, AP projections are taken as the patient externally and internally rotates the humerus (Fig. 51.15). The medical assistant must position the central ray perpendicular to a location about 1 inch below the coracoid process (Fig. 51.16). With clavicle x-rays, the patient can be

standing or recumbent. An upright PA and PA axial projections are done with the patient standing. A recumbent AP and AP axial projects can also be done.

When x-rays of the humerus are taken, the patient usually is standing but could be recumbent. When the patient is standing, the AP projection requires the supination of the hand (Fig. 51.17). The lateral projection requires the patient to place the hand on the hip, fingers pointing to the feet, and the elbow bent at 45 degrees. The central ray is positioned at the midpoint of the humerus.

X-rays of the structures from the elbow to the fingertips usually require the patient to be sitting alongside or lying on the radiographic table. The area to be x-rayed is placed on the table. Forearm and elbow x-rays include lateral and AP views. Wrist x-rays may include PA, lateral, and PA oblique-lateral rotation projections (Fig. 51.18). The medical assistant should position the central ray so it is perpendicular to the area being x-rayed (e.g., midcarpal area for the wrist, midpoint of the forearm, and elbow joint).

Hand x-ray views include the PA, PA oblique-lateral rotation, and the lateral projections. The fingers should be spread for a PA projection (Fig. 51.19). With the PA oblique projection, the anteromedial aspect of the hand is on the image receptor. For the lateral projection, the medial aspect of the hand rests on the image receptor with the fingers spread apart (Fig. 51.20). For the PA oblique and PA projections, the central ray is perpendicular to the third metacarpophalangeal joint and to the second metacarpophalangeal joint for the lateral projection.

For a finger x-ray, PA, lateral, and PA oblique views can be done (Fig. 51.21). The fingers not being x-rayed are spread away from the one that is. AP, lateral, and PA oblique projections can be done with thumb x-rays.

CRITICAL THINKING 51.6

Timmy fell off his bike and injured his left arm. He is crying and refuses to position his arm for the x-ray. How would you handle this situation?

Lower Extremities. The lower extremities are made up of:
- Pelvic girdle (coxal bone), which includes the ilium, ischium, and pubis.
- Femur (thigh bone) and the patella (kneecap).
- Tibia (shin bone), which is the larger bone and is on the inner side of the leg. The medial malleolus is on the inner side of the ankle, and the posterior malleolus is on the back of the ankle.
- Fibula (lower outer leg bone); the lateral malleolus is located on the outer side of the ankle.
- Tarsals, which include the calcaneus (heel bone), talus, navicular, cuboid, medial cuneiform, intermediate cuneiform, and the lateral cuneiform (Fig. 51.22).
- Metatarsals (feet bones) and the phalanges (toe bones).

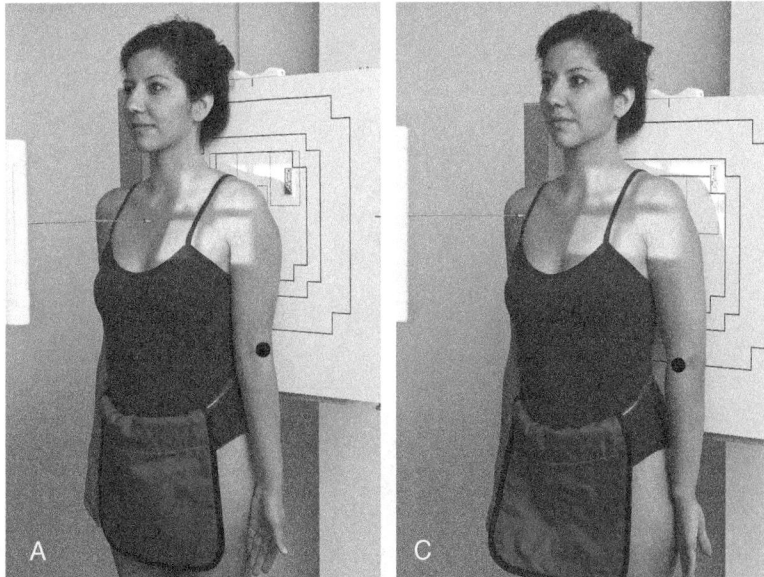

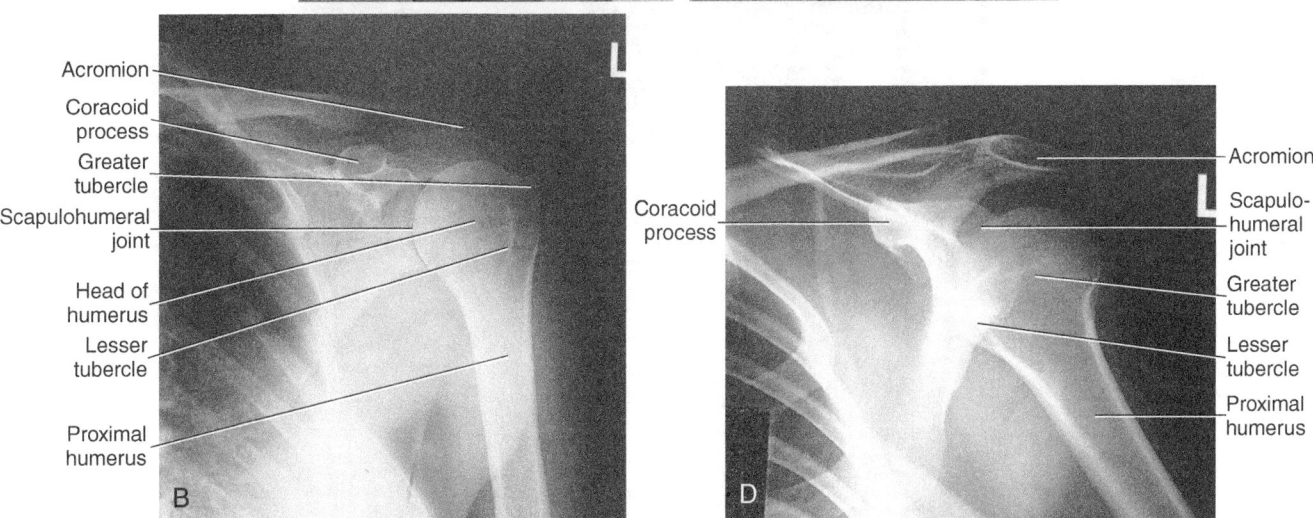

Fig. 51.15 Shoulder Views. A, Positioning for anteroposterior (AP) projection – external rotation. B, AP projection – external rotation. C, Positioning for AP projection – internal rotation (lateral). D, AP projection – internal rotation (lateral). (From Lampignano J, Kendrick L: *Bontrager's textbook of radiographic positioning and related anatomy,* ed 9, St. Louis, 2018, Elsevier.)

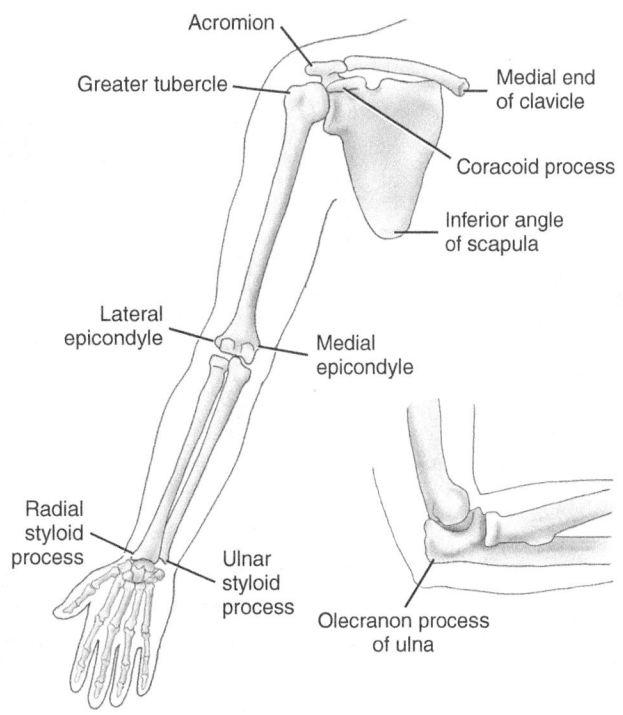

Fig. 51.16 Palpable Bony Landmarks of Upper Limb. (From Long B, Frank E, Ehrich A: *Radiography essentials for limited practice,* ed 5, St. Louis, 2017, Elsevier.)

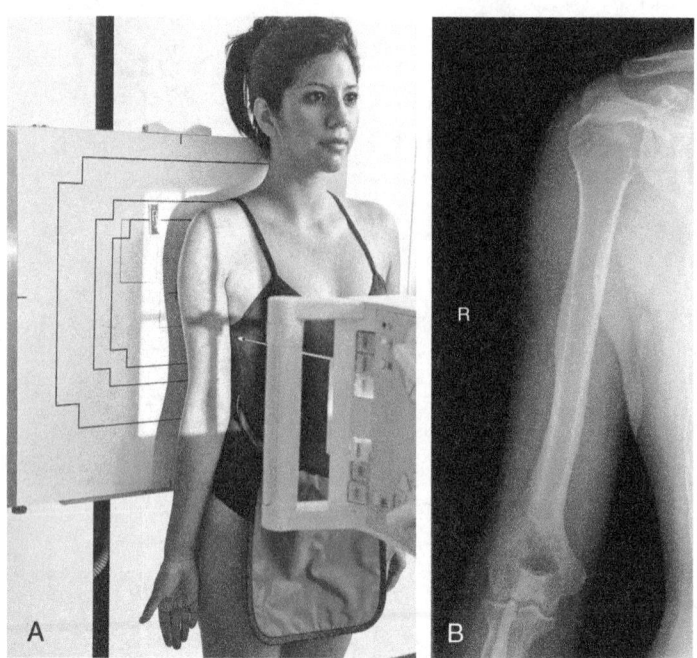

Fig. 51.17 A, Anteroposterior (AP) – erect. B, AP humerus projection. (From Lampignano J, Kendrick L: *Bontrager's textbook of radiographic positioning and related anatomy,* ed 9, St. Louis, 2018, Elsevier.)

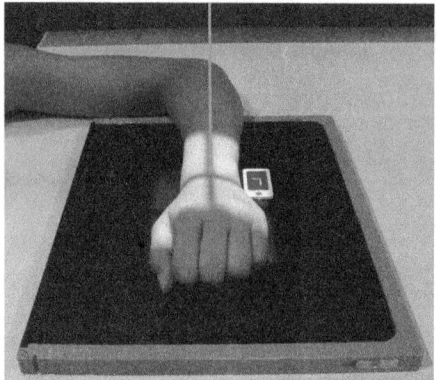

Fig. 51.18 Positioning for Posteroanterior Wrist. (From Long B, Rollins J, Smith B: *Merrill's atlas of radiographic positioning and procedures,* ed 14, St. Louis, 2020, Elsevier.)

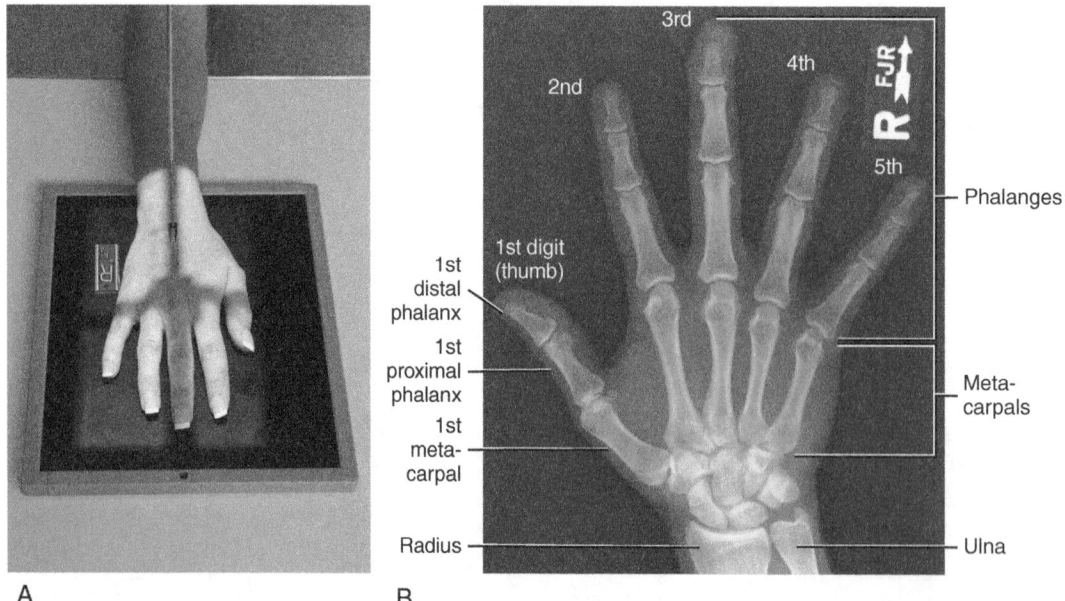

Fig. 51.19 A, Posteroanterior (PA) hand (central ray to third metacarpal joint). B, PA of right hand. (From Lampignano J, Kendrick L: *Bontrager's textbook of radiographic positioning and related anatomy,* ed 9, St. Louis, 2018, Elsevier.)

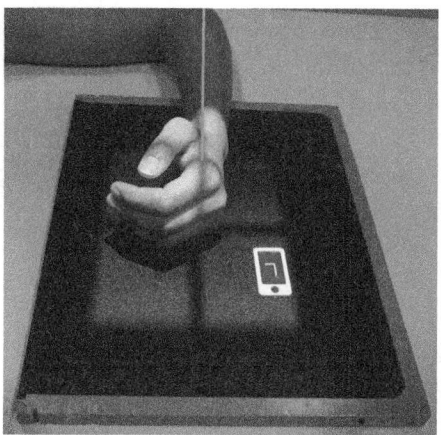

Fig. 51.20 Lateral Hand in Flexion. (From Long B, Rollins J, Smith B: *Merrill's atlas of radiographic positioning and procedures,* ed 14, St. Louis, 2020, Elsevier.)

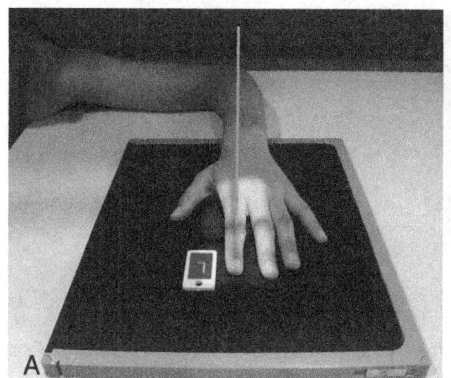
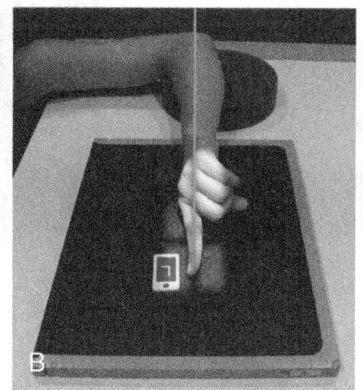
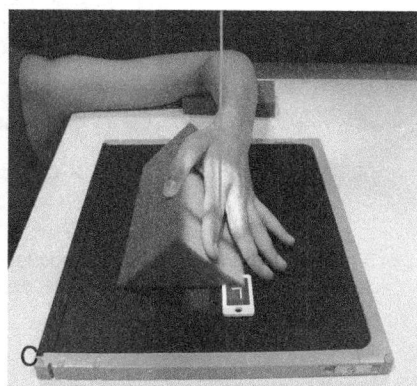

Fig. 51.21 A, Positioning for posteroanterior (PA) second digit. B, Positioning for lateral second digit. C, Positioning for PA oblique second digit. (From Long B, Rollins J, Smith B: *Merrill's atlas of radiographic positioning and procedures,* ed 14, St. Louis, 2020, Elsevier.)

Positioning. When the lower extremities are imaged, the patient should be resting on the radiographic table. It is very important to assist patients onto and off the table, because their injury will likely make it difficult for them to easily move themselves.

For pelvic x-rays, the AP projection is done. The patient is supine on the table. The femur may be rotated, and the heels are apart (Fig. 51.23). When the thigh (femur), knee, and lower leg are x-rayed, AP and lateral projections are done. With the AP view, the back of the leg is against the IR and the foot is dorsiflexed (Fig. 51.24). The lateral side of the leg is against the IR when a lateral projection is done (Fig. 51.25). The medical assistant should position the central ray at the midpoint of the structure being x-rayed.

The ankle x-ray views can include lateral, AP, and AP oblique. Depending on the view, the central ray position can differ. With the lateral projection, it should be perpendicular to the medial malleolus. With the AP and AP oblique views, the central ray is positioned midway between the lateral and medial malleoli (Fig. 51.26). The foot x-ray views can include the AP oblique, lateral, and AP axial. Usually the patient is sitting or lying on the table. For the AP axial view, the bottom of the foot (*plantar surface*) is next to the image receptor, and with the lateral view, the lateral aspect is against the IR (Fig. 51.27). With the AP oblique projection, the medial aspect of the foot is against the image receptor. The central ray is positioned at the base of the third metatarsal. There are many different types of x-ray projections used to image the bones of the feet. Just like the finger x-rays, the toe x-rays are done in several projections, such as AP and AP oblique. The toe being imaged should be centered over the IR. The image should include the distal portion of the metatarsal to the tip of the toe. The central ray is positioned at the metatarsophalangeal (MTP) joint.

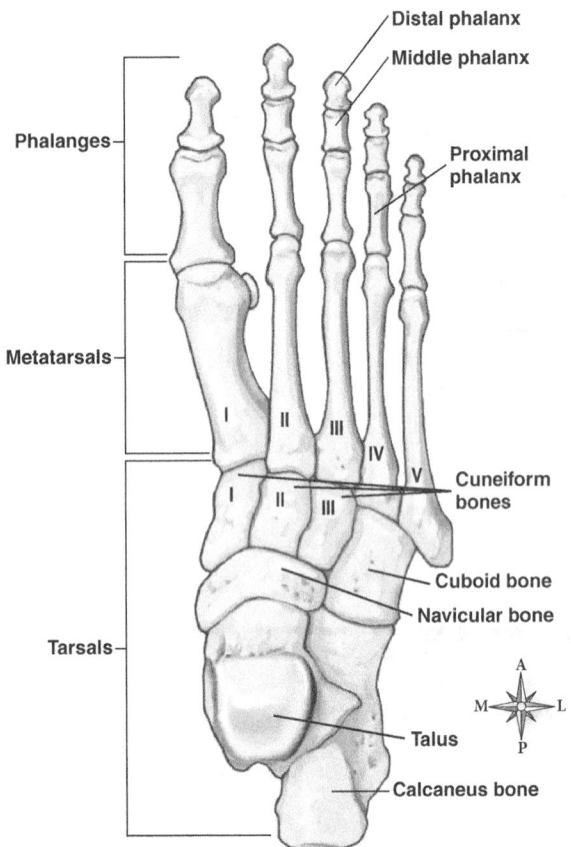

Fig. 51.22 Right Foot. (From Patton KT, Thibodeau GA: *The human body in health and disease,* ed 7, St. Louis, 2018, Elsevier.)

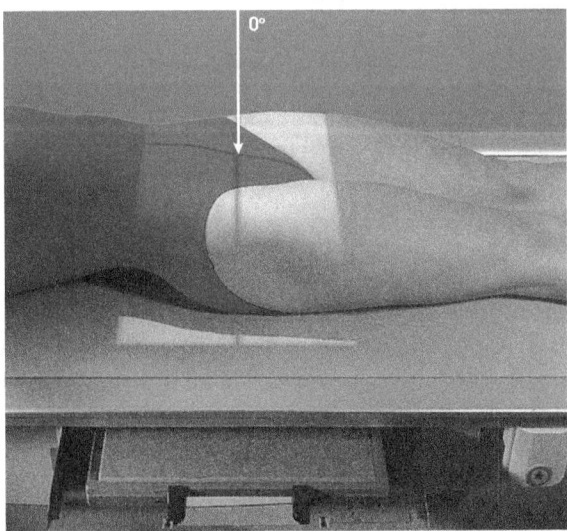

Fig. 51.23 Positioning for Anteroposterior Pelvis. (From Long B, Rollins J, Smith B: *Merrill's atlas of radiographic positioning and procedures,* ed 14, St. Louis, 2020, Elsevier.)

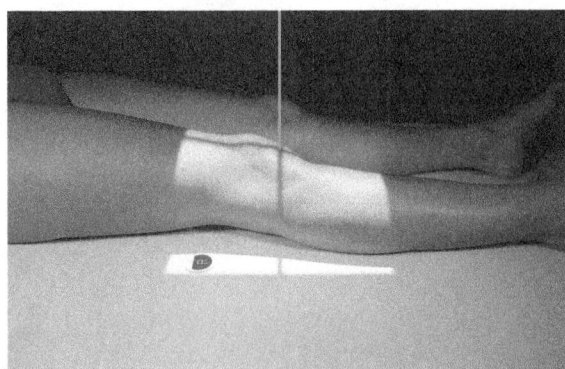

Fig. 51.24 Position for Anteroposterior Knee. (From Long B, Rollins J, Smith B: *Merrill's atlas of radiographic positioning and procedures,* ed 14, St. Louis, 2020, Elsevier.)

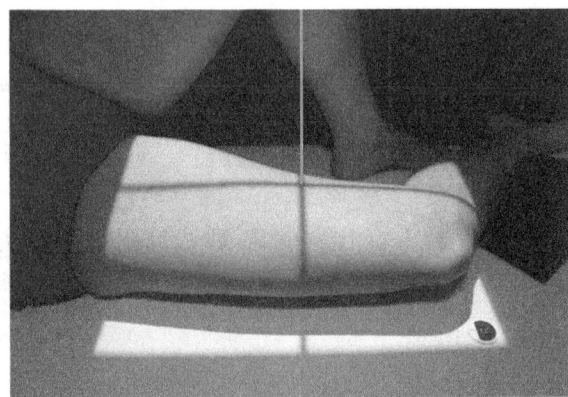

Fig. 51.25 Lateral Distal Femur, Unaffected Extremity Positioned Posterior. (From Long B, Rollins J, Smith B: *Merrill's atlas of radiographic positioning and procedures,* ed 14, St. Louis, 2020, Elsevier.)

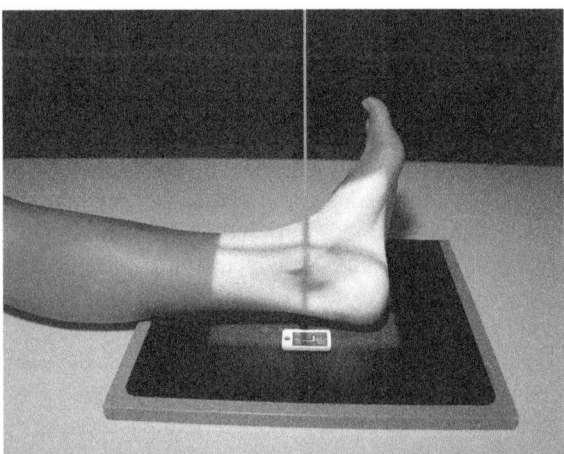

Fig. 51.26 Anteroposterior Oblique Ankle, Lateral Rotation. (From Long B, Rollins J, Smith B: *Merrill's atlas of radiographic positioning and procedures,* ed 14, St. Louis, 2020, Elsevier.)

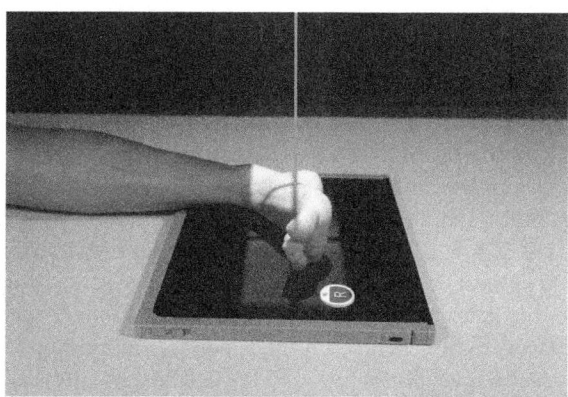

Fig. 51.27 Position for Lateral Foot. (From Long B, Rollins J, Smith B: *Merrill's atlas of radiographic positioning and procedures,* ed 14, St. Louis, 2020, Elsevier.)

CRITICAL THINKING 51.7

Taylor has been asked to take a patient back for an x-ray of his foot. The provider thinks John may have broken his foot and wants an x-ray image to confirm this diagnosis. Taylor notices the order asks for three x-rays from different angles. One from the front, one from the side, and one at an angle. Taylor wonders why so many x-rays are needed and worries about unnecessary radiation exposure to the patient. Why might a provider need multiple x-rays from different angles? How might this help in the diagnosis?

CLOSING COMMENTS

Every state has different laws regarding who can perform a radiographic procedure. Each facility will also have its own rules and regulations regarding radiography. It is becoming more common to see assistants working as limited x-ray technicians. Medical assistants working in this capacity assist in the diagnostic process by obtaining x-ray images of the patients in the ambulatory care setting. Proper patient positioning is vital to ensure the x-ray is clear and meets the needs of the provider in order to reach a diagnosis.

Medical assistants can actively participate in the radiography process even when they are not the individual taking the actual x-ray images. Medical assistants can coordinate patient care, explain the x-ray process to patients, address patients' questions and concerns about the procedure, and prepare the patient for the procedure. Preparing the patient for the procedure involves assisting the patient to the x-ray room and helping them to get into the proper position for the x-ray.

Images most commonly taken in the ambulatory care setting include chest, spine, and extremity views. In some cases head x-rays may also be ordered, but when they are, specialized equipment is commonly needed. When x-rays are needed, it is common to see a set of x-rays ordered together using different projections; this allows the provider to view the area of concern from all angles.

PATIENT-CENTERED CARE

Medical assistants have a responsibility to patients to ensure that they receive the best patient experience possible. Taking the time to communicate effectively is essential when working with a patient to position them for an x-ray procedure. It may be quick to bring patients in, set them in position, and tell them to hold still, but this will do nothing for their peace of mind or comfort. It is important for the medical assistant to:

- Take time to explain the procedure to the patient
- Allow the patient time to change positions and assist the patient to do so, if needed
- Help ensure the patient is comfortable and can hold the position until the x-ray is taken
- Never force an affected (injured) extremity into proper position

The process of having an x-ray taken is not always comfortable but helping the patient to get as comfortable as possible is important. If a patient moves during an x-ray, usually it needs to be repeated. This increases the amount of radiation the patient receives and the overall discomfort of the patient.

BEING PROFESSIONAL

Because there are so many considerations for a medical assistant working in radiology, it can be quite challenging. It is very important that the patient be placed in each radiologic position correctly. Patients needing x-rays are often nervous about the procedure, anxious as to what the image may show, and uncomfortable with the strange positions they will be asked to hold while the image is being taken. It is important for the medical assistant to take the time necessary to ease patients' concerns, answer any questions they have, and show patience with patients as they help them get into position for the x-ray.

Taylor is working with Mr. Green. He needs a chest x-ray. He is very nervous and states, "I have never had an x-ray. What does a chest x-ray show?" Role-play this scenario with a peer.

CHAPTER REVIEW

A medical assistant performing limited scope radiology must be knowledgeable about body positions, planes, and directional terms. The anatomic position means the body stands erect with the face forward, arms at the sides, palms forward, and toes pointed forward. The body can be divided into the coronal or frontal plane, the midsagittal or median plane, and the transverse or horizontal plane.

Body positioning in radiographic procedures depends on the path the x-ray will need to take through the body to get the best image. The following projections were discussed in the chapter:

- Anteroposterior (AP) projection: The primary x-ray beam passes from the front (anterior surface) to the back (posterior surface).
- Posteroanterior (PA) projection: The x-ray beam passes from the back (posterior surface) to the front (anterior surface) to reach the image receptor.
- Lateral projection: The primary x-ray beam passes from the side of the person to the other side of the person.
- Oblique projection: The x-ray beam passes through the body at an angle or a slant.
- Axial and tangential projections: The primary x-ray beam passes through the body at an angle.

Chest x-rays are very common in the ambulatory care setting. Most commonly chest x-rays are taken as an AP view, though they can also be taken as a PA or lateral view. Specific patient education must be given prior to the procedure. The patient should take a deep breath just before the image is obtained.

When rib x-rays are taken, an AP projection shows the posterior portion of the ribs. A PA projection shows the anterior portion of the ribs. Ribs in the axillary area are seen using an oblique projection; the RPO position is used for the right ribs, and the LPO position is used for the left ribs.

With spinal x-rays, the specific type of spinal x-ray will determine the location of the central ray. The cervical spine requires two different x-rays to capture all of the cervical vertebrae. With thoracic, lumbar, and sacral x-rays, patients must hold their breath after exhaling. The central ray should be at the midpoint of the sternum at the level of T7 for the lateral projection of the thoracic spine. For the lumbar spine, the center ray should at the level of the iliac crest. For the AP and PA projections the center ray is at the midline, and with the lateral projection the center ray is at the midaxillary line. For the sacral spine, the central ray should be at the midline about an inch below the anterior superior iliac spine.

With upper and lower extremity x-rays, the patient's position can vary, depending on the situation and the x-ray order. Usually, the central ray needs to be positioned at the midpoint of the structure being imaged. When fingers and toes are x-rayed, the digits not being x-rayed are usually fanned away from the one being x-rayed. The medical assistant should use the landmarks on the extremities when positioning the patient and the central ray.

SCENARIO WRAP-UP

During his time training, Taylor has learned a lot about how a patient needs to be positioned for each x-ray. He has also realized how important it is to be familiar with common fractures and disease processes that will be seen on x-rays and how to position the patient to ensure the proper areas are clear in the final image.

Because the x-ray equipment is new to his clinic, Taylor is working with his teacher and manager to create a procedure manual to outline specifics for patient positioning for each x-ray that will likely be ordered in the facility. This will ensure that all medical assistants who are involved in patient positioning and taking x-ray images are consistent and are properly positioning the patient to ensure the final x-ray image clearly shows the necessary structures.

PROCEDURE 51.1 Prepare and Position a Patient for a Chest X-Ray

Tasks
Position and shield the patient for a posteroanterior x-ray of the chest and document the procedure in the patient's health record.

Equipment and Supplies
- Patient's health record
- Upright Bucky and x-ray machine
- Patient gown
- Lower body shield
- Gloves
- Disinfectant wipes
- X-ray calipers

Procedural Steps
1. Wash your hands or use hand sanitizer.
   Purpose: Hand sanitization is an important step for infection control.
2. Greet the patient. Identify yourself. Verify the patient's identity with full name and date of birth. Explain the procedure to be performed in a manner that is understood by the patient. Answer any questions the patient may have on the procedure. If the patient is female, ask if she could be pregnant. If she answers yes, check with the provider before continuing.
   Purpose: Explanations help gain the patient's cooperation and alleviate apprehension.

3. Give the patient a gown. Explain what clothing must be removed and also jewelry, including neck chains and piercings on the chest. Provide assistance as needed. Allow the patient to use a changing room and give the patient privacy while changing. Knock on the door before reentering to make sure the patient has completed undressing and gowning. If the patient is female, ask if she could be pregnant. If she answers yes, check with the provider before continuing.
   Purpose: Metal and other highly dense materials will obscure the x-ray. Pregnant patients are considered at increased risk with radiologic procedures, and verification from the provider is required before an x-ray is performed on a patient who could be pregnant.
4. Review the provider's orders for the exact x-ray image that needs to be taken. Measure the patient's chest cavity from front to back with x-ray calipers.
   Purpose: Accurate measurement of the area involved in the x-ray is necessary to ensure proper settings on the x-ray machine.
5. Review the technique chart for a posteroanterior (PA) chest x-ray and set the mA, kVp, and exposure time appropriate for the image and the patient's size.
6. Stand the patient with the anterior surface of the chest against the upright Bucky. Ask patients to place the tops of their hands near the waist. The patient's shoulders should be rotated or moved forward. *Optional:* Patients who are unsteady can wrap their hands around the Bucky to improve stability and reduce the potential for a fall.

PROCEDURE 51.1   Prepare and Position a Patient for a Chest X-Ray—cont'd

Purpose: This position will rotate the scapulae out of the way so that they will not obscure the lungs in the final image.

7. As indicated by facility policy and procedure, secure the lower back x-ray shield to prevent scatter radiation from affecting the sensitive gonad area.
   Purpose: This will protect the sensitive tissue from scatter radiation.

8. Position the x-ray machine. The central ray should be at the level of T7. Place the marker in the field.

9. Ask the patient to hold as still as possible and move to the x-ray control panel. If using a portable x-ray unit, move at least 6 feet away.
   Purpose: If the patient moves before the image is taken, the final x-ray may have structures showing in inappropriate places, which could obscure the areas that need to be seen. Standing at the control station or at least 6 feet away will protect the medical assistant from unnecessary radiation exposure.

10. Tell the patient to take a deep breath in, blow it out, then take another deep breath and hold it. Once patients are holding their breath, activate the machine to take the image. Inform patients as soon as the image is complete that they can exhale and breath normally.

Purpose: Ensuring the chest cavity is filled with air will make the structures within the chest wall, in addition to the lungs, clearer in the final image.

11. Complete any other x-rays as ordered by the provider. Once all required x-rays are completed, provide a comfortable place for the patient to rest. Then review the images for clarity, looking specifically at density, contrast, and for distortions. If there are abnormalities, repeat the image.
    Purpose: If an x-ray image is unclear, it will be necessary to take another image to obtain appropriate results for the provider to use for diagnostics.

12. After the images are completed, remove the shield and assist the patient as needed to get dressed. Return patients to their room and inform the provider the images are available.

13. Put on gloves and use disinfectant wipes to clean the Bucky and all potentially contaminated surfaces. Dispose of the used gloves and sanitize hands.
    Purpose: This ensures infection control and prevents the transmission of pathogens from one patient to another.

14. Document completion of the imaging procedure in the patient's health record. Document the ordering provider's name, the order, and how the patient tolerated the procedure, or elements indicated by the facility's policies and procedures.

PROCEDURE 51.2   Prepare and Position a Patient for an Extremity X-Ray

Tasks

Position and shield the patient for an x-ray image of an extremity and document the procedure in the patient's health record.

Equipment and Supplies

- Patient's health record
- Radiographic table and x-ray machine
- Patient gown (optional)
- Radiation shield
- Gloves
- Disinfectant wipes
- Caliper

Procedural Steps

1. Wash your hands or use hand sanitizer.
   Purpose: Hand sanitization is an important step for infection control.

2. Greet the patient. Identify yourself. Verify the patient's identity with full name and date of birth. Explain the procedure to be performed in a manner that is understood by the patient. Answer any questions the patient may have on the procedure. If the patient is female, ask if she could be pregnant. If she answers yes, check with the provider before continuing.
   Purpose: Explanations help gain the patient's cooperation and alleviate apprehension. Pregnant patients are considered at increased risk with radiologic procedures, and verification from the provider is required before an x-ray is performed on a patient who could be pregnant.

3. Give the patient a gown. Explain what clothing must be removed. Specifically mention that any metal must be removed, such as pants with zippers and buttons, in addition to jewelry, including watches, bracelets, or any piercings that would be in the x-ray field. Allow the patient to use a changing room and give the patient privacy while changing. Knock on the door before reentering to make sure the patient has completed undressing and gowning.
   Purpose: Metal and other highly dense materials will obscure the x-ray.

4. Review the provider's orders for the exact x-ray image that needs to be taken. Measure the appropriate body part from front to back and side to side with an x-ray caliper.
   Purpose: Accurate measurement of the area involved in the x-ray is necessary to ensure proper settings on the x-ray machine.

5. Review the technique chart for the appropriate image and set the mA, kVp, and exposure time appropriate for the image and the patient's size.

6. Have the patient sit on or next to the x-ray table (depending on the patient's need for support and the specific image that will be taken). Ensure that the extremity is positioned consistent with the provider's order and the radiographic projection needed. Provide support or restraint devices as needed.
   Purpose: Proper positioning is necessary for a clear image of the structures needed. If a patient needs support or restraint to assist them in holding still, this should be provided.

7. Secure the x-ray shield to prevent scatter radiation from affecting the sensitive tissue, including thyroid, genital, breast, and abdominal tissues, as indicated by the facility's policies and procedures. Place the marker in the field.
   Purpose: This will protect the sensitive tissue from scatter radiation.

8. Position the x-ray machine directly in line with the patient, with the center placed directly over the center of the bone structure being imaged. Ask the patient to hold as still as possible and move to the x-ray control panel. If using a portable x-ray unit, move at least 6 feet away.
   Purpose: If the patient moves before the image is taken, the final x-ray may have structures showing in inappropriate places, which could obscure the areas that need to be seen. Standing at the control station or at least 6 feet away will protect the medical assistant from unnecessary radiation exposure.

9. Complete any other x-rays as ordered by the provider. Once all required x-rays are completed, provide a comfortable place for the patient to rest. Then review the images for clarity, looking specifically at density, contrast, and for distortions. If there are abnormalities, repeat the image.
   Purpose: If an x-ray image is unclear, it will be necessary to take another image to obtain appropriate results for the provider to use for diagnostics.

10. After the images are completed, remove the shield and assist the patient as needed to get dressed. Return patients to their room and inform the provider the images are available.

11. Put on gloves and use disinfectant wipes to clean the Bucky and all potentially contaminated surfaces. Dispose of the used gloves and sanitize hands.
    Purpose: This ensures infection control and prevents the transmission of pathogens from one patient to another.

12. Document completion of the imaging procedure in the patient's health record. Document the ordering provider's name, the order, and how the patient tolerated the procedure, or elements indicated by the facility's policies and procedures.

52

Assisting in the Clinical Laboratory

LEARNING OBJECTIVES

1. Discuss the personnel in the clinical laboratory, including the medical assistant's role.
2. Describe the departments of the clinical laboratory.
3. Explain the three regulatory categories established by the Clinical Laboratory Improvement Amendments (CLIA) and identify CLIA-waived tests associated with common diseases.
4. Identify quality assurance practices in healthcare, document the results on a laboratory flow sheet, and discuss quality control guidelines.
5. Summarize laboratory safety procedures for chemical hazards, including the use of Safety Data Sheets (SDS), signs, and chemical labels.
6. Summarize safety techniques to minimize biological and physical hazards in the clinical laboratory.
7. Describe the essential elements of a laboratory requisition.
8. Discuss specimen collection, including the importance of labeling containers and using the correct collection containers.
9. Discuss specimen handling, processing, storage, and the importance of the chain of custody.
10. Name common units used for measuring time, temperature, liquid volume, distance, and mass.
11. Describe the components of a microscope and how to use a microscope.
12. Describe the safe use of a centrifuge.
13. Discuss the use of an incubator.

OUTLINE

OPENING SCENARIO

John Stuart, CMA (AAMA), graduated from a medical assisting program 4 years ago and has been working at Walden-Martin Family Medical (WMFM) Clinic ever since. He enjoys working with patients and providers. Recently WMFM Clinic providers decided to expand their physician office laboratory (POL). John transferred into the phlebotomy laboratory area a few weeks ago and has really enjoyed it so far. He loves the patient contact during the phlebotomy procedures, and every day is just a little different. He really liked the laboratory portion of his medical assistant coursework in school and wanted a new challenge at work. It has been fun to brush up on his phlebotomy skills, and he has found that he has a real talent for putting people at ease.

He is working with another laboratory CMA, Macyn, as he trains in the laboratory. Macyn has worked in the POL for about 8 years and is happy to expand the services that are provided at WMFM Clinic. Today she is going to reintroduce John to the laboratory.

YOU WILL LEARN

1. To describe the role of the clinical laboratory in patient care and the medical assistant's role in performing laboratory tests.
2. To discuss the three regulatory categories established by the Clinical Laboratory Improvement Amendments (CLIA).
3. To identify the CLIA-waived tests used to screen for common diseases.
4. To identify quality assurance practices in healthcare.
5. To perform quality control testing and record results on a laboratory flow sheet.
6. To discuss the purpose and content requirements of a Safety Data Sheet (SDS).
7. To summarize safety techniques to minimize physical hazards, chemical hazards, and biohazards in the clinical laboratory.
8. To discuss specimen collection, including sensitivity to patients' rights and feelings when collecting specimens.
9. To identify the metric units used for measuring liquid volume, distance, and mass.
10. To recognize parts of a microscope and describe their functions.

INTRODUCTION

Clinical Laboratory and Patient Care

Laboratory medicine is part of the field of clinical laboratory science. Blood and other potentially infectious materials (OPIMs) are tested to aid in the diagnosis, treatment, and monitoring of patients. Patient specimens can be collected at the laboratory or in an ambulatory care facility. Once in the laboratory, the specimen is processed and directed to the proper laboratory department. Each department of the lab will assess the acceptability of the specimen based on specific tests ordered by the provider. If suitable, the specimen will be analyzed. Tests can be performed manually (by hand) or with a variety of specialized automated (AW tuh meyt ed) instruments. Once test results are completed, they are reported to the provider.

> **VOCABULARY**
> **automated** Measured by a machine or instrument. May involve human manipulation, coordination, or control.
> **specimen** A sample of blood, body fluid, waste product, or tissue collected for analysis.

Personnel in the Clinical Laboratory

Medical laboratories are in hospitals, ambulatory care facilities, public health departments, health maintenance organizations, and referral laboratories. The clinical laboratory could be staffed with:

- A director, who may be a pathologist (pah THOL uh jist) or a clinical laboratory scientist with a doctorate degree
- Certified medical laboratory scientists (MLS), medical technologists (MTs), and certified medical laboratory technicians (MLTs)
- Medical laboratory assistants (MLAs), medical assistants (CMAs, RMAs), and *phlebotomists* (fluh BOT uh mists)

Phlebotomists and laboratory assistants have received specialized training in the collection of blood samples and the preparation and processing of laboratory specimens. The agencies granting certifications and titles are listed in Table 52.1.

In ambulatory care facilities, the lab director may be the physician. These labs are referred to as *physician office laboratories*. Medical assistants are trained to collect and perform specific testing procedures in the POL. They are also trained to collect and process specimens that are sent to outside reference laboratories for testing.

Laboratory tests may be used for four main purposes:

- To document the good health of a patient
- To screen patients for diseases such as diabetes, high cholesterol, or urinary tract infection (UTI)
- To help the provider diagnose a medical disease, disorder, or condition
- To help the provider decide the most appropriate treatment and to monitor the effects of medications or a disease process

Only licensed healthcare practitioners (physicians, nurse practitioners, physician assistants) can order laboratory tests for a patient. The medical assistant may perform CLIA-waived laboratory tests. To assume this responsibility, the medical assistant must be properly trained in:

TABLE 52.1 Certifying Agencies for Laboratory Personnel

Certifying Agency	Title	Position
American Society for Clinical Pathologists (ASCP)	MLS (ASCP)CM	Medical laboratory scientist
	MT (ASCP)	Medical technologist
	MLT (ASCP)	Medical laboratory technician–certificate
	MLT-AD (ASCP)	Medical laboratory technician–associate's degree
American Medical Technologists (AMT)	MT (AMT)	Medical technologist
	MLT (AMT)	Medical laboratory technician
	MLA	Medical laboratory assistant
	RMA	Registered medical assistant
American Association of Medical Assistants (AAMA)	CMA (AAMA)	Certified medical assistant
National Healthcareer Association (NHA)	CCMA	Certified clinical medical assistant
	CPT	Certified phlebotomy technician
	CMLA	Certified medical laboratory assistant

TABLE 52.2 Comparison of Qualitative and Quantitative Testing

	Qualitative Test	Quantitative Test
Definition	A numeric value is not attached to the test results. May be used as a screening test.	Tests results represent the amount or quantity of an analyte in a certain volume of specimen.
Reported as	Positive or negative.	The test result is expressed as a number with units of measure attached.
Example	Negative fecal occult blood (FOB) –normal result; no blood found in the stool. Positive FOB – abnormal result; blood is found in the stool. Could indicate a cancerous colon lesion.	RBCs, 5 million per cubic millimeter ($5 \times 10^6/mm^3$) Hemoglobin 15 g per deciliter (15 g/dL) Hematocrit 45%

RBCs, Red blood cells.

- Proper patient preparation
- Testing procedures common to the provider's practice
- Normal range of results for common testing

The medical assistant must carefully follow all laboratory instructions. This includes properly collecting, assessing, and labeling patient specimens. Specimens not tested at the POL will be processed and sent to the clinical laboratory for testing. Excellent communication between the team members and the patient is very important. The medical assistant should make the patient feel at ease with these procedures and hopefully gain the patient's cooperation and trust.

VOCABULARY

analyte The substance or chemical being analyzed or detected in a specimen.
pathologist A physician specially trained in the nature and cause of disease.
profile testing A series of laboratory tests associated with a particular organ or disease; also referred to as a "panel" of tests.
reference range The upper and lower limits of test values expected for a healthy group individuals in the general population.
referral laboratory A laboratory that performs testing not done by the original laboratory. The tests may require special instrumentation or training not available at the original laboratory. Also called *reference, diagnostic,* or *commercial testing laboratories.* Often privately owned.

Clinical Laboratory Testing

The patient's health history and a physical examination are required to determine the appropriate tests for screening, diagnosis, or management of a patient's condition. The body is healthy when a state of equilibrium exists in the internal environment. This healthy state of equilibrium is called *homeostasis.* It occurs when the physical and chemical characteristics of body substances are within a certain acceptable range known as the *normal range,* or reference range. A change in the internal environment of the body often results in abnormal test values that are outside the reference range. The patient's results are compared with the reference range of values to determine if an illness or a disease is present. Reference values are also useful for assessing the progress of a patient's course of treatment.

Abnormal values for a particular test may be seen with more than one pathologic condition. For example, a decrease in the hemoglobin (HEE muh gloh bin) level in red blood cells (RBCs) is seen in iron-deficiency anemia, but also in hyperthyroidism and cirrhosis of the liver. Therefore providers cannot rely solely on one laboratory test to make a diagnosis. They must use all information from the history, physical exam, and diagnostic and laboratory tests.

Clinical laboratory tests range from simple screening tests of one analyte (AN e lit), such as glucose, to profile testing (also called a panel of tests), in which more than one analyte related to an organ system is tested, such as a liver panel. A *screening test* examines a specimen for the presence of an analyte that may indicate a disease state. Screening tests are not diagnostic for one particular disease, but rather indicate that the disease state may exist. The provider will use the patient's clinical presentation, along with the test results, to do further testing or to make a diagnosis. The results are often *qualitative* (KWOL I tey tiv), which means that a numeric value is not attached to the result.

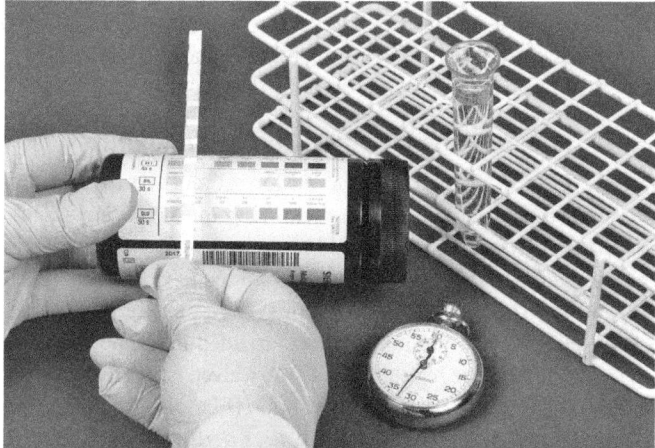

Fig. 52.1 Urinalysis.

Qualitative tests are reported as positive or negative. A *fecal occult blood (FOB)* test checks for blood in a stool specimen. An FOB test is an example of a screening test; if the test is positive, further testing is needed to diagnose the condition.

In a *quantitative* (KWON ti tey tiv) test, the test result is expressed as a number and unit of measure, such as mg/dL. Table 52.2 presents a comparison of qualitative and quantitative testing.

Departments of the Clinical Laboratory

Large laboratories are divided into two main areas:
- Clinical pathology: Includes phlebotomy, specimen processing, urinalysis, hematology, chemistry, special chemistry, toxicology (tok si KOL oh jee), microbiology, blood bank, coagulation, and immunology/serology
- Anatomic and surgical pathology: Includes histology (hi STOL oh jee), cytopathology (sahy to path oh LO jee), and cytogenetics (si to je NET ics)

A POL generally performs test procedures in urinalysis, hematology, chemistry, and microbiology.

Urinalysis. *Urinalysis* (yoo r uh NAL uh sis) is the physical, chemical, and microscopic examination of urine (Fig. 52.1). The physical examination assesses the color, clarity, and specific gravity of urine. Urine is tested with a multiple test strip, also called a *dipstick*, which examines the following analytes in urine: glucose, protein, *ketones* (KEE tohns), blood, *bilirubin* (BIL ih roo bin), *urobilinogen* (YUR o bi lin e jen), *nitrites* (NAHY trahyts), and pH. We will go into the details of urinalysis in Chapter 53. The provider may examine urine microscopically for the presence of RBCs, white blood cells (WBCs), and epithelial cells, in addition to mucus, casts, crystals, and microorganisms.

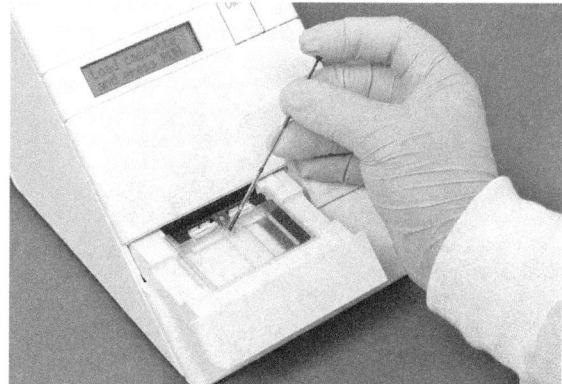

Fig. 52.2 Waived Chemistry Analyzer. (From Niedzwiecki B, et al: *Kinn's the medical assistant,* ed 14, St. Louis, 2020, Elsevier.)

Additional quantitative tests may be performed in the urinalysis department of a reference laboratory to confirm routine screening test results.

Hematology. *Hematology* (hee muh TOL uh jee) is the study of blood cells and *coagulation* (koh AG yuh ley shun). Laboratory testing in the hematology department may be qualitative or quantitative. In a POL, screening tests for hemoglobin, *hematocrit* (hi MAT uh krit), and the prothrombin time with the International Normalized Ratio (INR) (a coagulation test) are typically performed in the ambulatory setting. Reference laboratories perform blood cell counts that determine the number of RBCs, WBCs, and platelets in a blood sample. A differential is a microscopic test to determine the characteristics of cells, such as size, shape, and maturity. In addition, the hematology department performs tests to determine the ability of blood to clot.

Chemistry. The clinical chemistry department analyzes the chemical constituents found in blood, cerebrospinal fluid (CSF), urine, and joint fluid (synovial fluid). Specimen testing may be done manually or with complex chemistry instruments. In a POL, procedures may include single analyte tests (blood glucose) or multitest profiles. Chemistry profiles include tests for related analytes. Lipid profiles, for example, include assessments of total cholesterol, triglycerides, low-density lipoprotein (LDL), and high-density lipoprotein (HDL). POL chemistry analyzers are becoming more common in ambulatory care as technology becomes more compact and easier to use (Fig. 52.2).

Microbiology. Microbiology involves the study of very small, infectious organisms, such as bacteria, fungi, yeasts, parasites,

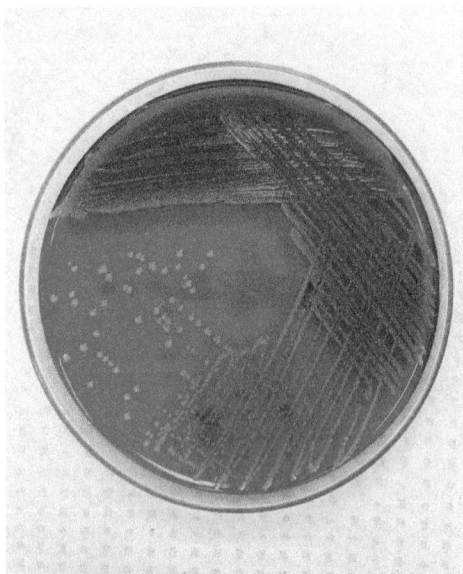

Fig. 52.3 Pure Culture Growing on Culture Medium.

and viruses. Specimens used in microbiology include blood, urine, sputum, CSF, stool, wound, and other biologic sources. Specimens used for microbiology testing must be collected aseptically (ey SEP tick all ee) in sterile containers.

The goal of the microbiology department is to identify the microorganism that is causing the infection. The staff will also determine the most effective antimicrobial (an tee mahy KROH bee uh l) medications, which include antibiotics. This process is *sensitivity* (or susceptibility) testing.

Microbiology specimens may be grown on culture media. Once the organism is growing and in pure culture, it can be identified. Organism identification tests have changed with technology and will continue to change in the future. Various methods and technologies are used to identify microorganisms, including biochemical, molecular, and antigen-antibody complex testing.

Sensitivity testing is performed on organisms to establish an appropriate antibiotic therapy for that specific bacterium or fungus. Once again, a variety of techniques and technologies may be used to help determine which antibiotic would be most effective.

The following actions may be applied in a POL:
- Rapid strep testing may be performed to screen for strep throat.
- Microbiological specimens may be aseptically collected and then sent to a reference laboratory.
- Microscope slides may be prepared for the provider to examine.

Identification and sensitivity testing is usually performed in larger centralized ambulatory care, hospital, or reference laboratories (Fig. 52.3).

CRITICAL THINKING 52.2

John and Macyn have reviewed the different areas that are common in a POL. WMFM Clinic is now doing testing in microbiology, a new area that has been added to the POL in the past 6 months. As they talk about microbiology Macyn asks the question, "Why do microbiology samples need to be collected aseptically in a sterile container?" How would you answer this question in your own words?

GOVERNMENT LEGISLATION AFFECTING CLINICAL LABORATORY TESTING

In 1988 Congress passed the Clinical Laboratory Improvement Amendments. This law established quality standards for all clinical laboratory testing. CLIA is designed to ensure the accuracy, precision, reliability, and timeliness of patient test results, regardless of which laboratory performed the testing. A clinical laboratory is defined as any facility that performs laboratory testing on human specimens to provide information about the diagnosis, prevention, and treatment of disease or the impairment of health.

Clinical Laboratory Improvement Amendments

Under CLIA, all laboratories that perform even one type of test must meet certain federal requirements. They must register with the Centers for Medicare and Medicaid Services (CMS) as a laboratory. The registration application must be submitted to CMS with information about the laboratory's operations. The type of certificate that is issued is based on the information provided in the application. (*Note:* Most POLs are registered as CLIA-waived laboratories.)

The US Food and Drug Administration (FDA) is responsible for categorizing commercially marketed tests performed in vitro (in VEE troh), based on the CLIA guidelines. The FDA has assumed primary responsibility for determining the CLIA complexity of all laboratory tests. Every laboratory test product is assigned to one of three CLIA categories based on the product's potential risk to public health. The CLIA categories are waived tests, moderate-complexity tests, and high-complexity tests. Table 52.3 lists common government acronyms used in the clinical laboratory.

> **VOCABULARY**
> **aseptically** Free from living pathogenic organisms.
> **culture media** A solid, liquid, or semisolid medium designed to support the growth of microorganisms, especially bacteria and fungus.
> **in vitro** A Latin term meaning "in glass"; it refers to a process that takes place outside the body in a test tube or culture plate.
> **pure culture** The growth of only one microorganism in a culture or on a nutrient surface.
> **sterile** Free of all living organisms.

CLIA-Waived Tests and Laboratories. CLIA-*waived* (WEY ved) tests are defined as laboratory tests and procedures that have been approved by the FDA for home use or that are simple laboratory tests and procedures to perform. Waived tests are designed to have straightforward directions and procedures so that they have a minimal risk of incorrect results. Waived tests include tests that:
- Use methodologies that are simple and accurate so that the likelihood of incorrect user results is negligible
- Pose no unreasonable risk of harm to the patient if performed incorrectly

Table 52.4 shows some common CLIA-waived tests performed in ambulatory care facilities registered as CLIA-waived laboratories.

The FDA's CLIA-waived database of tests is available to the public on the internet. This database contains the commercially

TABLE 52.3 Common Government Acronyms in the Clinical Laboratory

Acronym	Term	Application
BBPS	Bloodborne Pathogens Standard	OSHA standard that established precautions for dealing with all blood specimens
CDC	Centers for Disease Control and Prevention	Provides information for CLIA-waived laboratories in *Ready? Set? Test!* booklet
CLIA	Clinical Laboratory Improvement Amendments	Law that regulates all clinical laboratory testing products and sites
CMS	Centers for Medicare and Medicaid Services	Agency with which all labs must register and pay a biannual fee based on the complexity of tests performed in the lab
CoW	Certificate of waiver	The most common CLIA lab classification for physician office laboratories (POLs)
HHS	Department of Health and Human Services	Federal department that oversees the CMS, FDA, and CDC
FDA	Food and Drug Administration	Approves and categorizes CLIA-waived tests
HCS	Hazard Communication Standard	Standard regulated by OSHA that requires employers to communicate hazards to employees
HIPAA	Health Insurance Portability and Accountability Act	Law that enforces regulations for protected health information
HMIS	Hazardous Materials Information System	Identifies four color-coded chemical hazards (health, flammable, reactive, and other)
OPIM	Other Potentially Infectious Materials	Other materials related to bloodborne pathogens
OSHA	Occupational Safety and Health Administration	Regulates BBPS and HCS to ensure the safety of healthcare workers
PEP	Postexposure prophylaxis	Steps taken if a person is exposed to blood or OPIM
PHI	Protected health information	All test results are considered PHI and must be confidential
POL	Physician office laboratory	Located in ambulatory care facilities
PPE	Personal protective equipment	Gloves, gowns, and face protection worn when dealing with specimens
PPM	Provider-performed microscopy	CLIA moderate to complex microscopy tests available to POLs
QA	Quality assurance	Process-oriented policies to ensure a high level of accuracy and proficiency
QC	Quality control	Ensures analytical testing is error free and test results are reliable
SDS	Safety Data Sheet (formerly MSDS)	Must be in a uniform format with 16 section numbers, headings, and associated information to inform employees of chemical hazards in the laboratory

marketed laboratory test systems categorized as CLIA waived by the FDA since January 31, 2000, and tests categorized by the Centers for Disease Control and Prevention (CDC) before that date. The database can be searched by test system name, specialty or subspecialty, analyte, document number, qualifier, effective date, and complexity.

Moderate- and High-Complexity Tests and Laboratories.

The CLIA program oversees the quality of nearly 200,000 different laboratory procedures. Most laboratory tests are categorized by the FDA as moderate-complexity tests. Some moderate-complexity tests that are performed in POLs include:

- Hematology and chemistry: Testing done on an automated analyzer
- Microbiology: Gram stain procedures
- Urinalysis: Microscopic analysis of urine sediment

Moderate-complexity tests must be performed by qualified personnel as described by CLIA. High-complexity tests are generally not performed in a POL, but rather in a hospital or reference laboratory.

Laboratories that perform moderate- to high-complexity testing must meet rigorous CLIA regulations and are subject to surprise inspections every 2 years. Each laboratory that performs these tests must:

- Establish a system to maintain the identification of patients' specimens throughout the testing process and ensure accurate reporting of results.
- Establish and follow written quality control and quality assurance procedures, in addition to standard operating procedures (SOPs).
- Participate in *proficiency testing*, which is a form of external quality control. Three times a year, the laboratory must

test samples provided by an approved proficiency testing agency. The proficiency samples are tested in the same way as patient samples. Results are then reported to the proficiency testing agency, and test results are reviewed for accuracy and precision.

- Employ personnel that meet CLIA regulations and specific qualifications for a moderate- to high-complexity laboratory. Requirements are most rigorous for high-complexity testing.

Medical assistants can perform all CLIA-waived tests and some specific moderate-complexity tests. Additional training will be required to perform moderate-complexity tests, depending on the certification of the POL where they work. Although medical assistants cannot perform high-complexity tests, they can be involved in preparing patients, sharing provider-directed patient education, collecting specimens, and documenting results in the patient's health record.

VOCABULARY

standard operating procedures (SOP) A set of step-by-step instructions to help employees carry out routine operations efficiently with high quality and uniformity of performance.

CRITICAL THINKING 52.3

The laboratory at WMFM Clinic is a registered waived facility. List five commonly performed waived tests. What is the difference between waived testing and moderate- or high-complexity testing? List three differences and be ready to share them in the classroom.

TABLE 52.4   CLIA-Waived Tests and Their Purposes

Specimen and Test	Purpose
Dipstick or tablet reagent urinalysis (manual or automated)	Urine screening to assess or diagnose diseases such as diabetes mellitus, kidney disease, and urinary tract infection
Urine pregnancy tests: visual color comparison tests	Diagnose pregnancy
Fecal occult blood	Colorectal screening to detect hidden blood in the stool
Erythrocyte sedimentation rate, nonautomated	Diagnose inflammatory process; increases in arthritis, infection, leukemia, and most cancers
Spun microhematocrit	Measures red blood cells; screening for certain types of anemia
STAT-CRIT hematocrit	Screening for certain types of anemia
Hemoglobin	Measure hemoglobin level in whole blood
Blood glucose by glucose-monitoring devices cleared by the FDA specifically for home use	Monitor blood glucose levels
Hemoglobin A_{1c} by single analyte instruments with self-contained or component features to perform specimen-reagent interaction	Measure A_{1c} levels to assess and manage long-term care of patients with diabetes
Cholestech LDX	Measures total blood cholesterol, triglycerides, HDL, and glucose levels
Whole-Blood i-STAT Chem8+ Cartridge	Measures ionized calcium, carbon dioxide, chloride, creatinine, glucose, potassium, sodium, urea nitrogen, and hematocrit in whole blood
Whole-blood thyroid-stimulating hormone (TSH) assay	Qualitative determination of TSH in whole blood
Blood mononucleosis antibodies	Rapid whole-blood test to detect heterophile antibodies to help diagnose infectious mononucleosis
Helicobacter pylori antibodies	Rapid whole-blood test to detect *H. pylori* antibodies to determine the cause of peptic ulcer
Borrelia burgdorferi antibodies	Rapid whole-blood test to detect *B. burgdorferi* antibodies to diagnose Lyme disease
Trinity Biotech Uni-Gold Recombigen HIV Test	Detects HIV-1 in a blood specimen
Nasal influenza A and B	Quick qualitative diagnosis of influenza antigens in nasal secretions or swab
Streptococcus A throat swab	Rapid strep test
Urine or blood drug tests	Multiple tests for the presence of a variety of substance abuse agents
Urine fertility and menopause tests	Detect follicle-stimulating hormone in urine
Ovulation tests; visual color comparison tests for luteinizing hormone	Detect ovulation

CLIA, Clinical Laboratory Improvement Amendments; *FDA*, US Food and Drug Administration; *HDL*, high-density lipoprotein; *HIV-1*, human immunodeficiency virus type 1.
From the Centers for Medicare and Medicaid Services. https://www.cms.gov/CLIA/downloads/waivetbl.pdf.

QUALITY ASSURANCE GUIDELINES

Quality assurance (QA) are written policies and procedures that ensure monitoring of all of the processes involved before, during, and after a laboratory test to produce reliable test results. QA is the promise of healthcare professionals to achieve the highest degree of excellence in patient care. It is a process that monitors instruments and methodologies to ensure accurate results. QA establishes standard operating procedures to enable the laboratory to assess, verify, and document the quality of the laboratory process. This documentation is a way of comparing what is happening with what should be happening.

As mandated by law, QA programs monitor all aspects of laboratory activity, from collecting specimens through processing, testing, and reporting steps. Programs check supplies, reagents, machinery, and actual test performance. QA monitors quality control, personnel orientation, laboratory documentation, knowledge of laboratory instrumentation, and enrollment in a proficiency testing program (if the lab performs moderate- or high-complexity tests).

Three Stages of Quality Assurance in the Laboratory

The overall process required to ensure QA in the laboratory is divided into three stages. These three stages must be applied to each test or procedure performed in the laboratory. If any of these steps are missed or performed incorrectly, QA has been broken.

Preanalytic Stage

1. The provider orders a test to screen, monitor, or diagnose a patient's condition.
2. A written or electronic requisition is filled out, showing the test requested, the specimen required, and where the specimen will be tested.
3. The specimen is collected, labeled, and processed.
4. The specimen is transported to the laboratory in the POL or properly prepared for offsite laboratory pickup.

Analytic Stage

1. Instruments are maintained and calibrated.
2. Controls are run and analyzed for each test method (part of ongoing quality control).
3. The specimen is tested, and the results are compared with reference ranges.
4. The test results are logged and documented in the patient's health record.

Postanalytic Stage

1. Specimens are properly discarded.
2. Analyses of control results are compared over time.
3. Patient reports from outside laboratories are logged or documented.
4. The provider interprets and signs all lab reports.
5. The patient is notified of the results in the office or is contacted by laboratory personnel.
6. The final report and all communication with the patient are documented in the patient's health record.

Accurate record keeping is one of the key responsibilities of a medical assistant. Some POLs still use paper records, in which case the primary source of documentation is the *laboratory master logbook*. The logbook contains a written record for each procedure performed, the patient's identification number, results obtained, date performed, and personnel initials. The results are then sent to the provider for verification.

The test results are then transferred into the patient's electronic health record. POLs are also required to have a procedure manual that describes how each test is performed and how the patient results are reported to the provider. Personnel are required to perform calibration or opticschecks on laboratory instruments that use light detection or color change as part of the reaction process. In addition, they must run quality control (QC) testing each day before patient testing. QC uses special control materials designed to mimic the matrix of patient sample and constituents being tested. Each manufacturer includes instructions for running control materials for its kit, procedure, or instrument. Quality control results must be documented. If errors or problems occur while quality control is performed, the POL must perform and document remedial actions to correct errors or problems as they are identified. Patient tests cannot be run until the QC issue is resolved.

Finally, preventive maintenance schedules must be followed and documented. Preventive maintenance prolongs the life of equipment and reduces breakdown. Preventive maintenance includes daily cleaning and adjustment, in addition to replacement of parts when necessary. Each instrument should have a paper or electronic log or worksheet for recording all changes, including daily maintenance details.

Ready? Set? Test! is an excellent online resource provided by the CDC for setting up and maintaining a CLIA-waived laboratory. Fig. 52.4 shows the checklist summary of the steps needed to assure proper CLIA-waived testing in a POL.

QUALITY CONTROL GUIDELINES

A crucial step in the QA process is running QC specimens (Procedure 52.1). The purpose of QC in the laboratory is to ensure the reliability of test results while detecting and eliminating error. Here are two important terms to remember:

- *Accuracy* is a measure of how close a test result is to the true value of the control material, as established by the manufacturer.
- *Precision* is the ability to consistently reproduce a test result.

When a series of control results show both accuracy and precision, the instrument is considered *reliable* and may be used for testing patients. QC monitoring is crucial because patient treatment is often based on or reinforced by the results of laboratory tests. Without QC monitoring, laboratory error is difficult to detect. Undetected laboratory errors may result in harm to the patient.

Quality Control Testing

Prepared control samples are tested daily, along with patient samples. Control test results must fall within a preestablished range of results before patient results can be reported. QC samples are called *controls*. They are usually supplied with the manufacturer's prepackaged kits and are intended for use in a POL. Controls should be analyzed at specified intervals as recommended by the manufacturer. Examples of routine quality control testing in a physician office laboratory (POL) include:

- Positive and negative controls supplied with pregnancy test kits are performed with each patient specimen.
- Urinalysis dipstick controls (used for chemical examination of urine) should be checked daily before patient testing and each time a new reagent (re AY jent) container is opened.
- Controls for automated chemistry analyses should be performed before patient testing and at specified intervals during the day, depending on the number of tests run per day and the manufacturer's recommendations.

Consistent control results ensure constant conditions throughout the daily testing process.

On every day that patient tests are performed, QC tests must also be performed and the results entered onto a paper or electronic graph or flow sheet. (Box 52.1 provides more information on graphing QC results.) When new control materials are opened and used, the results and dates must be entered on a new flow sheet, along with the expiration dates of the controls. These records must be retained for several years; the exact number of years is determined by state law and CLIA mandates.

VOCABULARY

calibration The process of checking the precision, accuracy, and limits of an instrument by comparing measurements of the instrument with that of a known standard or reference instrument.

control materials Manufacturer-prepared samples that have a known quantity of a specific analyte. Used for quality control purposes. Testing results should fall within a manufacturer-defined range of results. Also called *controls* or *quality controls*.

optics checks A specific type of calibration that assesses the optics of an electronic testing instrument or system.

preventive maintenance Regularly scheduled care of equipment, which will reduce the likelihood of failure. Performed and documented at regular intervals while the equipment is in good working order.

quality control (QC) A process applied to ensure the reliability of test results, using manufactured samples with known values.

reagent A substance used in a chemical reaction.

shift(s) Data results on a graph that make an abrupt change in value.

trend(s) Data results on a graph that are obtained over time and which continue to go upward or downward in value.

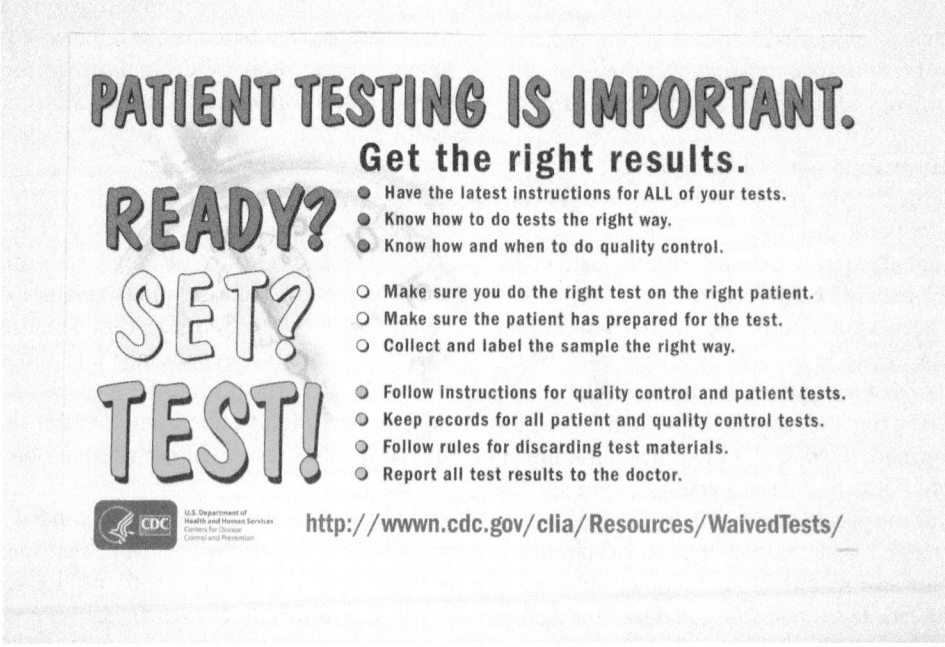

Fig. 52.4 Summary Checklist from Ready? Set? Test! (From Niedzwiecki B, et al: *Kinn's the medical assistant,* ed 14, St. Louis, 2020, Elsevier.)

BOX 52.1 Using a Graph for Quality Control Results

Many laboratories will use a graph to display daily quality control results. A paper graph or electronic graph file can be updated with daily quality control (QC) values. Graphing advantages include:

- A graph is a physical representation of QC results that can display data irregularities in an easy-to-see format.
- It displays possible **trends** and **shifts** in data over time. See the labeled graph.

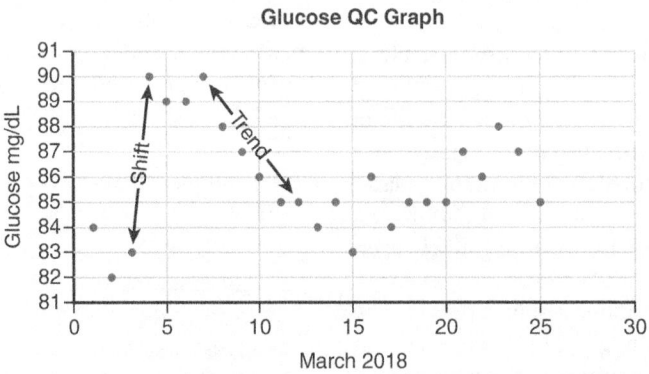

Routine Preventive Maintenance

Another part of quality control is routine preventive maintenance. All laboratory equipment should be on a routine preventive maintenance schedule so that equipment is serviced before a breakdown occurs. Any time equipment cannot be used is an inconvenience to the patient. Tips on preventive maintenance in the clinical laboratory include:

- Follow the manufacturer's instructions for calibrating instruments.
- Read and understand the instructions for routine instrument care.
- Perform all preventive maintenance specified by the manufacturer's instructions.

- Keep spare parts available for immediate use.
- Record the name, address, and phone number of a contact person for maintenance or repair.
- Create a maintenance form or use the one provided by the manufacturer.

CRITICAL THINKING 52.4

As John and Macyn are reviewing quality assurance and quality control, John asks Macyn to clarify the difference between QA and QC. In your own words, define QA and QC. How are they different? Be ready to discuss your answer with the class.

LABORATORY SAFETY

The importance of safety in the laboratory cannot be overemphasized. Most laboratory accidents can be prevented by using proper techniques and common sense. Following safe practices in the laboratory requires a personal commitment and concern for others. An unsafe act may harm an innocent bystander without harming the person who performs the act. Box 52.2 presents some common safety signs and symbols seen in the laboratory.

Several important safety standards in place by federal agencies that help protect the healthcare workers. In Chapter 19, the Occupational Safety and Health Administration (OSHA) standards were discussed. The standards that relate to the medical laboratory include:

- *Hazard communication:* Requires employers to provide information about the chemical hazards in the workplace. The General Duty Clause states that any equipment that can pose a health danger must be considered a hazard.

- *Laboratory standards or occupational exposure to hazardous chemicals in laboratories:* Agencies must have a written Chemical Hygiene Plan (CHP) in place, which addresses policies, procedures, and responsibilities that protect employees from hazardous chemicals. The CHP describes the appropriate handling of chemicals in the laboratory.

- *Bloodborne pathogen:* Protects healthcare workers against the hazards caused by bloodborne pathogens.

The CDC also established recommendations and resources, in Standard Precautions and Transmission Precautions, as they relate to specimen collection. (These recommendations were discussed in Chapter 32.)

The following sections will describe laboratory safety and the safety standards that must be followed.

VOCABULARY

Standard Precautions A set of infection control practices used to prevent the transmission of diseases that can be acquired by contact with blood, body fluids, nonintact skin, and mucous membranes.

BOX 52.2   Common Workplace Safeguards – Signs and Symbols – Used in the Laboratory

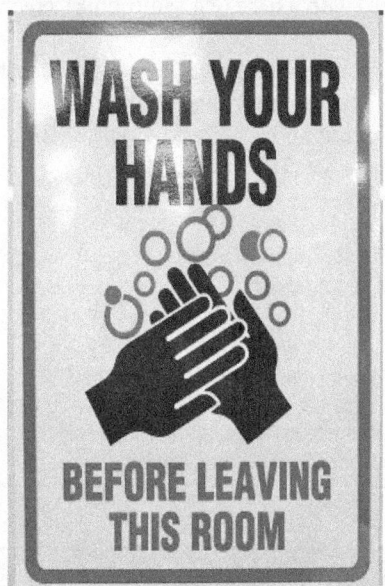

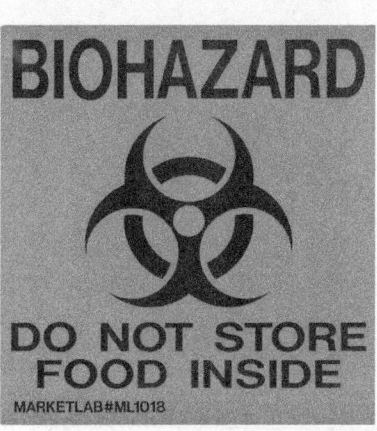

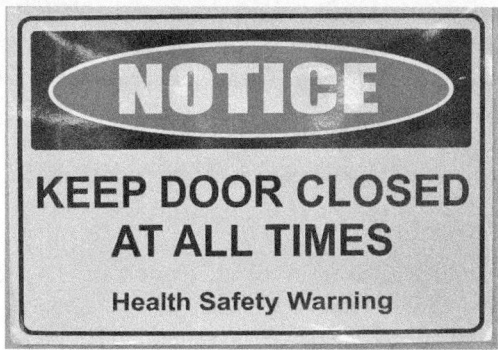

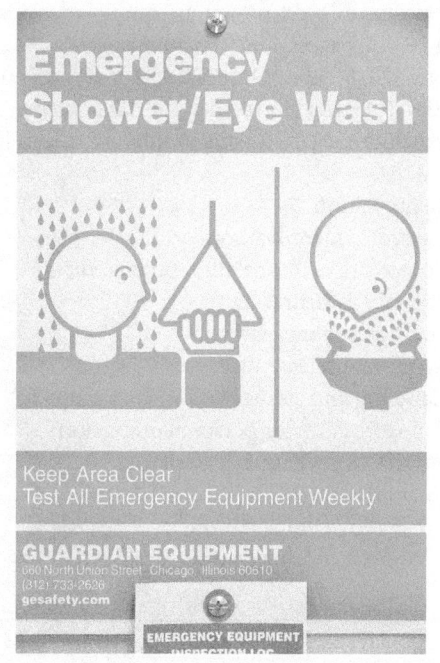

Chemical Hazards

The clinical laboratory may have chemicals that are flammable, caustic (KAW stik), and/or potentially poisonous. Exposure to these dangerous chemicals can occur by breathing in fumes, direct absorption by contact with the skin, ingestion, direct contact with a mucous membrane, or entry through a cut, abrasion, or burn on the skin. OSHA is involved in regulating the standards directed at minimizing occupational exposure to hazardous chemicals in laboratories. OSHA's Hazard Communication Standard (HCS; known as the employee "right to know" rule) became law in 1991. It ensures that laboratory workers are made fully aware of the hazards associated with their workplace. The law requires employers to design and implement protective programs for any employees who may be exposed to hazardous chemicals with the goal of reducing workplace injury and illnesses. All workers must be provided with information and training. A Safety Data Sheet (SDS) must also be on file for all chemicals used in the laboratory.

Common Hazardous Chemicals. In the POL, the most common hazardous chemicals are:

- *Sodium hypochlorite* (hahy puh KLAWR ahyt), commonly known as bleach, which is used for disinfecting laboratory work areas
- *CaviWipes* (KAH vee wahyps) and *glutaraldehyde* (gloo tuh RAL duh hahyd), which are disinfectants
- *Acetone* (AS i tohn) and dyes, which are used for staining slides

It should be noted that all of these disinfectants and dyes are available in premixed sprays or wipes to reduce chemical exposure during dilution.

Safety Data Sheet. An SDS supplies information about chemical safety and hazard information in case of an accident, spill, or fire, to the user or emergency personnel. OSHA requires the manufacturer of the chemical to make these sheets available, usually as a package insert or online. Employers must ensure that SDSs are readily accessible to employees.

Since June 2015, the Occupational Safety and Health Administration (OSHA) has required all SDSs to use a uniform format that includes the following section numbers, headings, and information:

Section 1. Identification
Section 2. Hazard(s) identification
Section 3. Composition/information on ingredients
Section 4. First-aid measures
Section 5. Fire-fighting measures
Section 6. Accidental release measures
Section 7. Handling and storage
Section 8. Exposure controls/personal protection
Section 9. Physical and chemical properties
Section 10. Stability and reactivity
Section 11. Toxicologic information
Section 12. Ecologic information[a]

Section 13. Disposal considerations[a]
Section 14. Transport information[a]
Section 15. Regulatory information[a]
Section 16. Other information

Chemical Labels. Chemicals should be tightly sealed and properly labeled with the original manufacturer's labels. A hazard identification system, developed by the National Fire Protection Association (NFPA), provides information at a glance on the potential health, flammability, and chemical reactivity hazards of materials. This identification system consists of four small, diamond-shaped, colored symbols grouped into a larger diamond shape.

- The top diamond is red and indicates flammability (the potential to catch on fire).
- The diamond on the left is blue and indicates a health hazard such as a dangerous inhalant or corrosive acid.
- The bottom diamond is white and provides special hazard information, including recommended personal protective equipment (PPE) if biohazards are present and other dangerous situations.
- The diamond on the right is yellow and indicates a reactivity or stability hazard. An example of reactivity is mixing an acid (e.g., bleach) with a base (e.g., ammonia), creating a dangerous gas.

The four-color system also indicates the severity of the hazard by using numbers imprinted in the diamonds from 0 to 4, with 0 representing no hazard and 4 representing an extremely hazardous substance (Fig. 52.5).

VOCABULARY

caustic Capable of burning, corroding, or damaging tissue by chemical action.
corrosive Causing or tending to cause the gradual destruction of a substance by chemical action.
inhalant Any substance that can be breathed into the lungs.
protective personal equipment (PPE) Clothing, eye protection, face shields, gloves, gowns, or other garments or equipment designed to protect the worker from workplace hazards. In healthcare these hazards include blood and body fluids.

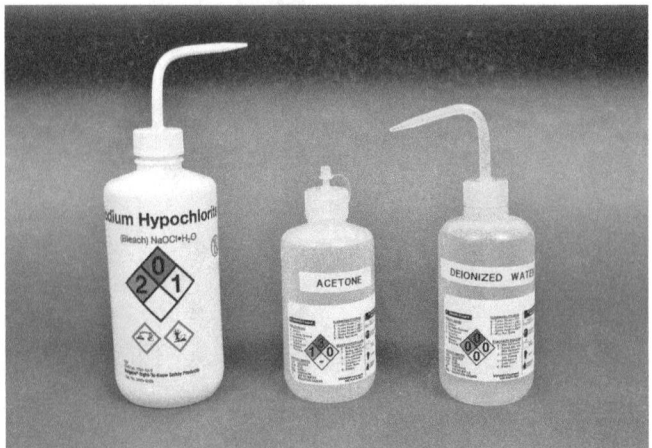

Fig. 52.5 Laboratory bottles with chemical labels are a common workplace safeguard. (From Niedzwiecki B, et al: *Kinn's the medical assistant*, ed 14, St. Louis, 2020, Elsevier.)

---

[a]Sections 12 to 15 are regulated by agencies other than OSHA and are required of the manufacturers, not the employees.

Proper Chemical Handling. Following principles of proper chemical handling reduces the risk of harmful effects. Examples of proper chemical handling include:

- If a chemical produces toxic or flammable vapors, work under a fume hood that exhausts air to the outside.
- In case of accidental exposure of the skin, rinse the affected area under cool running water for at least 10 minutes. Remove any contaminated clothing.
- If chemicals are splashed in the eyes, flush the eyes with water from an eyewash station (Fig. 52.6) for a minimum of 15 minutes. (Complete instructions on how to use an eyewash station are given in Procedure 52.2.)

Prompt medical attention must be given to victims of chemical exposure.

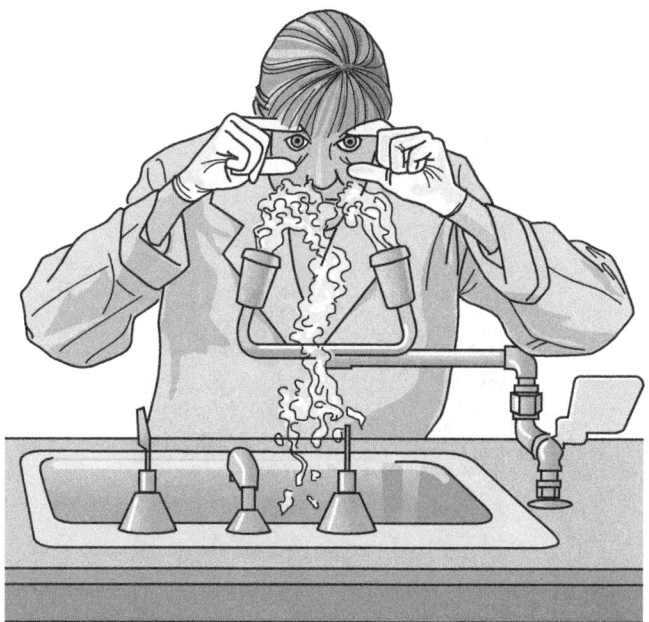

Fig. 52.6 Eyewash Station. (From Niedzwiecki B, et al: *Kinn's the medical assistant,* ed 14, St. Louis, 2020, Elsevier.)

CRITICAL THINKING 52.5

John has a few hours to review WMFM Clinic's current laboratory safety policies and procedures on his own. There are policies that apply to the laboratory only, but there are also many policies that apply to the entire facility. Why is it so important for employees to be aware of safety policies and procedures? Write down five reasons for being safety aware in the laboratory to be shared with the class.

Biohazards and Infection Control

Biohazards, or biological hazards, are materials or situations that present the possible risk of infection. Infection with biohazardous material can occur during specimen collection, handling, transportation, or testing. Specimens with the potential to be infectious include blood, body fluids, biological specimens, exudates (EKS yoo deyts), bacterial cultures, and smears. Infection can be introduced into the body in many ways, including:

- Breathing in a pathogen
- Accidental inoculation by a needlestick or a sharps injury
- Aerosols created by uncapping specimen tubes
- Centrifuge accidents
- Entry of pathogens through a cut, abrasion, burn, or break in the skin

---

VOCABULARY

exudates Fluids with high concentrations of protein and cellular debris that have escaped from the blood vessels and have been deposited in tissues or on tissue surfaces.

sharps Medical term for devices with sharp points or edges that can puncture or cut skin. Examples include needles, scalpels, or broken glass.

Standard Precautions. As described in Chapter 32, the CDC continuously monitors infection and disease in the United States. The CDC developed a single set of precautions called *Standard Precautions* to reduce the risk of transmission of bloodborne pathogens and other pathogens in the healthcare setting. These precautions apply to all patient care, regardless of the suspected or confirmed infection status of the patient. Standard Precautions include five elements:

- Hand hygiene: According to the CDC, the single most effective means of preventing the spread of infection. Wash hands

with soap, running water, and friction at the beginning of the day, when hands are visibly soiled, and after using the restroom. (See Chapter 32 for additional information.) Medical aseptic hand washing or alcohol-based hand sanitizer should be used:

- Before and after contact with the patient
- Before *donning* (putting on) gloves and after removing gloves
- After contact with blood, OPIM, or contaminated surfaces
- Before leaving the facility
- Before and after eating
- Use of personal protective equipment (PPE) (Fig. 52.7)
- Safe needle practices
- Safe handling of potentially contaminated equipment or surfaces in the patient environment
- Respiratory hygiene/cough etiquette

The precautions are designed both to protect the healthcare provider and to prevent the healthcare provider from spreading infections among patients.

Bloodborne Pathogens Standard. In 1991 OSHA published the Bloodborne Pathogen Standard in response to the significant health risk associated with workplace exposure to blood and other potentially infectious materials. Urine is not specifically included in the standard unless it is visibly bloody.

The Bloodborne Pathogen Standard requires employers to protect workers from occupational exposures to blood or other potentially infectious materials (OPIM). (See Chapter 32 for additional information.). Bloodborne pathogens are transmitted through exposure to blood and body fluids, which are the primary substances handled in the laboratory. The Bloodborne Pathogens Standard requires that the laboratory employer have a written exposure control plan that proves the following steps have been taken to protect employees:

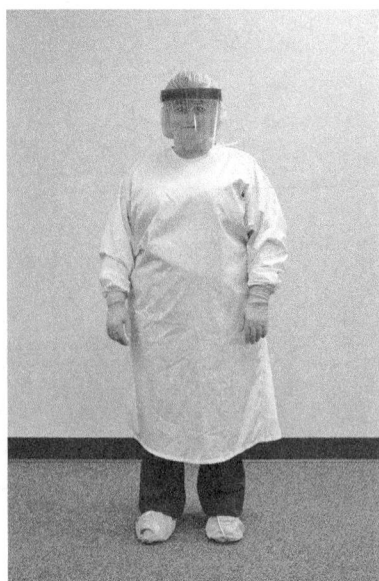

Fig. 52.7 Personal Protective Equipment. (From Niedzwiecki B, et al: *Kinn's the medical assistant,* ed 14, St. Louis, 2020, Elsevier.)

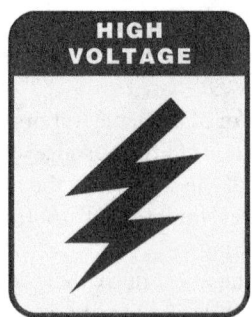
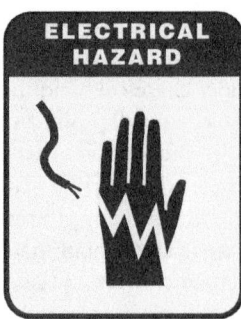

Fig. 52.8 High-Voltage and Electrical Hazard Labels. (From Niedzwiecki B, et al: *Kinn's the medical assistant,* ed 14, St. Louis, 2020, Elsevier.)

- Written job categories of employees at risk of exposure to blood (laboratory workers are considered "high risk")
- HBV vaccination guidelines and records for each employee at risk
- Record of initial and annual Standard Precautions training for bloodborne pathogens and safety training for each employee (including proper use of safety needles)
- Definition and listing of safe work practices and PPE for all lab personnel (fluid-impermeable lab coats that do not leave the laboratory area, gloves, face protection and labeling of biohazardous sharps and waste containers and their proper disposal)
- Sharps injury log of all work-related needlesticks and exposures to blood, with medical intervention after exposure incidents
- Written plan to maintain the privacy of the individual exposed to blood

Safety Guidelines for Other Potentially Infectious Materials.

The following guidelines are required for handling OPIM:

- Handle and process all specimens as if they contained infectious material.
- Wipe the outside of specimen containers with a germicide.
- Dispose of all infectious materials according to state and federal guidelines. Infectious agents may be inactivated (such as using the autoclave) before disposal. Blood and potentially infectious materials mixed with chemicals are considered mixed waste. If possible, the infectious material should be inactivated, and the disposal should follow the chemical waste procedure. Many Safety Data Sheets contain disposal information.
- Clean up spills using a disinfectant (see Chapter 32).
- Immediately dispose of any chipped or broken glassware into a sharps container using appropriate safety methods to prevent accidental punctures.

Physical Hazards

Physical hazards in the laboratory can be classified as electrical, fire, and mechanical hazards. Electric shock is a threat when any electrical equipment is in use. It is imperative to keep all electrical equipment in proper repair and to always to follow manufacturers' instructions.

Use these procedures for electrical hazards:

- Use surge protectors.
- Inspect all cords and plugs frequently.
- Never use extension cords.
- Do not overload circuits.

Unplug the electrical device before servicing and never operate electrical instruments with wet hands. If a sink is nearby, make sure electrical cords do not come in contact with the water supply. Signs and labels should be placed on specific electrical hazards (Fig. 52.8, Procedure 52.3).

Open flames are rarely used in a laboratory anymore, but the potential for fire still exists. Fires may be ignited by smoking, heating elements, and sparks from electrical connections. Flammable materials should not be stored near any source of ignition. All laboratory personnel should be familiar with the locations of fire extinguishers and fire safety blankets. Fire extinguishers should be the carbon dioxide (CO_2), dry chemical, or *halon* (HAY lohn) type, known as the ABC type of extinguisher. ABC extinguishers can be used on all types of fires. Extinguishers should be inspected regularly by a licensed inspector and replaced or recharged if used. The medical assistant may be responsible for maintaining records on the care and maintenance of fire extinguishers.

Fire safety blankets can be used to smother flames on burning clothing. However, a victim should not be wrapped in a fire blanket, because this may intensify burns. Instead, the flames should be patted out or the victim directed to stop, drop, and roll on the blanket.

Emergency phone numbers should be posted on the wall near the telephone, and all personnel should know the locations of fire alarms, the fire escape routes, and procedures to follow if exits are blocked. Periodic fire drills should be conducted, and hallways and exits should be kept free of clutter.

Mechanical hazards arise from the use of laboratory equipment. Care should be exercised when using equipment with moving parts, such as *centrifuges* (SEN truh fyooj es). Centrifuges are devices that separate liquids from solids, such as separating blood cells from serum or plasma or preparing urine sediment for examination. Centrifuges present a hazard not only from moving parts but also from glassware that might break during centrifugation and from aerosols that might be created if tubes are not capped tightly.

Care should also be exercised when using pieces of equipment that rely on pressure, such as *autoclaves* (AW tuh kleyv). Autoclaves are used to sterilize metal instruments, microbiological media, and some microbiological waste. Autoclaves present a danger if opened before the pressure has come down to a safe level.

Although centrifuges and autoclaves often have built-in safeguards, such as locks that prevent entry until the environment is safe, improper care of the equipment can cause the safety measures to fail.

SPECIMEN COLLECTION, PROCESSING, AND STORAGE

Laboratory Requisitions and Reports

When the provider orders laboratory testing, an electronic or a paper requisition must be generated. Patient information on the requisitions must be complete, accurate, and legible. The patient is then directed to the POL, where the specimen is collected, processed, prepared, and sent to an outside laboratory. Patients may also go to an outside laboratory if they so choose.

Fig. 52.9 shows the electronic lab requisition form used in SimChart for the Medical Office. The following information typically is required on the requisition when specimens are sent to a reference laboratory:

- Provider's name, account number, address, and phone number
- Patient's full name, age, date of birth, sex, address, and insurance information
- Source of specimen

- Date and time of collection, and initials of the person collecting the specimen
- Specific test (or tests) requested
- Medications the patient is taking
- Whether the patient fasted or followed dietary restrictions if required; time of last intake
- Possible diagnosis
- Indication of whether the test is to be performed STAT

When the results of the tests are obtained, a laboratory report is sent to the office. The laboratory reports can be distributed as follows:

- Sent directly from the referral laboratory to the patient's electronic health record (EHR)
- Sent electronically to the facility and then uploaded by staff to the EHR or printed out to be included in the paper medical record

A medical assistant is frequently responsible for making sure that all outside laboratory reports have been received and given to the provider for review. Test results cannot be given to a patient until the provider has reviewed them. Any testing that is completed outside the POL at a reference lab must be tracked. This can be done by maintaining a master laboratory specimen log sheet or electronic file, which can be used to track patient specimens, tests ordered, designated lab, results, and provider response.

VOCABULARY

STAT The medical abbreviation for the Latin term *statum*, meaning immediately; at this moment.

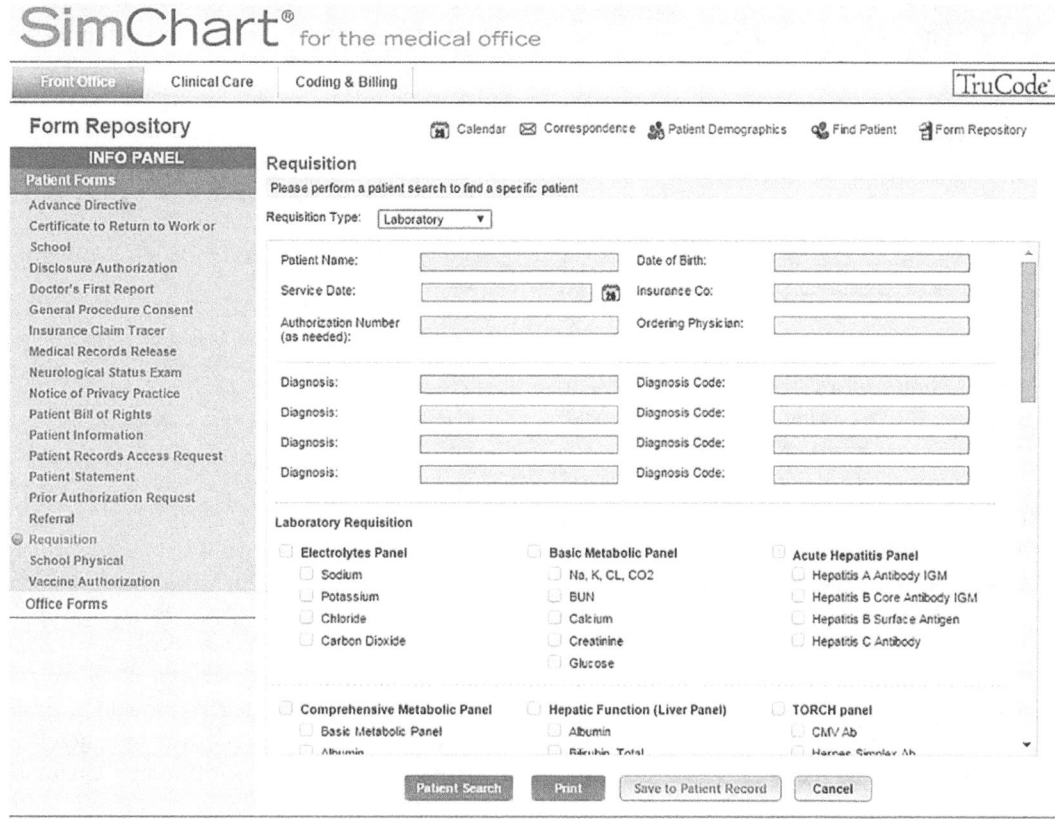

Fig. 52.9 Electronic Laboratory Requisition Form.

Specimen Collection

The medical assistant is responsible for the collection of many different types of specimens. It is important to recognize that laboratory results are only as good as the specimen collected. The importance of proper specimen collection cannot be overemphasized. To ensure that test results are accurate indicators of the patient's state of health, it is critical that proper specimen collection is understood and followed exactly. The most common specimens are blood, urine, and swab samples collected from wounds or mucous membranes. Specimens that may be collected less frequently include feces, gastric contents, CSF, tissue samples, semen, and aspirates (AS puh reyts).

Verifying the patient's identity before the specimen collection is a critical step in the collection process. Patient identification should follow the written procedure for your institution. Using a minimum of two patient identifiers before specimen collection is standard. If the patient is not identified properly, the laboratory results that are generated will be useless.

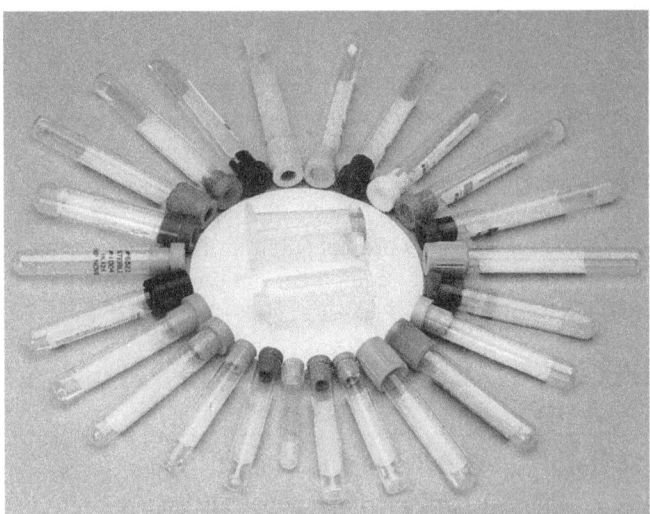

Fig. 52.10 Vacutainer Tubes With Colored Stoppers. (From Niedzwiecki B, et al: *Kinn's the medical assistant,* ed 14, St. Louis, 2020, Elsevier.)

Labeling Containers. The container must be labeled properly at the time of collection. Unlabeled containers are not acceptable for laboratory testing and must be rejected. When labeling a sample container, make sure you only use a black waterproof marker or pen, never pencil. All labels should include the following information, at a minimum:

- Patient's name; surname first, then middle initial
- Identification number
- Date (MM/DD/YYYY) and time of collection
- Phlebotomist or collector's initials
- Specimen type

If affixing a computer-generated label, make sure to write the time and initial the specimen after the venipuncture has been completed.

CRITICAL THINKING 52.6

As John has been working in phlebotomy, he has been reminded of the importance of patient identification. Write down three reasons patient identification is critical to laboratory specimens. Be ready to share your reasons with the class.

Collection Containers. Another important step in specimen collection is the proper choice of a collection container. For example, blood may be collected using a vacuum tube system. Blood collection tubes are available in a variety of sizes, depending on the collection needs. Blood collection tubes are also available with and without preservatives and anticoagulants (an tee koh AG yuh luh nts). The tube stoppers are color coded. The color of the stopper indicates which additive is present, if any (Fig. 52.10). Collection in an incorrectly colored tube may result in an unacceptable specimen, and recollection may be necessary.

If a specimen will be tested for the presence of microorganisms, a sterile container must be used. If patients are to collect the specimen at home, they should be provided with the appropriate container and complete instructions for collection. Patient education is an important role for the medical assistant. Each patient should receive clear instructions for proper home collection. Make sure your patients listen to the directions and ask them to repeat instructions back to you, so you know they understand the information. Remember to be sensitive to individual patient factors (e.g., hearing, sight, primary language, cognitive capacity). These can affect the patient's understanding of the instructions, in addition to their ability to follow through. Giving patients written directions to take home can also be helpful and reassuring.

The medical assistant should always check the laboratory's specimen requirements manual or reference laboratory website for any unfamiliar tests. A clear understanding of the specimen and collection requirements is very important. Any unanswered questions should be resolved by calling the reference laboratory before collecting the specimen.

VOCABULARY

anticoagulants Substances (i.e., medications or chemicals) that prevent clotting of blood.

aspirate To withdraw fluid using suction, such as occurs when a specimen has been removed from the body using a needle and syringe.

identifiers Information unique to an individual. Common identifiers used for patient identification include the full name, including middle initial; date of birth; medical identification number; or patient's address.

preservatives Substances added to a specimen to prevent the deterioration of cells or chemicals.

Preventing Contamination. Medical assistants must take care to prevent contamination of specimens and themselves. Expiration dates on swabs, tubes, transport media, and other collection containers should be checked before the items are used. Any expired materials should not be used and should be properly discarded. An improperly handled specimen may become contaminated or may contaminate the surrounding environment. Standard

Precautions should be followed. All blood and body fluids from all patients should be considered infectious.

The specimen collected must be a true representative sample. A swab for a wound culture collected from the surface of the wound generally does not yield the same results as one taken from the depths of the wound. A hemolyzed (HEE muh lahyz d) blood specimen shows marked differences in many tests (Fig. 52.11). If a large volume of specimen is collected (e.g., a 24-hour urine specimen), the total volume or weight must be carefully measured and recorded. The specimen must be well mixed before an aliquot (AL i kwuh t) is removed and submitted for testing.

> **VOCABULARY**
> **aliquot** A portion of a well-mixed sample removed for testing.
> **hemolyzed** Refers to a blood sample in which the red blood cells have ruptured.

Handling, Processing, and Storing Specimens

Specimens must be handled, processed, and stored according to the test manufacturer's guidelines to prevent any changes that would affect test results. In Chapters 53 through 56, specimen handling, processing, and storage will be discussed for each specific area of the laboratory. Each department in the lab has unique types of testing and specimen requirements. Some general guidelines to keep in mind include:

- The storage temperature of the specimen should follow the manufacturer's testing requirements. The manufacturer's package inserts should be consulted to ensure that each specimen is handled and processed properly.
- Serum must be separated from red blood cells as soon as possible after the specimen has clotted to prevent changes caused by the metabolism of the blood cells.
- Specimens for chemistry and liver panels may need to be protected from light.
- Specimens may need to be frozen to prevent chemical constituents from changing.

Most offices have a laboratory courier service that picks up specimens periodically throughout the day. Specimens should be properly stored (some may require refrigeration) until the courier arrives. Instructions for properly obtaining, processing, and preparing a specimen for transport are usually supplied by the testing laboratory. If the instructions are not clear or if you have a question about a particular test collection, the reference laboratory should answer the question over the phone. An understanding of the following criteria is necessary for the safe shipment of specimens:

- Length of time acceptable for transport
- Recommended temperature range to maintain the specimen
- Appropriate packaging material if the specimen needs to be protected from light

If the specimen is to be mailed, it must be carefully packaged to prevent breakage, damage, or contamination during handling. Follow the instructions for transport supplied by the reference laboratory. Do not ship specimens without proper packaging and labeling as specified by the test laboratory.

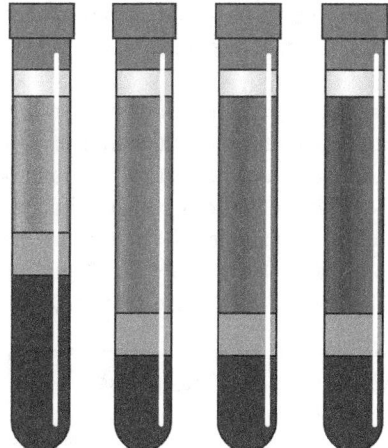

Fig. 52.11 Normal and Hemolyzed Blood Sample Graphic.

Chain of Custody. When a specimen may be needed as evidence in a court case, certain procedures must be followed when the specimen is collected and handled. Forensic, or legal, specimens should be collected, handled, and stored in a way that will allow them to be acknowledged in a court of law. Specimen processing must be documented precisely, ensuring that no tampering with evidence has occurred. *Chain of custody* refers to the stepwise method used to collect, process, and test a specimen. The documentation must be signed by every person who has any contact with the specimen, from collection to the final reporting of results. Blood alcohol level testing and drug screening often require chain of custody handling. Everything needed to collect the specimen is provided in a kit – the gloves, the vacuum tube, and the needle used to collect the blood specimen. Documentation is included and must be signed by all personnel. Medical assistants and phlebotomists can be subpoenaed (suh PEE nuhd) to testify in court about specimens they have collected. It is always in your best interest to follow chain of custody procedures exactly.

> **CRITICAL THINKING 52.7**
> What is the difference between a patient specimen and a forensic specimen? In your own words, describe *chain of custody*.

LABORATORY MATHEMATICS AND MEASUREMENT

All laboratory testing relies on the accurate use of values, units, and measurements. For example, values are used to report the time the sample was collected, the volume of the specimen, the amount of analyte found in a specimen, and dilutions used in sample preparation, and to record QC results. Some test results are measured in g/dL (grams per deciliter) and others as IU/mL (international units per milliliter).

Measuring Time

Time of day is a critical factor in patient care. Specimens must be collected on a timed schedule. Many laboratories use the 24-hour clock or military time when recording time. This method avoids the confusion that comes with the 12-hour clock, which uses a.m. (morning) and p.m. (afternoon) designations.

Military time uses four digits. The first two digits show the hour and the last two digits reflect the minutes. Noon is referred to as 1200 (twelve hundred) hours and midnight is 0000 (zero hundred), or 2400 hours. Before 1 p.m., the hours are the same as 12-hour clock. For examples, 10:10 am is 1010 in military time. After 1 p.m., add the hour to the 12. For example, 6:23 p.m. would be 1823 and 10:00 p.m. would be 2200.

CRITICAL THINKING 52.8

If the time on the clock is 10:00 a.m., how would you write it in military time? If the time is 10:00 p.m., how would you write it in military time? If the time on a document were written as 1900 hours, how would you write it using the 12-hour clock? What if it were written as 0800 hours?

Measuring Temperature

Two scales are currently used for measuring temperature; each is divided into units called *degrees* (Table 52.5). The *Fahrenheit* (FAHR uhn hahyt) scale is considered part of the *English system* of measurement and is the scale most commonly used in the United States. The *Celsius* (SEL see uh s) *scale* is used in countries that apply the *metric system*. On the Celsius (C) scale, water freezes at 0°C and boils at 100°F. On the Fahrenheit (F) scale, water freezes at 32°F and boils at 212°F. Almost all laboratories in the United States use the Celsius scale for temperature.

The following steps show how to convert a Fahrenheit temperature to a Celsius temperature.

98.6°F = _____ °C
Step 1: Subtract 32 from °F temp   98.6 – 32 = 66.6
Step 2: Divide number by 1.8   66.6 ÷ 1.8 = 37°C

The following steps show how to convert a Celsius temperature to a Fahrenheit temperature.

100°C = _____ °F
Step 1: Multiply °C temp by 1.8   100 × 1.8 = 180
Step 2: Add 32 to that number   180 + 32 = 212°F

Units of Measurement

The units of measurement that we commonly use in the United States differ from those used in the laboratory. In everyday life, we use the English system of measurement:

- Weight is measured in ounces and pounds.
- Length is measured in inches and feet.
- Volume is measured in cups and quarts.

In the laboratory, the metric system and the Système International (SI) are used. It is important that medical assistants memorize and practice these systems so that they can communicate professionally (Table 52.6).

The metric system is based on a decimal system, which consists of basic units and prefixes that indicate a system of division

TABLE 52.5   Common Laboratory Temperature Settings

	Fahrenheit	Celsius
Refrigerator	35°–46°	2°–8°
Freezer	32°	0°
Room	59°–86°	15°–30°
Incubator	98.6°	37°
Body temperature	98.6°	37°
Autoclave	254°	121°

TABLE 52.6   Comparing the English System of Measurement With the Metric System

	English System	Metric System	Common Units of Measure Seen in Healthcare
Weight	Ounces (oz) and pounds (lb)	Grams (g)	Gram (g) Kilogram (kg) Milligram (mg) Microgram (mcg)
Length	Inches and feet	Meters (m)	Meter (m) Centimeter (cm) Millimeter (mm)
Volume	Cups and quarts	Liters (L)	Liter (L) Milliliter (mL or ml) Cubic centimeter (cc) cc = mL

in multiples of 10. Prefixes are added to each symbol to reduce or enlarge them by units of 10. Table 52.7 present an overview of the metric system measurements.

International organizations, such as the World Health Organization (WHO), officially recognize SI units. Many countries have adopted this system, but the United States has not completely converted to it. The SI is an adaptation of the metric system that uses several of the basic units, although some units are different for reporting results. For example, blood glucose is reported in *millimoles* (MIL uh mohls) per liter (mmol/L) using the SI system, but it is reported as mg/dL using the metric system. Therefore it is very important for the medical assistant to double-check the laboratory's standard and include the appropriate units of measurement when reporting test values.

CRITICAL THINKING 52.9

If you have 3.2 g of salt and you want to express it in milligrams, how will you write it? If the length of an item is 455 cm and you want to express it in meters, how will you write it?

Measuring Liquid Volume

Test tubes are used to test or hold liquid reagents, samples, or aliquots. Test tubes come in many sizes and are typically disposable. Test tubes may be sterile for use in microbiology.

TABLE 52.7 Metric System: Prefixes of Measurements

Prefixes	Size	Or Another Way to Look At It	
Kilo (k)	1000 base units	1 kilo = 1000 base units	Larger than the base unit
Hecto	100 base units	1 hecto = 100 base units	
Deka	10 base units	1 deka = 10 base units	
Base Units (Meter, Liter, or Gram)			
Deci	0.1 unit	10 deci = 1 base unit	Smaller than the base unit
Centi (c)	0.01 unit	100 centi = 1 base unit	
Milli (m)	0.001	1000 milli = 1 base unit	
Micro (mc)	0.000001	1,000,000 micro = 1 base unit	

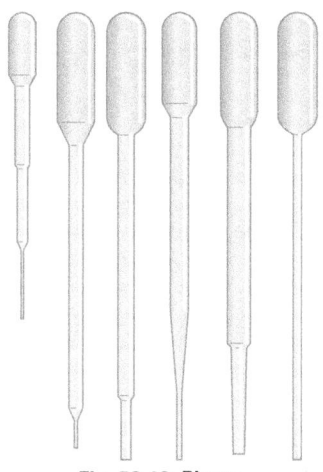

Fig. 52.12 Pipets.

When liquids are measured into test tubes, the most common piece of glassware used is the pipet (pie PET). A pipet is a hollow tube that can be made from glass or plastic. Pipets often have lines called *graduation marks* to indicate volume on the length of the tube. Some plastic pipets have a built-in bulb to help transfer fluids and are known as *transfer pipets*. This type of pipet usually may or may not have any measurement lines on the tube. Fig. 52.12 shows a variety of transfer pipets that are used in the laboratory. *Micropipets* are used to deliver very small volumes of liquid (Fig. 52.13). These pipetting devices must be fitted with an appropriate disposable tip. The device is equipped with a piston at the top, which must be depressed before the pipet is filled and when the pipet is drained. It is important to follow the manufacturer's instructions for use with all pipets and micropipets. Each type of pipet may be slightly different.

> **VOCABULARY**
> **pipet** A slender tube attached to or including a bulb that is used for transferring or measuring small amounts of a liquid; it is often used in a laboratory.

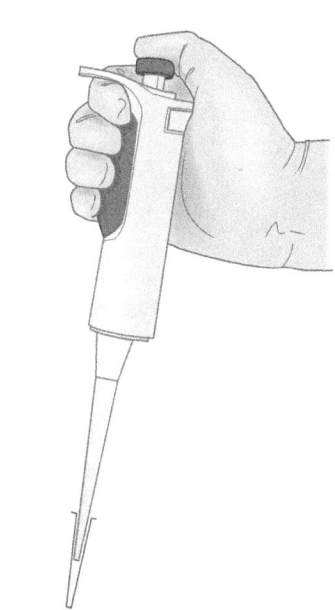

Fig. 52.13 Micropipet With Disposable Tips. (From Niedzwiecki B, et al: *Kinn's the medical assistant*, ed 14, St. Louis, 2020, Elsevier.)

LABORATORY EQUIPMENT

Microscope

Nearly every medical laboratory is equipped with a *microscope*. This indispensable instrument is used to view objects too small to be seen with the naked eye (Fig. 52.14). The microscope is used to evaluate stained blood smears, urine sediment, vaginal secretions, and smears made from body fluids and microorganisms.

Provider-Performed Microscopy Procedures. Microscopic procedures are not considered CLIA waived because they require judgment and additional training. In addition, an error in reading microscopic tests may have a detrimental effect on the patient's care. Providers petitioned the CMS to create a new laboratory category that would allow them to perform a set of simple microscopic tests in the ambulatory setting (Table 52.8). CMS approved the list and created an additional CLIA category called *provider-performed microscopy procedures (PPMP)*. Certified CLIA-PPMP laboratories must meet the same quality standards as laboratories that perform moderate-complexity tests, including passing three proficiency tests from an outside agency per year. The medical assistant is taught how to prepare the microscope slide and bring it into focus. The final analysis of a microscope slide must be made by one of the following personnel:

- Physician (medical doctor, doctor of osteopathy, or doctor of podiatric medicine)
- Midlevel practitioner (nurse midwife, nurse practitioner, or physician assistant)
- Dentist (doctor of dental surgery or doctor of dental medicine)
- Trained laboratory professional with CLIA moderate- or high-complexity training

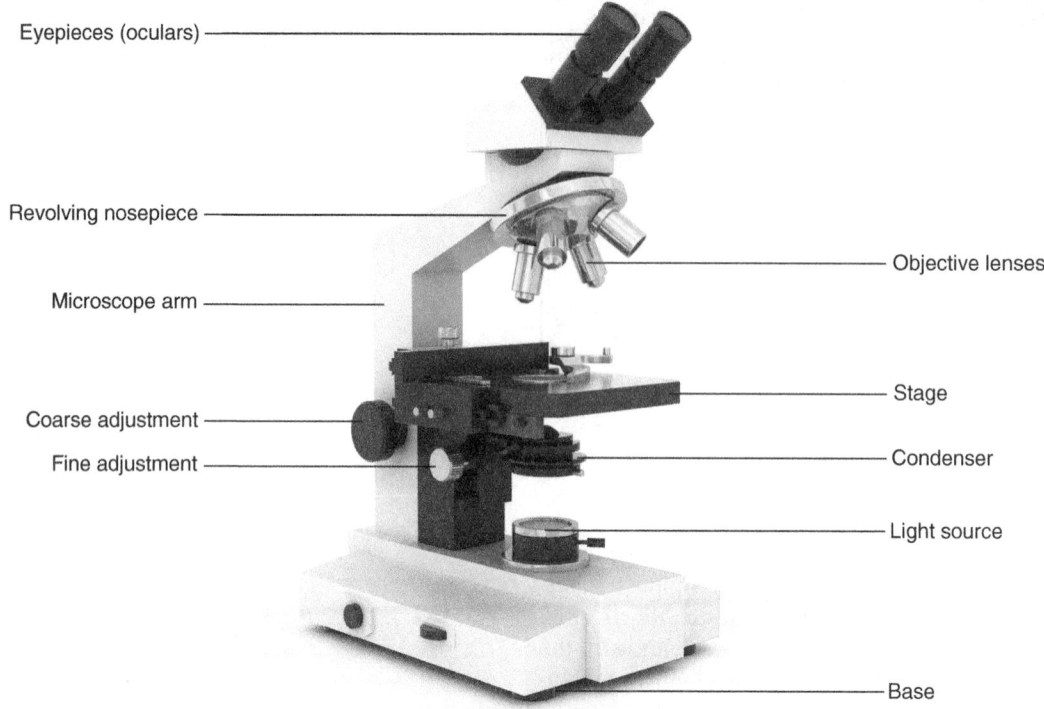

Eyepieces (oculars)

Revolving nosepiece

Microscope arm

Coarse adjustment

Fine adjustment

Objective lenses

Stage

Condenser

Light source

Base

Fig. 52.14 The Microscope. (Courtesy urfinguss/iStock/Thinkstock.)

TABLE 52.8	CLIA-Approved Procedures for Provider-Performed Microscopy (PPM)	
Test	**Description**	**Example**
Direct wet mount	Examination of specimens for the presence or absence of bacteria, fungi, parasites, and human cellular elements	Observing vaginal secretions for the presence of yeast to assist with diagnosis of vulvovaginal candidiasis
KOH preparation	Any preparation using potassium hydroxide	Observing skin scrapings for the presence of fungi
Fecal leukocyte examination	Simple stain of fecal specimen; assists in diagnosis of diarrheal disease	Leukocytes are found in stool in antibiotic-associated colitis, ulcerative colitis, shigellosis, and salmonellosis
Pinworm examination	Preparations are observed for the presence or absence of *Enterobius vermicularis* eggs	Performing a cellulose tape collection for pinworms
Postcoital direct, qualitative examinations	Vaginal or cervical mucus is examined 4–10 hours after intercourse for the presence of live, motile sperm	Assists in the diagnosis of infertility
Qualitative semen analysis	Semen is examined for the presence or absence of spermatozoa; motility of the sperm is noted	Assists in postvasectomy semen analysis and in the diagnosis of infertility
Urine sediment examination	Urine sediment is examined for the presence or absence of formed elements	Part of a routine urinalysis (see Chapter 53)

CLIA, Clinical Laboratory Improvement Amendments; *KOH,* potassium hydroxide.

Components of a Microscope. Microscopes have several major components:
- *Magnification* (mag nuh fi KAY shuhn) system, which provides visual enlargement of the object being viewed.
- Mechanical parts, including stage/clips to hold the slide; forward/back and left/right movement knobs to allow viewing of different areas of the slide; coarse and fine adjustor knobs allowing for clearer resolution of the specimen for viewing.
- *Illuminator* (ih loo muh NEY tor) system, which provides a steady light source that shines up through the slide. It includes the light source, condenser, and iris diaphragm.
- Framework, which is the structural parts of the microscope. It includes the head, the arm, and the base.

Microscopes may be *monocular* (muh NOK yuh ler) or *binocular* (bahy NOK yuh ler). A monocular microscope has one eyepiece for viewing, and a binocular microscope has two. Most laboratories use a binocular microscope.

The usual magnification in the ocular or eyepiece is 10 times (10×). In addition to the ocular, compound microscopes have objective lenses that increase the magnification of the specimen. The objectives are attached to the revolving nosepiece. Most microscopes have four objectives, each with a different magnifying power:
- The shortest objective has the lowest power (4×) and is called the *scanning lens.* This lens is used to scan the field of interest and then focus on a particular object.
- Greater detail is observed with the next longest objective, which is low power (10×).

- The high or high dry objective usually has a magnification of 40× or 45×.
- The longest objective, oil immersion (100×), allows the finest focusing of the object and requires the use of a special oil that is placed directly on the slide. This special oil, called *immersion oil,* prevents refraction of the light and improves the resolution (clarity) of the magnified image. Oil immersion is used to view cells and extremely small materials (e.g., bacteria and platelets) and to examine stained specimens.

The total magnification of the specimen is determined by multiplying the magnification of the objective lens by 10 (the magnification of the ocular lens). Therefore if you have the 10× objective in place when observing blood cells, you are magnifying the image 100 times. Just above the base are the focusing knobs. The coarse adjustment is used only with scanning and low-power lenses, and the fine adjustment is used with high-power and oil immersion lenses.

The arm of the microscope connects the objectives and the oculars to the base, which supports the microscope and contains its light source. The stage of the microscope is equipped with clips that hold the slide to be viewed. Under the stage is the light source, the condenser, and the iris diaphragm, which make up the illumination system. The condenser directs light up through the slide, and the iris diaphragm regulates the amount of light passing through the specimen.

Routine Maintenance. Microscopes are precise and expensive instruments that require careful handling. The amount of routine maintenance required depends on the amount of daily use. Dirt is the enemy of the microscope, which must be kept very clean at all times. Oil, makeup, dust, and eye secretions can all obstruct vision through the lens and may transmit infective organisms. The microscope should always be stored in a plastic dust cover when not in use. Lenses should be cleaned before and after each use with lens paper and lens cleaner. Any other type of tissue scratches the lenses or leaves lint residue behind. Routine use of solvent cleaners, such as xylene, is not recommended, because these cleaners may loosen a lens. The body of the microscope should be dusted with a soft cloth.

The microscope should be placed in a permanent location in the laboratory, on a sturdy table in an area where it cannot be bumped. If a microscope must be moved, it should be carried securely, with one hand supporting the base and the other holding the arm. When the microscope is stored, it should be left covered and with the low-power objective engaged or locked in place on the revolving nosepiece. The stage should be centered.

Using a Microscope. Using a microscope involves focusing and illumination (Procedure 52.4). The image is focused by moving the objectives closer to the specimen using the fine and coarse knobs. Proper focusing begins with the objective at lowest power. The coarse adjustment moves the objective quickly. This knob is used first to bring the specimen into approximate focus. The fine adjustment focus knob then brings the specimen into

precise focus. The fine focus moves the objective more slowly to allow the viewer to zero in on the specimen with greater accuracy. Illumination is accomplished by raising or lowering the condenser and by opening and closing the diaphragm on the condenser.

If the microscope is a binocular model, the eyepieces may need to be adjusted to accommodate the distance between the pupils and the individual's point of greatest visual acuity. A gentle push inward or pull outward adjusts the distance between the eyepieces.

Centrifuge

A centrifuge is an instrument that is used to separate solids from liquids. A centrifuge works by rapidly spinning the specimen, which increases the gravitational (grav i TEY shuhn uhl) force. The increased force pushes the heavier solids to the bottom of the specimen and lets lighter liquids remain at the top of the specimen. *Centrifugation* (SEN truh fyoo gahy shun) is used to separate blood cells from serum or plasma. It is also used to separate solid materials, such as cells and crystals, in urine specimens.

Centrifuges (Fig. 52.15) are designed for specific uses. They may be bench-top or floor models; some may be refrigerated. Some may have rotors or heads that are interchangeable to accommodate different-sized sample tubes. Centrifuge configurations vary with the laboratory task that needs to be done. Three common configurations are used in the clinical laboratory:

- A centrifuge that has a fixed-angle rotor, in which specimen cups are held in a rigid position at a fixed angle
- A centrifuge that has a horizontal head with buckets that swing out horizontally during centrifugation
- A centrifuge used for centrifuging capillary tubes for microhematocrit testing (see Chapter 55)

Directions for using a centrifuge usually are given in terms of revolutions per minute (rpm). Spinning generates centrifugal force, causing the heaviest particles in a liquid to migrate

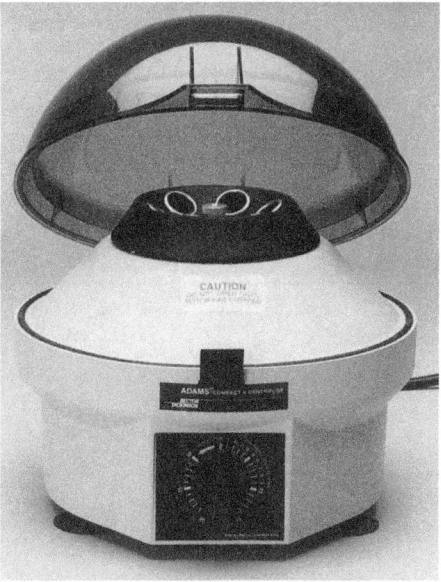

Fig. 52.15 A Centrifuge. (From Niedzwiecki B, et al: *Kinn's the medical assistant,* ed 14, St. Louis, 2020, Elsevier.)

to the bottom of the tube. Centrifuges can be dangerous if not used correctly. The most important rule is to ensure that the centrifuge is balanced so that tubes of equal size and containing equal volume are directly across from one another in the rotor holders or buckets. Therefore there must always be an even number of tubes in the centrifuge. If a second specimen of the same volume in the same-sized tube is not available for balance, a tube of water may be used to balance the load. Tubes being centrifuged should be capped to prevent samples from creating aerosols during spinning. Rubber cups should be placed in the bottom of the carrier cups to keep the glass tubes from breaking.

Centrifuges should never be opened while they are in operation, nor should you attempt to slow a centrifuge with your hands. Most centrifuges are equipped with a brake, which should be used only in an emergency, the most common of which is a broken glass tube. In this case, wait until the centrifuge comes to a complete stop and follow the manufacturer's instructions for disinfecting the unit; also follow Standard Precautions to prevent injury and disease transmission.

Centrifuges should be checked, cleaned, and lubricated regularly to ensure proper operation. A certified technician must ensure the centrifuge's speed to comply with quality assurance guidelines set forth by the College of American Pathologists (CAP).

> **VOCABULARY**
> **rotor** The rotating member of a machine or device.

Incubator

Incubators (IN kyuh bey ters) are cabinets that maintain constant temperatures (Fig. 52.16). They generally are used

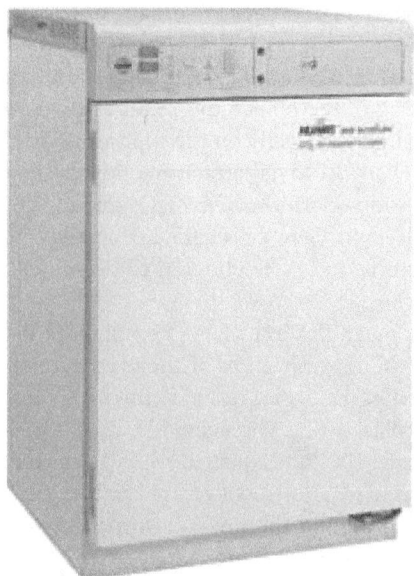

Fig. 52.16 An Incubator. (Courtesy NuAire, Plymouth, MN.)

in the microbiology laboratory. An incubator can be set to a specific temperature. Microbiology departments usually maintain a constant temperature of 95°F to 98.6°F (35°C to 37°C), although other temperatures may also be appropriate. Incubators usually have warning alarms that sound if the temperature exceeds or falls below a specified range. The temperature should be checked daily, and the interior and exterior should be cleaned regularly with a disinfectant approved by the manufacturer.

Table 52.9 presents an example of a laboratory maintenance log. All laboratory equipment that is temperature sensitive should have temperatures checked and recorded daily.

TABLE 52.9 Laboratory Maintenance Log

Medical Clinic

Daily Maintenance Control Chart

	MONTH					YEAR			
Day	Daily Refrig 2°–8°C	Freezer 0°–20°C	Room 15°–30°C	Incubator 34°–36°C	Bleach Counters	Monthly Eyewash Checked	Shower Checked	By	
1									
2									
3									
4									
5									

CLOSING COMMENTS

All health and safety risks to laboratory workers cannot be anticipated or eliminated. However, the risks are greatly reduced when safety guidelines are adhered to by everyone.

Use common sense and document everything. If it is not documented, in the eyes of the law it did not happen. If you have questions about a safety procedure, ask your supervisor. If you are aware of a potential safety problem, report it to the person in charge. Your welfare, the welfare of the patient, and the welfare of co-workers may depend on your commitment to safety.

If diseases did not exist, there would be little need for clinical laboratories. The fact that the human body is susceptible to disease creates a need for laboratory testing. The next four chapters discuss common CLIA-waived tests performed in the POL. They cover patient education, preparation, specimen collection, testing procedures, and proper documentation. All of these skills are aspects of a medical assistant's scope of practice within the laboratory.

PATIENT-CENTERED CARE

For many testing procedures, patients must be given a specific set of instructions to follow. Providers often communicate the instructions to the patient, but they may also ask the medical assistant to reinforce the information. For example, patients may be required to fast 8 to 12 hours before blood samples are collected.

Often the medical assistant is responsible for communicating the provider's directions that need to be followed before laboratory testing. Make sure you have reviewed the provider's orders correctly before explaining the procedure to the patient. The patient should be given verbal and written instructions prior to testing. Also include a phone number on the instruction sheet so that patients can call if they have questions after returning home. Maintaining a patient's privacy and confidentiality is a crucial factor that must be considered when dealing with test results.

BEING PROFESSIONAL

Role-play this scenario with your peer: You have just started working at a provider's office that also performs CLIA-waived laboratory testing. One of the medical assistants was performing a laboratory test and accidently spilled some of the control solution onto exposed skin and asks for your help. What should you do?

You ask the medical assistant where the Laboratory Safety Manual is so you can look up the SDS for further treatment information on the chemical reagent, but there is no manual. What should you say and/or do next?

CHAPTER REVIEW

In this chapter, you were introduced to the clinical laboratory and the role it plays in patient care. There are various categories of personnel who work in the laboratory. Categories are based on the education and certification of the individuals. Together, laboratory personnel work toward several key purposes in patient care: to document good health and to aid in the diagnosis, prognosis, prevention, treatment, and monitoring of disease.

Laboratory testing is one part of the information providers need to help patients maintain good health. We learned the definition for the term *homeostasis,* which is a state of internal balance the body needs to maintain proper function. This term is also applied to laboratory testing in defining a reference range. When testing for any particular analyte, a healthy person should test within the reference range of a test. Any test results that are out of the reference range should be investigated further to return the person to health, if possible. Laboratory tests can be quantitative, which means they have numeric values associated with testing, or qualitative, which means they provide a positive or negative result.

There are different departments within the laboratory, but the areas most commonly seen in physician office laboratories are urinalysis, hematology, chemistry, and microbiology. We also learned that government legislation affects the laboratory. The Clinical Laboratory Improvement Amendments established quality standards for clinical laboratories, and the FDA categorizes all laboratory tests. There are three designations for testing: waived, moderate-complexity, and high-complexity testing. Each type of testing has designated personnel who can perform the tests. Medical assistants can perform waived testing of all types.

This chapter defined and discussed laboratory quality assurance, comprehensive policies and procedures designed to ensure excellent documentation and the reliability of laboratory testing. The three stages of QA are preanalytic, analytic, and postanalytic. Each stage is designed to ensure reliable patient testing results and documentation. Quality control was also defined and discussed in this chapter. QC includes the procedures that should be followed to ensure there are no analytical errors in the testing process and thus documents the accuracy of test results. QA, QC, and preventive maintenance all work together to ensure that patient results are accurate and can be used by the provider with confidence.

This chapter also emphasized laboratory safety and safety standards regarding chemicals, biohazards, infection control, Standard Precautions, bloodborne pathogens, other potentially infectious materials, and physical hazards.

As a continuation of safety and patient care, specimen collection, processing, and storage were discussed. Part of specimen handling is the process of documentation and maintaining accurate patient identification and tracking throughout specimen testing. The importance of patient identification cannot be stressed enough. Without proper identification, all testing results are questionable. Specimen storage is also important so that the integrity of the sample is maintained until testing can be completed.

In the laboratory documentation of test results, appropriate units of measurement must be included. In this chapter, we discussed mathematics as it relates to measuring and documenting time, temperature, volume, length, and weight.

Laboratory equipment is necessary to properly test and store samples or testing materials. The laboratory equipment discussed in this chapter included microscopes, centrifuges, and incubators. A good example of a daily maintenance control chart that can be used as part of an instrument quality assurance program was presented.

This chapter wrapped up with a brief discussion about patient education and legal/ethical issues for the medical assistant related to the laboratory. Maintaining confidentiality and giving excellent patient care must be the focus of the medical assistant's work.

SCENARIO WRAP-UP

John has had a busy day in the laboratory. He has reviewed safety policies and procedures, reacquainted himself with waived laboratory testing, and had a refresher on units of measure. He is looking forward to another day of training in the lab tomorrow; he will be running some urinalysis tests.

There is a lot to remember and learn, but with some extra effort, review with Macyn, and hands-on testing practice, John will become more comfortable in his new department. He thinks the change will be a good move for him.

PROCEDURE 52.1   Perform a Quality Control Measure on a Glucometer and Record the Results on a Flow Sheet

Tasks

Test and analyze the results of glucometer controls to see whether a glucometer is producing reliable test results and to record the results on the laboratory flow sheet.

Equipment and Supplies

- Fluid-impermeable lab coat, gloves, and protective eyewear
- Glucometer
- Coded test strips designed for the glucometer used
- Control solution provided by the manufacturer
- Package insert showing directions on how to run the glucometer
- Biohazardous waste container
- Waste container
- Glucose test control flow sheet

The three color-coded bottles of controls (1, 2, and 3) in the figure will produce high, low, and normal test results. The test strip is to the right of the glucometer, and the container for the test strips is on the far right (Fig. 1).

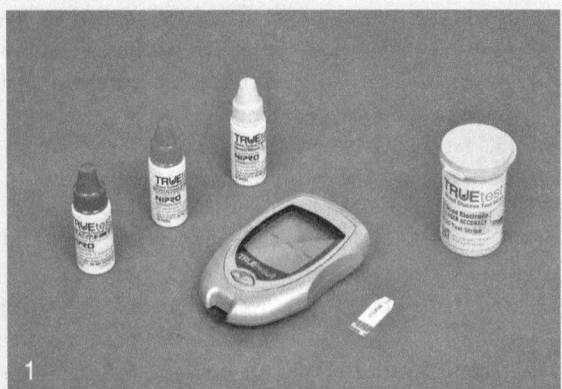

Procedural Steps

1. Put on a lab coat. Wash your hands or use hand sanitizer. Put on gloves and eye protection. Comply with safety practices during the procedure.

    Purpose: Hand sanitization is an important step for infection control. Personal protective equipment (PPE) is necessary when working with any control or specimen material.

2. Take a coded strip out of the bottle and note the control level and range listed on the control bottle or the strip container. Close the coded strip bottle.
3. Review the directions on the glucometer package insert. Calibrate the meter by inserting the precoded test strip into the monitor or by manually inserting the code number into the monitor (Fig. 2).

    Purpose: Manufacturers must provide directions on how to calibrate light-sensitive meters every time a new container of test strips is used. *Note:* The newer test strips will code themselves when inserted into the meter.

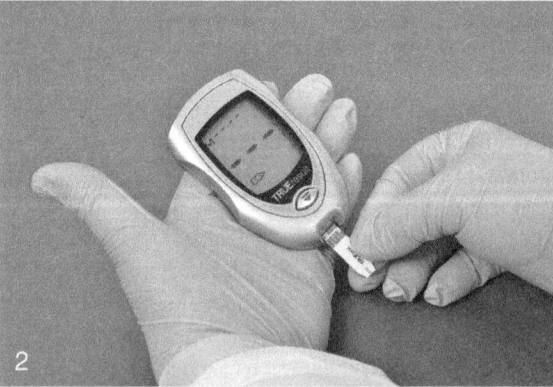

4. Check the expiration date on the liquid control bottle and mix well by inverting and rolling the bottle between the palms of your hands.

    Purpose: If the control bottle date is expired, the control cannot be run. And it is crucial to have all the reagents in the bottle in suspension to produce reliable results.

5. Complete the top portion of the control log sheet with the test name, control lot number, expiration date, and the control's reference range based on whether it is a low-level, normal, or high-level control.

    Purpose: All of this information is checked each time a control is run to compare the results of the same control.

6. Insert the strip into the glucometer and apply a drop of the liquid control to the strip according to the directions.

    Purpose: The manufacturer must supply clear directions that are consistent every time a control or patient specimen is run.

PROCEDURE 52.1 Perform a Quality Control Measure on a Glucometer and Record the Results on a Flow Sheet—cont'd

7. Record the result on the glucose test control flow sheet and note whether it falls within the manufacturer's reference range. If not, the test should be repeated with a new strip.

   Purpose: An occasional "out of range" result can occur. If the repeated test with a new strip is back in range, proceed with patient testing. If the second strip falls outside of the range, the patient cannot be tested until the cause of the error is determined.

8. When you have finished running the controls, properly dispose of the strips as recommended by the manufacturer.

9. Remove your gloves and eyewear. Dispose of the gloves in the waste container. Wash your hands or use hand sanitizer.

10. Review the control results for the following:
    - *Accuracy:* Did all the results fall near the middle of the reference range?
    - *Precision:* Were the results consistently close to each other (without extreme highs and lows)?
    - *Reliability:* If both of the previous points are affirmed, the test is reliable and the glucometer may be used to test patient samples.

GLUCOSE TEST CONTROL FLOW SHEET					
Control Lot #: _____			Expiration Date: _____		
Control Range: _____			Level: Low/Normal/High		
Date	Student/ MA Initials	Result	Accept	Reject	Corrective Action

PROCEDURE 52.2 Perform an Emergency Eyewash

Task
Minimize the risk of occupational exposure to pathogens if body fluids contact the eyes. Immediate flushing of the eyes is imperative to prevent eye injury or minimize exposure.

Equipment and Supplies
- Plumbed or self-contained eyewash unit

Procedural Steps
1. If a hazardous substance enters the eye, immediately go to the eyewash station and push the activation lever to discharge water into both eyes. If using an eyewash unit, follow the manufacturer's directions.

   Purpose: To ensure flushing of all material from the eyes.

2. Quickly remove your gloves once irrigation has begun and is in uninterrupted flow. Then hold the eyelids open with the thumb and index finger to ensure adequate rinsing of the entire eye and eyelid surface (Fig. 1). If you have contacts in, gently remove during the flushing process

   Purpose: The normal reflex is to close the eyes tightly, which prevents removal of all of the contaminated material. Failure to remove contacts can result in improper irrigation of the eyes. It is important to NOT delay irrigating the eyes by first stopping to wash hands, donning gloves, and then take them out. Immediately to the eyewash, activate it, and then remove contacts once flushing has begun.

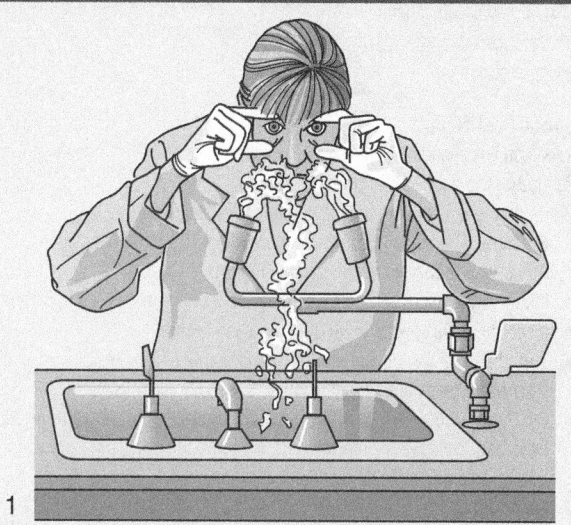

1

3. Flush the eyes and eyelids for a minimum of 15 minutes, rolling the eyes periodically to ensure complete removal of the foreign material.

   Purpose: To completely remove the potentially dangerous substance from the eyes.

4. After completion of the eyewash, wash your hands and complete the postexposure follow-up procedures.

   Purpose: Depending on the type of exposure, the facility's policies may include provider completion of an exposure incident form and provider follow-up.

PROCEDURE 52.3   Evaluate the Laboratory Environment

Tasks
Evaluate the laboratory environment and identify unsafe working conditions. Identify compliance with safety signs, symbols, and labels.

Equipment and Supplies
- Laboratory environment evaluation form
- Pen

Procedural Steps
1. Observe the use of safety signs, symbols, and labels in the laboratory setting. Document what each sign, symbol, and label means. Document your findings on the work environment evaluation form.

Purpose: Safety signs, symbols, and labels must be used in the laboratory setting.
2. Explain if the laboratory personnel are complying with the safety signs, symbols, and labels.
3. Observe the environment for safety risks. Document your findings.
   Purpose: Identifying and correcting safety risks is important in the workplace environment.
4. Based on your observations, summarize your findings. If risks are present, create a list of issues that need to be addressed. Describe what needs to be done for each risk.

PROCEDURE 52.4   Perform Routine Maintenance on Clinical Equipment (Microscope)

Tasks
Focus the microscope properly by using a prepared slide under low power, high power, and oil immersion. Then perform routine maintenance on the microscope before storing it.

Equipment and Supplies
- Microscope
- Lens cleaner
- Lens tissue
- Slide containing specimen
- Immersion oil
- Waste container

Procedural Steps
1. Wash your hands or use hand sanitizer.
2. Gather the needed materials.
3. Clean the lenses with lens tissue and lens cleaner.
   Purpose: Dust on lenses can obscure elements in the microscopic field.
4. Adjust the seating to a comfortable height.
5. Plug the microscope into an electrical outlet and turn on the light switch.
6. Place the slide specimen on the stage and secure it.
7. Turn the revolving nosepiece to engage the 4× or 10× lens.
   Purpose: Always begin microscopic observations at low power.
8. Carefully raise the stage while observing with the naked eye from the side.
   Purpose: Observing from the side prevents the slide from breaking if the coarse adjustment knob is advanced too far.
9. Focus the specimen using the coarse adjustment knob.
   Purpose: The coarse adjustment knob quickly brings the specimen into focus.
10. Adjust the amount of light by closing the iris diaphragm, by bringing the condenser up or down, or by adjusting the light from the source.

Purpose: Too much light when the low-power objective is used can be irritating to the eyes.
11. Switch to the 40× lens. Use the fine adjustment knob to focus the specimen in detail.
12. Turn the revolving nosepiece to the area between the high-power objective and oil immersion.
13. Place a small drop of oil on the slide.
   Purpose: Immersion oil has nearly the same refractive index as glass and prevents refraction of the light, thus improving resolution.
14. Carefully rotate the oil immersion objective into place. The objective will be immersed in the oil.
15. Adjust the focus with the fine adjustment knob.
   Purpose: The fine adjustment knob moves the objective slowly, preventing damage to the microscope and the slide.
16. Increase the light by opening the iris diaphragm and raising the condenser.
   Purpose: Lighting is crucial to microscopy – the higher the magnification, the more light needed.
17. Identify the specimen.
18. Return to low power, but do not drag the 40× lens through the oil.
19. Remove the slide and dispose of it in a biohazardous sharps container. Lower the stage.
20. Center the stage.
   Purpose: Returning the microscope to this position protects it during storage.
21. Switch off the light and unplug the microscope.
22. Clean the lenses with lens tissue and remove any oil with the lens cleaner.
   Purpose: Dust and oil must be removed from the lenses after a procedure.
23. Wipe the microscope with a cloth. Cover the microscope.
24. Place the trash in the waste container. Sanitize the work area.
25. Wash your hands or use hand sanitizer.

53

Assisting in the Analysis of Urine

LEARNING OBJECTIVES

1. Discuss the formation and elimination of urine.
2. Describe how to collect urine specimens, including supplies required, methods used, and timing.
3. Describe the three types of urine specimens and their diagnostic use.
4. Instruct patients on collecting urine specimens, including a 24-hour urine specimen and a clean-catch midstream urine specimen, while demonstrating sensitivity to their rights and feelings.
5. Discuss labeling, handling, and transporting specimens, along with assessing the acceptability of the specimen.
6. Discuss physical, chemical, and microscopic examination of urine.
7. Perform a physical examination of a urine specimen: color, foam, clarity/turbidity, volume, odor, and specific gravity by refractometry.
8. Perform chemical analysis of urine using a urine dipstick.
9. Discuss the limitations of reagent strip testing.
10. Explain quality control and quality assurance as they relate to urinalysis.
11. Describe the significance of casts, cells, crystals, and miscellaneous findings in the microscopic report.
12. Describe how to perform the following Clinical Laboratory Improvement Amendments–waived urine tests: urine pregnancy test, ovulation and menopause tests, and urine toxicology and drug tests.
13. Describe precautions to take for drug testing and the chain of custody rules.

OUTLINE

OPENING SCENARIO

Becca Rundle is a medical assistant student who is observing at the Walden-Martin Family Medical (WMFM) Clinic physician office laboratory (POL) today. As part of an assignment, Becca needs to shadow an experienced medical assistant in an area that interests her. Becca is curious about the laboratory, so she will be spending a few hours with Macyn, a certified medical assistant (CMA) (AAMA). Macyn is going to explain the tests that she will be performing in the urinalysis department. She has even saved a few interesting samples that came in earlier in the week.

YOU WILL LEARN

1. To describe urine collection procedures and discuss the choices of collection containers.
2. To instruct a patient in the proper collection of a 24-hour urine specimen and a clean-catch midstream urine specimen.
3. To examine and report on the physical and chemical aspects of urine.
4. To test and record quality control and chemical urinalysis using Clinical Laboratory Improvement Amendments (CLIA)-waived methods.
5. To prepare a urine specimen for microscopic evaluation.
6. To explain the following CLIA-waived urine tests: urine pregnancy test, ovulation and menopause tests, and toxicology/drug tests.

INTRODUCTION

Urine is the second most common specimen analyzed in the laboratory. Only blood is tested more frequently. Urine is analyzed for several reasons, including:

- To detect diseases or disorders in which the kidneys are working normally but are excreting abnormal substances. This occurs when there is an imbalance of homeostasis (hoh mee oh STEY sis) in the body. An example would be an individual with diabetes mellitus who is excreting glucose.
- To detect diseases or disorders of the kidneys or urinary tract. An example would be the presence of kidney stones. This is a condition within the renal system. A urinary tract infection (UTI) is an infection in the urinary bladder; this is a postrenal condition.

> **VOCABULARY**
> **filtrate** Fluid and substances that are filtered out of the blood in the Bowman capsule. The fluid that remains after a liquid is passed through a filter.
> **homeostasis** The internal environment of the body that is compatible with life. A steady state that is created by all the body systems working together to provide a consistent and unvarying internal environment.
> **nephron** The functional unit of the kidney. It is responsible for creating urine and adjusting it to maintain homeostasis.

URINE FORMATION

Medical assistants must have a basic knowledge of kidney structure and urine formation to understand the results of a urinalysis (UA). For a helpful review of the urinary system, see Chapter 13.

The urinary tract consists of two kidneys, two ureters, one bladder, and one urethra (Fig. 53.1). Blood passes through microscopic structures in the kidneys called nephrons (Fig. 53.2). The nephron is made up of:

- *Glomerulus:* Filters the blood to create the filtrate, which normally contains water, urea, and electrolytes. Protein and blood cells are too large to be filtrated by the glomerulus. So, when these substances appear in the urine, it may indicate kidney damage.

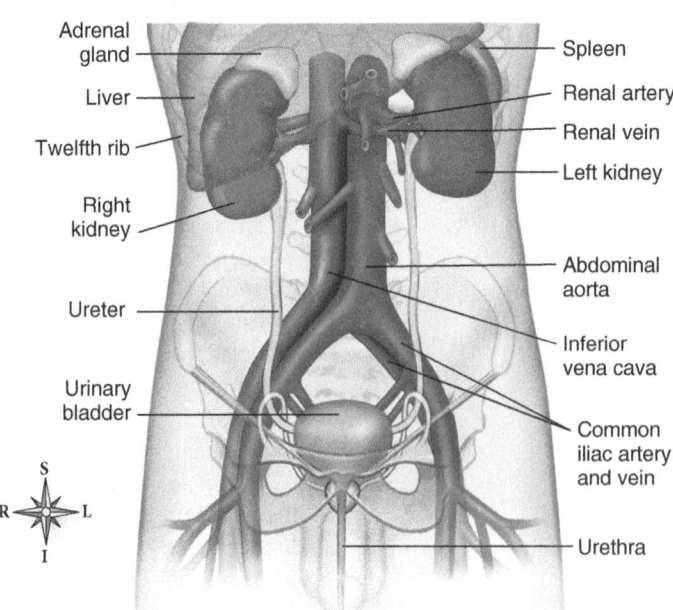

Fig. 53.1 Urinary System. Anterior view of urinary organs. (From Patton KT, Thibodeau GA: The *human body in health and disease*, ed 7, St. Louis, 2018, Elsevier.)

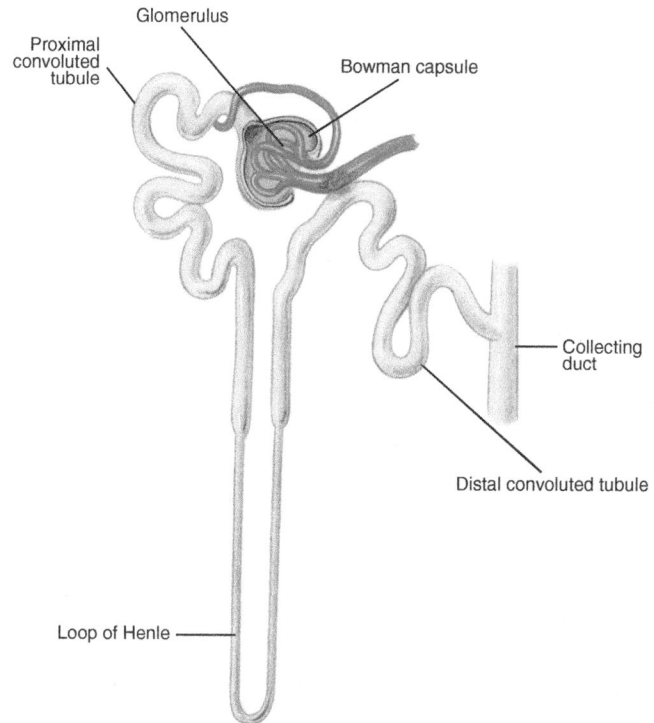

Fig. 53.2 **Nephron.** (From Applegate EJ: The *anatomy and physiology learning system*, ed 4, Philadelphia, 2011, Saunders.)

- *Bowman capsule:* Filtrate collects in this structure. The glomerulus and Bowman capsule together are called the renal corpuscle.
- *Proximal convoluted tubules and loop of Henle:* Reabsorb most of the water and glucose from the filtrate. See Box 53.1 for information on glucose reabsorption.
- *Distal convoluted tubules:* Blood vessels selectively secrete additional products into the urine, such as potassium and hydrogen.

The composition of the filtrate is adjusted as it passes through the renal tubules of the nephron. Selective reabsorption and secretion occur in the renal tubules until the filtrate reaches its final composition. The final filtrate is known as urine.

Elimination of Urine

Urine flows through a series of collection areas until it leaves the kidney through the ureter and is stored in the urinary bladder. Urine remains in the bladder until it is voided through the urethra. The average person voids about 1 to 2 liters of urine per day.

The largest component of urine is water. Normal waste products found in urine are:

- Urea (yoo REE uh) and uric (yoo RIK) acid
- Creatinine (kree AT n een)
- Electrolytes (e.g., chloride, sodium, and potassium)
- Urobilinogen (yoo roh by LIN uh jen) in small amounts only
Abnormal waste products that can be found in urine include:
- Protein
- Glucose and ketones (KEE tohns)
- Red blood cells, white blood cells, bacteria, and nitrites (NAHY trahyts)
- Bilirubin (BIL uh roo bin) and elevated urobilinogen levels

COLLECTING A URINE SPECIMEN: PATIENT SENSITIVITY

The request for a urine specimen may create an uneasy moment for the patient. The request should be made in a private area, such as the exam room, if possible. Patients should be given clear instructions so that they understand what is expected. The medical assistant should clearly communicate and explain the details of the procedure.

Be observant and ask patients to repeat the directions so you know they understand the procedure. Answer any questions with patience and clear directions to avoid confusion. If a language barrier exists, be creative but respectful of the patient's needs. Use an interpreter if one is available. Posting a picture with directions in a variety of languages in the patient restroom could also help.

CRITICAL THINKING 53.1

Becca and Macyn meet in the reception area and walk back to the POL. They talk about the need for proper PPE, and Macyn gives Becca a lab coat and protective eyewear. She also shows Becca where the gloves are near the UA counter. Becca will not be performing tests today, but anyone in the lab should wear proper PPE even if they are observing.

There are a few specimens on the counter waiting to be tested. Macyn asks Becca if she has practiced giving instructions for UA collection procedures in any of her classes. Becca replies that she has but thought it was a bit silly. Macyn talks about how patients can be embarrassed about collecting specimens and may not want to ask too many questions. Macyn asks Becca to write down three items that are important to include when explaining a UA collection procedure. Write down your own answer and be ready to share with your class.

Containers

The physician's office laboratory (POL) should provide the appropriate urine container for the patient. Patients should not use containers from home. Disposable, nonsterile, plastic, or coated paper containers are the most frequently used and are available in many sizes with tight-fitting lids. Most routine UA tests, pregnancy tests, and tests for abnormal analytes are performed on urine collected in nonsterile containers. Special flexible polyethylene (pol ee ETH uh leen) bags (Fig. 53.3) with adhesive are used to collect urine from infants and children who are not toilet trained. For specimens that must be collected over a stated time (24-hour urines), large, wide-mouth plastic containers with screw-cap tops are used (Procedure 53.1).

VOCABULARY

polyethylene A plastic material used mostly for containers and packaging.
renal threshold The blood level of a substance, above which the kidneys fail to reabsorb it, so the substance will appear in the urine.

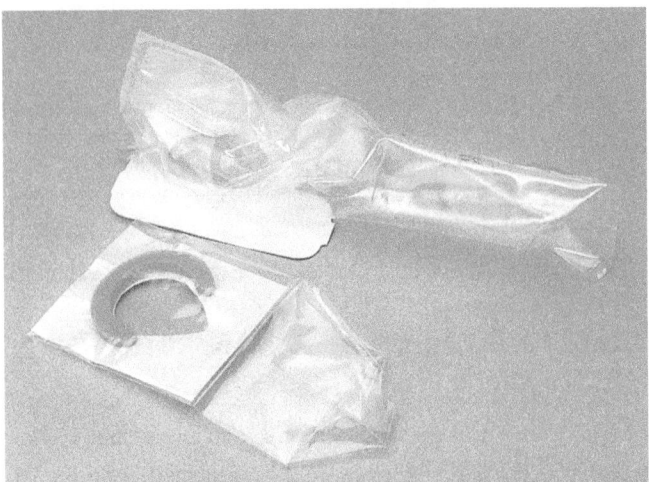

Fig. 53.3 Infant Urine Collection Bags. (From Niedzwiecki B, et al: *Kinn's the medical assistant,* ed 14, St. Louis, 2020, Elsevier.)

If the sample is being sent to the microbiology department of the laboratory for culture, it must be collected in a sterile container. Explain the collection procedure to the patient and make sure the patient understands how to collect the specimen and how to handle the sterile specimen cup. Sterile containers have a paper seal over the cap. If the seal is broken, the specimen cup may not be sterile and should be discarded. (Fig. 53.4).

When a clinic sends specimens to multiple laboratories, it is important to have a system in place that meets the labeling and collection needs of all facilities. Each laboratory may require specific information and specific specimen containers. To avoid mistakes and possible specimen recollection issues, double-check the laboratory name and specimen requirements before patient collection. Patient insurance may direct laboratory usage or affiliation.

The label on all specimens must be printed in permanent marker or ink and must include the patient's name, the date and time of collection, and the type of specimen. If available, computer-generated labels should be placed on the container so that the information is easy to read. The label should never be placed on the lid of a container because lids can easily be mixed up. Always put on gloves before handling filled specimen containers.

Types of Specimen Collection

Most routine urinalysis testing is performed on a *random specimen*. This specimen can be collected at any time during the day or evening in a clean (nonsterile) urine collection container.

The specimen of choice is a *first morning specimen*. This type of specimen is more concentrated than a random sample and is best used when testing for nitrite, protein, pregnancy, and microscopic examination. First morning samples are also the preferred sample for possible UTI testing, but this is not a requirement. A *second-voided specimen* usually is collected to determine glucose levels in urine. The first void of the morning is discarded, and the second void of the day is collected for testing.

There are several analytes that require timed specimen collection. *Two-hour postprandial urine specimens*, collected 2 hours after a meal, are used in diabetes screening and for home diabetes testing programs. A *24-hour urine specimen* is collected over

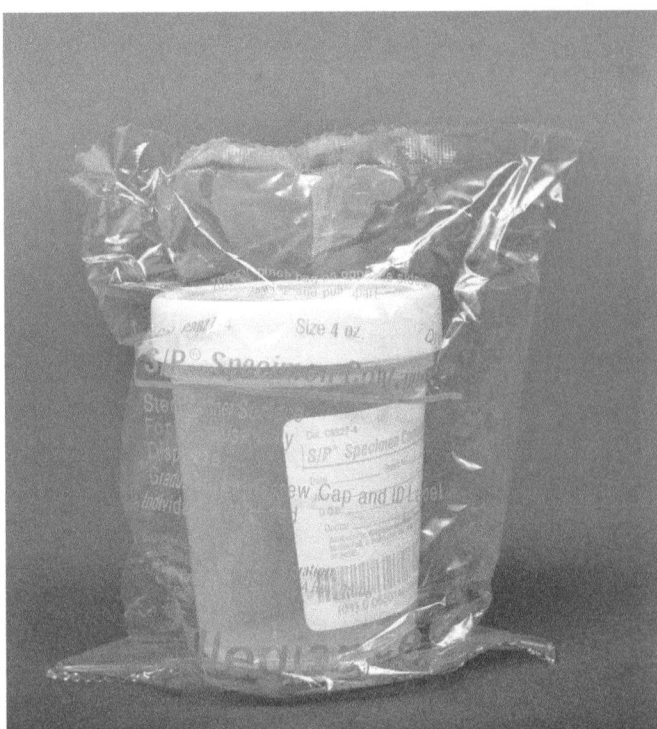

Fig. 53.4 Sterile Urine Container.

24 hours to provide a quantitative (KWON ti tey tiv) chemical analysis, such as hormone levels and creatinine clearance rates. The patient must understand the proper way to collect a 24-hour urine specimen (see Procedure 53.1; also Box 53.2).

VOCABULARY

creatinine clearance rates The result of a procedure used to evaluate the glomerular filtration rate of the kidneys.

culture and sensitivity (C&S) A procedure in which a specimen is cultured on microbiological media to detect bacterial or fungal growth. This is followed by screening for antibiotic sensitivity. C&S is performed in the microbiology department of a referral laboratory.

meatus A body opening or passage, especially the external opening of a structure.

quantitative Describes a test result that is expressed as a number, usually with units of measure attached to numeric values.

Methods of Specimen Collection

Urine specimens can be collected in different ways. As discussed in the prior section, random urine specimens are collected using nonsterile specimen containers. In the prior section, random specimens were discussed. The following sections will discuss other methods of collecting urine specimens.

Clean-Catch Midstream Specimen. A *clean-catch midstream specimen (CCMS)* is ordered when the provider suspects a urinary tract infection. When a UTI is possible, the provider will order a urine culture and sensitivity (C&S). The clean-catch technique is used to prevent contamination with microorganisms from the urinary meatus. Collection of CCMS samples starts by instructing the patient to thoroughly cleanse around the meatus and then urinate a small amount into the toilet. This is done to flush out the distal portion of the urethra where normal flora can accumulate. The patient then collects the middle portion in the cup and excretes the remainder in the toilet. Prior to collection, the medical assistant needs to give complete, understandable instructions to the patient on the method of collection (Procedure 53.2). Failure to do so may mean that the patient will have to return to the office to provide another specimen.

Pediatric Collection of Urine. Pediatric collection of urine can be performed in several ways. The easiest way to obtain a urine sample from a child who is toilet trained is to give the parent the container and instructions ahead of time. Then, when the child arrives at the office for the examination, the sample is available to be tested. If the sample is needed while the child is at the office, consult with the parent for the best method to use. If children are not toilet trained, a pediatric urine collection device can be put on them to collect the sample (see Fig. 53.3). This device is placed as soon as the child is checked in to increase the chance of obtaining the needed sample before the child leaves. Once the device is in place, the child can be diapered to help hold it properly. Make sure the adhesive sticks tightly so that the specimen collects in the device when the child urinates.

In some cases, the child may need to be catheterized to obtain the specimen. Pediatric catheterization kits contain all the supplies needed for this procedure. When preparing the kit, always remember that this is a sterile procedure. The provider usually asks the parent to help with the infant while the medical assistant labels and prepares the specimen for the laboratory. In some practices, a registered nurse (RN) or a specially trained medical assistant may perform a catheterization procedure to collect a pediatric urine sample.

Catheterized Specimen. Some patients may not be physically able to collect a routinely voided or clean-catch midstream specimen. A catheterized specimen is obtained after the insertion of a catheter. Any specimen type can be collected from a catheter reservoir by following appropriate collection procedures. For a catheterized (KATH I tuh rahyz ed) specimen, the provider, nurse, or specially trained medical assistant inserts a sterile catheter (KATH i ter) into the bladder to collect the specimen (Fig. 53.5).

Suprapubic aspiration is another urine collection technique. It may be performed in a urology office or other medical setting. This requires a physician to withdraw urine directly from the bladder through the abdominal wall using a syringe and needle. The procedure is used primarily for suspected anaerobic bacterial cultures.

Handling and Transporting a Specimen

Proper handling of specimens is essential. The chemical and cellular components of urine change if the urine warms to room temperature (Table 53.1). Urine specimens should therefore be kept refrigerated if they cannot be analyzed within 2 hours of collection. If the specimen must be transported to a referral laboratory, evacuated transport tubes are available (Fig. 53.6). These tubes contain preservatives and look like blood collection tubes. The preservatives in the tube prevent the overgrowth of bacteria and will prevent chemical changes in the urine that may affect test results. Chemical reagent strip testing can be performed on preserved specimens within 72 hours. Tubes may be held at room temperature during this time.

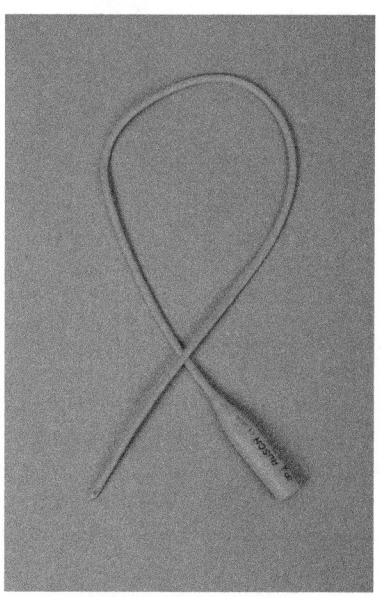

Fig. 53.5 Urinary Catheter.

TABLE 53.1   Changes in Urine After 1 Hour at Room Temperature

Constituent	Change
Clarity	Urine becomes cloudy as crystals precipitate, bacteria multiply
Color	Darkens due to oxidation or reduction of solutes
pH	Becomes alkaline as bacteria form ammonia from urea
Glucose	Decreases as it is metabolized by bacteria
Ketones	Decrease because of evaporation
Bilirubin Urobilinogen	Bilirubin undergoes degradation in light Urobilinogen decreases due to oxidation to urobilin
Blood	May lyse or disintegrate in alkaline or dilute urine
Nitrite	Test result may change from negative to positive as bacteria multiply and reduce nitrates to nitrites
Casts	Lyse or dissolve in alkaline or dilute urine
Cells	Lyse or dissolve in alkaline or dilute urine
Bacteria	Multiply twofold approximately every 20 minutes
Yeasts	Multiply
Crystals	Precipitate as urine cools; may dissolve if pH changes

From Niedzwiecki B, et al: *Kinn's the medical assistant,* ed 14, St. Louis, 2020, Elsevier.

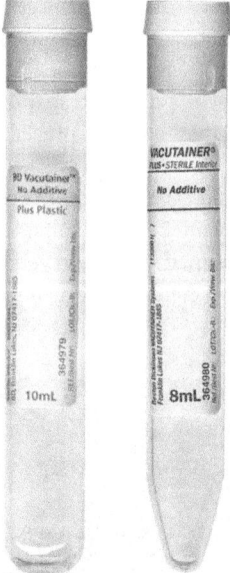

Fig. 53.6 Urine Transport Tubes. (Courtesy Becton, Dickinson & Co., Franklin Lakes, NJ.)

A different preservative must be used for urine culture specimens. The preservative used for culture specimens helps maintain the number of bacteria present at the time of collection. This type of transport system should be used only for urine specimens that will be cultured. Results on the chemical reagent strip may be altered by the alternative preservatives. Culture and sensitivity testing should be performed within 72 hours. The C&S tubes can be held at room temperature.

A laboratory request form, paper or electronic, must be completed for all specimens that will be transported to another site for analysis. Typical forms include the following information:
- Patient's name and the date
- Type of urinalysis ordered
- Name of the provider requesting the examination
- Appropriate Current Procedural Terminology (CPT) code for the diagnosis
- A line for the provider to sign after the results have been reviewed

Specimens are sent to the laboratory in a plastic biohazard bag that zips closed and has an outside pocket, where a paper laboratory request is placed. After the test has been performed, the lab physically sends a paper report or electronically sends the results to the provider.

ROUTINE URINALYSIS

The minimum volume needed for a routine UA usually is about 10 to 12 mL, but more is preferred. A complete UA is an assessment of:
- Physical properties of the urine including color, clarity, specific gravity, volume, odor, and foam. (Volume, odor, and foam may not always be assessed.)
- Selected chemical measurements that are important in the diagnosis of disease, including protein, glucose, ketones, bilirubin, blood, nitrite, pH urobilinogen, and leukocyte enzyme.
- Microscopic contents of the urine and its sediment

Physical Examination of Urine: Appearance

The physical examination of urine assesses the appearance of the specimen (Procedure 53.3). This includes the color, turbidity (TUR bid I tee), volume, foam, odor, and specific gravity.

Color. Normal urine is a shade of yellow that ranges from pale straw to yellow to amber (Fig. 53.7). The color depends on the concentration of the pigment urochrome (YOO R uh krohm) and the amount of water in the specimen. A dilute specimen should be a pale straw color, and a more concentrated specimen should be a darker yellow or amber color. First morning specimens will likely be amber in color due to the concentration of the urochrome during the night. Variations in color may also be caused by diet, medication, and disease. Abnormal colors may be related to pathologic or nonpathologic factors (Table 53.2).

VOCABULARY

turbidity A cloudy appearance; not clear.
urochrome The yellow pigment normally found in urine; it is described as straw, yellow, or amber based on its concentration.

Turbidity. Both normal and abnormal urine specimens may range in appearance from clear to very cloudy (Fig. 53.8). Turbidity may be caused by cells, bacteria, yeast, vaginal

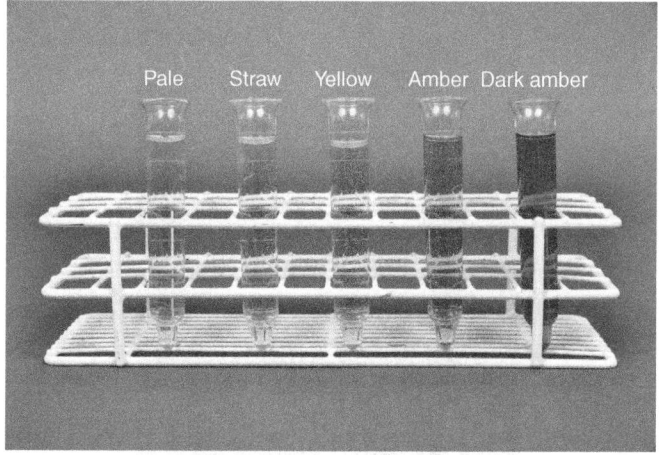

Fig. 53.7 Color of Urine Specimens.

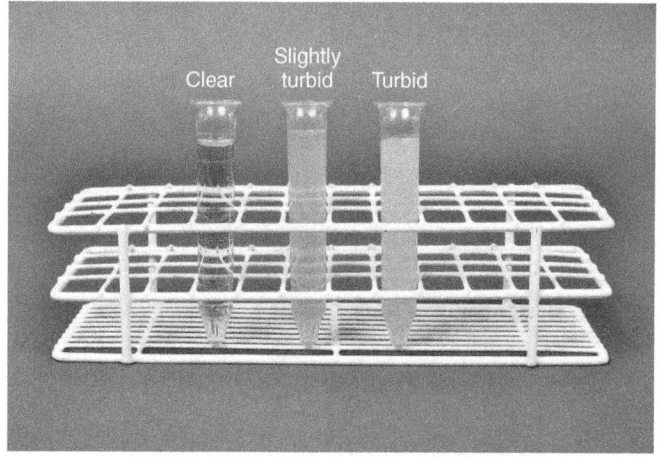

Fig. 53.8 Turbidity of Urine Specimens.

TABLE 53.2	Possible Causes of Urine Colors	
Color	Pathologic Cause	Nonpathologic Cause
Colorless to pale yellow	Polyuria due to diabetes insipidus or diabetes mellitus	Dilute urine; Fluid ingestion
Yellow/straw		Normal; due to urochrome, normal pigment of urine; uroerythrin and urobilin
Dark yellow to amber	Bilirubin; excessive urobilin; if shaken, foam is yellow	Concentrated first morning specimen; dehydration (excessive sweating, low fluid intake)
Bright yellow		Riboflavin, B vitamins, multivitamins
Red	Blood, red blood cells (RBCs) from kidney trauma; tumor, glomerulonephritis	Contamination from menstruation; beets, drugs, dyes, senna (brownish)
Red-purple	Porphyrins	
Orange-yellow		Food and drugs such as phenazopyridine (fen az oh PEER i deen) (Pyridium, Uristat), dyes, drugs (e.g., warfarin); high concentration of foods containing carotene
Dark yellow-green	Biliverdin	
Brown	Old blood, methemoglobin, myoglobin	Drugs
Brownish black	Methemoglobin, melanin, homogentisic acid	Carbidopa-levodopa (kar buh DOH puh-lee vuh DOH puh) (Sinemet)
Pink	Blood, RBCs, porphobilin	Amorphous urates
Blue-green	Urinary tract infection with Pseudomonas organisms	Breath deodorizers (Clorets), drugs, dyes

contaminants, or crystals. It is possible for a urine specimen to be clear when voided, but then as crystals form and precipitate (pre SIP i teyt) out of the liquid, this causes the urine to become cloudy as it cools.

> **VOCABULARY**
> **crystals** Solid substances formed from by the solidification of urinary solutes.
> **glomerulonephritis** A kidney disease affecting the glomeruli of the nephron. It is characterized by albumin in the urine, edema, and high blood pressure.
> **graduated cylinder** A narrow, tube-shaped container marked with horizontal lines to represent units of measurement used to precisely measure the volume of liquids.
> **precipitate** To separate a solid substance from a solution.

Volume. The amount of urine is rarely measured in a random specimen. With a timed specimen, volume is measured by pouring the complete collection into a large, graduated cylinder (Fig. 53.9). It is not accurate enough to use the markings on the side of the collection container. Once the volume has been measured and recorded, a portion of well-mixed specimen, called an *aliquot* (AL i kwuh t), is removed for testing. The remainder is discarded or stored, depending on the preference of the laboratory.

The normal volume of urine produced every 24 hours varies according to the age of the individual. Infants and children produce smaller volumes than adults. The normal adult volume of urine produced is approximately 800 to 2000 mL in 24 hours. Excessive production of urine is called *polyuria*. This is common in those who have diabetes mellitus, diabetes insipidus, and certain kidney disorders. *Oliguria* is an insufficient production of urine, which can be caused by dehydration, decreased fluid intake, shock, renal disease, or urinary tract infections. The absence of urine production, *anuria*, occurs when there is renal obstruction and renal failure.

CRITICAL THINKING 53.3

Write down in your own words definitions for the following terms: anuria, oliguria, and polyuria. Be ready to share with your class.

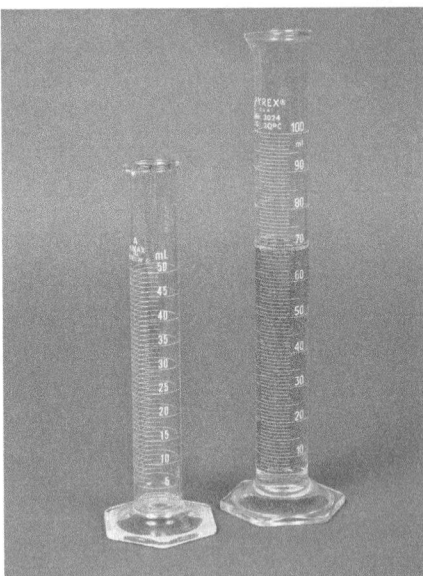

Fig. 53.9 Graduated Cylinder.

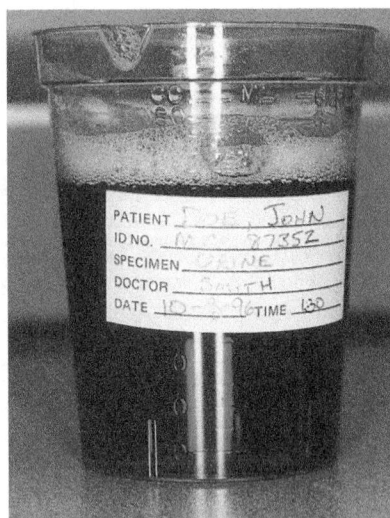

Fig. 53.10 Urine With Foam. (From Niedzwiecki B, et al: *Kinn's the medical assistant,* ed 14, St. Louis, 2020, Elsevier.)

Foam. Normally the presence of foam is not recorded, but careful observation of this property can be a significant clue to an abnormality. Foam consists of small bubbles that persist for a long time after the specimen has been shaken. Foam must not be confused with any bubbles that rapidly disappear. White foam can indicate the presence of increased protein (Fig. 53.10). Greenish yellow foam can mean bilirubinuria (bih lee ROO bin yuhr e uh). Care should be taken in handling such urine specimens because the greenish yellow color may indicate that the patient has viral hepatitis, which is highly contagious. Always observe Standard Precautions and wear appropriate personal protective equipment (PPE) when handling specimens. If foam is observed and seems significant, add a note in the comments field of a paper or an electronic test report.

Odor. As with foam, odor is not normally recorded but can be an important clue to metabolic disorders. Normal urine is said to be aromatic. Changes in the odor of urine may be caused by disease, the presence of bacteria, or diet. If odor seems significant, add a note in the comments field of a paper or electronic test report.

A diabetic patient whose blood sugar is not well controlled or a person who is eating a low-carbohydrate diet may pass ketones in the urine. Ketones are the products of fat metabolism and give urine a slightly sweet or fruity smell. The following chemical compounds are examples of ketones produced in the body: acetoacetate (ah see toh AS i teyt), acetone (AS i tohn), and beta hydroxybutyric (hayh DROK si byoo tir ik) acid; they are collectively called ketone bodies, or ketones.

An ammoniacal or putrid (PYOO trid) smell in the urine can be caused by an infection. A smell of ammonia may also be noticed in urine that has been at room temperature for too long before it is tested. In addition, foods such as asparagus and garlic can produce an abnormal odor in the urine. Urine from a child with *phenylketonuria* (fen l kee toh NOO r ee uh) *(PKU)* may smell musty. Phenylketonuria (PKU) is a rare hereditary

condition in which the amino acid phenylalanine (fe nil AHL uh neen) is not properly metabolized, or broken down in the body. PKU that is undiagnosed or untreated can lead to severe cognitive disabilities. Accumulation of phenylalanine in the blood and urine gives body fluids a musty odor. (Blood sampling for PKU is discussed in Chapter 54.)

VOCABULARY

aromatic Having a distinct, usually fragrant smell.

bilirubinuria The presence of bilirubin in the urine.

putrid Emitting a foul or decaying odor.

refraction Bending of light waves when they pass through one substance into another substance of different density.

Specific Gravity. *Specific gravity* is defined as the weight of a substance compared with the weight of an equal volume of distilled water. In UA, specific gravity is the approximate measurement of the concentration of substances dissolved in the urine. The specific gravity of distilled water is 1.000. The normal specific gravity of urine ranges from 1.005 to 1.030, depending on the patient's fluid intake. Most samples fall between 1.010 and 1.025. The urine's specific gravity indicates whether the kidneys can concentrate the urine. A change in urine specific gravity may be an indication of underlying disease, such as kidney disease. For example, glucosuria, diarrhea, and bladder infections may increase the specific gravity. Chronic renal insufficiency or diabetes insipidus may lower the specific gravity in urine.

To measure the specific gravity, laboratories may use a refractometer or a chemical reagent strip that has been waived by the Clinical Laboratory Improvement Amendments (CLIA). A *refractometer* (ree frak TOM ih ter) measures the refraction (ri FRAK shuh n) of light through solids in a liquid. The result is called the *refractive index,* which, for our purposes, is the same as *specific gravity.* The refractometer requires only a drop of urine. One drop of well-mixed urine is placed under the hinged cover of the instrument. Then the value is read directly from a scale viewed through the eyepiece. Fig. 53.11 shows the refractometer on the left and the visual results of the urine in the circle on the right. The scale on the left side of the circle shows a urine specific gravity of 1.020. The refractometer must be calibrated daily with distilled water, which should read 1.000 (Fig. 53.12). Note that specific gravity carries no unit of measure after the number.

The analysis that uses a reagent strip, also called a urine *dipstick,* is a CLIA-waived test. A reagent strip test is the most common method used for measuring specific gravity in the POL. The pad on the strip contains a chemical that is sensitive to ionized (AHY uh nized) analytes that are present in the urine. The pad detects the urine's specific gravity. Various color changes indicate values between 1.000 and 1.035, depending on the Multistix manufacturer (see the *specific gravity* row of colors in the second figure in Procedure 53.4).

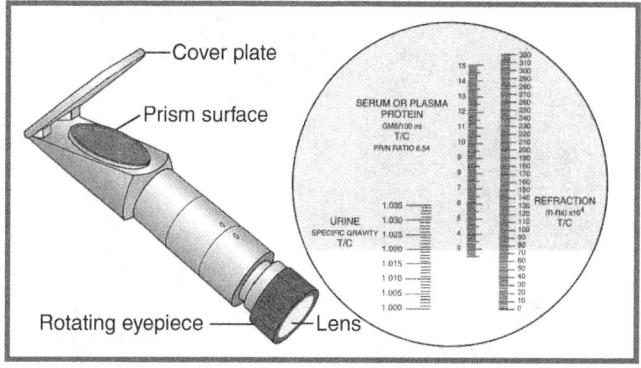

Fig. 53.11 Manual Refractometer. (From Niedzwiecki B, et al: *Kinn's the medical assistant,* ed 14, St. Louis, 2020, Elsevier.)

> **VOCABULARY**
>
> **ionized** Having an electrically charged atom or the smallest component of an element. (A cation has a positive charge, and an anion has a negative charge.)
>
> **reagent strip** A plastic strip with paper pads that contain chemical reagents. Reagents react with analytes in the urine and are read by looking for a color change.

> **MEDICAL TERMINOLOGY**
>
> | | |
> |---|---|
> | **chrom/o** | color or pigment |
> | **glomerul/o** | glomerulus |
> | **micr/o** | small |
> | **nephr/o, ren/o** | kidney |
> | **refract/o** | bend, deflect |
> | **ur/o** | urine |
> | **an-** | without |
> | **bio-** | life |
> | **oligo-** | a few, too little |
> | **poly-** | many |
> | **-itis** | inflammation |
> | **-meter** | instrument used to measure |
> | **-ology** | the study of |

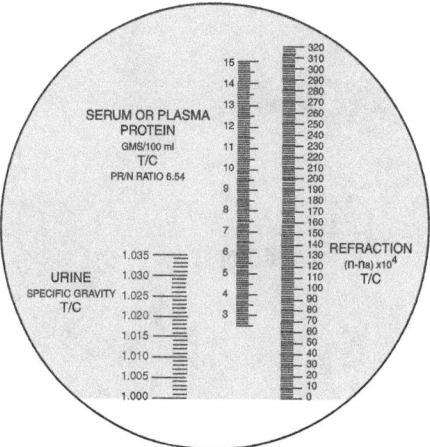

Fig. 53.12 Refractometer Reading With Distilled Water. (From Niedzwiecki B, et al: *Kinn's the medical assistant,* ed 14, St. Louis, 2020, Elsevier.)

Chemical Examination of Urine

Tests can be performed on urine to detect the presence of certain chemicals, which can provide valuable information to the provider. In certain situations, these chemical test results can be critical to a diagnosis. Also, some urine dipstick results will turn positive before a patient has specific symptoms of a disease or disorder. That is one reason a routine urinalysis can be a screening test for many conditions.

Reagent strip testing is the most widely used technique for detecting chemicals in the urine (Procedure 53.5). These strip tests are available in a variety of types (Fig. 53.13). Dipsticks are plastic strips with paper pads attached. The paper pads contain chemical reagents. The reagents react chemically with analytes in the urine. The chemical reaction is read by looking for a color change on each individual pad. The presence or absence of these chemicals in the urine provides information on the status of carbohydrate metabolism, kidney function, and the patient's acid-base balance.

Reagent strips are designed to be used once and then discarded in a biohazardous waste container. The directions for each type of reagent strip test are included inside the package. Instructions must be followed exactly if accurate results are to be obtained. A color comparison chart is provided on the label of the container. In addition to reagent strips, a few tablet tests are available for chemically testing urine.

All strips and tablets must be kept in tightly closed containers in a cool, dry area and should be removed just before testing. To prevent contamination of the bottle, never touch a strip that has been exposed to urine against the color comparison chart on the bottle. If both a UA and a C&S have been ordered for a specimen, separate the sample. The original sample in the sterile container will go to microbiology and be used for the C&S. Pour off an aliquot into a nonsterile urine tube for the UA. If you were to introduce a reagent strip into the sterile urine sample, it would contaminate the specimen and make it unfit for C&S testing.

pH. The pH is a measurement of acidity or alkalinity of the urine. A urine specimen with a pH of 7 is neutral (Fig. 53.14). A value below 7 indicates acidity, and a value above 7 indicates alkalinity. Normal, freshly voided urine may have a pH range of 5.5 to 8. The urinary pH varies with an individual's

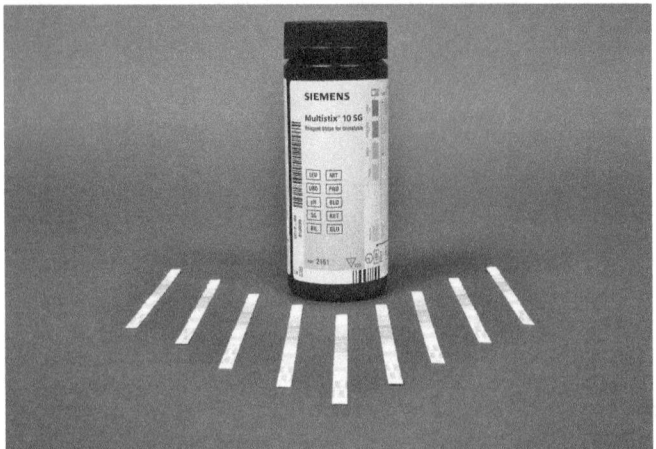

Fig. 53.13 Urine Reagent Strip Test.

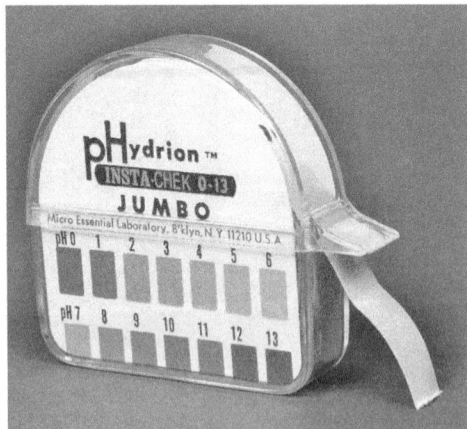

Fig. 53.14 pH Scale.

VOCABULARY

bacteriuria The presence of bacteria in the urine (possible infection).
cystitis Inflammation of the urinary bladder.
enzymatic reaction A specific chemical reaction controlled by an enzyme.
glycosuria An elevated urinary glucose level (possible diabetes mellitus).
intact Complete or whole. Not broken or altered.
ketonuria The presence of ketones in the urine.
lysed Broken apart or ruptured.
myoglobin A type of hemoglobin found in the muscle.
sediment An insoluble material that settles to the bottom of a urine specimen and to the bottom of centrifuged urine.

CRITICAL THINKING 53.4

Macyn performs routine urinalysis as Becca observes. One sample has a high glucose level and a low ketone level. Becca knows that both analytes are associated with diabetes. How would you explain a high urine glucose and low urine ketone result? Write down your answer. Could there be more than one explanation? Discuss this question with your class.

metabolic status, diet, drug therapy, and disease. In the case of gross bacteriuria (bak teer ee YOO r ee uh), the urine pH is usually alkaline. Knowing the pH of the sample also helps when identifying crystals that may be found in the urine sediment (SED uh ment).

Glucose. Glucose is filtered out of the blood in the glomerulus, and under normal conditions most glucose is reabsorbed in the tubules of the nephron. Detectable glycosuria (glahy kohs yoo REE uh) occurs when the filtered glucose in the renal tubules is so high it cannot be reabsorbed into the blood (see Box 53.1). A positive urine glucose may be the first indication that a patient is diabetic. The glucose pad on a reagent strip test is based on an enzymatic (en zahy MAT ik) reaction. It is specific for glucose, and no other sugar will cause a positive reaction.

Ketones. Ketones are the end product of fat metabolism in the body. Ketonuria (kee toh NOO r ee uh) is commonly seen in:
- Diabetes mellitus that is not well controlled
- Very-low-carbohydrate diets
- Excessive vomiting

Because ketones evaporate at room temperature, urine should be tested immediately or the specimen should be tightly covered and refrigerated.

Protein. Protein in the urine in detectable amounts is called *proteinuria* (proh tee NOO r ee uh) and is one of the first signs of renal disease. We normally excrete a very small amount of protein every day that is undetectable. Some causes of proteinuria may include:
- *Orthostatic* (awr thuh STAT ik) *proteinuria*: Protein is excreted only when the patient is in an upright position
- Pregnancy: Proteinuria is a common finding in pregnancy and must be monitored, along with excessive weight gain and increased blood pressure (three possible symptoms of preeclampsia; see Chapter 14)
- Heavy exercise
- Glomerular or tubular proteinuria

The reagent strip is highly sensitive to urinary albumin and is less sensitive to the other proteins.

MEDICAL TERMINOLOGY	
cyst/o	bladder
leuk/o	white
my/o	muscle
orth/o	straight, normal
glyco-	sugar
-cyte	cell
-globin	containing protein
-static	inhibiting

Blood. The presence of blood in urine may indicate infection or trauma to the urinary tract. The blood test pad on the reagent strip reacts with three different blood constituents: intact red blood cells, hemoglobin from lysed (lahys d) red blood cells, and myoglobin (mahy uh GLOH bin).

Hematuria (hee muh TOO r ee uh) is the presence of intact red blood cells in urine. The color reaction on the reagent strip ranges from yellow to green to dark green when hematuria is present, revealing a speckled appearance. Hematuria can be caused by irritation of the kidneys, ureters, bladder, or urethra. It also is a common finding in cystitis (si STAHY tis) and in individuals passing kidney stones. A random specimen may contain blood from vaginal contamination if the woman is menstruating.

Hemoglobinuria (hee muh gloh buh NOO r ee uh) is the presence of **hemolyzed** red blood cells in urine (Fig. 53.15). True hemoglobinuria is not common. True hemoglobinuria is the result of intravascular red blood cell destruction and can be caused by blood transfusion reactions, malaria, drug reactions, snakebites, and severe burns. The urine may have a clear red color due to lysis of the RBCs rather than a cloudy red color when intact RBCs are present. Urine specimens that contain blood may test positive for hemolyzed blood for a few reasons:

- The urine specimen has sat for too long at room temperature, causing the red blood cells (RBCs) to lyse. Freshly collected specimens give the most accurate testing results.
- The pH of the urine is highly alkaline, which can cause RBCs to lyse.
- The specific gravity of the sample is below 1.010; this can also cause RBCs to lyse.

The finding of blood or hemolyzed blood on the urine dipstick should be confirmed by microscopic examination of the urine. If intact RBCs are seen microscopically, it should be noted on the UA report to the provider.

Myoglobinuria occurs when muscle tissue is damaged or injured, as can occur with crushing injuries, myocardial infarctions, contact sports, or strenuous exercise. Patients with muscular dystrophy often have myoglobinuria. Hemoglobinuria cannot be distinguished from myoglobinuria by reagent strip testing. Both cause a uniform change in color from light green to dark green on the strip.

Bilirubin and Urobilinogen. *Bilirubin* is a product of the breakdown of hemoglobin. Hemoglobin is released from old red blood cells and is gradually converted to bilirubin in the liver. Bilirubin is converted to urobilinogen by intestinal bacteria in the duodenum (the first part of the small intestine). Bilirubin is a bile pigment not normally found in urine. Its presence in urine is one of the first signs of liver disease or other diseases in which the liver may be involved.

Bilirubinuria can occur even before jaundice (JAWN dis) or other symptoms of liver disease are evident. It is the result of liver cell damage or obstruction of the common bile duct by stones or tumors. Excessive bilirubin colors the urine yellow-brown to greenish orange. Because direct light causes bilirubin to break down, urine samples must be protected from light until testing is complete.

Urobilinogen normally is present in urine in small amounts. Elevated urobilinogen is seen with increased red blood cell destruction, liver disease, or total obstruction of the bile duct.

> **VOCABULARY**
> **esterase** Any enzyme that breaks down esters (a type of organic molecule) into alcohols and acids.
> **hemolyze** To cause the red blood cells in the sample to rupture.
> **jaundice** Yellow discoloration of the skin, whites of the eyes, and mucous membranes due to an increase of bilirubin in the blood.
> **myoglobinuria** The presence of myoglobin in the urine.

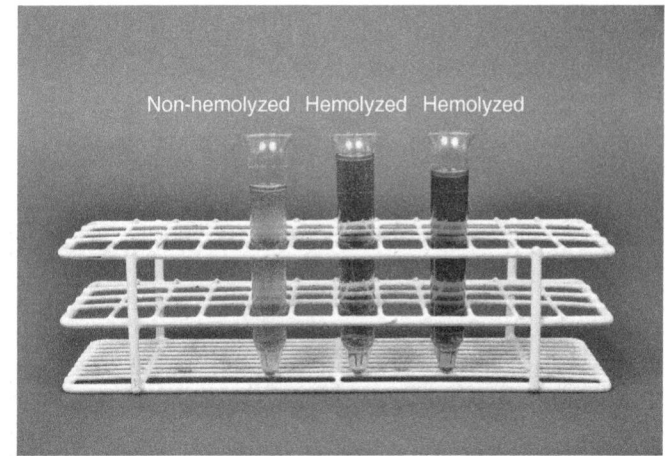

Fig. 53.15 Hemolyzed and Nonhemolyzed Blood in Urine Specimens.

Nitrite. Nitrate is a common component of normal urine. *Nitrites* occur in urine when bacteria break down nitrate. A positive nitrite test result may indicate the presence of a urinary tract infection. However, not all bacteria are able to break down nitrate to nitrite. A negative nitrite test can occur when bacteria are in small numbers or when the urine has not been in the bladder long enough for the chemical breakdown to occur. *Escherichia coli* (ESCH ur reek ee ah co lye) *(E. coli)*, the bacterium that is the most common cause of UTIs, does break down nitrate to nitrite. A positive reaction is any pink color on the nitrite dipstick pad.

Leukocyte Esterase. Leukocytes (white blood cells [WBCs]) are present in urine when a person has a UTI. The leukocyte esterase (ES tuh reys) test pad on the reagent strip takes 2 minutes to release esterase from white blood cells. Wait a full 2 minutes before reading the leukocyte esterase result. The test does not react with small numbers of white blood cells found in normal urine. A false-positive result could be caused by WBC contaminants from the vagina, especially if the sample is allowed to sit at room temperature. It is very important to refrigerate urine specimens if testing cannot be performed within 2 hours of collection or to test the samples as soon after collection as possible.

> **CRITICAL THINKING 53.5**
>
> One of yesterday's samples that Macyn saved in the laboratory refrigerator is ready to test. The sample gives a bright pink positive result for nitrites and a moderate positive result for leukocytes on the reagent strip test. What condition would give this result on a dipstick UA? Could there be more than one answer?

Limitations of Reagent Strip Testing

The reagent strip is a reliable method of testing urine if used properly. The normal urine reference ranges for a reagent strip are presented in Table 53.3. Errors can arise from several sources:

TABLE 53.3 Normal Urine Reference Ranges for Reagent Strips

Reference	Range
Color	Pale yellow to amber
Clarity	Clear to slightly turbid
Specific gravity	1.001–1.035
pH	4.6–8
Protein (mg/dL)	NEG
Glucose (mg/dL)	NEG
Ketone (mg/dL)	NEG
Bilirubin (mg/dL)	NEG
Blood (mg/dL)	NEG
Nitrite (mg/dL)	NEG
Urobilinogen (Ehrlich units)	0.1–1
White blood cells	NEG

From Niedzwiecki B, et al: *Kinn's the medical assistant,* ed 14, St. Louis, 2020, Elsevier.

- The test strip is soaked in the specimen, and chemicals in the pads may be overly diluted.
- The test strip is not held horizontally while read, and colors from one pad may bleed onto another.
- The test pads on the strip are not read at the proper time, or the chemical reaction may be read incorrectly.
- Certain chemicals, such as large amounts of vitamin C, also called *ascorbic acid*, may affect the results of nitrite, glucose, bilirubin, and blood tests. Normal levels of vitamin C do not interfere with routine urinalysis. A special strip can be used to detect interfering levels of vitamin C. If an elevated level is found, the patient should be instructed to discontinue vitamin C intake for 24 hours, and then another urine specimen should be collected for testing.

Urine reagent strip testing should also be performed as soon as possible after specimen collection, or if testing cannot be performed within 2 hours, samples should be refrigerated.

Visual interpretation of color on the reagent strip pads is likely to vary among individuals. Some laboratories use automated instruments to read the strips. Several companies manufacture instruments that detect the color change in the analysis of reagent strip. Once the strip has been placed in the instrument, a microprocessor controls the movement of the strip into the instrument. Light of a specific wavelength is beamed onto each of the test areas on the strip. The color change on each pad is analyzed by the microprocessor and converted into a digital reading, and the results are printed out (Fig. 53.16). The advantage of this method is that timing and color interpretation are consistent. The disadvantage is that the instrument is not able to identify and adjust for highly colored urine, leading to false results. The medical assistant should be aware of this and should manually test urine specimens that are darkly colored.

Quality Assurance and Quality Control in Urinalysis

The US Food and Drug Administration (FDA) categorizes the chemical analysis of urine performed by an instrument or a reagent strip as a CLIA-waived test. The chemical analysis includes the reagent strip (dipstick) tests for bilirubin, glucose, hemoglobin or blood, ketones, leukocyte esterase, nitrite, pH, protein, specific gravity, and urobilinogen. A commercially available control strip should be used to determine the reliability of the reagent strips used in chemical analysis. One such control strip is the Chek-Stix. The plastic control strip has seven pads, each of which contains synthetic ingredients that mimic human urine when reconstituted in water. After reconstitution, a reagent test strip is immersed in the control solution, and the results are compared with a chart that accompanies the Chek-Stix. Both positive and negative Chek-Stix controls are available (see Procedure 53.4). The positive reconstituted control shows positive (abnormal) results when a test strip is inserted and read. The negative reconstituted control shows negative test results, which are normal for urinalysis results. It is important to observe and record the abnormal and normal results produced by the positive and negative controls. Also, make sure the test results are consistent with the Chek-Stix charts provided by the manufacturer before testing patient urine specimens.

The Chek-Stix is one type of commercial control, but others strips and prepared liquid controls are also available. Each POL should investigate the best commercial control for its needs and quality control program.

MICROSCOPIC PREPARATION AND EXAMINATION OF URINE SEDIMENT

Microscopic examination of urine consists of categorizing and counting cells, casts, crystals, and miscellaneous constituents in the sediment of a urine sample. The sediment is obtained after a measured portion of urine is centrifuged. The sediment will be pushed to the bottom of the tube containing urine. The sediment will be prepared for a microscopic exam, and the remaining liquid urine will be poured off and disposed of properly.

Many formed elements are found in the urine. Some are significant, and others are not. Most important, the microscopic examination should correlate with the physical and chemical analyses. For example, if the physical examination of the urine appeared reddish in color and the chemical reagent strip tested positive for blood, then seeing red blood cells during the microscopic examination would be consistent with physical and chemical results. Medical assistants should be familiar with the preparation of urine specimens for this test and with the possible test results (Procedure 53.6).

Microscopic Preparation of Urine

To perform the microscopic UA procedure, a laboratory must be certified to perform CLIA Provider Performed Microscopy Procedures (PPMPs), a subcategory of CLIA moderate-complexity laboratories. Quality assurance is just as important in the microscopic examination as in the chemical analysis of urine. To ensure consistency and standardization, commercially available systems can be used, such as the KOVA System or the UriSystem. These systems may include specially designed, graduated centrifuge tubes with devices or pipets that allow easy

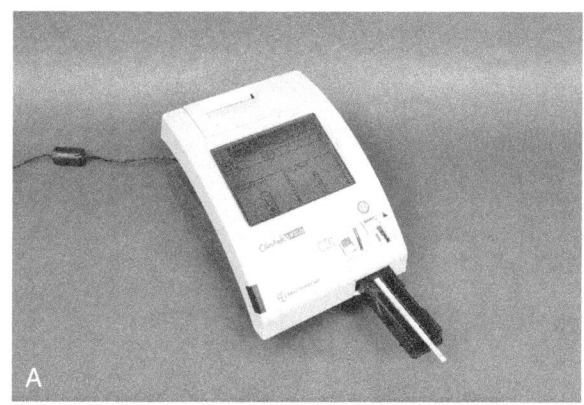

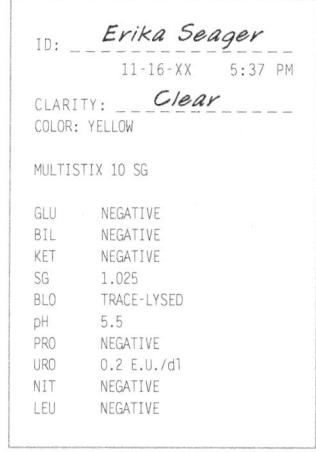

ID: *Erika Seager*

11-16-XX   5:37 PM

CLARITY: *Clear*

COLOR: YELLOW

MULTISTIX 10 SG

GLU	NEGATIVE
BIL	NEGATIVE
KET	NEGATIVE
SG	1.025
BLO	TRACE-LYSED
pH	5.5
PRO	NEGATIVE
URO	0.2 E.U./dl
NIT	NEGATIVE
LEU	NEGATIVE

Fig. 53.16 Clinitek 50 urine chemistry analyzer (A) and printout (B). (From Niedzwiecki B, et al: *Kinn's the medical assistant,* ed 14, St. Louis, 2020, Elsevier.)

decanting (dee KANT ihng) of supernatant (soo per NEYT nt) and retention of an exact amount of sediment. They also use specially designed plastic slides with wells or coverslips that accept only a given volume of sediment. Control solutions containing preserved cells are also available from KOVA. This type of solution also provides quality control for cell identification. Whatever system is used, the Clinical and Laboratory Standards Institute (CLSI) recommends:

- The urine volume should be 12 mL.
- The specimen should be centrifuged for 5 minutes at a relative centrifugal force of 400 *g* (i.e., 400 times normal gravity).
- A standardized slide should be used to view the sediment.
- A consistent reporting format should be used.

When a urine sample is centrifuged, the clear upper portion of the specimen is called the *supernatant*. It is poured off, and a drop of the well-mixed sediment at the bottom of the centrifuged tube is examined under a microscope. The sediment may be stained to give greater contrast to the formed elements. The stain assists in the identification of formed elements by improving the detail of cellular structures.

Microscopic Examination of Urine

The examination of urine is not categorized as CLIA waived; therefore it cannot be performed by a medical assistant without additional training, additional supervision, and rigid compliance with CLIA quality assurance protocols for the laboratory. Periodic proficiency testing must be successfully completed to maintain a PPMP laboratory certification (see Chapter 52 for CLIA moderate-complexity approved personnel).

The three main categories of microscopic findings are casts, cells, and crystals.

Casts. *Casts* are formed when protein accumulates and precipitates in the kidney tubules due to urinary stasis and is then washed into the urine. The protein takes on the size and shape of the tubules, which are called *casts*. Casts are cylindric, with flat or rounded ends, and are classified according to the

substances observed inside of them. Certain types of casts are connected to specific renal diseases and disorders. Other casts are physiologic and are generally caused by strenuous exercise (Table 53.4). Casts can dissolve in alkaline urine if the sample is not examined promptly. Microscopic exam should take place as soon as possible after specimen collection.

> **VOCABULARY**
> **crenate** Having a cell surface that is bumpy, scalloped, or indented.
> **decanting** Pouring a liquid gently so that it does not disturb the remaining sediment.
> **hyaline** Glassy or transparent.
> **nephrotoxic** Damaging or destructive to the kidneys.
> **renal ischemia** A blood flow deficiency to the kidney(s).
> **supernatant** The clear liquid above the sediment in a centrifuged urine specimen.

Cells. Cells found in the urine include epithelial cells, which come from the lining of the genitourinary tract. Red blood cells and white blood cells come from the bloodstream. Cells are classified and counted under high-power magnification.

Red blood cells may enter the urinary tract at any point of inflammation or injury. They may be found in normal urine in small numbers. Persistent hematuria should be investigated. Red blood cells are smaller than white blood cells and have no nucleus (Fig. 53.17). If they are in *hypotonic* (dilute) urine, they swell and burst. In *hypertonic* (concentrated) urine, they may crenate (KREE neyt) and wrinkle.

Yeast cells in the urine may indicate vaginal contamination or a urinary yeast infection (Fig. 53.18). Yeast is common in the urine of patients with diabetes. Yeasts cells are oval shaped and may show budding.

White blood cells may occasionally be found in normal urine, but increased numbers are associated with a UTI or with vaginal contamination during specimen collection. White blood cells are larger than red blood cells and have a granular appearance. They may have a multilobed nucleus. Most white blood cells in the urine are neutrophils (see Fig. 53.18).

TABLE 53.4 Types of Urinary Casts

Name of Cast	Description	Associated With Disease or Disorder	Additional Notes	Photographic Example
Hyaline casts (HAHY uh leen)	Formed from matrix of uromodulin; pale, transparent, cylinder shaped, rounded ends and parallel sides	Found in individuals with kidney disease or in people who have exercised heavily; fever, dehydration, stress; two or fewer found in healthy individuals	Easy to miss if lighting is too bright; adjust condenser to dim light	
White blood cell (WBC) casts	Formed from matrix of uromodulin; contain WBCs	Occur in patients with pyelonephritis (pahy uh loh nuh FRAHY tis)	WBCs usually have a multilobed nucleus	
Red blood cell (RBC) casts	Formed from matrix of uromodulin with embedded RBCs	Occur in patients with glomerulonephritis	They may appear brown	
Renal tubular epithelial cell casts[a]	Formed from matrix of uromodulin with embedded renal tubular epithelial cells	Associated with acute tubular necrosis, renal ischemia, heavy-metal poisoning, some allergic reactions, nephrotoxic drugs, and excessive renal damage	Can be confused with WBC casts if cells have started to break down	
Finely and coarsely granular casts[b]	Formed from matrix of uromodulin with coarse or fine granular inclusions	May indicate renal disease; normal healthy individuals may have occasional finely granular cast	Granules are caused by protein clumping or a breakdown of cellular inclusions	

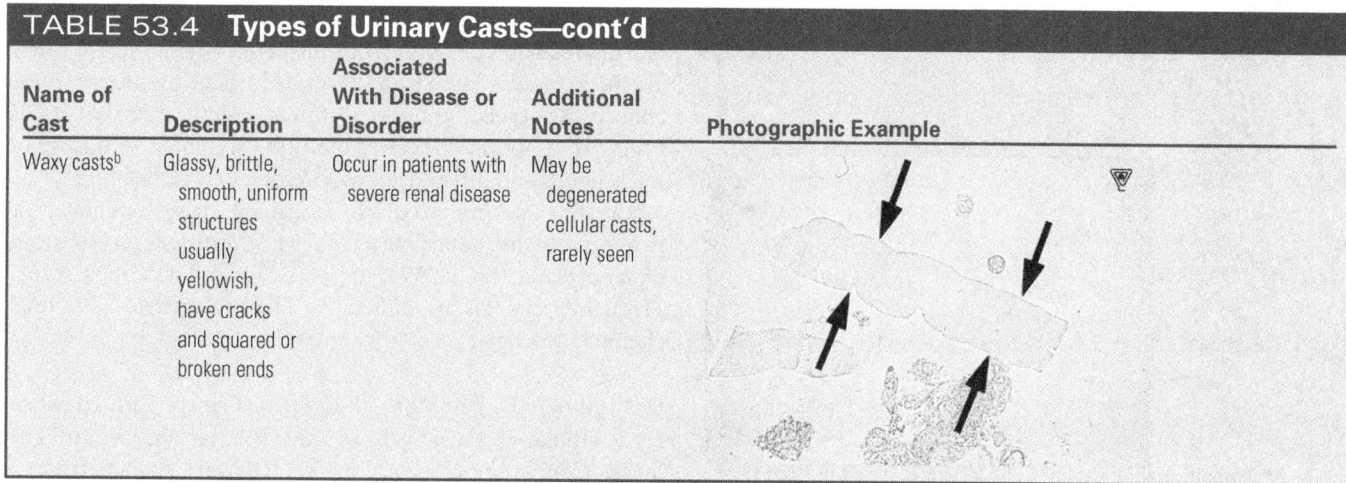

Name of Cast	Description	Associated With Disease or Disorder	Additional Notes	Photographic Example
Waxy casts[b]	Glassy, brittle, smooth, uniform structures usually yellowish, have cracks and squared or broken ends	Occur in patients with severe renal disease	May be degenerated cellular casts, rarely seen	

[a]From Brunzel NA: *Fundamentals of urine and body fluid analysis,* ed 3, Philadelphia, 2013, Saunders.
[b]From Stepp CA, Woods MA: *Laboratory procedures for medical office personnel,* Philadelphia, 1998, Saunders.

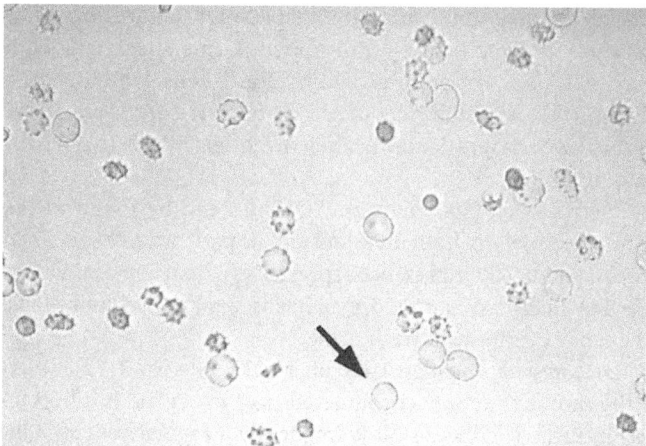

Fig. 53.17 Red Blood Cells in Urine. (From Stepp CA, Woods MA: *Laboratory procedures for medical office personnel,* Philadelphia, 1998, Saunders.)

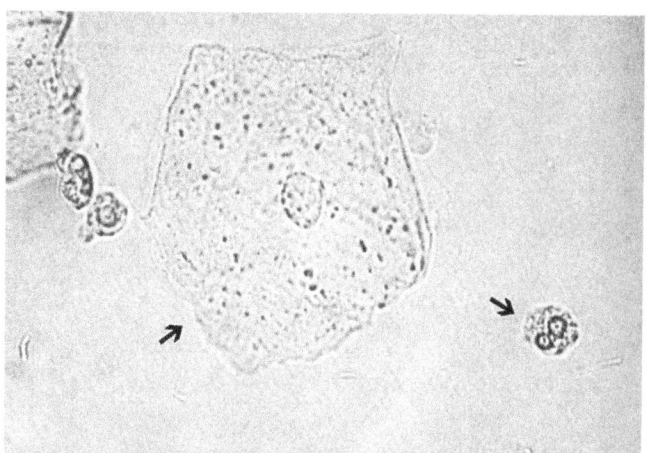

Fig. 53.19 Squamous Epithelial Cell *(Left)* and White Blood Cell *(Right)* in Urine. (From Ringsrud KM, Linne JJ: *Urinalysis and body fluids: a color text and atlas,* St. Louis, 1995, Mosby.)

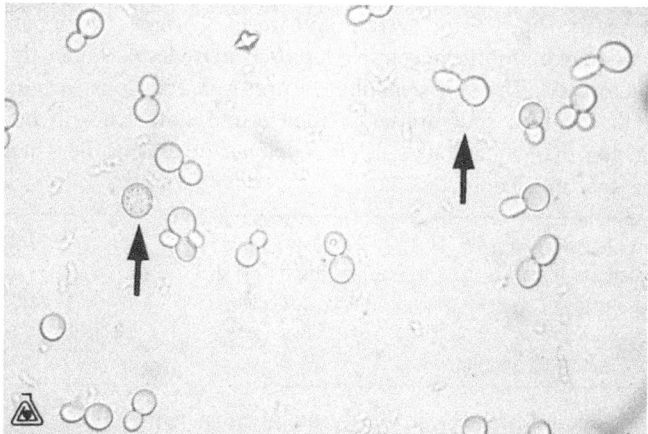

Fig. 53.18 Yeast Cells in Urine. (From Stepp CA, Woods MA: *Laboratory procedures for medical office personnel,* Philadelphia, 1998, Saunders.)

Squamous epithelial cells line the lower portion of the genito-urinary tract. When present in large numbers in female patients, they usually indicate vaginal contamination. Squamous epithelial cells are large, flat, and irregular. They have a single, small, round, centrally located nucleus and often occur in sheets or clumps (Fig. 53.19).

Transitional epithelial cells line most of the urinary tract. They are round or oval and may have a tail. Occasionally, two nuclei are seen. They may be seen in diseases of the urinary system (Fig. 53.20).

Renal tubular epithelial cells are somewhat larger than white blood cells, are round or oval, and have a nucleus that is single, large, oval, and sometimes eccentric. A few may be found in normal urine specimens, but their presence in increased numbers indicates tubular damage of the nephrons (Fig. 53.21).

MEDICAL TERMINOLOGY	
morph/o	form, shape, structure
nephr/o	kidney
tox/o	poison
a-	without, not
hyper-	over, above, beyond
hypo-	below, beneath, under
proto-	first formed, primitive, original
super-	above or superior
-ous	possessing
-zoa	animal, organism

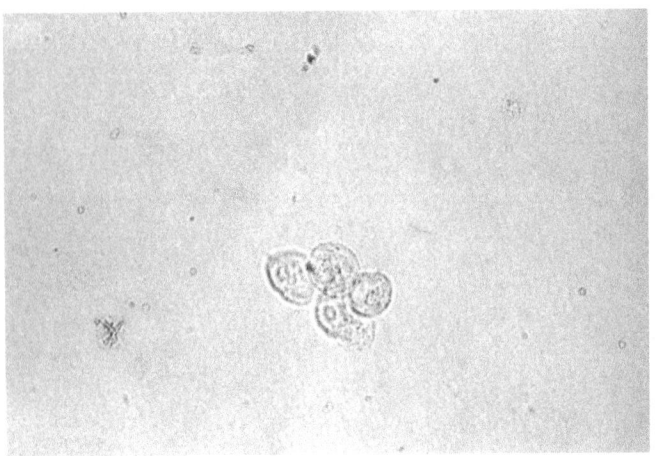

Fig. 53.20 Transitional Epithelial Cells in Urine. (From Ringsrud KM, Linne JJ: *Urinalysis and body fluids: a color text and atlas*, St. Louis, 1995, Mosby.)

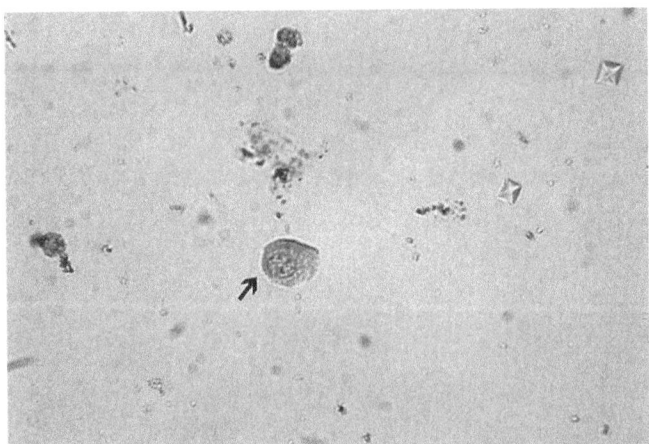

Fig. 53.21 Renal Epithelial Cells in Urine. (From Ringsrud KM, Linne JJ: *Urinalysis and body fluids: a color text and atlas*, St. Louis, 1995, Mosby.)

CRITICAL THINKING 53.6

Becca is excited to look in the microscope and see a urine sediment that has been prepared for the nurse practitioner at WMFM Clinic, Jean Burke. As Becca looks in the microscope's eyepiece, she sees quite a few red blood cells. What could cause red blood cells to be present in the urine? Discuss your thoughts with the class.

✴ STUDY TIP

When looking at the different types of epithelial cells in urine, it is helpful to remember the appearance of eggs:

- Squamous cells resemble fried eggs with a large nuclear "yolk" surrounded by the runny whites.
- Transitional cells are much smaller and resemble poached eggs.
- Renal tubular round epithelial cells resemble hard-boiled eggs that have been cut in half.

Crystals. Crystals are common in urine specimens, particularly if the specimen has been allowed to cool. Cooling causes solid crystals to precipitate out of the urine, which changes the urine's appearance from clear to cloudy. The presence of most crystals is not clinically significant unless the crystals are found in large numbers. With only rare exceptions, abnormal crystals are seen in acidic urine. Abnormal crystals may be present because of certain disease states or an inherited metabolic condition. They may also be *iatrogenic* (ahy a truh JEN ik), which means they are present because of medication or treatment. Identification of crystals begins with noting the pH of the urine specimen. A history of medications and recent diagnostic testing may be helpful too.

Crystals are reported as occasional, few, moderate, or many per high-power field (Table 53.5). At times, crystals can be *amorphous* (uh MAWR fuh s), or lacking a defined shape. Frequently crystals are difficult to identify without additional chemical testing.

Miscellaneous Findings. *Oval fat bodies* are formed when renal tubular epithelial cells or macrophages absorb fats. The fat droplets in the cells vary in size. They are characteristic of kidney distress (Fig. 53.22).

A few bacteria may be found in normal urine specimens. High bacterial counts in a urine specimen without white blood cells may indicate that the specimen sat at room temperature and the bacteria multiplied. Urine specimens with a putrid odor, numerous white blood cells, and bacteria (Fig. 53.23) are common in UTIs. Bacteria are seen under high-power magnification. They are often *motile* (MOH til) (moving).

Spermatozoa (spur mat uh ZOH uh) can be found in the urine specimens of both male and female patients. In a specimen from a female, their presence represents vaginal contamination. Sperm usually have pointed, oval heads and long, whiplike tails. They may be motile in fresh urine.

Trichomonas vaginalis (trik uh MOH nuhs vaj IH nal uhs) is the most commonly encountered protozoan (proh tuh ZOH un) in urine (Fig. 53.24). It is frequently a vaginal contaminant but may also be found in urine specimens from male patients. Trichomoniasis is the most commonly sexually transmitted disease in the United States, and its presence in urine must be reported. When urine is fresh and warm, *Trichomonas* organisms may be motile and move rapidly when viewed under the microscope. They are pear-shaped protozoa with four flagella (fluh JEL uh). They are larger than round epithelial cells but smaller than squamous cells. *Trichomonas* organisms die when the specimen cools.

VOCABULARY

flagella Threadlike or whiplike extensions of a cell that help the cell move.
protozoan A single-celled organism that is the most primitive form of animal life. Most are microscopic. Examples are amoebas, ciliates, flagellates, and sporozoans. (*pl.*, protozoa).

Mucous threads can be found in most urine specimens. They appear as pale, irregular, threadlike structures with tapered ends. Beginners often confuse hyaline casts with mucous threads. They are frequently seen in patients with inflammation and in specimens contaminated with vaginal secretions (Fig. 53.25).

Artifacts (AHR tuh fakts) and contaminants are often found in urine sediment. Training is required to tell them apart from significant structures. Fibers are common in the sediment and come from clothing, diapers, or digested plant material:

TABLE 53.5 Normal and Abnormal Crystals Found in Urine

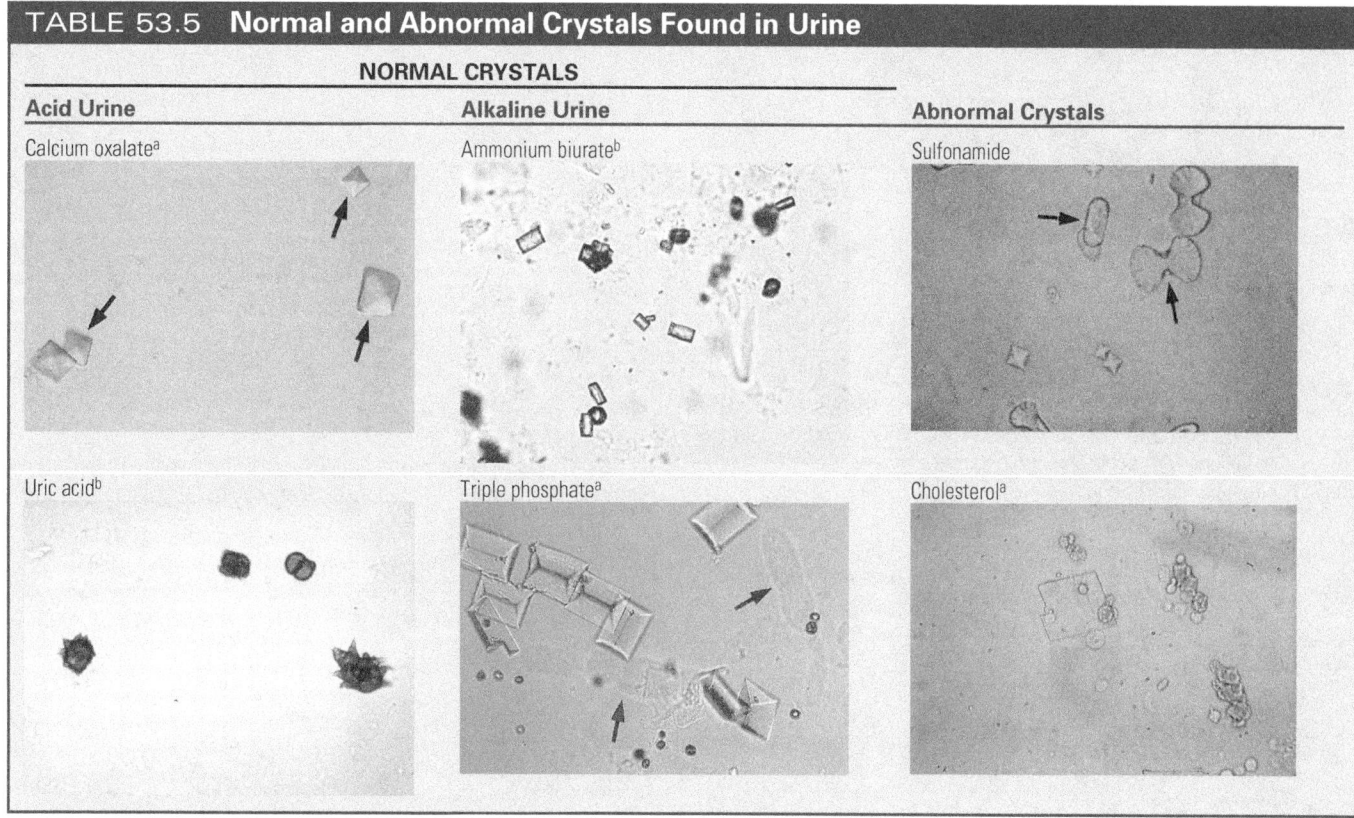

NORMAL CRYSTALS		
Acid Urine	**Alkaline Urine**	**Abnormal Crystals**
Calcium oxalate[a]	Ammonium biurate[b]	Sulfonamide
Uric acid[b]	Triple phosphate[a]	Cholesterol[a]

[a]From Stepp CA, Woods MA: *Laboratory procedures for medical office personnel*, Philadelphia, 1998, Saunders.
[b]From Brunzel NA: *Fundamentals of urine and body fluid analysis*, ed 3, Philadelphia, 2013, Saunders.

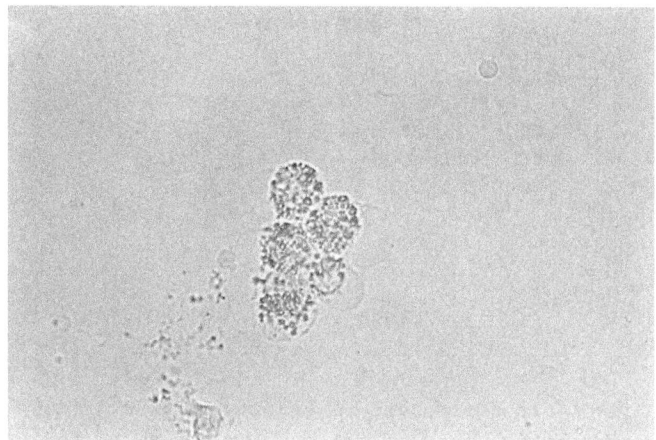

Fig. 53.22 Oval Fat Bodies in Urine. (From Ringsrud KM, Linne JJ: *Urinalysis and body fluids: a color text and atlas*, St. Louis, 1995, Mosby.)

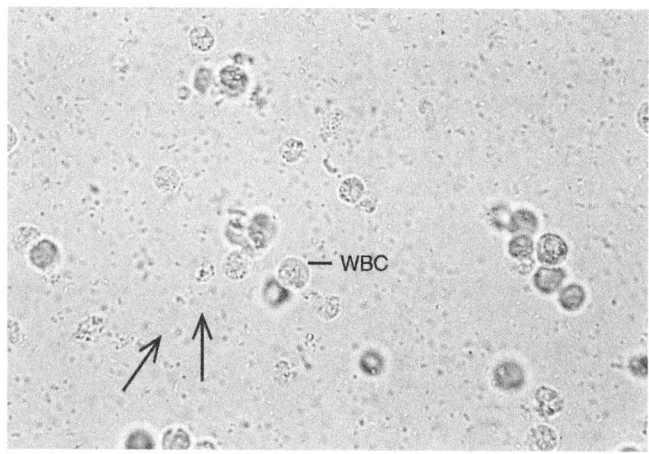

Fig. 53.23 Bacteria *(Arrows)* **and White Blood Cells (WBCs) in Urine.** (From Ringsrud KM, Linne JJ: *Urinalysis and body fluids: a color text and atlas*, St. Louis, 1995, Mosby.)

- Clothing fibers often are long and twisted and sometimes are colored. Diaper fibers can be confused with casts (Fig. 53.26).
- Plant fibers appear in the urine because of fecal contamination (Fig. 53.27).
- Hair is distinct not only because of the visible rough look to the strand, but also because of the large size (Fig. 53.28).
- Air bubbles are common if the coverslip was improperly placed over the sediment. Air bubbles are structureless and *refractile* (refracting light, causing a glow) and have a dark outline (Fig. 53.29).

Understanding the Results of Microscopic Examination

The medical assistant should understand how the microscopic findings of the sediment are reported. First, the sediment is examined under the low-power objective and low light to locate casts, which generally are found around the edges of the coverslip. The type of cast present is identified under high power (40×). From 10 to 15 low-power fields are scanned, and the number of casts is counted and reported.

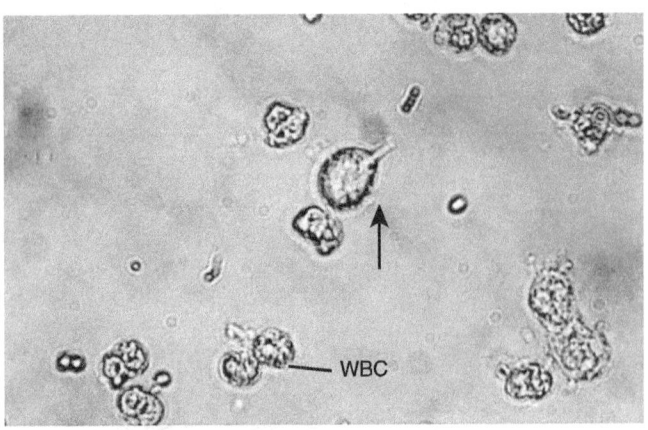

Fig. 53.24 *Trichomonas* **sp. in Urine.** *WBC,* White blood cell. (From Stepp CA, Woods MA: *Laboratory procedures for medical office personnel,* Philadelphia, 1998, Saunders.)

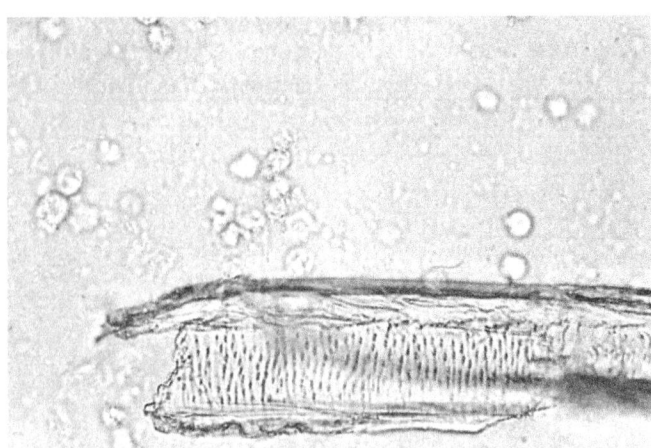

Fig. 53.27 **Plant Fiber from Fecal Contamination in Urine.** (From Ringsrud KM, Linne JJ: *Urinalysis and body fluids: a color text and atlas,* St. Louis, 1995, Mosby.)

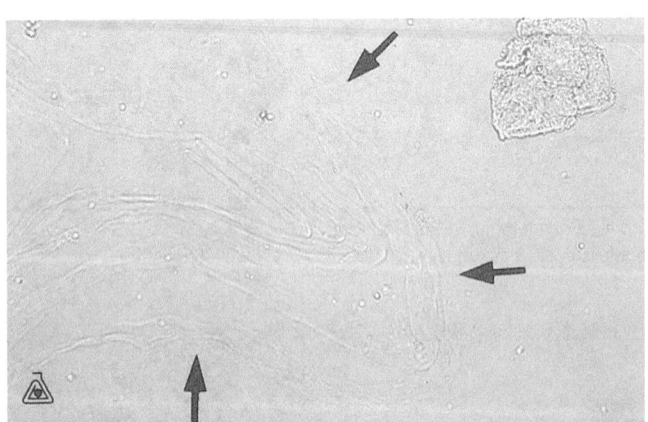

Fig. 53.25 **Mucous Threads in Urine** *(Arrows).* (From Stepp CA, Woods MA: *Laboratory procedures for medical office personnel,* Philadelphia, 1998, Saunders.)

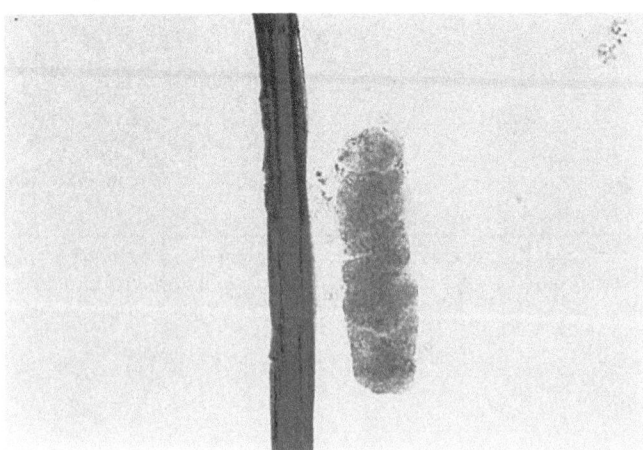

Fig. 53.28 **Fiber, Probably Hair** *(Left)* **and Waxy Cast** *(Right)* **in Urine.** (From Ringsrud KM, Linne JJ: *Urinalysis and body fluids: a color text and atlas,* St. Louis, 1995, Mosby.)

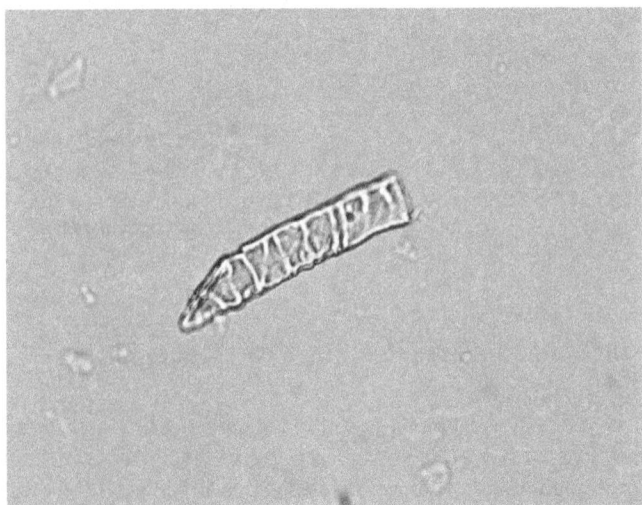

Fig. 53.26 **Diaper Fibers in Urine.** (From Brunzel NA: *Fundamentals of urine and body fluid analysis,* ed 3, Philadelphia, 2013, Saunders.)

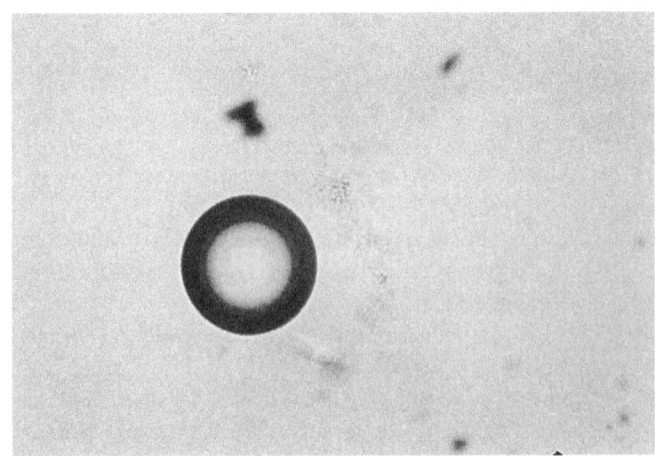

Fig. 53.29 **Large Air Bubble in Urine.** (From Ringsrud KM, Linne JJ: *Urinalysis and body fluids: a color text and atlas,* St. Louis, 1995, Mosby.)

Red and white blood cells, epithelial cells, yeasts, bacteria, and crystals are identified using the high-power objective and increased light. From 10 to 15 high-powered fields should be scanned and the number counted, averaged, and reported. The method of counting varies considerably among laboratories. It is important that all workers in the same laboratory use the same counting and reporting systems.

The results of the microscopic examination are reported as seen in Box 53.3.

ADDITIONAL CLIA-WAIVED TESTS PERFORMED ON URINE

Urine Pregnancy Testing

All pregnancy tests detect the presence of *human chorionic gonadotropin (hCG)*, a hormone produced by the placenta and present in urine during pregnancy (Procedure 53.7). After the fertilized egg has implanted in the uterus, the hCG levels in serum double every few days. This rapid rise occurs for approximately 7 weeks, and then the level begins to decline. Within 72 hours of delivery, the hormone disappears.

The most common type of test for pregnancy is the lateral flow immunoassay (im yuh noh uh SEY). Many brands are available for laboratory use and are also available over the counter (OTC) for home use. These tests are sensitive enough to detect the presence of hCG in urine as early as 1 week after implantation, or 4 to 5 days before a missed menstrual period. The tests can be performed in as little as 5 minutes and are easy to interpret. Waived pregnancy tests or home pregnancy tests are read following the manufacturer's instructions. Tests are easy to read and often are as simple as reading a color change. For optimum results, the test should be performed on a first morning urine specimen because it is the most concentrated urine of the day.

The test is based on reactions that occur between antibodies and antigens. Antibodies are proteins formed in response to antigens. Antibodies react against one specific antigen (e.g., like a lock and key). When antibodies and antigens come in contact, the antibody binds to the antigen. (See Chapter 9 for more information on antibodies and antigens.)

The pregnancy test cartridge contains a membrane with an absorbent pad. The urine sample is pipetted into the sample well of the test cartridge. The urine then moves along the absorbent pad, reaching the test area on the membrane. Reactions can occur:

- All samples (positive or negative) cause the control zone (C) line to turn blue. The presence of this line indicates that the test has been carried out correctly. If the C control zone does not show a color reaction, the test is considered invalid and must be repeated using another test device.
- In a positive sample, the hCG antigen attaches to the antibodies in the test zone (T), forming a pink line.
- In a negative sample, there is no hCG antigen to attach to the antibodies in the test zone (T), and no line forms.

The QuickVue test (see Procedure 53.7) is a lateral flow pregnancy test that can be performed on urine. It is used routinely in many POLs.

BOX 53.3 Microscopic Examination

Casts, RBCs, and WBCs

Casts, white blood cells (WBCs), and red blood cells (RBCs) are counted, totaled, and averaged. Casts, WBCs, and RBCs are reported using numeric ranges based on the average:

- 0
- 0–1
- 1–2
- 2–5
- 5–10
- 10–20 and so forth
- TNTC: too numerous to count

Epithelial Cells

Epithelial cells are counted, totaled, and averaged. They then are reported as occasional, few, moderate, or many (per high-powered field) as follows:

- 1–3: occasional
- 4–6: few
- 7–12: moderate
- >12: many

Miscellaneous

The miscellaneous elements are counted, averaged, and then estimated as occasional, few, moderate, or many as follows:

- Occasional: not seen in every field
- Few: covers less than a quarter of the field
- Moderate: covers approximately half of the field
- Many: covers the entire field

VOCABULARY

antibodies Protein substances, produced in the blood or tissues in response to a specific antigen, that destroy or weaken the antigen. Part of the immune system.

antigens Substances that stimulate the production of an antibody when introduced into the body. Antigens include toxins, bacteria, viruses, and other foreign substances.

artificial insemination The injection of semen into the vagina or uterus using a catheter or syringe. Nonsexual.

invalid Not valid. A process or outcome that is not correct.

lateral flow immunoassay A laboratory or clinical technique that uses the specific binding between an antigen and an antibody to identify and quantify a substance in a sample. The sample in this technique moves in a sideways motion, usually on an absorbent paper.

luteinizing hormone (LH) A hormone produced by the anterior pituitary gland. LH stimulates ovulation and the development of the corpus luteum in females and the production of testosterone in males.

Ovulation Testing

CLIA-waived lateral flow urine tests are available to predict ovulation for women attempting to conceive either naturally or using artificial insemination (in SEM uh ney shuhn). During the menstrual cycle, luteinizing (LOO tee uh nahyz ing) hormone (LH) remains at a relatively stable level. Approximately 14 days before menstruation, the body experiences the "LH surge," a brief, rapid increase in LH. This surge triggers the release of an ovum (egg) from the ovary. Two to 3 days after the surge, the LH level returns to the base level. Conception is most likely to occur within 36 hours after the LH surge. The principle behind this test is similar to that of the pregnancy test. The absorbent membrane contains anti-LH antibodies. A positive test result indicates a urine LH level of 20 mIU/mL or higher. Testing usually is performed for 5 consecutive days in the middle of a woman's cycle. Once the surge is detected, ovulation can be expected within 2 to 3 days.

Menopause Testing

A woman is said to have reached *menopause* when she has not had a menstrual period for at least 12 months. The time before menopause is called *perimenopause*. It can last for years, bringing with it uncomfortable symptoms such as irregular periods, hot flashes, vaginal dryness, and sleep problems. Some of this may be due to an increase in follicle-stimulating hormone (FSH). Levels of FSH increase temporarily each month to stimulate the ovaries to produce an ovum (egg). When a woman enters menopause, the ovaries stop producing eggs, and the levels of FSH rise. CLIA-waived lateral flow tests detect FSH in the urine. A positive test result indicates that a woman may be in menopause; a negative test result, along with symptoms of menopause, may indicate that a woman is in perimenopause.

The qualitative lateral flow test should never be used to direct a woman to stop using birth control methods if she does not want to conceive. Pregnancy is still possible during perimenopause.

CRITICAL THINKING 53.7

Becca thinks the immunoassays are so fun, watching the quality control samples flow through the kit and then seeing the results develop right in front of you. Take a few moments and in your own words describe how a lateral flow immunoassay works. What substances interact to create the reaction in the test kit?

Urine Toxicology

Toxicology (tok si KOL uh jee) is the study of poisonous substances and drugs and their effects on the body. The clinical laboratory performs testing on body fluids and tissues to monitor the use of therapeutic drugs such as antibiotics, anticonvulsants, antidepressants, and barbiturates.

They may also test for poisoning by herbicides, metals, animal toxins, and poisonous gases (e.g., carbon monoxide).

Laboratory testing for illegal drugs or alcohol is also done, most commonly due to an employment, insurance, or legal requirement (Table 53.6). A urine specimen is the most reliable choice for most routine screening procedures. Urine drug tests detect drug metabolites and not the drug themselves. Urine samples will remain positive even after the effects of the drugs are gone. For routine screening, a random specimen is usually collected.

Often, the following safeguards are used to ensure that a specimen is fresh and is truly from the patient:

- Water may be temporarily unavailable in the restroom.
- Bluing agents may be added to the toilets.
- A sealed container with a temperature-sensitive strip may be provided for collection.

TABLE 53.6 Commonly Abused Drugs and Body Retention Times

Drug	Retention Time
Alcohol	2–12 hours
Amphetamine	24–48 hours
Methamphetamine	2–3 days
Barbiturates	
Phenobarbital	2–6 days
Secobarbital	24 hours
Cocaine, cocaine metabolites	12 hours–3 days
Opiates, heroin, morphine	1–3 days
Phencyclidine (PCP)	3–7+ days
Marijuana (tetrahydrocannabinol metabolites)	1–7 days
Oxycodone	1–4 days

From Niedzwiecki B, et al: *Kinn's the medical assistant,* ed 14, St. Louis, 2020, Elsevier.

- Someone of the same gender may accompany the patient into the restroom during the collection.

Chain of custody protocol is required for any legal specimen. This means that everyone handling the specimen must document their interaction with the sample. The drugs and their metabolites often remain in urine much longer than the physical impairment lasts. This is one reason urine screening is favored over blood screening.

As a medical assistant, you may be responsible for collecting specimens for toxicology tests and for performing certain laboratory tests. Rapid drug screening devices are about the size and shape of a credit card (Fig. 53.30). The device is dipped into a urine sample, or urine is directly applied to the device. The results are read according to the manufacturer's instructions in just minutes. Negative results indicate that none of the targeted drugs were found in the urine sample at a detectable level. Inconclusive results indicate that the device reacted with something in the urine and confirmatory testing is needed.

Urine multidrug screening tests are a type of lateral flow immunoassay that tests for urine metabolites of a variety of drugs (Box 53.4). This type of testing is also an immunoassay in which antibodies and antigens react to form a readable test result. By using antibodies specific to different drug classes, some test cartridges can simultaneously detect up to 10 different drugs from a single sample in 5 minutes.

VOCABULARY

follicle-stimulating hormone (FSH) A glycoprotein hormone secreted by the anterior pituitary gland. It stimulates the growth of ovum (eggs) in the ovary and induces the formation of sperm in the testis.
metabolite A by-product of drug metabolism.

Adulteration Testing and Chain of Custody. Drug testing has legal consequences; therefore additional testing may be necessary to ensure that samples have not been *adulterated* (uh DUHL tuh reyt ed). Adulteration is the intentional manipulation of a

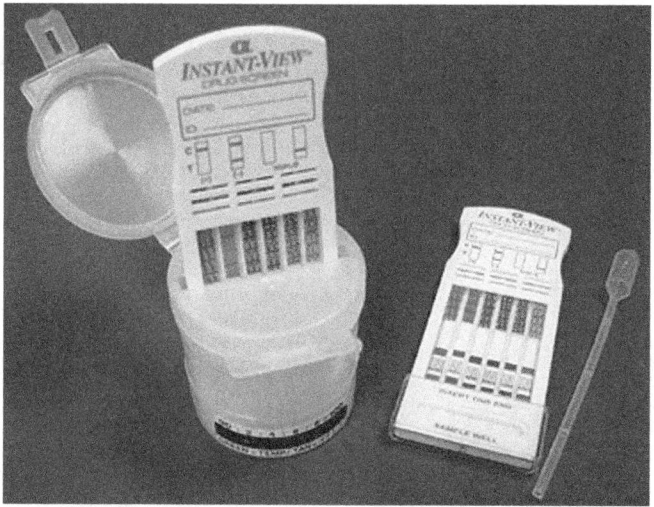

Fig. 53.30 Instant View Drug Screening Test. (Courtesy Alfa Scientific, Poway, CA.)

BOX 53.4 Detecting Drugs of Abuse

Urine multidrug screening tests may include the following drugs in a variety of combinations:

- Amphetamines
- Barbiturates
- Benzodiazepines (ben zoh dahy AZ uh peen)
- Cocaine
- Morphine
- Methadone
- Phencyclidine (PCP)
- Tricyclic antidepressants
- Marijuana
- Ecstasy
- Methamphetamines
- Oxycodone
- Opiates

---

urine sample that allows someone to falsely pass a drug screening test. It may involve using urine from another person or an animal, diluting the sample with water, or adding other substances that would compromise the test procedure.

Sensitivity limits for drug screening are set by the US Substance Abuse and Mental Health Services Administration (SAMHSA), the National Institute on Drug Abuse (NIDA), and the US Department of Health and Human Services (HHS). Positive results on urine drug samples should be confirmed with more specific confirmatory testing methods.

Chain of Custody Rules.

1. The collector gathers all supplies for Chain of Custody (COC) collection from a secured area in view of the subject.
2. The patient being tested (donor) must sign form giving permission to be tested and provide a photo identification.
3. The collector completes the top portion of the paperwork, including the donor's name, DOB, ID number, supervisor name (if needed), collection, date, time, and any medications being taken.

4. The donor signs the specimen label. The label is affixes it to the urine collection cup/vial and a matching label to the COC form in view of both the collector and the donor.
5. The donor should wash hands at a sink outside of the restroom if faucets disabled, so that any residue on hands that could neutralize drugs in a specimen would be removed.
6. The collector carries the supplies to the secured restroom with the subject.
7. Some states may allow for indirect observation of specimen collection. In this case it is important to make sure the patient being tested has provided the sample. Indirect methods of observation include:
   - Measuring the temperature of the urine specimen
   - Securing water faucets in the restroom so that urine cannot be diluted
   - Having the patient remove outer clothing, roll up sleeves, and leave personal belongings in the examination room
   - Not allowing water to be run or the toilet to be flushed in the restroom during the collection

Note: If you suspect the sample has been adulterated, the patient may be asked to provide another specimen.

8. If the state requires direct observation, then the collector must be positioned to view the urine exiting the body into the cup/vial.
9. Within 4 minutes of receiving the specimen, check its temperature (range should be 32° to 38°C [90° to 100°F]).
10. Some procedures require specific gravity to be tested to prevent subjects from trying to dilute specimen. Specific gravity must be in the range of 1.003 to 1.035.
11. Sample volume should be a minimum of 30 to 45 mL.
12. Inspect the sample for any indications of adulteration (e.g., an unusual color, the presence of foreign materials).
13. Seal the lid with the tamper-evident label/seal provided at the bottom of the chain-of-custody form. The donor should be present when this is done and should see collector write the date and initials on the label (Fig. 53.31). The donor the initials and signs as well.
14. Place the urine in a tamper-proof bag along with COC document an approved shipping container for COC specimens.
15. The specimen must be placed in a locked container until shipment.
16. Ship the specimen to the testing laboratory as soon as possible. It must be sent the same day it was collected.
17. Individual testing method results may vary. Some tests have lower limits of detection, which can make some results positive at lower substance levels. Also, a person's diet, the volume of urine flow, and recent fluid intake can affect some results.
18. Because of the legal implications of drug testing, chain of custody must be strictly followed. Each step from collection of the specimen to reporting the test results must be strictly monitored and documented. Requirements include sealed specimen containers, supervised laboratory analysis throughout the process, and authorized signatures at each step.

FEDERAL DRUG TESTING CUSTODY AND CONTROL FORM

SPECIMEN ID NO.   **1234567**   LAB ACCESSION NO.

OMB No. 0930-0158

STEP 1: COMPLETED BY COLLECTOR OR EMPLOYER REPRESENTATIVE

A. Employer Name, Address, I.D. No.   B. MRO Name, Address, Phone and Fax No.

C. Donor SSN or Employee I.D. No. _____

D. Reason for Test: ☐ Pre-employment   ☐ Random   ☐ Reasonable Suspicion/Cause   ☐ Post Accident
                       ☐ Return to Duty   ☐ Follow-up   ☐ Other (specify)_____

E. Drug Tests to be Performed: ☐THC, COC, PCP, OPI, AMP   ☐THC & COC Only   ☐ Other (specify)_____

F. Collection Site Address:

Collector Phone No. _____

Collector Fax No. _____

STEP 2: COMPLETED BY COLLECTOR

Read specimen temperature within 4 minutes. Is temperature between 90° and 100° F? ☐ Yes ☐ No, Enter Remark	Specimen Collection: ☐ Split ☐ Single ☐ None Provided (Enter Remark) ☐ Observed (Enter Remark)

REMARKS

STEP 3: Collector affixes bottle seal(s) to bottle(s). Collector dates seal(s). Donor initials seal(s). Donor completes STEP 5 on Copy 2 (MRO Copy)

STEP 4: CHAIN OF CUSTODY - INITIATED BY COLLECTOR AND COMPLETED BY LABORATORY

I certify that the specimen given to me by the donor identified in the certification section on Copy 2 of this form was collected, labeled, sealed and released to the Delivery Service noted in accordance with applicable Federal requirements.

X _____   AM / PM ►

Signature of Collector   Time of Collection

_____

(PRINT) Collector's Name (First, MI, Last)   Date (Mo./Day/Yr.) ►

SPECIMEN BOTTLE(S) RELEASED TO:

Name of Delivery Service Transferring Specimen to Lab

RECEIVED AT LAB:

X _____ ►

Signature of Accessioner

_____

(PRINT) Accessioner's Name (First, MI, Last)   Date (Mo./Day/Yr.) ►

Primary Specimen Bottle Seal Intact

☐ Yes
☐ No, Enter Remark Below

SPECIMEN BOTTLE(S) RELEASED TO:

STEP 5a: PRIMARY SPECIMEN TEST RESULTS - COMPLETED BY PRIMARY LABORATORY

☐ NEGATIVE   ☐ POSITIVE for: ☐ MARIJUANA METABOLITE   ☐ CODEINE   ☐ AMPHETAMINE   ☐ ADULTERATED
    ☐ DILUTE   ☐ COCAINE METABOLITE   ☐ MORPHINE   ☐ METHAMPHETAMINE   ☐ SUBSTITUTED
    ☐ REJECTED FOR TESTING   ☐ PCP   ☐ 6-ACETYLMORPHINE   ☐ INVALID RESULT

REMARKS _____

TEST LAB (if different from above) _____

I certify that the specimen identified on this form was examined upon receipt, handled using chain of custody procedures, analyzed, and reported in accordance with applicable Federal requirements.

X _____   _____   Date (Mo./Day/Yr.)

Signature of Certifying Scientist   (PRINT) Certifying Scientist's Name (First, MI, Last)

STEP 5b: SPLIT SPECIMEN TEST RESULTS - (IF TESTED) COMPLETED BY SECONDARY LABORATORY

Laboratory Name Laboratory Address	☐ RECONFIRMED ☐ FAILED TO RECONFIRM - REASON_____ *I certify that the split specimen identified on this form was examined upon receipt, handled using chain of custody procedures, analyzed, and reported in accordance with applicable Federal requirements.* X _____ _____ Date (Mo./Day/Yr.) Signature of Certifying Scientist (PRINT) Certifying Scientist's Name (First, MI, Last)

PEEL

1234567   A
SPECIMEN ID NO.

PLACE OVER CAP

1234567
SPECIMEN BOTTLE SEAL

Date (Mo. Day Yr.)

Donor's Initials

PEEL

1234567   B (SPLIT)
SPECIMEN ID NO.

PLACE OVER CAP

1234567
SPECIMEN BOTTLE SEAL

Date (Mo. Day Yr.)

Donor's Initials

COPY 1 - LABORATORY

PRESS HARD - YOU ARE MAKING MULTIPLE COPIES

0000-0000-0225

Drug Form Part 1
Face Inks: 000 BLK / 000 RED
Date: 05/09/00
Not To Use For Colormatch
Follow PMS Guide For Colors

Fig. 53.31 First page of the Five-Page Federal Drug Testing Custody and Control Form.

CLOSING COMMENTS

There is a lot involved in urine testing, and the results can help the provider to diagnose diseases and disorders. The beneficial attributes of a laboratory professional performing urinalysis include the following:

- A discreet, respectful attitude when communicating with patients, co-workers, and supervisors

- Good eyesight and manual dexterity
- Accountability, honesty, and integrity when performing a urinalysis
- The ability to multitask, manage time, pay attention to details, and problem-solve if test results are suspicious

PATIENT-CENTERED CARE

Frequently, a medical assistant is called on to explain specimen collection techniques to the patient. Patients want to do the procedure correctly but often lack the knowledge of urinary terminology. They may be embarrassed or may not know how to ask questions about cleaning the genital area. When explaining a urinary collection procedure, use pictures and words that the patient will understand. If the procedure is explained in terms the patient is familiar with, they will feel comfortable asking you about important details that may have an impact on treatment. Providing the patient with a clearly written instruction sheet is also helpful. The instruction sheet should be personalized with the patient's name, the time to begin collection or testing (if applicable), what supplies should be used, and a phone number to call if questions arise.

BEING PROFESSIONAL

Role-play this scenario with a peer: Today has been a really slow day for the laboratory in the office. It is 1630, and the nurse brings in a CCMS for a urinalysis. You have not had any urines to test today. It will take 30 minutes for the QC to be set up before you can even begin testing the specimen. Because the QC worked perfectly yesterday, can you just use those results and record them on the QC log for today, or do you need to set up new QC? Or can you just refrigerate it and test it in the morning? You decide to ask your co-worker what to do. Discuss the proper and professional way to handle this specimen for testing.

CHAPTER REVIEW

In this chapter, we covered urinalysis and the importance of this area of the laboratory. We started out with a brief review of the structure and function of the urinary system and how urine is formed and eliminated from the body.

Collecting a urine specimen is an important aspect of urinalysis. The testing is only as good as the specimen. A medical assistant often gives patients instructions on how to properly collect a urine sample. This can be a sensitive subject. Some patients may feel embarrassed talking about the topic, so we need to keep the feelings of our patients in mind. The medical assistant must be respectful, communicate clearly, and give patients a chance to ask questions and feel their concerns are important.

There are a variety of urine collection containers and methods. Being aware of which container is used for what method of collection is significant. Handling and transporting urine specimens are also areas that require the medical assistant to be detail oriented. Following proper labeling techniques is part of handling and transport. Also, sending samples in proper leak-proof containers is a necessary safety factor.

We looked at the procedures for performing a routine urinalysis. We first need to look at the physical characteristics and record our observations. Color, turbidity, volume, the presence of foam or odor, and specific gravity are all part of the physical analysis. Next, we looked at the chemical examination of urine. The most common urinalysis test is the reagent strip test, also called a urine dipstick. This test has 10 different analytes that can be analyzed simultaneously. The

provider gains information about the patient's kidney and liver function, pH, sugar metabolism, and possible bacterial urinary tract infection – all from one small reagent strip test. We also discussed the limitations of routine UA and the need for quality assurance and quality control to ensure reliable patient test results.

Medical assistants must learn to process and prepare urine specimens for microscopic examination. In this chapter, we learned how to prepare the specimens, set up the specimen, and focus the microscope. We also discussed what may be seen microscopically in a urine sample and why some of the structures that we can see under the microscope may be present.

In addition to routine urinalysis, the chapter covered other CLIA-waived tests that can be performed on a urine specimen. The urine pregnancy tests, ovulation tests, menopause tests, and urine toxicology testing can all be done on urine samples. Each different type of testing is important and useful to the provider.

We closed the chapter by highlighting the importance of remembering our patients. Patient education is a key role for the medical assistant. We can inform patients about collection procedures and answer their questions. The hope is that the medical assistant will put the patient at ease and their conversations will be helpful and informative.

Urine is the second most tested sample in the laboratory. It is important to be confident in your knowledge of the sample and its testing process.

SCENARIO WRAP-UP

Becca has had a fun and busy time in the laboratory at WMFM Clinic. She has enjoyed learning about the laboratory. She has had a chance to see some of the testing, PPE, quality assurance, and quality control processes that are part of a day in the lab. It was also nice to see the general workflow of the lab and the need for organization, attention to detail, and manual dexterity in laboratory testing. With these observations fresh in her mind, Becca will finish her assignment later today. She is looking forward to graduating soon and working as a medical assistant. There are so many areas in ambulatory care in which to work as a medical assistant. Becca is excited for the future.

PROCEDURE 53.1 Instruct a Patient in the Collection of a 24-Hour Urine Specimen

Task

Collect a 24-hour urine sample to test for creatinine clearance.

Equipment and Supplies

- Patient's health record
- 3-L urine collection container
- Plastic cup or specimen collection pan for collecting urine (which is then poured into the collection container)
- Printed patient instructions
- Laboratory requisition

Procedural Steps

1. Greet the patient. Identify yourself. Verify the patient's identity with full name, ask the patient to spell the first and last name, and give their date of birth. Explain the procedure to be performed in a manner that the patient understands. Answer any questions about the procedure.
   Purpose: It is important to identify the patient in two different ways to ensure that you have the correct patient. Explaining the procedure can make the patient feel more comfortable and reduces anxiety.
2. Label the container, not the lid, with the patient's name and the current date. Identify the specimen as a 24-hour urine specimen and include your initials.
   Purpose: Labeling the container prevents a possible mix-up of specimens.
3. Explain the following instructions to adult patients or to the guardians of pediatric patients.

Patient Instructions: Obtaining a 24-Hour Urine Specimen

  (1) Empty your bladder into the toilet in the morning without saving any of the specimen. On the label, record the time you first emptied your bladder.

  (2) For the next 24 hours, each time you empty your bladder, all the urine should be collected into the plastic cup or collection pan that is placed on the toilet (also called a nun's cap or toilet hat). Then pour all the collected urine directly into the large specimen container (Fig. 1).
   Purpose: Do not urinate directly into the large specimen container. It may contain a preservative that could be caustic. You do not want to splash any of the preservative while urinating.

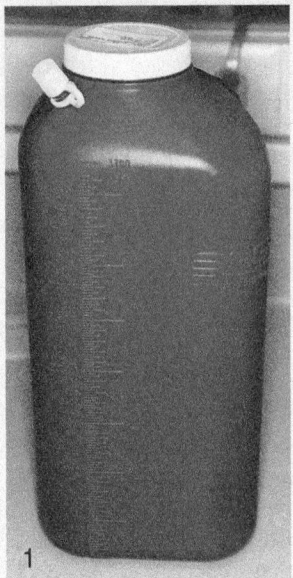

  (3) Put the lid back on the container after each urination and rinse out the plastic cup or collection pan; store the container in the refrigerator or at room temperature, as directed, throughout the 24 hours of the study.
   Purpose: Refrigeration or the preservative inhibits microbial growth in the specimen.

  (4) If at any time you forget to collect your specimen or if some urine is accidentally spilled, you must begin the test over again with a new container and a newly recorded start time.
   Purpose: The test will be inaccurate if you fail to collect all urine produced during the designated 24-hour period.

  (5) Collect the final urine specimen at the same time you started the collection process on the previous day. This last collected specimen is placed in the large container. Collection ends with the voided morning specimen on the second day, which completes the 24-hour period.

  (6) As soon as possible after completing collection, return the specimen container to the provider's office or the designated laboratory.

4. Give the patient the specimen container and supplies with written instructions to confirm understanding.

PROCEDURE 53.1   Instruct a Patient in the Collection of a 24-Hour Urine Specimen—cont'd

5. Document details of the patient education session in the patient's health record.

Processing a 24-Hour Urine Specimen

6. Ask patients whether they collected all voided urine throughout the 24-hour period or whether any problems occurred during the collection process.
   Purpose: To confirm the accuracy of the specimen.
7. Complete the laboratory request form. Make sure that all the information is filled out on the container label.

8. Wash your hands or use hand sanitizer. Put on a fluid-impermeable lab coat, protective eyewear, and gloves before preparing the specimen for transport if required.
9. Store the specimen in the refrigerator or at room temperature, as required for the test ordered, until the laboratory picks it up.
10. Remove your gloves and discard them appropriately. Remove protective eyewear and lab coat. Wash your hands or use hand sanitizer.
11. Document that the specimen was sent to the laboratory, including the type of test ordered, the date and time, the type of specimen, and your initials.

PROCEDURE 53.2   Collect a Clean-Catch Midstream Urine Specimen

Task

Collect a contaminant-free urine sample for culture or analysis using the clean-catch midstream specimen (CCMS) technique.

Equipment and Supplies

- Patient's health record
- Sterile container with a lid and label
- Antiseptic towelettes
- Fluid-impermeable lab coat, protective eyewear, and gloves
- Biohazard specimen bag label
- Biohazard specimen bag
- Laboratory requisition

Procedural Steps

1. Greet the patient. Identify yourself. Verify the patient's identity with full name, ask the patient to spell the last name, and give their date of birth. Explain the procedure to be performed in a manner that the patient understands. Answer any questions about the procedure.
   Purpose: It is important to identify the patient in two different ways to ensure that you have the correct patient. Explaining the procedure can make the patient feel more comfortable and reduce anxiety.
2. Label the sterile, sealed container and give the patient the towelette supplies (Fig. 1).
   Purpose: Labeling the container prevents a possible mix-up of specimens.

Patient Instructions: Obtaining a Clean-Catch Midstream Specimen (Female Patient)

(1) Wash your hands and open the towelette packages for easy access.
(2) Remove the lid from the specimen container, being careful not to touch the inside of the lid or the inside of the container. Place the lid, facing up, on a paper towel.
   Purpose: The lid and the container must be handled carefully to prevent contamination of the specimen cup and the urine sample.
(3) Lower your underclothing and sit on the toilet.
(4) Expose the urinary meatus by spreading apart the labia with one hand (Fig. 2A).
(5) Cleanse each side of the urinary meatus with a front-to-back motion, from the pubis toward the anus. Use a separate antiseptic wipe to cleanse each side of the meatus. Discard wipe in trash after use.
   Purpose: Cleansing the area around the urinary meatus prevents contamination of the urine sample. Wiping in one stroke from front to back prevents the passage of microorganisms from the anal region to the area around the urinary meatus.
(6) Cleanse directly across the meatus, front to back, using a third antiseptic wipe (see Fig. 2A). Discard wipe in trash after use.
(7) Hold the labia apart throughout this procedure.
(8) Void a small amount of urine into the toilet (Fig. 2B).
   Purpose: Allowing the initial flow of urine to pass into the toilet flushes the opening of the urethra.

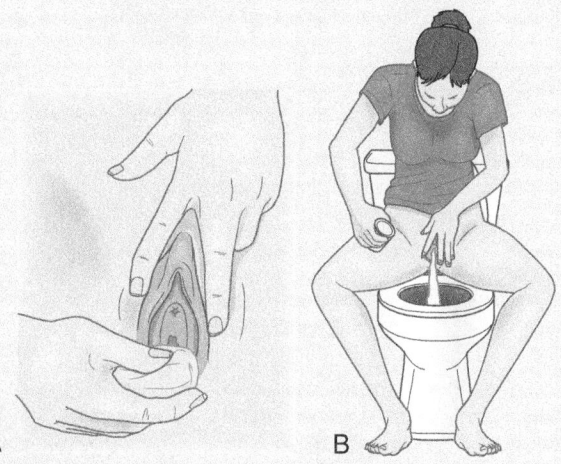

2 A   B

3. Explain the following instructions to adult patients or to the guardians of pediatric patients, making sure you show sensitivity to privacy issues.
   Purpose: Instructions must be understood if they are to be followed correctly. By talking to the patient, you can determine whether the patient understands or has any questions.

(9) Move the specimen container into position and void the next portion of urine into it. Fill the container halfway. Remember, this is a sterile container. Do not put your fingers on the inside of the container.

Continued

PROCEDURE 53.2   Collect a Clean-Catch Midstream Urine Specimen—cont'd

(10) Remove the cup and void the last amount of urine into the toilet. (This means that the first part and the last part of the urinary flow have been excluded from the specimen. Only the middle portion of the flow is included.)

(11) Place the lid on the container, taking care not to touch the interior surface of the lid. Wipe in your usual manner, redress, wash your hands, and return the sterile specimen to the place designated by the medical facility.

Patient Instructions: Obtaining a Clean-Catch Midstream Specimen (Male Patient)

(1) Wash your hands and expose the penis.

(2) Retract the foreskin of the penis (if not circumcised).

(3) Cleanse the area around the glans penis (tip of the penis) and the urethral opening (meatus) by washing each side of the glans with a separate antiseptic wipe (Fig. 3A). Discard wipe in trash after use.

(4) Cleanse directly across the urethral opening using a third antiseptic wipe. Discard wipe in trash after use.

(5) Void a small amount of urine into the toilet or urinal (Fig. 3B).

(6) Collect the next portion of the urine in the sterile container, filling the container halfway, without touching the inside of the container with the hands or the penis (Fig. 3C).

(7) Void the last amount of urine into the toilet or urinal.

(8) Place the lid on the container, taking care not to touch the interior surface of the lid. Wipe, wash your hands, and redress.

(9) Return the specimen to the designated area.

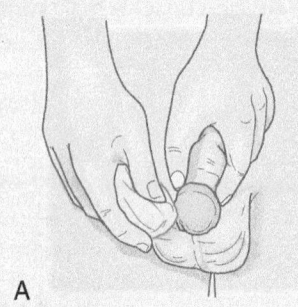 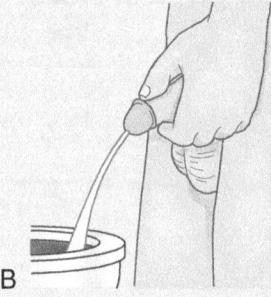 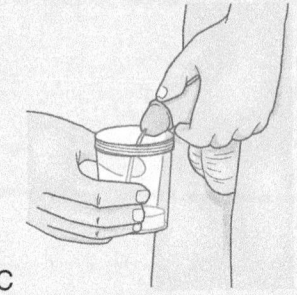

3 A   B   C

Processing a Clean-Catch Urine Specimen

4. Document the date, time, and collection type.

5. Wash your hands or use hand sanitizer. Put on the fluid-impermeable lab coat, protective eyewear, and gloves.
   Purpose: Hand sanitization is an important step for infection control. Personal protective equipment (PPE) is part of Standard Precautions.

6. Process the specimen according to the provider's orders. Perform urinalysis in the office or prepare the specimen for transport to the laboratory. If it is to be sent to an outside laboratory, complete the following steps:

- Make sure the label is properly completed with the patient's information and the date, time, test ordered, and your initials.
- Place the specimen in a biohazardous specimen bag.
- Complete a laboratory requisition and place it in the outside pocket of the specimen bag.
- Keep the specimen refrigerated until pickup.

7. Remove your gloves, protective eyewear, and lab coat. Dispose of the gloves appropriately. Wash your hands or use hand sanitizer. Document that the specimen was sent.

PROCEDURE 53.3   Assess Urine for Color and Turbidity: Physical Test

Tasks

Assess and record the color and clarity of a urine specimen.

Equipment and Supplies

- Patient's health record
- Urine specimen
- Centrifuge tube
- Fluid-impermeable lab coat, protective eyewear, and gloves
- Biohazardous waste container

Procedural Steps

1. Wash your hands or use hand sanitizer. Put on the fluid-impermeable lab coat, protective eyewear, and gloves. Comply with safety practices.
   Purpose: Hand sanitization is an important step for infection control. Wearing personal protective equipment (PPE) is part of Standard Precautions.

2. Mix the urine by gently and thoroughly swirling the specimen.
   Purpose: Suspended substances settle when urine stands. If urine is not mixed before its appearance is assessed, the finding will be incorrect.

3. Label a centrifuge tube.
   Purpose: If a complete urinalysis is to be done, a portion of the specimen will be centrifuged for microscopic examination. The centrifuged specimen must be labeled to prevent specimen confusion.

4. Pour the specimen into a standard-sized centrifuge tube.
   Purpose: Standard-sized containers are better for assessing color and clarity results.

5. Assess and record the color (see Fig. 53.7):
   - Pale straw or straw
   - Yellow
   - Amber or dark amber

6. Assess the clarity by placing a piece of white paper with fine black print behind the specimen and see if you can see the print:
   Clear – Able to read through the specimen; no cloudiness
   Slightly turbid – Can barely see fine print on white paper through the tube
   Turbid – Cannot see fine print, dark print possibly seen through the tube, or see no print at all through the tube

7. Clean the work area and dispose of procedure supplies in the biohazardous waste container.

8. Dispose of your gloves. Remove the lab coat and protective eyewear. Wash your hands or use hand sanitizer.
   Purpose: To ensure infection control.

9. Record the results in the patient's record.
   Purpose: A procedure is not considered done until it is recorded.

PROCEDURE 53.4   Perform Quality Control Measures: Differentiate Between Normal and Abnormal Test Results While Determining the Reliability of Chemical Reagent Strips

Tasks

Reconstitute a control sample and test the reliability of the urinalysis chemical testing strip.

Equipment and Supplies

- Chek-Stix Control Strips with reference ranges for urinalysis
- Distilled water
- Capped tube with milliliter markings
- Test tube rack
- Forceps
- Timer
- Urine chemical strips for urine testing
- Color chart for interpreting the chemical strip results
- Fluid-impermeable lab coat, protective eyewear, and gloves
- Biohazardous waste container
- Control reference sheet and control flow sheet

Procedural Steps

1. Assemble the equipment and supplies. Record the lot number and the expiration date of the Chek-Stix on the control log sheet.
   Purpose: Chek-Stix cannot be used if the expiration date has passed. Recording the lot number and expiration date is an important part of quality assurance.
2. Wash your hands or use hand sanitizer. Put on the fluid-impermeable lab coat, protective eyewear, and gloves. Comply with safety practices.
   Purpose: To ensure infection control. Personal protective equipment (PPE) is part of Standard Precautions.
3. Place a conical tube in a test tube rack and remove the cap.
4. Pour 15 mL of distilled water into the tube.

5. Using forceps, remove one strip from the Chek-Stix bottle. Inspect the strips for mottling or discoloration.
   Purpose: The control strips have chemicals that you should not handle or contaminate with your hands. Any mottling or discoloration may mean that the strips have been exposed to moisture, light, or solvents. Improperly stored control strips should not be used.
6. Place the strip into the water and tightly cap the tube.
7. Invert the tubes for 2 minutes.
   Purpose: Chemicals embedded in the pads must be thoroughly dissolved in the water.
8. Allow the tube to sit in the rack for 30 minutes.
9. Invert the tube one more time and remove the strip with forceps.
10. Discard the strip in the biohazardous waste container. Once reconstituted, the control solution is stable for 8 hours at room temperature.
    Purpose: To ensure integrity of the control solution.
11. Perform quality control of the chemical reagent strip by dipping it into the control solution according to Procedure 53.5.
12. Read and record the results.
13. Compare the results with the control reference ranges provided on the Chek-Stix package insert.
    Purpose: Results should fall within a given range provided by the manufacturer. If they do not, the chemical reagent strips cannot be used to test patients' urine.
14. Discard the chemical reagent strip and the control solution in the biohazardous waste container.
15. Clean up the work area and appropriately dispose of supplies and gloves in a biohazardous waste container. Remove protective eyewear and lab coat.
16. Wash you hands or use hand sanitizer. Document the results.

PROCEDURE 53.5   Test Urine With Chemical Reagent Strips

Tasks

Perform chemical testing on a urine sample.

Equipment and Supplies

- Patient's health record
- Urine specimen
- Reagent strips
- Timer
- Fluid-impermeable lab coat, protective eyewear, and gloves
- Biohazardous waste container

Procedural Steps

1. Wash or sanitize your hands. Put on the fluid-impermeable lab coat, protective eyewear, and gloves.
   Purpose: To ensure infection control. Personal protective equipment (PPE) is part of Standard Precautions.
2. Check the reagent strip container for the expiration date.
   Purpose: Do not use expired reagents.
3. Check requisition, specimen identification, the time of collection, the container, and the mode of preservation.
   Purpose: The validity of test results depends on proper specimen identification, collection, time, and preservation.
4. If the specimen has been refrigerated, allow it to warm to room temperature.

Purpose: Certain tests are temperature dependent. Testing cold specimens may cause false-negative results.
5. Label a conical tube with the specimen identification information.
6. Gently but thoroughly mix the specimen by swirling and/or gentle inversion of the specimen cup. Make sure the lid is secure prior to mixing.
   Purpose: If settling occurs, certain elements may not be detected.
7. Pour a 12-mL aliquot of the specimen into the correctly labeled tube.
8. Remove the reagent strip from the container. Hold it in your hand – do not lay it down – to prevent contamination. Recap the container tightly.
   Purpose: Test strips are sensitive to moisture and light and must be stored in tightly sealed containers. Contamination from chemical residues on countertops can affect the test results.
9. Following the manufacturer's directions, note the time, dip the strip immediately into the urine, and then remove it.
   Purpose: Tests are time dependent. Some pads darken over time.
10. Quickly remove the excess urine from the strip by pulling the edge of the strip across the lip of the specimen container and then blotting the edge of the strip on a paper towel.
    Purpose: Excess urine on the strip or prolonged dipping time affects test results.
11. Hold the strip horizontally (Fig. 1). At the required time, compare the strip with the appropriate color chart on the reagent container. *Do not touch the strip to the bottle.*

Continued

PROCEDURE 53.5   Test Urine With Chemical Reagent Strips—cont'd

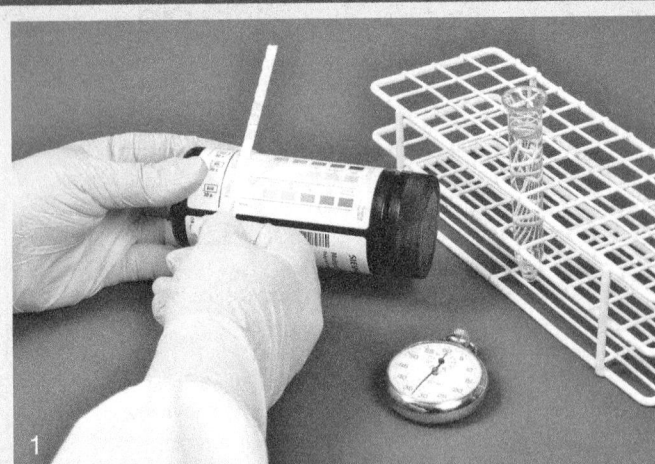

Purpose: Holding the strip horizontally prevents runover from one test pad to another and prevents interference from mixing chemicals in the test pads.

12. Read and record the first two results 30 seconds after dipping the strip (the indicated time to read the "Glucose" and "Bilirubin"). Compare the two reagent pads closest to your hand with the bottom two rows of the color chart (Fig. 2). Continue reading and recording each row of possible results with its appropriate reagent pad at its designated time.

Purpose: Timing is critical. Allowing the strip to touch the bottle contaminates the bottle.

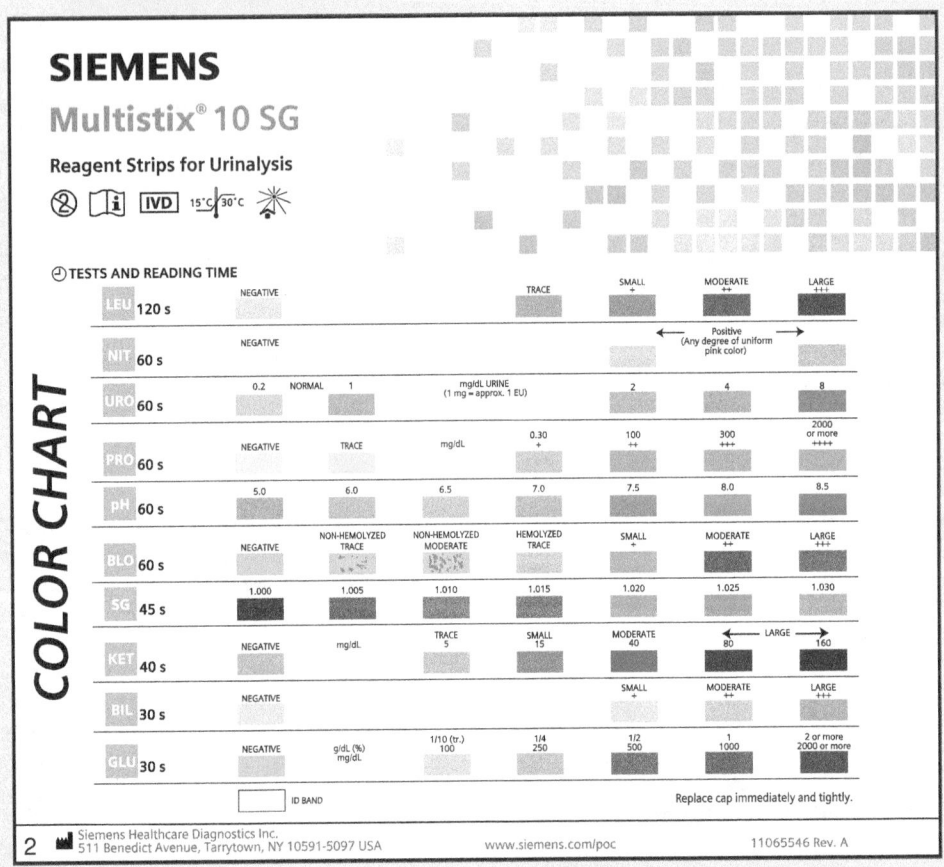

SIEMENS

Multistix® 10 SG

Reagent Strips for Urinalysis

COLOR CHART

TESTS AND READING TIME

2   Siemens Healthcare Diagnostics Inc.
511 Benedict Avenue, Tarrytown, NY 10591-5097 USA   www.siemens.com/poc   11065546 Rev. A

13. Clean the work area. If a paper towel was used, dispose of it and the reagent strip in an appropriate biohazardous waste container.

14. Remove your gloves and dispose of them appropriately. Remove protective eyewear and lab coat. Wash your hands or use hand sanitizer.

Purpose: To ensure infection control.

15. Document the results in the patient's health record.

Purpose: A procedure is not complete until it has been documented.

PROCEDURE 53.6 Prepare a Urine Specimen for Microscopic Examination

Task
Prepare a urine specimen for the provider's microscopic examination to determine the presence of normal and abnormal elements.

Equipment and Supplies
- Patient's health record
- Urine specimen
- Centrifuge tube
- Centrifuge
- Disposable pipet
- Sedi-Stain
- Microscope slide and coverslip
- Microscope
- Permanent marker
- Fluid-impermeable lab coat, protective eyewear, and gloves
- Biohazardous waste container

Procedural Steps
1. Wash your hands or use hand sanitizer. Put on the fluid-impermeable lab coat, protective eyewear, and gloves.
   Purpose: To ensure infection control. Personal protective equipment (PPE) is part of Standard Precautions.
2. Gently mix the urine specimen by swirling the covered specimen container.
   Purpose: If the urine is not well mixed, elements that have settled to the bottom of the specimen container will be missed.
3. Pour 12 mL of urine into a labeled centrifuge tube and cap the tube.
4. Place the tube in the centrifuge (Fig. 1).

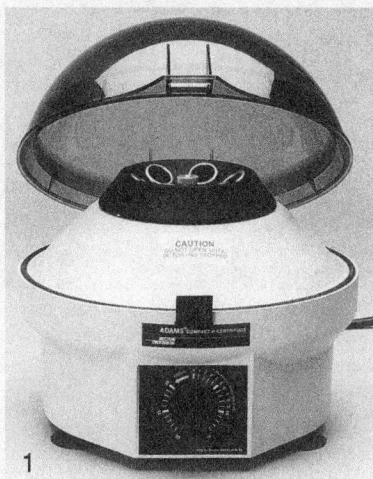

1

5. Place another tube containing 12 mL of urine or water in the opposite cup.
   Purpose: For proper operation, centrifuges must be carefully balanced. If not properly balanced, damage to the instrument can occur.
6. Secure the lid and centrifuge for 5 minutes or for the time specified for your instrument.
   Purpose: Timing varies according to the speed and the size of the centrifuge head.

7. Remove the tube from the centrifuge after the instrument has come to a full stop.
8. Pour off the clear supernatant from the top of the specimen by inverting the centrifuge tube over the sink drain while allowing the running water from the faucet to flush the urine down the drain.
9. Turn the tube upright when the supernatant has been decanted, allowing a small amount to return to the sediment on the bottom of the tube without losing sediment down the drain (Figs. 2-3).
   Purpose: The sediment will be examined under the microscope.

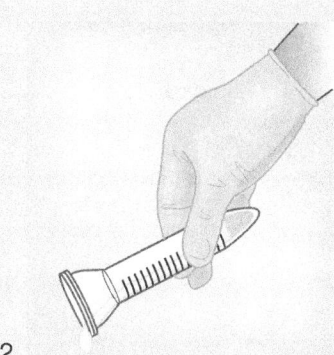

2

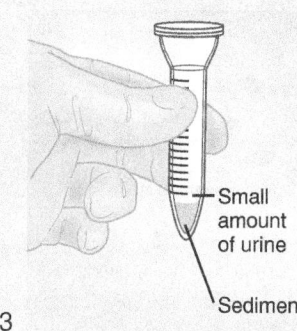

Small amount of urine

Sediment

3

10. Thoroughly mix the sediment with a drop of Sedi-Stain by grasping the tube near the top and rapidly flicking it with the fingers of the other hand until all sediment is thoroughly resuspended.
    Purpose: Elements centrifuge at different rates. Failure to mix the entire sediment completely may result in evaluation errors. Sedi-Stain colors the sediment for easier viewing.
11. Transfer 1 drop of sediment to a clean, labeled slide using a clean, disposable transfer pipet.
12. Place a clean coverslip over the drop and place the slide on the microscope stage. Remove your eye protection.
13. Focus under low power and reduce the light. *Note:* Once the slide is focused under low power, the remaining steps of this procedure are performed by the trained healthcare provider or moderate/highly complex–trained laboratory personnel.

From Stepp CA, Woods MA: *Laboratory procedures for medical office personnel,* Philadelphia, 1998, Saunders.

PROCEDURE 53.7   Perform a CLIA-Waived Urinalysis: Perform a Pregnancy Test

Task
Perform a pregnancy test on urine using the QuickVue pregnancy test method.

Equipment and Supplies
- Patient's health record
- Urine specimen
- QuickVue test kit
- Fluid-impermeable lab coat, protective eyewear, and gloves
- Biohazardous sharps container
- Biohazardous waste container

Procedural Steps
1. Wash your hands or use hand sanitizer. Put on the fluid-impermeable lab coat, protective eyewear, and gloves.
   Purpose: Hand sanitization is an important step for infection control. Personal protective equipment (PPE) is part of Standard Precautions.
2. Prepare the testing equipment (Fig. 1). Check the expiration date of the kit before proceeding.

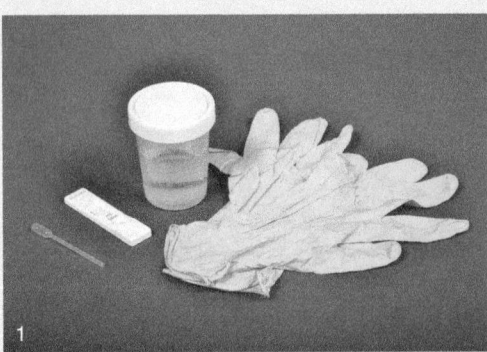

3. Collect the specimen (preferably a first morning specimen).
4. Remove the test cassette from the foil pouch.
5. Add 3 drops of urine using the transfer pipet (dropper) that accompanies the kit (Fig. 2).
   Purpose: To ensure accurate test results, the specimen amount must be added as indicated by the manufacturer's written procedure.

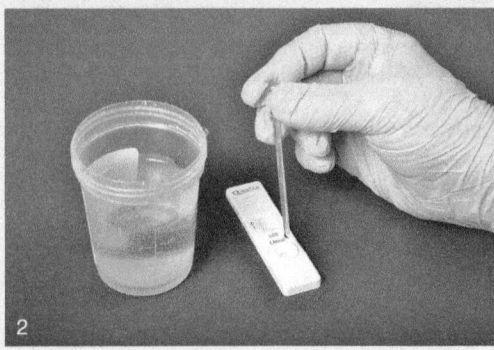

6. Dispose of the pipet in a biohazardous sharps container.
7. Wait 3 minutes and read the test results.
   Purpose: To ensure accurate test results, timing must be accurate.
8. Interpret the results as follows and record the results in the test logbook (see the following figure):
   - *Negative:* A blue control line is next to the letter C; no line is seen next to the letter T (see results in the middle).
   - *Positive:* A blue control line is next to the letter C; a pink line is next to the letter T (see results on the right).
   - *Invalid:* If a blue line does not appear in the C area, the test is invalid and the specimen must be retested using another kit. Check the expiration date of the kit before proceeding (Fig. 3).

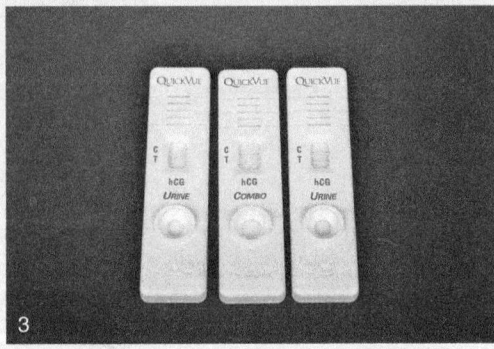

9. Discard the test cassette in the biohazardous waste container and clean up the testing area. Remove and discard your gloves in a biohazardous waste container. Remove the lab coat and protective eyewear.
10. Wash your hands or use hand sanitizer.
    Purpose: To ensure infection control.
11. Record the results in the patient's health record as either positive or negative for pregnancy.
    Purpose: A procedure is not considered finished until it is recorded.
    10/2/20XX 3:45 p.m.: Last menstrual period (LMP) 9/16/20XX. QuickVue pregnancy test: Positive._____ Macyn Black, CMA (AAMA)

PROCEDURE 53.8   Reassure a Patient of the Accuracy of Test Results

Tasks
Show empathy and communicate respectfully and professionally with the patient. Reassure the patient of the accuracy of the test result.

Directions: Role-play the following scenario with a peer. The peer is the patient, and you are the medical assistant. Your responses should include a discussion of what was different between the first and second test.

Scenario
Elyse is seeing Jean Burke, NP, at WMFM Clinic today. Elyse has been feeling tired and slightly nauseous for the last few weeks. She and her husband use birth control, but her menstrual periods are very irregular. She did a home pregnancy test one evening, and it was negative 2 weeks ago. But she is still feeling poorly. Jean orders a urine pregnancy test. The lab runs a CLIA-waived urine pregnancy test, and it is positive. Elyse does not believe the result. You need to reassure her about the accuracy of the test result.

54

Assisting in Blood Collection

LEARNING OBJECTIVES

1. Describe the personal protective equipment and the venipuncture equipment used to collect blood specimens
2. Explain the purpose of a tourniquet, when used, how to apply it, and the consequences of improper application.
3. Describes antiseptics used on the venipuncture site.
4. Describe the additives and uses of the different evacuated collection tubes.
5. Describe the order of the draw tubes.
6. Explain the effects of underfilling and the inversion required for the collection tubes.
7. Discuss the parts of a needles including safety features and the needle gauge.
8. Describe the needle holder, syringes, and needles used for blood collection.
9. Describe safety techniques to use to prevent needlestick injuries and postexposure needlestick follow-up.
10. Explain patient verification and preparation for the venipuncture.
11. Describe how to perform and complete the venipuncture.
12. Describe problems associated with venipunctures.
13. Describe capillary puncture procedure, include the sites used, the specimen collection, and specimen handling.
14. Discuss collection of blood from special populations: pediatric and geriatric patients.
15. Describe how to handle the specimen after collection and the chain of custody.

OUTLINE

▷ OPENING SCENARIO

Rosie Brandt, CMA (AAMA), has been a medical assistant with the Walden-Martin Family Medical (WMFM) Clinic for about 15 years. She has worked in many areas of the clinic, but for the past 8 years she has been the primary phlebotomist. Rosie has the right combination of skills to be a wonderful phlebotomist:

- She is warm, friendly, and can easily talk to patients.
- She is detail oriented, a stickler for safety practices, and very organized.

- She has good small motor skills and that certain quality that seems to make her venipunctures so smooth that you hardly feel the needle go through the skin.
- She can explain procedures well in understandable terms and is willing to listen to her patients and put them at ease.

It is Monday morning, and the phlebotomy area is usually busy with patients who have scheduled venipunctures in advance. Let's see what is happening in the phlebotomy area today.

YOU WILL LEARN

1. To assemble the equipment needed for a venipuncture and capillary puncture.
2. To discuss the different colored stoppers on vacuum tubes and correctly state the order of the draw.
3. To describe the types of safety needles and collection devices used in phlebotomy.
4. To summarize postexposure management of accidental needlesticks.
5. To perform a venipuncture using evacuated tubes, a syringe, and butterfly equipment, and also to perform a capillary puncture.
6. To discuss problem-solving strategies related to blood collection.
7. To discuss pediatric and geriatric phlebotomy, including behavior, parental involvement during phlebotomy, and general guidelines for blood collection in these special populations.

INTRODUCTION

Phlebotomy (fluh BOT uh mee) is the process of acquiring blood from a patient. Phlebotomy is performed primarily to:

- Aid in diagnosing disease
- Monitor a patient's condition, treatment, or medication levels
- Document the existing good health of a patient

According to the American Society of Clinical Pathology (ASCP), nearly 80% of providers base at least part of their diagnostic decisions on the results of laboratory tests. The most common specimen tested in the laboratory is blood. Phlebotomy requires highly trained individuals who can perform blood collection procedures. The procedures use special equipment to ensure the patient's comfort and safety.

When it comes to phlebotomy, safety is an important concern. There are several bloodborne viral diseases that can be spread by exposure to infected blood and body fluids. The bloodborne viruses identified as possible bloodborne pathogen risks are:

- Hepatitis B virus (HBV)
- Hepatitis C virus (HCV)
- Human immunodeficiency virus (HIV)

These viruses are not the only diseases that can be spread by contaminated blood or body fluids, but they are considered a risk for healthcare workers. The high standards necessary for the safe practice of phlebotomy led to the creation of the Bloodborne Pathogens Standard. These standards are overseen by the Occupational Safety and Health Administration (OSHA). Other guidelines, including Standard Precautions, also have

---

BOX 54.1   Phlebotomy Certifying Agencies

Phlebotomy certifying agencies include the following:
- American Society of Clinical Pathologists (ASCP) – gold standard
- American Allied Health, Inc.
- American Certification Agency for Healthcare Professionals (ACA)
- American Medical Technologists (AMT)
- American Society of Phlebotomy Technicians (ASPT)
- National Center for Competency Testing (NCCT)
- National Healthcareer Association (NHA)
- National Phlebotomy Association (NPA)

Continuing education often is required to maintain certification. It is important that medical assistants be familiar with the guidelines of the states in which they work because not all states require a certificate to perform phlebotomy. Other states require licensure, which differs from certification, to perform phlebotomy.

---

been designed to protect workers and patients (see Chapter 32 for more information on bloodborne pathogens).

Medical assistants are minimally trained to perform phlebotomy. To be certified as a phlebotomist (fluh BOT uh mist), they must complete phlebotomy course work and training at an accredited institution and perform a specified number of successful venipunctures (VEN uh puhngk chers). Once training is completed, they must pass a national phlebotomy certification examination (Box 54.1).

The most common method of obtaining a blood specimen is by *venipuncture*, blood that is taken directly from a surface vein. The vein is punctured with a needle, and the blood is collected directly into a stoppered vacuum tube or into a syringe. Once collected the blood is transferred into the vacuum tube. The procedure is safe when performed by a trained professional, but it must be performed with care. Practice is required to become skilled and confident in the technique of venipuncture.

VOCABULARY

syringe A device with a slender barrel and needle that is used to withdraw blood from a vein or an artery.

VENIPUNCTURE EQUIPMENT

Proper collection of blood requires specialized equipment. Phlebotomists in hospitals generally carry the equipment in a portable tray (Fig. 54.1). A physician office laboratory (POL) often has a permanent location where the same supplies are stored, and venipuncture is performed. In such cases, you may use a phlebotomy chair, which has an adjustable locking armrest to protect patients if they should faint (Fig. 54.2).

MEDICAL TERMINOLOGY

hepat/o	liver
phleb/o	vein
syncop/o	faint, cut off, cut short
ven/i-	vein
-itis	inflammation
-puncture	to pierce the surface
-tomy	the process of cutting

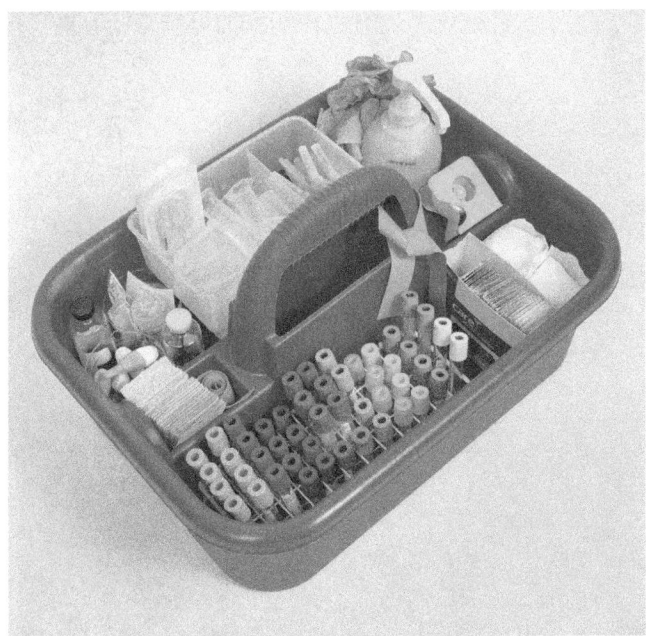

Fig. 54.1 A Stocked Venipuncture Tray. (From Niedzwiecki B, et al: *Kinn's the medical assistant*, ed 14, St. Louis, 2020, Elsevier.)

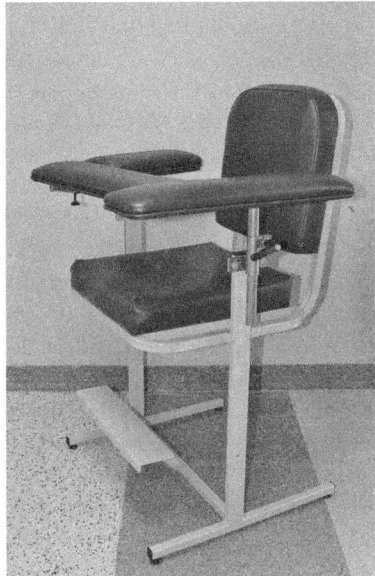

Fig. 54.2 A Phlebotomy Chair. (From Niedzwiecki B, et al: *Kinn's the medical assistant*, ed 14, St. Louis, 2020, Elsevier.)

Personal Protective Equipment

Employers must provide employees with personal protective equipment (PPE), such as gloves; disposable, fluid-impenetrable lab coats; protective eyewear; and face shields. All facilities must stock only latex-free supplies, including gloves and tourniquets, because of the potential for allergic responses in workers and patients. Some people with latex allergies can have life-threatening reactions with a latex exposure.

OSHA requires healthcare workers to wear gloves during venipuncture. Because veins can be difficult to locate with gloved fingertips, the site may be palpated before gloves are put on, as long as the hands have been washed or sanitized. According to the Clinical and Laboratory Standards Institute (CLSI), the standard procedure for venipuncture states that gloves may be put on after palpating the vein but before cleansing the site. Once the vein is cleansed, it is not to be touched prior to insertion of the needle. Touching the skin after cleansing contaminates the area. To help yourself find the vein after the area has been cleansed, make note of any skin markers, such as creases, freckles, or scars. If the area is touched, *it must be cleansed again*. Keep in mind that the tourniquet should be tied for no longer than 1 minute at a time.

CRITICAL THINKING 54.1

Rosie is in a little early on a Monday morning. She knows that Monday is usually busy, and she wants to make sure all her supplies are adequately stocked. Rosie cleans her protective eyewear and has it ready at the phlebotomy station. Why is it important to wear protective eyewear whenever drawing blood? Can you think of a few reasons and share them with your class?

Tourniquets

Before blood can be drawn, a vein must be located. Most venipunctures are done in the *antecubital* (an TEE kyoo bih tul) *region*, or inner bend in front of the elbow. Application of a tourniquet (TUR ni ket) is very helpful in locating veins in the antecubital region and any other area that may be drawn for venipuncture. Tourniquets prevent venous blood flow out of the site, causing the veins to bulge or plump up. If the antecubital area is drawn, a tourniquet is tied around the upper arm 3 to 4 inches above the puncture site. The tourniquet should be tight but still comfortable and easily released with one hand. Single use, nonlatex tourniquets are available (Fig. 54.3) and currently are recommended to:

- Reduce cross-contamination between patients and healthcare workers
- Help prevent nosocomial (nos uh KOH mee uh l) infections
- Prevent latex exposure

Other types of tourniquets with quick-release closures are available, but they must be disinfected after each use.

Tourniquets are applied immediately before the venipuncture procedure begins. Because a tourniquet slows blood flow, leaving it on for longer than 1 minute greatly increases the possibility of hemoconcentration (hee moe kon sen TRAY shun) and altered test results. The tourniquet should not be tied so tightly that it restricts arterial blood flow. If arterial blood flow is restricted, then venous blood return is also restricted. This will result in veins that will not plump up. Checking the pulse at the wrist ensures that arterial flow is not restricted. Tourniquets also are used when blood is drawn from hand and foot veins and are tied on the wrist or ankle, respectively.

Tourniquets can be uncomfortable for patients, especially those with heavy-set or hairy upper arms, if they are not applied correctly. Make sure the tourniquet is flat against the skin, and if necessary, tie it over the clothing if it is causing the patient discomfort. This may be especially important when blood is drawn on an elderly person because of the thinness or fragility of the skin.

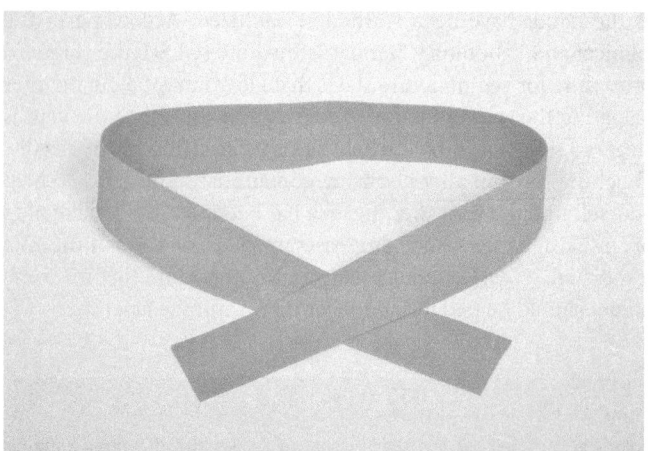

Fig. 54.3 A Latex-Free Tourniquet. (From Niedzwiecki B, et al: *Kinn's the medical assistant,* ed 14, St. Louis, 2020, Elsevier.)

> **VOCABULARY**
>
> **hemoconcentration** A condition in which the concentration of blood cells is increased in proportion to the volume of plasma.
>
> **nosocomial** An infection that is acquired in a healthcare setting. Also known as *healthcare acquired infections (HAI).*
>
> **tourniquet** A device for temporarily constricting blood flow.

CRITICAL THINKING 54.2

It is important to use a tourniquet to properly locate veins for phlebotomy. List three advantages of using a tourniquet to help locate veins. Be ready to share them with your class.

Antiseptics

To prevent infection, a venipuncture site must be cleansed with an antiseptic. The most commonly used antiseptic is 70% isopropyl (ahy suh PROH pil) alcohol, also known as *rubbing alcohol.* Prepackaged alcohol wipes are the product used most often. An alcohol wipe is used to clean the puncture site, which is then allowed to air dry. Alcohol does not sterilize the skin, but it kills many of the existing bacteria that might contaminate the sample. To achieve maximum bacteriostatic (bak TEER ee oh STAT ik) effect, the alcohol should remain on the skin for 30 to 60 seconds and be allowed to air dry. Isopropyl alcohol wipes should not be used to clean the venipuncture site when a blood alcohol test is drawn. Sterile soap pads, benzalkonium chloride, or povidone-iodine (Betadine) can be used instead.

> **VOCABULARY**
>
> **antiseptic** A substance, such as alcohol and povidone-iodine solution (Betadine), that inhibits the growth of microorganisms on living tissue. Used to cleanse the skin or wounds.
>
> **bacteriostatic** Prevents the growth of bacteria.

Blood Cultures

Blood cultures are ordered when a provider suspects that a bacterial infection in the blood is causing a fever of unknown origin

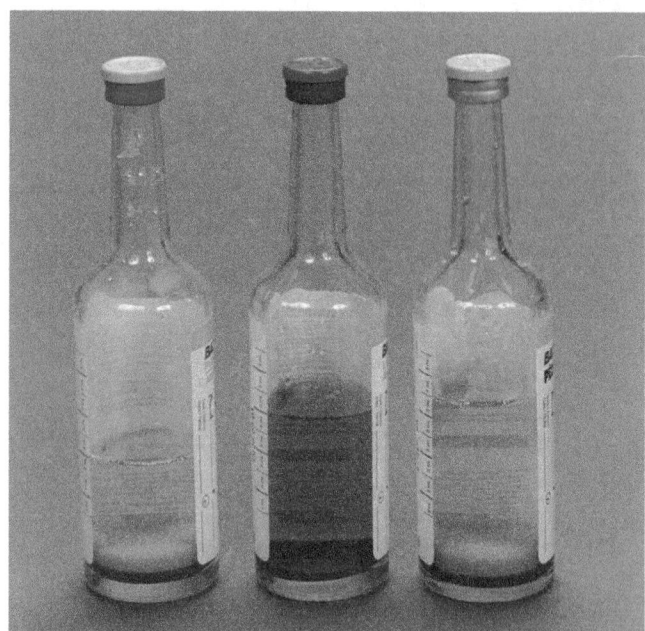

Fig. 54.4 An Example of Blood Culture Bottles. (From Niedzwiecki B, et al: *Kinn's the medical assistant,* ed 14, St. Louis, 2020, Elsevier.)

(FUO). A *blood culture* is a microbiological procedure in which a blood sample is placed in a nutrient medium and incubated at body temperature. If bacteria are in the blood sample, the culture medium will facilitate the growth of the bacteria, indicating *septicemia* (sep ti see me ah), which is a life-threatening infection.

If a blood culture is ordered, additional preparation is needed at the venipuncture site to eliminate contaminating bacteria. First, 70% isopropyl alcohol wipes are used to clean the area, which is allowed to air dry; then the area is wiped with an iodine solution. The iodine prep is also allowed to air dry. Benzalkonium (behn ZAHL koh nee uhm) chloride can be used for patients who are allergic to iodine. Alternatively, a chlorhexidine gluconate (klore HEKSI deen glue KON ate) prep kit can be used.

Once the venipuncture site is properly prepared, the blood cultures must be drawn into a sterile yellow-topped tube or bottle. These culture bottles are specifically designed to support the growth of any bacteria that might be present in the blood (Fig. 54.4). A yellow-topped tube can be drawn for blood cultures for mycobacteria, fungi, and acid-fast bacilli. These tubes are not drawn frequently in an ambulatory setting.

Evacuated Collection Tubes

The most common collection system is the evacuated tube system. (These tubes are also called *vacuum tubes;* a particular brand of vacuum tubes is the Vacutainer.) The system consists of evacuated tubes of various sizes that have color-coded stoppers. The colored stoppers indicate the tube's contents. Venipuncture tubes must be either shatter-resistant glass or plastic. More traditional rubber tube stoppers have been replaced by safer plastic *Hemogard* (HEE moh gahrd) colored tops. Hemogard tops have the advantage of not splattering blood when removed from the tube (Fig. 54.5). Table 54.1 lists the colored stoppers and the chemical additives, anticoagulants (AN tie koe ag yuh lahnt), clot activators, and/or thixotropic (THYH uh troh pik) gel that are contained in each type of tube. The different stopper colors indicate the unique contents of that color-coded tube. The vacuum in each tube draws a measured amount of blood into the tube. Tube volumes range from 2 to 15 mL.

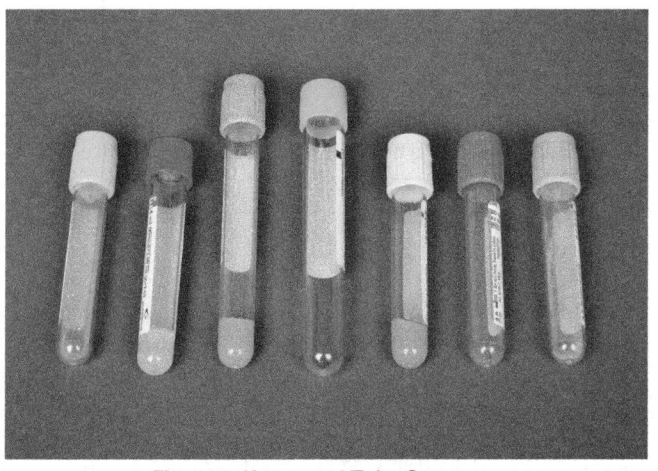

Fig. 54.5 Hemogard Tube Stoppers.

VOCABULARY

anticoagulants Substances (i.e., medications or chemicals) that prevent the clotting of blood.

clot activators Substances added to a venipuncture tube to enhance and speed up blood clotting.

evacuated tube A tube, flask, or reaction vessel in which a vacuum has been created.

thixotropic gel A chemically neutral gel added to evacuated blood tubes that creates a physical barrier between red blood cells and plasma or serum when the tube is centrifuged.

TABLE 54.1 Common Color-Coded Stoppers and Their Additives and Laboratory Uses

Vacuum Tube Color[a]	Color	Hemogard Color[b]	Additive and Its Function[c]	Laboratory Use
Blood culture bottles	No color for blood culture bottles (see Fig. 43.4)	Yellow / Pale yellow	Sodium polyanethol sulfonate (pohl ee AHN eh thawl SUHL fuh neyt) (SPS); prevents blood from clotting and stabilizes bacterial growth. Yellow-topped tubes have specific uses. They cannot be used to collect all blood culture specimens.	Blood culture bottles – blood or body fluid cultures. Yellow-topped tubes – mycobacteria (mahy koh bak TEER ee uh), fungus (FUHNG guh s), or acid-fast bacilli (buh SIL uh s) (AFB) blood cultures
Light blue		Light blue	Sodium citrate (SI treyt); removes calcium to prevent blood from clotting.	Coagulation (koh AG yuh ley shun) testing
Red		Red	None	Serum (SEER uh m) tests; chemistry studies, blood bank, immunology (im yuh NOL uh jee)
Red-gray (marbled)		Gold	No anticoagulant, but contains silica (SIL I kuh) particles to enhance clot formation, usually contain gel for serum separation.	Serum tests; chemistry studies, immunology
Green		Green	Heparin (HEP uh rin); inhibits thrombin (THROM bin) formation to prevent clotting.	Chemistry tests
Green-gray (marbled)		Light green	Lithium heparin and gel; for plasma separation.	Plasma (PLAZ muh) determinations in chemistry studies
Lavender		Lavender	Ethylenediaminetetraacetic (ETH uh leen DAHY uh meen TE truh uh SEE tik) acid (EDTA); removes calcium to prevent blood from clotting.	Hematology (hee muh TOL uh jee) tests
Gray		Gray	Potassium oxalate (OK suh leyt) and sodium fluoride; removes calcium to prevent blood from clotting; fluoride inhibits glycolysis (glahy KOL uh sis)	Chemistry testing, especially glucose and alcohol levels

[a]Stopper colors are based on BD Vacutainer tubes.
[b]Hemogard closures provide a protective plastic cover over the rubber stopper as an additional safety feature.
[c]Additives, additive functions, and laboratory uses are the same for both pediatric and adult tubes.
From Niedzwiecki B, et al: *Kinn's the medical assistant*, ed 14, St. Louis, 2020, Elsevier.

MEDICAL TERMINOLOGY

coagul/o	coagulation or clotting
comi/o	to care for
cubit/o	elbow, forearm
glyc/o	glucose or sugar
iatr/o	physician or treatment
nos/o	disease
ped/o	child or foot
ante-	forward, before
anti-	against
-al	pertaining to
-lysis	breakdown, destruction, separation
-sepsis	infection

The size of the tube to be drawn depends on several factors. Each test performed in the laboratory requires a specific amount of blood. Blood volumes can often be combined, which reduces the number of tubes that must be drawn. For example, both a complete blood count and an erythrocyte sedimentation rate test (discussed in Chapter 55) are performed on a sample from a lavender-topped tube. The combined volume for both tests can be drawn with one lavender-topped tube, so you do not need to draw two tubes. When in doubt, call the laboratory. Keep in mind that blood is approximately half cells and half liquid. If a test requires 2 mL of serum, at least 4 mL of blood must be collected.

PATIENT-CENTERED CARE

Patients often express great concern when several tubes of blood must be drawn. It seems like they are losing a lot of blood. You can put their fears to rest by explaining that the average adult has a little less than 5 L of blood (10 pints). Most adults can relate to donating a unit of blood, which is about 500 mL (1 pint). Because the red-topped tube may contain 5 mL, you would have to draw about 100 tubes to remove 500 mL of blood.

Tube Additives. Most vacuum tubes contain an additive. The glass plain red-topped tube contains nothing. It is a plain tube with no additives and no anticoagulants or clot enhancers. A plastic red-topped tube contains a clot activator in silicone-coated tubes. A gold-topped tube contains silica to activate clotting and an inert gel to separate serum and cells after the sample is centrifuged. All the other color-topped plastic tubes contain some form of anticoagulant, which prevents blood from clotting. The additive may be a powder, a liquid visible in the tube, or a liquid sprayed inside the tube by the manufacturer and allowed to dry. The choice of anticoagulant depends on the test to be completed.

Anticoagulant additives prevent blood from clotting, which allows the contents of the tube to be used in two ways. First, the sample can be used as whole blood. Second, the sample can be centrifuged, and the liquid portion, called plasma, can be used for testing. An example of a test that uses whole blood would be a complete blood count (CBC). An example of a test that uses plasma would be coagulation studies.

Ethylenediaminetetraacetic acid (EDTA) is the anticoagulant found in the lavender-topped tube. It prevents platelet clumping

and preserves the appearance of blood cells for microscopic examination.

Clot activators promote blood clotting in the tubes with either a plastic red top, a marbled red-gray top, or a gold top. For example, silica particles in the gold tubes enhance clotting by providing a surface for platelet activation. An orange-topped tube containing the additive thrombin promotes clotting within 5 minutes and is used for STAT (immediate) chemistry testing.

If blood clots and then is centrifuged, the liquid portion is referred to as serum. Without a clot activator, blood clots in 30 to 60 minutes at room temperature, after which it must be centrifuged. Clotting time in tubes containing clot activators allow clotting to occur with 30 minutes. The serum must be quickly separated from the cells because cells may continue to metabolize glucose or may release substances that interfere with testing.

Thixotropic gel can be found in some tubes, including *serum separator tubes (SSTs)*. SST tubes are identified by the marbled red-gray rubber stopper and the gold Hemogard top. The *plasma separator tube (PST)* also contains thixotropic gel. The glass tubes have a marbled green-gray top, and the Hemogard tubes have a light green top. Thixotropic gel, a synthetic gel, has a density between that of red cells and plasma or serum. The gel settles between the plasma/serum and cells during centrifugation. The gel forms a barrier that makes it easy to pour off the liquid portion of the sample without cells contaminating the specimen.

It is important to avoid a "short draw" (i.e., a tube that is not completely filled). Table 54.2 lists the consequences of underfilling tubes. Some tubes are designed to fill only partially, according to their preset vacuum. Having the proper ratio of blood to additive is crucial. Always check the tube for the expiration date. Outdated tubes may have a diminished vacuum, or the additive may have degraded and may not be as effective.

VOCABULARY

plasma The fluid portion of blood in the body. In an evacuated tube, it is the liquid portion of a whole-blood sample that has not clotted due to the presence of an anticoagulant. The liquid portion of the blood that contains clotting factors.

serum The liquid portion of a clotted blood specimen that no longer contains its active clotting agents.

CRITICAL THINKING 54.3

In your own words, define plasma and serum.

ORDER OF THE DRAW

If more than one tube must be drawn during a venipuncture, a specified order must be followed. Carryover of additives from one tube to the next could cause sample alteration and incorrect results. CLSI has established a set of standards outlining the order of draw for a multitube draw. The same order applies to the filling of tubes when blood is collected in a syringe.

1. *Blood culture bottles* are filled first because they are sterile and should not be contaminated by the other tubes.

TABLE 54.2 Effects of Underfilling and Inversion Mixing for Collection Tubes

Stopper Color	Effects of Underfilling	Mix by Gentle Inversion
Blood culture bottles or yellow	Reduces possibility of bacterial recovery	8–10 times
Light blue	Coagulation test results falsely prolonged	8–10 times
Gold (SST tubes), red, marbled red-gray	Poor barrier formation; insufficient sample	5–6 times
Green	False results because of excess heparin	8–10 times
Marbled green-gray, and light green (PST tubes)	False results because of excess heparin	8–10 times
Lavender	Falsely low blood cell counts and hematocrits; morphologic changes to red blood cells; staining changes	8–10 times
Gray	False results	8–10 times
Orange or marbled green-gray with gel		5–6 times
Orange or marbled green-gray without gel		8–10 times

Yellow-topped tubes would be drawn in the same place as blood culture bottles in the order of the draw.

2. *Light blue* top: These tubes, which contain sodium citrate, are next because other anticoagulants might contaminate the sample collected for coagulation studies. If no blood culture has been ordered, CLSI recommends that blood for the light blue–topped tube be drawn first if routine coagulation testing has been ordered (i.e., prothrombin time [PT] and activated partial thromboplastin time [APTT]).

   • Some laboratories recommend that a red-topped "waste" tube with no additives be partially filled before the light blue–topped tube, but this practice is slowly dying off. This is done to remove any tissue thromboplastin that was released during the venipuncture. Thromboplastin interferes with coagulation testing.

   • CLSI also recommends that when a winged infusion set (butterfly assembly) is used, blood be drawn into the red-topped tube even if the order does not call for it. This is done to fill the tubing's dead air space with blood before drawing the light blue–topped sodium citrate tube. A light blue tube must have an exact blood-to-citrate dilution. It is not necessary to completely fill the waste tube, because it will be discarded.

3. *Red* top: Glass red serum tubes without clot activator or plastic red tubes with clot activator are filled next. These clotted specimens are drawn to test the serum after the specimens have clotted and been centrifuged.

4. *Gold* or *marble* top: Gold top SS tubes with clot activator with thixotropic gel are also drawn at this time. SSTs have a marbled red-gray stopper or a gold Hemogard stopper.

5. *Green* top: These tubes are drawn next because the plasma in their anticoagulated specimen is used for testing when STAT results are needed (usually in chemistry). The dark green tops contain no thixotropic gel. The tubes with marbled green-gray tops and light green Hemogard tops both contain the gel to help separate the plasma from the cells when centrifuged.

6. *Lavender* top: These tubes are drawn next. They contain an EDTA anticoagulant that preserves blood cell morphology. EDTA tubes are drawn near the end of the draw because the additive interferes with chemistry and coagulation specimens.

7. *Gray* top: This tube is drawn last, and the blood is used to test glucose or blood alcohol levels. Its additives (potassium oxalate/sodium fluoride) may elevate electrolyte levels and damage cells if passed into the other tubes. The sodium fluoride is a glycolytic inhibitor and preserves glucose in whole blood.

To recap, Table 54.1 shows the order of draw of the colored tube tops, in addition to the additives, laboratory uses, and accepted volumes per tube. Table 54.2 lists the effects of underfilling the collection tubes. This table also shows how many times the various tubes need to be inverted after they have been filled with blood. It is important to gently mix the contents of the tubes well, after collection, by inverting them several times (do not shake the tubes).

VOCABULARY

STAT The medical abbreviation for the Latin term *statum*, meaning immediately; at this moment.

✳ STUDY TIP

Sometimes making up a saying or sentence can help you remember the order of a process. Here are a few sayings I have heard in the past to remember the order of the draw.

The order of the draw is: **St**erile (blood culture bottles/tubes) – **l**ight blue-**r**ed/gold-**g**reen-**l**avender-**g**ray. Use the first letter for each tube color and make up a sentence that helps you remember the order of the draw.

Examples: 1. Stop light red. Green light go. 2. Stan's light red glasses look gray. 3. Stella's lecture reading gives little giggles. 4. Street lights reveal green little gardens.

CRITICAL THINKING 54.4

Can you make up your own saying or sentence to remember the order of the draw? Work with a group in your class and come up with a few different ways to remember the order of the draw.

NEEDLES AND SUPPLIES USED IN PHLEBOTOMY

A critical part of phlebotomy is knowing which needle and which tube or syringe should be used in each situation. All needles used in phlebotomy are sterile and have a safety device that is activated immediately after withdrawal from the vein. The

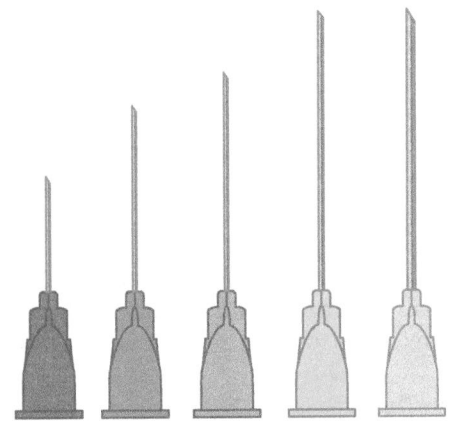

Fig. 54.6 Venipuncture Needles.

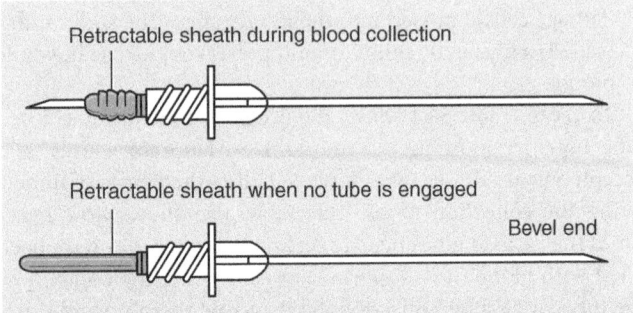

Retractable sheath during blood collection

Retractable sheath when no tube is engaged

Bevel end

Fig. 54.7 Bevel of a Venipuncture Needle. (From Niedzwiecki B, et al: *Kinn's the medical assistant*, ed 14, St. Louis, 2020, Elsevier.)

needle is then discarded in a biohazardous sharps container. Each needle is housed in a protected cover, which should be inspected before use to ensure that sterility has not been compromised (i.e., the seal should be intact). The needle itself should be inspected to make sure it has no manufacturing defects, such as burs, nicks, or bends.

Needles have several parts: the hub, the shaft, and the bevel. The hub of the needle is designed to attach the needle to the vacuum tube needle holder or a syringe. Shafts differ in length, ranging from ¾ inch to 1½ inches (Fig. 54.6). The length of the shaft has no bearing on the venipuncture procedure. Some phlebotomists prefer a longer needle, and others prefer a shorter needle because it makes patients less uneasy. One end of the shaft is cut at an angle and forms the *bevel*, which creates a very sharp point. The bevel of the needle prevents trauma to the tissue and makes the entry into the skin much smoother (Fig. 54.7).

The bore, or hollow space, inside the needle shaft is called the *lumen*. Lumen size is important and is referred to as the *gauge*. A numeric value designates the gauge of the needle. The higher the gauge number, the smaller the lumen. Be sure to match the needle gauge to the size of the tube. A large vacuum tube is more likely to hemolyze the blood if a high-gauge needle (i.e., small lumen) is used. For example, blood banks use a large, 16-gauge needle to collect pints of blood for transfusions. The lumen is wide, which reduces the chance of hemolysis (hee MOL i sis). A small, 23-gauge needle is used to collect blood from small or fragile veins, such as those in elderly and very young patients. Routine adult venipuncture requires a 20- to 21-gauge needle.

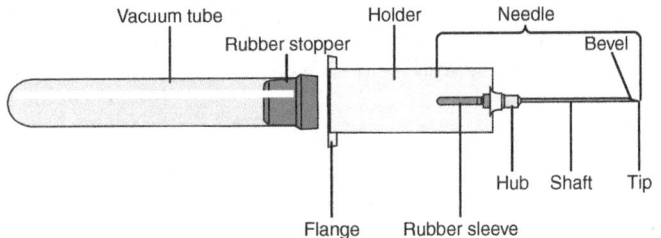

Fig. 54.8 Venipuncture Assembly. (From Hunt SA: Saunders *fundamentals of medical assisting*, revised reprint, St. Louis, 2007, Saunders.)

VOCABULARY
hemolysis The breakdown of red blood cells with the release of hemoglobin.

CRITICAL THINKING 54.5

Rosie has a few different-gauge needles to use in phlebotomy. Why would she need different-sized needles? The process is the same for each patient, why would the needle size be important? Share your ideas with the class.

Multisample Needles

Multisample needles are commonly used in routine adult venipuncture. They are used when several tubes need to be drawn during a single venipuncture. These needles are double pointed (Fig. 54.8). One point enters the patient's vein, and the other punctures the stopper of the collection tube. The point that enters the tube is sheathed with a retractable rubber sleeve that allows tubes to be changed without blood leaking into the needle holder or tube holder.

Needle Holders

Double-pointed needles must be firmly placed into a needle holder (see Fig. 54.8). Usually needle holders are translucent cylinders, and they come in different sizes to accommodate different-sized tubes. The holders often have a ring that indicates how far the tube can be pushed onto the needle without losing the vacuum. Once the safety shield has been activated on the needle, OSHA requires that the needle holder–needle unit be discarded into a biohazardous sharps container immediately after completing the venipuncture, to prevent needlesticks.

Syringes

Syringes are used when there is concern that the strong vacuum in a stoppered vacuum tube might collapse the vein. The syringe needle fits on the end of the syringe barrel. Syringe needles also come in different gauges. The size of the syringe indicates the amount of blood that the syringe can hold. For example, a 10-mL syringe indicates that 10 mL of blood can be drawn into the syringe. The size of the syringe selected for the venous draw, depends on how much blood needs to be collected for testing. When blood is drawn into a syringe, it must be transferred immediately to the evacuated tube(s). Blood that sits in the syringe barrel could clot if not transferred quickly. The syringe needle safety device must be activated and discarded in the sharps container. A special transfer tube device is then used to

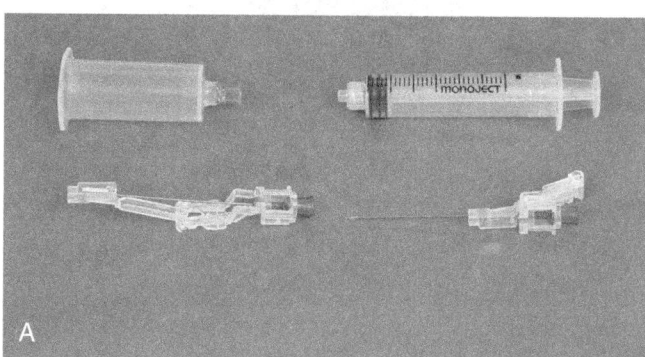

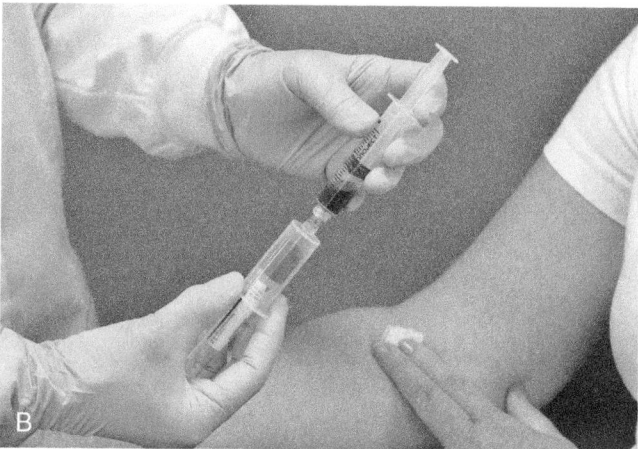

Fig. 54.9 A, Transfer tube device (top left), syringe (top right), and a safety needle (bottom right) and a covered safety needle (bottom left). B, Transferring the blood from the syringe to the evacuated tube.

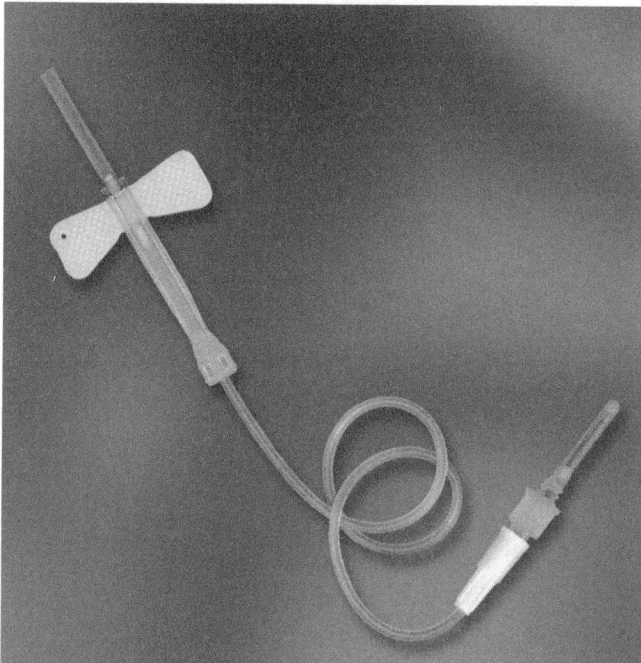

Fig. 54.10 Butterfly Assembly. (Courtesy Becton, Dickinson, Franklin Lakes, NJ.)

transfer the blood to the vacuum tubes. This device connects to the top of the syringe; it contains an enclosed needle that punctures the vacuum tube's stopper and delivers the blood into the tube (Fig. 54.9).

Winged Infusion Sets (Butterfly Assembly)

Butterfly assemblies (Fig. 54.10) are designed for use on small veins. Butterfly needles are often used to draw veins in the back of the hand or when drawing a pediatric patient. The most common butterfly needle size is a 22- or 23-gauge with a needle length of ½ to ¾ inch. A butterfly needle has a plastic, flexible, butterfly-shaped grip attached to a short length of tubing. The hub end is fitted into a syringe or a needle holder tube adapter. Syringes are frequently paired with butterfly needles because the syringe can create a gentle vacuum that can easily be controlled by the phlebotomist. The syringe blood sample must

be transferred to the evacuated tubes using the transfer device described previously.

CRITICAL THINKING 54.6

Describe the difference between a syringe and a winged infusion assembly. List two examples of when each type of equipment may be used.

NEEDLE SAFETY

Healthcare workers who use or may be exposed to needles are at increased risk of needlestick injury. Such injuries can lead to serious or fatal infections with bloodborne pathogens, such as HBV, HCV, and HIV. Needlestick injuries account for most accidental exposures to blood. As is discussed in Chapter 32, used needles should never be recapped. After use, needles should be covered with the appropriate engineered safety device that is part of the needle assembly.

According to OSHA, the best practice for preventing needlestick injuries after phlebotomy is to use safety needles that are activated with one hand immediately after use. The US Food and Drug Administration (FDA) has approved medical devices marketed and sold in the United States. They recommend devices that provide a barrier between the hands and the needle, after use, in which the phlebotomist's hands remain behind the needle at all times. Safety shields that can be activated before or immediately after removal of the needle from the vein should be an integral part of the device. Once activated the safety shield should lock in place. Finally, these devices should be as simple as possible, requiring little or no training to use. Some examples of needle safety devices are:

- *One-handed vacuum tube needle:* After the needle has been used and removed from the vein, the thumb holding the vacuum tube holder slides under the base of the pink safety device, causing it to snap over the contaminated needle (Fig. 54.11A). Or, an orange needle shield on the holder is activated by pressing the device against a hard, flat surface (Fig. 54.11B).
- *Syringe needle safety devices* (see Fig. 54.9): These devices have a spring-activated shield attached to a disposable

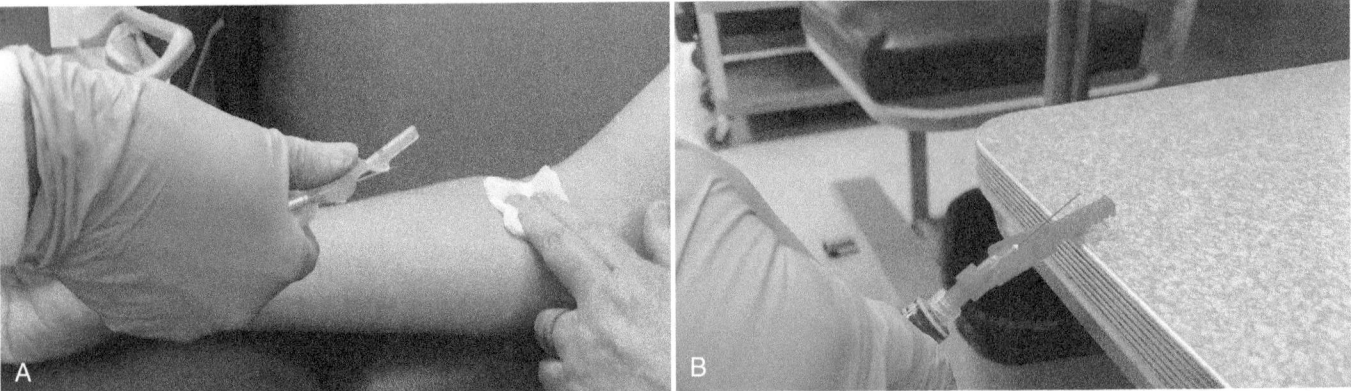

Fig. 54.11 One-Handed Safety Needles. A, Activated by sliding the thumb up at the base of the guard, causing it to cover the needle. B, Activated by pressing the orange guard (needle shield) against a solid surface, causing it to cover the needle.

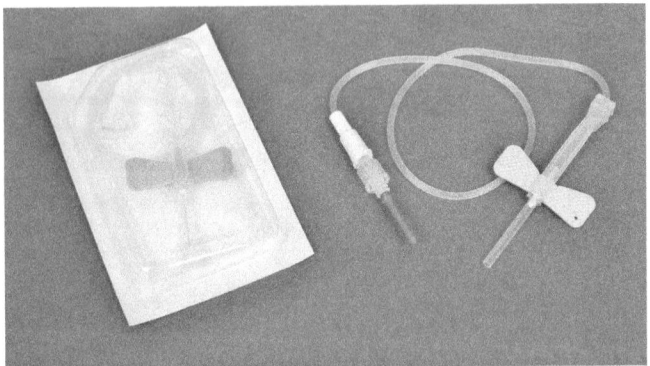

Fig. 54.12 Safety-Lok Butterfly Needle. (From Niedzwiecki B, et al: *Kinn's the medical assistant,* ed 14, St. Louis, 2020, Elsevier.)

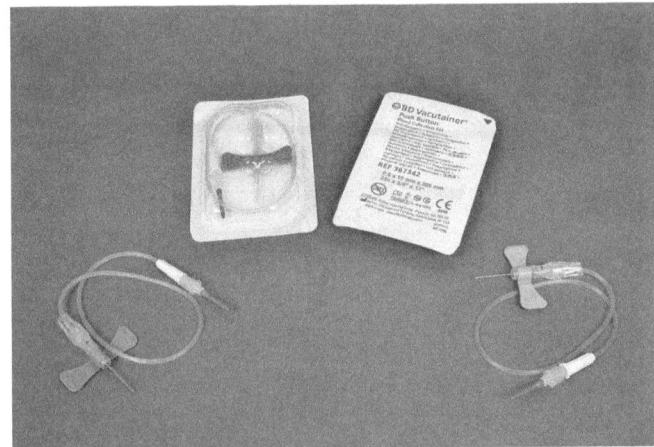

Fig. 54.13 Push-Button Butterfly Needle. (From Niedzwiecki B, et al: *Kinn's the medical assistant,* ed 14, St. Louis, 2020, Elsevier.)

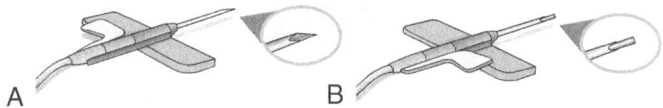

Fig. 54.14 Needle-Blunting Butterfly Needle. A, The sharp point is visible when the needle is inserted. B, Before the needle is removed, the third "wing" is rotated and a blunt needle moves down the shaft. (From Niedzwiecki B, et al: *Kinn's the medical assistant,* ed 14, St. Louis, 2020, Elsevier.)

syringe needle. After the venipuncture, the phlebotomist activates the device with the thumb holding the syringe, and a spring locks a protective plastic tip into place, protecting the needle. The needle can then be removed and discarded. The syringe is attached to the safety transfer device to deliver the collected blood into the appropriate vacuum tubes (see Fig. 54.9).

- *Butterfly needle safety lock* (Fig. 54.12): After the venipuncture, the dominant hand holds the butterfly tail while the nondominant hand pulls back on the tubing, causing the needle to slide into the tubing and lock into place.
- *Push-button butterfly safety device* (Fig. 54.13): With the needle still in the arm, the medical assistant grasps the tail of the butterfly with the dominant hand while the nondominant hand presses the button just below the wings, causing the needle to retract into the butterfly body as it leaves the vein.
- *Needle-blunting butterfly set* (Fig. 54.14): A third "wing" is rotated after collection and before removal of the needle from the vein. As the third wing is rotated, it moves the blunt needle down the shaft before it is removed from the patient.

OSHA requires employers to establish and maintain a sharps injury log for recording injuries from contaminated sharps. This log should contain information about the device involved in the incident and the department or work area where the incident occurred, in addition to an explanation of the incident. Employee confidentiality must be maintained.

Protect Against Needlestick Injuries

The Bloodborne Pathogens Standard, established by the Occupational Safety and Health Administration (OSHA), emphasizes that phlebotomists should have direct input on the type of safety needles they will be using. To protect against needlestick injuries:

- Help your employer evaluate and select devices with safety features.
- Use devices with safety features provided by your employer.
- Never recap a contaminated needle except with a safety device.
- Plan for safe handling and disposal before beginning any procedure using needles.
- Dispose of used needles and needle holders promptly in appropriate biohazardous sharps containers.
- Tell your employer about hazards from needles that you observe in your work environment.

- Participate in bloodborne pathogen training and follow recommended infection prevention practices, including vaccination against the hepatitis B virus (HBV).

Postexposure Needlestick Follow-Up

An accidental needlestick is a medical emergency. OSHA-recommended management procedures are discussed in Chapter 32. Postexposure needlestick management includes:

- Immediately after injury, the wound is inspected and washed for 10 to 15 minutes with soap, 10% iodine solution, or chlorine-based antiseptic.
- The injury is reported to the supervisor immediately after cleansing the site. An incident report is completed.
- The employee is referred to a physician for confidential assessment and follow-up.
- Baseline testing for hepatitis B virus (HBV), hepatitis C virus (HCV), and the human immunodeficiency virus (HIV) is recommended for both the employee and the source individual.
- Interim testing may be performed if the healthcare worker experiences symptoms of acute HIV exposure or hepatitis.
- Confidential follow-up care must include provisions for emotional support and counseling for the healthcare worker.

ROUTINE VENIPUNCTURE

Venipuncture involves a series of steps that are vital to collecting a good sample. In addition to learning good technique, we also want to be able to make our patients as comfortable as possible. As you read through the information you will start to become familiar with the venipuncture procedure and the details of the process.

The first step of the procedure is to select the proper method for venipuncture (evacuated tube, syringe, or butterfly assembly). Next, prepare your patient for the procedure. Then you are ready to collect the sample and process the specimen appropriately.

Patient Preparation

All blood collections begin with a requisition, a form from the patient's provider requesting a test. Requisitions may be computer generated or handwritten and at a minimum must include:

- Patient's identification: complete name, date of birth, and identification (ID) number
- Name of the provider submitting the order
- Type of test requested
- Test status (timed, fasting, STAT, and so forth)

A venipuncture starts with greeting the patient and verifying their identity. According to CLSI, proper identification includes asking outpatients to (1) state and spell their first and last names and (2) state their birth date. All the information must be compared and verified with the patient requisition. If communication with the patient is not possible, a family member, guardian, or medical translator must provide the required information. The name of the person assisting should be documented in the patient's medical record. Always follow your institution's

procedures for assisted communication before completing the venipuncture procedure.

Briefly explain the venipuncture procedure to your patient, and make sure to ask them the following questions:

- Do you have any questions or concerns?
- Do you have an arm, vein, or site preference?
- Were you given any special instructions prior to the venipuncture (e.g., does the person need to be fasting?)
- Have you taken any medication today?
- Have you ever experienced any problems or complications with a routine venipuncture in the past?

Answer patients' questions and address their concerns, and take steps to prevent any past problems from recurring. If you cannot answer all the questions, ask if they would like to talk to the provider for clarification. Obtain verbal consent to perform the venipuncture simply by asking whether you have permission to draw blood from the patient.

Your self-confidence in the procedure will help put your patient at ease. Act and speak professionally. Treat your patient with kindness and respect. Being pleasant and friendly is important. It makes your patients feel comfortable and shows that you take your role in their care seriously.

CRITICAL THINKING 54.7

Why is patient identification so very important in phlebotomy? List four reasons and be ready to share them with the class.

👪 PATIENT-CENTERED CARE

You may want to ask your patients how they would prefer to be addressed – by their first name? A nickname? Dr. Smith, Mr. Jones, Mrs. Blake, or Ms. Washington? – Don't assume that patients want to be called by their first name. Also, don't call patients "sweetie," "honey," or "dear." Be respectful.

Preparing for the Venipuncture

Seat the patient in a phlebotomy area. Ask the patient to extend an arm and position their other hand under the elbow to help straighten the elbow, if necessary. Inspect both arms and ask whether the patient has an arm or site preference. Veins in the antecubital area are most commonly used for venipuncture (Fig. 54.15). According to CLSI standards, the veins in the center of the antecubital area should be located as a first choice before alternative veins within the antecubital area are considered. The puncture site should be carefully selected after both arms have been inspected. Alternative sites may be chosen if the area is scarred, bruised, burned, or swollen. You may use the veins on the back of the hand if the patient gives permission. For any other alternative site, consult the provider and do not proceed without supervision.

When choosing the best available vein, palpate the area. Feel for a vein that has "bounce" when lightly palpated. The medial (MEE dee uh l) veins generally run at a slight angle to the fold in the antecubital area. The cephalic (se FAL ik) veins are on the thumb side of the antecubital area. These veins are the veins of choice. The

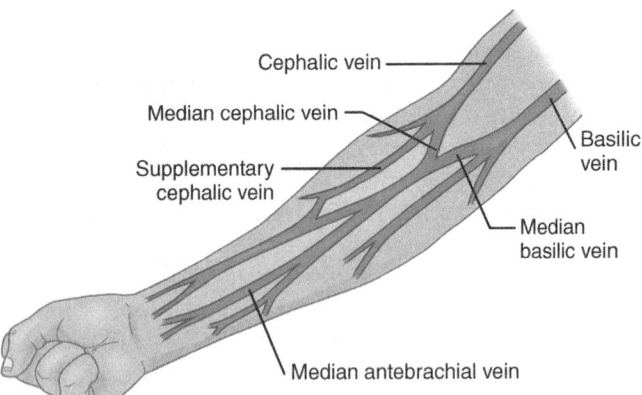

Fig. 54.15 Veins of the Forearm. (From Stepp CA, Woods MA: *Laboratory procedures for medical office personnel,* Philadelphia, 1998, Saunders.)

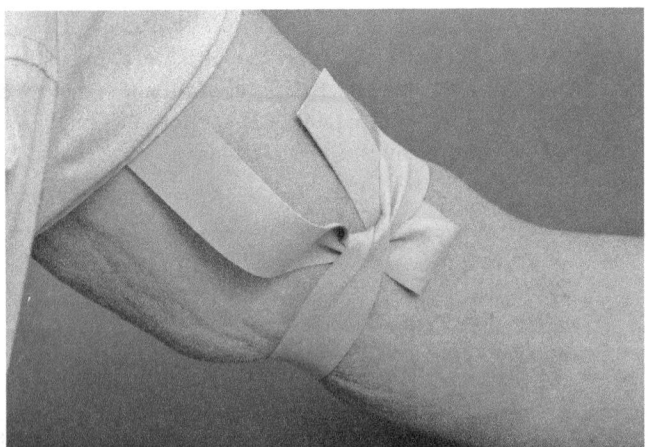

Fig. 54.16 Placement of the Tourniquet on the Arm. (From Niedzwiecki B, et al: *Kinn's the medical assistant,* ed 14, St. Louis, 2020, Elsevier.)

basilic (bah SIL ik) vein, which lies on the inside of the antecubital area (the little finger side), is very close to the brachial artery and median nerves and should *not* be used! If the medial or cephalic veins are not accessible, consult the provider. Only the most experienced phlebotomists should ever attempt a basilic venipuncture, since the chance for injury to the patient is too great.

The tourniquet should be placed about 3 to 4 inches above the patient's elbow. Make sure it is not twisted because that will cause discomfort to your patient (Fig. 54.16). Grasp the tourniquet ends, one in each hand, close to the patient's skin. Pull the ends apart to gently stretch the tourniquet, then cross one end over the other while maintaining the tension. Tuck the top portion of the tourniquet underneath the bottom portion, creating a loop with the upper flap free. The free end will be tugged on to release the tourniquet later in the draw. The tourniquet should be tight without being uncomfortable or pinching the patient's skin. Both ends of the tourniquet should be pointing upward on the arm. This way, the end of the tourniquet does not contaminate the venipuncture site.

When the tourniquet is in place, ask the patient to place their other hand or fist under the elbow of the arm that will be drawn if this aids in palpating the vein. Ask the person to just relax the arm. Palpate for an acceptable vein using your index finger. Palpate the vein through gloved fingers, and then continue with the phlebotomy process.

Performing the Venipuncture

When you have located a vein, remove the tourniquet. A tourniquet can remain in place for 1 minute. After its removal, wait 2 minutes before reapplying it. During this time, sanitize your hands and put on gloves (if they are not already on). Then cleanse the antecubital area with a 70% alcohol wipe. Clean the area by using a back-and-forth scrubbing motion per CLSI guidelines. Do not touch this area after cleaning with alcohol. Assemble the equipment and place it within easy reach of the patient's arm.

Reapply the tourniquet. The patient can make a fist but do not have the patient clench or pump the fist repeatedly. Relocate the vein. Anchor the vein by gently stretching the skin downward below the collection site with the thumb of the nondominant hand. Smoothly and quickly insert the needle into the vein at about a 15-degree angle, depending on the depth and position of the vein (Box 54.2). The bevel should be facing up. Push the evacuated tube onto the double-pointed needle or pull back on the syringe plunger with your nondominant hand.

Completing the Venipuncture

Continue to draw the specimens, checking periodically on the patient's condition. As you remove each tube from the needle holder, gently invert it several times before placing it in a collection rack. Tubes with clot activator should be inverted 5 times. Tubes with anticoagulant should be inverted 8 to 10 times (see Table 54.2). If the tubes are not inverted immediately after collection, small clots can form in the specimen. When the last tube has started to fill, carefully release the tourniquet. Gently tug on the short portion of the tourniquet, and it should just fall open. Remove the final vacuum tube. Cover the venipuncture area with gauze, then smoothly and quickly remove the needle. Once the needle is out of the arm, apply pressure to the site. At the same time, activate the safety device to cover the needle. Dispose of the entire venipuncture assembly into a biohazardous sharps container. Ask the patient to apply direct pressure to the gauze. *Do not* bend the arm.

While the patient applies pressure to the site, label the tubes with computer-generated labels or by writing the information in permanent marker. Make sure the label contains the following minimum information:

- Patient's identification, including complete name, date of birth, and ID number or insurance number
- Date and time of the draw, and the phlebotomist's initials
- Provider's name and whether patient was fasting (optional)

Before putting on a bandage, perform a two-point check to make sure the site is not leaking. Observe the site for 5 to 10 seconds after releasing pressure and removing the gauze. If visible bleeding occurs or if the tissue around the puncture site rises, continue applying pressure until the bleeding has stopped. Special precautions must be taken for patients taking anticoagulants because the phlebotomy site will bleed longer than normal. Once bleeding has stopped, put on a pressure bandage by placing a folded gauze (not a cotton ball) over the site and then applying hypoallergenic self-stick wrap, stretchy gauze, or a bandage. Never leave the room or release an outpatient until all the tubes have been labeled. Make sure patients are doing well, then escort them to the exit or to the reception area.

CRITICAL THINKING 54.9

At the end of Ken's venipuncture, Rosie asks Ken to hold pressure on the draw site. She puts the computer-generated labels on the three tubes she drew and writes her initials on the labels. Then Rosie checks Ken's arm and wraps a gauze around the site.

Why is it important to label the tubes immediately after finishing the venipuncture? List two reasons this is a good practice for a phlebotomist.

Procedures 54.1 and 54.2 outline the proper procedures for venipuncture using the evacuated tube method and the syringe method. Some patients may have small veins, and using a syringe or butterfly for venipuncture may work better than the standard evacuated assembly. Young children, chemotherapy patients, elderly patients, and people with veins that are difficult to draw may require syringe or butterfly equipment. Alternative equipment is always used to draw blood from hand veins (Procedure 54.3).

PROBLEMS ASSOCIATED WITH VENIPUNCTURE

Failure to obtain blood can occur due to several factors. Determining the cause of the problem may help you decide whether a second attempt would be successful. The first rule is to remain calm and professional. Remaining calm helps you think clearly about the situation and about the potential causes for not getting blood.

Hematoma

The most common injury patients suffer from phlebotomy is a hematoma (hee ma TOH muh). A *hematoma* is an abnormal buildup of blood in the tissues caused by a leak or cut in a blood vessel. It appears as a large, painful, bruised area at the puncture

site. This leakage causes the tissue around the puncture site to swell. The most common causes of hematoma formation during the draw are:

- Excessive probing with the needle to locate a vein
- Failure to insert the needle far enough into the vein
- Passing the needle through the vein

A hematoma can also form after a draw if:

- The tourniquet is not removed before the needle is removed.
- The vacuum tube is not removed from the hub of the needle before the needle is withdrawn.
- Adequate pressure is not applied at the puncture site.
- The elbow is bent while pressure is applied.
- The puncture reopens and bleeds into the tissue due to heavy lifting with the venipuncture arm. Instruct the patient to be careful with the arm for several hours after the procedure.

If a hematoma forms, discontinue the procedure immediately, apply pressure to the area for a minimum of 3 minutes, and then apply an ice pack to the area. Notify the provider and observe the site to determine whether the bleeding has stopped. Depending on the facility's policy, an incident report may have to be completed and documented in the patient's record.

Nerve Damage and Other Complications

The second most common injury is nerve damage. The risk of nerve damage is very small. If the patient complains of tingling, numbness, or a shooting pain, discontinue the procedure immediately. Preventive measures include:

- Avoiding the basilic vein for phlebotomy
- Refraining from "blind" probing if the vein is missed with the initial draw

Table 54.3 lists some workable solutions to complications. As a rule, it is wise to limit yourself to two venipuncture attempts for a patient. If a second attempt is unsuccessful, ask whether the patient would allow another phlebotomist to look at their arms. If another phlebotomist feels confident to attempt a venipuncture, that person will need to get permission from the patient first. If the patient doesn't give permission, it may be better to reschedule the venipuncture for another time. This strategy lets patients know that they have input into their care and some measure of control of the situation. At one time or another, everyone is unsuccessful in obtaining a blood sample, so do not feel badly. Make the best of the situation, learn from the experience, and treat the patient with kindness. We are all human, and our patients are usually quite understanding.

Fainting

Fainting, or syncope, can have serious consequences, so the phlebotomist must always be prepared to take action quickly. Positioning the patient in a blood collection chair (by turning the armrest pad in front of the patient) prevents bodily injury if the person faints. Making eye contact and observing patients before phlebotomy can help you estimate their level of comfort with the procedure. Constant light conversation with the patient during the venipuncture can help identify if the patient is distressed or anxious.

TABLE 54.3 **Managing Possible Blood Draw Complications**

Complication	Management Strategies
Burned area	Choose another site because these areas are prone to infection.
Convulsions	Stay calm. Remove the needle and quickly dispose of it in a biohazardous sharps container. Then help guide patients to the floor, protecting them from injury. Call for help.
Damaged or scarred veins or infected areas	Look for an alternative site; do not draw blood from scarred or infected areas.
Edema	Avoid the area; look for an alternative site.
Hematoma	Remove the needle and apply pressure.
Intravenous (IV) therapy or blood transfusion sites	Blood samples should not be drawn from an arm that is also the site for IV infusion or blood transfusion because of the dilution factor.
Mastectomy (ma STEK tuh mee)	Do not draw blood from the side of the mastectomy, because mastectomy surgery causes lymphostasis (lihm foh STEY sis), which may produce false results.
Nausea	Place a cold cloth on the patient's forehead, give patients a basin in case of vomiting, and instruct them to take deep breaths. Alert the provider.
No blood	Reposition the needle slightly or remove and replace the vacuum tube with a new tube in case the vacuum was compromised.
Collapsed vein	Caused by too much vacuum on a small vein or pulling on syringe plunger too fast. Remove needle and use a different vein with winged infusion (butterfly) system.
Petechiae (pih TEE kee uh)	Indicates the patient has a capillary wall or platelet disorder, and the site may bleed excessively once the needle is removed. Apply pressure until bleeding has stopped.
Syncope	Position the patient's head between the knees (if in a sitting position). Check and record the patient's pulse, blood pressure, and respiration rate and continue to observe the patient. Never leave the patient unattended.

From Niedzwiecki B, et al: *Kinn's the medical assistant,* ed 14, St. Louis, 2020, Elsevier.

Some medical conditions can cause the patient to faint during the venipuncture procedure. It is important to listen to patients when they say they faint with the procedure. Be proactive and place the patient in a safe position if fainting will occur. It is best to perform phlebotomy while the patient is lying on an examination table or in a reclining phlebotomy chair. Minimizing the patient's concern or just attributing the fainting to anxiety or distress is not providing patient-centered care and is frustrating for the patient.

As you finish the venipuncture, observe the patient's face, and assess the breathing rate if they seem anxious. Safety comes first. Make sure patients are not in a position in which they can be hurt. According to CLSI, the procedure for a fainting patient or one who is nonresponsive is:

1. If the patient begins to faint, quickly remove the tourniquet and needle from the arm, immediately activate the needle safety device, apply pressure to the site, and dispose of the unit in a biohazardous sharps container to prevent an accidental exposure.
2. Notify staff members for assistance.
3. Lay the patient flat or lower the head if the patient is sitting.
4. Loosen tight clothing.
5. Apply a cold compress or washcloth to the patient's forehead and back of the neck. Do not use ammonia inhalants/capsules because these are associated with adverse effects and are no longer recommended.
6. Stay with the patient until recovery is complete.
7. Document the incident according to facility policies.
8. When patients regain consciousness, they must remain in the facility for at least 15 minutes and should not operate a vehicle for at least 30 minutes.

> **VOCABULARY**
> **lymphostasis** Obstruction or interruption of normal lymph flow.
> **petechiae** Very small, round hemorrhage spots in the skin or mucous membrane.

Specimen Recollection

Sometimes problems with a sample cannot be determined until the specimen is analyzed in the laboratory. Rejected specimens must be recollected. The laboratory may reject a specimen for reasons that include:

- Unlabeled or mislabeled specimen
- Insufficient specimen quantity
- Defective tube
- Incorrect tube used for the test ordered (incorrect stopper color)
- Hemolysis (Table 54.4)
- Clotted blood in an anticoagulated specimen
- Improper handling

Hemolysis is the major cause of specimen rejection. It cannot be detected until the blood cells are separated from the plasma or serum. It is crucial to take steps to prevent red blood cell damage during collection. Hemolyzed serum or plasma appears rosy to bright red because of the release of hemoglobin from the cells. Some routine tests that are adversely affected by hemolysis are chemistry tests for electrolytes (e.g., potassium, sodium), bilirubin (BIL uh roo bin), total protein, and liver enzymes.

CAPILLARY PUNCTURE

Capillaries are connections between arteries and veins, so capillary blood is a mixture of the two. A *capillary puncture,* also called *dermal puncture,* and *fingerstick,* is an efficient means

TABLE 54.4 Major Causes of Hemolysis During Collection

Cause	Explanation	Prevention
Alcohol preparation	Transfer of alcohol into the specimen causes hemolysis.	Allow venipuncture site to dry completely.
Incorrect needle size	A high-gauge needle causes the blood to go through a small lumen with great force, causing hemolysis. A very-low-gauge needle causes a large amount of blood to suddenly enter the tube with great force, causing frothing.	Choose the correct needle for the job, aiming for a 21- to 23-gauge needle. Also angle tube so that blood flows down the side of the tube to prevent frothing and hemolysis.
Loose connections on the vacuum tube assembly	If the connection between the needle holder and the double-pointed needle or the syringe and the needle is loose, air can enter the sample and cause frothing.	Make sure all connections are tight before beginning the venipuncture.
Removing the needle from the vein with the tube intact	The remaining vacuum in the tube can cause air to be drawn forcefully into the tube, causing frothing. Also can indicate a short draw.	Make sure the tube is completely full and then remove the final tube from the needle holder before withdrawing the needle from the patient's vein.
Underfilled tubes	Underfilling tubes leads to an improper blood/additive ratio.	Permit blood to flow into the tubes until no more movement can be seen.
Syringe collections	Pulling back too rapidly on the plunger draws blood too quickly through the needle. This causes hemolysis or the vein to collapse.	Loosen the plunger before use. Use the smallest syringe possible. Gently draw the plunger to withdraw the amount of blood required for testing. When transferring blood into the vacuum tube, use a transfer device. *Never* push on the plunger when transferring blood. Allow blood to flow down the side of the tube.
Mixing tubes too vigorously	All tubes should be gently inverted (see Table 54.3).	Gently invert tubes immediately after the draw. Vigorous mixing can hemolyze cells.
Temperature and transport problems	Trauma and temperature extremes can damage cells. Freezing will cause hemolysis.	Tubes should be transported in the upright position with as little trauma as possible. Control the temperature.
Separation of plasma or serum from red blood cells (RBCs)	Removing the serum/plasma from cells lowers the risk of contaminating the specimen with RBCs and altered test results due to continued metabolism of RBCs.	Blood samples that are centrifuged should have cells and plasma/serum separated as soon as possible.
Prolonged tourniquet time	*Interstitial* (in ter STISH uhl) fluid can leak into the veins and hemolyze RBCs.	Only leave the tourniquet on for up to 1 minute.
Poor collection; blood flowing too slowly into the tube	The needle lumen may be blocked because it is too close to the inner wall of the vein.	Withdraw the needle slightly to center it within the vein.

From Niedzwiecki B, et al: *Kinn's the medical assistant,* ed 14, St. Louis, 2020, Elsevier.

of collecting a blood specimen when only a small amount of blood is needed. Capillary punctures are also used when a patient's condition makes venipuncture difficult, such as in a patient undergoing chemotherapy. Also, capillary punctures are performed on infants (as a heelstick) and some young children. The test requisition may not specify a capillary collection, so be familiar with the advantages, limitations, and appropriate uses of this technique. Capillary puncture is warranted in:

- Elderly patients or pediatric patients (especially younger than age 2)
- Patients who require frequent glucose monitoring
- Patients with burns or scars in venipuncture sites
- Obese patients
- Patients receiving intravenous (IV) therapy or chemotherapy
- Patients who have had a mastectomy
- Patients at risk for venous thrombosis
- Patients who are severely dehydrated
- Tests that require a small volume of blood (i.e., some Clinical Laboratory Improvement Amendments [CLIA]-waived tests)

Small volumes of tissue fluid also are present in capillary blood, especially in the first drop. Analyte levels are usually the same in capillary and venous blood, with a few exceptions. Hemoglobin and glucose values are higher in capillary blood; potassium, calcium, and total protein are higher in venous blood.

> **VOCABULARY**
> **interstitial** Between the cells.

Equipment

Capillary punctures are performed with specialized equipment. A look at the equipment is useful and can help you decide when a capillary puncture should be performed instead of a venipuncture.

Skin Puncture Devices. The device used to perform a dermal puncture is the *lancet*, which delivers a quick puncture to a preset depth (Fig. 54.17). OSHA has directed that lancets must have retractable blades. Safety lancets only puncture once and cannot be reused. Lancets are available as needle lancets and blade lancets. The choice of lancet should follow CLSI standards for

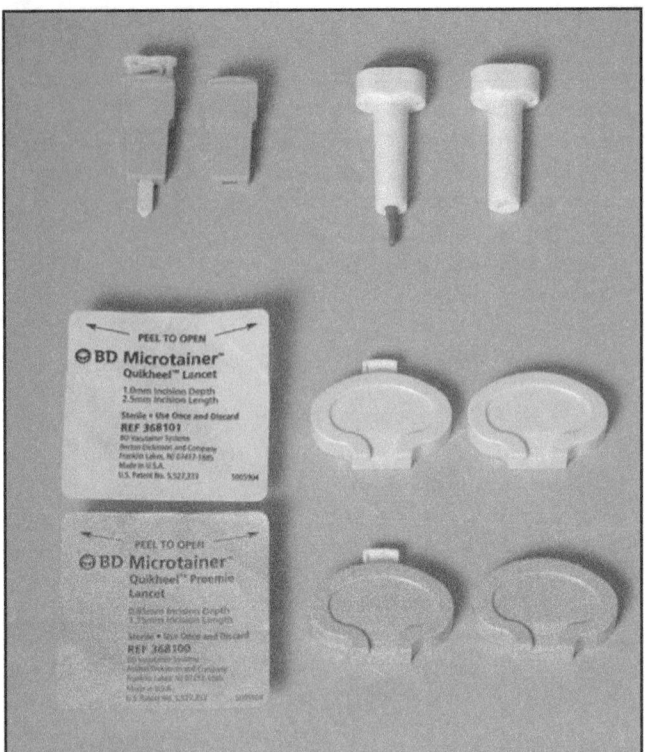

Fig. 54.17 Dermal Puncture Devices. (Courtesy Becton, Dickinson, Franklin Lakes, NJ.)

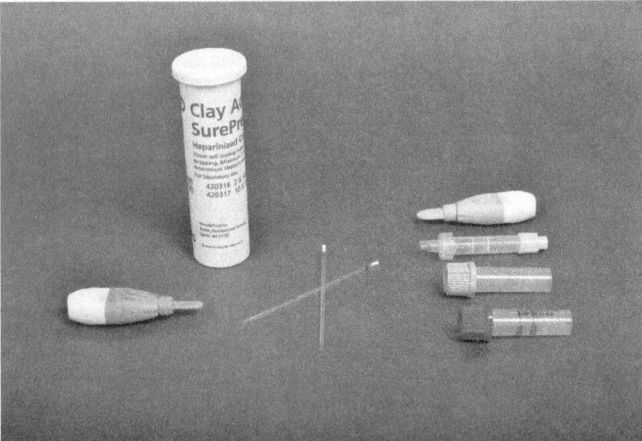

Fig. 54.18 Capillary Collection Containers, Microtainers, and Self-Sealing Microhematocrit Tubes. (From Niedzwiecki B, et al: *Kinn's the medical assistant,* ed 14, St. Louis, 2020, Elsevier.)

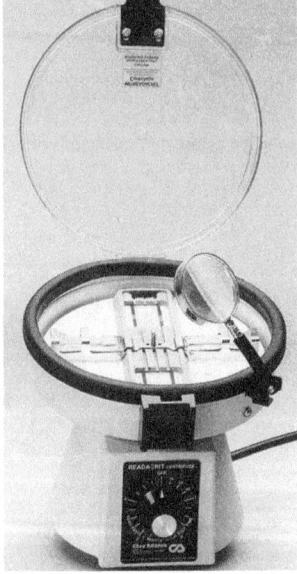

Fig. 54.19 Microhematocrit Centrifuge With Indicators for Capillary Tube Placement. (From Niedzwiecki B, et al: Kinn's *the medical assistant,* ed 14, St. Louis, 2020, Elsevier.)

puncture depth. Lancets should always be discarded in a biohazardous sharps container immediately after use.

Collection Containers. Different types of containers and collection devices are available, and the ones used depend on the test to be performed. The micro collection tubes most often used are Microtainers (MIE kroe TAE ner) (Fig. 54.18); these are available with a variety of anticoagulants and additives. Their color-coded tops indicate the same additives as evacuated tubes. Blood drops are collected into the Microtainers through a funnel-like device or scooplike opening.

Capillary tubes are another type of blood collection tube used to get a capillary sample. The blood is pulled into the tube by *capillary action*; this means that the blood fills these small, narrow tubes without the help of suction. If the capillary tube is coated with the anticoagulant heparin, a red band will be seen at the top of the tube. A common, heparin-coated capillary tube is the microhematocrit tube (Fig. 54.19). To reduce the risk of injury due to breakage of capillary tubes, the National Institute for Occupations Safety and Health (NIOSH), FDA, and OSHA recommend blood collection devices less prone to accidental breakage, such as:

- Plastic capillary tubes
- Glass capillary tubes wrapped in puncture-resistant film
- Self-sealing tubes without the need to push one end into putty to form a plug
- Products that do not require centrifugation to measure the blood hematocrit

Manufacturers often provide collection devices for obtaining small amounts of blood for point-of-care testing (POCT), such as glucose, hemoglobin A_{1C}, and cholesterol. Blood is pulled

into the collecting device by capillary action after the puncture, or it is applied to a reagent strip that has been inserted into the instrument to be analyzed.

Blood from a capillary puncture may also be deposited on paper cards. The Guthrie card (Fig. 54.20) is used to test babies for certain metabolic disorders, such as phenylketonuria (fen l kee toh NOOR ee uh) (PKU). Blood is deposited into circles on biologically inactive filter paper and is sent to a referral laboratory for analysis within 24 hours of sampling. Federal postal regulations for the mailing of biohazardous material must be followed.

VOCABULARY

suction The production of a partial vacuum by the removal of air to force fluid into a vacant space.

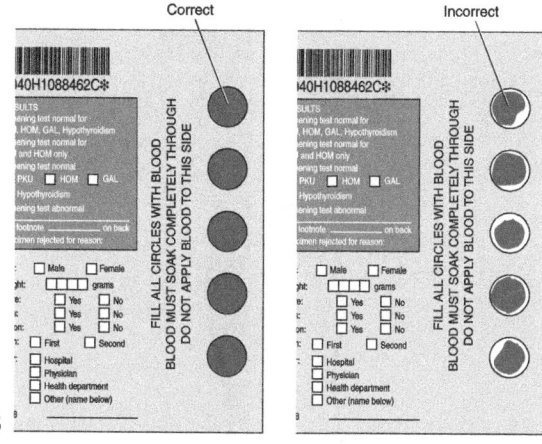

Fig. 54.20 A, Guthrie card used in neonatal screening. B, Correctly and incorrectly filled cards. (From Warekois RS, Robinson R, Primrose, P: *Phlebotomy: work text and procedures manual*, ed 5, St. Louis, 2020, Elsevier.)

ROUTINE CAPILLARY PUNCTURE

Site Selection

In adults and children (over 1 year old), capillary puncture sites include the ring or middle finger. The thumb usually is too callused, and the index finger has sensitive nerve endings that make the puncture more painful. The fifth finger (pinky finger) has too little tissue for a successful puncture.

Dermal puncture of an infant should be done on the heel of the foot (Fig. 54.21, Fig. 54.22, and Fig. 54.23). A capillary puncture is made on the palmar surface of the finger, near the tip and slightly to the side of the finger. Punctures should be made across the whorls of the finger. This helps to create a nice drop of blood to collect. Avoid areas that are callused, scarred, burned, infected, cyanotic, or edematous.

For children younger than 2 years of age, dermal puncture is performed on the medial or lateral areas of the *plantar* (PLAN ter) *surface* (bottom) of the heel or on the *palmar* (PAHL mer) *surface* of the ring or middle finger. Areas other than these are unsafe because bone or nerve damage to an infant may occur. Blood flow from an infant's heel can be increased by applying a warm, moist towel (or other warming device) at a temperature no higher than 108°F (42°C) for 3 to 5 minutes. Never place

bandages on the heel or anywhere on infants younger than age 2, because they may peel off and become a choking hazard.

MEDICAL TERMINOLOGY	
capillar/o	capillary, tiniest blood vessels
derm/o	skin
hem/o, hemat/o	blood
plant/o	sole of the foot
palm/o	anterior surface of the hand
thromb/o	clot
inter-	between
-oma	mass, fluid collection, tumor
-rrhage	bursting forth (of blood)
-sis	state of or condition
-stitial	pertaining to standing or positioned, to set

Patient Preparation

Preparation for a capillary puncture is similar to that for a venipuncture. Put on a fluid-impermeable lab coat, wash your hands or use hand sanitizer, and put on gloves and protective eyewear. If the patient's hands are excessively soiled, ask the person to wash them before the procedure. If the patient's hands are cold, warm them in warm water and dry them thoroughly, or ask the person to rub or shake them vigorously. You may also use a warming device to warm the hand and fingers. Cleanse the finger well with a 70% alcohol wipe.

You must work very efficiently when performing a capillary puncture because blood flow stops quickly. Be sure to have the supplies organized and within easy reach. Press the lancet firmly against the skin and quickly depress the plunger.

Collecting the Specimen

After the skin has been punctured, it is important to wipe away the first drop of blood with gauze. This drop contains tissue fluid that could interfere with test results. Fill the sampling containers according to the manufacturer's directions. Touch the container to the drop of blood as it is released from the puncture site, but do not touch the skin. Tap the container gently to move blood to the bottom of the Microtainer. Mix periodically during the collection by flicking the bottom of the tube with your finger. If blood flow stops, wiping the site with gauze may restart the flow. Because you are working with blood that is free flowing, make sure there are spare gloves, extra gauze, and disinfectant nearby. Be prepared if your gloves become contaminated with blood. After the containers have been filled, ask the patient to apply pressure to the gauze placed over the puncture site. Seal and mix the containers by gently inverting the tubes as recommended by the manufacturer.

CRITICAL THINKING 54.10

Rosie is performing a capillary puncture on Johnny Parker, who is 7 years old. She is looking at his fingers to choose a site, and his hands are chilly. Which fingers would be the best choice for a child? If Johnny's hands are chilly, what can Rosie do to make sure they warm up?

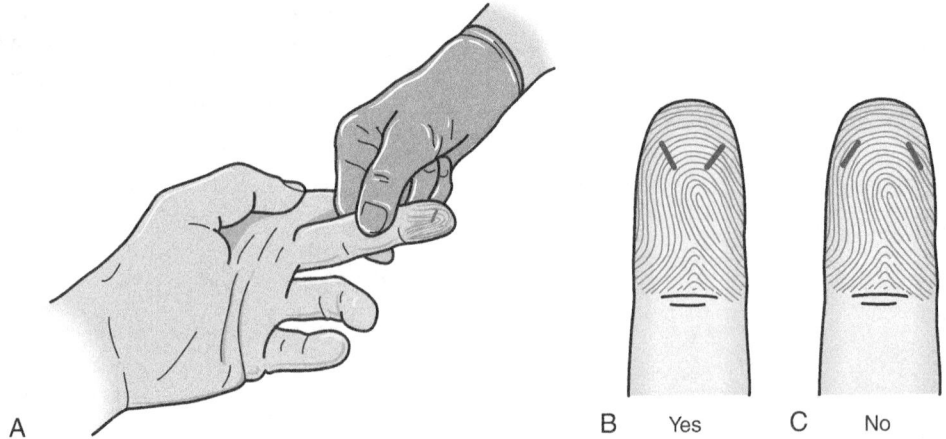

Fig. 54.21 A, A capillary puncture in adults and children is performed on the third (middle) or fourth (ring) finger. B, A capillary puncture is made on the palmar surface of the finger, near the tip and slightly to the side of the finger, perpendicular to the whorls. C, Never puncture in the same direction as the whorls. (From Warekois RS, Robinson R, Primrose, P: *Phlebotomy: work text and procedures manual*, ed 5, St. Louis, 2020, Elsevier.)

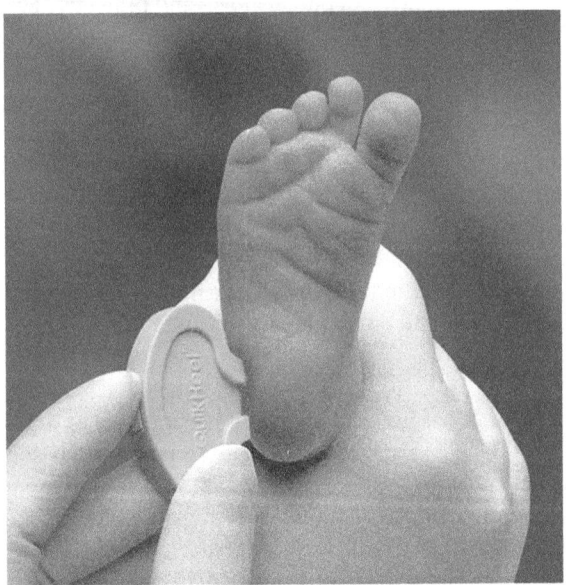

Fig. 54.22 BD Microtainer Quickheel Lancet. (Courtesy Becton, Dickinson and Co.; from Warekois RS, Robinson R, Primrose, P: *Phlebotomy: work text and procedures manual*, ed 5, St. Louis, 2020, Elsevier.)

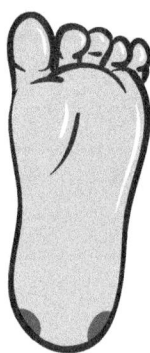

Fig. 54.23 Capillary puncture in infants is performed on the heel, on the medial and lateral borders only. (From Warekois RS, Robinson R, Primrose, P: *Phlebotomy: work text and procedures manual*, ed 5, St. Louis, 2020, Elsevier.)

Specimen Handling

Capillary collection containers are often too small for a label to be applied to the tube. The most efficient way to transport capillary tubes is to remove the stopper from a red-topped venipuncture tube, insert the capillary tubes, sealed-end down, replace the stopper, and label the red-topped tube. Microtainer tubes have plastic plugs that fit over the top. Due to the small size of Microtainer tubes, placement of the label will differ from other tubes. Fold the label across the tube like a flag, as close to the stopper as possible, making sure the volume in the lower part of the tube is visible. Write the date, time of collection, and your initials. Label the specimen in the presence of the patient. The Microtainer may then be placed in a labeled tube or in a labeled zipper-lock bag for transport. Always decontaminate collection

containers before delivering them to the laboratory if blood was deposited on the surface during collection. Procedure 54.4 presents an outline of the process for routine capillary collection.

PEDIATRIC PHLEBOTOMY

Obtaining blood from children and infants may be difficult and potentially hazardous. The procedure should be performed by personnel trained in pediatric phlebotomy. Successfully obtaining blood from children requires skill and an understanding of children and their development. Good communication skills are essential when dealing with children. The phlebotomist must gain the child's trust and often that of the parent or guardian. Parents frequently ask the phlebotomist to explain the tests being done and the reasons for testing. Be respectful when talking to parents. Defer to the provider if questions come up about specific information regarding possible diseases or conditions the child may have.

A parent or guardian may be helpful during phlebotomy. Ask the parent or guardian about the child's previous phlebotomy experiences and how cooperative the child has been in the past. Respectfully determine whether the parent or guardian seems

TABLE 54.5 Childhood Behavior and Parental Involvement During Phlebotomy

Age	Typical Mental State	Suggested Parental Involvement
Newborns (0–12 months)	Trust that adults will respond to their needs.	Parent should assist by cradling and comforting child.
Infants and toddlers (1–3 years)	Minimal fear of danger but fear of separation; limited language and understanding of procedure.	Parent should assist by holding the child and providing emotional support.
Preschoolers (3–6 years)	Fearful of injury to body; still dependent on parent.	Parent may be present to provide emotional support and to assist in obtaining child's cooperation.
School-aged children (7–12 years)	Less dependent on parent and more willing to cooperate; fear of loss of self-control (crying).	Child may not want parent present.
Teenagers (13–18 years)	Fully engaged in the process; embarrassed to show fear and may show hostility to cover emotions.	Teen may not want parent present.

From Niedzwiecki B, et al: *Kinn's the medical assistant,* ed 14, St. Louis, 2020, Elsevier.

comfortable assisting in restraint of an uncooperative child. Parental behavior greatly influences the child's behavior during the procedure. Children should never be restrained in a way that might cause physical injury or pain. If the parent or guardian is unable or unwilling to assist with the procedure, always refer to the office or laboratory policy on procedural holds for phlebotomy. Table 54.5 provides information on the typical fears and concerns of children during the procedure and suggested parental involvement.

Removing large amounts of blood, especially from premature infants, may result in anemia (Table 54.6). The amount of blood withdrawn must be recorded in the child's chart. Puncturing deep veins in children may result in cardiac arrest, hemorrhage, venous thrombosis, damage to the surrounding tissues, and infection.

In addition, the child could be harmed during restraint. To prevent these problems, blood should be collected only by dermal puncture from children younger than age 2 unless the procedure warrants venous collection (lead levels or blood culture). Venipuncture on children younger than age 2 should be performed only on surface veins, including the dorsal hand vein, using a 23-gauge winged infusion set coupled to a syringe or a pediatric vacuum tube collection set.

When the medical assistant is required to perform pediatric phlebotomy, remember to:
- Wear a colorful, fluid-impermeable jacket lab coat if possible
- Be truthful about the discomfort the child will feel
- Provide tokens and praise for bravery
- Try to lessen the child's fears

Topical anesthetics (e.g., ethyl chloride [EC] spray or EMLA cream) may be used to reduce pain at the puncture site. In most cases a calm, professional phlebotomist who understands children and relates to them on their level can gain the trust needed. Work to perform a successful venipuncture or capillary puncture with a minimum of restraint and frustration.

HANDLING THE SPECIMEN AFTER COLLECTION

The results of laboratory testing are only as good as the specimen sent for testing. Specimens handled improperly after collection may provide incorrect results. They may even

TABLE 54.6 General Guidelines for Pediatric Venipuncture

Weight (lb)	Single Draw Limit
8–10	3.5 mL
11–15	5 mL
16–40	10 mL
41–60	20 mL
61–65	25 mL
66–80	30 mL

From Niedzwiecki B, et al: *Kinn's the medical assistant,* ed 14, St. Louis, 2020, Elsevier.

compromise the patient's health. From the moment a specimen is collected, analytes in the blood begin to break down. By testing specimens as soon as possible, the laboratory tries to provide results that accurately represent the patient's condition at the time of blood collection. After collection, blood may need to be processed before the sample is tested. This may include separation of plasma or serum from the red blood cells. If the venipuncture tube contains no anticoagulant (i.e., tubes with a red, a marbled red-gray, or a gold stopper), blood starts the clotting process when it touches the tube. The "clot" tubes should sit upright in a rack for 30 to 60 minutes at room temperature while a solid clot forms. Tubes with clot accelerator should form a dense clot within 30 minutes. The presence of anticoagulants in the patient's blood, such as warfarin (Coumadin) or heparin, may delay clotting. Once the clot has formed, every effort should be made to remove the clot from the serum within 2 hours.

Removing the serum from a clot tube requires centrifugation. For thixotropic gel to form a barrier between the clot and the serum, certain requirements must be met. The tube must be centrifuged at a specified g-force, time, and temperature. A clinical centrifuge instruction manual should provide the appropriate settings for spinning blood specimens. The serum does not have to be removed from the tube after centrifugation because the gel has formed a barrier over the red blood cells. Once a tube with thixotropic gel has been centrifuged, it cannot be centrifuged again. The serum, however, can be decanted and centrifuged in another tube.

For tests that require plasma, the plasma should be removed from the cells as soon as possible. This can be done by centrifuging the tube and then aspirating the plasma off the cells using a transfer pipet. The plasma is then dispensed from the transfer pipet into another, properly labeled tube. You can also use a plasma separator tube with a marbled green-gray top or a PST with a light green top. Both contain lithium heparin anticoagulant and a thixotropic gel, which forms the necessary barrier when centrifuged and eliminates the need to transfer plasma to another tube.

Certain blood tests, such as a CBC, require whole blood. It is wise to check the specimen requirements of the laboratory that will perform the test and follow their instructions for transport and storage. The College of American Pathologists (CAP) recommends that whole blood for automated blood counts be refrigerated and tested within 72 hours.

Often specimens must be transported by courier to other facilities. The Hazardous Materials Shipping Regulations, established by the Department of Transportation, apply to the packaging and shipping of hazardous materials by ground transportation. POLs that ship human specimens must be trained to properly handle, pack, and ship biohazardous materials. Reference labs will frequently have couriers pick up specimens. The specimens and their requisitions are typically placed in individual biohazard bags and sorted according to which reference lab is affiliated with the patient's insurance.

VOCABULARY

aspirating Drawing off or removing by suction.
g-force A force acting on an object because of gravity. Example: A centrifuge spins and exerts g-force.

Chain of Custody

Blood samples may be collected as evidence in legal proceedings. Blood may be drawn for drug and alcohol testing, DNA analysis, or paternity testing. These samples must be handled according to special procedures to prevent tampering, misidentification, or interference with the test results.

Chain of custody is a legal term that refers to the ability to guarantee the identity and integrity of the specimen from collection to reporting of test results. It is a process used to maintain and document the history of a specimen. Documentation should include:

- Name or initials of the individual collecting the specimen
- Signature of each person who tests or transports the specimen
- Date and time the specimen was collected or transferred
- Employer or agency
- Specimen number and the patient's or employee's name
- Brief description of the specimen.

Collection kits are available that contain everything needed for the venipuncture, including the tube, the needle, the chain of custody forms and seals, the antiseptic, and even the tourniquet. Familiarize yourself with these kits before using them. Phlebotomists may be required to testify at legal proceedings if they are involved in the collection or testing of a legal sample.

▌CLOSING COMMENTS

Phlebotomy is an invasive procedure in which a sterile needle or lancet is inserted through the skin. When a venipuncture is performed, the rules and regulations must be obeyed with no exceptions. Be sure to follow the written procedures in the laboratory. Become familiar with the regulations and standards established by CLSI and OSHA and by state and local agencies. Deviations from the standards leave the medical assistant open to malpractice. Document any situations in which the standard of care comes into question.

PATIENT-CENTERED CARE

Provide as much explanation as needed to ease the patient's anxiety. Often the patient can help by identifying the site of the last successful blood venipuncture. Follow the patient's suggestion in choosing the site for obtaining a blood specimen. When patients become active participants in the procedure, they remain more relaxed, talkative, and confident in your expertise as a phlebotomist. It is important for the medical assistant to be aware of the patient's concern (Procedure 54.5).

BEING PROFESSIONAL

Role-play the following scenario with a fellow student: An EDTA tube filled with blood is found unlabeled on the counter. You check the log to see who had blood draws today, the tests performed in the POL, and those that are waiting for the courier to take to the reference lab. You have identified the person who is missing a labeled purple-stoppered tube. You talk with your friend, who is also a phlebotomist. What is your next step?

▌CHAPTER REVIEW

In this chapter we covered phlebotomy and the importance of proper technique, safety measures, collection equipment, specimen labeling, and specimen handling.

We started out with a brief overview of a venipuncture. We then discussed personal protective equipment and the role it plays in phlebotomy. When a healthcare worker is using a sharp and has the possibility of blood exposure, PPE is an important part of the procedure. Staying safe and protecting the patient are critical. Necessary PPE for venipunctures and capillary punctures includes gloves, a fluid-impermeable lab coat, and protective eyewear.

We also covered information about tourniquets: proper placement on the arm and how to tie a one-handed release tourniquet. The use of antiseptics was also discussed as it refers to phlebotomy. Most procedures use 70% isopropyl alcohol wipes, but blood cultures require additional antiseptic procedures.

Evacuated collection tubes and the additives they contain were discussed in detail. Each evacuated collection tube has a colored stopper. The stopper color indicates which additive, if any, has been put into the tube. Table 54.1 lists the different stopper colors, anticoagulants and other additives in the tubes, and laboratory uses for each colored tube.

Once we had discussed the types of anticoagulants and additives in venipuncture collection tubes, we discussed the order of the draw. Collection tubes are not filled in a random order. Their collection order is important so that there is no cross-contamination between tubes. This ensures the best specimen possible, with no carryover from one tube to another.

We talked about the different types of needles used in phlebotomy, in addition to the length and lumen size (or gauge) and needle holders. We learned about the different equipment available for delicate or more difficult draws, such as a syringe and a winged infusion set (butterfly assembly).

Needlestick safety and postexposure follow-up are important when you work with sharps on a regular basis. Safety should always be in the forefront of the medical assistant's mind, but if a needlestick occurs, it is important to know what to do.

We went through the procedural steps for a routine venipuncture, syringe venipuncture, and butterfly assembly venipuncture. Using different equipment requires different skills. Patient preparation, work area preparation, and performing and completing a venipuncture have many steps in common. We covered common problems associated with venipunctures.

Understanding what can go wrong and why, hopefully will give you insight into how to prevent problems. Common patient problems include hematoma formation, nerve damage, and fainting. Common specimen problems include hemolyzed blood, short samples, and improperly labeled tubes. When specimens are not acceptable, recollection may be necessary.

Another phlebotomy procedure we talked about is the capillary puncture. The equipment used for capillary puncture is different. The puncture device used for dermal puncture is a lancet. Collection tubes are called *Microtainer tubes* and *microhematocrit tubes*. Capillary punctures should be performed on the ring or middle finger on the palmar surface of the distal end of the finger. Patient preparation, collecting the specimen, and specimen handling are all part of a complete capillary procedure.

The pediatric phlebotomy technique is just a bit different from an adult phlebotomy, but the communication skills component is important. Knowing how to interact with children and gain their trust is a significant aspect of pediatric phlebotomy.

Handling venipuncture specimens after collection and properly directing specimens to laboratory departments or to a referral laboratory complete the process of phlebotomy. For any legal specimens, chain of custody documentation needs to be strictly followed.

Phlebotomy is a vital part of the laboratory. Phlebotomy that is done correctly and with compassion for the patient is a great benefit to the laboratory. Proper specimen collection, labeling, processing, and handling all add up to an efficiently functioning laboratory. Patient satisfaction and trust increase with kind and respectful laboratory contact. Phlebotomy can be a very rewarding area of the clinical laboratory.

SCENARIO WRAP-UP

Rosie has had a busy morning in the phlebotomy area! She likes it when it is busy—the morning seems to fly by. After the morning rush, Rosie restocks a few supplies and then is ready to sit down and take her lunch break. As she relaxes in the lunchroom for a few minutes, she thinks back on the morning with satisfaction. She helped a number of patients today. Norma Washington was in, and she is in her fourth week of chemotherapy. She was nervous about today's venipuncture. Rosie calmed her fears and was able to do a capillary puncture instead of a venipuncture. That made Norma's day! Every patient who came into the phlebotomy area this morning left with a smile.

PROCEDURE 54.1   Perform a Venipuncture: Collect a Venous Blood Sample Using the Vacuum Tube Method

Task
To collect a venous blood specimen by the vacuum tube technique.

Equipment and Supplies
- Patient's health record
- Provider's order and/or lab requisition
- Vacuum tube needle, needle holder, and proper tubes for requested tests
- 70% isopropyl alcohol wipes
- Gauze
- Nonlatex tourniquet
- Hypoallergenic self-stick wrap, tape, or bandage
- Permanent marking pen and/or printed labels
- Fluid-impermeable lab coat, protective eyewear, and gloves
- Biohazardous waste container
- Biohazardous sharps container

Procedural Steps
1. Check the provider's order and/or requisition form to determine the tests ordered. Gather the appropriate tubes and supplies. Put on a fluid-impermeable lab coat.
   Purpose: Each test requires a specific tube color that is indicated on the requisition. Putting on a lab coat is part of ongoing infection control.
2. Greet the patient. Identify yourself. Verify the patient's identity with full name; ask the patient to spell the first and last name and to give his or her date of birth. Explain the procedure to be performed in a manner that is understood by the patient. Answer any questions the patient may have on the procedure.
   Purpose: It is important to identify the patient in two different ways to ensure that you have the correct patient. It is important to identify the patient in two different ways to ensure that you have the correct patient. Explaining the procedure can make the patient feel more comfortable and helps to reduce anxiety.
3. Obtain permission for the venipuncture. Ask patients if they have a latex allergy.
   Purpose: According to CLSI standards, patients should be asked if they are allergic to latex if using latex products, such as tourniquet and gloves.
4. Wash your hands or use hand sanitizer, then put on gloves and protective eyewear.
   Purpose: To ensure infection control.
5. Have the patient sit with the arm well supported in a slightly downward position. Ask patients if they have a preference regarding which arm is used for the venipuncture.
   Purpose: The veins of the antecubital area are more easily located when the elbow is straight. Asking about a patient preference gives the patient a chance to participate in the procedure.
6. Apply the tourniquet around the patient's arm 3 to 4 inches above the elbow on the preferred arm. The tourniquet should never be tied so tightly that it

restricts blood flow in the artery (Fig. 1). Tourniquets should remain in place no longer than 60 seconds.
Purpose: The tourniquet is used to make the veins more prominent.

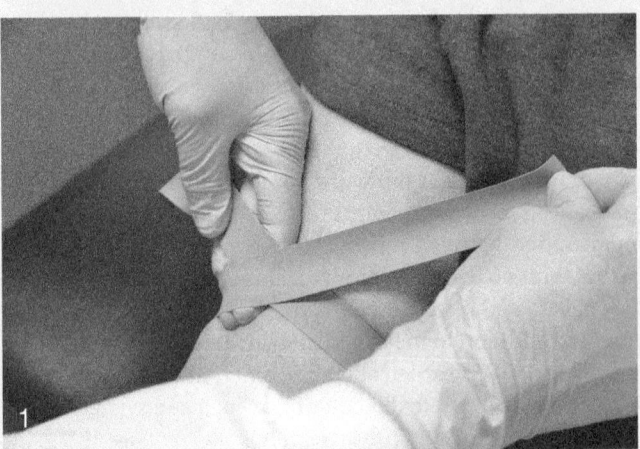

7. Select the venipuncture site by palpating the antecubital space. Use your index finger to trace the path of the vein and to judge its depth, direction, and width. Look at both arms and use your critical thinking skills to find the vein that will give you the greatest chance of success for the venipuncture.
   Purpose: The index finger is most sensitive for palpating the vein. Do not use the thumb because it has a pulse of its own. The veins most often used are the medial or cephalic veins, which lie in the middle of the elbow (Fig. 2).

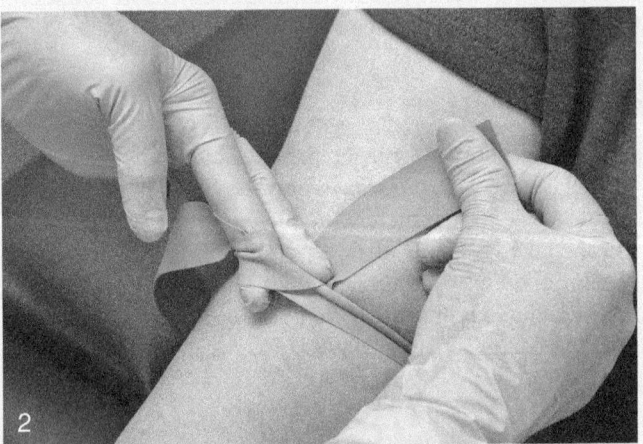

8. Remove the tourniquet and cleanse the site with a 70% alcohol wipe (Fig. 3).
   Purpose: The tourniquet should only be tied for 60 seconds.

PROCEDURE 54.1 Perform a Venipuncture: Collect a Venous Blood Sample Using the Vacuum Tube Method—cont'd

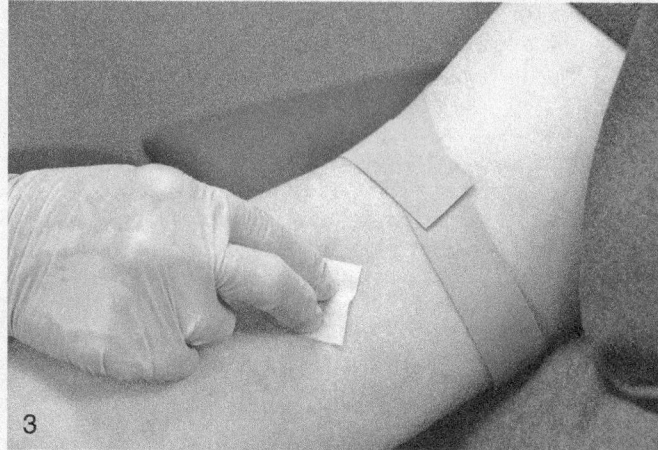

3

9. Assemble the equipment and supplies near your nondominant hand, next to the patient's arm for easy access during the procedure. Select an appropriate needle size and method of collection based on your inspection of the patient's veins. Attach the needle firmly to the vacuum tube holder. Keep the cover on the needle.

Purpose: If the needle is loose, it may turn during the procedure, causing the bevel of the needle to turn away from its upward position.

10. Reapply the tourniquet when the alcohol is dry.

Purpose: Puncturing an area that is still wet with alcohol stings and can cause hemolysis of the sample.

11. Hold the vacuum tube assembly in your dominant hand. Your thumb should be on top and your fingertips underneath (Fig. 4). You may want to lay the first tube to be drawn in the needle holder, but do not push it onto the double-pointed needle. Remove the needle sheath.

Purpose: Positioning the hand in this manner provides the best visibility of the needle entering the vein and accessibility to insert and withdraw tubes with the nondominant hand. Pushing the tube into the double-pointed needle before it is in the arm causes air to rush into the tube, destroying the vacuum.

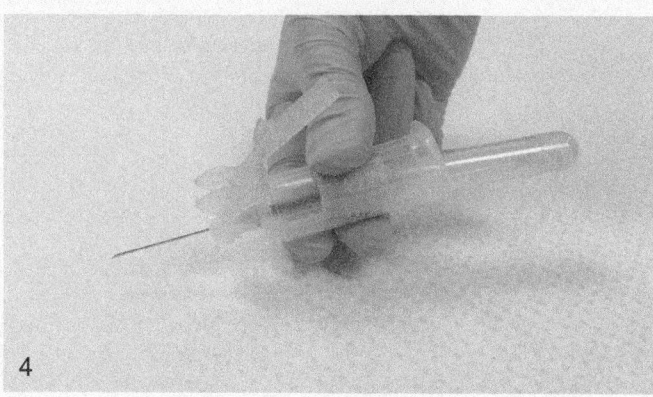

4

12. Grasp the patient's arm with the nondominant hand. Anchor the vein by gently stretching the skin downward below the collection site with the thumb of the nondominant hand.

Purpose: Failure to anchor the vein may cause the vein to move away from the needle as it enters the arm.

13. With the bevel up and the needle aligned parallel to the vein, insert the needle at a 15- to 20-degree angle through the skin and into the vein with a quick but smooth motion (Fig. 5).

Purpose: The sharpest point of the needle is inserted first. Inserting the needle quickly minimizes pain.

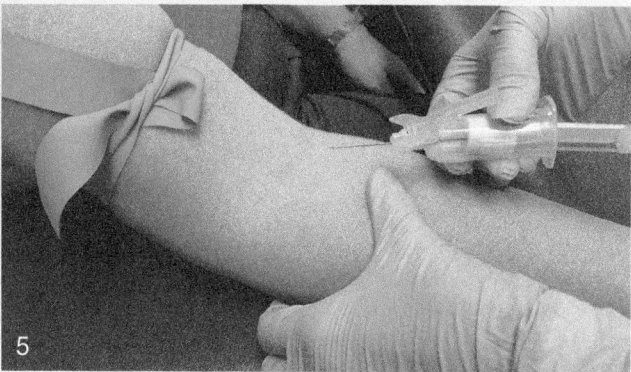

5

14. Hold the assembly in place and steady through the venipuncture. Steady the device by placing fingers of the dominant hand on the patient's arm. The dominant hand never lets go of the needle assembly once it is in the vein. Do not switch hands.

Purpose: Holding the needle assembly steady will keep the needle from moving in the vein.

15. Place two fingers of the nondominant hand on the flanges of the needle holder. Use the thumb to push the tube onto the double-pointed needle (Fig. 6). Make sure you do not change the needle's position in the vein.

Purpose: The thumb has the strength to push the needle swiftly through the stopper. Be careful and keep the position of the needle steady so it is not pushed farther into the site when the tube is pushed.

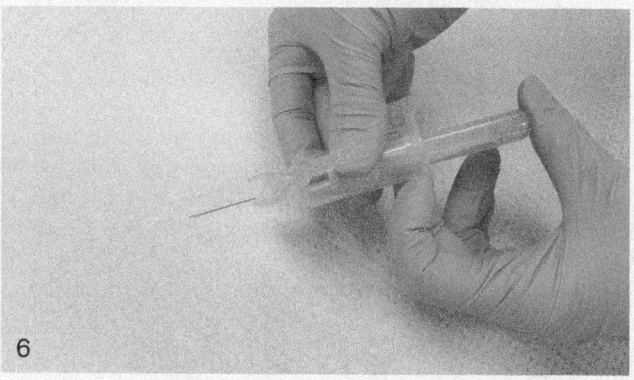

6

16. Allow the tube to fill to its maximum capacity. Remove the tube by placing the fingers at the end of the tube and pushing on the needle holder with the index finger (Fig. 7). Take care not to move the needle when removing the tube. Immediately after removing the tube from the needle holder, gently invert the tube to mix the additives and the blood.

Purpose: Tubes must be full to ensure the proper anticoagulant-to-blood ratio. Moving the needle may result in the needle advancing farther into the vein or slipping out of the vein. Gentle inversion prevents blood from clotting. Do not vigorously mix or shake the tubes, because this may cause hemolysis.

Continued

PROCEDURE 54.1   Perform a Venipuncture: Collect a Venous Blood Sample Using the Vacuum Tube Method—cont'd

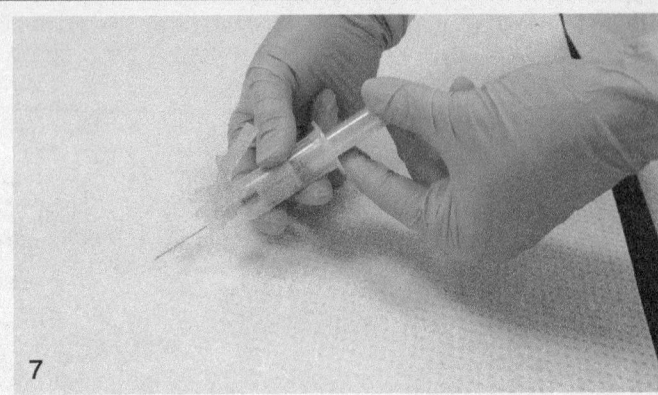

7

17. Insert the second tube into the needle holder, following the instructions in the previous steps. Continue filling tubes until the order on the requisition has been filled. Gently invert each tube after removing it from the needle holder. As the last tube begins filling, release the tourniquet. The tourniquet must be released before the needle is removed from the arm (Fig. 8).
   Purpose: The tourniquet should remain in place for no longer than 1 minute to prevent hemoconcentration.

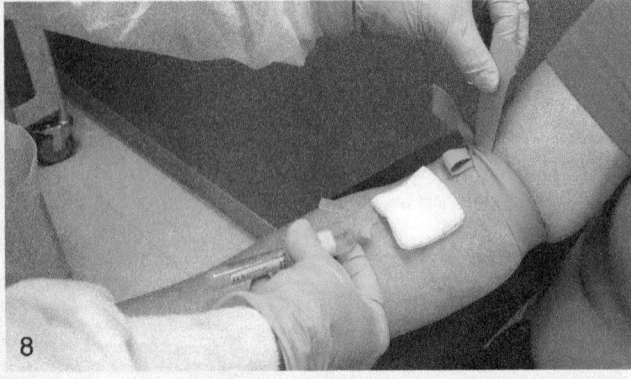

8

18. Remove the last tube from the holder. Place gauze over the puncture site and quickly remove the needle, engaging the safety device (Fig. 9). Dispose of the entire needle/holder assembly into the biohazardous sharps container.
   Purpose: The gauze over the puncture site and activation of the safety needle ensure infection control.

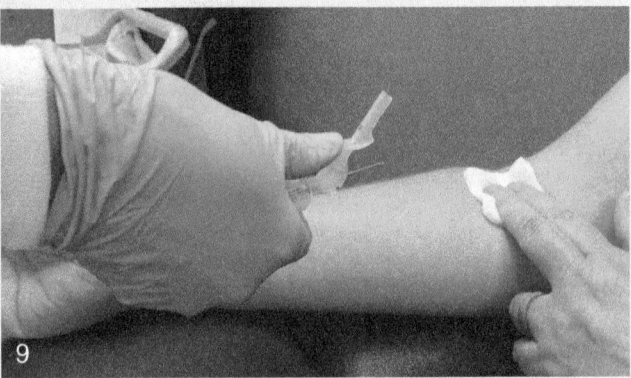

9

19. Apply pressure to the gauze or instruct the patient to do so. The patient may elevate the arm but should not bend the elbow.
   Purpose: Applying direct pressure and elevating the arm above the heart is the best method to stop bleeding.
20. While the patient is applying pressure to the site, label the tubes with the patient's name and the date, time, and your initials, or affix the preprinted tube labels and print your initials on the label.
21. Check the venipuncture site. Make sure bleeding has stopped. Apply a hypoallergenic self-stick wrap, gauze and tape, or bandage (Fig. 10).

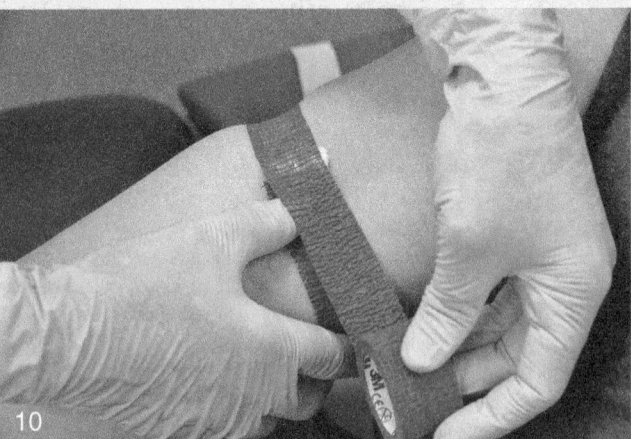

10

22. Disinfect the work area. Dispose of blood-contaminated materials (e.g., gauze and gloves) in the biohazard waste container. Remove your protective eyewear and gloves. Wash hands or use hand sanitizer.
   Purpose: To ensure infection control.
23. Complete the laboratory requisition form and route the specimen to the proper place. Record the procedure in the patient's record.
   Purpose: A procedure is not considered done until it is recorded in the patient record.

Documentation Example

10/05/20XX 1:45 p.m. Venous blood drawn from antecubital space of right arm. Lavender tube for CBC with differential, and red tube for Chemistry. Placed for pickup by Health Alliance Labs._____Rosie Brandt, CMA (AAMA)

PROCEDURE 54.2 Perform a Venipuncture: Collect a Venous Blood Sample Using the Syringe Method

Task
To collect a venous blood specimen using the syringe technique.

Equipment and Supplies
- Patient's health record
- Provider's order and/or lab requisition
- Syringe with 21- or 22-gauge safety needle
- Vacuum tubes appropriate for tests ordered
- 70% isopropyl alcohol wipes
- Gauze
- Nonlatex tourniquet
- Safety transfer device to transfer blood from syringe to vacuum tubes
- Hypoallergenic self-stick wrap, tape, or bandage
- Permanent marking pen or printed labels
- Fluid-impermeable lab coat, protective eyewear, and gloves
- Biohazardous sharps container
- Biohazardous waste container

Procedural Steps
1. Check the provider's order and/or requisition form to determine the tests ordered. Gather the appropriate tubes and supplies. Put on a fluid-impermeable lab coat.
   Purpose: To collect the specimen properly based on the tube requirements on the requisition. Putting on a lab coat is part of ongoing infection control.
2. Greet the patient. Identify yourself. Verify the patient's identity with full name; ask the patient to spell the first and last name and to give his or her date of birth. Explain the procedure to be performed in a manner that is understood by the patient. Answer any questions the patient may have on the procedure.
3. Obtain permission for the venipuncture. Ask patients if they have a latex allergy.
   Purpose: According to CLSI standards, patients should be asked if they are allergic to latex if using latex products, such as tourniquet and gloves.
4. Wash your hands or use hand sanitizer. Put on gloves and protective eyewear.
   Purpose: To ensure infection control.
5. Have the patient sit with the arm well supported in a slightly downward position. Ask patients if they have a preference regarding which arm is used for the venipuncture.
   Purpose: The veins of the antecubital area are more easily located when the elbow is straight. Asking about a patient preference gives the patient a chance to participate in the procedure.
6. Apply the tourniquet around the patient's arm 3 to 4 inches above the elbow on the preferred arm. The tourniquet should never be tied so tightly that it restricts blood flow in the artery (Fig. 1). Tourniquets should remain in place no longer than 60 seconds.
   Purpose: The tourniquet is used to make the veins more prominent.

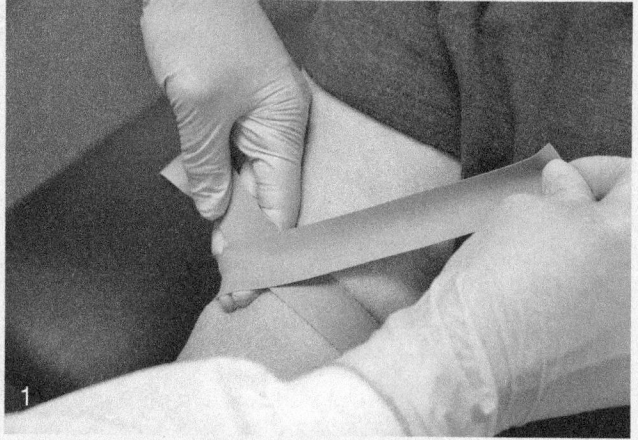

7. Select the venipuncture site by palpating the antecubital space. Use your index finger to trace the path of the vein and to judge its depth. Look at both arms and use your critical thinking skills to find the vein that will give you the greatest chance of success for the venipuncture.
   Purpose: The index finger is most sensitive for palpating the vein. Do not use the thumb because it has a pulse of its own. The veins most often used are the medial or cephalic veins, which lie in the middle of the elbow (Fig. 2).

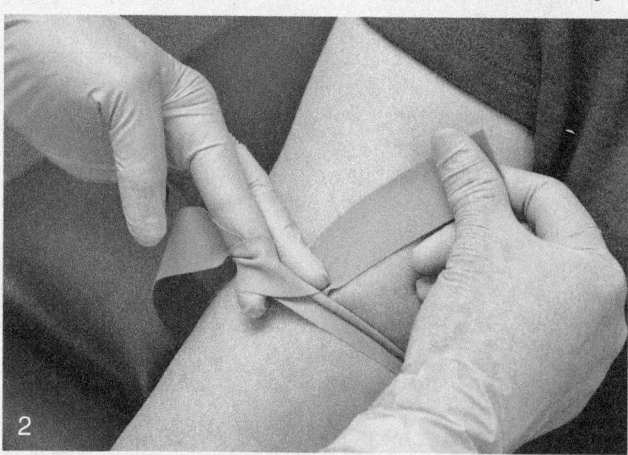

8. Remove the tourniquet and cleanse the site with a 70% alcohol wipe (Fig. 3).
   Purpose: The tourniquet should only be tied for 60 seconds.

Continued

PROCEDURE 54.2   Perform a Venipuncture: Collect a Venous Blood Sample Using the Syringe Method—cont'd

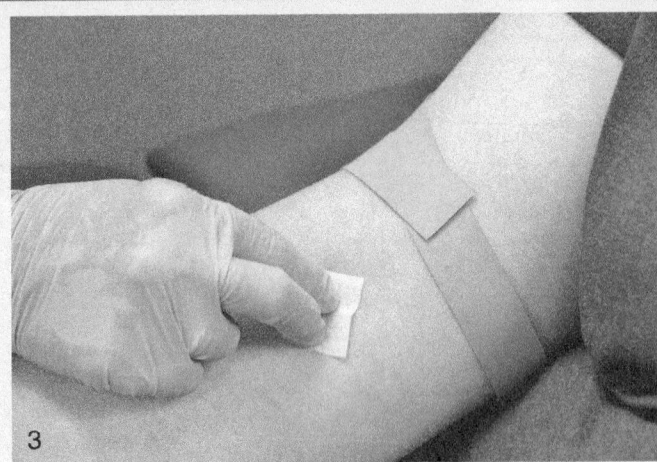

3

9. Assemble the equipment and supplies near your nondominant hand, next to the patient's arm for easy access during the procedure. Use your critical thinking skills to choose the proper syringe barrel size and needle size based on your inspection of the patient's veins.

   Purpose: The proper syringe barrel size and needle size depends on the amount of blood required for the ordered tests and your inspection of the patient's veins. Using the smallest syringe possible minimizes the chance of hemolysis.

10. Attach the needle firmly to the syringe. Pull and depress the plunger several times to loosen it in the barrel while keeping the cover on the needle (Fig. 4). The plunger must be pushed in completely after you have loosened it in the barrel.

    Purpose: Using the smallest syringe possible minimizes the chance of hemolysis. Engaging the plunger ensures that you will not have to use as much force to pull the blood into the barrel, thereby minimizing the chance of hemolysis.

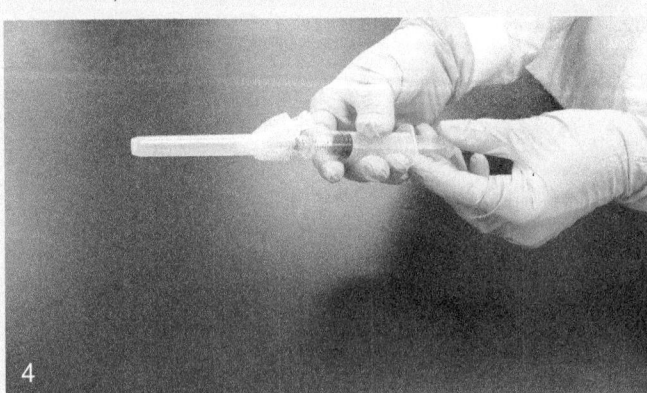

4

11. Reapply the tourniquet when the alcohol is dry.

    Purpose: Puncturing an area that is still wet with alcohol stings and can cause hemolysis of the sample.

12. Hold the syringe in your dominant hand. Your thumb should be on top and your fingers underneath, the same as in the vacuum tube method. Remove the needle sheath.

    Purpose: Positioning the hand in this manner provides the best visibility of the needle entering the vein and accessibility to the syringe plunger.

13. Grasp the patient's arm with the nondominant hand and anchor the vein by stretching the skin downward below the collection site with the thumb of the nondominant hand.

    Purpose: Failure to anchor the vein may cause the vein to move away from the needle when it is inserted, resulting in a missed vein.

14. With the bevel up and the needle aligned parallel to the vein, insert the needle at a 15- to 20-degree angle through the skin and into the vein with a quick but smooth motion (Fig. 5). Observe for a "flash" of blood in the hub of the syringe.

    Purpose: The sharpest point of the needle is inserted first. The angle ensures that the needle does not penetrate through the vein. The appearance (flash) of blood in the hub ensures that the needle is in the vein.

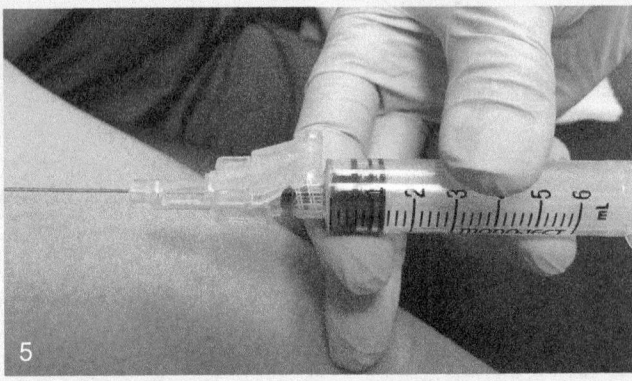

5

15. Slowly pull back the plunger of the syringe with the nondominant hand. Do not allow more than 1 mL of head space between the blood and the top of the plunger. Make sure you do not move the needle after entering the vein. Fill the barrel to the needed volume (Fig. 6).

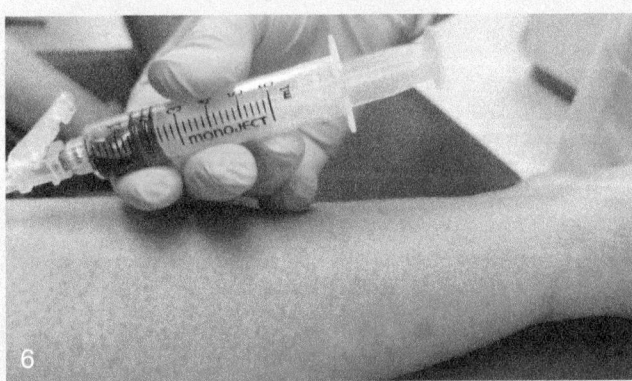

6

16. Release the tourniquet when the proper volume is reached. The tourniquet must be released before the needle is removed from the arm.

    Purpose: Removal of the tourniquet releases pressure on the vein and helps prevent blood from getting into adjacent tissues, causing a hematoma.

17. Place sterile gauze over the puncture site at the time of needle withdrawal. Then, immediately activate the needle safety device using the syringe hand and apply pressure to the site with the nondominant hand.

18. Instruct the patient to apply direct pressure on the puncture site with gauze (Fig. 7). The patient may elevate the arm but should not bend the elbow.

    Purpose: Applying direct pressure and elevating the arm above the heart is the best method to stop bleeding.

PROCEDURE 54.2 Perform a Venipuncture: Collect a Venous Blood Sample Using the Syringe Method—cont'd

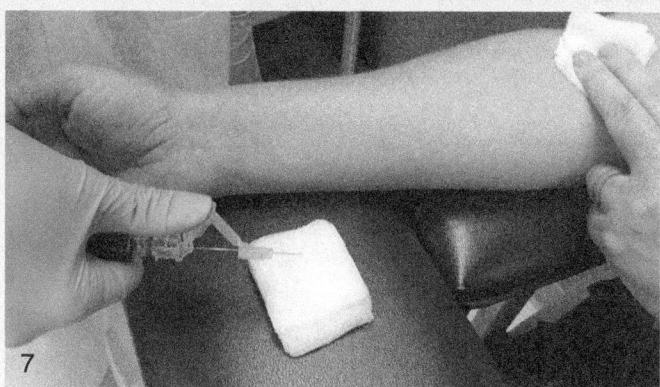

19. Remove the syringe safety needle and transfer the blood immediately to the required tube or tubes using a safety transfer device. Allow blood to freely flow down the side of the tube or tubes using a safety transfer device. Do not push on the syringe plunger during transfer. Discard the entire unit in the biohazardous sharps container when transfer is complete.
20. Gently invert each tube after the addition of blood.
21. Label the tubes with the patient's name and the date, time, and your initials, or affix the preprinted tube labels and print your initials on the label (Fig. 8).
    Purpose: The safety transfer device protects against accidental needlesticks and allows the correct amount of blood to be transferred into the tube by vacuum. Pushing the plunger hemolyzes the blood and may alter the amount of blood intended in each tube. Blood begins to clot shortly after collection, so it must be transferred into the vacuum tube and mixed with anticoagulant immediately after collection. Gently inverting the tubes ensures anticoagulation.

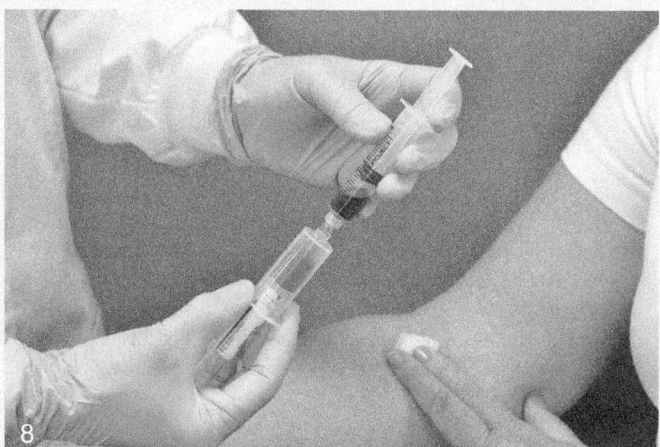

22. Check the venipuncture site. Make sure bleeding has stopped. Apply a hypoallergenic self-stick wrap, gauze and tape, or bandage (Fig. 9).

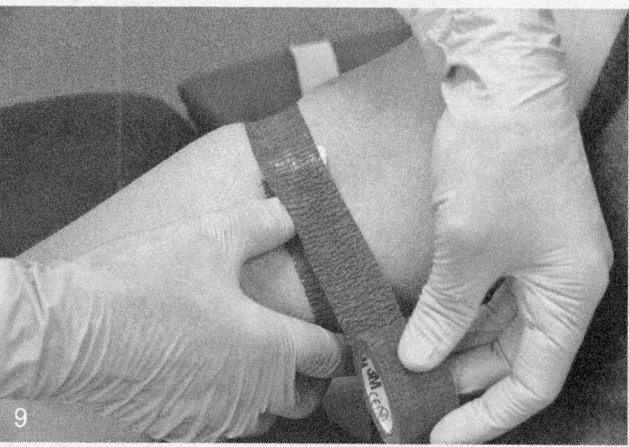

23. Disinfect the work area. Dispose of blood-contaminated materials (e.g., gauze and gloves) in the biohazard waste container. Remove your eyewear and gloves. Wash hands or use hand sanitizer.
    Purpose: To ensure infection control.
24. Complete the laboratory requisition form and route the specimen to the proper place. Record the procedure in the patient's record.
    Purpose: A procedure is not considered complete until it is recorded in the patient's record.

PROCEDURE 54.3 Perform Venipuncture: Obtain a Venous Sample With a Safety Winged Butterfly Needle Assembly

Task

To obtain a venous sample accurately from a hand or an arm vein using a butterfly needle and syringe.

Equipment and Supplies

- Patient's health record
- Provider's order and/or lab requisition
- Safety winged (butterfly) needle set
- Syringe of appropriate volume for testing
- Vacuum tubes appropriate for tests ordered
- 70% isopropyl alcohol wipes
- Gauze
- Nonlatex tourniquet
- Hypoallergenic self-stick wrap, tape, or bandage
- Permanent marking pen or printed labels
- Fluid-impermeable lab coat, protective eyewear, and gloves
- Biohazardous waste container
- Biohazardous sharps container

Procedural Steps

1. Check the provider's order and/or requisition form to determine the tests ordered. Gather the appropriate tubes and supplies. Put on a fluid-impermeable lab coat.

   Purpose: To collect the specimen properly based on the tube requirements on the requisition. Putting on a lab coat is part of ongoing infection control.

2. Greet the patient. Identify yourself. Verify the patient's identity with full name; ask the patient to spell the first and last name and to give his or her date of birth. Explain the procedure to be performed in a manner that is understood by the patient. Answer any questions the patient may have on the procedure.

3. Obtain permission for the venipuncture. Ask patients if they have a latex allergy.

   Purpose: According to CLSI standards, patients should be asked if they are allergic to latex if using latex products, such as tourniquet and gloves.

4. Wash your hands or use hand sanitizer. Put on gloves and protective eyewear.

   Purpose: To ensure infection control.

5. Ask patients if they have a preference which arm is used for the venipuncture. Position the arm correctly.

   - *If drawing from the antecubital region:* Have the patient sit with the arm well supported in a slightly downward position.
   - *If drawing from the back of the hand:* Have the patient place the venipuncture hand over the other, fisted hand with the fingers lower than the wrist.

   Purpose: Asking about a patient preference gives the patient a chance to participate in the procedure. The veins of the antecubital area are more easily located when the elbow is straight. When drawing from the back of the hand, these positions help blood fill the veins in the hand. It also makes it easier for you to identify the veins and choose the draw site.

6. Apply the tourniquet. The tourniquet should never be tied so tightly that it restricts blood flow in the artery. Tourniquets should remain in place no longer than 60 seconds.

- *If drawing from the antecubital region:* Apply the tourniquet around the patient's arm 3 to 4 inches above the elbow on the preferred arm.
- *If drawing from the back of the hand:* Apply the tourniquet above the wrist just proximal to the wrist bone (Fig. 1).

Purpose: The tourniquet is used to make the veins more prominent.

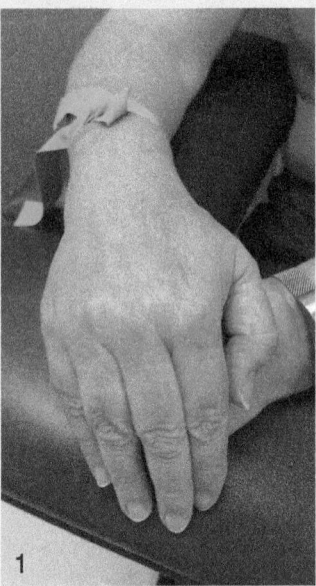

1

7. Select the venipuncture site. Use your index finger to trace the path of the vein and to judge its depth. Look at both arms/hands and use your critical thinking skills to find the vein that will give you the greatest chance of success for the venipuncture.

   - *If drawing from the antecubital region:* Select the venipuncture site by palpating the antecubital space.
   - *If drawing from the back of the hand:* Select a vein on the back of the hand that is prominent, stable, and as straight as possible.

   Purpose: The index finger is most sensitive for palpating the vein. Do not use the thumb because it has a pulse of its own. The veins most often used are the medial or cephalic veins, which lie in the middle of the elbow. Spend time to properly locate the best vein available.

8. Remove the tourniquet and cleanse the site with a 70% alcohol wipe.

   Purpose: The tourniquet should only be tied for 60 seconds.

9. Assemble your equipment and supplies on the nondominant side of the patient's arm. Remove the butterfly device from the package and stretch the tubing slightly. Take care not to activate the needle-retracting safety device accidentally.

   Purpose: To keep the butterfly tubing from recoiling.

10. Attach the butterfly device firmly to the syringe (Fig. 2) or vacuum tube holder. Keep the cover on the needle.

    - *If using a syringe:* Make sure to loosen the plunger a few times after the butterfly and syringe are attached.
    - *If using a vacuum tube holder:* Lay the first tube in the vacuum tube holder and place the unit carefully where it will not roll away.

    Note: When a vein on the back of the hand is used for the draw, a butterfly-syringe combination is almost always used.

PROCEDURE 54.3 Perform Venipuncture: Obtain a Venous Sample With a Safety Winged Butterfly Needle Assembly—cont'd

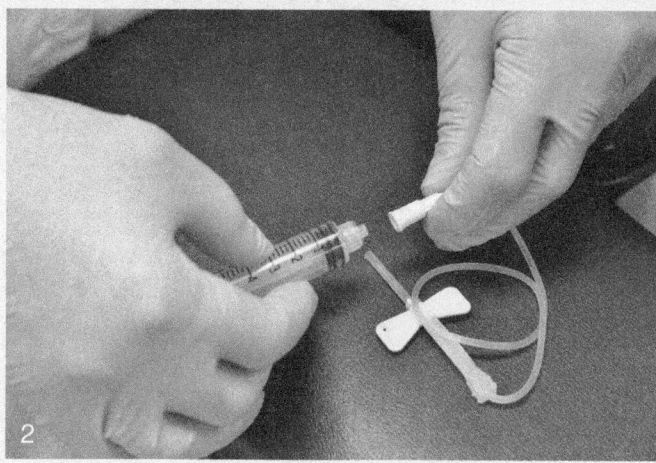

2

11. Reapply the tourniquet when the alcohol is dry.
    Purpose: Puncturing an area that is still wet with alcohol stings and can cause hemolysis of the sample.
12. Hold the butterfly wings pinched between your dominant hand thumb and index finger or hold the base of the needle (Figs. 3-4). Remove the needle sheath.
    Purpose: Positioning the hand in this manner provides the best visibility of the needle entering the vein and accessibility to insert and withdraw tubes with the nondominant hand.

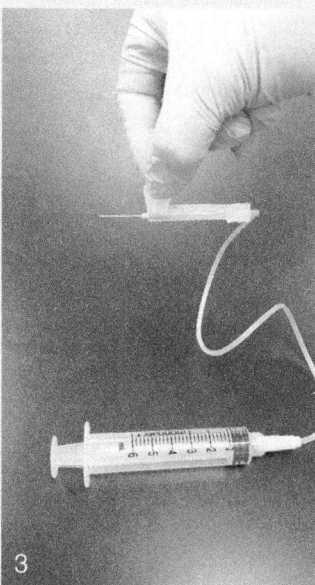

3

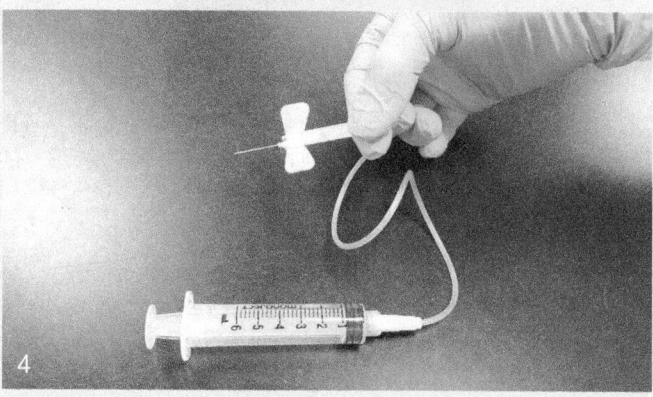

4

13. Anchor the vein with your nondominant hand.
    • *If drawing the antecubital region:* Grasp the patient's arm with the non-dominant hand and anchor the vein by stretching the skin downward below the collection site with the thumb.
    • *If drawing from the back of the hand:* Using your thumb, pull the patient's skin taut over the knuckles.
    Purpose: Failure to anchor the vein may cause the vein to move away from the needle when it is inserted, resulting in a missed vein. Stretching the skin prevents the veins from rolling underneath.
14. With the bevel up and the needle aligned parallel to the vein, insert the needle at a 10- to 15-degree angle through the skin and into the vein with a quick but smooth motion (Fig. 5). The wings should be held in place to keep the needle from moving until the butterfly needle is removed. Make sure the safety device is not activated.
    Purpose: The sharpest point of the needle is inserted first. The angle ensures that the needle does not penetrate through the vein. According to CLSI, after insertion of the needle, the wings should be held in place to keep the needle from moving until the butterfly needle is removed.

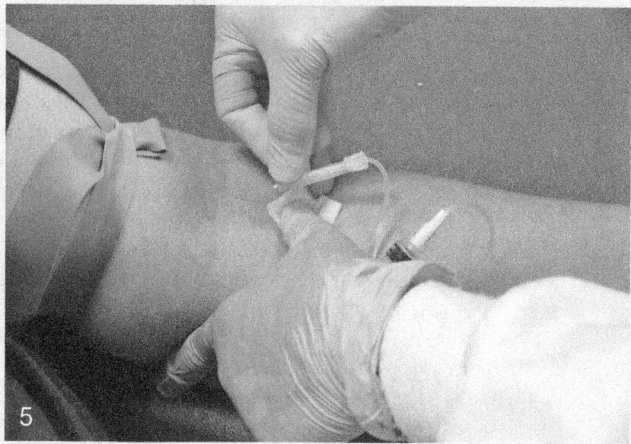

5

15. Start to withdraw the blood.
    • *If drawing with a needle holder assembly:* Push the blood collecting tube into the end of the holder with your nondominant hand.
    • *If drawing with a syringe:* Make sure the vacuum you create is slow and steady and that no more than 1 mL of head space exists between the blood and the plunger. Slowly pull back the plunger of the syringe with the nondominant hand. Fill the barrel of the syringe to the needed volume (Fig. 6).
    Purpose: Drawing blood too forcefully into the syringe may collapse the vein or hemolyze the blood.

PROCEDURE 54.3   Perform Venipuncture: Obtain a Venous Sample With a Safety Winged Butterfly Needle Assembly—cont'd

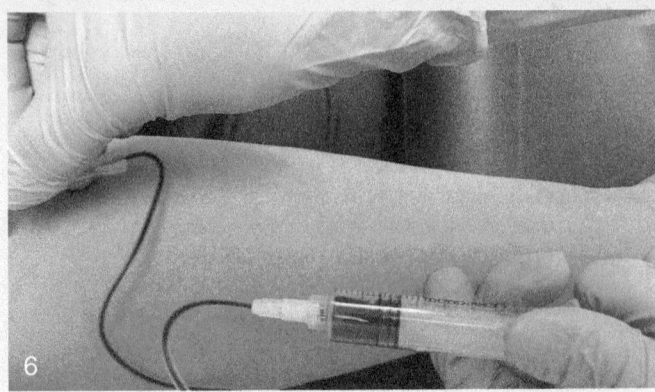

unit in the sharps container when transfer is complete. Gently invert each tube after the addition of blood.

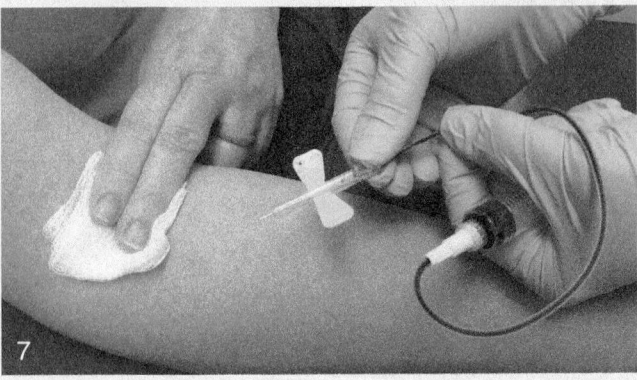

16. Always keep the tube and the holder in a downward position so that the tube fills from the bottom up. Release the tourniquet when the last tube begins to fill, or the syringe is almost to required blood volume for the draw.
    Purpose: To prevent hemoconcentration, the tourniquet should remain in place no longer than 1 minute.
17. Depending on the type of equipment:
    - *If drawing with a needle holder assembly:* Remove the last tube from the holder. Gently invert each tube after removing it from the needle holder. Place gauze over the puncture site and quickly remove the needle, engaging the safety device. Dispose of the entire needle/holder assembly into the sharps container. Apply pressure to the gauze or instruct the patient to do so (Fig. 7). The patient may elevate the arm but should not bend the elbow if the antecubital site was used.
    - *If drawing with a syringe:* Place sterile gauze over the puncture site at the time of needle withdrawal. Then, immediately activate the needle safety device using the syringe hand and apply pressure to the site with the nondominant hand. Instruct the patient to apply direct pressure on the puncture site with gauze. The patient may elevate the arm but should not bend the elbow if the antecubital site was used. Remove the safety needle and transfer the blood immediately. Allow blood to freely flow down the side of the tube or tubes using a safety transfer device. Do not push on the syringe plunger during transfer. Discard the entire

18. While the patient is applying pressure to the site, label the tubes with the patient's name and the date, time, and your initials, or affix the preprinted tube labels and print your initials on the label.
19. Check the venipuncture site. Make sure bleeding has stopped. Apply a hypoallergenic self-stick wrap, gauze and tape, or bandage.
20. Disinfect the work area. Dispose of blood-contaminated materials (e.g., gauze and gloves) in the biohazard waste container. Remove your protective eyewear and gloves. Wash hands or use hand sanitizer.
    Purpose: To ensure infection control.
21. Complete the laboratory requisition form and route the specimen to the proper place. Record the procedure in the patient's record.
    Purpose: A procedure is not considered done until it is recorded in the patient record.

Documentation Example

10/06/20XX 3:24 p.m. Venous blood drawn from antecubital space of ® arm. Lavender tube for CBC with differential, and red tube for Chemistry. Placed for pickup by Health Alliance Labs._____Rosie Brandt, CMA (AAMA)

PROCEDURE 54.4   Perform a Capillary Puncture: Obtain a Blood Sample by Capillary Puncture

Task

To collect a blood specimen suitable for testing using the capillary puncture technique.

Equipment and Supplies

- Patient's health record
- Provider's order and/or lab requisition
- Sterile, disposable safety lancet
- 70% alcohol wipes
- Gauze
- Hypoallergenic self-stick wrap, tape, or bandage
- Fluid-impermeable lab coat, protective eyewear, and gloves
- Appropriate collection containers (e.g., capillary tubes, Microtainer tubes)
- Permanent marking pen or printed labels
- Biohazardous sharps container
- Biohazardous waste container

Procedural Steps

1. Check the provider's order and/or requisition form to determine the tests ordered. Gather the appropriate tubes and supplies. Put on a fluid-impermeable lab coat.
   Purpose: To collect the specimen properly based on the tube requirements on the requisition. Putting on a lab coat is part of ongoing infection control.
2. Greet the patient. Identify yourself. Verify the patient's identity with full name; ask the patient to spell the first and last name and to give his or her date of birth. Explain the procedure to be performed in a manner that is understood by the patient. Answer any questions the patient may have on the procedure.
   Purpose: It is important to identify the patient in two different ways to ensure that you have the correct patient. It is important to identify the patient in two different ways to ensure that you have the correct patient.

PROCEDURE 54.4   Perform a Capillary Puncture: Obtain a Blood Sample by Capillary Puncture—cont'd

Explaining the procedure can make the patient feel more comfortable and helps to reduce anxiety.

3. Obtain permission for the venipuncture. Ask the patient if he or she has a latex allergy.

   Purpose: According to CLSI standards, patients should be asked if they are allergic to latex if using latex products, such as tourniquet and gloves.

4. Wash your hands or use hand sanitizer. Put on gloves and protective eyewear.

   Purpose: To ensure infection control.

5. Select a puncture site, depending on the patient's age and the sample to be obtained (e.g., palmar side of the middle or ring finger of the nondominant hand for an adult or child; medial or lateral curved surface of the plantar surface of heel for an infant).

   Purpose: The nondominant hand may have fewer calluses. The palmar side of the finger is less sensitive, and the skin usually is not as thick. Use great caution when performing capillary puncture on infants (see Fig. 54.21A and B).

6. Gently rub the finger or have your patient wiggle the fingers and open and close the hand.

   Purpose: To promote circulation. If the finger is very cold, you may immerse it in warm water or moisten it with warm towels or use an approved warming device.

7. Once the finger is warm, clean the site with a 70% alcohol pad and allow it to air dry (Fig. 1).

   Purpose: Puncturing skin that is wet with alcohol will sting and can hemolyze the specimen.

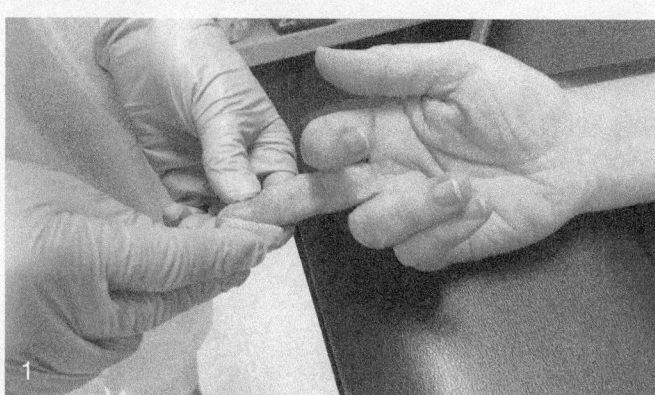

8. Hold onto the patient's finger just under the fleshy pad of the puncture site with your nondominant hand.

   Purpose: Firmly holding the finger allows control of the puncture and will not let the patient pull the hand away.

9. Hold the safety lancet firmly against the fleshy pad of the patient's finger, slightly to the side of the center, perpendicular to the whorls, and press down on the safety trigger that activates the needle or blade to penetrate the skin. The sharp will then automatically retract into the plastic housing of the lancet (Fig. 2).

   Purpose: Lancets are designed to puncture at specific depths that permit the free flow of blood.

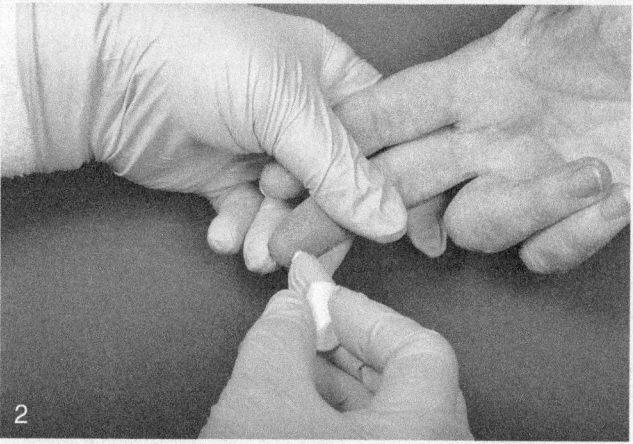

10. Dispose of the lancet in the biohazardous sharps container. Wipe away the first drop of blood with gauze (Fig. 3).

    Purpose: The first drop of blood contains tissue fluid, which may alter test results. If there is any residual alcohol on the finger, it will hemolyze the blood.

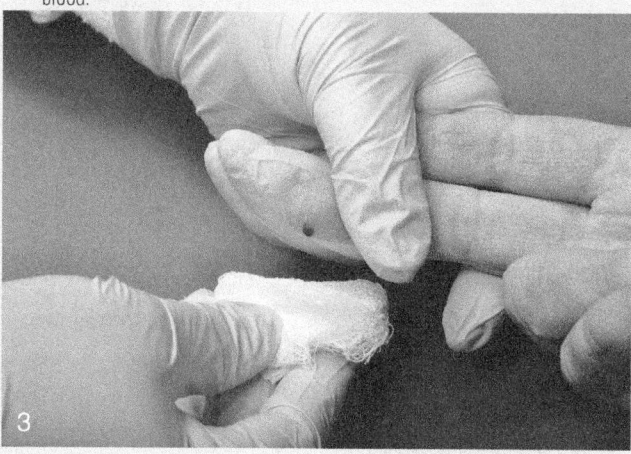

11. Apply gentle, intermittent pressure to cause the blood to flow freely (Fig. 4).

    Purpose: Forceful squeezing liberates fluid that dilutes the blood and causes inaccurate results. *Do not* milk the finger.

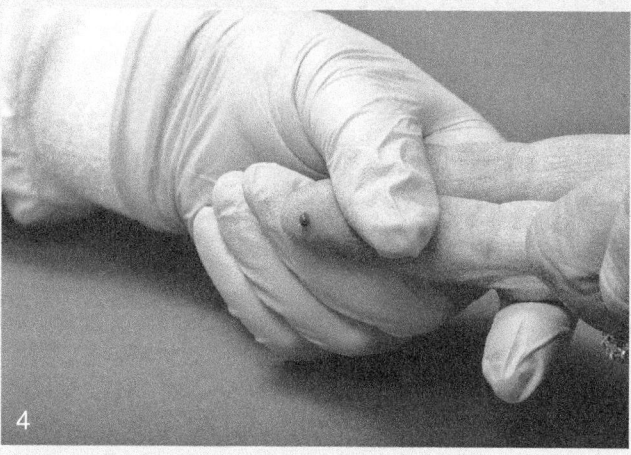

Continued

PROCEDURE 54.4   Perform a Capillary Puncture: Obtain a Blood Sample by Capillary Puncture—cont'd

12. Collect the blood samples. Gently apply pressure and release the finger two or three times to get a large drop of blood. Touch the capillary tube to the drop of blood. *Do not* scoop blood from the finger's surface. Fill the capillary to approximately three-fourths full or to the indicated line (Fig. 5). Then tip the tube with the presealed end down. When the blood flows down and touches the sealant, hold it for 30 seconds to allow it to seal automatically.
    Purpose: The specimen should be free of air bubbles and then sealed in preparation for centrifuging.

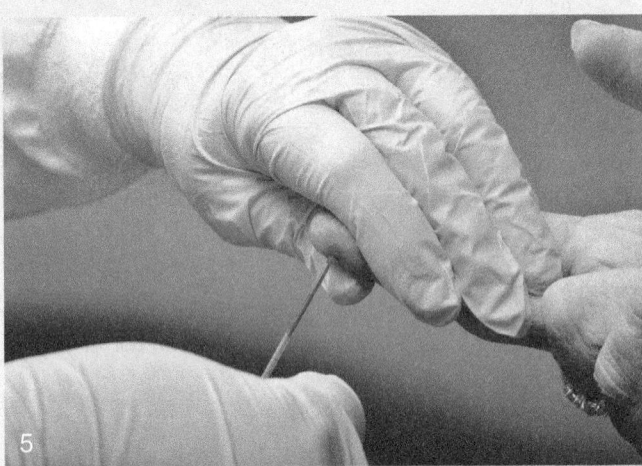

5

13. Wipe the patient's finger with gauze. Express another large drop of blood in the same way and fill a Microtainer (Fig. 6). Do not touch the container to the finger. If more blood is needed, gently apply pressure and release the finger to get another drop. Cap the Microtainer tube when the collection is complete.
    Purpose: Touching the container to the finger irritates the puncture site and may cause infection. Touching the container also smears the blood in the fingerprint and doesn't allow the blood to form a good hanging drop.

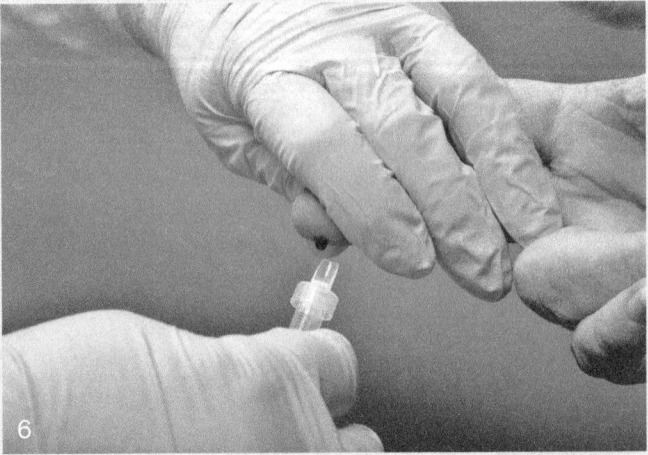

6

14. When collection is complete, apply pressure to the site with gauze (Fig. 7). The patient may be able to assist with this step.

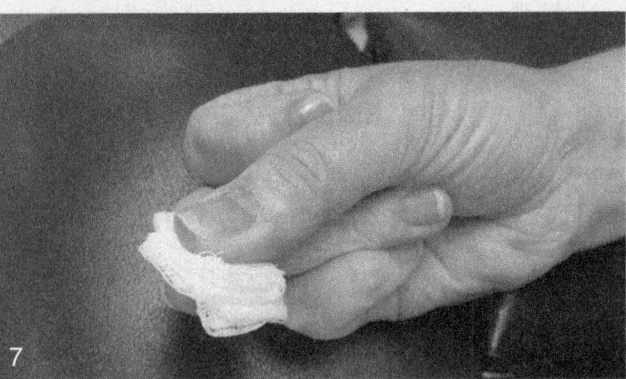

7

15. Select an appropriate means of labeling the containers. Sealed capillary tubes can be placed in a red-topped tube, which is then labeled. Microtainers can be labeled with a computer-generated label flag style and then placed in zipper-lock biohazardous bags that are subsequently labeled. Follow your institution's procedures for labeling.
16. Check the patient for bleeding and clean the site if traces of blood are visible. Apply a folded gauze square to the puncture site and wrap with hypoallergenic self-stick wrap, tape, or bandage (Fig. 8).

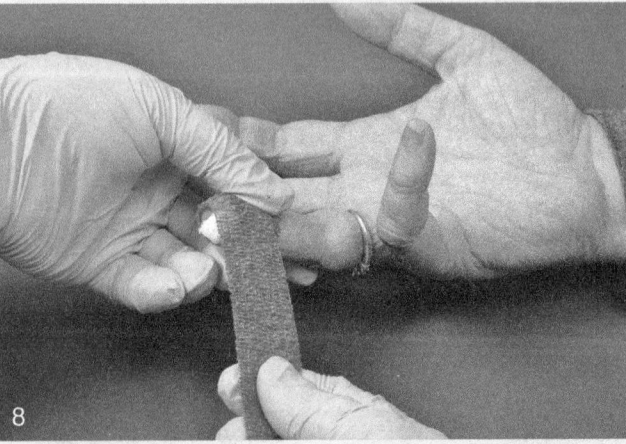

8

17. Disinfect the work area. Dispose of blood-contaminated materials (e.g., gauze and gloves) in the biohazard waste container. Remove your protective eyewear. Wash hands or use hand sanitizer.
    Purpose: To ensure infection control.
18. Complete the laboratory requisition form and route the specimen to the proper location. Record the procedure in the patient's record.
    Purpose: A procedure is not considered done until it is recorded in the patient's record.

PROCEDURE 54.5   Show Awareness of a Patient's Concern Related to a Procedure

Task
Show awareness of a patient's concern related to a venipuncture.

Scenario
You are a medical assistant working with Dr. Walden, who ordered bloodwork for Sam Brown. Your role includes performing venipuncture when bloodwork is ordered. You obtain the order, greet Sam, identify yourself, verify Sam's identity, and explain what you need to do. You notice that Sam appears to be uncomfortable and restless. Sam states he didn't really want the bloodwork done.

Directions
Role-play this scenario with a peer. The peer will play Sam and you are the medical assistant. During the role-play, address Sam's concerns regarding the procedure.

55

Assisting in the Analysis of Blood

LEARNING OBJECTIVES

1. Describe the components in the blood.
2. Describe the hematocrit test, including the purpose, collection method, and the testing procedures.
3. Describe the hemoglobin test, including the purpose, collection method, and the testing procedures.
4. Describe the erythrocyte sedimentation rate (ESR) test, including sources of testing errors and the testing procedure.
5. Describe the prothrombin time (PT) test, including the purpose, collection method, the testing procedures, and the international normalized ration (INR) value.
6. Identify the tests included in a complete blood count (CBC), the reference ranges, and differentiate between normal and abnormal test results.

7. Explain the reasons for performing a white blood cell (WBC) count and differential.
8. Differentiate between the ABO blood groupings and the Rh blood groupings.
9. Describe tests performed in chemistry panels.
10. Explain the clinical significance for testing blood glucose, hemoglobin A1c, cholesterol, liver enzymes, and thyroid hormones.
11. Discuss test sample required and perform tests for blood glucose, hemoglobin A1c, and cholesterol using Clinical Laboratory Improvement Amendments–waived test methods.

OUTLINE

OPENING SCENARIO

Michelle James, CMA (AAMA), has been working at the Walden-Martin Family Medical (WMFM) Clinic for 16 years. She loves her position as a medical assistant in a family medicine clinic. Every day is different. Each patient is unique. She has seen a number of children grow up over the years. Children who were toddlers when she started are now driving and thinking about college. The time has flown by.

Michelle is working with Dr. Perez today, and they have a busy schedule. A number of patients are in for follow-up visits, and a few new patients have appointments today, too.

YOU WILL LEARN

1. To identify the anticoagulant of choice for hematology testing and explain the purpose of the following tests: microhematocrit test, hemoglobin test, erythrocyte sedimentation rate (ESR).

2. To explain the purpose of the prothrombin time (PT) in coagulation testing.
3. To identify the tests included in a complete blood count (CBC) and their reference ranges, and to differentiate between normal and abnormal test results.
4. To describe the red blood cell (RBC) indices.
5. To explain the reasons for performing a white blood cell (WBC) count and differential.
6. To describe the medical assistant's role in blood transfusions.
7. To explain the reasons for testing blood glucose, hemoglobin A1c, cholesterol, liver enzymes, and thyroid hormones.
8. To summarize typical chemistry panels and the reason for performing each panel.

INTRODUCTION

The circulating blood supplies the body's cells with nutrients and oxygen. The blood also distributes enzymes, hormones, and other chemicals needed for regulation of body activities. In addition, the blood functions to maintain body temperature, keep body fluids in balance, and maintain pH. Maintaining a constant internal environment is called *homeostasis*.

Blood tests are done routinely in various departments of the laboratory identified as:

- Hematology (hee muh TOL uh jee)
- Immunohematology (im YUH noh hee muh TOL uh jee) (also known as blood bank)
- Chemistry
- Immunology (im yuh NOL uh jee) (also called serology)

Testing performed by medical assistants depends on the level of service offered by the ambulatory care facility. The tests performed fall under the regulations established by the Clinical Laboratory Improvement Amendments (CLIA). As a medical assistant, you are qualified to perform the CLIA-waived procedures described in the physician office laboratory (POL) sections of this chapter. Moderately and highly complex CLIA blood tests are performed at reference and hospital laboratories and are not performed by medical assistants. This chapter explains more complex procedures to provide background information important to an understanding of the analysis of blood.

> **VOCABULARY**
> **enzymes** Special proteins that speed up the chemical reaction in the body.
> **hormones** Chemical substances produced in an endocrine gland and transported in the blood to a specific tissue, where they have a specific effect.

HEMATOLOGY

Whole blood is composed of visible, formed elements suspended in *plasma* (a clear, yellow liquid). Plasma makes up approximately 55% of blood by volume. The remaining 45% consists of visible cellular elements:

- Erythrocytes (RBCs)
- Leukocytes (WBCs)
- Thrombocytes (platelets)

The characteristics of blood and cellular components are described in Chapter 9. A brief review of the components is presented in Table 55.1. Blood cells have a limited life span. Once

TABLE 55.1	**Review of Blood Components**			
Blood Component	**Function**	**Normal Values**	**Comments**
Plasma	Transports nutrients to cells and waste products away from cells	Approximately 55% of blood total volume	Plasma is the liquid portion of the blood inside the body
Red blood cells (RBCs)	Carry oxygen to the cells, help carry some carbon dioxide away from cells	Approximately 4–6 million/mm³; may be on slightly higher end for men and on slightly lower for women	About 120-day life span
Platelets	Help with the process of blood clotting	150,000–450,000/mm³	About 10-day life span
White Blood Cells (WBCs): Granular			
Neutrophils (NOO truh fils)	Engulf and destroy foreign substances, particularly bacteria	Most abundant WBC in the blood, about 40%–60%	Also called *polymorphonuclear cells, PMNs, segs,* or *polys*
Eosinophils (ee uh SIN uh fils)	Help in the destruction of parasites and fungi	About 1%–4% of WBCs in the blood	Also called *eos;* numbers increase when allergies present, skin infection, parasitic infections
Basophils (BEY suh fils)	Release histamine, resulting in swelling of tissues in response to allergic reactions; release heparin	About 0.5%–1% of WBCs in the blood	Also called *basos;* increased numbers associated with leukemia
WBCs: Agranular			
Monocytes (MON uh sahyts)	Engulf and destroy harmful pathogens (viruses, bacteria, fungi), senescent (si NES uhnt) cells or necrotic cells and malignant cells; help to active B cells to make antibodies	About 2%–8% of WBCs in the blood	Monocytes are found in the blood, but once they migrate into tissue, they are called *macrophages* (MAK ruh feyjs); also called *monos*
Lymphocytes (LIM fuh sahyts) B cell	Destroy foreign substances by producing antibodies	B and T cells combined are the second most abundant WBC in the blood, about 20%–40%	Looking under the microscope, you cannot see the difference between B- and T-cell lymphocytes; they look the same but function differently; also called *lymphs*
Lymphocyte T-cells	Immunity: Destroy foreign substances, particularly intracellular pathogens		

they become old and less efficient, they are broken down and the useful elements are recycled.

VOCABULARY

albumin Most abundant plasma protein in human blood. It is important in regulating the water balance of blood.

anemia A deficiency of hemoglobin in the blood. It is accompanied by a reduced number of red blood cells, pale skin, weakness, and shortness of breath, among other symptoms.

antibody A protein produced in the blood or tissues in response to a specific antigen that destroys or weakens the antigen. Part of the immune system.

buffy coat The layer of white blood cells and platelets that separates red blood cells and plasma in a centrifuged sample of whole blood.

centrifuge A machine that rotates at high speed and separates substances of different densities by centrifugal force. For example, a tube of blood is separated into plasma/serum, white blood cells, platelets, and red blood cells.

immunoglobulins A group of related proteins that function as antibodies. They are found in plasma and other body fluids.

intracellular pathogen A disease-causing organism that is inside of a cell.

malignant cell A cell with uncontrolled growth, rapidly spreading, and doing harm.

senescent cell An old or aging cell that can no longer divide and reproduce.

MEDICAL TERMINOLOGY

bas/o	base, opposite of acid
eosin/o	red, rosy, dawn colored
erythr/o	red
hemat/o	blood
immun/o	immune, protection, safe
leuk/o	white
neutr/o	neither, neutral, neutrophil
thromb/o	clot
intra-	within, into
-cyte	cell
-logy	study (process of)
-phil	attraction for

Plasma

Plasma is the highly complex liquid that carries the formed elements plus other substances, such as:

- Plasma proteins, including albumin (al BYOO min)
- Clotting proteins prothrombin (proh THROM bin) and fibrinogen (fie BRIN uh juhn)
- Immunoglobulins (im yuh noh GLOB yuh lins)
- Nutrients: carbohydrates, fats, and amino acids
- Hormones, enzymes, mineral salts, gases, and waste products

Plasma is composed of approximately 90% water, 9% protein, and 1% other chemical substances. The liquid portion of the blood in the body is plasma. Outside, the body plasma must have an added anticoagulant to remain part of whole blood, otherwise it will clot. The liquid that remains after blood has clotted is called *serum*.

HEMATOLOGY IN THE PHYSICIAN OFFICE LABORATORY (POL)

For many POL hematology tests, an adequate blood sample can be obtained from capillary puncture of the finger. If a larger sample is required, blood can be obtained via venipuncture. For a complete blood count (CBC), venous blood is collected

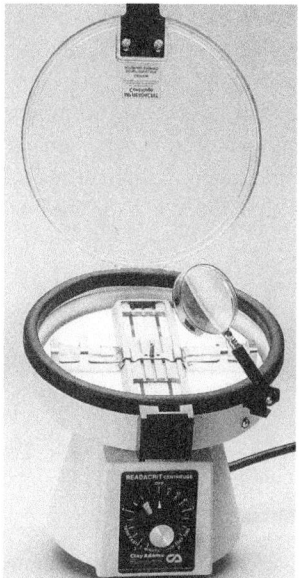

Fig. 55.1 Microhematocrit Centrifuge. (From Niedzwiecki B, et al: *Kinn's the medical assistant*, ed 14, St. Louis, 2020, Elsevier.)

in a lavender-topped tube containing *ethylenediaminetetraacetic* (ETH uh leen DAHY uh meen TE truh uh SEE tik) *acid* (EDTA), an anticoagulant that prevents whole blood from clotting. EDTA is the anticoagulant of choice for hematology testing because it also acts as a preservative for the blood cells. It is important to prevent blood from being *hemolyzed* (HEE muh lahyzd) during collection for hematology testing.

Hematocrit

The *hematocrit* (hee MAT uh krit) (Hct) is a measurement of the percentage of packed RBCs in a volume of blood. The spun microhematocrit test is based on the principle of separating the cellular elements from plasma using a centrifuge (SEN truh fyooj)(Procedures 55.1 and 55.2). Two or three drops of blood are collected from a capillary puncture in two microhematocrit tubes that are placed in a specially designed microhematocrit centrifuge (Fig. 55.1). Microhematocrit tubes can also be filled with EDTA-anticoagulated blood from a lavender-topped vacuum tube. As required by the Occupational Safety and Health Administration (OSHA), capillary tubes must be safe. They are made of either plastic or plastic-coated glass and allow for self-sealing at one end to avoid sharps injuries. The self-sealing microhematocrit tube must be tilted upright, causing the blood sample to flow down the tube and come into contact with the seal, and then held in place for 15 to 30 seconds prior to centrifugation.

After centrifugation, the packed RBCs are at the bottom of the tube against the sealant, the WBCs and platelets are in the center buffy coat, and plasma is on top (Fig. 55.2). The microhematocrit is determined by comparing the volume of RBCs to the total volume of the whole blood sample. The percentage is read by placing the tubes on a special microhematocrit reader. Some microhematocrit centrifuges have a built-in reading scale that reads the calibrated capillary tubes. Microhematocrits should be performed in duplicate and the average of the two results reported.

Normal Hct values vary with sex and age (Table 55.2). They range from a low of 36% in women to a high of 51% in men. Low microhematocrit values can indicate anemia or the presence of bleeding. High values may be caused by dehydration or polycythemia vera (pah lee sigh THEE mee uh VER uh). Values can be influenced by physiologic, pathologic, and even geographic factors and by collection techniques. Normal hematocrit (Hct) ranges are affected by a person's geographic location. For example, people living at high altitudes have a higher percentage of RBCs, to compensate for the lower oxygen levels in the atmosphere.

The microhematocrit is a commonly performed test requested by providers either separately or as part of the CBC. Because it is a simple procedure that requires only a small amount of blood, it is an ideal screening test and often is part of a routine physical examination. Quality assurance includes care and maintenance of the microhematocrit instrument.

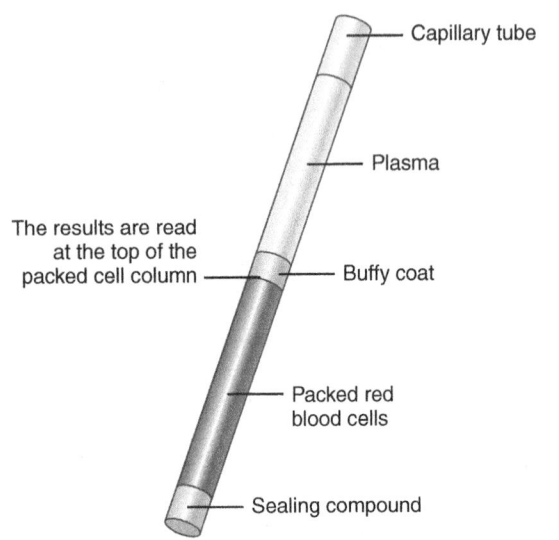

Fig. 55.2 Spun Microhematocrit Tube. (From Niedzwiecki B, et al: *Kinn's the medical assistant*, ed 14, St. Louis, 2020, Elsevier.)

VOCABULARY

pathologic Caused by or involving disease.
physiologic Consistent with the normal function of the body.
polycythemia vera A disorder characterized by an abnormal increase in the number of red blood cells in the blood.

MEDICAL TERMINOLOGY

cyt/o	cell
hem/o	blood
log/o	study
path/o	disease
physi/o	nature, physical
an-	no, not, without
auto-	self, own
micro-	small
poly-	many, much
-emia	blood condition
-globin	protein
-ic	pertaining to

TABLE 55.2   Reference Ranges for Complete Blood Count (CBC) Values[a]

Test	Neonates (Newborn–1 mo)	Infants (1 mo–23 mo)	Children (2–17 yr)	Men (>17 yr)	Women (>17 yr)
RBCs	3.2–5.7 million/mm³	2.9–5.1 million/mm³	3.8–5.7 million/mm³	4.4–5.7 million/mm³	3.9–5.1 million/mm³
Hematocrit (Hct)	31%–57%	27%–38%	31%–50%	38%–51%	36%–47%
Hemoglobin (Hgb)	10–20 g/dL	8.9–12.7 g/dL	10.2–16.9 g/dL	13.2–16.6 g/dL	11.6–15 g/dL
WBCs	7,800–15,900/mm³	6,000–15,000/mm³	3,800–13,400/mm³	3,400–9,600/mm³	
Platelets	144,000–586,000/mm³	206,000–597,000/mm³	139,000–320,000/mm³	150,000–450,000/mm³	
RBC Indices					
MCV	89–106 fL	70–96 fL	71–98 fL	80–100 fL	
MCH	30–42 pg			26–34 pg	
MCHC	30–34 g/dL			32–36 g/dL	
WBC Differential					
Neutrophils	25%–81%	15%–50%	20%–70%	55%–70%	
Bands	—	—	—	0%–7%	
Eosinophils	—	—	0%–3%	1%–4%	
Basophils	—	—	1%–3%	0.5%–1%	
Monocytes	0.2%–3.1%	0.2%–4%	0%–0.8%	2%–8%	
Lymphocytes	21%–70%	41%–77%	25%–74%	20%–40%	

[a]Lab reports, both electronic and paper, must supply their own reference ranges, along with each patient's results. This is because different methodologies may create different reference ranges and different units of measurement.
fL, Femtoliter; *MCH*, mean corpuscular hemoglobin; *MCHC*, mean corpuscular hemoglobin concentration; *MCV*, mean corpuscular volume; *pg*, picograms; *RBC*, red blood cell; *WBC*, white blood cell.

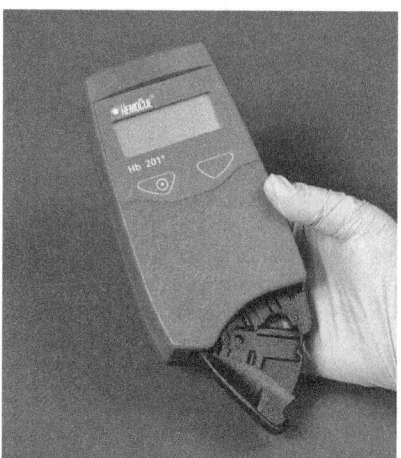

Fig. 55.3 Handheld Hemoglobin Monitor.

CRITICAL THINKING 55.1

One of Michelle's patients today is Carl Bowden. Carl retired recently and has been enjoying his new, less hectic schedule. Carl is in good health, but he did mention at his physical today that he was feeling a little tired and lacked energy. Dr. Perez ordered a microhematocrit for Carl. The lab just sent the results to Carl's electronic health record.

Michelle looks at the results and sees that his hematocrit is 38%. Is that value in the normal range for an adult male?

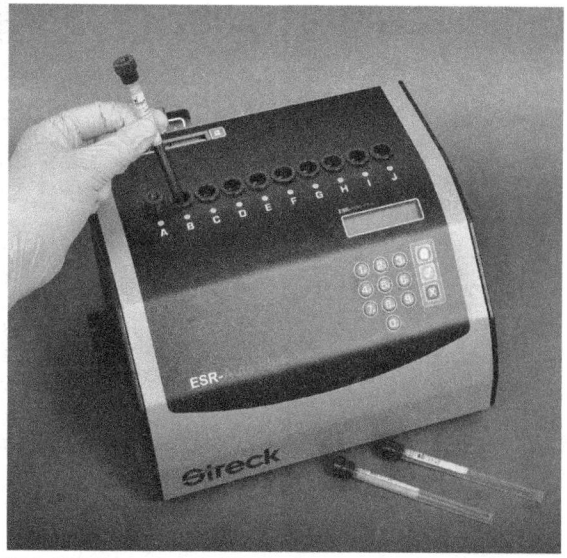

Fig. 55.4 30-Minute Streck ESR CLIA-Waived Test. (From Niedzwiecki B, et al: *Kinn's the medical assistant*, ed 14, St. Louis, 2020, Elsevier.)

VOCABULARY

autoimmune An immune response against a person's own tissues, cells, or cell parts.

dilution Reducing the concentration of a mixture or solution by adding a known volume of liquid.

hemoglobin The oxygen-carrying pigment of red blood cells.

microcuvette A small tube or vessel used in laboratory experiments.

pipet A slender tube, attached to or including a bulb, for transferring or measuring small amounts of a liquid, often used in a laboratory.

reagent A substance for use in a chemical reaction.

Hemoglobin

Hemoglobin (HEE muh gloh bin)(Hgb) determination is another way to measure the oxygen-carrying capacity of blood. The hemoglobin concentration can be part of the CBC or an individual test.

CLIA-waived methods include the STAT-Site M Hgb, HemoPointH2, and HemoCue, all portable, battery-operated hemoglobin analyzers that fit in the palm of the hand (Fig. 55.3 and Procedure 55.3). The HemoCue uses plastic microcuvettes (MAHY kroh koo VETs) that contain reagents (ree EY juh nts) that *lyse* (break apart) the RBCs in the sample, releasing the hemoglobin. The hemoglobin reacts with the reagents and forms a colored compound. The color is detected and measured in the instrument, producing a digital readout. Capillary, venous, or arterial blood can be used in the disposable microcuvette. The cuvettes have a long shelf life.

Normal hemoglobin values vary throughout a lifetime (see Table 55.2). Factors that affect the hemoglobin level include age, sex, diet, altitude, and disease.

Hemoglobin and hematocrit tests are often performed together and are referred to as an "H&H." A quick mental calculation should always be done before H&H results are reported: the hemoglobin value × 3 (± 3) should equal the hematocrit value. For example, if the hemoglobin is 15 g/dL, calculate the hematocrit as follows:

$$15\,g/dL \times 3 = 45 \pm 3 = 42\text{ to }48$$

The hematocrit should be between 42% and 48%.

Erythrocyte Sedimentation Rate

The *erythrocyte sedimentation rate* (ESR) is a laboratory test that measures the rate at which red blood cells gradually separate from plasma and settle to the bottom of a specially calibrated tube in 1 hour. The test is not specific for any disease in particular. An increased ESR is significant to the provider, since it indicates the presence of inflammation in the body. A lower-than-normal ESR is not considered clinically significant. Normal values for males under age 64 are 0 to 15 mm/hr. Normal values for males over 64 and females are 0 to 20 mm/hr. An increased ESR is seen in a number of conditions:

- Acute and chronic infections, such tuberculosis and hepatitis
- Autoimmune conditions such as rheumatoid arthritis, lupus erythematosus (er uh THEE muh toh sus), and rheumatic fever
- Multiple myeloma (mahy uh LOH muh) and other types of cancers

Several CLIA-waived methods of measuring the ESR are used, including the Sediplast procedure (Procedure 55.4). This closed system incorporates a pierceable stopper that ensures a leakproof seal when punctured by a pipet (pie PET). An automatic self-zeroing cap and reservoir accurately bring the blood level to the zero mark and prevent overfilling. A prefilled vial of sodium citrate reagent is provided for dilution of blood before testing. A closed-tube Streck ESR method uses a Streck black-topped Vacutainer sample of blood that is directly placed in a Streck rack that provides results in 30 minutes (Fig. 55.4).

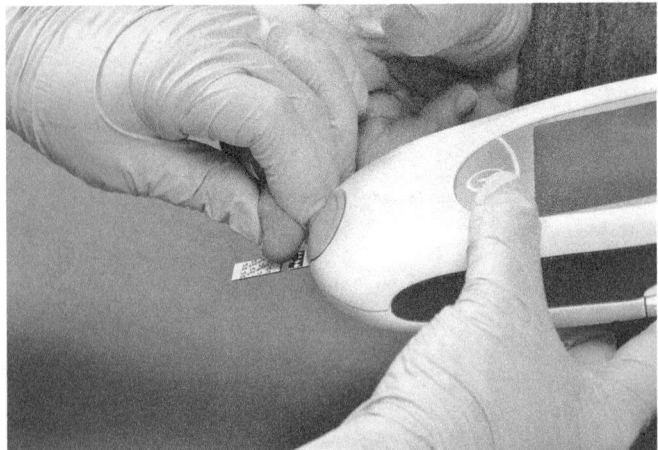

Fig. 55.5 Applying a Blood Sample to the CoaguChek XS PT Test Monitor.

Coagulation Testing

The medical assistant may be asked to perform a CLIA-waived test called a *prothrombin time* (PT; also called a protime). This test can be performed using a handheld, CLIA-waived instrument that uses whole blood from a fingerstick (Fig. 55.5). A PT is a method of measuring how long it takes blood to clot. Prothrombin is a protein in the liquid part of blood *(plasma)* that is converted to thrombin as part of the clotting process. Thrombin then causes fibrinogen to be converted to *fibrin* during the clotting process.

The PT is often used in combination with the partial thromboplastin (throm buh PLAS tin) time (PTT) to screen for hemophilia (hee muh FIL ee uh) and other clotting disorders. The PT is also used to monitor patients taking the anticoagulant drug *warfarin* (Coumadin) and similar anticoagulants. Warfarin is given to prevent clots in deep veins of the legs and to treat a pulmonary embolism (Box 55.1).

The CLIA-waived CoaguChek XS PT (see Fig. 55.5) measures the time it takes a blood sample to form a fibrin clot. A precise amount of capillary sample blood is dispensed into the channels of a testing strip. The blood is mixed with a thromboplastin reagent. The blood is pumped back and forth in the channel, and a series of light-emitting diodes (LEDs) detect formation of a clot when blood movement in the channels stop (Procedure 55.5).

PT test results are reported as the number of seconds blood takes to clot when mixed with the thromboplastin reagent. The international normalized ratio (INR) was created by the World Health Organization (WHO) because PT test results can vary, depending on the thromboplastin reagent used. The INR is a conversion unit that considers the different sensitivities of reagents. It is widely accepted as the standard unit for reporting PT results rather than actual clotting time. Many labs report

the time to the nearest tenth of a second along with the INR value for a PT/INR result. Normal PT values are 11 to 13.5 seconds, or an INR of 0.8 to 1.1. Patients who are taking warfarin to prevent the formation of blood clots or who have artificial heart valves should have an INR value of about 2 to 3. Their blood should take longer to clot than that of a normal healthy individual.

It is important that the medical assistant know how to accurately document INR follow-up and related warfarin dosages on a patient flow sheet. The provider will balance repeated INR levels with warfarin doses so the INR is maintained at about 2 throughout the anticoagulant treatment (Fig. 55.6). This particular instrument may also be used as a means of at-home monitoring of the patient's INR.

HEMATOLOGY IN THE REFERENCE LABORATORY

The most frequently ordered reference laboratory procedure for hematology is the CBC. This test requires a lavender-topped EDTA blood specimen. It gives a comprehensive look at the cellular components of blood and can provide a wealth of information about a patient's condition. It routinely includes:

- RBC and platelet counts
- Hematocrit and hemoglobin
- Red cell indices (IN duh seez)
- WBC count and differential

Complete Blood Count (CBC) Laboratory Reports

It is important that medical assistants understand the hematology laboratory reports that arrive from the reference

Walden-Martin Family Medical Clinic
Warfarin Anticoagulant Record

Patient's Name: _____   DOB:_____
Address: _____   SSN: _____

Patient's Phone:_____
Dx for Anticoagulation: _____   ICDM Code: _____
Date Warfarin Started: _____   INR Goal: _____
Phone for Outside Lab: _____

Date	Warfarin Dose Pre-Test	PT	INR	Warfarin Dose Order	Next INR/PT	Signature

Fig. 55.6 Warfarin Flow Sheet. (From Niedzwiecki B, et al: *Kinn's the medical assistant*, ed 14, St. Louis, 2020, Elsevier.)

laboratories. They should be able to distinguish between normal and abnormal results. Use the following references to complete the Critical Thinking exercise that follows:

- Hematology reference ranges (see Table 55.2).
- The patient report form (Fig. 55.7), a sample lab report, also identifies the lab's reference ranges. Lab reports, both electronic and paper, must supply their own reference ranges, along with each patient's results.

CRITICAL THINKING 55.3

Using the reference ranges in Table 55.2, decide if the following results are normal or abnormal.

1. Grace Sifuentes, age 4, has a hematocrit of 38%. Is that normal, high, or low?
2. Christian Washington, age 45, has a WBC count of 14,200/mm³. Is that normal, high, or low?
3. Brigitte Mulrooney, age 29, has a hematocrit of 32% and a hemoglobin of 10 g/dL. Are these results normal, high, or low?
4. Eleanor Jackson, age 81, has 23% bands in her white blood cell differential. Is that normal, high, or low?

Red Blood Cell Count. The RBC count is part of the CBC (see Table 55.2). It approximates the number of circulating RBCs in a person's blood. The function of RBCs is to transport oxygen to tissues. The RBC count often is decreased in patients with anemia. Increased RBC counts are found in people with dehydration, polycythemia vera, or severe burns, and those living at high altitudes.

Normal RBC values range from approximately 4 million to 6 million cells/mm³. RBC counts usually are higher in males than in females.

Red Blood Cell Indices. A variety of calculations can be performed using the information obtained from the CBC. The red cell *indices* provide information about RBC disorders. The indices are used to classify anemias and to select additional tests that may help determine the cause of anemia. Red cell indices are also helpful to monitor the treatment of anemia. Because indices may change in response to treatment, they can be used as an indicator in the evaluation of treatment. The indices are mathematical calculations using the three red cell tests: Hct, Hgb, and the RBC count.

- *Mean corpuscular volume (MCV):* MCV = (Hct/RBC) × 10. The average size of the RBCs is the most important index for classifying anemias. Abnormal RBC include:
  - *Macrocytic* (MAK ruh sih tik): Abnormally large RBCs and have a higher-than-normal MCV.
  - *Microcytic* (MAHY kruh sih tik): Small RBCs and have a lower-than-normal MCV. The reference range for adults is 80 to 100 femtoliters (fehm TOH lee turs) (fL).
- *Mean corpuscular hemoglobin (MCH):* MCH = (Hgb/RBC) × 10. The MCH is calculated to give the average weight of hemoglobin in the RBC. The reference range for adults is 26 to 34 picograms (PEE kuh grams) (pg).
- *Mean corpuscular hemoglobin concentration (MCHC):* MCHC = (Hgb × 100)/RBC. The MCHC indicates the average weight of hemoglobin compared with the cell size. The

	DATE & TIME RECEIVED	ACCESSION NUMBER
	I0/ 20/ 2013 20:45	
	LOCATION	DATE REPORTED
		I0/ 21/2000

PHYSICIAN		PATIENT INFORMATION

TEST		RESULTS	REFERENCE RANGE	UNITS
HEMOGRAM	LO	2.9	4. 5-10. 5	CU.MM.
WHITE BLOOD COUNT	LO	2. 39	4.40-5.90	CU.MM.
RED BLOOD COUNT	LO	7.4	14.0-18.0	GM/100ML
HEMOGLOBIN	LO	22.3	40. 0-52.0 %	
MEAN CORPUSCULAR VOLUME		93	80-100	fL
MEAN CORPUSCULAR HGB		31.0	27. 0-32.0	PG
MEAN CORPUSCULAR HgB CONC		33.2	31.0-36.0	%
DIFFERENTIAL, WBC				
SEGMENTED NEUTROPHILS		57	38-80	%
LYMPHOCYTE		29	15-45	%
MONOCYTES		7	1-10	%
EOSINOPHILS		1	0-4	%
BAND NEUTROPHILS	HI	6	0-5	%
ANISOCYTOSIS	ABN	SLIGHT		
HYPOCHROMIA	ABN	SLIGHT		
PLATELET ESTIMATE	ABN	DECREASED		
PARTIAL THROMBOPLASTIN TIME				
PARTIAL THROMBOPLASTIN TIME		31.7	20.0-40.0	SECONDS
CONTROL PTT		30.4	20.0-40.0	SECONDS
PROTHROMBIN TIME				
PROTHROMBIN TIME		12.2	10.0-13.5	SECONDS
CONTROL PT		12.0	11.0-13.0	SECONDS
FINAL Report (Summary)				

Fig. 55.7 Sample Lab Report with Normal and Abnormal Patient Results. (From Niedzwiecki B, et al: *Kinn's the medical assistant*, ed 14, St. Louis, 2020, Elsevier.)

reference range for adults is 32 to 36 g/dL. A decreased MCHC shows hypochromic RBCs in a stained blood smear. An increased MCHC is rare and should be flagged and brought to the attention of the provider.

> **VOCABULARY**
>
> **density** Describes how compact or concentrated something is.
> **hypochromic** Pale red blood cells. Lacking color.
> **morphology** The study of the form, shape, and structure of an organism or a cell.

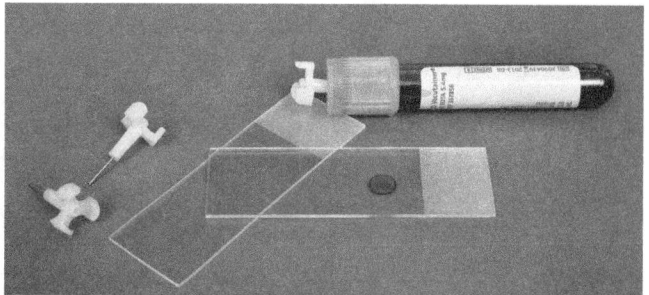

Fig. 55.8 DIFF-SAFE Device Used to Make a Blood Smear.

White Blood Cell Count. The WBC count gives an estimate of the total number of leukocytes in circulating blood. The count is performed to help the provider determine whether an infection is present or to aid in the diagnosis of leukemia. It also may be used to follow the course of a disease and indicate if patient is responding to treatment.

The normal WBC count varies with age. It is higher in newborns and decreases throughout a lifetime. The average adult range is 3,400 to 9,600 cells/mm^3. Many factors can affect the WBC count.

An increase in the number of normal WBCs is a condition called *leukocytosis* (loo koh sahy TOH sis). Increased WBC counts may normally be seen with pregnancy, stress, anesthesia, exercise, exposure to temperature extremes, and after treatment with corticosteroids. Pathologic causes of leukocytosis include many bacterial infections, leukemia, appendicitis, and pneumonia.

A decrease in the WBC count is called *leukopenia* (loo kuh PEE nee uh). This condition may be caused by viral infection or by exposure to radiation and certain chemicals and drugs.

Differential Cell Count. The purpose of the differential, or "diff," in the CBC is to analyze and count the types of WBCs found in a sample of blood. The differential can be manually performed using a stained blood smear and a microscope, or with an automated instrument. Automated cell counters have the ability to analyze the WBCs and gather information about cell size, internal structures, and density.

Preparation of Blood Smears for the Differential. A blood smear enables the examiner to view the preserved cellular structures of blood. The morphology (mawr FOL uh jee) of WBCs, RBCs, and platelets can be studied. Their size, shape, and maturity can also be evaluated.

A blood smear is prepared by placing a drop of blood from a fingerstick or an EDTA tube (using a DIFF-SAFE blood dispenser) onto a clean glass slide (Fig. 55.8). The slide must be free of dust and grease. The best specimen for a blood smear is capillary blood that has no anticoagulant added. EDTA-anticoagulated blood can be used, provided the smear is made within 2 hours of specimen collection. Because timing is important, the medical assistant may be asked to prepare a smear during collection of the CBC specimen.

The wedge smear is used most frequently and would follow these steps:

- Place a small drop of blood ½ inch from the frosted end (placed to the right) of a glass slide.

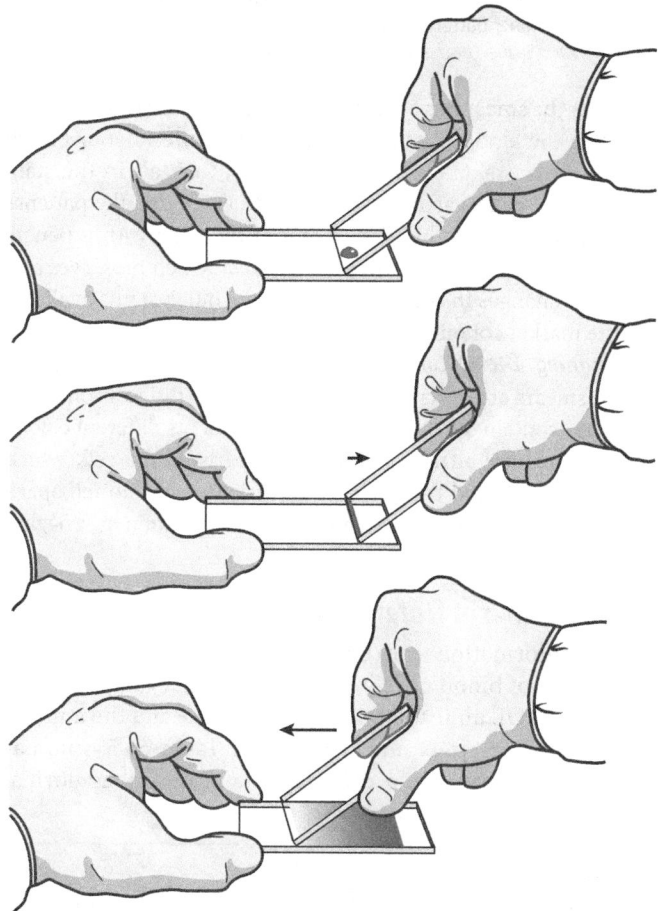

Fig. 55.9 Making a Differential Wedge Smear.

- The end of a second glass spreader slide is placed in front (to the left) of the drop of blood at an angle of 30 to 35 degrees.
- The spreader slide is brought back into the drop with a quick but smooth gliding motion until the blood spreads along the edge of the spreader slide.
- The spreader slide is then pushed to the left with a quick, steady motion, spreading the blood across the slide (Fig. 55.9).

A good wedge smear should cover one half to three fourths of the slide. It should show a gradual transition from a thick to a thin end with a feathered edge (Fig. 55.10). It should have a smooth appearance with no ridges, holes, lines, streaks, or clumps. On microscopic examination, the cells should be evenly distributed.

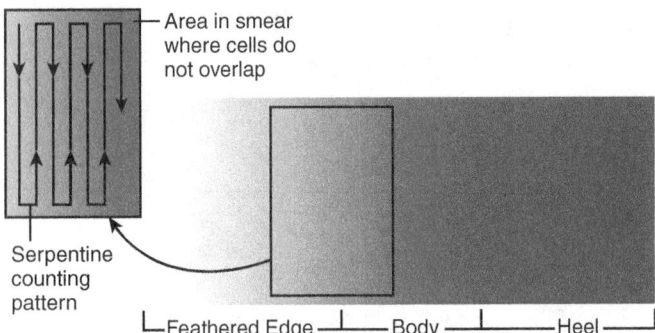

Fig. 55.10 *(Right)* Appearance of a properly prepared wedge smear. *(Left)* Serpentine pattern used to count the cells. (From Niedzwiecki B, et al: *Kinn's the medical assistant*, ed 14, St. Louis, 2020, Elsevier.)

After the smear has been made, it should be air dried. Do not blow on the blood slide to dry it. The moisture in your breath can cause artifacts to form on the slide. Crystals in the stain can also be seen as artifacts on the slide. Once dry, the patient's name is written on the frosted end of the slide with a pencil. After it has been labeled, the slide is *fixed,* which preserves and prevents changes in the cells. Many of the quick stains available on the market contain the fixative in the stain.

Staining Blood Smears. Stains commonly used to make blood smears are described as *polychromatic* (pol ee kroh MAR ik). They contain dyes that stain cell components different colors. These stains are attracted to different parts of the cell, which makes the cells and their structures easier to see and tell apart. The most commonly used differential blood stain is Wright's stain.

Identification of Normal Blood Cells

Useful information can be gathered from a microscopic evaluation of blood cells in a stained smear. Hematologists (hee muh TOL uh jists) look for the cell size and the appearance of the nucleus and cytoplasm. Table 55.3 summarizes the cells seen in a differential and describes normal characteristics.

> **VOCABULARY**
>
> **artifact** A substance, structure, or event that does not naturally occur in a situation. Examples include interference, or electrical "garbage," on an ECG, or crystals, lint, or contamination of a staining technique.
>
> **atypical lymphocytes** Large, misshaped lymphocytes, also called stimulated or reactive lymphocytes. Seen with many viral infections, including mononucleosis.
>
> **cytoplasm** The cell substance that fills the area between the nucleus and the cell membrane. It contains organelles of the cell.
>
> **hematologist** A person trained in the nature, function, and diseases of the blood and blood-forming organs. He or she can be a physician, trained laboratory personnel, or researcher.
>
> **nucleus** A structure in a cell that contains genetic material and controls the characteristics and growth of the cell.

Differential Examination

A specific area of a stained smear is examined under the microscope for a differential. The slide is examined near the feathered end of the smear, where cells are barely touching one another

and are easiest to identify. Cells are examined with the oil immersion objective of the microscope. The differential involves counting and classifying 100 consecutive WBCs while moving in a serpentine pattern through the smear (see Fig. 55.10). A count of the cells observed is kept on a differential cell counter or a computer.

Normal values for a differential vary with age. As mentioned previously, laboratory reports must include the lab's own reference ranges, along with each patient's results.

Disease states may give differential results that are unlike a normal diff. The types of leukocytes, their maturity, and the appearance of the differential can be very useful for the provider in making a diagnosis. The differential exam typically is performed in a reference laboratory.

Red Blood Cell Morphology. After the differential cell count has been determined, the RBCs are observed and evaluated. Normally, stained RBCs are the same size and shape and are well filled with hemoglobin. Any variations from the normal state are reported. Fig. 55.11 shows examples of abnormal cells. The appearance of the RBCs should correlate with the RBC indices.

Size. Normal-sized RBCs are said to be *normocytic.* If the cells are larger than normal, they are macrocytic; if the cells are smaller than normal, they are microcytic. The condition in which different sizes of RBCs are present is known as *anisocytosis* (ah nee soh sey TOH sis).

Shape. Normal RBCs are round or slightly oval. Cells may be shaped like sickles, targets, crescents, or burs. *Poikilocytosis* (poyh kee LOH sigh toh sis) is a significant variation in the shape of RBCs.

Content. An RBC with a normal amount of hemoglobin is said to be *normochromic.* Pale-staining cells are *hypochromic* and have less hemoglobin than normal. Any inclusions in red cells should be reported.

> ### CRITICAL THINKING 55.4
>
> Michelle checks Reuven Ahmad's CBC and differential results as she prepares information for Dr. Perez. Reuven's RBC count is 5.1 million/mm³. Is that a normal value for an adult male? In the notes from the differential, the laboratory technologist comments that Reuven's RBCs are normocytic and slightly hypochromic. Define normocytic and hypochromic in your own words. Be ready to share your definitions with the class.

Platelet Analysis

On a stained smear, the platelets are observed for any abnormalities. Platelets are small and irregularly shaped and may vary considerably in size. The normal platelet count for adults is 150,000 to 450,000/mm³, though normal value ranges may slightly vary. An increase in platelets is called *thrombocytosis,* and a decrease is called *thrombocytopenia.* A count less than 50,000/mm³ puts the person at a severe risk of bleeding. Excessive clumping of platelets is also reported in a platelet analysis.

TABLE 55.3 Cells in a Differential

Cell Name	Normal Characteristics	Photograph of Normal Cell
Red blood cell	Most numerous cell on diff. A small, red, biconcave disk with no nuclei.	
Platelet	Smallest cell on diff. May be round or oval. Has no nucleus. A fragment of cytoplasm from a large bone marrow cell called a *megakaryocyte*. (From *Mosby's dictionary of medicine, nursing, & health professions*, ed 8, St. Louis, 2009, Elsevier.)	
Neutrophil: mature	Most numerous white blood cell (WBC) on diff. Nucleus has many lobes. Increased numbers seen with bacterial infections.	
Neutrophil: immature	Called a *band* or *stab cell*. Horseshoe-shaped nucleus. Increased numbers seen with some types of leukemia, and infections.	
Eosinophil	Has large, red-orange granules. Increased numbers seen with allergies, asthma, and certain parasitic infections.	
Basophil	Has large, dark blue/purple granules. Granules contain histamine, which is involved in the inflammatory response. Natural anticoagulant.	
Lymphocyte	Smallest WBC, but most numerous in the blood. Large, dark blue/purple nucleus. Increased numbers seen with viral and some bacterial infections. Viral infections may show atypical lymphocytes.	
Monocyte	Largest WBC in the blood. Increased numbers seen with viral and some bacterial infections.	

MEDICAL TERMINOLOGY

chrom/o	color
morph/o	shape, form
norm/o	rule, order
thromb/o	clot
aniso-	unequal
hypo-	deficient, below, under, less than normal
macro-	large
micro-	small
poikilo-	varied, irregular
-osis	condition, usually abnormal
-penia	deficiency

during blood transfusions. *Compatibility testing* (also called cross-matching) is performed to prevent transfusion reactions in patients receiving blood from a donor. Identifying potential Rh incompatibility problems in expectant mothers is another procedure done in immunohematology. Rh incompatibility between an expectant mother and the unborn child may result in hemolytic disease of the fetus and newborn. (See Chapter 14 for more details on this condition.)

> **VOCABULARY**
>
> **antigen** A substance that stimulates the production of an antibody when introduced into the body. Antigens include toxins, bacteria, viruses, and other foreign substances.

IMMUNOHEMATOLOGY

The immunohematology department (blood bank) of the laboratory is responsible for blood typing. The major reason for performing immunohematology tests is to prevent problems caused by blood types that are not compatible

Blood Typing

The two major blood antigen systems are the ABO system and the Rh system. The ABO system has four major blood groups: A, B, O, and AB. Another major blood group is the Rh group. A person is either Rh-positive (Rh+) or Rh-negative (Rh−). Determinations of ABO and Rh blood groups

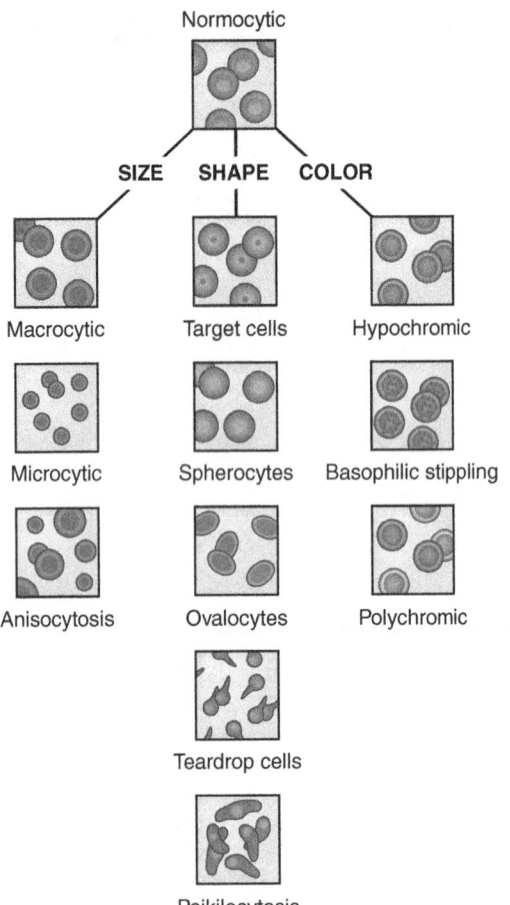

Fig. 55.11 Abnormal Red Blood Cells. (From Niedzwiecki B, et al: *Kinn's the medical assistant*, ed 14, St. Louis, 2020, Elsevier.)

TABLE 55.5   Blood Type Frequency by Population

Type	Caucasian	African American	Hispanic	Asian
O+	37%	47%	53%	39%
O–	8%	4%	4%	1%
A+	33%	24%	29%	27%
A–	7%	2%	2%	0.5%
B+	9%	18%	9%	25%
B–	2%	1%	1%	0.4%
AB+	3%	4%	2%	7%
AB–	1%	0.3%	0.2%	0.1%

Data from the American Red Cross. http://www.redcrossblood.org/learn-about-blood/blood-types.

BOX 55.2   Beyond ABO and Rh Typing

There are many blood types beyond ABO and Rh. Here are a few blood antigens or antigen systems, just so that you have seen the terms:
- Diego: Found only among East Asians and Native Americans.
- MNS: Useful in maternity and paternity testing.
- Duffy: The malarial parasite requires the Duffy antigen to enter the red blood cells. Lack of the antigen confers resistance to malaria. Duffy-negative blood is found only in descendants of African populations.
- Lewis: Antigens are soluble in blood rather than attached to the red blood cells. These are the only blood group antibodies that have never been implicated in hemolytic disease of the newborn.
- Other blood group systems: Colton, M, Kell, Kidd, Landsteiner-Wiener, P, Yt or Cartwright, XG, Scianna, Dombrock, Chido/Rodgers, Kx, Gerbich, Cromer, Knops, Indian, Ok, Raph, and JMH.

TABLE 55.4   Blood Compatibility

	RECIPIENT BLOOD	
RBC Antigen	**Plasma Antibodies**	**Compatible With Donor Types**
Type O (no antigens)	Anti-A and anti-B	O
Type A (type A antigen)	Anti-B	O and A
Type B (type B antigen)	Anti-A	O and B
Type AB (type AB antigen)	None	O, A, B, and AB

RBC, Red blood cell.
From Niedzwiecki B, et al: *Kinn's the medical assistant*, ed 14, St. Louis, 2020, Elsevier.

CRITICAL THINKING 55.5

Griffin Jones is in for a physical today, but she would also like to have her blood type tested. She and her husband are thinking of starting a family soon and would like to know her ABO/Rh type. She thinks she is A–. If Griffin is A–, what antigen or antigens are on her RBCs?

Other Blood Types

In addition to the A and B antigens that characterize the ABO blood grouping, more than 600 antigens and more than 20 other blood type systems are known. Many are named after the person or family in which the blood antigen system was discovered. Box 55.2 describes other blood systems.

Legal and Ethical Issues Related to Blood Transfusion

The Blood Safety Act was passed in 1991 to ensure that all donor blood is tested for the human immunodeficiency virus (HIV) and other bloodborne pathogens. The impact of this law can be seen in the ambulatory care environment. The law requires providers to explain to each elective surgery patient the chances that he or she may need a blood

are simple tests that can be performed easily. But because the consequences of performing the test incorrectly can be life threatening, blood typing is not a CLIA-waived test. See Table 55.4 for blood transfusion compatibility types. Patients with type AB blood are considered universal recipients. Patients with type O blood are considered universal donors. Table 55.5 shows the blood type frequency within ethnic populations in the United States.

transfusion. The discussion must include positive and negative aspects of *autologous* (aw TOL uh guh s) *transfusion* (i.e., transfusion with a person's own blood). The pros and cons of transfusions from family, friends, or other donors should also be discussed. The conversation must be documented in the patient's health record. Before the surgery, the patient must sign a form giving consent to any needed blood transfusions. The medical assistant should be aware that certain populations (e.g., Jehovah's Witnesses) do not believe in blood transfusions.

If the patient decides to use autologous transfusions, this may require the patient to donate blood several weeks before the procedure. Usually autologous transfusions are performed for stable patients undergoing major orthopedic, vascular, cardiac, or thoracic surgery. The medical assistant might need to help make arrangements for the blood donation. Another type of autologous transfusion can occur if the surgeon inserts an autologous drain in the surgical wound. The drain collects the blood from the surgical wound to prevent postoperative hematomas. The collected blood is then washed and reinfused into the patient.

MEDICAL TERMINOLOGY	
cardi/o	heart
glycos/o	glucose, sugar
log/o	speech, words
orth/o	straight, erect
ped/o	child, foot
thorac/o	chest
vascul/o	vessel (blood)
-ous	pertaining to

BLOOD CHEMISTRY IN THE PHYSICIAN OFFICE LABORATORY

CLIA-waived chemistry tests using whole blood from capillary punctures have become popular in ambulatory practices. With the increase in diabetes and cardiovascular disease in the United States, both metabolic diseases benefit from early diagnosis. Treatment is based on continued monitoring of glucose and hemoglobin A1c for diabetes and of cholesterol, lipid panels, and liver enzymes for cardiovascular diseases related to fatty plaque in the arteries.

> **VOCABULARY**
> **metabolic** Relating to or resulting from metabolism (the chemical process in which cells produce the substances and energy needed to sustain life).
> **plaque** Any small abnormal patch on or within the body. A deposit of fatty material.

Blood Glucose Testing

Glucose is used as a fuel by all body cells. Under normal circumstances, it is the only substance used to nourish brain cells. Maintenance of blood glucose levels within a normal range is vital to homeostasis of the human body. Understanding the importance of glucose can help the medical assistant understand

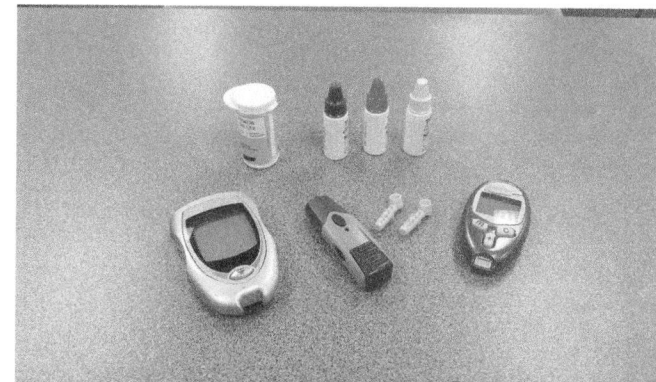

Fig. 55.12 Glucometer and Supplies.

why glucose is the most frequently tested chemical analyte in the blood.

Elevated blood glucose levels are most often associated with diabetes mellitus. They also may indicate pancreatitis, endocrine disorders, or chronic renal failure. Diabetes mellitus is a disorder of carbohydrate metabolism that results in elevated blood and urine glucose levels. In diabetes mellitus, either the pancreas is unable to produce sufficient insulin to meet the body's needs, or insulin resistance develops at the cellular level.

For the initial screening of a patient for type 2 diabetes, a fasting blood sample is usually taken in the morning, after a fast of 10 to 12 hours. The patient's fasting blood glucose (FBG) level should be less than 100 mg/dL. If it is higher than 105 mg/dL, the provider may request a blood *glucose tolerance test* (GTT). For this test, the fasting patient receives a sugary liquid to drink that contains 100 g of glucose. (The amount may be adjusted according to the patient's weight.) A blood sugar level of less than 140 mg/dL after 2 hours is normal. A reading of more than 200 mg/dL after 2 hours may indicate diabetes. A reading between 140 and 200 mg/dL indicates impaired glucose tolerance, or prediabetes.

The medical assistant can screen a patient's blood glucose levels by using a glucometer cleared for home use by the Food and Drug Administration (FDA) (Procedure 55.6). The blood glucose level is routinely monitored by patients with diabetes mellitus type 1 or type 2. Self-monitoring of blood glucose levels has become an important part of diabetes management. A very small amount of blood from a capillary puncture is drawn into a test strip in a glucose monitor. The test strip electronically calibrates the monitor and then tests the patient sample for blood glucose. These rapid-test glucose strips test the blood with the help of enzymes that convert glucose into a colored product that is measurable. The monitor detects and records the results and displays them on a small screen.

Glucose levels may also be monitored by women with *gestational diabetes*, a condition seen during pregnancy in which the effect of insulin is partially blocked by hormones produced by the placenta (Fig. 55.12).

TABLE 55.6   Relationship Between Glycosylated Hemoglobin Levels and Blood Glucose Levels

Glycosylated Hemoglobin A1c (%)	Blood Glucose (mg/dL)
14.0	355
13.0	326
12.0	298
11.0	269
10.0	240
9.0	212
8.0	183
7.0	154
6.0	125
5.0	97
4.0	68

Hemoglobin A1c Testing

Hemoglobin A1c is also described as *glycosylated* (glahy KOH suh lay ted) *hemoglobin* (sugar-coated hemoglobin). Glycosylated hemoglobin is the result of glucose irreversibly binding to the hemoglobin molecules in the RBCs. It is also referred to as the A1c.

RBCs have a life span of approximately 120 days. Measuring the amount of glucose that has been irreversibly bound to hemoglobin provides an assessment of the average blood sugar during the 60 to 90 days before the test. The A1c test is performed every 3 months in patients with diabetes to monitor the person's average blood glucose level during those months. An A1c value that is higher than normal indicates that the average blood sugar has been elevated during the past 2 to 3 months. A normal A1c level for a person without diabetes ranges from 4% to 5.7%. For patients with diabetes, the goal is to maintain the glycosylated hemoglobin level below 7%. See Table 55.6, which associates glycosylated hemoglobin A1c levels with blood glucose levels. The goal for people with diabetes type 2 is to have A1c levels of 7% or lower. With higher levels, the risk of developing complications from diabetes increases.

Several methods can be used to measure the A1c level, and the medical assistant can perform A1c testing using several CLIA-waived devices. The DCA A1cNOW+ for Professionals (Bayer Diagnostics) provides A1c values in 6 minutes from 1 drop of capillary blood obtained from a fingerstick. Patients also can perform A1c testing at home using FDA-approved instruments, such as the A1cNow SelfCheck (Bayer) and the in2it (II) Self-Test A1c System (Bio-Rad).

Cholesterol Testing

Cholesterol (kuh LES tuh rohl) is a fatlike substance (lipid) present in cell membranes. It is needed to form bile acids, steroid hormones, the coverings of our nerves, and some of our brain tissue. Cholesterol travels in the blood as distinct particles containing both lipid and proteins. These particles are called lipoproteins (lahy poh PROH teens). The cholesterol level in the blood is determined partly by inheritance and partly by acquired factors, such as diet, calorie and nutrient balance, and level of physical activity.

Patients often are confused by cholesterol testing. Cholesterol is often a catchall term for both the cholesterol a person eats and the cholesterol that is produced in the body. A high blood level of low-density lipoprotein, or LDL, cholesterol reflects an increased risk of heart disease. LDL cholesterol is often referred to as "bad" cholesterol. Lower levels of LDL cholesterol reflect a lower risk of heart disease. When too much LDL cholesterol circulates in the blood, it can slowly build up in the walls of arteries that feed the heart and brain. Together with other substances, it can form *plaque*, a thick and sticky deposit that can clog arteries. This condition is known as *atherosclerosis* (ath uh roh skluh ROH sis). If a clot (*thrombus*) forms at the site of plaque, blood flow can be blocked in the coronary arteries of the heart muscle, causing a heart attack. If a clot blocks blood flow to part of the brain, a stroke may result. LDL results are often interpreted as:

- LDL <100 mg/dL = Optimal
- LDL 100–129 mg/dL = Near or above optimal
- LDL 130–159 mg/dL = Borderline high
- LDL 160–189 mg/dL = High
- LDL 190+ mg/dL = Very high

About one-third to one-fourth of blood cholesterol is carried by high-density lipoprotein (HDL). HDL cholesterol is known as the "good" cholesterol. High levels of HDL cholesterol seem to protect against heart attack. HDL can carry cholesterol away from the arteries and back to the liver. It is believed that cholesterol is removed from the lining of the arteries when high levels of HDL exist. Low levels of HDL cholesterol (i.e., lower than 40 mg/dL) may result in a greater risk of heart disease.

Adults older than 20 years of age should have a cholesterol test at least once every 5 years. Total cholesterol and the combination of LDL and HDL typically are screened and monitored (Procedure 55.7). All three tests are considered screening tests, and elevated results require additional testing. In general, total cholesterol levels under 200 mg/dL are considered normal. Results over 240 mg/dL are considered elevated and may place a person in the high-risk category for coronary heart disease. An HDL cholesterol level of 40 mg/dL or higher is considered acceptable for men, and values of 50 or higher are acceptable for women. HDL levels below 40 mg/dL for men and below 50 mg/dL for women place a person at risk of coronary heart disease.

Although total cholesterol and HDL cholesterol levels are not significantly affected by food consumption, most providers prefer that patients fast from food and liquids, with the exception of water, for 12 hours before cholesterol levels are checked. If the total cholesterol is elevated, the provider is likely to order a *lipid profile,* which is a series of tests that measures the total cholesterol, HDL and LDL cholesterol levels, and triglyceride (try GLIS uh ride) levels. Triglycerides are fat in the blood related to caloric intake. Therefore the patient must be instructed to fast from all food and alcoholic beverages 12 hours before the triglyceride test or lipid profiles. Consistently high triglyceride levels may lead to heart disease, especially in people with low levels of HDL cholesterol and high levels of LDL cholesterol, and in people with type 2 diabetes. Elevated levels of triglycerides are typically stored in the belly and are associated with central obesity.

CLIA-waived cholesterol monitors can measure total cholesterol from a fingerstick specimen. The Cholestech LDX analyzer performs a lipid panel and provides a risk assessment using a capillary blood sample (see Procedure 55.7). This system uses a cassette testing device capable of measuring glucose, total cholesterol (TC), HDL, LDL, very-low-density lipoprotein (VLDL), triglycerides, and the TC/HDL ratio. It uses a combination of testing methods to detect the color changes caused by each of the lipid panel analytes.

CRITICAL THINKING 55.6

One of Michelle's favorite patients is in today, Sophie McCoy. She is 86 years young, still lives in her own home, and works in her garden every chance she gets. Sophie had a cholesterol screen at a local senior citizens health fair recently, and her results were as follows:
Total cholesterol 202 mg/dL, LDL 104 mg/dL, HDL 42 mg/dL
Given Sophie's age and general good health, are the cholesterol results concerning? Are they normal, high, or low?

Alanine Aminotransferase (ALT) and Aspartate Aminotransferase (AST) Testing

Certain drugs can impair liver function and require the monitoring of two liver enzymes:
- *Alanine aminotransferase* (AL uh neen uh mee noh TRANS fuh reys)
- *Aspartate* (uh SPAHR teyt) *aminotransferase*

These two liver enzymes will rise in the blood during liver damage. The following drugs cause liver damage:
- Statins, which are used to lower blood cholesterol
- Fibrates, a specific type of antidiabetic and antihypertensive drug

The provider will order liver function tests or panels to monitor the liver during therapy with drugs that have the potential to cause liver malfunction.

CLIA-waived liver enzyme testing for ALT and AST may be monitored on the same Cholestech LDX System using ALT/AST test cassettes.

Thyroid Hormone Testing

The thyroid gland is located anterior to the trachea in the throat. It produces the hormones *triiodothyronine* (trahy ahy oh doh THAHY ruh neen), or T₃, and *thyroxine* (thahy ROK seen), or T₄. These hormones are essential for life and regulate body metabolism, growth, and development. The thyroid gland is influenced by hormones produced by two other glands found in the brain, the pituitary gland and the hypothalamus. The pituitary gland produces thyroid-stimulating hormone (TSH), and the hypothalamus produces thyrotropin (thahy ruh TROH pin)-releasing hormone (TRH).

CLIA-waived rapid diagnostic tests are available to *qualitatively* (KWOL I tey tiv lee) measure TSH. These tests are available for point-of-care (POC) testing. Using whole blood from a fingerstick, CLIA-waived tests can screen patients for hypothyroidism. Hypothyroidism is indicated with elevated TSH levels. The tests use lateral flow immunoassay technology housed in a plastic cassette. One such commercially available test is the ThyroTest Whole Blood TSH Test.

VOCABULARY
hypothyroidism Deficient activity of the thyroid gland.
lateral flow immunoassay A laboratory or clinical technique that uses the specific binding between an antigen and an antibody to identify and quantify a substance in a sample. The sample in this technique moves in a sideways motion, usually on an absorbent paper.

REFERENCE LABORATORY CHEMISTRY PANELS AND SINGLE ANALYTE TESTING AND MONITORING

Automated blood chemistry analyzers are often used to perform blood chemistry testing in a reference laboratory. It is common for several analytes to be detected at once. A provider may order a chemistry panel, such as a renal or liver panel, to determine the levels of several related analytes (Fig. 55.13). Analytes commonly detected in the chemistry department are listed in Table 55.7. In general, serum from a clotted specimen is needed to perform these tests. Typical panels are shown in Table 55.8. As noted previously, laboratory reports, both electronic and paper, must provide their own reference ranges, along with each patient's results. Different methodologies may generate different reference ranges and may use different units of measurement.

Physician's Medical Center
77332 E. Capital Drive
Anytown, USA 11123

Ronald J. Haldor, M.D.
Kaye M. Jones, M.D.
Nicholas P. Stepp, M.D.

PATIENT – PLEASE NOTE

If this box is checked, don't eat or drink anything, except water, for 14 hours before going to the lab.

PATIENT NAME _____
           LAST   FIRST   M.I.

ADDRESS _____ DOB _____

CITY _____ STATE _____ ZIP _____ SEX: M F

TELEPHONE # _____ SOCIAL SECURITY # ____ – ____ – ____

ORDERING PHYSICIAN _____ DATE _____

BILLING: ☐ HMO ☐ MEDICARE ☐ MEDICAL ☐ OTHER # _____

    GUARANTOR (If other than patient) _____

☐ PHONE RESULTS TO _____

☐ SEND ADDITIONAL COPIES OF REPORT TO _____
    (Please attach copy of eligibility card.)

Patient Diagnosis _____

☐ 906 ARTERIAL BLOOD GASES
    ROOM AIR _____
    RESP. ASSIST _____
☐ 105 BLOOD CELL PROFILE (Hgb + Hct)
☐ 862 BILIRUBIN (NEONATAL)
☐ 868 BILIRUBIN (TOTAL & DIRECT)
☐ 100 CBC (Complete Blood Count & Diff)
☐ 3000 ELECTROLYTES
☐   (NA, K, CO2, Cl)
☐   FANA
☐   GLUCOSE
☐ 915 GLUCOSE, PRE-NATAL DIABETIC SCR.
    (1 Hour Post-Glucola)
☐   GLUCOSE TOLERANCE TEST
    # OF HOURS_____DOSE_____
☐ 3398 HEPATITIS PANEL
    (B-Surf Ag/Ab, B-Core Ab, A-Ab)
☐ 988 LIPID PROFILE
    (Chol, Trig, HDL, LDL, Cardiac Risk)
☐ 3380 LIVER PANEL
    (Alk Phos, Bili, TP, Alb, GGT, SGOT
    (AST) SGPT (ALT), & Consult)
☐ 3006 METABOLIC 7
    (Na, K, CO2, Cl, Glu, Mg)

☐ 3035 PANEL 17
    (Panel 13 + Na + K + Cl + CO2)
☐ 3020 METABOLIC 10
    (Na, K, CO2, Cl, Glu, BUN, Creat)
☐ 3015 METABOLIC 11
    (Met 10 & Phos)
☐ 3160 OBSTETRICAL PANEL 1
    (CBC, UA, ABO/Rh, Antibody
    Screen, Rubella, RPR)
☐ 3172 OBSTETRICAL PANEL 3
    (CBC, ABO/Rh, Antibody Screen,
    Rubella, RPR)
☐ 3445 OBSTETRICAL PANEL 7
    (ABO/Rh, Antibody Screen,
    Rubella, RPR)
☐ 3447 OBSTETRICAL PANEL 7A
    (ABO/Rh, Antibody Screen,
    Rubella, RPR, Hepatitis B Surt Ag)
☐ 3025 PANEL 13
    (Glu, BUN, Creat, Uric Acid, Ca,
    Tp, Alb, Bili, Chol, Alk, Phos,
    SGOT (AST), LDH, Phos)
☐ 3030 PANEL 15
    (Panel 13 + Na + K)

☐ 3010 METABOLIC 8
    (Na, K, CO2, Cl, Glu, BUN)
☐ 3040 PANEL 20 - SMAC
    (Panel 17 + SGPT (ALT) +
    GGT + Osmolality)
☐ 3043 S-1 Panel (Panel 20 + Triglyceride)
☐ 500 PROTHROMBIN TIME (PT)
☐ 505 Partial Thromboplastin Time (PPT)
☐ 7500 RPR
☐ 7515 RUBELLA
☐ 2030 THYROID SCREEN
    (T4, T3, Uptake, Adj T4)
☐ 704 URINALYSIS

BACTERIOLOGY

SPECIMEN SOURCE (REQUIRED)
COLLECTION DATE _____
☐ _____ ROUTINE CULTURE
☐ 8919 AFB CULTURE
☐ 8921 FUNGAL CULTURE

ADDITIONAL LABORATORY TESTS: _____
_____
_____
_____
_____

2804 (4/93)

LABORATORY OUTPATIENT REQUEST

OFFICE USE ONLY

Telephone Order per _____

Order Received by _____

Fig. 55.13 Panel Request Form. (From Niedzwiecki B, et al: *Kinn's the medical assistant*, ed 14, St. Louis, 2020, Elsevier.)

TABLE 55.7 Blood Chemistry Tests[a]

Test	Abbreviation	Normal Values	Description	Purpose
Alanine aminotransferase	ALT (SGPT)	8–20 units/L	Enzyme found predominantly in the liver but also in the kidney	To detect liver disease
Albumin		3.5–5 g/dL	Protein	To assess kidney function
Alkaline phosphatase	ALP	20–140 units/L	Enzyme found in several tissues	To detect liver and bone disease
Aspartate aminotransferase	AST (SGOT)	10–40 units/L	Enzyme found in several tissues	To detect tissue damage
Blood urea nitrogen	BUN	7–18 mg/dL or 2.5–6.4 mmol/L	Metabolic products of protein catabolism	To detect renal disease
Calcium	Ca	8.4–10.2 mg/dL or 2.1–2.6 mmol/L	Mineral	To assess parathyroid function and calcium metabolism
Chloride	Cl	95–105 mmol/L	Electrolyte	To determine acid-base and water balance
Cholesterol	CH, Chol	Total: <200 mg/dL LDL: <130 mg/dL HDL: >40 mg/dL (men); >50 mg/dL (women)	Lipid	To screen for atherosclerosis related to heart disease
Creatine phosphokinase	CPK or CK	Males: 25–90 U/L Females 10–70 U/L	Enzyme found in several tissues	To assess source of muscle damage (myocardial infarct)
Creatinine	Creat	0.6–1.2 mg/dL	Metabolic product of protein catabolism	To screen for renal function
Ferritin		Males: 40–400 ng/mL Females: 12–160 ng/mL	Iron-carrying protein	To detect amount of iron stored in the body
Gamma glutamyl transferase	GGT	0–45 units/L	Enzyme found mainly in liver cells	To detect liver disease
Globulin	glob, lg	Varies according to type	Protein	To detect abnormalities in protein synthesis and removal
Glucose fasting blood sugar	FBS	70–99 mg/dL	Carbohydrate	To detect disorders of glucose metabolism (diabetes)
Glucose tolerance test	GTT	Varies with time	Carbohydrate	To detect disorders of glucose metabolism (diabetes)
Iron	Fe	50–160 µg/dL	Mineral	To assist in diagnosis of anemia
Lactate dehydrogenase	LDH	45–90 U/L	Enzyme found in several tissues	To assist in confirmation of myocardial or pulmonary infarct
pH	pH	7.35–7.45	Measurement of the acid-base (acidity and alkalinity)	To assess acidity or alkalinity of blood
Phosphorus	P	3–4.5 mg/dL or 0.97–1.45 mmol/L	Mineral	To assist in proper evaluation of calcium levels and to detect endocrine system disorders
Potassium	K	3.5–5.0 mmol/L	Mineral	To assist in diagnosis of acid-base and water balance
Sodium	Na	135–145 mmol/L	Mineral	To assist in diagnosis of acid-base and water balance
Total bilirubin	TB	0.1–1 mg/dL or 2–17 mmol/L	Metabolic product of hemoglobin catabolism	To evaluate liver function and to aid in diagnosis of anemia
Total iron-binding capacity	TIBC	250–400 mcg/dL		A measure of the potential to transport iron
Total protein	TP	6–8 g/dL; 60–80 g/L		To assess the state of hydration; to screen for diseases that alter protein balance
Troponin I and T		<0.4	Cardiac-specific protein found only with heart muscle damage	To aid in diagnosis of myocardial infarct
Thyroid-stimulating hormone (thyrotropin)	TSH	0.5–6 milliunits/L	Hormone produced by the pituitary	To assess thyroid and pituitary gland function
Thyroxine	T4	5–12 mcg/dL	Hormone produced by the thyroid gland	To assess thyroid function
Triglycerides	Trig	30–190 mg/dL	Fats in the blood related to caloric intake.	To screen for atherosclerosis related to heart disease
Triiodothyronine (resin uptake)	T3	25%–35%	Hormone produced by the thyroid gland	To assess thyroid function
Uric acid	UA	Male: 3.4–7 mg/dL or 202–416 mcmol/L Female: 2.4–6 mg/dL or 143–357 mcmol/L	Metabolic product of protein catabolism	To evaluate renal failure, gout, and leukemia

[a]Lab reports, both electronic and paper, must supply their own reference ranges, along with each patient's results. This is because different methodologies may create different reference ranges and different units of measurement.

From Niedzwiecki B, et al: Kinn's the medical assistant, ed 14, St. Louis, 2020, Elsevier.

TABLE 55.8   Typical Chemistry Panels

Panel	Component	Panel	Component
Liver	Alkaline phosphatase (ALP) Gamma glutamyl transferase (GGT) Aspartate aminotransferase (AST) Alanine aminotransferase (ALT) Lactate dehydrogenase (LDH)	Cardiac	Creatine phosphokinase (CPK) Troponin I Troponin T
Anemia	Iron Total iron-binding capacity Ferritin Transferrin	Electrolyte	Sodium Potassium Chloride
Thyroid	Thyroid-stimulating hormone (TSH) Thyroxine (T_4) Triiodothyronine (T_3)	Renal	Creatinine Blood urea nitrogen (BUN) Uric acid Glucose

From Niedzwiecki B, et al: *Kinn's the medical assistant,* ed 14, St. Louis, 2020, Elsevier.

CLOSING COMMENTS

An ever-increasing number of CLIA-waived hematology and chemistry blood tests are relatively simple to perform and require minimal training. This has allowed the provider to share the results with the patient immediately. This results in greater patient compliance with the prescribed treatment plan. Proper patient care demands attention to detail in all three areas of the testing process:

- *Preanalytic:* Proper care of the testing supplies and equipment, and proper patient identification and specimen collection

- *Analytic:* Running the tests according to the specific manufacturer's instructions; recording and analyzing the controls and the test results
- *Postanalytic:* Proper disposal of biohazardous supplies; routing of test results to the provider and patient

The medical assistant is involved in all of these elements. He or she is responsible for the organization and documentation of each test performed on the appropriate lab flow sheet and in the patient's health record.

PATIENT-CENTERED CARE

As with all laboratory procedures, the test is only as good as the specimen! The medical assistant, as the provider's agent, is responsible for the authenticity of the sample when you instruct your patient regarding collection. You are also responsible for the patient results when you perform the test.

A medical assistant who is responsible for office laboratory testing must clearly understand the basic concepts of laboratory medicine. Therefore you must stay current with the rapid technological advances in laboratory medicine and help establish testing protocols best suited to your provider-employer.

You are responsible for properly collecting specimens and testing them accurately. Patient confidentiality is paramount when testing is performed, as is following all the established quality control procedures.

Excellent customer service comes from dedicated, detail-oriented healthcare workers!

BEING PROFESSIONAL

Michelle has been working at the office for a long time and has become well acquainted with many of the patients who frequent the office to have their PT/INR testing done. On this particular day, one of Michelle's patients refused to give the required patient identifiers prior to Michelle performing the test.

Role-play this scenario with a peer: Your peer will play a frequent patient who refuses to give the proper identification information required. You will be the medical assistant. In your role-play, address this situation.

CHAPTER REVIEW

Red blood cells, white blood cells, and platelets all have unique reference ranges that may change over a person's life span. Waived hematology testing performed in a POL consists of four tests: hematocrit, hemoglobin, erythrocyte sedimentation rate, and the prothrombin time, which is a coagulation test.

Hematology in the reference laboratory consists of mostly moderate-complexity tests, which include a complete blood count. A CBC has a number of individual tests included in this automated analysis. A CBC can include the following tests: RBC count, WBC count, platelet count, hemoglobin, and hematocrit. Other important values are the RBC indices, which are calculations based on the RBC analytes. The RBC indices include the mean corpuscular volume (MCV), the mean corpuscular hemoglobin (MCH), and the mean corpuscular hemoglobin concentration (MCHC). These calculated indices help the provider to determine the possible type of anemia present and possible mode of treatment.

Hematology white blood cell counts can indicate a variety of disease states, such as infection, leukemia, lymphoma, or viral infections. Abnormal platelet counts that are too low may cause easy bruising and bleeding and can be life threatening.

For the differential test, a drop of blood is spread out thinly on a glass microscope slide and allowed to air dry before a stain is added. The stained slide is then examined under the microscope to look at the cells of the blood. Their shape, size, content, and overall appearance are noted. This useful information should agree with the automated analysis of the blood and will give the provider additional clues to the person's health.

Blood typing and cross-matching blood for transfusion is precise work. Although type and crossmatch testing is not waived testing, the medical assistant may be involved in collecting the specimen and documenting the test results in the patient's electronic health record. ABO and Rh typing are the most common antigen systems in blood typing, but other blood systems do exist, and the medical assistant should easily recognize the terms.

There are many waived tests that can be performed in chemistry. They include blood glucose testing, hemoglobin A1c testing, cholesterol and lipid testing, alanine aminotransferase (ALT) and aspartate aminotransferase (AST) testing (i.e., liver enzyme testing), and thyroid hormone testing. Handheld chemistry monitors can do a variety of tests, and they have the added benefit of being quick and accurate. Patient samples can be tested in the provider's office, and results can be discussed in a timely manner. This may lead to better patient compliance.

Chemistry profiles or panels are groups of analytes that are common to a particular organ or body system. Examples of chemistry profiles include a cardiac profile, liver profile, thyroid profile, and electrolyte panel. Most profile or panel testing makes use of complex automated equipment and is generally not CLIA-waived testing. However, individual analytes may be available in a waived kit or monitor.

Proper patient care requires attention to detail in all three areas of the testing process: preanalytic, analytic, and postanalytic. From greeting a new patient to recording results and documenting laboratory results, the medical assistant must always remain detail oriented and patient focused.

SCENARIO WRAP-UP

It has been another busy day for Michelle at WMFM Clinic. She had a chance to see a variety of patients with a variety of concerns. It was a normal day at work! Michelle enjoys the variety. She also enjoys the work she does with the laboratory. Michelle prepares specimens for transport to the reference lab.

She checks on results once they are posted in patients' electronic health records. She knows that Dr. Perez and all the providers at WMFM Clinic rely on lab results as part of patient diagnosis and monitoring treatment.

PROCEDURE 55.1   Perform Preventive Maintenance for the Microhematocrit Centrifuge

Task
Perform daily, monthly, semiannual, and annual maintenance on a microhematocrit centrifuge.

Equipment and Supplies
- Microhematocrit centrifuge
- Maintenance logbook
- Utility gloves
- Fluid-impermeable lab coat, eye protection, and gloves
- Disinfectant
- Biohazard waste container

Procedural Steps
1. Wash hands or use hand sanitizer. Put on fluid-impermeable lab coat, eye protection, and gloves. In all maintenance procedures, gloves are worn under the utility gloves.
   Notes: These are generic recommendations. Always check the manufacturer's guidelines for specific instructions. Always unplug the power cord before cleaning or servicing the centrifuge.

Daily Maintenance
1. Clean the inside of the centrifuge and the gasket with a disinfectant recommended by the manufacturer. Plastic and nonmetal parts may be cleaned with a fresh solution of 5% sodium hypochlorite (bleach) mixed 1:10 with water.

Purpose: To remove any dried blood or shattered glass. Do not use bleach on the gasket because it may harden the rubber.

Monthly Maintenance
3. Check the reading device. Misuse and zeroing of the reading devices can result in considerable error. Always use a second, simple reading device as a cross-check. Use a ruler or a flat plastic card specially made for this purpose. To use these cards, lay the spun hematocrit tube on the card, and align the red cells with a line on the card to obtain the reading (Fig. 1).

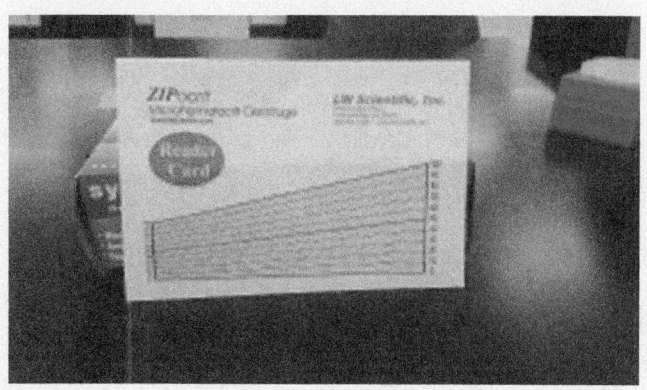

Continued

PROCEDURE 55.1   Perform Preventive Maintenance for the Microhematocrit Centrifuge—cont'd

4. Check the rotor for cracks or corrosion and check the interior for signs of white powder.

   Purpose: Cracks, corrosion, or powder may indicate impending rotor failure; these findings require the immediate attention of a service technician.

Semiannual Maintenance

5. Check the gasket for cuts and breaks.

   Purpose: Cut gaskets allow tubes to leak and must be replaced.
6. Check the timer with a stopwatch to verify timer accuracy.
7. Perform a maximum cell pack to verify the time required for complete packing by reading a sample after centrifugation and then recentrifuging for 1 minute. The results should be the same. If they are not, perform preventive maintenance or call the service technician.

   Purpose: If the cells compact further during recentrifugation, the centrifuge is not rotating at the proper speed, and hematocrit results will be falsely elevated.

Annual Maintenance (or Maintenance Performed as Needed)

8. The centrifuge functions and maintenance verification should be performed by qualified personnel. This includes checking the centrifuge mechanism, rotors, timer, speed, and electrical leads.
9. Record all preventive maintenance in the laboratory logbook.

   Purpose: Recording maintenance is necessary to maintain warranties and to comply with regulations established by CLIA and other regulatory agencies.

MICROHEMATOCRIT CENTRIFUGE MAINTENANCE LOG		
DATE	SERVICE	INITIALS
10/7/20XX	Performed routine daily and monthly preventive maintenance	AJ

PROCEDURE 55.2   Perform CLIA-Waived Hematology Testing: Perform a Microhematocrit Test

Tasks

Perform a microhematocrit test accurately. Document the result on the lab flow sheet and patient health record.

Equipment and Supplies

- Patient's health record
- Provider's order and/or lab requisition
- Microhematocrit lab log
- Fresh sample of blood collected in a tube containing ethylenediaminetetraacetic acid (EDTA) anticoagulant (or equipment for fingerstick specimen: lancet, alcohol wipe, gauze, bandage)
- Plastic-coated self-sealing capillary tubes, or plain capillary tubes (blue tipped)
- Sealing clay (if capillary tubes are not self-sealing)
- Gauze
- Microhematocrit centrifuge
- Fluid-impermeable lab coat, protective eyewear, and gloves
- Biohazard waste container
- Biohazard sharps containers

Procedural Steps

1. Wash hands or use hand sanitizer. Put on fluid-impermeable lab coat, protective eyewear, and gloves.

   Purpose: To control infection.
2. Assemble the materials needed.

   a. *If the capillary tubes are self-sealing:* Fill two tubes by inserting the end opposite the sealed end into the well-mixed EDTA blood sample. *Note:* If the capillary tube and the EDTA tube are held almost parallel to the table, the capillary tubes fill easily by capillary action. When the self-sealing capillary tubes are two-thirds to three-fourths filled, tilt them upright, causing the blood sample to flow down the tube and meet the sealant. Continue to hold the tube vertical when the blood contacts the sealant for an additional 15 seconds.

   Purpose: Duplicates should always be done as a means of quality control.

   b. *Alternative:* Fill two plain (blue-tipped) mylar-wrapped capillary tubes two-thirds to three-fourths full of a well-mixed EDTA blood sample. Tip the blood tube slightly, touching the capillary tube into the blood using the side that is opposite the blue band. When enough blood has filled

the capillary tube, tip the blue end of the tube down, causing the blood to flow toward the blue tip. Then readjust the tube horizontally while inserting the blue tip of the capillary tube into the clay sealant. Insert the tube as many times as needed to achieve a plug up to the blue band (Fig. 1).

Purpose: Duplicates should always be done as a means of quality control. Tubes are not filled completely to provide space for the sealing clay.

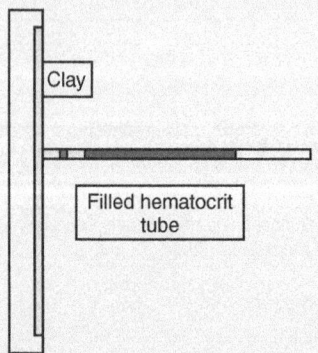

1

(From Keohane E et al: Rodak's hematology: clinical principles and applications, ed 5, St. Louis, 2016, Saunders.)

3. Wipe the outside of the tubes with clean gauze without touching the wet open end of the tube.

   Purpose: Wiping the outside of the capillary tube removes any blood. Touching the blood inside the capillary tube with absorbent material removes more plasma than blood cells and can alter the hematocrit.
4. Place the tubes opposite each other in the centrifuge with the sealed ends securely against the gasket (see Fig. 55.1).

   Purpose: The centrifuge must always be balanced to prevent damage. If the clay ends of the capillary tubes are not outermost against the gasket, the sample will spin out of the tubes, contaminating the centrifuge.

PROCEDURE 55.2 Perform CLIA-Waived Hematology Testing: Perform a Microhematocrit Test—cont'd

5. Note the numbers on the centrifuge slots and record the numbers on the log sheet, along with the patient's name
   Purpose: The sample must be identified throughout the entire procedure.
6. Secure the locking top, fasten the lid down, and lock it.
   Purpose: If the locking top is not firmly in place during the spinning cycle, the tubes will come out of their slots and break. The lid is always locked during centrifugation for safety purposes, to prevent the ejection of aerosols or broken glass.
7. Set the timer to 3 to 5 minutes and adjust the speed to 11,000 to 12,000 rpm, or as indicated by the manufacturer's instructions Note: Check the manufacturer's instructions for time and speed, since models vary.
8. Allow the centrifuge to come to a complete stop. Unlock the outer locking top, and then remove the inner lid.
   Purpose: Opening the centrifuge before it has stopped could result in harm to the user.
9. Remove the tubes immediately and read the results. If this is not possible, store the tubes in an upright position.
   Purpose: Tubes left in the centrifuge will show altered results because the red blood cell (RBC) layer will spread out horizontally.
10. Determine the microhematocrit values using one of the following methods:
    a. Centrifuge with built-in reader using calibrated capillary tubes:
       - Position the tubes as directed by the manufacturer's instructions.
       - Read both tubes.
       - The average of the two results is reported.
       - The two values should not vary by more than 2%.
    b. Centrifuge without a built-in reader:
       - Carefully remove the tubes from the centrifuge.
       - Place a tube on the microhematocrit reader.
       - Align the clay-RBC junction with the zero line on the reader. Align the plasma meniscus with the 100% line. The value is read at the junction of the red cell layer and the buffy coat. The buffy coat is not included in the reading (Fig. 2).
       - Read both tubes.
       - The average of the two results is reported.

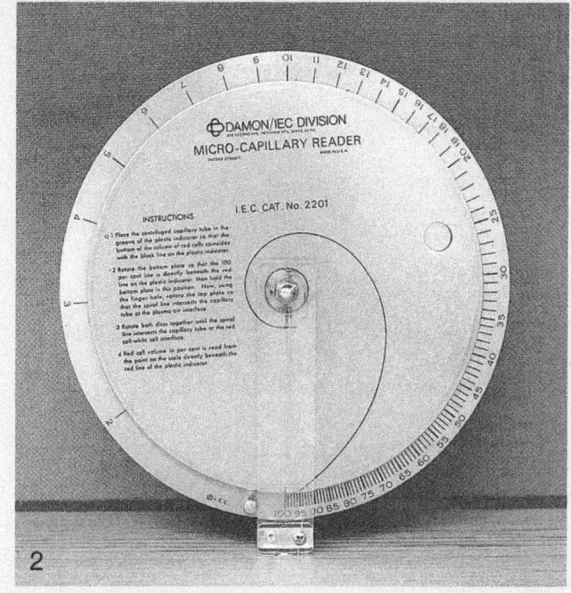

(From Keohane E et al: Rodak's hematology: clinical principles and applications, ed 5, St. Louis, 2016, Saunders.)

11. Dispose of the capillary tubes in a biohazard sharps container.
12. Disinfect the work area, and properly dispose of all biohazardous materials. Remove your gloves, eyewear, and lab coat.
13. Wash hands or use hand sanitizer.
    Purpose: To control infections.
14. Record the results in the Hematocrit Patient Log and document the results in the patient's health record. Using the normal range, identify if test result is normal or abnormal.
    Purpose: A procedure is not considered done until it is charted.

HEMATOCRIT—PATIENT LOG

Hematocrit expected values:
Adult Males = 42%–52%
Adult Females = 36%–48%
Infants = 32%–38%
Children = increase to adult

DATE	TECH	PATIENT I.D.	SLOT #	RESULT	CHARTED
10/7/20–	dc	# 12345	1 & 4	44% & 44%	✓

- The two values should not vary by more than 2%.

Documentation Example
10/07/20XX 11:25 a.m. Hct 55%._____Michelle James, CMA (AAMA)

PROCEDURE 55.3   Perform CLIA-Waived Hematology Testing: Perform a Hemoglobin Test

Tasks
Perform a capillary puncture and to accurately determine the level of hemoglobin present in a blood sample using the HemoCue B-Hemoglobin System. Document the result on the lab flow sheet and patient health record.

Equipment and Supplies
- Patient's health record
- Provider's order and/or lab requisition
- Hemoglobin laboratory log
- HemoCue monitor
- HemoCue microcuvette
- Safety blood lancet
- Alcohol wipes
- Gauze
- Fluid-impermeable lab coat, protective eyewear, and gloves
- Biohazard waste container
- Biohazard sharps containers

Procedural Steps
1. Perform an instrument quality control check by inserting the control cuvette into the instrument. Make sure the reading is within acceptable limits before proceeding.
   Purpose: Only instruments that record values within acceptable control limits can be used for patient testing. If the value is outside the control limits, refer to the troubleshooting guide for the instrument or contact the manufacturer.
2. Wash hands or use hand sanitizer. Put on fluid-impermeable lab coat, protective eyewear, and gloves.
   Purpose: To control infection.
3. Check the provider's order and collect the necessary equipment and supplies.
4. Greet the patient. Identify yourself. Verify the patient's identity with the full name, ask the patient to spell the first and last name and to give date of birth.
5. Explain the procedure to be performed in a manner that the patient understands. Answer any questions the patient may have on the procedure. Obtain permission for a capillary puncture.
   Purpose: It is important to identify the patient in two different ways to ensure that you have the correct patient. Explaining the procedure can make the patient feel more comfortable and reduces anxiety.
6. Examine the patient's fingers, and choose the site to be used to obtain the blood sample.
   Purpose: The site must be free of trauma, calluses, and scarring.
7. Clean the site with an alcohol wipe or another recommended antiseptic preparation.
8. Perform a capillary puncture, and wipe away the first drop of blood.
   Purpose: This drop may contain tissue fluid or antiseptic that may hemolyze the blood.
9. Obtain a large drop blood on the surface of the finger.
10. Touch the microcuvette to the drop of blood. Do not touch the finger. The correct volume is drawn into the cuvette by capillary action. Wipe off any excess blood from the sides of the cuvette (Figs.1 and 2).
    Purpose: Blood on the cuvette may alter the readings or contaminate the instrument.

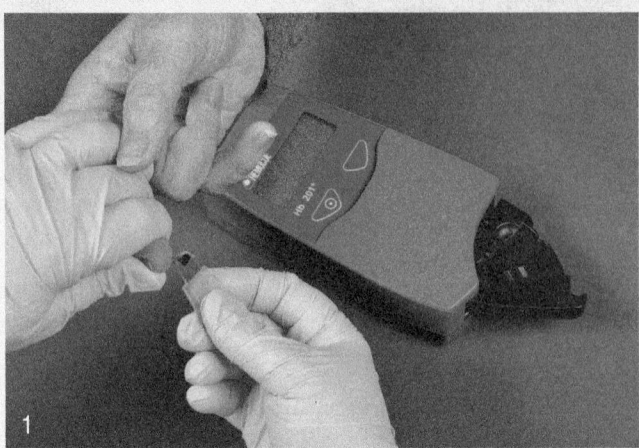

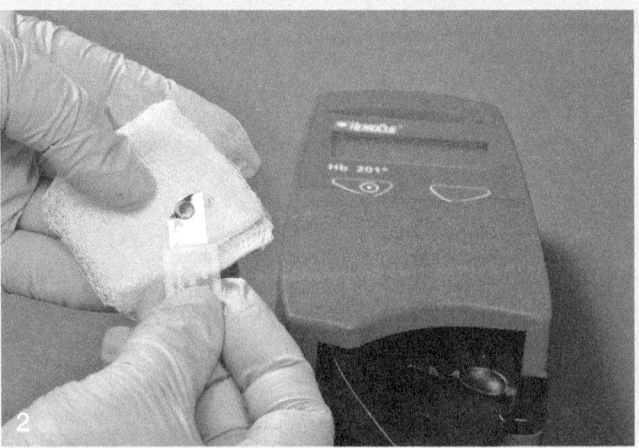

11. Place the cuvette in the cuvette holder of the HemoCue sample door, and close the door of the instrument (Fig. 3).

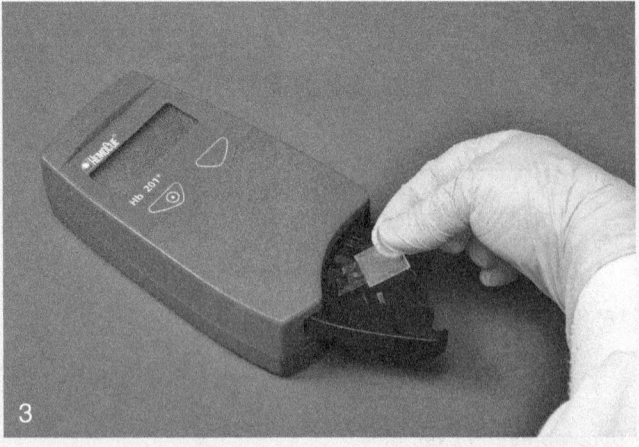

PROCEDURE 55.3 Perform CLIA-Waived Hematology Testing: Perform a Hemoglobin Test—cont'd

12. Read the result.
13. Dispose of biohazardous waste in biohazard waste containers and the sharps in the biohazard sharps container. Turn off the instrument. Properly disinfect the work area.
14. Remove your gloves and dispose of them in the biohazard waste container. Remove the lab coat and protective eyewear.
15. Wash hands or use hand sanitizer.
    Purpose: To control infection.

16. Record the result in the lab's hemoglobin log and the patient's health record. Using the normal range, identify if test result is normal or abnormal.
    Purpose: A procedure is not completed until the results are recorded.

HEMOCUE B HEMOGLOBIN SYSTEM PATIENT LOG

TEST: _____ KIT LOT # _____

Hemoglobin expected values= Adult Males = 13.0–18.0 g/dL
Adult Females = 12.0–16.0 g/dL
Infants = 10.0–14.0 g/dL
Children = increase to adult

DATE	TECH	PATIENT I.D.	RESULT	CHARTED
10/09/20–	DC	# 12345	15.5 g/dL	✓

Documentation Example
10/09/20XX 9:30 a.m. Hgb 15.5 g/dL._____ Michelle James, CMA (AAMA)

PROCEDURE 55.4 Perform CLIA-Waived Hematology Testing: Determine the Erythrocyte Sedimentation Rate Using a Modified Westergren Method

Tasks
Fill a Westergren tube properly and observe and record an erythrocyte sedimentation rate (ESR) obtained by using a modified Westergren method. Document the result on the lab flow sheet and patient health record.

Equipment and Supplies
- Patient's health record
- Provider's order and/or lab requisition
- Erythrocyte sedimentation rate (ESR) laboratory log
- Ethylenediaminetetraacetic acid (EDTA)–anticoagulated blood specimen
- Safety tube decapper (if tubes do not have Hemogard plastic tops)
- Disposable transfer pipet
- Sediplast ESR system (prefilled Sediplast vial)
- Sediplast rack
- Timer
- Fluid-impermeable lab coat, eye protection, and gloves
- Biohazard waste container
- Biohazard sharps container

Procedural Steps
1. Wash hands or use hand sanitizer. Put on a fluid-impermeable lab coat, eye protection, and gloves.
   Purpose: To control infection.
2. Assemble the materials needed.
3. Check the leveling bubble of the Sediplast rack.
   Purpose: The rack must be horizontal on the table or bench to ensure that the tube is vertical and free of any vibrations or movement.
4. Bring the blood sample to room temperature if it has been refrigerated and mix the sample well by gently inverting the tube 6 to 8 times, making sure the tube has no bubbles.

Continued

PROCEDURE 55.4   Perform CLIA-Waived Hematology Testing: Determine the Erythrocyte Sedimentation Rate Using a Modified Westergren Method—cont'd

Purpose: Cells settle when a specimen stands, and blood must always be well mixed before sampling. Test results will be altered if refrigerated blood is not brought to room temperature.

5. Remove the plastic Hemogard stopper on the blood sample by twisting and slowly pushing up on the stopper with your thumbs (or by using a tube decapper on rubber-stoppered blood tubes). Label with the patient's name and then remove the stopper on the prefilled Sediplast vial.

   Purpose: Using the Hemogard cover or removing the rubber cap with a protective device blocks blood splashes and helps prevent aerosolization of the specimen.

6. Fill the Sediplast vial with blood to the indicated line using a disposable transfer pipet (Fig. 1). Replace the stopper on the prefilled vial and invert it several times to mix. Recap the blood collection tube with its stopper.

   Purpose: This dilutes the blood in accordance with the Westergren procedure.

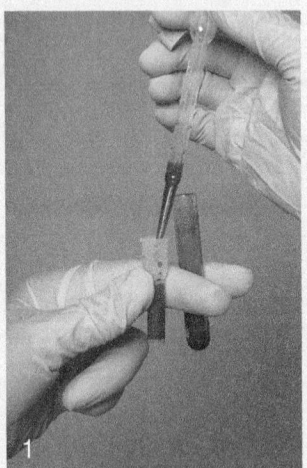

(Courtesy Polymedco, Cortland Manor, NY.)

7. Insert a Sediplast pipet through the pierceable stopper on the prefilled vial, and push down until the pipet touches the bottom of the vial. The pipet automatically draws the blood up and over the zero mark (Fig. 2).

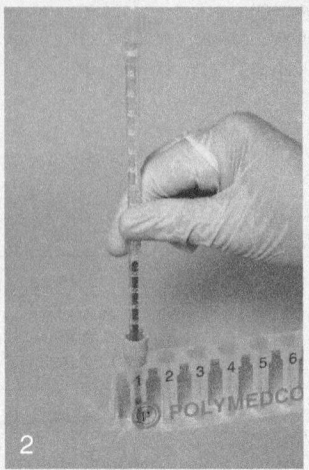

(Courtesy Polymedco, Cortland Manor, NY.)

8. Insert the filled Sediplast pipet and its vial into the Sediplast rack, making sure the vial is vertical.

   Purpose: A pipet that is not vertical produces incorrect results.

9. Note the start time on the ESR log sheet and allow the vial to stand undisturbed for 60 minutes.

   Purpose: Jarring or moving the vial increases the sedimentation rate.

10. After 60 minutes, measure the distance the erythrocytes have fallen at the top of the tube. The scale reads in millimeters—each line is 1 mm.

11. Properly dispose of all biohazardous materials. Dispose of the plastic Sediplast pipet and its vial into a biohazard sharps container. Disinfect the work area. Remove your gloves, protective eyewear, and lab coat. Wash hands or use hand sanitizer.

12. Record the findings in the lab's ESR log and the patient's health record. Remember, the Westergren ESR is reported in millimeters per hour (mm/hr). Using the normal range, identify if test result is normal or abnormal.

    Purpose: A procedure is considered not done until it is recorded.

ESR—SEDIPLAST—PATIENT LOG

ESR expected values: Adult Males < 50 years = 0–15 mm/hr
Adult Males > 50 years = 0–20 mm/hr
Adult Females < 50 years = 0–20 mm/hr
Adult Females > 50 years = 0–30 mm/hr

DATE	TECH	PATIENT I.D.	SLOT #	TIME	RESULT	CHARTED
10/09/20–	DC	# 12345	2	60 min	15 mm	✓

Documentation Example

10/09/20XX 9:30 a.m. ESR 15 mm in 60 minutes._____ Michelle James, CMA (AAMA)

PROCEDURE 55.5   Perform a CLIA-Waived PT/INR Test

Tasks

Perform a capillary puncture and perform a coagulation test to determine PT/INR using the CoaguChek XS instrument with built-in quality control. Document the result on the lab flow sheet and patient health record.

Directions

Perform a protime/INR test on Connie Lange STAT.

Equipment and Supplies

- Patient's health record or flowchart (see Fig. 55.6)
- Provider's order and/or lab requisition
- PT/INR lab log
- Gauze, alcohol wipes, bandage
- CoaguChek XS PT Test monitor (see Fig. 55.5)
- CoaguChek lancet
- CoaguChek test strip container and code chip
- Package insert or flowchart with directions
- Fluid-impermeable lab coat, protective eyewear, and gloves
- Biohazard waste container
- Biohazard sharps containers

Procedural Steps

1. Wash hands or use hand sanitizer. Put on fluid-impermeable lab coat, protective eyewear, and gloves.
   Purpose: For infection control.
2. Check the provider's order and collect the necessary equipment and supplies.
3. If you are using test strips from a new, unopened container, you must change the test strip code chip. The three-number code on the test strip container must match the three-number code on the code strip. To install the code strip, follow the instructions in the Code Chip section of the user's manual.
   Purpose: To ensure that the instrument is calibrated correctly, and to produce accurate, precise, and reliable results.
4. Place the meter on a flat surface so that it will not vibrate or move during testing.
   Purpose: The test results are based on the back-and-forth movement of the blood sample that stops when the clot has formed. Vibrations or other movements will result in an error message, and the test will have to be repeated.
5. Greet the patient. Identify yourself. Verify the patient's identity with full name, ask the patient to spell the first and last name, and give date of birth.
6. Explain the procedure to be performed in a manner that the patient understands. Answer any questions the patient may have on the procedure. Obtain permission for the capillary puncture.
   Purpose: It is important to identify the patient in two different ways to ensure that you have the correct patient. Explaining the procedure can make the patient feel more comfortable and reduces anxiety.
7. Examine the patient's fingers, and choose the site to be used to obtain the blood sample.
8. Prepare the site:
   - Warm the hand by placing it under the arm, using a hand warmer or washing the hand in warm water.
   - Have the patient hold his or her arm down to the side so that the hand is below the waist.
   - Massage the palm of the hand toward the base of the finger and toward the tip until the fingertip has increased color.
   Purpose: The hanging drop blood sample must be sufficient to travel down the three channels on the test strip. It must be free of contaminants, tissue fluids, and alcohol.

9. When you are ready to test, remove a test strip from the container, and immediately close the container. Make sure it seals tightly. *Do not open the container or touch the test strips with wet hands or wet gloves.*
   Purpose: Exposure to moisture damages the test strips.
10. Insert the test strip as far as you can into the meter. This powers the meter ON (Fig. 1).

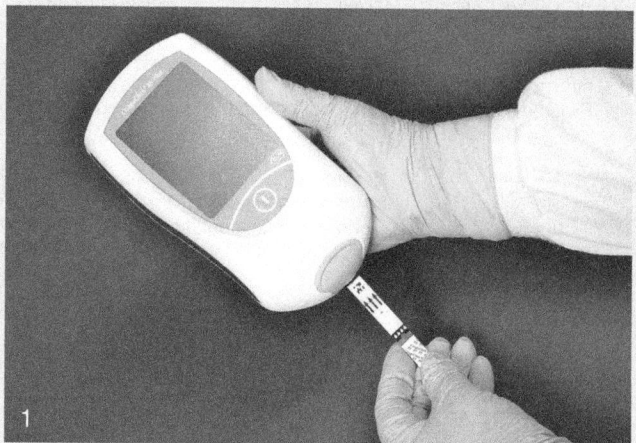

11. Disinfect the finger with an alcohol wipe, and allow the finger to air dry. Perform the fingerstick. If necessary, immediately after lancing, gently squeeze the finger to encourage blood flow. Do NOT wipe away the first drop of blood.
    Purpose: The hanging drop blood sample must be sufficient to travel down the three channels on the test strip. It must be free of contaminants, tissue fluids, and alcohol.
12. Hold the finger with a blood drop very close to the target (the clear area of the test strip). Apply 1 drop of blood to the top or side of the target area, and wait until you hear the beep. *You must apply a hanging drop of blood to the test strip within 15 seconds of the fingerstick. Do not add more blood. Do not touch or remove the test strip while the test is in progress.* The flashing blood drop symbol changes to an hourglass symbol when the meter detects a sufficient sample (see Fig. 55.5).
13. Read the results.
    Note: The result appears in approximately 1 minute. It may be displayed in three ways: as the international normalized ratio (INR), as the protime (PT) in seconds, or as %Quick (a unit used mainly in Europe). See the following chart.

Protime Expected Values for Normal and Therapeutic Whole Blood

	INR	PT (sec)
Normal	0.8–1.1	11.0–13.5 sec[a]
Low anticoagulation therapy	1.5–2.0	19.6–26.1 sec
Moderate anticoagulation therapy	2–3	26.1–39.2 sec
High anticoagulation therapy	2.5–4	32.6–52.2 sec

[a]Laboratory reports and manufacturers must supply their own reference ranges for PT results along with each patient's results. This is because different methodologies may create different reference ranges and different units of measurement.

Continued

PROCEDURE 55.5   Perform a CLIA-Waived PT/INR Test—cont'd

14. Dispose of the sharps into the biohazard sharps container. Dispose of regulated medical waste into the biohazard waste container. Disinfect the test area and remove your PPE.
15. Wash hands or use hand sanitizer.
    Purpose: For infection control.
16. Record the result in the lab's PT/INR log and in the patient's warfarin therapy flow sheet and/or patient health record. Using the normal range,

identify if test result is normal or abnormal. For the paper log and paper patient health record, circle any results that do not fall into the Desirable Ranges. Identify critical values and take appropriate steps to notify the provider. Document the steps taken.
Purpose: The provider needs to know the result while the patient is still in the office, for proper follow-up with the patient.

PROTIME—PATIENT LOG

Protime expected values for both normal and therapeutic whole blood:

	INR	PT seconds (ISI = 1.0)
Normal	0.8–1.2	10.4–15.7 sec
Low anticoagulation	1.5–2.0	19.6–26.1 sec
Moderate anticoagulation	2.0–3.0	26.1–39.2 sec
High anticoagulation	2.5–4.0	32.6–52.2 sec

DATE	TECH	PATIENT I.D.	INR	PT SECONDS	CHARTED
10/09/20–	DC	# 12345	1.0	19.7	✓

Documentation Example
10/09/20XX 9:30 a.m. INR = 1.0 and PT = 19.7 seconds. Patient is on low anticoagulation therapy._____Michelle James, CMA (AAMA)

PROCEDURE 55.6   Assist the Provider With Patient Care: Perform a Blood Glucose TRUEresult Test

Tasks
Perform a blood test for blood glucose accurately. Document the result in patient health record.

Equipment and Supplies
- Patient's health record
- Provider's order and/or lab requisition.
- TRUEresult glucometer or similar glucose monitoring device
- TRUEtest strip
- Lancet and autoloading finger-puncturing device
- Alcohol wipes
- Gauze
- Fluid-impermeable lab coat, protective eyewear, and gloves.
- Biohazard waste container
- Biohazard sharps containers

Procedural Steps
1. Check the provider's order and collect the necessary equipment and supplies. Perform quality control measures according to the manufacturer's guidelines and office policy.
2. Wash hands or use hand sanitizer. Put on a fluid-impermeable lab coat, protective eyewear, and gloves.

Purpose: For infection control.
3. Greet the patient. Identify yourself. Verify the patient's identity with full name, ask the patient to spell the first and last name, and give date of birth.
4. Explain the procedure to be performed in a manner that the patient understands. Answer any questions the patient may have on the procedure. Obtain permission for the capillary puncture.
   Purpose: It is important to identify the patient in two different ways to ensure that you have the correct patient. Explaining the procedure can make the patient feel more comfortable and reduces anxiety.
5. Ask the person to wash his or her hands in warm, soapy water, then rinse them in warm water, and finally dry them completely.
   Purpose: To clean the area that will be punctured; also, warming the fingers may increase peripheral blood flow.
6. Check the patient's middle and ring fingers, and select the site for puncture (both forearm and fingertip testing can be done).
   Purpose: To make sure the site of puncture is free of trauma.
7. Turn on the TRUEresult glucometer by pressing the ON button (Fig. 1). No coding is necessary with this monitor; you do not have to match the code on the test strip vial with the code on the glucometer. See manufacturers coding instructions for each individual brand of glucose testing system.

PROCEDURE 55.6   Assist the Provider With Patient Care: Perform a Blood Glucose TRUEresult Test—cont'd

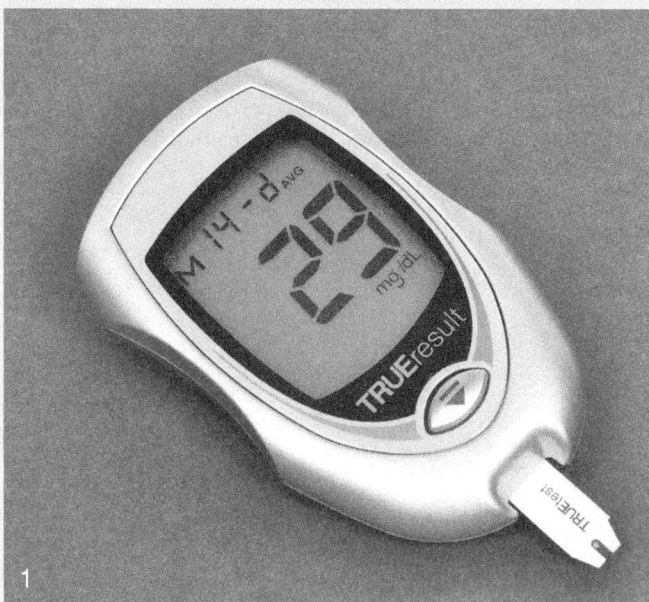

8. Check the expiration date on the test strip container. Take out a test strip, and insert it into the glucometer. (The glucometer may be preloaded with test strips, depending on the manufacturer.)
9. Cleanse the selected site on the patient's fingertip with an alcohol wipe, and allow the finger to air dry.
10. Perform the capillary puncture and wipe away the first drop of blood.
    Purpose: Tissue fluid may be present in the first drop of blood.
11. Apply a small blood sample (0.5 mL) to the end of the test strip (Fig. 2).

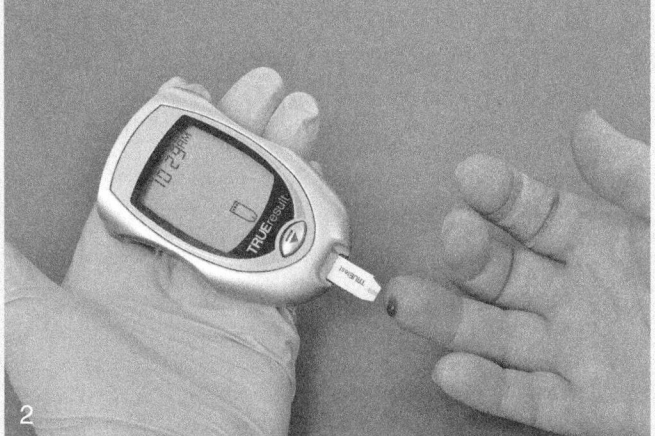

12. Give the patient gauze to hold securely over the puncture site; apply a hypo-allergenic bandage or wrap if needed.
13. Read the test results before the glucometer turns off.
    Notes: The glucometer automatically begins the measurement process, and results are obtained as soon as 4 seconds. The test result is shown in the display window in milligrams per deciliter (mg/dL) for most glucometers. Read manufacturer's instruction on how the result is displayed. The glucometer will likely turn off automatically.
14. Dispose of biohazardous waste in biohazard waste container and the sharps in the biohazard sharps container.
    Purpose: To control infection.
15. Clean the glucometer according to the manufacturer's guidelines. Disinfect the work area.
16. Remove your gloves and dispose of them properly. Remove protective eyewear.
17. Wash hands or use hand sanitizer
    Purpose: For infection control.
18. Record the test results in the patient's health record.
    Purpose: A procedure is not done until the patient results are recorded.

Documentation Example
08/16/20XX 1:00 p.m. Glucometer screening completed as ordered by Dr. Misha. NFBS 155. Pt took routine dose of 10 units Humalog insulin at noon. Pt had no questions._____Michelle James, CMA (AAMA)

PROCEDURE 55.7   Perform a CLIA-Waived Chemistry Test: Determine the Cholesterol Level or Lipid Profile Using a Cholestech Analyzer

Tasks
Perform a Cholestech test for total cholesterol level or a lipid panel, and accurately report the results. Document the result on the lab flow sheet and patient health record.

Directions
Perform a total blood cholesterol level or lipid panel on Connie Lange STAT.

Equipment and Supplies
- Patient's health record
- Provider's order and/or lab requisition
- Cholestech analyzer
- Package insert or flowchart with directions
- Optics check cassette
- Test cassettes (provided by Cholestech)

PROCEDURE 55.7   Perform a CLIA-Waived Chemistry Test: Determine the Cholesterol Level or Lipid Profile Using a Cholestech Analyzer—cont'd

- Levels 1 and 2 liquid controls
- Capillary tubes and plungers for fingerstick sample (provided by Cholestech)
- Mini-Pet pipet and pipet tips for venipuncture sample (provided by Cholestech)
- Lancet, gauze, alcohol wipes, bandage for capillary blood, *or* lithium heparin (green-topped) tube for venous blood
- Safety tube decapper (if tubes do not have a Hemogard plastic top)
- Fluid-impermeable lab coat, protective eyewear, and gloves
- Biohazard waste container
- Biohazard sharps containers

Procedural Steps

1. Check the provider's order and collect the necessary equipment and supplies. Allow refrigerated testing cassettes to come to room temperature (at least 10 minutes before opening).
   Purpose: The test is temperature and time sensitive when reading results.
2. Perform quantitative quality control by performing a calibration check with the optics check cassette (Fig. 1). Then test level 1 and level 2 liquid controls if using a new set of cassettes.
   Purpose: To ensure instrument is reading results accurately, precisely, and reliably.

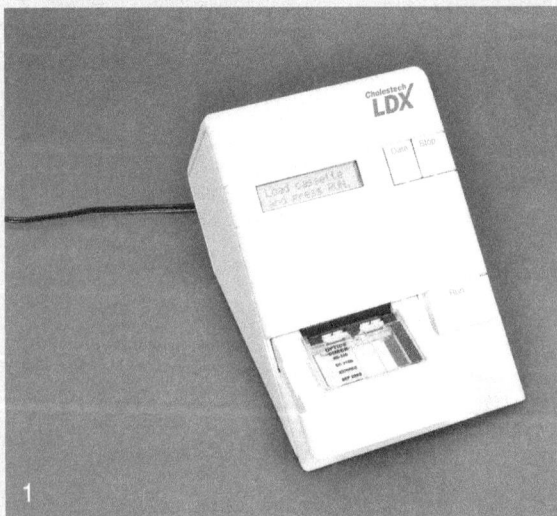

3. Wash hands or use hand sanitizer. Put on a fluid-impermeable lab coat, protective eyewear, and gloves.
   Purpose: For infection control.
4. Greet the patient. Identify yourself. Verify the patient's identity with full name, ask the patient to spell the first and last name, and give date of birth.
5. Explain the procedure to be performed in a manner that the patient understands. Answer any questions the patient may have on the procedure. Obtain permission for a capillary puncture.
6. Remove cassette from its pouch and place it on a flat surface without touching the black bar or magnetic strip.
   Purpose: The black bar is the testing area, and the magnetic strip must be read by the analyzer. Touching either may interfere with test results.
7. Press RUN on the analyzer (you may wait to press RUN until you have collected the patient's specimen), allowing it to do a self-test; this will be followed by OK on the screen, and then the test drawer will open. The drawer will stay open for 4 minutes while the specimen is prepared.
8. Perform a fingerstick and collect the capillary blood to the black line of the Cholestech capillary tube with its plunger inserted into the red end of the tube. *Or* collect the fresh venous whole blood with the Cholestech Mini-Pet pipet.

Purpose: Cholestech provides both collecting devices to ensure that the exact volume of blood necessary is tested.

9. Place the whole blood sample into the well of the cassette. *Note:* The capillary specimen must be in the cassette within 5 minutes of collection (Fig. 2).
   Purpose: Fingerstick blood will clot if not tested within 5 minutes.

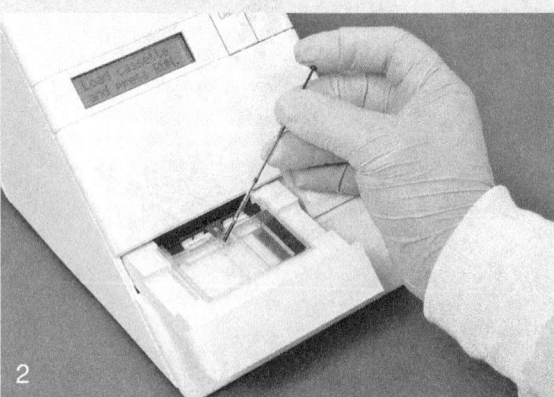

10. Immediately put the cassette into the drawer of the analyzer, and press RUN. (*Note:* If the drawer has closed, press RUN again to open the drawer; load the specimen into the drawer and then press RUN to close the drawer.) When the test is complete, the analyzer beeps. The screen displays and then prints out the results (Fig. 3).
    Purpose: This is a test with a color reaction that continues to change over time.

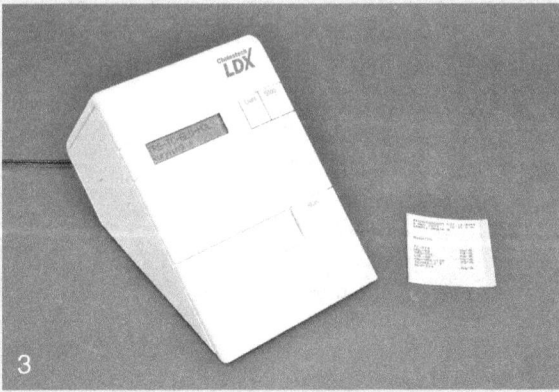

11. Dispose of all sharps in the biohazard sharps container. Place all regulated medical waste into the biohazard waste container.
12. Disinfect test area, remove PPE, and dispose of gloves in biohazard waste container.
13. Wash hands or use hand sanitizer.
    Purpose: To control infection.
14. Record the findings in the laboratory log and in the patient's health record. Using the normal range, identify if test result is normal or abnormal. If using paper health records, circle the results that do not fall within the Desirable Ranges column of the following table. Identify critical values and take appropriate steps to notify the provider. Document steps taken.
    Purpose: A procedure is considered not done until it is recorded. The provider needs to know the results while the patient is still in the office, for proper follow-up with the patient.

PROCEDURE 55.7   Perform a CLIA-Waived Chemistry Test: Determine the Cholesterol Level or Lipid Profile Using a Cholestech Analyzer—cont'd

CHOLESTECH LDX PATIENT/CONTROL LOG

Cassette Lot #: _____   Expiration Date: _____   LDX Serial #: _____

DATE	TECH	PT ID	TC	HDL	LDL	TRG	TC/HDL	GLU	CHARTED
10/09/20–	DC	#12345	190	50	120	135	4.3	80	✓

Documentation Example

Attach printed readout, or record results in the electronic chart:

Test	Results	Desirable
Total cholesterol (TC)	190	<200 mg/dL
HDL cholesterol	50	>40 mg/dL (men); >50 mg/dL (women)
LDL cholesterol	120	<130 mg/dL
Triglycerides	135	30–190 mg/dL
TC/HDL ratio	4.3	≤4.5
Other		
Glucose	80	Fasting: 70–99 mg/dL Nonfasting: <125 mg/dL

Note: Laboratory reports and manufacturers must supply their own reference ranges, along with each patient's results. This is because different methodologies may create different reference ranges and different units of measurement.

56

Assisting in Microbiology and Immunology

LEARNING OBJECTIVES

1. Discuss the classification of microorganisms, including how to name them.
2. Describe various characteristics of bacteria, including their staining properties, shapes, oxygen requirements, and physical structures.
3. Describe the unusual characteristics of chlamydia, mycoplasma, and rickettsia organisms.
4. Identify the characteristics of common diseases caused by fungi, protozoa, parasites, helminths, and viruses.
5. Describe procedures for handling and transporting specimens.
6. Describe specimen collection for stool, pinworm, nasopharyngeal, sputum, and throat swab specimens.

7. Explain how to perform Clinical Laboratory Improvement Amendments (CLIA)-waived microbiology testing for strep, influenza A and B, and respiratory syncytial virus.
8. Explain how to perform CLIA-waived immunology testing for mononucleosis, *Helicobacter pylori*, Lyme, and human immunodeficiency syndrome.
9. Discuss the staining process and identification of pathogens in the microbiology reference, including throat and urine cultures.
10. Describe stool-based tests, including the patient preparation, collection, and testing process.

OUTLINE

Lena Swartz, CMA (AAMA), has worked at Walden-Martin Family Medical (WMFM) Clinic for 6 years. She has seen many infectious diseases diagnosed over that time. Bacterial and viral infections are common, but Lena also knows that not all microorganisms are bad. Some diseases have been controlled using vaccines. Other infections can be treated with antibiotics. Not all infectious diseases can be treated with antibiotics, and improper use of antibiotics can lead to bacteria that are resistant to these useful drugs. Lena knows that it is important to identify pathogens quickly so that proper treatment can begin. The identification of pathogens can involve various types of tests, many of which can be performed in the physician office laboratory (POL) where she works.

YOU WILL LEARN

1. To describe various bacterial shapes, oxygen requirements, and physical structures.
2. To describe the unusual characteristics of *Chlamydia, Mycoplasma,* and *Rickettsia* organisms.
3. To describe the characteristics of common viral diseases.
4. To describe the common methods for the collection, transport, and processing of microbiology and immunology specimens.
5. To describe three CLIA-waived microbiology tests that use a rapid identification technique.
6. To discuss the purpose of indirect immunology testing.
7. To describe three CLIA-waived immunology tests that could be done in the physician office laboratory.
8. To discuss the importance of the Gram stain and acid-fast stains in microbiology.
9. To describe the reference laboratory assessment of a throat culture and a urine culture.

INTRODUCTION

Infectious diseases caused by microorganisms and infectious agents have gotten a lot of publicity. We have heard news stories about COVID-19, Ebola, influenza, Zika, and more. With news of foodborne illnesses, contaminated water supplies, tick-borne diseases, and communicable infections, it appears all microorganisms are harmful and can cause disease. Healthcare-associated infections (HAIs) such as the following are becoming increasingly difficult to control:

- methicillin-resistant *Staphylococcus aureus* (staf uh luh KOK uhs AWR ee uhs) (MRSA)
- *Clostridium difficile* (klo STRID ee uhm dif i SEEL) (C. diff) infections.

New strains of drug-resistant microorganisms are difficult to treat with existing antibiotics. Bioterrorism has become a real concern worldwide. Antimicrobial products line the pharmacy and supermarket shelves and are going to keep us "germ free." It is no wonder many people have the impression that all microorganisms are harmful. In reality, less than 1% of known microorganisms are pathogens.

Most microorganisms are good. For example, *saprophytes* are beneficial microorganisms that are responsible for breaking down organic matter, such as plants and organic waste in farming, water purification, composting, and gardening. Without microorganisms, we could not survive. The normal flora in and on our bodies is needed for the following processes:

- Digesting food and making nutrients available to the body.
- Forming blood clots. Vitamin K is used in the clotting process and is made by bacteria in our intestines.
- Preventing pathogens from invading our skin, mucous membranes, and gastrointestinal and genitourinary tracts.

Normal flora takes up space, requires nutrients, and excretes waste. When pathogens try to populate the skin or areas of the body that have normal flora, they must compete with the existing organisms. This makes it harder for pathogens to cause disease. Normal flora discourages pathogen populations.

When the body's normal flora is weakened (e.g., by antibiotic overuse or hormonal changes), certain *opportunistic organisms* that are normally present in low numbers can overgrow. An example is *Candida albicans* (KAN di duh AHL bi kanz), which is a yeast that is normally found in mucous membranes in the body. When a patient has been on broad-spectrum antibiotics for an infection, the antibiotics kill pathogens, along with some of the normal flora. For example, *Candida albicans* is not normally a problem in the vagina. If enough normal flora in the vagina is killed off, *Candida albicans* can increase in numbers, which causes a vaginal yeast infection.

As a medical assistant, you need to understand basic microbiology (mahy kroh bahy OL uh jee) and the role of microorganisms in both health and disease. The main objective in medical microbiology is to identify the organisms responsible for illness so that the provider can properly treat the patient. Your responsibilities will also include preventing HAIs by following infection control policies. Microbiology testing procedures may be performed in the physician office laboratory (POL) or in the microbiology department of a medical referral laboratory.

Immunology (im yuh NOL uh jee) is the study of the immune system, which is closely tied to microbiology. Invasive microorganisms stimulate an immune response, leading to the production of antibodies that come to our defense. Often a bacterial or viral infection is diagnosed by testing for a specific antibody that is produced to fight the infectious agent.

This chapter covers the following topics related to microbiology and immunology:

- Major categories of infectious agents
- Quality control issues regarding the collection and handling of microbiological specimens
- Common CLIA-waived microbiology and immunology testing

The chapter concludes with an overview of the more complex microbiology procedures and tests performed in hospitals and reference laboratories.

CLASSIFICATION OF MICROORGANISMS

Although the medical assistant is not responsible for identifying microorganisms, a working knowledge of the terminology used in naming microorganisms is essential.

Microorganisms are too small to be seen without magnification. Bacteria, fungus, and protozoa are all microorganisms that can be seen with a light microscope. Parasitic worm infections are also identified in the microbiology laboratory because their eggs are visible under the microscope. Viruses are the smallest microbe and are visible only with a highly magnified electron microscope.

Naming Microorganisms

Swedish botanist Carl Linnaeus developed the binomial system of nomenclature to name all living organisms: animals, plants, fungi, protozoa, and bacteria. Scientists use the binomial (bahy NOH mee uhl) system of nomenclature (NOH muh KLAY cher). This binomial system assigns two names:

- *Genus*: The first name, which begins with a capital letter. After the organism's full genus and species names are given once in a report, subsequent references can just use a single letter to represent the genus. For example, *Escherichia coli* (eh shu REEK e ah KOH lahy) is commonly referred to as *E. coli*.
- *Species*: The second name, which begins with a lower-case letter.

Both names are either *italicized* or underlined when written.

When microbiology laboratory results are reported, it is essential that both the genus and species names be recorded. Different species may cause different symptoms or require different antibiotic treatment. For example, *Streptococcus pyogenes* (strep tuh KOK uhs PAHY uh jen eez) causes strep throat, whereas *Streptococcus viridans* (VEER uh denz) is normal flora in the throat.

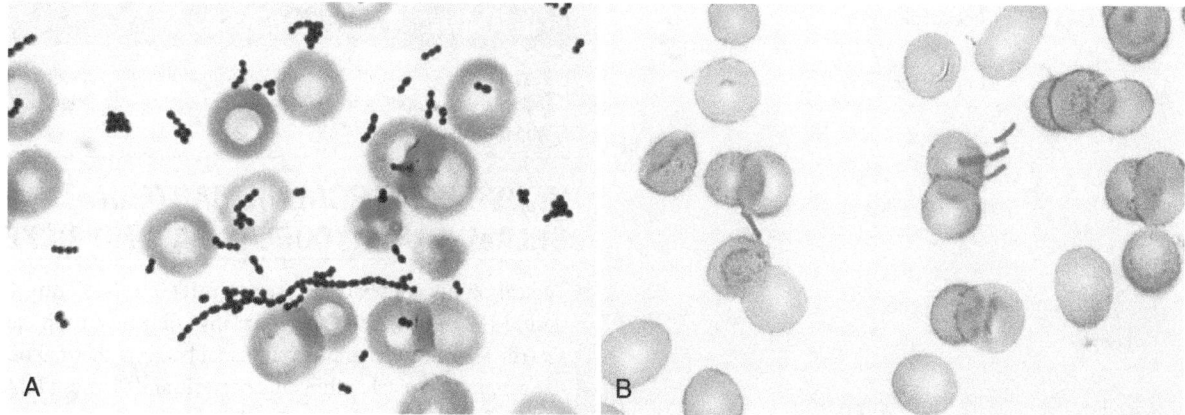

Fig. 56.1 A, Gram stain A—red blood cells (RBCs) and gram-positive cocci. B, RBCs with gram-negative bacilli. (From De la Maza LM, Pezzlo MT, Baron EJ: *Color atlas of diagnostic microbiology*, St. Louis, 1997, Mosby.)

CHARACTERISTICS OF BACTERIA

Bacteria are single-celled prokaryote (proh KAR ee oht) organisms that reproduce asexually, by binary fission. This process of reproduction results in large numbers of bacteria being formed from a single cell. Because bacteria reproduce quickly, bacterial infections can swiftly overwhelm a person's immune system. Some bacteria reproduce in as little as 14 minutes, whereas other bacteria may take days. For example, a single *E. coli* cell, which reproduces about every 30 minutes, to produce about 3.5 trillion offspring in 24 hours.

Bacteria often are classified according to their staining characteristics, shape, and the environmental conditions in which they thrive. Both shape and staining characteristics are direct results of their cell wall composition.

Bacterial Staining Properties

Three types of cell wall structures are found among pathogenic bacteria: gram-positive, gram-negative, and acid-fast structures. These labels are based on reactions in specialized stains used to visualize the bacteria under the microscope. Bacterial cell walls are composed of *peptidoglycan* (pep tih DOH glahy kan) (PG), a molecule composed of carbohydrate and protein.

- *Gram-positive cells* contain a thick layer of PG, which produces a deep blue/violet when stained with Gram stain (Fig. 56.1A).
- *Gram-negative cells* contain a thin layer of PG, which produces a pinkish red color when stained with Gram stain (Fig. 56.1B).
- *Acid-fast cells* contain a thin layer of PG surrounded by a thick layer of waxlike lipids. Acid-fast bacteria do not stain well with a Gram stain, but they stain pink with the acid-fast stain (Fig. 56.2).

> **VOCABULARY**
> **molecule** The simplest unit of a chemical compound that can exist, consisting of two or more atoms held together with chemical bonds.
> **stains** Reagents or dyes used to treat specimens for microscopic examination.

Bacterial Shapes

Bacteria assume three different shapes:
- Round bacteria are called *cocci* (KOK sahy).

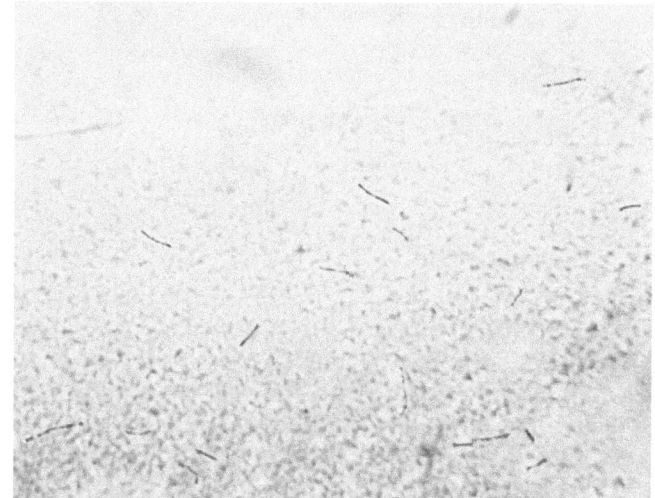

Fig. 56.2 Acid-Fast Stain. (From De la Maza LM, Pezzlo MT, Baron EJ: *Color atlas of diagnostic microbiology*, St. Louis, 1997, Mosby.)

- Rod-shaped bacteria are called *bacilli* (buh SIL ahy).
- Spiral-shaped bacteria are called *spirilla* (spahy RIL ah). Tightly coiled spirilla are called *spirochetes* (SPAHY ruh keets).

Certain arrangements are also seen with different bacteria. For example, when bacteria are in a chain formation, the prefix *strepto-* is used. When bacteria are found in pairs, the prefix *diplo-* is used, and when they are found in grapelike clusters, the prefix *staphylo-* is used. Cocci in packets of 4 are called *tetrads,* and in packets of 8 or 16 they are called *sarcinae* (SAHR suh nay) (Fig. 56.3).

Bacterial Oxygen Requirements

Bacteria are also classified according to oxygen requirements:
- *Aerobes* (AIR ohbs): Bacteria that require oxygen to live. An aerobic example is *Mycobacterium tuberculosis,* which thrives in white blood cells in the lungs
- *Anaerobes* (an AIR ohbs): Bacteria that die in the presence of oxygen. An anaerobic example is *Bacteroides fragilis,* a gram-negative rod-shaped bacterium. *B. fragilis* is part of the normal flora in the colon.
- *Facultative* (FAK uhl tey tiv) *anaerobes*: Bacteria that are flexible regarding their oxygen needs; they can survive in the presence of oxygen but prefer to live without oxygen. *E. coli,* which also found in the intestine, is an example of a facultative anaerobe.

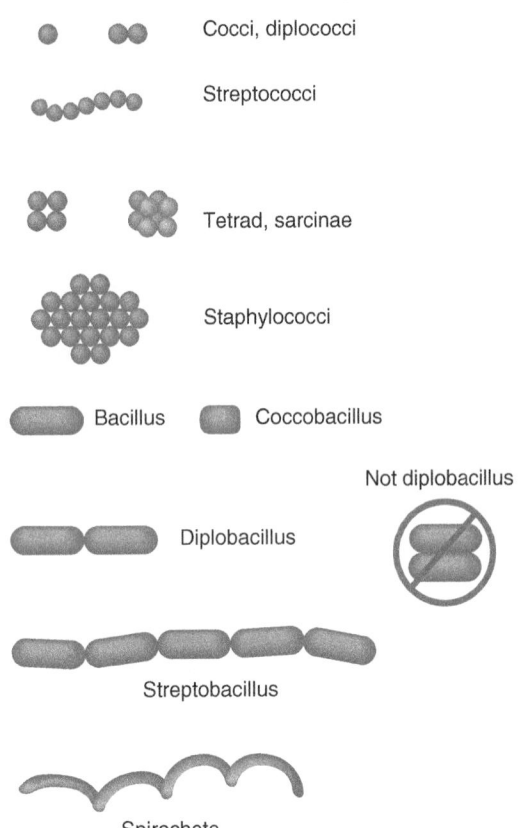

Cocci, diplococci

Streptococci

Tetrad, sarcinae

Staphylococci

Bacillus   Coccobacillus

Not diplobacillus

Diplobacillus

Streptobacillus

Spirochete

Fig. 56.3 Typical Bacterial Arrangement. (From Niedzwiecki B, et al: *Kinn's the medical assistant*, ed 14, St. Louis, 2020, Elsevier.)

MEDICAL TERMINOLOGY	
aer/o	air
dipl/o	double or two
an-	no, not, without
tetra-	four
bacillus (singular), **bacilli** (plural)	
coccus (singular), **cocci** (plural)	
spirillum (singular), **spirilla** (plural)	

Bacterial Physical Structures

Bacteria can be classified and identified according to additional physical structures. Some bacteria have long thin flagella that help them move. Some bacteria have a thick, jelly-like substance that surrounds the cell wall called a *capsule*, which can make the bacteria more pathogenic. Other bacteria form intracellular structures called an endospore. An endospore allows the bacteria to remain viable when environmental conditions are poor. *Clostridium tetani* (klo STRID ee uhm TET uh nee) produces spores; if spores enter a wound and grow, they cause the disease known as *tetanus*.

See Table 56.1 for a list of some important infectious diseases caused by pathogenic bacilli, cocci, and spirilla.

> **VOCABULARY**
> **endospore** An inactive form of certain bacteria that can withstand poor environmental conditions. When conditions improve, the bacteria become functional again.
> **flagella** A long, whip-like outgrowth from a cell that helps the cell move.
> **viable** Able to live and grow.

CRITICAL THINKING 56.1

In your own words, write a brief description of the term *capsule*. What advantage does a bacterium have if a capsule surrounds it? Share your thoughts with the class.

UNUSUAL PATHOGENIC BACTERIA: CHLAMYDIA, MYCOPLASMA, AND RICKETTSIA

Typical pathogenic bacteria measure 1000 to 5000 nm. *Chlamydia* (kluh MID ee uh), *mycoplasma* (mahy koh PLAZ muh), and *rickettsia* (rih KET see uh) are tiny, unusual bacteria that fall between the size ranges of typical pathogenic bacteria and viruses (Table 56.2).
- *Chlamydia*: Require host cells for growth.
- *Rickettsia*: Transmitted by blood-sucking insects and cannot multiply outside a living host cell.
- *Mycoplasmas*: Do not contain peptidoglycan in their cell wall. For example, *Mycoplasma pneumonia*, which causes "walking pneumonia," is a gram-negative bacterium that does not have a cell wall.

PATHOGENIC FUNGI

Mycology (mahy KOL uh jee) is the study of fungi and the diseases they cause (Table 56.3). Fungi are eukaryotes (yoo KAR ee ohts) that are larger than bacteria and have a nucleus. Fungi include yeasts and molds. Fungi are present in the soil, air, and water, but only a few species cause disease. They are transmitted by the following:
- Direct contact with infected persons
- Prolonged exposure to a moist environment
- Inhalation of contaminated dust or soil

Some fungal infections affect the skin, hair, or nails. Tinea infections, such as ringworm and athlete's foot, are examples of these types of fungal infections. Some fungi can penetrate the tissues of the internal body structures and cause serious diseases of the mucous membranes, heart, and lungs.

A diagnosis of a fungal skin infection is usually based on culturing skin scrapings or microscopic observation of skin scrapings. Before microscopic observation, the samples are treated with potassium hydroxide (KOH) to dissolve nonfungal material, making the fungal elements easier to observe. Fungal infections must be treated with antifungal medications.

> **VOCABULARY**
> **eukaryote** Any single-celled or multicellular organism that has genetic material contained in a distinct membrane-bound nucleus.
> **mold** A growth of tiny fungi forming on a substance. Often looks downy or furry and is associated with dampness or decay.

CRITICAL THINKING 56.2

Fungi include two other types of organisms. Name these organisms. Share your answers with the class.

PATHOGENIC PROTOZOA

Protozoa are single-celled parasitic organisms that contain a nucleus. They range in size from microscopic to *macroscopic*

TABLE 56.1 Common Diseases Caused by Bacilli

Caused By	Disease State	Causative Agent	Transmission
Bacilli	Botulism	*Clostridium botulinum*	Improperly cooked canned foods
	Clostridium difficile (C. diff)	*Clostridium difficile*	May be a healthcare-acquired infection (HAI); frequent antibiotic use increases likelihood; idiopathic
	Diphtheria	*Corynebacterium diphtheriae*	Inhalation
	Legionnaire's disease	*Legionella pneumophilia*	Grows readily in air conditioning systems (standing water)
	Pertussis (whooping cough)	*Bordetella pertussis*	Respiratory secretions
	Salmonella infection	*Salmonella species*	Foodborne illness
	Tetanus (lockjaw)	*Clostridium tetani*	Open fractures, soil-contaminated wounds, open wounds, puncture wounds
	Tuberculosis	*Mycobacterium tuberculosis*	Airborne, inhalation
	Urinary tract infection (UTI)	Various, most common include: *Escherichia coli* *Proteus species* *Klebsiella species* *Pseudomonas aeruginosa*	Bacteria contaminate urethra, catheterization
Cocci	Gonorrhea	*Neisseria gonorrhoeae*	Sexually transmitted
	Meningococcal meningitis	*Neisseria meningitidis*	Respiratory tract secretions
	Methicillin-resistant *Staphylococcus aureus* (MRSA) infection	Methicillin-resistant *Staphylococcus aureus*	Healthcare-acquired infection (HIA), direct contact, fomites, carriers, poor hand washing technique
	Pneumonia	*Streptococcus pneumoniae*	Direct contact, droplets
	Staphylococcal food poisoning	*Staphylococcus aureus*	Poor hygiene, improper refrigeration of foods
	Strep throat	*Streptococcus pyogenes*, also known as Group A Strep	Direct contact, droplets, fomites
	Wound infections, abscesses, boils	*Staphylococcus aureus*	Direct contact, fomites, carriers, poor hand washing technique
Spirilla	Foodborne illness (most commonly seen in the United States)	*Campylobacter jejuni*	Contaminated and under cooked food, contaminated water and milk
	Lyme disease	*Borrelia burgdorferi*	Tick bite
	Pyloric ulcers	*Helicobacter pylori*	Unknown, possible food/water-borne
	Syphilis	*Treponema pallidum*	Sexually or congenitally from infected mother

TABLE 56.2 Common Diseases Caused by Rickettsia, Mycoplasma, and Chlamydia

Disease State	Causative Agent	Transmission
Atypical or walking pneumonia	*Mycoplasma pneumoniae*	Respiratory secretions
Inclusion conjunctivitis or pneumonia	*Chlamydia trachomatis*	During the birth process from infected mother
Nongonococcal urethritis or vaginitis	*Chlamydia trachomatis*	Sexually
Rocky mountain spotted fever	*Rickettsia rickettsii*	Tick bite
Typhus (epidemic)	*Rickettsia prowazekii*	Body lice bite
Typhus (endemic)	*Rickettsia typhi*	Flea bite

on the patient's signs and symptoms and on microscopic examination of stool or blood.

PATHOGENIC PARASITES

Parasitology includes the study of all parasitic organisms that live on or in the human body (see Table 56.4). In a parasitic relationship, the host is harmed and the parasite thrives. Parasites are transmitted by ingestion, direct penetration of the skin, and injection by an arthropod also referred to as a vector. A parasite cannot be identified accurately based on a single test or specimen. Parasites are frequently identified in feces, blood, urine, sputum, tissue fluid, or tissue biopsy samples.

> **VOCABULARY**
> **arthropod** Any animal that lacks a spine, such as insects, crustaceans, arachnids, and others.
> **sputum** Thick mucus often referred to as phlegm. It is coughed up from the lungs; not saliva that originates in the mouth.
> **vector** Arthropod (mosquito, tick, flea) that carries disease and transmits to another organism through a blood meal.

(visible to the naked eye) (Table 56.4). They are present in moist environments and in bodies of water, such as lakes and ponds. Protozoa are transmitted through contaminated feces, food, and drink. Some pathogenic protozoa inhabit the bloodstream; others inhabit the intestines and genital tract. Diagnosis usually is based

TABLE 56.3   Common Diseases Caused by Fungi

Disease State	Causative Agent	Transmission
Candidiasis, vulvovaginal, monilial (vaginal yeast)	Candida species (yeast)	Opportunistic: After antibiotic therapy, using hormonal birth control, diabetes-type I, II, gestational, acquired immunodeficiency syndrome (AIDS)
Cryptococcosis	Cryptococcus neoformans	Contact with poultry droppings
Fungal infections; athlete foot, jock itch, ringworm	Tinea species and others	Direct contact with an infected person or animal, damp surfaces
Histoplasmosis	Histoplasma capsulatum	Inhaling dust contaminated with bird or bat droppings
Pneumocystis pneumonia	Pneumocystis jirovecii	Contact with animals, most likely in immune-compromised patients, common in AIDS patients
Thrush (in the mouth)	Candida species (yeast)	Opportunistic: Possibly during birth process, after antibiotic therapy, diabetes, or weakened immune system

TABLE 56.4   Common Diseases Caused by Protozoa and Parasites

Disease State	Causative Agent	Transmission
Amoebic dysentery	Entamoeba histolytica	Fecal contamination of food or water
Giardiasis	Giardia lamblia	Contaminated water, opportunist in intestinal tract
Lice	Pediculus humanus (head and body lice), Pthirus pubis (pubic lice)	Direct contact, contaminated clothing, bedding, furniture, personal items (combs, hats, etc.)
Malaria	Plasmodium species	Bite of the Anopheles mosquito
Pinworm	Enterobius vermicularis	Fecal-oral contamination
Scabies	Sarcoptes scabiei	Direct contact, contaminated clothing, bedding
Tapeworm—beef or pork	Taenia species	Eating undercooked beef or pork
Tapeworm—fish	Diphyllobothrium latum	Eating undercooked fish
Toxoplasmosis	Toxoplasma gondii	Ingestion of fecal oocysts—from fecal contamination of cat litter, congenitally
Trichinosis	Trichinella spiralis	Eating undercooked pork or bear

---

MEDICAL TERMINOLOGY

arthr/o	joint
kary/o	nucleus
pod/o	foot
eu-	good, normal

fungus (singular), **fungi** (plural)
protozoan (singular), **protozoa** (plural)

PATHOGENIC HELMINTHS

Helminths (HEL mihn th s) are parasites called worms. Helminths live on or in another living organism. They sustain themselves at the expense of the host organism. They can live in animals or humans. Worms are usually transmitted through the soil, by infected clothing or fingernails, contact with infected persons, or contaminated food/water. Helminths go through the same life cycle as other worms. The adult worm lays eggs (ova). The ova develop into larvae, which grow into adult worms, and the cycle begins again. Diagnosis usually is based on microscopic examination of feces for ova (eggs) and parasites, and on patient signs and symptoms (Fig. 56.4).

PATHOGENIC VIRUSES

Many scientists do not consider viruses to be microorganisms because they are not alive. Viruses are not able to metabolize or reproduce unless they are inside of a host cell. Viruses have their own enzymes but must use the host cell organelles and

macromolecules to reproduce and metabolize. Because of the absolute need for a host cell, a virus can be considered an *obligate intracellular pathogen*.

Viruses consist of a genetic core covered by a protein coat called a *capsid*. Some viruses have an additional spiked layer of protection over the capsid called an *envelope*. A viral genetic core is made up of either ribonucleic acid (RAHY boh noo klee ik as id) (RNA) or deoxyribonucleic acid (dee auk see RAHY boh noo klee ik as id) (DNA). The RNA or DNA contains information about how and what the host cell needs to produce to form a new virus. The genetic material is like a recipe for a new viral particle.

A virus cannot be cultured on solid nutrient media, such as those used to culture bacteria and fungi. Viruses must be cultured in fertilized eggs or in a tissue culture, which is done by referral, research, or large hospital laboratories.

Usually, instead of culturing a specimen for a virus, the patient's blood sample is tested for a specific antibody related to the possible viral infection. For example, in the diagnosis of Lyme disease, patient serum is tested for the specific antibody produced in response to the Lyme antigen. This form of testing is referred to as *serology* or *immunology testing* (discussed later in the chapter). Table 56.5 lists common diseases caused by viruses.

VOCABULARY

antigen A substance that stimulates the production of an antibody when introduced into the body. Antigens include toxins, bacteria, viruses, and other foreign substances.

larvae Immature free-living forms of many animals; develop into the adult form.

macromolecules The molecules needed for metabolism carbohydrates, lipids, proteins, amino acids, and nucleic acids.

organelles Structures inside of the cell.

tissue culture The technique or process of keeping tissue alive and growing in a culture medium.

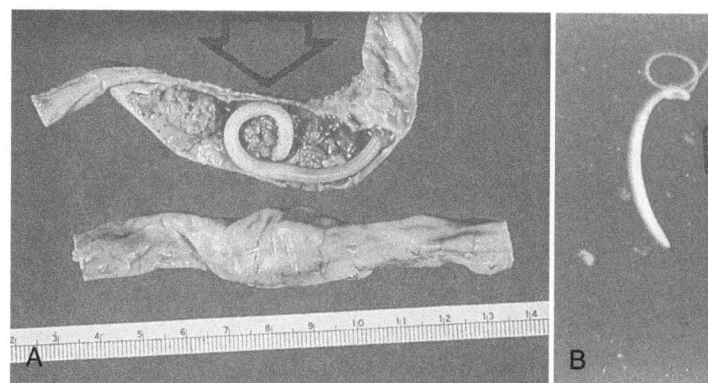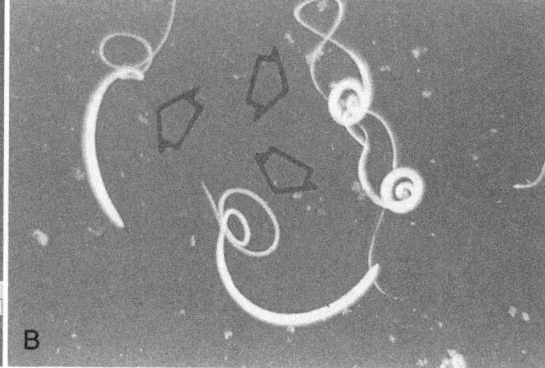

Fig. 56.4 A, Roundworms. B, Whipworms. (From Stepp CA, Woods MA: *Laboratory procedures for medical office personnel*, Philadelphia, 1998, Saunders.)

TABLE 56.5 Common Diseases Caused by Viruses

Disease State	Causative Agent	Transmission
Acquired immunodeficiency syndrome (AIDS)	Human immunodeficiency virus (HIV)	Sexual intercourse/contact, sharing needles, at risk behavior
Common cold	Rhinovirus most common among many possible	Direct contact, inhaling droplets, fomites
Coronavirus disease (COVID-19)	Severe acute respiratory syndrome coronavirus 2 (SARS-CoV-2)	Airborne
Ebola	Ebola virus species (five identified)	Direct contact with infected blood or body fluids (bloodborne)
Human papillomavirus (HPV) infection	Human papillomavirus	Sexually, direct skin to skin and indirect contact
Infectious mononucleosis	Epstein-Barr virus	Direct contact and airborne saliva/body fluids—kissing, same eating utensils
Influenza	Myxovirus, influenza A and B	Droplet and fomites—cough, sneeze, or talk
Measles	Paramyxovirus—measles virus	Direct contact, inhaling droplets
Molluscum contagiosum warts	Molluscipox virus	Direct contact with an infected person—skin to skin
Mumps	Paramyxovirus—mumps virus	Inhaling droplets, shared utensils with infected person
Polio	Poliovirus	Direct contact, feces, via mouth (saliva), sneeze, cough
Rubella (German measles)	Rubella virus	Direct contact, inhaling droplets from sneeze or cough, congenitally from mother

CRITICAL THINKING 56.3

Looking at Table 56.5, pick four viral diseases that you are familiar with. Write down the disease, the virus that causes it, and two ways to prevent the infection. Be ready to share your answers with the class.

SPECIMEN COLLECTION AND TRANSPORT IN THE PHYSICIAN OFFICE LABORATORY

Specimen collection and handling are important considerations in patient care because the results are only as good as the quality of the sample. Ideally, specimens should be collected during the acute phase of an illness and before antibiotics are prescribed. Specimens for microbiology testing can include urine, stool, sputum, and blood. Sterile swabs can be used to collect samples from wounds and the upper respiratory tract.

Guidelines for Specimen Collection

Specimens must be collected carefully so that contaminating microorganisms are not introduced into the specimen. This means not only using sterile collection and transport devices,

but also taking steps to prevent contamination. To prevent from contaminating the specimen, the person should:

- Wash hands before collecting the sample.
- Cleanse the area involved with an antiseptic, if appropriate. For example, when obtaining a clean-catch midstream urine specimen, antiseptic wipes are used.
- Open sterile containers only when necessary and avoid touching the inside surfaces.
- Never touch a sterile swab or collection device to a nonsterile surface.

If patients are expected to collect a sample, it is crucial that they receive clear instructions on how to perform the procedure correctly and without contaminating the sample. The referral laboratory is responsible for providing a manual of written instructions to the POL. The POL is responsible for providing clear oral

VOCABULARY

antiseptic A substance, such as alcohol and povidone-iodine solution (Betadine), that inhibits the growth of microorganisms on living tissue. Used to cleanse the skin or wounds.

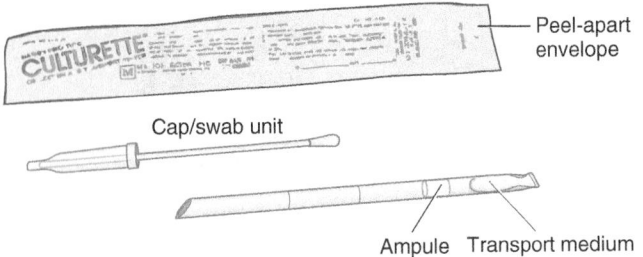

Fig. 56.5 Collection and Transport System. (From Niedzwiecki B, et al: *Kinn's the medical assistant*, ed 14, St. Louis, 2020, Elsevier.)

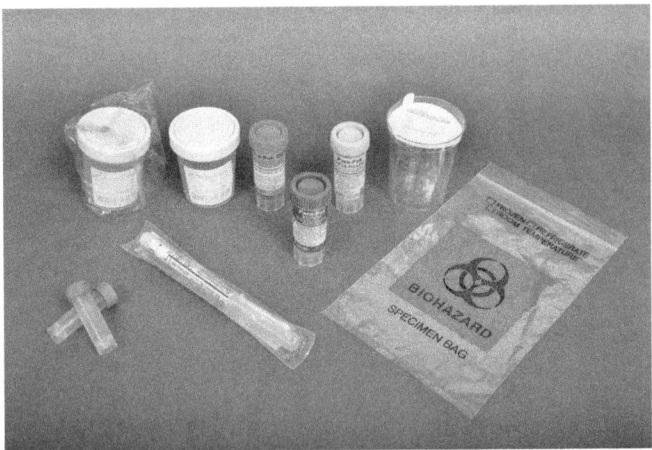

Fig. 56.6 Microbiology Specimen Containers. (From Niedzwiecki B, et al: *Kinn's the medical assistant*, ed 14, St. Louis, 2020, Elsevier.)

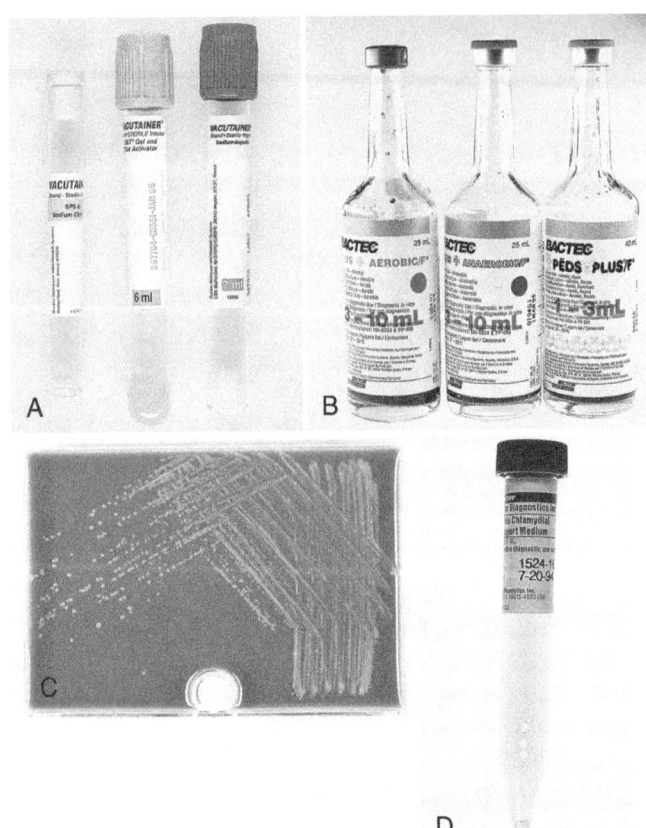

Fig. 56.7 A, Blood collection Vacutainer tubes, one for aerobic and one for anaerobic. B, BACTEC blood culture bottles. C, JEMBEC plate. D, Viral-chlamydial transport media. (From De la Maza LM, Pezzlo MT, Baron EJ: *Color atlas of diagnostic microbiology*, St. Louis, 1997, Mosby.)

and written instructions to the patient. If the patient will be collecting the sample in private or at home, written instructions that are simple and straightforward should be supplied.

To protect from pathogen exposure, the medical assistant should wear the appropriate personal protective equipment (PPE) when collecting, handling, and processing specimens. The medical assistant should wear gloves, a fluid-impermeable lab coat, a surgical mask (for droplet or airborne pathogens), and protective eyewear or a face shield. Proper hand washing techniques are also important before and after the procedure.

The following sections will discuss transporting specimens and how to collect different types of specimens. Collecting a specimen from a wound for a culture was discussed in Chapter 40.

Guidelines for Handling and Transporting Specimens

The transport of specimens to referral laboratories is also crucial. Different types of transport devices are available. Close attention must be given to their proper use. Microorganisms are living organisms, so they must be given conditions that ensure their survival. Care must also be taken so that any normal flora in the sample will not multiply and overgrow possible pathogens. The type and number of microorganisms in the sample should reflect the type and number of microorganisms at the site of collection and at the time of collection.

Specialized transport media are often included with specimen collection swabs or devices (Fig. 56.5). Collection devices typically consist of a plastic tube that encases a sterile Dacron swab and a sealed vial of transport medium. After the specimen has been collected on the swab, it is placed in the plastic tube with the transport medium. It is essential to follow the manufacturer's directions to prevent the swab and specimen from drying out. Transport system swabs also have a label that must be filled out completely, indicating the patient's full name, the date and time of collection, the collector's initials, and the source of the specimen (e.g., deep wound sample from left leg abscess).

If possible, a specimen should be placed on culture media immediately after collection. If this is not possible, then the transport device must be sent to a referral laboratory or held in the POL until it can be cultured. For specimens that will be transported by a courier, make sure the specimen is safely packaged in a leak-proof container marked with warning labels (Fig. 56.6). The proper time and temperature of storage are vital. Most

---

VOCABULARY

transport medium A medium used to keep an organism alive during transport to the laboratory.

TABLE 56.6 Collection, Transport, and Processing of Specimens Commonly Collected in the Physician Office Laboratory[a]

Specimen	Container	Patient Preparation	Special Instructions	Storage Before Processing
Throat	Transport swab (see Fig. 56.5)	Have patient sitting with head tilted back	Swab pharynx and tonsils, not mouth, tongue, or teeth	Transport and plate within 24 hr; room-temperature storage
Superficial wound	Aerobic transport swab (see Fig. 56.5)	Moisten area with sterile saline and pat dry before collection	Rotate swab while gently swiping wound	Transport swab stored at room temperature
Eye	Aerobic transport swab (see Fig. 56.5)	Pull lower lid down while gently collecting exudate along rim	N/A	Transport swab may be stored up to 24 hr at room temperature
Ova and parasite (O&P)	O&P transport containers (with formalin and PVA) (see Fig. 56.6)	See Procedure 56.1 for collection of a stool specimen for ova and parasites	Wait 7–10 days if patient has been taking Pepto-Bismol, Kaopectate, or milk of magnesia	Store at room temperature and deliver to laboratory within 24 hr
Stool	Clean, leak-proof containers (see Fig. 56.6)	Outpatients: At minimum, three specimens are collected every other day	Transport to laboratory within 24 hr if storing at 4°C (39.2°F)	Laboratory must plate within 72 hr if storing at 4°C (39.2°F)
Sputum	Sterile, screw-cap container (see Fig. 56.6)	Patient should rinse or gargle with water before collection	Have patient collect from deep cough; do not collect saliva	Store at 4°C (39.2°F); laboratory must plate within 24 hr
Urine	Vacutainer collection system or sterile, screw-cap container (see Fig. 56.6)	Instruct patient in clean-catch midstream collection	Hold at 4°C (39.2°F) and deliver to laboratory within 24 hr	Hold at 4°C (39.2°F) and plate within 24 hr
Skin scraping (fungal culture)	Clean, screw-top tube (see Fig. 56.6)	Wipe skin with alcohol wipe	Scrape skin at leading edge of lesion	Can be held indefinitely at room temperature but best to process within 72 hr of collection
Blood	Blood culture tube with SPS medium (see Fig. 56.7A) or Vacutainer blood culture medium (see Fig. 56.7B)	Disinfect venipuncture site with alcohol wipe and Betadine or chlorhexidine gluconate prep kit	Draw blood during febrile episodes	Deliver to laboratory within 2 hr; incubate at 37°C (98.6°F) on receipt in the laboratory
Gonorrhea culture	JEMBEC transport system (see Fig. 56.7C)	Wipe away exudate before obtaining culture specimen, obtain culture specimen with swab	Do not refrigerate	Transport to laboratory within 2 hr
Chlamydia culture	Specialized antibiotic Chlamydia transport medium (see Fig. 56.7D)	Urogenital swabs preferred; necessary to obtain epithelial cells, not exudate	Transport immediately on ice to laboratory	Store up to 24 hr at 4°C (39.2°F); inoculate cultures within 15 min of collection if swab is not on ice
Body fluids (e.g., peritoneal, synovial, pleural)	Sterile, screw-cap container or anaerobic transporter	Disinfect aspiration site with alcohol wipe and Betadine	Needle aspirations are preferable to swab collections	Transport immediately to laboratory
Rectal swab	Swab placed directly into enteric transport medium	N/A	Insert swab approximately 1 inch past anal sphincter	Store at 4°C (39.2°F), transport within 24 hr to laboratory and plate within 72 hr
Deep wound or abscess	Anaerobic transport device	Wipe area with sterile saline or alcohol wipe before collection	Aspirate material, excise tissue, or insert swab deep into wound	Store at room temperature; transport to laboratory and plate within 4 hr

O&P, Ova and parasites; PVA, polyvinyl alcohol; SPS, sodium polyanethole sulfonate.
[a]Reference laboratories also have specific directions for collecting specimens based on their testing methods.
Modified from Forbes BA, Sahm DF, Weissfeld AS: *Bailey and Scott's diagnostic microbiology*, ed 11, St. Louis, 2002, Mosby.

pathogenic organisms prefer body temperatures, approximately 37°C (98.6°F). They will remain viable for up to 72 hours if held at room temperature or refrigerator temperature (4°C [39.2°F]). Some organisms die if exposed to cold temperatures. Always check the referral laboratory's procedure manual for directions regarding sample time and temperature of storage. See Fig. 56.7 for some commonly used microbiology collection devices.

Devices used for both aerobic and anaerobic blood collection are shown in Fig. 56.7A, and BACTEC blood culture bottles are pictured in Fig. 56.7B. Two other commonly used transportation devices are the JEMBEC plate for transporting *Neisseria*

gonorrhoeae (see Fig. 56.7C) and a viral-chlamydial transport medium (see Fig. 56.7D).

See Table 56.6 for a description of the specimens, containers, patient preparation processes, and storage of specimens commonly collected or handled by medical assistants.

CRITICAL THINKING 56.4

Each time Lena collects a wound swab that needs to be sent to the reference laboratory, she needs to put the swab in a transport medium. List three reasons why we use transport media when wound specimens cannot be tested immediately. Be ready to share your ideas with the class.

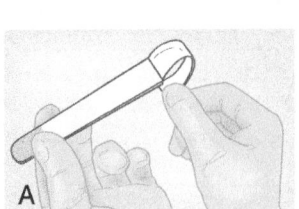
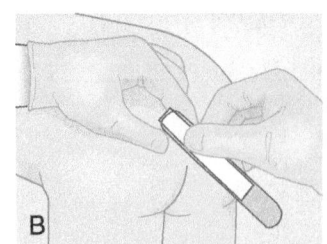
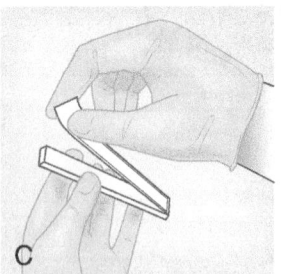

Fig. 56.8 The Three Steps for Collecting a Pinworm Specimen From a Child. A, Place cellulose tape over a tongue depressor with the sticky side out. B, Press the tape firmly against the right and left anal folds. C, Place the tape with adhesive side down on to the microscope slide. (From Niedzwiecki B, et al: *Kinn's the Medical Assistant*, ed 14, St. Louis, 2020, Elsevier.)

Stool Specimen Collection

Stool specimens are commonly examined for parasitic protozoa and helminths. The specimen is collected and placed into two vials, each with a preservative. From these preparations, a wet mount slide is made to observe moving organisms. A stained smear is made from a concentrated specimen. The smear is looked at under a microscope to observe protozoal cysts and helminth eggs. The medical assistant should always consult the procedure manual provided by the referral laboratory when an ova and parasites stool examination (O&P) is ordered to make sure that proper specimen collection and transport takes place (Procedure 56.1).

> **VOCABULARY**
>
> **nasopharyngeal** Describes the part of the throat behind and above the soft palate and connected to the nasal passages.
> **protozoal cyst** A thick-walled protective membrane enclosing a cell, larva, or organism.
> **wet mount** A glass slide that holds a specimen suspended in a drop of liquid for microscopic examination.

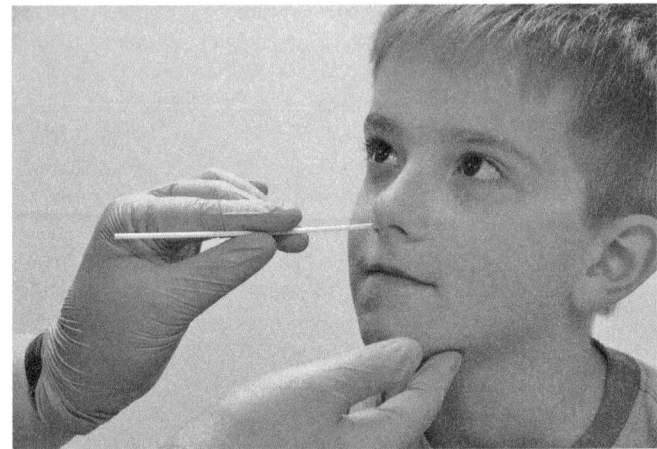

Fig. 56.9 For an anterior nasal specimen, the swab is inserted no more than 0.5 of an inch in the nostril for adults and less for a child. (From Niedzwiecki B, et al: *Kinn's the medical assistant*, ed 14, St. Louis, 2020, Elsevier.)

Pinworm Collection

Enterobius vermicularis (ehn tuh ROH bee uhs ver MIK yoo ler uhs) is commonly known as pinworm. The eggs hatch in the small intestine, and the females migrate out of the anus, usually at night, to deposit the eggs. The eggs adhere to the skin and hair surrounding the anus, sleeping garments, and other clothing. Pinworms cause itching in the anal area, which may cause the eggs to come in contact with the hands and fingernails of the host.

Pinworm infection is spread by the fecal-oral route. The infective pinworm eggs are transferred to the mouth directly by the hand or indirectly through contaminated clothing, food, liquids, and other articles. Since the pinworm eggs are so small, they can sometimes become airborne and are ingested while breathing.

In children, specimens are best collected late at night or early in the morning. Paraffin swabs impregnated with petroleum jelly or cellulose tape may be used to collect the eggs deposited by the adult worm during the night. The diagnosis is based on laboratory detection of the eggs in fecal smears. If the parent does not feel comfortable collecting the specimen, instruct parents to bring children to the office as soon as they wake up in the morning. Instruct the parent not to change the child's clothing or diaper before coming into the office. When the child arrives, have all the needed supplies ready to use, and perform the procedure immediately (Fig. 56.8).

Nasal and Nasopharyngeal Specimen Collection

Nasal and nasopharyngeal (ney zoh FAR in jee ahl) specimens are obtained for several respiratory tests, including COVID-19. Depending on the state's medical assistant scope of practice, a medical assistant may be able to perform nasal and nasopharyngeal specimen collection (Procedure 56.2). The types of swabs used depend on the test and the collect site.

Three types of specimens can be collected:
- *Anterior nasal specimen*: The swab is inserted no more than 0.5 of an inch (1 cm) into the nostril (Fig. 56.9).
- *Mid-turbinate nasal specimen*: With the patient's head tilted back at a 70-degree angle, the swab is inserted parallel to the nostril floor until resistance is met at the nasal turbinates. The swab is usually inserted no more than 1 inch (2 cm). This specimen is taken deeper into the nose than the anterior nasal specimen.
- *Nasopharyngeal (NP) specimen*: When obtaining the specimen, the patient's head should be tilted back at a 70-degree angle. The minitip swab needs to be inserted through the nostril. Insert the swab so it is parallel to the palate, continue to insert until resistance is encountered. The swab needs to be inserted the same distance as the nostril to the outer opening of the ear.

The swab should be gently rolled and then left in place for several seconds to allow it to absorb secretions. A specimen is obtained from both nostrils unless the swab is saturated with secretions from the first nostril. If the patient has a nasal blockage or deviated septum, the unobstructed nostril should be used for the collection.

Sputum Specimen Collection

Sputum cultures may be ordered when patients have symptoms that may be related to infectious respiratory diseases. Examples of other sputum tests include:

- Legionella testing for legionnaires' disease
- Acid-fast bacillus (AFB) testing for tuberculosis
- Gram stain for bacterial or fungal infections

The medical assistant may be responsible for coaching patients on how to collect sputum specimens. Many times, sputum specimens are collected in the morning. For some tests, three sputum samples may be collected over 3 days. When collecting a sputum specimen, patients should:

1. Avoid food for 1 to 2 hours before collecting the sputum specimen.
2. Rinse your mouth well to remove food particles.
3. Open the container and avoid touching the inside of the container and cover.
4. Inhale two to three times, breathing out hard each time, then cough deeply.
5. Collect the sputum from the cough. Do not spit oral secretions into the cup.
6. Cover the container when enough sputum is collected.

The medical assistant should discuss how the specimen should be stored and brought to the healthcare facility for testing.

CRITICAL THINKING 56.5

Lena needs to collect sputum from patient who needs a sputum culture. Lena tells the patient that she needs the sputum to come from the lungs. The patient asks why she cannot just use "spit" from her mouth. How might Lena respond?

Throat Swab Specimen Collection

A throat swab specimen collection is a common procedure in the ambulatory care facility. This type of specimen is used to identify the cause of throat infections, such as strep throat. It is important that patients resist gagging and closing their mouth while the swabbing occurs. Procedure 56.3 describes the collection process. Patients should not use antiseptic mouthwash prior to the collection.

CLIA-WAIVED MICROBIOLOGY TESTING

Often, growing a pathogen on a nutrient media plate is difficult, and it takes time to grow and isolate the pathogen. A rapid direct immunology test demonstrates the presence of the antigen in a specimen that is placed in a test kit containing its specific antibody. If the pathogen is present, it produces a colored reaction, indicating a positive result.

POLs with appropriate CLIA-waived certification can perform many rapid identification tests for a variety of infectious diseases. Rapid tests are designed to give the provider positive test results quickly and efficiently so that treatment can be started. If the test result is negative, the provider may need to order additional referral laboratory tests.

- The first step in performing these tests is to review the package insert provided by the manufacturer. This gives valuable information about the test:
  - Principle on which the test is based
  - Reagents and equipment needed
  - Proper specimen collection techniques
  - Patient preparation requirements
  - Test procedures
  - Any precautions or warnings pertaining to the procedure

The insert also provides information about quality control, interpretation of results, limitations of the procedure, and references.

Rapid Strep Testing

Rapid strep testing is commonly performed in the POL and can be completed while the patient waits. The patient's throat is swabbed. The test swab is placed in an extraction well, and the extract is tested for antigens found on the surface of *S. pyogenes* (also referred to as group A strep, or GAS). The test kit uses a *lateral flow immunoassay*. This means that the specimen "flows" into the test area. If the strep A pathogen is present, there will be an antigen-antibody reaction with the group A strep antibodies in the testing area. The reaction of the strep A antigen and the strep A antibodies cause a color change that can be seen (Procedure 56.4).

Negative test results should be confirmed with a throat culture performed in the microbiology laboratory (explained later in the chapter). The rapid strep tests are highly specific, so if the test results are positive, there is confidence that *S. pyogenes* is present in the sample. If the test results are negative, the organism may not have been present in high enough numbers to be detected. Then a transport swab should be sent to the microbiology reference laboratory to be cultured.

VOCABULARY

extract A certain substance that is taken out of a group or solution and is in a concentrated form.

extraction A process by which a specific substance is separated from a group or solution.

CRITICAL THINKING 56.6

Frankie Burns, a 10-year-old, has a raw, sore throat, a fever of 101°F (38.3°C), and just feels awful. Lena is going to collect a throat swab for a rapid strep test from Frankie. What bacteria cause strep throat? What is the scientific name of the bacteria? Which of the two names is the genus, and which of the two names is the species? Write down your answers and share them with your classmates.

Influenza A and B Testing

The *influenza* (in floo EN zuh) virus causes influenza, or "the flu." This is a highly contagious, acute viral infection of the respiratory tract. The infection is highly communicable through the respiratory route, and outbreaks are typically seen in the fall and winter. Type A viruses usually are more common than type B viruses. Type A viruses typically are associated with epidemics, and type B viruses cause a milder infection. A rapid diagnosis of influenza can help with the decision to give antiviral medications. They should be given early in the infection cycle to be the most effective. CLIA-waived rapid lateral flow immunoassays detect both influenza A and influenza B antigens from **nasopharyngeal** swabs or nasal washes.

Respiratory Syncytial Virus Testing

Respiratory *syncytial* (sin SISH ee ahl) virus (RSV) is a major cause of upper and lower respiratory tract infections. It is the major cause of bronchiolitis and pneumonia in children and infants. Outbreaks typically occur yearly in the fall, winter, and spring and can be severe for very young children. The CLIA-waived rapid direct immunoassay for RSV uses a nasopharyngeal swab specimen or nasal washings to detect the virus. Because antiviral agents are available to treat RSV infection, rapid diagnosis can lead to:

- Shorter hospital stays
- Reduced need for antibiotic therapy to treat secondary bacterial infection
- Lower cost for hospital care

The tests are intended for children under age 5.

CLIA-WAIVED IMMUNOLOGY TESTING

Immunology testing provides information about past or present infections with bacteria or viruses. It also detects certain types of cancers. Testing done in the immunology department is designed to demonstrate the reaction between an antigen and its specific antibody. Antibodies are formed when the body encounters a foreign agent. In the acute stage of a disease, the antibody level starts to rise and increases fourfold over the next several weeks. Paired testing of sera from the acute stage of illness and 2 weeks later that demonstrate a fourfold increase indicate the presence of the disease. During the later convalescent stage, the antibody level begins to decline for the next 3 to 6 months. Once the immune system recognizes an antigen, then antibodies are made. The antibody will remain in the blood at a low but detectable level for a lifetime. The amount of antibody can be measured with serologic (si ROL uh jik) testing called a titer.

Most serologic/immunologic testing performed in the ambulatory care center is done using individual test kits (e.g., strep, influenza, mononucleosis, and HIV tests). The difference is the source of the specimen and what the test is looking for.

The direct immunologic tests discussed in the previous section (strep test and influenza test) used a throat swab and nasal swab specimen. The test kits were detecting the antigen or pathogen causing the disease directly. In the indirect immunologic tests, the specimen is the patient's blood or serum. The blood or serum is tested to see whether the patient has produced the specific antibody to the pathogen in question. CLIA-waived immunology tests that can be performed by a medical assistant to detect antibodies to a pathogen include infectious mononucleosis, *Helicobacter pylori* (hee lih koh BAK tur pahy LAWR ee), Lyme disease, and human immunodeficiency virus (HIV) tests.

> **VOCABULARY**
> **acute stage** The phase during which rapid multiplication of the pathogen takes place. Symptoms are very distinct. A strong response of the immune system takes place during this stage.
> **bronchiolitis** Occurs when the small airways of the lungs become inflamed because of a viral infection.
> **convalescent stage** The phase during which the host recovers gradually and returns to baseline or normal health.
> **heterophile antibody** An antibody that has an affinity for an antigen other than the specific antigen that stimulated its production.
> **nasal wash** Also called a nasal aspirate. A syringe is used to gently squirt a small amount of sterile saline into the nose, and the resulting fluid is collected into a cup (for a wash). Or after the saline is squirted into the nose, gentle suction is applied (for the aspirate).
> **pneumonia** Inflammation of the lungs with congestion of the air sacs (alveoli). Can be caused by a bacterium or virus.
> **serologic** Pertaining to the science involving the immune properties and actions of serum.
> **titer** The lowest concentration of a serum solution containing a specific antibody where the antibody is still able to neutralize (or precipitate) an antigen.

Infectious Mononucleosis Testing

Infectious mononucleosis, commonly called mono, is an acute infectious disease caused by the Epstein-Barr virus (EBV). EBV is one of the many herpes viruses. The virus is especially common in teenagers. It is found most frequently in people 10 to 25 years of age and is seen occasionally in adults over the age of 25. In the United States, about 95% of adults between 35 and 40 have already been infected.

In children, the infection may pass unrecognized or result in a mild illness lasting only a few days. It is marked by sore throat, fever, swollen tonsils, and enlarged lymph nodes in the neck. In young people, some of the most common complications include the abrupt onset of fatigue, headaches, very swollen tonsils, enlarged lymph glands, and loss of appetite often associated with nausea. There may be a short or prolonged period (days or weeks) after the initial illness when the fatigue continues. Occasionally, complications occur, including the development of a swollen spleen or liver, referred to as *hepatosplenomegaly*.

Testing for mononucleosis involves a complete blood count (CBC) and immunology tests. The CBC should reveal an increased number of lymphocytes that appear atypical on the blood smear. Due to the abnormally high number of mononuclear leukocytes in the blood, the illness was called mononucleosis. Most patients exposed to EBV produce a nonspecific heterophile (HET er uh fihl) antibody response to the virus. These heterophile antibodies in the patient's blood react with the heterophile antigens supplied in the test kit, resulting in a positive color reaction in the testing area of the kit (Procedure 56.5).

CRITICAL THINKING 56.7

Allyson Anderson is 15 years old. She came into the clinic today with signs and symptoms of infectious mononucleosis. Lena is going to do a fingerstick on Allyson and do a mono test. What are the typical signs and symptoms of mono in a teenager? What is the mono test checking for in Allyson's blood?

MEDICAL TERMINOLOGY

hepat/o	liver
heter/o	another, different
ser/o	serum
splen/o	spleen
-phile	to love, be attracted to

Helicobacter pylori Testing

H. pylori is a spiral-shaped bacterium that can infect the stomach's mucous layer or lining. *H. pylori* causes more than 90% of duodenal ulcers and more than 80% of stomach ulcers. Several methods can be used to diagnose *H. pylori* infection. Serologic tests that measure specific *H. pylori* antibodies can determine whether a person has been infected. CLIA-waived rapid immunoassay tests use whole blood applied to a well in a test cartridge. The blood migrates from the well through the testing area of the cartridge. The presence of a line in the test area of the cartridge indicates the presence of antibodies to the pathogen *H. pylori*.

Lyme Disease Testing

Lyme disease is the most common insect-borne infectious disease in North America, and it is a significant public health concern. The spirochete bacterium *Borrelia burgdorferi* (buh REL ee uh buhrg DOR fuh rih) is the causative agent in Lyme disease.

The disease is contracted from an infected tick that bites a person. The bacteria are in the saliva of the tick. These ticks typically are found on deer, mice, dogs, horses, and birds. Infection occurs when the bacteria enter the tick bite. A characteristic bull's-eye rash, known as *erythema migrans* (MAHY grahns) (EM), develops at the bite site in 60% to 80% of patients. Lyme disease progresses in three stages. If the person is not treated, the disease progresses. The spirochete bacterium invades the skin, joints, central nervous system (CNS), heart, and other locations. Arthritic or CNS syndromes often accompany late-stage disease and may be the only clinical symptoms that indicate the infection.

Lyme disease can be detected early with a CLIA-waived test, such as the Wampole PreVue *B. burgdorferi* test. This immunoassay tests for antibodies in whole blood. A sample of blood is applied to a test cartridge, a diluent is added, and the results are read in 20 minutes. The microbiology reference laboratory should verify any positive results.

VOCABULARY

duodenal Describes the first section of the small intestines after the stomach.

diluent A liquid substance that dilutes or lessens the strength of a solution or mixture.

heterophile antibody An antibody that has an affinity for an antigen other than the specific antigen that stimulated its production.

opportunistic infections Microorganisms that normally do not cause disease but become pathogenic when the body's immune system is impaired and unable to fight off infection, as occurs with AIDS, malnutrition, and certain other diseases.

HIV Testing

HIV attacks and destroys the *T-helper (CD4) lymphocytes*. The T-helper lymphocytes play a critical role in protecting the body against infection. They work with the B lymphocytes to produce the specific antibodies that fight infections. As the HIV infection destroys more T-helper cells, the body becomes less able to fight off infections and more susceptible to opportunistic infections. If HIV is not treated with antiretroviral (ARV) medications, acquired immunodeficiency syndrome (AIDS) eventually develops. HIV infections become AIDS when life-threatening infections and cancers begin to appear.

In 2013 the Centers for Disease Control and Prevention (CDC) and the World Health Organization (WHO) both advised preventive measures to control the disease. This requires early detection and early treatment of individuals infected with HIV. The sooner the virus is detected via immunology testing, the sooner treatment with ARV medications may begin.

Two CLIA-waived HIV tests are readily available to detect the presence of HIV antibodies in blood and in oral specimens. Patients at risk of HIV infection are now strongly encouraged to take a blood test available in POLs or outpatient clinics. Note that HIV is a bloodborne pathogen. The medical assistant should always follow the Bloodborne Pathogens Standard established by the Occupational Safety and Health Administration (OSHA) when collecting and testing all patient blood and body fluids. Remember, all patients are treated the same when it comes to the Bloodborne Pathogens Standards and Standard Precautions.

The patient may also choose to perform an oral self-test from a kit that is available at pharmacies (Fig. 56.10). The test kit includes a testing device that is rubbed once over the upper and lower gums. It then is inserted into the test vial, which is placed in a plastic stand. The test results are read in 20 minutes. The test includes an internal control band that verifies a specimen was added and that the test was run correctly (Box 56.1).

MICROBIOLOGY REFERENCE LABORATORY: IDENTIFICATION OF PATHOGENS

After receiving the specimens collected in the POL described in the Specimen Collection and Transport in the Physician Office Laboratory section presented earlier in this chapter, the

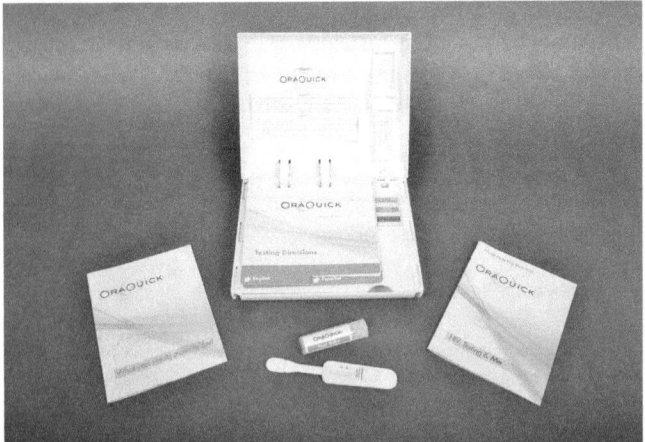

Fig. 56.10 Human Immunodeficiency Virus Home Testing Kit. (From Niedzwiecki B, et al: *Kinn's the medical assistant*, ed 14, St. Louis, 2020, Elsevier.)

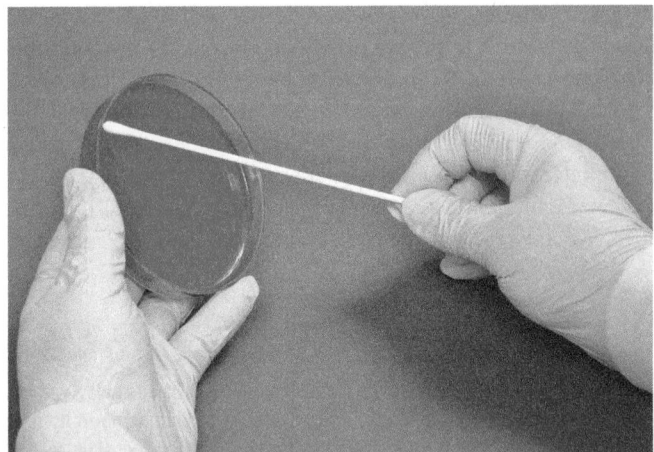

Fig. 56.11 Inoculating a Blood Culture Plate with a Swab.

BOX 56.1   HIV Testing

For both HIV testing methods, it is important to provide the patient with information or counseling regarding HIV infection and its relationship to AIDS. Be aware that patients being tested may be fearful; therefore proper knowledge presented in a therapeutic way can help them dispel the fear and take positive action toward preventive behavior and treatment. Positive HIV test results must be verified at a reference laboratory.

---

microbiology laboratory promptly inoculates the appropriate culture media first and then prepares a smear of the specimen on a slide to be stained (Fig. 56.11). This ensures that the swab is not contaminated by the slide. If two swabs are received from the same source, one may be used for the culture and the other to make the smear. The equipment and supplies in a microbiology laboratory vary with the size of the facility. Most laboratories have a refrigerator, an autoclave, a safety cabinet, a microscope, and an incubator.

Staining

Pathogenic microorganisms generally are colorless, and a microscope is needed to see them. Special stains (e.g., Gram stain and acid-fast stain) are used to differentiate bacteria based on cell membrane differences. As discussed previously, Gram stain differentiates bacteria into two categories according to chemical makeup of the cell wall. The acid-fast stain differentiates bacteria into two categories based on the presence or absence of a waxy lipid in the cell wall.

Before staining can be done, the specimen must be applied to a labeled slide. The slide is then air-dried and fixed or adhered to the slide. Both heat (e.g., from a Bunsen burner or an incinerator) and methanol can be used to fix the sample to the slide. The heat and methanol cause protein in the sample to break down and stick to the slide. Note, overheating the slide can cause cell distortion.

Gram Stain

The Gram stain, developed by Dr. Hans Christian Gram in the late 1800s, is still the most commonly used stain in microbiology. This procedure involves applying a sequence of reagents: a primary stain, *mordant*, *decolorizer*, and counterstain to the slide. The dyes are taken up differently according to the

chemical composition of the bacterial cell walls. Bacteria react best in the Gram stain when they are less than 24 hours old. Gram-positive bacteria stain purple, and gram-negative bacteria stain pink or red (see Fig. 56.1). It is useful for the medical assistant to understand the procedures and the microscopic results obtained. For example, when a Gram stain report is called in, the terms *GPCs* and *GNBs* mean "gram-positive cocci" (deeply blue-stained circular cells) and "gram-negative bacilli" (pink/red stained rod-shaped cells).

VOCABULARY
decolorizer A liquid that has the ability to wash out color.
mordant Having the ability to fix or set colors.

CRITICAL THINKING 56.8

What are the four reagents used in the Gram stain? What color are gram-positive organisms? What color are gram-negative organisms? Share your answers with the class.

Acid-Fast Stain

The acid-fast stain is used in the identification protocol for *Mycobacterium species*. *M. tuberculosis* causes tuberculosis and can be isolated from sputum or tissue samples. *M. avium* complex (MAC) is a common soil organism that enters through the respiratory tract and spreads throughout the body. MAC is one of the causes of death among patients with AIDS. An overview of the acid-fast stain is listed here:

- A red primary dye, *carbolfuchsin* (kar BOL fyoo shin), is applied first
- Then the decolorizer, acid-alcohol, is applied
- Followed by a counterstain, *methylene* (meth uh leen) blue

Acid-fast positive microbes stain fuchsia-red. Acid-fast negative microbes stain baby blue. Bacilli that are acid-fast positive often are referred to as *acid-fast bacillus (AFB)* (see Fig. 56.2).

Inoculating Equipment

Next, the specimen must be spread on specific culture media based on the source of the specimen. The inoculated culture

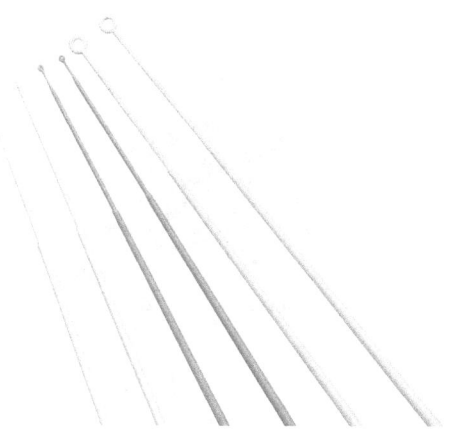

Fig. 56.12 *(Left)* Inoculating needles. *(Right)* Inoculating loops. (From Niedzwiecki B, et al: *Kinn's the medical assistant*, ed 14, St. Louis, 2020, Elsevier.)

media are placed in a body temperature incubator to grow overnight. Inoculating needles and loops (Fig. 56.12) are used to transfer samples to culture media or microbes to slides for staining. Needles and loops may be disposable and presterilized. They may also be made of wire and can be heat sterilized before and after each transfer (Fig. 56.13). An inoculating loop is shaped like a bubble wand, and a thin film of liquid adheres to the loop. The amount of fluid held by the loop can be calibrated. For example, a urine culture uses a loop that delivers a 1-mcL sample. The urine in the loop is spread across the culture medium and allowed to grow overnight. The next day, each bacterium becomes a visible colony. Colonies can then be counted and analyzed to determine the cause of a urinary tract infection.

Assessing a Culture

When the original (primary) culture has incubated at the appropriate temperature for 18 to 24 hours, it is examined for evidence of pathogens. Because normal flora is often present in samples in addition to pathogens, a trained eye is required to spot the organisms that might be causing an infection. Suspicious colonies are subcultured onto the appropriate medium to isolate them in pure culture. When the organism is in pure culture, staining and additional biochemical testing can be done to identify the organisms. Throat and urine cultures may be performed in POLs that have been CLIA certified to perform moderately-complex testing.

> **VOCABULARY**
> **colony** A discrete group of organisms, such as a group of bacteria, growing on a solid nutrient surface.
> **pure culture** The growth of only one microorganism in a culture or on a nutrient surface.
> **5% sheep's blood agar plate (BAP)** A solid agar medium that contains nutrients and 5% washed sheep's blood. The blood is added as an extra nutrient source for bacteria.
> **streaked for isolation** To have produced isolated colonies of an organism on an agar plate. Using an inoculating loop, pick one colony and methodically spread it out onto solid nutrient media. The goal is to have colonies that are separate from other colonies.
> **subcultured** Occurs when an organism (a bacterium) has been cultivated again on a new nutrient surface.

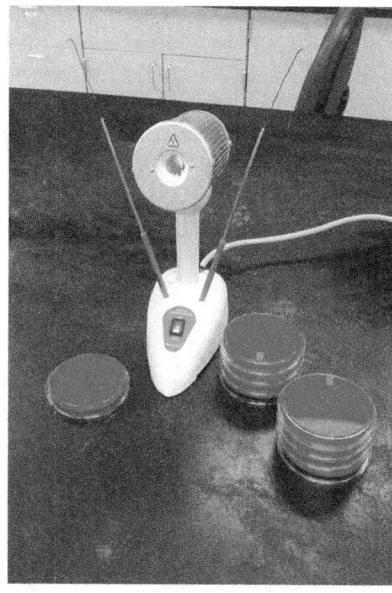

Fig. 56.13 Incinerator for Sterilizing Wire Loops and Needles.

Throat Cultures. *Streptococcus pyogenes,* also known as *group A strep (GAS)* or *beta hemolytic streptococcus,* causes strep throat. If not diagnosed and treated promptly, this infection can cause severe complications, including scarlet fever, rheumatic fever, and glomerulonephritis. A throat swab is collected from the patient's throat. Then the swab is streaked for isolation on a 5% sheep's blood agar plate (BAP) (Box 56.2). An antibiotic disk is placed on the first quadrant of the streaked plate (Fig. 56.14) and incubated overnight at 37°C (98.6°F). The antibiotic disk contains *bacitracin* (bas ih TREY sin), which prevents the growth of *S. pyogenes.* Complete clearing of the agar around the colonies indicates *beta hemolysis,* which is caused by a toxin produced by *S. pyogenes.* The toxin breaks down the red blood cells in the agar, causing the agar to be a clear golden color around the colonies. The presence of beta hemolysis and a zone of no growth around the disk indicate that the patient has strep throat (see Fig. 56.14). Additional testing may be needed to confirm the identity of the organism.

Urine Cultures. With urine cultures, the bacterial colonies that appear after incubation are counted. A calibrated inoculating loop is dipped into a well-mixed urine sample that was collected by the CCMS method or by catheterization. The urine from the loop is spread on solid culture media and incubated for 18 to 24 hours at 37°C (98.6°F). Each colony that grows on the plate represents 1000 colony-forming units (cfu) per milliliter. The final cfu results are interpreted as follows:

- Normal: <10,000 cfu/mL of urine; no urinary tract infection (UTI) present.
- Borderline: 10,000 to 100,000 cfu/mL of urine; a chronic or relapsing infection may be present, and the test should be repeated.
- Positive: >100,000 cfu/mL of urine; a UTI is likely.

BOX 56.2   Streaking for Isolation

Streaking for isolation is also called a four-quadrant streak. It is a procedure that is performed with most microbiology specimens. By distributing bacteria across the agar plate and isolating bacterial colonies, laboratory personnel can see characteristics of the bacteria that are useful in the identification process.

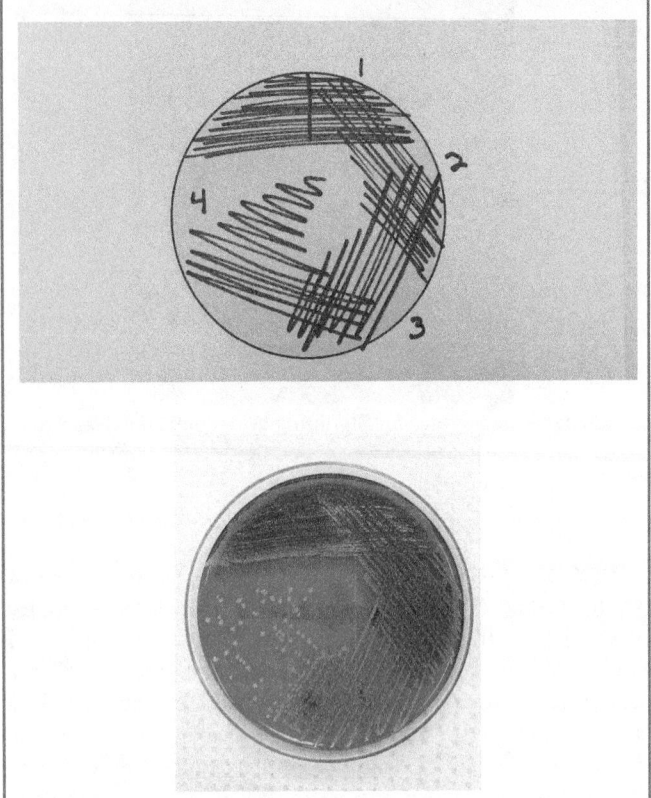

The medical assistant needs to be aware of the terminology and values reported for urine cultures.

CRITICAL THINKING 56.9

Lena is looking over the reference laboratory results from the day. Mrs. Liz Darcy was in for an office visit yesterday and collected a urine specimen for C&S. Her preliminary culture report came back as 82,000 cfu/mL, pure culture. The identification and susceptibility report is due to follow tomorrow.

- Does Mrs. Darcy have a urinary tract infection?
- Does Mrs. Darcy need any additional testing for this condition?
- In your own words, define pure culture.
- Describe C&S in your own words.

Microbiology Culture and Sensitivity Testing

Once a bacterial infection has been identified, additional steps are required for successful treatment. To determine the appropriate antibiotic to destroy the pathogen, the provider will order a culture and sensitivity (C&S) test. *Culture* refers to growing the organisms, and *sensitivity* refers to the organism's susceptibility to antibiotics.

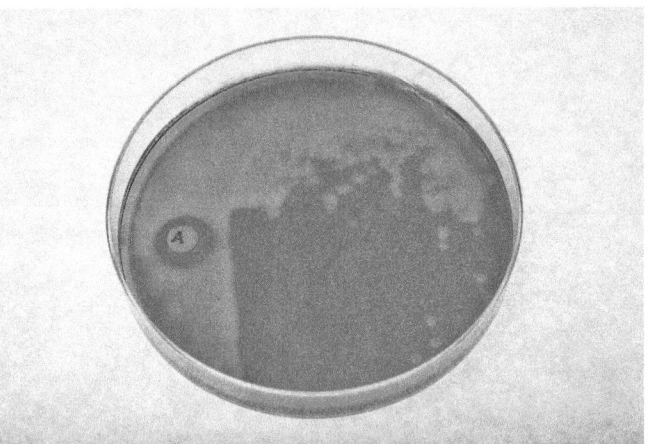

Fig. 56.14 Positive strep test result on blood agar (*left side of plate*); group A Streptococcus (GAS) shows beta hemolysis (clearing) of the blood agar below the growing colonies. Notice there is no hemolysis, or clearing of the blood around the white bacitracin disk. That is because bacitracin can destroy GAS. (From Niedzwiecki B, et al: *Kinn's the medical assistant*, ed 14, St. Louis, 2020, Elsevier.)

The healthcare provider must decide which medication to order based on initial test results and the patient's physical examination. C&S test results provide vital information about which specific antibiotics work best against the particular infective pathogen.

There are many methods of performing sensitivity testing. Some methods involve culture media and antibiotic disks. Other methods are fully automated and require a very small amount of the pure culture to be tested. No matter what method is used, sensitivity testing is reported to the provider in one of three categories for each antibiotic tested:

S means that the pathogen is *susceptible*, or that the antibiotic is effective in destroying that particular organism.

R means that the pathogen is *resistant*, or that the antibiotic is not effective in destroying that particular organism.

I means *intermediate*, or that additional testing must be performed to determine the dosage of antibiotic necessary for successful treatment.

Some testing methods may give additional information regarding the dosage tested in vitro. This information may be helpful as the providers choose the appropriate antibiotic for treatment. The appropriate antibiotic agent meets the criteria:

- Destroys the infectious agent with a reasonable level of the drug
- Is the least toxic to the patient and has the least impact on normal flora of the body
- Has the desired pharmacologic characteristics (preparation, route of delivery, effectiveness)
- Is the most economical

STOOL-BASED TESTS

There are several stool-based tests on the market used to screen for colorectal cancer. The fecal occult blood test (FOBT) checks a sample of stool for occult blood. Blood in the stools can be caused by hemorrhoids, diverticulosis, ulcers, colitis, and polyps. There are two main types of FOBT: the guaiac fecal occult blood test (gFOBT) and the fecal immunochemical test (FIT). Besides the FOBT, the multitargeted stool DNA test (MT-sDNA) may also be used. It detects abnormal DNA, along with the presence of occult hemoglobin in the stool. These three tests will be discussed in more depth in the following sections. Keep in mind the exact directions for the tests are in the kits and must be followed by the patient.

Fecal Occult Blood Tests

Guaiac Fecal Occult Blood Test.

The guaiac fecal occult blood test is a stool test that looks for the presence of occult blood. This is a common test in the ambulatory care environment. The medical assistant needs to coach the patient on both the preparations for the gFOBT and how to collect the stool specimens (Procedure 56.6). Usually, the patient is asked to collect samples from two or three stools on consecutive days. Each Hemoccult card has two locations (A and B) for samples. One card should be used on each day.

When the Hemoccult test cards are returned to the lab, the company recommends that the test be developed no sooner than 3 days after the stool sample was applied. If immediate testing is required, wait 3 to 5 minutes for the sample to penetrate the test paper. Open the back of the slide and apply 2 drops of the Hemoccult developer to the guaiac paper over each smear (Procedure 56.7). The medical assistant should read the results within 60 seconds. Any trace of blue on the specimen smear or near the edge is considered a positive test result for occult blood (Fig. 56.15). The medical assistant must also apply 1 drop of the developer between the positive and negative Performance Monitors areas, for quality control. The results must be read within 10 seconds. The Hemoccult card and the developer are functioning if a blue color appears in the positive Performance area and no blue appears in the negative Performance Monitors area.

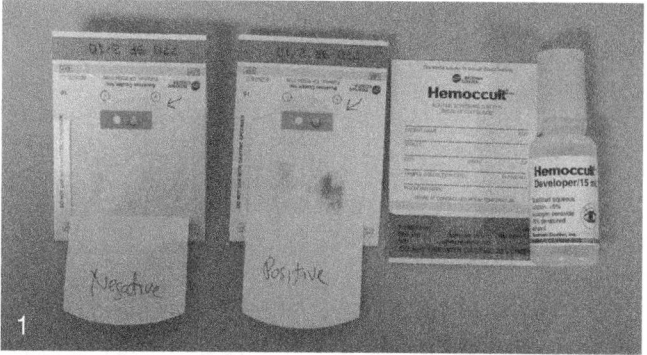

Fig. 56.15 Negative and Positive Hemoccult Results. (From Roberts J, Hedges J: *Clinical procedures in emergency medicine*, ed 5, Philadelphia, 2010, Saunders.)

Fecal Immunochemical Test.

The fecal immunochemical test (FIT), also called the *immunochemical fecal occult blood test* (iFOBT), is a screening test for colon cancer. It only detects human hemoglobin from the large intestine (e.g., cecum, colon, or rectum). Hemoglobin from bleeding occurring from the mouth to the small intestine is generally degraded by the digestive and enzyme processes. Food and medications do not affect this test, so it tends to have fewer false-positive results than the gFOBT.

InSure ONE. InSure ONE is a FIT that detects human hemoglobin in samples of toilet bowel water collected around the feces. The toilet bowl water is collected after the person brushes the surface of the feces to release any blood into the water. The patient is given the test to take home with instructions:

1. Do not collect samples 3 days before or during, or 3 days after the menstrual period; if the patient has bleeding hemorrhoids; or if there is visible blood in the urine.
2. Store the collection kit at room temperature away from heat and direct sunlight.
3. There are no preparations for the test.
4. Label the card as indicated.
5. Flush the toilet before starting. After having the bowel movement, put the used toilet paper in the wastebasket instead of the toilet.
6. Follow the kit instructions.
   a. Use the brush from the kit to brush the surface of the feces/stool for about 5 seconds.
   b. Then dip the brush into the toilet water before touching the brush to the space indicated on the test card.
   c. Wrap the brush in toilet paper and discard it in the wastebasket.
7. Seal the test card, and return as directed to your provider or the laboratory.

> **VOCABULARY**
>
> **guaiac fecal occult blood test** A test for fecal occult blood where glacial acetic acid and guaiac are mixed with the specimen.
>
> **Hemoccult test** A modified guaiac test using filter paper impregnated with guaiacum that turns blue if occult blood is present.
>
> **in vitro** Latin term meaning "in glass" and commonly known as "in the laboratory."
>
> **occult** Not visibly apparent or seen.

Multitargeted Stool DNA Test

An example of a multitargeted stool DNA test (MT-sDNA) is the Cologuard, which tests stool for cancer and pre-cancerous cells. Cologuard screens for DNA markers and the presence of occult hemoglobin in stool. The patient is asked to obtain the sample at home and mail the test to the laboratory.

The patient is given the test to take at home with directions:

1. Do not obtain the sample if you have diarrhea or obvious blood in the urine or stool (e.g., bleeding hemorrhoids, bleeding wounds on the hands, or menstruation).
2. There is no preparation required for this test.
3. Store the kit at room temperature, away from heat, direct sunlight, children, and pets.

4. The kit contains a bracket, sample container, tube, bottle of preservative, shipping label, and sample labels.
5. The bracket is placed in the toilet. The lid is removed from the stool sample container, and the container is placed into the bracket.
6. When having the bowel movement, the person must avoid getting toilet paper and urine in the stool sample container.
7. Following the test directions, the person must scrape the stool sample with the probe to get a small sample. In addition, the preservative must be poured onto the stool in the stool sample container.
8. Both samples (probe tube and sample container) must be sealed tightly, labeled, packed in the special shipping box, and mailed to the lab within a day. The lab must get the sample within 3 days.

■ CLOSING COMMENTS

Maintaining a laboratory in the office increases the physician's liability. By testing patients' specimens in the office, the physician assumes responsibility for the interpretation and accuracy of the results. As the person in the facility who runs the lab tests, you are responsible for maintaining accuracy in testing. A quality assurance program should include running, reading, and recording the controls supplied in each test kit. Both microbiology and immunology tests allow the patient to benefit from the convenience of POL testing. Strict confidentiality is essential. Never release information to anyone other than the patient or legal guardian.

Also note that certain infectious diseases must be reported to the CDC or to the local board of health. Each state legislature determines what diseases must be reported. Additional data for nationally notifiable diseases are published weekly in the CDC in the *Morbidity and Mortality Weekly Report* (MMWR). For additional information on infectious disease reporting, please review the reporting procedure presented in Chapter 19.

PATIENT-CENTERED CARE

Microorganisms such as bacteria, viruses, fungi, and parasites are responsible for most human infectious diseases. Patient education plays an important role in helping the patient and family control the spread of infection. The teaching topics can help you educate a patient about infection control:

- An explanation of the patient's type of infection: bacterial, viral, fungal, or parasitic
- How infections spread
- Hand washing and sanitization, proper storage and cleaning of personal items, and disposal of contaminated supplies
- Risk factors for infection, such as poor nutritional habits or poor ventilation with airborne pathogens present
- The patient's role in specimen collection

- Patient preparation for laboratory tests, imaging tests, and other needed procedures

Explain to the patient that an infection can be transferred from person to person in many ways. Reinforce the importance of following directions for taking any medication. If patients do not follow the directions given to them by the provider or pharmacist, there is a real chance of:

- Developing complications
- Having a relapse of an infection
- Allowing an infection to spread to other areas or becoming systemic

Always listen to the patient. Be sure to answer all the patient's questions. Notify the provider of the patient's concerns so that he or she can give further details or instructions before the patient leaves the facility.

BEING PROFESSIONAL

Lena and Anita take turns working the POL at WMFM Clinic. You overhear them discussing a patient who routinely comes in for HIV testing every 3 months and is coming in today. They talk about double-gloving when they perform the venipuncture and washing their hands for 15 minutes after drawing the patient. Do you agree or disagree? Role-play with several of your classmates and discuss the professionalism and validity of this behavior.

CHAPTER REVIEW

Microorganisms are any microscopic organisms, such as bacteria, protozoa, fungi, parasites, and helminths (eggs). Because viruses are not alive, most scientists refer to them as infectious agents or infectious particles.

There is a system of binomial nomenclature that gives names to all living organisms. The names consist of a genus, or more general name, and a species name, which is a specific name.

Characteristics of bacteria include:

- Staining properties: including the Gram stain and acid-fast stain
- Bacterial shapes: cocci, bacilli, and spirilla
- Oxygen requirements: aerobic, anaerobic, and facultative anaerobic
- Physical structures: flagella and endospores

Some bacteria do not have all of the typical characteristics. This group includes chlamydia, mycoplasma, and rickettsia. These organisms have unique characteristics and therefore must be identified and treated differently. All three types of bacteria are pathogenic and must be considered when certain conditions and symptoms exist.

Pathogenic fungi, protozoa, parasites, helminths, and viruses have unique characteristics and can cause disease. Microbiology includes all types of microorganisms, so we have to think beyond just bacteria when discussing possible pathogens.

Specimen collection is an important part of the medical assistant's job. If they are collecting a sample, medical assistants need to be aware of PPE and proper techniques to collect and not contaminate specimens. They also need to be aware of proper infection control. Proper collection, handling, and transport are critical to getting the correct specimen to its location safely and in a viable state.

The microbiology testing methods discussed include rapid strep testing, influenza A and B testing, and respiratory syncytial virus (RSV) testing. The types of immunology testing discussed include infectious mononucleosis testing, *Helicobacter pylori* testing, Lyme disease testing, and HIV testing.

Testing that needs to be done in a reference laboratory related to microbiology and immunology includes:

- Gram and acid-fast stains
- Use and choices of inoculating equipment
- Assessing a culture: throat and urine
- Antibiotic sensitivity testing

SCENARIO WRAP-UP

Lena has had another busy day at Walden-Martin Family Medical (WMFM) Clinic. Once again, she has seen infectious diseases in some of her patients today. Lena knows that most microorganisms are harmless but knowing the signs and symptoms of common infectious diseases is important.

Lena knows how important it is to diagnose and treat infectious diseases. She knows that proper specimen collection is essential. She is also aware that rapid CLIA-waived tests can identify pathogens and help treat patients in a timely manner.

Microbiology and immunology tests have become useful in the physician office laboratory. Meeting the needs of patients and quickly addressing their concerns are benefits of CLIA-waived testing. Lena feels comfortable collecting specimens, testing patient samples, and reporting the results for the provider to review. As a certified medical assistant, she knows that the work she does throughout the day is helping every one of her patients.

PROCEDURE 56.1 Instruct Patients in the Collection of Fecal Specimens to Be Tested for Ova and Parasites

Task

Instruct a patient in the proper collection of stool for an ova and parasite microscopic examination.

Equipment and Supplies

- Patient's health record
- Provider's order or lab requisition
- Clean, dry container for stool collection
- Plastic biohazard zipper-lock bag
- Two parasitology collection vials

Please note that several types of preservatives are available for the parasitology collection vials. Check with the referral laboratory to make sure the patient is given the proper vials for collection. Preservatives include low-viscosity polyvinyl alcohol (LV-PVA), zinc sulfite polyvinyl alcohol (ZN-PVA), sodium acetate acetic acid formalin (SAF), and 10% neutral buffered formalin.

Procedural Steps

1. Greet the patient. Identify yourself. Verify the patient's identity with full name, then ask the patient to spell first and the last name and to state his or her date of birth.
2. Explain the procedure in a manner that the patient understands. Answer any general questions the patient may have about the collection procedures before you give detailed instructions.
3. Instruct the patient not to take any antacids, laxatives, or stool softeners before collecting the specimen.
   Purpose: Laxatives increase fecal transit time and may lead to a false-negative test result.
4. Instruct the patient to urinate before collecting the specimen.
   Purpose: This eliminates the possibility of the stool becoming contaminated by urine.
5. Instruct the patient or parent/guardian how to collect the stool specimen.

Continued

PROCEDURE 56.1   Instruct Patients in the Collection of Fecal Specimens to Be Tested for Ova and Parasites—cont'd

a. *Adults:* Instruct the patient to defecate into the container provided. Stool cannot be retrieved from the toilet bowl.

b. *Children:* Instruct parents/guardians to loosely drape the toilet rim with plastic wrap and lower the seat. The child should have a bowel movement into the toilet, onto the wrap. Remove the stool using a disposable plastic spoon.

Purpose: The stool cannot be contaminated by or diluted with water.

c. *Infants:* Fasten a "diaper" made of plastic wrap over the child using tape. Remove the plastic wrap immediately after a bowel movement, and remove the stool using a plastic spoon. *Never leave the child unattended with the plastic wrap in place because of the risk of suffocation.*

Purpose: Stool cannot be collected in a diaper.

6. Instruct the patient or parent/guardian to add stool to the collection container.

a. If the stool is formed, use the scoop on the lid of the container to add a large, jelly bean–sized piece of stool to the liquid in the containers (Fig. 1).

b. If the stool is liquid, pour it into the container.

c. In both of the previous cases, keep adding the specimen until the liquid preservative in the vial reaches the indicated level on the containers.

7. Instruct the patient or parent/guardian to tighten the caps completely and wipe the outside of the vials with alcohol wipes or to wash carefully with soap and water.

Purpose: To ensure infection control.

8. The vials should be labeled, placed in a biohazard bag with a zippered closure, and transported to the laboratory immediately, if possible. *The vials should not be refrigerated.*

9. Instruct the patient or parent/guardian to wash his or her hands after the specimen collection process.

Purpose: To ensure infection control.

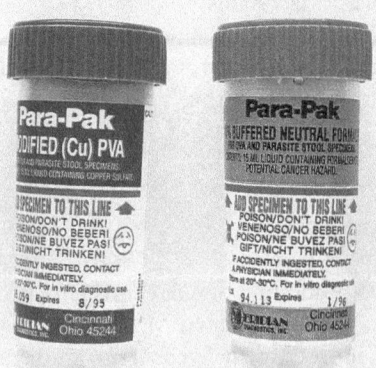

1

Courtesy Meridian Bioscience, Cincinnati, Ohio.

PROCEDURE 56.2   Collect a Nasal or Nasopharyngeal Specimen Using a Swab

Task
Collect an anterior nasal specimen, a mid-turbinate nasal specimen, or a nasopharyngeal specimen using a swab.

Equipment and Supplies
- Patient's health record
- Provider's order/or laboratory requisition
- Fluid-impermeable lab coat, mask, face shield, and gloves (or as indicated by healthcare facility)
- Collection kit or appropriate swab for test (e.g., sterile flocked or spun polyester tipped swab with a flexible shaft) and transport media tube
- Biohazard waste container

Procedural Steps
1. Wash hands or use hand sanitizer. Put on a fluid-impermeable lab coat, mask, and face shield.

   Purpose: To ensure infection control.

2. Review order and gather the supplies needed.

3. Greet the patient. Identify yourself. Verify the patient's identity with full name, then ask the patient to spell first and the last name and to state his or her date of birth.

4. Explain the procedure in a manner that the patient understands. Answer any questions the patient may have about the procedure.

   Purpose: It is important to identify the patient in two different ways to ensure that you have the correct patient. Explaining the procedure can make the patient feel more comfortable and reduces anxiety.

5. Obtain permission to perform the swab on the patient. Ask the patient if he or she has any nasal obstructions or a deviated septum. Have the patient blow his or her nose, if indicated.

   Purpose: If the patient has a nasal obstruction or a deviated septum, the opposite nostril should be used for the procedure.

6. Put on gloves.

7. Remove the sterile swab from the sterile wrap with your dominant hand.

8. Collect the specimen:

   a. For an anterior nasal swab:
   - Using the appropriate swab, insert the tip of the swab into the nostril, no more than 0. 5 inch (1 cm).
   - Slowly rotate the swab, gently pressing against the nasal wall. Rotate 4 times for a total of 15 seconds. Remove the swab and insert it into the other nostril. Repeat the process.

   Purpose: Allows for the swab to absorb the secretions.

   b. For a mid-turbinate nasal specimen:
   - Have patients tilt their head back 70 degrees.

PROCEDURE 56.2 Collect a Nasal or Nasopharyngeal Specimen Using a Swab—cont'd

Purpose: Tilting the head helps the medical assistant position the swab in the correct location.

- Using a tapered swab, rotate the swab while inserting it. Insert it less than 1 inch (2 cm) into the nostril along the nasal floor until resistance is met at the nasal turbinates. Rotate the swab for about 10 to 15 seconds. Hold in place for 5 seconds. Remove swab. Repeat process on the other nostril.

c. For a nasopharyngeal specimen:
- Have patients tilt their head back 70 degrees.

Purpose: Tilting the head helps the medical assistant position the swab in the correct location.

- Using the unobstructed nostril, insert the swab parallel to the palate until resistance is encountered. The swab should be inserted the same distance as the distance from the nose to the outer opening of the ear.

Purpose: The swab needs to be inserted far enough back to be in the correct position.

- Roll the swab gently and then leave the swab in place for several sections. Rotate the swab as it is slowly removed. If the swab is not saturated with secretions, repeat the process using the other nostril if indicated by the testing procedure. The same swab can be used.

Purpose: Leaving the swab in place allows it to absorb the nasopharyngeal secretions.

9. Place the swab in the transport medium. Snap or cut of the applicator stick if needed. Label the tube and send it to the laboratory.

Purpose: A transport medium prevents the swab from drying. Labeling immediately after collection prevents specimens from getting mixed up.

10. Dispose of contaminated supplies in the biohazard waste container. Disinfect the work area.

Purpose: To prevent the spread of infection.

11. Remove your gloves and discard them in the biohazard waste container. Remove face shield.

12. Wash hands or use hand sanitizer.

Purpose: To ensure infection control.

13. Document the procedure in the patient's health record.

Purpose: Procedures are not done until they are recorded.

Documentation Example:

8/14/20XX 8:55 a.m. Nasopharyngeal specimen collected via swab. Sent to University Laboratories for strep testing. _____ Lena Swartz, CMA (AAMA)

PROCEDURE 56.3 Collect a Specimen for a Throat Culture

Task

Collect a throat culture, using sterile technique, for immediate testing or for transportation to the laboratory.

Equipment and Supplies
- Patient's health record
- Provider's order or laboratory requisition
- Fluid-impermeable lab coat, face shield, and gloves
- Sterile swab if transporting to a reference laboratory, or sterile swab from the rapid strep test kit if testing patient in the POL
- Sterile tongue depressor
- Transport medium
- Biohazard waste container

Procedural Steps

1. Wash hands or use hand sanitizer. Put on fluid-impermeable lab coat and face shield. Put on a mask if required by the facility.
   Purpose: To ensure infection control.
2. Review order and gather the supplies needed.
3. Greet the patient. Identify yourself. Verify the patient's identity with full name, then ask the patient to spell the first and last name and to state his or her date of birth.
4. Explain the procedure in a manner that the patient understands. Answer any questions the patient may have about the procedure.
   Purpose: It is important to identify the patient in two different ways to ensure that you have the correct patient. Explaining the procedure can make the patient feel more comfortable and reduces anxiety.
5. Obtain permission to perform the throat culture on the patient.
6. Put on gloves. Position the patient so that the light shines into the mouth.
   Purpose: To ensure infection control and to illuminate the area to be swabbed.
7. Remove the sterile swab from the sterile wrap with your dominant hand, and grasp the sterile tongue depressor with your nondominant hand.
   Purpose: To achieve better control of the swabbing process.
8. Instruct the patient to open the mouth and say, "Ah." Depress the tongue with the depressor.

Purpose: Saying "Ah" helps elevate the uvula and reduces the tendency to gag. The tongue is depressed so that you can see the back of the throat and prevent contamination of the sterile swab.

9. Swab the back of the throat between the tonsillar pillars in a figure 8 pattern, especially any reddened, patchy areas of the throat, white pus pockets, purulent areas, and the tonsils; take care not to touch any other areas in the mouth (Fig. 1).

Purpose: Pathogenic organisms are found in the back of the throat and on the tonsils.

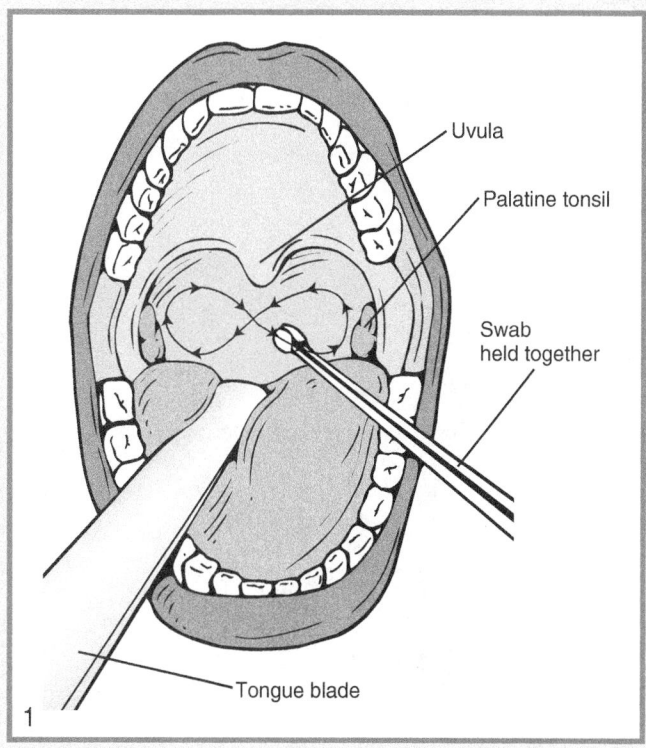

Uvula

Palatine tonsil

Swab held together

Tongue blade

1

Continued

PROCEDURE 56.3   Collect a Specimen for a Throat Culture—cont'd

10. Place the swab in the transport medium, label it, and send it to the laboratory (Fig. 2). If rapid strep testing is requested, return the labeled swab to the laboratory.

    Purpose: A transport medium prevents the swab from drying. Labeling immediately after collection prevents specimens from getting mixed up.

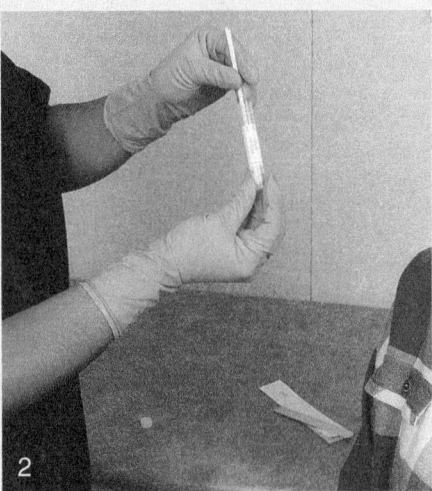

11. Dispose of contaminated supplies in the biohazard waste container. Disinfect the work area.

    Purpose: To prevent the spread of infection.

12. Remove your gloves and discard them in the biohazard waste container. Remove face shield.

13. Wash hands or use hand sanitizer.

    Purpose: To ensure infection control.

14. Document the procedure in the patient's health record.

    Purpose: Procedures are not done until they are recorded.

Documentation Example:

8/14/20XX 8:35 a.m. Throat specimen collected via swab from tonsillar area. Sent to University Laboratories for strep testing. _____

_____Lena Swartz, CMA (AAMA)

PROCEDURE 56.4   Perform a CLIA-Waived Microbiology Test: Perform a Rapid Strep Test

Task

Perform a rapid strep screening test to assist in the diagnosis of strep throat.

Equipment and Supplies

- Patient's health record
- Provider's order or lab requisition
- QuickVue In-Line Strep A test kit contents (Fig. 1):
  - One extraction solution bottle
  - One individually packaged test cassette
  - One individually wrapped sterile rayon swab, provided in the kit
  - One positive (+) control swab, provided in the kit
  - A visual flow chart outlining the steps of the test
- Rapid Strep Test Log Sheet
- Stopwatch
- Fluid-impermeable lab coat, face shield or protective eyewear, gloves
- Biohazard waste container

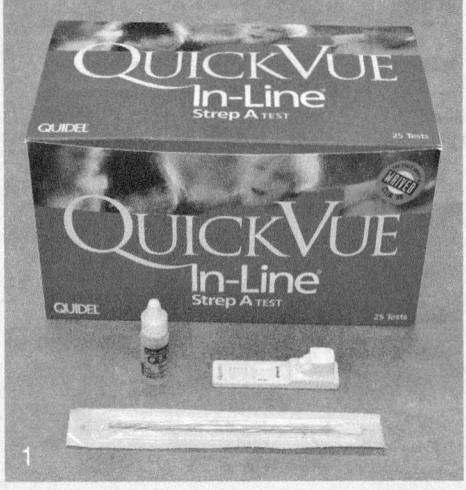

Procedural Steps

1. Wash hands or use hand sanitizer. Put on fluid-impermeable lab coat and face shield. Put on a mask if required by the facility.

   Purpose: To ensure infection control.

2. Collect all necessary supplies and equipment. Bring all reagents to room temperature. Check the expiration date on the test kit package.

   Note: Before running the first patient test from a new test kit, positive and negative controls must be run using the control swabs provided in the kit. Confirm that both controls reacted correctly and record the control results on the log sheet.

   Purpose: Both control swabs must be checked before patients are tested. If the controls show the appropriate results, the test kit is reliable.

3. Greet the patient. Identify yourself. Verify the patient's identity with full name, then ask the patient to spell the first and last name and to state his or her date of birth.

4. Explain the procedure to be performed in a manner that is understood by the patient. Answer any questions the patient may have on the procedure. Obtain permission to collect a throat culture

   Purpose: It is important to identify the patient in two different ways to ensure that you have the correct patient. Explaining the procedure can make the patient feel more comfortable and reduces anxiety.

5. Put on gloves. Collect a throat specimen using the rayon swab provided in the test kit.

   Purpose: The test kit provides a rayon swab to avoid the use of cotton swabs, which can kill bacteria, possibly causing a false-negative result.

6. Remove the test cassette from the foil pouch, and place it on a clean, dry, level surface. Using the notch at the back of the chamber as a guide, insert the patient's swab completely into the swab chamber (Fig. 2).

PROCEDURE 56.4   **Perform a CLIA-Waived Microbiology Test: Perform a Rapid Strep Test—cont'd**

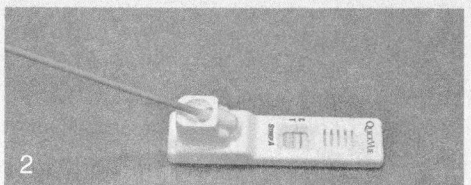

7. Place the extraction bottle between your thumb and forefinger and squeeze once to break the glass ampule inside the extraction solution bottle. Vigorously shake the bottle five times to mix the solutions. The solution should turn green.

   Purpose: The color change is an indicator of extraction reagent integrity and that the extraction procedure was performed correctly.

8. Immediately remove the cap on the extraction solution bottle, hold the bottle vertically over the chamber, and quickly fill the chamber to the rim (approximately 8 drops).

   Purpose: The liquid extract reacts with the swab and then flows into the test cassette, passing through the test area (T) and then through the internal control area (C).

9. Remove your face shield. Wait 5 minutes to read the results and record it in the lab log.

   Positive result: A pink line shows in the T area, indicating the presence of *Streptococcus pyogenes* antigen; a blue line appears in the C area, indicating that the fluid activated the internal control.

   Negative result: No pink line appears in the T test area; a blue line appears in the C control area, indicating that the internal control worked.

   Invalid result: The blue control line does not appear next to the letter C at 5 minutes. The test result cannot be reported.

10. Discard all the test materials in the appropriate biohazard waste container. Disinfect the work area.

    Purpose: Items that come in contact with samples are considered potentially infectious.

11. Remove your gloves. Wash hands or use hand sanitizer.

    Purpose: To ensure infection control.

12. Record the test results in the patient's health record.

    Purpose: A procedure is not done until the results are properly recorded.

13. If the test results are negative, a second throat swab should be obtained and sent to the reference laboratory for a throat culture. Often two swabs are used simultaneously when the sample is initially collected from the throat to prevent the need to re-collect a specimen.

    Purpose: Negative rapid strep test results should be confirmed with a throat culture.

Qualitative Control/Patient Log Sheet

TEST: ____STREP A TEST____

KIT NAME AND MANUFACTURER: QuickVue In-Line Strep A Test – Quidel

LOT # ___12356___ EXPIRATION DATE: ____11/22/20XX____

STORAGE REQUIREMENTS: _Room Temp_ TEST FLOWCHART __yes__

Date	Specimen I.D. (Control/ Patient)	Result (+ or –)	Internal Control Passed (Y or N)	Charted in Patient Record	Tech Initials
7/11/20XX	POSITIVE CONTROL	+	Y		LP
7/11/20XX	NEGATIVE CONTROL	–	Y		LP
7/11/20XX	PT ID: 5432	+	Y	✓	LP

Documentation Example:

10/9/20XX 9:30 a.m. Rapid Strep A Test performed with a positive result.
————————————————Lena Swartz, CMA (AAMA)

PROCEDURE 56.5   **Perform a CLIA-Waived Immunology Test: Perform a QuickVue+ Infectious Mononucleosis Test**

Tasks

Perform a capillary puncture. To perform and interpret a rapid CLIA-waived test for infectious mononucleosis.

Equipment and Supplies

- Patient's health record
- Provider's order and/or lab requisition
- CLIA-waived QuickVue+ test kit for infectious mononucleosis and blood collecting supplies (Fig. 1):
  - Package with supplies for 20 tests
  - Color-coded bottles of positive and negative controls and the developer
  - Test cassette in its foil-wrapped protective pouch
  - Alcohol wipes, gauze, and bandage
  - Pipets supplied in kit with black line indicating the amount of capillary blood to collect
  - Lancet
- Timer or wristwatch with sweep second hand
- Fluid-impermeable lab coat, protective eyewear, gloves
- Biohazard waste container

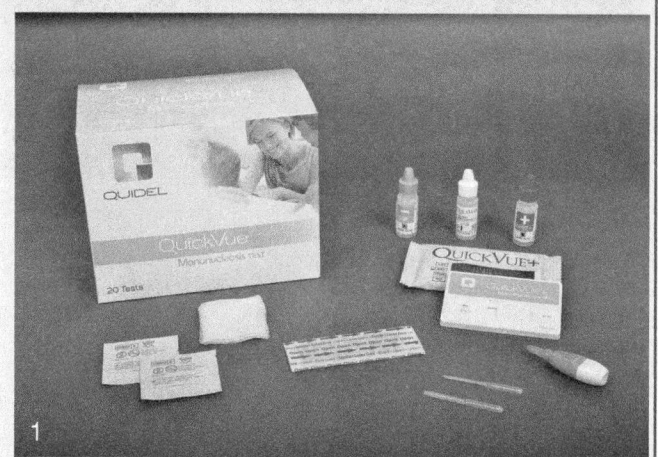

Continued

PROCEDURE 56.5 Perform a CLIA-Waived Immunology Test: Perform a QuickVue+ Infectious Mononucleosis Test—cont'd

Procedural Steps

1. Wash hands or use hand sanitizer. Put on the fluid-impermeable lab coat.
   Purpose: To ensure infection control.
2. Remove the test kit from the refrigerator and allow the reagents to warm to room temperature. Check the expiration date of the kit.
   Purpose: Outdated or cold reagents do not react as expected.
3. Before running the first patient test from a new test kit, run the positive and negative liquid controls provided in the kit to see whether they react correctly. Record your control results on the log sheet.
   Purpose: Both control samples must be checked before patients are tested. If the controls show the appropriate results, the test kit is reliable.
4. Greet the patient. Identify yourself. Verify the patient's identity with full name, then ask the patient to spell the first and last name and to state his or her date of birth.
5. Explain the procedure in a manner that the patient understands. Answer any questions the patient may have about the procedure.
6. Obtain permission for the capillary puncture.
   Purpose: It is important to identify the patient in two different ways to ensure that you have the correct patient. Explaining the procedure can make the patient feel more comfortable and reduces anxiety.
7. Put on gloves and protective eyewear. Remove the test device from its protective pouch, and label it with the patient's identification.
   Purpose: To ensure infection control. Label the test kit to ensure proper identity of the test being run.
8. Disinfect the patient's finger with an alcohol wipe. Allow it to dry, and then perform a capillary puncture.
9. Wipe away the first drop of blood, and then fill the disposable pipet provided in the kit to the calibration mark with capillary blood (Fig. 2).
   Purpose: The plastic capillary tube measures the exact amount of sample, for accurate testing.

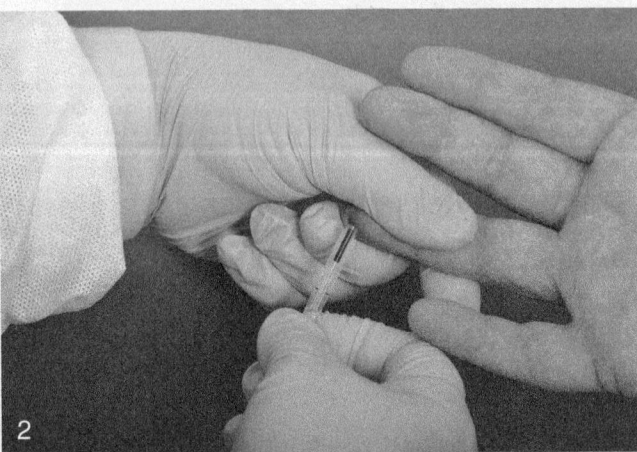

2

10. Dispense all the blood from the capillary tube into the "Add" well of the testing device. (Or, if you are using venous blood, transfer a large drop from the venous whole blood specimen using the longer capillary pipet provided in the kit.)
11. Hold the developer bottle vertically above the "Add" well, and allow 5 drops to fall freely.
    Purpose: Holding a dropper vertically ensures delivery of the same-size drop. If the dropper touches other materials, it becomes contaminated and the results will be inaccurate.

12. Read the results at 5 minutes. Note: The "Test Complete" box must be visibly colored by 10 minutes.
    Positive result: A vertical line in any shade of blue forms a plus sign in the "Read Result" window, along with a blue "Test Complete" line. Even a faint blue plus sign should be reported as a positive.
    Negative result: No vertical blue line appears, leaving a minus sign in the "Read Result" window, along with a blue "Test Complete" line.
    Invalid result: After 10 minutes, no line is visible in the "Test Complete" window, or a blue color fills the "Read Result" window. If either of these occurs, the test must be repeated with a new testing device. If the problem continues, request technical support.
13. Properly dispose of biohazardous waste material in the proper container, and disinfect the work area.
    Purpose: To ensure infection control.
14. Remove your gloves and protective eyewear. Wash hands or use hand sanitizer.
15. Document the patient's result and the control sample results in the lab logs and in the patient's health record.
    Purpose: A procedure is not done until the results are properly recorded.

Quality Control Procedures

External positive and negative liquid controls are provided with each new kit. Each new operator of the test should perform liquid positive and negative external controls once to confirm that his or her testing technique is correct. Also, external controls should be tested and charted when a new kit is used.

The *internal* control occurs in the "Test Complete" window built into each reaction unit. Chart the control results on the control log with the operator's initials.

Qualitative Control/Patient Log Sheet

TEST: ____MONONUCLEOSIS RAPID TEST_____
KIT NAME & MANUFACTURER: QUICK VUE+ Infectious Mononucleosis Test –QUIDEL
LOT # __12356_____ EXPIRATION DATE: ____11/22/20XX_____
STORAGE REQUIREMENTS: _REFRIGERATOR___ TEST FLOWCHART ___yes_____

Date	Specimen I.D. (Control/ Patient)	Result (+ or −)	Internal Control Passed (Y or N)	Charted in Patient Record	Tech Initials
7/11/20XX	POSITIVE CONTROL	+	Y		LP
7/11/20XX	NEGATIVE CONTROL	−	Y		LP
7/11/20XX	PT ID: 5432	−	Y	✓	LP

Documentation Example:

10/9/20XX 9:30 a.m. Mononucleosis rapid test performed with a negative result. Lavender-topped (EDTA) blood sample sent to lab for CBC and differential. ____
_____Lena Swartz, CMA (AAMA)

PROCEDURE 56.6   Coach Patient on Guaiac Fecal Occult Blood Test

Tasks

Coach a patient on the guaiac fecal occult blood test (gFOBT), while considering the patient's developmental life stage. Document the coaching in the health record.

Background

When coaching patients, it is important to consider their developmental life stage. When working with older adults, it is important to communicate with dignity and respect. Use simpler language. Speak clearly and allow time for the patient to respond. It is important to find out what patients know about the topic and respectfully correct any inaccuracies. Make sure to listen to their concerns and provide resources as needed.

Scenario

You work at WMFM Clinic. You are working with Dr. David Kahn, who asked you to coach Charles Johnson (date of birth [DOB] 03/03/19XX) on the gFOBT. He is to receive three Hemoccult cards for stool smears.

Directions

Role-play the scenario with a peer, who is the patient. Your instructor is the provider.

Equipment and Supplies

- Hemoccult test kit (Hemoccult cards, applicator sticks, and if available flushable collection tissue)
- Patient instructions
- Patient's health record
- Pen

Procedural Steps

1. Wash hands or use hand sanitizer.
   Purpose: Hand sanitization is an important step for infection control.
2. Greet the patient. Identify yourself. Verify the patient's identity with full name and date of birth. Explain what you will be doing.
   Purpose: It is important to identify the patient in two different ways to ensure that you have the correct patient. Explaining the procedure can make the patient feel more comfortable and reduces anxiety.

3. Use simpler language when talking. Speak clearly. Communicate with dignity and respect. Allow time for the patient to respond. Listen to the patient's concerns.
   Purpose: When working with older patients, it is important to treat them with respect and dignity. Listening is important.
4. Ask the patient if he has ever taken a guaiac fecal occult blood test. If so, ask him what he remembers about it.
   Purpose: It is important to find out what the patient already knows about the topic.
5. Discuss the purpose of the test and the supplies needed (e.g., Hemoccult cards, applicator kits, and, if available, flushable collection tissue). Show the supplies to the patient.
   Purpose: It is important that the patient knows what supplies will be used.
6. Discuss how the patient needs to prepare for the tests, and refer to the written instructions.
   Purpose: Referring to the written directions that will be sent home with the patient helps eliminate confusion.
7. Discuss how the patient should collect and return the Hemoccult cards. Use the written directions when coaching the patient. Write the patient's name, date of birth, and address on the Hemoccult cards if required by the agency.
   Purpose: The cards need to be labeled with the patient's information. Having the medical assistant label the cards ensures this step is completed.
8. Ask the patient to teach back the preparation and the collection to you. Clarify any misconceptions or inaccuracies. Answer any questions the patient may have.
   Purpose: Using the "teach back" method to evaluate the patient's understanding will help identify any misunderstandings the patient may have.
9. Document the coaching in the patient's health record. Include the provider's name, what was taught, and how the patient responded, and indicate the supplies and written directions sent home with the patient.
   Purpose: It is important to document the procedure in the health record to show it was done.

Documentation Example:

08/14/20XX 1105 Per Dr. Kahn's order, instructed patient on the gFOBT test including the preparation and collection. Patient taught back the instructions accurately. Gave the patient the Hemoccult testing kit and the Hemoccult Patient Directions booklet. Patient will return the cards to the clinic later this week.
_____Lena Swartz, CMA (AAMA)

PROCEDURE 56.7   Develop a Hemoccult Card and Perform Quality Control

Tasks

Develop a stool specimen using a Hemoccult card, and perform a quality control test. Document the test results in the patient's health record.

Scenario

Charles Johnson (date of birth [DOB] 03/03/19XX) returns his Hemoccult card(s). Dr. David Kahn is his provider. You need to develop (test) the sample.

Equipment and Supplies

- Hemoccult card with stool smear applied
- Hemoccult developer
- Gloves
- Biohazard waste container
- Waste container
- Patient's health record
- Timer

Procedural Steps

1. Wash hands or use hand sanitizer. Put on gloves.
   Purpose: Hand sanitization is an important step for infection control.
2. Identify when the specimen was applied and if testing can be done.
   Purpose: The company recommends a wait time of 3 days from when the sample was applied. This allows for the degradation of fruit and vegetable peroxidases from the sample. If immediate testing is required, wait 3 to 5 minutes to allow the sample to penetrate the test paper.
3. Open the back of the card and apply 2 drops of the Hemoccult developer to the guaiac paper directly over each smear.
4. Within 60 seconds, read the result accurately.
   Purpose: Any trace of blue on or near the edge of the sample is considered positive for occult blood.
5. Perform quality control on the card by applying 1 drop of the Hemoccult developer between the positive and negative Performance Monitors area.
   Purpose: This quality control test will indicate if the card and developer are functional.
6. Within 10 seconds, accurately read the results.
   Purpose: A blue color in the positive Performance Monitors area and no blue in the negative Performance Monitors area means the card and the developer are functional.
7. Discard the Hemoccult card in the biohazard bag. Clean up the area. Remove gloves and discard in the waste container.
   Purpose: It is important to discard the Hemoccult card in the biohazard bag for infection control.
8. Wash hands or use hand sanitizer.
9. Document the test result and the provider notified in the patient's health record.
   Purpose: It is important to document the procedure in the health record to show it was done.

Documentation Example:

08/18/20XX 1105 Hemoccult card × 3 developed. All results were negative. Dr. Kahn notified. _____ Lena Swartz, CMA (AAMA)

57

Career Development

LEARNING OBJECTIVES

1. Describe personality traits important to employers.
2. Discuss personality traits, technical skills, and transferable job skills.
3. Describe how to develop a career objective and identify your personal needs.
4. Explain job search methods.
5. Create a resume and cover letter.
6. Complete an online profile and job application.
7. Describe how to create a career portfolio.
8. Practice interview skills during a mock interview.
9. List legal and illegal interview questions.
10. Create a thank-you note for an interview.
11. Explain common human resource hiring requirements for those starting a new job.

OUTLINE

OPENING SCENARIO

Michelle, Krysia, and Zacarias (or "Zac" to his friends) met during their first semester of college. They have developed a great friendship over the past few months. They will be graduating from the medical assistant program in less than 6 weeks. Michelle just graduated from high school a year ago. Krysia entered the military just after her high school graduation. She spent 10 years in the Marines. Zac has been out of high school for several years and worked in a factory. He started as a line worker and gradually advanced to supervisory positions. Due to downsizing, his position was eliminated. He went back to school. These friends are looking forward to graduation and getting jobs as medical assistants.

As these three friends discuss finding a job, Michelle is hesitant about the job search experience. Her only work experience is 2 years as a waitress at a local restaurant. She has never created a resume or a cover letter. She had only an informal interview with the restaurant owner before she was given the job. Krysia is concerned about her military career. The positions she held were not related to healthcare. She managed inventory and supervised others. She was also deployed to many hot spots around the world. Zac has a lot of experience in the factory setting, but he feels that that world is so different from healthcare. As they talk with each other, it is clear that each person has a unique situation, and they all must take a closer look at their past experiences as they prepare for their job search adventure.

YOU WILL LEARN

1. The personality traits important to employers.
2. The best job search methods.
3. To develop a resume and cover letter.
4. To complete a job application.
5. How to prepare for an interview.

INTRODUCTION

As you move toward graduation, you may be experiencing many emotions. You might be excited about finishing your medical assistant program. You might be scared of the future changes. The thought of finding a job might be overwhelming. These are common feelings of all graduates. The important step before graduation is to prepare for the next phase: getting a job.

Preparing for the job-seeking phase is very important. This chapter will help you to:
- Understand the characteristics that employers want
- Identify your strengths, experiences, and skills
- Develop your career objectives

When you have done these things, you are ready to market yourself to potential employers. You will market yourself through your resume and interview experiences. Remember that an early job search, even before graduation, can be the key to landing a job soon after graduation.

UNDERSTANDING PERSONALITY TRAITS IMPORTANT TO EMPLOYERS

It is important to understand what employers are looking for in employees. Employers spend money and time training new employees. It is critical that they initially find the right employees. Many employers will agree that they can help refine technical skill proficiencies. It is more difficult to help grow or change personality traits. We will examine the five personality traits that are most important to employers. These include collaboration, interpersonal skills, professionalism, compassion, and a sincere interest in the job.

Collaboration and Interpersonal Skills

Collaboration (kuh lab uh RAY shun) and interpersonal skills are crucial to the efficiency of the healthcare environment. Employers look for people who can blend well with the current staff. New employees need to be flexible, dependable, supportive of peers, and remain calm under pressure. Employers want employees who will provide excellent customer service by having outstanding interpersonal skills, including:

- *Effective verbal communication*: Involves using clear, thoughtful, and easily understood language.
- *Professional nonverbal communication*: Relays more information to patients and peers than any words you could use. Eye contact, posture, voice, and gestures provide insights into a person's attitude. Being focused, calm, polite, and interested in the other person are traits of effective nonverbal communication.
- *Good listening skills*: Critical when working with peers and patients. For effective communication to occur, listening must occur. Appropriate questions can draw others into the conversation and show others you are listening and care. Communication techniques such as reflecting, paraphrasing, summarizing, and asking for clarification are also excellent ways of demonstrating active listening skills.
- *Good manners*: Are essential, along with a basic understanding of the diversity of your patient population.

> **VOCABULARY**
> **clarification** Allows the listener to get additional information by explaining a specific statement or topic.
> **collaboration** The act of working with another or other individuals.
> **interpersonal skills** The ability to communicate and interact with others; sometimes referred to as "soft skills."
> **paraphrasing** Rewording a statement to check the meaning and interpretation; also shows you are listening to and understanding the speaker.
> **reflecting** Putting words to the patient's emotional reaction, which acknowledges the person's feelings.
> **summarizing** Allowing the listener to recap and review what was said.

Professionalism

A person's professionalism is being evaluated from the cover letter to the interview and beyond. Employers are looking for employees

<table><tr><td>

BOX 57.1   Dignity and Respect Example

Imagine being a patient in your 70s. You have a walker. You spent 4 months in a wheelchair recovering from a stroke. You are proud to be walking today, even if you are slow. You know that walking is important, so that you do not get stiff and then cannot walk.

The medical assistant calls you in for the visit. You slowly walk to her and then she takes you down the hall. She is far ahead of you as you slowly make your way. It appears the room is at the end of the long hall. You hear the medical assistant calling to a peer to get a wheelchair. She looks back at you and states, "We have a wheelchair for you to speed things up." How do you feel? Do you feel that she values you? Is she showing you respect?

If you reverse the roles, how could you, as a medical assistant, show that you respect and value the patient?

</td></tr></table>

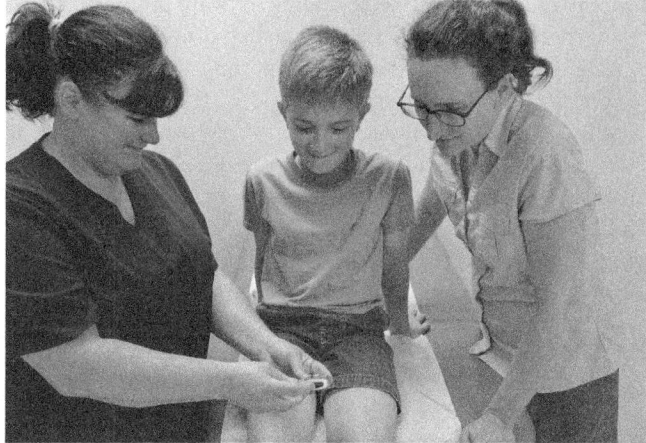

Fig. 57.1 Enjoyment of the job is paramount. Medical assistants should enjoy their work and give compassionate, friendly care to all patients. (From Niedzwiecki B, et al: *Kinn's the medical assistant*, ed 14, St. Louis, 2020, Elsevier.)

who project a professional image in all situations. Professionalism includes a person's appearance (i.e., dress and grooming habits) and behaviors. The behaviors include a person's flexibility, punctuality, honesty, attention to detail, time management skills, ability to following directions, and ability to prioritize.

Compassion

Compassion is another trait employers look for. *Compassion* means to have a deep awareness of another's suffering and the desire to lessen it. Dignity and respect are part of providing compassionate care to others (Box 57.1). Many people go into healthcare to help others. They may like the technical skills involved with patient care. Providing dignity and respect during patient care is just as important. Compassion and respect help healthcare employees connect to patients and their families. Patients welcome acts of kindness and thoughtfulness that lessen stress.

> **VOCABULARY**
> **dignity** The inherent worth or state of being worthy of respect.

Genuine Interest

Employers also look for people genuinely interested in the job. This trait can be seen during the interview. Does the person ask thoughtful questions regarding the position and the facility? Genuine interest in the job extends beyond the hiring phase into day-to-day operations. Being interested in one's job is critical. Looking for ways to improve procedures and provide better patient care is an important behavior to demonstrate to the employer. This genuine interest is reflected in your attitude and performance in the workplace (Fig. 57.1). It helps ease your transition into a new job and promotes your success.

ASSESSING YOUR STRENGTHS AND SKILLS

As you prepare to market yourself to potential employers, you need to examine your strengths and skills in three different areas. What personality traits do you possess? What technical skills are your strengths? What transferable job skills do you possess?

Personality Traits

In addition to the typical personality traits required by employers, the job posting may list extra traits, including personality traits. Which of these skills and strengths do you possess? Many people will tell potential employers what they think employers want to hear. They claim to be "a team player," to "communicate well," to be "dependable," and so on. Listing these phrases on your resume or during the interview is not enough to convince the potential employer that you truly have those characteristics. They like "supporting evidence"!

Early on in the preparation phase, make a list of the qualities that you believe you possess. For each quality provide one or two pieces of "evidence" to support your claims. Your "evidence" may be a past job review or the evaluation from your student clinical experience (e.g., practicum, internship, apprenticeship, or externship). The review or evaluation may indicate your strengths and characteristics. These are excellent documents to include in your portfolio, which will be discussed later in the chapter. Using stories of situations in which you portrayed those characteristics is another way to illustrate your qualities. It is important to share these during the interview, if pertinent to the questions asked.

<table><tr><td>

CRITICAL THINKING 57.1

Think of the three friends in the scenario. Michelle just graduated from high school and has 2 years of waitressing experience. Krysia has 10 years in the military, where she managed inventory, supervised others, and was deployed to many hot spots around the world. Zac has been working in a factory, advancing to supervisory positions. Now think about the personality traits that employers want. What personality traits might each friend possess? Explain your answer.

- Create your own list of the personality traits that employers want, and you possess.

</td></tr></table>

Technical Skills

Employers are also interested in your technical skills. Technical skills for medical assistants can be related to clinical procedures, such as phlebotomy, injections, electrocardiograms (ECGs), and obtaining vital signs. Technical skills can also be related to administrative procedures, including software proficiency, keyboard speed, reception duties, and coding procedures.

You may be able to provide supporting documentation of your technical skills through the use of the student clinical experience skill checklists or through a portfolio. Technical skills might also include skills that you developed outside the medical assistant program but that still relate to your chosen career. For instance, if you worked as a pharmacy technician at a local hospital, several of the technical skills you acquired may relate to a clinic position.

Transferable Job Skills

Transferable job skills are the last area to examine. A person develops these skills in one job or experience. The skills can be "transferred" to another job. This means the person will use these skills in other jobs. Many of these skills may sound familiar. They are also characteristics employers are looking for. Potential transferable skills include:

- Customer service
- Compassion and empathy
- Strong communication and listening skills
- Computer skills
- Leadership skills
- Organizational skills
- Teamwork
- Time management and prioritizing skills
- Creativity
- Grace under pressure
- Problem-solving skills

Identifying transferable job skills can be difficult for many people. Job descriptions for past experiences can be useful. To start, make a list of your past jobs, military experience, and volunteer opportunities. Make a list of potential transferable skills you developed and used for each experience. Here are some examples of transferable skills for different jobs and situations:

- Wait staff jobs: Strong communication and listening skills, prioritizing, and customer service skills
- Factory jobs: Communication skills, teamwork, and problem solving
- Military experience: Strong communication skills, grace under pressure, and prioritizing
- Stay-at-home parent: Organization, prioritizing, budgeting, time management, and problem solving

This list of transferable job skills will be used as you create your resume and prepare for your interview.

CRITICAL THINKING 57.2

What might be some transferable skills that the three friends, Michelle, Krysia, and Zac, possess? Explain your answer.
- Using the list you have already started, add on the personality traits, technical skills, and transferable job skills that you possess. Also, indicate why you believe you have these skills (e.g., which job or experience helped you develop the skill).

DEVELOPING CAREER OBJECTIVES

Each medical assistant has a reason for entering the healthcare field. This basic desire should influence decisions concerning his or her career choices. Because medical assisting is such a versatile profession, a medical assistant has numerous options after graduation.

Medical assistant students should take some time to think about what they want from their careers. While the medical assistant is attending school and subsequently completing the student clinical experience, ideas may surface about the area of healthcare or a specific facility in which she or he most wants to work.

When developing career objectives, the medical assistant should start by asking several questions:
- What areas and skills did I enjoy in the student clinical experience?
- Where do I want to be in 5 years?
- Where do I want to be in 10 years?
- What additional skills do I need to get where I want to go?

Write down the questions and answers and go into specific detail. Set realistic goals and develop a plan as to how and when they will be reached. Remember, career objectives are reached over time. It is important to know where you want to be, so you can start down the right path to reach your goals. Keep your list of goals available and visible so you can revisit it frequently.

CRITICAL THINKING 57.3

For the following four questions, write down your answers and explain them. These answers will help you as you start the job search process.
- What areas and skills did I enjoy in the student clinical experience?
- Where do I want to be in 5 years?
- Where do I want to be in 10 years?
- What additional skills do I need to get where I want to go?

IDENTIFYING PERSONAL NEEDS

The next step in the process is to identify personal needs. What do you need in a job? Do you need a specific wage to meet your living expenses? What benefits do you need? What hours do you need to work? Some people need to consider day care and school hours for their children. How far are you willing to travel for a job? Do you have a reliable mode of transportation? Evaluating your personal needs will help you find a job that matches your requirements.

CRITICAL THINKING 57.4

What are your personal needs? Make a list identifying your needs that must be considered when seeking a new position.

FINDING A JOB

Finding employment and staying employed in healthcare are typically not difficult. Usually healthcare employment needs remain high, even in a poor economy. However, graduation from a medical assisting program does not guarantee employment. Completion of the program gives the medical assistant the job skills needed to work. A good attitude and positive outlook are essential for success in the job search. The medical assistant should always be open to new and better opportunities.

Depending on the location, some job seekers assume that potential employers will not interact with students until they have passed a credential examination. Common credential examinations for medical assistants include:

- Certified Medical Assistant (CMA) through the American Association of Medical Assistants (AAMA)
- Registered Medical Assistant (RMA) through the American Medical Technologists (AMT)
- Certified Clinical Medical Assistant (CCMA) through the National Healthcareer Association (NHA)
- National Certified Medical Assistant (NCMA) through the National Center for Competency Testing (NCCT)
- Clinical Medical Assistant Certification (CMAC) through the American Medical Certification Association (AMCA)

Searching for a job before graduation is a smart idea. Some employers do not require credentialing examinations. Others may hire a medical assistant before the exam is taken. They may have an agreement that the medical assistant obtain the credential within a specified period of time. Many employers are interested in hiring new graduates. They consider new graduates "teachable." This means they can train and "mold" them into the employee they require. Employers recognize that new graduates have more current knowledge and skills.

Two Best Job Search Methods

There are many ways to find employment. Networking and checking job boards are the best and most effective methods.

> **VOCABULARY**
> **job boards** Websites where employers post jobs; job seekers can use them to identify open positions.

Networking. *Networking* is the exchange of information among others in your field. For medical assistant graduates or students searching for a job, networking involves meeting individuals in healthcare. It also involves sharing information on available opportunities. Through the medical assistant program, a student forms a network of friends and acquaintances (Fig. 57.2). Staying in contact with these people allows for networking opportunities. Email, LinkedIn, Facebook, Twitter, and other social networking advances make staying in touch easy.

The student clinical experience gives medical assistant students opportunities to network. During the experience, you will be working with many healthcare professionals. It is crucial that you look at the clinical experience as a continuous job interview (Box 57.2). It is important to be professional, follow the

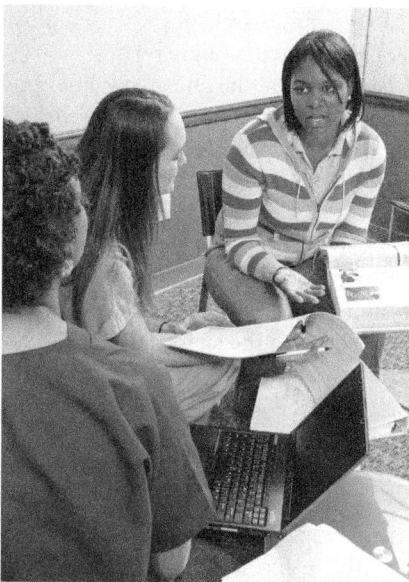

Fig. 57.2 Stay in Touch with Classmates. They are excellent networking contacts and may be able to provide job leads. (From Niedzwiecki B, et al: *Kinn's the medical assistant*, ed 14, St. Louis, 2020, Elsevier.)

> **BOX 57.2   Strategies Medical Assistants Can Use in the Clinical Experience to Assist With Job Seeking**
>
> During the student clinical experience, medical assistant students can:
> - Inquire about potential job openings, either through their mentor, supervisor, or the facility's human resource department.
> - Ask their mentors if they would be willing to provide a reference or a letter of recommendation.
> - Show their gratitude by formally thanking their mentors for the opportunity. In most cases, the clinical agencies provide assistance to help train the medical assistant student. It is important to send a thank-you note to the mentor, the supervisor, and to the department.
> - Provide the supervisor with a resume and cover letter.

guidelines, and strive to do your very best. It is not uncommon that when staff members find a student who portrays the characteristics of a professional medical assistant, they are willing to help the student find a job.

Another networking technique is to join a medical assistant organization. The members who attend regular meetings often know about job leads in the area. Creating connections with currently employed medical assistants can be helpful in the job search process.

> **CRITICAL THINKING 57.5**
>
> Michelle, Krysia, and Zac know that networking is a great way to find employment. They make a list of people with whom they can share their resume or whom they can inform that they are now ready to seek employment as a medical assistant.
> - Who among your relatives would be good prospects for networking?
> - Who among your professional contacts would be good prospects for networking?

Job Boards. Job boards are websites where employers post job openings. There are two types of job boards:

- *Facility job boards*: Larger healthcare facilities post job openings on their websites. The employment website can use different tools that make the process easier for the job seeker and the employer. Some sites allow the job seeker to register for a specific type of job. The software will generate emails to job seekers when new jobs are posted. Some websites allow job seekers to complete online profiles or applications and upload a resume and cover letter. These tools are useful to both the job seeker and the facility.
- *Public job boards*: These job boards include jobs from a variety of employers. The job boards can be local, state, or national. Local job boards may be found through your school or your community's media (i.e., newspaper, television, radio) agencies. These websites target the local audience. They are usually cheaper for employers. Smaller healthcare organizations tend to advertise using these boards. The Department of Workforce Development in each state addresses unemployment. It provides a job board for job seekers. National job boards provide job seekers the ability to search for openings across the country. Examples include:
  - https://www.monster.com/
  - https://www.indeed.com/
  - https://www.alliedhealthjobcafe.com/
  - https://www.glassdoor.com/index.htm
  - https://www.usajobs.gov/ (federal government jobs)

Many positions for medical assistants use alternative job titles. Some agencies may use "technician" or "coordinator" for medical assistant jobs. It is important to research the local job titles that are used for medical assistants. If you do not know the local job title, try looking at the allied health positions. Look at a job posting. What are the educational requirements? Are the duties skills you have? Make a list of job titles related to medical assisting, and search by those as you identify potential openings.

CRITICAL THINKING 57.6

Michelle, Krysia, and Zac make a list of possible job boards to review frequently for medical assistant postings. They know that sometimes the postings are only available for a short time, so they develop a schedule to review the sites.

- Make a list of five job boards you would like to check for potential jobs.
- What other titles are used for medical assistants in your area?

Additional Job Search Methods

Besides using networking and checking job boards, the medical assistant can find job postings by other, more traditional methods. The school's placement office resources, newspaper ads (online and print), and employment agencies also can have medical assistant job postings.

School Career Placement Offices. Students usually have lifetime access to their school placement offices. Students and graduates should take advantage of the opportunities offered.

Many schools offer resume building, job search classes, and interviewing assistance. School placement offices may also work with local employers to advertise their openings online to graduates. The school has a vested interest in helping you find employment. The placement office should be the first resource for the student's job search.

Newspaper Ads. Smaller healthcare facilities usually use newspaper ads to find potential employees. Many newspaper companies post their ads online. This allows more job seekers to view those positions.

Employment Agencies. Employment agencies hire staff to fill in at healthcare facilities. The facility pays the employment agency to staff different positions. Some employment agencies hire and pay the medical assistant. The medical assistants work in a healthcare facility as employment agency employees. After a period of time, if the medical assistant proves to be a good employee, the healthcare facility then hires that person. This allows the employment agency to do the hiring, firing, and managing of employees until the employees "prove themselves" to the healthcare facility.

Being Organized in Your Job Search

As you submit your resume and cover letter for various positions, it is important that you stay organized and track the jobs you applied for. You should also keep the original electronic files of your customized documents.

Create a handwritten or an electronic log of the jobs you apply for. Include the job title, number, and facility name. When you submit your resume and cover letter, update the log with the date of those activities. As you are notified about an interview, add the interview information (e.g., date, time, location, interview team members) to your log. Continually update the status of each job in the log.

It is important for you to save the customized documents for each job position. If you are called for an interview, it is important to bring copies of your customized resume and cover letter. The easiest method is to create a job-seeking folder on your computer. For each job you apply for, create a subfolder in the job-seeking folder. Save your customized resume and cover letter in the subfolder. Save any other documents related to that job in that subfolder, including the job posting. If you get called for an interview, print the customized resume and cover letter for your interview portfolio and for the interviewer(s). You may also want to print the job posting as a reference during the interview.

One of the most important things to remember with job searching is that it takes time, stamina, and persistence to find a job. Do not expect to get a job with the first resume and cover letter you send or with the first interview you have. By keeping good records, you will not apply for the same job twice or overlook job opportunities because you thought you had applied for them already.

DEVELOPING A RESUME

The purpose of a resume is to "market" yourself. You want an employer interested in you. You want your resume to be

Michelle Marison

1234 Cedar Way, Mytown, OH 45458
Home phone: 715.555.1899
Cell phone: 715.555.1355
mmarison@elsevier.net

Education
Community College, Mytown, OH
Medical Assistant Diploma, 20XX
- GPA 3.6

Healthcare Experience
Family Practice Associates, Mytown, OH
Medical Assistant Practicum, April 20XX to May 20XX (220 hours)
- Performed injections, electrocardiogram, wound care, phlebotomy, throat swabs, and waived tests.
- Obtained vital signs and measurements on children and adults.
- Utilized an electronic health record to document patients' histories, test results, and treatments.
- Answered calls, checked-in patients, and updated patients' demographic and insurance information.

Mytown Hospital, Mytown, OH
Volunteer, January 20XX to May 20XX
- Provided hospital information to visitors.
- Maintained confidentiality of patients.
- Assisted with deliveries of mail and flowers to patients.
- Assisted nursing staff as needed.

Work Experience
Mytown Family Diner, Mytown, OH
Waitress, June 20XX to present
- Provide efficient, accurate, and timely service to customers.
- Prioritize duties to meet customer needs.
- Provide exceptional customer service.

Special Skills
Fluent in Spanish.
Keyboarding speed: 73 wpm
Proficient in word processing and spreadsheet software

Credentials
Certified Medical Assistant, American Association of Medical Assistants (expires May 20XX)
BLS for Healthcare Providers, American Heart Association (expires March 20XX)

Fig. 57.3 Chronologic Resume.

Zacarias Garcia
523 River Way, Mytown OH 45459

Cell phone: 715.555.5472
ZacGarcia@elsevier.net

Education
Community College, Mytown, OH
Medical Assistant Diploma, 20XX
- Medical Assistant Practicum at Mytown Orthopedic and Massage Center, Mytown, OH
  o Obtained and charted history and vital signs in electronic health record.
  o Assisted providers with tests and treatments.

Credentials
Certified Medical Assistant, American Association of Medical Assistants, expires May 20XX.
BLS for Healthcare Providers, American Heart Association, expires March 20XX.

Skills and Achievement
Strong communication skills
- Supervised 60 employees in a factory setting for over 3 years.
- Initiated procedures to improve communication between employees and management.
- Promoted in union to assist with negotiations with upper management.
- Fluent in Spanish.
Excellent problem-solving skills
- Problem-solved factory issues that delayed shipments to customers.
- Initiated solutions to expedite shipments and increased the profit margin of the company.
Excel in Teamwork
- Assisted team on assembly line, helping fill in when others were absent.
- Promoted to Team Lead within 6 months of hire.
- Received "Outstanding Employee" award in 20XX, 20XX, and 20XX.

Work Experience
Mytown Doors, Mytown, OH
Supervisor, (March 20XX – January 20XX)
Team Lead – Door Assembly, (January 20XX – March 20XX)
Door Assembler, (August 20XX – January 20XX)

Fig. 57.4 Combination Resume.

included in those selected for an interview. A resume summarizes your qualifications, education, and experience. Medical assistants must determine what to include in the resume. The resume should be developed before the cover letter is written. Strengths for the posted job must be identified and emphasized on all documents. These documents include the resume, cover letter, and application.

Resume Formats

There are three commonly used resume formats: chronologic, combination, and targeted resumes. The resume format used will depend on the medical assistant's situation.

A *chronologic resume* is the most popular format used. It is useful when people are seeking employment in the same field as the one in which they have their education or previous experience. The chronologic resume focuses on the person's employment history. Job duties for each position are bulleted out (Fig. 57.3). See Procedure 57.1 for the steps in creating a chronologic resume.

The *combination resume* is sometimes called a hybrid resume. A combination resume lists a person's abilities and skill sets, along with listing the employment history. A combination resume may be used:

- If a person is switching careers.
- By new medical assistants, so they can indicate the skills they practiced during their student clinical experience, such as vital signs, injections, and obtaining patient information.

- By applicants who have a gap in their work history.

If using a combination resume, the person should also emphasize the transferable skills that related to the new position. The focus is on the person's skills and ability, rather than the employment history (Fig. 57.4).

The third type of resume is the *targeted resume*. This type of resume is customized to a unique job posting (Fig. 57.5). A targeted resume:

- Detail key skills required for the position
- Indicate how the applicant has demonstrated those skills
- Take longer to create, but can be the most effective format

CRITICAL THINKING 57.7

The three friends have very different backgrounds. Michelle has the waitressing experience, Krysia was in the military, and Zac worked in a factory. What type of resume might each use? Explain your answers.
- What type of resume would work best for you with your experience and background?

Resume Content

Between the resume formats, there are similarities and differences in the information presented. The following discussion describes the content found in the different sections of a resume. See Procedure 57.1 for the steps in creating a chronologic resume.

Krysia Debski

111 Mall Drive • Mytown, OH 45457
Cell phone: 715.555.6956 • Email: KDebski@elsevier.net

Education

Community College, Mytown, OH
A.S. in Medical Assisting, 20XX
- Medical Assistant Practicum at Mytown Associates, Mytown, OH
  o Obtained and charted patients' histories and vital signs in the electronic health record.
  o Assisted providers with tests and treatments in a busy internal medicine practice.
  o Performed injections, throat swabs, and phlebotomy.

Skills

ORGANIZATION SKILLS
- Organized supplies to expedited restocking procedures and decrease financial loss.
- Exceptional organizational and filing skills utilized to maintain purchase and delivery records from over 300 suppliers.
- Assisted with the install and training for inventory tracking software for warehouse.

TEAMWORK
- Refined teamwork skills with over ten years in the U.S. Marines.
- Taught teambuilding courses.
- Promoted teamwork among staff by incorporating incentives.

COMMUNICATION SKILLS
- Assertive when working with suppliers to meet deadlines.
- Utilized excellent listening skills to identify needs of various teams that impact the warehouse.
- Composed frequent emails and letters for supervisors.
- Fluent in Spanish and Polish.

Credentials

Certified Medical Assistant, American Association of Medical Assistants, (expires May 20XX)

BLS for Healthcare Providers, American Heart Association (expires March 20XX)

Work Experience

United States Marines
Supply Administration and Operations Specialist (May 20XX – September 20XX)
Warehouse Clerk (August 20XX – May 20XX)

Fig. 57.5 Targeted Resume Customized for a Medical Assistant Posting. The medical assistant should possess strong organizational skills, experience with teamwork, and exceptional communication skills. The posting indicated it required a person with a Certified Medical Assistant (CMA) credential and a current Basic Life Support (BLS) certification.

Header. The person's contact information is found in the header of the document. This includes the person's name, mailing address, professional email address, phone number, and personal websites (e.g., LinkedIn). This information or a variation of the information should appear on each sheet if the resume is more than one page long.

Professional email addresses may include your first and last name or first initial and last name. Email addresses that include expressions such as "one_hot_chick" or "party_dude" are not professional and are not used on resumes. An old email format may indicate that you are not knowledgeable about the current technology. If you do not have a professional email address or have an old email address, free email sites are available (e.g., gmail.com). Like professional emails, personal websites should be professional and contain a professional image of you

Before you give out your phone number to potential employers, make sure your voice mail message is appropriate and professional sounding. State your name clearly in the message so that the caller knows he or she has reached the right person.

Education. The education section includes information on the schooling that the person has received after high school. The information should appear in reverse chronologic order. Information should include:

- *If a diploma was obtained*: List the school's name, city, and state, the degree, and the year it was obtained.
- *If no degree was obtained*: Summarize the coursework completed. List the school's name, city, and state, and the years of the coursework.

- *Student clinical experience information*: Include the location, dates, and duties performed during the experience. This is optional. Some will include this information in the Healthcare Experience section, discussed later in the chapter.
- *Academic recognition*: Include such things as academic awards and scholarships.

The location of the education section can differ based on the person's situation. For new graduates, the education section should appear toward the top of the resume. If the degree is not related to the position or the degree is older, the education section would come toward the end of the resume. Moving education to the end allows the person's achievements and work history to be emphasized.

> **VOCABULARY**
>
> **reverse chronologic order** The most recent item is on top and the oldest item is last.

Work Experience. This section can be titled several different ways. If a person is strictly including job information, then "Work Experience" or "Job Experience" can be used. Using the word "job" or "work" implies the person got paid for the position. If a person wants to include volunteer positions with job positions, then the section should be titled "Related Experience" or "Other Experience." "Related" means it relates to the position the person is applying for. If the section contains unrelated experience, then use "Other Experience." For those with military experience, it is recommended to add a special section to discuss the military experience.

If you have prior healthcare experience, you may want to separate your volunteer and job experiences into two sections. First, use "Healthcare Experiences." Include any healthcare jobs and volunteer positions you have had. Some students may opt to include their student clinical experience in this section. Second, use a topic header, such as "Other Experience" or "Additional Experience." Include all of your non-healthcare jobs and volunteer positions. Do not repeat information you included in prior sections.

The information in this section should be presented in reverse chronologic order. For each position, all three resumes discussed require:

- Name of the facility
- City and state of the facility
- Title of position or positions held at that facility
- Dates in that position (include start date [month and date] and end date [month and date]; for a current position, include the start date and use "to present")

For those in the workforce for 10 years or longer, employers want to see 10 years of employment information. For those working at the same facility for over 10 years, it is important to list changes and advancements in the position over the duration of employment. Any gaps in the employment history should be explained to the potential employer during the interview or discussed in the cover letter.

For the chronologic resume, the most relevant job duties need to be listed. For instance, if you worked as a housekeeper

in a motel, making beds is not related to medical assisting. Providing customer service would be relevant.

The statements regarding the duties should be bulleted and begin with an active verb. For present positions, use active verbs in the present tense (e.g., administer, provide). For past positions, use active verbs in the past tense (e.g., administered, provided) (Box 57.3).

The position of the work experience section is dependent on the resume format. Chronologic resumes typically have work experience near the top, whereas combination and targeted resumes list it toward the end of the resume.

Summary and Skills. A "Summary" section appears at the top in the targeted resume. This section summarizes why the applicant is the best candidate for the job. It is helpful to use key words from the job posting when describing skills one possesses. This helps the reader to make the connection of why the person is the best candidate for the job.

A "Skills" or "Skills and Achievements" section is found in combination resumes. It showcases specific transferable skills that relate to the new position. These transferable skills may have been obtained in the military, by a stay-at-home parent, or by a person switching careers. This section can also include the skills learned during the student clinical experience.

A "Special Skills" section is found in a chronologic resume. Information that may appear in this section includes:

- Fluency in another language (e.g., fluent in Spanish)
- Keyboarding speed (e.g., keyboarding speed: 85 wpm)
- Computer skills and experiences (e.g., used electronic health records during the student clinical experience)

Certifications. Many employers may require specific certifications or credentials for a job position. It is important to include those that relate to the job position. When listing the information, include:

- Title of the certification or license
- Awarding agency
- Expiration date

An example for all resume formats would be "BLS for Healthcare Providers, American Heart Association, expires 10/2027."

BOX 57.3 Action Verbs in the Past Tense

Administered	Composed	Listened	Provided
Advocated	Computed	Logged	Purchased
Aided	Contacted	Mailed	Reconciled
Answered	Coordinated	Maintained	Restocked
Arranged	Copied	Monitored	Reviewed
Assigned	Developed	Operated	Scanned
Assisted	Distributed	Ordered	Scheduled
Balanced	Documented	Organized	Sorted
Calculated	Established	Performed	Supported
Cared	Filed	Posted	Taught
Coded	Guided	Prepared	Trained
Collected	Helped	Processed	Wrote
Compiled	Instructed		

Appearance of the Resume

As you create your resume, keep in mind the eye appeal, or interest the resume will create for the reader. It is recommended to boldface only important information. A job title should be bold, whereas the facility should not be bold. Simple bullets help organize information and provide a neat appearance to the resume. Changing the font size in certain areas can emphasize more important elements and help keep content on one page.

Spacing is crucial to the appearance of a resume. A lot of spacing creates too much "white space." This can give the reader a negative impression of the resume. Too little spacing creates a busy, text-heavy resume that is difficult to read. Make sure to use the same spacing between the sections. Use less spacing, but be consistent between subsections (e.g., different employment positions).

It is important to have resume paper available. Even if you submit your resume online, you should bring copies of your resume on resume paper to the interview. Use a light solid-colored resume paper (e.g., cream, light gray). The light colors will duplicate better than a pattern or dark-colored paper.

Before submitting your resume, have another person review it. Obtain the person's initial impression of the resume's appearance. Is there too much white space? Does the resume look too wordy? Does it look too plain? Does it look too busy? Then have the person read the content in the resume and provide you with feedback. Use the feedback to revise your resume.

Here are some tips for creating a resume:

- Do not add clipart or other pictures.
- Do not include personal information (e.g., married, children, and religious affiliation).
- Do not lie or exaggerate the truth.
- Do not add unrelated content, such as hobbies and interests.
- Do not include "References available upon request" or a similar statement, because it is understood references will be requested and required.
- Do not use personal pronouns, such as "I."
- Do not repeat content.
- Do not include any pay/salary information.
- Always keep the resume to one page unless you have been in the workforce for multiple years. Then use an additional page, but your content must fill both pages.
- Be concise and clear.
- Use key terms found in the job posting or job description in your resume.
- Put important details first.
- Perform a grammar and spelling check on your resume.
- Limit abbreviations to only the abbreviations used in the job posting (e.g., BLS for basic life support or CPR for cardiopulmonary resuscitation).

CRITICAL THINKING 57.8

Zac, Michelle, and Krysia drafted their resumes. They read each other's and provided feedback. Who else might they give their resumes to for proofreading and feedback?

- Think of your circle of family and friends. List three people who might be great candidates to provide feedback on your resume.

DEVELOPING A COVER LETTER

A cover letter should always accompany the resume (Fig. 57.6). The cover letter is a critical tool that gains the reader's attention. The goal is to have the cover letter create enough interest that the reader wants to look at the resume. The cover letter gives the reader more information on the applicant's personality than the factual resume. Cover letters allow applicants to express themselves.

Strategies When Writing a Cover Letter

To create a professional cover letter, it is important to follow these strategies:

- Match the appearance of the cover letter and resume.
  - Headers on both documents should be identical.
  - Font type and margins should be identical.
  - If using paper, use the same paper for both documents.
- Address the inside address and the salutation (greeting) to a specific person.
  - Address the letter to the person who is hiring the new employee. This shows that you took time to find out the details.
  - Use the person's name and job title in the inside address.
  - Use a formal salutation (e.g., Dear Mr. Jones:).
  - Call the healthcare facility or use online resources, such as LinkedIn, to find out the information.
- Start the body of your cover letter off with a bang!
  - In the first paragraph: Show enthusiasm as you summarize why you believe you are the best candidate for the job. Also include the job title and the number for easy reference for the reader.
  - For example: "Having a strong customer service background and a degree in medical assisting, I am confident that I can fulfill your expectations for the family practice medical assistant position (#123)."
- Sell yourself to the reader.
  - In the second paragraph: Provide a snapshot of your experiences.
  - Weave in the key "requirement" words from the job posting. Address the requirements first, followed by the lesser requirements or "would like" qualities. Some experts recommend using bold font for these key words.
  - You can bullet your qualifications and abilities but limit the bullets to four or five points.
  - Be concise, yet clear. Do not repeat the resume. You want the reader to move onto the resume for the details.
- Reaffirm that you are an excellent match for the job.
  - In the final paragraph: Use such phrases as "I believe I have the qualities you require" or "I am confident I will meet your expectations."
  - If you include an action you will take (e.g., "I will call the week of…"), do not be overly aggressive in your tone.
  - Finish the paragraph by expressing your interest in and enthusiasm for an interview (e.g., "I am very excited about this opportunity and would enjoy meeting with you to explore how my qualifications could meet your needs.").
- Be professional.
  - Express your thanks to the reader for his or her consideration.

Michelle Marison

1234 Cedar Way, Mytown, OH 45458
Home phone: 715.555.1899
Cell phone: 715.555.1355
mmarison@elsevier.net

May 15, 20XX

Ms. Alex Brown
Medical Assistant Supervisor
Mytown Medical Clinic
555 Clover Drive
Mytown OH 45457

Dear Ms. Brown:

I was excited to see the posting on the Mytown Telegram job board for the medical assistant position (#1243) and would like to be considered for that position. I am graduating from Community College on May 30, 20XX and will be taking my AAMA CMA exam June 2, 20XX.

With two years of customer service experience and five months of being a hospital volunteer, I have learned the importance of prioritizing, teamwork, and communication. During my medical assistant practicum, I have utilized these skills along with my attention to detail and my medical assistant knowledge, as I assist providers with procedures and treatments. The knowledge and skills I am learning in practicum combined with the skills I have developed as a waitress and volunteer will help me provide the best care to my future patients.

I have heard excellent things about Mytown Medical Clinic and would love to be a part of the staff of such a caring agency. I am available for interviews whenever it is convenient for you. I am available either by phone or email.

Thank you so much for considering me for this position.

Sincerely,

Michelle Marison

Enclosure: 1

Fig. 57.6 Basic Cover Letter. (From Niedzwiecki B, et al: *Kinn's the medical assistant*, ed 14, St. Louis, 2020, Elsevier.)

Proofreading the Cover Letter

After writing the cover letter, review it for inaccuracies. Use the spell-check tool in your word processing software to help identify errors. Also proofread your letter. Make sure your spelling, punctuation, grammar, and sentence structure are correct. Avoid common cover letter weaknesses:

- Starting a majority of sentences with "I."
- Introducing yourself in the first sentence (for instance, "Hi, I am Sally Green.")
- Spelling, grammar, punctuation, and sentence structure errors.
- Missing parts of the letter (e.g., date, inside address).
- Not including the position title and posting number.
- Too busy (overuse of font styles), too wordy, or too much white space.
- Inappropriate spacing that leads to the body of the letter being too high or too low on the page. Remember, the body should be centered vertically on the page.

- Creating a generic letter that does not contain the key requirement words from the job posting. (Many larger employers use software to screen letters and resumes for key words. Those with key words are reviewed more closely. Those that lack the key words are discarded.)

Create an error-free cover letter. It must have a professional tone and appearance. Also, have a few people proofread your letter. Use their advice as you make your changes. Refer to Chapter 25 if you need assistance with composing a business letter. Procedure 57.2 will help guide you in writing a professional cover letter.

> **VOCABULARY**
> **proofread** To read and mark corrections.

COMPLETING ONLINE PROFILES AND JOB APPLICATIONS

Many healthcare agencies use the internet during the employment process. The online human resource software may require

APPLICATION FOR EMPLOYMENT

Date: _____

Name: (First, Middle Initial, Last) _____

Social Security No.: _____   Phone: _____

Address: _____

EDUCATION

	Name, City, State	Graduation Date	Degree Obtained
High School:			
College:			
Other:			

LICENSURE/CERTIFICATION/REGISTRATION

Type of Certification, License or Registration	Agency/State	Registration Name

List any special skills or qualifications which you possess and feel are relevant to health care and the position for which you are applying. _____

_____

EMPLOYMENT HISTORY
May we contact and communicate with your present employer? ☐ Yes ☐ No

Employer:	Phone:
Address:	Supervisor:
Employed	Hourly Pay:
Position title and responsibilities:	
Reason for leaving:	

Fig. 57.7 Application for Employment. (From Niedzwiecki B, et al: *Kinn's the medical assistant,* ed 14, St. Louis, 2020, Elsevier.)

applicants to create a profile before applying for open positions. The online profile collects the information that previously was collected by paper applications.

Online profiles have many advantages over paper applications for both the employer and the applicant. An applicant completes the profile once and updates the information as needed. Typically, the agencies keep the profiles active for years. Employers can take several actions:

- Track the activities of applicants.
- Easily read a person's information.
- Advertise new postings to potential applicants whose profiles meet certain requirements.

If a healthcare facility does not use online profiles, then the applicant will need to complete a job application (Fig. 57.7). Some organizations require the application to be submitted with the cover letter and resume. Others have applicants arriving for interviews complete the application. If you need to complete an application before an interview, come prepared with your information. Arrive at least 20 minutes before the interview so you can complete the application. See Procedure 57.3 for the steps in completing a job application.

Regardless of whether you need to complete a profile or an application, you will need to provide the same information. Even if you have the information on your resume, you still need to add it to the application or profile. Having the reference information in a word-processed document will save you time. If you are providing the information online, the copy-and-paste feature will speed up completion time. You should include certain information in the word-processed document:

- *Education*: Institution's name and address; dates and titles of coursework or diploma
- *Past and present jobs*: Facility name and address; supervisors' names, titles, and contact information; job title, duties, start and end salary, start and end dates; and reason for leaving

- *Certifications and credentials*: Certifying agency's name and address; certification/credential; expiration date (a copy of your certification and BLS card may be required by the employer)
- *References*: Name, title, facility, address, phone number, and email address (Box 57.4)

When filling out the application or profile, answer the questions carefully. When addressing your current and past employment, keep these points in mind:

- When giving your availability date, make sure you know how long you have to give notice at your current position. Most employers have a 2-week notice policy. If you are hired, your new employer will understand that you need to give a 2-week notice.
- When giving the reason you left prior positions, make sure to write the reason using a positive tone. For instance, "Obtained a position that would advance my skill set" or "Resigned to focus on my education" sounds more professional than "I hated the job."

If you have a unique situation (e.g., sick parent, new baby), ask the advice of your school's placement counselor if you are unsure what to say in these sections. Most employers require an explanation for time not employed.

As you complete the online profile or paper application, you will be required to read important legal statements and add your signature (or electronic signature). This is a legal document. It should be filled out accurately and completely.

CAREER PORTFOLIOS

Many job seekers claim to have the skill sets required by the potential employer. Very few actually show the employer evidence of those qualifications. A career portfolio is a fantastic tool to show that you have the skills required for the job.

The portfolio should be developed along with the cover letter and resume. Creating a different portfolio for each type of job applied for is a great strategy. A receptionist portfolio would look different from a phlebotomy portfolio. There will be similarities in the information for all portfolios, but different "evidence" of skills will be in each. The medical assistant should be prepared to leave the portfolio with the interviewer, so no originals should be included.

Just before an interview, the medical assistant should customize the portfolio for that employer (Procedure 57.4). A copy of the cover letter and resume sent to the employer should be in the portfolio. A list of references should also be included. All three of these documents should be printed on the same type of resume paper. The medical assistant should do additional customization of the portfolio. The examples of work or the summary of projects should reflect the skills required and key words in the job posting.

Creating a Career Portfolio

The documents placed in the career portfolio binder should be positive and helpful to you in your mission of getting a job. Using a three-ring binder with plastic sheet protectors and divider tabs, put together a career portfolio that includes:

- Table of contents at the beginning with identified tabbed sections
- Cover letter and resume (a copy of what was sent to that facility)
- References
- Certifications (e.g., copy of BLS card, copy of credentials [e.g., CMA or RMA card])
- Education-related documents
  - Copies of letters of recommendation
  - Copies of transcripts, awards, and honors (optional)
  - A list of the courses successfully completed with a short description of each course (optional, but consider doing this if you are moving to another location where your institution may not be known)
  - Copies of student clinical experience evaluation forms and skill document form
  - Documentation of scholarships awarded
  - Copies/details of school-related activities (e.g., officer in student medical assistant group, athlete, volunteer activities)
- Prior employment documents
  - Copies of past employment evaluations
  - Copies of letters of recommendations
- Documentation showing the student balancing work and education (this can help exhibit a strong work ethic, organizational skills, and prioritizing skills)
- Examples of work or summaries of projects that can provide evidence of abilities and skills
- Criminal background documentation, blood titers, vaccination history, and current tuberculosis (TB) skin or blood tests results (optional)

Be creative as you prepare your portfolio, keeping the appearance professional and neat.

JOB INTERVIEW

Interviewers can consist of one or two people or a panel of employees. The job seeker may interview with a human resource employee, the office manager, the provider, or potential peers. The job seeker may have a number of interviews before the actual decision is made.

For many people, the interview is a stressful part of the job search. Some individuals dread job interviews and become extremely nervous at the prospect of interviewing. Others are very comfortable and consider the interview to be as much for their own purposes as for the employer's. The more interviews people do, the more comfortable they become with each subsequent interview.

We will examine the four phases of an interview. These include preparation for the interview, the interview itself, the follow-up, and the negotiation.

Preparation for the Interview

When preparing for an interview, the job seeker needs to:
- Research the facility.
- Practice answering potential questions.
- Select interview attire.
- Prepare for the day of the interview.

We will discuss each of these in depth. The better prepared the job candidate is, the more comfortable he or she will be during the interview.

Research the Healthcare Facility.
The job seeker should learn everything possible about the employer. The organization's website is an excellent source of information. A job seeker should research:
- Mission and value statements
- Size of the organization
- Size of the department with the open position
- Names and types of providers in the department

It is important to ask questions at the interview. Possible questions can relate to your research on the facility:
- "I see that there are two providers in this department. Would I be working with both of them?"
- "There are three locations for your clinic on your website; how will I interact with the other locations?"
- "Given the size of your organization, is there an opportunity to interact with the other departments?"

Questions that relate to your research show the interviewer you are truly interested in the position. They also show that you prepared for the interview.

Practice Answers to Questions.
Organizations need to follow federal and state hiring laws. The agencies cannot discriminate. During the interview phase, most organizations use a preset list of questions. All candidates are asked the same questions. You will not know the exact questions that will be asked. It is important to practice answering some standard interview questions (Fig. 57.8). This practice will help you prepare for the interview and also appear more confident during the actual interview.

When practicing your answers to standard interview questions, start by writing down your answer. Review your answer. Does it answer the question? What perception might you be giving to the interviewers by your answer? Is it the perception you want to be giving? How might you strengthen your answer? Is it really short or does it ramble on? Be clear and concise. Expand on the topic, but do not get too wordy. Provide examples to support what you say. When you have refined your answers, practice your answers before the interview.

Decide on Your Interview Attire.
Prior to the interview, it is important to select an interview outfit. Be conservative with wardrobe choices.
- Females: Business suit; skirt or dress pants and blouse. Skirt or dress should be of modest length (i.e., at the knee or longer). Blouse should not be sheer or show cleavage.
- Males: Business suit; dress pants and shirt. Conservative tie.

Be sure clothing is clean, wrinkle free, and well fitting, and that shoes are clean and shined. For a medical assistant, scrubs may be acceptable for an interview. (It is appropriate to ask the person arranging the interview if scrubs can be worn.) Take care in washing and pressing your scrubs, and use a lint roller on them, before wearing them on an interview.

Pay particular attention to other aspects of appearance. Make sure your hair is clean and styled attractively, your teeth are clean, and your breath is fresh. Nails should be clean and well-groomed. Nails should not be excessively long or painted in highly visible colors. Do not wear perfumes or colognes. Do not wear excessive jewelry or makeup. Do not chew gum during the interview. Do not smoke in your interview attire. Remember the appearance guidelines that applied to the student clinical experience. Some employers will react negatively to tattoos, piercings, extravagant hairstyles, unnatural hair colors, or other excessive wardrobe choices. Always dress appropriately and conservatively for an interview. Once hired, the new employee may be allowed to wear more diverse styles that comply with the employee handbook or procedures manual.

Prepare for the Interview Day.
Do a test run before the day of the interview to identify the travel time if the interview is in person. Always arrive 15 minutes early for the interview. Never take anyone along on a job interview, especially children. Expect to be a little nervous. Any interview can be a stressful situation. If necessary, practice stress-relieving strategies (e.g., deep breathing) that you can use before the interview. The better prepared a person is, the more successful the interview will be.

You should also prepare what you need to bring for the interview:
- An interview portfolio
- A copy of your cover letter and resume for each interviewer
- A notepad and pen to take notes
- A list of references on resume paper
- A list of questions for the interviewer

If you will be completing an application, bring the information discussed in the prior section regarding completing online profiles and applications.

Types of Interviews

Face-to-face interviews have been the normal method for interviewing job candidates until the recently. Over the last years, phone interviews have gained in popularity. These are common for prescreening candidates for face-to-face or virtual interviews. Virtual interviews also became popular over the last years.

Phone Interview.
Phone interviews are usually done by the supervisor or the human resource representative. A phone interview may be the selected option in order to:
- Screen applicants and narrow the candidate pool

1. Tell me about yourself.	16. What do you know about this facility and our competitors?
2. Why do you want to work for this company?	17. What has been your most rewarding experience at work?
3. Why should I hire you?	18. What was your single most important accomplishment for the company on your last job?
4. How do you work under pressure?	19. What was the toughest problem you have ever solved and how did you do it?
5. How do you handle criticism?	20. How do you see yourself fitting in with our company?
6. What do you think your co-workers think about you?	21. What skills did you learn on your last job that can be used here?
7. Describe your last supervisor.	22. What immediate contribution could you make if you came to work for us today?
8. What would you like to change about yourself?	23. Do you prefer working with others or by yourself?
9. What is your best asset?	24. Can you take instructions or criticism without being upset?
10. What adjectives would you use to describe yourself?	25. What job in this company would you choose if you could?
11. How would you describe the perfect job?	26. What have you done that shows initiative and willingness to work?
12. Why did you leave your last job?	27. What will previous supervisors say about you?
13. Why did you choose this type of profession?	28. Why would you be successful in this job?
14. What are your strongest and weakest personal qualities?	29. Can you explain the gap in your employment history?
15. What personal characteristics are necessary for success in your chosen field?	30. Are you a member of any professional organizations?

Fig. 57.8 Top 30 Interview Questions. (From Niedzwiecki B, et al: *Kinn's the medical assistant*, ed 14, St. Louis, 2020, Elsevier.)

- Provide additional information (e.g., benefits, job description) and verify that the applicant wants an interview
- Replace a face-to-face interview, especially if the candidate is from out of town

Phone interviews are becoming more prevalent. It is important to treat a phone interview like a face-to-face interview. Here are some tips for a phone interview:

- Prepare for the interview just as you would for a face-to-face interview.
- Take the call in a quiet environment. Make sure no dogs or children are in the room. Be alone in the room.
- Pay attention to the caller. Do not use other electronic devices or use the bathroom during the call.
- Have a copy of your resume and cover letter.
- Have your list of questions.
- Have a glass of water available should you need it.
- Make sure to thank the interviewer at the end of the call.

Face-to-Face Interview. When you meet the interviewers, greet each person and shake hands. A firm handshake is recommended. Ensure each person has a copy of your resume and cover letter before the interview begins.

During the actual interview, maintain good eye contact. Many supervisors refuse to hire people who seem uncomfortable looking them directly in the eyes. Never take control of the interview. Allow the supervisor or panel members to ask questions at their own pace. Do not fidget in the chair or display any nervous habits (e.g., tapping your pen) (Procedure 57.5).

Virtual Interview. Virtual or video interviews use technology such as Skype or Zoom. As with a phone interview, a virtual interview works well when the candidate is from out of town or if face-to-face interviews are not being held. There is a certain amount of technology needed for a virtual interview. Your school's placement office may be able to help you with that. The organization may have contacts for you to arrange your end of the interview. The benefit of a virtual interview over a phone interview is that the interviewer can actually see the interviewee. This allows the interviewer to assess the body language and the verbal message being presented.

Tips for a virtual interview include:

- Prepare like you would for a face-to-face interview. Research the company and create a list of questions to ask.
- Dress like you would for a face-to-face interview.
- Practice with the technology. Be familiar with the software that will be used for the interview.
- Identify an appropriate location for the interview. During the interview, the microphone and camera will be on. Choose a quiet area without pets and other people. Choose a neutral background, such as a blank wall. If this is not available, select the least distracting environment. Limit the distractions behind you that will be visible to the interviewer. Cluttered counters with dirty dishes, inappropriate pictures, dirty laundry, and so on do not help to create the professional image you are striving for.
- Make sure the camera is positioned appropriately. The interviewer should be able to see your head and shoulders. Make sure you are not sitting too close or too far from the camera. The camera should be positioned so you can appear to be making eye contact with the interviewer. Make sure there is no glare. Adjust the light source if needed.
- Just like the phone interview, have the same materials ready to access during the interview process.
- Refrain from nervous habits during the interview that can be observed by the interviewer.

During the Interview

During the interview it is important to be professional. Your professionalism may be tested if the interviewer asks illegal questions. We will discuss how to answer interview questions. We will also discuss professionalism during the different types of interviews.

Answering Interview Questions. It is important to give the interviewers a good impression of you. As discussed in a prior section, it is important to practice answering questions before the interview. This will help you to prepare and to feel more confident during the interview (Box 57.5).

Many times, the interview will start with a question such as "Tell me about yourself." The temptation is to answer the question focusing on your personal life. For example, "I'm a recent graduate, and I am married and have two children." The answer to this question should not reflect information about personal issues. Answer instead with "I am a recent graduate and completed a 6-week clinical experience in a family practice." Focus all answers on your career, your strengths and attributes, and what skills you have to bring to the healthcare setting. Be able to prove the skills you claim. You can provide examples either by relating professional situations you have handled well or by using your interview portfolio. Before the interview ends, the medical assistant should ask when a decision will be made and if it would be acceptable to call to follow up (Procedure 57.5).

Illegal Interview Questions. The interviewer should not ask any illegal questions. Table 57.1 lists such topics and potential illegal questions. Employers may either intentionally or accidentally ask illegal questions. The way that the medical assistant answers the questions can influence the employer's hiring decision. Here are some points to consider:

BOX 57.5 Tips for All Interviews

- For simple, straightforward questions, do not pause before you answer. Any pause would hint at insincerity.
- For complex questions, pause for a few seconds as you think about your answer. Write down some key words to help you focus and answer the question.
- Refrain from saying "um."
- Do not volunteer any negative information.
- Be honest, and do not exaggerate experiences or lengths of employment.
- Never speak negatively about former employers.
- Write down the names of the interviewers to help you as you follow up after the interview.
- Avoid a "know-it-all" attitude, which indicates overconfidence and a reluctance to take direction.
- Express a sincere interest in the employer and his or her projects, rather than in what the employer can do for the employee.
- Ask intelligent questions at the end of the interview if given the opportunity. Your first question should never be, "How much will I be paid?" Money, although important, cannot appear to be your primary concern.

TABLE 57.1 Illegal versus Legal Interview Questions

Topic	Examples of Illegal Questions	Examples of Legal Questions
Birthplace, ancestry, or national origin	When did you move to the United States?	Are you eligible to work in this state?
Marital status, children, or pregnancy	Who will look after your child when he or she is born?	Are you able to work an 8 a.m. to 5 p.m. schedule?
Physical disability, health or medical history	What medications are you on?	Can you perform the essential job functions of a medical assistant with or without reasonable accommodation?
Religion or religious days observed	Where do you attend church services?	Can you work on weekends?
Age, race, ethnicity, gender, or color	How old are you?	Are you 18 or older? (or whatever the minimum age is for the facility)
Criminal record	Have you ever been arrested?	Have you ever been convicted of a crime?

- If the medical assistant is openly offended: Employers may negatively conclude that the applicant will be offended by abrasive comments from patients.
- If the illegal question is answered: Discrimination may occur in the hiring process. The employer may use the information to weed out the medical assistant as a candidate.

The best approach is to politely address the question. Either answer the question or redirect the interviewer back to the job requirements. For example, an interviewer asks if the candidate plans to put his or her children in day care. This may be a way of determining the age of the dependent children. It could also provide information on the likelihood of absenteeism because of the children's illnesses. The medical assistant could answer, "I will be able to meet the work schedule and the responsibilities that this job requires."

Some questions that might normally be considered illegal, such as "What organizations are you a member of?" might be job related. The employer may be interested in knowing if the medical assistant is a member of various professional organizations, such as the AAMA or the AMT.

CRITICAL THINKING 57.9

Krysia is enjoying a good interview when the interviewer, a male supervisor, asks her if she is married. When Krysia replies that she is not, he asks if she has a steady boyfriend.

- What might the supervisor's motive be with this line of questioning?
- How should Krysia respond?
- Are these questions inappropriate or do they serve a purpose?

Follow-Up After the Interview

Follow-up is critical after an interview. Always send a thank-you note, letter, or email to the person who conducted the interview (Procedure 57.6). It can be challenging to figure out what to send to the interviewer.

- *Send an email if* the decision is going to be made quickly. Send an email later the day of the interview.
- *Send a written thank-you note or a letter if* the facility is more conservative and formal. Also, it can be sent if the decision is going to be made in a week or two. Send the thank-you note within 24 hours of the interview.

Many employers see the thank-you as an expression of gratitude and professionalism. Even if you do not see yourself in that position, it is still important to send a thank you. This may be their last perception of you, and it may help you in the future at that facility.

Typically, at the end of the interview, there will be a discussion of how quickly the decision will be made. Many agencies using online hiring software will indicate the status of the job on the posting. Candidates not selected for the position usually receive an email or letter.

After the initial interviews are completed with all the candidates, several things can occur. With some employers, the list of interviewed candidates will be narrowed. The top two or three may be asked to come back for a second interview with additional team members (e.g., providers, medical assistants). With other employers, the top candidate is selected, and references are checked. These processes take time, and the deadline may be extended if vacations or out-of-office times occur.

If the interviewer indicates a decision would be made in 2 weeks, wait to hear from the facility. Allow a few days after the deadline before you follow up. At that time, you can call and ask the status of the job. Remember, following up prior to the deadline may not be in your best interest. The employer may perceive that you do not follow directions if you make extra phone calls. If you receive a job offer from another facility but are waiting for a decision on your favorite position, it is appropriate to contact the interviewer. Explain that you were offered another position and wondered about the status of this position. Many employers will let you know if you are in the running for the position.

Never place all your hope in one job. Make sure to continue to search and interview until an offer is made and accepted. In addition, always be on the lookout for the next job opportunity.

Negotiation

The negotiation stage of job acceptance can be as stressful as the actual interviews. The salary and benefits must be considered when determining whether to accept a position or not. When a job offer is made, there should also be a discussion of the other benefits. If the salary offered is a bit lower than expected, but the employee's share of the health insurance premium is less than expected, the salary offer becomes more attractive. Medical assistants should know the lowest salary/benefit combination they can afford. They should ask for a little more than that figure.

Bracket salary requests or providing salary ranges are often helpful. Before doing this, it is important to know the typical wage in the area for the position. Let the employer mention a figure or a range of salary first. Usually the person who mentions a salary range first has the disadvantage. For example, if the medical assistant requests $15 per hour, but the facility was willing to pay $18 per hour, the medical assistant probably will get $15.

Many organizations have a starting pay level for new medical assistants. If you hope to get a higher pay level, you may need to:

- Obtain a national medical assistant credential (e.g., CMA [AAMA] or RMA)
- Show an advanced skills level acquired from previous work experience in healthcare. Having a well-designed interview portfolio will allow you to show the interviewer all that you have accomplished.

Never say no to a job offer on the spot. Request at least 24 hours to consider the offer. Before accepting or rejecting a job offer, consider whether the position carries any authority, the benefits, the hours, the distance from home, and the potential for advancement. People accept jobs for reasons other than the salary; remember the value of experience.

CRITICAL THINKING 57.10

Michelle has been on several interviews and likes the prospect of working for three different physicians. If each office makes an offer, how can Michelle decide which to accept? What will help Michelle make this decision?

IMPROVING YOUR OPPORTUNITIES

We will examine ways to improve your opportunities for finding a job.

Finding Job Postings

Some students and graduates may not find job postings. This can be stressful, but it is important not to give up. Those who are not having success with the job search may want to reevaluate their search methods. Consider these questions:

- Am I looking for a selective opportunity? For instance, are you looking for a dermatology medical assistant position in a specific facility? Those positions may be limited. Try to broaden your search to other possible opportunities.
- Am I looking for the correct job title? Remember, employers may use a wide range of titles for a medical assistant.
- Am I looking at all agencies that potentially could hire a person with my skill sets? Depending on your area, medical assistants can be in many agencies besides a medical clinic, including a nursing home, hospital, school, assisted-living facility, and insurance company.
- Can I increase the geographical search area for employment opportunities? Can I relocate to an area with greater employment opportunities?
- Where can I network to increase my awareness of job openings?
- What job boards are local employers using?

Increasing Interview Opportunities

People who apply for jobs but never get calls for interviews must reevaluate the information given to employers. Consider these questions:

- *Is your cover letter, resume, online profile, or application negatively affecting the job search?* It may be important to get another opinion on the content and presentation. Often the school career placement officer will provide improvement tips.
- *Do you have spelling and grammar errors in your information?* Some employers may perceive that details are not important to you, and so they may not be interested in hiring you.
- *Do your cover letter and resume need to be reformatted or revised?* Applicants need their letter and resume to stand out from the crowd. People get very creative in how they make this occur.
- *Are your cover letter and resume customized to the job posting?* Do your documents reflect the key words in the posting? Or do your documents look generic? Generic-looking documents lead employers to perceive that the person is not into details and was not interested enough to spend the time to customize the documents.
- *Are you following the directions in the job posting?* For instance, an employer may want a handwritten cover letter to be included. Sometimes the employer provides a mailing address and states that no calls or visits will be allowed. If applicants do not follow the directions, they may not be considered for the job.
- *Are you providing a professional image with your email address and on social media sites, such as Facebook?*

Graduates struggling to find positions may want to review their social media sites. Consider tighter security settings to limit outside viewers. You may want to remove any questionable content and pictures.

Increasing Job Offers

If you are getting interviews but no job offers, reevaluate your interview strategies. Again, the school's career placement office may have interview assistance. Mock interviews can help you refine your interview skills and behavior.

The following is a ranked list of reasons interviewers do not hire job candidates, as expressed by surveyed career consultants and reported on the website http://careers.workoplis.com:

- Based on social media postings
- Bad attitude, not interested, or appeared not to care
- Not researching a potential employer/company
- Smelled bad: heavy cologne or perfume use, reeked of cigarette smoke
- Sloppy documents: misused and misspelled words, inappropriate grammar and punctuation, and failed to proofread the resume and cover letter
- Appeared desperate for the job
- Failed to have references that provided work and professionalism information
- Unrealistic salary expectations

It is always important to prepare for the interview, show enthusiasm for the position, and ask the right questions. Other factors may have negatively affected the decision as well:

- Inappropriate interview attire and grooming: The outfit was too tight, neckline was too low, pants dragged on the ground, or the shoes were too casual (e.g., flip-flops). The perfume or cologne was too strong. The hairstyle or color was too extreme.
- Did not fit in the environment: Each facility has a corporate environment. The interviewer looks to see which candidate would fit best. If a person is too shy, too talkative, or too loud, he or she might not be the best fit. Or, a person may have worn too many piercings, or too many tattoos were visible.
- Used poor grammar: Some employers correlate good grammar with intelligence. Employers look for candidates who sound intelligent and who will positively represent their facility.

If you have heard or feel that your resume lacks skills needed for specific positions you want to obtain, you may want to improve your skill sets. This can occur through education and experience. Some people improve their job history and skill sets by obtaining temporary employment through temp agencies. Temporary jobs can provide experience and also help you refine your skills. Another way to better your skill sets through experience is by volunteering at a healthcare facility or free clinic. Depending on the volunteer position, it may help enhance your skill sets and provide you with potential job leads. Volunteer activities should be added to the resume because these valuable experiences often can be used in a healthcare setting. It does not matter that the position was not a paid job; experience counts, whether paid or not.

VOCABULARY

mock Simulated; intended for imitation or practice.
skill set A person's abilities, skills, or expertise in an area.

TABLE 57.2 Forms to Complete When Hired

Form	Description
Form I-9: Employment Eligibility Verification Form	Form I-9 is used to verify a person's identity and employment authorization. All US employers must ensure the form is completed by both the new hire and the employer. The form requires the new hire to provide the employer with documents that prove identity and employment authorization proof.
Form W-4: Employee's Withholding Certificate	New hires must provide their tax status (e.g., single) and how many withholding allowances they are claiming. This information is used when the employer withholds money from their paycheck for income taxes.
Insurance benefit form	Most agencies have health and life insurance benefits that the new hire can participate in. Completion of paperwork is required as part of the enrollment activities.
Background check form	Many healthcare providers will pay for background checks on new hires. Some hiring may be contingent based on a clean background check. Some types of background checks include criminal, sexual offender registry, and caregiver.
Emergency contact form	The new employee gives the employer information on whom to contact in case of an emergency.
Handbook acknowledgement form	Some agencies have handbooks for each employee. They may require that the employee sign a form to acknowledge receiving the handbook.
Direct deposit form	Most healthcare agencies will pay the employees using the direct deposit method. Funds are transferred into the employee's bank account instead of the employee receiving a paper paycheck.
Agreement forms	The newly hired employee must sign agreement forms related to the Health Insurance Portability and Accountability Act (HIPAA) and computer security.

YOU GOT THE JOB!

Human Resource Requirements

When you obtain a job, you will be required to complete a number of documents (Table 57.2). You will be asked to bring in proof of identity and employment authorization (e.g., US passport, Social Security card, and driver's license). These documents are required for the employer's portion of the Form I-9. Form I-9 must be completed within the set time period to meet governmental regulations. Make sure to complete all the required forms in a timely manner. Meet the deadlines given to you by the human resource representative.

Getting Started

When you get your first job, it can be an exciting and scary time. You may feel excited for the new opportunities yet scared of the new responsibilities. With any job, it takes time to learn the position. Most healthcare agencies have *probationary periods* for new employees. This time frame can vary. The purpose of the probationary period is to see if the new employee is the right fit for the job. If the employee is not able to do the job or is not the right person for the job, the employer can terminate the employee during the probationary period.

It is important for the medical assistant to do well during the probationary period. The first weeks to months of the job are usually devoted to orientation. The new employee learns the processes and becomes efficient and confident in the role. To be successful it is important for the medical assistant to adopt the following practices:

- Arrive 10 to 15 minutes prior to the start of the day. Limit absences, especially during the probationary period.
- Be groomed appropriately according to the facility's dress code.
- Be honest, trustworthy, and respectful in all interactions with peers, patients, and providers.
- Be willing to try new things and ask questions.
- Take feedback professionally and with a positive attitude.

- Be motivated to do a good job and be willing to keep learning.
- Be a team player and be willing to help others.
- Provide safe care to patients, always working within the medical assistant scope of practice.
- Be open to new ideas, concepts, and procedures.
- Attempt to resolve simple differences with peers before involving the supervisor.
- Work with the supervisor to improve oneself and the department.
- Finish all assigned tasks in a timely manner and look for additional duties if time is available.

Maintaining Your Job

For the medical assistant to continue with the facility, it is important to be a reliable employee. It is also important to improve one's weaknesses. The medical assistant will get regular feedback from supervisors through performance appraisals. The performance appraisals inform employees of their strengths and weaknesses on the job. These appraisals are done after the probationary period and annually thereafter. Types of performance appraisals include:

- *180-degree style*: Supervisors evaluate their employees based on their observations of job performance over a given time period.
- *360-degree style*: Supervisors gather input from your co-workers and others whom you interact with on a regular basis.

Do not expect to receive a perfect appraisal. Employees are seldom perfect in all aspects of their jobs. If the supervisor gives perfect scores to an employee, there is no room for growth or improvement. The areas for growth are usually discussed during a meeting with the supervisor. You may be asked where you want to grow or improve and your goals for the coming year. It is important to consider these topics prior to the meeting with the supervisor.

Professional development is also important in maintaining one's job. Medical assistants must keep updated and current in the healthcare industry. It is important to meet the continuing education units (CEUs) needed to maintain your certification or registration. Information on the requirements can be found on the credentialing agency's website.

Leaving a Job

Always offer at least 2 weeks' notice when resigning from a job, since you would want a 2 week notice from your employer if your job was terminated. Prepare a written notice of resignation and take it to the supervisor in person. Do not just leave it on a desk or place it in the interoffice mail.

Resigning from a job just as an attempt to get a salary increase is a dangerous practice. Once the employer doubts the employee's loyalty, the future is not usually bright for the employee at that facility. Resign only after a final decision has been made. If the medical assistant is resigning to take another position, the current employer may be expected to make a counteroffer. However, be wary about accepting counteroffers. What led you to look for a new job in the first place? Has the situation been resolved? Ask yourself these questions before agreeing to stay with the current employer. Often employees who accept a counteroffer and stay at their original job find that few changes are made, and the employee ends up leaving the position in the long run.

> **VOCABULARY**
> **counteroffer** Return offer made by one who has rejected an offer or a job.

CLOSING COMMENTS

As you finish your medical assistant program, embrace the challenge of finding a job. Spend time preparing for the search. Design a professional resume and cover letter that positively set you apart from the other graduates. Network and check job boards for job openings. Apply for any jobs that interest you. Keep organized in your search so you do not overlook opportunities. Work with employment resources at your school to increase your confidence in interviewing. Your preparation and hard work will help you find your first medical assistant job!

BEING PROFESSIONAL

In many ambulatory care facilities, the supervisor will have medical assistants in the department participate on the interview team. The interview team members ask each interviewee the same set of questions. At the end of the interviews, the interview team members provide feedback to the supervisor about the interviewees. The information discussed is confidential. The interview team members should not discuss the interview process with others.

Role-play this scenario with a peer: You and Sam are medical assistants and work in different departments. Sam knows you were part of the interview team for a new medical assistant in your department. Sam's best friend Sally was being interviewed. Sam asks you how the interviews went and what the final decision was. Respond to Sam in a respectful, professional manner, yet protect the confidential interview information.

CHAPTER REVIEW

Employers spend a lot of time and money training their staff. It is important that they select the right employee initially. Employers look for specific personality traits when interacting with potential new employees. They seek people who already have collaboration and interpersonal skills, professionalism, compassion, and a sincere interest in the job.

Prior to job seeking, medical assistants need to prepare. They should identify the personality traits, technical skills, and transferable job skills that they possess. Medical assistants must consider what they want from their career and a job. What are their personal needs (e.g., wage, benefits, hours, locations)?

The two best methods to identify jobs are through networking and using job boards. Networking involves the medical assistant exchanging information with other professionals in hopes of obtaining possible job leads. Job boards are online sites that list positions posted by employers. Traditional job search methods include school career placement offices, newspaper ads, and employment agencies.

The three commonly used resume formats are chronologic, combination, and targeted resumes. As you create your resume, keep in mind the eye appeal, or interest, the resume will create in the reader. A cover letter should always accompany a resume, and much attention to detail is necessary.

The four phases of the interview process are the preparation, the actual interview, the follow-up, and the negotiation. It is important to write a thank-you note for an interview. It is a way to make you stand out from the other people who have interviewed for the same position. It shows that you are a courteous and conscientious person and also gives you another opportunity to show why you are the right person for the job.

SCENARIO WRAP-UP

Before graduation, Michelle was offered a job at Walden-Martin Family Medical (WMFM) Clinic. She took her instructor's advice and sent a thank-you note to those who interviewed her. When she was offered the job, the supervisor mentioned how thoughtful the note was. During the call, the supervisor summarized the benefits and the starting salary. She mentioned to Michelle that all medical assistants start at the same wage, but after they pass the CMA (AAMA) certification examination, they get a raise. Michelle took 2 days to consider the position and decided to accept the job offer. The wage was lower than what she was hoping for, but the benefits were much better.

Krysia interviewed for several medical assistant positions over the past few weeks. She found that employers respected her service to her country and valued the skills she learned in military service. She just received her third job offer within the last few days and has decided to accept the position at the local Veterans Affairs (VA) clinic. It is a full-time position with great benefits. The higher wage will help offset the extra mileage that she will be driving to work. She is very excited to be working with other veterans.

Zac has struggled to identify what type of clinic he wants to work for. With his strong leadership skills, he hopes to find a position where he can advance to a supervisory position. He has interviewed for job positions at small and large clinics. He is finding that he is more interested in working with surgeons than with family practitioners. He likes the complexity involved with surgical patients. He is hoping to receive a job offer shortly after graduation. He has decided that if his dream job is not offered to him, he will pursue a position in family medicine or internal medicine. This will give him a solid foundation for his new career, and then someday he can move into orthopedics or surgery.

PROCEDURE 57.1 Prepare a Chronologic Resume

Task
Write an effective resume for use as a tool in obtaining employment.

Equipment and Supplies
- Computer with word processing software and a printer
- Current job posting
- Resume paper
- Paper and pen

Procedural Steps
1. Apply critical thinking skills as you create a list of the personality traits (wanted by employers), technical skills, and transfer job skills that you possess. Also write down your career goal(s).
   Purpose: To determine the strongest aspects of your abilities so that you can emphasize them on your resume.
2. Using the current job posting, identify the required and recommended qualifications and credentials needed for the position.
   Purpose: Identifying what the employer requires and would like will help you tailor your resume to address these qualifications and credentials.
3. Using the computer with word processing software, create a professional-looking header for your document. Include your name, address, telephone number(s), and email address. Select an appropriate font style for your name and a smaller font size for your contact information.
   Purpose: To make sure potential employers have a means of contacting you. Using a font style that is bold and a larger size for your name will help your name stand out. Make sure to have your contact information in a smaller, nonbold style so it will not detract from your name.
4. Create a section header for "Education." For the learning institution(s) you attended, list the school's name, city and state, degree obtained or coursework successfully completed, and the year. Include any additional educational information, such as awards and the student clinical experience information.
   Purpose: It is important to provide the school's name, city, and state, along with the degree. Some employers may need to verify the information.
5. Create a section header for "Healthcare Experience" and/or "Work Experience." Provide details about your work experience, including the facility's name, city and state, title of your position, start and end date (month and year), and job duties. The job duties must start with an active verb using

the appropriate tense (e.g., a past job would have past tense verbs and a current job would include present tense verbs).
   Purpose: The potential employer will need to know your employment history and all the details.
6. Create a section header for "Special Skills," and list your special language skills, computer proficiencies, and other unique skills you possess that relate to the position.
   Purpose: This section can be a "marketing" area where you emphasize unique skills you possess.
7. Create a section header for "Certifications and Credentials," and list the active credentials and certifications you have. Include the title of the certification, awarding agency, and the expiration date.
   Note: You may want to consider adding in the date you are taking a credential examination. Employers like to know the status of your credential examination.
   Purpose: Employers need to know if you have your medical assistant credential (CMA or RMA). They also might like to know if you have an active cardiopulmonary resuscitation (CPR) card.
8. All information on the resume needs to appear in reverse chronologic order (i.e., newest information is on top). Work experiences should include both the start and end month and year.
   Purpose: Employers need to know how long you worked at a specific place. If the position was seasonal or temporary, it is important to note that.
9. The resume needs to look professional and interesting. Use font styles (e.g., bold, underline, italic) to emphasize important words and phrases. Use professional-looking bullets to list job duties and other information. Use the key words from the posting throughout the resume.
   Purpose: The more professional and interesting a resume appears, the better the chance that the potential employer will review it.
10. Proofread the resume. Correct any spelling, grammar, punctuation, or sentence structure errors you find. If time allows, have another person review your resume, and use the feedback to revise it.
    Purpose: Resumes submitted with errors often are discarded without consideration.
11. Print the resume on resume paper, and proofread it one final time. Any errors should be corrected, and the document should be reprinted or emailed to the instructor.

PROCEDURE 57.2   Create a Cover Letter

Task
Write an effective cover letter that will accompany the resume.

Equipment and Supplies
- Computer with word processing software and a printer
- Current job posting
- Resume paper
- Pen

Procedural Steps
1. Using the job posting, read through the job description. With a pen, circle the position requirements and the key phrases.
   Purpose: Your letter should contain the key phrases and position requirements that are found in the job posting.
2. Using the computer with word processing software, create a professional-looking header in the document's header that matches your resume header. Include your name, address, telephone number(s), and email address.
   Purpose: To ensure potential employers have a means of contacting you. You can enhance the professional appearance of your documents by having the same header on each document.
3. Type the date in the correct location using the correct format. Have one blank line between the date line and the last line of the letterhead.
   Purpose: All letters require a date for legal purposes. The correct format would be month date, year (e.g., May 14, 2025).
4. Type the inside address using the correct spelling, punctuation, and location for the information. Leave 1 to 9 blank lines between the date and the inside address, depending on the location of the body of the letter.
   Purpose: The body of the letter needs to be centered vertically from top to bottom of the document. More blank lines can be added to move the body to the correct location.
5. Starting on the second line below the inside address, type the salutation using the correct format. Use a colon after the person's name.
   Purpose: A proper greeting helps set the tone of the letter.
6. Type the message in the body of the letter using the proper location and format. There should be a blank line after the salutation and between each paragraph. The message should be clear, concise, and professional. Use proper grammar, punctuation, capitalization, and sentence structure.
   Purpose: Proper grammar usage helps convey the message more accurately and professionally.
7. The first paragraph should contain the title and number of the job posting. The middle paragraph(s) should summarize your strengths and include key phrases from the posting. The final paragraph should discuss your availability for an interview. The body should end with an expression of gratitude to the reader.
   Purpose: It is important to thank the reader for considering you for the position.
8. Type a proper closing, leaving one blank line between the last line of the body and the closing. Use the correct format and location.
   Purpose: The closing helps end the message with a proper tone.
9. Type the signature block using the correct format and location. There should be four blank lines between the closing and the signature block.
   Purpose: The four blank lines will provide you with space to sign your name.
10. Spell-check and proofread the document. Check for proper tone, grammar, punctuation, capitalization, and sentence structure. Check for proper spacing between the parts of the letter.
    Purpose: The spell-check tool will identify only certain errors; proofreading will help to identify incorrect word usage, improper tone, and errors in formatting. The tone of the letter should be professional, but not aggressive.
11. Make any final corrections. Print the document on resume paper and sign the letter, or email the document to your instructor or employer.
    Purpose: It is professional to use resume paper when submitting a resume and cover letter to an employer.

PROCEDURE 57.3   Complete a Job Application

Task
Complete an accurate, detailed job application legibly so as to secure a job offer.

Equipment and Supplies
- Pen
- Application form
- Information regarding your past education, job experiences, and the skill sets you have developed (e.g., computer skills, keyboarding speed)
- Contact information for former supervisors and references
- Current resume

Procedural Steps
1. Read the entire job application before completing any part of the document.
   Purpose: Reading through the entire application helps prevent errors when filling out the document.
2. Refer to your information on past jobs, education experiences, and skill sets you have developed as you complete the application. Answers to the questions need to be accurate and honest.
   Purpose: The application is a legal document, and the answers must be correct and true.
3. Use proper grammar, sentence structure, punctuation, spelling, and capitalization. Handwriting should be legible to the reader.
   Purpose: Errors on the application or illegible sections may affect whether you are hired.
4. Do not leave any space blank. Answer each question on the document. If the question does not apply, write "not applicable."
   Purpose: Leaving a space blank on the application may suggest that the candidate did not want to answer a certain question or accidentally overlooked it. By writing "not applicable" on such questions, the candidate demonstrates competence and attention to detail.
5. Do not write "See resume" anywhere on the document.
   Purpose: Many supervisors view this practice as laziness. Always fill out the job application completely, and do not leave blank spaces.
6. Include information on the application that exhibits dependability, punctuality, teamwork, attention to detail, a positive work ethic and initiative, the ability to adapt to change, a responsible attitude, and use of technology.
   Purpose: These phrases send an important message to employers. It is important to use words they are looking for.
7. Sign the document and date it.
   Purpose: Because this is a legal document, read the fine print before signing the document and dating it.
8. Proofread the document, and make sure none of the information conflicts with the resume.
   Purpose: Proofreading helps the candidate to catch any errors before submitting the application.

PROCEDURE 57.4 Create a Career Portfolio

Task

Create a custom portfolio that provides potential employers evidence of your skills and knowledge as a medical assistant.

Equipment and Supplies

- Three-ring binder or folder
- Plastic sleeves for the three-ring binder
- Dividers with tabs for the three-ring binder
- Current resume and cover letter
- Documents providing evidence of your skills and knowledge (e.g., transcripts, job evaluations, student clinical experience evaluation forms and skill checklist, projects completed in school, letters of recommendation, and copies of certifications [e.g., CPR card])

Procedural Steps

1. Group documents in a logical manner, putting similar documents together. Identify the arrangement for the portfolio. An arrangement could include cover letter and resume, education section (e.g., transcript, evaluation form and skills checklist, awards), prior job-related documents (e.g., evaluations), reference letters, and work products (e.g., projects you created in your medical assistant program).

Purpose: Organizing the documents in a logical manner will help the reader identify the important documents. The arrangement will also show the reader your ability to organize content.

2. Insert one document per plastic pocket. Place all documents in plastic pockets.

Purpose: The plastic pockets will keep the documents clean and neat.

3. Neatly write the topic area on the tab of the dividers. Insert the tabbed dividers in the binder or folder.

Purpose: This will help the reader find the content easier.

4. Place all documents in the binder or folder behind the correct divider. Place your cover letter and resume in the front of all the other documents.

Purpose: The reader can review the letter and resume as needed before looking at the other documents in the portfolio.

5. Create a table of contents to identify the tabbed areas.

Purpose: Organizing the documents in a logical manner will help the reader identify the important documents. The arrangement will also show the reader your ability to organize content.

6. After the portfolio is assembled, review the entire portfolio to ensure it looks professional and the documents provide positive support of your skill set and knowledge.

Purpose: Minimize the negative documents in your portfolio. They will not help you obtain a job as much as the positive, supporting documents.

PROCEDURE 57.5 Practice Interview Skills During a Mock Interview

Tasks

Project a professional appearance during a job interview, and be able to express the reasons the medical assistant is the best candidate for the position.

Equipment and Supplies

- Current job posting
- Resume
- Cover letter
- Interview portfolio (optional)
- Application (optional)
- Interviewer
- Mock interview questions

Procedural Steps

1. Wear interview-appropriate attire, and be groomed professionally.

Purpose: Your appearance will influence the first impression made on this potential employer. Most medical facilities prefer conservative dress.

2. Portray a professional image by shaking hands firmly prior to the start of the interview. Ensure that each interviewer has a copy of your resume and cover letter. Refrain from nervous behaviors (e.g., saying "um," tapping a pen or your foot) during the interview.

Purpose: Many employers feel a firm handshake is important. Each interviewer may need a copy of your documents to reference during the interview.

3. Answer introductory questions by providing only professional information. This may include information about your education, experience, and career goals.

Purpose: Many people are tempted to answer with personal information (e.g., if they are married, have children). Personal information should not be discussed during the interview.

4. Answer interview questions with open, honest, and positive responses. Completely answer questions, provide information or examples, and do not answer in single sentences or with limited responses.

Purpose: The goal of the interview is for the employer to get to know you. Limited responses negatively affect this goal.

5. Use key words from the job posting when answering the interview questions.

Purpose: This helps to prove the interviewee has exactly what the organization is looking for.

6. Ask the interviewer two to three appropriate questions about the facility or the position.

Purpose: This demonstrates an interest in the organization and the position.

7. Express interest in the job, and politely complete the interview by shaking hands and thanking the interviewer for the opportunity for the interview.

Purpose: The employer wants to know that you are interested in the job. It is professional to thank the interviewer for the interview opportunity.

PROCEDURE 57.6   Create a Thank-You Note for an Interview

Task

Create a meaningful, thank-you note to be sent after the interview process.

Equipment and Supplies

- Computer with word processing software and a printer
- Job description
- Contact name from interview

Procedural Steps

1. Using word processing software, compose a professional letter using the business letter format. Include all of the required elements in the letter. Use correct spacing between the elements.

   Purpose: Creating a letter that reflects a professional business letter shows the employer you pay attention to detail.

2. Emphasize the particulars of the interview in the body of the letter.

   Purpose: Providing highlights of the interview will assure the employer that you took the time to write an individual thank-you letter.

3. Include positive information you wish you had covered in the interview.

   Purpose: This allows you to present any missed skills or details in a professional manner.

4. Create a message that is concise and to the point.

   Purpose: Keep the letter short and concise. Employers look for employees who can summarize a message and communicate that message.

5. Proofread the letter and make any revisions as needed. Sign and send the thank-you note.

   Purpose: It is important to make sure your note is written correctly. You want to leave a positive perception with the employer.

A

abortion Termination of pregnancy before the fetal age of viability through miscarriage or spontaneous or elective abortion.

abstract To collect important information from the health record.

abuse An action that purposely harms another person.

accessory muscles Muscles in the neck, abdomen, and back that assist in breathing.

accounts payable Money owed by a company to other companies for services and goods; pertains to paying the facility's bills.

acetylcholinesterase An enzyme that destroys acetylcholine and counters its action.

acronym An abbreviation formed from the first letter of each word of a phrase and pronounced as a word.

actinic keratosis A wartlike growth that can become malignant. Usually seen in middle to older adults due to excessive exposure to the sun. Also called senile or solar keratosis.

acuity Test of the clearness or sharpness of vision.

acute infection A disease with a rapid onset of symptoms that can be quite severe but lasts a relatively short time.

acute stage The phase during which rapid multiplication of the pathogen takes place. Symptoms are very distinct. A strong response of the immune system takes place during this stage.

addiction A disease that occurs when a person cannot stop or limit the use of a drug, even after negative consequences have been experienced.

adenosine triphosphate (ATP) A high-energy molecule, found in every cell, that supplies large amounts of energy for various biochemical processes.

adherence The act of sticking to something.

adhesions Bands of scar tissue that can bind anatomic structures together.

adjudicate To settle or determine judicially.

adjustment A credit or debit modification on an account.

advance directives Written instructions about healthcare decisions in case a person is unable to make them.

aerobic Occurring in the presence of oxygen

affect The external emotional expression.

afferent Pertaining to carrying toward a structure.

age of majority The age at which the law recognizes a person to be an adult; it varies by state.

age-related macular degeneration A condition in which the cells of the macula lutea degenerate, causing blurred vision and ultimately blindness.

age spots Hyperpigmented flat dark areas on the skin that occur in irregular shapes; also called liver spots, sunspots, and senile lentigo.

airborne transmission Pathogens exit the reservoir host and remain suspended in the air, often carried by dust, and are inhaled by a susceptible host. Airborne pathogens are known to travel through air ducts and ventilation systems.

albumin Most abundant plasma protein in human blood. It is important in regulating the water balance of blood.

aliquot A portion of a well-mixed sample removed for testing.

alphabetic filing Any system that arranges names or topics according to the sequence of the letters in the alphabet.

alphanumeric Describes systems made up of combinations of letters and numbers.

Ambu bag A self-refilling bag-valve-mask unit used for artificial respiration that is effective for ventilating and oxygenating intubated patients.

ambulatory care Medical services provided by healthcare professionals in an outpatient setting.

amenorrhea Lack of menstrual flow.

amino acids Found in protein-containing foods and released during the digestion process in the intestines; carried by the blood to cells, where they are used to make proteins. Used for growth, maintenance, and repair of cells; they also transport nutrients.

amnesia Memory loss.

amygdala A small mass of gray matter found in each temporal lobe of the cerebrum and involved with memories, emotions, and activating the fight-or-flight response; part of the limbic system.

amyloid plaques Masses or clumps of proteins that form between neurons and disrupt cellular function.

anaerobic Occurring without the presence of oxygen

analgesic A drug that reduces or eliminates pain.

analyte The substance or chemical being analyzed or detected in a specimen.

anaphylaxis A rapidly progressing, life-threatening allergic reaction; characterized by hives, swelling of the mouth and airway, difficulty breathing, wheezing, and loss of consciousness.

anaplastic A rapidly dividing cancer cell that has little to no similarity to normal cells.

anastomosis The surgical connection of separate or severed tubular hollow organs to form a continuous channel.

androgens Usually thought of as male sex hormones, such as testosterone or androsterone, that cause the male secondary sex characteristics. Females produced a small amount of androgen in the ovaries and other organs.

anemia A deficiency of hemoglobin in the blood. It is accompanied by a reduced number of red blood cells, pale skin, weakness, and shortness of breath, among other symptoms.

anencephaly Congenital absence of part or all of the brain.

anesthetic An agent that causes partial or complete loss of sensation.

aneurysm An abnormal blood-filled sac formed from a localized dilation of the wall of a vein, artery, or heart.

anhedonia The inability to feel or experience pleasure during a pleasurable activity.

aniridia A condition in which the iris in the eye is partially formed or fails to form.

anorexia Loss of appetite for food.

anovulation Failure of the ovaries to release an ovum at the time of ovulation.

answering service A commercial service that answers telephone calls for its clients.

anteroposterior (AP) projection The central ray passes from the front of the patient to the back of the patient.

antiarrhythmic A drug that prevents or alleviates heart arrhythmias.

antibiotic A substance or medication that can destroy or inhibit the growth of bacteria.

antibodies Protein substances produced in the blood or tissues in response to a specific antigen, that destroy or weaken the antigen. Part of the immune system.

anticoagulant A substance (i.e., a medication or chemical) that prevents clotting of blood.

anticonvulsant A drug used to prevent or treat seizures.

antigen A substance that stimulates the production of an antibody when introduced into the body. Antigens include toxins, bacteria, viruses, and other foreign substances.

antihyperlipidemic A substance (i.e., medication) that lowers the lipid levels in the blood.

antihypertensive A substance (i.e., medication) that reduces high blood pressure.

antimalarial A drug used to treat or prevent malaria.

antimicrobial A general term used to describe drugs, chemicals, or other substances that can destroy or inhibit the growth of microorganisms. Can be antibiotics or antiviral, antifungal, and antiparasitic drugs or agents (e.g., there are chemical antimicrobial additives in hand soap).

antioxidant Synthetic or natural substances found in food and supplements; may prevent or delay some types of cell damage.

antipyretic A drug that is used to reduce a fever.

antiseptic A substance that inhibits the growth of microorganisms on living tissue (e.g., alcohol and povidone-iodine solution [Betadine]); it is used to cleanse the skin, wounds, and so on.

aphasia Partial or complete loss of the ability to articulate ideas or understand written or spoken language.

apnea Abnormal, periodic cessation of breathing.

approximated   Near, close together.

arbitration   The process in which conflicting parties in a dispute submit their differences to a court-appointed person (arbitrator), who submits a legally binding decision.

arcus senilis   A white or gray opaque ring around the cornea that commonly occurs in people over age 50 years. Can be caused from fat deposits or hyaline degeneration.

aromatic   Having a distinct, usually fragrant, smell.

arrhythmia   An abnormal heart rate or rhythm.

arterioles   Small arteries.

arteriosclerosis   Thickening, decreased elasticity, and calcification of the arterial walls.

arteriovenous fistula   An abnormal joining of an artery and a vein.

arteriovenous graft   A synthetic tube that connects an artery to a vein; also called AV graft.

arthropod   Any animal that lacks a spine, such as insects, crustaceans, arachnids, and others.

articulate   To pronounce distinctly, concisely, and carefully; enunciate.

artifact   A substance, structure, or event that does not naturally occur in a situation. Examples include interference, or electrical "garbage," on an electrocardiogram (ECG), or crystals, lint, or contamination of a staining technique.

artificial insemination   The injection of semen into the vagina or uterus using a catheter or syringe.

asepsis   The condition of being free of infection or infectious material.

aseptic   Free from living pathogenic organisms.

asexually   Describes reproduction that does not involve the fusion of male and female sex cells, such as in plant reproduction, fission, or budding.

aspirate   To withdraw fluid using suction; for example, when a specimen is removed from the body using a needle and syringe.

aspiration   (1) The process of removing fluids or gases from the body using a suction device. (2) Inhalation of a liquid (e.g., blood and vomitus) or a foreign object into the respiratory tract.

ataxia   Loss of the ability to coordinate muscular movement.

atypical lymphs   In many viral infections, stimulated or reactive lymphs are called *atypical lymphs*. They are commonly seen in infectious mononucleosis, commonly called *mono*.

audiologist   An allied healthcare professional who specializes in the evaluation of hearing function, detection of hearing impairment, and determination of the anatomic site of impairment.

audit   A process completed before claims submission in which claims are examined for accuracy and completeness.

audit trail   Record of computer activity used to monitor users' actions within software, including additions, deletions, and viewing of electronic records.

auscultate   To listen to with a stethoscope.

auscultatory gap   A period during which Korotkoff sounds fade away and reappear later at a lower pressure point as the cuff deflates.

authorized agent   A person who has written documentation that they can accept a shipment for another individual.

autoimmune   An immune response against a person's own tissues, cells, or cell parts, as in autoimmune disease, leading to the deterioration of tissue.

autoimmune disease   Illness caused by the immune system mistakenly attacking structures or systems within the body.

automated   Measured by a machine or instrument. May involve human manipulation, coordination, or control.

autonomy   The ability to function independently.

axial projection   The central ray passes through the long axis of the body at an angle.

axon   A long extension of a nerve fiber that conducts the impulse away from the nerve cell body; white matter.

B

backordered   An order placed for an item that is temporarily out of stock and will be sent later.

bacteria   A large group of microorganisms that are single celled, lack a nucleus, reproduce asexually, or can form spores. Some can cause disease. The most abundant life form on earth.

bacteriostatic   Prevents the growth of bacteria.

bacteriuria   The presence of bacteria in the urine (may indicate infection).

Bartholin cyst   Caused from a blockage of the Bartholin's gland resulting in fluid backing up into the gland, causing a painless swollen area on the side of the vaginal opening

basal metabolic rate   The rate at which the body burns calories while a person is at rest.

baseline   An observation or value that represents the normal or beginning level of a measurable quality; used for comparison.

belligerent   Hostile and aggressive.

beneficiary   A designated person who receives funds from an insurance policy.

biconvex   Having two outward-curving surfaces on a lens.

bilingual   The ability to communicate effectively in two languages.

bilirubinuria   The presence of bilirubin in the urine.

billable service   Assistance (i.e., service) that is provided by a healthcare provider and can be billed to the insurance company or patient.

binary fission   Asexual reproduction in single-celled organisms during which one cell divides into two daughter cells.

binomial   A name consisting of a generic and a specific term.

bioethicists   People who study the ethical effect of biomedical advances (e.g., drugs and genetic engineering).

biomarkers   Detectable cellular indicators used as a marker for a substance or disease process.

biopsy   Process of viewing living tissue that has been removed for the purpose of diagnosis or treatment.

bipolar   Having two poles or electrical charges.

blood culture   A microbiological procedure in which a blood sample is placed in a nutrient medium and incubated at body temperature. If bacteria are in the blood sample, the culture medium will facilitate the growth of the bacteria, indicating septicemia.

bloodborne pathogen   A pathogen present in blood that can be transmitted to an individual who is exposed to the blood or body fluids of an infected individual. Can include HIV, hepatitis B virus (HBV), and hepatitis C virus (HCV).

bloodborne transmission   Occurs when pathogens are transferred through contact with blood or other contaminated body fluids.

bonded   A term describing employees for whom an employer has obtained a fidelity bond from an insurance company, which will cover losses from any dishonest acts (e.g., embezzlement, theft) committed by those employees.

boot   The process of starting or restarting a computer when the operating system is loaded.

bounding   Describes a pulse that feels full because of the increased power of cardiac contraction or as a result of increased blood volume.

bradycardia   A slow heartbeat; a pulse below 60 beats per minute.

bradypnea   Abnormally slow breathing.

breach   Disclosure of protected health information without a reason or permission, which compromises the security or privacy of the information.

bremsstrahlung   The radiation produced when an electron decelerates (slows down).

broad-spectrum antibiotics   Antibiotics that act against a wide range of disease-causing bacteria, including both gram-positive and gram-negative bacteria.

bronchiolitis   A condition in which the small airways of the lungs become inflamed because of a viral infection.

bronchodilator   A drug that relaxes smooth muscle contractions in the bronchioles to improve lung ventilation.

bruit   An abnormal sound or murmur heard on auscultation of an organ, vessel (e.g., carotid artery), or gland.

Bucky   Contains a moveable grid device that absorbs scatter radiation and also contains the image receptor.

buffy coat   The layer of white blood cells and platelets that separates red blood cells and plasma in a centrifuged sample of whole blood.

business associate   A person or business that provides a service to a covered entity that involves access to protected health information (PHI). Examples include legal, billing, and management services; accreditation agencies; consulting firms; and claims processing organizations.

buying cycle   Refers to how often an item is purchased; the cycle depends on how frequently the item is used and the storage space available for it.

C

calcify Harden by deposition of or conversion into calcium compounds.

calcium A naturally occurring element that is necessary for many body functions, including strong bones and teeth, proper blood clotting, nerve conduction, and muscle contractions.

calibrated Determined by or checked against a standard (as in readings).

calibration The process of checking the precision, accuracy, and limits of an instrument by comparing measurements of the instrument with those of a known standard or reference instrument.

caliper A pocket-sized tool used for measuring the height and width of the ECG waves and intervals.

callus Hard bony tissue that forms at the ends of fractured bones during the healing process.

candidiasis An infection caused by a yeast that typically affects the vaginal mucosa and skin.

cannula A hollow, flexible tube that can be inserted into a vessel, organ, or cavity of the body to withdraw or instill fluid, monitor information, and visualize a vessel or cavity

canthus The inner or outer corner of the eye where the upper and lower eyelids meet.

capitation A payment arrangement for healthcare providers. The provider is paid a set amount for each enrolled person assigned to them, per period of time, whether or not that person has received services.

cardiopulmonary resuscitation (CPR) The application of manual chest compressions and ventilations (also called *rescue breathing*) to patients who are not breathing or do not have a pulse; also known as *basic life support (BLS)*.

carrier A person who does not have a disease but can transmit it, spreading microorganisms to others.

cartilage Flexible connective tissue that covers the ends of many bones at the joint.

cash flow Movement of cash into and out of the healthcare facility.

cash on hand The amount of money the healthcare facility has in the bank that can be withdrawn as cash.

cataplexy A sudden loss of muscle strength and tone associated with an emotional stimulus.

cataract Progressive loss of transparency (clouding) of the lens of the eye, leading to decreased vision.

catheter A hollow, flexible tube that can be inserted into a vessel, organ, or cavity of the body to withdraw or instill fluid, monitor information, and visualize a vessel or cavity.

catheterized To have had a catheter inserted into a vessel, an organ, or a cavity of the body (e.g., the urinary bladder).

caustic Capable of burning, corroding, or damaging tissue by chemical action.

cauterize To destroy tissue through burning. Used to remove tissue and/or close off blood vessels.

centrifuge A machine that rotates at high speed and separates substances of different densities by centrifugal force. Example: A tube of blood

is separated into plasma/serum, white blood cells, platelets, and red blood cells.

cerumen A waxy secretion in the ear canal; commonly called *earwax*.

cessation Bringing to an end.

charge The cost for goods or services that is owed.

charting by exception (CBE) A method of documentation based on established standards of practice. Only abnormal findings or exceptions to the predefined normal findings are documented.

chief complaint A statement in the patient's own words that describes the reason for the visit to the medical facility.

cholecystitis Inflammation of the gallbladder.

cholelithiasis The presence of stones in the gallbladder.

choroid plexus A network of capillaries found in the lateral ventricles and the third and fourth ventricles that secrete cerebrospinal fluid.

chromosomes Rod-shaped structures found in the cell's nucleus; they contain genetic information.

chronic Developing slowly and lasting for a long time, generally 3 or more months.

chronic infection A disease that persists for a long period of time, sometimes for life.

chronic obstructive pulmonary disease (COPD) A progressive, irreversible lung condition that results in diminished lung capacity.

chronologic Arranged in the order of time.

chyle A mix of lymph and triglyceride fats that create a milky fluid, which is taken up by the lacteals from the intestine and transported to the bloodstream via the thoracic duct.

claim An itemized statement of services and costs from a healthcare facility submitted to the health (insurance) plan for payment.

claim scrubbers Software that finds common billing errors before the claim is sent to the insurance company.

claims clearinghouse An organization that accepts the claim data from the provider, reformats the data to meet the specifications outlined by the insurance plan, and submits the claim.

clarification (1) Gathering additional information to make a concept or idea easier to understand. (2) Allows the listener to get additional information by explaining a specific statement or topic.

Clostridium difficile (C. diff) A bacterium that can cause symptoms that range from diarrhea to severe inflammation of the colon (can be fatal). This condition is most commonly seen after antibiotic use.

clot activators Substances added to a venipuncture tube to enhance and speed up blood clotting.

clubbing Abnormal enlargement of the distal phalanges (fingers and toes) associated with chronic tissue hypoxia due to cyanotic heart disease or advanced chronic pulmonary disease.

CMS-1500 Health Insurance Claim Form (CMS-1500) The standard insurance claim

form used for all government and most commercial insurance companies.

coaching Providing information in a supportive environment that allows people to grow, change, or improve their situation.

code A term used in healthcare settings to indicate an emergency situation and to summon the trained team to the scene.

coding system A system designed to use characters (i.e., numbers and letters) to represent something, such as a medical procedure or a disease.

coinsurance After the deductible has been met, the policyholder may need to pay a certain percentage of the bill and the insurance company pays the rest. A typical split is 80/20; the insurance company pays 80%, and the policy holder pays 20%.

collaboration The act of working with another or other individuals.

collagen The most abundant structural protein found in skin and other connective tissues. It provides strength and cushioning to many parts of the body.

colony A discrete group of organisms, such as a group of bacteria, growing on a solid nutrient surface.

colostomy A surgical procedure in which the large intestine is brought though the abdominal wall, creating either a temporary or a permanent opening (stoma) to allow stool to pass out of the body.

coma A state of deep, often prolonged unconsciousness, usually the result of a head injury, neurologic disease, intoxication, or metabolic abnormalities.

common law Unwritten laws that come from judicial decisions based on societal traditions and customs.

communicable diseases Diseases spread from person to person by either direct contact or indirect contact (e.g., insects).

compact bone Consists of tightly packed osteons; denser and heavier compared to spongy bone.

compartment syndrome A serious condition that involves increased pressure, usually in the muscles; it leads to compromised blood flow and muscle and nerve damage.

compassion Having a deep awareness of the suffering of another and the wish to ease it.

compliance The act of following through on a request or demand. "Patient compliance" sounds negative; thus *patient adherence* is now being used. Also, meeting the standards and regulations of the practice's established policies and procedures. Can also mean cooperation.

computer network A system that links personal computers and peripheral devices to share information and resources.

computerized physician/provider order entry (CPOE) The process of entering medication orders or other provider instructions into the electronic health record.

conception Formation of a viable zygote by the union of the ovum from the female and the sperm from the male; also called *fertilization*.

concise   Using as few words as possible to express the message.

concussion   A type of brain injury resulting from a hit to the head or body that causes the brain to move rapidly back and forth.

congruence   Agreement; the state that occurs when the verbal expression of the message matches the sender's nonverbal body language.

conscientious   Meticulous, careful.

continuity of care   The smooth continuation of care from one provider to another. This allows the patient to receive the most benefit with no interruption or duplication of care.

contraindicate   Suggest that something should not be used.

contrast   The difference between the light areas and dark areas in an x-ray, which allows for detail to be seen.

control materials   Manufacturer-prepared samples that have a known quantity of a specific analyte. Used for quality control purposes. Testing results should fall within a manufacturer-defined range of results. Also called *controls* or *quality controls*.

controlled substances   A behavior-altering or addictive drug or chemical substance whose possession and use are prohibited by or regulated under the federal Controlled Substances Act.

convalescent stage   The phase during which the host recovers gradually and returns to baseline or normal health.

copayment   A set dollar amount that the patient must pay for each office visit. There can be one copayment amount for a primary care provider, a different copayment amount (usually higher) to see a specialist or to be seen in the emergency department.

coping mechanisms   Behavioral and psychological strategies used to deal with or minimize stressful events.

correlate   To establish an orderly relationship or connection.

corrosive   Causing or tending to cause the gradual destruction of a substance by chemical action.

corrugated   Shaped with alternating ridges and grooves.

corticosteroids   A group of steroid hormones produced in the body or given as a medication. Some have metabolic functions, and others reduce tissue inflammation. Glucocorticoids and mineralocorticoids are two types.

counterfeit   An imitation intended to be passed off fraudulently or deceptively as genuine; a forgery.

counteroffer   Return offer made by one who has rejected an offer or a job.

covered entity   A healthcare facility, healthcare provider, pharmacy, health (insurance) plan, or claims clearinghouse that transmits protected health information electronically.

CPT Assistant   An online CPT coding journal, supported by the American Medical Association (AMA), which addresses subjects such as appealing insurance denials, validating coding to auditors, training staff members, and answering day-to-day coding questions.

crash cart   Medications and equipment (e.g., oxygen, intravenous [IV] and airway supplies) stored in a cart and ready for an emergency.

creatinine clearance rates   Result from a procedure used to evaluate the glomerular filtration rate of the kidneys.

crenate   Describes a cell surface that is bumpy, scalloped, or indented.

crepitation   A dry, crackling sound or sensation.

cryopreservation   To preserve by freezing.

cryotherapy   Use of an extremely cold liquid or instrument to freeze and destroy abnormal tissue.

crystals   Solid substances formed from by the solidification of urinary solutes.

culture and sensitivity (C&S)   A procedure in which a specimen is cultured on microbiologic media to detect bacterial or fungal growth. This is followed by screening for antibiotic sensitivity. C&S is performed in the microbiology department of a referral laboratory.

culture medium   A solid, liquid, or semisolid medium designed to support the growth of microorganisms, especially bacteria and fungus.

cyanosis   Abnormal blue coloration to tissues caused by an excess of carbon dioxide.

cyst   A small, capsulelike sac that is filled with a semisolid material, such as a keratinous or sebaceous cyst.

cystic fibrosis (CF)   A disorder that affects all the exocrine cells but affects the respiratory system the most. Mucus is abnormally thick and blocks the alveoli, causing dyspnea.

cystitis   Inflammation of the urinary bladder.

cytopathology   The study of cells using microscopic testing methods.

cytoplasm   A jellylike substance the surrounds the nucleus and fills the cells. Organelles (structures in the cell) are suspended in the cytoplasm.

D

damages   A monetary settlement the defendant pays the plaintiff in a civil case for loss or injury. Also, one of the 4 Ds of negligence, meaning the patient suffers a legally recognized injury.

database   The record of the patient's demographic information, along with the history, physical examination, and initial laboratory findings.

debridement   The surgical removal of dead, damaged, or infected tissue to improve the function of healthy tissue.

debris   The remains of anything broken down or destroyed; ruins, rubble.

decanting   Pouring a liquid gently so that it does not disturb the remaining sediment.

declaratory judgment   A court judgment that defines the legal rights of the parties involved.

decolorizer   A liquid that has the ability to wash out color.

decongestant   A drug that is used for nasal congestion.

decryption   The computer process of changing encrypted text to readable or plain text after a user enters a secret key or password.

decubitus ulcers   Sores or ulcers that develop over a bony prominence as the result of ischemia from prolonged pressure; also called *bed sores* or *pressure sores*.

deductible   A set dollar amount that the policyholder must pay before the insurance company starts to pay for services.

de-escalating   To reduce the level or intensity; bringing down a person's anger or elevated emotions.

defendant   An individual or a business against which a lawsuit is filed.

defense   A strategy used by the defendant to avoid liability in a lawsuit.

defense mechanisms   Unconscious mental processes that protect people from anxiety, loss, conflict, or shame.

degenerative disease   Illness caused by cells or tissues that have deteriorated over time.

delusion   Unshakable belief in something untrue; may be accompanied by hallucinations and/or paranoia.

dementia   Loss of cognitive abilities, including memory, concentration, communication, planning, and abstract thinking. May also cause emotional disturbance and personality changes. Results from brain injury, Alzheimer disease, Parkinson's disease, and other conditions.

demographics   Statistical data of a population. In healthcare this includes the patient's name, address, date of birth, employment, and other details.

density   (1) Describes how compact or concentrated something is. (2) Overall darkness or lightness of the radiographic image related to the number of x-rays that pass through the tissue.

deoxygenated   Oxygen deficient; oxygen was removed.

dependent adults   People between the ages of 18 and 64 who have a mental or physical impairment that prevents them from doing normal activities or from protecting themselves.

depersonalization   Alternative perception of the self; a person's own reality is lost. The person feels they are not in control of their own actions or speech.

deposition   A sworn testimony made before a court-appointed officer; it is used in the discovery process and may be used at trial.

depreciate   To diminish in value (e.g., the value of an item) over a period of time; a concept used for tax purposes.

derealization   Loss of sensation of the reality of one's surroundings.

dextrocardia   A condition in which the heart is located on the right side of the chest and the apex is pointing to the right.

dextrose   A glucose solution administered intravenously.

diabetic retinopathy   Diabetes mellitus damages the blood vessels in the retina, leading to loss of vision and eventual blindness.

diagnosis Determination of the disease or condition that is causing a patient's signs and symptoms.

diagnostic procedures Tests and procedures used to help diagnose or monitor a condition.

diagnostic statement Information about a patient's diagnosis or diagnoses that has been taken from the medical documentation.

diaphragm A broad, dome-shaped muscle used for breathing that separates the thoracic and abdominopelvic cavities.

diastolic The lowest pressure level in the arteries; it occurs when the heart is relaxed and is the last sound heard when taking a blood pressure.

dictation To say something aloud for another person to write down.

differentiated Describes how malignant tissue or cells looks like the normal tissue or cells it came from; poorly differentiated means it does not look like the normal tissue or cells, and well differentiated means it looks like the normal tissue or cells.

diffuse To spread, scatter, disperse, or move.

dignity The inherent worth or state of being worthy of respect.

diluent A liquid substance that dilutes or lessens the strength of a solution or mixture; it is added to vials of powdered medications to create a solution of the drug for injection.

dilution Reducing the concentration of a mixture or solution by adding a known volume of liquid.

direct filing system A filing system in which materials can be located without consulting another source of reference.

direct patient identifiers Used to link the information back to a specific person; can include payment, insurance, and personal demographic information

direct transmission The spread of a pathogen from a reservoir to a susceptible host by direct contact or droplet spread.

discipline A branch of knowledge, learning, or instruction; for instance, medicine, nursing, social work, and physical therapy.

discrepancy A lack of similarity between what is stated and what is found; for instance, the computer inventory count is different from the physical count.

discretionary income Money in a bank account that is not assigned to pay for any office expenses.

discrimination Unfair treatment of another person based on the person's age, gender (sex), ethnicity, sexual orientation, disability, marital status, or other selective factors.

disinfect The process of cleaning to destroy or prevent the growth of disease-causing microorganisms.

disinfectant Any chemical agent used on nonliving objects to destroy or inhibit the growth of harmful organisms; not effective against bacterial spores.

disinfection The process of eliminating most to all pathogenic microorganisms except for spores.

dissect To cut or separate tissue with a cutting instrument or scissors.

distortion The difference between the actual subject and the radiographic image.

diuretic A substance (i.e., medication) that increases the amount of urine produced.

diurnal variation Fluctuations that occur during each day.

docking station Also known as a *universal port replicator;* this hardware device allows laptops to connect with other devices, making them into a desktop computer.

donning Putting on.

dosage The quantity of medication to be administered at one time.

douche Irrigating the vagina for hygienic reasons. Usually water is used, and occasionally other substances for cleaning or odor control are also used.

Down syndrome A genetic disorder in which abnormal cell division results in an extra chromosome 21.

downtime The interval of time during which something, such as hardware or software, is not functioning.

drive A computer device that reads data from and may write data to a storage medium.

droplet transmission The spread of pathogens through respiratory droplets.

duodenal Describes the first section of the small intestines after the stomach.

dynamic equilibrium Relating to balance when moving at an angle or rotating.

dysphagia Difficulty swallowing.

dyspnea Difficult or painful breathing.

E

echocardiography (ECHO) The use of ultrasonic waves directed through the heart to study the structure and motion of the heart. The visual record produced is called an *echocardiogram.*

ectopic pregnancy Implantation of the embryo in any location other than the uterus.

efferent Pertaining to carrying away from a structure.

egress Leaving a place; exit route.

elastin A highly elastic protein in connective tissue that allows tissues to resume their shape after stretching or contracting. It is found abundantly in the dermis of the skin.

elective abortion A procedure for the planned termination of a pregnancy. Also called a *therapeutic abortion.*

electrocardiogram (ECG, EKG) A record or recording of electrical impulses of the heart as produced by an electrocardiograph.

electrodes Adhesive patches that conduct electricity from the body to machine wires (e.g., ECG and transcutaneous electrical nerve stimulation [TENS] unit).

electrodessication Destruction of lesions or sealing off of blood vessels using electric current.

electrolyte A chemical substance that separates into ions in solution (water) and is capable of conducting an electric current. Electrolytes found in body fluids include sodium, potassium, calcium, magnesium, chloride, bicarbonate, and phosphate.

electron A tiny particle of matter with a negative charge, which circles around the center of an atom.

electron energy (kVp) The speed at which the electrons travel, or the total energy of those electrons.

electronic health record (EHR) An electronic record that conforms to nationally recognized standards and contains health-related information about a specific patient. It can be created, managed, and consulted by authorized clinicians and staff from more than one healthcare organization.

electronic medical record (EMR) An electronic record of health-related information about an individual that can be created, gathered, managed, and accessed by authorized clinicians and staff members within a single healthcare organization. An EMR is an electronic version of a paper record.

electronic transaction The electronic exchange of information between two agencies to accomplish financial or administrative healthcare activities.

eligibility Meeting the stipulated requirements to participate in the healthcare plan.

emancipated minor A minor who has been granted emancipation by the court; the minor can assume the rights and responsibilities of adulthood.

embezzlement The misuse of funds for personal gain.

embolus An air bubble, blood clot, or foreign body that travels through the bloodstream and blocks a blood vessel.

embryo A developing organism from the moment of conception through the eighth week of development.

emergency An unexpected, life-threatening situation that requires immediate action.

empathy The ability to understand another's perspective, experiences, or motivations.

emphysema Thinning and eventual destruction of the alveoli; a type of chronic obstructive pulmonary disease (COPD).

emulsifies When a substance suspends tiny droplets of one liquid in a second liquid. By creating an emulsion, you can mix two liquids that usually do not mix well, such as oil and water.

EMV chip technology Global technology that includes imbedded microchips that store and protect cardholder data; also called *chip and PIN* and *chip and signature.*

encoder Software that will apply diagnostic or procedure codes to medical conditions or procedures.

endocrine A glandular secretion that is released into the blood or lymph directly (does not go through a duct).

endolymph Fluid found in the membranous labyrinth of the inner ear.

endoscope A scope with a camera attached to a long, thin tube that can be inserted into the body.

endoscopy A nonsurgical procedure that uses an endoscope to view the inside of the body.

endospore An inactive form of certain bacteria that can withstand poor environmental conditions. When conditions improve, the bacteria become functional again.

endotracheal (ET) tube   A catheter that is inserted into the trachea through the mouth; provides a patent airway.

enema   Fluid introduced into the rectum for a therapeutic or diagnostic purpose.

enriched   Nutrients are added back into a food after they were lost during food processing.

enunciation   The use of articulate, clear sounds when speaking.

enzymatic reaction   A specific chemical reaction controlled by an enzyme.

enzymes   Special proteins that speed up a chemical reaction in the body.

epidemiologic   Pertaining to the branch of medicine dealing with the incidence, distribution, and control of disease in a population. It also involves the prevalence of disease in large populations, in addition to detection of the source and cause of epidemics of infectious disease.

epiglottis   The lidlike structure over the glottis that prevents food and liquids from entering the trachea when swallowing occurs.

epiphyseal plate   A thin layer of cartilage located at the ends of a long bone where new bone forms. Also called the *growth plate*.

epithelial cells   Form cellular sheets that cover surfaces, both inside and outside the body. Epithelial cells are closely packed, take on different shapes, and strongly stick to each other.

eponym   In medical terms, a medical diagnosis or procedure named for the person who discovered it.

e-prescribing   The use of electronic software to communicate with pharmacies and send prescribing information. It takes the place of writing a prescription by hand and giving it to a patient. Most new or refill prescriptions can be submitted electronically, cutting down on fraud and errors.

ergonomics   An applied science concerned with designing and arranging things needed to do a job in an efficient and safe way.

erythropoietin   A hormone that is produced by the kidney cells and travels to the bone marrow to stimulate red blood cell formation.

essential hypertension   Elevated blood pressure of unknown cause that develops for no apparent reason; sometimes called *primary hypertension.*

established patient   A patient who has been treated by the healthcare provider within the past 3 years.

esterase   Any enzyme that breaks down esters (a type of organic molecule) into alcohols and acids.

Ethernet   A communication system for connecting several computers so information can be shared.

ethics   Rules of conduct that differentiate between acceptable and unacceptable behavior.

ethics committee   A group composed of members from a variety of disciplines that analyze ethical issues.

etiology   The cause or origin of a disease.

eukaryote   Any single-celled or multicellular organism that has genetic material contained in a distinct membrane-bound nucleus.

euphoria   An exaggerated sense of physical and mental well-being.

evacuated   A tube, flask, or reaction vessel in which a vacuum has been created.

evidence-based practice   Healthcare practice that incorporates the most current and valid research results, thus allowing the best patient care.

evoked potential test   A nerve response test that uses electrodes placed on the scalp to measure brain reaction to a stimulus.

excised   Surgically removed.

exclusivity   The sole right to market an approved medication granted by the FDA.

excoriation   Inflammation and irritation of the skin.

executor   An individual assigned to make financial decisions about the estate of a deceased patient.

exhalation   The act of breathing out. The diaphragm relaxes, allowing air to be expelled from the lungs.

exocrine   A glandular secretion released through a duct.

exocrine gland   A gland that secretes substances through a duct.

expectorate   To cough up and spit out mucus from the lower respiratory tract.

expediency   A means of achieving a particular end, as in a situation requiring urgency or caution.

expert witnesses   People who are educated and knowledgeable in the area of concern; they testify in court and provide an expert opinion on the topic of concern.

expiration   Exhaling; movement of waste gases from the alveoli into the atmosphere.

explanation of benefits (EOB)   A document sent by the insurance company to the provider and the patient explaining the allowed charge amount, the amount reimbursed for services, and the patient's financial responsibilities.

exploitation   The act of using another person for one's own advantage.

extension   The process of stretching out; increasing the angle of a joint.

external respiration   The exchange of oxygen and carbon dioxide between the body and the atmosphere that occurs within the lungs.

extract   A certain substance that is taken out of a group or solution and is in a concentrated form.

extraction   A process by which a specific substance is separated from a group or solution.

exudates   Fluids with high concentrations of protein and cellular debris that have escaped from the blood vessels and have been deposited in tissues or on tissue surfaces.

F

fact witnesses   People who observed the situation and testify in court about the facts of the case.

familial   Occurring in or affecting members of a family more than would be expected by chance.

family history (FH)   A summary of the health of the patient's parents and siblings, including information on age and cause of death, in addition to the general health status of living relatives.

fascia   A tough, fibrous covering of the muscles.

fatty acids   The result when fats are broken down; they are used by the body for energy and tissue development.

febrile   Pertaining to an elevated body temperature.

fee schedule   A list of fixed fees for services.

fenestrated drape   A surgical drape with an opening in the center. The size of the opening depends on the size of the surgical field.

fever   Abnormally high body temperature

fidelity bond   An insurance policy that protects an employer from loss resulting from a fraudulent or dishonest act by an employee.

file   A collection of data or program records stored as a unit with a specific name.

filter   A device placed below the focal spot that absorbs low-energy radiation and reduces the total radiation exposure to the patient.

filtrate   Fluid and substances that are filtered out of the blood in the Bowman capsule. The fluid that remains after a liquid is passed through a filter.

fire doors   Doors made of fire-resistant materials; they close manually or automatically during a fire to prevent it from spreading.

fiscal year   An accounting period of 12 months during which a company determines earnings and profit; the business determines the beginning of its fiscal year.

fissure   A groove that divides an organ into lobes or parts.

flagella   A long, whiplike outgrowth from a cell that helps the cell move.

flare   An area of redness on the skin that surrounds the wheal.

flexion   The process of reducing the angle of a joint.

flow rate   The number of drops (gtt) in 1 minute required to infuse the ordered solution; also called the drip rate.

fluctuate   To shift back and forth.

focal spot   A point below the anode used to allow the x-ray beam to be focused.

follicle-stimulating hormone (FSH)   A glycoprotein hormone secreted by the anterior pituitary gland. It stimulates the growth of ovum (eggs) in the ovary and induces the formation of sperm in the testis.

fomite   Objects that are likely to carry infectious organisms.

fontanel   A soft membranous gap between the incompletely formed cranial bones of an infant; also called a *soft spot.*

food-borne transmission   The spread of pathogens by consuming contaminated foods or beverages.

foramen magnum   A large opening in the base of the skull. It forms a passageway for the spinal cord.

forensic   Concerning the use of scientific tests or techniques regarding the detection of a crime.

form   Physical characteristics of a medication (e.g., tablet and suspension).

fortified   Describes food to which one or more substances have been added to increase the food's nutrient density.

frequency   Urination at short periods without increase in the daily volume of urine output.

fundus   The top of the uterus.

fungus   Any of a diverse group of single-celled organisms, including mushrooms, molds, mildew, smuts, rusts, and yeasts and classified in the kingdom Fungi.

G

gait   The manner or style of walking.

gamete   A mature sexual reproductive cell; spermatozoon or ovum.

gatekeeper   The primary care provider, who is in charge of a patient's treatment. Additional treatment, such as referrals to a specialist, must be approved by the gatekeeper.

genetic immunity   An inherited ability to resist certain diseases because of one's species, race, gender, or individual genetic makeup.

germicides   Agents that destroy pathogenic organisms.

germline cells   Sperm and egg cells.

g-force   A force acting on an object because of gravity. Example: A centrifuge spins and exerts g-force.

girth   The measurement around something; when referring to mail, it is the measurement around the middle of the package that is being shipped.

Glasgow Coma Scale   A scale used to measure the level of consciousness and severity of a head injury; the ability to open the eyes, verbal response, and motor response are evaluated and the score is determined based on the findings.

glaucoma   A condition in which the fluid pressure in the eye increases; this can lead to blindness if not treated.

global services   For purposes of Current Procedural Terminology (CPT) coding, medical services and procedures, performed for the patient before, during, and after a surgical procedure, that are included with the assigned CPT code.

glomerulonephritis   A kidney disease affecting the glomeruli of the nephron. Characterized by albumin in the urine, edema, and high blood pressure.

glucagon   A hormone produced by the alpha cells in the pancreas; it works in the liver to release glycogen and thereby prevent dangerously low blood glucose levels.

glucose   A simple sugar, which results when carbohydrates are broken down, that is absorbed by the intestines and found in the blood. Used by cells for energy, and the extra is stored in the liver as glycogen.

glycolysis   The chemical breakdown of carbohydrates (glucose) by enzymes, with the release of energy.

glycosuria   An elevated urinary glucose level (may indicate diabetes mellitus).

gonad   Organs that produce sex cells in both males and females.

graduated cylinder   A narrow, tube-shaped container marked with horizontal lines to represent units of measurement used to precisely measure the volume of liquids.

graft   Tissue taken from one area of the body and inserted into another area or person.

gravida   Number of pregnancies.

gray matter   Nerve tissue that lacks the insulation that gives a white appearance to other nerves; thus gray matter looks gray.

grid   A device placed behind an x-ray cassette that is used to absorb scatter radiation.

gross   The amount earned before any tax deductions or adjustments.

guaiac test   A test for fecal occult blood in which glacial acetic acid and guaiac are mixed with the specimen.

guarantor   The person legally responsible for the entire bill. This is usually the patient, but in the case of a minor it would be a parent or legal guardian.

gyri   Folds or convolutions on the surface of the cerebral hemisphere that increase the gray matter surface area. *Gyrus* is the singular form.

H

hacker   An unauthorized user who attempts to break into computer networks.

hallucination   A sensory experience (e.g., a smell, sound, sight, touch, or taste) involving something that is not present.

hand hygiene   Cleaning of the hands in a way that substantially reduces pathogenic microorganisms.

harassment   Continued, unwanted, and annoying actions done to another person.

hardware   The physical equipment of the computer system required for communication and data processing functions.

headset   A combination earphone and microphone that is attached to the telephone by a cord or is wireless.

health insurance exchange   An online marketplace where people can compare and buy individual health insurance plans. State health insurance exchanges were established as part of the Affordable Care Act.

healthcare-associated infections (HAIs)   Infections that patients acquire while receiving treatment for other conditions in a healthcare setting (e.g., ambulatory care, long-term care, or rehabilitation facility).

helminth   A parasitic worm. Examples: tapeworms, roundworms, and flatworms.

hematologist   A person trained in the nature, function, and diseases of the blood and blood-forming organs. They can be a physician, trained laboratory personnel, or researcher.

hematoma   An abnormal buildup of blood in an organ or a tissue of the body, caused by a leak or cut in a blood vessel.

hematopoiesis   The formation of blood cells.

hemoccult test   A modified guaiac test using filter paper impregnated with guaiacum, which turns blue if occult blood is present.

hemoconcentration   A condition in which the concentration of blood cells is increased in proportion to the volume of plasma.

hemoglobin   The oxygen-carrying pigment of red blood cells.

hemolysis   The breakdown of red blood cells with the release of hemoglobin.

hemolytic uremic syndrome   A kidney disorder that can occur after a digestive infection with *Escherichia coli, Shigella,* or *Salmonella;* red blood cells are destroyed and block the kidneys' filtering system, causing acute kidney failure.

hemolyze   To cause the red blood cells in a blood sample to rupture.

hemophilia   A group of inherited blood disorders characterized by a deficiency of one of the factors necessary for the coagulation of blood.

hemostasis   The stoppage of bleeding.

hereditary   Passed from parents to offspring through the genes.

hereditary disease   Condition passed from parents to offspring through the genes.

hernia   Protrusion of a loop of intestine through a weakness in the abdominal wall.

hertz   The unit of measurement used in hearing examinations; a wave frequency equal to 1 cycle per second.

heterophile antibody   An antibody that has an affinity for an antigen other than the specific antigen that stimulated its production.

hierarchy   Things arranged in order and rank.

hippocampus   A ridge in the floor of the lateral ventricle composed of gray matter. It is involved with the limbic system and with creating and filing new memories.

histologic   Pertaining to the study of body tissues.

histology   The study of tissues.

history of present illness (HPI)   Describes the signs and symptoms from the time of onset.

holistic   Considering the patient as a whole; includes the physical, emotional, social, economic, and spiritual needs of the person.

homeostasis   The internal environment of the body that is compatible with life. A steady state that is created by all the body systems working together to provide a consistent and unvarying internal environment.

hormones   Chemical substances produced in an endocrine gland and transported in the blood to a specific tissue, where they have a specific effect.

hospitalist   A provider who oversees the general medical care of hospitalized patients; may include physicians, nurse practitioners, and physician assistants.

host   The living organism that a pathogen resides within.

hyaline   Glassy or transparent.

hydrocephalus   An abnormal accumulation of cerebrospinal fluid that causes enlargement of the skull and compression of the brain.

hyperbaric oxygen therapy   Treatment in which a patient is placed in a sealed chamber and breathes oxygen at higher-than-atmospheric pressure. The high-pressure oxygen can stop bacteria growth and increase the blood oxygen concentration, which can help with the healing process.

hyperkalemia   High potassium levels in the blood.

hyperlipidemia   An elevated level of lipids in the blood.

hyperpnea   Excessively deep breathing.

hypertension   Chronically high blood pressure; generally readings of more than 129/80 for an extended period of time.

hypertrophy   The enlargement of an organ or a tissue due to an enlargement of its cells.

hyperventilation   Abnormally increased breathing.

hypoalbuminemia   A decreased level of albumin (protein) in the blood.

hypocalcemia   Abnormally low level of calcium in the blood.

hypochromic   Pale red blood cells; lacking color.

hypospadias   A condition in which the urethral opening is on the underside of the penis.

hypotension   Blood pressure that is below normal (systolic pressure below 90 mm Hg and diastolic pressure below 50 mm Hg).

hypothyroidism   Deficient activity of the thyroid gland.

I

identifiers   Information unique to an individual. Common identifiers used for patient identification include the full name, including middle initial; date of birth; medical identification number; and patient's address.

idiopathic   Of unknown cause.

image receptor (IR)   A cassette or a digital image receptor that receives the energy from the remnant radiation and forms the image; found in the Bucky.

immunoglobulins   A group of related proteins that function as antibodies. They are found in plasma and other body fluids.

immunosuppressant   A drug used to suppress the immune system.

impervious   Not permitting penetration.

in vitro   A Latin term meaning "in glass" and commonly known as "in the laboratory."

in vitro fertilization   An assisted reproductive technology procedure that involves removing mature eggs from the ovaries and fertilizing the eggs with sperm outside of the body. The fertilized eggs are then transferred to the uterus.

incidence   How often something happens.

incompetence   The state of being incompetent or lacking the ability to manage personal affairs due to mental deficiency; an appointed guardian or conservator manages the person's affairs.

incompetent valves   Valves that do not close completely and allow blood to leak backward into the prior chamber; also called "leaky valves."

inconspicuous   Not noticeable or prominent.

incubation period   The period between exposure to an infection and the appearance of the first symptoms.

incurs   Acquires or sustains.

indigent   Poor, needy, impoverished.

indirect transmission   The process in which a pathogen leaves a reservoir host and is picked up by a susceptible host, often after some time.

infarction   Tissue death.

infectious agents   Living and nonliving pathogens (e.g., bacteria, viruses, fungi, protozoa, parasite, helminths, and prions) that can cause disease. Also called *infectious particles*.

infectious disease   Illness caused by microbes that can be spread from person to person.

infusion rate   The volume of fluid infused per hour; written as mL/hr.

ingested   Swallowed, as food, into the body.

inhalant   Any substance that can be breathed into the lungs.

inhalation   The act of breathing in. The diaphragm contracts and drops down, drawing air into the lungs.

initiative   The ability to determine what needs to be done and take action on your own.

injunction   A court order by which an individual or institution is required to perform or refrain from performing a certain act.

inpatient   A person who is admitted to a healthcare facility that requires at least one overnight stay.

international normalized ratio (INR)   A calculation used to adjust for variations in prothrombin time (PT) reagents and is used to standardize results so they are the same from one laboratory to the next.

inspiration   Inhaling; movement of oxygen (O_2) from the atmosphere into the alveoli.

insufficiency   A condition in which a valve does not close completely, and blood leaks backward across the valve into the prior chamber. Also called *regurgitation* or *incompetence*.

insulin   A hormone produced by the beta cells in the pancreas; it moves glucose into the cells so it can be used for energy.

intact   Complete or whole. Not broken or altered.

intangible   Something of value that cannot be touched physically.

integral   Essential; an indispensable part of a whole.

integrity   Adhering to ethical standards or right conduct standards.

intercellular   Located between cells.

intercostal muscles   Muscles located between the ribs that help with quiet respiration.

interest   Money that is paid in exchange for borrowing or using another person's or organization's money.

interface   An interconnection between systems.

interferon   A protein formed when a cell is exposed to a virus; the protein blocks viral action on the cell and protects against viral invasion.

intermittent   Occurring in intervals.

intermittent pulse   A pulse in which beats occasionally are skipped.

internal respiration   Exchange of oxygen and carbon dioxide between the bloodstream and body cells.

interoperability   The ability to work with other systems.

interpersonal skills   The ability to communicate and interact with others; sometimes referred to as "soft skills."

interrogatory   Written or oral questions that must be answered under oath.

interstitial   Between the cells.

interstitial cells   Testosterone-secreting cells of the testes that are found in the spaces between the seminiferous tubules.

interstitial fluid   Liquid found between the cells of the body.

interval   The space of time between events.

intracellular pathogens   Disease-causing organisms that are inside a cell.

intranet   A private computer network that can only be accessed by authorized people (e.g., employees of the facility that owns the network).

intraocular pressure   The pressure exerted against the outer layers by the content (e.g., humors) of the eyeball.

intraosseous   Within bone; the route for delivery of fluids and medications through a needle inserted into the marrow of certain bones (e.g., humerus, tibia, and femur).

intravenous   Through a vein; fluids and medications can be given through a vein.

intravenous therapy   Administration and monitoring of fluid and medication by intravenous infusion. Also called *IV therapy*.

intrinsic factor   Secreted by the parietal cells of the stomach; necessary for the absorption of vitamin B_{12} to prevent pernicious anemia.

invalid   Not valid. A process or outcome that is not correct.

inventory   A detailed list of equipment and supplies owned and stored; the process of counting the supplies in stock.

invoices   Billing statements that list the amount owed for goods or services purchased.

ion   An electrically charged atom or the smallest component of an element.

ionized   Having an electrically charged atom or the smallest component of an element. (A cation has a positive charge, and an anion has a negative charge)

J

jargon   The vocabulary of a particular profession, as opposed to common, everyday terms.

jaundice   Yellow discoloration of the skin, whites of the eyes, and mucous membranes due to an increase of bilirubin in the blood.

job boards   Websites where employers post jobs; they can be used by job seekers to identify open positions.

K

ketonuria   A condition caused by the presence of ketones in the urine.

L

laceration   A wound produced by the tearing of soft body tissue.

laparoscopy   A procedure used to visually examine the abdomen.

larynx   The voice box.

latent image   An invisible or hidden image created by x-rays that is made visible through processing.

latent infection   A persistent infection in which the symptoms cycle through periods of relapse and remission.

lateral flow immunoassay   A laboratory or clinical technique that uses the specific binding between an antigen and an antibody to identify and quantify a substance in a sample. The sample in this technique moves in a sideways motion, usually on an absorbent paper.

leakage   Radiation escaping from the x-ray tube that is not part of the primary x-ray beam.

lethargy   The state of being drowsy and dull, listless and unenergetic.

liability   The state of being liable or responsible for something.

liable   Legally responsible or obligated.

liaison   A person who interacts and communicates between different groups.

libido   Sexual drive or instinct.

licensure   A mandatory process established by state law that ensures a person has met the legal standards for practicing an occupation in that state.

ligaments   Supportive connective tissue that connects bones at a joint.

ligated   Tied or otherwise closed off.

light microscope   An instrument that uses focused light and lenses to magnify a specimen, usually a cell.

limbic system   Consists of several structures, including the amygdala, hippocampus, and hypothalamus; plays an important role in behavior, memories, and emotions.

limited radiography   A simplified role in radiography, usually in an outpatient setting; also called *practical radiography*. The limited radiographer may be referred to as a limited operator or basic machine operator.

litigious   Prone to lawsuits.

local   Affecting the area where applied.

localized   Restricted or limited to a specific spot.

locum tenens   A Latin term meaning "to substitute for"; the term refers to physicians or advanced practice professionals who temporarily contract to provide healthcare services when a facility has a vacancy, vacation, or a leave of absence.

lumen   The cavity, channel, or open space within a tube or tubular organ.

luteinizing hormone (LH)   A hormone produced by the anterior pituitary gland. LH stimulates ovulation and the development of the corpus luteum in females and the production of testosterone in males.

lymph   A clear, yellowish fluid containing white blood cells in a liquid similar to plasma. The fluid comes from the tissues of the body and is moved through the lymphatic vessels and the bloodstream.

lymphostasis   Obstruction or interruption of normal lymph flow.

lysed   Broken apart or ruptured.

M

macrophage   A very large monocyte that grows in size once it migrates out of the bloodstream and that lives in the tissues. It engulfs foreign particles, microorganisms, and cell debris.

malaise   A condition of general bodily weakness or discomfort, often marking the onset of a disease.

malignant   A cell with uncontrolled growth, rapidly spreading, and doing harm.

malpractice   A type of negligence in which a licensed professional fails to provide the standard of care, causing harm to a person.

malware   Malicious software designed to damage or disrupt a system (e.g., a virus).

mania   Abnormally elated mental state; the person may have feelings of euphoria, lack of inhibitions, sleeplessness, talkativeness, risk-taking behaviors, and irritability.

manipulation   Movement or exercise of a body part by means of an externally applied force.

matrix   The environment in which something is created or takes shape; a base on which to build.

mature minor   A person under the age of adulthood who demonstrates the maturity to make a personal healthcare decision and can give informed consent for treatment.

meatus   A body opening or passage, especially the external opening of a structure.

media   Types of communication (e.g., social media sites); with computers, the term refers to data storage devices.

mediastinum   The space in the thoracic cavity that lies between the lungs, containing the heart, trachea, and esophagus.

mediation   The process of facilitating conflicting parties to make an agreement, settlement, or compromise.

medical asepsis   The use of practices to reduce disease-causing organisms; also considered the clean technique.

medical aseptic technique   Strategies used to maintain medical asepsis (or to destroy disease-causing organisms); also called the clean technique.

medical necessity   Accepted healthcare services that are appropriate for the evaluation and treatment of a disease, condition, illness, or injury, and are consistent with the applicable standard of care. The service can also be called medically necessary.

medically necessary   Accepted healthcare services that are appropriate for the evaluation and treatment of a disease, condition, illness, or injury, and are consistent with the applicable standard of care. The service can also be called a medical necessity.

medication history   A summary of the patient's medication use, including over-the-counter (OTC) products, supplements, and herbal remedies.

menarche   The first menstrual period.

Ménière disease   A chronic disease of the inner ear that causes recurrent episodes of vertigo, progressive sensorineural hearing loss, and tinnitus.

meninges   A protective covering around the brain and spinal cord.

meningocele   The protrusion of the meninges through an opening in the spinal column or skull.

metabolic   Relating to or resulting from metabolism (the chemical process in which cells produce the substances and energy needed to sustain life).

metabolism   The chemical process that occurs within a living organism to maintain life; the process the body uses to obtain or make energy from the food eaten.

metabolite   A by-product of drug metabolism.

metastasize   To spread from one part of the body (the primary tumor) to another part of the body, forming a secondary tumor.

methicillin-resistant *Staphylococcus aureus* (MRSA)   A gram-positive pathogen that is resistant to multiple antibiotics.

microbes   Microscopic organisms, including bacteria, viruses, fungi, and parasites.

microcephaly   The condition of an abnormally small head, associated with impaired brain development.

microcuvette   A small tube or vessel used in laboratory experiments.

microorganisms   Any living organisms of microscopic size, such as bacteria, protozoa, fungi, parasites, and helminths. Some definitions include viruses, which are not alive.

minim   An apothecary unit of measurement for liquid; approximately equal to one drop.

minor   A person who has not reached adulthood, which is usually considered to be age 18 or 21, depending on the jurisdiction.

mock   Simulated; intended for imitation or practice.

modalities   Therapeutic treatments for a disorder.

modem   Peripheral computer hardware that connects to the router to provide internet access to the network or computer.

mold   A growth of tiny fungi forming on a substance. It often looks downy or furry and is associated with dampness or decay.

molecule   The simplest unit of a chemical compound that can exist, consisting of two or more atoms held together with chemical bonds.

monotone   A succession of syllables, words, or sentences spoken in an unvaried key or pitch.

morals   Internal principles that distinguish between right and wrong.

morbidity   The rate of a disease in a population.

mordant   Having the ability to fix or set colors.

morphology   The study of the form, shape, and structure of an organism or a cell.

mortality   The relative frequency of deaths in a specific population.

mucous membrane   A mucus-producing membrane that lines tracts and structures of the body (e.g., gastrointestinal tract, respiratory tract); also called *mucosa*.

multigravida   A woman who has been pregnant two or more times.

multipara   A woman who has carried two or more pregnancies to the age of fetal viability.

murmur   An abnormal sound heard during auscultation of the heart that may or may not have a pathologic origin; it is associated with valve disease or a congenital heart defect.

myelin sheath   A protective insulation that covers the axons and helps with the transmission of nerve impulses.

myoglobin A type of hemoglobin found in the muscle.

myoglobinuria The presence of myoglobin in the urine.

myxedema Advanced hypothyroidism in adulthood.

N

nasal wash The use of a syringe to gently squirt a small amount of sterile saline into the nose; the resulting fluid is collected into a cup (for a wash). Or, after the saline is squirted into the nose, gentle suction is applied (for the aspirate). Also called a *nasal aspirate*.

nasopharyngeal Describes the part of the throat behind and above the soft palate and connected to the nasal passages.

nasopharyngeal airway (NPA) A soft, flexible tube that is inserted into the nose and provides a patent airway; also known as a *nasal trumpet*.

National Provider Identifier (NPI) An identifier assigned by the Centers for Medicare and Medicaid Services (CMS) that classifies the healthcare provider by license and medical specialties.

necrosis Death of cells in an organ or a tissue, generally due to damage or lack of blood supply. Tissue death.

negative feedback loop A process in which a change from the normal ranges causes a response that opposes or decreases the change, thus helping to maintain homeostasis.

negative pressure A ventilation system designed so the air flows from the hallways into an isolation room. This prevents the contaminated air from passing from the isolation room to other parts of the building.

neglect Failure to provide proper attention or care to another person.

negligence Failure to act as a reasonably prudent person would under similar circumstances; such conduct falls below the standards of behavior established by law for the protection of others against unreasonable risk of harm.

negotiable instrument A document guaranteeing payment of a specific amount of money to the payer named on the document.

nephron The functional unit of the kidney; it is responsible for creating urine and adjusting it to maintain homeostasis.

nephrotoxic Damaging or destructive to the kidneys.

netback The amount collected by the collection agency less the agency's fee.

neuralgia Sharp, spasmlike pain in a nerve or along the course of one or more nerves.

neurofibrillary tangles Abnormal structures composed of twisted protein fibers within nerve cells.

neuropathy A nervous system disorder of the peripheral nerves that causes discomfort, numbness, and weakness, especially in the extremities.

neurotransmitter A chemical that helps a nerve cell communicate with another nerve cell or muscle.

nocturia Frequent urination at night.

nodules Small lumps, lesions, or swellings that are felt when the skin is palpated.

nomenclature A system of names or terms, used in science and art to categorize items.

noninfectious disease Illness that is not caused by pathogenic organisms.

noninvasive procedures Procedures that do not penetrate human tissue.

nonorganic Not having an organic or physiologic cause; a disorder that does not have a cause that can be found in the body.

nonverbal communication A type of communication that occurs through body language and expressive behaviors rather than with verbal or written words.

normal flora Microorganisms (mostly bacteria and yeast) that live on or in the body and usually do not cause disease. Normal microscopic residents of the body.

no-show A patient who fails to keep an appointment without giving advance notice.

nosocomial Describes an infection that is acquired in a healthcare setting. Also known as a *healthcare-acquired infection (HAI)*.

Notice of Privacy Practices (NPP) A written document describing the healthcare facility's privacy practices. The patient must be provided with the NPP and must sign an acknowledgment of receipt.

nucleus A specialized organelle of a cell that is encased in a membrane and directs growth, metabolism, and reproduction of the cell.

nulligravida A woman who has never been pregnant.

nullipara A woman who has not carried a pregnancy to the age of fetal viability.

nystagmus Unusual involuntary rapid eye movements.

O

oblique projection The patient is placed in such a way that the central ray passes through the transverse plane of the body at an angle.

obliteration To remove or destroy all traces of; do away with; destroy completely.

obturator A metal rod with a smooth, rounded tip that is placed in hollow instruments to reduce injury to body tissues during insertion.

occlude To close, shut, or stop up.

occult Hidden or unseen.

oncologist A specially trained physician who diagnoses and treats cancer.

online insurance web portal An online service provided by various insurance companies for providers to look up a patient's insurance benefits, eligibility, claims status, and explanation of benefits.

oocyte An immature ovum (egg).

operating system System software; it acts as the computer's software administrator by managing, integrating, and controlling application software and hardware. Windows is an example.

opportunistic Describes a microorganism that causes disease only in a person with a lowered resistance.

opportunistic infections Infections caused by microorganisms that normally do not cause

disease but that become pathogenic when the body's immune system is impaired and unable to fight off infection; for example, as occurs with acquired immunodeficiency syndrome (AIDS), malnutrition, and certain other diseases.

optics checks A specific type of calibration that assesses the optics of an electronic testing instrument or system.

organ of Corti Organ of hearing in the inner ear that contains hair cells, sensory epithelial cells.

organelle A structure within a cell that performs a specific function.

orientation Awareness of one's environment, with reference to people, place, and time.

orthopnea A condition of difficult breathing unless in an upright position.

orthostatic (postural) hypotension A temporary fall in blood pressure that occurs when a person rapidly changes from a recumbent position to a standing position.

osteoporosis Abnormal thinning of the bone structure, causing bones to become brittle and weak.

ototoxic A medicine or substance capable of damaging cranial nerve VIII (vestibulocochlear nerve) or the organs of hearing and balance.

outpatient A person who received healthcare services at a healthcare facility but is not admitted for an overnight stay.

output device Computer hardware that displays the processed data from the computer (e.g., monitors and printers).

P

packing slip A document that accompanies purchased merchandise and shows what is in the box or package.

palliative Describes treatments focused on relieving symptoms

palpation The use of touch during the physical examination to assess the size, consistency, and location of certain body parts.

para The number of pregnancies that have gone to the age of fetal viability (20 weeks' gestation).

paralysis A loss of muscle function and/or sensation, causing the inability to move or use a body part.

parameter A rule that controls how something should be done; guidelines or boundaries.

paranasal sinuses Hollow, air-filled cavities in the skull and facial bones. They lighten the weight of the skull and increase the tone, or resonance, of speech.

paranoia An unfounded or excessive suspicion of the motives of others.

paraphrasing Rewording a statement to check the meaning and interpretation; it shows that a person is listening to and understanding the speaker.

parasite An organism that lives in or on another organism. A parasite benefits from the host, but the host does not benefit from (and is often harmed by) the parasite.

parasitic Pertaining to a parasite.

parenteral To take into the body by any route other than the digestive tract.

participating provider A physician or other healthcare provider who enters into a contract with a specific insurance company or program and by doing so agrees to abide by certain rules and regulations set forth by that particular insurance company.

past medical history A summary of the patient's previous health, including details on medical and surgical events.

patency Open condition of a body cavity or canal.

patent (1) Open. (2) A grant from the government that gives a creator (or manufacturer) of an invention the sole right to produce, use, and sell the product for a set period of time.

pathogen A disease-causing organism or agent.

pathologic Caused by or involving disease.

pathologist A physician specially trained in the nature and cause of disease.

pathology The study of disease.

patient abandonment A form of medical malpractice, also called *negligent termination;* the provider ends the provider-patient relationship without reasonable or adequate notification.

patient account A running balance of all financial transactions for a specific patient.

patient navigator A person who identifies patients' barriers, works closely with the healthcare team and patients, and guides the patients through the healthcare system; may also be called a *patient advocate.*

patient portal A secure online website that gives patients 24-hour access to personal health information using a username and password.

payment The amount paid for goods, services, or a loan.

pegboard system A manual bookkeeping system that uses a day sheet to record all financial transactions for the date of service and maintains patient account balances by using physical ledger cards.

percussion Tapping or striking the body to create sounds, vibratory sensations, or involuntary reactions.

performance measurement The regular collection of data to assess whether the correct processes are being performed and desired results are being achieved.

perilymph A watery fluid found between the membranous labyrinth and the bony labyrinth in the inner ear.

perineal Pertaining to the area between the vaginal opening and the rectum (perineum).

peripheral Area outside of or away from an organ or structure.

peripheral neuropathy Occurs as a result of damage to the peripheral nervous system. The patient can experience multiple symptoms including tingling, numbness, weakness, burning pain, muscle wasting, and organ dysfunction.

peripheral resistance The resistance of the arteries to blood flow.

peristalsis Rhythmic contraction of involuntary muscles lining the gastrointestinal tract.

peritoneum A serous membrane lining the abdominal cavity that folds inward to enclose the viscera (internal organs).

peritubular capillaries Blood capillaries surrounding the proximal and distal convoluted tubules in the kidneys.

permeability A quality or characteristic of a material that allows another substance to pass through it.

permeable Allowing penetration.

permission A reason for releasing or disclosing patient information under the Health Insurance Portability and Accountability Act (HIPAA).

personal ethics An individual's code of conduct.

personal protective equipment (PPE) Clothing, eye protection, gloves, or other garments or equipment designed to protect the wearer's body from injury or infection.

petechiae Very small, round hemorrhage spots in the skin or mucous membrane.

pharyngitis Inflammation or infection of the pharynx, usually causing the symptoms of a sore throat.

phenylalanine An essential amino acid found in milk, eggs, and other foods.

phenylketonuria (PKU) A deficiency in the enzyme phenylalanine hydroxylase, which is responsible for converting phenylalanine into tyrosine.

phlebitis Inflammation of a vein.

physiologic Consistent with the normal function of the body.

pineal gland A small organ in the brain that secretes melatonin, a hormone that regulates the sleep/awake cycle.

pipet A slender tube attached to or including a bulb, used for transferring or measuring small amounts of a liquid; often used in a laboratory.

pitch The depth of a tone or sound; a distinctive quality of sound.

pitting edema Excessive fluid in the intercellular spaces in the tissue; when external pressure (e.g., socks, finger pressure) is relieved, a depression is seen in the tissue.

plaintiff An individual or a party who brings a lawsuit to court.

planes Imaginary cuts or sections through the body.

plaque Any small abnormal patch on or within the body. A deposit of fatty material. Also, a sticky substance made of mucus, food particles, and bacteria that builds up on the exposed part of the tooth.

plasma The fluid portion of blood in the body. In an evacuated tube, it is the liquid portion of a whole blood sample that has not clotted due to the presence of an anticoagulant. The liquid portion of the blood that contains clotting factors.

pneumonia Inflammation of the lungs with congestion of the air sacs (alveoli). Can be caused by a bacterium or virus.

pocket face mask A device used to deliver a rescue breath.

point-of-care Something designed to be used at or near where the patient is seen; point-of-care tools and apps are resources for the provider to use when working directly with the patient.

poised Having a composed and self-assured manner.

policy A written agreement between two parties in which one party (the insurance company) agrees to pay another party (the patient) if certain specified circumstances occur.

polycythemia vera A disorder characterized by an abnormal increase in the number of red blood cells in the blood.

polydipsia Extreme thirst.

polyethylene A plastic material used mostly for containers and packaging.

polyp A growth or mass protruding from a mucous membrane (e.g., nose, bladder, intestine).

polyphagia Excessive hunger.

polyuria High levels of urine output.

pores Tiny openings in the surface of the skin that allow gases, liquids, or microscopic particles to pass.

porous Having many small spaces or holes.

portrait orientation The most common layout for a printed page; the height of the paper is greater than its width.

positive feedback loop A process in which a change causes a response that enhances that change.

posteroanterior (PA) projection The central ray passes from the back of the patient to the front of the patient.

practice management software A type of software that allows the user to enter demographic information, schedule appointments, maintain lists of insurance payers, perform billing tasks, and generate reports.

preauthorization A process that requires the provider to submit documentation to the payer to show the service or treatment is medically needed and the payer determines if the service or treatment is medically necessary and covered under the insurance plan. Also called prior authorization.

precedence The top priority.

precedent A prior court decision that serves as a model for similar legal cases in the future.

precertification The process of determining if a procedure or service is covered by the insurance plan and what the reimbursement is for that procedure or service.

precipitate (1) Solid particles that settle out of a liquid. (2) To separate a solid substance from a solution.

preeclampsia A form of toxemia during pregnancy characterized by high blood pressure, fluid retention, and protein in the urine. May progress to eclampsia.

premenstrual dysphoric disorder (PMDD) A mood disorder that includes depression, irritability, fatigue, changes in appetite or sleep, and difficulty in concentrating; it occurs 1 to 2 weeks before the onset of the menstrual flow.

premenstrual syndrome (PMS)   A poorly understood group of symptoms that occur in some women on a cyclical basis; breast pain, irritability, fluid retention, headache, and a lack of coordination are some of the symptoms.

premium   The periodic (monthly, quarterly, or annual) payment of a specific sum of money to an insurance company, for which the insurer in return agrees to provide certain benefits.

presbycusis   Age-related hearing loss.

presbyopia   Far-sightedness caused by changes to the eye related to aging.

preservatives   Substances added to a specimen to prevent the deterioration of cells or chemicals.

preventive maintenance   Regularly scheduled care of equipment, which reduces the likelihood of failure. It is performed and documented at regular intervals while the equipment is in good working order.

primary care provider (PCP)   A general practice or nonspecialist provider or physician responsible for the care of a patient for some health maintenance organizations. Also called a *gatekeeper.*

primigravida   A woman who is pregnant for the first time.

primipara   A woman who has carried one pregnancy to the age of fetal viability.

privileged communication   Communication that cannot be disclosed without authorization of the person involved; includes provider-patient and lawyer-client communications.

process   A prominence or projection on a bone.

product   The number obtained by multiplying two or more numbers together.

productive   Producing mucus or sputum

productive cough   A cough that produces phlegm or mucus.

proficiency   The state of being skilled as a result of training or practice.

profile testing   A series of laboratory tests associated with a particular organ or disease; also referred to as a "panel" of tests.

prognosis   The likely outcome of a disease, including the chance of recovery.

progress notes   Documentation in the medical record that can be used to track the patient's condition and progress.

prokaryote   Any organism that is made up of at least one cell and has genetic material that is not enclosed in a nucleus. Bacteria are prokaryotes, primitive organisms.

Promoting Interoperability Program   Formerly known as Meaningful Use requirements. Requirements established by the Centers for Medicare and Medicaid Services (CMS) as part of the Electronic Health Records (EHR) Incentives Program. The program provides financial incentives for healthcare organizations that "meaningfully used" their certified EHR technology. The requirements include implementing security measures to ensure the privacy of patients' EHRs.

proofread   To read and mark corrections.

protected health information (PHI)   Individually identifiable health information stored or transmitted by covered entities or business associates; includes verbal, paper, or electronic information.

protozoa   Single-celled organisms that are the most primitive form of animal life. Most are microscopic. Examples are amoebas, ciliates, flagellates, and sporozoans.

provider network   An approved list of physicians, hospitals, and other providers.

provisional diagnosis   A temporary diagnosis made before all test results have been received.

pruritus   Itching.

psoriasis   A usually chronic, recurrent skin disease marked by bright red patches covered with silvery scales.

psychiatrists   Medical doctors who have been specially trained to diagnose and treat patients with mental, emotional, and behavioral conditions.

psychotherapy   The treatment of behavioral health disorders through the use of psychological techniques that encourage communication of conflicts and insights into the person's problems. The goals of this treatment include symptom relief, changes in behavior leading to improved social and vocational function, and personality growth.

puberty   The stage of life in which males and females become functionally capable of sexual reproduction.

pulmonary hypertension   High blood pressure that affects the pulmonary system (pulmonary arteries and the right side of the heart).

pulse   The palpable beat of the arteries throughout the body as they expand in response to contraction of the heart.

pulse deficit   A condition in which the radial pulse is less than the apical pulse; it may indicate a peripheral vascular abnormality.

pulse pressure   The difference between the systolic and diastolic blood pressures (30 to 50 mm Hg is considered normal).

pupil   The opening in the center of the iris through which light enters the eye.

purchase order number   A unique number assigned by the ordering facility that allows the facility to track or reference the order.

pure culture   The growth of only one microorganism in a culture or on a nutrient surface.

putrid   Emitting a foul or decaying odor.

pyrexia   A febrile condition or fever.

Q

Qualified Medicare Beneficiaries (QMBs)   Low-income Medicare patients who qualify for Medicaid for their secondary insurance.

quality assurance   Written policies and procedures that ensure monitoring of all of the processes involved before, during, and after a laboratory test is performed to produce reliable patient test results.

quality control   A process applied to ensure the reliability of test results, using manufactured samples with known values.

quantitative   Describes a test result that is expressed as a number, usually with units of measure attached to numeric values.

R

radiography   The process of creating an x-ray image to examine internal structures of the body.

radiologist   A physician who specializes in medical imaging or therapeutic applications of radiation.

radiopaque   Not allowing the passage of x-rays or other radiation.

rales   An abnormal lung sound heard on auscultation, characterized by discontinuous bubbling noises.

random specimen   A urine specimen that can be collected at any time of the day into a nonsterile container.

rapport   A relationship of harmony and accord between the patient and the healthcare professional.

Raynaud phenomenon   Cramping of small arteries in the fingers and toes in cold temperatures, causing limited blood flow to the area. The skin feels cold and looks white or bluish.

reagent   A substance used in a chemical reaction.

reagent strip   A plastic strip with paper pads that contain chemical reagents. Reagents react with analytes in the urine and are read by looking for a color change.

rebound pain   Pain felt when pressure on the abdomen is released.

receptors   Structures or sites on or in a cell that bind with substances such as hormones, antigens, or drugs.

recommended dietary allowance (RDA)   The average daily level of food intake needed to meet the nutrient requirements of most healthy people.

reconcile   To compare (an account or log) so that it is consistent or compatible with another.

reconciliation   To bring into agreement.

reconstituted   A dried substance (powder) that has been restored to a fluid form so it can be injected.

recovery position   A position in which the patient is on their side; this helps to keep the airway open and clear.

red bone marrow   Soft, gelatinous tissue that consists of blood stem cells that can become white or red blood cells or platelets. Found at the center of most bones.

reference range   The upper and lower limits of test values expected for a healthy group individuals in the general population.

referral   An order from a primary care provider for the patient to see a specialist or to get certain medical services.

referral laboratory   A laboratory that performs specialized testing. The tests may require special instrumentation or training not available at the original laboratory. Also called a *reference, diagnostic,* or *commercial testing laboratory.* Often privately owned.

referred pain *Pain that is felt at a site in the body at a distance from the cause (e.g., the injury or diseased part).*

reflecting Putting words to the patient's emotional reaction, which acknowledges the person's feelings.

reflexes Movements or processes caused by an automatic response; no thought is required.

refraction Bending of light waves when they pass through one substance into another substance of different density.

registered dietitian A credentialed healthcare professional who is trained in nutrition and is able to apply the information to the dietary needs of healthy and ill patients.

regular diet The food and drink a person typically consumes when there are no dietary limitations.

reimbursement To make repayment for an expense or a loss incurred.

relapse Recurrence of the symptoms of a disease after apparent recovery.

release of information A form completed by the patient that authorizes the medical office to release medical records to the insurance company for health insurance reimbursement.

reliable Dependable, able to be trusted.

remission The partial or complete disappearance of the clinical and subjective characteristics of a chronic or malignant disease.

renal ischemia A blood flow deficiency to the kidney(s).

renal threshold The blood level of a substance above which the kidneys fail to reabsorb it; thus the substance will appear in the urine.

replication The production of exact copies of a complex molecule, such as deoxyribonucleic acid (DNA).

res ipsa loquitur A Latin term meaning "the thing speaks for itself." A legal concept under which the plaintiff's burden to prove malpractice is minimal because the jury can clearly understand the details of the injury. For example, a surgical instrument was left in the body during surgery.

res judicata A Latin meaning "a thing decided." Once a case has been decided by the court, it cannot be litigated again.

resection Surgical removal of all or part of an organ.

resident A physician who has graduated from medical school and is finishing specialized clinical training.

residual urine Urine that remains in the bladder after micturition or urination.

resource-based relative value system (RBRVS) A system used to determine how much providers should be paid for services rendered. It is used by Medicare and many other health insurance companies.

respect Showing consideration or appreciation for another person.

respiration A metabolic process by which cells break down substances (e.g., carbohydrates, amino acids, and fats) to produce adenosine triphosphate (ATP).

respiratory arrest Stoppage of breathing.

respondeat superior A Latin term meaning "let the master answer"; a legal doctrine by which the employer/provider is legally responsible for the wrongful actions (or lack of actions) of employees if done within the scope of employment.

restock The process of replacing supplies that were used.

retaliation Getting back at others for something they did.

retention schedule A method or plan for retaining or keeping health records and for their movement from active to inactive to closed.

retractions The sucking in of tissues between the intercostal spaces and neck due to respiratory distress; a classic sign of severe asthma.

retribution Punishment inflicted on someone as vengeance for a wrong or criminal act; the act of taking revenge.

revenue Money collected for providing a product or service.

reverse chronologic order A system in which the most recent item is on top and the oldest item is last.

review of systems (ROS) A list of questions, arranged by organ system, designed to uncover dysfunction and disease.

rhonchi An abnormal rumbling sound heard on auscultation, caused by airways blocked by secretions or muscle contractions.

rotor The rotating member of a machine or device.

rugae Folds in the wall of an organ; when an organ (e.g., stomach, bladder, uterus) fills or needs to expand, the rugae unfold.

S

salary A fixed compensation periodically paid to a person for regular work.

sanitization Reducing the number of pathogens to a level at which they cannot be harmful.

sanitize The process of cleaning equipment and instruments with detergent and water to remove debris and reduce the number of microorganisms to a safe level.

scatter radiation Radiation produced when the primary x-ray beam encounters an object and some x-rays are bounced off or ejected; this creates an unpredictable path of scattered x-rays.

scope of practice Defines the procedures, actions, and processes that individuals in a specific occupation are permitted to perform.

scored tablet A tablet with a groove on the surface, used for splitting it in half.

seborrheic keratosis A benign epidermal tumor that ranges in color from light tan to black. It appears flat or slightly raised; waxy or scaly; round or oval. Typically appears on the face, shoulders, chest, and back.

secondary hypertension High blood pressure caused by another medical condition.

secondary storage devices Media (e.g., jump drive, flash drive, hard drive) capable of permanently storing data until they are replaced or deleted by the user.

sediment An insoluble material that settles to the bottom of a urine specimen and to the bottom of centrifuged urine.

senescent cell An old or aging cell that can no longer divide and reproduce.

sentinel lymph node First lymph node to which cancer cells are most likely to spread from the primary tumor.

septicemia A life-threatening infection caused by the growth of bacteria in the blood.

sequela An abnormal condition resulting from a previous disease.

serologic Pertaining to the science involving the immune properties and actions of serum.

serum The liquid portion of a clotted blood specimen that no longer contains its active clotting agents.

server Computer hardware and software that perform data analysis, storage, and archiving; accepts and responses to requests from devices (clients) made over a network. Also called a database server or data server.

sexual transmission Occurs when a pathogen is spread through intimate contact, specifically intercourse or other sexual acts.

shaken baby syndrome A condition resulting from internal head injuries that occur when a baby or young child is violently shaken.

sharps A medical term for devices with sharp points or edges that can puncture or cut skin. Examples include needles, scalpels, or broken glass.

shearing Occurs when two surfaces move in the opposite direction.

sheep's blood agar plate (BAP)–5% A solid agar medium that contains nutrients and 5% washed sheep's blood. The blood is added as an extra nutrient source for bacteria.

shift(s) Data results on a graph that mark an abrupt change in value.

sickle cell anemia An inherited anemia characterized by crescent-shaped red blood cells (RBCs). This causes RBCs to block capillaries, reducing the oxygen supply to the cells.

side effects Unpleasant effects of a drug in addition to the desired or therapeutic effect.

sign Something that is measured or observed by others; also called *objective data*. Examples of signs include redness, swelling or edema, blood pressure, and pulse.

sinus arrhythmia An irregular heartbeat that originates in the sinoatrial node (pacemaker).

skill set A person's abilities or expertise in an area.

small claims court A special court established to handle small claims or debts without the services of lawyers.

small talk Polite light conversation about uncontroversial matters.

social history A summary of the patient's lifestyle, including health habits and cultural influences on health.

software A set of electronic instructions to operate and perform different computer tasks.

solute A substance that is dissolved in a solvent (liquid) to form a solution

solvent A liquid that can dissolve other substances.

somatic cells Nonreproductive cells; they do not include sperm and egg cells.

source–image receptor distance (SID) The distance between the x-ray tube and the receptor.

spatial resolution The amount of detail that can be seen in the produced x-ray image.

special report Additional medical documentation required to confirm the need for the use of unlisted, unusual, or newly adopted medical procedures code.

specificity The quality or state of being specific.

specimen A sample of blood, body fluid, waste product, or tissue collected for analysis.

spermatozoa Mature male reproductive cells.

sphincter A circular muscle that either constricts and closes the opening or relaxes and allows substances to pass through the opening.

spina bifida A condition in which the spinal column has an abnormal opening that allows protrusion of the meninges and/or the spinal column.

spongy bone A type of bone that is lighter and less dense than compact bone; also called *cancellous bone*. It is usually found at the ends of bones and contains red bone marrow.

spontaneous abortion The natural death of an embryo or fetus before the fetal age of viability. Also called a *miscarriage*.

spore A thick-walled, dormant form of bacteria that is very resistant to disinfection measures.

sputum Thick mucus, often referred to as *phlegm*. It is coughed up from the lungs; not saliva that originates in the mouth.

stains Reagents or dyes used to treat specimens for microscopic examination.

standard of care The level and type of care an ordinary, prudent healthcare professional with the same training and experience in a similar practice would have provided under a similar situation.

standard operating procedure (SOP) A set of step-by-step instructions to help employees carry out routine operations efficiently, with high quality, and uniformity of performance.

Standard Precautions A set of infection control practices used to prevent transmission of diseases that can be acquired by contact with blood, body fluids, nonintact skin, and mucous membranes.

standing order An order that applies to all patients who meet specific criteria.

STAT The medical abbreviation for the Latin term *statum*, meaning immediately; at this moment.

static equilibrium Relating to balance when moving in a straight line.

statute of limitations The length of time legal action can be taken after an event has occurred.

stem cells Undifferentiated cells that can become specialized cells in the body.

stenosis Occurs when the heart valve flaps are stiff or fused together, thus narrowing the valve.

sterile Free of all microorganisms.

sterile field An area free of microorganisms which is used in a surgical procedure to reduce the risk of infection.

sterile technique A set of specific procedures performed to keep a sterile field, a surgical incision, and any other invasive procedure (e.g., injections) free of microorganisms; also called surgical aseptic technique.

sterilization The process that kills all microorganisms and any spores on surfaces.

sterilize The process of removing all microorganisms.

stertorous Heavy breathing causing a low-pitched sound on inspiration (snoring).

stillbirth Fetal death after 20 weeks' gestation. Also called *intrauterine fetal death (IUFD)*.

stoma A temporary or permanent surgically created opening used for drainage (i.e., urine, stool).

strata Naturally or artificially formed layers of material, usually multiple layers.

streaked for isolation To have produced isolated colonies of an organism on an agar plate. With an inoculating loop, one colony is picked and methodically spread out onto solid nutrient media. The goal is to have colonies that are separate from other colonies.

stretch receptor A sensory nerve ending that responds to a stretch stimulus.

stridor A high-pitched, wheezing sound noted on inspiration, caused by a disrupted airflow.

stroke volume The amount of blood that moves through the arteries when the heart beats.

stylus A metal probe that is inserted into or passed through a catheter, needle, or tube used for clearing purposes or to facilitate passage into a body orifice. Also, a pen-shaped device with a variety of tips that is used on touchscreens to write, draw, or input commands.

subcultured An organism (a bacterium) that has been cultivated again on a new nutrient surface.

subpoena A court order requiring a person to appear in court at a specific time to testify in a legal case.

subpoena duces tecum A legal document commanding a person to bring a piece of evidence (e.g., the plaintiff's health record) to court.

suction The production of a partial vacuum by the removal of air to force fluid into a vacant space.

sulci Grooves or depressions on the surface of the brain between the gyri. *Sulcus* is the singular form.

summarizing Allowing the listener to recap and review what was said.

supernatant The clear liquid above the sediment in a centrifuged urine specimen.

suppurative Characterized by the formation and/or discharge of pus.

surety bond A surety agency guarantees payment of a sum of money to a third part in the event the client fails to fulfill certain obligations.

surfactant A mixture of protein and fats that lines the alveoli and prevents the tissues from sticking together and collapsing during exhalation.

surgical asepsis The use of practices to eliminate all microorganisms.

surrogate A person who acts on behalf of another person or takes the place of another person. Examples include a surrogate mother or a healthcare agent.

susceptible Capable of supporting the growth of an infecting organism.

symmetric Similar in size, form, and arrangement of parts on opposite sides of the body.

symmetry Similarity in size, form, and arrangement of parts on opposite sides of the body.

sympathy Feeling sorrow or concern for what the other person has gone through.

symptom Something that is only perceived by the patient; also called *subjective data*. Examples include pain, headache, dizziness, and nausea.

synapse A point of communication between two cells.

syncope A loss of consciousness and postural tone caused by diminished blood flow to the brain.

syringe A device with a slender barrel and needle that is used to withdraw blood from a vein or an artery.

systemic Affecting the entire body.

systolic The highest pressure level in the arteries that occurs when the heart is contracting; it is the first sound heard when taking a blood pressure.

T

tachycardia A rapid but regular heart rate; one that exceeds 100 beats per minute.

tachypnea Rapid, shallow breathing.

tangential projection A type of axial projection in which the angle at which the central ray passes through the patient is very small. The central part of the beam skims the surface.

target cell A cell selectively affected by a specific agent, such as a drug, hormone, or virus.

target tissue The destination, or intended tissue, in the nervous impulse (e.g., a muscle).

telehealth Remote clinical services and nonclinical services, such as provider training, meetings, and continuing education.

telemedicine The use of telecommunication technology to provide healthcare services to patients at a distance; it is usually used in rural communities.

template A document or file that has a preset format; this is used as a starting point when composing something and saves the healthcare worker from having to recreate it each time it is used.

tendons Connective tissue that attaches muscles to bone.

termination letters Documents sent to patients explaining that the provider is ending the physician-patient relationship and the patient needs to see other providers.

testes Male gonads; also called *testicles*.

testosterone A male sex hormone produced by the interstitial cells in the testes.

therapeutic abortion A procedure for the planned termination of a pregnancy. Also called an *elective abortion*.

therapeutic range A value that is reached when blood concentrations of a medication are high enough for the therapeutic effect to occur.

thermionic emission The release of free electrons from the tungsten filament of a cathode that is heated by an electric current passing through it.

third-party administrator (TPA) An organization that processes claims and provides administrative services for another organization. Often used by self-funded plans.

thixotropic gel A chemically neutral gel added to evacuated blood tubes that creates a physical barrier between red blood cells and plasma or serum when the tube is centrifuged.

thoracentesis Aspiration of a fluid from the pleural cavity.

thready Describes a pulse that is thin and feeble.

thrombus A blood clot that blocks the flow of blood. (plural, thrombi)

tickler file A chronologic file used as a reminder that something must be dealt with on a certain date.

tinea Any fungal skin disease that results in scaling, itching, and inflammation. Examples include ringworm and athlete's foot.

tissue density Refers to how dense or solid a body part is.

titer A test that measures the amount of antibodies found in a person's blood.

tort A civil wrongdoing that causes harm to a person or property; excludes breach of contract.

tortfeasor The individual or entity who committed the tort, either intentionally or as a result of negligence.

touchpad A small flat surface chiefly found on laptops, which is sensitive to touch and pressure. Operates as a computer input device and an alternative to a mouse. Used to control the pointer on a display screen.

tourniquet A device for temporarily constricting blood flow.

toxicity The harmful and deadly effect of a medication that can develop due to the buildup of medication or by-products in the body.

toxicology The study and science dealing with the effects, antidotes, and detection of poisons or drugs.

toxins Substances created by microorganisms, plants, or animals that are poisonous to humans; can cause disease.

tract A system of tissues (e.g., neuronal axons) and/or organs (e.g., intestines) that function together.

transcription To make a written copy of dictated material.

transient flora Microbes inhabiting a body surface or cavity for a brief period of time.

transillumination Inspection of a cavity or organ by passing light through its walls.

transitional epithelium A type of cell found in the lining of hollow organs; it has the ability to stretch with the contraction and distention of the organ.

transmission To pass or spread disease.

transport medium A medium used to keep an organism alive during transport to the laboratory.

trauma A physical injury or wound caused by external force or violence.

trend(s) Data results on a graph, obtained over time, which continue to go upward or downward in value.

triage To sort out and classify the injured; used in the military and emergency settings to determine the priority of a patient to be treated.

triage flow map A written flow map for making triage decisions; based on answers to questions, the person moves through the map until a triage decision is made.

tripod position The standing position when crutches are used; crutch tips are 4 to 6 inches to the side and front of each foot.

trustee The coordinator of financial resources assigned by the court during a bankruptcy case.

tube current (mA) The total number of electrons in the x-ray tube traveling from the cathode to the anode.

turbidity A cloudy appearance; not clear.

turgor Refers to normal skin tension; the resistance of the skin to being grasped between the fingers and released. Turgor decreases with dehydration and increases with edema.

U

undescended testicles A condition in which one or both testicles do not descend into the scrotum.

unipolar Having one pole or electrical charge.

unique user identification Each employee is assigned a unique name or number for identifying and tracking user identify.

unit-dose packaging Holds a specified quantity of medication in a single-use container.

Universal Precautions Provisions for treating all human blood and certain human body fluids as if they were known to be infectious with bloodborne pathogens.

unsecured debt Debt that is not guaranteed by something of value; credit card debt is the most common type of unsecured debt.

urgency The sudden, almost uncontrollable need to urinate.

urgent An acute situation that requires immediate attention but is not life-threatening.

urochrome The yellow pigment normally found in urine; it is described as straw, yellow, or amber based on its concentration.

urostomy A surgically created opening on the abdominal wall used to drain urine.

utilization management A decision-making process used by managed care organizations to manage healthcare costs. It involves case-by-case assessments of the appropriateness of care.

V

valvulitis Inflammatory condition of a valve that results in valvular stenosis and obstructed blood flow; caused most commonly by rheumatic fever, bacterial endocarditis, or syphilis.

vascular Having (blood) vessels that conduct or circulate liquids (blood).

vascular access A surgical procedure that creates a vein to remove and return blood during the hemodialysis procedure.

vasoconstriction Contraction of the muscles causing the narrowing of the inside tube of the vessel.

vector An arthropod (mosquito, tick, flea) that carries disease and transmits it to another organism through a blood meal.

vector transmission The passing of pathogens from a reservoir host to a susceptible host though an outside agent, such as an insect.

vendors Companies that sell supplies, equipment, or services to other companies or individuals.

venules Very small veins.

verification of eligibility The process of confirming health insurance coverage for the patient.

vertebrae A series of small, irregularly shaped bones that form the spine. Each vertebra has several projections, joint surfaces, areas for muscle attachment, and a hole through which the spinal cord passes.

vertigo A false sensation that one or one's environment are spinning or moving.

vesicant medication A medication that can damage tissue and can produce blisters.

vested Granted or endowed with a particular authority, right, or property; to have a special interest in.

viable Able to live and grow.

viral Relating to or caused by a virus.

virile Having strength, energy, and a strong sex drive.

virus A microorganism that consists only of genetic material within a protein coat and can only multiply once it is within a living cell.

viscosity Resistance to flow; the thicker the liquid, the higher the viscosity.

vital signs Measurements of a patient's essential body functions, including temperature, pulse, respiratory rate, and blood pressure. Also referred to as *cardinal signs*.

void To urinate.

W

waiting period The length of time a patient waits for disability insurance to pay after the date of injury.

water deprivation test A test to measure the amount and concentration of urine produced when water is withheld from a patient for a period of time.

well approximated The margins or edges of the wound fit neatly together.

wheal A raised mark on the skin.

wheezing A whistling sound made during breathing.

whistleblower A person (usually an employee) who reports a violation of the law within the organization. The person reports the information to the public or to a person in authority.

whole blood Plasma and the formed elements of blood in a free-flowing liquid form.

workplace emergencies Unforeseen situations that threaten the employees and visitors; can disrupt services provided.

X

x-ray caliper A device used to measure the size of a body part to assist in determining proper x-ray settings.

Y

yeast A single-celled fungus that reproduces by budding and is able to ferment sugars.

Z

Zollinger-Ellison syndrome A rare condition that causes tumors to form in the pancreas or duodenum. The tumors secrete large amounts of gastrin, which causes an increase in acid production.

zone A region or geographic area used for shipping.

Page numbers followed by "*f*" indicate figures, "*t*" indicate tables, and "*b*" indicate boxes.

Interpersonal skills, 1212
Interrogatory, 342b
Interrupted baseline artifact, 992, 992f
Interstitial cells, 258
Interstitial cell–stimulating hormone (ICSH), 115
Interstitial cystitis (IC), 252
Interstitial fluid, 157, 965
Interval, 434, 984
Intervening cause, 341
Interventricular septal depolarization, 985
Interview questions, illegal, 1226–1227, 1226t
Interviews. *See* Job interviews; Patient interviews
Intestinal obstructions, 230
Intestines, disorders of, 227–231
Intimate partner violence screening, 827
Intimate space, 320
Intracerebral hemorrhage, 1024
Intramuscular injections, for medication administration, 938–941, 939f, 946b–948b
  air lock technique in, 938–939
  aspiration in, 938
  deltoid site for, 939–940, 940f
  giving, 961b–962b
  summary of, 939t
  techniques in, 938–939
  vastus lateralis site for, 940, 941f
  ventrogluteal site for, 940–941, 941f
  Z-track technique in, 939, 940f, 957b–959b
Intraocular lenses, 137t
Intraocular melanoma, 142
Intraosseous, 1013
Intrauterine device (IUD), 717, 717f
Intravenous (IV) therapy, 965
  additional supplies, 968, 968f
  catheters, 967–968, 968f
  complications, 972–974
    air embolism, 974
    extravasation, 973
    hypersensitivity, 973
    infiltration, 972–973
    local and systemic infections, 973
    phlebitis, 973
    pulmonary edema, 973
  discontinuing, 974
  infusions, 968–970
    catheter, inserting, 971–972
    documentation, 972
    gravity, 969–970, 970b
    identifying a vein, 970–971, 971f
    infusion pump delivery, 969, 969f, 969b
    maintaining, 972
    monitoring, 972
    primary infusion set, 970
    site preparation, 971, 971f
  supplies, 965–968, 965b
  tubing, 966–967, 967f

Intrinsic factor, 219
Invasion of privacy, 339
Inventory
  of equipment, 496–497, 497f
  records, 885
  of supplies
    control systems for, 499–500
    management for, 499
    taking, 500
Inversion, 36t–38t
In vitro fertilization, 261
Invoices, 501
Iodine, 846t
Ionized, 1101
Ions, 983
Iridotomy, 137t
Iris scissor, 768t
Iron, 846t
Irregular bones, 29
Irrigation routes, in medication administration, 925
Irritable bowel syndrome (IBS), 230
Ischemic stroke, 1024
Ishihara test, 694–695, 705b–706b
Islet cell carcinoma, 129
Isoelectric line, 984
Isometric contractions, 868
Isotonic contractions, 868
Isotonic solutions, 965

J
Jargon, 418
Jaundice, 232–233, 1103
Job applications, online profiles and, 1221–1223, 1232b
Job boards, 1216
Job interviews, 1223–1228
  answering questions in, 1226
  face-to-face, 1225
  follow-up after, 1227
  illegal interview questions in, 1226–1227
  interview day, 1224
  negotiation after, 1227–1228
  opportunities improving for, 1228
  on phone, 1224–1225
  preparation for, 1224
    attire decisions in, 1224
    healthcare facility, 1224
    interview day, 1224
    practice answers to questions in, 1224
  professionalism during, 1212–1213
  virtual or video, 1225–1226
Jobs, 1229–1230
  human resource requirements for, 1229
  leaving, 1230
  maintaining, 1229–1230
  starting, 1229
Job search, 1216
  employment agencies, 1216
  newspaper ads, 1216
  school career placement officers for, 1216
Joint Commission, 350

Joints, 34–35
  diarthrotic, 34–35
  stability, 60
J point, 985
Judicial branch, of government, 337t
Justice, ethics and, 379
Juvenile arthritis (JA), 45–46
  types of, 46t

K
Kaposi sarcoma, 81
K-Dur (potassium), 889t–893t
Kegel exercises, 249b
Keratin, 69
Keratitis, 142
Keratoplasty, 137t
Ketamine, 294t–296t
Ketoacidosis, 120
Ketones, 1102
Ketonuria, 120, 1102
Keyboards, 457, 457f
Khat, 294t–296t
Kidney
  anatomy of, 238–239, 238f
  blood flow, 239f
  cancer of, 245
    types of, 245t
  failure of, 246–248
  geriatrics changes in, 752
Klonopin (clonazepam), 889t–893t
Knee-chest position, 687, 703b
Knee walker, 870, 872f
Korotkoff sounds, 650–651
Kratom, 294t–296t
K-Tab (potassium), 889t–893t
Kübler-Ross, Elizabeth, 816
Kyphosis, 42

L
Labels, 920
Laceration, 769
Lactation
  labeling rule of drugs for, 846t
  nutrition needs for, 856
Lactose-intolerance diet, 855
Laparoscopy, 273
Laptop computers, 456
Large intestine, 221
Larvae, 1190
Laryngeal cancer, 209
Laryngeal mask airways, 1012
Laryngeal tubes, 1012
Laryngectomy, 225t
Laryngopharynx, 201
Laser in-situ keratomileusis, 137t
Laser surgery, 794
Laser therapy, 259–260
Lasix (furosemide), 889t–893t
Last menstrual period (LMP), 675
Latent image, 1039
Latent infections, 618
Lateral flow immunoassay, 1111, 1169
Lateral projections, 1053, 1055f
Latex-free tourniquet, 1125, 1126f
Latino patients, cultural differences with, 820b

Law, 337. *See also* Compliance reporting
  additional healthcare law and regulations, 361–364
  balance of power and, 337
  civil, 338
  consent and, 345–346
  contract, 343–345
    breach of contract, 345
    provider-patient relationship, 344–345, 344f
  criminal, 338
  drug, 362
    in ambulatory care setting, 883–886
    Controlled Substances Act, 362
    CSA, 884–886, 885t, 886b
    Food, Drug, and Cosmetic Act, 362, 883–884
  end-of-life issues and, 364
  Good Samaritan, 364
  insurance, 362
  medical laboratory regulations and, 362–363
  Patient's Bill of Rights and, 346–347
  practice requirements and, 347–350, 348t
    accreditation in, 350
    certification and registration, 349–350
    disciplinary action and, 349
    licensure and, 348–349
    practice acts and state boards, 347–349
    scope of practice and, 349, 349b
  privacy and confidentiality in, 356–361, 356f
    GINA and, 361
    HIPAA and, 356–361
    HITECH Act and, 361
  safe haven infant protection, 382–383
  sources of, 337–338
  tort
    damages in, 342–343
    defenses in, 340–341
    negligent, 339–343
    professional liability insurance and, 343
    proving malpractice in, 341–342
    types of, 337–338
    workplace safety, 363–364
LDLs. *See* Low-density lipoprotein
Leakage radiation, 1048
Learning
  domains and, 817–818
    affective, 817t, 818, 818f
    cognitive, 817, 817t
    psychomotor, 817–818, 817t
  teaching-learning process and, 817–822
Left bundle branch, 183
Left lateral position, 687, 701b–702b
Left lower quadrant (LLQ), 17
Left upper quadrant (LUQ), 17